The METABOLIC TREATMENT *of* FIBROMYALGIA

Dr. John C. Lowe

In collaboration with Jackie Grosch Yellin

McDowell Publishing Company
Boulder

Editor: Jackie Grosch Yellin
Associate Editor: Gail Arnold
Assistant Editor: Jan Calloway
Proofreader: Michael Yellin
Graphics: Gina Honeyman
Cover design: Brenda Howell
Cover illustration: John C. Lowe

The beliefs and advice in this book are based on the clinical and research experiences of the author and on his study of the relevant published research literature. The beliefs and advice are not meant as directions for the management of any individual case. Also, they are not intended to substitute for individualized or personalized care by a qualified, licensed, and competent health care professional. Care by such a professional is necessary in all cases due to the unique needs of many individuals that can be identified and allowed for only within the context of personal interaction with a health care professional. The information in this book should be applied in any particular case only after the patient and health care professional determine that the application is safe for the individual patient. Thus, the author, publisher, and others involved in the production and publication of this book do not recommend altering a treatment program devised by a health care professional without individualized guidance by that professional or another. Neither the author, publisher, nor any other party who has been involved in the preparation or publication of this book warrant that the information contained herein is indicated, applicable, effective, or safe in any individual case. The author, publisher, and others involved in the production and publication of this book also disclaim any liability resulting directly or indirectly from the use of the information contained in this book. In particular, it is advised that before it is concluded that a patient has fibromyalgia and/or that metabolic rehabilitation is the appropriate treatment in the individual case, a qualified, licensed, and competent health care professional should, by deductive differential diagnosis, rule out other conditions that would require other forms of treatment or that would contraindicate metabolic rehabilitation. It is also advised that when appropriate in the individual case, a qualified, licensed, competent health care professional should at proper intervals reevaluate the patient for such possible conditions.

Library of Congress Cataloging-in-Publication Data

Lowe, John C.
    The metabolic treatment of fibromyalgia/John C. Lowe FIRST EDITION 2000 (third printing 2007)
    Includes bibliographical references and index
    1. Fibromyalgia 2. Hypothyroidism 3. Metabolism
I. Yellin, Jackie Grosch II. Title

ISBN 0-914609-02-5

Printed in the United States of America

McDowell Publishing Company
Boulder, Colorado

For my fibromyalgia patients,
who collaborated over the years in my investigation of their illness.

For
Jackie, Michael, and Tammy

Acknowledgments

I would like to acknowledge the contributions of the following individuals, in alphabetical order.

Gail Arnold, for her extraordinary diligence in editing the language of the book.

Issam Awad, M.D., Ph.D., for discussions about his biopsy findings and for his encouragement during my early investigation of fibromyalgia.

Carol Burckhardt, Ph.D., for permission to reprint the updated Fibromyalgia Impact Questionniare and the instructions for scoring it.

Jan Calloway, for editing chapters of the book.

Bill Cohen, Publisher of Haworth Medical Press, for his kindness and integrity. Web site: <getinfo@haworthpressinc.com>

Ruth Crumley, M.D., for her enthusiasm for metabolic rehabilitation, and for her cooperation in helping to free patient after patient from their fibromyalgia.

Malford E. Cullum, Ph.D., for extremely helpful communications regarding biochemistry.

Professor J. Eisinger, whose biochemistry studies are without parallel in expanding our understanding of fibromyalgia, for voluminous and enriching communications over several years. Web site: <http://www.infomyalgie.com>

Steve Emerson, for providing me with references related to the effects of mercury on the thyroid system; and along with Gary Osborne, Anne Bradley, and one other person who wishes to remain nameless here, for being exemplary voices of reason and fair-mindedness in Internet communications about matters of logic, medical research, and fibromyalgia.

Richard Finn, C.T.P.M., for sharing his understanding of the relation of myofascial trigger points to fibromyalgia.

Richard L. Garrison, M.D., for his encouragement, favors, and continuing our line of research.

John Gedye, M.B., B.Chir., for serving as a model of tolerance, diplomacy, and rationality, and for many enriching conversations based on his extraordinary understanding of the philosophy and logic of science.

Jay A. Goldstein, M.D., for courageously crossing most basic science fields and all clinical specialties in his search for the links essential to understanding fibromyalgia—something he has been condemned for but for which I praise him—and for publishing his findings.

Lloyd H. Graf, Jr., Ph.D., for extremely helpful communications regarding biochemistry and molecular biology.

Sharland and Richard Grimes, for their generosity and support for our studies of fibromyalgia.

Arthur C. Guyton, M.D., for extremely helpful conversations about general physiological regulatory systems.

Lillian McConnell, musician and teacher who understands the flightiness of the Muses and generously provided a haven where they and I could meet.

William L. Mikulas, Ph.D., for teaching me so many years ago the value of informative feedback—an indispensable feature of the metabolic rehabilitation of fibromyalgia patients—within the context of behavioral psychology.

Garth Nicolson, Ph.D., for his exceptional generosity in making detailed and extensive recommendations for changes in the sections on mycoplasmal infection in Chapter 3.13. Web site: <www.immed.org>

Alan J. Reichman, M.D., for his extraordinary generosity, cooperation, and competence as my cotreating physician and as a member of our research team.

Mary Shoman, for important communications and for her tireless devotion to providing people with accurate, reasonable, and practical information through her Web site and newsletter, *Sticking Our Necks Out*, about their thyroid diseases. Web site: <http://thyroid.about.com>

David G. Simons, M.D., for valuable communications regarding fibromyalgia, myofascial pain syndromes, and the clinical use of T_3, and for lending his support to me in several circumstances.

Jim W. Spears, M.S.W., L.C.S.W., for reading Chapter 1.2 and providing useful suggestions for revisions.

Mervianna Thompson, R.N., M.S.N., A.P.N., for suggesting to me that a modified version of the rule of nines method for burn victims could be a method of measuring fibromyalgia patients' pain distribution, and for her help with our double-blind studies.

Steve Usala, M.D., Ph.D., for extremely valuable talks about thyroid hormone resistance syndromes and c-*erb*Aβ gene mutations, and for encouraging me to pursue the association between thyroid hormone resistance and fibromyalgia.

Fredrick Wolfe, M.D., for his preeminent role in providing us with criteria for identifying fibromyalgia patients—criteria which have enabled researchers the world over to study and further understand fibromyalgia patients, and for his helpful communications over the years.

Todd Yellin, B.S., for reading, editing, commenting on, and spending time with me working on concepts and language in the cell and genome chapters (Chapters 2.2. and 2.3).

PEOPLE FOR WHOM THANKS IS NOT ENOUGH

Jackie Yellin, my Collaborator, Editor, and best friend for 20 years.

Michael Yellin, one of the finest people I have ever met, for his friendship and his endless understanding, support, patience, and generosity.

Tammy Lewis Lowe, my wife, the mother of our lovely daughter, Michele, and the person who inspires me every day.

Preface

The symptoms and objective findings of inadequate thyroid hormone regulation of cell function and those of fibromyalgia are one and the same. To support this proposition, I drew heavily in this book from the plethora of published studies of hypothyroidism. When data were available, I also used published studies of patients with partial cellular resistance to thyroid hormone. However, compared to hypothyroidism, researchers have paid paltry attention to thyroid hormone resistance. Nonetheless, the symptoms and objective findings of hypothyroidism are virtually the same as those of thyroid hormone resistance. Therefore, I considered hypothyroidism our archetypal form of inadequate thyroid hormone regulation of cell function. Overall, the reader can assume what I write of hypothyroidism to also be true of thyroid hormone resistance.

To support the points I made in this book, I used thousands of studies from the research literature. In commenting on some of these studies, I found it necessary to describe all the groups of subjects included—for example, a hypothyroid group, a hyperthyroid group, and a control group of presumably healthy subjects. Many times, I declined to mention the control group. My reason was to save space in the book. Where I considered that the reader's understanding of the outcome of the study did not depend on my commenting on the control group, I described only the experimental groups.

All the conventions we chose to use in this book were intended to make comprehension of the text as easy as possible. We felt this was necessary because of the highly technical nature of the information the book contains.

For example, we chose to hyphenate some words that are not hyphenated in most dictionaries, such as the word "post-menopause." We based our decisions about hyphenation on one consideration—what could be most easily perceived at a quick glance at the text. If a hyphenated word appeared to cause one to pause at the word (perhaps making it harder to read), we chose not to hyphenate it. For this reason, as an example, we chose not to hyphenate "premenopause."

In many places in the text of the book, I defined terms within parentheses. I did so if I used the word only once in the book. For other terms used multiple times, I provided definitions in the Glossary to help the reader comprehend the text. In some places in the text, I followed a term with the word "Glossary" in parentheses. Usually, I did this when I thought the definition to be particularly important. Some words I included in the Glossary have two or more definitions in most medical dictionaries. Most often, however, I defined the term only according to my use of it in this book.

In most chapters, and usually in parentheses, I referred the reader to "sections" or "subsections" in other chapters. For example: (see Chapter 3.1, *section* titled "Decreased Density of β-Adrenergic Receptors"). The term "section" (italicized in the above statement in parentheses) means that the title "Decreased Density of β-Adrenergic Receptors" is positioned above the beginning of the paragraph. To illustrate:

Decreased Density of
β-Adrenergic Receptors
In addition, inadequate thyroid hormone transcription regulation of the adrenergic receptor genes results in decreased synthesis of this type of adrenergic receptor.

As another example: (see Chapter 4.2, *subsection* titled "Subclinical Hypothyroidism"). The term "subsection" (italicized in the above statement in parentheses) means that the title "Subclinical Hypothyroidism" is positioned to begin the text of the paragraph. To illustrate:

> **Subclinical Hypothyroidism.** Subclinical hypothyroidism is defined as an elevated TSH level and a low free T_4 level. Over time, the TSH level may decrease to within the normal range, or it may remain elevated despite the patient's free T_4 level remaining normal.

I chose to disregard the current political correctness that avoids the use of the masculine form to refer to people in general. My main reason for doing so is that I consider this recent convention of many authors a corruption of an elegant, concise, and reasonably precise language. I mean no slight to females by this decision; instead, it is a staunch refusal to "muck up" the English language. Thus, I did not further burden the reader of this highly technical book with grotesque conventions such as "he or she," "he/she," "his or hers," or "his/hers," nor with the convention I find utterly insufferable of mixing singular and plural for the sake of avoiding reference to gender. (For example, "Examine *the patient* when *they* come for *their* initial visit.") When I referred to "the clinician," I used the masculine form, referring to both the female and male clinician. On the other hand, when I referred to "the patient," I used the feminine rather than the masculine form. This seemed to me more practical in that the vast majority of fibromyalgia patients are females. Male fibromyalgia patients should take no offence at this; they, along with female fibromyalgia patients, would be strained by my making allowances hundreds of times in the book for the reality that fibromyalgia afflicts both sexes.

In Appendix A, we provided all the forms necessary to evaluate the fibromyalgia status of patients. The forms should be copied and used to assess the status at the initial evaluation and at intervals as patients progress through metabolic rehabilitation.

In Appendix B, we provided the papers on fibromyalgia that my colleagues and I have published. We included these to make the study results, as well as the methods we used in the studies, available to those with an interest in them.

In Appendix C, we reprinted a refutation I wrote of the conclusions of a neurologist who conducted a study involving fibromyalgia patients. We included this as a supplement to Chapters 1.1 and 1.2.

Appendix D contains a conversion table showing the equivalent amounts of T_4, T_3, and desiccated thyroid. We created this table for the convenience of the clinician when switching a patient's thyroid hormone medication from one form to another.

The first edition of a book of this size is likely to contain errors. Some information errors may have resulted from my finding it necessary to make judgments as to the meaning of the published statements of many researchers. The text may contain some typos, spelling, and grammatical errors despite my best efforts and the diligent work of my Editor and collaborator Jackie Yellin, my two English usage editors, Gail Arnold and Jan Calloway, and several proofreaders. In view of the likelihood of errors, we will be grateful if readers notify us of any they find. We will use the information to improve the quality of the book in its second edition.

The METABOLIC TREATMENT
of FIBROMYALGIA

Contents

SECTION I   FIBROMYALGIA: THE NEW IMPERATIVE

Chapter 1.1

Introduction ▪
Before the Rheumatology Fibromyalgia Paradigm ▪
   Perpetuation of Freudian Concepts By DSM Labeling ▪
Genesis of the Rheumatology Fibromyalgia Paradigm ▪
   Distinguishing Features of Fibromyalgia: Widespread Pain and Tender Points ▪
Fall of the Rheumatology Fibromyalgia Paradigm ▪
   Falsified Hypotheses of the Rheumatology Paradigm ▪
      Physical Deconditioning ▪
      Low Growth Hormone and Somatomedin C Levels ▪
      Stress ▪
      The Serotonin Deficiency Hypothesis ▪
   Anomalies and the Fall of the Rheumatology Paradigm ▪
      Failure of Treatments Based on the Serotonin Deficiency Hypothesis ▪

Chapter 1.2 _____

SECTION II   BACKGROUND: BASIC AND CLINICAL SCIENCES

Chapter 2.1

Chapter 2.4

Chapter 2.5

Chapter 2.6

SECTION III INTERPRETATION OF FIBROMYALGIA SYMPTOMS AND OBJECTIVE FINDINGS AS MANIFESTATIONS OF INADEQUATE THYROID HORMONE REGULATION

SECTION III-A SYSTEM MECHANISMS

Chapter 3.1

Chapter 3.2 _____

Chapter 3.3

Chapter 3.4

Chapter 3.5 _____

Chapter 3.6

SEX HORMONES: HYPOTHALAMIC-PITUITARY-GONADAL AXIS

Chapter 3.14 _____

Introduction ▪
Irritable Bowel Syndrome in Fibromyalgia ▪
Gastrointestinal Effects of Hypothyroidism ▪
    Impaired Intestinal Motility ▪
    Improper Treatment Following Misdiagnosis ▪
    Use of Fiber Supplements ▪
    "Irritable Bowel Syndrome" in Hypothyroidism ▪
    Mechanisms of IBS in Hypothyroidism ▪
    Amplification of Perceptions of Gastrointestinal Sensations by
      Elevated Substance P ▪

Chapter 3.15 _____

Introduction ▪
Pain in Fibromyalgia ▪
Pain in Hypothyroidism ▪
    Headaches ▪
Possible Pain Mechanisms in Hypothyroidism ▪
    Impaired CNS Pain Modulation System ▪
      Norepinephrine and Serotonin ▪

Chapter 3.16 _____

Introduction ▪
Paresthesia in Fibromyalgia ▪
Prevalence of Paresthesia in Hypothyroidism and Euthyroid Hypometabolism ▪
Possible Mechanisms of Paresthesia and Related Symptoms in Fibromyalgia ▪

Chapter 3.17 _____

Introduction ▪
Sicca-like Membranes and Dry Skin in Fibromyalgia ▪
Sicca-like Membranes and Dry Skin in Hypothyroidism ▪
Skin Discoloration in Fibromyalgia ▪
    Increased Capillary Permeability in Hypothyroidism ▪

Chapter 3.18 _____

Chapter 3.19 _____

Chapter 3.20 _____

SECTION IV DIAGNOSIS AND ASSESSMENT

Chapter 4.3

Chapter 4.4

SECTION V TREATMENT: METABOLIC REHABILITATION

Chapter 5.3

Chapter 5.4

Chapter 5.5

COMPLEMENTARY METHODS: INCREASING METABOLIC CAPACITY AND DECREASING METABOLIC DEMAND

APPENDICES

Appendix A

Appendix B

PUBLISHED PAPERS ON FIBROMYALGIA BY DR. JOHN C. LOWE AND COLLEAGUES *1077*

Lowe, J.C., Eichelberger, J., Manso, G., and Peterson, K.: Improvement in euthyroid fibromyalgia patients treated with T_3. *J. Myofascial Ther.*,1 (2):16-29, 1994. ■

Lowe, J.C.: T_3-induced recovery from fibromyalgia by a hypothyroid patient resistant to T_4 and desiccated thyroid. *J. Myofascial Ther.*, 1(4):26-31, 1995. ■

Lowe, J.C.: Results of an open trial of T_3 therapy with 77 euthyroid female fibromyalgia patients. *Clin. Bull. Myofascial Ther.*, 2 (1):35-37, 1997. ■

Lowe, J.C.: Thyroid status of 38 fibromyalgia patients: implications for the etiology of fibromyalgia. *Clin. Bull. Myofascial Ther.*, 2 (1):47-64, 1997. ■

Lowe, J.C., Cullum, M., Graf, L., Jr, and Yellin, J.: Mutations in the c-*erb*Aβ_1 gene: do they underlie euthyroid fibromyalgia? *Med. Hypotheses*, 48(2):125-135,1997. ■

Lowe, J.C., Garrison, R., Reichman, A., Yellin, J., Thompson, M., and Kaufman, D.: Effectiveness and safety of T_3 (triiodothyronine) therapy for euthyroid fibromyalgia: a double-blind, placebo-controlled response-driven crossover study, *Clin. Bull. Myofascial Ther.*, 2(2/3):31-57, 1997. ■

Lowe, J.C., Reichman, A., Yellin, J.: The process of change with T_3 therapy for euthyroid fibromyalgia: a double-blind placebo-controlled crossover study, *Clin. Bull. Myofascial Ther.*, 2(2/3):1997. ■

Honeyman, G.S.: Metabolic therapy for hypothyroid and euthyroid fibromyalgia: two case reports. *Clin. Bull. Myofascial Ther.*, 2(4):19-49, 1997. ■

Lowe, J.C., Garrison, R., Reichman, A., Yellin, J.: Triiodothyronine (T_3) treatment of euthyroid fibromyalgia: a small-n replication of a double-blind placebo-controlled crossover study. *Clin. Bull. Myofascial Ther.*, 2(4):71-88, 1997. ■

Lowe, J.C., Reichman, A., Honeyman, G.S., Yellin, J.: Thyroid status of fibromyalgia patients (abstract). *Clin. Bull. Myofascial Ther.*, 3(1):69-70, 1998. ■

Lowe, J.C., Reichman, A., Yellin, J.: A case-control study of metabolic therapy for fibromyalgia: long-term follow-up comparison of treated and untreated patients (abstract). *Clin. Bull. Myofascial Ther.*, 3(1):23-24, 1998. ■

Lowe, J.C. and Honeyman-Lowe, G.: Facilitating the decrease in fibromyalgic pain during metabolic rehabilitation: an essential role for soft tissue therapies. *J. Bodywork Movem. Ther.*, 2(4):208-217, 1998. ■

Appendix C ————————————————————————

Introduction ▪
Lowe, J.C.: Litigating-chronic pain syndrome: Weintraub's unproven entity. *American Journal of Pain Management*, 3(3):131-136, 1993. ▪
Lowe, J.C.: Litigating pain patients: Just greedy neurotics? *The Chiropractic Journal,* May 1993, pp.27 & 43. ▪

Appendix D ————————————————————————

Foreword

I am honored to be invited to write this Foreword to John Lowe's book, *The Metabolic Treatment of Fibromyalgia*, the more so because we have known each other for such a short time. We first met at the University of Texas Health Science Center in Houston, Texas, as co-organizers of a "Congress on Defining a New Paradigm for the Healing Arts, May 28-31, 1998." My colleagues and I were impressed by the account John gave to the Congress of his systematic approach to fibromyalgia research, particularly his practical use of the principles of formal logic, including Mill's Canons of Induction. This use of formal logic, in my experience, is as rare as it is potentially relevant to clinical research.

In spite of a quite extensive pre-conference e-mail discussion, there was a noticeable lack of consensus amongst participants at the Houston Congress on its purpose. This is not unusual at such gatherings, but amongst a small group of us a sense of purpose emerged quite quickly. We were there to try to characterize an increasingly perceptible paradigm shift in the healing arts of which we, and we felt many others, were becoming aware, and to try to discern and express some of its consequences.

After the conference, I reported to participants and observers that it now seemed clear to me that the nature of the paradigm shift itself had been presented to us—in slightly disguised form—on the very first day. Physicist Elizabeth Rauscher (one of our group) had shown the Congress a cartoon with two near-identical blob-like creatures with the caption "Have you con-sidered the possibility that your reality and my reality are not the same?" The shift itself can be expressed in the following terms: from "implicit acceptance of the view that all human beings have the same perceived reality" (old paradigm) to "explicit recognition that each human being has his or her own unique perceived reality" (new paradigm). The consequences of such a shift are profound and cover all aspects of human existence, including of course, the healing arts.

More recently, Virginia Postrel, in her book *The Future and Its Enemies*, characterized a static-dynamic, stasist-dynamist polarity in our present day society that reflects, but cuts across, traditional political boundaries. The framework provided by her approach helps us to capture very precisely what is wrong with current, essentially stasist, approaches to clinical practice and how the essentially dynamist approach advocated and illustrated by John Lowe in this book provides a remedy. Ultimately, it all comes down to making it possible for informative feedback to be effective in promoting continual learning in our humanly-created artificial systems, just as it is in natural systems.

One of the consequences of the new paradigm is that we are required to be explicit about things which previously we handled implicitly. This, it seems to me, is literally a change in human consciousness. Frank Lucatelli (one of our group) has pioneered the development of a formal general methodology for making explicit what is implicit in our language of common and technical discourse. It is commonly assumed, for example, that there is just one kind of scientific method; but Lucatelli's formal general methodology allows at least four types of science—operational, axiomatic, experimental, and exploratory—to be distinguished. At the present time, clinical science seems to be largely an operational science, and this suggests that there may be much to be gained from broadening its scientific base to include the other three types. As the work described in this book demonstrates, John Lowe has made significant progress in this direction.

But when, at the Houston Congress, we attempted to start to apply Lucatelli's methodology to the language of the healing arts in general, we were almost overwhelmed by the enormity of the task, and many of us were tempted to try to set it aside. The enormity of the task, however, is a pointer to its importance and to the profound consequences of accomplishing it successfully.

Nevertheless, the somewhat harrowing session conducted by Frank Lucatelli at the Congress bore fruit. It led to a realization that maybe one of the things that has been missing is the overt recognition by clinical scientists, that clinical science is, amongst other things, a behavioral science. The study of systems with feedback is, of course, a central preoccupation of behavioral scientists, and it is perhaps no accident that both John Lowe and I were psychologists—behavioral scientists—before we became clinicians.

As a teenager growing up in England in the immediate post WW-II period, I aspired to be a biological chemist. Amongst my heroes were A.J.P. Martin and R.L.M. Synge, who were awarded the Nobel Prize for Chemistry in 1952 "for their invention of partition chromatography." In his presentation speech on behalf of the Nobel Committee, Professor A. Tiselius asked: "How can it happen . . . that something apparently so commonplace as a separation method should be rewarded by a Nobel Prize? The answer is that from the very beginnings of chemistry until our own time, methods for separating substances have occupied a key position in this science. Even today, in Holland, chemistry is called 'Scheikunde' or 'the art of separation'. . . ."

When, in the mid 40s, I first became aware of Martin and Synge's work, I marveled at the power of their separation method. It made me realize—in a way that I had not up to that time—that one can contribute to the solution of a problem not just by solving it, but also by developing a method for solving it. Indeed, the latter may be a more profound way of contributing and may have the most lasting impact, as many other problems beyond the original one may be amenable to the

new method. This was already clearly the case with Martin and Synge's work in 1952. I therefore committed myself to learning not just how to solve problems, but how to develop methodologies for solving problems. From that time on, a project—to get my interest—had to provide opportunities for both.

But I also had an interest in chromatography as such. According to Tiselius, it was invented in 1906, as a technique of chemical separation, by the Russian-Polish scientist Michael Tsvett, although there are earlier examples of similar approaches. So what exactly did Martin and Synge contribute? Tiselius described it as follows: "The novelty in Martin and Synge's method is thus not the [specific techniques] but rather concerns the fundamental chromatographic process itself. This can now be formulated as the partition of a substance between two liquids . . . . Thus we have a rational basis for the method and enormously larger possibilities for choosing the experimental conditions which will be most suitable in any particular case." This is a clear example of the importance of knowing not only that something works but also why it works.

John Lowe's work illustrates these same principles. He has conducted systematic clinical research to gather evidence that his fibromyalgia protocol works for many patients, and he has developed a rational scientific explanation for how and why this protocol works when it works. This means that his techniques can be applied and, if necessary, adapted to meet the needs of any individual fibromyalgia patient. By starting from the working assumption that fibromyalgia is a manifestation of some form of "hypometabolism," a search for the underlying metabolic abnormality in any particular case can be conducted, and if it is found, a rational therapy can be instituted. Furthermore, in the context of this approach, the implications of the occurrence of hypometabolic signs and symptoms in various modern chronic conditions, such as chronic fatigue syndrome, silicone breast implant syndrome, and Gulf War Syndrome, can be seen.

In his Nobel presentation speech, Professor Tiselius described a common application—paper chromatography—of Martin and Synge's method as follows: "A drop of a liquid containing the substance to be investigated is allowed to fall onto a strip of paper, where it forms a little spot. This paper is then caused to draw up some suitable mixture of liquids . . . by capillary action. The spot begins to move, and one can see how it then gradually segregates into several spots, some of which follow the liquid which has been drawn up, while others lag behind. There thus results a resolution of the mixture into its component parts, a resolution which in the last analysis depends on the different partition of the substances between [the liquids in the mixture]."

To me, the most obvious thing about this account is that it describes a "behavioral" science. The components of the substance being investigated are separated because they behave differently in the liquid environment in which the spot is placed. One can imagine photographing the paper at regular intervals to show successive positions of the spot. This record would allow construction of a behavioral trajectory of the spot. Its final photograph—when the spot has come to rest—would correspond to the paper chromatograph as normally understood. In John Lowe's fibromyalgia protocol, the results of examinations (photographs) at intervals of various aspects of the status (spot positions) of the patient are recorded graphically to show the "behavioral trajectory" of the status of the patient, as she responds or fails to respond to therapy.

This kind of behavioral trajectory was pictured in my mind when I later became a behavioral scientist and started looking for opportunities to return the chemists' compliment and develop a "behavioral chromatography." There was no shortage of leads. Maze learning tasks—if the details of the learner's behavior in successive traverses of the maze are recorded, and this is a purely technical problem—can be regarded as generating a series of behavioral chromatographs. In 1966, my coworkers and I reported the application of a method based on this principle to the study of brain failure in elderly patients. We were later able to show that it yielded results of considerable predictive value in the management of the rehabilitation of patients with brain damage. It was found, for example, that irrespective of their performance on such a maze learning task on the day following admission to a rehabilitation unit, patients who had achieved an error-free performance by their third weekly re-test had a high likelihood of eventually making a good functional recovery. The task performance seemed to be reflecting not so much the patients' initial status as their ability to respond to the rehabilitation program. Back then there were technological barriers to the widespread use of this method. But nowadays an up-to-date version of the method could easily be made available as a computer game—downloadable over the Internet—and might well have a future role in the management of the metabolic rehabilitation of patients with fibromyalgia by allowing the regular monitoring of behavioral markers of hypometabolism.

The picture of chromatography that I have painted above led me to an interest in analogous processes of

many kinds. Stimulated by my own Cornish ancestry, I developed an interest in the history of tin mining—until quite late in the 19th century Cornwall was the world's leading producer of tin. I was particularly intrigued by the mechanical separation processes that had been developed to concentrate the relatively low grade cassiterite (SnO_2) ore found in Cornwall to a smeltable level. The processes involved mixing the pulverized ore with water to form a slurry which was then fed through a series of devices, including vibrating tables, which separated the cassiterite particles "behaviorally"—according to their relative density. Interestingly enough, mining engineers call these devices "classifiers." But I was initially mystified by the fact that the flow charts of the separation plants for different mines, while constructed of similar components, were quite different from each other. This turned out to be a reflection of the fact that while the cassiterite from different mines was quite similar, the other minerals from which the cassiterite had to be separated were characteristic of the specific mine from which the ore came. And so a unique process, adapted to the context of the cassiterite ore, had to be designed, implemented, and managed—using informative feedback—to maximize yield. The individualized nature of the metabolic treatment of fibromyalgia patients parallels the mining situation. John Lowe's protocol can be "adapted to the context" (to the variability of symptoms in patients with inadequate thyroid hormone regulation of transcription) by "using informative feedback—to maximize yield."

When, nowadays, we speak metaphorically of "data mining," we are acknowledging similarities between the mining engineer's physical processes and our own data processing techniques. We recognize both the extent to which our software processes model mining processes and the extent to which mining processes may be thought of as embodying a form of computation—witness the mining engineer's use of the term "classifier."

An account of a seminal experience which, to the best of my recollection, took place in the spring of 1965, will lead us to a discussion of the relevance of these considerations to the metabolic rehabilitation of fibromyalgia patients. In the fall of the previous year, I had been appointed to the faculty of the University of Cambridge, England, and had set up a Unit for Research on Medical Applications of Psychology (URMAP) under the joint auspices of the Departments of Medicine and Experimental Psychology. The general aim of the URMAP program was to develop a model of a behaviorally-oriented clinical science, while its specific focus was research on traumatic brain injury (TBI) rehabilitation. This implied taking a careful and thorough look at the nature of rehabilitation and re-habilitation research in general. We started by noting that people seemed quite prepared to discuss *re*-habilitation without first discussing habilitation. It raised the question, "Can one understand how to re-do something without first understanding how to do it?" In view of the fact that I ended up with an approach which placed regular clinical practice in a rehabilitation context, rather than the (traditional) reverse, I find it particularly significant that John Lowe has chosen the title "metabolic rehabilitation" for his approach.

At that time, I held an appropriate British National Health Service honorary (adjunct) appointment in the Department of Neurological Surgery at the university hospital (Addenbrooke's Hospital, Cambridge). This department was headed by a well-known neurological surgeon who had worked in Oxford during WW-II and had helped to pioneer modern surgical methods of treating traumatic brain injury.

Most weeks my URMAP colleagues and I attended the Department of Neurological Surgery rounds at Addenbrooke's Hospital. On the occasion in question, the director of the Department was out-of-town and his deputy officiated in his place. We reached the bedside of an unconscious young women who had been admitted some days previously. The deputy director went up to her and conducted a neurological examination, relaying his findings to the rest of us as he did so. On completion of his examination, he confessed that he was stymied; he could not recall having previously seen anything like the clinical picture the woman presented. Neither could anyone else present. The deputy director decided that the only thing to do was to maintain the necessary life support and wait until the director was back in town.

The following week the director was back in town. When the round reached the bedside of the unconscious woman, the deputy director summarized the situation for the director, who then conducted his own neurological examination. When he had finished, he stepped back from the bedside and said to the assembled company that he had seen a case like this when he was at Oxford in the fall of 1939 (over 25 years previously). The patient had died and on post-mortem examination it had been found that a small blood vessel had burst and bled into a mid-brain nucleus. He suggested, therefore, that in the present situation a radiological examination that would visualize the region of the woman's brain where the bleed had occurred in the previous case should be carried out.

This type of procedure had not been available in 1939, though in 1965, there were still many advances to come before reaching the days of modern radiological visualization techniques.

The radiological examination suggested by the director was carried out, and it revealed not a burst blood vessel but a tumor causing pressure on the same region of the midbrain nucleus that had been damaged in the earlier case.

The events described in this story had a profound effect on the direction of both the general and the specific URMAP program. The points to which it drew attention were as follows:

1. Until the director recalled the case he had seen in Oxford in 1939, the clinical team lacked the knowledge needed to take meaningful action on behalf of the patient in front of them.
2. The meaningful action that they took in 1965 had not been technically possible in 1939, but this did not make the earlier knowledge irrelevant.
3. When they did take meaningful action, the situation they found was not the same as in the earlier case, but the action suggested by the precedent case was nevertheless helpful.

Consideration of these three points makes it clear that the value of precedent cases in deciding what to do for a current case does *not* depend on there being exact matches between corresponding parts of the precedent case and the current case. It depends, rather, on there being what we might call a "sufficient connection" between corresponding parts.

The situation in legal reasoning is similar. In his *Introduction to Legal Reasoning*, Edward H. Levi wrote: "The basic pattern of legal reasoning is reasoning by example. It is reasoning from case to case. It is a three step process . . . similarity is seen between cases; next the rule of law inherent in the first case is announced; then the rule of law is made applicable to the second case." The judge's initial task is to determine similarity or difference between cases, deciding when it will be "just to treat different cases as though they were the same" and so allow a rule derived from consideration of a first case to be justly applied to a second case.

John Lowe started his work by studying the literature to find conditions that "matched" the symptoms of fibromyalgia. It appeared that rheumatologists had failed to recognize—or even to look for—known conditions that had a "sufficient connection" with fibromyalgia. So, like the deputy director of the Department of Neurological Surgery in the story above who had to wait for the director to come back to town to "recognize" the problem, clinicians have had to wait for someone to recognize fibromyalgia as hypometabolism. And this is what John Lowe has done. He saw the connection between inadequate thyroid hormone regulation of transcription and fibromyalgia signs and symptoms. He studied the literature further to see if most characteristics of both conditions "fit" together. And in Section III of this book, he shows that he has established a foundation for making such a "sufficient connection" a working hypothesis in individual cases.

Much of clinical practice is based on reasoning from case to case, and like the judge, the clinician's initial task is to determine similarity or difference between cases. If a clinician learns the science and follows the protocol in this book, he will be able to recognize fibromyalgia as a hypometabolic disorder and discern how to help fibromyalgia patients, even though they may vary from each other in the specific pattern of symptoms they exhibit (which is, in itself, evidence of a pathophysiology that can manifest with variable tissue responses). John Lowe has developed guidelines for determining when it is "just to treat different cases as though they were the same," so that fibromyalgia patients can be treated as hypometabolic by reason of either thyroid hormone deficiency or peripheral resistance to thyroid hormone. When he treated fibromyalgia patients this way, most of them recovered. The protocol chapter (Chapter 5.2) describes a set of rules derived from consideration of a set of "first cases" which can be justly applied to a "second case."

The story of the "out-of-town director" also raised the question of what would have happened if the director of the Department of Neurological Surgery had not seen a similar case previously, or if he had been out-of-town indefinitely, or if the patient had been admitted to a different hospital, and so on. The whole process of relying on the recalled personal experience of the individuals who happened to be on duty, or on call, seemed too haphazard and inefficient. It suggested a role for the then-emerging electronic information handling technology in health care—to store the experience gained by clinicians in handling each case in such a way that it could be retrieved to assist the same, or other, clinicians in handling a similar case at a later date.

A little reflection will show that pursuit of these seemingly modest goals will sooner or later raise all the key questions and drive a long-term R&D program. And that has certainly been the case up to the present time. One not immediately obvious consequence is that a patient might well benefit from the investigation of another patient seen later by the same,

or another, physician. To see something of the implications of this, just consider how the early history of AIDS or the Gulf War illnesses might have been different if such a system had been in place 20 years ago.

The above example introduces what is, essentially, a librarian-library model of clinical research. One can imagine a case library, each volume containing a clinical description, with a shelf-mark based on its contents. With each new case, baffling or not, an appropriate shelf-mark is determined using standard classificatory rules, and adjacent volumes on the shelf are examined for helpful suggestions on how best to help the new case. Easier said than done, but a very worthwhile goal nevertheless.

Nowadays, of course, the librarian-library metaphor is ubiquitous; it is the underlying metaphor of the Internet and the World Wide Web, with the Universal Resource Locator (URL) as the shelf mark. We can conceive of patient records being a part of such a library and accessible by the same means as any other document on the Web. Leaving aside issues of security and privacy—which may be best handled by infomediary agents buffering transactions—the main outstanding problem is how to address documents by content. The method used must determine similarity or difference between cases, allow a decision as to when it will be "just to treat different cases as though they were the same," and so allow a rule derived from consideration of a first case to be justly applied to a second case.

The issue of whether people should be treated as fundamentally all the same or as fundamentally all different has already been raised, and it has been suggested that the latter presumption underlies the emerging new healing arts paradigm. In practice, however, it comes down to a matter of finding an appropriate "resolution level" for the situation we are trying to deal with. At one extreme everyone is unique; at the other extreme everyone is the same. But for most problems, particularly clinical problems, we need a resolution level that will give us a picture between these extremes. This is the resolution level that will maximize the informative feedback needed for learning by both physician and patient. The following example brings out some of the relevant issues.

Imagine a black and white graphics display screen showing a 64 by 64 checkerboard. Overall there are equal numbers of black and white pixels, but they are distributed over the screen in such a way that the individual checkerboard squares appear as lighter and darker shades of gray. When we view this checkerboard from the right distance, we recognize a portrait of Abraham Lincoln. Now imagine what will happen if we progressively simplify the picture by merging adjacent pairs of rows and columns, replacing each 2 by 2 block of 4 squares by a single block which displays the average of their grayscale values. The number of squares in the picture will decrease from 4096 to 1024 to 256 to 64 to 16 to 4 to 1. At some point we will fail to recognize the President, and at some point we will fail to recognize a human head, until, with the portrait collapsed into a single gray square, we will have a picture of nothing.

If I ask the question, "This is a portrait of Abraham Lincoln—True or False?", the answer will obviously depend on the resolution level of the display. If I ask the more general question, "This is a portrait of a man —True or False?", it will usually be answerable at a relatively coarse minimum resolution level, while a more specific question, "This is a portrait of Abraham Lincoln wearing his double-breasted coat—True or False?" will usually require a relatively fine minimum resolution level.

But now imagine the 64 by 64 checkerboard resolved downward to the penultimate level, where it becomes a 2 by 2 picture containing just 4 squares. We cannot answer any of the questions about Abraham Lincoln simply by looking at such a picture using our unaided human senses. But we may be able to answer most, if not all of them—or at least narrow the possibilities—by using a technology of "pattern matching." Each of the four squares represents a shade, or value, of gray. If we reduce "reference" portraits of all American Presidents to such 2 by 2 pictures, the likelihood of any two portraits containing identical gray scale values for each of the four squares is small.

If we now similarly reduce an unknown portrait to the same 2 by 2 level, we can almost certainly identify it (or demonstrate that it does not belong to the reference set) by comparing it with each of the reference portraits until we find (or fail to find) a match. If we find multiple matches, we can resolve the uncertainty by moving to the next highest resolution level. If we find no matches, we can reasonably conclude that the unknown portrait does not belong to the reference set. This kind of pattern matching is possible because, in any set of portraits created under uniform conditions, even small patterns of gray scale ratios drawn at low (and therefore economical) resolution levels are likely to be unique for each individual portrait.

This use of a "portrait library" to identify an unknown portrait is an example of what, nowadays, is called "collaborative filtering." The "filtering" portion of the name refers to the pattern matching that sorts, or "filters," or classifies, the unknown portraits. The "col-

laborative" portion refers to the fact that the people who contribute portraits to the library collaborate to produce the result. We may apply collaborative filtering to clinical practice (and thus lift it beyond "anecdotal evidence," which is the rough equivalent of trying to recognize the 2 by 2 square portrait of Lincoln by unaided senses alone) by producing, electronically, "clinical portraits" based on such clinical data as patient and family histories, symptom profiles, standard laboratory blood test results, and so on. And in the future, this data will be augmented with relatively easily obtained "personality profiles," "behavioral chromatographs," and "biofield characterizations" of various kinds.

Such clinical portraits provide us with the informative feedback we need to manage the metabolic rehabilitation process. In this book John Lowe describes *manual* ways of doing this by plotting charts (behavioral chromatographs) of patients' progress based on changes in their symptoms. Our goal for the future is to develop and provide easy-to-use computer based aids that will bring this process electronically within the reach of all physicians treating fibromyalgia with this protocol.

I suggest that an important element in our description of the "new healing arts paradigm" is the idea that for each "clinical problem" there is a "clinical portrait" at an appropriate resolution level. This ensures that the informative feedback the physician uses is relevant and appropriate and so maximizes the opportunity for learning. A corollary is that many current problems result from adoption of inappropriate resolution levels, sometimes because the very concept of appropriate resolution level is itself unacknowledged. If, for example, the indications for a particular drug therapy are defined at too coarse a resolution level, the success rate at clinical trial could turn out to be less than that needed for the drug to become an accepted treatment. If the indications had been defined at a higher resolution level, it is likely that fewer patients would have met the criteria for the therapy but the success rate in those who did qualify would have been higher. One can even imagine a situation in which there are, say, 10 drugs which, when given to a random selection of the patients for whom they are indicated on the basis of a low resolution level clinical picture, each work in 10% of the patients treated—not an impressive outcome. But this situation is entirely compatible with the same 10 drugs being given to (random selections from) subsets of patients defined in terms of a higher resolution level clinical picture and working in 100% of the patients so selected, and together covering all patients, a 100% overall success rate.

Not very likely perhaps, but clinical trials of drugs and other therapies could be aimed at learning how to move closer and closer to such an outcome. By comparison, the current approach is enormously wasteful and ineffective.

One of our Houston Congress colleagues referred, in a nice turn of phrase, to "the much-worshiped double-blind study." In the present context, "taking the double-blind study seriously" is a convenient way of introducing some key issues of practical importance. We will conclude that the role of the double-blind study in the new healing arts paradigm will be a much more restricted one than is generally accepted at present, as it is possible to sketch the outlines of a plausible successor. The value of examining this issue in some detail is that it exposes the weaknesses of the current paradigm and leads to an appreciation of the strengths of possible successors.

Imagine the following situation. We have a pure chemical substance, PCS, and we have good *a priori* reason to believe that PCS, administered to patients according to a well-defined PCS protocol, could be an effective therapy for some, but not all, patients in a general diagnostic category known as CDC (Chronic Debilitating Condition), for which there is no known effective treatment. In the present context, it is acceptable to substitute "thyroid hormone" for PCS and "fibromyalgia" for CDC, and to note that the PCS example provides a model for understanding what John Lowe actually achieved with a *mental* inference engine in his early clinical trials and later double-blind studies.

We conduct a clinical study of PCS therapy by, initially, offering the treatment to ALL patients who meet the standards for diagnosing CDC. After a prespecified time, appropriate to the natural history of CDC, we evaluate each patient's response to the therapy and decide whether they are "better," "worse," or "neither" (this is, of course, a nontrivial task, but with computer aids it can be done with internal consistency). As soon as we have some patients who have been evaluated in this way, we build the first version of an inference engine that, given the data on which the original diagnosis of CDC was made, infers whether the outcome of PCS treatment will be better, worse, or neither.

We use this inference engine to predict the outcome in all patients who have started, or are about to start, PCS treatment but have not yet been evaluated. As each patient is evaluated, her data is added to the database and a new version of the inference engine is

built and applied to patients whose responses to PCS therapy have not yet been evaluated. Let us suppose that, after a time, the inference engine is predicting, with a consistently high level of performance, the outcome of PCS therapy in patients who have not been evaluated. Let us say, for illustrative purposes, that the engine is indistinguishable from 100% effective. We might now make a decision to offer PCS treatment only to patients for whom the inference engine predicted a "better" response, or perhaps, a "not-worse" response, depending on how cautious we want to be. An advantage of the latter would be that it would allow a more effective fine-tuning of the inference engine's discrimination of the boundary between "better" and "not-better."

The overall result of this approach is that the inference engine has allowed us to refine our diagnostic criteria to the point that PCS treatment is, for all practical purposes, 100% effective. A smaller proportion of CDC patients will be getting PCS treatment than originally, but those that do get it may be, with near certainty, expected to benefit. And the search for equally effective alternative therapies for those who do not qualify for PCS will be accelerated.

At this point a skeptic might ask, "OK, you have evolved this augmented PCS treatment protocol that is 100% effective, but how do you know that the pure chemical substance, as such, has anything to do with it?" Responses to such a question might take many forms, some best left to the imagination. But if PCS was a low cost, readily available, nutritional supplement with no known harmful effects, and given that CDC is what its name implies, a chronic debilitating condition for which there is no known treatment, we might be tempted to answer, "We don't, and it doesn't matter to us or to our patients; they are only too happy to be better, whatever the mechanism." (Such arguments are often put forward by practitioners of Traditional Chinese Medicine—"This therapy has worked for 4,000 years; who are we to question it?").

But mindful of the value of learning more about how such a successful therapy works we might be tempted, in our response to the skeptic, to add, "If you can provide us with a good enough reason for wanting to know the answer to this question (one that will make sense to us and our patients), and if you are willing to cover the cost, we will conduct a double-blind study for you." The study will be conducted as follows: Starting from a certain date, we will explain to each new patient meeting the requirements for being offered the augmented PCS treatment protocol, that we are conducting a study to determine what contribution the pure chemical substance in the PCS treatment protocol makes to its 100% effectiveness. We explain that if the patient agrees to volunteer to enter the study, she will have a 50% chance of having the pure chemical substance in her PCS treatment protocol, and neither she nor we, her doctors, will know whether she did or did not until after the evaluation of the treatment's effectiveness.

It should be noted at this point that whether or not the patient volunteers, the very introduction of this choice opportunity into the situation changes the doctor-patient relationship irrevocably. The doctor has revealed him or herself to be someone who is willing to put the patient in the position—potentially stressful—of having to decide whether to volunteer or not. If the doctor decides beforehand which patients to offer the choice to, he or she may later be accused of biasing the results of the study by manipulating the patient selection. I am not suggesting that putting the patient in this situation can never be justified; I am just making the point that such a step cannot be taken without consequences that may affect the outcome, one way or another.

If, for the moment, we assume that a double-blind study can be justified and that we have sufficient volunteers, the advantage of the approach I have outlined is that since all the volunteers are qualified under the augmented PCS treatment protocol, the expected success rate if treated is 100%. So if the pure chemical substance is indeed essential, the effects of its absence will show up quickly and definitely, and so a statistically significant result can be obtained with a small sample. Under the most favorable circumstances, this might mean that the placebo patients start on the genuine PCS treatment protocol after a modest delay, the research having been completed.

The key point is that *to use the double-blind approach legitimately, the treatment protocol must have already been optimized.* The double-blind method can then be used to detect differences in alternative approaches to the part of the therapy for which double-blind substitution is possible (such as PCS versus a lower cost alternative).

As I mentioned above, John Lowe's therapeutic research followed this model quite closely. In his double-blind studies, the "pure chemical substance" was indeed essential, and the effects of its absence in placebo phases showed up quickly and definitely. So a statistically significant result was obtained with small samples of patients. John's treatment was not quite 100% effective, but almost! His experience, however, raised an additional issue: If, in a double-blind study

of the above kind, the treatment works, the patient, the doctor, or both will tend to change their *a priori* expectations as to efficacy and outcome while the study is still in progress. It is clear that this happened in John's studies because the treatment was so effective. So in this extreme case the double-blind may be of limited duration.

So what, in a nutshell, is the message of this Foreword? There is a phrase in American political discourse that originates from the 1992 Presidential campaign. The ultimately victorious Democratic party campaign manager had a slogan over his desk to remind him of what it was all about, lest he be tempted to wander off target. The slogan was, "The economy, stupid!" I shall count my writing of this Foreword a success if just one reader makes him or herself a sign, physically or metaphorically, that says, "The feedback, stupid!" Let me, in conclusion, put this statement in a broader perspective.

One of my most persistent memories of the pathology course I took as an undergraduate at Cambridge in 1952—the year prior to the publication of James D. Watson and Francis H.C. Crick's paper on the "double helix" structure of DNA in the journal *Nature*—was Professor H.R. (Daddy) Dean's unstinting praise of Oswald T. Avery's work, published in 1944, which identified DNA as the purveyor of genetic information. This primed me to read, upon its publication in 1976 (nearly a quarter of a century after my course), Rene J. Dubos' fascinating book, *The Professor, The Institute, and DNA: Oswald T. Avery, His Life and Scientific Achievements.* In Chapter 5, "Avery's Life in the Laboratory," the book contained an account of a normal day. I was astonished to learn that, typically, research was conducted on a 24-hour cycle. I had not appreciated until then, that in this kind of laboratory research (because, in this case, of the relatively short incubation times needed to grow microorganisms) new hypotheses could be formulated and tested, and the resulting feedback digested and assimilated, in less than 24 hours. At that time, all my own research experience (apart from computer software development) had been in the human behavioral sciences, much of it in clinical research on possible therapies for Alzheimer's Disease, and the research was conducted on a minimal time cycle of months, if not years. No wonder progress was slow! Since this realization I have become increasingly interested in the whole question of how the minimum possible informative feedback cycle time affects the nature of research.

In her recent book, *Molecules of Emotion: The Science Behind Mind-Body Medicine*, Candace Pert made the very same points about feedback in describing what she found most effective in the conduct of her own laboratory research. She wrote: "This concept of the rapid feedback loop . . . explains the way I have done my science over the years. Most of the success my team and I have had resulted from a shortened feedback loop between performing an experiment and then using the results to make immediate changes or adjustments. In our AIDS research [my partner] and I cracked the mystery of the peptide that fit the AIDS virus receptors by initiating a new experimental question each morning, getting the results in the afternoon, and then pouring over the data every night for changes to be made the next day." This approach was part of her legacy from Solomon H. Snyder, in whose laboratory she did her Ph.D. research. She wrote of "[Snyder's] philosophy of the rapid, one-day turnaround, what he called the 'speedy flier.'"

The above quotation comes from a section, in Chapter 12 of her book, in which she described a visit and consultation with an "information doctor," a California physician, Dr. Robert Gottesman. Dr. Gottesman approvingly quoted Gregory Bateson's definition of information as "the difference that makes a difference" and went on to say to her: "'. . . I use the rapid feedback loop concept when treating patients. As you yourself have experienced during our consultation, I ask lots of questions to get my patients to pay attention to what's going on with them, to self monitor. It takes time, which most doctors won't spend, but I do it because I want my patients to become aware of the difference that makes a difference to them. Those who are able to respond in this way, to do their own self-monitoring, get well faster because they have more intelligence at work in their systems, more information to bring about changes that bring about improvement. So I think ultimately it saves time.'"

Dr. Gottesman is helping his patients to become co-researchers of their own health problems. But why do most of us regard this as new? Have not good physicians always done this? Yes, I think they have, but what may be new is that we now have the concepts of information science available to us to help us to describe and discuss, in behavioral terms, what may be going on in such doctor-patient relationships. It seems to have taken an inordinately long time for this to come about. When, in 1953, I was a beginning psychology student at Cambridge, there was incessant talk about "information theory" and the promise it offered for the development of a truly scientific psychology. Similar discussions were going on amongst students of other biological sciences, including the future molecular biologists. Information theory inspired the work described by British psychiatrist W. Ross Ashby in his well-known book *Design for a Brain*. This, and similar publications, formed our staple diet. When, in 1954, I arrived at University College Hospital Medical School, London, as a clinical student, one of my classmates, Oxford graduate Hugh B.G. Thomas had already made substantial progress in developing a quantitative information theoretic approach to the study of human behavior that could be applied to a wide range of clinical research problems. Later he was one of the earliest clinical researcher users of the computer time-sharing services that became available in the early 60s.

While I can think of quite a few possible reasons for this 50-year delay in adopting an information theoretic approach to clinical science, I suspect that the reasons are quite complex, a reflection of the static-dynamic, stasist-dynamist polarity described by Virginia Postrel (referenced above), and will need careful historical research to sort out. Such research would be very useful because it would help us, at this millennial moment, to better understand our present situation and future opportunities. Nevertheless, we already know enough to conjecture that the minimum informative feedback cycle time for clinical research can be lowered to close to the time it takes for a therapy to produce reportable change in individual patients. The technology of the Internet makes this possible by *allowing cases that previously had to be studied sequentially to be studied in parallel.* Instead of one physician studying 16 patients, 16 physicians—using an agreed upon protocol—can study one patient each. The results can be analyzed as they become available, and the information so obtained can be used, as necessary, to modify the protocol for the next cycle—a clinical "speedy flier." The development and promulgation of such a collaborative, parallel approach to clinical research are important aims of the new Academy for the Helping Professions. John Lowe, our colleagues, and I are currently working to bring the Academy into operational existence.

In this book John Lowe describes what appears to be a remarkably successful therapeutic approach to fibromyalgia, which is generally considered an "incurable" and largely "untreatable" condition. It is an approach based on well-tried principles that have, in times past, found expression in a wide variety of human endeavors, from jurisprudence to tin mining. These principles—as I have tried to show above—allow past experience to be justly brought to bear on new situations, even when those new situations are perceived to be unique. Taking the message of this book seriously is the first step in providing meaningful help, and a well-founded hope of recovery, to fibromyalgia patients. The book does not offer a "cure" for fibromyalgia, or give, or even try to give, all the "answers." But it asks and begins to answer the right questions—questions that change the underlying paradigm upon which fibromyalgia research is based, and thus help steer this research in a more promising direction.

—John L. Gedye, M.B., B.Chir.

Formerly, Squadron Leader, Royal Air Force Medical Branch and Junior Specialist in Aviation Physiology, Royal Air Force Institute of Aviation Medicine, Farnborough, England
Formerly, University Lecturer in Psychopathology, University of Cambridge, Cambridge, England
Formerly, Fellow, Lecturer, and Senior Lecturer, Department of Electrical Engineering Science, School of Physical Sciences, University of Essex, Colchester, England
Formerly, Research Associate Professor of Neurology, Baylor College of Medicine, Houston, Texas
Formerly, Professor of Neurology, School of Medicine, and Adjunct Professor of Electrical and Computer Engineering, College of Engineering, Wayne State University, Detroit, Michigan

Introduction

"As often in the history of science, the biggest obstacle in finding the truth is not the difficulty in obtaining data, but the bias of the investigators on what data to chase and how to interpret them."

—Peter H. Duesberg, PhD, *Inventing the AIDS Virus*
Washington, DC, Regnery Publishing, Inc., 1996

When I began to write this book several years ago, I did so because I knew it was essential if most fibromyalgia patients were ever to be relieved of their suffering. I had learned through clinical experience and research that most patients' fibromyalgia is little more than the symptoms and signs of one or both of two underlying conditions: (1) undiagnosed or undertreated hypothyroidism, and/or (2) untreated partial cellular resistance to thyroid hormone. I say "little more" because various other metabolism-impeding factors also influence most patients' signs and symptoms. Among the other factors are poor diet and nutritional deficiencies, physical deconditioning, various medications, and imbalances of other hormones. For patients to improve or recover, the influence of these other factors must be effectively reduced or eliminated. But for most patients, the use of the proper form and dosage of exogenous thyroid hormone is also indispensable.

Slowly, through trial and error, meticulous record-keeping, and data analysis, my colleagues and I evolved a treatment protocol, now called metabolic rehabilitation, that was highly effective and safe in enabling most fibromyalgia patients to markedly improve or completely recover. Later, we conducted various controlled studies which confirmed that the effects we obtained in the clinical setting were real—they were not due to misperceptions, nor were they placebo effects.

I gradually learned during this odyssey, which has lasted from 1986 until the present, that the greatest obstacle to the improvement or recovery of fibromyalgia patients (and other patients with too little thyroid hormone tissue regulation) is the adherence to four false yet dogmatic beliefs by most conventional medical clinicians: 1) that the only thyroid-hormone-related cause of the symptoms characteristic of thyroid hormone deficiency is hypothyroidism, 2) that no one should be permitted to use exogenous thyroid hormone unless laboratory test results confirm hypothyroidism, 3) that hypothyroid patients should be permitted to use only T_4, and 4) that the T_4 dosage should be adjusted according to TSH and possibly thyroid hormone blood levels.

These four beliefs are mandates of the current endocrinology paradigm. Conventional endocrinology touts them as scientifically established facts that apply to the entire human population. This, however, is simply not true. I have seen a small minority of fibromyalgia patients improve using the diagnostic and treatment protocol dictated by the mandates. But most patients improve or recover *only* when treated by a protocol that violates the mandates. As a result, to be effective and safe in helping fibromyalgia patients improve or recover, metabolic rehabilitation (as I describe and advocate it in this book) is by necessity a transgression against the endocrinology mandates.

Over the past 30 years, most conventional clinicians have unquestioningly accepted the endocrinology mandates. They obstinately believe that the mandates are true, and they comply with them as guidelines for diagnosis and treatment. Their doing so has created a major unrecognized public health problem—incalculable thousands of patients with chronic symptoms sustained by inadequate thyroid hormone regulation of their tissues. The epidemic of inadequate tissue regulation and chronic symptoms results from these clinicians undertreating patients with thyroid hormone or denying them treatment altogether. The clinicians' imperious belief in the truth of the mandates has led them to erroneously interpret patients' chronic symptoms as "new diseases." Of these new diseases, fibromyalgia and chronic fatigue syndrome are the two most publicized.

Most medical researchers, like most conventional clinicians, have narrow-mindedly refused to consider that the mechanism underlying these "new diseases" may be inadequate thyroid hormone regulation of patients' tissues. Blinded by their own beliefs, they have been unable—and will remain unable!—to solve the mystery before them. They remain baffled even though, as I describe in Section III, they themselves, through their studies, have generated a substantial body of evidence that points unequivocally to the mechanism I describe in this book.

My efforts to communicate with members of the rheumatology fibromyalgia research community regarding our findings have been largely ignored over the years. The notable exception is the eminent French rheumatologist and fibromyalgia researcher, Professor J. Eisinger, whose work I extensively cite throughout this book. His finding of glycolysis abnormalities in fibromyalgia patients that resemble those of hypothyroid patients was a landmark discovery. It is a finding that the serotonin deficiency hypothesis (the unifying concept of the rheumatology fibromyalgia paradigm) cannot explain. It therefore raises doubt that a serotonin deficiency could be the main underlying causative factor in fibromyalgia.

Over a 20-year period, the rheumatology paradigm was fruitful. It motivated researchers to conduct hundreds of studies of fibromyalgia patients, and the studies have provided vitally important information about the disorder. Gradually, however, progressively more studies have produced anomalies—research findings that the rheumatology paradigm cannot account for. Some of the anomalies are crucial blows to the paradigm, and show that it is inadequate for understanding fibromyalgia. The accumulation of anomalies has begun to dissolve the sense of cohesion the paradigm previously provided clinicians and researchers. Consequently, some researchers and clinicians have lost confidence in the paradigm.

At the same time, the anomalies, one after another, have strengthened the hypothesis that inadequate thyroid hormone regulation of tissues is the cause of most patients' fibromyalgia. During the years of my work on this book, the accumulating anomalies and continued suffering of fibromyalgia patients have kept me aware of the importance of making the information in the book available for patients and their clinicians. Now, however, just before the book goes to press, I realize that it is not only *important*—it is *imperative*! The accumulating anomalies are conspicuous signs that the rheumatology paradigm is crumbling. But it is the potentially ominous outcome of the fall of the paradigm that concerns me.

In conventional medicine, when there is no strong biologically-oriented paradigm to explain a disorder, many clinicians and researchers irrationally conclude that the symptoms of the disorder are psychogenic. This means, of course, that they come to believe, by default, that the symptoms are of mental or emotional origin. In recent years, in the field of fibromyalgia, this line of thinking has been developing into a trend. As the history of medicine teaches, this turn of events will not favor the interests of fibromyalgia patients. If the trend is not curtailed, their plight is likely to markedly worsen in years to come.

What has led to this trend? My assessment is as follows. Long-term studies show that rheumatology treatments, mainly the use of antidepressants, are ineffective—they have no beneficial effect whatever on the long-term status of fibromyalgia patients. In addition, the long-term use of the medications is far from benign for some patients. For example, amitriptyline, probably the most prescribed medication for fibromyalgia, may cause coronary artery constrictions. This is an adverse effect that could devastate some fibromyalgia patients who have, as most do, extremely low cardiovascular fitness levels. But such adverse effects from medications are not the only dangers patients face.

The cost of these currently prescribed medications is substantial. And so are the costs of other health care services fibromyalgia patients continue to use because they remain ill, even while taking the medications. Many patients remain so ill that they are unable to work, and as a result, a considerable percentage of them apply for and receive disability payments. The overall cost of the medications, other health care services, and disability has increased as fibromyalgia has become popularized (progressively more clinicians are diagnosing the disorder). Some members of the rheumatology research community continue to incorrectly report that amitriptyline and cyclobenzaprine are "effective" treatments for fibromyalgia. These reports influence clinicians to prescribe the medications for their newly diagnosed patients. Such patients have swollen the ranks of those using the medications on an indefinite basis and of those on the disability rosters. Hence, cumulative costs continue to escalate.

It should not come as a surprise that third party payers (mainly insurance companies) have become concerned about escalating costs for fibromyalgia treatments. Third party payers, whose job it is to pay the bills, are in business. All businesses, to succeed, must effectively curb costs that threaten to endlessly rise. But when the "business" of a business is paying health-care costs, cutting those costs is crucial to making a profit.

An effective tool for cost-containment is the accusation that the symptoms of the patients in question are psychogenic. There is no shortage of clinicians and researchers willing to brandish this sword against patients—and literally brand into the patients' records labels from the *Diagnostic and Statistical Manual* (*DSM*) of the American Psychiatric Association. The *DSM* label transmutes the accusation of psychogenesis into a "diagnosis," although a spurious one.

Probably most clinicians today earnestly believe that *DSM* labels are genuine diagnoses. Despite this, the labels are nothing more than descriptive terms applied to patients who have certain sets of symptoms, with no regard for the underlying biological causes. The labels are profitable to third party payers. Patients who use health care services based on the labels receive minimal third party reimbursement or none at all. The payoff from *DSM* labels is substantial enough to motivate third party payers to employ clinicians (usually called expert witnesses or independent medical evaluators) willing to ignore their Hippocratic or chiropractic oaths and assign these labels to patients. Thus, for third party payers, *DSM* labels are an effective remedy for the rising costs of the care of fibromyalgia patients.

Most clinicians and researchers who use *DSM* labels do not do so for this strategic financial purpose, as I explain in Chapter 1.2. It is my belief that for some researchers, resorting to the use of *DSM* labels serves as a psychological refuge from the harsh realization that they have failed to learn the biological basis of a health problem such as fibromyalgia. After all, if fibromyalgia is psychogenic, as *DSM* labels imply, one cannot be responsible for failing to have found a biological cause for the condition. One can stop searching without chagrin.

It is crucial that fibromyalgia patients, and the clinicians who are committed to care for them, not forget the facts about *DSM* labels and the putative psychogenic mechanisms they imply. No credible scientific study has ever verified a purely psychogenic cause of *any* disease, including fibromyalgia. There is no logical or scientific reason patients should ever receive these counterfeit "diagnoses." Fibromyalgia patients and concerned clinicians would best steadfastly refuse to accept *DSM* labels and take to task (based on information I provide in Chapter 1.2) any clinician who dares try to apply one.

Ultimately, it is the cost concerns of third party payers that make it imperative that a truly effective treatment for fibromyalgia come into widespread use.

I describe that treatment, metabolic rehabilitation, in this book. Most fibromyalgia patients who have undergone metabolic rehabilitation have markedly improved or completely recovered. My research colleagues and I have decisively demonstrated patient recovery in stringently controlled clinical trials. And we found in a 1-to-5-year follow-up study that patients maintained their improvement long term.

Fibromyalgia patients who have improved or recovered with metabolic rehabilitation require either minimal or no further health care services under the diagnosis of fibromyalgia. In the clinical sections of this book, I provide clinicians and their patients with a "how to" manual of metabolic rehabilitation. This includes a precise and detailed description of the treatment protocol. I am convinced that the widespread and proper use of this treatment will halt the rising costs for the clinical care of fibromyalgia patients and end the need for most disability applications. These results will remove the main motive for branding fibromyalgia patients with *DSM* labels.

My professional credentials are different from those of most researchers who are members of the rheumatology fibromyalgia community. On this basis, most of them (with a few notable exceptions), à la *ad hominem*, have dismissed the possibility that my view of fibromyalgia could possibly have merit. Quite the contrary—it is *because* of the differences in my educational background and clinical practice that I have been able to sidestep what Peter Duesberg called "the biggest obstacle in finding the truth"; that is, "the bias of investigators on what data to chase and how to interpret them." When Duesberg wrote, "As often in the history of science, the biggest obstacle in finding the truth is not the difficulty in obtaining data," he could have been referring to the field of fibromyalgia. A quick glance at the thousands of published papers I cite in this book will show that we have no shortage of data to interpret. My detractors may argue that most of the references are not to studies of fibromyalgia patients but to those of hypothyroid and thyroid hormone resistant patients. In retort, I conjecture that if these detractors were to scrupulously look for the differences between fibromyalgia patients and the other two groups (as I have been doing for well over a decade), they would soon discover that fundamentally, there are none.

I want to emphasize the most important feature of the clinical sections of this book. As I wrote above, the clinical sections are a manual on the proper use of metabolic rehabilitation. The clinical success rate is the same when different clinicians use precisely the same protocol. Using the protocol properly will require that most clinicians change their customary mode of practice to one of a rehabilitation model, even if they do so only with their fibromyalgia patients. To vary from the protocol as I describe it, is to compromise the therapeutic outcome.

The most critical component of the protocol is the feedback from objective measures of fibromyalgia status. The clinician must monitor the patient's fibromyalgia status at close intervals using objective measures, which I describe in Chapters 4.1, 4.3, and 5.2. He must also post the scores from the measures as data points to line graphs, which we provide in Appendix A. He must base therapeutic decisions on clinical judgment integrated with the trends of the data points on the graphs. Informative feedback is currently used in conventional medicine in places such as post-surgery and critical care wards, and in the care of patients with conditions such as hypertension. Otherwise, clinical practice usually lacks the use of informative feedback. As John Gedye explains in the Foreword, however, the use of such feedback is *essential* to the effective control of most any phenomena in our world, including fibromyalgia.

In Section IV, I describe the diagnostic protocol of metabolic rehabilitation. Chapter 4.1 includes information on diagnosing fibromyalgia and monitoring the fibromyalgia status of patients. The methods I describe in the chapter for quantifying the patient's status are critically important. Only by using these methods precisely is the clinician likely to effectively guide the patient through the rehabilitation process. For most patients, maximum improvement—which I consider complete and lasting relief from fibromyalgia symptoms—is possible *only* when the methods are used properly.

In Chapter 4.2, I describe and comment on the currently available laboratory tests for assessing the patient's thyroid status. My view is that: 1) these tests are useful only for initially establishing the thyroid status of the patient who appears to have inadequate thyroid hormone regulation of cell function, 2) the tests are useless for determining the patient's effective dosage of exogenous thyroid hormone, and 3) while some clinicians may use the tests during patients' treatment to comply with the current "standard of care," the cost of the tests during that time cannot be justified logically or scientifically.

What makes laboratory thyroid function tests useless for adjusting the thyroid hormone dosage? Simply that they do not measure what is most important in the treatment of hypothyroid and thyroid hormone resis-

tant patients—that is, how patients' tissues are responding to the hormone. In Chapter 4.3, I describe how to measure the responses of different tissues. Essentially, the chapter is an effort to revive a rational, safe, and highly effective clinical method of guiding patients to recovery. To the detriment of patients with inadequate thyroid hormone tissue regulation, conventional clinicians discarded this method some 30 years ago. On behalf of patient welfare, clinicians should resume use of the method.

I devote Chapter 4.4 to the possible adverse effects of the patient using dosages of exogenous thyroid hormone that are excessive for her. The chapter is an overview of available studies. One of the most pertinent points of the chapter is that the possible adverse effects have been highly exaggerated. At the same time, I emphasize that *the clinician must consider each patient on an individual basis*. To effectively do so, he must use measures that can accurately detect adverse *tissue* effects. These measures do not include laboratory thyroid function tests. Instead, the measures are those that assess tissue responses to thyroid hormone, as I describe in Chapter 4.3.

In Chapter 4.4, I also include a section on a tragically neglected subject: the adverse effects of too little thyroid hormone stimulation of tissues. The importance of this section is that the current practice of titrating thyroid hormone dosages by laboratory thyroid function tests typically restricts patients to dosages of thyroid hormone that are too low. The low dosages permit inadequate thyroid hormone regulation of tissues to continue apace. As a result, patients suffer from symptoms of hypometabolism, such as chronic fatigue, pain, stiffness, depression, and cognitive dysfunction. They are also at an increased risk for potentially lethal cardiovascular disease. As this section indicates, patient welfare is truly safeguarded only when clinicians have a balanced concern for excessive *and* deficient thyroid hormone tissue stimulation.

Section V is devoted to treatment. In Chapter 5.1, I review the studies of fibromyalgia treatments. Most of the treatments are intended to control the symptoms of fibromyalgia without an appreciation of the underlying cause of those symptoms. Other treatments are intended to relieve fibromyalgia symptoms by compensating for an objective fibromyalgia abnormality, such as a low growth hormone level. Such treatments may reduce or relieve the particular features of fibromyalgia caused by that abnormality. However, the treatments do not address the underlying cause of fibromyalgia in most cases—inadequate thyroid hormone regulation of cell function. Inadequate thyroid hormone regulation can account not only for the particular abnormality such a treatment addresses, it can also account for all the other symptoms and objectively verifiable abnormalities of fibromyalgia. Thus, predictably, none of the treatments described in Chapter 5.1 (exempting metabolic rehabilitation) were effective enough to provide any noteworthy improvement in the status of the average fibromyalgia patient.

Chapter 5.2 provides a detailed description of metabolic rehabilitation. Each component of the treatment protocol is included for one reason: trial and error and systematic testing have shown that the component is essential to most patients markedly improving or recovering.

In Chapter 5.3, I describe and critique the mandates of the current endocrinology paradigm for deciding who might or might not benefit from the use of exogenous thyroid hormone. I contend that these mandates are false propositions that are the root cause of the "new diseases" such as fibromyalgia and chronic fatigue syndrome. I also explain why T_4 alone is a poor choice for treating the hypothyroid patient, and I provide details on the therapeutic use of combinations of T_4 and T_3. In Chapter 5.4, I cover special considerations concerning the use of T_3 alone.

Chapter 5.5 addresses forms of treatment that are complementary to the use of exogenous thyroid hormone during metabolic rehabilitation. This chapter is a supplement to Chapter 5.2 (which describes the treatment protocol).

In Section II, I cover the basic science foundations of clinical thyroidology. Reading the chapters in this section is not essential before the clinician begins to use metabolic rehabilitation. However, as with any other special area of clinical practice, an understanding of the basic science underpinnings will give the clinician the edge in helping patients improve or recover. The clinician is most likely to acquire that understanding as he selectively uses information from the chapters in Section II when that information is relevant to cases under his care. Learning more about the science behind clinical thyroidology can also help the clinician troubleshoot any puzzling cases.

Section III is the bridge between the basic science foundations in Section II and the diagnostic and treatment protocols in Sections IV and V. In Section III, I interpret the main symptoms and objectively verified abnormalities of fibromyalgia as effects of inadequate thyroid hormone regulation of cell function. To the extent possible based on the available evidence, I describe and document plausible mechanisms by which fibromyalgia symptoms and objective findings develop from inadequate thyroid hormone tissue regulation. I suspect that most patients, clinicians, and researchers who read this book will take the most interest in this section. In some chapters, I show that it is plausible that the symptoms or objective findings are products of thyroid hormone deficiency or resistance. In most chapters, I show that this is highly probable.

In the chapters in Section I, I provide details of the argument I make in this introduction: that the plight of fibromyalgia patients in the future is likely to be worse than now, unless we avert developing trends. In my view, the only way to ward off the trends is to influence patients, clinicians, and researchers to accept, based on the evidence I present, the basic thesis of this book: that hypometabolism due to inadequate tissue regulation by thyroid hormone is the cause of fibromyalgia. To justify acceptance of this thesis, an acceptance which would change the direction of fibromyalgia research and clinical care, has been my main purpose in writing this book. Only through the widespread acceptance of this thesis—scientifically-derived, scrupulously tested, and able to plausibly explain all we know about fibromyalgia—will the suffering of most fibromyalgia patients finally come to an end.

Dr. John C. Lowe
drlowe@drlowe.com

Section I

Fibromyalgia:
The New Imperative

1.1

Fall of the Rheumatology Paradigm and the New Imperative

In the mid-1970s, medical practitioners learned that when the slow-wave sleep of sedentary subjects was disrupted, the subjects exhibited the same features as patients with fibromyalgia (then termed "fibrositis"). This observation soon led to the speculation that the symptoms resulted from a deficiency of serotonin. This conjecture is now expressed as the "serotonin deficiency hypothesis."

The serotonin deficiency hypothesis has been the unifying concept for most researchers who have contributed to the body of information now available on fibromyalgia. Researchers from a variety of disciplines and specialties have taken part and made valuable contributions. However, rheumatologists spearheaded and have been most active in sustaining the study of fibromyalgia. Because of their contributions, it is appropriate to refer to the overall research effort and the concepts that have emerged from it and guided continuing research as the "rheumatology fibromyalgia paradigm."

The serotonin deficiency hypothesis and several spin-off hypotheses have been highly productive. They have generated many studies that over the past 25 years have gradually provided patients, clinicians, and researchers with a descriptive understanding of fibromyalgia. To the credit of the rheumatology paradigm and its hypotheses, mainly the serotonin deficiency hypothesis, the most common symptoms and objectively verifiable features of the disorder are now well-known.

The main conceptual view of fibromyalgia described in this book is the "inadequate thyroid hormone regulation hypothesis." This hypothesis is a corollary of the broader "hypometabolism hypothesis" that will be elaborated elsewhere. The inadequate thyroid hormone regulation hypothesis was inspired in part by studies engendered by the rheumatology paradigm. However, the extraordinary productivity of this hypothesis has stimulated a line of research that diverges from the rheumatology paradigm. The hypothesis has, at this time, stimulated a small body of research, but its high productivity and its greater usefulness raise the probability that this hypothesis will lead to a second paradigm, one that will supplant the rheumatology paradigm. The most important product of the hypothesis is that it has provided a highly effective form of treatment, metabolic rehabilitation. This form of treatment provides marked improvement or complete recovery that is sustained long term for most patients who undergo it.

Objective verification of the biological abnormalities of fibromyalgia patients has made it obvious that fibromyalgia is an organic disorder, although, as most biological disorders, it may be modified by psychological factors. An enormously beneficial outcome for fibromyalgia patients of studies conducted within the rheumatology paradigm is the verification of objective abnormalities among patients.

A benefit in the verification of fibromyalgia as a biological disorder is that it potentially frees patients *from a particularly contentious subset of clinicians and researchers—those who, by default, ascribe health problems that have no generally accepted biological basis, such as fibromyalgia, to psychogenic processes.*

Before the researchers of the rheumatology paradigm began to unearth the biological abnormalities of fibromyalgia, many 20th century clinicians and researchers concluded that fibromyalgia patients' symptoms were psychogenic. These clinicians and researchers often described the patients as having "hysteria" or "psychogenic rheumatism."

The view that fibromyalgia was psychogenic was a lingering effect of Freudian thinking on many 20th century clinicians. Today, some quarter century after the genesis of the rheumatology paradigm, many clinicians and researchers continue to hold these Freudian-based views of fibromyalgia patients. However, the terms "hysteria" and "psychogenic rheumatism," which imply underlying psychogenesis, have been replaced with several newer labels taken from the Diagnostic and Statistical Manual *of the American Psychiatric Association (*DSM*).* DSM *labels imply the same underlying mechanisms as did the older labels.*

The rise of the rheumatology fibromyalgia paradigm and the studies that established the disorder as biological staved off the tendency of most clinicians to give fibromyalgia patients DSM *labels. However, this reprieve for patients was short-lived. In recent years, the failure of the rheumatology paradigm to provide an effective treatment for fibromyalgia has led to a crisis. The numbers of patients under active care has increased at an accelerated rate as clinicians make the diagnosis more often. In addition, many patients have applied for and received disability payments. These events have led to cost concerns by third party payers. Following these concerns, an increase in the number of papers and conference presentations favoring* DSM *labeling of fibromyalgia patients has occurred.*

At the same time, researchers have produced study results that the serotonin deficiency hypothesis cannot explain. The inadequate thyroid hormone regulation hypothesis adequately accounts for all the symptoms and objective findings of fibromyalgia. For several reasons, however, members of the rheumatology paradigm have ignored the hypothesis and the treatment derived from it. With no other hypothesis generally accepted as plausibly explaining the etiology of fibromyalgia, clinicians and researchers appear to be falling back on the traditional default hypothesis of conventional medicine—psychogenesis.

This has further contributed to the increase in DSM *labeling of patients.*

Rheumatology paradigm clinicians and researchers appear to have neglected the inadequate thyroid hormone regulation hypothesis for five reasons. (1) Studies based on the hypothesis have been blocked from publication in mainstream medical journals. This is a common obstacle to innovation in conventional medicine. Disingenuous tactics are often used by medical journal editors and peer reviewers to prevent the publication of views that may displease advertisers or against which conventional clinicians and researchers are prejudiced. This treatment is not limited to unknown researchers but also to Nobel Laureates who express unconventional views.

(2) Most conventional clinicians are not familiar with the rehabilitation model of clinical practice, or for various reasons, such as the dictates of managed care, they are not able to practice according to the model.

(3) Researchers appear to have a natural resistance to paradigm change. Due to this resistance, innovative ideas and practices may be ignored or rejected by the old guard of a long-standing paradigm. Acceptance of the innovative ideas and practices usually occurs gradually as younger researchers without vested interests in the older paradigm come to dominate in clinical and research settings.

(4) Most conventional clinicians today have a truncated knowledge of clinical thyroidology. This has resulted from an achievement of conventional endocrinology. This specialty successfully convinced other medical specialties to accept its mandates for which patients are to be permitted to use thyroid hormone and how they should use it. Practicing according to the mandates has diminished clinicians' and researchers' knowledge of thyroidology. With their knowledge truncated, most clinicians and researchers feel uncomfortable with protocols that violate the endocrinology mandates. Unfortunately, most patients with hypothyroidism or resistance to thyroid hormone improve or recover only when they are treated with a protocol that violates the mandates. Metabolic rehabilitation is such a protocol.

(5) The code of conduct in conventional medicine resembles that of the military or the church. It prescribes unquestioning acceptance of the beliefs of medical authorities, much of which is dogma. This code of conduct is appropriate for the military or the church and serves their purposes well. But it is not appropriate for those practicing health care, and it is the antithesis of the code of professional scientists.

Compliance with the code of conduct results in extreme resistance to the views of anyone not considered an authority within conventional medicine. And until a conventional medical authority endorses a new view, most conventional clinicians and researchers are not inclined to listen to it. The authorities, however, are usually prejudiced toward the views and practices they helped establish during their careers, and they tenaciously resist the introduction of new ideas and practices.

For most of the 20th century, many conventional medical clinicians believed that mental or emotional disturbance was the cause of the symptoms characteristic of fibromyalgia. Research by some medical clinicians that began in the mid-1970s established that fibromyalgia is a biologically-based disorder. The studies gave rise to the rheumatology paradigm of fibromyalgia. Over the years this paradigm has prevailed, the results of some studies inspired by the paradigm's predominant hypothesis, the serotonin deficiency hypothesis, showed that the hypothesis does not adequately explain fibromyalgia. Instead, these results, called anomalies (see Glossary) suggest that the hypothesis is false.

Study results that the rheumatology paradigm cannot explain have strengthened an alternate view of fibromyalgia, one that is outside the realm of the rheumatology model. I formulated this alternate view, which I term the hypometabolism hypothesis, over a span of 14 years of study of fibromyalgia, in collaboration with my research colleagues. This book is about a corollary of the hypometabolism hypothesis that I term the "inadequate thyroid hormone regulation hypothesis." This corollary hypothesis states that the main mechanism of the symptoms and objective findings of fibromyalgia is inadequate thyroid hormone regulation of fibromyalgia-specific tissues. By fibromyalgia-specific tissues I mean the set of tissues from which the symptoms and objective abnormalities of fibromyalgia arise when the metabolism of the cells of those tissues is sufficiently subnormal.

In this chapter, I overview the rise of the rheumatology paradigm of fibromyalgia. I also overview the inadequacies of that paradigm that account for its fall, which is now well underway. Throughout the overview, I describe the events that compelled me to formulate the inadequate thyroid hormone regulation hypothesis. The hypothesis is now stimulating research outside the domain of the rheumatology paradigm. This hypothesis is a rich source of testable predictions

that can contribute to a new body of studies more promising than those stimulated by the rheumatology paradigm. With the inadequate thyroid hormone regulation hypothesis, we have the likelihood of a second fibromyalgia paradigm, one that will replace the first. For some science historians, philosophers of science, and other observers of the advance of science, the time is exhilarating when a new and promising concept takes shape enough to suggest that it may supplant a formerly productive paradigm. The time is rich with promise for advanced understanding of the phenomenon under study and for our ability to control it. Those of us whose work is inspired by the inadequate thyroid hormone regulation hypothesis feel that exhilaration. The feeling derives from our knowledge that the hypothesis meets the ultimate test of medical theories—usefulness for patient care. The form of treatment that derives from the hypothesis, metabolic rehabilitation, effectively enables most patients who undergo it, within a few months, to markedly improve or completely recover from fibromyalgia long term. This result, which is rigorously documented, means that the inadequate thyroid hormone regulation hypothesis has succeeded where the serotonin deficiency hypothesis has failed.

In this chapter, I describe the events of the rise and fall of the rheumatology paradigm, and those that led to the formulation of the inadequate thyroid hormone regulation hypothesis and the development of metabolic rehabilitation. I have not attempted to provide here an encyclopedic coverage of historical events. I have included only those necessary for an understanding of my thesis in this chapter.

● BEFORE THE RHEUMATOLOGY FIBROMYALGIA PARADIGM

The symptoms of fibromyalgia were described by ancient medical writers, such as Maimonides, Galen, and Sidenham. Some of these writers expressed the view, which is correct, that a sedentary lifestyle can produce the symptoms. This observation, that sedentary people are prone to develop the symptoms, is a clue to the basis of perhaps most patients' fibromyalgia: Metabolism in certain tissues is slow enough to cause symptoms, which modern health psychology teaches us are signals to the affected individual that damage is threatened or occurring.

In the late 19th century, something happened that would prove to be a scourge to those who suffer from fibromyalgia. Surreal and fantastical ideas were prolifically generated by a neurologist-psychiatrist and cocaine addict named Sigmund Freud. His ideas, which became more bizarre as his addiction worsened and he suffered nose and brain damage, gave tremendous impetus to the perpetuation of the false Cartesian mind-body dichotomy (see Chapter 1.2, subsection titled "Delusional (Paranoid) Disorder").

In the 20th century, science philosophers and logicians have appropriately denounced Freud's ideas as metaphysical in some cases and pseudo-scientific in others. His ideas are properly termed metaphysical because they are incapable of scrutiny by objective scientific methods and thus must remain empirically unverified. Other of his ideas are properly termed pseudo-scientific because they are often promoted (at least by implication) as scientifically verified or verifiable concepts. As I explain in Chapter 1.2, the psychogenesis hypothesis is easily falsified and is to be excluded from the domain of scientific hypotheses.

Because *DSM* labeling (assignment of labels from the *Diagnostic and Statistical Manual of the American Psychiatric Association*) of fibromyalgia patients is increasing, the reader should be sensitized to a common logical fallacy of those who hypothesize that fibromyalgia is psychogenic. Those who promote the idea of psychogenesis argue that if a disorder does not have a generally accepted biological basis, it is therefore psychogenic. The use of this fallacious argument is common practice in conventional medicine. Its use is stimulated most often by those neurologists and psychiatrists who mimic Freud in embroidering elaborate tales of mental and emotional processes interacting to produce fibromyalgia patients' symptoms (see the case of K. Sharon Baillie in Chapter 1.2, subsection titled "One Illustrative Case"). They typically argue that we have no scientific proof of an underlying biological cause of fibromyalgia. To them, the presumed absence of proof proves that fibromyalgia is psychogenic. But where is the evidence that symptoms without a proven biological cause are, ergo, mentally or emotionally based? There simply is none. As I have learned from journal debates and personal communications, however, to reason with most of them is useless. By various convoluted misapplications of logic, they are unable to see that their argument is a *non sequitur*. To accept their argument would be to submit to a double standard—one in which we are required to prove through evidence that fibromyalgia is biologically caused, but in which no evidence is deemed necessary to prove fibromyalgia is psychogenic.

Why does this illogic continue to be used in con-

ventional medicine? There are several answers to this question (see Chapter 1.2), but only one is important to my purposes in this chapter. The public in general and many conventional medical clinicians believe a mistaken idea, one that is sustained by Hollywood, the news media, and the political wings of medical associations. The idea is that we live in an era in which the physician is also a scientist. Of the many published statements contradicting this idea is a recent one by Gunn: "Michael L. Millenson's well-documented book, *Demanding Medical Excellence: Doctors and Accountability in the Information Age*, is a wake up call to both medicine and nursing for somewhat different reasons. Millenson decries the lack of scientifically-based medical practice and medicine's failure to wake up due to its own historical studies. He cites data that 85% of current practice has not been scientifically validated despite medicine's claims of the physician-scientist."[101]

In general, conventional medical clinicians—unlike science philosophers, science logicians, and formally trained, professional scientists—lack an education and understanding of science. (I do not write this with pejorative intent; it is simply a fact. Medical clinicians are educated and trained in the diagnosis and treatment of disease, not in the practice of science.) Therefore, unless they have separate, extensive training in the practice of science and the mind-set of the professional scientist, physicians are not qualified to evaluate the scientific legitimacy of ideas such as Freud's. Largely because of this, I believe, many medical clinicians embraced Freudian ideas or their descendants and incorporated them into their medical practices. Some physicians then invented new terminology for old concepts such as "psychogenic rheumatism" (a former label applied to fibromyalgia patients). These old concepts now survive as today's *DSM* labels.

I have included in Chapter 1.2 a more detailed history of clinicians' believing that fibromyalgia is a psychogenic disorder (see section titled "Fibromyalgia Viewed as Psychogenic Pain"). This history begins well before the rheumatology paradigm came to prominence and before the American College of Rheumatology (ACR) diagnostic criteria were established.

PERPETUATION OF FREUDIAN CONCEPTS BY *DSM* LABELING

Today, the *DSM* perpetuates the Freudian line of thinking. It provides clinicians with convenient *DSM* labels they can apply to patients after ruling out a few of the main medical conditions that could account for the patients' symptoms.[1,p.111] At this time, few medical clinicians probably seriously believe Freudian ideas expressed in their original form. But as Walker recently wrote, the committee that writes the *DSM*, by "cowardly" attempting to placate both biological psychiatrists and psychoanalysts (the *crème de la crème* of *DSM* labelers), perpetuates the false mind-body dichotomy.[1p.110] As I point out in Chapter 1.2, the committee appears to be gradually distancing itself from Freudian terminology and concepts with successive editions of the *DSM*. But gradually distancing itself is not good enough. Despite the changes it has made, the committee still provides dubious criteria for clinicians to justify their applying labels to patients based ultimately on Freudian metaphysical and pseudo-scientific concepts. To my mind, this denies the *DSM* scientific credibility. But worse, it provides a broadsword, in the form of *DSM* labels, that some clinicians and attorneys can wield to drive fibromyalgia patients from insurance benefits, disability payments, and medical offices where they are perceived as a nuisance. (In a 1997 study, use of the "Difficult Doctor-Patient Relationship Questionnaire" showed that some rheumatologists included fibromyalgia patients among those the physicians found frustrating and difficult.[6] Use of *DSM* labels enables some physicians to rid themselves of the patients by referring them to mental health practitioners.) Unfortunately, during the fall of the rheumatology paradigm that we are now witnessing, the *DSM* broadsword is out of the scabbard, and not on behalf of the interests of fibromyalgia patients.

Freud's ideas about the mental or emotional basis of disease also survive today embedded in a belief of some bodywork practitioners. They believe that virtually every physical ailment, such as fibromyalgia, is the manifestation of some unresolved emotional matter. The therapeutic intention of these practitioners, who may use any of a vast array of bodywork techniques, is to help the client bring to the forefront of her mind the emotional conflict that underlies her physical ailment. Through re-experiencing the main conflict ("abreacting," in psychoanalytic terms), the client resolves the conflict, and is thereupon liberated from the ailment that is the conflict's physical expression. Undoubtedly, some clients acquire expectations of such emotional experiences from inadvertent hypnosis-like tutoring by the practitioners, and the clients may thus experience what appears to be abreactions. Yet equally undoubtedly, not one credible case of recovery from fibromyalgia through this sort of therapy can be documented. Such psychoanalytically-based bodywork often has value in temporarily reducing muscle tension and relieving stress. Otherwise, however, I believe it is as nonsensical and therapeutically fruitless as psychoanalysis itself. These practitioners are of concern today because, with the failure of the rheumatology paradigm to provide an effective treatment, many patients wisely seek relief from bodyworkers. The subset of bodyworkers I refer to here, in all likelihood, are sincere and well-intending, but they are misguided by Freudian concepts. Their *physical* treatments often temporarily benefit fibromyalgia patients, but nothing constructive is to be gained from providing the patients with a relabeled bottle of Freudian delusion.

I want to emphasize, regarding the previous paragraph, that when I denounce the Freudian notion that repressed emotions sneakily express themselves as socially-acceptable physical illness, I am not denouncing modern psychophysiology. My view is consistent with that of psychologist Robert Fried, who wrote: "The emergence of psychoimmunology, and health psychology in general, strongly attests to the 'symbiosis' of mind and body in both individual and community health behavior. No one questions the connection any longer. But the current view resembles nothing of the old mind-body constructs of psychoanalytic theory, where obscure unverifiable processes were held responsible for the 'conversion' of id-impulses into psychosomatic equivalents."[120,p.34]

● GENESIS OF THE RHEUMATOLOGY FIBROMYALGIA PARADIGM

In 1880, Beard, a U.S. psychiatrist, concluded that the stresses of modern life caused a syndrome of widespread pain, fatigue, and psychological disturbance, which he termed "neurasthenia."[102,p.7] In the 20th century, however, under the influence of Freudian thinking, many clinicians came to believe that psychiatric illness caused the symptoms. In 1989, Merskey stated that a trend had grown for some 60 years to attribute regional pain to psychiatric illness.[30,p.213] The concept was applied to soldiers who developed physical symptoms after experiencing battlefield stress. Some U.S. soldiers developed widespread pain and fatigue after being subjected to combat stress in World War II. From this observation, clinicians created the label "psychogenic rheumatism." From observing soldiers in English hospitals following combat stress, other clinicians created the label "fibrositis."[31,p.232]

Merskey wrote that although stress can aggravate pain, it is surprising how little evidence exists suggesting that stress causes pain. He also cited a study showing that stress did not exacerbate or promote facial pain. He wrote, "No authors have produced evidence that demonstrates that a pain disorder that is not due to a psychiatric illness might be due to environmental stress."[30,p.221] (Although I will not go into it here, there is also no evidence that any psychiatric illness is the cause of a pain disorder. The reader must bear in mind that "somatoform pain disorder" is not a diagnosis—it is only a *DSM* label some clinicians apply to patients who have pain that has no obvious or easily identified physical cause. See Chapter 1.2, section titled "Somatoform Pain Disorder.")

Moldofsky conjectured that stress causes disturbed sleep, and in turn, the disturbed sleep produces fibromyalgia symptoms.[31,p.232] Because of studies he had conducted with the rheumatologist Smythe, he came to believe that sleep disturbance was the basis of fibromyalgia. An introduction to these two important fibromyalgia researchers is proper at this point.

Hugh Smythe is the rheumatologist who first noted that fibromyalgia is not psychogenic rheumatism. In 1972, in a chapter in a rheumatology textbook, he tried to distinguish fibromyalgia (then termed fibrositis) from psychogenic rheumatism. Soon after, based on his collaboration with Moldofsky, Smythe ceased using the qualifier "psychogenic" at all in relation to fibromyalgia. Smythe is now considered the "Father of Fibromyalgia."[20] Over the next decade, other researchers, mainly rheumatologists, came to the same conclusion. In 1989, Goldenberg wrote that controlled studies had made it clear that fibromyalgia was not hysteria or psychogenic rheumatism, as some clinicians had thought in the 1950s and 1960s.[24] (See Chapter 1.2, section titled "Psychological Status of Fibromyalgia Patients.")

Harvey Moldofsky, a Canadian psychiatrist, developed an interest in musculoskeletal pain while he was in England in 1963 and 1964. When he returned to Canada, he became acquainted with Smythe who had been studying "fibrositis" patients. Because of his background in sleep physiology, Moldofsky was interested in the patients' complaints of nonrestorative sleep. He began sleep studies of the patients and is now well-recognized for his contributions to our understanding of the sleep abnormalities of fibromyalgia.[21]

Moldofsky et al. found that intentionally distur-

bing the sleep of healthy, sedentary individuals would cause fibromyalgia-like symptoms—both widespread pain and tender points—the next day. From this finding, he believed that combat and other stresses disturbed sleep, and the disturbed sleep caused fibromyalgia. However, I believe it is far more likely that while stress can cause sleep disturbance in anyone, disturbed sleep caused fibromyalgia only in individuals with borderline sufficient metabolism. The disturbed sleep further slows metabolism in these individuals enough to cause symptoms of hypometabolism. This hypothesis is suggested by the reports of Moldofsky, Smythe, and others in the mid-1970s and later[32][33] that individuals with high levels of aerobic fitness are resistant to developing fibromyalgia symptoms when they are subjected to disturbed sleep. Others later confirmed the observation.[34][35][36] This finding provides support for the view of ancient medical writers that sedentary individuals were more susceptible to the symptoms that today we consider typical of fibromyalgia.

It was this finding that in the late 1980s struck me as an important clue to the nature of fibromyalgia. Its importance is even more obvious now. If disturbed sleep precipitates fibromyalgia only in individuals predisposed by low or borderline sufficient metabolism, then metabolic insufficiency is the most fundamental factor in the development of symptoms. We would expect that disturbed sleep and many other factors that impede metabolism will most readily cause fibromyalgia symptoms in those whose metabolism is on the slower end of the bell curve.

In publications between 1976 and 1982, Moldofsky suggested that a serotonin deficiency might underlie fibromyalgia.[33][104][105] In 1978, Moldofsky and Warsh had found that free plasma tryptophan levels were normal in fibromyalgia patients. Within the normal range, however, the free plasma tryptophan levels correlated inversely with the severity of fibromyalgia patients' subjective estimate of morning pain: The higher the estimated pain, the lower the plasma tryptophan level. The researchers proposed that the lower plasma tryptophan levels caused reduced serotonin production, that reduced serotonin levels caused poor maintenance of slow-wave sleep, and in turn, reduced slow-wave sleep generated fibromyalgia symptoms.[104] That lower tryptophan levels would result in a clinical syndrome due to impaired slow-wave sleep was a plausible hypothesis. Its plausibility was based on the evidence that serotonin potently mediates pain perception and restorative slow-wave sleep,[106][107][108] and that inhibition of serotonin synthesis with *p*-chlorophenylalanine reduces slow-wave sleep and produces somatic symptoms.[107] Moldofsky and Warsh recognized the therapeutic potential and conducted a study to test the effects of exogenous tryptophan on fibromyalgia patients. When patients took 5 grams of tryptophan, their sleep improved but their pain and other musculoskeletal symptoms did not improve.[104][105] Moldofsky and Lue began a double-blind placebo-controlled study of the use of L-5-hydroxy-tryptophan and carbidopa (a decarboxylation inhibitor used in combination with levodopa to treat Parkinson's disease) at bedtime by fibromyalgia patients. The researchers ended the study because the medication caused nausea and vomiting that interrupted the patients' sleep, and there was no therapeutic effect.[109] In another study, researchers found that levels of total tryptophan (free + protein-bound) in the serum of fibromyalgia patients were significantly low.[110] Yunus et al. confirmed these findings.[43] In 1982, Yunus proposed that fibromyalgia is a syndrome of pain modulation.[105]

In 1988, researchers reported that the mean serum level of serotonin in 9 fibromyalgia patients was significantly lower than in matched controls.[42] Other groups also reported that the concentration of serotonin in the serum and on the platelets of fibromyalgia patients was lower than in controls.[39][40][41] These studies showed low peripheral levels of serotonin, but significantly low central nervous system levels have not been demonstrated. Thus, the serotonin deficiency hypothesis originated from the findings supporting Moldofsky's proposal.

DISTINGUISHING FEATURES OF FIBROMYALGIA: WIDESPREAD PAIN AND TENDER POINTS

In 1981, Yunus, another rheumatologist, and his colleagues compared patients with muscle pain to healthy control subjects. In this paper, they introduced the concept of fibromyalgia as a primary disorder. They also proposed diagnostic criteria for the condition.[95]

Yunus et al. concluded, "Primary fibromyalgia should be suspected by the presence of its own characteristic features, and not diagnosed just by the absence of other recognizable conditions." They also noted that fibromyalgia was "a poorly recognized condition."[95] In 1986, Wolfe wrote of fibromyalgia, "All patients have multiple areas of local tenderness called 'tender points' that are easily identified during physical examination and are diagnostic."[96]

Chronic widespread pain was the most prominent feature of fibromyalgia, and most patients had abnormal tenderness at predictable body sites. After the multicenter consensus study published in 1990, the presence of widespread pain and tender points became the American College of Rheumatology (ACR) criteria for distinguishing patients considered to have fibromyalgia.[37] These two criteria were a boon to the rheumatology paradigm of fibromyalgia. They enabled researchers to distinguish the group of patients they were studying. Regardless of the merit of the criteria for an understanding of the nature of fibromyalgia, they made it possible for researchers to begin identifying objective abnormalities common to patients who met the criteria.

Based on the ACR criteria, researchers have now compiled a vast amount of descriptive information on fibromyalgia. In Section III, I have included chapters on each of the most common symptoms and objectively verified abnormalities among fibromyalgia patients. Some symptoms and objective findings support the serotonin deficiency hypothesis. Most, however, do not. These have led to the falsification of the hypothesis. At the same time, the findings overall support the inadequate thyroid hormone regulation hypothesis. In fact, some of those that most effectively falsify the serotonin deficiency hypothesis are the strongest in support of the inadequate thyroid hormone regulation hypothesis. (See Table 1.1.1.)

● FALL OF THE RHEUMATOLOGY FIBROMYALGIA PARADIGM

A scientific paradigm is viable only as long as it spawns studies that provide understanding and/or control of the subject it conceptualizes. The viable time of the rheumatology fibromyalgia paradigm spanned some 20 years. From its beginning in the mid-1970s, the paradigm was fertile in generating studies that provided us with a descriptive understanding of fibromyalgia patients. By the mid-to-late 1990s, however, several events signaled that the paradigm was barren.

The signaling events were: (1) the publication of anomalous study results, research findings the paradigm could not plausibly account for, (2) the failure of the concepts of the paradigm to lead to an effective treatment, resulting in escalating costs to third party payers, and (3) a resurgence of the pseudo-scientific notion that fibromyalgia is psychogenic, providing an easy remedy for escalating costs and solace for some researchers who had failed to find a biological cause of fibromyalgia. I explore each of these events below. Before doing so, however, it is fitting to note the useful etiological hypotheses that the rheumatology paradigm generated during its two fertile decades. None of the rheumatology paradigm hypotheses plausibly account for all or even most of the fibromyalgia symptoms and objective findings. In addition, some objective findings falsify the hypotheses. Hence, none of the hypotheses are viable competitors against the hypometabolism hypothesis of fibromyalgia and its corollary, the inadequate thyroid hormone regulation hypothesis. (See Table 1.1.1.)

FALSIFIED HYPOTHESES OF THE RHEUMATOLOGY PARADIGM

Disturbed Slow-Wave Sleep

An initially good hypothesis, in that it generated useful fibromyalgia studies, was that fibromyalgia is the physiological and psychological effects of disturbed slow-wave sleep. Predictions from this hypothesis were tested and the hypothesis was falsified. Researchers determined that not all fibromyalgia patients have disturbed slow-wave sleep. Some researchers have reported that only a small percentage of fibromyalgia patients have disrupted slow-wave sleep, and the severity of the disruption does not correlate with the severity of fibromyalgia.[64] Moreover, medications and other therapeutic methods that enable patients to sleep sufficiently do not relieve patients' fibromyalgia. (See Chapter 3.18.)

Physical Deconditioning

A reasonable hypothesis when first proposed was that fibromyalgia is the effects of physical deconditioning Similarly, not all fibromyalgia patients were physically deconditioned, a high fitness level does not protect some individuals from having fibromyalgia, and patients guided through physical conditioning programs improve slightly at most. (See Chapter 5.1, section titled "Exercise.")

Low Growth Hormone and Somatomedin C Levels

Low levels of growth hormone and somatomedin C are not found in all fibromyalgia patients. Exogenous growth hormone appears to relieve the features of fibromyalgia mediated by low levels of the two hormones in those patients who are deficient, but exogenous growth hormone is not a generally effective treatment. Eisinger's findings of glycolysis abnormalities in fibromyalgia patients falsify the growth hormone hypothesis in that low growth hormone levels would be predicted to increase, rather than decrease, glycolysis. (See Chapter 3.12.)

Stress

It seems that at one time or another, someone hypothesizes that stress is the cause of any and every disease afflicting humans. Some researchers have proposed that abnormal hormonal measures in fibromyalgia patients result from the stresses associated with fibromyalgia. Bennett suggested to me that the pituitary-thyroid axis abnormalities my research group found were due to stress,[66] and Riedel et al. recently proposed that stress causes a host of endocrine abnormalities.[67] This stress hypothesis suffers from serious flaws. First, virtually everyone in modern society is stressed. Why stress would cause fibromyalgia in some patients and not others necessitates proposing some other factor that would render those who develop fibromyalgia in response to stress susceptible to do so. In that a history of stress—even chronic, severe stress—is not peculiar to those who develop fibromyalgia, stress alone cannot be the sole factor. The element that would render some individuals susceptible to fibromyalgia would be the responsible factor, not stress *per se*. Second, if stress were a significant contribution to the biological mechanisms underlying fibromyalgia, improved fibromyalgia status would result upon stress relief. However, the results of studies of stress-relief treatments such as cognitive-behavioral therapy show that these treatments do not improve fibromyalgia status. (See Chapter 5.1, section titled "Behavioral Treatments.")

Third, the stress mechanism does not explain many of the well-documented symptoms and objective findings in fibromyalgia. For example, Riedel et al. wrote that stress-related somatostatin release suppresses TSH response to TRH, and some of their 16 fibromyalgia patients had blunted TSH responses.[67] In the 38 fibromyalgia patients I studied, I found that 11 of 20 patients (55%) had blunted TSH responses to injected TRH. However, 9 of the 20 patients had exaggerated TSH responses to TRH.[68] And in a subsequent study my colleagues and I conducted of 54 additional fibromyalgia patients, we found TRH stimulation test results consistent with my testing of the original 38 patients.[69]

The failure to plausibly account for most of the

features of fibromyalgia is a crippling blow to the stress hypothesis. The three main faults of this hypothesis relegate it to the classification of easily falsifiable and discardable conjectures.

Serotonin Deficiency Hypothesis

The failure of most hypotheses of the etiology of fibromyalgia engendered by the rheumatology paradigm was not crucial. However, the falsification of the serotonin deficiency hypothesis is decisively important.

The serotonin deficiency hypothesis was the conceptual linchpin that unified the various researchers working within the rheumatology paradigm. Compared to the other hypotheses generated by the paradigm, the serotonin deficiency hypothesis has spawned more studies and has survived the longest. However, an accumulation of research findings are anomalous to the hypothesis, making it improbable that a serotonin deficiency is the main etiological factor in fibromyalgia. It is inevitable that these anomalies will dissolve confidence in the hypothesis and the paradigm that depends on it. Some researchers may continue for awhile testing predictions derived from the serotonin deficiency hypothesis. But it is now only a matter of time until enough researchers learn of the greater usefulness of the inadequate thyroid hormone regulation hypothesis, begin testing predictions derived from it, and abandon completely the serotonin deficiency hypothesis as a source of testable theorems.

Moldofsky et al. are responsible for the origin of the serotonin deficiency hypothesis. Russell, however, has been its foremost protagonist. In 1994, he described his working hypothesis as deceptively simple. He wrote: "Abnormal levels of or a disproportion of serotonin and substance P in the brain and the spinal cord result in a variety of neuroendocrine, biorhythm, and nociceptive abnormalities which explain the signs and symptoms of fibromyalgia syndrome."[123,p.109] At that time, a serotonin deficiency was still considered a plausible mechanism of the features of fibromyalgia.

In 1996, Russell wrote: "Our simplest model to explain these findings [the objectively verified abnormalities of fibromyalgia patients] would focus on the 'serotonin deficiency hypothesis' evidenced by a decrease in 5HT [serotonin] effect (failure to properly activate 5HT receptors) on 5HT regulated systems in the CNS."[122,p.85] A serotonin deficiency was still a component of the hypothesis, although Russell added "a decrease in serotonin effect."[122,p.85]

In another 1996 publication, he did not mention a serotonin deficiency but wrote, "Our simplest model to

explain these findings would focus on a decrease in serotonin effect (failure to properly activate serotonin receptors for whatever reason) on serotonin-regulated systems in the brain and/or spinal cord."[97,p.193]

In 1999, Russell argued for a serotonin deficiency again. He noted that studies have shown (1) a correlation between fibromyalgic pain and low plasma levels of tryptophan (the amino acid precursor of serotonin), (2) low cerebrospinal tryptophan levels, (3) low serum serotonin due to low levels of platelet serotonin, (4) low cerebrospinal 5-hydroxytryptophan (the immediate precursor of serotonin), and (5) low 24-hour urinary excretion of 5-hydroxyindoleacetic acid.[118,pp.185-186]

Russell also wrote that the cerebrospinal level of 5-hydroxyindoleacetic acid (the metabolite of serotonin) in fibromyalgia patients was lower than that in controls.[118,p.185] He cited a 1992 study by his research group.[103] The fact is, however, that he and his colleagues found that the mean cerebrospinal fluid level of fibromyalgia patients was "numerically" lower than that of control subjects, but the difference between the levels of the two groups was *not* statistically significant. This means that the small difference in the levels of the patients and controls was probably due to chance variation rather than to a real difference between the two groups.

Despite low platelet levels of serotonin, low urinary 5-hydroxyindoleacetic acid, and low plasma and cerebrospinal fluid levels of tryptophan, various other findings are contrary to what we would expect if patients' CNS serotonin levels were low. For example, several studies have documented reduced blood flow through the brain (see Chapter 3.2). Serotonin is a potent vasoconstrictor. If CNS levels of serotonin were low, we would expect increased rather than decreased brain blood flow. Also, if low serotonin levels were responsible for features of fibromyalgia, the antidepressant medications such as amitriptyline and cyclobenzaprine, by increasing serotonin levels, would relieve patients of those features. However, besides an extremely minor and brief improvement on a few measures of fibromyalgia status, the medications are no more effective than placebos. For all practical purposes, increasing patients' serotonin levels with the medications does not affect their fibromyalgia status. Because Russell and McCain have continued to report that the medications are effective, I have included the section below titled "Failure of Treatments Based on the Serotonin Deficiency Hypothesis" to clarify this important issue. Decreased brain blood flow and the failure of treatments based on the serotonin deficiency hypothesis are anomalies that falsify the hypothesis (see the next section).

To my knowledge, Russell has provided no evidence to support his hypothesis that a "decrease in serotonin effect" underlies fibromyalgia. The proposal may be what in science logic we call an *ad hoc* hypothesis. *Ad hoc* hypotheses are weak because they go as little as possible beyond the facts they are expected to explain.[25,p.232] This means that they provide few or no predictions that researchers can empirically test in an attempt to falsify the hypotheses. Hopefully, Russell will soon provide predictions derived from the decreased serotonin effect hypothesis that can be subjected to empirical testing. Without generating such predictions, a hypothesis risks being considered strictly *ad hoc* and thereby not worthy of serious consideration. Regardless, whether the hypothesis proposes a serotonin deficiency or decreased serotonin effect, it cannot plausibly account for many objective fibromyalgia findings (see the next section). At this time, the serotonin deficiency and decreased serotonin effect hypotheses cannot account for numerous research findings (see Table 1.1.1). Their failure to account for some findings effectively falsifies the hypotheses. In contrast, the inadequate thyroid hormone regulation hypothesis plausibly accounts for the findings the other two hypotheses can and cannot account for—including a peripheral serotonin deficiency itself (see Section III). The inadequate thyroid hormone regulation hypothesis, then, is the more useful scientifically, and it should supplant the serotonin deficiency and decreased serotonin effect hypotheses as guides to further fibromyalgia research.

Russell wrote in 1996, "We are currently unaware of any clinical findings or laboratory data that would specifically invalidate this model. . . ."[97,p.194] Table 1.1.1 lists numerous findings that the serotonin deficiency hypothesis and/or the decreased serotonin effect hypothesis cannot plausibly account for. The findings therefore do invalidate these hypotheses.

ANOMALIES AND THE FALL OF THE RHEUMATOLOGY PARADIGM

During the reigning years of the rheumatology paradigm, numerous anomalies have turned up, and some are crucial blows to the serotonin deficiency hypothesis. These include carbohydrate abnormalities, several connective tissue abnormalities, a positive response to the β-adrenergic agonist salbutamol, in-creased α-adrenergic receptors on platelets, cold intolerance, and decreased brain blood flow.

Two of the most important anomalies are that (1) antidepressant medications that increase serotonin levels do not benefit fibromyalgia patients and (2) most patients markedly improve or completely recover with metabolic rehabilitation involving the use of exogenous thyroid hormone. Several research groups, including my own, have shown a high incidence of primary and central hypothyroidism among fibromyalgia patients. In addition, my research group has documented that most euthyroid fibromyalgia patients have partial tissue resistance to thyroid hormone.

Inadequate thyroid hormone regulation can explain the disturbed slow wave sleep of fibromyalgia patients, but Carette et al. found that only a small percentage of fibromyalgia patients had sleep disturbance. They also found that amitriptyline did not relieve alpha intrusions into slow-wave sleep.[64] This suggests that a serotonin deficiency was not responsible for the slow-wave sleep anomaly. It is possible that inadequate thyroid hormone regulation of sleep regulation was. (See Chapter 3.18.)

Failure of Treatments Based on the Serotonin Deficiency Hypothesis

A crippling blow to the serotonin deficiency hypothesis of fibromyalgia is that treatments derived from the hypothesis are ineffective. (See Chapter 5.1, section titled "Antidepressant Drugs"). The use of amitriptyline and cyclobenzaprine provided no long-term benefits beyond those provided by placebos. Carette et al. published a preliminary report of this result of the only long-term study of the effectiveness of amitriptyline and cyclobenzaprine in *Arthritis and Rheumatism* in 1992.[58] They published their final report in the same journal in 1994.[59] Further, at a major fibromyalgia conference in Vancouver, Carette reiterated the same result. The following year, his report was published in the *Journal of Musculoskeletal Pain*. He wrote, "In the short-term (one-to-three months) these drugs provide significant clinical improvement in 15 to 20 percent of patients, which is statistically higher than what is observed in patients receiving a placebo. However, the superiority of these drugs over placebos for longer periods of intake has yet to be demonstrated and will require studies with total enrollment of a minimum of 250-300 patients."[60,p.134] He also wrote, "So far, no treatment has been shown to have any significant impact on the natural history of this condition."[60,p.133]

Evidence from epidemiological studies supports

this last statement by Carette regarding the natural history of fibromyalgia. Consider as an example a study by Wolfe et al. published in 1995. They conducted a follow-up study of 453 fibromyalgia patients 7 years after their first evaluation, and 85 other patients more than 10 years after their first assessment. The participants in this study were patients at 6 rheumatology centers where fibromyalgia patients were treated. It is therefore highly probable that most of the patients were treated with the medications that Russell and McCain continue to state are effective. Wolfe et al. concluded, "Values [of measures of fibromyalgia status] at the first assessment are predictive of final values."[70] Essentially, this means that whatever treatment they underwent did not improve their fibromyalgia status. This report is typical of others suggesting that conventional treatments derived from the rheumatology paradigm simply do not work.

Despite the reports by Carette and his colleagues, and epidemiological studies such as the one I referenced in the preceding paragraph, some high profile rheumatology paradigm researchers have continued to publish statements that amitriptyline and cyclobenzaprine are effective fibromyalgia treatments. I.J. Russell is a fibromyalgia researcher and the Editor of the *Journal of Musculoskeletal Pain* where Carette's report on fibromyalgia treatments was published in 1995. In 1994, two years after the preliminary report by Carette et al. was published in *Arthritis and Rheumatism*, and the same year their final report was published in that same publication, Russell wrote, "Several investigations have demonstrated that amitriptyline is helpful in very low doses, less than is usually needed to treat depression or other affective disorders," and "Another drug with demonstrated efficacy is cyclobenzaprine."[98,p.82] In 1996, Russell wrote, "This drug [amitriptyline] has been tested in many placebo-controlled research studies and does help the symptoms in some people with FMS."[97,p.37] In the same publication he wrote, "The drug has been tested and found effective in placebo-controlled FMS research trials."[97,p.38]

In 1994, in the same issue of the *Journal of Musculoskeletal Pain*, rheumatology paradigm researcher Glen McCain wrote, "Acceptable clinical trials have now been completed showing that both amitriptyline and cyclobenzaprine are effective in fibromyalgia."[99,p.95] In the same paper, he wrote, "Scientific evidence for the efficacy of amitriptyline, cyclobenzaprine and triazolam has recently emerged . . . ."[99,p.102] He did not reference the 1992 and 1994 reports by Carette et al.[58][59]

In 1995, at the Third World Congress on Myofas-

cial Pain and Fibromyalgia, McCain gave an update on studies of fibromyalgia treatments. His report was published in a 1996 issue of Russell's *Journal of Musculoskeletal Pain.* McCain reiterated his 1994 statement verbatim: "Acceptable clinical trials have now been completed showing that both amitriptyline and cyclobenzaprine are effective in fibromyalgia."[61,pp.17-18]

In the 1996 issue of the *Journal of Musculoskeletal Pain* where McCain's report was published, Russell wrote an Editorial introducing the papers published in the issue. He wrote, "It is fair to say that the contents of the resultant papers represent a current summary of the 'state of the art' in FS and MPS as of August 3, 1995."[99,p.xiii]

At the 1998 Myopain conference in Italy, McCain again reported that the two medications are effective for the treatment of fibromyalgia. His report was published the following year in the *Journal of Musculoskeletal Pain.* He wrote, "A number of clinical trials have now been completed showing that both amitriptyline and cyclobenzaprine are effective in FMS."[62,p.194] Neither in the 1996 nor the 1999 reports did McCain cite the 1992 or 1994 reports of Carette et al.,[58][59] and he did not reference Carette's 1994 report in the *Journal of Musculoskeletal Pain.*[60]

In a 1999 issue of the *Journal of Musculoskeletal Pain*, Russell again wrote an Editorial in which he introduced the papers published in the issue. He wrote a slightly altered version of his statement from the 1996 Editorial: "It is fair to say that the contents of the resultant papers represent a current summary of the 'state of the art' in fibromyalgia syndrome and myofascial pain syndrome as of August 1998."[63,p.xx]

McCain's failure to cite the 1992 and 1994 reports by Carette et al.[58][59] was a puzzling omission, considering two points: (1) the two reports concerned the only long-term study of amitriptyline and cyclobenzaprine as fibromyalgia treatments, and (2) the study conclusion was that long term, the medications were no more effective than placebos. McCain also did not mention the report by Carette presented at the 1994 Vancouver, British Columbia conference and subsequently published in the *Journal of Musculoskeletal Pain*, in which Carette wrote, "So far, no treatment has been shown to have any significant impact on the natural history of the condition."[60] This mystified me.

Overall, in the available studies, amitriptyline and cyclobenzaprine have provided very slight and short-term improvement on a minority of measures of fibromyalgia status. In a 1995 Editorial in the *Journal of Myofascial Therapy*, I discussed some of the findings of Carette et al. reported in 1994.[59] I wrote:

The majority of patients in Carette's study did *not* improve. Of the placebo patients, 100% failed to benefit. Of amitriptyline patients, 79%, and of cyclobenzaprine patients, 88%. Put another way, 21% of amitriptyline patients and 12% of cyclobenzaprine patients improved. The superiority of the drugs over the placebo, slight as it was, was only evident during the first month of the study. At three and six months, placebo patients had improved as much as the drug patients.

Carette speculated that more subjects in his study groups *might* have shown a real superiority of the drugs over the placebo. The main point at this time, however, is this: in the only long-term study, the results showed the drugs did *not* work any better than a placebo after one month. And during that first month, only a smidgen of the drug patients had improved somewhat. Moreover, 98% of patients taking cyclobenzaprine had adverse effects, and 13% of the patients stopped the drug because of adverse effects. This means more patients had bad side effects than improved: 13% to 12%.[65]

I ended the Editorial with the following conclusion: "Busy practitioners who don't read most original journal papers on treatment studies depend on the statements fibromyalgia authorities make in journals and lectures. Because of this, these authorities have an *obligation* to report precisely and accurately what science has told us. This isn't up to the authorities' discretion. It's a scientific and journalistic responsibility, and it has everything to with the question of credibility."[65]

I wrote that Editorial in 1995 because I felt compelled to object to these authorities continuing to publish statements saying that amitriptyline and cyclobenzaprine are effective. As I pointed out in the abstract that begins Chapter 5.1, studies may show a *statistically* significant difference between the effectiveness of a treatment and that of a placebo, but that does not mean that the treatment is *clinically* significant. I believe this distinction *must* be made regarding the outcome of studies of the effects of amitriptyline and cyclobenzaprine on fibromyalgia patients. Otherwise, practicing clinicians are likely to falsely believe that the medications enable patients to markedly improve or recover. They clearly do not.

As a result of my Editorial, I become *persona non grata* to rheumatology paradigm researchers and their affiliated fibromyalgia support groups. The rheumatologist who was on the advisory board of the Fibromyalgia Research Foundation, for which I am Director of Research, resigned in protest. My Editorial was published in April of 1995. In August of 1995, the Myopain '95 fibromyalgia conference was held in San Antonio, Texas. At that conference, Jackie Yellin, my editor and collaborator on this book, who is also Director of Education of the Fibromyalgia Research Foundation, was subjected to the disdain of the rheumatology paradigm researchers apparently in retaliation for my Editorial.

I consider banishment from the rheumatology fibromyalgia research community a negligible price to pay for standing up for truth. And regardless of any future adverse social consequences, I must protest Russell's and McCain's continuing their inaccurate reporting. It is proper here that I challenge them and any other rheumatology paradigm researchers to document that a single patient has ever recovered with the use of either or both of the medications they report to be effective—document with *credible* scientific evidence, not with *ex cathedra* assurances or pronouncements, nor with statistically significant but clinically insignificant study results.

The debatable reports that amitriptyline and cyclobenzaprine are effective is relevant to one of my theses of this chapter—that the trend toward more *DSM* labeling of fibromyalgia patients may soon worsen the patients' plight. This trend may be fueled in part by rheumatology paradigm researchers reporting that the medications are effective without properly qualifying that statistical significance does not in this case translate into clinical significance. If practicing clinicians are led to believe the drugs are effective, some may become suspicious of patients who do not appear to benefit from use of the medications. As I showed in a 1993 paper in the *American Journal of Pain Management*, some clinicians/researchers are all too willing to provide an answer to why these patients do not improve. A typical offered answer is that the fibromyalgia patients have psychogenic pain mixed with some degree of malingering (faking symptoms for financial profit) that is fueled by desires for financial or interpersonal gain. (See Appendix C, paper titled "Litigating-Chronic Pain Syndrome: Weintraub's Unproven Entity.") Regardless of the pseudo-scientific nature of this proposed answer, practicing clinicians may unwittingly come to agree with it because of the air of legitimacy of *DSM* labels. It is entirely reasonable to expect that some confused and misguided clinicians will apply *DSM* labels to fibromyalgia patients who fail to improve with "effective" medications such as amitriptyline and cyclobenzaprine.

Comparison of the Serotonin Deficiency Hypothesis and the Inadequate Thyroid Hormone Regulation Hypothesis

The failing usefulness of the serotonin deficiency hypothesis of fibromyalgia has unfortunately not yet resulted in a turn to the far more useful inadequate thyroid hormone regulation hypothesis. Instead, evidence suggests that increasing numbers of clinicians and researchers are returning to the notion of psychogenesis, the pseudo-scientific, default hypothesis of conventional medicine to explain disorders without generally accepted biological causes. Study of the contents of Table 1.1.1 (and Section III of this book) shows that the inadequate thyroid hormone regulation hypothesis accounts for virtually all the objectively verified abnormalities in fibromyalgia. The superior usefulness of this hypothesis must be considered in lieu of the notion of psychogenesis and the practice of *DSM* labeling.

CONTINUING RESEARCH STUDIES UNDER THE RHEUMATOLOGY PARADIGM

The falsification of the serotonin deficiency hypothesis, the main conceptual underpinning of the rheumatology paradigm, has resulted in the crumbling of the paradigm. Despite this, some rheumatology paradigm researchers who are passionate about helping fibromyalgia patients have pressed on conducting studies. However, a review of the studies being published indicates that any guidance once provided by the rheumatology paradigm is now absent. Studies that researchers are now conducting do not center around a conceptual line of thought. Kuhn wrote that studies done without the guidance of a paradigm seldom lead to any conclusions at all.[93,p.28] Certainly, the conclusions do not contribute to the economic use of manpower and resources to arrive at the implicit goal—relieving patients of their fibromyalgia.

Some might argue that the psychogenesis hypothesis, embodied by *DSM* labels, now provides a unifying concept for fibromyalgia research. However, this hypothesis cannot serve this purpose because it is not scientific. Instead, it enjoys the dual status of being both metaphysical and pseudo-scientific (see Chapter 1.2). Metaphysics is an acceptable form of epistemological inquiry, but pseudo-science certainly is not.[100]

Only a scientific hypothesis, such as the inadequate thyroid hormone regulation hypothesis, can serve a legitimate unifying role within a scientific paradigm.

OMINOUS AFTERMATH TO THE FALL OF THE RHEUMATOLOGY PARADIGM: RESURGENCE OF THE PSYCHOGENESIS HYPOTHESIS

To understand the ominous trends developing as the rheumatology fibromyalgia paradigm falls, it is useful to consider factors that have contributed to the fall. These include cost concerns of third party payers, and two main purposes of *DSM* labeling of patients.

The cost to third party payers for health care services and disability for fibromyalgia patients has escalated. Typically, when costs rise for the care of patients with a disorder lacking a generally accepted biological cause, clinicians increase their *DSM* labeling of the patients. (For an explanation of *DSM* labeling, see the section above titled "Perpetuation of Freudian Concepts by *DSM* Labeling.")

This trend in the field of fibromyalgia was expressed in 1998 by Hausotter in the journal *Versicherungsmedizin*. (Presumably, the somewhat awkward wording in the quoted material is due to English not being the author's native language.) He wrote that no one had scientifically proven that fibromyalgia is an organic disorder. Then: "Psychological causes are more and more considered to be responsible for this problem. Nowadays a psychosomatic disorder is assumed although as well a depression with somatization or a neurosis are discussed." He then mentioned what is at the crux of the motivation for *DSM* labeling: "Therapeutical problems and pain coping strategies are described just *as the medico-legal assessment for pension scheme* [italics mine]." He then recommended *DSM* nomenclature: "Because the term 'fibromyalgia' suggests an organic disorder which does not exist, it seems instead useful to prefer the terms 'somatization disorder' or 'pain disorder' to make easier the approach to early psychotherapy and to prevent a further chronification."[75]

Clinicians and researchers who recommend *DSM* labeling of fibromyalgia patients usually also state or insinuate, as the labels imply, that psychotherapy and the use of psychiatric drugs are the proper treatments for fibromyalgia. They do so despite substantial evidence of the ineffectiveness of psychological approaches, benzodiazepines, and antidepressant medications in fibromyalgia treatment studies. The risks of this *DSM*-and-drug approach are considerable. As Walker wrote, "A *DSM* label is not a diagnosis—and psychiatric patients whose disorders are caused by tumors, infections, toxic exposures, hormonal imbalances, or other physical ailments will suffer needlessly, or even die, if they are simply labeled, drugged, and psychoanalyzed."[1,p.viii] This is precisely the risk most fibromyalgia patients face if the trends I describe below are not curtailed.

COSTS FOR THE CARE OF FIBROMYALGIA PATIENTS

Fibromyalgia represents a continuing cost to third party payers. In a study published in 1997, researchers reported that 538 fibromyalgia patients averaged 10 outpatient visits to medical practitioners per year. The rate of hospitalization was once every 3 years. About 50% of hospitalizations were for fibromyalgia-associated symptoms. In each study period of 6 months, patients used an average of 2.7 fibromyalgia-related medications. Medical costs increased over the course of the 7-year study. The average yearly cost per patient was $2,274.00. Patients who used more medical services skewed the results; many patients used few services and costs for them were low. The total use of services and costs for patients were related to comorbid or associated conditions, functional disability, and disease severity. The researchers wrote, "Compared to patients with other rheumatic disorders, those with fibromyalgia were more likely to have lifetime surgical interventions, including back or neck surgery, appendectomy, carpal tunnel surgery, gynecologic surgery, abdominal surgery, and tonsillectomy, and were more likely than other rheumatic disease patients to report comorbid or associated conditions." They concluded: "Fibromyalgia patients have high lifetime and current rates of utilization of all types of medical services. They report more symptoms and comorbid or associated conditions than patients with other rheumatic conditions, and symptom reporting is linked to service utilization and, to a lesser extent, functional disability and global disease severity."[72]

Another study, also published in 1997, showed that over a quarter of fibromyalgia patients from 6 rheumatology centers received disability payments. The researchers determined that more than 16% of fibromyalgia patients at the 6 rheumatology centers had received U.S. Social Security disability (SSD) payments. This percentage compares with only 6% of

the U.S. population in general who received such payments. In one rheumatology center, 28.9% of patients received payments. When SSD and other sources of disability payments were considered, 26.5% of fibromyalgia patients had received payments. The researchers wrote, "In Wichita, less than 25% of SSD awards were made specifically for FM, but after 1988, that figure increased to 46.4%." They also wrote, "In addition, more than 70% of patients reporting being disabled did receive disability payments. On the other hand, 64% reported being able to work all or most days, and more than 70% were employed or were homemakers."[71]

CAUSES OF ESCALATING COSTS

In 1995, medical professor Anthony S. Russell wrote of the ACR criteria, "One great advantage of defining and codifying this problem is that at the level of the individual patient, it has called a halt to the never-ending searches for obscure organic disease—'Furor Medicus'—thus it allows a positive diagnosis to be made without the time and expense of a diagnosis of exclusion."[3,p.43]

Despite the ACR diagnostic criteria, however, the average fibromyalgia patient I have seen over the years had previously accumulated a considerable total cost for diagnostic and treatment services. Some patients' costs had mounted to $40,000.00 or more during the preceding 2 or 3 years before they came to me. Considering the available information, I believe that fibromyalgia represents an ongoing rise of costs in terms of insurance reimbursement and disability payments.

DSM LABELING AS A METHOD OF COST CONTAINMENT

The remedy that can appropriately reduce the costs for services and disability is two-fold: (1) adoption of the hypothetical view that fibromyalgia is mainly a result of inadequate thyroid hormone tissue regulation, and (2) the widespread use of expertly guided metabolic rehabilitation of fibromyalgia patients. Rather than this scientifically sound option, however, the recent trend toward *DSM* labeling of fibromyalgia patients suggests a growing tendency of clinicians and researchers to believe that fibromyalgia is psychogenic. Although this is detrimental to patients, the trend serves well the purposes of third party payers.

Table 1.1.1. Comparison of fibromyalgia symptoms and objective findings accounted for by major hypotheses of the etiology of fibromyalgia.

SYMPTOM OR OBJECTIVE FINDING	SD-H*	ITHR-H †	GHD-H§	D-Hᵒ	HPA-H ‡
↓ slow-wave sleep	X	X	X	X	X
irritable bowel syndrome	X	X			
↓ HPA axis function	X	X			X
urinary frequency	X	X			
↑ pain perception	X	X	X	X	X
↑ substance P	X	X			
depression	X	X	X		X
cognitive dysfunction	X	X	X		X
↓ muscle relaxation time		X			
exercise intolerance		X	X	X	X
↓ RBC ATP levels		X			
impaired glycolysis		X			
↑ hyaluronic acid		X			
↑ tissue proteoglycans		X			
↓ procollagen III		X			
↓ hydroxyproline		X			
↓ pyridinoline & deoxypyridinoline		X			
↓ brain blood flow		X			
↑ α-adrenergic receptors on platelets		X			
dysmenorrhea		X			
↓ serotonin secretion		X			
ineffectiveness of serotonin-increasing treatments		X			
effectiveness of thyroid hormone treatment		X			
effectiveness of β-adrenergic agonists		X			
joint hypermobility		X			
↓ growth hormone & somatomedin C		X			
stiffness & swelling		X		X	
sicca symptoms		X			
orthostatic hypotension		X			X
cold intolerance		X	X	X	X
paresthesia		X			
↑ mast cells		X			
anxiety		X	X		
fatigue		X	X	X	X

*SD-H = serotonin deficiency hypothesis.
†ITHR-H = inadequate thyroid hormone regulation hypothesis.
§GHD-H = growth hormone deficiency hypothesis.
ᵒD-H = deconditioning hypothesis.
‡HPA-H = HPA hypothesis. This has not been proposed as the underlying cause of fibromyalgia but only as a mechanism of some fibromyalgia features.

Increasing DSM Labeling: Fibromyalgia Conferences

The increase in *DSM* labeling is obvious from a consideration of the topics at fibromyalgia conferences over the last 10 years.

Minneapolis Conference (1989). The focus of this conference was on clinical features of fibromyalgia. The proceedings of the conference contain few references to proposed mental and emotional contributions to fibromyalgia.[4,p.xvi] Of 86 abstracts and poster presentations, only 2 (2%) focused on possible psychogenesis. But the authors of both papers concluded essentially that psychogenesis is not a causative factor in fibromyalgia. In one paper, Merskey, a psychiatrist, wrote: "The differential diagnosis of hysteria from physical states is examined, and it is concluded that many misdiagnoses have been made of hysteria, or conversion symptoms, particularly when organic illness was present but poorly understood. In some circles, the influence of compensation in promoting complaints of pain has been overemphasized."[18] In the other paper, Ahles et al. reported on a study they had conducted. They concluded, "These data do not support the hypothesis that [primary fibromyalgia syndrome] is a variant of a psychiatric disorder such as depression or somatization disorder."[19]

Copenhagen Conference (1992). The main focus of this conference was on the epidemiology of fibromyalgia.[4,p.xvi] Of 33 articles from the conference published in the *Journal of Musculoskeletal Pain*, 6 dealt with psychological aspects of fibromyalgia. In 4 of the 6 (12% of the 33 articles), the authors concluded that fibromyalgia is not primarily a psychologically-based disorder. Another article was a report of the use of psychological methods to help patients cope with their disability. The 6th article was by Wolfe. He wrote: "It has been argued that the issue is complex and that the severe pain and/or disability of fibromyalgia causes rather than is the consequence of psychological distress. My own view is that it is true in some patients, but not in others; and that, taken as a whole, psychological factors are more often causative rather than the consequence of fibromyalgia."[7,p.28]

As a result of the Copenhagen Conference, Csillage stated in 1992 that the Copenhagen Declaration would result in many fibromyalgia patients not being considered hypochondriacs any more and that they would be able to obtain disability awards.[2]

NIH (National Institutes of Health) Workshops (1993 and 1994). The main focus of the 1993 NIH Workshop was the pathogenesis of fibromyalgia.[4,p.xv] The focus of the 1994 NIH Workshop was the neuroscience and endocrinology of fibromyalgia.[20,p.xiii]

Vancouver Conference (1994). The Editor of the *Journal of Musculoskeletal Pain* wrote that the unique feature of this conference was its emphasis on disability and compensation. He wrote, "The importance of those issues was so substantial and opinions have traditionally varied so widely that there was much speculation about how the conference would proceed, what its outcome might be, and whether consensus really could be achieved on such divisive topics." He continued, "There were also differing opinions regarding the relative merits of involving the insurance industry as both participants and sponsors of debates on questions which so clearly affected their services and profit margins."[4,p.xv] Three of the listed sponsors of the conference were The Canadian Government, Health and Welfare Canada; The British Columbia Government, Ministry of Health; and Seaboard Life Insurance Co. One focus of the meeting, expressed in the formal title of the conference, was "cost containment."[5,p.2] The Editor also wrote that previous conferences paid some "obeisance," that is, courteous regard, "to psychological aspects." He continued, "But, with the Vancouver Conference, the pendulum seems to have perceptively swung back in the direction of viewing affective [psychological] pathology as a contributor to the underlying processes."[4,p.xvi]

Indeed, *DSM* labelers made a strong showing at the conference. Of the 23 articles published as a result of presentations at the conference, 4 dealt with psychological subjects but did not indicate that fibromyalgia is a psychogenic disorder. However, 10 papers (44%) included suggestions or direct arguments to the effect that fibromyalgia is psychogenic. Another 3 papers dealt with cost containment.

Anthony Russell described fibromyalgia as "a reflection of an inability to cope, often because of patterns of behavior or expectation set up in childhood." He continued, "As long as the rewards of this behavior pattern, provided by society, by doctors, etc., outweigh the debits, the pattern will be encouraged both at an individual and societal level."[3,pp.43-44]

At the end of his Preface describing the 1995 conference in the *Journal of Musculoskeletal Pain*, the Editor wrote, "It now falls to each participant and reader to evaluate issues that have been raised, and to embrace truth where it is found."[4,p.xvi]

San Antonio Conference (1995). Of the 165 abstracts published as a result of the San Antonio Conference, 10 dealt with psychological aspects of fibromyalgia. None of the 10 focused on mental or emotional factors as causes of fibromyalgia.

Bad Nauheim, Germany Conference (1997). Of the 15 papers from the Bad Nauheim Conference, the authors of 9 discussed psychological factors, and the authors of 4 (26%) directly related fibromyalgia to psychological abnormalities.

In summary, at the 1989 Minneapolis Conference, the first of the international conferences, none of the authors of papers, abstracts, or posters attributed fibromyalgia to psychogenesis. At the 1992 Copenhagen Conference, 12% dealt with psychogenesis. At the 1994 Vancouver Conference, the authors of 44% of the papers suggested or contended that fibromyalgia is psychogenic. At the 1995 San Antonio Conference none of the papers dealt with psychogenesis, but at the 1997 Bad Nauheim Conference, 26% of the papers directly related fibromyalgia to psychological abnormalities.

Increasing DSM Labeling: Published Papers

Recently, attention has turned even more to the influence of psychogenic and psychosocial factors in fibromyalgia. Goldenberg wrote in 1999 that it is important to determine the psychosocial differences between fibromyalgia patients who are being treated from other people in the community who meet the ACR criteria but who do not seek medical care. "Such factors," he wrote, "may be among the most important in long-term treatment."[8]

In 1998, Wolfe and Hawley wrote: "Psychosocial distress and psychological abnormality occur frequently in fibromyalgia patients. Patterns of decreased levels of education, and increased rates of divorce, obesity, and smoking have been noted in clinical and epidemiological studies. Links to physical and sexual abuse have been noted as well. Major depression as well as increased rates of depression, anxiety, and somatization are also commonly found in fibromyalgia."[9]

Meyer-Lindenberg and Gallhofer of the National Institute of Mental Health wrote: "We suggest that a subgroup of patients with this symptom combination may be pragmatically classified as suffering from somatized depression. Clinical indicators such as a family history of depressive disorders, circadian disturbances, pronounced loss of appetite or libido, and chronic psychosocial stressors should be assessed and, if present, prompt the initiation of psychiatric evaluation and treatment including pharmaco- and psychotherapeutic modalities."[10] Offenbaecher et al. have written of the high incidence of depression among fibromyalgia patients.[11] Netter and Hennig suggested

that fibromyalgia may be a manifestation of "neuroticism."[13] In 1998, Cathebras et al. wrote of the "striking comorbidity" between fibromyalgia and psychiatric disorders. They wrote of "abnormal illness behaviors" and cautioned, "The social consequences of the popularization of the diagnosis of fibromyalgia should not be neglected."[14] In 1998, Ackenheil reported looking for a gene relating fibromyalgia to "neurotic anxiety."[17] In a 1999 paper, researchers reported that functional impairment of fibromyalgia patients was predictable by psychiatric comorbidity and psychological variables. Patients had significant elevations in depression, anxiety, neuroticism, and hypochondriasis on self-rating scales. The patients had a high lifetime and current incidence of major depression and panic disorder, and the most common psychological disorders were major depression, dysthymia, panic disorder, and simple phobia.[16]

Recently, I searched Medline for papers published on costs for the care of fibromyalgia patients. The search turned up 80 papers published between 1986 and 1999. I also searched for published papers that mentioned both fibromyalgia and *DSM* somatoform diagnoses. The search turned up 33 papers published between 1986 and 1999. I separated these latter papers into those that favored *DSM* labels for fibromyalgia patients (21) and those that did not favor the labels (12). I then graphed the results as Figure 1.1.1. according to the years the papers were published. The trend line for publication dates of papers on costs for fibromyalgia care is interesting compared to that for publication dates for papers disfavoring and those favoring *DSM* labeling. The line for cost papers is moderately negatively correlated, although insignificantly, with the line for papers disfavoring *DSM* labeling (-0.29, p=0.32). In comparison, the line for cost papers is weakly positively correlated, albeit insignificantly, with the line for papers favoring *DSM* labeling (0.18, p=0.54). Although the correlations are not significant, observing the graph in Figure 1.1.1 raises the question as to whether surges in the number of papers published on costs for the care of fibromyalgia patients are shortly followed by an increase in the number of papers published favoring *DSM* labeling of the patients. I conjecture that an exhaustive inclusion of all papers presented at conferences and published in journals and trade publications will show a statistically significant positive correlation between the publication of papers on cost concerns and those favoring the *DSM* labeling of fibromyalgia patients.

Not all researchers are resorting to psychogenesis labels. Walter et al. wrote in 1998, "Affective distress is not a unique feature of FMS, but seems to be caused entirely by higher levels of pain severity. "[12] And in the same year, Hannonen et al. treated a group of fibromyalgia patients in whom psychiatric illness had been effectively ruled out.[15] Despite these exceptions, publication of papers attributing fibromyalgia to psychological abnormalities appears to be substantially increasing. It is to their credit that some researchers of the crumbling rheumatology paradigm, such as Russell, appear to be standing their ground on a biological basis for fibromyalgia.

Meaning of the Increase in DSM Labeling of Fibromyalgia Patients

As long as humans suffer from symptoms for which there are no unequivocally proven biological causes, some medical writers will relentlessly weave fanciful psychosocial explanations for the symptoms. But patients and clinicians should bear in mind the failure of such writers to offer credible scientific evidence for a psychogenic basis for any disease, including fibromyalgia. If there is any value whatever to the current resurgence of *DSM* labeling of fibromyalgia patients, it is that it signifies the fall of the rheumatology paradigm of fibromyalgia. While some researchers within that paradigm will seek cognitive refuge in psychogenic theorizing, others, upon realizing that the end of the paradigm is near, will question where the paradigm failed. If they do so open-mindedly, abandoning all previous beliefs in their search for answers, they will recognize the metabolic basis of the condition and see that the inadequate thyroid hormone regulation hypothesis has succeeded scientifically and clinically where the hypotheses of the rheumatology paradigm failed.

In the meantime, fibromyalgia patients are at risk from the increase in *DSM* labeling. Whenever third party payers wish to increase their profit margins, they do so by denying benefits to patients with whom they have contractual agreements. One way third party payers accomplish this is by employing clinicians as independent medical examiners and expert witnesses. If the clinicians do not fulfill the wishes of the third party payers by sufficiently reducing the claims the third party payers must pay, these clinicians find themselves without further employment by the third party payers. Some clinicians, however, maintain a lucrative relationship with third party payers by reducing, through giving patients *DSM* labels, the amount of claims paid.

My belief that *DSM* labels are used to reduce costs and increase profits is not armchair speculation.

In my years as an expert witness, I have had occasion to experience first hand the motives and methods of some insurance companies. I was dismissed by one insurance company as an independent medical examiner soon after I started because I provided accurate reports on my findings from examining patients, rather than giving reports that would justify refusing to pay the patients' health care claims. In addition, other expert witnesses, ones who regularly work for third party payers, have admitted to me in private conversations that they used *DSM* labels strategically. Taking me into their confidence, they admitted that they used the labels to put a stop to patients and their treating doctors bilking insurance companies. Some expressed a zeal in helping stop the "exploitation of insurance companies by patients and their doctors." Moreover, checking the record should make it obvious that the major promoters of *DSM* psychogenic labels are clinicians who earn a good portion of their income from third party payers, working as expert witnesses, record reviewers, or independent medical examiners.

Perhaps the specialty most actively employed by third party payers is board certified neurologists. Psychiatrists are useful to third party payers, but neurologists are more useful. Patients may be more willing to undergo an independent medical exam by a neurologist than by a psychiatrist, assuming while they do so, that the neurologist will perform a legitimate medical evaluation. However, for some neurologists, the evaluation is merely a pretext for rubber stamping the patients' medical records with *DSM* labels. For this slight of hand, these neurologists are well paid by third party payers.

I am not alone in my beliefs about the uses of *DSM* labels by clinicians and others for purposes other than helping suffering humanity. Neuropsychiatrist Sydney Walker recently wrote:

> *DSM-IV* does contain a disclaimer that 'there are significant risks that diagnostic information will be misused or misunderstood' in legal settings, and the manual's authors state that *DSM* labels, in and of themselves, are not a sufficient basis for legally determining competence, criminal responsibility, or disability. These warnings, however, have largely fallen on deaf ears—as anyone who has been a party in a court proceeding involving psychiatric expert witnesses knows all too well.[1,p.210]

Based upon my professional experiences with expert witnesses and independent medical examiners, I am convinced that the abuse of *DSM* labeling is so rampant that the plight of fibromyalgia patients can only be worsened by a progressive increase in the practice. This developing trend makes it imperative that the information in this book be put into use on behalf of patients.

● NEGLECT OF THE INADEQUATE THYROID HORMONE REGULATION HYPOTHESIS

My fundamental hypothesis of fibromyalgia is that in all cases, the condition results from hypometabolism of select tissues. In this book, I propose a corollary of this hypothesis. It states that in most cases, fibromyalgia is the clinical manifestation of inadequate thyroid hormone regulation due to thyroid hormone deficiency and/or resistance.

One might ask why conventional clinicians and researchers have not recognized the soundness of the hypothesis I describe in this book. This is a proper question, considering that my colleagues and I have propounded the hypothesis in several other publications over the past 6 years.[68][69][76][77][78][79][80][81][82][83][84][85][86] It is also an especially relevant question because we have repeatedly reported that most of our patients improve or recover, and their improvement and recovery last long term.

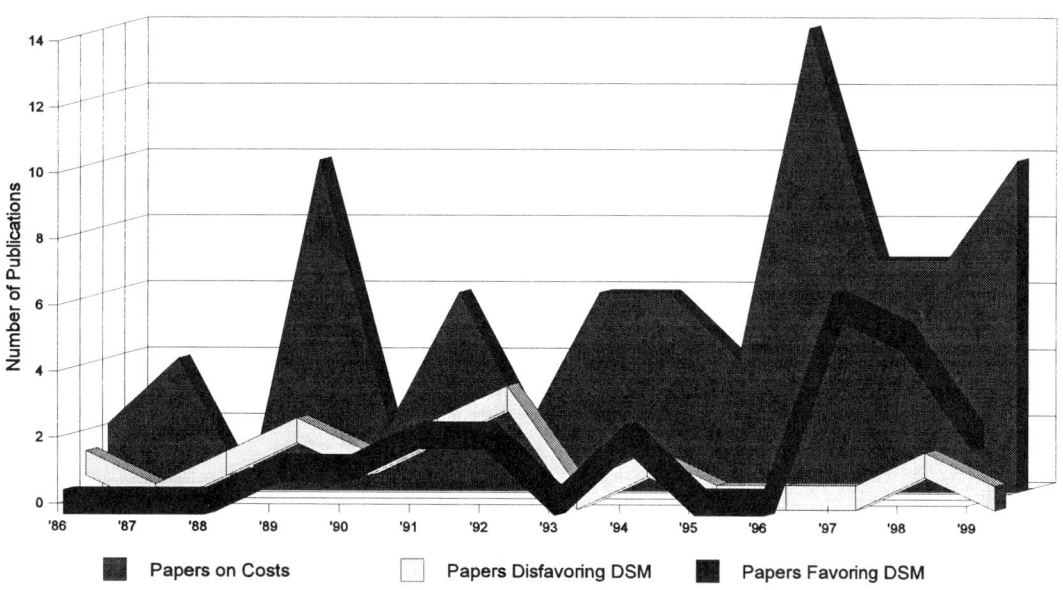

Figure 1.1.1 Trend of published papers on costs for fibromyalgia care, papers disfavoring *DSM* labeling, and papers favoring such labeling.

Patients, clinicians, and other researchers have posed variations of this question to me, and I believe it is important that I answer it forthrightly. Some medical clinicians and researchers will find my answers unpalatable. Nevertheless, I present my answers for two reasons. First, in my experience, patients and clinicians tend to assume that neglect of a treatment by conventional medicine means that the treatment really does not have merit. Otherwise, conventional medicine would surely embrace the treatment and the hypothesis it is founded on. Nothing, however, could be further from the truth.

My second reason for providing answers is that it is in the true spirit of science. To those who might take offense at some of my answers, I would point out that professional scientists consider criticism from colleagues *absolutely essential* to the advancement of science.[92] To abstain from criticizing each other's views and methods—as well as one's own, I might add as well—is to retard science. Criticism is the lifeblood of scientific advancement. It is with this in mind that I forthrightly describe what I consider to be the factors responsible for the neglect of our hypothesis and treatment. Not to do so would be a dereliction of my duty as a scientific thinker.

Parenthetically, I would remind members of the rheumatology paradigm that they have failed in the most important aim of their mission—to develop a truly effective treatment, one that enables most patients to markedly improve or completely recover. Twenty-five years is long enough for fibromyalgia patients to wait for that aim to be achieved. When it is obvious that a paradigm has failed in this way, the scientific and humanitarian responsibility of researchers is to leave no stone unturned until the causes of that failure are known and rectified. Not examining their own social psychology when searching for the causes of their failure may be the greatest form of negligence by any researchers. In this regard, rheumatology paradigm researchers would do well to model other medical physicians, such as Garrison[87] and Nobel Laureate Bernard Lown.[113] These two physicians/researchers have noted that the orthodox medical paradigm is crumbling, and they have encouraged self-scrutiny by its members. Lown pointed out that increasing numbers of patients have turned to alternative practitioners because his profession has failed to help them. "At present," he wrote in 1999, "about 25 percent of patients who visit an American doctor are successfully treated. The other 75 percent have problems that scientific medicine finds difficult to resolve."[113,p123] Garrison's and Lown's sincere and forthright examinations of their own discipline are exemplary examples of the scientific spirit.

I hold myself to the same scientific standard of self-scrutiny, thanks to the influence in my formative years of Professor William L. Mikulas, my mentor in behavioral and research psychology. What initiated my interest in fibromyalgia was, in fact, my recognizing and acknowledging that my use of myofascial therapy (which enabled me to promptly and reliably relieve most of my patients' pain) was ineffective with a subset of patients. I later learned that the subset of patients had fibromyalgia. Had I defensively ignored my failure to relieve their pain, I would not have begun the odyssey that led to the development of metabolic rehabilitation—the form of treatment that does effectively relieve the suffering of most fibromyalgia patients who undergo it. Therefore, the fruitful outcome of that odyssey is ultimately the product of my forthright

recognition and admission of my clinical failures and my determination to learn exactly why I had failed.

I believe that our hypothesis and treatment have not yet been embraced by conventional medicine, including rheumatology paradigm researchers, for at least 5 reasons: (1) conventional medical journals block publication of unconventional views, (2) clinicians' lack familiarity with, or the ability to use, a rehabilitation model of practice, (3) clinicians and researchers naturally resist paradigm change, (4) conventional clinicians have a truncated knowledge of clinical thyroidology, and (5) in general, conventional medical clinicians and researchers are inculcated with an unscientific code of conduct.

BLOCKING OF UNCONVENTIONAL VIEWS BY CONVENTIONAL MEDICAL PUBLICATIONS

Blocking of the publication of views unfavorable to special interests within the medical profession in the U.S. is well-known. Until recently, manuscripts from the doctor of chiropractic (D.C.) were not accepted by medical journals. Now, some journals devoted to subjects such as the spine, the musculoskeletal system, or pain take submissions from D.C.s and publish some of their papers. But most medical journals still politely find reasons not to publish papers of which chiropractic physicians are coauthors. This is especially true of journals that publish papers on subjects related to my field of research, thyroidology and metabolism. Experience with the various excuses and stall tactics of editors, and the sometimes bogus reasons "peer" reviewers give editors to reject our manuscripts, make it clear that submissions by my research team are not welcome in the editorial offices of conventional medical journals. This is an *ad hominem* phenomenon, of course, and it has forced my colleagues and me to publish our results in relatively obscure U.S. journals or in less prejudicial medical journals published outside the U.S.

Documenting for the reader the statements in the previous paragraph is difficult. The U.S. is a highly litigious society. Because of this, those who hold prejudices against a group (such as chiropractic physicians) have developed sophisticated methods for accomplishing the aims of prejudice while making the methods extraordinarily difficult to document, just in case the victims of the prejudice decide to litigate. In view of this and for supporting evidence, I cite published statements of a prominent scientist, two-time

Nobel Laureate Linus Pauling, whose views on nutrition were prejudicially suppressed by medical editors. Pauling described his experiences in a book he wrote for the general public.[111] He wrote the book believing, based on his experiences with medical journal editors, that it was a more effective way to get vital information to the public than depending on medical journals.

Pauling wrote that when he began studying nutrition and learned from published studies the possibilities for relieving human suffering, he believed that by presenting the facts in a simple, straightforward, and logical way, the public and physicians would listen to and accept them. "I was right, in this expectation," he said, "about the people but wrong about the physicians, or perhaps not about the physicians as individuals but about organized medicine."

Pauling described "orthomolecular medicine" (see Glossary: Orthomolecular) as the use of optimal amounts of vitamins and other nutrients, together with the use of other orthomolecular substances such as thyroid hormone. "Orthomolecular medicine," he wrote, "for some reason seems to be considered a threat to conventional medicine. Orthomolecular physicians are harassed by the medical establishment."[111,p.301]

In addition to harassment of orthomolecular physicians came censorship of information related to orthomolecular medicine. Pauling wrote, "Even after the appearance of *Vitamin C and the Common Cold* [which he authored] (7 December 1970), when the evidence was clearly brought to the attention of the medical authorities, they continued to deny the existence of the evidence. This denial was sometimes accompanied by statements that contradicted or misconstrued the facts."[111,p.305]

When sales of vitamin C soared after the publication of *Vitamin C and the Common Cold*, Charles E. Edwards, the physician who was chief of the FDA, asked Pauling to come to Washington for a meeting about the issue of vitamin C. The next day, Edwards told reporters that the sale of vitamin C after publication of the book was "ridiculous," and he stated, "There is no scientific evidence and [there] never have been any meaningful studies indicating that vitamin C is capable of preventing or curing colds." Pauling asked Edwards how he could reconcile that statement with the evidence summarized in his book. Edwards answered by criticizing some studies Pauling had summarized and then withdrew his invitation for Pauling to come to Washington. In addition, despite considerable evidence of the therapeutic potential of vitamin C, federal medical agencies continued to deny it had any value.[111,p.306]

The *Medical Letter* published an unsigned criticism of Pauling's book. The anonymous author wrote that Pauling had relied on uncontrolled studies and stated that no adequate testing had been done. According to Pauling, "I wrote a letter pointing out the falsity of this statement and showing the writer of the article how the Cowan, Diehl, and Baker study, for one, surely met all of his specifications [for an adequate study]. I concluded by asking the *Medical Letter* to publish my letter." The editor did not publish the letter. Instead, another article was published claiming that the Cowan et al. study was not controlled. Pauling wrote that in fact the study was randomized and double-blind, as Cowan himself confirmed to Pauling. Also in the article in the *Medical Letter*, the author dismissed another study Pauling cited on trivial grounds—because the authors of the study did not give the age and sex of the subjects. The authors, however, had described the subjects in the paper as schoolboys. The writer of the *Medical Letter* article suggested that the use of vitamin C might cause kidney stones but offered no evidence. *Reader's Digest* later published this suggestion as a fact. The Canadian physician Abram Hoffer wrote of this interaction: "[These critics] use two sets of logic. Before they are prepared to look at Dr. Pauling's hypothesis, they demand proof of the most rigorous kind. But when arguing against his views, they refer to evidence of the flimsiest sort for the toxicity of ascorbic acid."[111,pp.307-308]

JAMA published a paper in 1975 in which the author concluded that the use of vitamin C was clinically unimportant. Only select studies were used for evidence—those that supported the author's point of view. Pauling wrote: "In order to present to the readers of the *Journal of the American Medical Association* an account of all the evidence, I at once prepared a thorough but brief analysis of thirteen controlled trials and submitted it to the editor on 19 March. He returned it to me twice, with suggestions for minor revisions, which I made. Finally, on 24 September, six months after I had submitted the article to him, he wrote me that it was not wholly convincing and that he had decided to reject the article and not publish it in *JAMA*."[111,p.309] Another journal later published the paper. Pauling wrote of this incident:

> It is my opinion that it is quite improper for the editor of *JAMA* (or of any other journal) to follow the policy of publishing only those papers that support only one side of a scientific or medical question and also to interfere with the proper discussion of the question by holding a paper that had been submitted to him for half a

year, during which period, according to accepted custom, the paper could not be submitted to another journal.[111,p.310]

Pauling also pointed out that this was not the only incident of this sort involving *JAMA.* He wrote, "These actions suggest that the AMA works to protect American physicians from information that runs counter to its own prejudices. The evidence indicates that the AMA is prejudiced against vitamin C." Pauling noted that during these years, he was not permitted to speak in medical schools.[111,p.310]

Finally, Pauling wrote: "The most recent and the most outrageous action by organized medicine against the new science of nutrition and the well-being of the American people has been perpetrated by the Mayo Clinic. He described the action as "the publication of a fraudulent paper in the 17 January 1985 issue of the *New England Journal of Medicine*." He explained: "The principal author of the paper, Dr. Charles G. Moertel, and his five collaborators, deliberately misrepresented their investigation of the value of high doses of vitamin C for patients with metastatic cancer of the colon or rectum as a repetition of and check on the work by Dr. Ewan Cameron and his collaborators (of whom I was one)."[111,pp.312-313] Pauling described the incident: In the Mayo Clinic study,

The vitamin-C patients received the vitamin for only a short time (median 2.5 months). None of the vitamin-C patients died while taking the vitamin (amount somewhat less than 10 g per day). They were, however, studied for another two years, during which their survival record was no better than that of the controls, or even somewhat worse. The Moertel paper and a spokesman for the National Cancer Institute who commented on it (Wittes, 1985), both suppressed the fact that the vitamin-C patients were not receiving vitamin C when they died and had not received any for a long time (median 10.5 months). They announced vigorously that this study showed finally and definitely that vitamin C has no value against advanced cancer and recommended that no more studies of vitamin C be made.[111,p.234]

Pauling noted that the publication was considered to unfavorably reflect on his and Cameron's treatment of cancer patients. He explained, however, that the study results actually suggested that cancer patients should not stop taking large doses of vitamin C. He went on:

When this Mayo Clinic paper appeared, 17 January 1985, Cameron and I were angry that Moertel and his Mayo Clinic associates, the

spokesman for the National Cancer Institute, and also the editor of the *New England Journal of Medicine* had managed to prevent us from obtaining any information about their results until a few hours before their publication. Six weeks earlier Moertel refused to tell me anything about the work, except that their paper was going to be published. In a letter to me, he promised that he would arrange for me to have a copy of the paper several days before publication, but he broke that promise.[111,p.234]

Pauling wrote in conclusion: "The misrepresentation by Moertel and his associates and by the National Cancer Institute spokesman has done great harm. Cancer patients have informed us that they are stopping their vitamin C because of the 'negative results' reported by the Mayo Clinic." He concluded: "It is not often that unethical behavior of scientists is reported. Fraud committed by young physicians doing medical research has been turned up several times in the last few years. Improper representation of the results of clinical studies, as in the second Mayo Clinic report, is especially to be condemned because of its effects in increasing the amount of human suffering."[111,p.235]

LACK OF FAMILIARITY WITH, OR INABILITY TO USE, A REHABILITATION MODEL

As I explain in Chapters 4.1 and 5.2, metabolic rehabilitation entails the use of feedback from objective measures of fibromyalgia status. The use of feedback at intervals is inherent in the process of rehabilitation. Feedback as scores from the measures must be generated at the beginning of the patient's treatment, at weekly or biweekly intervals during the treatment, at the end of the treatment, and at various follow-up intervals afterward. The scores, posted to line graphs, give us accurate, objective information about the patient's status. Because of this, we have no delusions about the benefits or lack of them from our treatment for any individual patient. Also, we can make new therapeutic decisions based on ample objective evidence tempered by clinical judgment. The feedback is meaningful because our measures are valid and reliable, and comparison of the scores at any time with those at previous times permits us to see the effect on patient status of our current therapeutic interventions.

In the minds of some clinicians, the downside of this rehabilitation approach is data collection and the posting of scores to line graphs. Some clinicians who have been open to considering our clinical approach have expressed concern about the labor intensity of the data collection and posting. Their concerns are understandable, considering the pressures on clinicians to move quickly, especially on those whose schedules are dictated by managed care.

Having a trained assistant to collect data and post scores can reduce the labor-intensity for the clinician. Then, the clinician, before making appropriate clinical decisions, has only to examine and communicate with the patient and view the trend of the data points on the line graphs.

Work is now under way, with the company Zygotech, to develop a software package that will eliminate nearly all of the labor intensity involved. Rather than filling out forms with a pen or pencil, patients will do so on a computer. Zygotech will analyze the data instantly and forward the results and graphs to the office of the patient's clinician. Clinicians will only have to review the line graphs and data supplied by Zygotech, examine and communicate with the patients, and then make appropriate clinical decisions. These decisions should be based on the combination of the data and their own clinical judgment.

RESISTANCE TO PARADIGM CHANGE

Resistance to paradigm changes is well-known in science. Such resistance was poignantly expressed in a now famous statement by physicist Max Planck, the founder of the quantum theory: "A new scientific truth does not triumph by convincing its opponents and making them see the light, but rather because its opponents eventually die, and a new generation grows up that is familiar with it."[112]

Kuhn wrote that the change of allegiance from one paradigm to another cannot be forced. To him, lifelong resistance is inherent in the nature of science. He wrote:

The source of resistance is the assurance that the older paradigm will ultimately solve all its problems, that nature can be shoved into the box the paradigm provides. Inevitably, at times of revolution, that assurance seems stubborn and pigheaded as indeed it sometimes becomes. But it is also something more. That same assurance is what makes normal or puzzle-solving science possible. And it is only through normal science that the professional community of scientists succeeds, first, in exploiting the potential scope and pre-

cision of the older paradigm and, then, in isolating the difficulty through the study of which a new paradigm may emerge.[93,pp.151-152]

Ziman emphasized "the social obstacles to revolutionary changes of outlook, and the resistance of the scientific community to innovation." He added, "Yet the ethos of science is receptive in principle to such upheavals, and successful innovation is cherished and honored." (Ziman was referring, of course, to professional scientists, not physicians doing research. The latter group is generally not receptive to innovative ideas, often rejecting them with hostility.) Science begins, Ziman wrote, in the minds of men, where "conceptual mutations" arise. He asked, "Why does it require an extraordinary individual talent to recognize, for the first time, a pattern that can be made obvious to the dullest student once it has been pointed out?" His answer: "Habitual association of features inhibits the imagination. The current scientific map or picture bears with it conventional associations that are difficult to break," and "the current paradigm completely misinterprets a wide variety of facts, yet the truth cannot be immediately seen." Ziman noted that to make a paradigm switch, researchers must unlearn much that they thought they knew.[92,pp.151-152]

Garrison described resistance to change in his description of the five generations of American medical revolutions: "The fifth generation is identified by progressive accumulation of wealth and power, characteristic tactics in gaining and holding that wealth and power, and progressive decline into moral depravity."[87,p.284] He also described the fifth generation's mode of action regarding pressure for change: "They consolidate their stranglehold on those less ruthless than themselves. They oppose the emergence of new ideas of all kinds, knowing that change would displace them from their positions of power. Early on, they find it effective to simply ignore new ideas. Later, as the moral decay of the fifth generation advances and the urgency and appeal of new ideas grow, they recognize the need for more severe tactics and are willing to use them."[87,p.285]

I am not, of course, implying that members of the rheumatology fibromyalgia paradigm are ruthless and in moral decay. I quote Garrison's insightful observations mainly to show that resistance to change, including paradigm change in medical practice and research, is an inherent part of medical and scientific social dynamics. At the same time, as Garrison noted, members of a paradigm in its "corrupted last generation will take predictable steps as they struggle to hold on to the reins of power."[87,p.281] Often, power brokers within a crumbling paradigm will stretch the envelope of propriety in resisting change. I have witnessed this in what I consider unscrupulous acts by some members of the rheumatology fibromyalgia paradigm. An example is using bogus reasons, as "peer reviewers," to reject our grant proposals, or as editorial board members, misquoting our findings and conclusions so that our submitted reports are rejected for publication (see section above titled "Blocking of Unconventional Views by Conventional Medical Publications").

TRUNCATED KNOWLEDGE OF CLINICAL THYROIDOLOGY

Since the early 1970s, conventional clinicians have adopted the four propositions regarding hypothyroidism and its treatment promoted by conventional endocrinology. The propositions are 1) a thyroid hormone deficiency is the only cause of hypothyroid-like symptoms; 2) only patients whose thyroid function tests indicate hypothyroidism should be permitted to use exogenous thyroid hormone; 3) the only form of thyroid hormone clinicians should permit patients to use is T_4; and 4) patients should be permitted to use only "replacement dosages, dosages that keep the TSH within the normal range. (See Chapter 5.3, section titled "Mandates of the Conventional Medical Hypothyroidism Paradigm.")

In line with the military or church code of conduct in conventional medicine that was described so well by Robert S. Mendelsohn, M.D.(see next section, "Code of Unscientific Conduct within Conventional Medicine"), most conventional clinicians have taken these propositions as mandates and strictly adhered to them in patient management. Thus, the propositions have become the "official standard of care." One consequence of this compliance has been a narrowing of conventional clinicians' knowledge of clinical thyroidology down to the content of these four mandates.

I have attempted to discuss broader issues involved in clinical thyroidology with many conventional clinicians and researchers. Most have shown distinct discomfort with the discussions. They have made it clear to me that until the "standard of practice" is different, they would not consider practicing in a manner out of line with the endocrinology propositions. Since my views and those of my colleagues are in discord with the propositions, most conventional clinicians decline to consider the scientific validity of

our views. This is understandable considering the pressure exerted on conventional clinicians not to vary from the "standards of care" within conventional medicine (see next section, "Code of Unscientific Conduct within Conventional Medicine"). This conduct is diametrically opposed to the spirit of science; it is more characteristic of the military or church model of conduct Robert S. Mendelsohn, M.D. emphasized by referring to mainstream medicine as the "Church of Modern Medicine."[73] Due to this code of conduct, conventional clinicians generally fail to recognize patients in their practices who have symptoms characteristic of inadequate thyroid hormone tissue regulation. As a result, the treatments the clinicians prescribe for the patients do not address the underlying cause of the symptoms. Hence, the treatments are generally ineffective. As I explain in the next section, this method of practice is unscientific, and in my mind, it raises serious humanitarian concerns.

CODE OF UNSCIENTIFIC CONDUCT WITHIN CONVENTIONAL MEDICINE

The unscientific code of conduct of conventional medical clinicians and researchers begins with their entry into U.S. medical schools. The inculcation of the code during the school years is then reinforced by various pressures during the physicians' careers. Robert S. Mendelsohn, M.D., a medical educator for more than 30 years, described the purpose of education in non-medical doctoral programs:

> In all other areas of higher education, the purpose is to expose the student to information and ideas that he can use to develop the capacity to think rationally, to reason, to question, to create. He is encouraged to debate with his professors and, when he applies for approval of his doctoral dissertation, he is expected to defend his thesis.[88,p73]

Mendelsohn's view of the ideals of education in nonmedical programs is in line with Bertrand Russell's beliefs about education for the young. Russell wrote:

> I believe that the main object of education should be to encourage the young to question and to doubt those things which have been taken for granted. What is important is independence of mind. What is bad in education is the unwillingness to permit students to challenge those views which are accepted and those people who are in power. It is necessary for new ideas to emerge,

that young people have every encouragement to fundamentally disagree with the stupidities of their day. Most people who are respectable and most ideas which are considered to be fundamental are barriers to human achievement. I feel that it is not as important to learn large numbers of things as it is to feel passionately that one has the right to disagree and the obligation to develop new ideas.[88,p73]

Mendelsohn also described how education in U.S. medical schools differs from that in other educational programs, where students are encouraged "to develop the capacity to think rationally, to reason, to question, to create":

Not so in medical school. There, students are taught to absorb doctrine without argument or question. They are taught to respond to their teachers in a reflex manner. For example, when he hears the word 'streptococcus' the student is taught to respond with 'penicillin.' When the professor says 'right lower quadrant pain,' he is taught to respond 'appendectomy,' and God help him if he suggests that it might be a passing cramp. In short, medical school teaches the student a body of dogmatic material and restricts his right to exercise judgment to very narrow limits. He may be permitted to debate what kind of pertusis vaccine to use, but not to question whether whooping cough vaccine should be used at all. He may be allowed to disagree about the kind of antibiotic to use for ear infections, but not to question the use of antibiotics as standard treatment for infections, whatever the cause.[73,pp.24-25]

This form of education, in which students are trained to bow before the seat of authority, encourages the adoption on their part of a dogmatic and authoritarian manner. After entering clinical practice, some medical physicians impose on their doctor/patient relationships the same military/church code of conduct that Mendelsohn explained they learned in medical school. That many patients and clinicians of disciplines other than medicine find this conduct of some medical physicians abhorrent is legend. Yet I believe the physicians' conduct becomes second nature and largely unconscious. Most mean no harm by it, although I believe it does cause much harm.

Some harm results from the conduct blocking collaborative interaction between the physicians and their patients. My opinion, in line with that of Bernard Lown,[113] is that quality clinical care does not occur without collaborative interaction between the clinician and patient.

Harm also results because the code of conduct causes conventional clinicians and researchers to accept without question the beliefs of authorities within sister specialties. The code also dictates that clinicians conduct their practices according to the authorities' beliefs, the "standard of practice." The code of conduct is expressed in the old motto of the medical profession that prescribes conformity: "Be not the first by whom the new are tried, nor the last to lay the old aside."[114,p.153] Even today, the motto is enforced, especially within some specialties. John Dommisse, M.D. described the mode of enforcement in explaining the resistance of conventional physicians to the use of T_3 in clinical practice: "The . . . resistance has to do with the conservatism that many doctors are influenced or coerced to adopt because of the huge survival- and career-jeopardizing pressures that physicians who 'step out of line' are subjected to, by medical boards, plaintiff lawyers, other physicians, medical schools, etc., etc."[74] The fact that until very recently most physicians complied with this code of conduct led Linus Pauling in his last interview to comment: "I have a number of reports from people—scientists—that say, 'Well, I don't know anything about vitamin C or other vitamins, but Linus Pauling has been right so often in the past that I just accept what he says.' Physicians, of course, are a bit more skeptical and outspoken, and, in general, they don't have the background of knowledge. They don't know enough to say that he [Pauling] has been successful so often in the past that he's probably right this time. Physicians don't try to form opinions of this sort anyway. They just do what the medical authorities say to do. Of all the professions, the medical profession is the one in which the individual practitioners do the smallest amount of thinking for themselves."[115] Pauling had long held this view and had written in 1986, "Almost all physicians rely upon the statements made by authorities. This situation is inevitable. The practicing physician is too busy to make a thorough study of the complex and often voluminous original literature on every medical topic."[111,p.302]

Now, a few years later, with the rapid decay of the orthodox medical paradigm that Garrison has so well described[87] and that Lown has suggested,[113] many physicians no longer comply with this code of conduct. This is especially true of family physicians and those who are holistic- or nutrition-oriented. In contrast, the code still tightly regulates the conduct of other specialists, particularly endocrinologists and rheumatologists.

Psychologists Albert Ellis and Robert Harper

wrote that the most effective route to solving human problems is to question and challenge our own fundamental assumptions and beliefs, and when the rules of reason dictate, dispute and abandon the assumptions and beliefs, no matter how much we cherish them.[94] The military or church model of conduct of conventional medicine is the exact opposite of this rational, scientific approach to problem-solving. The military/church code of conduct is appropriate for, and serves well the purposes of, the military and the church. It is not appropriate for physicians in their interactions with patients and colleagues. Conventional physicians involved in research who abide rigidly by the code are hampered by their own conduct, reducing the probability that they will help solve medical problems such as fibromyalgia.

Why Research Moves So Slowly

In 1999, Clauw answered a question submitted by a reader of the *Syndrome Sentinel*: "Why does fibromyalgia/chronic fatigue syndrome research move so slowly?" One of his answers implied that research would move more quickly if more money were spent on studies of the illnesses. He noted that patient advocacy groups have been responsible for increasing government spending on research into the illnesses, and he urged patients and their friends to appeal to members of Congress.[28,p.2]

With all due respect, I disagree with Clauw's opinion that research will progress more quickly if, as a result of appeals to Congress, more government-allocated money is spent on fibromyalgia studies. I believe that allocating more money, especially through the National Institutes of Health (NIH), will actually stunt scientific progress. I say this because the record shows the piddling return the public gets for the tax dollars poured into the NIH. Conventional medical physicians are the decision-makers at the NIH, yet the code of conduct of conventional medicine is unscientific. Physicians who conform to that code are therefore more likely to impede than to advance our understanding and treatment of fibromyalgia patients.

Below, I discuss problems with NIH involvement in fibromyalgia research. First, though, let me explain what I see as the most fundamental cause of the failure of rheumatology paradigm researchers to learn that the weight of scientific evidence leans on the side of inadequate thyroid hormone tissue regulation being the mechanism underlying most cases of fibromyalgia. This is pertinent to my views on NIH involvement.

Failure to Search Among Entrenched Medical Beliefs for the Cause and Solution to Fibromyalgia.

Because of the military/church code of conduct of conventional medicine, rheumatology paradigm fibromyalgia researchers have failed, in their exploration of fibromyalgia, to clear their previous beliefs from their collective frame of reference. The beliefs within their frame of reference that have steered them off course from the start, and have kept them off course, are the four mandates of conventional endocrinology. Quite simply, rheumatology paradigm researchers have rigidly and unquestioningly accepted the endocrinology mandates as unequivocal truth. Due to that acceptance, they implicitly concluded that inadequate thyroid hormone regulation cannot possibly underlie fibromyalgia.

I sometimes ponder an intriguing speculation: If rheumatology paradigm researchers had followed the proper protocol of scientific inquiry, the current failing paradigm would not have emerged. Instead, they would have established another paradigm unified by the very hypothesis I posit in this book.

In the mid-1970s, Smythe, Moldofsky, Yunus, and others, through their studies of fibromyalgia patients, became the catalysts to the genesis and rise of the rheumatology paradigm. Already by then, however, conventional endocrinologists had reached illogical conclusions about two things: (1) who might and might not benefit from the use of thyroid hormone, and (2) how patients' dosages should be adjusted (see Chapter 2.5, subsection titled "Advent of the TSH Assay," and Chapter 5.3, subsection titled "Misinterpretation of Investigative Data and Its Gradual Acceptance as Scientific Fact"). These illogical conclusions soon led to the four mandates I describe in Chapter 5.3. Many medical writers have noted that the features of fibromyalgia are remarkably similar to hypothyroidism.[45][46][47][48][49][50][51][52][53][54][55][56] These papers alerting clinicians and researchers to a possible relation between hypothyroidism and fibromyalgia span the years from 1945 to 1998. Rheumatology paradigm researchers began using laboratory thyroid function tests in an attempt to identify and exclude hypothyroid patients from their fibromyalgia studies. Their belief that the laboratory tests reliably identified patients whose fibromyalgia symptoms were actually those of hypothyroidism was largely false. As a result, it is highly probable that many patients included in the studies were hypothyroid despite the laboratory test results, and that most other patients had partial cellular resistance to thyroid hormone. Trust in the veracity of the endocrinology mandates was well-intentioned. But it was precisely this trust, dictated by the code of unscientific conduct of conventional medicine, that misguided them in their search for the cause of fibromyalgia.

Their trust was a violation of a main rule of scientific inquiry, as described by most philosophers of science. Prominent philosophers of science have differed on whether scientific inquiry begins by inductive or deductive steps. Most, however, have shared one belief—that scientific inquiry should begin by clearing one's mind of previously held beliefs. For Francis Bacon, this involved proceeding purely inductively, laying aside all preconceived hypotheses or ideas, which he called "Idols," and identifying the errors in previous beliefs about the problem at hand. After giving up all previous beliefs, he argued that we should collect facts. For René Descartes, the beginning of scientific inquiry involved doubting all that could be doubted, leaving only the single or a few beliefs that were thoroughly beyond doubt. He recommended that we then reason deductively from the remaining undoubted beliefs. John Dewey, Morris Cohen, and Ernest Nagel also emphasized beginning our search for truth with doubt in our own beliefs.[1,pp.6-15]

I mentioned previously the medical writers who, over a span of 53 years, noted that the features of fibromyalgia are remarkably similar to those of hypothyroidism.[45][46][47][48][49][50][51][52][53][54][55][56] Unlike the rheumatology paradigm researchers, I did not dismiss the possibility that, in fact, fibromyalgia might be a clinical phenotype of hypothyroidism. I did not dismiss this possibility despite laboratory test results indicating, according to standard methods of interpretation, that most fibromyalgia patients were not hypothyroid. In the late 1980s, I suspended judgment as I read everything I could get my hands on about hypothyroidism and fibromyalgia. My aim was to learn how the two conditions differed or resembled one another. When my colleagues and I treated some fibromyalgia patients with replacement dosages of thyroid hormone, their fibromyalgia persisted, even though their symptoms might have diminished somewhat. But when some patients took TSH suppressive dosages of thyroid hormone, the fibromyalgia symptoms disappeared altogether. These observations convinced me that some patients' fibromyalgia symptoms were in fact mainly due to hypothyroidism. They also led me to suspect that the endocrinologists' mandates were wrong. When I found that the TRH stimulation test results of many of my fibromyalgia patients were consistent with central hypothyroidism, I became convinced that the endocrinology mandates were wrong.

Later, I discovered the subset of thyroidology literature on thyroid hormone resistance. My colleagues and I then began treating fibromyalgia patients who were euthyroid (according to conventional thyroid function test results) as though they had thyroid hormone resistance. They recovered dramatically when using T_3, if they also ceased certain metabolism-impeding medications, exercised to tolerance, changed to a wholesome diet, began using nutritional supplements, and underwent physical treatment. From this experience, I became convinced that most of my euthyroid patients had partial cellular resistance to thyroid hormone.

Throughout my research, over and over again I rejected the idea that fibromyalgia is related to thyroid hormone. Each time, however, the hypothesis forced itself upon me again. It did so when I thought of my fibromyalgia patients who had improved or recovered with the use of thyroid hormone. Eventually, I could no longer doubt the hypothesis that the patients' fibromyalgia symptoms were caused by hypometabolism of select tissues. The firmness of my belief increased each time rheumatology paradigm researchers reported finding a previously unknown objective abnormality among fibromyalgia patients. Inadequate thyroid hormone regulation plausibly explained each in succession. The general conclusion that I was compelled to accept, and that I present in this book, is that most patients' fibromyalgia is underlain mainly by inadequate thyroid hormone regulation, due either to primary or central hypothyroidism or thyroid hormone resistance. The results of the controlled studies my colleagues and I conducted (reprinted in Appendix B), combined with a subsequent stream of recovered patients under the care of my colleagues Gina Honeyman-Lowe and Richard Garrison, have left me with no doubt whatever that the inadequate thyroid hormone regulation hypothesis should begin the next paradigm upon which new fibromyalgia research is based.

Most researchers within the rheumatology paradigm did not pursue a possible link between fibromyalgia and inadequate thyroid hormone tissue regulation. The notable exception in this regard is the French rheumatologist, Prof. J. Eisinger. Although he and I have not yet reached a consensus in our theoretical views and clinical procedures, his diligent and often brilliant work has inspired me over the past several years. He continues to publish on the relation of fibromyalgia to thyroid hormone.[121] Eisinger's studies have produced important findings related to metabolism and thyroid hormone that are anomalous to the rheumatology paradigm. He is also a prolific and persuasive member of the avant-garde germinating the concepts that will serve to unify research into a second fibromyalgia paradigm. For these reasons, I consider Eisinger the most distingished researcher to have taken part in the rheumatology paradigm.

Except for Eisinger, rheumatology paradigm researchers did not consider an association between inadequate thyroid hormone and fibromyalgia. Instead, they complied with the military/church code of conduct of the conventional medical profession, a code of conduct which supports distinctly unscientific behavior. I expressed the problem succinctly in 1998 in the Internet communications that were a prelude to the First Congress on Defining a New Paradigm for the Healing Arts, held at the University of Texas-Houston Health Science Center. I made the point that a major fault of the orthodox medical paradigm, which is presently crumbling, is a failure to use the scientific method. By the scientific method, I meant the rigorous use of logical reasoning in the formation of our scientific beliefs. I wrote:

> My old friend, Robert S. Mendelsohn, M.D. (who, if still alive, would have enthusiastically taken part in this Congress), made this point back in the 1980s in several books (*Confessions of a Medical Heretic, Malepractice: How Doctors Manipulate Women,* and *How to Raise a Healthy Child in Spite of Your Doctor*). Bob argued that what the popular press calls medical science is more accurately described as the Church of Modern Medicine. In his analogy, physicians are the priests, and their aim is to persuade the congregation of patients to submit to the authoritarian dogma of the Church. His point was well taken: He catalyzed a movement of patients and heretical physicians who defiantly challenged the dogma. This movement contributed to the current widespread determined opposition to orthodox medical authority.
>
> Despite this opposition, I suspect that most people will continue to acquiesce to authoritarian medical dogma. They find it easier to accept without question the axioms, postulates, and other assumptions issued by others, and then let the chips fall as they may. This tendency is not all bad, of course. The volume of new information that flows forth necessitates that we often trust the judgments of those we consider authorities. But problems can develop when we take careless advantage of this convenience. Thus, for illustration, it appears that incalculable numbers of people have died of heart disease that could have been averted, had they taken enough supplemental B vitamins and lowered their homocysteine levels. But they failed to do so. Why? Their well-meaning but misguided physicians assured

them that medical science had proven that we get enough vitamins in our foods and that vitamin supplements are of no value.

> As another illustration, a medical researcher may ignore important clues to the solution to medical problems, delaying the solution for decades. The reason? Because he compliantly accepts as scientifically established a dogmatic belief of authorities in a field that overlaps his own—a belief falsely professing that a particular class of clues is irrelevant to the problem he is studying. Let me give a brief example of this. Richard Garrison, M.D., others, and I are actively studying the use of thyroid hormone as a treatment for fibromyalgia. More times than I can count, my particular efforts with this experimental treatment have been seriously hampered by authoritarian dogma accepted as scientific fact. The problem is the current clinical paradigm of endocrinology. This paradigm is expressed in a false proposition: that the serum basal TSH level is the "gold standard" for diagnosing thyroid hormone deficiency and for adjusting the patient's dosage of thyroid hormone. In line with this, those who believe this proposition make two pronouncements: (1) If the TSH level is within the normal range, then the patient cannot possibly have too little thyroid hormone regulation of cell function, and (2) taking enough thyroid hormone to suppress the TSH level is hazardous and possibly life-threatening. Based on these false beliefs, many physicians have actively opposed my use of our treatment that ignores these mandates yet helps patients get well.

> Acceptance of authoritative dogma is synonymous with a rejection of the first rule of reason of traditional rationalism. This rule says to examine the relevant evidence before accepting and acting on a belief. It is this that I believe is the fundamental fault of the current orthodox medical paradigm. It is also the reason philosophers of science generally consider medical science primitive and unsophisticated. I believe a novel solution would be a commitment by medical clinicians and researchers to a purely rational path to our beliefs. I believe we should: (1) question all preconceived ideas; (2) refuse to unquestioningly accept anyone's belief, except for temporary expedience, simply because he or she is considered an authority; (3) willingly, albeit cautiously, abandon beliefs that conflict with the available evidence; and (4) tentatively adopt, rather than dogmatically adhere to, beliefs that are the best supported. It seems to me that this approach is one we must accept, if the emerging new paradigm for the healing arts stands a chance of serving us better than the old one.[57]

Complying with the code of unscientific conduct of conventional medicine, researchers of the rheumatology paradigm obediently accepted the mandates of authorities of the endocrinology specialty. (See Chapter 2.5, subsection titled "Advent of the TSH Assay," and the section titled "Misbeliefs about the Serum TSH that have Diverted Fibromyalgia Researchers from an Understanding of Euthyroid Fibromyalgia." Also see Chapter 5.3, section titled "Mandates of the Conventional Medical Hypothyroidism Paradigm"). By doing so, they were thrown off track from the start. This misdirected beginning has been and remains costly. Northrop pointed out that scientific rigor later on will not correct a false start. "It is like a ship leaving port for a distant destination," he wrote. "A very slight erroneous deviation in taking one's bearings at the beginning may result in entirely missing one's mark at the end, regardless of the sturdiness of one's craft or the excellence of one's subsequent seamanship."[44,p.1] A scientifically correct start ensures economy of thought and effort, directing investigators to the key facts, and designating the proper study methods. Had the researchers of the rheumatology paradigm not been diverted at the start, I believe that fibromyalgia would no longer be a health problem of concern.

The continuing obstinate faith of rheumatology paradigm researchers in the truth of the mandates of conventional endocrinology has amazed and fascinated me. Some researchers with whom I have had close communication, and who I believe consider me an intellectually honest and credible thinker, have heard me describe in detail some of my patients' full recovery from fibromyalgia with metabolic rehabilitation involving the use of thyroid hormone. They listened politely, but their beliefs about fibromyalgia were as thoroughly unaffected as if I had not spoken to them.

Some of my patients who have fully recovered have written letters to the prominent researchers of the rheumatology paradigm who had previously treated them unsuccessfully. In these letters, the patients implored the researchers to consider their recovery and what had brought it about. The responses are typified by that of a prominent rheumatology paradigm researcher. In his return letter to the patient, he simply stated that if her symptoms had been related to a thyroid problem, someone other than Dr. Lowe would have determined it long before. He made no comment on her report of having recovered. This type of reaction, or lack of reaction, by rheumatology paradigm researchers brings to mind an observation once made by Chester Wilk: "A closed mind is like the iris of the eye: the more light you expose it to, the more it constricts."

Dubious Potential of NIH Involvement in Fibromyalgia Research

As I wrote above, I disagree with Clauw's opinion about how to accelerate advancement in the field of fibromyalgia research. He implied that research will progress more rapidly if, through appeals to Congress, more tax dollars are provided for fibromyalgia studies. If the money would be provided to independent researchers through some route exempt from NIH mediation, research probably would move along more rapidly. But if government money is allocated to researchers at the discretion of medical physicians appointed to "peer review" research grant proposals, progress is highly likely to stall.

NIH Involvement in Fibromyalgia Research. In its 1993 budget, the Senate Committee on Appropriations directed the National Institutes of Health (NIH) to become involved in various ways in fibromyalgia research. The NIH was directed to report on grants awarded, established contracts, intramural research, and research priorities on behalf of the fibromyalgia community. Fibromyalgia-related research was supported by several Institutes of the NIH. Pillemer and Shulman (physician-representatives of the National Institute of Arthritis and Musculoskeletal and Skin Diseases of the NIH [26,p.4]) wrote that the main means by which the National Institute of Arthritis and Musculoskeletal and Skin Diseases (NIAMS) supported research is "investigator initiated research." Researchers submit applications, and these are submitted to "quality review": "funding is on the basis of relative meritorious quality of these applications received by the institute." Pillemer and Shulman also wrote, "To further encourage research, the NIAMS convened a workshop of experts of FMS who would be charged with identifying future research priorities for fibromyalgia syndrome research. The goal of the workshop was to provide state-of-the-art knowledge, identify research gaps and opportunities, and recommend future directions for research on the cause, pathogenesis, diagnosis, and treatment of fibromyalgia syndrome."[26,p.2] Individuals who attended the workshop included: (1) representatives from various Institutes of the NIH; (2) the leaders of 3 of the major fibromyalgia support groups whose members derive their fibromyalgia-*Weltansicht* from the ideas propounded by core rheumatology paradigm researchers; and (3) 10 well-known veteran rheumatology paradigm researchers.

Many fibromyalgia patients have been heartened and reassured by the 10 researchers from the rheumatology paradigm finally becoming involved with the NIH on patients' behalf.[26,pp.2-3] In my view, however, their positive feelings about this turn of events are misguided. For NIH involvement is virtual assurance that the field will cease to advance. As Robert S. Mendelsohn, M.D. said: "The physicians who serve as surgeon general and at the NIH and CDC are the Keystone Cops of modern medicine. And this is why the NIH and CDC haven't solved a serious health problem in the fifty years of their existence."[116] Many people appear to still have confidence in the ability of the NIH to competently orchestrate the search for solutions to health problems such as fibromyalgia. I urge them to read at least two books: (1) *Osler's Web: Inside the Labyrinth of the Chronic Fatigue Syndrome Epidemic*, in which Hillary Johnson provides detailed accounts of NIH handling of chronic fatigue syndrome research,[117] and (2) *Inventing the AIDS Virus*, in which Peter Duesberg describes NIH handling of AIDS research.[27]

I see at least two reasons why NIH involvement is likely to impede progress in fibromyalgia research: (1) the predominant role of physicians over scientists at the NIH, and (2) the peer review system for approving grants.

Physicians Not Trained as Scientists Dominate the Professional Scientists at NIH. The main purpose of medical school in the U.S. is for students to learn to diagnose and treat according to conventional methods. Despite the popular belief, training to be a clinician is not training to be a scientist. It is true that many physicians take part in conducting studies using scientific methods. What most of them learn about research is essentially on-the-job training. And what they learn is usually a minimal amount of research procedure relevant to the studies they participate in.

Consider the opinion of Candace Pert, Ph.D. She is the neuroscientist who discovered the opiate receptor and, with her husband, confirmed that endorphins are our natural internal opiates. She conducted research at the National Institutes of Health (NIH) between 1977 and 1987. In *Molecules of Emotion*, she wrote that at the NIH, "A wise scientist will seek out a niche protected by a powerful M.D. and be content to stay there. No matter how smart or productive he or she may be, the scientist with a Ph.D. has absolutely no chance of ever rising to a position of controlling resources. M.D.s only need apply." She pointed out, "This intellectual imbalance creates a certain amount of friction between the two categories, scientist and medical doctor. Success often depends on a certain amount of sucking-up to your superiors, something

that doesn't come easy for a lot of brilliant scientists." Speaking from her personal experience, she notes: "During my years there, I saw more than a few who weren't willing to play the game, usually because they considered their boss an imbecile who wouldn't know an experimental breakthrough if it strolled into his office and burst into song. While most of the doctors high up in the Palace [her term for the NIH] had a passing familiarity with experimental science, few were experimenters, and they often had a difficult time evaluating data, particularly when two experiments conflicted." Of the M.D.s in charge, she wrote: "But they were in charge, the princes, the power-boy doctors, and I saw more than one frustrated scientist return to his basement lair to bang his head against the walls over a discrepancy between what his boss had learned in medical school and what he himself had just seen under his microscope."[119,p.96]

What I am saying here, however, is not limited to M.D.s doing research, but also to most D.C.s, D.O.s, and dentists who take part in research. The limited on-the-job-learning of clinicians doing research cannot be equated with the long, rigorous education and training of the scientist. To call physicians doing medical research "scientists" is to call short order cooks chefs. As a rule, clinicians, regardless of whether or not they are doing research, have no educational background in subjects such as the philosophy of science, research methodology, or logical methods of evaluating evidence. This lack of training of physicians in science and the code of unscientific conduct of conventional medicine do not add up to advancement of medical science. What we have inside and outside the NIH is practicing conventional physicians unquestioningly accepting the conclusions of conventional medical researchers who are poorly trained or not trained at all to evaluate scientific evidence. When the researchers' conclusions are incorrect (such as those of conventional endocrinology researchers regarding hypothyroidism), the clinical decisions of practicing conventional physicians are also likely to be incorrect. I am convinced that most conventional clinicians are sincere and well-intending in their beliefs and health care practices. But sincerity and good intentions cannot compensate for decisions based on false conclusions.

Peer Review System for Grant Approval. One reason for the failure of NIH-controlled research to solve health problems is the way it goes about selecting those who participate in deciding which researchers get NIH funding and which do not. To wit, consider the explanation of the eminent virologist

Peter H. Duesberg, Ph.D. of how the medical establishment maintains power and betrays public trust. One method is the peer review process, which enforces a consensus view about a disease. He wrote:

> The initial power base of the establishment is grant allocation. No medical scientist could even hope to make a career without a research grant from the NIH. Grant allocation selects and rewards conformism with the establishment view. Nonconformists are eliminated by the outwardly democratic 'peer review system' advertised by the orthodoxy as an independent jury system that provides checks and balances.
>
> However, a truly independent jury would be fatal for the establishment. Indeed, a grant awarded to test an unorthodox theory of AIDS that proved to be successful would be an end to the orthodoxy itself. Therefore, orthodox scientists (with NIH grants) are carefully selected as the 'peers' to review 'investigator-initiated' grant applications. The system works because the peers serve the orthodoxy by serving their own vested interests.[27,p.451]

Understanding how this system works can enable one to also understand why some independent researchers, such as my research group, with a treatment that obviously works for most patients, are ignored by establishment researchers or denied funds for further study of our point of view. As Duesberg also wrote:

> Under this review system, a scientist's access to funding, promotions, publication in journals, ability to win prizes, and invitations to conferences are entirely controlled by his peers. This absurd situation puts one's competitors in charge of one's career, a direct conflict of interest. Imagine if every new automobile or new computer had to be approved by competing corporations before being released to the market. *Products would cease improving, and the market would experience a steady decline in quality. Innovation and competition would die.* Such inherent problems have led to public criticisms of peer review over the past twenty years, with various congressmen and even the Office of Management and Budget voicing objections to the system [italics mine].[27,pp.452-453]

The italicized sentence in the last quoted paragraph explains my concerns about NIH involvement in fibromyalgia research, with the old guard researchers of the rheumatology paradigm sitting at the grant proposal review table. When decision makers see to it that funding sustains only those who share their views, ra-

ther than dispassionately deciding to fund only those whose conventional or unconventional ideas hold the most promise for advancing the field, we see another example of unscientific conduct in medical research. As Kohn, in describing the proper conduct of the scientist, wrote, "The scientist's activities and efforts should be directed towards the extension of scientific knowledge, and not towards the personal interests of an individual or a group of scientists."[89,p.2]

What is now needed in fibromyalgia research is innovation that can advance the field. This need is not likely to be filled once the old guard of the rheumatology paradigm grasps the reigns of power in deciding which studies are funded and which are not. Those who were instrumental in building a paradigm that is falling seldom become active in the paradigm that succeeds it, as Kuhn[93] and Garrison have shown.[87] The old guard has taken the field as far as it can, and others must now have the liberty and financing to advance the field. I do not mean this as a slight to the old guard in fibromyalgia research. It is their history of contributions that can now enable us, unless they impede the process, to advance to another paradigm that builds on the one they created. Their body of empirically-gathered information related to fibromyalgia patients must now give way to a more useful deductive hypothesis built around understanding that information. We should respect them for their praiseworthy accomplishments, but at the same time, thank them in advance for graciously abstaining from obstructing further progress.

The NIH spends a staggering amount of tax dollars, presumably pursuing solutions to diseases that afflict taxpayers. The record shows that taxpayers get little return from the NIH for the money it spends. This being the case, I seriously doubt that Clauw is right in his view that what is needed to hasten progress in fibromyalgia research is more money. More money will lead to a peer review process involving the old guard that is likely to hold the field in a state of stagnation. And when more money is available, more of the old guard are likely to come on board, with added problems. As Duesberg wrote:

> The stifling effect of peer review becomes worse as the number of peers increases, one of the direct effects of over-funded science. The growing number of researchers creates a herd effect, drowning out the voice of the lone scientist who questions official wisdom. Researchers begin spending more time networking and seeking to build coalitions of allies rather than stepping on toes by raising unpopular questions.[27,p.453]

On July 12, 1999, the U.S. Department of Health and Human Services released a report that NIAMS was funding multiple research grants for the study of fibromyalgia. Alas.

REFERENCES

1. Walker, S., III: *A Dose of Sanity.* New York, John Wiley & Sons, Inc., 1996.
2. Csillage, C.: Fibromyalgia: the Copenhagen Declaration. *Lancet,* 340:663-664, 1992.
3. Russell, A.S.: Fibromyalgia: a historical perspective. *J. Musculoskel. Pain,* 3(2):43-48, 1995.
4. Russell, I.J.: Preface: the Vancouver Conference. *J. Musculoskel. Pain,* 3(2):xv-xvi, 1995.
5. Introduction: *The Physical Medicine Research Foundation's 8th International Symposium*—fibromyalgia, chronic fatigue syndrome, and repetitive strain injury: current concepts in diagnosis, management, and cost containment. *J. Musculoskel. Pain,* 3(2):1-2, 1995.
6. Walker, E.A., Katon, W.J., Keegan, D., Gardner, G., and Sullivan, M.: Predictors of physician frustration in the care of patients with rheumatological complaints. *Gen. Hosp. Psych.,* 19(5):315-323, 1997.
7. Wolfe, F.: Fibromyalgia: on diagnosis and certainty. *J. Musculoskel. Pain,* 1(3/4):17-35, 1993.
8. Goldenberg, D.L.: Fibromyalgia syndrome a decade later: what have we learned? *Arch. Intern. Med.,* 159(8):777-785, 1999.
9. Wolfe, F. and Hawley, D.J.: Psychosocial factors and the fibromyalgia syndrome. *Z. Rheumatol.,* 57(Suppl.2):88-91, 1998.
10. Meyer-Lindenberg, A. and Gallhofer, B.: Somatized depression as a subgroup of fibromyalgia syndrome. *Z. Rheumatol.,* 57(Suppl.2):92-93, 1998.
11. Offenbaecher, M., Glatzeder, K., and Ackenheil, M.: Self-reported depression, familial history of depression and fibromyalgia (FM), and psychological distress in patients with FM. *Z. Rheumatol.,* 57(Suppl.2):94-96, 1998.
12. Walter, B., Vaitl, D., and Frank, R.: Affective distress in fibromyalgia syndrome is associated with pain severity. *Z. Rheumatol.,* 57(Suppl.2):101-104, 1998.
13. Netter, P. and Hennig, J.: The fibromyalgia syndrome as a manifestation of neuroticism? *Z. Rheumatol.,* 57 (Suppl.2):105-108, 1998.
14. Cathebras, P., Lauwers, A., and Rousset, H.: Fibromyalgia: a critical review. *Ann. Med. Interne.* (Paris), 149(7):406-414, 1998.
15. Hannonen, P., Malminiemi, K., Yli-Kerttula, U., Isomeri, R., and Roponen, P.: A randomized, double-blind, placebo-controlled study of moclobemide and amitriptyline in the treatment of fibromyalgia in females without psychiatric disorder. *Br. J. Rheumatol.,* 37(12):1279-1286, 1998.
16. Epstein, S.A., Kay, G., Clauw, D., et al.: Psychiatric disorders in patients with fibromyalgia. A multicenter investigation. *Psychosomatics,* 40(1):57-63, 1999.
17. Ackenheil, M.: Genetics and pathophysiology of affective disorders: relationship to fibromyalgia. *Z. Rheumatol.,* 57

(Suppl.2):5-7, 1998.
18. Merskey, H.: Psychosocial factors and muscular pain. *First International Symposium on Myofascial Pain and Fibromyalgia,* Meeting Program, May 8-10, 1989, p.27.
19. Ahles, T.A., Khan, S.A., Yunus, M.B., and Spiegel, D.A.: Psychiatric diagnoses among primary fibromyalgia (PFS) and rheumatoid arthritis (RA) patients and non-pain controls. *First International Symposium on Myofascial Pain and Fibromyalgia,* Meeting Program, May 8-10, 1989, p.78.
20. Russell, I.J.: Foreword: Second National Institutes of Health Fibromyalgia Conference. *J. Musculoskel. Pain,* 6(3):xiii-xiv, 1998.
21. Russell, I.J.: A tribute to Harvey Moldofsky, M.D.: *J. Musculoskel. Pain,* 4(1/2):1-2, 1996.
22. Bradley, L.A., Alcarcón, G.S., Triana, M., et al.: Health care seeking behavior in fibromyalgia: associations with pain thresholds, symptoms severity, and psychiatric morbidity. *J. Musculoskel. Pain,* 2(3):79-87, 1994.
23. Straus, S.E.: Chronic fatigue syndrome. *J. Musculoskel. Pain,* 2(3):57-63, 1994.
24. Goldenberg, D.L.: An overview of psychologic studies in fibromyalgia. *J. Rheum.,* 16(Suppl.19):12-13, 1989.
25. Popper, K.: *Realism and the Aim of Science.* London, Routledge, 1985.
26. Pillemer, S.R. and Shulman, L.E.: Introduction: fibromyalgia research planning workshop: future directions in fibromyalgia research. *J. Musculoskel. Pain,* 2(3):1-4, 1994.
27. Duesberg, P.H.: *Inventing the AIDS Virus.* Washington, D.C., Regnery Publishing, Inc., 1996.
28. Clauw, D.: Research in CFS and fibromyalgia: why do we move so slowly? *The Syndrome Sentinel,* 2(2):1-3, 1999.
29. United States Department of Health and Human Services: NIAMS funds multiple research grants in Fibromyalgia. July 12, 1999.
30. Merskey, H.: Psychosocial factors and muscular pain. In *Advances in Pain Research and Therapy,* Vol. 17. Edited by J.R. Fricton and E. Awad, New York, Raven Press, Ltd., 1990, pp.213-225.
31. Moldofsky, H.: The contribution of sleep-wake physiology to fibromyalgia. In *Advances in Pain Research and Therapy,* Vol. 17. Edited by J.R. Fricton and E. Awad, New York, Raven Press, Ltd., 1990, pp.227-240.
32. Moldofsky, H., Scarisbrick, P., England, R., and Smythe, H.: Musculoskeletal symptoms and non-REM sleep disturbance in patients with "fibrositis syndrome" and healthy subjects. *Psychosomat. Med.* 37(4):341-351, 1975.
33. Moldofsky, H. and Scarisbrick, P.: Induction of neurasthenic musculoskeletal pain syndrome by selective sleep stage deprivation. *Psychosom. Med.,* 38:35-44, 1976.
34. Moldofsky, H.: Sleep and fibrositis syndrome. *Rheum. Dis. Clin. North Amer.,* 15:91-103, 1989.
35. McCain, G.A., Bell, D.A., Mai, F.M., and Halliday, P.D.: A controlled study of the effects of a supervised cardiovascular fitness training program on the manifestations of primary fibromyalgia. *Arthritis Rheum.,* 31:1135-1141, 1988.
36. Bennett, R.M., Clark, S.R., Goldberg, L., Nelson, D., Bonafede, R.P., Porter, J., and Specht, D.: Aerobic fitness in the fibrositis syndrome: a controlled study of respira-

tory gas exchange and [133]xenon clearance from exercising muscle. *Arthritis Rheum.*, 32:454-460, 1989.

37. Wolfe, F., Smythe, H.A., Yunus, M.B., et al.: The American College of Rheumatology 1990 criteria for the classification of fibromyalgia: report of the multicenter criteria committee. *Arthritis Rheumatol.*, 33:160-172, 1990.

38. Simms, R.W. and Goldenberg, D.L.: Symptoms mimicking neurologic disorders in fibromyalgia syndrome. *J. Rheumatol.*, 15:1271, 1988.

39. Stratz, T., Schochat, T., Hrycai, P., et al.: The blockade of -HT3 receptors in fibromyalgia: a new therapy concept? *J. Musculoskel. Pain*, 3(Suppl.1):64, 1995.

40. Sprott, H., Kluge, H., Franke, S., and Hein, G.: Altered serotonin-levels in patients with fibromyalgia. *J. Musculoskel. Pain*, 3(Suppl.1):65, 1995.

41. Russell, I.J.: Abnormal laboratory findings related to pain and fatigue in fibromyalgia. *J. Musculoskel. Pain*, 3(2):59-65, 1995.

42. Russell, I.J., Bowden, C.L., Michalek, J., Fletcher, E., and Hester, G.A.: *Arthritis Rheumat.*, 30(Suppl.):S63, 1988.

43. Yunus, M.B., Dailey, J.W., Aldag, J.C., Masi, A.T., and Jobe, P.C.: Plasma tryptophan and other amino acids in primary fibromyalgia: a controlled study. *J. Rheumatol.*, 19:90-94, 1992.

44. Northrop, F.S.C.: *The Logic of the Sciences and the Humanities.* New York, Meridian Books, 1960.

45. Alajouanine, T. and Nick, J.: De l'existence d'une myopathie d'origine hypothyroidienne. *Paris Med.*, 35:346, 1945.

46. Wilson, J. and Walton, J.N.: Some muscular manifestations of hypothyroidism. *J. Neurol. Neurosurg. Psychiat.*, 22:320-324, 1959.

47. Bergouignan, M., Vital, C., and Bataille, J.M.: Les myopathies hypothyroidiennes: aspects cliniques et histopathologiques. *Presse Med.*, 75:1551, 1967.

48. Fessel, W.J.: Myopathy of hypothyroidism. *Ann. Rheumatic Dis.*, 27:590-596, 1968.

49. Golding, D.N.: Hypothyroidism presenting with musculoskeletal symptoms. *Ann. Rheum. Dis.*, 29:10-14, 1970.

50. Wilke, W.S., Sheeler, L.R., and Makarowski, W.S.: Hypothyroidism with presenting symptoms of fibrositis. *J. Rheumat.*, 8:627-630, 1981.

51. Delamere, J.P., Scott, D.L., and Felix-Davies, D.D.: Thyroid dysfunction and rheumatic diseases. *J.Royal Soc. Med.*, 75:102,1982.

52. Sonkin, L.S.: Endocrine disorders and muscle dysfunction. In *Clinical Management of Head, Neck and TMJ Pain and Dysfunction.* Edited by B. Gelb, Philadelphia, W.B. Saunders Co., 1985, pp.137-170.

53. Awad, E.A.: Pathological changes in fibromyalgia. *First International Symposium on Myofascial Pain and Fibromyalgia*, Minneapolis, Minnesota, May 9, 1989.

54. Awad, E.A.: Histopathological changes in fibrositis. In *Advances in Pain Research and Therapy*, Vol.17. Edited by J.R. Fricton and E.A. Awad, New York, Raven Press, Ltd., 1990, pp.249-258.

55. Aaarflot, T. and Bruusgaard, D.: Association of chronic widespread musculoskeletal complaints and thyroid autoimmunity: results from a community survey. *Scand. J. Prim. Health Care*, 14(2):111-115, 1996.

56. Rodolico, C., Toscano, A., Benvenga, S., et al.: Myopathy as the persistently isolated symptomatology of primary autoimmune hypothyroidism. *Thyroid*, 8(11):1033-1038, 1998.

57. Lowe, J.C.: If the new paradigm for the healing arts is going to serve us better than the old one—*First Congress on Defining a New Paradigm for the Healing Arts*, University of Texas, Health Science Center Houston, Texas, May 28-31, 1998.

58. Carette, S., Bell, M., Reynolds, W.J., et al.: A controlled trial of amitriptyline, cyclobenzaprine, and placebo in fibromyalgia. *Arthritis Rheum.*, 35(Suppl.9):112, 1992.

59. Carette, S., Bell, M., Reynolds, W.J., et al.: Comparison of amitriptyline, cyclobenzaprine, and placebo in the treatment of fibromyalgia. *Arthritis Rheum.*, 37(1):32-40, 1994.

60. Carette, S.: What have clinical trials taught us about the treatment of fibromyalgia? *J. Muscloskel. Pain*, 3(2):133-140, 1995.

61. McCain, G.A.: A clinical overview of the fibromyalgia syndrome. *J. Muscloskel. Pain*, 4(1/2):9-34, 1996.

62. McCain, G.A.: Treatment of the fibromyalgia syndrome. *J. Muscloskel. Pain*, 7(1/2):193-208, 1999.

63. Russell, I.J.: Preface: Myopain '98. *J. Muscloskel. Pain*, 7(1/2):xix-xxi, 1999.

64. Carette, S., Oakson, G., Guimont, C., and Steriade, M.: Sleep electroencephalography and the clinical response to amitriptyline in patients with fibromyalgia. *Arthritis Rheumatol.*, 38(9):1211-1217, 1995.

65. Lowe, J.C.: Reliable scientific reporting. Editorial. *J. Myofascial Ther.*, 1(4):3, 1995.

66. Bennett, R.: Personal written communication. Feb. 27, 1996.

67. Riedel, W., Layka, H., and Neeck, G.: Secretory pattern of GH, TSH, thyroid hormones, ACTH, cortisol, FSH, and LH in patients with fibromyalgia syndrome following systemic injection of the relevant hypothalamic-releasing hormones. *Z. Rheumatol.*, 57(Suppl.2):81-87, 1998.

68. Lowe, J.C.: Thyroid status of 38 fibromyalgia patients: implications for the eitiology of fibromyalgia. *Clin. Bull. Myofascial Ther.*, 2(1):36-40, 1996.

69. Lowe, J.C., Reichman, A., Honeyman, G.S., and Yellin, J.: Thyroid status of fibromyalgia patients (Abstract). *Clin. Bull. Myofascial Ther.*, 3(1):69-70, 1998.

70. Wolfe, F., Ross, K., Anderson, J., Russell, I.J., and Hebert, L.: The prevalence and characteristics of fibromyalgia in the general population. *Arthritis Rheum.*, 38(1):19-28, 1995.

71. Wolfe, F., Anderson, J., Harkness, D., et al: Work and disability status of persons with fibromyalgia. *J. Rheumatol.*, 24(6):1171-1178, 1997.

72. Wolfe, F., Anderson, J., Harkness, D., et al.: A prospective, longitudinal, multicenter study of service utilization and costs in fibromyalgia. *Arthritis Rheumat.*, 40(9):1560-1570, 1997.

73. Mendelsohn, R.S.: *MalePractice: How Doctors Manipulate Women.* Chicago, Contemporary Books, Inc., 1981.

74. Shomon, M.: An interview with John Dommisse, M.D., F.R.C.P.: Sept.22, 1999, <http://thyroid.about.com/health/thyroid/library/ weekly/aa092299.htm>

75. Hausotter, W.: Fibromyalgia--a dispensable disease term? *Versicherungsmedizin*, 50(1):13-17, 1998.

76. Lowe, J.C., Eichelberger, J., Manso, G., and Peterson, K.: Improvement in euthyroid fibromyalgia patients treated with T$_3$. *J. Myofascial Ther.*,1 (2):16-29, 1994.

77. Lowe, J.C.: T$_3$-induced recovery from fibromyalgia by a hypothyroid patient resistant to T$_4$ and desiccated thyroid. *J. Myofascial Ther.*, 1(4):26-31, 1995.

78. Lowe, J.C.: Results of an open trial of T$_3$ therapy with 77 euthyroid female fibromyalgia patients. *Clin. Bull. Myofascial Ther.*, 2(1):35-37, 1997.

79. Lowe, J.C., Garrison, R., Reichman, A., Yellin, J., Thompson, M., and Kaufman, D.: Effectiveness and safety of T$_3$ therapy for euthyroid fibromyalgia: a double-blind, placebo-controlled response-driven crossover study. *Clin. Bull. Myofascial Ther.*, 2(2/3):31-57, 1997.

80. Lowe, J.C., Reichman, A., and Yellin, J.: The process of change with T$_3$ therapy for euthyroid fibromyalgia: a double-blind placebo-controlled crossover study, *Clin. Bull. Myofascial Ther.*, 2(2/3):91-124, 1997.

81. Lowe, J.C., Cullum, M.E., Graf, L.H., Jr., and Yellin, J.: Mutations in the c-*erb*Aβ$_1$ gene: do they underlie euthyroid fibromyalgia? *Med. Hypotheses*, 48(2):125-135, 1997.

82. Honeyman, G.S.: Metabolic therapy for hypothyroid and euthyroid fibromyalgia: two case reports. *Clin. Bull. Myofascial Ther.*, 2(4):19-49, 1997.

83. Lowe, J.C., Garrison, R., Reichman, A., and Yellin, J.: Triiodothyronine (T$_3$) treatment of euthyroid fibromyalgia: a small-n replication of a double-blind placebo-controlled crossover study. *Clin. Bull. Myofascial Ther.*, 2(4): 71-88, 1997.

84. Lowe, J.C., Reichman, A., and Yellin, J.: A case-control study of metabolic therapy for fibromyalgia: long-term follow-up comparison of treated and untreated patients (Abstract). *Clin. Bull. Myofascial Ther.*, 3(1):23-24, 1998.

85. Lowe, J.C. and Honeyman-Lowe, G.: Facilitating the decrease in fibromyalgic pain during metabolic rehabilitation: an essential role for soft tissue therapies. *J. Bodywork Movem. Ther.*, 2(4):208-217, 1998.

86. Web site: <www.drolwe.com> 1997-to-present.

87. Garrison, R.L.: The five generations of American medical revolutions. *J. Fam. Pract.*, 40(3):281-287, 1995.

88. Feinberg, B. and Kasrils, R.: *Dear Bertrand Russell: A Selection of His Correspondence with the General Public, 1950-1968.* New York, Simon and Schuster, 1969.

89. Kohn, A.: *False Prophets: Fraud and Error in Science and Medicine.* New York, Barnes and Nobel Books, 1988.

90. Bell, David S.: *The Doctor's Guide to Chronic Fatigue Syndrome: Understanding, Treating, and Living with CFIDS.* Redding, Perseus Books, 1995.

91. Cournance, A. and Zuckerman, H.: The code of science. In *Knowledge in Search of Understanding.* Edited by P. Weiss, New York, Mt. Kisco Publishing, 1975, pp.126-147.

92. Ziman, J.: *Reliable Knowledge: An Exploration of the Grounds for Belief in Science.* Cambridge, Cambridge University Press, 1978.

93. Kuhn, T.S.: *The Structure of Scientific Revolutions*, 2nd edition. Chicago, University of Chicago Press, 1970.

94. Ellis, A. and Harper, R.A.: *A New Guide to Rational Living.* N. Hollywood, Wilshire Book Company, 1975.

95. Yunus, M., Masi, A.T., Calabro, J.J., Miller, K.A., and Feigenbaum, S.L.: Primary fibromyalgia (fibrositis): clinical study of 50 patients with matched normal controls. *Semin. Arthritis Rheum.*, 11:151-171, 1981.

96. Wolfe, F.: The clinical syndrome of fibrositis. *Amer. J. Med.*, 81(3A):7-14, 1986.

97. Fransen, J. and Russell, I.J.: *The Fibromyalgia Help Book: Practical Guide to Living Better with Fibromyalgia.* Saint Paul, Smith House Press, 1996.

98. Russell, I.J.: Pathogenesis of fibromyalgia: the neurohormonal hypothesis. *J. Musculoskel. Pain*, 2(1):73-86, 1994.

99. McCain, G.A.: Treatment of the fibromyalgia syndrome. *J. Musculoskel. Pain*, 2(1):93-104, 1994.

100. Popper, K.R.: *The Logic of Scientific Discovery.* London, Routledge, 1980.

101. Gunn, I.P.: A critique of Michael L. Millenson's book, *Demanding Medical Excellence: Doctors and Accountability in the Information Age*, and its relevance to CRNAs and nursing. *A.A.N.A. J.*, 66(6):575-582, 1998.

102. Reilly, P.A. and Littlejohn, G.O.: Fibromyalgia: the wheel reinvented? *J. Musculoskel. Pain*, 1(2):5-17, 1993.

103. Russell, I.J., Vaeroy, H., Javors, M., and Nyberg, F.: Cerebrospinal fluid biogenic amine metabolites in fibromyalgia/fibrositis syndrome and rheumatoid arthritis. *Arthritis Rheum.*, 35:550-556, 1992.

104. Moldofsky, H. and Warsh, J.J.: Plasma tryptophan and musculoskeletal pain in non-articular rheumatism ("fibrositis syndrome"). *Pain*, 5:65-71, 1978.

105. Moldofsky, H.: Rheumatic pain modulation syndrome: The interrelationship between sleep, central nervous system, serotonin, and pain. *Adv. Neurol.*, 33:51-57, 1982.

106. Harvey, J.A., Schlosberg, A.J., and Yunger, L.M.: *Fed. Proc.*, 34:1796-1801, 1975.

107. Morgane, P.J.: Serotonin: twenty years later—monoamine theory of sleep: the role of serotonin: a review. *Psychopharmacol. Bull.*, 17:13-17, 1981.

108. Chase, T.N. and Murphy, D.L.: Serotonin and central nervous system function. *Ann. Rev. Pharmacol.*, 13:181-197, 1973.

109. Moldofsky, H. and Lue, F.A.: Unpublished observations. Reported in: Moldofsky, H.: The contribution of sleep-wake physiology to fibromyalgia. In *Advances in Pain Research and Therapy*, Vol. 17. Edited by J.R. Fricton and E. Award, New York, Raven Press, Ltd., 1990, pp.227-240.

110. Russell, I.J., Michalek, J.E., Vipraio, G.A., Fletcher, E.M., and Wall, K.: Serum amino acids in fibrositis/fibromyalgia syndrome. *J. Rheumatol.*, 19:158-163, 1989.

111. Pauling, L.: *How to Live Longer and Feel Better.* New York, Avon Books, 1986.

112. Planck, M.: *Scientific Autobiography and Other Papers.* Trans. F. Gaynor, New York, 1949, pp.33-34.

113. Lown, B.: *The Lost Art of Healing: Practicing Compassion in Medicine.* New York, Ballantine Books, 1999.

114. Nichols, J.D.: *"Please Doctor, Do Something!"* Atlanta, Natural Food Associates, 1972.

115. Kauffman, G.B. and Kaufman, L.M.: Linus Pauling: reflections. *Amer. Scientist*, 82:522-524, 1994.

116. Mendelsohn, R.S.: Personal communication, 1987.

117. Johnson, H.: *Osler's Web: Inside the Labyrinth of the*

Chronic Fatigue Syndrome Epidemic. New York, Penguin Books, 1996.

118. Russell, I.J.: Neurochemical pathogenesis of fibromyalgia syndrome. *J. Musculoskel. Pain*, 7(1/2):183-191, 1999.

119. Pert, C.: *Molecules of Emotion.* New York, Scribner, 1997.

120. Fried, R.: Dr. John Sarno's psychology: not fact but theory—and discredited theory at that. *J. Myofascial Ther.*, 1(1):32-34, 1994.

121. Eisinger, J.: Hypothyroïdie et fibromyalgie: indications d'une double hormonothérapie thyroïdienne. *Méd. Sud-Est*, Avril-Mai-Juin, 2:31-36, 1999.

122. Russell, I.J.: Neurochemical pathogenesis of fibromyalgia syndrome. *J. Musculoskel. Pain*, 4(1/2):61-92, 1996.

123. Russell, I.J.: Biochemical abnormalities in fibromyalgia syndrome. *J. Musculoskel. Pain*, 2(3):101-115, 1994.

124. Russell, I.J.: Preface: Myopain '95. *J. Muscloskel. Pain*, 7(1/2):xi-xiii, 1996.

1.2

Fibromyalgia is Not a "Somatoform Disorder"

The old paradigm of a separation of the mental and physical aspects of the human being (referred to as the Cartesian split) has been debunked. The split was formerly a matter of convention and convenience, but it is contrary to what has been learned during the past century about the biopsychological/psychobiological functioning of the human being. Because there is no psychological function independent of organic function, symptoms of disease are never purely a product of psychological factors—that is, symptoms are never purely psychogenic. Conversely, no physical disease is entirely independent of psychological factors and all are modulated to some degree by them. Nevertheless, the Diagnostic and Statistical Manual (DSM) of the American Psychiatric Association currently still publishes diagnostic criteria for the diagnosis of "somatoform disorders." These diagnoses are given to patients who meet at least three criteria: their symptoms suggest a physical disorder, an organic basis for the symptoms is not established, and the clinician has at least a strong suspicion that the symptoms are linked to psychological factors. The authors of the DSM specify that the somatoform symptoms are not volitional. They classify somatoform disorders as mental disorders because the specific pathophysiology of each somatoform disorder is undetermined, not understandable by current laboratory methods, and is " . . . conceptualized most clearly by means of psychological constructs."

Fibromyalgia should be excluded from the classification of mental disorders for at least two reasons. First, documented objective biochemical, endocrine, and physiological abnormalities clearly establish that fibromyalgia is an organic (biological) disorder. Second, the increased prevalence of psychological disturbance in patients as chronicity progresses is a reasonable expectation (rather than detection of a higher incidence of primary mental disorders among the subset of longer-duration patients).

Of the six somatoform diagnoses, fibromyalgia patients are most likely to receive one or more of five. These include conversion disorder, hypochondriasis, somatization disorder, somatoform pain disorder, and undifferentiated somatoform disorder.

At least two related hypotheses underlie the interpretation of fibromyalgia as a somatoform disorder: (1) bodily symptoms for which there is no proven organic mechanism are of psychological origin, and (2) purely or largely psychogenic mechanisms are capable of generating symptoms that falsely indicate an underlying organic cause. These hypotheses are shown to be false beyond reasonable doubt through logical analyses of predictions derived from them.

The following four methods recommended for diagnosing somatoform disorders are invalidated by major problems:

(1) Failing to find a physical lesion to account for the patient's symptoms. Such a failure never proves conclusively that an organic mechanism is not responsible for the symptoms. In some cases, the clinician fails to find an organic lesion because of his diagnostic incompetence. Examples of incompetence are failing to perform a proper physical examination and neglecting to order a necessary laboratory test or imaging procedure.

(2) Failure of the patient to respond to physical

exam procedures as the clinicians expects. There is no scientific evidence to indicate that when a patient fails to respond to a physical exam procedure as expected that the patient's symptoms are psychological in origin. Clinicians who subscribe to this diagnostic method ignore well-established explanations for the patients' unexpected responses to the test procedures.

(3) Positive findings from valid, objective psychological tests should be required for the diagnosis of psychological disorders. Clinicians who use diagnoses of somatoform disorders seldom base the diagnoses on psychological testing. Even if they wished to do so, however, there are no psychological tests that validly and reliably identify patients whose physical symptoms are of psychological origin.

(4) Exhibition by the patient of an "hysterical" personality. As described in the literature, the "hysterical personality" is all-inclusive; the clinician intent on making a somatoform diagnosis may use any predominant personality feature of the patient as evidence that he or she has such a disorder.

The use of somatoform diagnoses results in adverse effects on many patients. The diagnoses subject many patients to iatrogenic distress, detain some patients from proper care for physical abnormalities, interfere with the patient/doctor relationship (encouraging duplicity by clinicians and exaggeration of symptoms by patients), and impede patients from receiving benefits they contracted to receive under specific conditions from third party payers.

Clinicians who tend to use somatoform diagnoses can generally be grouped into one of three categories. One category is clinicians who are indifferent to the validity or invalidity of the diagnoses. They use them mainly for purging from their practices patients who are confusing, frustrating, or annoying. This category includes clinicians/researchers who, having failed to determine the cause of a disorder they have been studying, resort to the default conclusion that the disorder must be psychogenic. Their conclusion is false because it is based on the false proposition that any disorder not underlain by a physical mechanism is psychogenic. Their conclusion is a default conclusion.

A second category of clinicians continues to believe that fibromyalgia and similar syndromes are somatoform disorders. Some of these clinicians are merely deficient in critical thinking skills. Others appear to have what Yunus has termed "disturbed physician syndrome." The appropriate DSM diagnosis is "delusional (paranoid) disorder." Some of the clinicians in category two appear to be unable to rationally deal with their inability to determine the physical

cause of patients' symptoms. This inability conflicts with their self-image which includes the features of omniscience and omnipotence. They tend to use somatoform diagnoses as quasi-diagnoses that essentially get them off the hot seat. There is a sociopathic component inherent in this pattern of conduct: The physician, in the effort to sidestep the conflict with his self-image, disregards any adversity to the patient from the somatoform diagnosis. The conduct of category two clinicians toward patients constitutes a public health problem. This problem should be studied (probably by sociologists, psychologists, social workers, and public health and judicial officials) and steps taken to safeguard patients from these clinicians.

A third category of clinicians uses somatoform diagnoses for business purposes. Clinicians within this category include some independent medical examiners, expert witnesses, and company doctors. By using these diagnoses, they strategically impede patients in their efforts to be reimbursed for health care services or to receive disability compensation or settlements. Impeding patients in this way favors the financial interests of the third party payers that employ the clinicians. In turn, favoring the financial interests of the employers favors the clinicians' own financial interests by increasing the likelihood of continued employment by the third party payers.

Fibromyalgia has been diagnosed by some clinicians through much of the 20th century as a psychogenic disorder. This misdiagnosis has derived mainly from the false premises held by many clinicians even today that any symptoms without proven physical causes are of psychological origin. Studies using modern psychological tests have shown that the incidence of psychological disturbance among fibromyalgia patients is proportional to the incidence in other groups of chronic pain patients. The prevalence of psychological disturbance is higher among patients whose fibromyalgia is of longer duration. The higher prevalence among patients at speciality clinics may result from the tendency of primary care clinicians to refer their most difficult fibromyalgia cases to these facilities. The higher incidence among long-duration patients can also be explained by the persistence of their pain, financial distress, insufficient social support, and other people's reactions that the patients find discouraging or disturbing. Among the adverse reactions of others is the issuance of somatoform diagnoses by some clinicians. These diagnoses can be especially disturbing when made under the guise of independent medical examinations by clinicians employed by third party payers.

The use of somatoform diagnoses should be abandoned for scientific and humane reasons. The psychogenesis hypothesis of physical illnesses (the theoretical underpinning of somatoform diagnoses) is false beyond a reasonable doubt. There are no logical or scientific grounds for concluding that physical symptoms without a demonstrated, or even probable, organic etiology are psychogenic. And there are no logical or scientific grounds for making a somatoform diagnosis because clinicians cannot determine an organic cause of a patient's symptoms. Attorneys and expert witnesses employed by third party payers commonly use somatoform diagnoses for purposes of financial profit without regard for the adverse effects upon patients. Fibromyalgia patients are poorly prepared to cope with these common abuses. The authors of the DSM *can help safeguard the well being of patients subjected to this abuse by publicly conceding the illogicality of somatoform diagnoses and renouncing their use altogether.*

In the 3rd edition of the *Diagnostic and Statistical Manual (DSM-III-R)* of the American Psychiatric Association, the authors provided a description of the putative "Somatoform Disorders." According to them, "The essential features of this group of disorders are physical symptoms suggesting physical disorder (hence, Somatoform), (1) for which there are no demonstrable organic findings or known physiologic mechanisms, and (2) for which there is positive evidence, or a strong presumption, that the symptoms are linked to psychological factors or conflicts [numbering mine]."[77,p.255] The authors specified that the patient does not intentionally produce the symptoms.

The authors of the *DSM-III-R* also justified their classifying somatoform disorders as mental disorders: "Although the symptoms of Somatoform Disorders are 'physical,' the specific pathophysiologic processes involved are not demonstrable or understandable by existing laboratory processes and are conceptualized most clearly by means of psychological constructs."[77,p.255] In the 4th edition of the *DSM (DSM-IV)*, published in 1994, the authors stated in their introduction to somatoform disorders:[107,p.445] "The grouping of these disorders in a single section is based on clinical utility (i.e., the need to exclude occult general medical conditions or substance-induced etiologies for the bodily symptoms) rather than on assumptions regarding etiology or mechanism. These disorders are often encountered in general medical settings."

● WHY FIBROMYALGIA SHOULD BE EXCLUDED FROM ANY CLASSIFICATION OF MENTAL DISORDERS

The authors of the *DSM* wrote that the pathophysiologic processes of somatoform disorders are "conceptualized most clearly by means of psychological constructs."[77,p.255] I argue in this chapter, however, that fibromyalgia should be excluded from any classification of mental disorders. Exclusion is justified on two counts: One, by the organic findings documented in patients with fibromyalgia; and two, by the reasonable expectation of an increased prevalence of emotional disturbance among patients who have suffered from the condition for a prolonged time.

EXCLUSION BASED ON ORGANIC FINDINGS IN FIBROMYALGIA

For a diagnosis of a somatoform disorder to be proper, the quoted criteria clearly stipulate, (1) the patient's symptoms cannot be accounted for by demonstrable pathophysiologic processes, and (2) the patient's physical symptoms must suggest a physical disorder ". . . for which there are no demonstrable organic findings . . . ." These stipulations exclude fibromyalgia from the diagnostic category of somatoform disorders and thus from the classification of mental disorders. Throughout this book, I site the objectively verified organic findings in fibromyalgia. Among these are low peripheral serotonin levels, low central nervous system levels of norepinephrine and dopamine metabolites, elevated central nervous system substance P levels, and low cerebral blood perfusion. It is arguable what the cause of these abnormalities is. Nonetheless, such objective abnormalities, as features of abnormal physiological processes, are capable of generating the fibromyalgia symptoms such as chronic pain, fatigue, sleep disturbance, anxiety, cognitive dysfunction, and depression.[97] These symptoms are likely to lead some clinicians to give the patient a somatoform disorder diagnosis. Yet the symptoms are predictable from the documented organic physiological abnormalities in fibromyalgia that are listed above. In fact, the objectively confirmed organic abnormalities in fibromyalgia constitute more than sufficient "demonstrable organic findings" to exclude fibromyalgia from the list of somatoform disorders and thus from the classification of mental disorders.

EXCLUSION BASED ON THE EXPECTATION OF EMOTIONAL DISTURBANCE FROM LONG-DURATION FIBROMYALGIA

In defining "mental disorder," the authors of the *DSM* wrote: "In *DSM-III-R*, each of the mental disorders is conceptualized as a clinically significant behavioral or psychological syndrome or pattern that occurs in a person and that is associated with (1) present distress (a painful symptom) or (2) disability (impairment in one or more important areas of functioning) or (3) a significantly increased risk of suffering death, pain, disability, or an important loss of freedom [numbering mine]."[77,p.xxii]

According to this definition, it might appear appropriate to classify fibromyalgia as a mental disorder. This might be justified by all of the three criteria enumerated in the previous paragraph. Indeed, many fibromyalgia patients (1) are distressed, (2) are disabled and unable to work, and (3) lose their freedom to engage in both family, occupational, and recreational activities. Many are also at risk of suicide.

Despite meeting these three criteria for a mental disorder, however, a qualification of the authors of the *DSM-III-R*[77,p.xxii] should exempt most patients with fibromyalgia from somatoform disorders diagnoses. The qualification is, "In addition, this syndrome or pattern [the 'clinically significant behavioral or psychological syndrome or pattern' they describe in their definition] must not be merely an expected response to a particular event, e.g., the death of a loved one." The psychological symptoms of fibromyalgia patients constitute a pattern that we can reasonably expect as a response to not one, but many adverse events. A recent description by Starlanyl illustrates the types of events typical fibromyalgia patients are subjected to: "These patients have usually experienced extreme frustration trying to get doctors to listen to them and take their symptoms seriously. Previous encounters with such frustration may cause them to seem hostile and moody. They are probably in great pain, and past experiences with the medical establishment may have included ridicule and abuse. When dysregulated neurotransmitters (which control mood) and chronic sleep deprivation are added to this volatile mix, you cannot expect to find a cheerful, happy person."[73,p.2]

Studies using psychological testing have shown a higher incidence of psychological disturbance among fibromyalgia patients than in the general population. However, the prevalence of psychological disturbance among fibromyalgia patients is tantamount to that among other chronic pain patients.

The prevalence of psychological disturbance among fibromyalgia patients is greatest among those referred to tertiary specialty facilities (see section below titled "Studies of the Psychological Status of Fibromyalgia Patients"). The higher prevalence of psychological disturbance among fibromyalgia patients in these facilities may be due to the tendency of clinicians to refer their most psychologically disturbed patients to the facilities. This would suggest that the higher incidence within such facilities is not representative of the more general population of fibromyalgia patients. In addition, however, the symptoms of those reaching these facilities are more severe, prolonged, and treatment-resistant. The patients experience frustration, fear of an uncertain prognosis, a sense of hopelessness from failed treatment and continued suffering, and adverse social consequences from having fibromyalgia. It is highly probable that these experiences increase the incidence of measurable psychological disturbance among these patients. As I describe below, there is experimental evidence to support this conjecture. Under these conditions, a resulting " . . . clinically significant behavioral or psychological syndrome or pattern . . ." is a reasonable and ". . . expectable response . . ."[77,p.xxii] for many patients. (Below, I describe the experiences many fibromyalgia patients are subjected to that may tax their psychological wherewithal to the limit. See section titled "Factors that May Account for Psychological Disturbance Among Fibromyalgia Patients.")

SOMATOFORM DIAGNOSES FIBROMYALGIA PATIENTS ARE MOST LIKELY TO RECEIVE

Many clinicians diagnose fibromyalgia as a somatoform disorder. Of the six somatoform disorders, clinicians most often diagnose fibromyalgia as one or a mixture of five: (1) conversion disorder (conversion type hysterical neurosis), (2) hypochondriasis (hypochondriacal neurosis), (3) somatization disorder, (4) somatoform pain disorder, or (5) undifferentiated somatoform disorder.[77,pp.257-267] According to the authors of the *DSM-III-R*, "The essential features of this group of disorders are physical symptoms suggesting physical disorder (hence, Somatoform) for which there are no demonstrable organic findings or known physiologic mechanism, and for which there is positive evidence, or strong presumption, that the symptoms are linked to psychological factors or conflicts."[77,p.255] The authors give specific criteria for the diagnosis of each of disorder.

For each of these putative disorders, the diagnostic criteria include some of the symptoms and signs typical of fibromyalgia and related syndromes. Diagnosis of each disorder depends on the inability or failure of the clinician to find evidence of a physical mechanism for the patient's complaints. In this sense, all of the diagnoses are default diagnoses—they are used by default when lack of diagnostic skill or technological ability result in a failure to identify the organic mechanism of the patient's signs and symptoms (see section below titled "Problems with the Methods for Diagnosing Somatoform Disorders: Absence of Physical Findings").

Conversion Disorder (or Conversion Type Hysterical Neurosis)

The authors of the *DMS-III-R* give the following definition of conversion disorder: "The essential feature of this disorder is an alteration or loss of physical functioning that suggests physical disorder, but that instead is apparently an expression of a psychological conflict or need." They stipulate that after appropriate testing, the symptoms " . . . cannot be explained by any physical disorder or known pathophysiologic mechanism."[77,p.257] The authors of *DSM-IV* changed the description of how psychological factors presumably relate to the patient's physical condition. They wrote, "Psychological factors are judged to be associated with the symptoms or deficit . . . ."[107,p.452]

After 100 years of use, the hypothesis of hysterical conversion still has only anecdotal support. Nevertheless, some clinicians argue that the pain of fibromyalgia is psychogenic, and authors such as Merskey[1] and Weintraub[2] have proposed that the psychogenic mechanism is "hysteria." The International Association for the Study of Pain favors hysteria as a mechanism of psychogenic pain.[4]

In his comments on hysteria, Slater wrote, ". . . as a diagnosis it is used at peril. Both on theoretical and on practical grounds it is a term to be avoided."[5,p.1396] He also wrote, ". . . like all unwarranted beliefs which still attract credence, it is dangerous."[5,p.1399] Slater's admonition is justified for several reasons. I cover these in the sections below titled "Adverse Effects to the Patient from the Use of Somatoform Disorders Diagnoses," "Adverse Legal and Financial Results," and "Iatrogenic Psychological Distress."

Those who subscribe to the hypothesis of hysteria unfortunately still often prevail over fibromyalgia patients in the courtroom. (This is not always the case. See the section below titled "Financial Incentives for Insurance Companies and Their Expert Witnesses to Define Fibromyalgia and Similar Disorders as Somatoform.") In an Alberta, Canada court in 1995, a psychiatrist testified that fibromyalgia is accurately explained as a personality disorder known as "hysterical conversion." The judge stated: "The evidence satisfies me that the symptoms diagnosed as fibromyalgia are a relabeling by rheumatologists of a condition . . . that has been with mankind for hundreds of years and represents a personality disorder. This particular disorder is often found in individuals who will not or cannot cope with everyday stresses of life but convert this inability into acceptable physical symptoms to avoid dealing with reality."[94]

The authors of the *DSM-III-R* stated that the patient does not intentionally produce the symptoms of this disturbance, as occurs in factitious disorder or malingering.[77,p.257] Despite this, Wilbourn[109,p.399] and Weintraub[110] in *Neurologic Clinics* and Weintraub[7] in the *American Journal of Pain Management* blended the diagnoses of hysteria and malingering in accusations about fibromyalgia patients. Weintraub wrote, for example, that the litigating chronic pain patient's symptoms of hysterical conversion reaction (HCR) ". . . arise because the patient wishes to obtain some gain (financial or interpersonal)." In addition, he wrote: "It must be recognized that malingering and HCR are on a continuum; most patients who malinger have some degree of suggestibility that might be labeled hysterical. Conversely, most patients with HCR have at least some vague conscious knowledge that the symptom is not all that it appears to be."[7,p.199] Such blending of the two diagnoses brings to mind those 3-D pictures in which, with a slight turning of the picture, a smiling face transforms into a horrifying skull, and back again with another slight turn. Such glib description violates the criteria in the *DSM*, but it enables the expert witness or independent medical examiner employed by insurance companies to conveniently convert the diagnosis of hysteria into that of malingering and vice versa, whichever bests serves his need at the time.

Weintraub implied that a high prevalence of chronic pain patients deceptively perpetuate their pain for ulterior motives. He wrote that 11% of the people in the general population have chronic pain, and although ". . . not all chronic pain patients are in litigation," regardless of the medical treatment they undergo, their pain persists. He then attributed the persistence of their pain to motives of gain: "It appears that, in all too many cases, the advantages of illness far outweigh the advantages of health."[7,p.202]

Weintraub's preconceived notion of a high prevalence of malingering and deception among chronic pain patients for the purpose of secondary gain is not supported by the evidence. Bedard pointed out that this concept, originated by Freud, has never been rigorously examined for validity. While the possibility of secondary gain has been given considerable attention, Bedard also noted the issue of secondary losses to the chronic pain patient. These may include loss of physical mobility, career, friendships, and social life. The patient may also suffer divorce, financial ruin, homelessness, and the extreme stresses of prolonged litigation.[69,p.3] One wonders whether Weintraub considered such losses when he wrote, ". . . in all too many cases, the advantages of illness far outweigh the advantages of health."[7,p.202]

Considerable evidence indicates that the motivation of secondary gain is not common among litigating chronic pain patients. As I detailed in another book,[120,pp.44-46] numerous studies show that the chronic pain of many patients does not cease after they settle compensation claims.[8][74][82][114][121] Thomas and Aidinis noted that psychological and medico-legal factors may obscure the validity of pain perception in patients with musculoskeletal pain related to traumatic or work injuries. They administered Pentothal to 45 patients with musculoskeletal injuries.[42] Pentothal or thiopental sodium is a short-acting barbiturate injected to induce anesthesia. The drug has been called "truth serum." While the patients were under the influence of the anesthetic, the researchers subjected the presumably injured tissues to the stress of stretching, and they measured the pressure/pain thresholds of the tissues by algometry. The results confirmed that a total of 40 patients had genuine, organic pain. The researchers judged 1 patient's pain to be "equivocal." Four patients' findings were negative. The researchers concluded that the pain of these 4 patients was "non-organic." It is possible, however, that the tissues these patients reported to be painful were actually pain referral zones for anatomically distant myofascial trigger points. Patients would perceive the tissues as painful, but they would not react to the stimuli of stretching and pressure in such a way as to indicate tissue injury. In this case, their pain would be organic.

No Evidence for Psychogenic Pain Due to Hysteria. Merskey wrote that hysteria is probably the most common psychological mechanism of pain.[17][18][19] Weintraub argued that psychogenic pain is the most common form of hysteria.[2][7,p.199]

Weintraub, an outspoken proponent of the concept of hysterical pain, stated that hysterical conversion re-

action ". . . is not readily suited to direct experimentation . . . ."[21,p.123] As Copi[22,p.426] wrote: "Few propositions of science are *directly* verifiable as true. In fact, none of the important ones are." The hypothetical construct of hysteria is also not directly verifiable. But if hysteria is to be considered a scientific hypothesis, it must be testable, at least indirectly.[22] This can be accomplished through experimental tests of predictions deduced from the hypothesis,[23] yet the hypothesis has never been subjected to experimental tests. Merskey[16] reviewed the evidence for hysterical pain; it consisted only of reports of clinical observations and a number of descriptions of associations between pain presumably not underlain by physical lesions and other "hysterical" symptoms. We can predict, however, that the outcome of experimental tests would be negative in that logical analysis does not support but rather falsifies the hypothesis (see section below titled "Logical Analysis of the Putative Somatoform Disorders and Their Hypothesized Underlying Psychogenic Mechanisms").

Slater wrote: ". . . to suppose that one is making a diagnosis when one says that a patient is suffering from 'hysteria' is to delude oneself. The justification for accepting 'hysteria' as a syndrome is based entirely on tradition and lacks evidential support. No clearly definable meaning can be attached to it . . . ."[5,p.1396] In fact, hysterical conversion reaction is pure psycho-silliness. The construct of hysteria: (1) began as a speculative fiction by Freud, based partly on fraudulent claims of clinical success through use of the construct; (2) is antiquated, obsolete, and no more scientifically credible than the demonology of the middle ages; (3) is a mechanism of inadvertent disservice to the patient when used by clinicians who believe the construct to be real; and (4) is a device used inhumanely for strategic business advantage by some clinicians in a profit-generating alliance with insurance companies.

Continued use of the construct of hysteria by some neurologists, psychiatrists, and psychologists compromises their credibility. The same is true of the authors of successive editions of the *DSM*. As I wrote above, the authors of the *DSM* have changed their wording pertaining to the role of psychological factors in generating physical illnesses. In the *DSM-III-R* they wrote that a conversion disorder was an ". . . expression of a psychological conflict or need."[77,p.257] In the *DSM-IV* they wrote, "Psychological factors are judged to be associated with the symptoms or deficit . . . ."[107,p.452] This change may be an attempt to cleanse the *DSM* of association with the construct. It would be a humanitarian gesture toward patients and a credit to the authors to forthrightly denounce the construct as having no scientific validity or clinical value.

Hypochondriasis

Hypochondriasis is defined in the *DSM-III-R* as a preoccupation with a fear of having or developing a serious disease based on the patient's interpretation of physical sensations or signs as evidence for the disease.[77,p.261] The patient typically has brought his or her concerns to the attention of numerous medical personal, but the fear persists regardless of negative medical tests and assurance from clinicians.

Patients who are likely to get this diagnosis are those whose fibromyalgia has not yet been diagnosed. Negative diagnostic tests despite severe, and in some cases debilitating, symptoms leaves many patients deeply troubled, frightened, and in continual pursuit of a medical explanation for their symptoms. A diagnosis of fibromyalgia and an explanation that the condition is not lethal tends to substantially reduce patients' distress.[118] This is indicated by the results of a study by Vlaeyen et al. They assessed changes in fibromyalgia patients' status in response to one of three different conditions: combined cognitive/educational intervention, group education, or a waiting-list control group.[119] The researchers evaluated patients' status 2 weeks before treatment, at the initiation of treatment, immediately after treatment, and at 6- and 12-month follow-ups. Compared to patients on the waiting list, patients who underwent cognitive training were better able to cope with their pain and had a better understanding of fibromyalgia. Patients who underwent education were better able to cope with pain, controlled pain better, and had less fear than patients who were on the waiting list or who only had cognitive training. Therefore, education about fibromyalgia produced better results than cognitive behavioral therapy. Psychological testing showed that patients improved in several respects: (1) the severity of their pain, (2) affective distress (tension, irritability, mood, depression), and (3) the interference their pain caused during their daily activities. Patients also enhanced their sense of control and mastery over their life circumstances.

In addition to quelling distress, receiving the diagnosis of fibromyalgia has been found to reduce patients' pursuit of diagnostic and treatment services. Cathey et al. found that the 81 fibromyalgia patients they studied had a very high hospitalization rate prior to receiving the diagnosis of fibromyalgia.[117] The patients had been hospitalized mainly for depression, general pain, and other skeletal, neck, back, and joint symptoms. During the year following the patients'

diagnoses of fibromyalgia, their hospitalization rate dropped. The investigators wrote, ". . . it seems possible that diagnosis leads to a reduction in hospitalization and, hence, to a significant reduction in the lifetime cost of the disease."[117,p.83]

Until a clinician diagnoses the patient's condition as fibromyalgia, however, the patient is likely to continue pursuing a medical diagnosis. During the pursuit, the patient may reiterate multiple nonspecific symptoms to different clinicians and show fear over an uncertain prognosis. As a consequence, one or more clinicians are likely to misdiagnose the patient's condition as hypochondriasis.

Incidentally, during my clinical experiences over a 20-year period involving many hundreds of patients, including those with fibromyalgia, I encountered only 1 patient who appeared to me to be truly hypochondriacal—and I would not bet my life that this patient's signs and seemingly interminable complaints were not of organic origin. This patient did not have fibromyalgia.

Somatization Disorder

The essential feature of somatization disorder, according to the *DSM-III-R*, is that the patient, over several years, seeks medical attention for multiple recurrent somatic complaints that are apparently not due to a physical disorder.[77,pp.261-262] The patient's pursuit of medical care from a number of clinicians, sometimes simultaneously, is apparently important to the diagnosis. Frequent symptoms include anxiety and depression. Patients commonly have antisocial behavior and occupational, interpersonal, and marital troubles. Invariably, the patient's complaints include pain. The patient often complains of pain in the joints and back, during urination, and especially in the extremities, but she seldom complains of headaches. The patient may also have what the *DSM* authors term conversion or pseudo-neurologic symptoms. Those listed in the *DSM-III-R* are paralysis or blindness, gastrointestinal symptoms such as abdominal pain, female symptoms such as menstrual pain, sexual problems such as indifference toward sex, and cardiopulmonary symptoms such as dizziness.

Goldstein, a psychiatrist and family physician who specializes in chronic fatigue syndrome, wrote: "It is not difficult for me to distinguish the patient with somatization disorder from one with chronic fatigue syndrome. Patients with somatization disorder should not have recurrent flu-like illnesses with sore throat, specific encoding problems (trouble making new memories), fibromyalgia tender points, laboratory results suggesting immune activation, or characteristic findings on brain functional imaging. The symptoms of somatization disorder must begin prior to age 30 in order to be diagnosed by *DSM-III-R* criteria. The average age of onset of chronic fatigue syndrome is the mid-30s. I thus find patients with somatization disorder to be rare, although the diagnosis is made frequently."[72,p.57]

Many fibromyalgia patients do not meet the exact criteria for the diagnosis of somatization disorder detailed in the *DSM*. Other patients do, but this does not validate the diagnosis. Instead, it shows that the criteria are so poorly conceived that the symptoms and signs of patients with a serious organic illness such as fibromyalgia can be misdiagnosed as somatization disorder.

Somatoform Pain Disorder

The authors of the *DSM-III-R* specify that the essential feature of somatoform pain disorder is the patient's preoccupation with pain despite no physical findings to account for the pain or its intensity.[77,p.264] The patient's description of the pain (1) does not conform to the anatomical distribution of the nervous system, or (2) it mimics the distribution of pain such as that of classic angina or sciatica, but an organic source of the pain cannot be confirmed despite adequate testing. The patient may also have paresthesias, muscle spasms, and a prior history of hysterical conversion. In about 50% of cases, the pain begins immediately after physical trauma.[77,p.264]

Numerous researchers have confirmed that referred somatic pain does not follow a simple "segmental" pattern, and the distribution of pain referred from most myofascial trigger points is anatomically distant from the muscle that contains the trigger points. Travell published these facts over 50 years ago.[112] Also, referral from some myofascial trigger points mimics the pain patterns typical of angina, sciatica, and other clinical pain conditions. When these pain patterns are caused by myofascial trigger points, tests are likely to be negative for lesions that mediate the pain of conditions such as angina and sciatica. As a result, some clinicians, using the two *DSM* criteria in the previous paragraph, will diagnose the patient's pain as somatoform pain disorder.

Undifferentiated Somatoform Disorder

Through the diagnosis of undifferentiated somatoform disorder, the *DSM* allows the diagnosis of somatization disorder even when a patient does not meet the diagnostic criteria. The *DSM* explains that this diagnosis ". . . is for clinical conditions that resemble Soma-

tization Disorder, but do not meet the full criteria for that disorder."[77,p.255] Clinicians use this alternative diagnosis more often than they do somatization disorder, "Although Undifferentiated Somatoform Disorder is defined here as residual to Somatization Disorder, it is far more common than Somatization Disorder itself."[77,p.266] Even if diagnostic tests confirm that the patient's signs and symptoms are undergirded by organic mechanisms, the clinician can still assign this diagnosis. This is permitted through a qualification in the *DSM*: "When there is related organic pathology, the physical complaints or resulting social or occupational impairment is grossly in excess of what would be expected from the physical findings."[77,p.267]

I am confident that the motivation for these liberal allowances in diagnosis is well-intended. But the essential message in them is this: If the patient meets the criteria for somatization disorder, fine; if the patient does not, then diagnose it anyway, in the form of undifferentiated somatoform disorder (or as another alternative, somatoform disorder not otherwise specified). The *DSM* thus provides clinicians with an officially sanctioned justification for diagnosing fibromyalgia as a somatoform disorder—despite the patient's well-documented organic abnormalities and regardless of the patient failing to meet other *DSM* criteria for somatization disorder.

LOGICAL ANALYSIS OF THE PUTATIVE SOMATOFORM DISORDERS AND THEIR HYPOTHESIZED UNDERLYING PSYCHOGENIC MECHANISMS

In considering the interpretation of fibromyalgia as a somatoform disorder, there are at least two related hypotheses to consider. One hypothesis states that bodily symptoms for which there is no confirmed organic mechanism are of psychological origin. This hypothesis can be stated as the following categorical syllogism:

> (*a*) Illnesses that have no confirmed organic cause are
> (*b*) illnesses that are of psychological origin.
>
> (*c*) Fibromyalgia is (*a*) an illness that has no confirmed organic cause.
> _____
> Therefore, (*c*) fibromyalgia is (*b*) an illness that is of psychological origin.

The argument says that all members of class *c* are members of class *a* which are all members of class *b*. For two reasons the conclusion of the argument is false beyond reasonable doubt: First, there is no credible evidence for the truth of the first premise, that illnesses without confirmed organic causes are of psychological origin; second, although the organic cause(s) of fibromyalgia has not been confirmed, overwhelming objective evidence indicates that its features are products of underlying pathophysiological processes.

I include arguments against this first hypothesis in two sections below. The first is the section titled "Traditional Rationalism and the Somatoform Disorders." The second is the section titled "Problems with the Methods for Diagnosing Somatoform Disorders: Absence of Physical Findings."

The second hypothesis underlying the interpretation of fibromyalgia as a somatoform disorder, specifically conversion disorder, states this: In some patients, psychogenic mechanisms, either alone or through interacting with organic mechanisms, generate physical symptoms and signs that falsely indicate an underlying organic cause. I include arguments against this hypothesis above in the section titled "Somatoform Diagnoses Fibromyalgia Patients are Most Likely to Receive," subsection titled "Conversion Disorder (or Conversion Type Hysterical Neurosis)."

The authors of the *DSM-III-R* wrote that the etiologies of most of the disorders in the book are not known. Because of this, they take an atheoretical approach and do not discuss possible mechanisms of the disorders. Instead, they classify disorders on the basis of their clinical manifestations.[77,p.xxii] They also wrote that although somatoform disorders are "physical," they are most clearly conceptualized by means of psychological constructs.[77,p.255] Under conversion disorder, for example, they wrote that the altered or lost physical functioning suggests a physical disorder, but " . . . instead is apparently an expression of a psychological conflict or need."[77,p.257] In the *DSM-IV*, the authors altered their statement regarding conversion disorder to read, "Psychological factors are judged to be associated with the symptoms or deficit, a judgement based on the observation that the initiation or exacerbation of the symptom or deficit is preceded by conflicts or other stressors."[107,p.452] Similarly in the *DSM-IV*, under pain disorder (termed somatoform pain disorder in the *DSM-III-R*), they stated that "Psychological factors are judged to play a significant role in the onset, severity, exacerbation, or maintenance of this pain."[107,p.458] These revisions suggest an attempt to avoid the implication that the patient's complaints are purely or largely psychological in origin. This contrasts with Freud and Breuer's original hypothesis that hysteria is a purely psychogenic mechanism of some

physical illnesses.[33,pp.3-17] Despite the revisions in the *DSM-IV*, writers such as Weintraub[2][7][110] and Ford[70] have continued to promote hysterical conversion reaction as the psychogenic mechanism of somatoform disorders.

In the philosophy of science, there are two main methods for deciding whether a hypothesis is useful. The method that has dominated is traditional rationalism. The less known and appreciated, yet the more decisive, is critical rationalism. The hypothesis that psychogenic mechanisms underlie and give rise to signs and symptoms of physical disorders (somatoform disorders) does not stand up to either method. According to traditional rationalism, the hypothesis is highly improbable, and according to critical rationalism, it is false.

Traditional Rationalism and the Somatoform Disorders

Traditional rationalism requires that a hypothesis be supported or justified by evidence. Traditional rationalism also stipulates that the reliability of a hypothesis depends on the quality of the evidence that supports or justifies it. When the lack of evidence renders a hypothesis false beyond reasonable doubt, the hypothesis can be rejected in favor of a more probable one.

A problem with traditional rationalism is that the theorist can virtually always muster at least some meager evidence to support his hypothesis. This has enabled the hypotheses of theorists such as Freud to persist despite their lack of scientific fruitfulness. By contrast, Einstein formulated hypotheses and made predictions in a manner that made them entirely capable of being refuted and dismissed.[55,p.26] By virtue of this approach, he was practicing critical rationalism. The scientific fertility of Einstein's hypotheses is testimony to the relative value of critical rationalism over traditional rationalism. However, the hypotheses of Freud, re-clothed today as somatoform disorders, do not stand up even to the highly permissible traditional rationalism.

The absence of scientific support for psychoanalytic hypotheses and the diagnoses that have stemmed from them is well-established. Scientists and philosophers of science have protested the implication that psychoanalytic thinking is scientific. "Truth" within the framework of psychoanalytic thought is a matter of faith, as in religion. In contrast, truth within science is a matter of testable generalizations about regularities in the empirical world.[96,p.314][106,pp.10,20&41] The meaning of truth within the framework of psychoanalytic thought is also inherent in the concept of somatoform disorders and the psychogenic mechanisms that are presumed to underlie them. As a practice of metaphysics—which is a legitimate form of inquiry—these concepts are acceptable within the *un*scientific search for knowledge. But when the impression is encouraged that these concepts are generalizations that have been subjected to credible testing through scientific methodology, the concepts and their use in clinical practice are *pseudo*-scientific.

Eysenck provides an explanation for the lack of science underlying these concepts. The lack appears to be a product of the personality of Freud himself.[106,p.41] Freud's attitude toward the experimental approach to pursuing truth was shown in a famous postcard he sent in 1934 to a researcher who was attempting to study repression experimentally. Freud wrote, "I cannot put much value on these confirmations because the wealth of reliable observations on which these assertions rest make them independent of experimental verification." Regarding this comment of Freud's, Eysenck wrote: "Nothing could demonstrate more clearly the nonscientific character of Freud's thinking; in his view, experiments were not needed to confirm his hypotheses, nor could they influence them. No other discipline claiming attention has so clearly and decisively cut itself off from experimental testing of its theories—even astrology and phrenology make claims which are empirically testable and have been tested, albeit unsuccessfully."[106,pp.149-150] Freud's rejection of rational and scientific methods imbues the attitudes and thinking of those today who have relabeled the old bottle of psychoanalytic notions with terms such as somatoform disorders.

Szasz provides an explanation of how the use of these concepts began: "It is important to understand clearly that modern psychiatry—and the identification of new psychiatric diseases—began not by identifying such diseases by means of the established methods of pathology, but by creating a new criterion of what constitutes disease. To the established criterion of detectable alteration of *bodily structure* was now added the fresh criterion of alteration of *bodily function*; and, as the former was detected by observing the patient's body, so the latter was detected by observing his behavior. This how and why of conversion hysteria became the prototype of this new class of disease—appropriately named 'mental' to distinguish it from those that are 'organic,' and appropriately called 'functional' in contrast to those that are 'structural.' Thus, whereas in modern medicine new diseases were *discovered,* in modern psychiatry they were *invented.*

Paresis was *proved* to be a disease; hysteria was *declared* to be one."[3,p.267] Szasz continued, "Psychiatric diagnoses are stigmatizing labels. They are phrased to resemble medical diagnoses, and applied to persons whose behavior annoys or offends others."[3,p.267]

Many clinicians today are under the spell of the psychoanalytic mode of thought. When faced with a patient whose complaints have no obvious organic source, these clinicians reflexly attribute the complaints to some psychogenic mechanism. The clinicians explain the patients' complaints with terms such as hysterical conversion, somatization, emotional disturbance, psychogenic pain, or an array of others. This practice is so common among clinicians that most fibromyalgia patients probably have been subjected to such accusations.

In the first half of this century, many people assumed that psychoanalysis was an effective form of psychotherapy. Even the eminent rationalist Bertrand Russell assumed this. He wrote a short story that ". . . was inspired by a psycho-analytic doctor in America who was somewhat dissatisfied by the use commonly made of psycho-analysis. He felt that everyone might be brought to humdrum normality, so I tried portraying Shakespeare's more interesting heroes after they had undergone a course of psycho-analysis. In the dream, a head of Shakespeare speaks, ending with the words, 'Lord, what fools these mortals be.' I had an approving letter from the American doctor."[30,pp.34-35] As it turns out, Shakespeare's words are more accurately applied to those who still assume today that psychoanalysis or concepts derived from it have any basis in empirical reality. Eysenck published the data available for the effectiveness of psychoanalysis and psychotherapy. In his conclusions he wrote that no positive studies were available to support the claims of psychoanalysis. He pointed out, as other researchers had, an important finding: While the available evidence did not indicate that psychoanalysis improved the status of patients, there was evidence that it might actually make patients worse![108,pp.93-99] In this publication, Eysenck quoted O.H. Mowrer, a former president of the American Psychological Association. Mowrer had also been a leading psychoanalyst and psychotherapist for more than 30 years. He said, "From testimony now available from both friends and foes of analysis, it is clear that, at best, analysis casts a spell but does not cure."[108,p.94]

More important to the consideration of the concept of somatoform disorders and their psychogenic underpinnings, Mowrer also said, " . . . there is not a shred of evidence that psychoanalyzed individuals permanently benefit from the experience, and there are equally clear indications that psychoanalysis, *as a common philosophy of life,* is not only nontherapeutic but actively pernicious [italics mine]." Moreover, ". . . as a result of a succession of personal and professional experiences, I have become increasingly convinced, during the last ten or fifteen years, of *the basic unsoundness of Freud's major premises* [italics mine]."[108,p.94] The italics I have added emphasize an important point: The foundations of Freud's psychoanalytic system of thought—including the hypothesis that underlying psychological mechanisms generate physical symptoms and signs—have given rise to concepts that are "pernicious." "Somatoform Disorders" are merely the most recent repackaging of these harmful psychoanalytically-based concepts.

In 1985, Eysenck wrote, ". . . over eighty years after the original publication of Freudian theories, there still is no sign that they can be supported by adequate experimental evidence, or by clinical studies, statistical investigations, or observational methods."[106,p.170] Those who have criticized psychoanalytic thinking and the diagnoses that have arisen from it, such as somatoform disorders, have never been answered in credible scientific terms. Instead, the critics have largely been answered with *ad hominem* arguments that Eysenck notes are repugnant to logicians and scientists. He wrote that the defenders of psychoanalytic thinking have accused critics of ". . . hostility towards psychoanalysis, produced by neurotic and other infantile repressed wishes and feelings."[106,p.170]

In short, there is no scientifically acceptable evidence to support, confirm, corroborate, or justify Freud's hypothesis that psychogenic mechanisms generate physical symptoms and signs.[106,p.170] By extension, the concept of somatoform disorders that stems from his hypothesis also lacks scientifically credible evidential support. The hypothesis and the diagnoses therefore fail to meet the fundamental requirement of traditional rationalism.

Critical Rationalism and the Somatoform Disorders

Critical rationalism stipulates that a hypothesis is acceptable until it can be shown to be false. When it is shown to be false, we must reject it as a scientific hypothesis. The best method for attempting to falsify a hypothesis (such as the hypothesis that fibromyalgia is psychogenic) is to use a prediction that follows from it, stated as a proposition and used as the major premise of a hypothetical syllogism.[96,p.41] If the conclusion (the deductive inference) of the argument is that the prediction is false, then the hypothesis from which the

prediction followed is also false. This is a valid form of deductive argument called *modus tollens.*[96,p.76] For reference, I describe the form of *modus tollens* in Figure 1.2.1.

(Written form)	(Symbolic form)
If *a*, then *c*	$a \supset c$
Not *c*	$\sim c$
Therefore, not *a*	$\therefore \sim a$

Figure 1.2.1. The structure of the valid deductive argument form called *modus tollens.* According to the rules of deductive inference, conclusions in all arguments of this form are validly inferred or deduced from the premises. The conclusion always states that since c derives from a, and c is false, then a is also false. Symbols: $\supset$ (if, then), $\sim$ (not), and $\therefore$ (therefore).

The form is easily understood by a simple example:

If it is raining (*a*), then the streets are wet (*c*).

The streets are not wet ($\sim c$).

Therefore, it is not raining ($\sim a$).

An example relevant to somatoform diagnoses involves a claim made by Freud and Breuer. They wrote that the form of psychotherapy they invented, psychoanalysis, has "a curative effect" on symptoms caused by the mechanism of hysteria.[33,p.17] They published cases in which they claimed psychoanalysis enabled patients to recover from their symptoms (although there is evidence to doubt this claim[106]). They offered these reported successes as evidence for an hysterical mechanism of the patients' symptoms (while ignoring that this constitutes a *post hoc ergo propter hoc* fallacy). Their argument can be stated as this:

If symptoms are caused by hysteria (*a*), then psychoanalysis cures the symptoms *(c).*

Psychoanalysis does not cure symptoms ($\sim c$).

Therefore, symptoms are not caused by hysteria ($\sim a$).

The evidence for the truth of the second premise, which denies c, is that the symptoms of patients who undergo psychoanalysis tend to worsen.[108,pp.93-99] According to critical rationalism, the hypothesis that symptoms are caused by hysteria is falsified.

The more predictions from a hypothesis that are falsified in this way, the less useful we consider the hypothesis. We say that the outcomes of the predictions (which are negative) diverge from the hypothesis.[101,pp.57,59] At some point in the logical analysis of competing hypotheses, the number of diverging outcomes for a hypothesis make it clear that the hypothesis is not useful compared to one or more competitors. At that point, the hypothesis should be dismissed from the class of scientific hypotheses.

Table 1.1.1 contains three examples of the falsification of predictions from the psychogenesis hypothesis of fibromyalgia (and thus the hypothesis itself) by means of *modus tollens*. Each of these examples of the valid deductive argument, along with others not included here, supports the argument that the psychogenesis hypothesis of fibromyalgia is adequately falsified to be excluded from the class of scientific hypotheses. In the examples, keep in mind (see Figure 1.2.1) that the symbol ⊃ represents the statement "If *a*, then *c*"; the symbol ∴ is read "therefore."

The propositions that state the conclusions of the three hypothetical syllogisms in Table 1.2.1 diverge from the predictions. Diverging propositions deny predictions that would be true if the hypothesis they follow from were true.[101,pp.57&59] The propositions simultaneously diverge from the hypothesis from which the predictions follow. An accumulation of diverging propositions, such as these, progressively decreases the reliability of the psychogenesis hypothesis. I use the three examples of *modus tollens* only to illustrate the falsification of the psychogenesis hypothesis of fibromyalgia. The outcomes of these predictions, as well as other such outcomes, diverge sufficiently from the psychogenesis hypothesis of fibromyalgia to make it false beyond reasonable doubt. A diagnosis based on the hypothesis is thus, beyond reasonable doubt, a misdiagnosis.

When a clinician appeals to the hypothesis of psychogenesis in diagnosing fibromyalgia as a somatoform disorder, he implies that the hypothesis is scientifically acceptable. But because the hypothesis does not stand up to analysis by traditional or critical rationalism, it is unreasonable to consider it scientific. Its use by the clinician therefore constitutes the practice of pseudo-science.

PROBLEMS WITH THE METHODS FOR DIAGNOSING SOMATOFORM DISORDERS

In this section, I detail problems with four criteria recommended by different writers for the diagnosis of somatoform disorders, either by this term or by synonyms such as hysteria and psychogenesis. These problems invalidate the diagnoses, rendering them misdiagnoses. This information may be especially helpful to clinicians in counseling the patient who is distressed by another clinician's diagnosis of a somatoform disorder.

According to Sternback, a diagnosis of psychogenic pain can be justified only when there are no physical findings and there are positive findings from psychometric tests and a psychological evaluation.[24,p.290] Weintraub contended that psychogenesis is demonstrated by a patient reacting to physical exam procedures in ways that are inconsistent with what the clinician expects.[2,p.7] And Merskey wrote that the diagnosis can be made, at least tentatively, when the patient exhibits features of the hysterical personality.[19,p.323] None of these criteria, however, provide logical grounds for concluding that a patient's symptoms are somatoform. I will discuss each of the criteria separately.

Absence of Physical Findings

Clinicians who make somatoform diagnoses often assert that they have excluded, conclusively or with a high degree of probability, all possible physical abnormalities that could be generating a patient's symptoms. This assertion implies an irrational belief in the diagnostic capability. The notion that all possible abnormalities can be effectively ruled out may have begun with Joseph Francois Felix Babinski in 1896. Babinski was a French neurologist; the great-toe reflex is named after him. Normally, when the bottom of the foot is stimulated, all the toes reflexly flex. In a positive Babinski reflex, however, the big toe extends and the other toes abduct in response to plantar stimulation. Vidal et al. wrote that Babinski had in mind, in the development of the Babinski test, "practical applications of the sign, particularly in the differential diagnosis of hysteria and in medico-legal areas."[100] More recently, Weintraub (see below: "Diagnosing Hysteria Through Patients' Reactions") has carried this notion to a high point of irrationality.

Some authors have reported their patients had both organic lesions and "hysteria."[5,p.1398][7] And Slater[5,p.1398] noted that some authors have described their patients as having "hysterical exaggeration of organically determined symptoms."

Limitations in Diagnostic Skill or Technology. There are, and probably always will be, limitations to diagnostic skill and technology. Consequently, it is unlikely that clinicians will ever be able to exclude all possible organic lesions that may be causing a patient's symptoms. The symptoms can thus be diagnosed as somatoform as long as the authors of the *DSM* continue to publish their current criteria for this putative class of disorders. The following cases and studies are illustrative.

Individual Cases

In some cases, a patient's diagnosis of a somatoform disorder is a product of outright misdiagnosis. One example shows diagnostic negligence by Breuer, Freud's colleague and coauthor. Fräulein Anna O is a pseudonym for a young woman with classic "hysteria" whom Breuer claimed he completely cured with psychoanalysis circa 1880.[33,pp.21-47] He maintained that her "hysterical" symptoms were precipitated by the emotional trauma of caring for her father. He was sick and eventually died from a virulent form of tuberculosis. The father had an abscess that was surgically drained. Anna was probably exposed to materials contaminated by her father's abscess while she closely nursed him. Years later, case notes were found in the Bellevue Sanatorium in the Swiss town of Kreuzlingen. The notes proved that after her treatment by Breuer had ended, she still had precisely the symptoms of which he claimed to have cured her. Her "hysterical" symptoms were actually those of tuberculous meningitis, a serious physical ailment that she likely contracted from her father.[106,pp.31-32] In addition to the misdiagnosis, the documentation in this case shows that Breuer was also either deceitful or self-deluded about the outcome of Anna O's psychoanalysis.

Alvarez and Low reported the case of a woman with foot and ankle swelling who had seen 3 doctors in 24 hours. The diagnosis she received was swelling due to depression or "hysteria." Her symptoms progressed to respiratory arrest. An emergency room specialist determined that she had distal renal tubular acidosis. With proper medical treatment, she recovered rapidly from her "hysterical" symptoms.[31]

Travell stopped symptoms previously diagnosed as "hysterical" in several patients by effectively treating myofascial trigger points.[25] Myofascial lesions such as trigger points are the most common sources of musculoskeletal pain.[10][11] Features of these lesions can be demonstrated objectively, and until they are ruled out, no patient's symptoms, especially pain, should be attributed to psychological causes.

Some physical lesions are not observable until autopsy. Strecker described an Irish girl, a devout Catholic, who had epileptic-like convulsions. Physicians found no physical lesions. Because of this, and because she had convulsions only on Fridays when she smelled burning meat, the physicians diagnosed her

symptoms as "hysterical." When she died of a convulsion, autopsy revealed a tumor in the olfactory center of her brain. The intense odor of burning meat was the stimulus that had induced the convulsions.[29]

In 1962, Slater and Glitero did an 11-to-13 year follow-up study of 85 patients previously diagnosed as

Table 1.2.1. Three examples of the falsification of predictions from the psychogenesis hypothesis of fibromyalgia (FMS) by means of the *modus tollens.*

HYPOTHESIS		PREDICTION
Example 1:		
FMS is psychogenic	⊃	some of the various forms of psychotherapy would enable patients to recover from FMS.

Clinical experience and studies have shown that psychotherapies do not enable patients to recover from FMS.

∴ FMS is not psychogenic.

Example 2:		
FMS is psychogenic	⊃	chemical and/or physical treatments that do not improve, correct, or eliminate the underlying psychological abnormality will not enable patients to recover from FMS.

Some patients do in fact completely recover from FMS with metabolic therapy.[102][103][104]

∴ FMS is not psychogenic.

Example 3:		
FMS is psychogenic	⊃	recovery from FMS through forms of treatment that do not improve, correct, or eliminate the underlying psychogenic mechanism will result in the mechanism generating symptoms of some other physical disease as a substitute for its expression as FMS.*

Follow-up at 1-5 years has shown that patients who recovered from FMS with metabolic therapy did not in the interim develop symptoms of another physical disease. In fact, the patients' health was in general better than it had been before they developed FMS.[105]

∴ FMS is not psychogenic.

---

*Symptom substitution is an argument of psychoanalytic theorists. They argue that if therapies (such as cognitive treatment or medication) effectively eliminate symptoms produced by an underlying psychogenic mechanism, the mechanism will generate symptoms of another disease. Supposedly, a boiling cauldron of conflicts within the psyche relentlessly generates new symptoms that elicit social approval and possibly financial rewards. Also termed the "pressure cooker" theory by critics.[65]

having symptoms due to "hysteria." Most of the patients were shown to have physical diseases or non-hysterical psychological abnormalities that well accounted for their previously diagnosed "hysterical" symptoms.[6]

Group Studies

Gould et al. attempted to validate the claim of some clinicians that the best indicators of hysteria are various "positive" findings during a neurological exam. The investigators assessed 30 consecutive patients undergoing neurological evaluation because of acute nervous system damage. They looked for seven of the features claimed by hysteria-oriented clinicians to be the most accepted features of hysteria. The features were: history of hypochondriasis, pursuit of secondary gain, *la belle indifference* (inappropriate lack of concern about others' perceptions of one's illness), non-anatomical sensory loss, split of midline by pain or vibratory stimulation, changing boundaries of hypalgesia, and give-way weakness. All 30 patients had at least one of the seven findings; most patients had three or four features. The researchers wrote, "The presence of these 'positive' findings of hysteria in patients with acute structural brain disease invalidates their use as pathognomonic evidence of hysteria." Gould et al. also presented another interesting finding. They wrote, "A second, retrospective study on the misdiagnosis of hysteria demonstrated that women, homosexual men, the psychiatrically ill, and patients presenting plausible psychogenic explanations for their illness are most liable to be misdiagnosed. Certain disorders, particularly movement disorders and paralysis, are most often mislabeled as hysteria."[35] This finding suggests that some clinicians use the diagnosis pejoratively. This is consistent with my experience with clinicians who use the diagnosis. The only shortcoming of the report by Gould et al. is their final caution to clinicians: "A diagnosis of hysteria must be made with great caution as it so often proves incorrect." This caution presupposes that the diagnosis of hysteria is at least sometimes correct. The available evidence shows that this presupposition is false.

Wallis et al. recently conducted a pertinent study. Their aim was to determine whether eliminating the organic source of chronic neck pain following whiplash injuries would have any effect on the well-recognized psychological distress exhibited by such patients. With a randomized, double-blind, placebo-controlled design, they studied 17 patients, each of whom had a single painful cervical zygapophyseal joint. The researchers treated the patients with percu-

taneous radio-frequency neurotomy. They evaluated the patients' pain and psychological status before surgery and 3 months afterward. The evaluation involved a medical interview and examination, a visual analogue pain scale, the McGill Pain Questionnaire, and the SCL-90-R psychological questionnaire. At follow-up, the 16 patients whose pain was completely relieved had no psychological distress. The 1 patient who still had pain continued to suffer psychological distress. The researchers concluded, "Because psychological distress resolved following a neurosurgical treatment which completely relieved pain, without psychological co-therapy, it is concluded that the psychological distress exhibited by these patients was a consequence of the chronic somatic pain."[76]

Hendler, Zinreich, and Kozikowski recently studied 3 litigating patients diagnosed by neurosurgeons or orthopedic surgeons as having "psychogenic pain." The rationale for the diagnoses was the absence of physical lesions: the surgeons had failed to identify lesions through CT, MRI, myelography, X-rays, bone scans, EMG, nerve conduction velocity, and thermography. When three-dimensional (3-D) reconstructed CT images of the patients' lumbar spines were obtained, however, the physical lesions responsible for the patients' pain were "unequivocally documented."[27]

Hendler and Kozikowski followed the course of 60 chronic pain patients. The patients were referred to a pain diagnostic center and complete diagnoses were made. The most common "diagnoses" patients had received before being referred were, according to Hendler and Kozikowski, "really descriptions or vague explanations, such as 'chronic pain,' 'psychogenic pain,' 'cervical strain,' or 'lumbar strain.'" Examinations and testing showed that five diagnoses were most often missed by previous clinicians: (1) myofascial disease, (2) facet disease, (3) peripheral nerve entrapment, (4) radiculopathy, and (5) thoracic outlet syndrome. Of the laboratory tests ordered at the pain clinic, 70% revealed significant organic abnormalities that had not previously been diagnosed. The investigators concluded that the overall rate for inaccurate or incomplete diagnosis among the patients was 66.7%.[57]

In a similar study, Hendler et al. followed 120 chronic pain patients referred to a multidisciplinary pain center. The patients' diagnoses upon referral, such as "chronic pain," "psychogenic pain," or "lumbar strain," were incomplete or inaccurate in 40% of the cases. Patients underwent a multidisciplinary evaluation at the pain center. The appropriate diagnostic tests included MRI, computed tomography, nerve blocks, and qualitative flowmeter. Of the tests performed, 76% revealed significant physical abnormalities in the patients. Pain was determined to be of organic origin in 98% of the patients. The researchers wrote, "The patients were discharged with objective verification of diagnoses including facet disease, nerve entrapment, temporomandibular joint disease, thoracic outlet syndrome, and herniated discs."[113]

Such studies as those in the above paragraphs lead to a firm conclusion: As diagnostic technology advances and as patients eventually reach clinicians with high levels of diagnostic competence, symptoms claimed by some clinicians to be somatoform are likely to confirmed to be of organic origin.

Future of the Diagnosis of Somatoform Disorders Through the Exclusion of Organic Lesions. Despite studies such as those in the section above, Weintraub has argued that the cornerstone of an accurate diagnosis of hysteria depends upon two procedures: (1) the clinician making a careful examination followed by (2) sensitive objective tests, such as MRI, CAT, EMG, SSEP, and myelography.[7] He wrote in 1977 that such tests provide the physician with highly accurate (99%) screening for organicity.[2] Were he correct, this would mean that the tests are 99% accurate in detecting lesions subject to being identified by the particular test. This estimate, which Weintraub cannot justify, shows that confidence vastly exceeds competence in diagnostic capability. It is nonsense to posit that the use of even our most highly sensitive and accurate diagnostic tools can rule out all or even most lesions that may be causing a patient's symptoms. At no point in the history of diagnostics, including the present, have diagnosticians had this ability. This is especially true regarding soft tissue lesions that are capable of generating pain at a disabling intensity.[98,p.1823]

Slater has pointed out that the ". . .absence of physical findings applies universally to a stage in the development of all diseases."[5,p.1399] As a result, when using the negative protocol of ruling out physical lesions, symptoms of many budding diseases may be diagnosed as somatoform.

As some of the studies I mentioned in the previous section show, as diagnostic technology becomes more sophisticated, clinicians are better able to confirm the presence of physical lesions responsible for symptoms previously diagnosed as somatoform. Some of the evidence I present in this book indicates that symptoms such as pain may be underlain by molecular lesions. So that we can effectively rule out such lesions, re-searchers will have to advance our diagnostic technology and make it available for practical clinical use. In the interim, in that molecular lesions cannot conveniently be ruled out, complaints of patients that cannot be related to more gross physical lesions should not be assumed, despite the *DSM*, to be of psychological origin. If a somatoform diagnosis is given to explain the symptoms, the presumption is that psychological treatment is in order. Yet the authors of the *DSM* cannot logically justify recommending psychotherapy, even through implication, as a method of treatment for symptoms that are possibly caused by molecular abnormalities.

Unless we somehow acquire omniscience—which some clinicians assume they already have—the probability approaches nil that ruling out organic lesions will ever become a fail-safe diagnostic endeavor. In the future, even if organic lesions cannot be found with diagnostic methods far more advanced than those we have today, a comment by Hachinski will still ring true: "Absence of proof is no proof of absence."[32]

Neglect in Testing for Physical Sources of Patient Complaints. In some cases, clinicians simply neglect to order or perform tests capable of determining whether there is a physical basis for a fibromyalgia patient's complaints. To illustrate, I quote part of a letter I wrote protesting a *DSM* diagnosis by an endocrinologist. I referred a patient to this specialist specifically for a TRH stimulation test. He and I had only recently met. We concurred in the interpretation of the result of a TRH stimulation test of a patient we already had in common. He and I also agreed that clinicians often misinterpret the results of this test. He agreed to perform the test for my fibromyalgia patients whose basal TSH, T_4, T_3 uptake, and free T_4 index test results were within the normal reference range. The patient I then referred to him promptly returned to me and was obviously exasperated. She complained that the endocrinologist had declined to perform the TRH stimulation test. Instead, he had diagnosed her condition as "cyclothymic personality disorder." The patient, an astute banker, was appropriately appalled. The endocrinologist had made the diagnosis "off-the-cuff," after only a 15-minute interview, without excluding through proper testing the suspected physical cause of her symptoms, and without the benefit of the results of objective psychological tests.

By the dictates of the patient's managed care plan, her family physician had been required to approve referral to the endocrinologist. In a letter to the family physician, which I copied to the endocrinologist, I wrote:

As I wrote to you previously, there are reasons to suspect that this patient has pituitary hypothyroidism. It is mainly because of these reasons that I must take issue with the endocrinologist's conclusion that the patient has a "cyclothymic personality disorder." Dysthymia, of course, refers to chronic, mild depression on more days than not, for at least two months. The patient may also have (as this patient does) poor appetite, impaired concentration, and feelings of hopelessness. But there is one essential requirement for the diagnosis that the endocrinologist failed to comply with. According to the *DSM-III-R*, ". . . the diagnosis is not made if the disturbance is . . . sustained by a specific organic factor . . . ."[77,p.230] Also, the diagnosis shouldn't be made unless: ". . . it cannot be established that an organic factor initiated and maintained the disturbance."[77,p.232] By declining to do the TRH stimulation test, he also declined to determine definitively whether her symptoms are the manifestation of an organic factor. That possible factor, pituitary hypothyroidism, is well-documented to cause the four symptoms (mild depression, poor appetite, impaired concentration, and feelings of hopelessness) that are included in the criteria for diagnosing dysthymia.

The patient was offended that the endocrinologist give her an "off-the-cuff" psychological diagnosis, despite her symptoms, without properly ruling out pituitary hypothyroidism as a cause and without the benefits of psychological testing. With all due respect for the endocrinologist's expertise in his specialty, he did not follow proper protocol to arrive at his psychological diagnosis. There is reason to suspect that the patient has pituitary hypothyroidism. To deny the patient a TRH stimulation test, a simple procedure that could have distinguished whether her complaints were of an endocrine origin, cannot be justified—especially in that so much is possibly at stake for her not having the test result.

In addition, my professional experiences in medico-legal interactions convince me that assigning the patient a questionable diagnosis of a psychological disorder places her at risk: The diagnosis in her medical records will render her unnecessarily vulnerable to abuse in the future by claims adjusters, attorneys, and physicians employed by insurance companies. Because of this, I believe she has a right to a retraction of the psychological diagnosis by the endocrinologist.

As in this case, when a clinician has made an improper or questionable diagnosis of psychogenesis, it is advisable to request that the clinician retract the diagnosis. If the clinician does not comply, the patient (possibly with the cooperation of some other clinician

who *is* sympathetic) should take the steps necessary to have the diagnosis expunged from the patient's health care records. This may require a complaint with the state board of examiners for the clinician's health care discipline requesting a hearing. In some cases, it may be necessary to seek recourse through civil litigation with the guidance of a reputable attorney.

Absence of Positive Findings from Psychological Tests

Sternback recommended that the clinician make a diagnosis of psychogenic pain when there are no physical findings, but only with positive findings from psychometric tests and a psychological evaluation.[24,p.290] I do not believe, as I have stated elsewhere in this chapter, that an organic etiology for symptoms can ever be conclusively ruled out. That aside, however, I believe there are two minimum requirements for concluding that it is probable that psychological factors play a prominent role in a patient's symptoms. First are positive results from objective psychological tests, and second is a psychological evaluation by a qualified mental health practitioner. The practitioner, such as a psychologist or social worker, should be specifically trained to interpret the test results and perform the psychological evaluation. Few psychiatrists have these qualifications.

I believe mental health practitioners should at most render an opinion as to the probability that psychological factors play a prominent role in the patient's symptoms. This qualification is based on an absence of scientific evidence of any purely psychogenic mechanism of pain. Biochemical and physiological correlates of psychological experiences such as fear can modulate features of virtually all diseases. And hypnotic suggestion in rare susceptible individuals can transiently alter physiology and produce some minor physical lesions. *But it is scientifically unjustified to extrapolate from such phenomena that purely psychological factors produce medically diagnosable diseases such as fibromyalgia.*

In his comments about headache and "hysteria," Merskey wrote, "There is no easy way to diagnose hysterical headache. There are no positive signs of hysteria which would help." He then stated, "The practitioner who feels that he is dealing fundamentally with a problem of emotional conflict or personality disorder should establish this for himself, but he can rarely write down firmly and with confidence that a particular headache is hysterical."[16,p.117]

The necessity for the clinician to "feel" that the patient has hysterically-based headache, as opposed to objectively confirming it, would not be the case if "hysteria" were a well-defined entity with clearly identifiable and objectively verifiable features. But it is not. Instead, it is a loose-knit hypothetical construct that no one has ever objectively verified.

Consider the trouble a conscientious clinician has in trying to distinguish between a patient who is faking and one who has hysterical symptoms. Ullman and Krasner reviewed some supposed clinical rules of thumb. "Clinically," they wrote, "the hysteric is reported to display *la belle indifference*: that is, he does not seem upset. A malingerer is more likely to appear cautious. The hysteric gladly, voluminously, and endlessly welcomes an opportunity to talk about his symptoms, his physical complaints, and what they are doing to him. The malingerer is likely to view an interview with a physician as a challenge and a threat and therefore to be far more guarded." They concluded, "The behavioral distinctions boil down to the hysteric's playing a role that is accepted by the labeler [the one who diagnoses him as hysterical] and the malingerer's not successfully playing such a role."[44,p.279] In other words, the clinician, based upon his preconceived ideas, arbitrarily decides whether to label the patient hysteric or a malingerer.

In a similar vein, Henderson and Batchelor wrote: "To distinguish sharply between hysteria and simulation is in fact arbitrary. Simulation is the voluntary production of symptoms by an individual who has full knowledge of their voluntary origin. In hysteria, there is typically no such knowledge, and the production of symptoms is the result of processes that are not fully conscious. Kretchmer pointed out, however, that the criteria 'conscious or unconscious' will not serve to distinguish simulation from hysteria, for not all motives of a healthy mind are conscious, and not all hysterical ones are unconscious. There are all gradations between hysteria and simulation."[45,p.155]

Merskey wrote that diagnosing hysterical pain is a "difficult matter." He specified that the diagnosis can be made with confidence only when three criteria are met: (1) a conflict has been found in the patient's life, (2) the patient himself has established a relationship between the conflict and the development of pain, and (3) resolution of the conflict has led as well to resolution of the pain.[19,p.323] These criteria are consistent with those in the *DSM-III-R*.[77,p.265] As Slater remarked, however, "Unfortunately we have to recognize that trouble, discord, anxiety, and frustration are so prevalent at all stages of life that their mere occurrence near to the time of onset of an illness does not mean very much."[5,p.1399]

Inappropriate Psychological Testing. That a patient's scores on some psychological tests suggest psychopathology may not mean that the patient has a psychological disorder. Ranges of normal for some psychological tests are based on patients with psychological disorders. These test are appropriate only for patients with such disorders. They are not appropriate for individuals without the disorders for despite the normal psychological status of these individuals, the test results may falsely indicate some degree of psychopathology.[47]

Diagnosing Hysteria
Through Patients' Reactions

Weintraub's method for diagnosing hysterical pain is to use physical neurological exam procedures that he believes test sensory and motor function. He claims that hysteria is demonstrated by a patient reacting to the procedures in ways that are inconsistent with anatomical and physiological principles. He is more confident of the diagnosis when a patient's pain pattern is inconsistent with textbook segmental patterns.[2,p.7] Others agree with him.[34]

The essence of Weintraub's hypothesis is this: The clinician should subject the patient to various physical exam procedures. If the patient's reactions to the procedures are not what the clinician expects, then the patient's symptoms are not of organic origin and instead must be of psychological origin. I have found no scientific evidence to support this hypothesis. Moreover, patients' reactions that are not consistent with Weintraub's expectations can usually be explained by documented phenomena such as referral from myofascial trigger points.[20][25][36][37][38][39][40][41,p.16] As I noted under "Somatoform Pain Disorder" above, pain referred from myofascial trigger points does not follow a simple "segmental" pattern. Numerous researchers have documented this, and Travell published the fact over 50 years ago.[112] Travell eliminated "hysterical" symptoms in several patients by effectively treating trigger points.[25]

Weintraub admonished clinicians to diagnose hysteria only when there is positive evidence for it.[2] However, he violated his own admonition by recommending that clinicians diagnose hysteria when patients fail to respond to exam procedures as the clinicians expect them to. Failure of patients to respond as expected no more positively demonstrates a psychogenic mechanism than it does the Medieval theorists' demons swimming through the patient's blood.

The All-Inclusive "Hysterical Personality" as a Diagnostic Criterion

Merskey wrote that the hysterical personality type seems to have a significant link with "hysterical" symptoms. According to him, the tentative diagnosis of hysterical personality disorder can be made in the presence of: (1) labile or shallow affect, (2) histrionic behavior, (3) dependency in human relationships, (4) attention-seeking behavior, (5) over-reaction to minor events, and (6) a readiness to be helpful to others, often found in those who work in service occupations.[19,p.323]

In a review of hysterical personality, however, Merskey wrote that almost any personality type, including a normal personality, may be associated with hysterical symptoms.[16,pp.112-113] This can be taken to mean that the clinician can consider any prominent personality feature evidence that the patient's symptoms are hysterical. If the latter is the case, Merskey provided a broad brush criterion for clinicians prone to make somatoform diagnoses. A personality study of Swedish women with fibromyalgia indicated that they tended to be pedantic, perfectionistic, and had a great need for order, planning, and cleanliness.[78] Otherwise, they were no different from a normative Swedish female population. According to Merskey's broad brush criterion, the Swedish patients' need for order, planning, and cleanliness could be used as evidence that their fibromyalgia symptoms are hysterical.

Critiquing the concept of the hysterical personality, Slater wrote: "All these phenomena seem to be entirely irrelevant to the formulation of a trustworthy diagnosis. People with, say, a histrionic temperament naturally lend the stamp of their personality to their symptoms, whether they are suffering from an organic or a neurotic disorder."[5]

ADVERSE EFFECTS TO THE PATIENT FROM THE USE OF SOMATOFORM DISORDERS DIAGNOSES

There are at least four potentially adverse effects to patients from the use of diagnoses of somatoform disorders. These include iatrogenic distress, delays in proper treatment for physical lesions, harmful effects to the patient/doctor relationship, and legal consequences.

Iatrogenic Psychological Distress

Clinicians often diagnose physically-based pain as hysterical.[5][6] The distress experienced by some patients over the diagnosis of physically-based pain as hysterical constitutes iatrogenic psychological disturbance. Macnab wrote of clinicians inducing "litigation neurosis."[12] They may do so, for example, by failing to diagnose and properly treat whiplash injuries because they believe *a priori* the patients are neurotic and just out for a financial settlement.[13][14]

Teasell stated that psychogenic factors undoubtedly play a role in claims made for soft tissue injuries. He wrote: "In some cases the litigation or welfare system creates an environment where recovery from disability may be discouraged or delayed. However, these factors play a role in any illness behavior following disease whether it be stroke, multiple sclerosis, or systemic lupus erythematosus."[98,p.1823] Teasell was referring to the threshold for willingness to file claims. According to him: "The most likely cause for increased claims is an increased willingness to submit the claim. This is likely related to an attitudinal shift regarding rights to compensation rather than an inherent dishonesty and as such could be regarded primarily as a societal influence." Regarding the threshold, he wrote, "If the threshold for compensation is low, more people will claim compensation, and if the threshold is increased, only more severely injured or disabled individuals will choose to claim compensation." He also stipulated, however, that only the tendency to file claims is sensitive to the threshold, not the incidence of soft tissue injuries following accidents nor the degree of suffering or disability. Reilly, Travers, and Littlejohn essentially agreed. They wrote, ". . . we feel it quite clear that chronic pain syndromes are markedly influenced by the threshold for compensation . . . ."[99,p.1823] Ergo, Teasell and these other authors raise the possibility of a *societo*genic or *litigo*genic phenomenon as opposed to a *psycho*genic one.

A tenaciously rational fibromyalgia patient might rebuff the clinician who has a pejorative attitude toward the condition and walk away unscathed. But many fibromyalgia patients have compromised cognitive function and emotional disturbance due to their impaired metabolism. They simply do not have the cognitive and emotional wherewithal to stand up to negative authoritative dogma. In addition, for some patients, the ability to assertively resist may be diminished by distress over too little or no social or familial support. In one study, 50% of fibromyalgia patients who had suffered from pain for a mean of 6.7 years were dissatisfied with the responses of their families to their health needs.[46] It is easy to understand their having high levels of stress[53][60][61] when we consider Wessely's description of their common experiences with some clinicians. He pointed out that many clinicians equate "psychological disorder" with "unreal disorder."[81,p.114] He wrote: "The reluctance to accept suffering perceived as being of psychological origin as genuine is shared, and often initiated, by the medical profession. A doctor agreed that it is important that psychiatric patients are separated from ME [myalgic encephalomyelitis, a British term for chronic fatigue syndrome] patients because 'some neurotic patients devalue the tales of genuine sufferers.'" He mentioned clinicians who consider patients with chronic fatigue after Lyme disease as malingerers and who refer many of the patients to psychiatrists. The referrals are based on the clinicians' prejudice that "psychiatrists treat imaginary, malingered, or non-existent diseases."[81,p.114]

Detaining Proper Care for Physical Lesions

Merskey wrote that one of the criteria for diagnosis of hysteria is resolution of the patient's physical symptoms with resolution of a concomitant psychological conflict.[19,p.323] However, Slater wrote: "The difficulty for the clinician comes from the fact that these symptoms are very striking, and can often be removed by simple psychotherapeutic measures. Unfortunately, as it seems, the symptom may go, while the disordered state of the nervous system which made it possible persists unrecognized."[5,p.1399]

Slater's observation indicates that Merskey's criterion for the diagnosis of hysteria (simultaneous resolution of a psychological conflict) is potentially hazardous. Hypnotherapists such as Barber have cautioned against removing pain with psychological techniques without thoroughly ruling out physical lesions.[15] To use an extreme example, the hazards are obvious in using suggestion to temporarily reduce or stop pain caused by a brain tumor.

Adverse Effects on the Patient/Clinician Relationship

The relationship between the patient and the clinician may be damaged by at least two phenomena that may result from somatoform disorders diagnoses. First, a clinician may be duplicitous in his relationship with the patient. Second, the patient may feel a need to exaggerate to convince the clinician of the reality of her symptoms.

Duplicity by the Clinician. Merskey wrote: "It is counterproductive to tell the patient that the diagnosis is hysteria, because the word itself is subject to many misinterpretations and may produce an unfavorable reaction. For his own purposes, the physician will need to be aware, however, that he is dealing with a patient whose personality or tendency to symptom-formation is hysterical in type."[16,p.117]

Merskey thus advises the clinician to interact duplicitously with the patient. Following this advice is fraught with potential problems. One problem is that such double-dealing may enable the clinician to avoid protests of the diagnosis by some patients. In the absences of protests, the clinician may feel no need to rationally consider the grounds for making somatoform diagnoses. The clinician's deceit with patients may therefore result in continuing self-deception.

Exaggeration by the Patient. Regarding exaggeration by fibromyalgia patients, Reilly, Travers, and Littlejohn wrote: "We also agree that malingering is as rare as exaggeration is common, and patients with no demonstrable pathology on a clinical, radiological, or serological basis are prone to exaggerate symptoms *in an attempt to be believed by the medical profession.* Unfortunately, such exaggeration is likely to be counterproductive [italics mine]."[99,p.1823] Indeed, many clinicians are likely to detect the exaggeration. They are then also likely to consider the exaggeration to be evidence for any of the somatoform disorders they prefer to diagnose. They are encouraged to do so by statements in the *DSM*. According to the authors of the *DSM-III-R*: The patient with hypochondriasis ". . . may be exaggerating the extent of the feared disease . . . ."[77,p.260] The patient with somatization disorder may have complaints that " . . . are often presented in a dramatic, vague, and exaggerated way . . . ."[77,p.261] The patient with somatoform pain disorder may exhibit ". . . preoccupation with pain in the absence of adequate physical findings to account for the pain or its intensity."[77,p.264] The patient with undifferentiated somatoform disorder is likely to have ". . . physical complaints or resulting social or occupational impairment [that] is grossly in excess of what would be expected from the physical findings."[77,p.267] The patient with body dysmorphic disorder responds to a slight physical anomaly in such a way that is ". . . grossly excessive."[77,p.256] And the patient with conversion disorder is predisposed to the disorder by "histrionic" tendencies[77,p.258] which involve ". . . excessive emotionality and attention-seeking . . . ."[77,p.348] and may result in ". . . the dramatic presentation of organic pain, which may seem excessive to an observer because of minimal physical findings . . . ."[77,p.266]

Adverse Legal and Financial Results

Clinicians and defense attorneys representing third party payers often use the concept of psychogenesis strictly to sabotage the patient's chances of success in litigation and claims for compensation.[8][9] If these clinicians and attorneys successfully convince decision-makers, the third party payer involved is required to pay less or nothing at all as a result of the decision. As Goldstein wrote, ". . . health insurance often will not pay for psychiatric care, and disability will reimburse less, or not at all, for a 'nervous and mental disorder.'"[72,p.150] As a result of their testimony leading to a verdict favorable to the third party payer, the clinicians and attorneys are likely to be rewarded with further business interaction with the payer. The clinicians, the attorneys, and the third party payers that employ them thus engage in a mutually profitable business enterprise at the cost of the patients, most of whose claims I am convinced are authentic. Patients on the losing end are left to cope with an occupational and private life burdened by their continuing symptoms. For some, the burden is so great that they cannot maintain a tolerable quality of life and opt for suicide as a last resort.

A somatoform diagnosis in the patient's health records can adversely affect her in future circumstances. I base this statement on my experiences giving expert testimony on the behalf of fibromyalgia patients. In my experiences, attorneys and expert witnesses for third party payers have used prior somatoform diagnoses to attribute patients' present symptoms to psychological disorders. They have done so even though there was no relationship between the prior somatoform diagnoses and the patients' current conditions. In using such prior diagnoses, the main purpose of attorneys and expert witnesses for third party payers is to mislead the judiciary into deciding that patients' current symptoms are of psychological origin. It has usually proven difficult to counter their sophisticated maneuvering. Because of this, I believe it is best to preempt such maneuvering entirely by keeping patients' records free from somatoform diagnoses. Clinicians should abstain from making the diagnoses, and patients should refuse to accept them. (See previous section titled "Neglect in Testing for Physical Sources of Patient Complaints.")

THREE CATEGORIES OF CLINICIANS WHO ARE LIKELY TO DIAGNOSIS FIBROMYALGIA AS A SOMATOFORM DISORDER

Clinicians who are likely to diagnosis fibromyalgia as a somatoform disorder generally fit into one of three categories: those who are indifferent to whether the concept is scientifically established, those who believe it is established, and those who are mostly concerned with the potential business benefits of the concept.

Clinicians Who Use the Diagnosis with Indifference

Some clinicians who diagnose fibromyalgia as a somatoform disorder are not concerned with the scientific validity or invalidity of the concept of somatoform disorders. They leave the discretion up to mental health professionals. At most, for these clinicians a somatoform diagnosis serves as a convenient conduit for purging confusing, frustrating, or annoying patients from their practices. Such clinicians are likely to make the diagnosis tentatively and refer the patients to mental health practitioners.

Clinicians Who Continue to Believe that Fibromyalgia is a Somatoform Disorder

Some writers continue to publish journal papers describing conditions such as fibromyalgia as somatoform disorders. These papers contain the presumption that fibromyalgia has been scientifically established to be a manifestation of psychogenic mechanisms. Some of the writers express a fervent, religious-like faith in the hypothesis of psychogenesis, and they violate the fundamental rules of critical thinking to justify their faith.

A recent example is a 1997 paper by Ford. First, he pronounces that a phenomenon he describes as "nondisease" dates back at least 4000 years to some of the earliest descriptions of hysteria. He writes, "Somatization can serve as a rationalization for psychosocial problems or as a coping mechanism and for some illness, becomes a way of life." He describes fibromyalgia, multiple chemical sensitivities, dysautonomia, and "reactive hypoglycemia" as "fashionable diagnoses." They are, to him, ". . . phenomenologically related to environmental or occupational syndromes and mass psychogenic illness." He states further: "They are final common symptomatic pathways for a variety of influences including environmental factors, intrapersonal distress and solutions to social problems. A fashionable diagnosis allows psychosocial distress to be comfortably hidden from both the patient and the physician . . . ."[70]

According to Ford, the features of "fashionable illnesses" include (1) multiple vague, subjective complaints, (2) an absence of objective laboratory findings, (3) "quasi-scientific explanations," (4) an overlap between the various fashionable illnesses, (5) symptoms indicating depression or anxiety or both, and (6) denial by the patient that he or she is psychosocially distressed or that the illness can be attributed to distress. He concluded, "Hysteria remains alive and well and one contemporary hiding place is fashionable illness."[70]

Unfortunately, papers such as Ford's tend to reinforce some clinicians' presumption that a psychogenic basis for fibromyalgia is scientifically established. I know from my communications with some of these clinicians that the consistent irrationality of the arguments for the hypothesis escapes them. I have become convinced that for many of these clinicians the responsible factor is a lack of training in the principles of critical thinking and argument analysis. By this, I do not mean that the clinicians are lacking requisite intelligence. Instead, I am concurring with a view of de Bono, a leading authority on thinking skills. "It has always seemed to me," he wrote, "that the most dangerous and obstructive fallacy in education has been the belief that intelligent people are good thinkers. Implicit in education is the notion that thinking is simply intelligence in action, just as traffic is cars in motion."[28,p.3] He stated that this fallacy is dangerous because if one has high intelligence, he tends to believe that nothing needs to be done to improve his thinking. De Bono concluded: "Highly intelligent people may turn out to be rather poor thinkers. They may need as much or more training in thinking skills than other people."[28,p.4]

Regardless of the reason for some clinicians unquestioningly accepting the psychogenesis hypothesis of fibromyalgia, their uncritical acceptance renders the hypothesis dogma. For those of us who strive to abstain from reaching conclusions until we critically examine relevant evidence, it is clear that the hypothesis cannot be justified scientifically and neither can the diagnosis of fibromyalgia as a somatoform disorder.

"Disturbed Physician Syndrome." In a recent interview, rheumatologist and fibromyalgia researcher Muhammad Yunus took a bold and laudable position: He proposed a diagnostic term, "disturbed physician syndrome," for physicians who continue to attribute fibromyalgia to psychological disturbance.[71] Yunus is to be praised for taking this position. It may be the first step in bringing to an end the abominable practice of diagnosing fibromyalgia as a somatoform disorder. Because of the importance of the passage from the Yunus interview, I quote it *verbatim et literatim* from the Internet document.

Ten years after Dr. Yunus published the first controlled study of the clinical characteristics of FM [fibromyalgia], the role of psychological factors is still being debated. There are people who, according to Yunus, are inclined to say that 'FM is nothing; it's all psychological.' Then refuting these blame-it-on-the-patient theories, he points to the pain of cancer.

"I do not know of a more organic (visible under the microscope) cause of pain than that of cancer, and it is definitely known to be increased and aggravated by psychological factors—including depression, anxiety and stress. FM is no exception."

Yunus took 103 FM patients and classified them into three psychological subgroups using the MMPI [Minnesota Multiphasic Personality Inventory]: (1) normal profile, (2) typical chronic pain profile, and (3) psychological disturbance profile. Categories (1) and (3) each accounted for one fourth of the patient group while most patients were found to fit into the chronic pain profile. Dr. Yunus reasoned that if the patient's psychological status was playing a major role in her condition, then those in category (3) should have more severe or frequent symptoms or a greater number of tender points than those in the other two categories.

As it turned out, the central features of FM, namely the number of tender points, fatigue and poor sleep did not correlate with psychological status. The same held true for the associated symptoms of swollen tissues in the extremities and paresthesias (numbness and tingling feelings). Given that all participants were selectively referred to Dr. Yunus' clinic because their primary care physician was unable to help them, there is an inherent problem of referral bias in this study (perhaps over-representing those with psychological problems)—a situation that even Yunus openly acknowledges. Such a bias may explain why a quarter of the patients had significant psychologic distress. However, the report of Yunus' study published in the January 1991 issue of *Arthritis & Rheumatism* stated the following conclusion: "The central features of FM are independent of the psychological status and are more likely related to the FM itself. However, pain severity may be influenced by psychological factors."

So often FM patients are labeled as having a stress-related sleep disorder—once again implying that stress is at the root of their problems. While more experiments are needed in the area of sleep, a 1989 article by Yunus (*J. Rheumatol.* 16:62-71, suppl. 19) casts doubt on this claim. "In this paper," says Yunus, "we analyzed the patient-administered questionnaire about poor sleep, and actually, anxiety and stress did not correlate with the poor sleep . . . . That doesn't mean that stress does not play a role. Stress may be important, but it does not play the primary or predominant role.

It's not an invariable cause, that's for sure."

For patients who are tired of being told that their symptoms are all stress-related, Dr. Yunus' comments are most welcome and serve to reinforce what most patients believe in their hearts. However, there is a very important message that Yunus wished to relay: "You shouldn't ignore stress or depression because they both may be acting as aggravating factors . . . . This is true of all chronic pain disorders."

Referring back to Dr. Yunus' 1989 report in which two control groups were used (77 patients with rheumatoid arthritis and 67 healthy individuals), he made an interesting point: "Anxiety and stress aggravated the pain symptom of FM, but the same results were also found in the rheumatoid arthritis group without any significant differences between the two groups. You can plug in almost any of the chronic diseases, including cancer, and come up with similar results."

Dr. Yunus has combed through the cancer literature because many physicians cling to this notion that FM is a predominantly psychological illness in a disturbed group of people. He has even come up with a new name for these doctors: Disturbed Physician Syndrome, or DPS for short.

"DPS people are trouble because of their preoccupation that FM patients are psychologically disturbed. It is not the FM patients who are disturbed, it is the physicians who are psychologically disturbed because they ignore the data, and whatever data there is, they manipulate it to say what they want it to say."

Dr. Yunus suspects that DPS is less common among rheumatologists and those physicians who have taken the time to learn more about FM— although only time will tell.

Summing it up, the history of FM has been colored by false accusations that this syndrome is none other than a problem of stress, anxiety or depression. These all are aggravating factors and have been used to camouflage the real cause of FM, which Yunus and several other modern-day researchers believe to be aberrant neurotransmitter mechanisms, perhaps in genetically predisposed individuals.[71]

I am entirely sympathetic to Yunus' view. According to some psychological theorists,[95] neurosis is underlain largely by the habitual tendency toward faulty reasoning and irrational conclusions. The irrational conclusions result in emotional disturbances such as inappropriate and excessive anger, anxiety, and depression. This operational definition of neurosis has led to forms of psychotherapy in which the therapist reeducates the patient to think more rationally and thereby emote more appropriately. At least theoretically, the rational thinking and sane emoting benefits society: The reeducated patient tends to behave more adaptively, and he tends to contribute to rather than impede the betterment of society.

In line with the view of these theorists and with that of Yunus, I firmly believe that the Freudian-derived hypothesis of some clinicians that unresolved emotional tensions or conflicts manifest as physical illnesses such as fibromyalgia, and their liberal use of somatoform-type diagnoses, are neurotic tendencies of the clinicians. The unfettered exercise of this neurosis in the clinicians' professional activities has serious public health implications. I recognize that there are disadvantages to labeling the behavior of others as neurotic, dysfunctional, or abnormal. In some instances, however, such labeling may enable us to recognize and take corrective action toward a behavioral pattern that does not serve well the best interests of society. I believe this is the case with clinicians who continue to believe that fibromyalgia is psychogenic and that it is sane to diagnose it as such—all the while ignoring the total lack of scientific evidence justifying these beliefs and the scientific evidence that the beliefs are false.

Delusional (Paranoid) Disorder. Some physicians believe fervidly that syndromes such as fibromyalgia are caused purely by psychological processes. And some of these physicians irresistibly promote this psychogenic hypothesis. The behavior of some of the physicians may constitute "delusional (paranoid) disorder." The authors of the *DSM-III-R* describe the disorder and provide a diagnostic code for it, 297.10. According to them, the essential feature of delusional disorder is the persistent expression of a non-bizarre delusion that is not due to any other mental disorder. Aside from the delusion, the person's behavior is not otherwise odd or bizarre.[77,pp.192-199]

There are several reasons to suspect that the belief of some of these physicians in the psychogenesis of physical illnesses is delusional. First, they deny that conditions such as fibromyalgia and myofascial pain syndromes exist. While doing so, they ignore the published documentation of such conditions, and they decline other clinicians' and researchers' offers to demonstrate for them that the conditions do in fact exist. Second, the physicians are apparently unable to recognize the thorough absence of credible evidence for an hysterical basis for physical illnesses. They also appear unable to acknowledge the available scientific evidence that some illnesses they diagnosis as somatoform are clearly organic. Their irrational behavior is similar to that of a spouse with delusional jealousy (classified by the *DSM-III-R* as jealous type delusional disorder[77,p.200]). The jealous spouse appears unable to recognize the complete absence of evidence for the other spouse's presumed infidelity, and the jealous spouse also ignores overwhelming evidence of the other spouse's complete loyalty. Third, despite the presumably high intelligence levels of the physicians, they ignore *DSM* criteria for differentiating various somatoform disorders, jumbling and mixing the criteria as needed to support their arguments that fibromyalgia (or other syndromes) is psychogenic.

In the grandiose type of delusional disorder, the person believes he possesses some extremely important insight that others do not recognize.[77,p.200] He usually takes the insight to various government agencies, such as the FBI or the U.S. Patent Office. The physician whose delusion consists of a belief in hysteria-based somatoform disorders may confidently express that belief to other official bodies: to medical audiences through lectures and published papers, and to insurance companies and the courts through written reports and expert testimony.

People with grandiose delusions of a spiritual nature often become leaders of religious cults. In a similar pattern, those with delusions of a psycho-medical nature may become medical "authorities." In their role as "authority," they proselytize other physicians to accept the false belief of hysteria-based physical illnesses and to use somatoform diagnoses. In *DSM-III*, delusional disorder was termed "delusional paranoid disorder." The authors changed the name of the disorder in the subsequent *DSM-III-R* because a delusion is the primary symptom of the disorder and the term paranoid has multiple meanings.[77,p.199] Some members of the small cadre of physicians I refer to here, however, do exhibit paranoia. Their paranoia consists of an obstinate belief that the patients whom they designate as having hysteria-based complaints are faking their symptoms and conniving to get undeserved money from third party payers. These physicians will debate at length that *most* patients who report chronic symptoms and litigate for settlements or other benefits are faking. The physicians almost always include in the putative profit-making plot clinicians who treat and testify on behalf of litigating patients. The physicians steadfastly stand by their paranoid accusations despite overwhelming contradictory evidence. The very boldness of their paranoid assertions can convince readers or listeners. But careful logical analysis usually shows that their assertions consist of multiple logical fallacies fluidly woven together to convince others of the truth of the paranoid assertions.

The major problem in applying the diagnosis of delusional paranoid disorder is the same as applying somatoform diagnoses to fibromyalgia patients: The authors of the *DSM* specify that the diagnosis of delusional disorder should be used only when it cannot be shown that the disturbance is the product of an organic mechanism.[77,p.199] As a student of applied logic, this qualification makes the diagnosis abhorrent to me. But if we are to apply labels for social purposes, we would do better to apply that of delusional disorder to these physicians rather than somatoform disorders to fibromyalgia patients—*for it is the physicians' behavior and not the patients' that is problematic.* The physicians' problematic behavior may or may not have an organic basis. Regardless, labeling their behavior can serve as a starting point for rectifying the public health problems this type of behavior tends to generate. If labeling the physicians' behavior safeguards patients and their relationships with their treating clinicians, then the labeling is a humane and worthwhile practice.

The judiciary can contribute to rectifying the public health consequences of the physicians' neurotic behavior. One way is to require the physicians, in their testimony in written reports and as expert witnesses, to conform to at least minimal standards of rational, scientific thinking. Not to require this leaves these physicians free to mislead judges and juries.

The problem would perhaps best be studied by a combination of sociologists, psychologists, social workers, public health professionals, and judicial officials. An investigation could begin with an appeal to the descendants of Sigmund Freud (the fountainhead of the notions underlying somatoform diagnoses) to permit examination of some of his potentially telling written communications. In the 1890s, Freud underwent an extreme personality change that appears to have resulted from a cocaine addiction. Eysenck wrote, "Until the change, his scientific contributions had been lucid, concise, and conformed to the state of knowledge as it existed at the time, but now his style became extraordinarily speculative and theoretical, strained, and contrived."[106,p.38] There is evidence that Freud suffered nose and brain damage from long-term cocaine use. As Eysenck indicated, the brain damage apparently accounts for the progressively bizarre quality of Freud's theories.[106,p.39] The irrationality inherent in modern physicians' use of fantastical psychoanalytically-based interpretations of fibromyalgia is a fitting legacy from the cocaine-addicted Freud. Regardless, a hundred years of adversity for patients from such irrationality is simply too much. It is time that we recognize these physicians' delusions for what they are and take all necessary steps to end the doctors' pernicious impact on patients.

Clinicians Whose Main Concern with Somatoform Diagnoses is Their Business Benefits

Some clinicians who work for third party payers are not concerned with whether so-called somatoform disorders are fact or fiction. Instead, their chief concern is the business benefits of using the diagnoses. For these clinicians, the diagnoses are a useful ploy for denying or minimizing patients' benefits such as reimbursement for health care services or disability compensation.

Third party reimbursement for health care services became widespread in the U.S. during the 20th century. Before then, clinicians presumably gave patients psychological diagnoses because they believed psychological processes underlay some patients' health problems. The patients were encouraged to undergo psychoanalysis or psychotherapy. The aim was for the patients to overcome their psychological problems. With the advent of widespread third party payment for health services, however, psychological diagnoses took on a cost-saving purpose. Some clinicians came to make part or all of their income from third party payers by functioning as company doctors, records reviewers, independent medical examiners, and expert witnesses during litigation. Many insurance policies exclude payment for treatment of psychological diagnoses, or they reimburse at a far lower rate than for physical diagnoses. For clinicians working for third party payers, diagnosing a patient's condition as psychogenic became a method by which they could favorably affect the financial interests of the third party payers. This in turn benefitted the clinicians because third party payers tended to continue employing them. The qualification in the *DSM* that somatoform diagnoses can be used whenever an organic mechanism for a patient's complaints cannot be proven was a boon to these clinicians. The qualification legitimized their use of the diagnoses for any health condition for which the cause is not confirmed.

In this enterprise, many clinicians have abandoned the Hippocratic caution to "do no harm." Instead, they use their professional licenses in a nefarious business alliance with third party payers. In such cases, the problem is one of professional ethics. Pressure by the judiciary could impose a much-needed control over the use of somatoform diagnoses by these clinicians.

Financial Incentives for Insurance Companies and Their Expert Witnesses to Define Fibromyalgia and Similar Disorders as Somatoform. The goal of many insurance companies is to adjudge, through the expert witnesses they employ, that conditions such as fibromyalgia and chronic fatigue syndrome are manifestations of psychogenic mechanisms. These conditions can then be classified as "psychiatric illnesses." Regardless of the adverse effects on the patient, this ploy provides a substantial financial advantage for insurance companies: Many insurance policies either specifically exclude benefits for psychiatric illnesses, or they curtail them compared to those for physical diseases. One major medical policy stipulates under its limitations: "After application of the deductible, the policy will pay 25% of Covered Expenses for mental or nervous disorders. Must be incurred while hospital confined as an overnight bed patient. Lifetime benefit for each insured person for all mental or nervous disorders may not exceed $2,500. Coverage is not provided for outpatient mental or nervous disorder treatment."[111] The $2,500 allowance could well be expended during a 1- or 2-day stay in a hospital psychiatric ward.

One Illustrative Case. The attorney representing a fibromyalgia patient would best bear in mind the inconsistency in the arguments typically given by expert witnesses employed by insurance companies. They often argue that organic causes of fibromyalgia, chronic fatigue syndrome, and similar conditions have not been scientifically established. Ergo, they reason, the conditions are the products of psychogenic mechanisms. As I pointed out earlier in this chapter, the diagnosis of psychogenesis by default is a false conclusion: There is no scientific evidence that syndromes without demonstrable physical causes are therefore psychological in origin. Nonetheless, these expert witnesses ignore this and imply that the psychogenic basis of the syndromes is scientifically established. This is patently false. But rather than offering scientific evidence to support their argument, they merely express their opinions. The expert witnesses usually buttress their opinions with *ex cathedra* pronouncements, specious references to a consensus among psychiatrists or neurologists, and various other logical fallacies. The attorney should demand of these expert witnesses the same standards of evidence that the witnesses require of those who maintain that fibromyalgia is an organic disorder.

In the case of K. Sharon Baillie, Crown Life Insurance Company argued that chronic fatigue syndrome is a psychiatric illness and was therefore excluded from disability coverage.[47] The Honorable C. P. Clarke wrote in his decision: "The Blue Book [of the insurance company] does not contain a section purporting to define terms. However, under limitations it states a set of circumstances where the Defendant [the insurance company] will not pay for any disability including, for example, certain types of sickness related to a pregnancy and includes one relevant limitation, 'psychoneurotic disorders or behavioral disorders.' The policy itself in the definition section defines sickness as being 'an organic disease or a psychosis as defined under psychosis but does not include psychoneurotic disorders or behavioral disorders.'" Judge Clarke noted: "Both the Blue Book [the employee's information booklet describing medical benefits] and the [insurance] Contract exclude as a cause of total disability a psychoneurotic disorder. The only witness called on behalf of the Defendant was Dr. Keith Pearce, a psychiatrist who has diagnosed the Plaintiff as suffering from conversion disorder, which is a type of psychoneurotic disorder. Thus, if the Defendant's position is correct, the Plaintiff does not meet the requirements necessary to establish total disability."

The judge also pointed out: "The Plaintiff's position was that the Plaintiff was suffering from a condition known as CFS [chronic fatigue syndrome], that she had been unable to engage not only in her own occupation, but in fact in any occupation, as that term is understood since the fall of 1989. The origin of this problem was organic and it fell within the requirements of both the Blue Book and the Contract."

Judge Clark quoted the testimony of another witness, neuropsychiatrist Dr. Flora-Henry, regarding the psychiatrist, Dr. Pearce. Dr. Pearce testified that K. Sharon Baillie's chronic fatigue syndrome was a "conversion disorder." Dr. Flora-Henry wrote, "The opinion of Dr. Pearce that such an illness [chronic fatigue syndrome] does not exist is bizarre, since the illness has been recognized by the Atlanta Center for Disease Control, by the American Medical Association, is recognized and is being studied in the United Kingdom, and there is an enormous medical literature related to it." He continued: "It is a debilitating and complicated illness which involves pathological dysregulation of at least three fundamental physiological systems: the central nervous system, the hypothalamic-pituitary axis, and the immunological system." He mentioned fibromyalgia as a related syndrome.

Judge Clarke's comments on Dr. Pearce's testimony show an exemplary keenness of observation: "I was troubled by the evidence of Dr. Pearce," he wrote. "My first concern is that his diagnosis of the Plaintiff was done on the basis of a preconceived notion of what that diagnosis should be. It seems from his publi-

cations that Dr. Pearce is in the process of building a career on the idea that there is no such thing as CFS and that people who claim to have that condition really have psychiatric problems. Dr. Pearce produced a 67-page report. When those portions of the report served his purposes, he was quite definite in cross-examination that he chose his words carefully. When parts of his report were put to him in cross-examination that did not serve his purposes, he was quick to indicate that he had chosen the wrong word but did have an explanation for it. In addition, he was prepared to recognize the expertise of a witness, such as Dr. Butcher, but when it appeared that Dr. Butcher might be saying something different with respect to Dr. Pearce's areas, his answer was that 'Well, Dr. Butcher is not an expert in that area.'"

Judge Clarke also pointed out an error often made by expert witnesses who offer the results of psychological tests to support their opinions that fibromyalgia patients have somatoform disorders: "In addition, one of the important tests used by Dr. Pearce was the MCM-II and III test. This is a test which is administered to persons who are being treated for a psychiatric illness. Because the norms in the test are based on such persons, the instrument is not appropriate for use with a non-clinical patient. In other words, as I understand it, even a person who might otherwise be 'normal' in psychiatric terms, who took this test, would produce a result that showed that person had at least some psychiatric problems." Clarke commented that Dr. Flora-Henry, who specializes in neuropsychiatry and clinical neuropsychology, disagreed with the appropriateness of the MCM-II and III test in this case and with Dr. Pearce's interpretation of the patient's test result.

Judge Clarke ruled in the patient's favor, arguing that she was healthy and normally-functional until contracting giardiasis in 1989. He concluded that the patient did not have a psychiatric illness, that chronic fatigue syndrome is an organic disorder, and that the patient therefore met the requirements for total disability. (The full written judgement of Judge Clarke is available on the Internet.[47])

Psychology of a Subset of Clinicians Who Use Somatoform Diagnoses on Behalf of Third Party Payers. I have observed that some clinicians who use their professional licenses to protect the financial interests of insurance companies go through an interesting psychological process. They invested many years in acquiring an education and license they intended to use to benefit patients. Then they find themselves in a new role: using their education and license to prevent patients from collecting financial benefits they contracted to receive from third party payers under specified conditions. The clinicians' business relationships with third party payers continues only if they successfully impede patients in the collection of benefits. They find that making the accusation that a patient's complaints are somatoform is in many cases an effective impediment.

To believe in the reality of somatoform disorders strains the credulity of some of these clinicians. To use the diagnoses liberally without self-reproach, some adopt a change in attitude soon after they begin working for third party payers. The change converts them from advocates of patients to advocates of third party payers. They soon become distrustful of all patients, not only those who file for compensation or engage in litigation, but almost any patient who submits a claim. The attitude becomes one of distrust and progresses to one of scorn and hostility toward patients. The attitude is similar to that of some IRS personnel toward taxpayers. They assume that all taxpayers are guilty of evasion until proven innocent, and innocence simply means that the IRS is not able to prove how the taxpayer in question has cheated. Some clinicians who continue a profitable relationship with third party payers come to label (in private conversation to which I have been privy) patients and their treating clinicians with terms such as "cheating scoundrels." These clinicians have established in their minds justification for vigorously impeding patients in their efforts to collect benefits. The psychology appears to be similar to that of others who have conscience-wrenching jobs to do. The invading soldier in a foreign country, for example, may find his job easier when he labels the defenders of the country "subhuman."

In line with this psychology, some clinicians who work for third party payers and use somatoform diagnoses hold patients in contempt and accuse them of litigating because of greed. (The clinicians often suggest or accuse patients outright of faking and litigating for financial gain.) As Wessely wrote of the chronic fatigue syndrome patient who receives a somatoform diagnosis, "Being referred to a psychiatrist is 'being blackballed,' 'being imprisoned for a crime I didn't do,' or being on trial."[81,p.113] He also wrote that the atmosphere surrounding the condition is adversarial: "Others speak of bitterness and anger. The accusation is not just that the sufferer is guilty of being depressed, or of having a psychiatric disorder, but of not being ill at all—of having an imaginary disease."[81,pp.113-114]

Clinicians and attorneys who argue, and may actually believe, that most litigating fibromyalgia pa-

tients are faking for financial gain are likely to be encouraged by authors such as Weintraub. Weintraub is a neurologist who attributes much litigating by chronic pain patients to hysterical conversion mixed with a desire for financial gain. In one paper, he termed this "chronic pain-litigation syndrome."[7] In this paper, he reported conclusions that support his view from a study he conducted. As I have argued elsewhere, the study did not approach even the minimal standards for modern clinical research.[26] In reaching his conclusions, he violated the most elementary rules of logic. Despite this, publication of his fallacious conclusions in the otherwise reputable *American Journal of Pain Management* lends credibility to these conclusions. Probably because this journal published the report, the *New York Times* publicized his conclusions as though they were derived through sound reasoning. A number of authorities in pain management, myself among them, were outraged that this journal had published such a substandard report. But our protests were to no avail. Publication of my detailed rebuttal[9] was delayed by the journal for unexplained reasons for the better part of a year (see Appendix C).

When false conclusions such as Weintraub's appear in reputable journals, an *ad hominem* fallacy tends to come into play. Some clinicians and attorneys infer that the conclusions *must* be correct because they are published in reputable peer-reviewed journals. The unquestioned conclusions then become embedded in the clinicians' frame of reference as dogma that influences their conduct toward litigating patients.

● FIBROMYALGIA VIEWED AS PSYCHOGENIC PAIN

Some physicians have used the term fibromyalgia, or its predecessor fibrositis, to denote musculoskeletal pain they believed was psychological in origin.[50,p.876][115][116] Other authors, when referring to fibromyalgia, have used the terms "hysteria"[83] or "psychogenic rheumatism"[84] as synonyms for the different somatoform disorders described in the *DSM*. Due to such references in the medical literature and the continuing propaganda of some neurologists and psychiatrists, many clinicians still mistakenly believe that fibromyalgia symptoms are somatoform.

I quote here a physician whose opinion is typical of clinicians misled by somatoform advocates. The physician wrote the statement in the progress notes of a young woman who, unbeknownst to the physician, had fibromyalgia. Subsequently, the patient completely recovered by undergoing our metabolic rehabilitation protocol. Under the heading "Psychophysiologic symptoms," the physician wrote: "I had a long discussion with her, telling her my opinion that I felt the symptoms were mostly due to unconscious conflicts or feelings of some sort, and that she would need to face those before she would be free of symptoms. Otherwise, she is apt to remain chronically restricted in her life and relationships for her lifetime." I am convinced that most clinicians such as this one intend no malice in interpreting fibromyalgia symptoms as somatoform. An absence of malice, however, does not make the misdiagnosis of value to the patient nor does it minimize the potential harm. It is critical to the welfare of fibromyalgia patients that their clinicians come to understand the pseudo-scientific nature of somatoform diagnoses.

HISTORY

In 1955, Lowman wrote: "Psychogenic rheumatism is a muscular response to the stress of emotional tensions and physiologically is probably a manifestation of muscular fatigue." He continued, "When the muscular system is called upon for sustained reaction, the result is a dysfunction of the responding system; psychogenic rheumatism is the result."[43,pp.222-223] This was a testable proposition, one that could be confirmed or shown to be false by proper experimental testing. But Lowman promptly moved, through quoting Ruesch,[48] into a psychoanalytic conceptual quagmire that virtually defies meaningful scientific scrutiny. Lowman wrote: "Ruesch has pointed out that these vegetative or visceral neuroses are manifestations of an infantile personality. Such persons are unable to dispense emotional tensions through adult interpersonal relationships and other mature vents, and as a consequence, suffer the cumulative effects of this closed system viscerally."[43,p.223] Where is the evidence to support this proposal? There was none in 1955, and although I have diligently searched, I find none today.

Lowman was confident about the appropriate course of action for patients with "rheumatism" (fibromyalgia), which he considered a totally subjective disorder: "With the removal of the precipitating emotional stresses, the muscular system is released from tension and the visceral symptoms dissipate. Understanding by the patient of the underlying mechanism causing the muscular symptoms is important, lest the

patient's concern over the 'rheumatism' add further emotional stress to the system. The definitive approach to treatment obviously is the alleviation or elimination of the psychic stresses while palliatively treating the distressing subjective symptoms."[43,p.224] His approach to therapy was, again, based on a psychoanalytic conjecture of Ruesch.[48] "Ruesch points out," Lowman wrote, "that the treatment of the infantile personality as seen in psychogenic rheumatism is actually child psychology for a chronologically adult person, and that therapy is a protracted undertaking in an endeavor to effect maturity. Such an individual has not regressed from a mature to a less mature state of reaction, but is exhibiting a facet of his personality that has not matured. Not only must he develop insight into his immaturity, but he must then be helped to grow and develop adult reaction mechanisms much as a child is helped in its progress towards a mature mind."[43,p.225]

The view of fibromyalgia as a form of "malingering and conversion reaction" continues to be perpetuated by some neurologists and psychiatrists. In 1995, *Neurology Clinics* published a paper by neurologist T.W. Bohr in which he attributed fibromyalgia and myofascial pain syndromes to psychogenic mechanisms.[93] As is typical of such papers, Bohr's was chock-full of logical fallacies. "It is in the healing business," he wrote, "that the temptations of junk science are the strongest and the controls against it the weakest. Despite their subjective nature, these syndromes have little reliability and validity. Despite a legacy of poor quality science, enthusiasts continue to cite small, methodologically flawed studies reporting to show biological variables for these syndromes."[93] What is amazing is how neurologists such as Bohr fail to comprehend the illogic that pervades their writings on fibromyalgia and myofascial pain syndrome. They argue that these syndromes are fictitious. It is truly astonishing that a physician can make such a statement publicly in view of the overwhelming scientific evidence that it is false. For whatever strange reason, however, these authors ignore the evidence and conclude that these syndromes are actually manifestations of psychogenesis. It is truly bizarre that these physicians ignore the fact that there is not one iota of scientific evidence that fibromyalgia or any other such syndrome is caused or underlain by a psychogenic mechanism.

Some commentators on fibromyalgia have exhibited more practicality than those such as Bohr. They do not attribute fibromyalgia to psychoanalytic fictions such as hysteria, but they still attribute fibromyalgia to purely speculative *psycho*social factors. Wessely surmised, for example, that chronic fatigue syndrome serves social purposes. He wrote that the diagnosis gives "legitimacy to distress that would otherwise be unacceptable to the patient, relative, employer, doctor, and insurer." According to this view, the syndrome enables sufferers to make lifestyle changes without condemnation by others. For example, overworked patients can cut back on their work burden and adopt a more leisurely way of life. Through the "metaphor of illness," the patient's responsibility for the changes she must make are limited to the "relatively blameless (and indeed praiseworthy) habit of overwork, of struggling on beyond the limits of what is physiologically tolerated."[81,pp.118-120] Some patients may indeed make lifestyle changes due to their symptoms of fibromyalgia/chronic fatigue syndrome. But it is pure speculation that some patients conjure their symptoms, consciously or subconsciously, so as to justify making the needed or desired lifestyle changes. The evidence for biological abnormalities in fibromyalgia makes it highly improbable that the socio-cultural "purposes" listed by Wessely give rise to or sustain fibromyalgia. It is far more likely that patients make lifestyle changes as adaptations to make their largely biogenic symptoms more tolerable.

Confusion Based on Lack of Proven Pathophysiological Mechanisms

In recent years, substantial evidence has accumulated that fibromyalgia is an organic illness. Still, though, the research community has not come to an agreement as to the underlying abnormality or abnormalities.[79,p.230][85,p.210] This has left many clinicians free to view fibromyalgia as a somatoform disorder. Since Freud and Breuer began to interpret physical illnesses as psychogenic, some clinicians continue to attribute any and every condition without a proven organic cause to this hypothetical mechanism. Fibromyalgia has taken its turn. Even some clinicians who thoughtfully and compassionately care for fibromyalgia patients still maintain that the condition is psychogenic. Reilly and Littlejohn are examples. They recently wrote: "We believe that fibromyalgia is not a distinct entity like gout or rheumatic fever, but that, as with many illnesses, the presentation is influenced by attitudes, beliefs, and mood states. *It can be considered as truly psychosomatic, with features being of a functional, rather than anatomic, nature* [italics mine]."[68,p.11] These authors lamented the current negative connotation of the diagnosis, "It is unfortunate that terms such as functional, psychosomatic, and psychogenic are now interpreted in a pejorative fashion,

implying that the patient's complaints are not genuine, and certainly not worth the skills of a real doctor." Despite negative connotations, however, they point out that the patient's "symptoms remain very real."[68,p.11]

Reilly and Littlejohn noted that fibromyalgia patients have been considered not to be "psychologically robust, or that they manifest somatic complaints when confronted by intolerable psychological trauma." They also wrote, "When confronted by a tearful, unhappy woman with widespread pain, multiple non-specific complaints, who has been treated by numerous other medical and paramedical professionals, and who withdraws when palpated even gently, then physicians initially feel justified in seeking a psychological cause for the symptoms."[68,p.12] Next they cited some of the evidence I have referenced above as a way of conceding that studies do not support a psychogenic mechanism of fibromyalgia.

PSYCHOLOGICAL STATUS OF FIBROMYALGIA PATIENTS

Hugh Smythe is a rheumatologist who has been highly active in fibromyalgia research. In 1972, a chapter he wrote on fibromyalgia (then called fibrositis) was published in a rheumatology textbook. In that chapter, Smythe cautiously considered psychogenesis as a contributing factor in fibromyalgia. He wrote: "The use of the term 'psychogenic rheumatism' as a synonym for fibrositis has drawn attention to an important contributing factor . . . but has not served the patients well. Most patients and many doctors have understood this term to imply that the pain is imaginary or hysterical in origin, which is very rarely the case."[50,pp.874-875]

Smythe made some distinctions between fibromyalgia and what might be considered psychogenic pain: "The fibrositis syndrome lacks the bizarre features of symbolic psychogenic regional pain. The symptoms are similar from patient to patient, and the tender points predictable and relatively constant in location. The term 'tension rheumatism' more accurately describes the psychogenic mechanism involved, but fails to account for the pain and tenderness found over bony prominences and other non-muscular areas."[50,p.875] In 1977, in collaboration with Moldofsky, Smythe dropped the word "psychogenic" even as a conservatively applied qualifier, and redefined fibromyalgia as a nonrestorative sleep syndrome.[66]

In 1989, Goldenberg wrote that in the 1950s and 1960s, some clinicians considered fibromyalgia a manifestation of hysteria and termed it "psychogenic rheumatism." He pointed out, however, that recent controlled studies had made it obvious that the symptoms and signs of fibromyalgia patients were stable and reproducible rather than bizarre and changeable as in hysteria.[80,p.12]

Smythe's decision to drop the psychogenic qualifier from the diagnosis of fibromyalgia and Goldenberg's notation that the signs and symptoms of fibromyalgia differ from those presumed to be of hysterical origin, are now supported by the results of studies. These studies were done to determine the psychological status of fibromyalgia patients.

Studies of the Psychological Status of Fibromyalgia Patients

Three studies in the 1980s using the Minnesota Multiphasic Personality Inventory (MMPI) showed that about ⅓ of the fibromyalgia patients had significant psychological disturbance.[53][58][59] In one of the studies, investigators showed that the patients' fibromyalgia symptoms (pain, fatigue, and sleep disturbance) do not explain the abnormal MMPI test results.[59]

Psychological profiles of fibromyalgia patients did not correlate with a number of fibromyalgia features: number of painful sites, number of tender points, sleep disturbance, fatigue, feeling swollen, paresthesias, or the description "I hurt all over." The severity of pain, however, was greater in more psychologically disturbed fibromyalgia patients.[56] This is consistent with the higher pain intensity in more psychologically disturbed rheumatoid arthritis patients.[67]

All groups of patients with chronic pain have more psychological disturbance than subjects without chronic pain.[51][64][85][86] Psychological testing has shown no difference in psychopathology between fibromyalgia patients and other chronic pain patients.

The incidence of psychological disturbance among fibromyalgia patients is correlated with increased chronicity. This is also true of other types of chronic pain patients.[87][88][89][90][91][92] Researchers found no significant difference between fibromyalgia and rheumatoid arthritis patients in any lifetime psychological abnormality. This included anxiety, depression, and somatization.[62] (In one study, for example, 31.0% of rheumatoid arthritis patients had depression compared to only 28.6% of fibromyalgia patients.[63]) These results justify the conclusion of those who published studies in 1985[51] and 1991[56] that psychological disturbance is not essential to the diagnosis of fibromyalgia.

In a 1994 overview of psychological factors in fibromyalgia, Yunus distinguished the condition from psychogenic rheumatism by two factors: the consistent finding of tender points and a demonstrably aberrant central pain mechanism in fibromyalgia patients.[52][54] He pointed out that some 25%-to-35% of patients in specialty rheumatology clinics have significant psychological distress. Patients referred to these clinics are those who do not find some relief at primary care facilities (see below: "Referral Bias"). He noted that the only study in a primary care internal medicine clinic that assessed the psychological status of fibromyalgia patients showed no differences between them and clinic control subjects. He concluded, "Presently available data indicate that [fibromyalgia] is not a psychiatric condition."[52]

FACTORS THAT MAY ACCOUNT FOR PSYCHOLOGICAL DISTURBANCE AMONG FIBROMYALGIA PATIENTS

The reported increase in psychological disturbance among fibromyalgia patients at specialty or tertiary clinics may result from one or more of several factors. These include referral bias, the effects of persistent pain, financial distress, and the reactions of other people to the patient.

Referral Bias

Yunus wrote that the higher incidence of psychological distress among speciality clinic patients may represent referral bias.[52] Perhaps clinicians more readily refer psychologically troubled fibromyalgia patients to specialty facilities.

Persistent Pain

That the persistent pain of fibromyalgia eventually leads to a higher prevalence of psychological disturbance is suggested by a recent World Health Organization study. Oye et al. conducted the study to assess the impact of persistent pain on primary care patients. The researchers included 15 primary care centers in the study. The centers were located in Asia, Africa, Europe, and the Americas. Of 25,916 patients, ranging in age from 18-to-65 years, 5,438 were interviewed. Across the 15 centers, 22% of patients reported persistent pain. (The researchers defined persistent pain as the experience of pain most of the time for 6 months or more during the previous year.) The incidence of pain varied from 5.5%-to-33.0%. Standard tests were conducted to assess the incidence of psychological disturbance, disability, and limitation of activity among the patients. Compared to patients without persistent pain, those with persistent pain had a significantly higher incidence of anxiety and depression, limited activity, and perceptions of poor health. The relationship between persistent pain and anxiety and depression occurred among patients in all 15 centers.[49]

The increase in psychological disturbance with persisting pain may result from the taxing emotional and social effects. It is common for fibromyalgia patients to report that the adverse psychological effects of their continuing pain are worsened by the frustration and sense of hopelessness they experience after successive treatments fail to provide relief.

Financial Distress

Among the population of patients with chronic pain, fibromyalgia patients are especially likely to be subjected to a condition that appears to engender psychological disturbance. That condition is financial distress. In my experience, many fibromyalgia patients find themselves impecunious for one or both of two reasons: they have expended so much or all of their money in the pursuit of relief through clinical care, or they have not been able to work because of their fibromyalgia symptoms. Weich and Lewis, in a study of 7,726 adults in England, Wales, and Scotland, recently found that financial strain was strongly associated with the maintenance of common mental disorders. The investigators wrote that unemployment and poverty increased the prevalence of mental disorders by sustaining them. This result supports the anecdotal observation that anxiety and depression are commonly experienced by those who are unemployed and in poverty.[75] Dwindling financial status and the inability to work may also help prolong psychological disturbances associated with the fibromyalgia patient's extended illness, failed treatment, and lack of social support by friends, relatives, and clinicians.

Reactions of Other People to the Patient

Another possible contribution to the increased incidence of psychological disturbance among fibromyalgia patients who reach specialty facilities is that they have had more time to accumulate more adverse social experiences. This is understandable when considering some of the psychologically traumatic experiences many fibromyalgia patients experience. Goldstein wrote of the marital relations of some chronic fatigue syndrome patients, "Husbands have beaten their wives because they thought they were lazy, and divorces have occurred because the spouse did not understand

the illness and/or could not handle the pressures of living with a person who had a chronic, disabling illness which could not be authentically demonstrated to much of the medical profession."[72,p.54] He also wrote of their other social relations: "The general public, relatives, friends, and neighbors may be afraid of 'catching it.' Patients may withdraw from social interactions not just because of fatigue but because friends do not understand chronic fatigue syndrome, and the patient gets tired of making up excuses for unavailability."[72,p.54]

The account of chronic fatigue syndrome/fibromyalgia patient, K. Sharon Baillier, reported by Judge C.P. Clarke, illustrates the social experiences that may adversely affect a patient's psychological status.[47] (I have included other details of her disability case in a previous section: "Financial Incentives for Insurance Companies and Their Expert Witnesses to Define Fibromyalgia and Similar Disorders as Somatoform.") This patient contracted giardiasis while vacationing in Florida and the Caribbean in September, 1989. Judge C. P. Clarke wrote his decision in her disability case in 1998. He described her health and functional status prior to the infection, as expressed in her testimony: "She testified that during this time [before the infection], her health was basically good. She had no serious complaints. She played squash three times a week, she could go on 25-to-30 km hikes, she enjoyed sailing and canoeing and lifted weights as part of her exercise program. She did volunteer work in the community, and she worked within her church in an outreach program. She testified that she worked usually between 40-to-60 hours per week."

Judge Clarke wrote that the illness that began on her vacation initiated symptoms from which the patient had not recovered in 1998, 9 years later. Her initial symptoms included diarrhea, fever, nausea, exhaustion, and arm and leg aches. Despite taking medication for the infection, she continued to suffer from fatigue. In addition, she began to have headaches, muscle weakness, and night sweats. She had been an avid reader before becoming ill, but soon memory problems began interfering with this activity. For example, upon reaching the 3rd page of a document, she was not able to remember what she had read on page 1.

Prior to her illness, she had seldom taken days off from work. But since the illness began, her exhaustion made it difficult to work, and she began missing days. Her primary physician referred her to a psychiatrist who referred her for relaxation therapy. She stopped seeing the psychiatrist when he told her she was "too healthy and she should get out and go back to work."

(Judge Clarke indicated that this psychiatrist's diagnosis was correct: The patient did not have psychiatric problems, and therefore, psychiatric illness could not be the reason for her inability to work.)

After she relocated to another city in Canada, her new general practitioner diagnosed her condition as chronic fatigue syndrome. Another physician subsequently told her that there was no such condition. The general practitioner then, according to Judge Clarke, ". . . counseled her further about the stressors associated with the diagnosis and had to reassure her that CFS [chronic fatigue syndrome] was recognized as a disease by the medical community." Another physician, a specialist in industrial health medicine, subsequently confirmed the diagnosis of chronic fatigue syndrome. An internist with expertise in diagnosing chronic fatigue syndrome also confirmed the diagnosis.

Around 1990, her former Alcoholics Anonymous sponsor employed her to provide pictures for a science text he was helping produce. He testified that in his previous experiences with her, she had been a high-energy, positive, goal-oriented person whose job was important to her. But after hiring her, he had to terminate her employment because of her inability to meet deadlines and attend meetings. He testified that when he saw her again in 1992, he was shocked at her deterioration.

The patient wrote of her condition: "It is very demoralizing for me not to be able to even cook my meals and clean my house. I now have to depend on others' help just to get through a day at home." Judge Clarke noted that the insurance company hired a private investigator to try to persuade the patient to take part in activities that would show she was "faking." This surreptitious enterprise showed instead that the patient required several months to complete a simple task. It also revealed that she did not complete tasks satisfactorily. For obvious reasons, the defendant (Crown Life Insurance Company) declined to show medical experts a video tape of the patient made during the investigation.

Judge Clarke wrote, "Undoubtedly, the most distressing thing to the Plaintiff [K. Sharon Baillier] was not knowing why, in medical terms, this was happening and [how] to stop it." In my experience, patients are often further distressed by two classes of professionals: (1) physicians employed by insurance companies to testify that the cause of the patient's symptoms is emotional disturbance or greed, and (2) insurance company attorneys who argue that the patient is not honest about her condition. In the Baillier

case, counsel for the insurance company ". . . strongly urged the Court to find that the Plaintiff was not a credible witness." Judge Clarke replied to their accusative request. He wrote, in effect, that despite substantial evidence to the contrary, the defendant suggested that the plaintiff did not tell the truth to two government agencies in applying for disability and did not tell the truth to the court. He disagreed and denied the request to find the patient not credible.

In summary of this case, applying for disability when the patient was not able to work resulted in (1) treatment that provided no relief; (2) progressive deterioration; (3) uncertainty about the nature of her condition; (4) instruction by a psychiatrist that she was healthy and should go back to work; (5) baffling disagreement between her physicians, some telling her that she had chronic fatigue syndrome, others telling her that no such syndrome exists; and (6) insurance company attorneys arguing in court essentially that she was lying about her disability, despite evidence from a private investigator with a secretly recorded video tape showing this to be false.

I contend that few seriously ill and debilitated individuals could withstand such adverse social consequences without developing—as a *consequence*—some degree of psychological disturbance.

● ABANDONING SOMATOFORM DIAGNOSES FOR SCIENTIFIC AND HUMANE REASONS

Somatoform diagnoses are default diagnoses. They are made when limits in diagnostic skill or technology result in failure to identify an organic mechanism of a patient's complaints. There is no credible scientific evidence that psychological processes purely or largely generate physical illnesses. In addition, the psychogenesis hypothesis of physical illnesses, which undergirds somatoform diagnoses, does not stand up to logical analysis by either traditional rationalism or critical rationalism. The hypothesis is therefore false beyond reasonable doubt. It should be excluded from the class of scientific hypotheses. On scientific grounds, then, fibromyalgia should never be diagnosed as a somatoform disorder.

Somatoform diagnoses are commonly used for unscrupulous business purposes to the detriment of fibromyalgia patients and others. On humanitarian grounds, then, clinicians should abandon the practice of making diagnoses of somatoform disorders, and the authors of future editions of the *DSM* should exclude these diagnoses from the classification of mental disorders.

There is no logical or scientific justification for assigning a mental disorder diagnosis to symptoms and signs that indicate a physical disorder but for which no organic basis can be established. The best solution would be for the diagnosis to only describe the patient's physical and psychological symptoms and signs and contain a modifier such as "etiology not known."

REFERENCES

1. Merskey, H.: *The Analysis of Hysteria.* London, Bailliere Tindall, 1979.
2. Weintraub, M.: Hysteria: A clinical guide to diagnosis. *Clin. Symposia*, 29:1-31, 1977.
3. Szasz, T.S.: *The Myth of Mental Illness.* New York, Harper Colophon Books, 1974.
4. International Association for the Study of Pain: Classification of chronic pain syndromes. *Pain*, Suppl. 3, 1986.
5. Slater, E.T.O.: Diagnosis of "hysteria." *Brit. J. Med.*, 1: 1395-1399, 1965.
6. Slater, E.T.O. and Glitero, E.: A follow-up of patients diagnosed as suffering from "hysteria." *J. Psychosomatic Res.*, 9:9-13, 1965.
7. Weintraub, M.: Chronic pain-litigation syndrome. *Amer. J. Pain Manag.*, 2(4):198-204, 1992.
8. Mendelson, G.: Not "cured by a verdict." *Med. J. Australia*, 2:132-134, 1982.
9. Lowe, J.C.: Litigation-chronic pain syndrome: Weintraub's unproven entity. *Am. J. Pain Manag.*, 3(3):131-136, 1993.
10. Lowe, J.C.: The neglected mechanism. *Dyn. Chiro.*, Aug. 29, 1990, p.35.
11. Lowe, J.C.: The most common source of pain. *North Carolina Chiro. Assoc. J.*, Aug., 1992, pp.26-27.
12. Macnab, I.: The whiplash syndrome. *Clin. Neurosurg.*, 20: 232-241, 1972.
13. Institute of Medicine: *Pain and Disability: Clinical, Behavioral and Public Policy Perspectives.* Washington, D.C., National Academy Press, 1987.
14. Simons, D.G. and Simons, L.S.: Chronic myofascial pain syndrome. In *Handbook of Chronic Pain Management.* Edited by C.D. Tollison, Baltimore, Williams and Wilkins, 1989, pp.509-529.
15. Barber, T.X.: Toward a theory of pain: relief of chronic pain by prefrontal leucotomy, opiates, placebos, and hypnosis. *Psychol. Bull.*, 56:430-460, 1959.
16. Merskey, H.: Headache and hysteria. *Cephalagia*, 1:109-119, 1981.
17. Merskey, H.: The characteristics of persistent pain in psychological illness: psychiatric patients with persistent pain. *J. Psychosomatic Res.*, 9:299, 1965.
18. Merskey, H.: Psychiatry and pain. In *Psychology of Pain*, 2nd edition. Edited by R.A. Sternback, New York, Raven Press, 1986, pp.97-120.
19. Merskey, H.: Chronic pain and psychiatric illness. In *The Management of Pain.* Edited by J.J. Bonica, Malvern, Lea & Febiger, 1990, pp.320-327.
20. Merskey, H.: Regional pain is rarely hysterical. *Arch.*
21. Weintraub, M.I.: *Hysterical Conversion Reactions: A Clinical Guide to Diagnosis and Treatment.* New York, SP Medical & Scientific Books, 1983.
22. Copi, I.M.: *Introduction to Logic*, 4th edition. New York, Macmillan Publishing Co., Inc., 1972.
23. Northrop, F.S.C.: *The Logic of the Sciences and the Humanities.* New York, Meridian Books, Inc., 1960.
24. Sternback, R.A.: Psychophysiologic pain syndrome. In *The Management of Pain.* Edited by J.J. Bonica, Malvern, Lea & Febiger, 1990, pp.287-290.
25. Travell, J.G. and Bigelow, N.H.: Role of somatic trigger areas in the patterns of hysteria. Paper presented at the Annual Meeting of the American Society for Research in Psychosomatic Problems, Inc., Atlantic City, May 3, 1947.
26. Lowe, J.C.: Litigating pain patients: just greedy neurotics? *Chiro. J.*, May, 1998, pp.27 & 43.
27. Hendler, N., Zinreich, J., and Kozikowski, J.G.: Three-dimensional CT validation of physical complaints in "psychogenic pain" patients. *Psychosomatics*, 34(1):90-96, 1993.
28. de Bono, E.: *de Bono's Thinking Course.* New York, Facts on File, Inc., 1985.
29. Strecker, E.A.: *Basic Psychiatry.* New York, Random House, Inc., 1952.
30. Russell, B.: *The Autobiography of Bertrand Russell: 1944-1969.* New York, Simon and Schuster, 1969.
31. Alvarez, J. and Low, R.B.: Acute respiratory arrest due to hypokalemia. *Ann. Emerg. Med.*, 17:288-289, 1988.
32. Hachinski, V.: The nature of regional pain. *Arch. Neurol.*, 45:918, 1988.
33. Strachey, J.: *Josef Breuer and Sigmund Freud: Studies on Hysteria.* New York, Basic Books, Inc., (year of publication not given).
34. Bangash, I.H., Worley, G., and Kandt, R.S.: Hysterical conversion reactions mimicking neurological disease. *Am. J. Dis. Child.*, 142:1203-1206, 1988.
35. Gould, R., Miller, B.L., and Goldberg, M.A,: The validity of hysterical signs and symptoms. *J. Nerv. Ment. Dis.*, 174: 23-28, 1986.
36. Jaeger, B. and Skootsky, S.A.: Letter to the Editor. *Pain*, 29:263-264, 1987.
37. Fishbain, D.A. and Rosomoff, H.: Letter to the Editor. *Pain*, 29:265, 1987.
38. Bonica, J.J.: Myofascial syndromes with trigger mechanism. In *The Management of Pain.* Edited by J.J. Bonica, Philadelphia, Lea and Febiger, 1150-1151, 1953.
39. Kendall, H.O., Kendall, F.P., and Wadsworth, G.E.: *Muscle Testing and Function.* Baltimore, Williams and Wilkins, 1971.
40. Inman, V.T., Saunders, J.B., deCamp, M.: Referred pain from skeletal structures. *J. Nerv. Ment. Dis.*, 99:660-667, 1944.
41. Travell, J.G. and Simons, D.G.: *Myofascial Pain and Dysfunction: The Trigger Point Manual.* Baltimore, Williams and Wilkins, 1983.
42. Thomas, D. and Aidinis, S.: Objective documentation of musculoskeletal pain syndrome by pressure algometry during thiopentone sodium (Pentothal) anesthesia. *Clin. J. Pain*, 5(4):343-350, 1989.
43. Lowman, E.W.: Psychogenic rheumatism. *Arch. Phys.*

(Reference 20 continued) *Neurol.*, 45:915-918, 1988.

Med. Rehab., 36:222-226, 1955.

44. Ullman, L.P. and Krasner, L.: *A Psychological Approach to Abnormal Behavior.* Englewood Cliffs, Prentice-Hall, Inc., 1969.

45. Henderson, D. and Batchelor, I.R.C.: *Henderson and Gillespie's Textbook of Psychiatry*, 9ᵗʰ edition. London, Oxford University Press, 1962.

46. Moral, R.R., Alamo, M.M., Detorres, L.P., and Galeote, M.: Biopsychosocial features of patients with widespread chronic musculoskeletal pain in family medicine clinics. *Fam. Pract.*, 14(3):242-248, 1997.

47. Clarke, C.P.: Reasons for judgement of the Honorable Mr. Justice C. Philip Clarke. *K. Sharon Baillie vs. Crown Life Insurance Company.* Court of the Queen's Bench of Alberta, Canada, Judicial District of Edmonton, Judgement March 2, 1998, filed March 3, 1998. Nightingale Research Foundation web site: http://www.nightingale.ca.

48. Ruesch, J.: The infantile personality. *Psychosom. Med.*, 10:134, 1948.

49. Oye, G., Korff, M.V., Simon, G.E., and Gater, R.: Persistent pain and well-being: a World Health Organization study in primary care. *J.A.M.A.*, 280:147-151, 1998.

50. Smythe, H.A.: Non-articular rheumatism and the fibrositis syndrome. In *Arthritis and Allied Conditions*, 8ᵗʰ edition. Edited by J.L. Hollander and D.J. McCary, Philadelphia, Lea & Febiger, 1972, pp.874-884.

51. Clark, S., Campbell, S.M., Forehand, M.E., Tindall, E.A., and Bennett, R.M.: Clinical characteristics of fibrositis. II. A "blinded" controlled study using standard psychological tests. *Arthritis Rheum.*, 28:132-137, 1985.

52. Yunus, M.B.: Psychological factors in fibromyalgia syndrome: an overview. *J. Musculoskel. Pain*, 2(1):87-91, 1994.

53. Ahles, T.A., Yunus, M.B., Railey, S.D., et al.: Psychological factors associated with primary fibromyalgia syndrome. *Arthritis Rheum.*, 27:1101-1106, 1984.

54. Yunus, M.B.: Towards a model of pathophysiology of fibromyalgia: aberrant central pain mechanisms with peripheral modulation. *J. Rheumatol.*, 19:846-850, 1992.

55. Corvi, R.: *An Introduction to the Thought of Karl Popper.* London, Routledge, 1997.

56. Yunus, M.B., Ahles, T.A., Aldag, J.C., and Masi, A.T.: Relationship of clinical features with psychological status in primary fibromyalgia. *Arthritis Rheum.*, 34:15-21, 1991.

57. Hendler, N.H. and Kozikowski, J.G.: Overlooked physical diagnoses in chronic pain patients involved in litigation. *Psychosomatics,* 34(6):494-501, 1993.

58. Wolfe, F., Cathey, M.A., Kleinheksel, S.M., et al.: Psychological status in primary fibrositis and fibrositis associated with rheumatoid arthritis. *J. Rheumatol.*, 11:500-506, 1984.

59. Leavitt, F. and Katz, R.S.: Is the MMPI invalid for assessing psychological disturbance in pain related organic conditions? *J. Rheumatol.*, 16:521-526, 1989.

60. Dailey, P.A., Bishop, G.D., Russell, I.J., and Fletcher, E.M.: Psychological stress and the fibrositis/fibromyalgia syndrome. *J. Rheumatol.*, 17:1380-1385, 1990.

61. Uveges, J.M., Parker, J.C., Smarr, K.L., et al.: Psychological symptoms in primary fibromyalgia syndrome: relationship to pain, life stress, and sleep disturbance.

Arthritis Rheum., 33:1279-1283, 1990.

62. Ahles, T.A., Khan, S.A., Yunus, M.B., et al.: Psychiatric status of primary fibromyalgia and rheumatoid arthritis patients and nonpain controls: a blinded comparison of *DSM-III* diagnoses. *Am. J. Psychiat.*, 148:1721-1726, 1991.

63. Ahles, T.A., Yunus, M.B., and Masi, A.T.: Is chronic pain a variant of depressive disease? The case of primary fibromyalgia syndrome. *Pain*, 29:105-111, 1987.

64. Birnie, K.J., Knipping, A.A., Van Rijswijk, M.H., et al.: Psychological aspects of fibromyalgia compared with chronic and nonchronic pain. *J. Rheumatol.*, 18:1845-1848, 1991.

65. Yates, A.J.: Symptoms and symptom substitution. *Psychol. Rev.*, 65(6):371-374, 1958.

66. Smythe, H.A. and Moldofsky, H.: Two contributions to understanding of the "fibrositis" syndrome. *Bull. Rheum. Dis.*, 28:928-931, 1977.

67. Parker, J., Frank, R., Beck, N., et al.: Pain in rheumatoid arthritis: relationship to demographic, medical, and psychological factors. *J. Rheumatol.*, 15:433-437, 1988.

68. Reilly, P.A. and Littlejohn, G.O.: Fibromyalgia: the wheel reinvented? *J. Musculoskel. Pain*, 1(2):5-17, 1993.

69. Bedard, M.E.: Bankruptcies of the heart: secondary losses from disabling chronic pain. *Syndr. Sentin.*, 1(4):3-5, 1998.

70. Ford, C.V.: Somatization and fashionable diagnoses: illness as a way of life. *Scand. J. Work Environ. Health*, 23 (Suppl. 3):7-16, 1997.

71. Jackson, B.: Psychological status in fibromyalgia and associated syndromes: based on an interview with Muhammad B. Yunus, M.D., pioneer FM researcher from the Univ. of Illinois College of Med. at Peoria. http://www/sunflower.org/~cfsdays/yunus.htm, 1996.

72. Goldstein, J.A.: *Chronic Fatigue Syndromes: The Limbic Hypothesis.* New York, Haworth Medical Press, 1993.

73. Starlanyl, D.: What everyone on your health care team should know, part 1. *Syndr. Sentin.*, 1(4):1-3, 1998.

74. Kelly, R. and Smith, B.N.: Post-traumatic syndrome: another myth discredited. *J. Royal Soc. Med.*, 74:275-277, 1981.

75. Weich, S. and Lewis, G.: Poverty, unemployment, and common mental disorders: population based cohort study. *Brit. Med. J.*, 317(7151):115-119, 1998.

76. Wallis, B.J., Lord, S.M., and Bogduk, N.: Resolution of psychological distress of whiplash patients following treatment by radiofrequency neurotomy: a randomized, double-blind, placebo-controlled trial. *Pain*, 73(1):15-22, 1997.

77. *Diagnostic and Statistical Manual of Mental Disorders*, 3ʳᵈ edition. Washington, D.C., American Psychiatric Association, 1987.

78. Johannsson, V.: Does a fibromyalgia personality exist? *J. Musculoskel. Pain*, 1(3/4):245-252, 1993.

79. Schuessler, G. and Konermann, J.: Psychosomatic aspects of primary fibromyalgia syndrome. *J. Musculoskel. Pain*, 1(3/4):229-236, 1993.

80. Goldenberg, D.L.: An overview of psychologic studies in fibromyalgia. *J. Rheum.*, 16(suppl. 19):12-13, 1989.

81. Wessely, S.: Social and cultural aspects of chronic fatigue syndrome. *J. Musculoskel. Pain*, 3(2):111-122, 1995.

82. Hohl, M.: Soft-tissue injuries of the neck in automobile

accidents: factors influencing prognosis. *J. Bone Joint Surg.*(Amer.), 56-A(8):1675-1682, 1974.

83. Ellman, P., Savage, D.A., Wittkower, E., and Rodger, T.F.: "Fibrositis"—a biographical study of fifty civilian and military cases. *Ann. Rheumatol. Dis.*, 3:56-76, 1942.

84. Boland, E.W.: Psychogenic rheumatism: the musculoskeletal expression of psychoneurosis. *Ann. Rheumatol. Dis.*, 6:195, 1947.

85. Roth, R.S. and Bachman, J.E.: Pain experience, psychological functioning, and self-reported disability in chronic myofascial pain and fibromyalgia. *J. Musculoskel. Pain*, 1 (3/4):209-216, 1993.

86. Birnie, D.J., Knipping, A.A., vanGrijswijk, M.H., deBlecourt, C., and deVoogd, J.: Psychological aspects of fibromyalgia compared with chronic and non-chronic pain. *J. Rheumatol.*, 18:1845-1848, 1991.

87. Merskey, H.: Chronic muscular pain—a life stress syndrome? *J. Musculoskel. Pain*, 1(3/4):61-69, 1993.

88. Woodforde, J.M. and Merskey, H.: Personality traits of patients with chronic pain. *J. Psychosom. Res.*, 16:167-172, 1972.

89. Atkinson, J.H., Slater, M.A., Grant, I., Patterson, T.L., and Garfin, S.R.: Depressed mood in chronic low back pain: relationship with stressful life events. *Pain*, 35:45-55, 1988.

90. Sternbach, R.A., Wolf, S.R., Murphy, R.W., and Akeson, W.H.: Traits of pain patients: the low-back "loser." *Psychosomatics*, 13:226-229, 1973.

91. KuKull, W.A., Koepsell, T.D., Inui, T.S., Borson, S., Okimoto, J., Raskind, M.A., and Gate, J.L.: Depression and physical illness among elderly general medicine clinic patients. *J. Affect. Dis.*, 10:153-162, 1986.

92. Radnov, F., Bogdan, P., Stefano, G., Schnidrig, A., and Ballinari, P.: Role of psychosocial stress in recovery from common whiplash. *Lancet*, 338:712-715, 1991.

93. Bohr, T.W.: Fibromyalgia syndrome and myofascial pain syndrome: do they exist? *Neurol. Clinics*, 13:365-384, 1995.

94. Capen, K.: The courts, expert witnesses and fibromyalgia. *Canadian Med. Ass. J.*, 15:206-208, 1995.

95. Ellis, A.: *Reason and Emotion in Psychotherapy*. Secaucus, N.J., The Citadel Press, 1979.

96. Popper, K.R.: *The Logic of Scientific Discovery*. New York, Routledge, 1980.

97. Mountz, J.N., Bradley, L.A., Modell, J.G., Alexander, R.W., et al.: Fibromyalgia in women: abnormalities of regional cerebral blood flow in the thalamus and the caudate nucleus are associated with low pain thresholds. *Arthritis Rheumatol.*, 38:926-938, 1995.

98. Teasell, R.W.: Letter to the Editor. Epidemiology of soft tissue rheumatism. *J. Endocrinology*, 19:1823, 1992.

99. Reilly, D.A., Travers, R., and Littlejohn, G.O.: Letter to the Editor: response to Teasell. Epidemiology of soft tissue rheumatism. *J. Endocrinology*, 19:1823-1824, 1992.

100. Vidal, B.E., Diaz, E.H., and Ramos, G.G.: One hundred years of the Babinski sign. *Revista de Investigacion Clinica*, 49(2):141-144, 1997.

101. Moore, W.E.: *Creative and Critical Thinking*. New York, Houghton Mifflin Company, 1967.

102. Lowe, J.C., Garrison, R.L., Reichman, A.J., Yellin, J., Thompson, M., and Kaufman, D.: Effectiveness and safety of T₃ (triiodothyronine) therapy for euthyroid fibromyalgia: a double-blind placebo-controlled response-driven crossover study. *Clin. Bull. Myofascial Ther.*, 2(2/3):31-58, 1997.

103. Lowe, J.C., Reichman, A.J., and Yellin, J.: The process of change during T₃ treatment for euthyroid fibromyalgia: a double-blind placebo-controlled crossover study. *Clin. Bull. Myofascial Ther.*, 2(2/3):91-124, 1997.

104. Lowe, J.C., Garrison, R.L., Reichman, A.J., and Yellin, J.: Triiodothyronine (T₃) treatment of euthyroid fibromyalgia: a small-N replication of a double-blind placebo-controlled crossover study. *Clin. Bull. Myofascial Ther.*, 2(4):71-88, 1997.

105. Lowe, J.C., Reichman, A.J., and Yellin, J.: A case-control study of metabolic therapy for fibromyalgia: long-term follow-up comparison of treated and untreated patients. *Clin. Bull. Myofascial Ther.*, 3(1):23-24, 1998.

106. Eysenck, H.J.: *Decline and Fall of the Freudian Empire*. London, Penguin Books, 1985.

107. *Diagnostic and Statistical Manual*, 4th edition. Washington, D.C., American Psychiatric Association, 1994.

108. Eysenck, H.J.: *The Effects of Psychotherapy*. New York, International Science Press, 1966.

109. Wilbourn, A.J.: The electrodiagnostic examination with hysteria-conversion reaction and malingering. *Neurologic Clinics*, 13(2):385-404, 1995.

110. Weintraub, M.I.: *Neurologic Clinics: Malingering and Conversion Reactions*, 13(2), 1995.

111. Universal Advantage: *Comprehensive Medical Insurance Form 12A-B (OK)*. Continental General Insurance Company, 8901 Indian Hills Drive, Omaha, NE 68124-7007, August 1996.

112. Travell, JG.: Referred somatic pain does not follow a simple "segmental" pattern. *Red. Proc.*, 5:106, 1946.

113. Hendler, N., Bergson, C., and Morrison, C.: Overlooked physical diagnoses in chronic pain patients involved in litigation, part 2. The addition of MRI, nerve blocks, 3-D CT, and qualitative flow meter. *Psychosomatics*, 37(6):509-517, 1996.

114. Macnab, I.: The whiplash syndrome. *Clin. Neurosurg.*, 20:232-241, 1972.

115. Halliday, J.L.: The concept of psychosomatic rheumatism. *Ann. Intern. Med.*, 15:666-677, 1941.

116. Graham, W.: Fibrositis and non-articular rheumatism. *Phys. Ther. Rev.*, 35:128-133, 1955.

117. Cathey, M.A., Wolfe, F., Kleinheksel, S.M., and Hawley, D.J.: Socioeconomic impact of fibrositis: a study of 81 patients with primary fibrositis. *Am. J. Med.*, 81:78-84, 1986.

118. Yunus, M.B. and Masi, A.T.: Juvenile primary fibromyalgia syndrome: a clinical study of thirty-three patients and matched normal controls. *Arthritis Rheum.*, 28:138-145, 1985.

119. Vlaeyen, J.W.S., Teeken-Gruben, N.G., Goossens, M.E.J.B., Rutten, M.P.M.H., Pelt, H., vanEek, H., and Heut, P.H.G.T.: Cognitive-educational treatment of fibromyalgia: randomized clinical trials. *J. Rheumatol.*, 23:1237-1245, 1996.

120. Lowe, J.C.: *Documentary Evidence*. Houston, Mc Dowell Publishing Company, 1991.

121. Thompson, G.N.: Post-traumatic psychoneurosis: a statistical survey. *Am. J. Psychiatry*, 121:1043-1048, 1965.

Section II

Background:
Basic and Clinical Sciences

2.1

Thyroid Hormone Physiology

Maintenance of normal amounts of T_4 and T_3 in the blood depends upon a normal interaction between the hypothalamus, the pituitary gland, and the thyroid gland. TRH from the hypothalamus stimulates the thyrotrophs of the anterior pituitary gland to secrete TSH. The hypothalamus and TRH function as a fine control mechanism for TSH secretion. TSH in turn stimulates the thyroid gland to release thyroid hormones. Circulating transport proteins bind the thyroid hormones and deliver them to cells. Delivery of sufficient amounts of thyroid hormones to hypothalamic cells inhibits their synthesis and secretion of TRH. Similarly, sufficient amounts of thyroid hormones reaching anterior pituitary cells inhibit their synthesis and release of TSH. The normal interaction of the hypothalamic-pituitary-thyroid axis constitutes a negative-feedback system. This system, when functioning normally, maintains normal blood levels of thyroid hormones.

The thyroid hormones T_4 and T_3 are synthesized in the colloid of the secretory follicles of the thyroid gland. The follicles, which make up the bulk of the gland, store the hormones until they are released into the circulation. The hormones, largely T_4, circulate bound to transport proteins. When T_4 enters cells, the enzyme 5'-deiodinase catalyzes release of an iodine atom from the outer ring of the T_4 molecule, converting it to the most metabolically active thyroid hormone, T_3. Deiodination (removal of an iodine atom) of the inner ring of T_4 produces reverse-T_3 (rT_3). Reverse-T_3 has little or no biologic activity. This step is considered the thyroid hormone deactivating reaction. Other deiodinating enzymes convert T_3 and rT_3 successively to T_2, T_1, and the non-iodinated molecule T_0. The released iodide may be used by the thyroid gland to synthesize more thyroid hormone.

A major prerequisite to normal cellular metabolism is adequate delivery through the blood of the two thyroid hormones, T_4 (thyroxine, or tetraiodo-thyronine) and T_3 (triiodothyronine). Delivery alone, however, is not sufficient for a normal metabolic rate. Thyroid hormones must, without hindrance, enter cells, undergo processing, and exert their intracellular actions. Initially, however, normal metabolism is dependent upon adequate production of thyroid hormones by the thyroid gland and delivery of the hormones in sufficient quantities to cells. Adequate production and delivery of the hormones depends upon a normally functioning hypothalamic-pituitary-thyroid axis (see Figure 2.1.1).

● THE HYPOTHALAMIC-PITUITARY-THYROID AXIS

The thyroid gland synthesizes thyroid hormones and secretes them into the blood. Normally, the gland performs these functions only when exposed to a sufficient quantity of thyroid-stimulating hormone (thyro-

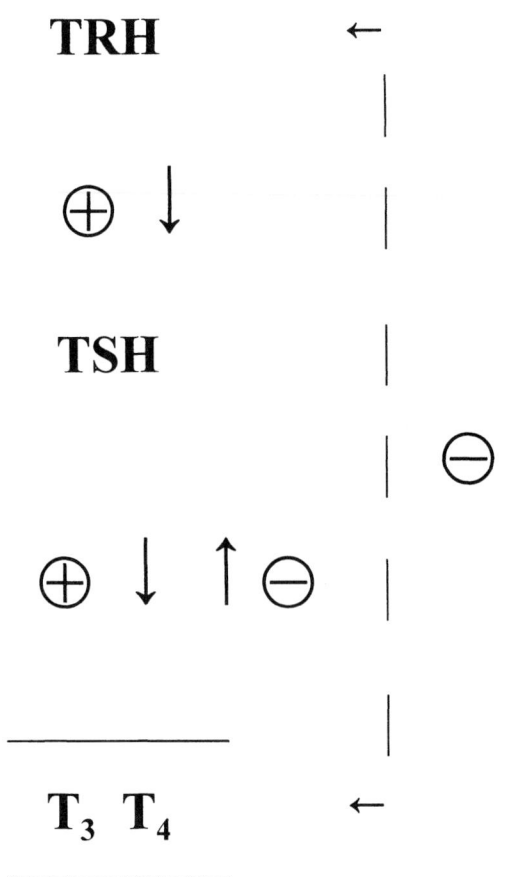

Figure 2.1.1. Schematic representation of the stimulatory and inhibitory interactions of the components of the hypothalamic-pituitary-thyroid axis. These components make up the primary system for regulation of the axis. The basic interactions involve: 1) TRH stimulation of TSH secretion, 2) TSH stimulation of thyroid hormone secretion, and 3) powerful negative-feedback inhibition of TSH and TRH secretion by the thyroid hormones. (After figure 12-1, p.231, by Scanlon, M.A.: Neuroendocrine control of thyrotropin secretion. In *Werner and Ingbar's The Thyroid: A Fundamental and Clinical Text*, 6th edition. Edited by L.E. Braverman and R.D. Utiger, New York, J.B. Lippincott Co., 1991.[21, pp.230-256])

tropin, or TSH). The anterior pituitary gland cells termed thyrotrophs synthesize and secrete TSH. The amount of TSH the thyrotrophs produce and release into the circulation is regulated by the amount of thyroid hormones circulating through the anterior pituitary gland. As the amount of thyroid hormones circulating through the pituitary increases, thyrotroph function becomes progressively more inhibited. The thyrotrophs reduce their production and release of TSH and the circulating TSH level decreases. As the amount of TSH reaching the thyroid gland decreases, the gland reduces the amount of thyroid hormones it synthesizes and releases into the blood. The decreasing level of thyroid hormones in the blood circulating through the pituitary gland disinhibits the thyrotrophs. The thyrotrophs then increase the amount of TSH they synthesize and secrete into the blood. In turn, the increased amount of TSH reaching the thyroid gland increases the synthesis and secretion of thyroid hormones by the gland. In this interaction, when the pituitary-thyroid axis functions normally, TSH and thyroid hormone production and release rhythmically counterpoise one another. The equilibrating ebb and flow keeps levels of circulating thyroid hormones sufficient to maintain normal metabolism in cells that are properly responsive to thyroid hormones.

Another hormone, thyrotropin-releasing hormone (TRH), is secreted by the hypothalamus. TRH directly influences the pituitary thyrotroph cells, stimulating them to produce and secrete TSH. TRH also decreases the number of T_3 receptors in the thyrotrophs. The decrease minimizes the inhibition of the thyrotrophs by T_3.

Thyroid hormones reaching the hypothalamus through the blood decrease the secretion of TRH. This reduces the amount of TRH that reaches and stimulates the pituitary thyrotrophs. Thus, thyroid hormones indirectly inhibit TSH secretion by reducing TRH secretion. Thyroid hormones also decrease the count of TRH receptors in the thyrotrophs. The reduced receptor count decreases the ability of TRH to stimulate the thyrotrophs to synthesize and secrete TSH.

The hypothalamus, pituitary gland, and thyroid gland, and the hormones the three secrete, constitute a negative feedback system. Figure 2.1.1 is a schematic representation of the interactions of the hypothalamic-pituitary-thyroid axis. Figure 2.1.2 is a summary of the feedback mechanisms. When structurally and functionally intact, the hypothalamic-pituitary-thyroid axis maintains a normal amount of thyroid hormone in the blood. Barring defects in the cellular processing and actions of the thyroid hormone, this amount should be adequate to keep the metabolic rate properly apace.

The hypothalamic-pituitary-thyroid axis is not, however, a closed circuit: Neural innervation, neurotransmitters, and other hormones influence the synthesis and secretion of thyroid hormones, TSH, and TRH. As these influences alter the activity of one or more of the three components of the axis, the levels of thyroid hormones in the blood may also be altered.

● STIMULATION OF THYROID HORMONE SYNTHESIS BY TSH

After TSH attaches to TSH-receptors on thyroid gland cell membranes, the gland releases T_3 and T_4 into the circulating blood, typically within 30 minutes. TSH also accelerates nearly all aspects of thyroid gland metabolism, including synthesis of thyroid hormones. The latency of these effects may be hours- to-weeks.[1,p.903]

Binding of TSH to TSH-receptors in thyroid gland cell membranes activates the enzyme adenylate cyclase inside the membranes. In the presence of magnesium, the activated enzyme induces conversion of ATP to 3',5'-adenosine monophosphate (cyclic-AMP).[19,p.29] Through various biochemical routes, the cyclic-AMP stimulates production of T_3 and T_4.[2][11]

First, cyclic-AMP, functioning as a second messenger, activates the enzyme protein kinase. At this point, the enzyme phosphodiesterase inactivates cyclic-AMP by catalyzing its conversion to 5'-AMP.[19,p.30] The kinase activated by cyclic-AMP sets off the reversible phosphorylation of multiple "control" proteins throughout the cell. The phosphorylated proteins induce the gland to immediately increase its secretion of thyroid hormones. This process is a major mechanism of metabolism regulation.[19,p.29]

The main hormones the gland manufactures and secretes are T_4 and T_3. It is mainly through the cellular action of T_3, however, that thyroid hormone potently regulates cell metabolism. Through regulating metabolism, the hormones have widespread and profound effects throughout the body. Complete absence of thyroid hormones (for example, after the entire thyroid gland is surgically removed) slows the metabolic rate to some 40% below normal. An extreme excess of thyroid hormones (as in severe, untreated Graves' disease) can increase the metabolic rate as high as 60%-to-100% above normal.[1,p.897] When the metabolic rate decreases or increases sufficiently in humans, cells begin to dysfunction. If the dysfunction continues, signs and symptoms of either hypometabolism or hypermetabolism eventually develop.

● THYROID GLAND SYNTHESIS AND SECRETION OF THYROID HORMONE

The production and secretion of thyroid hormones by the thyroid gland are complex processes. This sec-

tion describes only the minimal steps necessary to understand the processes.

THYROID HORMONE PRODUCTION IN THE THYROID GLAND

The thyroid gland consists of a mass of minute, rounded follicles of various sizes. The follicles function as secretory sacs. A fibrous connective tissue capsule encloses groups of the follicles, forming lobules.

Actions of TRH

Increases TSH release by stimulating anterior pituitary cells.

Indirectly increases TSH release by decreasing T_3- receptors in the anterior pituitary (binding of T_3 to these receptors inhibits TSH release).

Actions of TSH

Directly stimulates the thyroid gland to produce and release thyroid hormones.

Actions of Thyroid Hormones

Directly inhibit TSH release by the pituitary gland through binding to T_3-receptors.

Directly inhibit TRH release by the hypothalamus.

Indirectly inhibit TSH release by decreasing TRH-receptors on TSH-secreting pituitary cells.

Figure 2.1.2. Summary of the effects of TRH, TSH, and thyroid hormones on different components of the hypothalamic-pituitary-thyroid axis.

The fibrous tissue, called stroma, passes from the outer capsule down between the follicles, forming a framework that supports them. The stroma is also continuous externally with the capsule that encases the whole gland. Lymph vessels, veins, and a rich supply of arteries course through the sheets of stroma.

The thyroid gland has an extensive blood supply. The supply is so extensive that it stimulated some debate at the beginning of the last century. Someone proposed, as Haynes pointed out, that the abundant paths of blood vessels through the thyroid gland indicated that the gland was a vascular shunt for the brain. Then in 1820, Rush reasoned that the larger size of the gland in women was "necessary to guard the female system from the influence of the more numerous causes of irritation and vexation of mind to which they are exposed than the male sex." That same year, Hofrichter objected, "If it were indeed true that the thyroid contains more blood at some times than at others, this effect would be visible to the naked eye; in this case women would certainly have long ceased to go about with bare necks, for husbands would have learned to recognize the swelling of this gland as a danger signal of threatening trouble from their better halves."[20,p.1361]

In addition to blood vessels, nerves course through the thyroid gland. These are non-myelinated post-ganglionic sympathetic fibers, and their source is the superior and middle cervical sympathetic ganglia. These nerves are vasomotor; they influence thyroid gland secretion indirectly by their effects on blood vessels, especially the gland's arteriovenous anastomoses.[26,pp.566-567] The neuroanatomical structure of the gland is a clue to the possible role of spinal and paraspinal myofascial manipulation in the treatment of hypothyroid patients (see Chapter 5.2, subsection titled "Manipulative Therapies: Spinal and Myofascial Manipulation").

The various-sized secretory follicles make up the bulk of the thyroid gland. They hold a jelly-like substance called colloid. A layer of epithelial cells form the walls of each follicle. From these walls, many microvilli project into the lumen of the follicle. These projections increase the surface area in contact with the colloid. An extensive network of capillaries course through the follicles, providing an abundant blood supply.[47,p.23]

The follicles store thyroid hormones dispersed uniformly in the colloid. The amount of colloid in the follicles depends on the activity of the gland. When the secretory activity of the gland is low, the follicles contain more colloid. When the gland is highly active, the follicles contain less colloid and may actually become depleted.

The ribosomes in the epithelial cells of the follicle walls synthesize the carbohydrate-protein compound termed thyroglobulin. Thyroglobulin is then packaged in the Golgi apparatus of the cells and secreted into the colloid. Thyroglobulin, the main constituent of the colloid, attaches to the thyroid hormones in the colloid and keeps them uniformly suspended.[47,p.23]

It is in the colloid, rather than the follicular cells, that thyroid hormones form.[27] This extracellular site of synthesis makes thyroid hormone unique among hormones produced by endocrine glands; all other hormones are produced intracellularly.[47,p.23]

Residing in the microvilli and other components of the follicular cells is the most important enzyme in the synthesis of thyroid hormone, human thyroid peroxidase.[48] Once the colloid traps iodide ions that have entered the follicular cells, peroxidase oxidizes the iodide to the higher valency form, iodine (the active form of the iodide molecule). Hydrogen peroxide is produced in the process.[49] Next, one active iodine atom combines with the amino acid tyrosine. This forms mono-iodotyrosine (T_1). In addition, two active iodine atoms combine with tyrosine to form di-iodotyrosine or (T_2). Through another oxidative step, triggered by peroxidase functioning as a coupling enzyme, T_1 and T_2 couple to form the iodothyronines. (Coupling of tyrosines produces thyronines.) In this step, thyroid peroxidase combines T_1 and T_2 to form T_3, and combines two T_2 molecules to form T_4.[47,p.30] These are the thyroid hormones, *per se*.[29]

To summarize—the thyroid hormones form by a three-step process: (1) the colloid traps iodide that is then converted to an active form (iodine), (2) iodine impregnates the amino acid tyrosine forming iodotyrosine, and (3) iodotyrosine molecules couple to form iodothyronines.[28]

SECRETION OF THYROID HORMONES

Until the thyroid gland secretes its T_3 and T_4, the hormones remain attached to thyroglobulin and suspended in the colloid of the follicles. Near the time of secretion, thyroglobulin moves from the colloid into the epithelial cells of the follicles by endocytosis. (Endocytosis is the process in which the cell's outer wall invaginates around and encloses small amounts of thyroglobulin.) In the epithelial cells, the thyroglobulin is held within vesicles called "colloid droplets." Lysosomes next move toward and fuse with the colloid droplets. As the fused lysosomes move to the secretory edge of the cell, lysosomal enzymes (both proteases and peptidases) break down the thyroglobulin and the colloid disappears. This frees the iodine-containing amino acid hormones (the iodothyronines) and releases them to the circulation.[36,p.84-85][45][46] During their release, T_3 and T_4 diffuse from the follicles' epithelial cells into the capillaries that course through the gland's stroma. The capillary blood carries the hormones to larger vessels through which they enter the general circulation.

Hormone Production
Rate of the Thyroid Gland

The mean daily thyroid gland production of T_4 has been estimated to be 101 μg (56.2 μg/m²)[73,p.2500] and 96 μg.[74] The mean daily production rate of T_3 has been reported as 6 μg (3.3 μg/m²).[73,p.2500] Pilo et al. calculated the molar ratio of T_4 to T_3 secreted by the human thyroid gland as 14:1.[75]

The amount of T_3 in the circulation is approximately 4 times the amount produced daily by the thyroid gland. The additional ¾ is released into the circulation by tissues other than the thyroid gland following the deiodination of T_4.[73,p.2500] Thus, the thyroid gland is a relatively minor source of T_3.[76,p.2828] Utiger reported that the concentration of T_4 in the circulation is more than 30 times that of T_3.[23]

Sources of Cellular T_4 and T_3

T_4 inside cells is derived exclusively from the thyroid gland. However, the T_3 inside cells is derived from both the pool of circulating T_3 and the local intracellular conversion of T_4 to T_3.[76,p.2828] Studies by Escobar-Morreale et al. indicate that the T_3 generated from T_4 in nonthyroidal tissues does not rapidly and completely exchange with circulating T_3. Because of this, a normal circulating T_3 level does not ensure a normal cellular T_3 concentration.[77][78]

Metabolic Activity of the Iodotyrosines and Iodothyronines

T_4, the thyroid hormone that circulates through the blood in greatest quantity, is generally considered a prohormone for T_3. According to this view, T_4 is considered metabolically inactive until converted to T_3. T_3 is considered the metabolically active thyroid hormone. However, as Chopra wrote of iodotyrosines and iodothyronines, ". . . T_3 is the predominant but not unique mediator of biologic activity."[56,p.137] There is some evidence that T_4 also has some cellular functions independent of T_3. Depending on how the overall thyroid hormone effect in humans is calculated, the contribution of T_4 ranges from 35%-to-0.[56,p.137]

Reverse-T_3 is a major by-product of the peripheral cell metabolism of T_4 (see below, "Enzymatic Conversion of T_4 to T_3"). Reverse-T_3 is reported to have calorigenic activity that is 5% that of T_4[55] and is therefore relatively inert.[56,p.137]

Various other iodothyronines have some biologic activity *in vitro*, but it is not certain that they do so *in vivo*.[56,p.138] Money et al. reported that in some animals, 3,3'-T_2 has 25%-to-70% the biologic activity of T_4. 3,5-T_2 has about 40%.[57] 3,3'T_2 and T_3 are some 4 times more effective than T_4 in stimulating the uptake of amino acids by rat thymocytes.[62]

Recent data suggest that the iodothyronine, T_2 (3,5-diiodo-l-thyronine), has selective cellular activity. *In vivo*, T_2 suppressed TSH levels. The dosages of T_2 that suppressed TSH levels were not enough to produce the significant peripheral effects of thyroid hormone. Ball et al. found that T_2 stimulated growth hormone mRNA in GH₃ cells, but with 100-fold less potency than T_3. However, T_2 and T_3 were almost equally effective in down-regulating β₂ T_3-receptor mRNA levels. *In vivo*, T_2 and T_3 were equally effective in inducing hepatic malic enzyme mRNA. T_2 was more effective in inducing malic enzyme mRNA than in suppressing TSH levels. The researchers found that T_2 was only 27% as effective as T_3 in suppressing circulating TSH levels. Also, *in vitro*, in displacing ^{125}I-T_3 from T_3-receptors and GH₃ nuclear extracts, T_2 was 500 times less potent than T_3.[64]

DEIODINASES THAT BREAKDOWN THE IODOTYROSINES (T_1 AND T_2) AND THE IODOTHYRONINES (T_3 AND T_4)

Different enzymes break down T_1, T_2, T_3, and T_4, liberating iodide. Other enzymes convert T_4 to the highly metabolically active T_3.

Enzymatic Breakdown of T_1, T_2, T_3, and T_4

Powerful enzymes in the thyroid gland called thyroid iodotyrosine deiodinases break down T_1 and T_2 that are not combined into T_3 and T_4. The breakdown frees iodide molecules. The thyroid gland reuses most of the liberated iodide by later combining it with additional tyrosine molecules.[30] Some of the iodide, however, is lost from the gland. This is called the "iodide leak."[36,p.86]

The same type of thyroid iodotyrosine deiodinase that decomposes T_1 and T_2 in the thyroid gland is also present in the cells of peripheral tissues. Presumably, the enzyme breaks down T_1 and T_2 in these tissues as it does in the cells of thyroid tissue.[44]

Other types of deiodinases decompose T_3 and T_4. T_1 and T_2 are liberated when T_3 and T_4 are broken down in peripheral tissues. Released and uncombined T_1 and T_2 molecules may circulate in the blood stream and eventually inhibit synthesis of the catecholamine norepinephrine.[34,p.229] This may be a negative feedback mechanism: It may diminish the increased metabolism caused by binding of norepinephrine to the increased numbers of β-adrenergic receptors on cell membranes induced by T_3.

DEIODINASES THAT CONVERT T₄ TO T₃ AND REVERSE-T₃

The conversion of T_4 involves the removal of an iodine atom from the outer (phenolic) ring (5'-) of T_4 by deiodination. Conversion of T_4 to reverse-T_3 (rT_3) involves the removal of an iodine atom from the inner (tyrosyl) ring (5-) by deiodination.[65,p.144] It is not certain whether the same enzyme, T_4 5'-deiodinase, catalyzes conversion to both by-products. It is possible that T_4 5'-deiodinase converts T_4 to T_3 and T_4 5-deiodinase converts T_4 to rT_3. Regardless, conversion of T_4 to T_3 occurs by enzymatic removal of an iodine atom from the 5-' position of the outer ring. This is called 5'-deiodination. Conversion of T_4 to rT_3 occurs by enzymatic removal of an iodine atom from the 5- position on the inner ring. This is termed 5-deiodination. 5'-Deiodination is also called phenolic ring deiodination, and 5-deiodination is also termed tyrosyl ring deiodination. 5'-Deiodination is an activating enzymatic reaction; it generates T_3 which has high bioactivity. 5-Deiodination is a thyroid hormone inactivating reaction; it produces rT_3, which has minimal if any bioactivity. This inactivating path is essential to the recycling of iodide. Increased rT_3, however, is time-limited (see Chapter 2.5, section titled "Proposal of a Sustained Euthyroid Sick Syndrome . . . .") For detailed coverage of deiodination, I refer the reader to the excellent presentation by Kohrle, Hesch, and Leonard in the 6th edition of *Werner's The Thyroid*.[65,pp.144-189]

T₄ 5'-Deiodinases

Through T_4 5'-deiodination (removal of an iodine atom from the 5'- position of the outer ring of T_4), cells of different tissues generate T_3 for local use.[19,pp.170-171][63,p.376] Most of the T_3 that binds to T_3-receptors in cell nuclei is derived from 5'-deiodination.[65,p.146] According to Larsen and coauthors, T_3 produced locally within cells does not appear to be exchanged with T_3 circulating in the blood.[67] The 5'-deiodinases occupy cell membranes; in liver cells, they are stationed in the membrane of the endoplasmic reticulum.[66]

Kohrle et al. wrote that in mammals, deiodination involves removal of iodine atoms from the inner and outer rings of T_4 in a stepwise fashion: an atom is removed from either the outer or inner ring and then the other in an alternating sequence. The researchers also pointed out that of the T_4 secreted daily by the thyroid gland, about 70% is deiodinated to T_3 and rT_3. Deiodination of T_4 outside the thyroid gland accounts for 70%-to-90% of the daily production of T_3. The thyroid gland provides the remaining T_3. The thyroid gland produces only a small amount of rT_3; deiodination in other tissues is responsible for 95%-to-98% of the daily production. Deiodination of T_3 and rT_3 yields various T_2 isoforms. Deiodination of T_2 isoforms yields T_1 isoforms, and removal of the single iodine atom of T_1 yields T_0, the iodine-free thyronine molecule.[65,p.147]

Reverse-T_3 is a competitive substrate for 5'-deiodination of T_4. This substrate may thus be important in the regulation of metabolism through altering the availability of T_3.[65,p.148]

There are at least two 5'-deiodinase isoenzymes, type I and type II.

Type I 5'-Deiodinase. Type I 5'-deiodinase catalyzes conversion of T_4 to T_3 and of rT_3 to T_2 through 5'-deiodination. The membranes of most tissues of the body contain this Type I isoenzyme of 5'-deiodinase, although organ content varies considerably. In humans, the thyroid gland, liver, and kidneys have the highest activity levels of the Type I isoenzyme. Other tissues, such as pituitary tumors, placenta, and white fat cells; and other cells, such as fibroblasts and peripheral mononuclear blood cells, have much lower activity levels.[65,p.149]

Type I 5'-deiodinase is a selenium-dependent enzyme. Selenium deficiency in rats reduced activity of the isoenzyme in liver, kidney, and brain by 90%. Providing abundant selenium normalized activity of the enzyme.[72] The activity of Type I 5'-deiodinase is completely inhibited by the antithyroid medication propylthiouracil.[66]

Type II 5'-Deiodinase. *In vitro* studies indicate that the tissue content and enzymatic activity of type II 5'-deiodinase is more limited than that of type I 5'-deiodinase. Type II 5'-deiodinase preferentially acts on T_4 rather than rT_3. Its activity increases the amounts of T_3 available for local cellular use, and it is most active in membranes of the anterior pituitary, central nervous system, placenta, and brown fat.[65,p.159] In the cerebral cortex, neurons appear to contain most of the type II 5'-deiodinase.[71] It is resistant to inhibition by propylthiouracil.[69]

Studies indicate that local cellular production of T_3 is especially important in the pituitary and brain. T_3-receptors are plentiful in the brain, and the T_3 that interacts with them appears to be derived mainly through type II 5'-deiodinase-catalyzed conversion of T_4 to T_3.[67] This is indicated by the failure of propylthiouracil to inhibit T_4 to T_3 conversion in the brain and pituitary using amounts that block type I 5'-deiodinase in the kidneys, liver, and brain.[67][70]

T_4 5-Deiodinases

Conversion of T_4 to rT_3 by removal of an iodine atom of the 5- position of the inner ring is a major pathway for inactivating T_4. It is also a major route for degrading T_3. This conversion can be catalyzed by 5'-deiodinase (especially type I 5'-deiodinase in liver cells[68]). But there is evidence that 5-deiodinases selectively deiodinate the inner ring of T_4. Activity of the enzymes is high in tissues such as the brain, liver, and placenta. The enzymes are active in almost all other tissues except the pituitary.[65,p.163] The 5-deiodinases occupy membranes; in liver cells, they are most active in the endoplasmic reticulum membrane.[68] One function of these enzymes may be to prevent an adverse accumulation of T_3 in cells. For example, 5-deiodinases are active in the chorionic membranes of the placenta. This activity may explain the high levels of rT_3 in amniotic fluid. Conversion of the mother's T_4 and T_3 to rT_3 in the placenta may reduce the amounts of the active hormones the fetus receives and liberate iodide to be used by the fetus's thyroid gland.[65,p.164]

● THYROID HORMONE TRANSPORT PROTEINS

Most of the thyroid hormone secreted by the thyroid gland attaches to transport proteins in the blood to travel to peripheral tissue cell sites. Robbins stated that it is necessary to understand thyroid hormone transport to properly evaluate and manage patients whose carrier proteins are being influenced by physiological changes, pharmacologic agents, or disease.[50,p.122]

Upon entering the blood, most T_3 and T_4 bind to one of three transport proteins: thyroxine-binding globulin, albumin, or transthyretin (thyroxine-binding prealbumin).[18] These circulating proteins act as stabilizing carriers and eventually deliver the hormones to cells. More than 99% of circulating thyroid hormones are bound to proteins.

Thyroxine-binding globulin binds about 70% of the circulating thyroid hormones. It does so because of its high affinity for T_3 and T_4. Albumin binds 15%-to-20% of the circulating thyroid hormones, but it does so with an affinity lower than that of transthyretin. As a result, the complex of albumin and the hormones also dissociates promptly. Transthyretin binds to only about 10% of the hormones because its affinity for T_3 and T_4 is lower than that of thyroxine-binding globulin. Since the hormones detach readily from transthyretin, it delivers much of the T_3 and T_4 to cells.[50,p.111]

Like the other transport proteins, transthyretin is synthesized by liver cells. Unlike the others, however, it is also synthesized at a high rate[51] by the epithelium of the choroid plexus.[52][53] The high rate of production by the choroid plexus results in a higher concentration of transthyretin, compared to the other transport proteins, in the cerebrospinal fluid.[54] Transthyretin, therefore, is the main thyroid hormone-binding protein in the cerebrospinal fluid.[50,p.111] It is the protein that transports T_4 across the choroid plexus and distributes it throughout the brain.[25]

Bound thyroid hormones are not active physiologically. Only a minute fraction of circulating thyroid hormones are unbound or free at any one time. It is the free hormones, however, that diffuse into cells.[33,p.744] Under normal conditions, the hormones release rapidly to enter cells.[50,p.111] Once inside, the cells convert T_4 to T_3, the metabolically active form which stimulates cellular metabolism (see section above, "Enzymatic Conversion of T_4 to T_3").

Transport proteins bind T_3 far more tenuously than T_4. This enables T_3 to detach from its carrier proteins more easily. It also accounts in part for the shorter biological half-life of T_3 (about 1 day in humans, compared with about 1 week for T_4).[23]

● THYROID-STIMULATING HORMONE (TSH)

When the amount of thyroid hormones in the blood decreases below a certain level, thyrotroph cells in the anterior pituitary gland detect the decrease. These cells are elongated, medium-to-large-sized, and constitute from 1%-to-5% of the cells in the anterior pituitary. They are concentrated in the anteriomedial portion of the anterior pituitary which is a considerable distance from the posterior pituitary.[24] Thyrotroph nuclei are centrally located. The Golgi complex is close to the nucleus, and its prominence varies with the hormonal activity of the thyrotrophs. TSH can be seen in the secretory granules by immunoelectron microscopy.[40,pp.40-41]

In the pituitary glands of rats, some cells contain both immunoreactive TSH and growth hormone.[12] Kovacs, Horvath, and Stefaneau write that these results indicate a close link between somatotrophs (the cells that secrete growth hormone, which is also called somatotropin) and thyrotrophs, and that one may transform to the other. They point out that these two types of anterior pituitary cells cannot be conclusively differentiated. Under special circumstances, one cell type may transform to another cell type and begin secreting the hormone peculiar to that cell type. "Thus," they write, "the 'one cell, one hormone' theory that dominated our thinking for several decades, which recognized five distinct cell types producing the six adenohypophysial hormones, is no longer accepted."[8][40,p.42]

In response to a lowered thyroid hormone level in the blood circulating through the anterior pituitary, the thyrotrophs secrete TSH into the blood. When TSH reaches the thyroid gland, it attaches to TSH-receptors on the membrane surface of thyroid cells.[9] The thyroid gland responds by increasing its synthesis and release of T_3 and T_4. When the thyroid hormone blood level rises above normal, the thyrotrophs respond by reducing their secretion of TSH. This may occur because the increased concentration of thyroid hormone stimulates the thyrotrophs to synthesize a protein or peptide that inhibits the release of TSH.[10]

Effective action of T_3 in the nuclei of the thyrotrophs is partly dependent on the presence of cortisol, a glucocorticoid secreted by the cortices of the adrenal glands. The affinity of T_3-receptors for T_3 in the nuclei of the thyrotrophs is reduced over 50% in the absence of cortisol. This may explain why in Addison's disease (deficient glucocorticoid secretion by the adrenal cortices) serum TSH levels rise even though the circulating T_3 level is normal. A normal T_3 level should inhibit excessive release of TSH by the thyrotrophs, but without sufficient cortisol to act as a synergist, T_3 loses some of its potency in suppressing the thyrotrophs. As a result, they continue to secrete TSH and the blood level rises. The TSH level returns to normal when Addison's patients begin corticosteroid replacement.[39]

The main negative regulator of TSH secretion is direct inhibition of the pituitary thyrotrophs by thyroid hormone. But dopamine and somatostatin (the hypothalamic hormone that inhibits pituitary secretion of growth hormone) also inhibit TSH release.[43,p.9]

The amount of TSH secreted in the body is fairly stable. Strong and persistent stimuli (such as high levels of cortisol or prolonged exposure to cold) are necessary to cause small changes in secretion. By contrast, secretion of ACTH (the anterior pituitary hormone that stimulates cortisol secretion by the adrenal cortices) changes dramatically in response to minor stimuli.[38,p.807]

VARIATIONS IN TSH BIOACTIVITY

The "bioactivity" of TSH refers to its potency in stimulating the synthesis and secretion of thyroid hormones by the thyroid gland. Investigators have found that in some pathophysiological conditions, the bioactivity of TSH is at variance with what has traditionally been considered normal. The two main conditions are general resistance to thyroid hormone and hypothalamic hypothyroidism.[61] TSH bioactivity is increased in some patients with general resistance to thyroid hormone, and it is decreased in some with hypothalamic hypothyroidism. However, the bioactivity of TSH also varies in normal individuals. In such cases, the variability may be a device for transiently altering the amount of thyroid hormone secreted by the thyroid gland. The variation may be pathogenic in some conditions, but a normal physiologic adaption in others.

General Resistance to Thyroid Hormone

In general resistance, the pituitary thyrotrophs and peripheral tissues are partially resistant to thyroid hormone. Because the thyrotrophs are resistant, their secretion of TSH can be inhibited only when the level of circulating thyroid hormones is abnormally high. As a result, some patients (although not all) with general resistance have elevated TSH levels. Both sets of patients, those with elevated TSH levels and those with normal levels, usually have goiter and elevated thyroid hormone levels. Goiter and elevated thyroid hormone levels indicate excess TSH stimulation of the thyroid gland. This is expected in the patient with an elevated TSH, but not in the patient with a normal TSH. Recently, Persani and colleagues[58] found that in general resistance patients with normal TSH levels, the TSH has increased bioactivity. Normal amounts of the high-bioactivity TSH are sufficiently potent to induce goiter and increase thyroid hormone secretion. The bioactivity of the TSH normalizes after patients begin using exogenous T_3.

Hypothalamic Hypothyroidism

The typical patient with hypothalamic (and possibly pituitary) hypothyroidism has a normal basal serum TSH level. However, the TSH may not adequately stimulate thyroid hormone secretion. As a result, the patient's thyroid hormone levels may be improperly low for the normal TSH level.[59,p.297] In such cases, the structure of the patient's TSH molecules varies from normal; this reduces the bioactivity of the molecules.[60] Structurally altered TSH does not bind normally to TSH-receptors on thyroid gland cell membranes. Due to this, normal levels of the altered TSH do not adequately stimulate the gland to secrete normal amounts of thyroid hormones. As a result, the patient has some degree of hypothyroidism despite normal basal TSH levels.

There is currently a myth almost ubiquitous in the medical profession that the basal TSH is sufficient for identifying hypothyroid patients. Until this myth is abandoned, most patients with central hypothyroidism and low-bioactivity TSH are likely to continue to be misdiagnosed as euthyroid.

Other Groups of Individuals with TSH of Low Bioactivity

Beck-Peccoz and Persani pointed out that TSH, like other pituitary glycoprotein hormones, is produced as a mixture of isoforms. The different isoforms have variable degrees of bioactivity. They wrote, "The secretion of TSH molecules with altered bioactivity plays an important pathogenic role in various thyroid disorders, while in some particular physiological conditions, the bioactivity of TSH may vary in order to adjust thyroid hormone secretion to temporary needs."[61] Accordingly, researchers have reported finding low bioactive TSH in patients with thyroid hormone resistance and hypothalamic hypothyroidism, and in some patients with primary hypothyroidism, nonthyroidal illness, and TSH-secreting pituitary adenomas. In addition, researchers have found TSH of low bioactivity in normal subjects during the nocturnal TSH surge and normal fetuses during the first trimester of pregnancy.[61]

● THYROTROPIN- RELEASING HORMONE (TRH)

The hypothalamus helps maintain a normal metabolic rate by secreting thyrotropin releasing hormone (TRH). Nerve endings in the medial eminence of the hypothalamus secrete the TRH.[14] From the medial eminence, the TRH travels through the portal venous system traversing the stalk that joins the hypothalamus and pituitary glands. Upon reaching the anterior pituitary, the TRH directly stimulates the thyrotrophs to secrete TSH. The TSH then, in turn, induces the thyroid gland to release T_3 and T_4.

Completely blocking the portal blood system *diminishes* TSH secretion by the thyrotrophs. They continue, however, to secrete at least small amounts. This shows that the pituitary secretes TSH in response to low levels of T_3 and T_4 independently of TRH stimulation.

TRH Effects in Thyrotroph Cells

Upon binding to a TRH-receptor on a pituitary thyrotroph cell membrane, TRH stimulates activity of phospholipase C. Phospholipase C rapidly catalyzes the hydrolysis of phosphatidyl-inosital 4,5-bisphosphate to inositol 1,4,5-bisphosphate and 1,2-diacylglycerol. In turn, 1,2-diacylglycerol activates intracellular protein kinase C.[21,p.235] This enzyme stimulates production of TSH.

Calcium is also an activator of TSH production. In response to TRH, the free calcium concentration in the thyrotrophs promptly rises. The calcium concentration quickly decreases, but it remains somewhat elevated for an extended time. The rapid rise in the calcium concentration results from two processes: (1) the release of intracellular calcium stores, and (2) the sustained but somewhat lower elevation that results from the influx of calcium into the cell.[21,p.236]

TRH also induces in the pituitary a dose-related decrease in T_3-receptors, and this reduces responsiveness of the thyrotrophs to T_3.[22] The reduced T_3-receptor density disinhibits the thyrotrophs and increases their secretion of TSH.[21,p.234]

Effects of Thyroid Hormone on TRH

An excess or deficiency of thyroid hormone has little effect on the entire TRH content of the hypothalamus. However, thyroid hormone decreases TRH secretion as part of a negative feedback mechanism.[3,p.261][16][17][21,p.234]

TRH gene expression increases TRH mRNA in the paraventricular nuclei of the hypothalamus. The nuclei are targets of thyroid hormone. During thyroid hormone deficiency, TRH mRNA levels increased in the paraventricular nuclei; thyroid hormone replacement lowered the mRNA levels.[31][32] In rats with bilateral lesions of the paraventricular nuclei, induced hypothyroidism did not result in a normal rise in serum TSH and TSH-subunit mRNA.[41] *In vitro*, T_3 acutely induced the hypothalamus to release somatostatin,[42] the hormone that inhibits growth hormone and TSH secretion by the pituitary.[43,p.9] By affecting the hypothalamus in these ways, thyroid hormone *indirectly* inhibits secretion of TSH by the pituitary. These indirect inhibitory effects are in addition to the *direct* effect of thyroid hormone on the pituitary thyrotrophs.[3,p.261] Thyroid hormone also changed the number of TRH receptors on the thyrotrophs. In hypothyroid animals, TRH-binding to anterior pituitary membranes increased twofold.[21,p.234] TRH-binding to the membranes was reduced by thyroid hormone replacement.[4][5] T_3 also reduced the density of TRH receptors in TSH-secreting mouse tumors and in the GH_3 strain of pituitary cells in culture.[6][7]

THE HYPOTHALAMUS AND TRH AS A FINE CONTROL FOR TSH SECRETION

High levels of T_3 and T_4 inhibit secretion of TSH in two ways. The main way is direct inhibition of the thyrotrophs. A weaker way is inhibition of TRH secretion by the hypothalamus. The hypothalamus and the TRH it secretes act as a fine control device that adjusts how sensitively the thyrotrophs respond to thyroid hormone.[13] This fine control function clearly operates when individuals are exposed to a cold environment.[15] The metabolic rates of military personnel increase when they live in Arctic regions for several months. Eskimos have unusually high basal metabolic rates. There is also a comparatively high rate of toxic thyroid goiters in people living in cold climates.[35,p.804] Nerve signals originating in chilled skin activate the anterior hypothalamus to increase its secretion of TRH. The TRH raises the set-point of the thyrotrophs for responding to thyroid hormone, much like adjusting a thermostat. As a result, amounts of thyroid hormone circulating through the pituitary that would normally suppress TSH secretion are less effective in doing so. More TSH than normal is secreted. The increased amounts of TSH reaching the thyroid gland stimulate the release of greater than normal amounts of thyroid hormone. The exposure of cells to the increased amounts of thyroid hormone causes a sustained acceleration of the metabolic rate. *It is important to note that the increased metabolic rate is not uniform in all body tissues.* The rate increases to some degree in most tissues. The degree of increase, however, varies with the sensitivity of each tissue to thyroid hormone.

This fine control function of the hypothalamus and TRH, however, is not as predictable as some physiology texts might suggest. In 1986, for 42 weeks researchers studied humans residing in Antarctica. During that time, total and free T_4 levels in their serum did not change, while the total and free T_3 in their serum fell significantly. Basal TSH values did not change, but TSH responses to TRH injections increased by 50%. It is of interest that the subjects' serum cortisol levels rose through the first 21 weeks of the study. By the end of the study, cortisol levels had

fallen back to baseline. Elevated cortisol levels ordinarily suppress the TSH response to injected TRH, and decrease T_3 levels by blocking conversion of T_4 to T_3. While the subjects' T_3 levels were reduced, suggesting inhibited T_4 to T_3 conversion, their TSH responses to TRH *increased*.[37] These results are puzzling.[38,p.807] It is possible, however, that the exaggerated TSH responses to injected TRH could have resulted from two mechanisms. First, the elevated cortisol may have blocked conversion of T_4 to T_3 in the anterior pituitary. This would have reduced the amount of T_3 available to inhibit TSH synthesis, allowing some TSH reserve to accumulate. Second, the cold-induced increase in TRH secretion may have reduced the T_3-receptor count in the thyrotrophs. This could have further impeded T_3 suppression of TSH synthesis (the proposed increased set-point of the thyrotrophs) and favored accumulation of a TSH reserve. The reserve TSH could have been liberated by the injected TRH, causing the exaggerated post-injection increases.

REFERENCES

1. Guyton, A.C.: *Textbook of Medical Physiology,* 7th edition. Philadelphia, W.B. Saunders Co., 1986.
2. Field, J.B.: Studies on the mechanism of action of thyroid-stimulating hormone. *Metabolism,* 17:226-245, 1968.
3. Wondisford, F.E., Magner, J.A., and Weintraub, B.D.: Thyrotropin: chemistry and biosynthesis of thyrotropin. In *Werner and Ingbar's The Thyroid: A Fundamental and Clinical Text,* 6th edition. Edited by L.E. Braverman and R.D. Utiger, New York, J.B. Lippincott Co., 1991, pp.257-276.
4. De Lean, A., Ferland, L., Drouin, J., et al.: Modulation of pituitary thyrotropin releasing hormone receptor levels by oestrogens and thyroid hormones. *Endocrinol.,* 100:1496, 1977.
5. Hinkle, P.M., Perrone, M.H., and Schonbrunn, A.: Mechanism of thyroid hormone inhibition of thyrotropin-releasing hormone action. *Endocrinol.,* 108:199, 1981.
6. Hinkle, P.M. and Goh, K.B.C.: Regulation of thyrotropin-releasing hormone receptors and responses by L-triiodothyronine in dispersed rat pituitary cell cultures. *Endocrinol.,* 110:1725, 1982.
7. Hinkle, P.M. and Tashjian, A.H.: Thyrotropin-releasing hormone regulates the number of its own receptors in the GH3 strain of pituitary cells in culture. *Biochemistry,* 14: 3845, 1975.
8. Kovacs, K., Horvath, E., Asa, S.L., Stefaneau, L., and Sano, T.: Pituitary cells producing more than one hormone: human pituitary adenomas. *Trends Endocrinol. Metab.,* 1: 95, 1989.
9. Pastan, I., Roth, J., and Macchia, V.: Binding of hormone to tissue: the first step in polypeptide hormone action. *Proc. Natl. Acad. Sci.,* 56:1802-1809, 1966.
10. Hershman, J.M. and Pittman, J.A.: Control of thyrotropin

secretion in man. *N. Eng. J. Med.*, 285(18):999, 1971.

11. Degroot, L.J. and Niepomniszcze, H.: Biosynthesis of thyroid hormone: basic and clinical aspects. *Metabolism*, 26 (6):665-718, 1977.

12. Losinski, N.E., Horvath, E., and Kovacs, K.: Double-labeling immunogold electron-microscopic study of hormonal colocalization in nontumorous and adenomatous rat pituitaries. *Am. J. Anat.*, 185:236, 1989.

13. Sterling, K. and Lazarus, J.H.: The thyroid and its control. *Ann. Rev. Physiol.*, 39:360, 1977.

14. McKelvy, J.F., Sheridan, M., Joseph, S., Phelps, C.H., and Perrie, S.: Biosynthesis of thyrotropin-releasing hormone in organ cultures of the guinea pig median eminence. *Endocrinol.*, 97:908-913, 1975.

15. Reichlin, S., Martin, J.B., Mitnick, M.A., Boshans, R.L., Grimm, Y., Bollinger, J., Gordon, J. and Malacara, J.: The hypothalamus in pituitary thyroid regulation. *Rec. Prog. Horm. Res.*, 28:229-286, 1972.

16. Joseph, S.A., Scott, D.E., Vaala, S.S., Knigge, K.M., and Krobisch-Dudley, G.: Localization and content of thyrotropin releasing factor (TRH) in median eminence of the hypothalamus. *Acta Endocrinol. Copenhagen*, 74:215-225, 1973.

17. Knigge, K.M. and Joseph, S.A.: Neural regulation of TSH secretion: sites of thyroxine feedback. *Neuroendocrinol.*, 8:273-288, 1971.

18. Oppenheimer, J.H.: Role of plasma proteins in the binding, distribution and metabolism of the thyroid hormones. *N. Engl. J. Med.*, 278:1153-1162, 1968.

19. Tepperman, J. and Tepperman, H.M.: *Metabolic and Endocrine Physiology*, 5th edition. Chicago, Year Book Medical Publishers, Inc., 1987.

20. Haynes, R.C., Jr.: Thyroid and antithyroid drugs. In *Goodman and Gilman's The Pharmacological Basis of Therapeutics*, 8th edition. New York, Pergamon Press, 1990, pp.1361-1383.

21. Scanlon, M.F.: Neuroendocrine control of thyrotropin secretion. In *Werner and Ingbar's The Thyroid: A Fundamental and Clinical Text*, 6th edition. Edited by L.E. Braverman and R.D. Utiger, New York, J.B. Lippincott Co., 1991, pp.230-256.

22. Kaji, H. and Hinkle, P.M.: Regulation of thyroid hormone receptors and responses to thyrotropin-releasing hormone in GH_4C_1 cells. *Endocrinol.*, 121:1697, 1987.

23. Utiger, R.D.: Serum triiodothyronine in man. *Ann. Rev. Med.*, 25:289, 1974.

24. Kovacs, K. and Horvath, E.: Cytology. In *Tumors of the Pituitary Gland: Atlas of Tumor Pathology*, 2nd series, fascile 21. Washington, D.C., Armed Forces Institute of Pathology, 1986, p.16.

25. Dickson, P.W., Aldred, A.R., Mentiny, J.G.T., Marley, P.D., Sawyer, W.H., and Schreiber, G.: Thyroxine transport in the choroid plexus. *J. Biol. Chem.*, 262:13907, 1987.

26. Romanes, G.J.: *Cunningham's Textbook of Anatomy*, 11th edition. London, Oxford University Press, 1972.

27. Doniach, I.: The structure of the thyroid gland. *J. Clin. Pathol.*, Supplement 20:309-317, 1967.

28. Pitt-Rivers, R.: The biosynthesis of thyroid hormones. *J. Clin. Pathol.*, Supplement 20, 318-322, 1967.

29. DeGroot, L.J.: Physiological precepts in thyroid diagnosis. In *Diagnosis and Treatment of Common Thyroid Diseases*. Edited by H.A. Selenkow and F. Hoffman, Amsterdam, *Excerpta Medica*, 1971, pp.3-14.

30. Halmi, N.S. and Pitt-Rivers, R.: The iodine pools of rat thyroid. *Endocrinol.*, 70:660-668, 1962.

31. Koller, K.J., Wolff, R.S., Warden, M.K., and Zoeller, R.T.: Thyroid hormones regulate levels of thyrotropin-releasing hormone mRNA in the paraventricular nucleus. *Proc. Natl. Acad. Sci.*, 84:7329, 1987.

32. Segerson, T.P., Kauer, J., Wolfe, H.C., et al.: Thyroid hormone regulates TRH biosynthesis in the paraventricular nucleus of the rat hypothalamus. *Science*, 238:78, 1987.

33. Davidsohn, I. and Henry, J.B.: *Clinical Diagnosis by Laboratory Methods*, 15th edition. Philadelphia, W.B. Saunders Company, 1974.

34. Cooper, J.R., Bloom, F.E., and Roth, R.H.: *The Biochemical Basis of Neuropharmacology*, 5th edition. New York, Oxford University Press, 1986.

35. Guyton, A.C.: *Textbook of Medical Physiology*, 8th edition. Philadelphia, W.B. Saunders Co., 1991.

36. Taurog, A.: Hormone synthesis: thyroid iodine metabolism. In *Werner and Ingbar's The Thyroid: A Fundamental and Clinical Text*, 6th edition. Edited by L.E. Braverman and R.D. Utiger, New York, J.B. Lippincott Co., 1991, pp.51-97.

37. Reed, H.L., Burman, K.D., Shakir, K.M.M., and O'Brian, J.T.: Alterations in the hypothalamic-pituitary-thyroid axis after prolonged residence in Antarctica. *Clin. Endocrinol.* (Oxford), 25:55, 1986.

38. Christy, N.P.: The adrenal cortex in thyrotoxicosis. In *Werner and Ingbar's The Thyroid: A Fundamental and Clinical Text*, 6th edition. Edited by L.E. Braverman and R.D. Utiger, New York, J.B. Lippincott Co., 1991, pp.806-815.

39. DeNayer, P., Dozin, B., Vandeput, Y., Bottazzo, F.C., and Crabbe, J.: Altered interaction between triiodothyronine and its nuclear receptors in the absence of cortisol: a proposed mechanism for increased thyrotropin secretion in thyroid deficient states. *Eur. J. Invest.*, 17:106, 1987.

40. Kovacs, K., Horvath, E., and Stefaneau, L.: Anatomy and pathology of the thyrotrophs. In *Werner and Ingbar's The Thyroid: A Fundamental and Clinical Text*, 6th edition. Edited by L.E. Braverman and R.D. Utiger, New York, J.B. Lippincott Co., 1991, pp.40-50.

41. Taylor, T., Wondisford, F.E., Blaine, T., and Weintraub, B.D.: The paraventricular nucleus of the hypothalamus has a major role in thyroid hormone feedback regulation of thyrotropin synthesis and secretion. *Endocrinol.*, 126:317, 1990.

42. Berelowitz, M., Maeda, K., Harris, S., and Frohman, L.A.: The effect of alterations in the pituitary-thyroid axis on hypothalamic content and *in vitro* release of somatostatin-like immunoreactivity. *Endocrinol.*, 107:24, 1980.

43. Pintar, J.E. and Toran-Allerand, C.D.: Normal development of the hypothalamic-pituitary-thyroid axis. In *Werner and Ingbar's The Thyroid: A Fundamental and Clinical Text*, 6th edition. Edited by L.E. Braverman and R.D. Utiger, New York, J.B. Lippincott Co., 1991, pp.7-21.

44. Stanbury, B.J. and Morris, M.L.: Deiodination of diiodotyrosine by cell-free systems. *J. Biol. Chem.*, 233:106, 1958.

45. Yoshinari, M., Taurog, A., and Krupp, P.P.: Purification of thyroid lysosomes by colloidal silica density gradient centrifugation. *Endocrinol.*, 117:580, 1985.

46. Yoshinari, M. and Taurog, A.: Lysosomal digestion of thyroglobulin: role of cathepsin D and thiol proteases. *Endocrinol.*, 117:1621, 1985.

47. Capen, C.C.: Anatomy, comparative anatomy, and histology of the thyroid. In *Werner and Ingbar's The Thyroid: A Fundamental and Clinical Text*, 6th edition. Edited by L.E. Braverman and R.D. Utiger, New York, J.B. Lippincott Co., 1991, pp.22-40.

48. Tice, L.W. and Wollman, S.H.: Ultrastructural localization of peroxidase on pseudopods and other structures of the typical thyroid epithelial cell. *Endocrinol.*, 94:1555, 1974.

49. Kimura, T., Okajima, F., Sho, K., Kabayashi, I., and Kondo, Y.: Thyrotropin-induced hydrogen peroxide production in FRTL-5 thyroid cells is mediated not by adenosine 3',5'-monophosphate, but by Ca^{2+} signaling followed by phospholipase-A2 activation and potentiated by an adenosine derivative. *Endocrinol.*, 136(1):116-123, 1995.

50. Robbins, J.: Thyroid hormone transport proteins and the physiology of hormone binding. In *Werner and Ingbar's The Thyroid: A Fundamental and Clinical Text*, 6th edition. Edited by L.E. Braverman and R.D. Utiger, New York, J.B. Lippincott Co., 1991, pp.111-125.

51. Dickson, P.W. and Schreiber, G.: High levels of messenger RNA for transthyretin (prealbumen) in human choroid plexus. *Neurosci. Lett.*, 66:311, 1986.

52. Soprano, D.R., Herbert, J., Soprano, K.J., Schon, E.A., and Goodman, D.S.: Demonstration of transthyretin mRNA in the brain and other extrahepatic tissues in the rat. *J. Biol. Chem.*, 260:1793, 1985.

53. Dickson, P.W., Aldred, A.R., Marley, P.D., Bannister, D., and Schreiber, G.: Rat choroid plexus specializes in the synthesis and the secretion of transthyretin (prealbumin). *J. Biol. Chem.*, 261:3475, 1986.

54. Bartalena, L.: Recent achievements in studies on thyroid hormone binding proteins. *Endocr. Rev.*, 11:47, 1990.

55. Pittman, H.A., Brown, R.W., and Register, H.B., Jr.: Biological activity of 3,3',5'-triiodo-DL-thyronine. *Endocrinol.*, 70:79, 1962.

56. Chopra, I.J.: Nature, sources, and relative biologic significance of circulating thyroid hormones. In *Werner and Ingbar's The Thyroid: A Fundamental and Clinical Text*, 6th edition. Edited by L.E. Braverman and R.D. Utiger, New York, J.B. Lippincott Co., 1991, pp.126-143.

57. Money, W.L., Kimaoka, S., Rawson, R.W., and Kroc, R.L.: Comparative effects of thyroxine analogues in experimental animals. *Ann. N.Y. Acad. Sci.*, 86:512, 1960.

58. Persani, L., Asteria, C., Tonacchera, M., et al.: Evidence for the secretion of thyrotropin with enhanced bioactivity in syndromes of thyroid hormone resistance. *J. Clin. Endocrinol. Metab.*, 78(5):1034-1039, 1994.

59. Toft, A.D.: Thyrotropin: assay, secretory physiology, and testing of regulation. In *Werner's The Thyroid: A Fundamental and Clinical Text*, 5th edition. Edited by S.H. Ingbar and L.E. Braverman, Philadelphia, J.B. Lippincott Co., 1986, pp.287-305.

60. Beck-Peccoz, P., Acr, S., Menezes-Ferreira, M., Faglia, G., and Weintraub, B.: Decreased receptor binding of biologically inactive thyrotropin in central hypothyroidism. *N.*

Engl. J. Med., 312:1085, 1985.

61. Beck-Peccoz, P. and Persani, L.: Variable biological activity of thyroid-stimulating hormone. *Euro. J. Endocrinol*, 131(4):331-340, 1994.

62. Goldfine, O., Smith, G.J., Simmons, G.C., et al.: Activities of thyroid hormones and related compounds in an *in vitro* thymocyte assay. *J. Biol. Chem.*, 251:4233, 1976.

63. Larsen, P.R., and Silva, J.E.: Intrapituitary mechanism of control of TSH secretion. In *Molecular Basis of Thyroid Hormone Action*. Edited by J.H. Oppenheimer and H.H. Samuels, New York, Academic Press, Inc., 1983, pp.351-385.

64. Ball, S.G., Sokolov J, and Chin, W.W.: 3,5-Diiodo-L-thyronine (T_2) has selective thyromimetic effects *in vivo* and *in vitro*. *J. Mol. Endocrinol.*, 19(2):137-147, 1997.

65. Kohrle, J., Hesch, R.D., and Leonard, J.L.: Intracellular pathways of iodothyronine metabolism. In *Werner and Ingbar's The Thyroid: A Fundamental and Clinical Text*, 6th edition. Edited by L.E. Braverman and R.D. Utiger, New York, J.B. Lippincott Co., 1991, pp.144-189.

66. Visser, T.J., van der Does-Tobe, I., Docter, R., and Hennemann, G.: Conversion of thyroxine into triiodothyronine by rat liver homogenate. *Biochem. J.*, 150:489, 1975.

67. Larsen, P.R., Silva, J.E., and Kaplan, M.M.: Relationship between circulating and intracellular thyroid hormones: physiological and clinical implications. *Endocr. Rev.*, 2:87, 1981.

68. Fekkes, D., van Overmeeren-Kaptein, E., Docter, R., Hennemann, G., and Visser, T.J.: Location of the rat liver iodothyronine deiodinating enzymes in the endoplasmic reticulum. *Biochim. Biophys. Acta*, 587:12, 1979.

69. Kaplan, M.M. and Shaw, E.A.: Type II iodothyronine 5'-deiodination by human and rat placenta *in vitro*. *J. Clin. Endocrinol. Metab.*, 59:253, 1984.

70. Maeda, M. and Ingbar, S.H.: Evidence that the 5'-monodeiodinases for thyroxine and 3,3',5'-triiodothyronine in the rat pituitary are separate enzymes. *Endocrinol.*, 114:747, 1984.

71. Gavin, L.A., Moeller, M., McHahon, F., Gulli, R., and Cavalieri, R.R.: Cyclic adenosine 3',5'-monophosphate and glucose stimulate thyroxine 5'-deiodinase type II in cultured mouse neuroblastoma cells. *Metabolism*, 39:474, 1990.

72. Arthur, J.R., Nichol, F., and Beckett, J.: Hepatic iodothyronine 5'-deiodinase: the role of selenium. *Biochem. J.*, 272:537, 1990.

73. Escobar-Morreale, H.F., Escobar del Rey, F., Obregón, M.J., and Morreale de Escobar, G.: Only the combined treatment with thyroxine and triiodothyronine ensures euthyroidism in all tissues of the thyroidectomized rat. *Endocrinol.*, 137(6):2490-2502, 1996.

74. DiStefano, J.J.: Modeling approaches and models of the distribution and disposal of thyroid hormones. In *Thyroid Hormone Metabolism*. Edited by G. Henneman, New York, Marcel Dekker, 1985, pp.39-76.

75. Pilo, A., Iervasi, G., Vitek, F., Ferdeghini, M., Cazzuola, F., and Bianchi, R.: Thyroidal and peripheral production of 3,5,3'-triiodothyronine in humans by multicompartmental analysis. *Am. J. Physiol.*, 258:E715-E726, 1990.

76. Escobar-Morreale, H.F., Obregón, M.J., Escobar del Rey, F., and Morreale de Escobar, G.: Replacement therapy for

hypothyroidism with thyroxine alone does not ensure eu-thyroidism in all tissues, as studied in thyroidectomized rats. *J. Clin. Invest.*, 96:2828-2838, 1995.

77. Obregón, M.J., Roelsema, F., Escobar del Rey, F., Morre-ale de Escobar, G., and Querido, A.: Are there hidden pools of tri-iodothyronine? (Abstract) *Acta Endocrinol.*

Suppl., 204:30A, 1976.

78. Obregón, M.J., Roelsema, F., Morreale de Escobar, G., Escobar del Rey, F., and Querido, A.: Exchange of triiodo-thyronine derived from thyroxine with circulating triiodo-thyronine as studied in the rat. *Clin. Endocrinol.*, 10:305-315, 1979.

2.2

Cellular Actions of Thyroid Hormones

The plasma membrane is the outer wall of the cell. Substances enter or exit the cell through this membrane. Thyroid hormone transport across the plasma membrane is energy-dependent, and the hormone crosses mainly by endocytosis. Thyroid hormone also appears to diffuse into the plasma membrane and interact there with proteins involved in hormone and sugar transport into the cell.

The cytoplasm is held between the plasma membrane and the nuclear membrane. The nuclear membrane walls off and contains the nucleoplasm. In the cell's nucleus, the codes contained in the DNA molecules of the chromosomes are transcribed to messenger RNA (mRNA) for protein synthesis. mRNA carries the code in its base sequence to the ribosomes in the cytoplasm. tRNAs bring amino acids to the ribosomes where enzymes catalyze linkage of the amino acids in a specific order according to the base sequence of the mRNA. The resulting peptide or protein has one of two initial destinations. It may move to sites in the cell where it is immediately used, or it may travel to the Golgi complex. The protein destined for the Golgi complex is inserted into the endoplasmic reticulum while undergoing synthesis; after modification in the reticulum, it proceeds to the Golgi complex. The Golgi complex processes the protein and releases it for its next destination. Most often, the destination is the cell surface, either for deposit in the membrane or excretion from the cell.

The cell is a site of constantly interacting anabolic and catabolic chemical processes. The general term for these processes is metabolism. Thyroid hormone is a major regulator of cell metabolism. The hormone

regulates cell metabolism mainly by controlling transcription of specific genes. However, the hormone may also influence translation of mRNAs independently of its genomic effects.

The metabolic processes included in this chapter are those most relevant to an understanding of the cellular actions of thyroid hormone. Among the processes most potently affected by thyroid hormone is energy production. The hormone controls transport of energy-yielding substances across the plasma membrane and processing of the substances in the cytoplasm and the mitochondria. Thyroid hormone increases sugar uptake by cell membranes and transport of amino acids across the membranes.

The breakdown of glucose and glycogen and the synthesis of glycogen from glucose occur in the cytoplasm. Thyroid hormone regulates these processes mainly by controlling (1) the availability of various enzymes involved in the processes and (2) the ratio of α- to β-adrenergic receptors on cell membranes.

The mitochondria carry out functions that are regulated either directly or indirectly by thyroid hormone: (1) oxidation of some of the end products of glycolysis and the citric acid cycle, (2) oxidation of fatty acids, (3) creation of high-energy ATP molecules from ADP, (4) breakdown of amino acids, and (5) synthesis of non-essential amino acids.

Thyroid hormone also contributes to cell homeostasis by increasing the level and activity of Na^+/K^+-ATPase and increasing activity of the Na^+/K^+ pump. By these effects, the hormone contributes to the transport of substances by the Na^+ gradient, and helps maintain cell volume, the electrical potential of mem-

branes, and the ionic composition of the cytoplasm. Thyroid hormone also increases the levels of the mitochondrial enzyme α-glycerophosphate dehydrogenase. The parallel increase in α-glycerophosphate dehydrogenase and Na⁺/K⁺-ATPase may largely account for the heat-producing effect of thyroid hormone.

Thyroid hormone regulates the levels of various enzymes and electron carriers necessary for the metabolism of substrates for ATP production. The enzymes and carriers take part in glycolysis, the citric acid cycle, and the electron transport system. Thyroid hormone affects metabolic processes in the cytoplasm, but its major metabolism-regulating effects occur in the mitochondria. The hormone directly and indirectly influences mitochondrial structure and function; it increases both the size and activity of mitochondria as well as their oxygen consumption and ATP production.

A number of micronutrients play synergistic roles in the metabolic processes regulated by thyroid hormone. Folic acid, vitamin B₁₂, and the amino acid glycine are essential to the synthesis of adenine, the base component of the ATP molecule. Vitamin B₁ as thiamine pyrophosphate is also a component of the multienzyme complex pyruvate dehydrogenase. Pyruvate carboxylase, which converts pyruvate to the citric acid cycle intermediate oxaloacetate, contains four molecules of the vitamin biotin. Each of the four subunits of the enzyme also binds one manganese ion. Niacin (vitamin B₃) is a constituent of NADH, a compound that transports electrons to the electron transport chain for generation of ATP. Riboflavin (vitamin B₂) is a constituent of FADH₂ which also transports electrons to the electron transport system. Four vitamins take part in the decarboxylation of pyruvate to acetyl-CoA: niacin, thiamine, riboflavin, and pantothenic acid. Magnesium and lipoic acid (a coenzyme that contains two sulfur atoms) are also involved. Magnesium and vitamin B₆ must be present for the normal interactions of malate in the malate-aspartate shuttle involved in the transfer of electrons across the mitochondrial membrane. Coenzyme Q (ubiquinone) and the heme-containing cytochromes also take part in electron transport within the electron transport system. (The iron of the heme group is synthesized from glycine and succinyl-CoA.)

All patients taking exogenous thyroid hormone should also take supplemental nutrients. Supplementation is important for two reasons. First, supplements can help provide sufficient cellular levels of the nutrients for optimum synergism with thyroid hormone.

Second, taking supplements can avert nutritional deficiencies that might be induced by thyroid hormone accelerating the chemical pathways that the nutrients take part in.

To write separately of the cellular and molecular aspects of thyroid hormone action is to make an artificial distinction. To explain thyroid hormone action, however, the distinction must be made. In *Werner's The Thyroid*, Davis[1] and Oppenheimer[2] made a distinction between cellular and molecular aspects. Davis explained the basis of their distinction: molecular aspects are genomic—they involve the interaction of thyroid hormone with the genes in cell nuclei.[1,p.190] Cellular aspects are nongenomic—they involve the plasma membrane, cytoplasm, and mitochondria, but not the nucleus. In this and the following chapter, I maintain their distinction for the most part, but some overlap is unavoidable between the cellular and molecular aspects of thyroid hormone action. Some of these aspects are virtually impossible to tease into purely cellular or purely genomic components for the sake of discussion. Malic enzyme and Na⁺/K⁺-ATPase are two examples. I include information on these genomic products (as well as some others) in this chapter for one reason: Understanding certain aspects of cell function critically depends upon familiarity with the cellular roles of these enzymes. So I include some T₃-induced gene transcription products in this chapter. Nonetheless, the chapter is largely an overview of the influence of thyroid hormones on cellular structures and processes, emphasizing the sites of action of the hormones.

● METABOLISM

Metabolism is the sum of all the chemical reactions that occur in the cell. From a biochemical point of view, cell life can be defined as a network of highly integrated and carefully regulated metabolic pathways. Each pathway contributes to the activities the cell must carry out.[31,p.315][34,p.178] In that the cell is the functional unit of the body, cell metabolism is the underpinning of whole body structure and function. The state of health of the individual and his continued biopsychological existence are ultimately dependent upon the status of his cell metabolism.[34,p.178] Psychological factors can alter physiology to a considerable extent. However, all human functions, both physical and psychological, are most potently regulated by the chemical processes in cells that we call metabolism. Interpreting our social environment as threatening or hopeless, for example, is accompanied by biochemical, hormonal, and physiological changes that may eventually adversely affect our health. But alteration of cell metabolism by food, water, or oxygen deprivation will cause a more immediate and extreme change in our biopsychological state.

Metabolic pathways are divided into two types. Pathways in which compounds are synthesized are termed anabolic, from the Greek word for "up." Pathways concerned with degradation of compounds are called catabolic, from the Greek word for "down."[34,p.178] Thyroid hormone is unusual among hormones in that it influences both anabolic and catabolic pathways.[88,p.48]

Anabolic pathways provide for growth and repair; catabolic pathways furnish the energy that drives anabolic pathways. Energy-requiring and energy-yielding reactions must be efficiently coupled. (Coupling is a process in which one or more products of a chemical reaction are the subsequent substrates of a second reaction.) Coupling of energy-requiring and energy-yielding reactions is accomplished in the cell by adenosine triphosphate (ATP). ATP is a high-energy phosphorylated compound. It stores and conserves energy derived from catabolized food substances, and it releases the energy at proper times to drive anabolic reactions. Essentially, as Marks wrote, "ATP transfers energy from the processes that produce it to those that use it."[156,p.108] ATP is involved in virtually every cellular energy-based reaction. Therefore, it is appropriate to cover its role in relation to the actions of thyroid hormones. I also include information on the role of vitamins and minerals in energy metabolism because they are synergists to thyroid hormone—the combined metabolism-regulating effects of the hormone and these micronutrients are greater than that of either when the other is deficient.

All chemical pathways of metabolism must be carefully regulated to ensure that their activity levels correspond closely to cellular needs.[34,pp.178&224] Otherwise, cell dysfunction and eventually cellular structural abnormalities may result. Two common causes of inadequate regulation of metabolism are (1) a deficiency of thyroid hormone in the cell and (2) inadequate cellular action of normal concentrations of the hormone. Thyroid hormone is central to metabolism. In fact, Guyton terms them "thyroid *metabolic* hormones."[33,p.831] How a deficiency or inadequate action of thyroid hormone in cells can cause and sustain fi-

bromyalgia is best explained against a background understanding of the normal action of thyroid hormone within the cell.

Another factor that can cause careful regulation of chemical pathways to fail and contribute to fibromyalgia is inadequate glucose breakdown due to deficiencies of various B complex vitamins. B complex vitamins (and other nutrients) are expended during chemical reactions in the cell, especially during carbohydrate metabolism. Exogenous thyroid hormone, in dosages sufficient to improve fibromyalgia status, accelerates the rate of the reactions in carbohydrate metabolism. Because of the acceleration, in an individual with a marginally-adequate intake of B complex vitamins, the use of exogenous thyroid hormone may induce B vitamin insufficiencies or frank deficiencies. It is important, therefore, for the patient taking exogenous thyroid hormone to also take B vitamin supplements.

● **THE EFFECTS OF THYROID HORMONE ON CELL STRUCTURE AND FUNCTION**

Table 2.2.1 displays the cell structures I describe in this section. To the right of the name of each structure is a list of the metabolic processes that occur in that structure. In the sections below, I describe the structures, the processes they host, and the effects of thyroid hormone on those structures and processes.

An organelle is a membrane-confined particle of living substance in the cell. Mitochondria, endoplasmic reticulum, ribosomes, and lysosomes are organelles. Each organelle provides a function vital to the health and productivity of the cell. Below, I briefly describe those organelles that are relevant to understanding how inadequate thyroid hormone regulation of cell function may mediate the symptoms and signs of fibromyalgia.

PROTOPLASM

Protoplasm is the general name for the semiliquid inside the cell that is considered the essential material of all plant and animal cells. It is a viscous colloidal suspension composed of water and a vast array of other chemicals. Its composition varies in different types of cells. In brain cells, for example, it contains a high concentration of lipids. In skeletal muscles, it contains a high percentage of the contractile proteins, actin and myosin. Most cell protoplasm contains "inclusions," temporarily inactive stored cell products such as droplets of lipid and granules of glycogen.

Table 2.2.1. The cell structures included in this chapter and the processes that occur in each.

Structure	Process
CYTOPLASM	Glycogen synthesis and breakdown Glycolysis Protein and fatty acid synthesis Suspension of lipid droplets and glycogen
GOLGI APPARATUS	Packaging and secretion of proteins
LYSOSOMES	Breakdown of organic compounds
MITOCHONDRIA	Citric acid cycle Cell respiration Electron transport chain Nonessential amino acid synthesis
NUCLEUS	RNA synthesis
ROUGH ENDOPLASMIC RETICULUM	Protein synthesis
SMOOTH ENDOPLASMIC RETICULUM	Synthesis of membranes Synthesis of cholesterol Metabolism of drugs

The protoplasm inside the double-layered membranous wall of the nucleus is called the nucleoplasm. The protoplasm held within the cell's plasma membrane, excluding the nucleoplasm, is called the cytoplasm or cytosol. The endoplasmic reticulum is suspended in the cytoplasm. The chemical constituents of protoplasm engage in metabolic activities, such as release of energy from nutrients, production of body heat, and growth and repair of tissues.

Cytoplasmic Proteins and Thyroid Hormones

Considerable evidence shows that thyroid hormones interact with solubilized cytoplasmic proteins.[1,p.195] Binding of thyroid hormones to cytoplasmic proteins may impede the hormones from entering the nucleus.[27] In rat kidney, nicotinamide-adenine dinucleotide phosphate (NADP) facilitates entry into the nucleus of T_3 combined with cytoplasmic binding protein.[28] Some evidence shows that the cytoplasmic proteins that bind thyroid hormone in the rat kidney contain ribonucleoprotein.[27] This finding raises the possibility that in some tissues, thyroid hormone has a direct effect on the translation of messenger RNA (mRNA).[1,p.194] Thyroid hormone increases the quantities of many mRNAs in the cell by activating transcription of their genes. Maintaining adequate amounts of other mRNAs depends on thyroid hormone stabilizing the mRNAs after their transcription.[29] Davis has written that thyroid hormone may stabilize mRNA by regulating the activity of enzymes that decompose the mRNA, or by compartmentalizing in some way those enzymes so they do not have access to mRNA.[1,p.194]

CELL MEMBRANES

Cell and organelle membranes serve specialized functions: the plasma membrane releases wastes from the cell; the membrane of the sarcoplasmic reticulum releases calcium from the sarcoplasmic fluid, takes it up again, and temporarily stores it; and the membrane of the lysosome incarcerates lysosomal enzymes that would, if released, lyse the organic compounds that make up the structures of the cell.

Most membranes share the function of the regulation of cellular concentrations of electrically charged particles (ions). Sodium (Na^+), potassium (K^+), and calcium (Ca^{++}) are particularly important ions. Ions are in a free state, unattached to other particles or molecules. A proper concentration of ions is critical to a number of cell functions such as fluid regulation, protein synthesis, activation of enzymes, nerve conduction, and muscle contraction.

Some materials are *actively* transported into the cell; cellular energy is expended in the process. Energy released from ATP is required, for instance, to fuel the transport mechanism that brings the sugars glucose and galactose into the cell. Active transport also brings iron, calcium, vitamin B_{12}, folic acid, and amino acids into the cell. Other materials *passively* diffuse through membranes without the cell expending energy in the process. Fructose, monoglycerides, and glycerol are examples.

Thyroid hormone affects various functions of cell

membranes. These functions include transport of sodium, potassium, calcium, glucose, and amino acids across the membranes.

PLASMA, ENDOPLASMIC RETICULUM, AND MITOCHONDRIAL MEMBRANES

The plasma and endoplasmic reticulum membranes, and possibly the mitochondrial membranes, are structural sites where thyroid hormone exerts substantial effects on the homeostasis and metabolism of cells.

Plasma Membrane

Our word "cell" derives from the Latin word for room. The plasma membrane is the elastic outer wall of this biological room. It encapsulates the cytoplasm. A similar membrane inside the cells, the nuclear membrane, holds the nucleoplasm and separates it from the cytoplasm in which the nucleus is suspended.

The plasma membrane consists of a lipid bilayer (a thin sheet of lipids two molecules thick). The lipid bilayer, consisting mostly of phospholipids and cholesterol, makes up the continuous wall of the cell. The lipid bilayer is fluid rather than solid, and substances dissolved or floating in it can move about liberally. Globulin proteins, for example, float in the plasma membrane. Some serve as ion channels, others serve as carrier systems for membrane transport of substances, and still others function as enzymes.[33,pp.11-12]

Selected materials enter and leave the cell through the membrane. Some materials become part of substances manufactured within the cell that are destined for export from the cell through the membrane. "Waste" materials also leave through the plasma membrane.

The plasma membrane also contains proteins that act as receptors. These receptors are "attachment" sites for hormones and transmitter substances such as peptides that influence the chemical processes within the cell. Essentially, receptors mediate the transfer of information (inherent in the structure of the hormone or transmitter) from the outside to the inside of the cell. This function is termed *signal transduction*. A cell may have from 200-to-10,000 receptors studding its surface.

Mechanisms of Transport of Thyroid Hormone Across the Plasma Membrane. Thyroid hormone crosses the plasma membrane by more than one route. The hormone crosses by binding to membrane receptors. The high affinity and specificity with which the hormone binds to the receptors implies some biologic role for the binding sites.[1,p.190] The hormone also

enters the cell by endocytosis. In this process, the cell ingests a thyroid hormone molecule. First, the plasma membrane invaginates to form a space with membranous walls, called a "coated pit,"[107] for the molecule. Once the hormone enters the outer opening, the opening closes, trapping the hormone. The hormone then escapes the pit and enters the cytoplasm. Treating a number of different cell types with a chemical that inhibits endocytosis reduces their uptake of thyroid hormones.[5]

Thyroid hormone also diffuses into the plasma membrane. However, the hormones may not pass into the interior of the cell by this mechanism. Upon dissolving into the plasma membrane, the hormones may laterally diffuse within the lipid bilayer of the membrane. The lipid bilayer may force thyroid hormone into a specific structural orientation that promotes attachment of the hormone within the membrane to proteins involved in transporting other hormones and glucose across cell membranes.[1,p.191][4] Treating cells with a chemical that inhibits the mitochondrial electron transport system (which supplies the cell with its major source of energy, ATP) decreases entry of thyroid hormone into the cell. Therefore, at least some routes of thyroid hormone entry into the cell are energy-[6] and ATP-dependent.[7]

Endoplasmic Reticulum Membrane

The endoplasmic reticulum is a system of hollow tubes that network though the cytoplasm. The tubes contain a fluid matrix of different composition than the cytoplasm. The space inside the walls of the endoplasmic reticulum is connected to the space between the double layers of the nuclear membrane. The walls of the reticulum, composed of lipoprotein membranes, are channels through which substances travel within the cell. Upon entering the cell through the plasma membrane, for example, the phosphoric acid, sugars, and bases that will unite to form DNA and RNA travel to the nucleus through the endoplasmic reticulum. Once a genetic code in the form of mRNA reaches a ribosome, ribosomal enzymes translate the code into proteins. Some of the ribosomes are free in the cytoplasm, but others are attached to the endoplasmic reticulum. The proteins synthesized by these latter ribosomes may be released into the lumen of the reticulum. Through the lumen, they travel to the Golgi complex to be packaged and possibly excreted from the cell.

Mitochondrial Membranes

The mitochondrion, the energy-production organelle, has an outer and inner membrane. The outer membrane is rich in cholesterol and contains several enzymes that initiate the lysis of fats and amino acids. Other outer membrane proteins are called "porins" because they form sieve-like channels. They are not highly selective in the substances they permit to pass through the membranes. But while small molecules such as amino acids pass through, enzymes and other proteins do not.[83,pp.345-346]

The inner mitochondrial membrane is virtually devoid of cholesterol. It does, however, contain a high concentration of cardiolipin, a phospholipid that makes up part of the fatty framework of the membrane. Except in bacteria, cardiolipin is either absent or low in concentration in cell membranes such as the outer membrane of the mitochondrion. The inner membrane holds the carriers and complexes of the electron transport system, ATPases, and proteins that help transport metabolites across the inner membrane.[83,pp.345-346]

Important Cell Membrane Effects of Thyroid Hormone

Thyroid hormone mediates several particularly important effects at cell membranes. These effects include increased sugar and amino acid transport; increased activity of Na^+/K^+-ATPase, Ca^{2+}-ATPase, and adenylate cyclase; and possible alteration of the lipid content of the mitochondrial membranes.

Thyroid Hormone and Sugar Uptake by Cell Membranes. Thyroid hormone increases cellular uptake of sugars. Several research groups have shown that T_3 increases the uptake of 2-deoxyglucose by rat thymocytes.[4][8][9][71] Kvetny and Matzen found that both T_4 and T_3 in physiologic doses rapidly stimulated glucose uptake. The effects of T_4 and T_3 were quantitatively identical.[70] In promoting sugar uptake, thyroid hormones appear to act at plasma membrane receptors.[70][71]

Thyroid hormone induces sugar uptake even in the absence of insulin or cortisone.[70,p.719] The mechanism by which thyroid hormone stimulates sugar uptake is different from that of insulin,[72] and the mechanism does not entail T_3 stimulation of insulin receptors.[73] Kvetny and Matzen wrote that the mechanism appears to be a direct effect on glucose carriers at the time when thyroid hormones bind to membrane proteins. The effect on glucose carriers is probably not genomic. If the effect were mediated by thyroid hormone-activated transcription, one or more proteins would be produced in the process. But thyroid hormones induced rapid sugar uptake despite the administration of

tiothepa, a protein synthesis inhibitor.[70,p.719]

Of parenthetical interest, Davis wrote that membrane sugar transport does not contribute substantially to the production of ATP by thyroid hormones.[1,p.192][143]

Thyroid Hormone and Membrane Amino Acid Transport. T_3 stimulates amino acid transport across the cell membrane.[108] This effect is not genomic: it occurs rapidly and without synthesis of RNA or protein.[46,p.172] Also, supraphysiologic amounts of thyroid hormones increase the net amount of amino acids in rat thymocytes by inhibiting amino acid membrane outflow.[23] This shows that the effect of T_3 on amino acid transport into thymocytes is exerted at the plasma membrane and does not require action in the nucleus of the cell (where T_3 exerts its principle effects).[109]

Adenylate cyclase activity also increases in rat thymocytes in response to thyroid hormone.[24] The effect requires calmodulin[25] (a Ca^{2+}-activated regulatory protein) and involves a guanine nucleotide regulatory unit (G protein).[26]

Thyroid Hormone and Membrane Na^+/K^+-ATPase Activity. Sodium-potassium-activated ATPase (Na^+/K^+-ATPase) is a membrane enzyme vital to cellular homeostasis. The enzyme increases the rate of transport of both sodium (Na^+) and potassium (K^+) through cell membranes. It assures low Na^+ and high K^+ concentrations inside the cell, thus maintaining electrical potential of the membrane. The enzyme also maintains cell volume, transport of substrates into the cell by the Na^+ gradient, and proper ionic composition of the cytoplasmic fluid.[60,p.C295]

The Na^+/K^+ pump (see Glossary: sodium-potassium pump), whose activity is catalyzed by Na^+/K^+-ATPase, uses cytoplasmic ATP. In fact, the pump is one of the main energy-users of the cell. The pump is inactive part of the time, yet it accounts for 5%-to-40% of steady-state energy expenditure.[61] In an individual with normal metabolism, a large portion of the total ATP produced (and oxygen consumed) provides energy for the Na^+/K^+ pump. Edelman and Ismail-Beigi wrote that they were surprised when they found how much this pump contributes to resting metabolism.[120]

Activity of the Na^+/K^+ pump increases promptly in response to subtle moment-to-moment changes in the ionic balance of the cytosol. When activated, the pump works vigorously to maintain an uneven distribution of ions on the opposing sides of cell membranes, with potassium high inside the cells and sodium high outside.[60,p.C296]

In skeletal muscle, heart, liver, fat, and kidney, thyroid hormone is a primary factor regulating steady-state activity of Na^+/K^+-ATPase.[62] In kidney and muscle, the concentration of the enzyme is low in hypothyroidism and high in hyperthyroidism.[63][64] Activity of the enzyme increases in the livers of both normal and hypothyroid rats when treated with thyroid hormone.[67] Na^+/K^+-ATPase activity is increased in hyperthyroid animals.

Thyroid hormone controls genomic expression of Na^+/K^+-ATPase.[62] When T_3 binds to a high percentage of T_3-receptors on the chromosomes in the nucleus, the concentration of Na^+/K^+-ATPase in the cell increases.[46,p.174] Thyroid hormone regulates transcription of Na^+/K^+-ATPase mRNA isoforms and the proteins translated from these mRNAs. Isoforms of Na^+/K^+-ATPase vary from tissue-to-tissue.[63][64] Radioactively labeled amino acids incorporated in the enzyme are high in hyperthyroid patients, low in hypothyroid patients, and intermediate in euthyroid subjects.[120]

Thyroid hormone also appears to exert nongenomic control over Na^+/K^+-ATPase by regulating translational or post-translational processes.[65][66] This non-genomic control is indicated by the lower concentration of α_2-subunit (a translation product) than its corresponding mRNA (a transcription product) in hypothyroid rats. Both the mRNA and the α_2-subunit it codes for are lowered, but the α_2-subunit is disproportionately lower. This finding of disproportionately lower α_2-subunit indicates that during a thyroid hormone deficiency, although transcription is repressed, translation is suppressed even more so.[65][66] In addition, in hypothyroid rats treated with thyroid hormone, the increases in mRNAs and the resulting proteins were disproportional: α_2-mRNA increased 5-fold, but the level of the corresponding translation product (proteins) increased 14-fold. In contrast, while β_1-subunit mRNA increased 12-fold, its protein increased only by 2.5-fold.[65][66] This finding of disproportionately higher mRNA indicates that for the β_1-subunit, thyroid hormone impacts transcription far more than translation.

Skeletal muscle α_1-subunit and β_1-subunit mRNAs and the resulting proteins were not changed in rats treated with thyroid hormone.[62] However, levels of α_2-mRNA increased 5-fold, and the resulting proteins increased 3-fold. Also β_2-mRNA increased 4-fold, and the resulting proteins increased 2-fold.[63] On the other hand, in kidney, 8 days of thyroid hormone administration were followed by a 1.6-fold increase in α_1-mRNA, β_1-mRNA, and their resulting proteins.[64] In skeletal muscle[63] and kidney,[64] both mRNA isoforms and their respective proteins increased proportionately to one another after thyroid hormone treatment. The proportional increases in mRNAs and their proteins

demonstrated a transcriptional effect of thyroid hormone.

Thyroid Hormone, Membrane Ca^{2+}-ATPase Activity, and the Cell Content of Calcium. An important nongenomic effect of thyroid hormone is its activation of membrane Ca^{2+}-ATPase.[1,p.192][18] Thyroid hormone does not, however, directly interact with Ca^{2+}-ATPase.[19] The mechanism may instead entail phosphatidylinositol[20] and protein kinase C.[21] Davis wrote[1,p.192] that an activation sequence is possible because thyroid hormone can activate red cell protein kinase C,[21] and protein kinase C can increase the activity of membrane Ca^{2+}-ATPase.[22]

Researchers have repeatedly shown that T_4 and T_3 activate Ca^{2+}-ATPase in mature nonnucleated human red cells.[3][11][12][13] The activation requires calmodulin,[10] a Ca^{2+}-activated regulatory protein. Activation occurs *in vivo*, as shown in red blood cells from hyperthyroid and hypothyroid humans[15] and in erythrocytes, liver, and muscle of T_3-treated rabbits.[14] By activating membrane Ca^{2+}-ATPase, T_4 increased Ca^{2+} outflow from human red cells[15][17] and, *in vitro*, reduced the amount of Ca^{2+} in red cells.[16] Sarcoplasmic reticulum, the endoplasmic reticulum in muscle, is responsive to T_3 and T_4 with activation of Ca^{2+}-ATPase.[1,p.193]

Davis suggested that the influence of thyroid hormones on Ca^{2+}-ATPase is to set the enzyme's basal level of activity. By doing so, the hormones participate with other factors in controlling the resting activity level of Ca^{2+} in hormone-responsive cells.[1,p.193]

Hyperthyroidism and Changes in Mitochondrial Membrane Lipid Content. Paradies and Ruggiero found that hyperthyroidism (and therefore an excess of thyroid hormone) substantially altered the lipid composition of mitochondrial membranes in rat liver.[146] Total cholesterol decreased and phospholipids significantly increased. In particular, the negatively charged phospholipid cardiolipin, peculiar to the inner membrane, increased by more than 50%. Minor changes occurred in the pattern of fatty acids. Hyperthyroidism also increased the rate of citrate (a constituent of the citric acid cycle) uptake into the mitochondrion, measured as the exchange of citrate for malate (via the mitochondrial tricarboxylate carrier[83,p.353]). The authors wrote, "The thyroid hormone-induced change in the activity of the tricarboxylate carrier can be ascribed either to a general modification of membrane lipid composition, which increases membrane fluidity and in turn the mobility of the carrier, or to a more localized change of the lipid domain (cardiolipin content) surrounding the carrier molecules in the mitochondrial membrane."[146]

RIBOSOMES AND PROTEIN SYNTHESIS

Ribosomes are small angular or bead-shaped particles composed of protein and ribosomal RNA (rRNA). When actively synthesizing protein, many ribosomes may cluster together attached to a single molecule of mRNA. The clustering forms coils or helices called polysomes or polyribosomes.[45,p.7][156,p.81] Ribosomes that produce proteins for use within the same cell float freely in the cytoplasm. Ribosomes that synthesize proteins for export from the cell are attached to the rough endoplasmic reticulum. In the synthesis of proteins bound for secretion, a hydrophobic signal sequence coded by the gene is included at the N-terminus of the protein. The signal sequence causes the protein to enter the reticulum after synthesis. Upon entry, the sequence is cleaved and the protein travels in a vesicle to the Golgi apparatus. There, the protein is incorporated into a secretory vesicle that is secreted from the cell by exocytosis.[156,p.85]

mRNA (which serves as a blueprint for production of a type of protein) travels from the nucleus and reaches the ribosome. At this time, other RNA molecules, called transfer RNA or tRNA, take part in the process. They bind amino acids in the cytoplasm and transport them to the ribosomal site of protein synthesis. Each tRNA binds an amino acid that is specific to it. A highly specific enzyme (aminoacyl-tRNA synthetase) induces binding of an amino acid specific to each tRNA.[156,p.81]

Each amino acid is delivered to the ribosome where the protein is synthesized. The amino acid is inserted into the growing polypeptide chain based on matching of the codon of the mRNA and the anticodon of the tRNA. A codon is a three base sequence that is a code for a specific amino acid. The sequence of codons of mRNA determines the sequence of amino acids in the protein being synthesized. An anticodon is a tri-nucleotide sequence that is complementary to a codon. Insertion of a specific amino acid is dictated by the codon of the mRNA, and incorporation of the amino acid results from the codon-anticodon interaction.[156,p.81] Synthesis of the protein according to the code inherent in the structure of the mRNA is termed *translation*. Essentially, at the ribosome the genetic code is translated into the new protein.

Each protein synthesized at the ribosome is composed of some combination of the 22 amino acids derived from the proteins humans consume in their food.

DNA nucleotide sequences called exons code for the precise sequence of amino acids necessary for a particular protein. mRNA is a template of the DNA code and functions as an intermediate between DNA and the ribosome.

A sufficient quantity of proteins is essential to cell structure and function. For example, proteins are components of cell membranes and the contractile filaments of muscle cells. As components of enzymes (apoenzymes), proteins are vital to the normal rate of biochemical reactions. To function normally, enzymes must be synthesized with structural exactitude, for their structure determines their function.

Altering the structure of a protein that acts as an enzyme also alters its functional properties. A structural alteration may render a protein completely inactive as an enzyme. A chemical reaction may occur without the proper enzyme to trigger it, but the rate of the reaction may be too slow to adequately serve its intended biological purpose.[35,p.33] A reaction in the absence of the appropriate enzyme may decelerate by a factor of a million.[31,p.177] Faltering of a chemical pathway results in signs and symptoms. In a lactase deficiency, for example, the individual cannot digest lactose and develops painful and distressing abdominal symptoms such as bloating, cramps, and watery stools.

An enzyme relevant to the subject of this book is T_4 5'-monodeiodinase.[47,p.376] This enzyme converts T_4 to the metabolically active thyroid hormone T_3.[46,pp.170-171] If one amino acid necessary for its complete synthesis is not available during translation at the ribosomes, production of the enzyme may decrease. As a result, a deficiency of the enzyme may result, and too little T_4 will be converted to T_3. The inadequacy of T_3 that follows, if severe enough, will result in hypometabolism of susceptible tissues.

If an improperly structured protein functions as a receptor for a hormone or neurotransmitter, the receptor may have a low affinity for binding of the hormone or neurotransmitter. With improperly structured T_3-receptors, for example, low affinity for its ligand, T_3, impairs normal regulation of transcription. Failed transcription of many genes occurs, resulting in a variety of abnormalities. This condition is termed thyroid hormone resistance syndrome (see Chapter 2.6).

ENERGY-YIELDING PROCESSES IN THE CYTOPLASM AND MITOCHONDRIA

Carbohydrates, fats, and proteins are electron sources to cells. These macronutrients are first split into their component subunits in reactions that precede their being oxidized. During oxidation, the subunits forfeit their electrons. Oxidation of the subunits occurs in one or both of two major stages. The first occurs in the cytoplasm and the second in the mitochondria.

Glycogen (animal starch) is split into monosaccharides which then follow a path of oxidation through both stages. First, sugar breakdown (glycolysis) takes place in the cytoplasm; second, complete oxidation of the short carbon chains to carbon dioxide and water (pyruvate oxidation and the citric acid cycle) occurs inside the mitochondria. Fats are split into alcohol, glycerol, and fatty acids. The glycerol enters the glycolytic pathway in the cytoplasm, and the fatty acids undergo oxidation in the mitochondria. Proteins are first hydrolyzed to amino acids. The amino, or —NH_2, group is then removed, a process termed deamination. The deaminated molecules may undergo oxidation at either of the two stages.

Both stages produce a small amount of ATP by substrate-level phosphorylation. Most ATP, however, is produced as the electrons released from substrates during these two oxidative stages pass through the electron transport system.[34,pp.244-245][83,pp.311-312] Thyroid hormones potently influence mitochondrial electron transfer and thereby play a major role in regulating energy metabolism.[144]

Energy Processes in the Cytoplasm

The cytoplasm serves as a medium for glycolysis, the breakdown of glucose. The enzymes, reactants, and products of glycolysis are suspended in the cytoplasm outside the mitochondria. They are organized loosely by attachment to the cytoskeleton and interact through random collisions.[83,p.315] Glycolysis is a ten-step sugar-splitting reaction sequence. It is the single most common pathway in all of energy metabolism, occurring in virtually every living cell, and it is one of the major metabolic activities that occurs in the cytoplasm.[34,p.187] Glycolysis produces a small amount of ATP.[34,p.199] Most importantly, glycolysis yields electrons and the three-carbon substance pyruvate. The pyruvate molecule is the main fuel substance for the second stage of oxidative reactions.[83,p.312]

Glycolysis. The presence of thyroid hormone in the cytoplasm affects the rate of glycolytic activity. During 11 days in a culture absent of thyroid hormone, the glucose depletion rate in neonatal rat heart cells decreased by 32%, indicating reduced glycolytic activity.[150] In hypothyroid rats, the activity of glucokinase was decreased. (Glucokinase, also called hexokinase, is the enzyme that catalyzes the first reaction in gly-

colysis, transferring a phosphate group from ATP and generating glucose-6-phosphate.) Also, activity of enzymes in the glycolytic pathway below phosphofructokinase (Figure 2.2.1) was reduced.[152] Increased or decreased levels of thyroid hormone therefore significantly increase or decrease the rate of glycolysis.

Mitochondrial cell respiration, however, is substantially more responsive (than the rate of glycolysis) to increased and decreased thyroid hormone levels. This response shows that the stimulation of cell metabolism by thyroid hormone is mediated mainly by its effects on mitochondrial processes[143] (see sections below).

The building blocks of glycogen are molecules of the simple sugar glucose. The glucose molecule has a structural backbone of six carbon atoms. As the molecule is degraded, it splits into two three-carbon molecules.[35,p.29]

(1) One molecule of glucose with its six carbon atoms
↓
(2) Two molecules of three-carbon atoms
↓
(3) Two molecules of pyruvic acid

Catabolism of glucose in the cytoplasm proceeds only to pyruvic acid.[31,p.351] Subsequent catabolic stages take place in the mitochondria. Oxidation occurs in four steps in glycolysis, and once during the conversion of pyruvate to acetyl-CoA. During oxidation (loss of electrons), electrons are tranferred from the successive breakdown products of glucose to electron carriers. During one step, electrons are transferred to the oxidized electron carrier flavin adenine dinucleotide (FAD). At the other steps, electrons are transferred to nicotinamide adenine dinucleotide (NAD^+), another oxidized electron carrier.[34,p.216] Because of the negative charge of electrons, acquisition of electrons by the carriers is defined as reduction. By virtue of the electrons they carry, the reduced molecules are considered high-energy substances. The reduced carriers shuttle the electrons between reaction systems. When sufficient oxygen is available, the electrons carried by these molecules are exchanged for oxygen (oxidation of the carriers) and the electrons enter the transport system in mitochondria. Much of the energy of the electrons is captured in the third phosphate bond of ATP when the molecule is produced from the two-phosphate molecule ADP.[83,p.314] Addition of the third phosphate to ADP is oxygen-dependent and therefore termed oxidative phosphorylation.[34,p.190] Along with the citric acid cycle, oxidative phosphorylation is central to the production of most ATP derived from the oxidation of food.[156,p.108]

The sixth step in glycolysis, shown in Figure 2.2.1, is catalyzed by the enzyme glyceraldehyde 3-phosphate dehydrogenase. Eisinger found that the level of this enzyme was abnormally low in hypothyroid patients and in 18% of fibromyalgia patients. The level was normal in control subjects.[90]

A Note to Clinicians. Chemical reactions by which food is oxidized cannot occur rapidly enough without all components of enzymes (apoenzymes and cofactors) to catalyze the reactions. For many enzymes, minerals and compounds derived from vitamins are necessary as cofactors.[156,p.109] (A cofactor is a nonprotein element of an enzyme necessary for the enzyme to efficiently catalyze reactions.) For example, a number of substances take part in the breakdown of glucose to pyruvic acid, including oxygen, the sugars glucose and ribose, and niacin (vitamin B_3). Magnesium is involved as a cofactor.[35,p.34] Clinicians should bear in mind that the increase in the rate of glycolysis stimulated by exogenous thyroid hormone increases the amount of nutrients expended in the pathway of reactions. Patients taking exogenous thyroid hormone should also take nutrient supplements that increase the availability of expendable nutrients such as vitamin B_3 and magnesium. Otherwise, the increased rate of reactions by thyroid hormone may induce deficiencies of the cofactors. Travell and Simons pointed out that when a patient has a vitamin B_1 inadequacy, taking exogenous thyroid hormone even in small dosages may precipitate symptoms of acute thiamine deficiency. *In some respects, the symptoms resemble thyrotoxicosis and the clinician may misinterpret them as intolerance to thyroid medication.* In most cases, after the patient corrects the vitamin B_1 deficiency, she tolerates well the same small dose or even larger dosages of thyroid hormone.[119,p.120]

Lactate Formed from Pyruvate in Contracting Muscle: Converted into Glucose by the Liver. Lactate is produced by active muscles and erythrocytes. During strenuous exercise, oxygen is limited in contracting skeletal muscle. At this time, the rate of pyruvate production by glycolysis exceeds the rate of oxidation of pyruvate in the citric acid cycle. Also, the rate of production of NADH during glycolysis is higher than its rate of oxidation by the respiratory chain. (NADH is a compound reduced by accepting electrons during glycolysis. It then contributes the electrons to the electron transport system, being oxidized in the process to NAD^+.) As a result, pyruvate and NADH accumulate during the low oxygen availability. Their accumula-

tion, however, is reversed by lactate dehydrogenase. This enzyme reduces pyruvate to lactate while it oxidizes NADH to NAD^+.[31,p.444] In other words, lactate dehydrogenase catalyzes reduction of pyruvate to lactate by oxidizing NADH.[31,p.263] The purpose of the conversion of pyruvate to lactate is production of NAD^+. NAD^+, as an electron acceptor, oxidizes glyceraldehyde 3-phosphate (Figure 2.2.1), thereby enabling glycolysis to continue. Lactate diffuses out of skeletal muscle cells and into liver cells where it is oxidized first to pyruvate then to glucose. After entering the blood, the glucose is taken up by skeletal muscles where it eventually enters the glycolytic pathway again when sufficient oxygen is available.[31,p.445]

Lactate Dehydrogenase in Fibromyalgia and in Hypothyroidism. Eisinger et al. reported that in fibromyalgia patients, the muscle isoenzyme lactate dehydrogenase is 23% lower than in control subjects. The investigators also found that the isoenzyme level was lower in hypothyroid patients. The difference from control subjects, however, was significant only for fibromyalgia patients.[90] Eisinger also found an increase in blood pyruvic acid levels in fibromyalgia patients and a normal-to-decreased production of lactate during the forearm ischemic exercise testing.[91][92] The experimentally-induced ischemia reduced the oxygen supply to the exercising muscles. The reduced oxygen supply should have increased lactate production, but pyruvate-to-lactate conversion did not appear to increase. It occurred at the normal rather than increased rate probably because of the low lactate dehydrogenase levels. These findings are similar to those in patients with hypothyroidism and McArdle's disease.[93] (In McArdle's disease, the enzyme myophosphorylase B is deficient. The deficiency results in an abnormal accumulation of glycogen in muscle. Symptoms include pain, fatigue, and muscle stiffness after sustained exertion.)

Thiamine Deficiency. Eisinger pointed out that an increased pyruvate-to-lactate ratio, as he found in fibromyalgia patients, has also been reported in patients deficient in thiamine.[90] For example, in beriberi, a thiamine deficiency disease, the level of pyruvate in the blood is elevated.[31,p.383]

Thiamine (as thiamine pyrophosphate) serves as a catalytic cofactor in the conversion of pyruvate to acetyl-CoA. After pyruvate combines with thiamine, the enzyme pyruvate dehydrogenase catalyzes the decarboxylation of pyruvate (its first carbon atom is liberated as CO_2).[34,p.216] Pyruvate dehydrogenase functionally bridges glycolysis and the citric acid cycle. It does so by converting pyruvate, the end point of glycolysis, to acetyl-CoA, the starting point of the citric acid cycle.[34,p.216] The positively charged ring nitrogen of thiamine pyrophosphate functions as an electron sink to stabilize formation of the negative charge necessary for decarboxylation.[31,pp.379-380]

Glycogenesis. Glycogenesis (the opposite of glycogenolysis) is the formation of glycogen from glucose in the cytoplasm. Upon entering the cell, glucose is converted to glucose 6-phosphate. Glucose 6-phosphate is critically important for the initiation of several metabolic pathways. One of these pathways is the synthesis of glycogen which can proceed after glucose 6-phosphate is converted to UDP-glucose.[156,p.141]

Glycogenesis proceeds by the addition of glucose to a glycogen chain. Energy for the bonds holding glucose molecules to the glycogen molecule is contributed by uridine triphosphate (UTP). When insulin facilitates entry of glucose into the cell, it also activates the enzyme glycogen synthase. This enzyme catalyzes glycogenesis, binding to glycogen molecules the glucose that is available in excess of the immediate needs of the cell. This mechanism is important to understand because the inhibition of glycogen synthase activity by exogenous female sex hormones (as in birth control pills) appears to be a factor underlying treatment-resistant myofascial trigger points and pain in some women.[75][76] In most cases, myofascial pain underlain by this mechanism affects multiple muscles and may be misinterpreted as fibromyalgia.

Liver Cell Glycogenesis and Thyroid Hormone. In hyperthyroidism, glycogen synthase activity is increased in liver cells. Also increased are activity levels of two other enzymes (synthase phosphatase and phosphorylase phosphatase) that favor glycogen deposition. Paradoxically, hyperthyroidism is associated with low liver glycogen stores.[77][78][79][80] Betley, Peak, and Agius suggested an explanation. They pointed out that in euthyroid humans, T_3 has an anabolic role in the control of liver glycogen after food consumption. They found that T_3 stimulated glycogen synthase, increased glycogen synthesis, and through these effects, was additive with the long-term stimulating effects of insulin on glycogen synthesis. However, they also found that 10 times the physiologic dose of T_3 decreased liver cell responsiveness to insulin. It appears, then, that glycogen synthesis is favored by physiologic doses of T_3 and disfavored by excessive T_3. The authors proposed that the well-documented low glycogen content of hepatocytes exposed to excessive amounts of T_3 results from either a secondary metabolite and/or impaired responsiveness to insulin.[81]

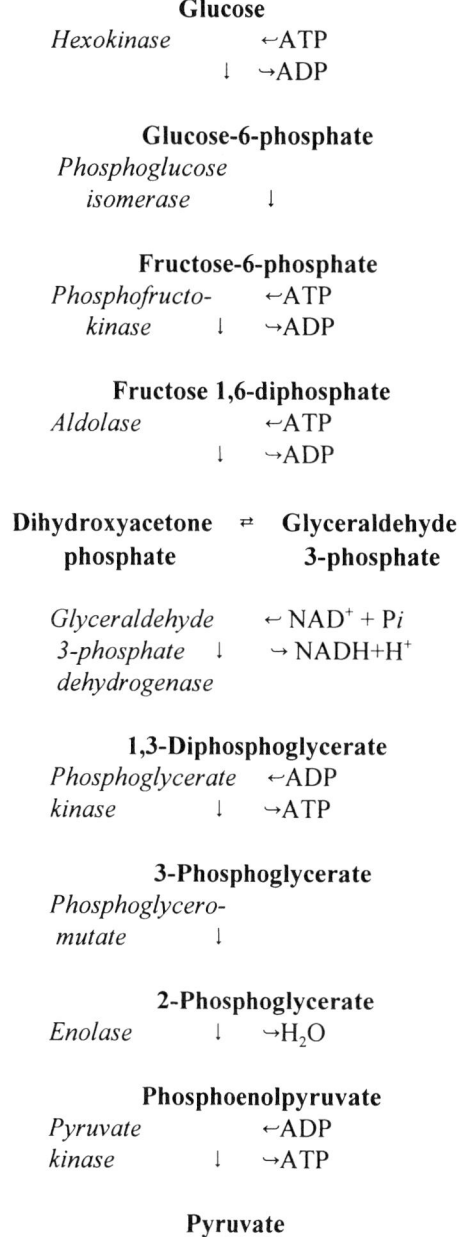

Figure 2.2.1. The glycolytic pathway. Glucose and the subsequent intermediate compounds are in bold, and catalyzing enzymes are in italics. Pyruvate is subsequently oxidized in the mitochondria.

Glycogenolysis. Glycogenolysis is the conversion of glycogen to glucose. For cells to meet their needs for ATP, they must carefully and continuously adjust the functioning of the glycolytic pathway so that glucose is converted to pyruvate at the proper rate. The glucose molecules that undergo glycolysis are derived from glycogen. Glycogen consists of a long chain of glucose subunits. During glycogenolysis, the enzyme phosphorylase catalyzes the phosphorylation of glucose, and the phosphorylation separates the glucose molecule from glycogen.[156,p.185] The cleavage reaction is represented below for a glycogen chain with x glucose subunits:[110]

$$(\text{glucose})_x + P_i \ (\text{inorganic phosphate})$$
$$\rightarrow$$
$$\text{glucose-1-phosphate} + (\text{glucose})_{x-1}$$

(Enzymatically combining P*i* with a glucose molecule separates the molecule from glycogen, resulting in glucose 1-phosphate and glycogen minus one glucose molecule.)

The phosphorylation of glucose produces glucose 1-phosphate. After one molecule of glucose 1-phosphate is released, the remainder of the glycogen chain remains intact until all glucose molecules are released in the same fashion. Glucose 1-phosphate is next converted to glucose 6-phosphate by the enzyme phosphoglucomutase.[156,p.156] (See below in this section for the fate of glucose 6-phosphate.)

This glycogenolytic process is stimulated in liver cells by the hormone glucagon. Glucagon is secreted by the α cells of the pancreas when the blood glucose level decreases sufficiently. The hormone promptly induces release of glucose from hepatic glycogen. The glucose is secreted from the cells to help maintain the blood glucose concentration. When the glucagon level increases, the enzyme glucose 6-phosphatase is induced. This enzyme cleaves inorganic phosphate from glucose 6-phosphate; this frees the glucose to be released into the blood.[156,pp.170&173]

Glycogenolysis is stimulated in liver and muscle cells by the catecholamines epinephrine and norepinephrine when they bind to β-adrenergic receptors.[34,p.200][156,p.157] The glucose released from glycogen in liver cells is secreted into the blood to help maintain the blood glucose level. Glucose release in muscle cells provides energy for contraction and relaxation. This catecholamine-β-adrenoceptor effect is especially potent during stress.[34,p.300] Binding of catecholamines to α-adrenergic receptors inhibits the process. This important concept explains why exercise and other catecholamine-releasing stresses can worsen the symptoms of fibromyalgia when the condition is a manifestation of inadequate thyroid hormone regulation of adrenergic gene transcription.

Figure 2.2.2 shows the sequence of steps in catecholamine-β-adrenoceptor-induced glycogenolysis. The figure shows that norepinephrine or epinephrine, upon binding to a β-adrenergic receptor, stimulates adenylate cyclase. Adenylate cyclase increases the concentration of cyclic AMP inside the cell. Cyclic AMP activates protein kinase, which then activates phosphorylase kinase. This enzyme catalyzes phosphorylation of phosphorylase *b* (the inactive form), transforming it to phosphorylase *a* (the active form). Next, this active form of the enzyme promotes the breakdown of glycogen to glucose 1-phosphate through the phosphorolytic cleavage of glucose. Glucose 1-phosphate is then enzymatically changed (by phosphoglucomutase) to glucose 6-phosphate.[31,p.359]

The catecholamine-induced increase in cyclic AMP also inactivates glycogen synthase. When active, this enzyme catalyzes glycogen synthesis. When inactive, glycogen accumulation decreases in the cell. Catecholamines therefore both mobilize glycogen and inhibit its synthesis.[34,pp.200-201]

Glucose 6-Phosphatase: Catalytic Activity Increased by Thyroid Hormone. In liver, kidney, and intestinal cells, glucose is not a major fuel. The luminal side of the membrane of smooth endoplasmic reticulum in these cells contains glucose 6-phosphatase. This enzyme, the activity of which is increased by thyroid hormone,[56][57][58][59] is critical to the release of glucose from liver cells. Phosphorylated glucose is held in the liver cells. During muscle activity and between meals, glucose 6-phosphatase dephosphorylates the liver cell glucose, separating inorganic phosphate from glucose. The freed glucose then enters the blood and travels to other cells.

The following represents the conversion by the enzyme of glucose 6-phosphate to glucose, which is then free to enter the glycolytic pathway.[34,p.324]

$$\text{Glucose 6-phosphate} + H_2O \rightarrow \text{glucose} + P_i$$

(Glucose 6-phosphatase catalyzes the hydrolysis of glucose 6-phosphate to glucose and inorganic phosphate, freeing the glucose for secretion from the cell.)

In contrast with the liver cells, muscle and brain cells require large amounts of glucose to generate ATP. Muscle and brain cells do not contain glucose 6-phosphatase. As a result, glucose is not freed from glucose 6-phosphate within these cells. Instead, the glucose 6-phosphate generated from glucose 1-phosphate enters the pathway of glycolysis[31,p.359][156,p.156] (see Figure 2.2.1).

Thyroid Hormone Regulation of Glycogenolysis. Thyroid hormone influences glycogenolysis by several mechanisms. One is the genomic regulation of adrenergic receptor type (see the following chapter). To understand the role thyroid hormone appears to play in fibromyalgia, it is critical to understand the mechanism by which adrenergic receptors influence cell metabolism.

The type of adrenergic receptor that predominates on cell membranes dictates the metabolic effects catecholamines have on the cell. Adrenergic receptors are classified as alpha (α) and beta (β). Each has isoforms. When α-adrenergic receptors predominate on the cell membranes of most cell types, exposure to catecholamines inhibits intracellular metabolic processes. When β-adrenergic receptors predominate, exposure to catecholamines accelerate metabolic processes. Whether α- or β-adrenergic receptors predominate in membranes depends largely upon whether thyroid hormone is properly regulating transcription of the adrenergic genes. When transcription of the adrenergic genes is properly regulated by the hormone, the balance of α- and β-adrenergic receptors favors normal cell metabolism. But with inadequate thyroid hormone regulation, transcription shifts: in most cells, α-adrenergic receptors come to predominate. As a result, exposure of the cells to catecholamines impedes metabolic processes. Among the impeded processes is liberation of glucose from glycogen through glycogenolysis and the breakdown of glucose through glycolysis. Adequate regulation of the adrenergic genes shifts the β-adrenergic receptor count back toward normal so that exposure of cell membranes to catecholamines facilitates glycogenolysis and glycolysis.

In hypothyroidism, the intracellular effects of a shift from a balance of adrenergic receptor types toward predominance of the α-adrenergic receptor type are measurable. Guttler et al. found that when hyperthyroid men engaged in physical activity, their 24-hour urinary cyclic-AMP excretion increased. Also, giving the men infusions of epinephrine over a 2-hour period increased their urinary cyclic-AMP excretion and augmented their cardiovascular responses to activity. These reactions in hyperthyroid men were similar to but more intense than that of euthyroid men. In hypothyroid men, however, epinephrine infusions did not significantly increase urinary cyclic-AMP excretion. Moreover, the cardiovascular responses that hyperthyroid men had to activity were virtually absent in the hypothyroid men.[68]

Phosphorylase Kinase: A Direct Mediator of Thyroid Hormone-Induced Release of Metabolic Fuels. Nebioglu et al. found that a single injection of T_3 severely diminished glycogen accumulation in rat liver cells.[55,p.E109] They noted that one mechanism by which

thyroid hormone stimulates metabolism is synthesis of enzymes that catalyze reactions that increase consumption of ATP.[55,p.E115] The increase in these enzymes also increases the rate of oxidative phosphorylation and oxidative metabolism, drawing on stored fuels such as glycogen. The researchers also reported, however, that T_3 induced two other liver enzymes that more directly cause release of stored fuels. The two enzymes are phosphorylase kinase and lysosomal α-1,4-glucosidase. (For details on lysosomal α-1,4-glucosidase, see the section on lysosomes below.)

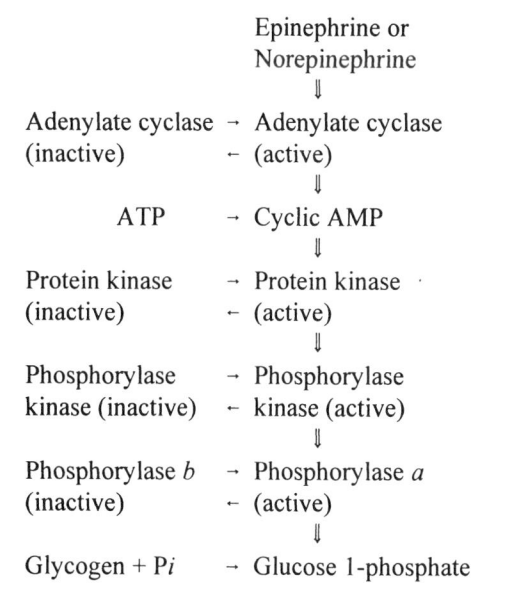

Figure 2.2.2. Steps in glycogen phosphorylase activity during glycogenolysis under the regulatory control of catecholamines (Pi = inorganic phosphate).

The function of phosphorylase kinase, induced by T_3, can be seen in Figure 2.2.2 above. The fourth reaction involves activation of phosphorylase kinase by protein kinase. Activated phosphorylase kinase, in the subsequent fifth reaction, catalyzes conversion of the less active phosphorylase b to the more active phosphorylase a. Phosphorylase a is more active because its serine is phosphorylated; phosphorylase b is less active because it lacks a phosphate on the serine. Activated phosphorylase kinase catalyzes phosphorylation of the serine by ATP.[34,p.200]

Phosphorylase a catalyzes the breakdown of glycogen to glucose-1-phosphate. Glucose-1-phosphate may then be converted to glucose-6-phosphate, the second substrate in the glycolytic pathway.

Lysosomal Enzymes: Their Role in the Availability of Glucose for ATP Production. The lysosome is a storage unit for digestive enzymes in the cytoplasm. The organelle has a single layer lipoprotein membrane that protects the cell's organic compounds outside the lysosomes from its powerful enzymes. Some consider the lysosome the cell's digestive system. None of the lysosomal enzymes, however, are able to digest the lysosomal membrane. The enzymes break down proteins to amino acids, glycogen to glucose, and nucleic acids to nucleotides.

The lysosome engulfs substances by endocytosis. When the lysosome approaches a substance, the part of its membrane closest to the substance falls back, forming first a depression and then an invagination. The invagination provides a space in the edge of the lysosome that the substance occupies. Next, the space sinks further into the lysosome, allowing the outer rim of the space to completely encircle the substance, enclosing it in a sphere within the lysosome. Once inside, vesicles containing lysosomal enzymes approach the sphere. The membrane of the vesicles fuse with the one containing the engulfed substance, and an opening forms between them. The enzymes then pass into the sphere and break down the substance it contains.

Because the lysosomes both ingest and digest substances, the process is considered phagocytosis. If the ingested and digested substance is a protein, the released amino acids are ejected out of the lysosome and back into the cytoplasm. There, they attach to their specific tRNAs which transport them to ribosomes. At the ribosomes, the amino acids are again incorporated into proteins. The lysosome has been called the cell's "cup of hemlock." De Duve called it the "suicide bag" and later bemoaned the term. He considered it "unfortunately catchy" because the lysosome's biological role is greater than being a cell assassin.[48,p.533] Nevertheless, if its membrane ruptures, the enzymes that escape digest the entire cell.[35,pp.26-27]

Vitamins E and A are stabilizers of lysosomal membranes. Vitamin E stabilizes the lysosomal membrane by preventing lipid peroxidation. In this form of peroxidation, oxygen combines with a polyunsaturated fatty acid in the membrane, producing free radicals. The free radicals then oxidize to peroxides. Peroxides can damage the membrane, but vitamin E, as an antioxidant, blocks the peroxidation chain reaction. It also protects vitamin A from oxidation. Vitamin A inadequacy[49] or excess [50] tends to disrupt the lysosomal membrane. Excess vitamin A may accomplish this by entering the membrane and expanding its lipoprotein component, rendering the membrane unstable.[51]

Lysosomal Enzymes are Direct Mediators of Thyroid Hormone-Induced Breakdown of Glycogen. Nebioglu et al. found that a single injection of T_3 induced the release of stored fuel and severely diminished glycogen accumulation in rat livers. They wrote that one mechanism of this action is induction by T_3 of the enzyme lysosomal α-1,4-glucosidase.[55,p.E109] This enzyme thoroughly hydrolyzes all glycogen that enters the lysosomes. During starvation, the enzyme becomes active, providing glucose for ATP production. During feeding, however, the enzyme becomes markedly less active. But during feeding in T_3-treated rats, the enzyme is more active than normal. According to Nebioglu et al., this greater-than-normal activity of lysosomal α-1,4-glucosidase during feeding at least partly accounts for the previously reported T_3-induced reduction in glycogen accumulation during feeding.[55,p.E114]

The activity of lysosomal proteolytic enzymes also increases under the influence of excessive amounts of thyroid hormone. Examples are cathepsin-B_1 and cathepsin-D.[74] As with α-1,4-glucosidase, the normal decrease in the activity of these enzymes during feeding does not occur in rats treated with T_3.[55,p.E115] This indicates that T_3 is a potent stimulator of the activity of these enzymes.

Energy Processes in the Mitochondria

The mitochondria are organelles in the cytoplasm of the cell. The mitochondrion is called the "power house of the cell." This name fits because the mitochondrion's metabolic processes effectively transfer energy from the chemical bonds of nutrients to the high-energy bonds of ATP. A cell may have 50-to-2500 mitochondria, depending on its demands for energy. The mitochondria can be spherical or elongated, but they are ordinarily kidney-shaped. The organelle is about the size of a bacterium (0.5 μm in diameter and 1-to-2 μm in length), although it may be much larger in some cells.[83,p.321] Mitochondria may move about in the cytoplasm, change their shape, and enlarge or shrink, depending on the demands or influences imposed on them.

A mitochondrion contains from 500-to-10,000 sets of oxidative enzymes. Each of these sets contains 15 or more molecules, essential constituents of mitochondrial structure, arranged in a tightly ordered manner.[48,p.491]

Pike and Brown's words highlight the magnificent structure/function interaction of this organelle:

The exquisite precision with which the mitochondrion performs its intricate biochemical procedures implies a corresponding precision in organization. Such coordinated and efficient function could not occur by random meeting of enzymes and substrates; it could only occur with an architectural design elegantly integrated with function.[48,p.531]

The chemical pathways within the mitochondrion and across its membranous borders provide energy for cell functions in the form of ATP molecules. The ATP molecule stores and transports large amounts of energy in its phosphate bonds. After ATP is synthesized in the mitochondrion, it exits the organelle and travels to various other sites within the cell. When energy is required at a site, the energy of an ATP phosphate bond is transduced into some active process. Among the energy-expending processes powered by ATP are synthesis of large molecules, myofibril contraction, and active transport through membranes.[48,p.531]

Like the plasma membrane, the mitochondrial membrane is double-layered. The outer membrane is smooth and constitutes one continuous outer layer. The inner membrane, as though it is too big for its container (the outer membrane), folds with alternate furrows and ridges into the interior of the mitochondrion.[83,p.320] Some folds are short; others almost reach the opposite inner wall of the mitochondrion.

The corrugated shape of the inner mitochondrial membrane provides a larger surface area for contact with the chemicals interacting in the mitochondrion. The surface area of the inner membrane is especially expansive in cells such as myocytes that must conserve and release large amounts of energy. The inner mitochondrial membrane permits free passage of both ions and simple and complex compounds.[35,p.36]

Effect of Thyroid Hormone on the Mitochondrion. Thyroid hormones directly and indirectly influence mitochondrial structure and function. The hormones stimulate mitochondrial physiology and increase the RNA and protein content of mitochondria. A series of mitochondrial genes that encode mitochondrial proteins is controlled by thyroid hormones.[131][132][133][134] These mitochondrial genome influences may account for the very rapid mitochondrial effects of thyroid hormone with both intact cells and isolated mitochondria.[127,p.999]

Exposure to excess thyroid hormone may increase the number, size, and surface area of mitochondria.[84][85][86] This increase is consistent with the increase in oxygen consumption *in vivo* in experimental thyrotoxicosis.[87,p.845] In thyroid hormone deficiency, the total mass of mitochondria in the cell increases.

Despite the increase in mass, the concentration of oxidative enzymes in the mitochondria is low. Production of the protein component of enzymes may be low due to inadequate exposure of mitochondrial DNA or cell nucleus DNA to T_3. The inadequacy reduces the rate of transcription which reduces protein synthesis at the ribosomes.

Intake of T_3 or T_4 increases the size and number of mitochondria in most cells. The total membrane surface area of mitochondria increases in almost direct proportion to the increased metabolic rate of the whole body. The increased size and activity of mitochondria may be either a cause or a result of the increased cellular activity. It is possible that the mitochondrial changes are a result of the actions of T_3 and T_4. The mitochondrial changes may be a prerequisite to thyroid hormones increasing ATP formation to energize cellular functions.

Sterling et al. found that mitochondria from myocardium, striated skeletal muscle, liver, and kidney, bind T_3 with high specificity. T_3 was bound with a higher association constant than T_4. But mitochondria from spleen, testis, and rat brain did not show specific, saturable binding.[82,p.998] We do know, however, that the metabolism of brain mitochondria is sensitive to thyroid hormones.[89]

Mitochondrial Energy Processes. Mitochondrial energy metabolism involves the production of ATP by the citric acid cycle and the electron transport chain. Sufficient oxygen is critical to the process. Thyroid hormone potently regulates mitochondrial energy metabolism. It does so mainly by regulating the enzymes that catalyze various chemical reactions involved in ATP production.

Production of ATP. Inside the mitochondrion, pyruvic acid is converted to acetyl coenzyme A (acetyl-CoA). Acetyl-CoA enters the citric acid cycle where its electrons are transferred to carriers (NADH and $FADH_2$). These carriers deliver the electrons to the electron transport chain in the inner membrane of the mitochondrion. The carriers pass the electrons to molecular oxygen through a series of other carriers. The transfer of the electrons to oxygen results in the production of ATP molecules.[156,p.128] Below is a written version of the structure of ATP:

$$\text{adenine—ribose—P—P*P}$$

$$\text{(ATP)}$$

The ATP molecule is composed of adenine, ribose, and three phosphates groups.

Adenine is a purine (an aromatic base) present in DNA and RNA. It is synthesized with the aid of the amino acid glycine and the vitamins folic acid and B$_{12}$.[35,pp.29-30] Linking adenine with the sugar ribose forms adenosine. The phosphorylation of adenosine forms monophosphate (AMP), adenosine diphosphate (ADP), or adenosine triphosphate (ATP).[34,p.179] AMP contains one phosphate group, ADP contains two, and ATP contains three.

The asterisk in the written version of the structure of ATP represents a high-energy phosphate bond. As glycogen is decomposed and its energy relinquished, the energy is employed to bind an inorganic phosphate (consumed in the diet as phosphorus) group to an ADP molecule. The energy is essentially the glue that binds the phosphate group to ADP in the ATP molecule.[1,p.195] Binding of the phosphate group transforms the ADP molecule to ATP. The binding of ADP to a molecule of inorganic phosphate (PO$_4$) traps 7.6 Kcal of energy (a kilocalorie is 1000 times the energy in a calorie) per mole of ATP produced. This process is called substrate-level phosphorylation because a substrate transfers a phosphate group to ADP.[35,p.31] During substrate-level phosphorylation, ATP is formed from ADP by the energy released from another chemical such as glucose.

Oxidative phosphorylation occurs in the mitochondria. In this process, high energy phosphoric bonds are formed from energy released by the oxidation of various substrates. (Oxidation is also known as dehydrogenation. The term dehydrogenation refers to the removal of a pair of hydrogen atoms with their electrons from a compound by the action of dehydrogenases or other enzymes.)

During oxidative phosphorylation, hydrogen ions (H$^+$) pass through ATP synthase molecules to form ATP. The direction of flow is from the space between the outer and inner mitochondrial membranes to the matrix of the mitochondrion. The ATP synthase complex is a large protein that forms a channel in the inner mitochondrial membrane. The terminal of the protein that projects into the mitochondrial matrix synthesizes ATP.[156,p.128] Synthesis occurs as hydrogen ions flow through the channel into the matrix. The ATP synthase uses energy derived from the hydrogen ion flow to catalyze the binding of inorganic phosphate to ADP, forming ATP.[33,p.750]

In 1984, Sterling and coauthors wrote that the rate at which mitochondria produce ATP from ADP correlates with the amount of T$_3$ that mitochondrial T$_3$-receptors are exposed to.[117] Studies in the 1970s had indicated that thyroid hormone binding sites existed in the mitochondrial membrane.[82][115] Since then, other researchers have reported finding thyroid hormone binding sites in isolated mitochondria.[154][155] Others did not find such sites.[153] In fact, other researchers have not been able to demonstrate a direct action of thyroid hormone on mitochondrial function *in vitro*.[37][38]

Normally, mitochondria form three ATP molecules for every atom of oxygen used, giving a phosphate-to-oxygen (P:O) ratio of 3:1. When the ratio is 3:1, physiologists say the system is "tightly coupled." "Coupling" is the term for converting the energy in other chemical bonds to that in phosphate bonds.[111] Tight coupling means the energy from other molecules is efficiently transferred to the phosphate bonds of ATP, with little loss of energy as heat. Until recently, some physiologists believed body heat resulted from uncoupling during oxidative phosphorylation. In other words, in uncoupling, or poor coupling, energy was not efficiently transferred from oxygen bonds to phosphate bonds. Theoretically, enough energy escaped during the process to warm the body.

Physiologists generally agree now, however, that body heat largely derives from other processes. Hydrolysis of ATP in a variety of cellular processes contributes to heat production. The processes include ion transport (as with the Na$^+$/K$^+$ pump and the Ca^{2+} pump in muscle cells), synthesis of various compounds (proteins, DNA, RNA, complex carbohydrates, and lipids), muscle contraction, secretion and absorption, and various metabolic pathways.[123,p.294]

When T$_3$ increases Na$^+$/K$^+$-ATPase concentration,[112] and the enzyme is active, it catalyzes conversion of ATP to ADP by breaking a phosphate bond. Breaking of the bond liberates energy. Part of the energy fuels the pump that moves sodium and potassium ions across membranes, such as those of nerve and muscle cells. Some energy also escapes as heat and warms the body. Some physiologists contend that this pump accounts for much,[121] although not all,[122] of the energy expenditure and heat production caused by thyroid hormones.

Another heat-producing mechanism involves the enzyme α-glycerophosphate dehydrogenase that functions in liver cell mitochondria. T$_3$ increased the concentration of this enzyme in rat liver cells. The increase in enzyme concentration was proportional to the degree of occupation of liver cell nuclear T$_3$-receptors by T$_3$.[113] Activity of the enzyme in hepatic cells was also increased by a higher occupation of T$_3$-receptors by T$_3$; activity of the enzyme is markedly amplified with progressively increased occupation of T$_3$-receptors.[125] When hypothyroid rats were given T_3, the increased concentration of α-glycerophosphate dehydrogenase was similar to that of Na^+/K^+-ATPase.[114] Shambaugh wrote that the parallel increase in these two enzymes accounts for the calorigenic (heat producing) action of thyroid hormones —even though oxidative phosphorylation remains tightly coupled[42,p.207] as in hypothyroidism.[116] Estimates vary concerning the amount of energy that becomes stored in ATP and how much is released as body heat. Davis wrote that about 50% of the energy is conserved in the phosphate bonds of ATP, and 50% escapes as heat.[1,p.195] Mason et al. wrote that only 40% of the energy released from foods is transferred to ATP, and that roughly 60% escapes as heat and contributes to body temperature.[35,p.44]

By virtue of its phosphate bonds, ATP is an energy storage and transport unit. It leaves the mitochondrion and migrates through the cell. When energy is required for a chemical reaction in the cell, the enzyme adenosine triphosphatase (ATPase) cleaves a phosphate group from the ATP molecule. Breaking of the phosphate bond converts the molecule back to ADP and releases 7.6 Kcal of energy per mole of ATP converted. Part of the energy is released as heat. The remainder is either expended or transferred to another molecule during the chemical reaction.[35,p.31]

Nicotinamide and Flavin Adenine Dinucleotide. Nicotinamide adenine dinucleotide and flavin adenine dinucleotide take part in energy metabolism by serving as electron transport devices.

Nicotinamide adenine dinucleotide is a compound that contains niacin (vitamin B_3). The glycolytic pathway generates two molecules of reduced nicotinamide adenine dinucleotide (NADH) by transferring a hydrogen atom with its electrons to oxidized nicotinamide adenine dinucleotide (NAD^+).

$$H^- + NAD^+ \rightarrow NADH$$

(Hydride ion) (Oxidized) (Reduced)

In the cytoplasm, NADH is important in forming other compounds such as fatty acids. In the mitochondrion, the reduced compound contributes to energy conservation by donating its hydrogen atom with its electrons within the electron transport chain.[35,p.33] When NADH releases its electrons, it again becomes NAD^+ (nicotinamide adenine dinucleotide), the oxidized form. NAD^+ is then available to undergo reduction again by accepting a hydrogen atom with its electrons.

Flavin adenine dinucleotide is a compound that contains riboflavin (vitamin B_2). Like nicotinamide adenine dinucleotide, flavin adenine dinucleotide is capable of accepting and donating electrons. The compound becomes reduced by accepting two hydrogen atoms with their electrons. The reduced form, $FADH_2$, releases the electrons within the electron transport chain. It then becomes FAD, the oxidized form.[35,pp.23&37][156,p.115]

Pyruvate. The membrane of the mitochondrion is permeable to pyruvate, the salt of pyruvic acid. Once pyruvate enters the mitochondrion, an enzyme removes one of its carbon atoms as CO_2 and adds coenzyme A. This reaction, called decarboxylation, yields acetyl coenzyme A (acetyl-CoA). Oxidation (the removal of electrons) also occurs with the shift of two electrons from pyruvate to the coenzyme acceptor, NAD^+.[34,p.216]

Four vitamins take part in the reaction: niacin (present in NAD), thiamine (as thiamine pyrophosphate, a coenzyme), riboflavin or vitamin B_2 (present in flavin adenine dinucleotide or FAD, part of the enzyme catalyzing the reaction), and pantothenic acid (as part of the acetyl-CoA molecule).[34,p.216] NAD^+ and FAD, the two most common coenzymes involved in energy metabolism, are derivatives of vitamins. Niacin is a part of NAD^+, and riboflavin is a part of FAD. These coenzymes function as electron-acceptors in most biological oxidations, and as electron donors in most biological reductions.[34,p.184] The other components in the reaction are a protein, magnesium (Mg^{2+}), and lipoic acid (a coenzyme that contains two sulfur atoms).[35,p.37]

Fatty Acid Oxidation. Triglycerides are composed of three fatty acids and glycerol, an alcohol. The fatty acids and glycerol easily dissociate from one another. Glycerol can be catabolized through glycolysis, but fatty acids cannot. Fatty acids vary in size and shape. They may have from 2-to-24 carbon atoms and may have various numbers of double bonds.

Like glucose, fatty acids are metabolized to CO_2, H_2O, and energy. Like pyruvate, fatty acids are first converted to acetyl-CoA. But unlike pyruvate, fatty acids are converted to acetyl-CoA through a series of chemical reactions called β-oxidation. A fatty acid with 20 carbon atoms yields 10 molecules of acetyl-CoA. A fatty acid with 16 carbon atoms produces 8 acetyl-CoA molecules. At this metabolic step (conversion to acetyl-CoA), further breakdown of fatty acids is the same as that of glucose. Glucose and fatty acids join their common final pathway,[35,p.41] the citric acid cycle, at this step.

The nutrients needed to convert fatty acids to

acetyl-CoA are the same as those necessary to break down glucose to acetyl-CoA: riboflavin (FAD), niacin (NAD), pantothenic acid (CoA), and magnesium ions (enzymatic conversion of fatty acids to acetyl-CoA). These agents are not a part of the enzymes; rather they are cofactors that bind to the enzymes and enable them to work properly.[110]

Citric Acid Cycle. The citric acid cycle (also called the Krebs or tricarboxylic acid cycle) is the major energy-generating pathway in cells. The cycle occurs in mitochondria. Breakdown products of fats, proteins, and carbohydrates are converted to acetyl-CoA, which is then oxidized in the citric acid cycle. The cycle is a series of repetitive chemical reactions that continue as long as the necessary enzymes and intermediates are available in the mitochondrion. The cycling of the reactions varies, depending on the supply of the reaction components or the demand for their end products.[35,p.43]

During the cycle, oxaloacetate (a four-carbon compound), acquires two carbons from acetyl-CoA, forfeits two carbons as CO_2, and finally reproduces oxaloacetate. During the cycle, acetyl-CoA is oxidized to CO_2. During the oxidation, electrons pass to the oxidation-reduction coenzymes FAD and NAD^+. The electrons transferred during the cycle result in the production of three molecules of NADH + H^+, one of $FDHH_2$, and one GTP (guanosine 5'-triphosphate; a compound similar to ATP). ATP forms when NADH and $FDHH_2$ contribute their electrons to CO_2 during oxidative phosphorylation. ATP is also generated from GTP. One round of the cycle produces 12 ATP molecules.[156,p.121] In addition to oxidizing the by-produces of fats, proteins, and carbohydrates, the citric acid cycle synthesizes fatty acids, amino acids, and glucose.

Steps in the Citric Acid Cycle and Production of Electron Carriers. The cycle passes through eight steps: citric acid→ isocitrate → α-ketoglutaric acid → succinyl-CoA → succinate → fumarate → malate → oxaloacetate → citric acid. Figure 2.2.3, simplified after Mason et al., shows only four of the intermediates of the cycle.[35,p.42] Reactions involving these intermediates produce carriers that transfer electrons to the electron transport chain. An NADH is produced when isocitrate is converted through oxidative decarboxylation to α-ketoglutaric acid; another NADH is produced when α-ketoglutaric acid is converted through oxidative decarboxylation to succinyl-CoA; GTP is generated from GDP when a thioester bond of succinyl-CoA is cleaved; FAD is converted to $FADH_2$ when succinyl-CoA is oxidized to fumarate, with removal of two hydrogens with their electrons; fumarate

is converted to malate; and malate is oxidized to oxaloacetate, with removal of two hydrogens and their electrons and production of NADH.[156,p.123]

As Figure 2.2.3 shows, each turn of the citric acid cycle generates three NADH, one $FADH_2$, and one GTP. ATP is generated from GTP, and the NADH and $FADH_2$ transport electrons to the electron transport chain where additional ATP molecules are produced.

Citric Acid Cycle and Thyroid Hormone. Davis wrote that the activity of the citric acid cycle is not directly affected by thyroid hormones, but theoretically, thyroid hormone regulates the availability of citric acid cycle intermediates.[1,p.197] In part, the hormone does so by regulating the activity of various enzymes.

Pyruvate Dehydrogenase and Thyroid Hormone. To form acetyl-CoA, pyruvate dehydrogenase catalyzes the oxidative decarboxylation of pyruvate.[31,p.379] Activity of pyruvate dehydrogenase is increased in the adipose tissue of hyperthyroid rats, whereas it is decreased in adipose tissue of hypothyroid rats.[95] Holness and Sugden found increased activity of renal pyruvate dehydrogenase in hyperthyroid rats.[96] Weinberg and Utter found that liver pyruvate dehydrogenase activity was normal in hyperthyroid rats, but that in hypothyroid rats, activity was reduced by a third.[97] While thyroid hormone status affects the activity level of pyruvate dehydrogenase, O'Reilly and Murphy concluded that the enzyme is not *stringently* controlled by thyroid hormone status.[94]

In the brain, activity of pyruvate dehydrogenase is also influenced by thyroid hormone status, but in a direction opposite to that in peripheral tissues. Murthy and Baquer[88] found that thyroid hormone deficiency increased the activity of pyruvate dehydrogenase in the cerebrum, cerebellum, and brain stem. After thyroidectomy, activity gradually increased in the cerebral hemispheres. Activity reached a maximum at 21 days, and remained constant at 30 and 60 days. Enzyme activity was also maximum in the cerebellum and brain stem at 21 days. In contrast to the constant activity in the cerebral hemispheres, activity diminished in the cerebellum at 30 days and in the brain stem at 60 days. T_3 injections brought the activity level in the cerebral hemispheres to normal at 60 days. But despite T_3 injections, activity in the brain stem continued at 25% above normal at 60 days.[88,p.49]

Thyroid hormone increased the activity in the brain of the insulin-dependent enzyme hexokinase type II.[140] Hexokinase catalyzes the first reaction in glycolysis in which a phosphate is transferred from ATP to glucose, forming glucose 6-phosphate[83,p.315] (see Figure 2.2.1). The enhanced ability of the brain to metabolize glucose is presumably a mechanism to stabilize, within narrow homeostatic limits, the functions of this organ that are critical to survival.

The apparent heightened ability of the brain to metabolize glucose during thyroid hormone deficiency differs from the diminished ability of insulin-sensitive tissues such as liver and adipose.[88,p.52] For example, in liver, decreased pyruvate flux was associated with decreased pyruvate dehydrogenase activity.[135] In liver and adipose, thyroid hormone deficiency decreases the activity of enzymes of the glycolytic and pentose phosphate pathways and of the citric acid cycle.[135][136] These effects are part of the diminished responsiveness of tissues in hypothyroidism to the rapidly-acting hormones epinephrine, glucagon, and insulin[137][138][141][142] (despite normal circulating levels of insulin[88,p.52][139]).

Vitamin B_1, as thiamine pyrophosphate, is also a component of the multienzyme complex pyruvate dehydrogenase.[31,p.379] It functions primarily as a required coenzyme to pyruvate decarboxylase. This enzyme decarboxylates pyruvate to CO_2 and acetaldehyde. Mg^{2+} is also required as a cofactor.[98,p.804][99,pp.336-337]

Pyruvate Carboxylase and Thyroid Hormone.
Conversion of pyruvate to the citric acid cycle intermediate oxaloacetate is catalyzed in the mitochondrion by pyruvate carboxylase. Pyruvate carboxylase contains four molecules of the vitamin biotin. The biotin serves as an intermediate carrier of the carboxyl group (activated CO_2). Biotin transfers the activated CO_2 to the pyruvate molecule, forming oxaloacetate.[31,p.441][156,p.118] Also, each of the four subunits of the enzyme binds one manganese ion (Mn^{2+}).[99,p.464]

Pyruvate is converted to oxaloacetate whenever intermediates are deficient. This conversion, then, is considered a "filling up" enzymatic reaction that replenishes a citric acid cycle intermediate.[99,p.464] Pyruvate carboxylase thus plays a critical role in maintaining proper levels of citric acid cycle intermediates.[31,p.441]

Unless acetyl-CoA is present, pyruvate carboxylase activity is minimal. An increasing concentration of acetyl-CoA, however, stimulates pyruvic carboxylase to generate more oxaloacetate.[99,p.464] The B vitamin biotin is involved in the carboxylation of acetyl-CoA. (This carboxylation forms malonyl coenzyme A. Malonyl-CoA, is the condensation product of malonic acid and coenzyme A. Malonyl-CoA is an intermediate in the synthesis of fatty acid.)[156,p.118] Biotin is carboxylated only when acetyl-CoA is bound to pyruvate carboxylase, allosterically activating it.[31,p.441] The activation produces more oxaloacetate as the product of

the pyruvate carboxylase reaction, and enables the citric acid cycle to oxidize more acetyl-CoA.[99,p.464] This physiological control mechanism is important because oxaloacetate is an intermediate in gluconeogenesis and in the citric acid cycle.[31,p.441]

Weinberg and Utter found that liver from hyperthyroid rats had twice the pyruvate carboxylase activity of normal rats. By contrast, liver from hypothyroid rats had only two-thirds the activity of normal rats.[97]

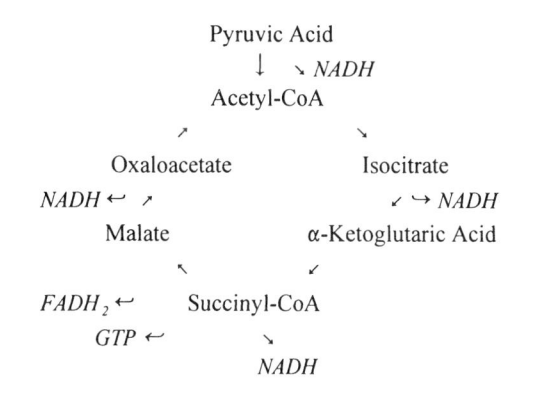

Figure 2.2.3. The citric acid cycle. Each turn generates three NADH, one $FADH_2$, and one GTP.

Malate in the Citric Acid Cycle. Malate is derived from foods and from synthesis in the citric acid cycle.[104,p.52] It is involved in the transfer of the electrons of oxaloacetate across the mitochondrial membrane.[31,p.441] It is also an intermediate in the citric acid cycle.[31,pp.377&388]

Oxidation of malate to oxaloacetate is another "filling up" enzymatic reaction. When citric acid cycle intermediates are deficient, malate dehydrogenase (malic enzyme)[99,p.464] catalyzes the oxidation of malate to oxaloacetate. This replenishes the available supply of oxaloacetate.[99,p.342] First, malate dehydrogenase binds its coenzyme, the electron acceptor NAD^+. Next, the enzyme catalyzes removal of hydrogen atoms with their electrons from malate and converts malate to oxaloacetate.[99,p.203] The reaction also occurs in the opposite direction, with malate dehydrogenase catalyzing reduction of oxaloacetate to malate.[31,p.488]

Malate-Aspartate Shuttle. Malate, as part of the malate-aspartate shuttle, transfers the electrons of the reducing agent NADH from the cytoplasm into mitochondria. This transfer involves two membrane carriers and four enzymes. The shuttle is necessary because the inner mitochondrial membrane is impermeable to

NADH and NAD⁺. For NADH to be oxidized by the mitochondrial respiratory chain (its electrons donated to the chain), the electrons from NADH, rather than NADH itself, are carried by electron shuttles across the mitochondrial membrane. The hydrogens with their electrons are transported across the mitochondrial membranes by three main shuttles: the α-glycerophosphate, malate-aspartate, and malate-citrate shuttles. Thyroidectomy reduced the activity of all three shuttles in rat liver and kidney cell mitochondria.[151]

In the cytoplasm, malate dehydrogenase[31,p.488] catalyzes transfer of electrons from NADH to oxaloacetate. The electron transfer reduces oxaloacetate to malate. Malate then traverses the inner mitochondrial membrane.[31,pp.417-418] In the mitochondrial matrix, malate is reoxidized by NAD⁺ to form NADH and oxaloacetate. Oxaloacetate does not readily pass out through the mitochondrial membrane. It must first undergo transamination to form aspartate. Aspartate is then transported to the cytoplasm. There, the aspartate is changed back to oxaloacetate ready to receive more electrons from NADH. This shuttle is reversible and requires no energy expenditure. The shuttle occurs only if the NADH/NAD⁺ ratio is higher in the cytoplasm than in the mitochondrial matrix.[31,pp.417-418]

For the normal interactions of malate in the malate-aspartate shuttle, Mg^{2+}[105] and vitamin B_6[106] must be present.

Thyroid Hormone Regulates Malic Enzyme Synthesis through Genomic Action. Liver cell malate dehydrogenase (malic enzyme) is considered a biomarker of thyroid hormone action.[124,p.156] Kohn and coauthors[147] found that adding TSH to thyroid cells induced a 7-to-8-fold increase in steady levels of malic enzyme. T_3 increases malic enzyme synthesis at the nuclear level by inducing transcription and increasing the level of cellular malic enzyme mRNA.[100][101][103] Expression of the malic enzyme gene in the liver is a function of thyroid state.[148] Two hours after T_3 administration, there is a modest increase in two malic enzyme mRNA levels. mRNA levels surge to a several-fold increase 18-to-24 hours later.[126]

Katyare et al. measured the effects of thyroid hormones, administered for 4 consecutive days, on the respiratory activity of isolated brain mitochondria from euthyroid rats. The researchers found a 2-fold increase in primary mitochondrial hydrogenases, including glutamate, succinate, and malate dehydrogenase. (These enzymes catalyze reactions in the citric acid cycle.[83,p.325]) Mitochondrial but not cytosolic malate dehydrogenase activity increased.[144] Mooradian and coauthors, however, found that T_3 increased mRNA

levels for and activity of malate dehydrogenase in hepatic cell cytosol of rats. The response of aged rats was only 50% that of young rats. The age-related diminished response was not due to reduced food intake and was mediated at a pretranslational level.[145]

Activity of liver cell malic enzyme is increased by occupation of T_3-receptors by T_3. Enzyme activity is markedly amplified with progressively increased occupation of T_3-receptors.[125] Mooradian found that 3-month old hypothyroid rats had a significantly lower malic enzyme level than control (euthyroid) rats. Euthyroid rats had 17.1±2.3 malic enzyme units per mg of protein; hypothyroid rats had 4.8±0.6 units per mg of protein (only 28% of the units per mg of euthyroid rats).[124,p.157]

Insulin has effects similar to those of T_3 on malic enzyme. Low insulin levels in diabetic rats were accompanied by low malic enzyme mRNA levels and reduced synthesis of the enzyme. In diabetic rats, transcription rates were 64% of normal. Malic enzyme mRNA levels were 39% of normal values. In diabetic animals, insulin treatment increased to normal the transcription rate, mRNA levels, and enzyme synthesis. Transcription rates and mRNA levels were restored to normal 8 hours after treatment with insulin; enzyme production returned to normal after 4 days of treatment. The researchers concluded that insulin plays a role at the stages of transcription, translation, and/or accumulation of malic enzyme. Administering T_3 increased transcription of the gene for the enzyme even at low insulin levels, partially restoring enzyme synthesis even in diabetic animals. During T_3 treatment of diabetic rats, the transcription rate increased by 65%, enzyme mRNA increased by 36%, and enzyme production increased by 29%.[103,p.116]

Interaction of Carbohydrates and T_3 in the Induction of Malate Dehydrogenase. Macronutrients also influence malic enzyme levels. They do so through post-translational regulation. Malic enzyme mRNA levels in liver cells increased in rats fed a high-carbohydrate diet. Transcription of the mRNA was not increased, however, indicating that carbohydrates had a regulatory effect in the cytoplasm.[101][102] Dozin, having found that a high-carbohydrate diet increased malic enzyme mRNA, suggested that carbohydrate stabilizes transcript for the enzyme.[101] Stabilization could occur by inhibition of mRNA degrading enzymes or by a decrease in the rate of translation. Dietary fat decreased mRNA levels but did not decrease the rate of transcription. This suggests that dietary fat destabilizes mRNAs.[102]

Mariash and Oppenheimer found a synergistic relationship between carbohydrate feeding and dosing with T_3. Their studies with hepatocytes indicate that glucose is the main factor inducing hepatic malate dehydrogenase. Glucose induced the enzyme in the absence of hormones, including absence of T_3. But T_3 amplified the carbohydrate-induced increase in production of the enzyme. This amplification of enzyme production does not necessarily mean that carbohydrates and T_3 acted in unison; they could have influenced enzyme production through independent steps, resulting in a compound effect. The researchers wrote that studies of aging animals have shown a reduced induction responsiveness of hepatic malate dehydrogenase to both carbohydrates and T_3.[149]

Electron Transport System. The electron transport system carries out oxidative phosphorylation. The efficiency of this process (at least in brown fat) is improved by thyroid hormone.[37][82,p.996] In the process, ADP and inorganic phosphate are combined to form ATP. The energy released upon oxidation of compounds in this system is not used directly to synthesize ATP. Instead, the energy fuels the pumping of protons (H^+ ions) across the inner mitochondrial membrane to the space between the inner and outer membranes. This creates an electrochemical gradient ($\Delta\psi$). The gradient causes protons to move back across the membrane to reduce the potential difference between the two sides of the membrane. To move back, the protons must flow through the ATP synthase complex. The passage of protons through the synthase catalyzes formation of ATP from ADP and P_i.[110]

In oxidation-reduction (redox) reactions, one compound is reduced by another. The first compound becomes reduced because it acquires an electron from the second compound. The second compound, which donates the electron, is called the reducing agent. During the reaction, the second compound becomes oxidized by the first compound, which is called the oxidizing agent for the reaction. In most biological redox reactions, electrons are directly transferred by the use of metal cations, via H^- (hydride ions), by formation of a covalent bond with oxygen (resulting in sharing of electron pairs with oxygen), or by loss or addition of H^+.[110] In the most common oxidation-reduction reactions in biology, hydrogen atoms with their electrons are either donated or accepted by various compounds. In oxidation, compounds give up their hydrogen atoms (protons) and their electrons.[34,p.183] In reduction, compounds accept hydrogen with its electrons.

The reduced form of nicotinamide adenine dinucleotide (NADH), for example, contains a hydrogen

atom. In the presence of ADP and inorganic phosphate, NADH releases the hydrogen, and the energy of its electron is used to bind the phosphate to the ADP molecule, forming ATP. (Keep in mind, though, that the energy is indirectly used for this. The energy is used directly to pump protons across the inner mitochondrial membrane, creating the $\Delta\psi$ that drives protons through the ATP synthase complex, catalyzing formation of ATP.)

In the process, NADH is converted to its oxidized form, NAD^+. NADH dehydrogenase is the enzyme that catalyzes transfer of electrons from NADH to flavin mononucleotide (FMN) in the electron transport chain. FMN is complexed with proteins and extends through the inner mitochondrial membrane. It operates as an electron carrier in biological oxidative reactions,[83,pp.70&333] shuttling electrons from NADH and $FADH_2$ to oxygen.[83,p.327] The NADH dehydrogenase that catalyzes the electron transfer from NADH to FMN is under the transcriptional control of T_3.

Freerksen et al. studied the enzymes that catalyze the shuttle that transfers NADH (reduced in glycolysis outside the mitochondrion) to FAD inside. They found that T_3 added to cultured rat heart cells decreased NAD-linked α-glycerol-3-phosphate dehydrogenase activity by 35%. The decreased activity showed a strong inverse relationship between T_3 and activity of the enzyme. Activity decreased by 65% when the medium also contained hydrocortisone and insulin. T_3 produced the classic elevation of FAD-linked α-glycerophosphate dehydrogenase,[150] the enzyme that catalyzes transfer of electrons to FAD and forms $FADH_2$.[83,p.352] However, Tobin et al. found that thyroidectomy reduced the activity of the α-glycerophosphate, malate-aspartate, and malate-citrate shuttles in rat liver and kidney mitochondria.[151]

This transcriptional control of NADH dehydrogenase by T_3 is exerted in the genome of the mitochondrion. T_3 exerts genomic effects by binding with high affinity to T_3-binding sites on the chromosomes of the mitochondria[127,p.999][129][130] (see Chapter 2.3). Iglesias and coworkers isolated a DNA fragment in cerebrum, hippocampus, and heart mitochondria that clones a mRNA that is regulated *in vivo* by T_3. Through sequencing, they characterized this clone as part of the NADH dehydrogenase subunit 3 (ND3) gene in mitochondria.[127,p.996] In early postnatal hypothyroid rats, but not adult hypothyroid rats,[128] ND3 mRNA was reduced by 40%-to-60%.

Cytochromes. Cytochromes are proteins that contain a central iron atom.[83,p.329] The iron of the heme group of the cytochromes is synthesized from glycine and succinyl-CoA. The iron can both give up electrons (oxidation) and accept them (reduction).[156,p.116]

$$Fe^{3+} \rightleftharpoons Fe^{2+}$$

By doing so, the cytochromes perform electron transport and contribute to ATP formation. Cytochromes are among the compounds whose genes in the mitochondrial genome are under thyroid hormone control.[131][132][133][134] Thyroid hormone increases levels of mRNAs for cytochrome c oxidase subunits and cytochrome b.[131][132][133]

Cytochrome b is a component of complex III of the electron transport system. Complex III picks up electrons from the ubiquinone (coenzyme Q) pool and delivers them to cytochrome c, a relatively small protein and highly mobile carrier that shuttles electrons from complex III and complex IV.[83,pp.328&334] Ubiquinone, popularly known as coenzyme Q, can be produced endogenously and is not derived from a vitamin.[156,p.116] It can also be taken as a nutritional supplement.

Cytochrome c oxidase (also called cytochrome c-O_2-oxidoreductase) is the final complex (complex IV) in the electron transport system. It conducts electrons from cytochrome c to oxygen along with H^+ (which is taken up from the matrix) to form H_2. Complex IV functions as the electron carrier that donates the electrons to O_2 in the mitochondria, and by doing so, is responsible for 90% of the oxygen consumed by living organisms. (Cyanide is a deadly poison because it impairs complex IV in transporting electrons to oxygen.[83,p.334]) Regulation by thyroid hormone of mRNA levels for cytochrome c oxidase subunits highlights the importance of this hormone for oxidative processes and energy metabolism.

T_3 Appears to Affect ATP⇌ADP Exchange Across the Mitochondrial Membrane. The electron transport system is highly efficient in transferring energy to ATP molecules. Nonetheless, only about 41% of the energy in foods is conserved in ATP.[35,p.44] The rest is released as heat and contributes to body temperature. As I pointed out above, after being synthesized, ATP migrates to various locations of energy-requiring processes in the cell. There, the enzyme adenosine triphosphatase (ATPase) cleaves a phosphate group from the molecule. Energy is released and used to fuel the process peculiar to that location. The work may be physical, as in myofibril contraction, or metabolic, as in shifting the equilibrium of a reaction to the forward direction.[110]

When the phosphate group is removed from ATP, the molecule then constitutes ADP. When ADP enters the mitochondrion again, it stimulates stage III respiration. During respiration, ADP again takes part in oxidative phosphorylation, resulting in the formation of new ATP.[42,p.207] The rate at which ADP re-enters the mitochondrion is regulated by ADP-ATP translocase. Translocase is the most abundant protein in the mitochondrion and constitutes about 14% of the mitochondrial membrane protein.[31,p.419] This specific transport protein enables ADP and ATP to traverse the mitochondrial membrane, which is a permeability barrier. The flow of ADP and ATP is a precisely coupled exchange: ADP enters the mitochondrion when ATP exits, and translocase catalyzes the exchange.[31,pp.418-419] T_3 appears to increase translocase[38] and translocator[39][69] activity. Translocase may[40] or may not[41] be the mitochondrial protein that binds T_3.

ADP must be present for ATP to form. Because of this, how quickly the putative T_3-translocase combination imports ADP partly controls the rate of oxidative phosphorylation in mitochondria. In hypothyroidism, the transport of ADP into mitochondria is lower than normal. As a result, the mitochondria receive too little ADP to convert to ATP as a form of stored energy.[46,p.172] Consequently, the mitochondria produce fewer ATP molecules.[118,p.1208]

Mitochondrial phosphate transporter is a compound that ferries inorganic phosphate into the mitochondrion. The activity of the transporter was increased in thyrotoxic rat liver.[43] The increase was due to an effect of thyroid hormone on the lipid component of the phosphate transporter. Horrum suggested that thyroid hormone increases proton transfer at the inner mitochondrial membrane.[44] This indicates that thyroid hormone increases the production of ATP through promoting proton transfer.[1,p.197]

Harper and Brand studied the mechanism of changes in resting oxygen consumption in liver cells from hypothyroid and hyperthyroid rats compared to euthyroid rats. They reported that 50% of the change in oxygen consumption resulted from changes in the rate of movement of protons across the inner mitochondrial membrane. In hypothyroid mitochondria, there was a decrease in oxygen consumption due to a decrease in proton leak.[53] The decrease may have resulted from effects on ATP synthase and ADP-ATP translocase. These two enzymes are a part of the ATP-synthesizing complex. ATP synthase is a spherical particle that protrudes upon a short stalk from the inner mitochondrial membrane. At this location, ADP is phosphorylated (an inorganic phosphate, P_i, is added to the molecule) to form ATP.[34,p.238] ADP-ATP trans-locase brings ADP into the mitochondrion in exchange for ATP, which exits the organelle.[31,pp.418-419] Harper and Brand also showed that hyperthyroid mitochondria had increased mitochondrial proton movement[53] and ATP turnover.[54] The other 50% change in resting oxygen consumption, according to Harper and Brand, resulted from (1) changes in nonmitochondrial-dependent oxygen consumption in hypothyroid rats and (2) ATP turnover-dependent oxygen consumption in hyperthyroid rats.[53]

Many nutrients are involved in the metabolic pathways in the cytoplasm and mitochondria. The vitamin biotin, for example, is necessary as an enzyme cofactor in fatty acid synthesis. The active form of vitamin B_6, pyridoxal phosphate, is a cofactor necessary to transamination (as in the breakdown of amino acids).[35,pp.50-51] Listing all the nutrients that are needed in the cell is beyond the scope of our concerns. The reader should note, however, that they all ultimately interact and must be available in sufficient quantifies for optimal cell function.

Table 2.2.2. Summary of the cellular actions and effects of thyroid hormone.

- Plays major roles in the regulation of cell metabolism.

- Affects cell functions mainly by regulating transcription of specific genes but may also influence translation of mRNAs.

- Appears to diffuse into the plasma membrane and interact with proteins involved in hormone and sugar transport into the cell. Increases sugar uptake by cell membranes and transport of amino acids across the membranes.

- Increases the level and activity of Na^+/K^+-ATPase and increases activity of the Na^+/K^+ pump.

- Increases the levels of the mitochondrial enzyme α-glycerophosphate dehydrogenase.

- Increases body temperature largely through parallel increases in α-glycerophosphate dehydrogenase and Na^+/K^+-ATPase.

- Regulates the levels of various enzymes and electron carriers necessary for the metabolism of substrates for ATP production. The enzymes and carriers take part in glycolysis, the citric acid cycle, and the electron transport system.

- Affects metabolic processes in the cytoplasm but more so in mitochondria.

- Directly and indirectly influences mitochondrial structure and function. Increases both size and activity of mitochondria; increases mitochondrial oxygen consumption, ATP production, and lipid content of mitochondrial membrane.

- Regulates the balance of α- and β-adrenergic receptors that is necessary for proper catecholamine regulation of cell metabolism.

Oxygen, Thyroid Hormone, and the Mitochondrion. Oxygen is particularly important in metabolism. An adequate quantity is essential if the energy requirements of the body are to be met. All but a tiny fraction of the total oxygen use in the body occurs in mitochondria.[87,p.845] Oxygen is essential to the oxidation of carbohydrates, fats, and proteins.[34,pp.185-186] Through

oxidation, the energy of the chemical bonds of these foods is transferred to the phosphate bonds of ATP. Cells continually adjust their rates of glucose oxidation to meet their needs for ATP.[34,pp.185-186]

As Becker details,[34,p.209] the availability of oxygen and the respiratory metabolism it permits is the crucial component that allows cells to move beyond glycolysis. Oxygen is the electron acceptor by which the carbon atoms of glucose (and other substrates) are oxidized fully to carbon dioxide.[110] All the electrons that are removed from these substrates ultimately transfer to oxygen. Oxygen makes this transfer possible, yet it serves only as a terminal acceptor of electrons. Serving this role, oxygen enables continuous reoxidation of the reduced coenzyme molecules NADH and $FADH_2$. In their oxidized form, these coenzymes act as cofactors in the stepwise oxidation of organic intermediates (components of the system produced at one step and used by another step in the same pathway[53,p.229]) derived from pyruvate. In respiratory metabolism, electrons (actually hydrogen ions and their electrons) are transferred from organic substrates to the coenzyme carriers NADH and $FADH_2$. These reduced coenzymes are then reoxidized; their electrons are transferred to oxygen with the production of ATP.

The rate of oxygen consumption by the body, called the metabolic rate, is powerfully affected by thyroid hormone status. In thyroid hormone deficiency, oxygen consumption decreases; correcting the hormone deficiency increases consumption.[89,p.220]

Thyroid hormone appears to increase the amount of oxygen available for metabolic processes by mobilizing it through enzyme regulation. In mature human red blood cells *in vitro*, thyroid hormone increased synthesis of 2,3-diphosphoglycerate.[30] This compound binds to hemoglobin and lowers its affinity for oxygen by a factor of 26. The decreased affinity enables the hemoglobin to unload oxygen in tissue capillaries.[31,p.157] The red cells of hyperthyroid patients contain increased amounts of 2,3-diphosphoglycerate.[32] The unloading of oxygen by hemoglobin makes more available for the increased oxidation rate in hypermetabolic tissues.

Thyroid Hormone Increases Mitochondrial Oxygen Consumption. It has long been known that T_3 promptly increases mitochondrial oxygen consumption. The rapidity of the increase makes it likely that this initial effect of T_3 results from direct action at the mitochondrion rather than the nucleus.[82,p.999] The increase in oxygen consumption occurs with physiological dosages of T_3 and T_4 and in a dose-dependent manner.[36][70] In the presence of glucose, the respiratory rate of liver cells from hyperthyroid rats was 1.4 times that of hepatocytes from euthyroid rats; the rate was twice that of hepatocytes from hypothyroid rats. The relatively faster rate of liver cell respiration in hyperthyroid rats indicates that mitochondrial respiration is more potently affected by variations in thyroid status than is cytoplasmic glycolysis.[143] The site of thyroid

hormone action in increased respiration appears to be mitochondrial receptors.[70]

The rapid increase in mitochondrial oxygen consumption following T_3 administration[36][70] may be independent of a nuclear genomic effect of T_3. A nuclear genomic effect of T_3 would increase the presence of proteins that could serve as enzymes.[1,p.196] The cell nucleus, through gene *transcription*, is responsible for protein synthesis. When protein synthesis is chemically blocked, however, T_3 still stimulates liver cell respiration.[36] In incubated liver cells, a physiologic dosage of T_3 increased oxygen consumption by 121%. A greater than physiologic dosage increased consumption by 138%. Blockage of protein synthesis with cycloheximide did not impede the stimulating effect of T_3 on oxygen consumption. This suggests that the effect of T_3 was not nuclear.[52] Table 2.2.2 summarizes the cellular actions and effects of thyroid hormone.

THE CELL NUCLEUS

Nucleus in Latin means "seed" or "kernel." The term is fitting because the structure and function of the cell are determined by processes that occur within the nucleus. The membrane of the nucleus separates the nucleoplasm from the cell cytoplasm. Within the nucleus are the chromosomes where T_3, upon binding to T_3-receptors, regulates the expression of a vast array of genes. These genomic actions of thyroid hormone are the subject of the next chapter.

REFERENCES

1. Davis, P.J.: Cellular actions of thyroid hormone. In *Werner and Ingbar's The Thyroid: A Fundamental and Clinical Text*, 6th edition. Edited by L.E. Braverman and R.D. Utiger, New York, J.B. Lippincott Co., 1991, pp.190-203.

2. Oppenheimer, J.H.: Thyroid hormone action at the molecular level. In *Werner and Ingbar's The Thyroid: A Fundamental and Clinical Text*, 6th edition. Edited by L.E. Braverman and R.D. Utiger, New York, J.B. Lippincott Co., 1991, pp.204-224.

3. David, P.J. and Blas, S.D.: *In vitro* stimulation of human red blood cell Ca^{2+}-ATPase by thyroid hormone. *Biochem. Biophys. Res. Commun.*, 99:1073, 1981.

4. Segal, J. and Ingbar, S.H.: 3,5,3'-tri-iodothyronine enhances sugar transport in rat thymocytes by increasing the intrinsic activity of the plasma membrane sugar transporter. *J. Endocrinol.*, 124:133, 1990.

5. Peavy, D.E., Edmondson, J.W., and Duckworth, W.C.: Selective effects of inhibitors of hormone processing on insulin action in isolated hepatocyles. *Endocrinology*, 114:753, 1984.

6. Goncalves, E., Lakshmanan, M., Pontecorvia, A., and Robbins, J.: Thyroid hormone transport in a human glioma cell line. *Mol. Cell. Endocrinol.*, 69:157, 1990.

7. Centanni, M. and Robbins, J.: Role of sodium in thyroid hormone uptake by rat skeletal muscle. *J. Clin. Invest.*, 80:1068, 1987.

8. Segal, J. and Ingbar, S.H.: Stimulation by triiodothyronine of the *in vitro* uptake of sugars by rat thymocytes. *J. Clin. Invest.*, 63:507, 1979.

9. Segal, J. and Ingbar, S.H.: Studies on the mechanism by which 3,5,3'-triiodothyronine stimulates 2-deoxyglucose uptake in rat thymocytes *in vitro*: role of calcium and 3':5'-monophosphate. *J. Clin. Invest.*, 68:103, 1981.

10. Davis, F.B., Davis, P.J., and Blas, S.D.: The role of calmodulin in thyroid hormone stimulation *in vitro* of human red blood cell Ca^{2+}-ATPase activity. *J. Clin. Invest.*, 71:579, 1983.

11. Constante, G., Sand, G., Connart, D., and Glinoer, D.: *In vitro* effects of thyroid hormones on red blood cell Ca^{2+}-ATPase activity. *J. Endocrinol. Invest.*, 9:15, 1986.

12. Galo, M.G., Unates, L.E., and Farias, R.N.: Effect of membrane fatty acid composition on the action of thyroid hormones on $(Ca^{2+} + Mg^{2+})$-adenosine triphosphate from rat erythrocyte. *J. Biol. Chem.*, 256:7113, 1981.

13. Segal, J., Hardiman, J., and Ingbar, S.H.: Stimulation of calcium-ATPase activity by 3,5,3'-triiodothyronine in rat thymocyte plasma membranes: a possible role in the modulation of cellular calcium concentration. *Biochem. J.*, 261:749, 1989.

14. Nassi, P., Liquri, G., Nediani, C., Taddei, N., and Ramponi, G.: Increased acylphosphatase levels in erythrocytes, muscle and liver of triiodothyronine treated rabbits. *Horm. Metab. Res.*, 22:33, 1990.

15. Dube, M.P., Davis, F.B., Davis, P.J., Schoenl, M., and Blas, S.D.: Effects of hyperthyroidism and hypothyroidism on human red blood cell Ca^{2+}-ATPase activity. *J. Clin. Endocrinol. Metab.*, 62:253, 1986.

16. Baskurt, O.K., Levi, E., Temizer, A., et al.: *In vitro* effects of thyroxine on the mechanical properties of erythrocytes. *Life Sci.*, 46:1471, 1990.

17. Davis, P.J., Davis, F.B., and Lawrence, W.D.: Thyroid hormone regulation of membrane Ca^{2+}-ATPase activity. *Endocr. Res.*, 15:651, 1989.

18. Warnick, P.R., Davis, P.J., Davis, F.B., Cody, V., Galindo, J., Jr., and Blas, S.D.: Rabbit skeletal muscle endoplasmic reticulum Ca^{2+}-ATPase activity: stimulation *in vitro* by thyroid hormone analogues and bipyridines. *Biochem. Pharmacol.*, 45:1091, 1991.

19. Davis, P.J., Davis, F.B., and Blas, S.D.: Studies on the mechanism of thyroid hormone stimulation *in vitro* of human red cell Ca^{2+}-ATPase activity. *Life Sci.*, 30:675, 1982.

20. Davis, P.J., Davis, F.B., and Blas, S.D.: Components of the phosphatidylinositol cycle modulate thyroid hormone stimulation of human red cell Ca^{2+}-ATPase activity. Abstract 114, Program of the Annual Meeting of the Endocrine Society, Anaheim, California, 1986.

21. Lawrence, W.D., Schoenl, M., and Davis, P.J.: Stimulation *in vitro* of rabbit erythrocyte cytosol phospholipid-dependent protain kinase activity: a novel action of thyroid hormone. *J. Biol. Chem.*, 264:4766, 1989.

22. Smallwood, J.I., Gugi, B., and Rasmussen, H.: Regulation of erythrocyte Ca^{2+} pump activity by protein kinase C. *J. Biol. Chem.*, 263:2195, 1988.

23. Goldfine, I.D., Simons, C.G., Smith, G.J., and Ingbar, S.H.: Cycloleucine transport in isolated rat thymocytes: *in vitro* effects of triiodothyronine and thyroxine. *Endocrinology*, 118:207, 1975.

24. Segal, J. and Ingbar, S.H.: 3,5,3'-triiodothyronine increases cellular 3',5'-monophosphate concentration and sugar uptake in rat thymocytes by stimulating adenylate cyclase activity: studies with the adenylate cyclase inhibitor MDL 12330A. *Endocrinology*, 124:2166, 1989.

25. Segal, J. Rehder, M.C., and Ingbar, S.H.: Calmodulin mediates the stimulatory effect of 3,5,3'-triiodothyronine on adenylate cyclase activity in rat thymocyte plasma membranes. *Endocrinology*, 199:2629, 1989.

26. Segal, J.: Calmodulin modulates thymocyte adenylate cyclase activity through the guanine nucleotide regulatory unit. *Mol. Cell. Endocrinol.*, 64:95, 1989.

27. Yoshida, K. and Davis, P.J.: Dissociable and nondissociable cytoplasmic protein-thyroid hormone interaction. *Biochem. Biophys. Acta*, 582:332, 1979.

28. Hasizume, K., Miyamoto, T., Kobayashi, M., et al.: Cytosolic 3,5,3'-triiodo-L-thyronine (T_3)—binding protein (CTBP) regulation of nuclear T_3 binding: evidence for the presence of T_3-CTBP complex-binding sites in nuclei. *Endocrinology*, 124:2851, 1989.

29. Narayan, P. and Towle, H.C.: Stabilization of a specific nuclear mRNA precursor by thyroid hormone. *Mol. Cell. Biol.*, 5:2642, 1985.

30. Schoenl, M. and Davis, P.J.: Unpublished observation, December, 1990.

31. Stryer, L.: *Biochemistry*, 3rd edition. New York, W.H. Freeman and Co., 1988.

32. Alvarez-Sala, J.L., Urban, M.A., Sicilia, J.J., DiazFdez, A.J., FdezMendieta, F., and Espinos, D.: Red cell 2,3-diphosphoglycerate in patients with hyperthyroidism. *Acta Endocrinol.* (Copenh.), 3:424, 1980.

33. Guyton, A.C.: *Textbook of Medical Physiology*, 8th edition. Philadelphia, W.B. Saunders Company, 1991.

34. Becker, W.M.: *The World of the Cell*. Menlo Park, Benjamine/Cummings Publishing Co., Inc., 1986.

35. Mason, M., Mackin, J.L., Harrison, G.G., and Seubert, S.A.: *Nutrition and the Cell: The Inside Story*. Chicago, Year Book Medical Publishers, Inc., 1973.

36. Sterling, K.: Direct triiodothyronine (T_3) action by a primary mitochondrial pathway. *Endocr. Res.*, 15:55, 1989.

37. Tulp, O.L. and Krupp, P.P.: Thermogenesis in thyroidectomized, protein-malnourished rats. *J. Nutr.*, 114:2365, 1984.

38. Sterling, K.: Direct thyroid hormone activation of mitochondria: the role of adenine nucleotide translocase. *Endocrinology*, 119:292, 1986.

39. Mowbray, J. and Corrigall, J.: Short-term control of mitochondrial adenine nucleotide translocator by thyroid hormone. *Eur. J. Biochem.*, 139:95, 1984.

40. Sterling, K.: Direct thyroid hormone activation of mitochondria: identification of adenine nucleotide translocase (AdNT) as the hormone receptor. *Trans. Assoc. Am. Physicians*, 100:284, 1987.

41. Rasmussen, U.B., Kohrle, J., Rokos, H., and Hesch, R.D.:

Thyroid hormone effect on rat heart mitochondrial proteins and affinity labeling with N-bromoacetyl-3,3'-5-triiodo-L-thyronine: lack of direct effect on the adenine nucleotide translocase. *FEBS Lett.*, 255:385, 1989.

42. Shambaugh, III, G.E.: Biologic and cellular effects. In *The Thyroid: A Fundamental and Clinical Text*, 5th edition. Edited by S.C. Werner and S.H. Ingbar, New York, Harper and Row, Publishers, 1986.

43. Paradies, G. and Ruggiero, F.M.: Stimulation of phosphate transport in rat liver mitochondria by thyroid hormones. *Biochem. Biophys. Acta*, 1019:113, 1990.

44. Horrum, M.A., Tobin, R.B., and Ecklund, R.E.: Thyroid hormone effects on the proton permeability of rat liver mitochondria. *Mol. Cell. Endocrinol.*, 68:137, 1990.

45. Warwick, R. and Williams, P.L.: *Gray's Anatomy*, 35th British edition. Philadelphia, 1973.

46. Tepperman, J. and Tepperman, H.M.: *Metabolic and Endocrine Physiology*, 5th edition. Chicago, Year Book Medical Publishers, Inc., 1987.

47. Larsen, P.R. and Silva, J.E.: Intrapituitary mechanism of control of TSH secretion. In *Molecular Basis of Thyroid Hormone Action*. Edited by J.H. Oppenheimer and H.H. Samuels, New York, Academic Press, Inc., 1983, pp.351-385.

48. Pike, R.L. and Brown, M.L.: *Nutrition: An Integrated Approach*, 2nd edition. New York, John Wiley & Sons, Inc., 1975.

49. Roels, O.A.: The influence of vitamins A and E on lysosomes. In *Lysosomes in Biology and Pathology*. Edited by J.T. Dingle and H.B. Fell, New York, Wiley-Interscience, 1969, pp.254-275.

50. Dingle, J.T.: Vacuoles, vesicles and lysosomes. *Brit. Med. Bull.*, 24:1968, pp.141-145.

51. Weissman, G. and Thomas, L.: Studies on lysosomes. II. The effect of cortisone on the release of acid hydrolases from storage granule fraction of rabbit liver induced by an excess of vitamin A. *J. Clin. Invest.*, 42:661-669, 1963.

52. Sterling, K., Tsuboyama, G.K., and Brenner, M.A.: Rapid thyroid hormone action *in vitro* in the absence of new protein synthesis. *Trans. Associa. Am. Physicians*, 97:332-336, 1984.

53. Harper, M-E. and Brand, M.D.: Use of the top-down elasticity analysis to identify sites of thyroid hormone-induced thermogenesis. *Proc. Soc. Experi. Biol. Med.*, 208:228-237, 1995.

54. Harper, M-E. and Brand, M.D.: Hyperthyroidism stimulates mitochondrial proton leak and ATP turnover in rat hepatocytes but does not change the overall kinetics of substrate oxidation reactions. *Can. J. Physiol. Pharmacol.*, 72:899-908, 1994.

55. Nebioglu, S., Wathanaronchai, P., Nebioglu, D., Pruden, E.L., and Gibson, D.M.: Mechanisms underlying enhanced glycogenolysis in livers of 3,5,3'-triiodothyronine-treated rats. *Am. J. Physiol.*, 258(1 Pt.1):E109-E116, 1990.

56. Ashmore, J. and Weber, G.: The role of hepatic glucose-6-phosphatase in the regulation of carbohydrate metabolism. *Vitam. Horm.*, 17:91-132, 1959.

57. Batterbee, H.D.: The effects of thyroid state on rat liver glucose-6-phosphatase activity and glycogen content. *Proc. Soc. Exp. Biol. Med.*, 147:337-343, 1974.

58. Holness, J.J. and Sugden, M.C.: Hepatic carbon flux after refeeding. *Biochem. J.*, 247:627-634, 1987.

59. Nordlie, R.C.: Metabolic regulation by multifunctional glucose-6-phophatase. *Curr. Top. Cell. Regul.*, 8:33-117, 1974.

60. Ewart, H.S. and Klip, A.: Hormonal regulation of the Na+-K+-ATPase: mechanisms underlying rapid and sustained changes in pump activity. *Am. J. Physiol.*, 269(Cell Physiol.38):C295-C311, 1995.

61. Ismail-Beigi, F. and Edelman, I.S.: The mechanism of the calorigenic action of thyroid hormone: stimulation of Na+-K+-activated adenosinetriphosphatase activity. *J. Gen. Physiol.*, 57:710-722, 1971.

62. Ismail-Beigi, F.: Thyroid hormone regulation of Na^+-K^+-ATPase expression. *Trends Endocrinol. Metab.*, 4:152-155, 1993.

63. Azuma, K.K., Hensley, C.B., Tang, M.-J., and McDonough, A.: Thyroid hormone specifically regulates skeletal muscle Na^+-K^+-ATPase α_2- and β_2-isoforms. *Am. J. Physiol.*, 265(Cell Physiol.34):C680-C687, 1993.

64. McDonough, A.A., Brown, T.A., Horowitz, B., Chiu, R., Schlotterbeck, J., Bowen, J., and Schmitt, C.A.: Thyroid hormone coordinately regulates Na^+-K^+-ATPase α- and β-subunit mRNA levels in kidney. *Am. J. Physiol.*, 254(Cell Physiol.23):C323-C329, 1988.

65. Hensley, C.B., Azuma, K.K., Tang, M.-J., and McDonough, A.A.: Thyroid hormone induction of rat myocardial Na^+-K^+-ATPase α_1-, α_2-, and β_1-mRNA and protein levels at steady state. *Am. J. Physiol.*, 262(Cell Physiol.31):C484-C492, 1992.

66. Horowitz, B., Hensley, C.B., Quintero, M., Azuma, K.K., Putnam, D., and McDonough, A.A.: Differential regulation of Na^+-K^+-ATPase α_1-, α_2-, and β-mRNA and protein levels by thyroid hormone. *J. Biol. Chem.*, 265:14308-14314, 1990.

67. Nobes, C.D., Lakin-Thomas, P.L., and Brand, M.D.: The contribution of ATP turnover by the Na^+-K^+-ATPase to the rate of respiration of hepatocytes: effects of thyroid status and fatty acids. *Biochem. Biophys. Acta*, 979:241-245, 1989.

68. Guttler, R.B., Shaw, J.W., Otis, C.L., and Nicoloff, J.T.: Epinephrine-induced alterations in urinary cyclic AMP in hyper- and hypothyroidism. *J. Clin. Endocrinol. Metab.*, 41(4):707-711, 1975.

69. Verhoeven, A.J., Kamer, P., Groen, A.K., and Tager, J.M.: Effects of thyroid hormone on mitochondrial oxidative phosphorylation. *Biochem. J.*, 226:183-192, 1985.

70. Kvetny, J. and Matzen, L.: Thyroid hormone stimulated glucose uptake in human mononuclear blood cells from normal persons and from patients with non-insulin-dependent diabetes mellitus. *Acta Endocrinol.* (Copenh.), 120:715-720, 1989.

71. Segal, J. and Ingbar, S.H.: *In vivo* stimulation of sugar uptake in rat thymocytes. An extranuclear action of 3,5,3'-triiodothyronine. *J. Clin. Invest.*, 76(4):1575-1580, 1985.

72. Helderman, J.H.: Role of insulin in the intermediary metabolism of the activated thymic-derived lymphocyte. *J. Clin. Invest.*, 67:1636-1642, 1981.

73. Caro, J.F., Cecchin, F., Folli, F., Marchini, C., and Sinha, M.K.: Effect of T_3 on insulin action, insulin binding, and insulin receptor kinase activity in primary cultures of rat

hepatocytes. *Horm. Metab. Res.*, 20:327-332, 1988.

74. DeMartino, G.N. and Goldberg, A.L.: Thyroid hormones control lysosomal enzyme activities in liver and skeletal muscle. *Proc. Natl. Acad. Sci.* (USA), 75:1369-1373, 1978.

75. Lowe, J.C.: Oral contraceptives and myofascial pain. *Dig. Chiro. Econ.*, 34:100-101, 1991.

76. Lowe, J.C.: Myofascial pain and "the Pill." *J. Nat. Assoc. Trigger Point Myother.*, 5.1:5, 1992.

77. Malbon, C.C. and Campbell, R.: Thyroid hormone administration *in vivo* regulates the acivity of hepatic glycogen phosphorylase phosphatase. *Endocrinology*, 111:1791-1796, 1982.

78. Malbon, C.C. and Campbell, R.: Thyroid hormones regulate hepatic glycogen synthase. *Endocrinology*, 115:681-686, 1984.

79. Bollen, M. and Stalmans, W.: The effect of the thyroid status on the activation of glycogen synthase in liver cells. *Endocrinology*, 122:2915-2919, 1988.

80. Remesar, X. and Alemany, M.: Glycogen and glycogen enzymes in the liver and striated muscle of rats under altered thyroid states. *Horm. Metab. Res.*, 14:179-182, 1982.

81. Betley, S., Peak, M., and Agius, L.: Triiodo-L-thyronine stimulates glycogen synthesis in rat hepatocyte cultures. *Molec. Cell. Biochem.*, 120:151-158, 1993.

82. Sterling, K., Milch, P.O., Brenner, M.A., and Lazarus, J.H.: Thyroid hormone action: the mitochondrial pathway. *Science*, 197:996-999, 1977.

83. Wolfe, S.L.: *Molecular and Cellular Biology.* Belmont, Wadsworth Publishing Co., 1993.

84. Douglas, J.E.: Thyroxine-induced alterations in the fine structure of rat liver cells. *Johns Hopkins Med. J.*, 114:253, 1964.

85. Engel, A.G.: Electron microscopic observations in thyrotoxic and corticosteroid-induced myopathies. *Mayo Clin. Proc.*, 41:785, 1966.

86. Paget, G.E. and Thorp, J.M.: An effect of thyroxine on the fine structure of the rat liver cell. *Nature*, 199:1307, 1963.

87. Loeb, J.N.: Metabolic changes in thyrotoxicosis. In *Werner and Ingbar's The Thyroid: A Fundamental and Clinical Text*, 6th edition. Edited by L.E. Braverman and R.D. Utiger, New York, J.B. Lippincott Co., 1991, pp.845-853.

88. Murthy, A.S.N. and Baquer, N.Z.: Changes in pyruvate dehydrogenase in rat brain with thyroid hormones. *Enzyme*, 28:48-53, 1982.

89. Dembri, A., Belkhiria, M., Michel, O., and Michel, R.: Effects of short- and long-term thyroidectomy on mitochondrial and nuclear activity in adult rat brain. *Molec. Cell. Endocrinol.*, 33:211-223, 1983.

90. Eisinger, J., Plantamura, A., and Ayavou, T.: Glycolysis abnormalities in fibromyalgia. *J. Am. Coll. Nutr.*, 13:144-148, 1994.

91. Eisinger, J., Mechtouf, K., Plantamura, A., et al.: Anomalies biologiques au cours des fibromyalgies: I. Lactacidemie et pyruvicemie. *Lyon Méditerranée Med.*, 28:851-854, 1992.

92. Valen, P.A., Flory, W. Pauwel, M., et al.: Forearm ischemic testing and plasma ATP degradation products in primary fibromyalgia. *Arthritis Rheum.*, 31:115, 1988.

93. Mathur, A.K., Gatter, R.A., Bank, W.J., et al.: Abnormal P-NMR spectroscopy of painful muscles of patients with fibromyalgia. *Arthritis Rheum.*, 31:523, 1988.

94. O'Reilly, I. and Murphy, M.P.: Studies on the rapid stimulation of mitochondrial respiration by thyroid hormones. *Acta Endocrinol.*, 127(6):542-546, 1992.

95. McKenzie, M.L., Thomaskutty, K.G., Swift, M.L., and Pointer, R.H.: Interaction between insulin and thyroid hormones on the control of carbohydrate and lipid metabolism in rat adipose tissue. *Biochem. Med. Metab. Biol.*, 38(1):81-87, 1987.

96. Holness, M.J. and Sugden, M.C.: Regulation of renal and hepatic pyruvate dehydrogenase complex on carbohydrate re-feeding after starvation: possible mechanisms and a regulatory role for thyroid hormone. *Biochem. J.*, 241(2):421-425, 1987.

97. Weinberg, M.B. and Utter, M.F.: Effect of thyroid hormone on the turnover of rat liver pyruvate carboxylase and pyruvate dehydrogenase. *J. Biol. Chem.*, 254(19):9492-9499, 1979.

98. Orten, J.M. and Neuhaus, O.W.: *Biochemistry*, 8th edition. Saint Louis, C.V. Mosby Co., 1970.

99. Lehninger, A.L.: *Biochemistry*, 2nd edition. New York, Worth Publishers, Inc., 1975.

100. Back, D.W., Wilson, S.B., Morris, S.M., Jr., and Goodridge, A.G.: Hormonal regulation of lipogenic enzymes in chick embryo hepatocytes in culture. Thyroid hormone and glucagon regulate malic enzyme mRNA level at post-transcriptional steps. *J. Biol. Chem.*, 261(27):12555-12561, 1986.

101. Dozin, B., Rall, J.E., and Nikodem, V.M.: Tissue-specific control of rat malic enzyme activity and messenger RNA levels by a high carbohydrate diet. *Proc. Natl. Acad. Sci.* (USA), 83(13):4705-4709, 1986.

102. Katsurada, A., Iritani, N., Fukuda, H., Noguchi, T., and Tanaka, T.: Influence of diet on the transcriptional and post-transcriptional regulation of malic enzyme induction in the rat liver. *Eur. J. Biochem.*, 168(3):487-491, 1987.

103. Katsurada, A., Iritani, N., Fukuda, H., Noguchi, T., and Tanaka, T.: Transcriptional and post-transcriptional regulation of malic enzyme synthesis by insulin and triiodothyronine. *Biochem. Biophys. Acta*, 950:113-117, 1988.

104. Abraham, G.E. and Flechas, J.D.: Management of fibromyalgia: rationale for the use of magnesium and malic acid. *J. Nutri. Med.*, 3:49-59, 1992.

105. Taroni, F. and Donato, S.: Purification and properties of cytosolic malic enzyme from human skeletal muscle. *Int. J. Biochem.*, 20(8):857-866, 1988.

106. Cheeseman, A.J. and Clark, J.B.: Influence of the malate-aspartate shuttle on oxidative metabolism in synaptosomes. *J. Neurochem.*, 50:1559-1565, 1988.

107. Cheng, S-Y, Maxfield, F.R., Robbins, J., Willingham, M.C., and Pastan, I.H.: Receptor-mediated uptake of 3,3',5-triiodo-L-thyronine by cultured fibroblasts. *Proc. Natl. Acad. Sci.* (USA), 77:3425, 1980.

108. Goldfine, I.D., Simons, C.G., and Ingbar, S.H.: Stimulation of uptake of aminoisobutyric acid in rat thymocytes by L-triiodothyronine: a comparison with insulin and dibutyryl cyclic AMP. *Endocrinology*, 96:802, 1975.

109. DeGroot, L.J., Larsen, P.R., Refetoff, S., and Stanbury, J.B.: *The Thyroid and Its Diseases*, 5th edition. New York, John Wiley & Sons, Inc., 1984.

110. Yellin, T.: Personal communication, Dec. 1996.

111. Loomis, W.F. and Lipman, F.: Reversible inhibitions of the coupling between phosphorylation and oxidation. *J. Biol. Chem.*, 173:807, 1948.

112. Lin, M.H. and Akera, T.: Increased (Na⁺,K⁺)-ATPase concentrations in various tissues of rats caused by thyroid hormone treatment. *J. Biol. Chem.*, 253(3):723-726, 1978.

113. Oppenheimer, J.H., Silva, E., Schwartz, H.L., and Surks, M.I.: Stimulation of hepatic mitochondrial alpha-glycerophosphate dehydrogenase and malic enzyme by L-triiodothyronine. *J. Clin. Invest.*, 59:517-527, 1977.

114. Somjen, D., Ismail-Beigi, F., and Edelman, I.S.: Nuclear binding of T_3 and effects of QO2, Na-K-ATPase and alpha-GPDH in liver and kidney. *Am. J. Physiol.*, 240(2): E146-E154, 1981.

115. Sterling, K. and Milch, P.O.: Thyroid hormone binding by a component of mitochondrial membrane. *Proc. Natl. Acad. Sci.* (USA), 72:325, 1975.

116. Bronk, J.R. and Bronk, M.S.: The influence of thyroxine on oxidative phosphorylation in mitochondria from thyroidectomized rats. *J. Biol. Chem.*, 237:897, 1962.

117. Sterling, K, Campbell, G.A., and Taliadouros, G.S.: Mitochondrial binding of triiodothyronine (T_3). *Cell Tiss. Res.*, 236:321, 1984.

118. Loeb, J.N.: Metabolic changes. In *The Thyroid: A Fundamental and Clinical Text*, 5th edition. Edited by S.C. Werner and S.H. Ingbar, New York, Harper and Row, Publishers, 1986.

119. Travell, J.G. and Simons, D.G.: *Myofascial Pain and Dysfunction: The Trigger Point Manual*, Vol. 1. Baltimore, Williams & Wilkins, 1983.

120. Edelman, I.S. and Ismail-Beigi, F.: Thyroid thermogenesis and active sodium transport. *Recent Prog. Horm. Res.*, 30: 235-257, 1974.

121. Edelman, I.S.: Thyroid thermogenesis. *New Engl. J. Med.*, 290:1303, 1974.

122. Fain, J.N. and Rosenthal, J.W.: Calorigenic action of triiodothyronine on white fat cells: effects of ouabain, oligomycin, and catecholamines. *Endocrinology*, 89:1205, 1971.

123. Guernsey, D.L., and Edelman, I.S.: Regulation of thermogenesis by thyroid hormones. In *Molecular Basis of Thyroid Hormone Action*. Edited by J.H. Oppenheimer and H.H. Samuels, New York, Academic Press, Inc., 1983, pp.293-324.

124. Mooradian, A.D.: Metabolic fuel and amino acid transport into the brain in experimental hypothyroidism. *Acta Endocrinol.* (Copenh.), 122(2):156-162, 1990.

125. Oppenheimer, J.H., Coulombe, P., Schwartz, H.L., and Gutfeld, N.W.: Nonlinear (amplified) relationship between nuclear occupancy by triiodothyronine and the appearance rate of hepatic α-glycerophosphate dehydrogenase and malic enzyme in the rat. *J. Clin. Invest.*, 61 (4):987-997, 1978.

126. Strait, K.A., Kinlaw, W.B., Mariash, C.N., and Oppenheimer, J.H.: Kinetics of induction by thyroid hormone of the two hepatic mRNAs coding for cytosolic malic enzyme in the hypothyroid and euthyroid states. Evidence against an obligatory role of S14 protein in malic enzyme gene expression. *J. Biol. Chem.*, 264(33):19784-19789, 1989.

127. Iglesias, T., Caubin, J., Zaballow, A., Bernal, J., and Muñoz, A.: Identification of the mitochondrial NADH dehydrogenase subunit 3 (ND3) as a thyroid hormone regulated gene by whole gene PCR analysis. *Biochem. Biophys. Res. Comm.*, 210(3):995-1000, 1995.

128. Iñiquez, M.A., Rodriquez-Peña, A., Ibarrola, N., Morreale de Escobar, G., and Bernal, J.: Adult rat brain is sensitive to thyroid hormone. Regulation of RC3/neurogranin mRNA. *J. Clin. Invest.*, 90(2):554-558, 1992.

129. Sterling, K., Lazarus, J.H., Milch, P.O., Sakurada, T., and Brenner, M.A.: Mitochondrial thyroid hormone receptor: localization and physiological significance. *Science*, 201 (4361):1126-1129, 1978.

130. Sterling, K., Brenner, M.A., and Sakurada, T.: Rapid effect of triiodothyronine on the mitochondrial pathway in rat liver *in vivo*. *Science*, 210(4467):340-342, 1980.

131. Mutvei, A., Kuzela, S., and Nelson, B.D.: Control of mitochondrial transcription by thyroid hormone. *Eur. J. Biochem.*, 180(1):235-240, 1989.

132. Van Itallie, C.M.: Thyroid hormone and dexamethasone increase the levels of a messenger ribonucleic acid for a mitochondrially encoded subunit but not for a nuclear-encoded subunit of cytochrome c oxidase. *Endocrinology*, 127(1):55-62, 1990.

133. Wiesner, R.J., Kurowski, T.T., and Zak, R.: Regulation by thyroid hormone of nuclear and mitochondrial genes encoding subunits of cytochrome-c oxidase in rat liver and skeletal muscle. *Mol. Endocrinol.*, 6(9):1458-1467, 1992.

134. Luciakova, K. and Nelson, B.D.: Transcript levels for nuclear-encoded mammalian mitochondrial respiratory-chain components are regulated by thyroid hormone in an uncoordinated fashion. *Eur. J. Biochem.*, 207(1):247-251, 1992.

135. Walters, E. and McLean, P.: Effect of thyroidectomy on pathways of glucose metabolism in lactating mammary gland. *Biochem. J.*, 109:737-741, 1976.

136. Baquer, N.A., Cascales, M., McLean, P., and Greenbaum, A.L.: Effects of thyroid hormone deficiency on distribution of hepatic metabolites and control of pathways of carbohydrate metabolism in liver and adipose tissue. *Eur. J. Biochem.*, 68:403-413, 1976.

137. Waldstein, S.S.: Thyroid-catecholamine interaction. *Annu. Rev. Med.*, 17:123-132, 1966.

138. Caldwell, A. and Fain, J.N.: Triiodothyronine stimulation of cyclic adenosine 3',5'-monophosphate accumulation in fat cells. *Endocrinology*, 89:1195-1204, 1971.

139. West, T.E.T., Owens, D., Sonkenson, P.H., Srivastava, M.C., Tompkins, C.V., and Nabarro, J.D.N.: Metabolic responses to monocomponent human insulin infusion in normal subjects and patients with liver and endocrine disease. *Clin. Endocrinol.*, 4:573-584, 1975.

140. Ali, F. and Baquer, N.Z.: Effect of thyroid hormones on hexokinase isoenzymes in rat brain and heart. *Indian J. Biol.*, 18:406-409, 1980.

141. Coulombe, P., Dussult, J.H., Letarte, J., and Simard, S.J.: Catecholamine metabolism in thyroid disease. I. Epinephrine secretion rate in hyperthyroidism and hypothyroidism. *J. Clin. Endocrinol. Metab.*, 42:125, 1976.

142. Coulombe, P., Dussault, J.H., and Walker, P.: Plasma catecholamine concentration in hyperthyroidism and hypothyroidism. *Metabolism*, 25:973, 1976.

143. Gregory, R.B. and Berry, M.N.: The influence of thyroid state on hepatic glycolysis. *Eur. J. Biochem.*, 229(2):344-348, 1995.

144. Katyare, S.S., Bangur, C.S., and Howland, J.L.: Is respiratory activity in the brain mitochondria responsive to thyroid hormone action? A critical reevaluation. *Biochem. J.*, 302(Pt.3):857-860, 1994.

145. Mooradian, A.D., Deebaj, L., and Wong, N.C.: Age-related alterations in the response of hepatic lipogenic enzymes to altered thyroid states in the rat. *J. Endocrinol.*, 128(1):79-84, 1991.

146. Paradies, G. and Ruggiero, F.M.: Enhanced activity of the tricarboxylate carrier and modification of lipids in hepatic mitochondria from hyperthyroid rats. *Arch. Biochem. Biophys.*, 278(2):425-430, 1990.

147. Kohn, A.D., Chan, J., Grieco, D., Nikodem, V.M., Aloj, S.M., and Kohn, L.D.: Thyrotropin increases malic enzyme messenger ribonucleic acid levels in rat FRTL-5 thyroid cells. *Mol. Endocrinol.*, 3(3):532-538, 1989.

148. Usala, S.J., Young, W.S., III, Morioka, H., and Nikodem, V.M.: The effect of thyroid hormone on the chromatin structure and expression of the malic enzyme gene in hepatocytes. *Mol. Endocrinol.*, 2(7):619-626, 1988.

149. Mariash, C.N. and Oppenheimer, J.H.: Thyroid hormone-carbohydrate interaction at the hepatic nuclear level. *Fed. Proc.*, 41(10):2671-2676, 1982.

150. Freerksen, D.L., Schroedl, N.A., and Hartzell, C.R.: Triiodothyronine depresses the NAD-linked glycerol-3-phosphate dehydrogenase activity of cultured neonatal rat heart cells. *Arch. Biochem. Biophys.*, 228(2):474-479, 1984.

151. Tobin, R.B., Berdanier, C.D., and Ecklund, R.E.: Effect of thyroidectomy upon the activity of three mitochondrial shuttles in rats. *J. Environ. Pathol. Toxicol.*, 3(1-2):307-314, 1979.

152. Baquer, N.A., Cascales, M., McLean, P., and Greenbaum, A.L.: Effects of thyroid hormone deficiency on the distribution of hepatic metabolites and control of pathways of carbohydrate metabolism in liver and adipose tissue of the rat. *Eur. J. Biochem.*, 68(2):403-413, 1976.

153. Greif, R.L. and Sloane, D.: Mitochondrial binding sites for triiodothyronine. *Endocrinology*, 103:1899, 1978.

154. Hashizume, K. and Ichikawa, K.: Localization of 3,5,3'-L-triiodothyronine receptor in rat kidney mitochondrial membranes. *Biochem. Biophys. Comm.*, 106:920, 1982.

155. Goglia, F., Torresani, J., Bugli, P., Barletta, A., and Liverni, G.: *In vitro* binding of triiodothyronine to rat liver mitochondria. *Pflügers Arch.*, 390:802, 1981.

156. Marks, D.B.: *Biochemistry*. Baltimore, Williams & Wilkins, 1990.

2.3

Genomic Actions and Molecular Biology of Thyroid Hormones

Hypothyroidism is the prototypical model of hypometabolism. In attempting to understand fibromyalgia as a form of hypometabolism, it is therefore instructive to review the biochemical and physiological effects of thyroid hormone, its excess, and especially its deficiency, as mediated by its genomic actions. This chapter provides a brief overview of the cell nucleus, the genes of the chromosomes, thyroid hormone receptors, and the effects on gene transcription of the interaction of T_3 with T_3-receptors. The effects of this interaction on the functioning of the body are far-reaching.

The material in this chapter is limited to those effects that appear at this time relevant to the objectively verified abnormalities in fibromyalgia. These include changes in the levels of several molecular products (caused by inadequate T_3 transcription regulation) that cause the hypometabolism of hypothyroidism: a shift toward α-adrenergic dominance, and increases in phosphodiesterase and inhibitory G_i proteins. The adrenergic receptors and the catecholamines (dopamine, norepinephrine, and epinephrine) are especially emphasized because it is through the adrenergic system that thyroid hormones exert most of their metabolism-regulating effects on the body. And, there is evidence that fibromyalgia patients have an increased concentration of $α_2$-adrenergic receptors on their platelets, a positive therapeutic response to a β-adrenergic agonist, and low central nervous system levels of dopamine and norepinephrine.

Information is also included on other molecular products of transcription regulation by T_3 that have been found to be abnormal in fibromyalgia. Researchers have reported changes in levels of mRNA that code for these products, changes in levels of the products themselves, and changes in the activity levels of the products. These products include serotonin. The synthesis and secretion of serotonin is inhibited by α-adrenergic receptors. The density of α-adrenergic receptors increases in serotonergic cell membranes when thyroid hormone regulation of the α-adrenoceptor gene is inadequate. The products also include growth hormone, substance P, and corticotropin releasing hormone. Transcription of the genes for these products is also under the regulatory control of T_3.

This chapter also contains information on monoamine oxidase (MAO), the enzyme that catabolizes the neurotransmitters serotonin, dopamine, norepinephrine, and epinephrine. Thyroid hormone regulates MAO activity through production of MAO inhibitors. Inadequate regulation of transcription by T_3 disinhibits MAO. The disinhibition increases the catabolic activity of the enzyme which perhaps partly accounts for low central nervous system levels of the metabolites of norepinephrine and dopamine in fibromyalgia patients. Levels of serotonin or its end metabolite 5-hydroxyindole acetic acid have not been found to be low in the central nervous systems of fibromyalgia patients. Studies have shown, however, that peripheral circulating levels of serotonin were low (though not significantly) in fibromyalgia patients.

Thyroid hormones have sweeping and profound effects on the biological functions of cells and tissues. The hormones are major regulators of development, metabolism, and homeostasis in vertebrates.[283,p.995] Many of the effects are mediated by thyroid hormone stimulating the production of mRNAs that code for specific proteins,[263] and by the hormone's changing the rate of synthesis of specific proteins.[1] As production of a given protein (such as an α- or β-adrenergic receptor) is related to the degree of activation or repression of its gene, the thyroid hormone-stimulated increase in the cellular levels of proteins suggests that the hormone exerts profound genomic effects. In fact, the major actions of thyroid hormone occur at the genes.

It is T_3 that acts in the cell nucleus to regulate the expression of specific genes. T_3 regulates genes and exerts most of its cellular effects by binding with high affinity to nuclear[8] and mitochondrial genomic T_3-receptors.[283] The T_3-receptor is a protein encoded by different genes of the c-erbA family.[265][266] The T_3-receptor interacts with distinct DNA sequences known as thyroid hormone response elements (TREs) in order to control gene expression.[34,p.587] The interaction increases or decreases the rate of mRNA synthesis.[1][8]

T_3 attaches to the ligand-binding domain of the T_3-receptor. In the presence of an appropriate auxiliary protein, attachment of T_3 to this domain of the receptor increases transcription of some target genes (such as the growth hormone gene[14]) and represses transcription of others (such as the pituitary TSH gene[15]). When T_3 is absent, the unliganded thyroid hormone receptor induces opposite expression of target genes from that induced by T_3-activated thyroid hormone receptors.[16][17]

Despite extensive *in vitro* studies during the past several years characterizing T_3-receptors, researchers have thus far identified few genes known to be regulated by T_3 *in vivo*.[283,p.995] Nevertheless, some of the genes known to be regulated by thyroid hormone could, when inadequately regulated, mediate virtually all the symptoms and objective findings of fibromyalgia.

For example, it is plausible that inadequate transcription regulation by T_3 underlies the neuroendocrine abnormalities identified in fibromyalgia patients. T_3-receptors are present in neurons of the developing and adult rat brain with irregular distribution.[8] The hypothalamus contains T_3-receptors,[267] especially in the paraventricular region.[268] Both α- and β-thyroid hormone receptors have been identified in the parvocellular part of the paraventricular nucleus.[269][270] The nucleus raphe dorsalis and limbic areas such as the cortex and hippocampus have high levels of expression of the genes for the three types of α thyroid hormone receptors (α_1, α_2, and rev-erbA) and the β_1 thyroid hormone receptor.[91][92] The metabolism of the nervous system is substantially affected by thyroid gland ablation,[172,p.701] and even peripheral humoral and metabolic effects of thyroid hormone inadequacy affect the central nervous system.[8]

As I detail in this chapter, these sites of thyroid hormone action and influence may underlie the neuroendocrine abnormalities of fibromyalgia. Exploring this possibility leads to the hypothesis that (1) inadequate thyroid hormone regulation of transcription produces fibromyalgia by direct actions in the brain and peripheral tissues, and (2) by indirect actions exerted through other chemical messengers (such as catecholamines) which mediate many effects of thyroid hormone adequacy, inadequacy, and excess.[271][272]

Before discussing the genomic action and effects of thyroid hormone, a review of the cell nucleus, its contents, and their functions is in order.

● **THE NUCLEUS AND DNA**

Nucleus in Latin means "seed" or "kernel." The term is fitting because it is from the nucleus that most cell activities generate. Its membrane separates its nucleoplasm from the cytoplasm of the cell.

The nucleus contains the chromosomes made of DNA (deoxyribonucleic acid). Early researchers called DNA "chromatin" because it has an affinity for stains. The chromosomes carry the genetic code for the individual. Every cell in the body carries the same genetic code. The code is written in a language whose alphabet is composed of the arrangement of molecules called nucleotides. Each nucleotide consists of a deoxyribose sugar, a phosphate group, and a nitrogenous base. The chromosome is a combination of four different nucleotides. Nucleotides bond to one another and form a long nucleotide chain, which constitutes single-strand DNA. The sequence of nucleotides in a segment of a chromosome contains information for a number of purposes. Two purposes are particularly pertinent to this chapter: (1) sequences of nucleotides serve as hormone binding sites, such as the T_3-receptor; and (2) sequences constitute a code that is transcribed to mRNAs. The mRNAs then deliver the code to the ribosome in the cytoplasm for assembly of a particular protein.

The nitrogen bases of the nucleotides contain various arrangements of nitrogen, oxygen, carbon, and hydrogen atoms. Some of the carbon and nitrogen atoms are contributed by the B vitamin folic acid and the amino acids, glycine, aspartic acid, and glutamic acid.[362,p.16] Adequate amounts of pyridoxine (vitamin B_6), folic acid, and vitamin B_{12} are critical to the normal structure and function of genes. Their importance in nuclear DNA metabolism is clear from the abnormalities in cell-mediated immunity when these nutrients are deficient.[363]

Pyridoxine deficiency is the most common cause of inadequate cell-mediated immune responses in laboratory animals.[364] Among other immune abnormalities caused by folic acid deficiency is a low T lymphocyte count.[365,p.539] Most folic acid in the body is in the form of methyltetrahydrofolic acid (5-methyl THFA). But it must be converted to other forms to serve as a coenzyme in four functions: (1) catabolism or interconversion of amino acids, (2) purine synthesis, (3) protein synthesis, and (4) formation of thymidylate, the rate-limiting compound in DNA synthesis. So that folic acid is not locked into the form of 5-methyl THFA and can serve as a coenzyme in these other functions, a transmethylase catalyzes transfer of the methyl group from THFA to homocysteine, forming methionine. The transmethylase requires vitamin B_{12} to perform this transmethylation. The methionine is required for formation of S-adenosylmethionine, which is the most common methyl-group donor in vertebrate cells (see Chapter 5.1, subsection titled "Non-steroidal Anti-inflammatory Drugs (NSAIDs): S-adenosylmethionine"). Transfer of the methyl group from 5-methyl THFA to homocysteine regenerates THFA, which then takes part in DNA synthesis. In a vitamin B_{12} deficiency, the transmethylase does not catalyze the methyl transfer, and folic acid accumulates in the form of 5-methyl THFA. This form of folic acid does not favor DNA synthesis, and cell proliferation decreases.[366,p.142]

DNA AND mRNA

DNA consists of two chains of nucleotides, connected by their bases, that twist about one another, forming a double-stranded helix. The helix resembles a long twisted ladder, its nucleotide pairs forming the rungs.

DNA's code for the structure of a protein must be transmitted to the ribosomes in the cytoplasm, where proteins are manufactured. This transfer occurs through the formation of a substance in the nucleus called messenger ribonucleic acid (mRNA). mRNA is essentially a blueprint for protein synthesis, and DNA is the template from which the blueprint is drawn.

To prepare for the production of mRNA, DNA first splits down its middle. The enzyme RNA polymerase causes the split. (Polymerases are enzymes that catalyze the joining together of long chains of subunits.[394,p.348] DNA polymerase, for example, catalyzes the synthesis of DNA. The enzyme copies a DNA template in one direction (3' to 5') and the freshly synthesized DNA strand is produced in the other direction (5' to 3').[395,p.65]) RNA polymerase binds to a promoter nucleotide sequence on the DNA. Binding to the promoter induces unwinding of the double helix DNA, partially separating the two strands. The RNA polymerase initiates transcription of the template strand. The polymerase then moves along the DNA, inducing the next region of DNA to unwind, leaving the single-stranded region that has been transcribed to rejoin the other strand. The process ends when the polymerase encounters a special region with a termination code.[395,p.73] During the process, each single strand of the DNA ladder retains its nucleotides. Free ribose-containing nucleotides suspended in the nucleoplasm—waiting in the wings as it were—move over to one of the split DNA strands. They attach to the proper complementary sites on the DNA strand based on the positions of the DNA's exposed nucleotides. During this process, the free nucleotides link together in a sequence complementary to the sequence of nucleotides of the DNA strand, forming a mRNA molecule. The sequence codes for the amino acid line-up of a particular protein. DNA has essentially transcribed its codes for the protein by creating a specific mRNA. The mRNA consists of a precise arrangement of nucleotides complementary to that of the DNA strand. The process is called *transcription*.

The rate at which transcription occurs at certain chromosome segments is dictated to a great extent by two factors: whether T_3 is present and whether a normal T_3-receptor is stationed in the gene. T_3 deficiency or failure of T_3 to bind to the T_3-receptor either stimulates or inhibits transcription of that particular gene. Binding of T_3 to a normal receptor has the opposite transcriptional effect.

After mRNA forms, DNA zips itself back up so that its two loose single strands bind again. mRNA leaves the nucleus and carries the code in its sequence to a ribosome in the cytoplasm. The ribosome translates the code so that the proper sequence of amino acids is assembled to form the protein. This process is called, of course, *translation*.

In summary, the complement of the DNA code, or mRNA, is formed in the process called transcription. The process called translation results in the formation of a particular protein by the ribosome from the code in the mRNA.

NUCLEAR T₃-RECEPTORS

Discovery of Nuclear T₃-Receptors

Relation of the Human Thyroid Hormone Receptor to the v-erbA Oncogene

Our understanding of nuclear T₃-receptors and thyroid hormone action at the nuclear level results from efforts to identify the ligand specific for the gene that is homologous (similar in origin and structure, but not necessarily function) to the *v-erbA* oncogene. This viral gene (in a retrovirus) causes erythroblastosis in chickens. The cellular version of the *v-erbA* gene is c-*erbA*. The structural homology between the glucocorticoid receptor and the v-*erbA* gene prompted two research groups to search complementary DNA (cDNA) libraries for the cellular homologues of v-*erbA*. In 1986, one group isolated a cDNA from a chick embryonic library.[131] The other isolated cDNA from a human placental library.[132] It was shown then that these cDNAs encode proteins with thyroid hormone binding properties similar to that of nuclear extracts, as shown in previous studies.[133]

When tested, a wide array of steroid hormones failed to specifically bind to the proteins. The researchers were aware, however, that the estimated size of the yet unidentified thyroid hormone receptor corresponded to that of the translational product of the cloned cDNAs. They tested radioactive T₃ and found that it had highly specific binding. The finding that the translational product of c-*erbA* mRNA cloned from the chicken library was located in the nucleus supported the view that the T₃-receptor is coded by a cellular homologue of the v-*erbA* gene.[139,pp.205-210] It was indeed appropriate to label this cellular homologue c-*erbA*.

Identification of Nuclear Thyroid Hormone Receptors. The translational products (proteins) of *c-erbA* mRNAs contained the specific T₃-binding sites in rat liver and kidney that in 1972 Oppenheimer and coworkers had reported and proposed as nuclear thyroid hormone receptors.[130] It was established that the c-*erbA* gene encodes a thyroid hormone receptor,[132] a protein that attaches to specific chromosome se-

quences[36,p.61][39] that we now know are TREs (thyroid hormone response elements). The cDNA from chicken embryos and that from human placenta had significant differences in their nucleotide sequences that coded for the amino-terminal segments. It was obvious that there were two different genes that code for T₃-nuclear binding proteins.

Researchers designated the gene isolated from chicken embryo α and that from the human placenta β.[139,p.210] In 1989, Sakurai and coworkers reported mRNA sequences derived from both α- and β-genes in humans.[146] They found that in humans, the α-gene (c-*erbA*α) is located on chromosome 17, and the β-gene (c-*erbA*β) on chromosome 3.[147][148]

The two thyroid hormone receptor genes, c-*erbA*α and c-*erbA*β, are structurally similar.[149][150] Both spawn more than one isoform of thyroid hormone receptor. They do so through alternative splicing of the initial transcript from each gene.[129,p.353] This is a process by which alternate introns (the noncoding spaces between discrete coding regions called exons of the DNA of a gene) are removed from mRNAs. Alternative splicing allows the same gene to give rise to different but related mRNAs and, subsequently, to different but related proteins. The related yet distinct proteins have different functions or are routed to different final locations.[45,pp.599-600] The β thyroid hormone receptor gene gives rise to the c-*erbA*β₁ and c-*erbA*β₂ mRNAs and the corresponding isoforms of thyroid hormone receptor,[151][152] and the α gene generates the c-*erbA*α₁ and c-*erbA*α₂ mRNAs and isoforms of receptors.[153][154][155][156] Both β isoforms bind T₃. The c-*erbA*β₂ receptor is specifically expressed in the pituitary.[151] When it binds T₃, it represses transcription of the genes for the α- and β-subunits of TSH.[157][158] This is indicated by a dramatic reduction in the amount of mRNAs for the subunits, causing TSH synthesis and secretion to decrease.

Terms used for the thyroid hormone receptor differ in the thyroidology literature. Some authors such as Refetoff, Weiss, and Usala use the term thyroid hormone receptor, abbreviated TR.[129] Others such as Oppenheimer use the term T₃-receptor.[139,p.208] That T₄ may attach to the nuclear receptors is implied by statements such as: the receptor is ". . . not functional until activated by thyroid hormone (mainly T₃)."[129,p354] I will use the term T₃-receptor because it is more concise, and as a visual symbol, it contrasts well with the mass of written text, possibly easing my readers' burden of comprehension.

Two Functional Domains of Thyroid Hormone Receptors. The c-*erbA*β₁, β₂, and α₁ thyroid hormone receptors have two functional domains in common. One is a DNA binding domain at their amino (NH_2) terminus, and the other is a ligand (mainly T_3) binding domain at their carboxy (COOH) terminus.[129,pp.353-354] The DNA binding domain of the receptor attaches to specific DNA sequences termed thyroid hormone response elements (TREs). To exert transcriptional actions, the T_3-receptor binds to these TREs located in the genes regulated by T_3 as a heterodimer with the 9-cis retinoic acid receptor.[284][285][286] The TREs are degenerate versions of the motif AGGTCA and exist either singly or in direct, inverted, or everted repeats.[283,p.995] TREs are typically located upstream from the transcription start sites of genes that are regulated by T_3.[129,p.353] In 1991, it was reported that binding of a T_3-receptor to a TRE is stabilized by a number of proteins (including retinoic acid[162]) called auxiliary proteins.[159]

Activation of the T_3-Receptor—Effects on Transcription. T_3-receptors, stationed on TREs, are usually not functional unless they bind T_3, which activates them. A receptor is activated when T_3 binds to the ligand-binding domain. This is assumed to modify the steric configuration of the receptor. *The changed configuration alters the rate of transcription of the gene that contains the TRE occupied by the T_3-receptor.*[129,p354] As I describe in Chapter 2.6, mutations in the T_3-binding domain have been discovered. These account for the syndrome of general resistance to thyroid hormone.

Binding of T_3 to a T_3-receptor in the presence of an auxiliary protein activates transcription of some genes. Examples relevant to fibromyalgia are the genes for growth hormone,[43][163] dopamine,[164] β-adrenergic receptors,[13,p.1117] and corticotropin-releasing hormone.[168] Binding of T_3 to a T_3-receptor also represses transcription of some genes, such as the genes for TSH subunits[15] and α-adrenergic receptors.[13,p.1117]

C-erbAα₂ Receptor and Rev-erbA Do Not Bind T₃. The c-*erb*Aα₂ receptor does not bind T_3. The receptor's carboxy terminus (the ligand-binding domain) is distinctly different from that of the other three receptors due to substituted nucleotides in the DNA that code for the carboxy terminus. This makes it impossible for the c-*erb*Aα₂ receptor, the translation product of the c-*erb*Aα₂ gene, to bind T_3. Because of this, Oppenheimer wrote that this protein is not a T_3-receptor but a "receptor variant."[139,p.210] The DNA strand opposite to the strand that codes for c-*erb*Aα mRNA codes for another mRNA termed rev-*erb*A. The translational product of rev-*erb*A, like the c-*erb*Aα₂ re-

ceptor variant, does not bind T_3.[160]

Although the c-*erb*Aα₂ receptor does not bind T_3, it has a DNA binding domain. Oppenheimer proposes that rev-*erb*A and the c-*erb*Aα₂ receptor variants may serve as regulators of gene expression.[139,p.211] There is evidence that the c-*erb*Aα₂ receptor variant competes with active c-*erb*Aα₁ and c-*erb*Aβ₁ receptors for binding sites at the TREs of genes.[161] Also, rev-*erb*A and c-*erb*Aα₂ may block transcription of each other's gene.[160]

Nature of T₃-Receptors

Unlike steroids, thyroid hormones do not require a transport protein to move through the cytoplasm to reach their receptors in the nucleus. T_3 passes through the cytoplasm to reach the nucleoplasm and attaches directly to a receptor in the nucleus.[36,p.61][38] There is, however, a stereospecific T_3 transport system in the nuclear membrane that has not yet been characterized. It results in a 10-fold-to-100-fold higher concentration of free T_3 in the nucleoplasm than in the cytoplasm.[134]

T_3-receptors are confined to the nucleus[142] and mitochondrion,[283][290] both of which contain α and β isoforms. Investigators have found nuclear T_3-receptors in many tissues, including pituitary, liver, brain, kidney, lung, bone, and heart. Rat pituitary tissue has the highest concentration—some 10,000 per cell. Liver tissue has the next highest concentration at some 5000 per cell.[135][136][137][138][139,p.208] Brain tissue has a T_3-binding capacity per mg of DNA about 50% that of liver.[135] In the rat, the c-*erb*Aβ₁ receptor has been shown to have a six times higher affinity for T_3 than the c-*erb*Aα₁ receptor.[139,p.211]

In the cells of most tissues, about 50% of the T_3-receptors are occupied. In brain[140] and pituitary,[141] however, some 95% of receptors are occupied. In general, full occupancy of the receptors in a cell produces a maximal cellular response to the hormone,[143][144] but receptor occupancy and cellular response are not always linear.[139,p.209] The activities of hepatic malic enzyme (which is regulated transcriptionally and post-transcriptionally by T_3[311][378]) and hepatic α-glycerophosphate dehydrogenase, however, are substantially increased with progressively higher occupancy of T_3-receptors.[145] Also, the more thyroid hormone receptors occupied by T_3, the greater the activity of tyrosine hydroxylase, production of which is induced at the transcriptional level by T_3.[379,p.1408] (For the role of these enzymes in the cell, see Chapter 2.2.)

A small fraction of T_3-receptors may be located in transcriptionally active regions of the chromosomes. Such regions actively transcribe their codes to mRNA to promote protein synthesis. The majority of the receptors, however, appear to be concentrated in inactive regions. A receptor's location within chromosomes indicates that it binds directly to DNA.[37,p.95] The receptor has a half-life of about 5 hours. The complete population of nuclear receptors is replaced within a 24-hour period. New receptors do not appear at fixed chromosomal sites. Instead, the chromosomal sites they occupy vary through loss of receptors from some locations and replacement in others.[35,pp.134-135]

Thyroid hormones may regulate the synthesis of their own receptors. During hypothyroidism, the number of T_3-receptors increases with changes in the receptors' binding properties.[357][358][359][360] When the number of thyroid hormone receptors is low in hypothyroidism, one dose of T_3 tends to temporarily increase their numbers.[40]

PROTEIN BYPRODUCTS OF THYROID HORMONE/T_3-RECEPTOR BINDING

The processes controlled in the nucleus by the thyroid hormone/thyroid hormone receptor complex appear to involve DNA transcription and/or post-transcription activities. These processes increase the number of mRNA molecules that code for specific proteins.[41][42]

Some of the proteins, once synthesized, are exported from the cell to regulate the functions of other tissues. Growth hormone is one such protein.[43] Others, such as malic acid, are soluble enzymes that regulate specific metabolic events in the cells that synthesize them.

Other proteins become membrane-bound as receptors in their cell of origin. An example is the enzyme sodium/potassium ATPase (Na^+/K^+-ATPase). Na^+/K^+-ATPase enables nerves and muscles to conduct electrochemical impulses. Thyroid hormone contributes to cell homeostasis by increasing the level and activity of Na^+/K^--ATPase and increasing activity of the Na^+/K^+ pump.[310][399] Adrenergic (catecholamine) receptors are another example of proteins that become membrane-bound in cells where they are synthesized. Adrenergic receptors bind to and mediate the cellular effects of epinephrine and norepinephrine. *Thyroid hormone regulates transcription of mRNA for the adrenergic receptors* (see subsection below titled "Adrenergic Receptor Isoform in Hypothyroidism and Hyperthyroidism").

Still other proteins are enzymes located in other cellular organelles. An example is α-glycerophosphate in mitochondria.[36,p.61-62] An increase in protein production probably also accounts for the greater enzymatic activity in skeletal muscles and mitochondria exposed to thyroid hormones.[44]

T_3-Regulated Proteins Involved in Energy Metabolism. It is worth noting that many of these proteins are enzymes that make energy available to the cell by degrading carbohydrates. In hypothyroidism, the number of these enzymes decreases, and less energy is released from carbohydrates. This is one reason a thyroid hormone deficiency impairs muscle energy metabolism in susceptible individuals.

For example, NADH dehydrogenase is the protein that enzymatically catalyzes transfer of an electron from NADH to flavin mononucleotide. Both NADH and flavin mononucleotide form complexes with proteins that extend through the inner mitochondrial membrane. They function there as electron carriers in biological oxidative reactions.[45,pp.70&333] The NADH dehydrogenase that catalyzes the electron transfer is under the transcriptional control of T_3. Iglesias and co-workers[283,p.996] have isolated a DNA fragment in cerebrum, hippocampus, and heart mitochondria that codes for a mRNA transcript which is regulated *in vivo* by T_3. Through sequencing, they characterized this clone as part of the NADH dehydrogenase subunit 3 (ND3) gene in mitochondria. Hypothyroidism induced in 10-to-30-day postnatal rats caused a 40%-to-60% reduction in ND3 mRNA (the effect did not occur with adult-onset hypothyroidism in 60-day old rats[287]). The researchers proposed that T_3 affects the expression of mitochondrial genes as it does nuclear genes: by binding as T_3/c-*erb*A receptor complexes that directly activate transcription. High affinity T_3-binding sites in the mitochondrion were reported in 1978[288] and 1980.[289] The finding of c-*erb*A receptor binding sites in the mitochondrial ND3 gene, and regulation of the gene by T_3, shows the nature of these binding sites and strongly supports the view of Iglesias and colleagues.[283,p.999]

A series of nuclear and mitochondrial genes that encode mitochondrial proteins are under thyroid hormone control.[291][292][293][294] In addition to mRNAs that code for the protein subunits 1, 5, and 6 of NADH dehydrogenase discussed above, thyroid hormone increases levels of several other mRNAs encoded by the mitochondrial genome. These include cytochrome c oxidase subunits, and cytochrome b.[291][292][293]

● WHICH THYROID HORMONE EFFECTS ARE GENOMIC AND WHICH ARE NOT

Much remains to be learned about which cellular effects of thyroid hormones are genomic and which are not. As an example, T_3 and T_4 both rapidly increase sugar intake by the plasma membrane.[18][19][20][21][22] The administration of a protein synthesis inhibitor (tiothepa) before thyroid hormone is used to increase sugar uptake shows that neosynthesis of protein is not essential to the process.[21] Because protein synthesis requires activation of gene transcription or ribosomal translation, this finding indicates that increased sugar uptake is not dependent on a nuclear effect of thyroid hormone. Kvetny and Matzen pointed out, however, that finding that new protein is not necessary for thyroid hormone-induced glucose uptake does not obviate binding of thyroid hormone to nuclear structures as a prerequisite.[21,p.719] There are two reasons for this view. First, although protein synthesis is chemically blocked, the doses of T_3 and T_4 used to stimulate glucose uptake saturate the high-affinity T_3-receptors in the nuclei of the tested cells.[23] Also, sugar uptake may be dependent on nuclear or genomic T_3-receptor binding but not require protein synthesis.[21,p.718]

There are, nevertheless, well-established genomic effects of the presence or absence of thyroid hormone at specific genes. I include below only those that appear relevant to fibromyalgia.

● MOLECULAR BYPRODUCTS OF THYROID HORMONE-REGULATED TRANSCRIPTION: RELEVANCE TO FIBROMYALGIA

MOLECULAR BYPRODUCTS THAT MEDIATE HYPOMETABOLISM: α-ADRENERGIC RECEPTORS, PHOSPHODIESTERASE, AND G_i PROTEINS

Thyroid hormones exert a profound influence on adrenergic receptor isoform balance and, through this mechanism, control cellular responsiveness to catecholamines.[2,p.387] In thyroid hormone deficiency, the balance of adrenergic receptors shifts toward the α isoform, which in general has inhibitory cellular effects. Thyroid hormones also regulate the concentration in cells of the inhibitory compounds phosphodiesterase[3][343] and G_i proteins.[4][5][6]

When properly regulated by thyroid hormones, phosphodiesterase and G_i proteins—like a proper balance of α- and β-adrenergic receptors—help maintain normal metabolism. In hypothyroidism, however, the levels of phosphodiesterase[3] and G_i proteins[4][5][6] increase and excessively inhibit cell processes. (In hyperthyroidism, the balance of adrenergic receptors shifts toward the β isoform.)

The combined inhibitory effects of α-adrenergic receptors, phosphodiesterase, and G_i proteins account for the majority of the metabolism-inhibiting effects of thyroid hormone deficiency. Most features of fibromyalgia can be accounted for by the impact of these inhibitory molecules. They probably also mediate the inhibitory effects of thyroid hormone resistance, although there is limited experimental data to confirm this. If fibromyalgia is a manifestation of inadequate thyroid hormone regulation of gene transcription, these inhibitory compounds are likely to be molecular mediators of the clinical features of fibromyalgia.

Adrenergic System: Receptors and Catecholamines

In this section, I discuss the effects of thyroid hormone on the balance of adrenergic receptor isoforms and norepinephrine levels. In several subsequent sections, I will describe the impact of the two isoforms of adrenergic receptor on various cell functions, hormones, neurotransmitters, and neuromodulators.

Adrenergic Receptor Isoform in Hypothyroidism and Hyperthyroidism. For the most part, the cellular and physiological effects of hyperthyroidism are mediated by enhanced adrenergic activity,[9][10][11] and those of hypothyroidism are mediated mainly by diminished adrenergic activity.[12] These effects result largely from a shift toward β-adrenergic receptor dominance in hyperthyroidism and a shift toward α-adrenergic receptor dominance in hypothyroidism.

Both α- and β-adrenoceptor genes contain thyroid hormone response elements.[13,p.1118] There is an inverse relationship between relative concentrations of α- and β-adrenoceptor mRNA and between adrenoceptor subtypes: generally, when one type increases, the other decreases. This suggests that in various tissues, when T_3 binds to the T_3-receptor stationed on the TRE of each gene, this activates the β-adrenoceptor gene and represses the α-adrenoceptor gene.[13,p.1117] (In some tissues, as I discuss below, the opposite effect on adrenergic receptor isoforms prevails.) Conversely, when the T_3-receptor is not occupied by T_3, the effect is opposite from that induced by T_3-activated thyroid hormone receptors.[16][17] That is, the β-adrenoceptor gene is repressed and the α-adrenoceptor gene is activated. Correspondingly, when thyroid hormone is present, β-adrenergic receptor count increases and α-adrenergic receptor count decreases in various tissues. When thyroid hormone is deficient, α-adrenergic receptor count increases and β-adrenergic receptor count decreases.

In a variety of physiological and pathological conditions, the gene expression of α-adrenoceptors and β-adrenoceptors is inversely regulated.[101][102][103][104][105] In general, alterations in mRNA levels for these two receptor types correlate with changes in cell adrenoceptor density and reactivity.[104][105][106][107][108] [109][110][111][112][113] Hypothyroidism reduces β-adrenoceptor density and reactivity in a number of tissues including the heart[104][105][106][107][108][109][113] and lungs.[114] Increases in α_{1B}-adrenoceptor mRNA in hypothyroid rat heart correlates with the potentiation of inotropic and chronotropic heart responsiveness mediated by α_{1B}-adrenoceptors.[104][107][113] Conversely, administration of thyroid hormone increases β-adrenoceptor mRNA and the membranous population of β-adrenoceptors,[115,p.15867][117,p.539][95] and decreases α-adrenoceptor density in most tissues.[108][113][116]

Apparent Contradictions. Thyroid hormone's effects on adrenergic receptor type and density are not completely clear at this time, and there are some apparent contradictions in the research literature. Gross, for example, found that after 6 weeks of propylthiouracil treatment to induce hypothyroidism in Wistar rats, there was a significant reduction of β-adrenergic receptors in the cerebral cortices of the rats.[125] This is contrary to the finding of Atterwill after he treated rats for 2 weeks with propylthiouracil,[126] and of Mason and coworkers who found no change in the binding of ligand to β-adrenergic receptors 28-to-42 days after thyroidectomy.[95]

These seemingly contradictory findings of researchers may be due to a number of factors. These include the use of different strains of rats, different experimental manipulations of the hypothalamic-pituitary-thyroid axis, different methods of measuring receptor binding,[59,p.266] and other differing methodological options taken by researchers. Some of the apparent contradictions, however, have resulted from differential responsiveness of adrenergic receptors in various locations of the brain studied. Perumal,[127] Atterwill,[126] Mason,[95] and their coworkers have documented regional differences in the effects of thyroid hormone on brain β-adrenergic receptors. Mason and coworkers, for illustration, found a dose-related in-

crease in β-adrenergic receptor binding in the cerebral cortex with large doses of thyroid hormone,[95] as did Perumal.[127] Mason and coauthors stated that the increased binding more likely resulted from an increased number of β-adrenergic receptors rather than enhanced affinity for the ligand.[95,p.264] They found no effect, however, of thyroidectomy or large doses of thyroid hormone on the status of β-adrenergic receptors in striatal tissue. They found a 16% decrease in β-adrenergic receptor binding in cerebellar membranes after thyroidectomy, and an increase in binding in the hippocampus only after large doses (in line with the stability of the thyroid hormone status of the brain, and its resistance to small fluctuations in peripheral thyroid hormone levels[128]) of T_3 or T_4.[95,p.267]

The confusion over such regional differences is akin to that invoked from the finding that in the liver, T_3 represses the β-adrenoceptor gene and activates the α-adrenoceptor gene, exactly the reverse of the T_3-induced genomic effect in most other peripheral tissues.[13,p.1117] Confusion will eventually give way to comprehension as (1) researchers catalog regional and tissue differences in thyroid hormone impact on adrenoceptor isoform, and (2) genetic studies reveal the distinct molecular actions of thyroid hormone at specific genes. But for now, in attempting to understand the probable thyroid hormone-mediated adrenergic effects, we must conjecture based on the current state of knowledge. To insist that we abstain from making judgments until the results of blinded studies are in, as many clinicians do today, is to ignore the method of exploration by which virtually all important scientific developments occur—not by the accumulation of inductive data from blinded studies, although this is an important preliminary step, but through the hypothetico-deductive method of testing the best explanation based on the available, yet always incomplete, data.

Interpretation of Fibromyalgia Features as Manifestations of Low β-Adrenergic Receptor and High α-Adrenergic Receptor Density

It is important to understand the concept that, for the most part, thyroid hormone induces inverse changes in α- and β-adrenoceptor gene expression and α- and β-adrenergic receptor count.[13] This phenomenon provides a plausible explanation for many findings from fibromyalgia studies. Eisinger and colleagues, for example, reported improved fibromyalgia status, especially reduced pain and increased exercise tolerance, in 7 of 10 patients with the use of salbutamol.[312] This medication is a selective β_1-adrenergic receptor agonist. It is typically used for symptomatic relief of bronchospasm in asthmatic patients. The cardiovascular effects are considerably milder than those of isoproterenol (a potent agonist of all β-adrenergic receptors) at doses sufficient to relieve bronchospasm.[380,pp.201-205] The study patients' positive responses to it suggest that their symptoms were mediated by insufficient β-adrenergic receptor density in cell membranes and possible α-adrenoceptor dominance. The responses also provide an explanation for the glycolytic abnormalities (low lactate production and increased pyruvate-to-lactate ratio) Eisinger found in fibromyalgia patients that resemble those in hypothyroid patients,[345][346][347] as I explained in the previous chapter.

Some fibromyalgia patients were found to have increased α_2-adrenoceptors on platelets.[51] Activated α_2-adrenergic receptors could account for a span of fibromyalgia features. The sedation associated with α_2-adrenoceptors[295][296][297][298] could account in part for patients' fatigue. The hypothermia[299] and cooling of the skin due to α_2-adrenoceptor-induced cutaneous vasoconstriction[300] may be responsible for the cold sensitivity and Raynaud's symptoms of fibromyalgia patients.

Binding of norepinephrine to α_2-adrenergic receptors in the central and peripheral systems can induce hypotension and bradycardia,[53] cardiovascular conditions common in fibromyalgia patients. This effect is possibly mediated in part by an increase in prejunctional α_2-adrenoceptor activity in the sympathetic ganglia. Use of clonidine as an α_2-adrenergic receptor agonist has shown that increased α_2-adrenoceptor activity hyperpolarizes sympathetic ganglionic cells, increasing their resistance to the generation of action potentials.[280]

α_2-Adrenergic receptors, when exposed to agonists, are antinociceptive.[301] It may appear to be a paradox that the fibromyalgia patient has chronic widespread pain if her nervous system has a high density of α_2-adrenergic receptors. The answer to the paradox is possibly that α_2-adrenergic receptors also have pain-*increasing* effects in the central nervous system that may override their antinociceptive effects. Norepinephrine and serotonin interact at the spinal cord to make the antinociceptive effect of each more potent.[302][303] In addition, administration of clonidine (an α_2-adrenergic receptor agonist) at doses too low to have antinociceptive effects simultaneously with a serotonin 5-HT$_2$ or 5-HT$_{1B}$ receptor agonist induced "supra-additive" antinociceptive effects against visceral pain.[304] In the spinal cord, therefore, α_2-adrenergic receptors and serotonin 5-HT$_2$ or 5-HT$_{1B}$ receptors act synergistically to suppress pain.[301] Norepinephrine

also appears to interact with cholinergic systems in spinal nociception.[305] On the other side of the ledger, α_2-adrenergic receptors inhibit both norepinephrine[50] and serotonin[92] secretion. Thus, if the count of α_2-adrenergic receptors is increased in the norepinephrine- and serotonin-secreting regions of the central nervous system of fibromyalgia patients, the increase in pain due to decreased secretion of norepinephrine and serotonin may override the antinociceptive effects of α_2-adrenergic receptors at sites of antinociception in the dorsal horns.

Effects of Thyroid Hormone on α- and β-Adrenergic Receptor Isoforms are Tissue Specific. In most tissues, increased binding of thyroid hormone to wild type (non-mutated) T$_3$-receptors at the chromosomes increases β-adrenergic receptor count and decreases α-adrenergic receptor count. In some tissues, however, the reverse is true.

In the liver, thyroid hormone increases α-adrenergic receptors and decreases β-adrenergic receptors, the opposite effect from that in most other cells.[13,p.1117] The phenomenon is similar to that with neurons in the hypothalamus that secrete corticotropin releasing hormone (CRH). When norepinephrine or epinephrine binds to α_1- and α_2- adrenergic receptors in these neurons, they secrete more CRH.[178] In hyperthyroidism, CRH secretion increases, and in hypothyroidism, it decreases,[168][172][173][174][175][176][177] indicating that hyperthyroidism increases the count of α-adrenergic receptors in CRH-secreting hypothalamic neurons.

This may also be true of the hypothalamic cells that secrete growth hormone releasing hormone (GHRH). GHRH stimulates the pituitary gland to release growth hormone. Norepinephrine induces secretion of GHRH upon binding to α_2-adrenergic receptors in the hypothalamus. The GHRH in turn stimulates pituitary growth hormone secretion.[234] The α_2-adrenergic receptor agonist clonidine increases secretion of GHRH. Drugs that interfere with α-adrenergic receptors, such as phentolamine, decrease secretion of GHRH.[247,p.1585] GHRH secretion decreases in hypothyroidism and recovers to normal with thyroid hormone administration,[251] suggesting that α_2-adrenergic receptor count in the hypothalamus decreases in hypothyroidism and increases when thyroid hormone is administered. This possibility is supported by reports of *in vivo* studies in which β-adrenergic receptor agonists inhibited growth hormone release, especially during narco-analgesia[281][282] and administration of GHRH.[235] Jaffer and coauthors suggested that this inhibitory effect on growth hormone secretion resulted from an effect of the β-adrenergic receptor agonist on the hypothalamus, possibly from an increase in somatostatin[276,p.1258] or a decrease in GHRH. Since growth hormone secretion is increased by administration of thyroid hormone[163][238][251] and decreased in hypothyroidism,[43][242][243][247][248][249][250][251][254][255][256] this raises the possibility that thyroid hormone decreases β-adrenergic receptors in the hypothalamic cells that secrete GHRH. This is diagrammatically displayed as the following:

---

norepinephrine binds to α₂ › stimulates GHRH in hypothalamus
› stimulates pituitary to release GH

↓

decreases in hypothyroidism

∴

thyroid hormone increases α₂ receptor count in hypothalamus
(this is opposite from most tissues)

Norepinephrine

Norepinephrine metabolite levels in the cerebrospinal fluid of fibromyalgia patients has been reported to be low,[123] with levels in 24-hour urine samples high.[118][119][381] In both the central nervous system and the periphery, these findings may result from inadequate regulation of transcription by thyroid hormone, as I detail below.

Tissue Specific Changes in Norepinephrine Production in Altered Thyroid Status. In contrast to the normal plasma concentration and clearance rate of epinephrine, in hypothyroidism[348][349] the concentration and clearance of norepinephrine are typically increased.[349][350] The increased norepinephrine level has been attributed to increased release from sympathetic nerves.[351] However, whether hypothyroidism or hyperthyroidism increases or decreases norepinephrine synthesis and secretion depends on the region of the brain or peripheral tissue in question. Thyroid hormone regulates synthesis rates of the catecholamines dopamine and norepinephrine by controlling the activity of tyrosine hydroxylase, the rate-limiting enzyme in catecholamine biosynthesis.[306] In the following four sections, I present studies of the relations between thyroid status, tyrosine hydroxylase, and catecholamine synthesis.

Effects of Hypothyroidism on Tyrosine Hydroxylase, Norepinephrine, and Dopamine Synthesis in Various Tissues. Tyrosine hydroxylase catalyzes conversion of the amino acid tyrosine to DOPA, the precursor of dopamine. As a result of hypothyroidism modulating tyrosine hydroxylase activity, catecholamine synthesis decreased in the striatum, the heart, and the interscapular brown adipose tissue in neonatal rats.[307] Hypothyroidism increased tyrosine hydroxylase activity in the mesencephalon[308] and in several hypothalamic nuclei,[309] and increased catecholamine synthesis in the brainstem and adrenal glands.[307] Thyroid hormone deficiency also increased adrenal tyrosine hydroxylase activity in hypothyroid post-natal rats.[313] As would be predicted from these findings, hypothyroidism increased norepinephrine synthesis in the adrenal glands.[98] Norepinephrine synthesis also increased in the heart.[98] (For norepinephrine findings in fibromyalgia, see section above titled "Norepinephrine.")

Effects of Hyperthyroidism or T₄ Treatment on the Tyrosine Hydroxylase, Norepinephrine, and Dopamine Synthesis in Various Tissues. In whole brain of adult rats, T₄ administration decreased dopamine and norepinephrine synthesis.[99] But in the mediobasal hypothalamus, T₄ treatment increased dopamine and norepinephrine synthesis.[272] As a result, in primary hypothyroidism, elevated prolactin secretion results from impaired dopaminergic inhibition of the pituitary lactotropic cells.[396] Hyperthyroidism decreased norepinephrine synthesis in the heart.[99] Hyperthyroid post-natal rats had decreased tyrosine hydroxylase activity in the adrenal gland.[314]

Effect of Thyroid Status on Tyrosine and Dopamine-β-Hydroxylase Induction in the Superior Cervical Ganglion. An increase in phosphorylated tyrosine hydroxylase in the superior cervical ganglion is associated with an increase in the activity of the enzyme, with conversion of tyrosine to DOPA, which can progress to sequential synthesis of dopamine and norepinephrine.[354][355] Dopamine-β-hydroxylase is the enzyme that converts dopamine to norepinephrine.[94,p237] In young and adult rats, thyroid hormone deficiency or administration did not change the ganglion synthesis of tyrosine hydroxylase[352][353] or dopamine-β-hydroxylase.[353] Rats made hypothyroid in infancy, however, had lower basal tyrosine hydroxylase activity in the superior cervical ganglion at 30, 50, and 110 days. The basal dopamine-β-hydroxylase activity was markedly lower at 50 days.[353][356] Even more important, rats made hypothyroid at birth showed no evidence of induction of either enzyme at any age. This indicates that thyroid hormones are absolutely essential for induction of these enzymes.[353,p.36]

De Lonlay et al. wrote that action of thyroid hormones during infancy appears to be important for development of the capacity for induction of tyrosine hydroxylase and dopamine-β-hydroxylase in the superior cervical ganglion. They also stated, "Indeed, there may be a 'critical period' during development when the action of thyroid hormone is particularly important for the complete functional organization of the superior cervical ganglion."[353,p.37] Hypothyroidism probably inhibits production of tyrosine hydroxylase and dopamine-β-hydroxylase at the transcriptional level,[353,p.37] and thyroid hormone probably increases transcription rate in infant rats.

These findings raise an interesting question. Is it likely that inadequate thyroid hormone regulation in some human infants, with consequently deficient induction of these catecholamine-inducing enzymes in the superior cervical ganglion, predisposes to the "hypo-sympathetic" features of fibromyalgia, such as low norepinephrine secretion during exercise, low neuropeptide Y levels (see Chapter 3.1), low cerebral and peripheral blood flow, slow and weak heart contractions, and low blood pressure?

Effects of T_3 on Catecholamine Enzymes in Cultured Neuroblastoma Cells. A relationship between thyroid hormone and catecholamines is certain.[1,p.1405] The exact nature of the relationship has been confused, as the above three sections indicate. One reason is that depending on the region of the brain studied, hypothyroidism has been shown to increase,[90][93][99][370] decrease,[96][372] or leave unchanged,[98] catecholamine levels. In addition, tyrosine hydroxylase has been shown to increase[374][375][376] or decrease[90][327][377] in different brain areas with varying thyroid status.

Most studies have been conducted using *in vivo* systems. The effects on catecholamine synthesis may have been direct. But a lingering question has been whether the effects have been indirect, with variable thyroid status exerting its effects through complex interacting biological systems. Safaei and Timiras[379] side-stepped this problem by studying the effects of thyroid hormone on neuroblastoma cell lines cultured in euthyroid and hypothyroid media, *in vitro*. Neuroblastomas are malignant tumors made up mainly of cells similar to neuroblasts (embryonic cells derived from the neural tube or neural crest that give rise to neurons). Cells of the sympathetic system are derived from neuroblasts, especially in the adrenal medulla.

The researchers measured the effects of thyroid hormone deficiency and T_3 administration on the activity of two catecholamine enzymes: tyrosine hydroxylase (which catalyzes conversion of tyrosine to DOPA) and monoamine oxidase (which degrades norepinephrine and serotonin through oxidative deamina-

tion[94,p.245]). Hypothyroidism decreased activity of both enzymes and slowed the growth rate of the cells. This reflected a decreased rate of protein synthesis, a possible genomic effect. The researchers also found that the higher the dose of T_3 administered, the further tyrosine hydroxylase activity increased. Enzyme activity was dose-dependent and correlated with the number of nuclear T_3-receptor sites occupied by the hormone. Safaei and Timiras concluded that thyroid hormone directly affects through nuclear receptors the activity of tyrosine hydroxylase and monoamine oxidase in cultured, immature neurons. They also concluded that as long as cells are immature, catecholamine transmission is highly dependent on the presence of thyroid hormone.[379,p.1409]

Effects of Thyroid Status on Amino Acid Transport Across the Blood Brain Barrier: Possible Relation to Low Cerebrospinal Norepinephrine Levels in Fibromyalgia. The blood brain barrier is the site of transport systems for a number of cerebral substrates.[315] These systems are located in the plasma membrane of the endothelial cells of brain capillaries. Tight junctions between the endothelial cells block the diffusion of any molecules between the cells.[316][317] Hypothyroidism in neonatal rats decreases the density of blood vessels of the brain.[318][319] The reduction may decrease the total area available for transport of substrates into the brain and be a means by which thyroid hormone controls the transport of amino acids into the central nervous system as well as other tissues.[320][321][322][371]

In 16-day old rats, hypothyroidism decreased the blood-brain influx of phenylalanine.[323] Thyroidectomy in *adult* rats decreased the influx of leucine.[324] This latter finding may indicate that the influx of tyrosine also is decreased in adult hypothyroidism in that leucine and tyrosine share the same transport system.[326] The transport of tyrosine across the blood brain barrier is important in fibromyalgia because tyrosine is the precursor of the three catecholamines—dopamine, norepinephrine, and epinephrine.[325]

Norepinephrine-Mediated Secretion of Serotonin, Dopamine, and Growth Hormone. Norepinephrine-secreting neurons that originate in the locus ceruleus control the firing rate of serotonergic neurons in the nucleus raphe dorsalis.[50,p.R5] The serotonin content of the hypothalamus is also regulated by norepinephrine. The major provision of noradrenergic fibers innervating the hypothalamus, however, originate from the A_1 and A_2 nuclei of the pons-medulla, with a more modest contribution of noradrenergic fibers from the locus ceruleus. These fibers contribute to the medial forebrain bundle situated in the lateral hypothalamus.[274][275] Many medial forebrain bundle fibers terminate in nuclei of the hypothalamus.[275] Bilateral injections of 6-hydroxydopamine, which is neurotoxic and lesions the medial forebrain bundle, significantly reduced the concentration of norepinephrine, dopamine, and serotonin in the hypothalamus. The injections also decreased the concentration of norepinephrine by 52% and serotonin by 47.5% in the hypothalamic paraventricular nucleus. There was a substantially greater reduction in norepinephrine in the hippocampus (91%) and frontal cortex (86%).[276] This study showed lesioning of the medial forebrain bundle disrupts noradrenergic input from the brain stem locus ceruleus and A_1 and A_2 nuclei, which reduces secretion of several neurotransmitters whose levels have been shown to be abnormal in many fibromyalgia patients.[277][278]

Depletion of catecholamines in the hypothalamus by injection of the neurotoxin 6-hydroxydopamine into the third ventricle stopped growth hormone secretion for 7 days. After this time, normal growth hormone secretion resumed despite continuing low catecholamine levels.[279]

Dopamine

Dopamine is a catecholamine. It is the second intermediate in a series of conversions: tyrosine to L-DOPA to dopamine to norepinephrine to epinephrine.[94,pp.224-226] Thyroid hormone stimulates dopamine production by the hypothalamus.[180,p.585] Dopamine in turn indirectly lowers thyroid hormone levels by inhibiting TSH secretion by the anterior pituitary gland[181][182] upon binding to dopamine receptors in the anterior pituitary gland.[184] The dopamine agonist L-dopa lowers serum TSH.[181][180] The dopamine antagonist sulpiride increases plasma TSH in humans,[181] and the drug metoclopramide, which blocks dopamine receptors of anterior pituitary cells, raises serum TSH.[180] These effects (decreased secretion of TSH by dopamine and its agonists, and increased secretion of TSH by dopamine antagonists) are more pronounced in patients with subclinical hypothyroidism (high TSH but normal T_4 levels) than in those with overt primary hypothyroidism (high TSH and low T_4 levels).[180] The more pronounced effects in subclinical hypothyroid patients support the concept that declining thyroid hormone levels decrease dopaminergic inhibition of TSH secretion,[183] and demonstrate that thyroid hormone stimulates dopamine production.

Hypothyroidism reduces the rate of catecholamine

synthesis in the striatum where dopamine is the main catecholamine synthesized.[307][330] Some researchers report that thyroid hormone regulates dopamine synthesis in the brain by controlling the concentration of the dopamine precursor 3,4-dihydroxyphenylalanine (DOPA).[94,p.227] Jacoby and coworkers administered a chemical to hypothyroid rats that inhibits decarboxylase, the enzyme that removes a carboxyl (COOH) group from DOPA,[93] converting it to dopamine.[94,p.227] This procedure causes DOPA to accumulate. After the researchers administered the inhibitor, hypothyroid rats accumulated DOPA at a decreased rate. After treatment with enough T_4 to induce hyperthyroidism, DOPA accumulated faster than would be expected merely from blocked conversion to dopamine by the decarboxylase inhibitor.[93] These results are consistent with those reported by Engstrom[96] and Strombom[97] and their colleagues. The results are strong support for the regulation of DOPA, and therefore dopamine synthesis, by thyroid hormone.

Fetal dopamine neurons have T_3 nuclear receptors. Puymirat and coworkers found that 64% of the neurons had T_3-receptors.[164] Based on these findings, they wrote that hypothalamic dopamine neurons are target cells for T_3. Noting that numerous studies have clearly shown the sensitivity of fetal hypothalamic dopaminergic neurons to thyroid hormones, they proposed that T_3 has a direct effect on the maturation of hypothalamic dopamine neurons.[164,p.443] There is a decrease in dopamine and its metabolite, dihydroxyphenyl acetic acid (DOPAC), in the hypothalamus of hypothyroid neonatal rats. And neonatal hyperthyroidism increases the rate of dopamine synthesis in the rat diencephalum.[165] In addition, T_3 was found to increase the morphological and biochemical differentiation of fetal mouse hypothalamic dopamine neurons.[166][167]

Dopamine stimulates growth hormone secretion.[233][273] This finding raises the possibility— relevant to findings in fibromyalgia patients—that low dopamine levels, resulting from inadequate thyroid hormone regulation of dopamine synthesis and release, may contribute to low growth hormone levels, and in turn, low somatomedin C levels (see Chapter 3.5).

Decreased Dopamine Due to Hypothyroidism Lowers Locomotor Drive and Activity. The locomotor activity of young rats (their movement or power to move) is decreased by hypothyroidism.[327] It is well-established that dopaminergic neurons in the meso-limbic and nigro-striatal pathways control locomotor activity.[328][329][336][337][338][339][340][341] Hypothyroidism decreases catecholamine synthesis in the striatum where dopamine is the main catecholamine produced,[307][330] and evidence indicates that reduced synthesis of dopamine in the striatum accounts for impaired locomotor activity of developing hypothyroid rats.[307] This could partly account for the fatigue and low motor drive of fibromyalgia patients.

Modulation of the Effect of Decreased Dopamine on Locomotor Activity by α-Adrenergic Receptors. Lowered locomotor drive or activity, from reduced dopamine due to inadequate T_3 regulation of transcription, may be compounded by a concurrently increased population of α_2-adrenergic receptors. The α_2-adrenoceptor agonist clonidine inhibited both normal[331][332][333] and amphetamine-driven[334] locomotor activity. Whether this compounding effect occurs, however, would depend on the isoform of α-adrenergic receptor increased by inadequate T_3 regulation. In contrast with the inhibiting effect of α_2-adrenoceptor activation, α_1-adrenergic receptor agonists (phenylephrine and methoxamine) increased locomotor activity.[331][335][342] The finding of increased α_2-adrenoceptors on the platelets of fibromyalgia patients[51] makes this an enticing line of investigation.

Catecholamine Synthesis in Hypothyroidism, Hyperthyroidism, and Fibromyalgia. Some researchers report an increase in catecholamine synthesis in hyperthyroidism and a decrease in hypothyroidism. Jacoby et al., for example, reported that hypothyroid rats accumulated DOPA (the precursor to the catecholamine dopamine) at a decreased rate (see section above). After rendering the rats hyperthyroid with T_4, DOPA accumulated at an exaggerated rate.[93] Other investigators have reported similar results.[96][97]

Such studies have led to confusion because the results are inconsistent with outcomes of other studies.[98][99][100] The other studies indicate that catecholamine (particularly norepinephrine) synthesis and turnover in the brain is increased in hypothyroidism and decreased in hyperthyroidism. The problem appears to be lack of sufficient data. The sequence of conversions in catecholamine synthesis produces from the amino acid tyrosine, DOPA, dopamine, norepinephrine, and epinephrine,[94,p.227] in that order. The increase in DOPA in hyperthyroidism reported by Jacoby[93] presumably forecasts increased norepinephrine and epinephrine as descendants of DOPA. The apparent inconsistency (increased DOPA, but decreased norepinephrine and epinephrine) has two possible explanations: first, tissue specific differences in thyroid hormone-induced catecholamine production, and second, differential effects of thyroid status on DOPA and dopamine as opposed to norepinephrine and epinephrine.

In one small study, 14 fibromyalgia patients had higher levels of norepinephrine (in a 24-hour sample) than did 14 matched control subjects without musculoskeletal pain.[381] Mean level of norepinephrine per 24 hours for patients was 38.57±5.71 μg, and for controls was 24.61±3.46 μg. The difference was almost statistically significant (p=0.06, Wilcoxin test for paired data) despite the small number of study subjects. Caffeine consumption was correlated with elevated norepinephrine levels in fibromyalgia patients.[118][119] In other reports, 20% of fibromyalgia patients were reported to have elevated norepinephrine levels.[118][119] *This is consistent with increased activity of tyrosine hydroxylase[98] and norepinephrine synthesis[313] in the adrenal glands in hypothyroidism.* In another study, fibromyalgia patients compared to rheumatoid arthritis patients and control subjects had significantly lower levels of the breakdown product of norepinephrine, homovanillic acid (HVA), in the cerebrospinal fluid.[123] *This finding is consistent with inhibition of norepinephrine secretion in the central nervous system by α_2-adrenergic receptor activation.* Activation of α_2-adrenergic receptors on neurons by catecholamines or their analogs increases membrane potassium conductance. This hyperpolarizes the nerves,[120,p.119] reducing their spontaneous neural firing rate.[7,p.94][122]

Researchers have shown this effect in norepinephrine-secreting neurons of the locus ceruleus in the brain stem. α_2-Adrenergic receptor agonists hyperpolarize the neurons, and receptor antagonists reduce polarization.[121] Norepinephrine-containing neurons in the locus ceruleus secrete norepinephrine, and they also respond to norepinephrine via presynaptically stationed α_2-adrenergic receptors on the cell bodies of their neurons.[120,p.120] When stimulated, neurons of the locus ceruleus secrete norepinephrine. The norepinephrine binds to α_2-adrenergic receptors (which act as inhibitory autoreceptors), and this hyperpolarizes the neurons and reduces their excitability.[121] As a result, α_2-adrenergic autoreceptors on noradrenergic nerve terminals inhibit norepinephrine release,[50,p.R6] and chemical blockade of α_2-adrenergic autoreceptors increases norepinephrine secretion.[50] The antidepressant Org 3770, which blocks α_2-adrenergic autoreceptors on noradrenergic nerve terminals, has been found to increase the rat hippocampal dihydroxyphenyl acetic acid (a measure of norepinephrine activity) by 80%.[50] Thus, an increase in α_2-adrenoceptor autoreceptors on noradrenergic neurons due to inadequate thyroid hormone regulation of the α-adrenergic receptor gene[13] would be expected to lower norepinephrine levels in the central nervous system. A predominance of α_2-adrenergic receptors on locus ceruleus neurons due to inadequate thyroid hormone regulation of transcription might account for the low concentration of the metabolite of norepinephrine in fibromyalgia patients' cerebrospinal fluid.

Catecholamine Catabolism: Monoamine Oxidase and Catechol-O-methyltransferase

The actions of biogenic amines, such as the neurotransmitters serotonin, dopamine, norepinephrine, and epinephrine, are terminated by three processes: (1) reuptake into nerve terminals, (2) dilution by diffusion from the synaptic cleft and uptake at extraneuronal sites, and (3) catabolic transformation. The amines are catabolized by two enzymes: monoamine oxidase (MAO) and catechol-O-methyltransferase.[264][344][368,p.106][390,pp.414-418] In addition to the catabolic termination of catecholamine action, MAO also plays a crucial defensive role in the liver where it inactivates circulating monoamines and monoamines that are absorbed into the portal circulation from the gut, such as the sympathomimetic amine tyramine.[390,p.415] Thyroid hormone-related abnormalities of these enzymes, particularly MAO, may play a role in the pathogenesis of fibromyalgia.

Thyroid Hormone-Inducible Monoamine Oxidase (MAO) Inhibitor. It is possible that the low central nervous system levels of norepinephrine and serotonin in fibromyalgia patients result in part from overly active MAO, a flavin-containing enzyme. This overactivity could be due to inadequate thyroid hormone stimulation of the synthesis of MAO inhibitor.

MAO is located in the outer mitochondrial membrane,[229] whether in nerve terminals, liver, or other tissues.[390,p.415] There are two forms of the enzyme, classified according to their specificity for different substrates and sensitivity to inhibitors. MAO-A catalyzes the breakdown of serotonin and is inhibited by clorgyline; MAO-B catalyzes breakdown of β-phenylethylamine and is inhibited by deprenyl.[216][217][218] Stress increased the amount of MAO inhibitor in the urine of rats. Presumably, the increase in MAO inhibitor in responses to stress delays the breakdown of biogenic amines after they are secreted. The resulting sustained "life-span" of the amines probably contributes to the heightened physiological arousal associated with stress. Benzodiazepines, a group of tranquilizing compounds, reduce the quantity of urinary MAO inhibitor.[222]

Numerous researchers have reported that administration of thyroid hormone is accompanied by decreased MAO activity[219][224][230] in the kidney[221] and

liver.[225][226][227] Others have reported that hyperthyroidism increases cardiac MAO activity.[220][226][228] This conflicts with the findings of Ichikawa and coworkers.[223] They found that activity of three cardiac MAO inhibitors was increased in hyperthyroidism, indicating that thyroid hormone regulates MAO activity in the mitochondrial membrane through production of the inhibitors.[223,p.1808]

The activity of one inhibitor was much lower in the hepatic cytoplasm of thyroidectomized rats.[227,p.814] In concordance with this, MAO activity was increased in hypothyroid neonatal rats.[392] Thyroid hormone markedly reduced hepatic MAO activity by inducing an endogenous MAO inhibitor.[227] The inhibitor's activity increased in T_4 treated rats. The inhibitor induced by thyroid hormone was more potent for the A-form MAO (which breaks down serotonin) than for the B-form. Obata and colleagues proposed that because thyroid hormone controls the level of the MAO inhibitory modulator, the hormone regulates mitochondrial MAO activity by gene induction.[227,p.814]

Pharmaceutical MAO inhibitors have potentially high toxicity. Because they potentiate the actions of both endogenous and exogenous sympathomimetic amines,[389][397] overdosage may occur within hours, although signs of their effects are initially largely inconspicuous.[252][264] These include agitation, hallucinations, hyperreflexia, hyperpyrexia, and convulsions. The possible toxicity is more variable and potentially more serious than that of other drugs used with psychiatric patients.[390,p.416] All the MAO inhibitors cause orthostatic hypotension. Having the patient lie down usually relieves this promptly, but the patient may have to reduce the dosage or stop the drug to completely relieve the hypotension. Other less severe adverse effects include constipation, vertigo, headache, inhibited ejaculation, difficulty urinating, weakness, fatigue, dry mouth, blurred vision, and skin rashes.[390,p.416]

When norepinephrine and serotonin levels are low due to inadequate thyroid hormone regulation of MAO inhibitors, treatment with thyroid hormone should be used instead of pharmaceutical MAO inhibitors. I mention this because there is a tendency among fibromyalgia researchers to intervene with therapy that reverses a single documented abnormality. Examples are the use of tricyclic antidepressants or serotonin reuptake inhibitors in an attempt to raise low serotonin levels, and the use of growth hormone to increase low levels of somatomedin C.

Catechol-O-methyltransferase (COMT). Whereas MAO catabolizes catecholamine transmitters released *within* nerve terminals, COMT, located mainly in the cytoplasm, catabolizes most of the norepinephrine and epinephrine that enter the circulation from the adrenal medulla or from exogenous administration.[368,p.106] The enzyme is especially active in the liver, breaking down endogenous circulating and administered catecholamines.[368,p.106][390,p.417] MAO and COMT are widely distributed throughout the body, including the brain, although the liver and kidney have the highest concentrations.[368,p.106][391] COMT is also present in the epithelial cells of the stomach, duodenum, and ileum of the gastrointestinal tract, the insulin-generating β-cells, somatostatin-producing D-cells (but not the glucogon-forming α-cells of the islets of Langerhans of the pancreas), the posterior and anterior pituitary gland, epithelial cells of the thyroid gland, the zona glomerulosa of the adrenal gland, ependymal cells of the cerebral ventricles and choroid plexus, the neurophils of the striatum and cortex, and the spinal sensory ganglion. The widespread presence of this protein indicates that it is important in the inactivation of catecholamines.[391]

Coulombe and coworkers reported that there was no significant difference between COMT activity in the red blood cells of euthyroid, hypothyroid, or hyperthyroid humans.[393] COMT activity was also normal in brown fat of hyperthyroid neonatal rats, but in hypothyroid rats, COMT activity was significantly increased.[392] These inconsistent findings are heuristic; more studies of both neonates and adults are necessary to establish whether thyroid status significantly affects COMT activity in various tissues.

Phosphodiesterase

Phosphodiesterase is the enzyme that has a high affinity for and inactivates cAMP. Thyroid hormone represses phosphodiesterase to a proper level.[12] Inadequate thyroid hormone regulation of transcription in adipose cells enhances membrane activity of phosphodiesterase.[12][343] When catecholamines bind to β-adrenergic receptors, this increases the level of cAMP inside the membrane. The increase in cAMP initiates a cascade of metabolic reactions in the cell. Phosphodiesterase in turn inactivates the cAMP. When the phosphodiesterase level is increased in hypothyroidism, metabolic activities such as glycolysis that are stimulated by catecholamines are impaired. High levels of phosphodiesterase in fibromyalgia patients, combined with a decreased density of β-adrenergic receptors, may account for the glycolytic abnormalities reported by Eisinger et al., including low lactate production and high pyruvate-to-lactate ratio.[345][346][347]

Eisinger et al. found increased pyruvate and decreased lactate in the circulation of both fibromyalgia and hypothyroid patients.[367]

G_i Proteins

Inhibitory G proteins (G_i proteins) reduce cyclic adenylate formation in the cell membrane. Thyroid hormones negatively regulate G_i proteins at the nuclear level, inhibiting transcription of mRNA for the β subunit common to all G-proteins. In thyroid hormone deficiency, β subunit transcription increases.[13][398] Inadequate thyroid hormone regulation of transcription also enhances expression of the α subunit of inhibitory G-proteins and G_β-subunits common to all G-proteins and their mRNA levels in adipose cells. When thyroid hormone is deficient, G_i protein synthesis increases, resulting in higher concentrations in cell membranes.[13][14][15] By inhibiting adenylate cyclase activity, and as a result, reducing cAMP formation, G_i proteins contribute to the hypometabolism of hypothyroidism.

OTHER MOLECULAR PRODUCTS OF THYROID HORMONE REGULATION OF TRANSCRIPTION

Serotonin

Control of Serotonin Synthesis and Secretion by Adrenergic Receptors: Thyroid Hormone Controls Serotonin Secretion by Controlling Transcription of α- and β-Adrenergic Receptors. The low serotonin levels found in fibromyalgia patients[57][58][59][60][61][62] would be expected from the model I propose in this book, as the model predicts adrenergic alterations that reduce serotonin levels. When activated by norepinephrine secreted by neighboring noradrenergic neurons,[96] α_2-adrenoceptors located presynaptically on serotonergic nerve terminals inhibit secretion of serotonin[92] in the rat hippocampus,[94] rat medullary nucleus tractus solitarii,[95] rat and rabbit brain cortex,[95] and human neocortex. This inhibitory effect of α_2-adrenoceptors on serotonin secretion,[92] and a possible shift toward increased α_2-adrenergic receptor dominance in fibromyalgia,[51] makes plausible the hypothesis that inadequate transcription regulation by thyroid hormone mediates the low serotonin levels in fibromyalgia patients.

Interaction of the Noradrenergic and Serotonergic Systems. Norepinephrine-secreting neurons that originate in the locus ceruleus control the firing rate of serotonergic neurons in the nucleus raphe dorsalis.[50,p.R5] Also, the serotonin content of the hypothalamus is regulated by norepinephrine. The major norepinephrine-secreting neurons that innervate the hypothalamus originate from the A_1 and A_2 nuclei of the pons-medulla, and these contribute to the medial forebrain bundle situated in the lateral hypothalamus.[274][275] Many of the fibers from the medial forebrain bundle, accompanying other noradrenergic fibers from the locus ceruleus, terminate in nuclei of the hypothalamus.[275] Bilateral lesioning of the medial forebrain bundle with injected 6-hydroxydopamine significantly reduced the concentration of serotonin in the hypothalamus. The procedure also reduced the concentration of serotonin by 47.5% in the hypothalamic paraventricular nucleus.[276][277][278]

The concurrent participation of the noradrenergic and serotonergic systems in physiology and pathophysiology suggests that the two systems interact. Both systems are activated, for example, during arousal induced by stressful sound and immobilization.[60][61] There are a number of reasons to suspect that the noradrenergic system takes part in the control of serotonin release.

First, anxiety, aggression, sleep/waking cycle, arousal, and depression are mediated by the serotonergic system,[61][67][69] but they are also affected by drugs that affect adrenergic receptors.[68][70][71] For example, depression, which is thought to be partly related to dysfunction of serotonergic transmission, is often relieved by β_2-adrenergic receptor agonists. Hallberg et al. found that the β_2-adrenergic receptor agonist salbutamol increased the concentration of 5-hydroxytryptophan, the precursor of serotonin, in the limbic forebrain, the corpus striatum, and the cerebral cortex of rats.[59] Such activation of the brain serotonergic system in humans may have an antidepressant and pain-diminishing effect. Eisinger found that salbutamol increased exercise tolerance and decreased pain in 7 of 10 fibromyalgia patients.[312]

Second, normal levels of norepinephrine and interaction with β-adrenergic receptors are important to the excitability of the cortical and thalamic neurons. In cortical pyramidal cells,[54] activation of β-adrenergic receptors by norepinephrine enhances excitability and responsiveness to depolarizing neural input. In the thalamus, normal interaction of norepinephrine with β- and α_1-adrenergic receptors invokes the single spike firing mode of action potential generation. McCormick and coauthors wrote, "Together with the actions of other neuromodulatory neurotransmitters (i.e., acetylcholine, histamine, serotonin) these effects of norepinephrine facilitate switching of these neurons from a state of rhythmic oscillation and low excitability during drowsiness and slow-wave sleep, to a state of increased excitability and responsiveness during periods of waking, attentiveness, and cognition."[54] Yet activation of the serotonergic system may contribute to the arousal, or it may serve to prevent hyperarousal.[61]

To help define the nature of interaction between the two systems, Clement and coworkers administered to rats, α_1-, α_2-, and β-adrenergic receptor agonists and antagonists. They measured the resulting changes in DOPAC (3,4-dihydroxyphenylacetic acid), an index of norepinephrine metabolism in the locus ceruleus, and 5-HIAA (5-hydroxyindoleacetic acid), the major metabolic breakdown product of serotonin.[55] Reductions of DOPAC levels indicated decreased firing of norepinephrine neurons and a reduced norepinephrine release in the locus ceruleus (the primary site of noradrenergic neurons in the brain stem). Reductions of 5-HIAA levels indicated decreased firing of serotonergic neurons in the nucleus raphe dorsalis (the main site of serotonergic neurons in the brain stem) and reduced serotonin secretion.

In the nucleus raphe dorsalis, which receives noradrenergic input from the locus ceruleus, the effects of the α_2-adrenergic receptor agonist clonidine were different, depending on the dosage used. A low dose of clonidine decreased the concentration of 5-HIAA; a high dose of clonidine increased its levels.[55] This is consistent with the findings of other researchers.[62][63] The increase in 5-HIAA levels with high-dose clonidine, suggesting increased serotonin release in the nucleus raphe dorsalis, is consistent with the finding that high-dose clonidine has been found to induce sleep.[64] A decrease in 5-HIAA with low-dose clonidine, suggesting reduced serotonin release in the nucleus, is consistent with the findings that low-dose clonidine reduces deep slow wave sleep and rapid eye movement sleep.[65][236] Other investigators have reported that α_1-adrenergic receptor antagonists reduce the firing rate of serotonergic neurons.[55,p.47][66]

Clement[55] concluded that the β-adrenergic receptor agonist isoproterenol increased serotonin metabolism in the nucleus raphe dorsalis. So did high doses of the α_1-adrenergic receptor agonist methoxamine. In contrast, adrenergic receptor antagonists decreased serotonin metabolism in the nucleus. The researchers concluded that there is a close functional relationship between the noradrenergic and serotonergic systems, with serotonin neurotransmission in the nucleus raphe dorsalis stimulated by the noradrenergic system of the locus ceruleus. In addition, the researchers shared the speculation of others[61] that increased metabolism of serotonin with higher doses of the α_2-adrenergic receptor agonist clonidine serves to avoid hyper-arousal from excessive serotonin levels.[55,p.47]

Inhibition of Serotonin Synthesis and Secretion by α_2-Adrenergic Receptors. It is well-established that in the brain, presynaptic α_2-adrenergic receptors occupy serotonergic neurons, and these receptors, upon binding to norepinephrine released from neighboring noradrenergic neurons.[81,p.474] inhibit serotonin release.[73][74][75][76][77][78][79][80] The receptors are termed heteroreceptors because also they interact with norepinephrine to control release of another type of transmitter.[72,p.25] They are identical pharmacologically to the α_2-adrenergic receptors (called autoreceptors) that interact with norepinephrine to inhibit norepinephrine secretion by noradrenergic neurons.[72] In the cerebral cortex, inhibitory α_2-adrenergic heteroreceptors were found to up-regulate (become supersensitive) when noradrenergic nerves neighboring serotonergic nerves were destroyed with 6-hydroxydopamine. The α_2-adrenergic receptors also down-regulated (became subsensitive) when the norepinephrine reuptake blocker desipramine was administered, providing more norepinephrine to bind to the receptors on serotonergic neurons. Low doses of the α_2-adrenergic receptor agonist clonidine, upon binding to α_2-adrenergic autoreceptors on noradrenergic neurons, reduced secretion of norepinephrine. The reduced secretion decreased norepinephrine inhibition of serotonergic neurotransmission. High doses of clonidine, upon binding to α_2-adrenergic heteroreceptors on serotonergic neurons, inhibited serotonergic neurotransmission.[81][82][369][373]

Other researchers have also found that α_2-adrenergic receptors inhibit serotonin synthesis and secretion by serotonergic neurons[46] in various brain tissues. Benkirane and coworkers[47] reported that α_2-adrenergic receptors, located presynaptically on serotonergic nerve terminals, inhibit the release of serotonin. They demonstrated that in the rat hippocampus, electrically-evoked calcium-dependent release of serotonin was inhibited by 6-fluoronoradrenaline, an α_2-adrenergic receptor agonist. They also showed that application of β-phenylethylamine, which causes an outflow of norepinephrine, activates α_2-adrenergic receptors and thereby inhibits the electrically-evoked release of serotonin.

Numazawa confirmed that α_2-adrenergic receptors located on serotonergic nerve terminals in the rat hippocampus inhibit serotonin release.[48] Numazawa and colleagues[49] found that perfusion of rat hippocampus with potassium evoked a three-fold increase in serotonin secretion. But addition of the α_2-adrenergic receptor agonist UK14,304 to the perfusion solution

significantly inhibited the potassium-evoked release of serotonin. The inhibitory action of UK14,304 was reversed (with increased secretion of serotonin) by the addition of an α_2-adrenergic receptor antagonist. Feuerstein and colleagues[52] showed that endogenous norepinephrine (levels of which are increased at serotonergic neurons by norepinephrine uptake blockers) activates α_2-adrenoceptors on serotonergic nerve endings and inhibits electrically-invoked serotonin release in slices of human and cat neocortex.

β-Adrenergic and α_1-Adrenergic Receptors Increase Serotonin Synthesis. β-Adrenergic receptor antagonists reduce serotonin synthesis.[56] The antagonists also diminish serotonin-induced behavioral effects such as the head-twitch response[57] and serotonin-induced sleep.[58] Clement and coauthors wrote that the antidepressant effects of some β-adrenergic receptor agonists may result from increased neuronal serotonin activity.[55,p.47] An increase in serotonin may also have mediated the improvement in 7 of 10 fibromyalgia patients (especially exercise tolerance and reduced pain) when Eisinger had them take the β_2-adrenergic receptor agonist salbutamol.[312] This agonist increases brain serotonin synthesis.[59]

In contrast to the effect of α_2-adrenergic receptor agonists, indirect α_1-adrenergic receptor agonism increases serotonergic nerve firing and increases the extracellular concentration of serotonin.[50] When stimulated by the agonist methoxamine, α_1-adrenergic receptors increase extraneuronal 5-hydroxyindoleacetic acid (5-HIAA),[55,p.47] the major metabolite of serotonin. α_1-Adrenergic receptor antagonists decrease extracellular serotonin levels in the rat hippocampus.[83]

Thyroid Hormone Status and Serotonin. Synthesis and turnover of serotonin is decreased in hypothyroid neonatal animals and increased in hyperthyroid animals,[42][43][44] and central serotonin function is decreased in hypothyroidism.[88][89][90] Thyroxine has been shown to increase serotonin levels in rat skin and ilium,[39] and urinary levels of 5-HIAA were found to increase in thyrotoxicosis and decrease in hypothyroidism.[40]

Tóth and Csaba measured the serotonin levels, minus the blood serotonin content, in brain stems of rabbits that had either been thyroidectomized or fed thyroxine. Brain stem serotonin increased in thyroxine treated rabbits 56.5% and decreased in thyroidectomized animals 21.7%. Blood content of serotonin increased by the same amount in thyroxine-treated rabbits, but decreased markedly more in the thyroidectomized group. *The researchers proposed that peripheral symptoms of hyperthyroidism and hypothy-*

roidism are in part the effects of thyroid hormone on the central nervous system metabolism of tryptophan and serotonin.[245]

Serotonin Metabolism in Mature Rat Brain is Critically Dependent on Thyroid Hormone Adequacy During Early Life. Rastogi and Singhal induced hypothyroidism in 1-day old rats.[361] Subsequently, the mid-brain was found to have a low level of tryptophan hydroxylase, the enzyme that hydroxylates tryptophan to 5-hydroxytryptophan, the stage preceding formation of serotonin.[94,p.262] Serotonin levels were reduced in the cerebellum by 22%, the mid-brain by 29%, and the striatum by 31%. When T_3 was administered 5 days after the beginning of thyroid hormone deficiency and continued for 25 days, tryptophan hydroxylase activity and tryptophan and serotonin levels returned to normal values. The concentration of 5-hydroxyindoleacetic acid also increased.

However, when the researchers postponed T_3 replacement until the rats reached adulthood, none of the serotonin-related abnormalities improved. Rastogi and Singhal stated, "Our data demonstrate that deficiency of thyroid hormone in early life disrupts the normal upsurge of 5-hydroxytryptamine [serotonin] metabolism in brain. A critical period exists in early life of rats during which thyroid hormone must be present for the optimal development of 5- hydroxytryptamine metabolizing systems in maturing brain."[361] This finding raises an interesting question: Does suboptimal thyroid status in susceptible humans at a critical early stage in life predispose them to permanent adverse effects of low serotonin levels, such as depression, hypersensitivity to pain, and disturbed sleep?

Regulation of 5-Hydroxytryptophan by Thyroid Hormone. Thyroid hormone regulates serotonin synthesis in the brain partly through controlling the concentration of the serotonin precursor tryptophan. Jacoby and coworkers[93] administered to hypothyroid rats a chemical that inhibits 5-hydroxytryptophan decarboxylase, the enzyme that removes a carboxyl (COOH) group from 5-hydroxytryptophan, converting it to serotonin.[94,pp.343-344] This procedure caused the accumulation of 5-hydroxytryptophan. Rats in the hypothyroid state accumulated this serotonin precursor at a lower rate than controls. After treatment with enough T_4 to induce hyperthyroidism, 5-hydroxytryptophan accumulated at a rate greater than would be expected merely from administration of the decarboxylase inhibitor.[93] This implies that thyroid hormone exerts an influence on brain tryptophan levels.

Changes in 5-HT_{1A} Receptor Binding with Varying Thyroid States. Among the types of serotonin receptors in the brain, the 5-HT_{1A} receptor appears to be principally involved in mediating anxiety and depression.[86] This receptor is abundant in the nucleus raphe dorsalis and limbic areas such as the cortex and hippocampus.[87] These brain areas also have a high level of expression of the genes for the three types of α thyroid hormone receptors and the β_1 thyroid hormone receptor.[91][92]

Mason and colleagues found that thyroidectomy decreased 5-HT_2 (serotonin) receptor binding in the striatum. *Peripheral administration of large doses of T_4 or T_3 for 7 days increased 5-HT_2 receptor binding in the cortex, striatum, and hippocampus in the limbic system.*[95] The researchers stated that the increased binding probably resulted from an increased number of receptors.[95,p.264]

Similarly, Tejani-Butt and coworkers found that at 7 and 35 days after rats were thyroidectomized, there was a significant increase in binding of a highly specific radioactive ligand to 5-HT_{1A} receptors in the cortex and hippocampus. Thyroidectomy did not increase 5-HT_{1A} receptor binding in the hypothalamus where there is a low density of the receptors. It also did not increase binding in the nucleus raphe dorsalis. High doses of T_4 for 28 days returned binding to normal levels in the cortex. Binding also increased in the hippocampus and hypothalamus, but it did not change in the dorsal raphe nucleus.[85] The authors wrote, "These results suggest that a neuromodulatory link may exist between the hypothalamic-pituitary-thyroid axis and 5-HT_{1A} receptors in the limbic regions of the rat brain. Depending on the brain region examined, a differential response to circulating levels of thyroid hormone was observed."[85,p.1011]

The question arises as to whether the increased binding of the 5-HT_{1A} serotonin receptor resulted from a thyroid hormone-induced reduction in serotonin level. Tejani-Butt and coauthors pointed out that the mechanism by which thyroid hormone treatment increases selective binding of ^{3}H-PAT (a compound that selectively binds with the 5-HT_{1A} receptor) to 5-HT_{1A} receptors in limbic regions is not clear. The most immediate answer is that thyroid hormone decreases the local release of serotonin, and the receptors adapt by coming to supersensitively bind serotonin. This may not be the complete answer, however, because studies indicate that drugs that alter serotonin neurotransmission do not modify 5-HT_{1A} receptors in the brain.[84] Tejani-Butt and coauthors propose that the increased binding may have been mediated by compounds endogenous to the cells whose concentrations may depend on thyroid state. Alternately, they suggest that the increased binding might result from thyroid hormone receptors in serotonergic neurons that mediate changes in 5-HT_{1A} receptors through various intraneuronal processes.[85] Regardless, an increase in 5-HT_{1A} receptor binding due to a reduction in serotonin upon administration of thyroid hormone is incompatible with the evidence I presented above indicating that thyroid hormone regulation increases serotonin synthesis and secretion and that inadequate regulation decreases synthesis and release.

Growth Hormone and Somatomedin C (Insulin-like Growth Factor-I)

In an early study, researchers found a loss of the normal diurnal variation in fibromyalgia patients' growth hormone levels.[382] Later, other researchers reported that patients had low levels of somatomedin C, a growth factor whose levels are directly induced in the liver by growth hormone. Investigators inferred from the latter finding that growth hormone levels were also low.[383][384][385][386][387] Buchwald and colleagues, however, did not find the disruption of the growth hormone-somatomedin C axis reported previously in fibromyalgia patients.[257] As with most other abnormalities reportedly characteristic of fibromyalgia, it is likely that a certain percentage of fibromyalgia patients have low levels of growth hormone and somatomedin C, although levels may only be mildly decreased. For example, Beaufort and colleagues concluded from their study of somatomedin C levels in fibromyalgia patients, "Even if not significantly, growth hormone is decreased in fibromyalgia, peculiarly in a subgroup (36% of fibromyalgia patients)."[239] The low levels may result from inadequate thyroid hormone regulation of growth hormone synthesis and secretion.

Growth hormone and somatomedin C control mammalian growth. Release of growth hormone by the somatotroph cells[237] of the pituitary gland is regulated by growth hormone releasing hormone (GHRH) and somatostatin, both of which are released from the hypothalamus. GHRH stimulates release of growth hormone, and somatostatin inhibits its release and blunts tissue responses to growth hormone.[231][232] Somatomedins (insulin-like growth factors-I and -II) are both anabolic and stimulate mitotic cell division[238,p.239] (the process by which the body grows and somatic cells are replaced).

Other neurotransmitters and hormones also inhibit or stimulate growth hormone secretion. They do so mainly by modulating hypothalamic release of GHRH or somatostatin.[231][233] For example, dopamine stimu-

lates growth hormone secretion,[233] and low dopamine levels due to inadequate thyroid hormone regulation may contribute to low growth hormone and in turn, low somatomedin C levels.

Krieg et al. found that the β-adrenergic agonist isoproterenol, acting on the pituitary gland, induced a rapid but brief release of GH. However, isoproterenol indirectly inhibited growth hormone release by stimulating the secretion of somatostatin by the hypothalamus.[235][237] Somatostatin, also called "somatotropin release-inhibiting factor," inhibits the release of growth hormone by the somatotrophs of the anterior pituitary gland. The α_2-adrenergic agonist clonidine increases secretion of GHRH, and α-adrenergic antagonists, such as phentolamine, decrease secretion of GHRH.[247,p.1585]

Effect of Thyroid Status on Growth Hormone and Somatomedin C. Thyroid hormone exerts a powerful influence over the levels of growth hormone and somatomedin C. Hypothyroidism impairs growth hormone secretion directly through inhibiting the somatotroph cells of the pituitary gland.[242][243] The resulting low growth hormone levels decrease secretion of somatomedin C by the liver and impede the response of cartilage to somatomedin.[241,p.1041] This is clearly shown by dramatic growth retardation in hypothyroid children.[241,p.1040] In hypothyroid adults, there are few manifestations.[240,p.974] Hypothyroid patients were found in one study to have growth hormone levels that did not differ from controls, although patients' somatomedin C levels were significantly decreased.[239] Rodriquez-Arnao[259] and Beaufort[239] and their co-workers also found low plasma levels of somatomedin C in hypothyroid patients.[259]

Thyroidectomy induced a 61%-to-65% reduction in hypothalamic growth hormone-releasing hormone (GHRH) mRNA levels. Levels were reversed with T_4 replacement. Pituitary growth hormone levels varied parallel to GHRH after thyroidectomy and T_4 supplementation.[251] Thyroid hormone is important in regulating growth hormone synthesis by increasing the amount of growth hormone mRNA in the cytoplasm. T_3 and T_4 increased expression of growth hormone receptor mRNA and potentiated the expression of somatomedin C mRNA in the presence of growth hormone.[238] In the absence of thyroid hormone, growth hormone mRNA synthesis and accumulation dropped more than 98%.[43][248][249][250][254][255][256] Hypothyroid patients had a blunted growth hormone response to insulin-induced hypoglycemia.[247]

Thyroid Hormone Regulation of the Growth Hormone Gene. The growth hormone gene has an extensively studied thyroid hormone response element, a nucleotide sequence bound by the DNA binding domain of the thyroid hormone receptor.[139,pp.214&215] [163][170][171] *Measurements of the rate of accumulation of labeled mRNA molecules have shown that the transcriptional rate of the growth hormone gene is proportional to the concentration of T_3-occupied nuclear thyroid hormone receptors.*[169] Thyroid hormone binding to the T_3-receptor positioned at the TRE activates the growth hormone gene[163] and stimulates production of growth hormone mRNA.[43] T_3 induction of synthesis of new growth hormone mRNA[43] leads to synthesis of growth hormone.

Brameld and coworkers demonstrated that T_3, T_4, and dexamethasone (a synthetic adrenocortical steroid[388,p.1449]) stimulate growth hormone receptor expression, and the increase in growth hormone receptors enhances somatomedin C gene expression in response to growth hormone administration.[238,p.244] The induction of growth hormone mRNA is potentiated by the simultaneous presence of adrenal glucocorticoids.[244,p.174] Although glucocorticoids facilitate production of growth hormone mRNA, chronic use of exogenous glucocorticoids inhibits growth hormone release.[246,p.126]

Ikeda and colleagues reported that T_3 but not T_4 increased somatomedin C release by perfused rat livers.[260] Latimer reported, however, that T_4 replacement in hypophysectomized fetal pigs increased liver somatomedin C (IGF-I), but not IGF-II, concentrations.[261] Brameld reported that both T_3 and T_4 stimulate growth hormone receptor expression induced by dexamethasone. Thyroid hormones appear to have at least a minor *direct* effect on somatomedin C expression. *When thyroid hormone was administered, cells responded to growth hormone with greater expression of somatomedin C than when growth hormone was added without thyroid hormones.*[238,pp.243-244] This corresponds to the finding of Freyschuss and colleagues that somatomedin C expression increased in the liver when combinations of dexamethasone, T_3, and growth hormone were administered to hypophysectomized rats.[262]

Westermark and coworkers investigated the influence of thyroid hormone levels on two growth factors: serum levels of somatomedin C and urine levels of epidermal growth factor. The investigators concluded: "Data from the present study thus demonstrate that the hyper- and hypothyroid states are accompanied by changes in serum and urine levels of growth factors and that these are affected by the treatment for these conditions. This conforms to the view that the growth promoting effect of thyroid hormones involves a stim-

ulated synthesis or release of the classic growth factors."[258,p.420]

Precautions Regarding Growth Hormone Injections as a Treatment for Fibromyalgia. The clinician should bear in mind that when low growth hormone/somatomedin C levels result from inadequate thyroid hormone regulation, the proper treatment is administration of thyroid hormone, not growth hormone. Though the above is likely the case in fibromyalgia, growth hormone injections are being used as a fibromyalgia treatment.[384] This treatment, without proper thyroid hormone therapy, may result in long-term adverse effects from the inadequate thyroid hormone regulation. Furthermore, injections of exogenous growth hormone may have adverse effects, such as antibodies to growth hormone,[194] lipoatrophy at injections sites,[186,p.1342] inhibited iodine uptake by the thyroid gland,[253] and important impairing alterations in thyroid hormone metabolism.[128,p.E192] Growth hormone injections have caused hypothyroidism in children.[186,p.1342] (See Chapter 5.1, subsection titled "Growth Hormone Injections" for a more detailed discussion of growth hormone injections as a treatment for fibromyalgia.)

Substance P

Several studies have shown elevated levels of substance P in the cerebrospinal fluids of fibromyalgia patients,[24][31][190] although two unpublished studies found normal levels in serum and urine.[25,p.74] One author stated that elevated cerebrospinal substance P in fibromyalgia ". . . is the most dramatically abnormal laboratory measure yet documented in these patients. It clearly distinguishes patients selected by the ACR criteria from healthy normal individuals." He also stated that fibromyalgia is the only clinical disorder in which patients have profoundly elevated levels of cerebrospinal substance P.[25,p.76]

Substance P is a small neuropeptide that is excitatory to centripetal nociceptive and centrifugal motor neurons.[33][203][204][205][206][207] Evidence indicates that in the spinal cord, substance P acts in a background manner to facilitate transmission through powerful synaptic pathways that subserve reflex activity.[203] Also, substance P facilitates sensory processing.[207][208][209] Because of this, high concentrations of substance P in the dorsal horns of the spinal cord (see below) of hypothyroid animals are possibly related to their hypersensitivity.[197,p.266]

Thyroid Hormone Regulation of Substance P in Widespread, Discrete Nuclei of the Brain. Dupont and colleagues[198] measured changes in substance

P content in discrete brain nuclei from various regions of the brain of neonatal rats after thyroidectomy and after T4 replacement. They found very marked increases in substance P after thyroidectomy, and the effect was completely reversed by T4 therapy. Increases in substance P in thyroidectomized rats was 2.5 times the concentration in the same brain areas in control animals. The increases were statistically significant in 19 of the 32 brain nuclei dissected.[198,p.2042] By far, the greatest increase in substance P occurred in the substantia nigra zona reticulata.

Thyroid Hormone Regulation of Substance P in the Anterior Pituitary Gland. Substance P is synthesized by cells in the anterior pituitary gland,[187][195] where the neuropeptide may act locally as an autocrine or paracrine agent in controlling pituitary secretions.[189,p.393][195] A subset of thyrotroph cells that synthesize and release TSH also contain substance P.[215] Decreased thyrotroph exposure to thyroid hormone activates transcriptional activities that increase both TSH and substance P. Substance P in the rat pituitary gland has also been shown to be negatively regulated by thyroid hormone.[189,p.396] Thyroid hormone administration decreases substance P mRNAs, and thyroidectomy increases substance P mRNAs.[187][188][189][195][196]

Thyroid Hormone Regulation of the Preprotachykinin Gene and Preprotachykinin-A mRNA. Thyroid hormone directly regulates transcription of the preprotachykinin gene.[187][193,p.2913][195,p.339] The preprotachykinin-A gene encodes both preprotachykinin-A (PPT-A), the precursor of substance P, and the cognate receptor, the substance P receptor.[191][192] The gene gives rise to several preprotachykinins from which substance P derives through alternative mRNA splicing.[213][214] Thyroidectomy increased PPT-A mRNA in the anterior pituitary.[187] Jonassen and coworkers reported an 800% increase in PPT-A mRNA levels in hypothyroidism.[187] T4 replacement after thyroidectomy decreased PPT-A mRNA levels relative to thyroidectomized controls.[188] Excess T4, enough to cause hyperthyroidism, significantly reduced substance P levels.[189]

Thyroid Hormone Regulation of Substance P in the Lumbar Spinal Cord. In the spinal cord, substance P is present in the descending projections of the intermediolateral horn cells, and moderate amounts are present in the ventral horns.[26][28] It is more concentrated, however, in the dorsal horns.[30][199][200] The dorsal root ganglia and primary sensory neurons that connect to the dorsal horns also contain substance P.[199][210][211][212] In the dorsal horns, substance P is located principally in the superficial layers.[201] Some substance P has also been found in the somata of spinal sensory ganglia.[30][199][200] When Savard and colleagues made neonatal rats hypothyroid, the substance P content in the dorsal horns increased by 100%.[197]

Serotonin-Stimulated Secretion of Substance P: Possibly Controlled by Thyroid Hormone. Inadequate thyroid hormone regulation of transcription may also increase substance P by impairing serotonin secretion (see serotonin section above). A population of serotonergic raphe nucleus neurons contain substance P.[26][27][28] Substance P is present in the raphe nucleus cell bodies, the descending projections of the intermediolateral horn cells, and the ventral horn of the spinal cord, where it coexists with serotonin.[26][28] Gilbert and coworkers identified a substance P/serotonin pathway that originates in the nucleus raphe magnus and projects to the ventral horns.[202] Serotonin stimulates the release of substance P in the ventral spinal cord.[29] Because of this, during a serotonin deficiency, as proposed in fibromyalgia, one might expect the substance P level to decrease, at least in the ventral cord. But when p-chlorophenylalanine was used to inhibit serotonin synthesis in euthyroid neonatal rats, substance P levels in the dorsal horns of the spinal cord increased by 90%.[197,p.265]

Both substance P elevation and serotonin deficiency up-regulate pain perception.[32,p.81] The substance P elevation and the proposed CNS serotonin deficiency in fibromyalgia may thus constitute a dual amplifier of pain perception in these patients and may account for their chronic widespread pain (see Chapters 3.15 and 3.19). Inadequate thyroid hormone regulation can account for both a substance P elevation and a serotonin deficiency.

Corticotropin-Releasing Hormone (CRH)

Demitrack and Crofford wrote that CRH serves as a principal stimulus to the hypothalamic-pituitary-adrenal axis. Administering CRH to the central nervous system of animals and non-human primates induces signs of physiological and behavioral arousal. The researchers conjectured that a relative or absolute deficiency of hypothalamic CRH could contribute to the profound lethargy and fatigue of 'atypical' depressive syndromes, fibromyalgia, and chronic fatigue syndrome, either through direct effects upon the central nervous system or indirectly by causing glucocorticoid deficiency.[124,p.69]

CRH is secreted by the hypothalamic paraventricular nucleus. Expression of the CRH gene is mainly controlled by glucocorticoids,[185] and secretion of

CRH is especially stimulated by the stress-induced release of norepinephrine.[179] Shi and colleagues found that making rats hypothyroid with propylthiouracil decreased CRH gene transcripts in the paraventricular nucleus. The hypothyroidism induced a concomitant decrease in both proopiomelanocortin (the precursor of ACTH) gene transcription in the anterior pituitary and circulating corticosterone. The researchers also found that thyroid hormone deficiency significantly reduced CRH gene transcripts and decreased CRH mRNA in the hypothalamic paraventricular nucleus of male rats. As a result of these findings, the authors wrote, "We conclude that circulating levels of thyroid hormones have a major effect on the central regulation of the hypothalamic-pituitary-adrenal axis."[168] Ceccatelli and coworkers found that after surgical ablation of the thyroid gland, CRH mRNA decreased in the hypothalamic paraventricular nucleus of adult rats, and administering T_4 up-regulated CRH mRNA levels. They pointed out that thyroid hormone acts directly on CRH-secreting neurons.[172]

This genomic, molecular action of thyroid hormones most likely accounts for the decreased levels of cortisol in hypothyroidism[173] and the increases in ACTH-like activity[176][177] and cortisol levels in hyperthyroidism[174][175][176] (see Chapter 3.5). Circulating levels of thyroid hormones are a major central regulator of the hypothalamic-pituitary-adrenal axis.[168,p.1577] Hypothyroidism profoundly depresses activity of this axis while hyperthyroidism slightly increases it.[168,p.1579]

REFERENCES

1. Lavin, T.N.: *Endocrinology,* 2nd edition. Edited by L.J. DeGroot, New York, Grune & Stratton, 1988, pp.562-573.
2. Bilezikian, J.P. and Loeb, J.N.: The influence of hyperthyroidism and hypothyroidism on α-and β-adrenergic receptor systems and adrenergic responsiveness. *Endoc. Rev.*, 4:378-388, 1983.
3. Goswami, A. and Rosenberg, I.N.: Effects of thyroid status on membrane-bound low K_m cyclic nucleotide phosphodiesterase activity in rat adipocytes. *J. Biol. Chem.*, 260:82-85, 1985.
4. Milligan, G., Spiegel, A.M., Unson, C.G., and Saggerson, E.D.: Chemically induced hypothyroidism produces elevated amounts of the α subunit of the inhibitory guanine nucleotide binding protein (G_i) and the β subunit common to all G-proteins. *Biochem. J.*, 247:223-227, 1987.
5. Rapiejko, P.J., Watkins, D.C., Ros, M., and Malbon, C.C.: Thyroid hormones regulate G-protein β-subunit mRNA expression *in vivo. J. Biol. Chem.*, 264:16183-16189, 1989.
6. Ros, M., Northup, J.K., and Malbon, C.C.: Steady-state levels of G-proteins and β-adrenergic receptors in rat fat cells. *J. Biol. Chem.*, 263:4362-4368, 1988.
7. Schmidt, R.F.: Synaptic transmission. In *Fundamentals of Neurophysiology.* Edited by R.F. Schmidt, New York, Springer-Verlag, pp.69-102.
8. Oppenheimer, J.H.: The nuclear receptor-triiodothyronine complex: relationship to thyroid hormone distribution, metabolism, and biological action. In *Molecular Basis of Thyroid Hormone Action.* Edited by J.K. Oppenheimer and H.H. Samuels, New York, Academic Press, 1983, pp.1-35.
9. Roncari, D.A.K. and Murthy, V.K.: Effects of thyroid hormones on enzymes involved in fatty acid and glycerolipid syntheses. *J. Biol. Chem.*, 250(11):4134-4138, 1975.
10. Van Inwegen, R.G., Robison, G.A., Thompson, W.J., Armstrong, K.J., and Stouffer, J.E.: Cyclic nucleotide phosphodiesterases and thyroid hormones. *J. Biol. Chem.*, 250(7):2452-2456, 1975.
11. Wildenthal, K.: Studies of isolated fetal mouse hearts in organ culture. Evidence for a direct effect of triiodothyronine in enhancing cardiac responsiveness to norepinephrine. *J. Clin. Invest.*, 51(10):2702-2709, 1972.
12. Kunos, G., Vermes-Kunos, I., and Nickerson, M.: Effects of thyroid state on adrenoceptor properties. *Nature*, 250: 779-781, 1974.
13. Lazar-Wesley, E., Hadcock, J.R., Malbon, C.C., Kunos, G., and Ishac, J.N.: Tissue-specific regulation of α_{2B}, β_1, and β_2-adrenergic receptor mRNAs by thyroid state in the rat. *Endocrinology*, 129(2):1116-1118, 1991.
14. Brent, G.A., Larsen, P.R., Harney, J.W., Koening, R.J., and Moore, D.D.: Functional characterization of the rat growth hormone promoter elements required for induction by thyroid hormone with and without a co-transfectant β type thyroid hormone receptor. *J. Biol. Chem.*, 264:178-182, 1989.
15. Carr, F.E., Burnside, J., and Chin, W.W.: Thyroid hormones regulate rat thyrotropin β gene promoter activity expressed in GH3 cells. *Mol. Endocrinol.*, 3:709-716, 1989.
16. Brent, G.A., Dunn, M.K., Harney, J.W., Gulick, T., Larsen, P.R., and Moore, D.D.: Thyroid hormone aporeceptor represses T_3-inducible promoters and blocks activity of the retinoic acid receptor. *New Biol.*, 1:329-336, 1989.
17. Damm, K., Thompson, C.C., and Evans, R.M.: Protein encoded by v-*erbA* functions as a thyroid hormone receptor antagonist. *Nature*, 339:593-597, 1989.
18. Segal, J. and Ingbar, S.H.: 3,5,3'-tri-iodothyronine enhances sugar transport in rat thymocytes by increasing the intrinsic activity of the plasma membrane sugar transporter. *J. Endocrinol.*, 124:133, 1990.
19. Segal, J. and Ingbar, S.H.: Stimulation by triiodothyronine of the *in vitro* uptake of sugars by rat thymocytes. *J. Clin. Invest.*, 63:507, 1979.
20. Segal, J. and Ingbar, S.H.: Studies on the mechanism by which 3,5,3'-triiodothyronine stimulates 2-deoxyglucose uptake in rat thymocytes *in vitro*: role of calcium and 3':5'-monophosphate. *J. Clin. Invest.*, 68:103, 1981.
21. Kvetny, J. and Matzen, L.: Thyroid hormone-stimulated glucose uptake in human-mononuclear blood cells from normal persons and from patients with non-insulin-dependent diabetes mellitus. *Acta Endocrinologica* (Copenh.), 120:715-720, 1989.

22. Segal, J. and Ingbar, S.H.: *In vivo* stimulation of sugar uptake in rat thymocytes. *J. Clin. Invest.*, 76:1575-1580, 1985.

23. Kvetny, J.: Nuclear thyroxine binding in human mononuclear blood cells. *Scand. J. Clin. Lab. Invest.*, 46 (Suppl.182):7-64, 1986.

24. Russell, I.J., Orr, M.D., Michalek, J.E., Nyberg, F., and Eridsson, U.: Substance P (SP), SP endopeptidase activity (SP_{1-7}) in fibromyalgia syndrome (FS) cerebrospinal fluid (CSF). (Abstract) *J. Musculoskel. Pain*, 3(Suppl.1):5, 1995.

25. Russell, I.J.: Neurochemical pathogenesis of fibromyalgia syndrome. *J. Musculoskel. Pain*, 4(1/2):61-92, 1996.

26. Appel, N.M., Wessendorf, M.W., and Elde, R.P.: Thyrotropin-releasing hormone in spinal cord: coexistence with serotonin and with substance P in fibers and terminals apposing identified preganglionic sympathetic neurons. *Brain Res.*, 415:137-143, 1987.

27. Sasek, C.A., Wessendorf, M.W., and Helke, C.J.: Evidence for coexistence of thyrotropin-releasing hormone, substance P, and serotonin in ventral medullary neurons that project to the intermediolateral cell column in the rat. *Neuroscience*, 35:105-119, 1990.

28. Wessendorf, M.W., Appel, N.M., Molitor, T.W., and Elde, R.P.: A method for immunofluorescent demonstration of three coexisting neurotransmitters in rat brain and spinal cord, using the fluophores fluoescein, lissamine rhodamine, and 7-amino-4-methylcoumarin-3-acetic acid. *J. Histol. Cytol.*, 38: 1859-1877, 1990.

29. Iverfeldt, K., Peterson, L.-L., Brodin, E., Ogren, S.-O., and Bartfai, T.: Serotonin type-2 receptor-mediated regulation of substance P release in the ventral spinal cord and the effects of chronic antidepressant treatment. *Naunyn-Schmiedeberg's Arch. Pharmacol.*, 333:1-6, 1986.

30. Hökfelt, T., Kellerth, J.O., Nilsson, G., and Pernow, B.: Substance P: localization in the central nervous system and in some primary sensory neurons. *Science*, 190:889-890, 1975.

31. Russell, I.J., Orr, M.D., Littman, B., et al.: Elevated cerebrospinal levels of substance P in patients with the fibromyalgia syndrome. *Arthritis Rheum.*, 37:1593-1601, 1994.

32. Russell, I.J.: Pathogenesis of fibromyalgia: the neurohormonal hypothesis. *J. Musculoskel. Pain*, 2(1):73-86, 1994.

33. Malmberg, A. and Yaksh, T.: Hyperalgesia mediated by spinal glutamate or substance P receptor blocked by spinal cyclooxygenase inhibition. *Science*, 257:1276-1279, 1992.

34. Pescovitz, O.H., Cutler, G.B., and Loriaux, D.L.: Synthesis and secretion of corticosteroids. In *Principles and Practice of Endocrinology and Metabolism*. Edited by K.L. Becker, J.P. Bilezinkian, W.J. Bremner, W. Hung, C.R. Kahn, D.L. Loriaux, R.W. Rebar, G.L. Robertson, and L. Wartofsky, Philadelphia, J.B. Lippincott Co., 1990, pp.579-591.

35. Samuels, H.H., Perlman, A.J., Raaka, B.M., and Stanley, F.: Thyroid hormone receptor synthesis and degradation and interaction with chromatin components. In *Molecular Basis of Thyroid Hormone Action*. Edited by J.K. Oppenheimer and H.H. Samuels, New York, Academic Press, Inc., 1983, pp.99-137.

36. Samuels, H.H.: Identification and characterization of thyroid hormone receptors and action using cell culture tech-niques. In *Molecular Basis of Thyroid Hormone Action*. Edited by J.K. Oppenheimer and H.H. Samuels, New York, Academic Press, Inc., 1983, pp.35-65.

37. Apriletti, J.W., David-Inouye, Y., Baxter, J.D., and Eberhardt, N.L.: Physiochemical characterization of the intranuclear thyroid hormone receptor. In *Molecular Basis of Thyroid Hormone Action*. Edited by J.K. Oppenheimer and H.H. Samuels, New York, Academic Press, Inc., 1983, pp.67-97.

38. Oppenheimer, J.K., and Dillmann, W.H.: Molecular mechanisms at the tissue level in hyperthyroidism. *Clin. Endocrinol. Metab.*, 7:145-165, 1978.

39. Samuels, H.H., Tsai, J.S., and Casanova, J.: Thyroid hormone action: *in vitro* demonstration of putative receptors in isolated nuclei and soluble nuclear extracts. *Science*, 184:1188-1191, 1974.

40. Nakamura, M., Hamada, S., and Imura, M.: Sequential changes in rat liver nuclear triiodothyronine receptors and mitochondrial alpha-glycerophosphate dehydrogenase activity after administration of triiodothyronine. *Biochem. J.*, 182:377-382, 1979.

41. Tata, J.R., and Widnell, C.C.: Ribonucleic acid synthesis during the early action of thyroid hormones. *Biochem. J.*, 98:604-620, 1966.

42. Dillmann, W.H., Mendecki, J., and Koerner, D.: Triiodothyronine (T_3) stimulated formation of poly(A)-containing nuclear RNA and mRNA in rat liver. *Endocrinology*, 102: 568-575, 1978.

43. Seo, H., Vassart, G., Bocas, H., and Refetoff, S.: Triiodothyronine stimulates specifically growth hormone in RNA in rat pituitary tumor cells. *Proc. Natl. Acad. Sci. (USA)*, 74:2054-2058, 1977.

44. Tata, J.R., Ernster, L., and Lindberg, O.: The action of thyroid hormones at the cell level. *Biochem. J.*, 86:408-428, 1963.

45. Wolfe, S.L.: *Molecular and Cellular Biology*. Belmont, Wadsworth Publishing Co., 1993.

46. Frankhyzen, A. and Muller, A.: *In vitro* studies on the inhibition of serotonin release through α-adrenoreceptor activity in various regions of the rat CNS. *Abstract of 5th Catecholamine Symposium*, 1983, p. 137.

47. Benkirane, S., Arbilla, S., and Langer, S.Z.: Newly synthesized noradrenaline mediates the α_2-adrenoceptor inhibition of [3H]5-hydroxytryptamine release induced by β-phenylethylamine in rat hippocampal slices. *Eur. J. Pharmacol.*, 131(2-3):189-198, 1986.

48. Numazawa, R.: Pharmacological characterization of α_2-adrenoceptor regulated serotonin release in the rat hippocampus. *Hokkaido Igaku Zasshi—Hokkaido J. Med. Sci.*, 69(4):927-939, 1994.

49. Numazawa, R., Yoshioka, M., Matsumoto, M., Togashi, H., Kemmotsu, O., and Saito, H.: Pharmacological characterization of α_2-adrenoceptor regulated serotonin release in the rat hippocampus. *Neuroscience Letters*, 192(3):161-164, 1995.

50. De Boer, T., Nefkens, F., and Van Helvoirt, A.: The α_2-adrenoceptor antagonist Org 3770 enhances serotonin transmission *in vivo*. *Eur. J. Pharmcol.*, 253(1-2):R5-R6, 1994.

51. Bennett, R.M., Clark, S.R., Campbell, S.M., et al.: Symptoms of Raynaud's syndrome in patients with fi-

bromyalgia: a study utilizing the Nielsen test, digital photoplethysmography and measurements of platelet α_2-adrenergic receptors. *Arthrit. and Rheumat.*, 34:264-269, 1991.

52. Feuerstein, T.J., Muschler, A., Lupp, A., Van Velthoven, V., Schlicker, E., and Gothert, M.: Endogenous noradrenaline activates α_2-adrenoceptors on serotonergic nerve endings in human and cat neocortex. *J. Neurochem.*, 61 (2):474-480, 1993.

53. Head, G.A. and Burke, S.: Importance of central noradrenergic and serotonergic pathways in the cardiovascular actions of rilmenidine and clonidine. *J. Cardiovascular Pharmacol.*, 18(6):819-826, 1991.

54. McCormick, D.A., Pape, H.C., and Williamson, A.: Actions of norepinephrine in the cerebral cortex and thalamus: implications for function of the central noradrenergic system. *Prog. Brain Res.*, 88:293-305, 1991.

55. Clement, H-W., Gemsa, D., and Wesemann, W.: The effect of adrenergic drugs on serotonin metabolism in the nucleus raphe dorsalis of the rat, studied by *in vivo* voltammetry. *Eur. J. Pharmacol.*, 217:43-48, 1992.

56. Hallberg, H., Almgren, O., and Svensson, T.H.: Reduced brain serotonergic activity after repeated treatment with β-adrenoceptor antagonists. *Psychopharmacology*, 76:114, 1982.

57. Deakin, J.F.W. and Green, A.R.: The effects of putative 5-hydroxytryptamine antagonists on the behavior produced by administration of tranylcypromine and L-tryptophan or tranylcypromine and L-DOPA to rats. *Br. J. Pharmacol.*, 64:201, 1978.

58. Weinstock, W., Weiss, C., and Gitter, S.: Blockade of 5-hydroxytryptamine receptors in the central nervous system by β-adrenoceptor antagonists. *Neuropharmacology*, 16:273, 1977.

59. Hallberg, H., Almgren, O., and Svensson, T.H.: Increased brain serotonergic and noradrenergic activity by the β_2-agonist salbutamol: a putative antidepressant drug. *Psychopharmacology*, 73:201-204, 1981.

60. Wesemann, W., Grote, C., and Clement, H.W.: Rhythmicity of 5-HT releases in rat brain and the effect of antidepressant treatment. 7th International Symposium on Neuronal Control of Bodily Function, Mainz, 1990.

61. Trulson, M.E. and Jacobs, B.L.: Raphe unit activity in freely moving cats: correlation with level of behavioral arousal. *Brain Res.*, 163:135, 1979.

62. Aslanian, V. and Renaud, B.: Changes in serotonin metabolism in the rat raphe magnus and cardiovascular modifications following systemic administration of clonidine and other central α_2-agonists: an *in vivo* voltammetry study. *Neuropharmacology*, 28:387, 1989.

63. Svensson, T.H., Bunney, B.S., and Aghajanian, G.K.: Inhibition of both noradrenergic and serotonergic neurons in brain by the α-adrenergic agonist clonidine. *Brain Res.*, 92:291, 1975.

64. Monti, J.M.: Catecholamines and the sleep-wake cycle. I. EEG and behavioral arousal. *Life Sci.*, 30:1145, 1982.

65. Hilakivi, I.: The role of β- and α-adrenoceptors in the regulation of the stages of the sleep-waking cycle in the cat. *Brain Res.*, 277:109-118, 1983.

66. Marwaha, J. and Aghazanian, G.K.: Relative potencies of α_1 and α_2 antagonists in the locus coeruleus, dorsal raphe, and dorsal lateral geniculate nuclei: an electrophysiological study. *J. Pharmacol. Exp. Ther.*, 222:287-293, 1982.

67. Jacobs, B.L., Fornal, C.A., and Wilkinson, L.O.: Neurophysiological and neurochemical studies of brain serotonergic neurons in behaving animals. In *Neuropharmacology of Serotonin*. Edited by P.M. Whitaker-Azmitia and S.J. Peroutka, New York, New York Academy of Sciences, 1990, p.447.

68. Unnerstall, J.R., Kopajtic, T.A., and Kuhar, M.J.: Distribution of α_2 agonist binding sites in the rat and human central nervous system: analysis of some functional and anatomical correlates of the pharmacologic effects of clonidine and related adrenergic agents. *Brain Res. Rev.*, 7:69, 1984.

69. Wauquier, A. and Dugovic, C.: Serotonin and sleep-wakefulness. In *Neuropharmacology of Serotonin*. Edited by P.M. Whitaker-Azmitia and S.J. Peroutka, New York, New York Academy of Sciences, 1990, p. 447.

70. Dourish, C.T., Hutson, P.H., and Curzon, G.: Putative anxiolytics 8-OH-DAT, buspirone, and TVXQ 7821 are agonists at 5-HT_{1A} autoreceptors in the raphé nuclei. *Trends Pharmacol. Sci.*, 7:212, 1986.

71. Frances, H. and Simons, P.: The effect of a β-adrenergic agonist on behaviors mediated by 5-HT_{1A} and 5-HT_{1B} receptors. *Biol. Psychiatry*, 21:1072, 1986.

72. Trendelenburg, A-U., Trendelenburg, M., Starke, K., and Limberger, N.: Release-inhibiting α_2-adrenoceptors at serotonergic axons in rat and rabbit brain cortex: evidence for pharmacological identity with α_2-autoreceptors. *Naunyn-Schmiedeberg's Arch. Pharmacol.*, 349:25-33, 1994.

73. Starke, K. and Montel, H.: Involvement of α-receptors in clonidine-induced inhibition of transmitter release from central monoamine neurons. *Neuropharmacol.*, 12:1073-1080, 1973.

74. Frankhuzen, A.L. and Mulder, A.H.: Noradrenaline inhibits depolarization-induced ^{3}H-serotonin release from slices of rat hippocampus. *Eur. J. Pharmacol.*, 63:179-182, 1980.

75. Göthert, M. and Huth, H.: α-Adrenoceptor-mediated modulation of 5-hydroxytryptamine release from rat brain cortex slices. *Naunyn-Schmiedeberg's Arch. Pharmacol.*, 31:21-26, 1980.

76. Maura, G., Gemignani, A., and Raiteri, M.: Noradrenaline inhibits central serotonin release through α_2-adrenoceptors located on serotonergic nerve terminals. *Naunyn-Schmiedeberg's Arch. Pharmacol.*, 320:272-274, 1982.

77. Galzin, A.M., Moret, C., and Langer, S.Z.: Evidence that exogenous but not endogenous norepinephrine activates the presynaptic α_2-adrenoceptors on serotonergic nerve endings in the rat hypothalamus. *J. Pharmacol. Exp. Ther.*, 228:725-732, 1984.

78. Feurestein, T.J., Hertting, G., and Jackisch, R.: Endogenous noradrenaline as modulator of hippocampal serotonin (5-HT)-release. *Naunyn-Schmiedeberg's Arch Pharmacol.*, 329:216-221, 1985.

79. Limberger, N., Bonanno, G., Späth, L., and Starke, K.: Autoreceptors and α_2-adrenoceptors at the serotonergic axons of rabbit brain cortex. *Naunyn-Schmiedeberg's Arch. Pharmacol.*, 332:324-331, 1986.

80. Göthert, M. and Schlicker, E.: *Regulation of Serotonin Release in the Central Nervous System by Presynaptic Heter-*

oreceptors of Neurotransmitter Release: A Handbook, Vol. 2. Freund, Tel Aviv, 1991, pp.845-876.

81. Feuerstein, T.J., Mutschler, A., Lupp, A., Van Velthoven, V., Schlicker, E., and Göthert, M.: Endogenous noradrenaline activates α_2-adrenoceptors on serotonergic nerve endings in human and rat neocortex. *J. Neurochem.*, 61 (2):474-480, 1993.

82. Mongeau, R., Blier, P., and De Montigny, C.: *In vivo* electrophysiological evidence for a tonic inhibitory action of endogenous noradrenaline on α_2-adrenoceptors on 5-hydroxytryptamine terminals in the rat hippocampus. *Naunyn-Schmiedeberg's Arch. Pharmacol.*, 247:266, 1993.

83. Rouquier, L., Claustre, Y., and Benavides, J.: Centrally acting α_1-adrenergic antagonists decrease extracellular serotonin levels in the rat hippocampus: a microdialysis study. *Proceedings 7th International Catecholamine Symposium*, Amsterdam, 1992, p.277.

84. Hensler, J.G., Kovachich, G.B., and Frazer, A.: A quantitative autoradiographic study of 5-HT$_{1A}$ receptor regulation: effect of 5,7-dihydroxytryptamine and antidepressant treatments. *Neuropsychopharmacology*, 4:131-143, 1991.

85. Tejani-Butt, S.M., Yang, J., and Kaviani, A.: Time course of altered thyroid states on 5-HT$_{1A}$ receptors and 5-HT uptake sites in rat brain: an auto-radiographic analysis. *Neuroendocrinology*, 57:1011-1018, 1993.

86. Hamon, M., Gozlan, H., Mestikawy, S.E., Emerit, M.B., Gozlan, H., and Schechter, L.: The central 5-HT$_{1A}$ receptors: pharmacological, biochemical, functional, and regulatory properties. *Ann. N.Y. Acad. Sci.*, 600:114-131, 1990.

87. Gothert, M.: 5-Hydroxytryptamine receptors: an example for the complexity of chemical transmission of information in the brain. *Arzneimittelforschung*, 2:238-249, 1992.

88. Savard, P., Merand, Y., Paolo, T.D., and Dupont, A.: Effect of neonatal hypothyroidism on the serotonin system of the rat brain. *Brain Res.*, 292:99-108, 1984.

89. Vaccari, A.: Decreased central serotonin function in hypothyroidism. *Eur. J. Pharmacol.*, 82:93-95, 1982.

90. Singhal, R.L., Rastogi, R.B., and Hedina, P.D.: Brain biogenic amines and altered thyroid function. *Life Sci.*, 17: 1617-1626, 1975.

91. Bradley, D.J., Young, W.S., III, and Weinberger, C.: Differential expression of α and β thyroid hormone receptor genes in rat brain and pituitary. *Proc. Natl. Acad. Sci. (USA)*, 86:7250-7254, 1989.

92. Cook, C.B. and Koenig, R.J.: Expression of erbAα and β mRNAs in regions of adult rat brain. *Mol. Cell. Endocrinol.*, 70:13-20, 1990.

93. Jacoby, J.K., Mueller, G., and Wurtman, R.J.: Thyroid state and brain monoamine metabolism. *Endocrinology*, 97:1332-1335, 1975.

94. Cooper, J.R., Bloom, F.E., and Roth, R.H.: *The Biochemical Basis of Neuropharmacology*, 6th edition. New York, Oxford University Press, 1991.

95. Mason, G.A., Bondy, S.C., Nemeroff, C.B., Walker, C.H., and Prange, A.J., Jr.: The effects of thyroid state on beta-adrenergic and serotonergic receptors in rat brain. *Psychoneuroendocrinology*, 12:261-270, 1987.

96. Engstrom, G., Svensson, T.H., and Waldeck, B.: Thyroxine and brain catecholamines: increased transmitter synthesis and increased receptor sensitivity. *Brain Res.*, 77:

471-483, 1974.

97. Strombom, U., Svensson, T.H., Jackson, R.M., and Engstrom, G.J.: Hyperthyroidism: specifically increased response to central NA-(alpha)-receptor stimulation and generally increased monoamine turnover in brain. *J. Neural Transm.*, 41:73-92, 1977.

98. Lipton, M.A., Prange, A.J., Jr., Dratman, W., and Undenfriend, S.: Increased rate of norepinephrine biosynthesis in hypothyroid rats. *Proc. Fed. Am. Soc. Exp. Biol.*, 27:399, 1968.

99. Prange, A.J., Jr., Meek, J.L., and Lipton, M.A.: Catecholamines: diminished rate of synthesis in rat brain and heart after thyroxine pretreatment. *Life Sci.*, 9:901-907, 1970.

100. Parker, L.N.: The turnover of norepinephrine in brain stems of dysthyroid rats. *J. Neurochem.*, 19:1611-1613, 1972.

101. Kunos, G., Vermes-Kunos, I., and Nickerson, M.: Effects of thyroid state on adrenoceptor properties. *Nature*, 250: 779-781, 1974.

102. Kunos, G. and Ishac, E.J.N.: Mechanism of inverse regulation of α_1- and β-adrenergic receptors. *Biochem. Pharmacol.*, 36:1185-1191, 1987.

103. Ishac, E.J.N., Lazar-Wesley, E., and Kunos, G.: Rapid inverse changes in α_{1B}- and β_2-adrenergic receptors and gene transcripts in acutely isolated rat liver cells. *J. Cell. Physiol.*, 152:79-86, 1992.

104. Kunos, G.: Thyroid hormone-dependent interconversion of myocardial α- and β-adrenoceptors in the rat. *Brit. J. Pharmacol.*, 59:177-189, 1977.

105. Kupfer, L.E., Bilezikian, J.P., and Robinson, R.B.: Regulation of alpha- and beta-adrenergic receptors by triiodothyronine in cultured rat myocardial cells. *Naunyn-Schmiedeberg's Arch. Pharmacol.*, 334:275-281, 1986.

106. Kunos, G.: Modulation of adrenergic reactivity and adrenoceptors by thyroid hormone. In *Adrenoceptors and Catecholamine Action*. Edited by G. Kunos, New York, John Wiley & Sons, 1981, part A, pp.297-333.

107. Williams, L.T., Lefkowitz, R.J., Watanabe, A.M., Hathaway, D.R., and Besch, H.R., Jr.: Thyroid hormone regulation of β-adrenergic receptor number. *J. Biol. Chem.*, 252: 2787-2789, 1977.

108. Sharma, V.K. and Banerjee, S.P.: α-Adrenergic receptor in rat heart. *J. Biol. Chem.*, 253:5277-5279, 1978.

109. Ishac, E.J.N., Pennefather, J.N., and Handberg, G.M.: Effect of changes in thyroid state on atrial α- and β-adrenoceptors, adenylate cyclase activity, and catecholamine levels in the rat. *J. Cardiovasc. Pharmacol.*, 5:396-405, 1983.

110. Preiksaitis, H.G. and Kunos, G.: Adrenoceptor-mediated activation of liver glycogen phosphorylase: effects of thyroid state. *Life Sci.*, 24:35-42, 1979.

111. Malbon, C.C.: Liver cell adenylate cyclase and beta-adrenergic receptors: increased β-adrenergic receptor number and responsiveness in the hypothyroid rat. *J. Biol. Chem.*, 255:8692-8699, 1980.

112. Preiksaitis, H.G., Kan, W.H., and Kunos, G.: Decreased α_1-adrenoceptor responsiveness and density in the hypothyroid rat. *J. Biol. Chem.*, 257:4320-4326, 1982.

113. Kunos, G., Mucci, L., and O'Regan, S.: The influence of hormonal and neuronal factors on rat heart adrenoceptors. *Brit. J. Pharmacol.*, 71:371-386, 1980.

114. Baker, S.P.: Effects of thyroid status on beta-adreno-receptors and muscarinic receptors in the rat lung. *J. Autonom. Pharmacol.*, 1:269-277, 1981.

115. Bahouth, S.W.: Thyroid hormone transcriptionally regulates the β_1-adrenergic receptor gene in cultured ventricular myocytes. *J. Biol. Chem.*, 266(24):15863-15869, 1991.

116. Williams, L.T. and Lefkowitz, R.J.: Thyroid hormone regulation of alpha-adrenergic receptors: studies in rat myocardium. *J. Cardiovasc. Pharmacol.*, 1:181-189, 1979.

117. Sharma, V.K. and Banerjee, S.P.: β-adrenergic receptors in rat skeletal muscle: effects of thyroidectomy. *Biochim. Biophys. Acta*, 539:538-542, 1978.

118. Russell, I.J., Vipraio, G.A., Morgan, W.W., et al.: Catecholamine excretion in fibromyalgia syndrome. Unpublished material, 1988.

119. Russell, I.J.: Neurohormonal aspects of fibromyalgia syndrome. *Rheu. Dis. Clinics North Am.*, 15:149-168, 1989.

120. Nichols, A.J. and Ruffolo, R.R., Jr.: Functions mediated by α-adrenoceptors. In *α-Adrenoceptors: Molecular Biology, Biochemistry and Pharmacology*. Basel, Karger, 1991, pp.113-179.

121. Williams, J.T., Surprenant, A.-M., and North, R.A.: Inhibitory synaptic transmission mediated by catecholamines. VI. Adrenergic neuron electrophysiology and behavior. In *Epinephrine in the Central Nervous System*. Edited by P. Stolk, E. U'Prichard, and J. Fuxe, New York, Oxford University Press, 1988, pp.252-258.

122. Simson, P.E., Cierpial, M.A., Heyneman, L.E., and Weiss, J.M.: Pertussis toxin blocks the effects of α_2-agonists and antagonists on locus coeruleus activity *in vivo. Neurosci. Lett.*, 89:361-366, 1988.

123. Russell, I.J., Vaeroy, M., Jabors, M., and Nyberg, F.: Cerebrospinal fluid biogenic metabolites in fibromyalgia/fibrositis syndrome in rheumatoid arthritis. *Arthritis Rheum.*, 35:550-556, 1992.

124. Demitrack, M.A. and Crofford, L.J.: Hypothalamic-pituitary-adrenal axis dysregulation in fibromyalgia and chronic fatigue syndrome: an overview and hypothesis. *J. Musculoskeletal Pain*, 3(2):67-73, 1995.

125. Gross, G., Broddee, O.E., and Schumann, H.: Decreased number of β-adrenoceptors in cerebral cortex of hypothyroid rats. *Eur. J. Pharmacol.*, 61:191-194, 1980.

126. Atterwill, C.K., Bunn, S.J., Atkinson, D.J., Smith, S.L., and Heal, D.J.: Effects of thyroid status on presynaptic α_2-adrenoceptor and β-adrenoceptor binding in rat brain. *J. Neural Transm.*, 59:43-55, 1984.

127. Perumal, A.S., Halbreich, U., and Barkai, A.I.: Modifications of β-adrenergic receptor binding in rat brain following thyroxine administration. *Neurosci.*, 48:217-221, 1984.

128. Dratman, M.B., Crutchfield, F.L., Gordan, J.T, and Jennings, A.S.: Iodothyronine homeostasis in rat brain during hypothyroidism and hyperthyroidism. *Am. J. Physiol.*, 245:E185-E193, 1983.

129. Refetoff, S., Weiss, R.E., and Usala, S.J.: The syndromes of resistance to thyroid hormone. *Endocrin. Reviews*, 14 (3):348-399, 1993.

130. Oppenheimer, J.K., Koerner, D., Schwartz, H.L., and Surks, M.I.: Specific-nuclear triiodothyronine binding sites in rat liver and kidney. *J. Clin. Endocrinol. Metab.*, 35:330-333, 1972.

131. Sap, J., Muñoz, A., Damm, K., et al.: The *c-erb-*A protein is a high-affinity receptor for thyroid hormone. *Nature*, 324:635-640, 1986.

132. Weinberger, C., Thompson, C.C., Ong, E.S., Lebo, R., Gruol, D.J., and Evans, R.M.: The *c-erb-*A gene encodes a thyroid hormone receptor. *Nature*, 324:641-646, 1986.

133. Samuels, H.H., Tsai, J.S., and Casanova, J.: Thyroid hormone action *in vitro*: demonstration of putative receptors in isolated nuclei and soluble extracts. *Science*, 184:1188, 1974.

134. Oppenheimer, J.K. and Schwarz, H.L.: Stereospecific transport of triiodothyronine from plasma to cytosol and from cytosol to nucleus in rat liver, kidney, brain, and heart. *J. Clin. Invest.*, 75:147, 1985.

135. Oppenheimer, J.K., Schwartz, H.L., and Surks, M.I.: Tissue differences in the concentration of triiodothyronine nuclear binding sites in the rat: liver, kidney, pituitary, heart, brain, spleen, and testis. *Endocrinology*, 95:897, 1974.

136. Morishige, W.K. and Guernsey, D.L.: Triiodothyronine receptors in rat lung. *Endocrinology*, 102:1628, 1978.

137. Krieger, N.S., Stappenbeck, T.S., and Stern, P.H.: Characterization of specific thyroid hormone receptors in bone. *J. Bone Miner. Res.*, 3:473, 1988.

138. Lee, J.T., Lebenthal, E., and Ping-Cheung, L.: Rat pancreatic nuclear thyroid hormone receptor: characterization and postnatal development. *Gastroenterology*, 96:1151, 1989.

139. Oppenheimer, J.K.: Thyroid hormone action at the molecular level. In *Werner and Ingbar's The Thyroid: A Fundamental and Clinical Text*, 6th edition. Edited by L.E. Braverman and R.D. Utiger, New York, J.B. Lippincott Co., 1991, pp.204-224.

140. Crantz, F.R., Silva, J.E., and Larsen, P.R.: An analysis of the sources and quantity of 3,5,3'-triiodothyronine specifically bound to nuclear receptors in rat cerebral cortex and cerebellum. *Endocrinology*, 110:367, 1982.

141. Silva, H.E., Dick, T.E., and Larsen, P.R.: Contribution of local tissue monodeiodination to the nuclear 3,5,3'-triiodothyronine in pituitary, liver, and kidney of euthyroid rats. *Endocrinology*, 103:1196, 1978.

142. Surks, M.I., Koerner, D., Dillman, W., et al.: Limited capacity binding sites for L-triiodothyronine (T_3) in rat liver nuclei: localization to the chromatin and partial characterization of the T_3-chromatin complex. *J. Biol. Chem.*, 248:7066, 1973.

143. Oppenheimer, J.K., Schwartz, H.L., and Surks, M.I.: Nuclear binding capacity appears to limit the hepatic response to L-triiodothyronine (T_3). *Endocr. Res. Commun.*, 2:309, 1975.

144. Oppenheimer, J.K., Silva, E., Schwartz, H.L., et al.: Stimulation of hepatic mitochondrial α-glycerophosphate dehydrogenase and malic enzyme by L-triiodothyronine: characteristics of the response with specific nuclear thyroid hormone binding sites fully saturated. *J. Clin. Invest.*, 59:517, 1977.

145. Oppenheimer, J.K., Coulombe, P., Schwartz, H.L., et al.: Nonlinear (amplified) relationship between nuclear occupancy by triiodothyronine and the appearance rate of hepatic α-glycerophosphate dehydrogenase and malic en-

zyme. *J. Clin. Invest.*, 61:987, 1978.

146. Sakurai, A., Nakai, A., and DeGroot, L.J.: Expression of three forms of thyroid hormone receptor in human tissues. *Mol. Endocrinol.*, 3:392, 1989.

147. Soloman, E. and Barker, D.F.: Report of the committee on the genetic constitution of chromosome 17 (HGH10). *Cytogenet. Cell. Genet.*, 51:319-337, 1989.

148. Naylor, S.L. and Bishop, D.T.: Report of the committee on the genetic constitution of chromosome 3 (HGH10). *Cytogenet. Cell. Genet.*, 51:106-120, 1989.

149. Sakurai, A., Nakai, A., and DeGroot, L.J.: Structural analysis of human thyroid hormone receptor β gene. *Mol. Cell. Endocrinol.*, 71:83-91, 1990.

150. Laudet, V., Begue, A., Henry-Duthoit, C., et al.: Genomic organization of the human thyroid hormone receptor α (c-erbA-1) gene. *Nucleic Acid Res.*, 19:1105-1112, 1991.

151. Hodin, R.A., Lazar, M.A., Wintman, B.I., et al.: Identification of a thyroid hormone receptor that is pituitary-specific. *Science*, 244:76-79, 1989.

152. Yen, P.M., Sunday, M.E., Darling, D.S., and Chin, W.W.: Isoform-specific thyroid hormone receptor antibodies detect multiple thyroid hormone receptors in rat and human pituitaries. *Endocrinology*, 130:1539-1546, 1992.

153. Nakai, A., Seino, S., Sakurai, A., Szilak, I., Bell, G.I., and DeGroot, L.J.: Characterization of a thyroid hormone receptor expressed in human kidney and other tissues. *Proc. Natl. Acad. Sci.*, 85:2781-2785, 1988.

154. Miyajima, N., Horiuchi, R., Shibuya, Y., et al.: Two erbA homologs encoding proteins with different T_3 binding capacities are transcribed from opposite DNA strands of the same genetic locus. *Cell*, 57:31-39, 1989.

155. Izumo, S. and Mahdavi, V.: Thyroid hormone receptor α isoforms generated by alternative splicing differentially activate myosin HC gene transcription. *Nature*, 334:539, 1988.

156. Mitsuhashi, T., Tennyson, G.E., and Nikodem, V.M.: Alternative splicing generates messages encoding rat c-erbA proteins that do not bind thyroid hormone. *Proc. Natl. Acad. Sci. (USA)*, 85:5804, 1988.

157. Gurr, J.A. and Kourides, I.A.: Thyroid hormone regulation of thyrotropin α and β subunit gene transcription. *DNA*, 4:301, 1985.

158. Shupnik, M.A., Greenspan, S.L., and Ridgway, E.C.: Transcriptional regulation of thyrotropin subunit genes by thyrotropin-releasing hormone and dopamine in pituitary cell culture. *J. Biol. Chem.*, 261:12675, 1986.

159. Darling, D.S., Beebe, J.S., Burnside, J., Winslow, E.R., and Chin, W.W.: 3,5,3'-triiodothyronine (T_3) receptor-auxiliary protein (TRAP) binds DNA and forms heterodimers with the T_3 receptor. *Mol. Endocrinol.*, 5:73-84, 1991.

160. Lazar, M.E., Hodin, R.A., Darling, D.S., et al.: Identification of a rat-c-erbA-α-related protein which binds deoxyribonucleic acid but does not bind thyroid hormone. *Mol. Endocrinol.*, 2:893, 1988.

161. Koenig, R.J., Lazar, M.A., Hodin, R.A., et al.: Inhibition of thyroid hormone action by a non-hormone binding c-erbA protein generated by alternate mRNA splicing. *Nature*, 337:659, 1989.

162. Glass, C.K., Lipkin, S.M., Devary, O.V., and Rosenfeld, M.G.: Positive and negative regulation of gene transcrip-

tion by a retinoic acid-thyroid hormone receptor heterodimer. *Cell*, 59:697-708, 1989.

163. Brent, G.A., Larsen, P.R., Harney, J.W., Koenig, R.J., and Moore, D.D.: Functional characterization of the rat growth hormone promoter elements required for induction by thyroid hormone with and without co-transfectant β type thyroid hormone receptor. *J. Biol. Chem.*, 264:178-182, 1989.

164. Puymirat, J., Luo, M., and Dussault, J.K.: Immunocytochemical localization of thyroid hormone nuclear receptors in cultured hypothalamic dopaminergic neurons. *Neuroscience*, 30(2):443-449, 1989.

165. Puymirat, J.: Effects of dysthyroidism on central catecholaminergic neurons. *Neurochem. Int.*, 7:969-978, 1985.

166. Puymirat, J., Barret, A., Picart, R., et al: Triiodothyronine enhances the morphological maturation of dopaminergic neurons from fetal mouse hypothalamus cultured in serum-free medium. *Neuroscience*, 10:801-810, 1983.

167. Puymirat, J., Barret, A., Faivre-Bauman, A., and Tixier-Vidal, A.: Biochemical characterization of the uptake and release of ^{3}H-dopamine by dopaminergic neurons: a developmental study using serum-free cultures. *Devel. Biol.*, 119:75-84, 1987.

168. Shi, Z-X, Levy, A., and Lightman, S.L.: Thyroid hormone-mediated regulation of corticotropin-releasing hormone messenger ribonucleic acid in the rat. *Endocrinology*, 134(3):1577-1580, 1994.

169. Yaffe, B. and Samuels, H.H.: Hormonal regulation of the growth hormone gene: relationship of the rate of transcription to the level of nuclear thyroid hormone-receptor complexes. *J. Biol. Chem.*, 259:6284, 1984.

170. Glass, C.K., Franco, R., Weinberger, C., Albert, V.R., Evans, R.M., and Rosenfeld, M.G.: A c-erb-A binding site in rat growth hormone gene mediates trans-activation by thyroid hormone. *Nature*, 329(6141):738-741, 1987.

171. Wight, P.A., Crew, M.D., and Spindler, S.R.: Sequences essential for activity of the thyroid hormone responsive transcription stimulatory element of the rat growth hormone gene. *Mol. Endocrinol.*, 2:536, 1988.

172. Ceccatelli, S., Giardino, L, and Calzá, L.: Response of hypothalamic peptide mRNAs to thyroidectomy. *Neuroendocrinology*, 56:694-703, 1992.

173. Brien, T.G.: The adrenocortical status of patients with thyroid disease. *Clin. Endocrinol. (Oxf.)*, 5:97-99, 1976.

174. Gallagher, T.F., Helmann, L., Finkelstein, J., et al.: Hyperthyroidism and cortisol secretion in man. *J. Clin. Endocrinol. Metab.*, 34:919-927, 1972.

175. Bigos, R., Ridgeway, E.C., Kourides, A., and Maloof, F.: Spectrum of pituitary alterations with mild and severe thyroid impairment. *J. Clin. Endocrinol. Metab.*, 2:317-325, 1978.

176. Sanchez-Franco, F., Fernandez, L., Fernandez, G., and Cacicdeo, L.: Thyroid hormone action on ACTH secretion. *Horm. Metab. Res.*, 21:550-552, 1989.

177. Hilton, J.G., Black, W.C., Athos, W., McHugh, B., and Westermann, C.D.: Increased ACTH-like activity in plasma of patients with thyrotoxicosis. *J. Clin. Endocrinol. Metab.*, 22:900-905, 1962.

178. Calogero, A.E., Gallucci, W.T., Chrousos, G.P., and Gold, P.W.: Catecholamine effects upon rat hypothalamic corticotropin-releasing hormone secretion *in vitro*. *J. Clin. In-*

vest., 82(3):839-846, 1988.

179. Koibuchi, N., Gibbs, R.B., Suzuki, M., and Pfaff, D.W.: Thyroidectomy induces Fos-like immunoreactivity within thyrotropin-releasing hormone-expressing neurons located in the paraventricular nucleus of the adult rat hypothalamus. *Endocrinology*, 129(6):3208-3216, 1991.

180. Feek, C.M., Sawers, J.S.A., Brown, N.S., Seth, J., Irvine, W.J., and Toft, A.D.: Influence of thyroid status on dopaminergic inhibition of thyrotropin and prolactin secretion: evidence for an additional feedback mechanism in the control of thyroid hormone secretion. *J. Clin. Endocrinol. Metab.*, 51(3):585-589, 1980.

181. Sasaki, A., Hanew, K., Sato, S., and Yoshinaga, K.: Evidence for endogenous dopaminergic regulation of thyrotropin (TSH) secretion in man. *Tohoku J. Exp. Med.*, 139 (1):1-7, 1983.

182. Besses, G.S., Burrow, G.N., Spaulding, S.W., and Donabedian, R.K.: Dopamine infusion acutely inhibits the TSH and prolactin response to TRH. *J. Clin. Endocrinol. Metab.*, 41:985, 1975.

183. Scanlon, M.F., Weightman, D.R., Mora, B., et al.: Evidence of dopaminergic control of thyrotropin secretion in man. *Lancet*, 2:421, 1977.

184. Brown, G.M., Burrow, G.N., and Spaulding, S.W.: Dopamine/neuroleptic receptors in the basal hypothalamus and pituitary. *Endocrinology*, 99:1407, 1976.

185. Young, W.S.: Regulation of gene expression in the hypothalamus: hybridization histochemical studies. *Ciba Foundation Symposium*, 168:127-138, 1992.

186. Kuret, J.A. and Murad, F.: Adenohypophyseal hormones and related substances. In *The Pharmacologic Basis of Therapeutics*, 8th edition. Edited by A.G. Gilman, T.W. Rall, A.S. Nies, and P. Taylor, New York, Pergamon Press, 1990, pp.1334-1360.

187. Jonassen, J.A., Mullikin-Kirkpatrick, D., McAdam, A., and Leeman, S.E.: Thyroid hormone status regulates preprotachykinin-A gene expression in male rat anterior pituitary. *Endocrinology*, 121(4):1555-1561, 1987.

188. Lam, K.S., Lechan, R.M., Minamitani, N., Segerson, T.P., and Reichlin, S.: Vasoactive intestinal peptide in the anterior pituitary is increased in hypothyroidism. *Endocrinology*, 124:1077-1084, 1989.

189. Jones, P.M., Ghatei, M.A., Wallis, S.C., and Bloom, S.R.: Differential response to neuropeptide Y, substance P, and vasoactive intestinal polypeptide in the rat anterior pituitary gland to alterations in thyroid hormone status. *J. Endocrinol.*, 143:393-397, 1994.

190. Vaerøy, H., Helle, R., Øystein, F., Kåss, E., and Terenius, L.: Elevated CSF levels of substance P and high incidence of Raynaud phenomenon in patients with fibromyalgia: new features for diagnosis. *Pain*, 32:21-26, 1988.

191. Mendelson, S.C. and Quinn, J.P.: Characterization of potential regulatory elements within the rat preprotachykinin-A promoter. *Neuroscience Letters*, 184(2):125-128, 1995.

192. Too, H.P., Marriott, D.R., and Wilkin, G.P.: Preprotachykinin-A and substance P receptor (NK1) gene expression in rat astrocytes *in vitro*. *Neuroscience Letters* 182(2):185-187, 1994.

193. Aronin, N., Coslovsky, R., and Chase, K.: Hypothyroidism increases substance P concentrations in the het-erotopic anterior pituitary. *Endocrinology*, 122(6):2911-2914, 1988.

194. Marshak, D.R. and Liu, D.T. (Editors): *Banbury Report 29: Therapeutic Peptides and Proteins: Assessing the New Technologies.* New York, Cold Spring Harbor Laboratory, 1988.

195. Jones, P.M., Ghatei, M.A., O'Halloran, D., et al.: Evidence for neuropeptide Y synthesis in the rat anterior pituitary and the influence of thyroid hormone status: comparison with vasoactive intestinal peptide, substance P, and neurotensin. *Endocrinology*, 125(1):334-341, 1989.

196. Aronin, N., Morency, K., Leeman, S.E., Braverman, L.E., and Coslovsky, R.: Regulation by thyroid hormone of the concentration of substance P in the rat anterior pituitary. *Endocrinology*, 114(6):2138-2142, 1984.

197. Savard, P., Mérand, Y., Bédard, P., Dussault, J.K., and Dupont, A.: Comparative effects of neonatal hypothyroidism and euthyroidism on TRH and substance P content of lumbar spinal cord in saline and PCPA-treated rats. *Brain Res.*, 277:263-268, 1983.

198. Dupont, A., Dussault, J-H., Rouleau, D., et al.: Effect of neonatal thyroid deficiency of the catecholamine, substance P, and thyrotropin-releasing hormone contents of discrete rat brain nuclei. *Endocrinology*, 108(6):2039-2045, 1981.

199. Hökfelt, T., Kellerth, J.O., Nilsson, G., and Pernow, B.: Experimental immunohistochemical studies on the localization and distribution of substance P in cat primary sensory neurons. *Brain Res.*, 100:135-252, 1975.

200. Hökfelt, T., Elde, R., Johansson, O., Luft, R., Nilsson, G., and Arimura, A.: Immunohistochemical evidence for separate populations of somatostatin-containing and substance P-containing primary afferent neurons in the rat. *Neurosci.*, 1:131-136, 1976.

201. Jancso, G., Hökfelt, T., Lundberg, J.M., et al.: Immunohistochemical studies of the effect of capsaicin on spinal and medullary peptide and monoamine neurons using antisera to substance P, gastrin/CCK, somatostatin, VIP, enkephaline, neurotensin, and 5-hydroxytryptamine. *J. Neurocytol.*, 10:963-980, 1981.

202. Gilbert, R.F.T., Bennet, G.W., Marsden, C.A., and Emson, P.C.: The effects of 5-hydroxytryptamine-depleting drugs on peptides in the ventral spinal cord. *Europ. J. Pharmacol.*, 76:203-210, 1981.

203. Nicoll, R.A.: Excitatory action on TRH on spinal motoneurons. *Nature* (Lond.), 265:242-243, 1977.

204. Nicoll, R.A.: The action of thyrotropin-releasing hormone, substance P, and related peptides on frog spinal motoneurons. *J. Pharmacol. Exp. Ther.*, 207:817-824, 1978.

205. Henry, J.L., Krnjevic, K., and Morris, M.E.: Excitatory effects of substance P in the spinal cord. *Fed. Proc.*, 33:548, 1974.

206. Henry, J.L., Krnjevic, K., and Morris, M.E.: Substance P in spinal neurons. *Canad. J. Physiol. Pharmacol.*, 33:423-432, 1975.

207. Henry, J.L., Sessle, B.J., Lucier, G.E., and Hu, J.W.: Effects of substance P on nociceptive and non-nociceptive trigeminal brain stem neurons. *Pain*, 8:33-45, 1980.

208. Henry, J.L.: Effects of substance P on functionally identified units in rat spinal cord. *Brain Res.*, 114:439-451, 1976.

209. Randic, M. and Miletric, V.: Effect of substance P in rat dorsal horn neurons activated by noxious stimuli. *Brain Res.*, 128:164-169, 1977.

210. Theriault, E., Otsuka, M., and Jessell, T.: Capsaicin-evoked release of substance P from primary sensory neurons. *Brain Res.*, 170:209-213, 1979.

211. Harmar, A. and Keen, P.: Chemical characterization of substance P-like immunoreactivity in primary afferent neurons. *Brain Res.*, 220:203-207, 1981.

212. Hökfelt, T., Lundberg, J., Schultzberg, M., Johansson, O., Ljungdahl, A., and Rehfeld, J.: Co-existence of peptides and putative transmitters in neurons. In *Neural Peptides and Neuronal Communications*. Edited by E. Costa and M. Trabucci, New York, Raven Press, 1980, pp.1-23.

213. Nawa, H., Kotani, H., and Nakanishi, S.: Tissue-specific generation of two preprotachykinin mRNAs from one gene by alternative splicing. *Nature*, 312:729, 1984.

214. Krause, J.E., Chirgwin, J.M., Carter, M.S., Xu, Z.S., and Hershey, A.D.: Three rat preprotachykinin mRNAs encode the neuropeptides substance P and neurokinin A. *Proc. Natl. Acad. Sci.* (USA), 84:881, 1987.

215. DePalatis, L.R., Fiorindo, R.P., and Ho, R.H.: Substance P immunoreactivity in the anterior pituitary gland of the guinea pig. *Endocrinology*, 110:282, 1982.

216. Neff, N.H. and Yang, H.-Y.T.: Another look at the monoamine oxidase and the monoamine oxidase inhibitor drugs. *Life Sci.*, 14:2061-2074, 1974.

217. Johnstoe, J.P.: Some observations upon a new inhibitor of monoamine oxidase in brain tissues. *Biochem. Pharmacol.*, 17:1285-1297, 1968.

218. Knoll, J. and Maagyar, K.: Some puzzling pharmacological effects of monoamine oxidase inhibitors. *Adv. Biochem. Psychopharmacol.*, 5:393-408, 1972.

219. Assad, M.M. and Clarke, D.E.: Modulation *in vitro* monoamine oxidase activity by thyroid hormones. *Biochem. Pharmacol.*, 27:751-756, 1978.

220. Lyles, G. and Callingham, B.A.: The effects of thyroid hormones on monoamine oxidase in the rat heart. *J. Pharm. Pharmacol.*, 25:921-930, 1974.

221. Moonat, L.B.S., Assad, M.M., and Clarke, D.E.: L-thyroxine and monoamine oxidase activity in the kidney and some other organs of the rat. *Res. Commun. Chem. Path. Pharmacol.*, 12:765-779, 1975.

222. Glover, V., Bhattachary, S.K., and Sandler, M.: Benzodiazepines reduce stress-augmented increase in rat urine monoamine oxidase inhibitor. *Nature* (Lond.), 292:347-349, 1981.

223. Ichikaw, K., Hashizume, K., and Yamad, T.: Monoamine oxidase inhibitory modulators in rat heart cytosol: evidence for induction by thyroid hormone. *Endocrinology*, 111:1803-1809, 1982.

224. Egashira, T. and Yamanaka, Y.: Changes in MAO activity in several organs of rats after administration of *l*-thyroxine. *Jap. J. Pharmacol.*, 45:135-142, 1987.

225. Zile, M. and Lardy, H.A.: Monoamine oxidase activity in liver of thyroid-fed rats. *Arch. Biochem. Biophys.*, 82:411-421, 1959.

226. Utley, H.G.: Effect of thyromimetic compounds on myocardial and hepatic monoamine oxidase activity in the rat. *Endocrinology*, 75:975-977, 1964.

227. Obata, T., Tamura, M., and Yamanaka, Y.: Thyroid hor-

mone-inducible monoamine oxidase inhibitor in rat liver cytosol. *Biochem. Pharmacol.*, 40(4):811-815, 1990.

228. Tong, J.K. and D'Iorio, A.: Differential effects of *l*-thyroxine on cardiac and hepatic monoamine oxidase activity toward benzylamine and serotonin. *Endocrinology*, 98:761-766, 1976.

229. Brucke, R. and Cohen, P.P.: Alterations in enzyme and cytochrome profiles of *Rana catesbeiana* liver organelles during thyroxine-induced metamorphosis, and cytochrome levels in response to *in vivo* thyroxine administration. *J. Biol. Chem.*, 251:6161, 1976.

230. Obata, T. and Yamanaka, Y.: Leakage of thyroid hormone-inducible monoamine oxidase inhibitor from rat liver cytosol. *Res. Commun. Chem. Path. Pharmacol.*, 68(1):65-71, 1990.

231. Lesch, K.P. and Rupprecht, R.: Psychoneuroendocrine research in depression. II. Hormonal responses to releasing hormones as a probe for hypothalamic-pituitary-end organ dysfunction. *J. Neural Transm.*, 75:179-194, 1989.

232. Terry, L.C. and Martin, J.B.: The effect of lateral hypothalamic medial forebrain stimulation and somatostatin antiserum on pulsatile growth hormone secretion in freely behaving rats: evidence for a dual regulatory mechanism. *Endocrinology*, 109:622-627, 1981.

233. Tuomisto, J. and Männisto, P.: Neurotransmitter regulation of anterior pituitary hormones. *Pharmacol. Rev.*, 37:249-332, 1985.

234. Krulich, L., Mayfield, M.A., Steele, M.K., McMillen, B.A., McCann, S.M., and Koenig, J.I.: Differential effects of pharmacological manipulations of central α_1-adrenergic and α_2-adrenergic receptors on the secretion of thyrotropin and growth hormone in male rats. *Endocrinology*, 110:796-804, 1982.

235. Krieg, R.J., Perkins, S.N., Johnson, J.K., Rogers, J.P., Aarimura, A., and Cronin, M.J.: β-Adrenergic stimulation of growth hormone (GH) release *in vivo*, and subsequent inhibition of GH-releasing factor-induced GH secretion. *Endocrinology*, 122:531-537, 1988.

236. Makela, J.P. and Hilakivi, I.T.: Evidence for the involvement of α_2-adrenoceptors in the sedation but not REM sleep inhibition by clonidine in the rat. *Med. Biol.*, 64(6):355-360, 1986.

237. Krieg, R.J., Johnson, J.K., and Adler, R.A.: Growth hormone (GH) secretion in the pituitary-grafted male rat: *in vivo* effects of GH-releasing hormone and isoproterenol and *in vitro* release by individual somatotropes. *Endocrinology*, 125:2273-2278, 1989.

238. Brameld, J.M., Weller, P.A., Saunders, J.C., Buttery, P.J., and Gilmour, R.S.: Hormonal control of insulin-like growth factor-I and growth hormone receptor mRNA expression by porcine hepatocytes in culture. *J. Endocrinology*, 146:239-245, 1995.

239. Beaufort, M.C., Rinaldi, J.P., Gandolfo, C., Plantamura, A., and Eisinger, J.: Growth hormone and fibromyalgia. Unpublished summary of study results, April 17, 1996.

240. Pinchera, A., Martino, E., and Faglia, G.: Central hypothyroidism. In *Werner and Ingbar's The Thyroid: A Fundamental and Clinical Text*, 6th edition. Edited by L.E. Braverman and R.D. Utiger, Philadelphia, J.B. Lippincott Co., 1991, pp.968-984.

241. Snyder, P.J.: The pituitary in hypothyroidism. In *Werner*

and Ingbar's The Thyroid: A Fundamental and Clinical Text, 6th edition. Edited by L.E. Braverman and R.D. Utiger, Philadelphia, J.B. Lippincott Co., 1991, pp.1040-1044.

242. Valcavi, R., Dieguez, C., Preece, M., Taylor, A., Portioli, I., and Scanlon, M.F.: Effect of thyroxine replacement therapy on plasma insulin-like growth hormone releasing factor in hypothyroid patients. *Clin. Endocrinol.,* 27:85, 1987.

243. Williams, T., Maxon, H., Thorner, M.O., and Frohman, L.A.: Blunted growth hormone (GH) response to GH-releasing hormone in hypothyroidism resolves in the euthyroid state. *J. Clin. Endocrinol. Metab.,* 61:454, 1985.

244. Tepperman, J. and Tepperman, H.M.: *Metabolic and Endocrine Physiology,* 5th edition. Chicago, Year Book Medical Publishers, Inc., 1987.

245. Tóth, S. and Csaba, B.: The effect of thyroid hormone on 5-hydroxytryptamine (5-HT) level of brain stem and blood in rabbits. *Experientia,* 22:755-756, 1966.

246. Merimee, T.J. and Grant, M.B.: Growth hormone and its disorders. In *Principles and Practice of Endocrinology and Metabolism.* Edited by K.L. Becker, J.P. Bilezinkian, W.J. Bremner, W. Hung, C.R. Kahn, D.L. Loriaux, R.W. Rebar, G.L. Robertson, and L. Wartofsky, Philadelphia, J.B. Lippincott Co., 1990, pp.125-134.

247. MacGillivary, M.H.: Disorders of growth and development. In *Endocrinology and Metabolism,* 2nd edition. Edited by P. Felig, J.D. Baxter, A. Broadus, and L.A. Frohman, New York, McGraw-Hill Book Co., 1987, pp.1581-1628.

248. Frohman, L.A.: Diseases of the anterior pituitary. In *Endocrinology and Metabolism,* 2nd edition. Edited by P. Felig, J.D. Baxter, A. Broadus, and L.A. Frohman, New York, McGraw-Hill Book Co., 1987, pp.247-337.

249. Noel, G.L., Dimond, R.C., Wartofsky, L., Earl, J.M., and Frantz, A.G.: Studies of prolactin and TSH secretion by continuous infusion of small amounts of thyrotropin-releasing hormone. *J. Clin. Endocrinol. Metab.,* 39:6, 1974.

250. Martial, J.A., Baxter, J.D., and Goodman, H.M.: Regulation of growth hormone messenger RNA by thyroid and glucocorticoid hormones. *Proc. Natl. Acad. Sci.,* 74:1816, 1977.

251. Miki, N., Ono, M., Murata, Y., et al.: Thyroid hormone regulation of gene expression of the pituitary growth hormone-releasing factor receptor. *Biochem. Biophys. Res. Comm.,* 217(3):1087-1093, 1995.

252. Hansten, P.D.: *Drug Interactions,* 5th edition. Philadelphia, Lea & Febiger, 1985.

253. Root, A.W., Bongiovanni, A.M., and Eberlein, W.R.: Inhibition of thyroidal radioiodine uptake by human growth hormone. *J. Pediatr.,* 76:422-429, 1970.

254. Seo, H., Refetoff, S., Martino, E., Vassart, G., and Brocas, H.: The differential stimulatory effect of thyroid hormone on growth hormone synthesis and estrogen on prolactin synthesis due to accumulation of specific messenger ribonucleic acid. *Endocrinology,* 104:1083, 1979.

255. Martial, J.A., Baxter, J.D., and Goodman, H.M.: Regulation of growth hormone messenger RNA by thyroid and glucocorticoid hormones. *Proc. Natl. Acad. Sci.,* 74:1816, 1977.

256. Shapiro, L.E., Samuels, H.H., and Yaffe, B.M.: Thyroid and glucocorticoid hormones synergistically control growth hormone mRNA in cultured GH-1 cells. *Proc. Natl. Acad. Sci.,* 75:45, 1978.

257. Buchwald, D., Umali, J., and Stene, M.: Insulin-like growth factor-I (somatomedin C) levels in chronic fatigue syndrome and fibromyalgia. *J. Rheumatol.,* 23:739-742, 1996.

258. Westermark, K., Alm, J., Skottner, A., and Karlsson, A.: Growth factors and the thyroid: effects of treatment for hyper- and hypothyroidism on serum IGF-I and urinary epidermal growth factor concentrations. *Acta Endocrinologica* (Copenh), 118:415-421, 1988.

259. Rodriquez-Arnao, J., Miell, J.P., and Ross, R.J.M.: Influence of thyroid hormones on the GH-IGF-I axis. *Trends in Endocrinology and Metabolism,* 4:169-173, 1993.

260. Ikeda, T., Fujiyama, K., Hoshino, T., et al.: Stimulating effect of thyroid hormone on insulin-like growth factor-I release and synthesis by perfused rat liver. *Growth Regulation,* 1:39-41, 1991.

261. Latimer, A.M., Hausman, G.J., McCusker, R.H., and Buonomo, F.C.: The effects of thyroxine on serum and tissue concentrations of insulin-like growth factors (IGF-I and -II) and IGF-binding proteins in the fetal pig. *Endocrinology,* 133:1312-1319, 1993.

262. Freyschuss, B., Sahlin, L., Masironi, B., and Eridsson, H.: The hormonal regulation of the oestrogen receptor in rat liver: an interplay involving growth hormone, thyroid hormones, and glucocorticoids. *J. Endocrinology,* 142:285-298, 1994.

263. Samuels, H.H., Forman, B.M., Horowitz, Z.D., and Ye, Z-S.: Regulation of gene expression by thyroid hormone. *Annu. Rev. Physiol.,* 51:623-639, 1989.

264. Axelrod, J.: Methylation reactions in the formation and metabolism of catecholamines and other biogenic amines: the enzymatic conversion of norepinephrine (NE) to epinephrine (E). *Pharmacol. Rev.,* 18:95-113, 1966.

265. Strait, K.A., Schwartz, H.L., Perez-Castillo, A., and Oppenheimer, J.K.: Relationship of c-*erb*A mRNA content to tissue triiodothyronine nuclear binding capacity and function in developing and adult rats. *J. Biol. Chem.,* 265:10514-10521, 1990.

266. Weinberger, C., Thompson, C.C., Ong, E.S., Lebo, R., Gruol, D.J., and Evans, R.M.: The c-*erb*A gene encodes a thyroid hormone receptor. *Nature,* 324:641-646, 1986.

267. Ruel, J., Faure, R., and Dussault, J.K.: Regional distribution of nuclear T3 receptors in the rat brain and evidence for preferential localization in neurons. *J. Endocrinol. Invest.,* 8:343-348, 1985.

268. Ford, D.H. and Gross, J.: The metabolism of ^{131}I-labeled thyroid hormones in the hypophysis and brain of the rabbit. *Endocrinology,* 62:416-436, 1958.

269. Bradley, D.J., Young, W.S., III, and Weinberger, C.: Differential expression of α and β thyroid hormone receptor genes in rat brain and pituitary. *Proc. Natl. Acad. Sci.* (USA), 86:7250-7254, 1989.

270. Mellström, B., Narano, J.R., Santos, A., Gonzales, A.M., and Bernal, J.: Independent expression of the α and β c-*erb*A genes in developing rat brain. *Mol. Endocrinol.,* 5:1339-1350, 1991.

271. Andersson, K. and Eneroth, P.: Thyroidectomy and central

catecholamine neurons of the male rat. *Neuroendocrinology*, 45:14-27, 1987.

272. Harris, P.E., Dieguez, C., Lewis, B.M., Hall, R., and Scanlon, M.F.: Effects of thyroid status on brain catecholamine biosynthesis in adult rats: assessment by a steady-state method. *J. Endocrinol.*, 111(3):383-389, 1986.

273. Ericksson, E. and Modigh, K.: Depression, α_2-receptors, and sex hormones: neuroendocrine studies in the rat. In *Frontiers in Biochemical and Pharmacological Research in Depression.* Edited by E. Usdin, M. Äsberg, L. Bertilsson, and F. Sjögvist, New York, Raven Press, 1984, pp.161-178.

274. Niewenhuys, R., Geeraedts, L.M.G., and Veening, J.G.: The medial forebrain bundle of the rat. I. General introduction. *J. Comp. Neurol.*, 206:49-81, 1982.

275. Swanson, L.W., Sawchenko, P.E., and Lind, R.W.: Regulation of multiple peptides in CRF parvocellular neurosecretory neurons: implications for the stress response. *Prog. in Brain Res.*, 68:169-190, 1986.

276. Jaffer, A., Daniels, W.M.U., Russell, V.A., and Taljaard, J.J.F.: Effects of α_2- and β-adrenoceptor agonists on growth hormone secretion following lesion of the noradrenergic system of the rat. *Neurochem. Res.*, 17(12):1255-1260, 1992.

277. Jonsson, G., Hallman, H., Ponzio, F., and Ross, S.: DSP$_4$ N-(2-chloroethyl)-N-ethyl-2-bromobenzylamine: a useful denervation tool for central and peripheral noradrenaline neurons. *Eur. J. Pharmacol.*, 72:173-188, 1981.

278. Lookingland, K.J., Chapin, D.S., McKay, D.W., and Moore, K.E.: Comparative effects of the neurotoxin N-chloroethyl-N-2-bromobenzylamine hydrochloride (DSP$_4$) and 6-hydroxy-dopamine on hypothalamic noradrenergic, dopamine, and 5-hydroxytryptaminergic neurons in the male rat. *Brain Res.*, 365:228-234, 1986.

279. Willoughby, J.O. and Day, T.A.: Central catecholamine depletion: effects on physiological growth hormone and prolactin secretion. *Neuroendocrinology*, 32:65-69, 1981.

280. Brown, D.A. and Caulfield, M.P.: Hyperpolarizing α_2-adrenoceptors in rat sympathetic ganglia. *Br. J. Pharmacol.*, 65:435-445, 1979.

281. Bluet-Pajot, M.T., Schaub, C., and Nasiet, J.: Growth hormone response to hypoglycemia under gamma-hydroxybutyrate narcoanalgesia in the rat. *Neuroendocrinology*, 26:141-149, 1978.

282. Bluet-Pajot, M.T., Durand, D., Mounier, F., Schaub, C., and Kordon, C.: Interaction of β-adrenergic agonists and antagonists with the stimulation of growth hormone release induced by clonidine or by morphine in the rat. *J. Endocrinol.*, 94:327-331, 1982.

283. Iglesias, T., Caubin, J., Zaballow, A., Bernal, J., and Muñoz, A.: Identification of the mitochondrial NADH dehydrogenase subunit 3 (ND3) as a thyroid hormone regulated gene by whole gene PCR analysis. *Biochem. Biophys. Res. Comm.*, 210(3):995-1000, 1995.

284. Brent, G.A.: The molecular basis of thyroid hormone action. *New Engl. J. Med.*, 331(13):847-853, 1994.

285. Lazar, M.A.: Thyroid hormone receptors: multiple forms, multiple possibilities. *Endocr. Rev.*, 14(2):184-193, 1993.

286. Yen, P.M. and Chin, W.W.: *Trends Endocrinol. Metab.*, 5:65-72, 1994.

287. Iñiguez, M.A., Rodriguez-Peña, A., Ibarrola, N., Morreale de Escobar, G., and Bernal, J.: Adult rat brain is sensitive to thyroid hormone. Regulation of RC3/neurogranin mRNA. *J. Clin. Invest.*, 90(2):554-558, 1992.

288. Sterling, K., Lazarus, J.K., Milch, P.O., Sakurada, T., and Brenner, M.A.: Mitochondrial thyroid hormone receptor: localization and physiological significance. *Science*, 201 (4361):1126-1129, 1978.

289. Sterling, K., Brenner, M.A., and Sakurada, T.: Rapid effect of triiodothyronine on the mitochondrial pathway in rat liver *in vivo*. *Science*, 210(4467):340-342, 1980.

290. Ardail, D., Lerme, F., Puymirat, J., and Morel, G.: Evidence for the presence of alpha and beta-related T$_3$ receptors in rat liver mitochondria. *Eur. J. Cell Biol.*, 62(1):105-113, 1993.

291. Mutvei, A., Kuzela, S., and Nelson, B.D.: Control of mitochondrial transcription by thyroid hormone. *Eur. J. Biochem.*, 180(1):235-240, 1989.

292. Van Itallie, C.M.: Thyroid hormone and dexamethasone increase the levels of a messenger ribonucleic acid for a mitochondrially-encoded subunit but not for a nuclear-encoded subunit of cytochrome-c oxidase. *Endocrinology*, 127(1):55-62, 1990.

293. Wiesner, R.J., Kurowski, T.T., and Zak, R.: Regulation by thyroid hormone of nuclear and mitochondrial genes encoding subunits of cytochrome-c oxidase in rat liver and skeletal muscle. *Mol. Endocrinol.*, 6(9):1458-1467, 1992.

294. Luciakova, K. and Nelson, B.D.: Transcript levels for nuclear-encoded mammalian mitochondrial respiratory chain components are regulated by thyroid hormone in an uncoordinated fashion. *Eur. J. Biochem.*, 207(1):247-251, 1992.

295. Virtanen, R., Savola, J.-M., Saano, V., and Nyman, L.: Characterization of the selectivity, specificity, and potency of medetomidine as an α_2-adrenoceptor agonist. *Eur. J. Pharmac.*, 150:9-14, 1988.

296. Savola, J.-M. and Virtanen, R.: Central α_2-adrenoceptors are highly stereoselective for dexmedetomidine. *Eur. J. Pharmac.*, 195:193-199, 1991.

297. Stenberg, D., Salven, P., and Miettinen, M.V.J.: Sedative action of the α_2-agonist medetomidine in cats. *J. Vet. Pharmac. Ther.*, 10:319-323, 1987.

298. Aransten, A.F. and Leslie, F.M.: Behavioral and receptor binding analysis of the α_2-adrenergic agonist, 5-bromo-6 [2-imidazoline-2-YL amino] quinoxaline (UK-14304): evidence for cognitive enhancement at an α_2-adrenoceptor subtype. *Neuropharmacology*, 30:1279-1289, 1991.

299. Scheinin, H., MacDonald, E., and Scheinin, M.: Behavioural and neurochemical effects of atipamezole, a novel α_2-adrenoceptor antagonist. *Eur. J. Pharmac.*, 157:35-42, 1988.

300. Flavahan, N.A.: The role of vascular α_2-adrenoceptors as cutaneous thermosensors. *News Physiol. Sci.*, 6:251-255, 1991.

301. Pertovaara, A.: Antinociception induced by α_2-adrenoceptor agonists, with special emphasis on medetomidine studies. *Prog. Neurobiol.*, 40:691-709, 1993.

302. Archer, T., Arwestrem, E., Jonsson, G., Minor, G., and Post, C.: Noradrenergic-serotonergic interactions and nociception in the rat. *Eur. J. Pharmac.*, 120:295-307, 1986.

303. Nakagawa, I., Omote, K., Kitahata, L.M., Collins, J.G., and Murata, K.: Serotonergic mediation of spinal analges-

ia and its interaction with noradrenergic systems. *Anesthesiology*, 73:474-478, 1990.

304. Danzebrink, R.M. and Gebhart, G.F.: Intrathecal coadministration of clonidine with serotonin receptor agonists produces supra-additive visceral antinociception in the rat. *Brain Res.*, 555:35-42, 1991.

305. Gordh, T., Jansson, I., Hartvig, P., Gillberg, P.G., and Post, C.: Interactions between noradrenergic and cholinergic mechanisms involved in spinal nociceptive processing. *Acta Anaesthesiol. Scand.*, 33:39-47, 1989.

306. Levitt, M., Spector, S., Sjoerdsma, A., and Udenfriend, S.: *J. Pharmacol. Exp. Ther.*, 148:1-8, 1965.

307. Diarra, A., Lefauconnier, J.M., Valens, M., Georges, P., and Gripois, D.: Tyrosine content, influx, and accumulation rate, and catecholamine biosynthesis measured *in vivo*, in the central nervous system and in peripheral organs of young rats: influence of neonatal hypo- and hyperthyroidism. *Arch. Intern. de Physiologie et de Biochem.*, 97:317-332, 1989.

308. Kizer, J.S., Palkovits, M., Zivin, J., Brownstein, M. Saavedra, J.M., and Kopin, I.J.: The effect of endocrinological manipulations on tyrosine hydroxylase and dopamine-beta-hydroxylase activities in individual hypothalamic nuclei of the adult male rat. *Endocrinology*, 95(3):799-812, 1974.

309. Nakahara, T., Uchimura, H., Hirano, M., Saito, M., and Ito, M.: Effects of gonadectomy and thyroidectomy on the tyrosine hydroxylase activity in individual hypothalamic nuclei and lower brain stem catecholaminergic cell groups of the rat. *Brain Res.*, 117(2):351-356, 1976.

310. Ismail-Beigi, F. and Edelman, I.S.: The mechanism of the calorigenic action of thyroid hormone: stimulation of Na$^+$/K$^+$-activated adenosinetriphosphatase activity. *J. Gen. Physiol.*, 57:710-722, 1971.

311. Back, D.W., Wilson, S.B., Morris, S.M., Jr., and Goodridge, A.G.: Hormonal regulation of lipogenic enzymes in chick embryo hepatocytes in culture. Thyroid hormone and glucagon regulate malic enzyme mRNA level at post-transcriptional steps. *J. Biol. Chem.*, 261(27):12555-12561, 1986.

312. Eisinger, J., Dupond, J.L., and Cozzone, P.J.: Anomalies de la glycolyse au cours des fibromyalgies: étude biologique et thérapeutique. *Lyon Méditerranée Méd.*, 32:35-39, 1996.

313. Lau, C. and Slotkin, T.A.: Maturation of sympathetic neurotransmission in the rat heart. VIII. Slowed development of noradrenergic synapses resulting from hypothyroidism. *J. Pharmacol. Exp. Ther.*, 220(3):629-636, 1982.

314. Gripois, D., Klein, C., and Valens, M.: Tyrosine hydroxylase activity and catecholamine content in the adrenals of young hypo- and hyperthyroid rats. *Biol. Neonate*, 37(3-4):165-171, 1980.

315. Oldendorf, W.H. and Szabo, J.: Amino acid assignment to one of three blood-brain barrier amino acid carriers. *Amer. J. Physiol.*, 230(1):94-98, 1976.

316. Bertler, A., Falck, B., Owman, C., and Rosengrenn, E.: The localization of monoaminergic blood-brain barrier mechanisms. *Pharmacol. Rev.*, 18(1):369-385, 1966.

317. Reese, T.S. and Karnovsky, M.J.: Fine structural localization of a blood-brain barrier to exogenous peroxidase. *J. Cell Biol.*, 34(1):207-217, 1967.

318. Eayrs, J.T.: *J. Anat.*, 88:164-173, 1954.

319. David, S. and Nathaniel, E.J.: Development of brain capillaries in euthyroid and hypothyroid rats. *Exp. Neurol.*, 73(1):243-253, 1981.

320. Guidotti, G.G., Borghetti, A.F., and Gazzola, G.C.: The regulation of amino acid transport in animal cells. (Review) *Biochim. Biophys. Acta*, 515(4):329-366, 1978.

321. Shotwell, M.A., Kilberg, M.S., and Oxender, D.L.: The regulation of neutral amino acid transport in mammalian cells. (Review) *Biochim. Biophys. Acta*, 737(2):267-284, 1983.

322. Riggs, T.R., Pote, K.G., Im, H.S., and Huff, D.W.: Developmental changes in the neutral alpha-amino acid transport systems of rat brain over the first three weeks after birth. *J. Neurochem.*, 42(5):1251-1259, 1984.

323. Lefauconnier, J.M., Lacombe, P., and Bernard, G.: Cerebral blood flow and blood-brain influx of some neutral amino acids in control and hypothyroid 16-day-old rats. *J. Cereb. Blood Flow Metab.*, 5(2):318-326, 1985.

324. Daniel, P.M., Love, E.R., and Pratt, O.E.: Hypothyroidism and amino acid entry into brain and muscle. (Letter) *Lancet*, 2(7940):872, 1975.

325. Coupland, R.E.: *The Natural History of the Chromaffin Cell*. London, Longmans, 1965.

326. Wade, L.A. and Katzman, R.: Synthetic amino acids and the nature of L-DOPA transport at the blood-brain barrier. *J. Neurochem.*, 25(6):837-842, 1975.

327. Rastogi, R.B., Lapierre, Y., and Singhal, R.L.: Evidence for the role of brain biogenic amines in depressed motor activity seen in chemically thyroidectomized rats. *J. Neurochem.*, 26(3):443-449, 1976.

328. Heffner, T.G. and Seiden, L.S.: Synthesis of catecholamines from [3H] tyrosine in brain during the performance of operant behavior. *Brain Res.*, 183(2):403-419, 1980.

329. Plaznik, A. and Kostowski, W.: The interrelationship between brain noradrenergic and dopaminergic neuronal systems in regulating animal behavior: possible clinical implications. (Review) *Psychopharmacol. Bull.*, 19(1):5-11, 1983.

330. Bertler, A. and Rosengren, E.: *Experientia*, 15:10-11, 1959.

331. Clinescmidt, B.V., Flataker, L.M., Faison, E., and Holmes, R.: An *in vivo* model for investigating α_1-and α_2-receptors in the CNS: studies with mianserin. *Arch. Int. Pharmacodyn. Ther.*, 242:59-76, 1979.

332. Delini-Stula, A., Baumann, P., and Buch, O.: Depression of exploratory activity by clonidine in rats as a model for the detection of relative pre- and postsynaptic central noradrenergic receptor selectivity of α-adrenolytic drugs. *Naunyn-Schmiedeberg's Arch. Pharmacol.*, 307:115-122, 1979.

333. Drew, G.M., Gower, A.J., and Marriott, A.S.: α_2-Adrenoceptors mediate clonidine-induced sedation in the rat. *Br. J. Pharmacol.*, 67:133-141, 1979.

334. Mueller, K. and Nyhan, W.I.: Modulation of the behavioral effects of amphetamine in rats by clonidine. *Eur. J. Pharmacol.*, 83:339-342, 1982.

335. Pifl, Ch.F. and Hornykiewicz, O.: α-Noradrenergic involvement in locomotor activity. *Naunyn-Schmiedeberg's Arch. Pharmacol.*, 330(Suppl.):R71, 1985.

336. Creese, I. and Iversen, S.D.: The pharmacological and an-

atomical substrates of the amphetamine response in the rat. *Brain Res.*, 83:419-436, 1975.

337. Jackson, D.M., Anden, N.-E., and Dahlstrom, A.: A functional effect of dopamine in the nucleus accumbens and in some other dopamine-rich parts of the rat brain. *Psychopharmacology*, 45:139-149, 1975.

338. Kelly, P.H., Seviour, P.W., and Iversen, S.D.: Amphetamine and apomorphine responses in the rat following 6-OHDA lesions of the nucleus accumbens septi and corpus striatum. *Brain Res.*, 94:507,1975.

339. Pijnenburg, A.J.J., Honig, W.M.M., and Van Rossum, J.M.: Effects of antagonists upon locomotor stimulation induced by injection of dopamine and noradrenaline into the nucleus accumbens of nialamide-pretreated rats. *Psychopharmacology*, 41:175-180, 1975.

340. Costall, B., Marsden, C.D., Maylor, R.J., and Pycock, C.J.: Stereotyped behavior patterns and hyperactivity induced by amphetamine and apomorphine after discrete 6-hydroxydopamine lesions of extrapyramidal and mesolimbic nuclei. *Brain Res.*, 123:89-111, 1977.

341. Makanjuola, R.O.A., Dow, R.C., and Ashcroft, G.W.: Behavioural responses to stereotactically controlled injections of monoamine neurotransmitters into the accumbens and caudate-putamen nuclei. *Psychopharmacology*, 71: 227-235, 1980.

342. Dickinson, S.L., Gadie, B., and Tulloch, I.F.: α_1- and α_2-Adrenoreceptor antagonists differentially influence locomotor and stereotyped behaviour induced by *d*-amphetamine and apomorphine in the rat. *Psychopharmacology*, 96:521-527, 1988.

343. Stouffer, J.E., Armstrong, K.J., Inwegen, R.V., Thompson, W.J., and Robison, G.A.: *Program of the Endocrine Society*, 1974, p.A-122.

344. Kopin, I.J.: Metabolic degradation of catecholamines, the relative importance of different pathways under physiological conditions and after administration of drugs. In *Catecholamines: Handbuch der Experimentellen Pharmakologie*, Vol. 33. Edited by H. Blaschko and E. Muscholl, Berlin, Springer-Verlag, 1972, pp.271-282.

345. Eisinger, J., Geoffroy, M., Plantamura, A., Zakarian, H., and Ayavou, T.: Energy metabolism, antioxidant status, and myalgias: II. Fibromyalgia. *Lyon Méditerranée Méd.*, 32:2171-2174, 1996.

346. Eisinger, J.: Personal written communication, April 17, 1996.

347. Eisinger, J., Arroyo, P., Calendini, C., Rinaldi, J.P., Combes, R., and Fontaine, G.: Anomalies biologiques au cours des fibromyalgies. III. Explorations endocriniennes. *Lyon Méditerranée Méd.*, 28(5/6):858-860, 1992.

348. Coulombe, P., Dussult, J.K., Letarte, J., and Simard, S.J.: Catecholamine metabolism in thyroid disease. I. Epinephrine secretion rate in hyperthyroidism and hypothyroidism. *J. Clin. Endocrinol. Metab.*, 42:125, 1976.

349. Coulombe, P., Dussault, J.K., and Walker, P.: Plasma catecholamine concentration in hyperthyroidism and hypothyroidism. *Metabolism*, 25:973, 1976.

350. Coulombe, P., Dussault, J.K., and Walker, P.: Catecholamine metabolism in thyroid disease. II. Norepinephrine secretion rate in hyperthyroidism and hypothyroidism. *J. Clin. Endocrinol. Metab.*, 44:1185, 1977.

351. Polikar, R., Kennedy, B., Ziegler, M., et al.: Plasma norepinephrine kinetics, dopamine-β-hydroxylase, and chromgranin-A, in hypothyroid patients before and following replacement therapy. *J. Clin. Endocrinol. Metab.*, 70:277, 1990.

352. Wang, P.S., Gonzales, H.A., Reymond, M.J., and Porter, J.C.L.: Mass and in situ molar activity of tyrosine hydroxylase in the median eminence. *Neuroendocrinology*, 49: 659-663, 1989.

353. de Lonlay, A., Blouquit, M.F., Valens, M., Chami, N., Edwards, D.A., and Gripois, D.: Tyrosine hydroxylase and dopamine β-hydroxylase inductions evoked by reserpine in the superior cervical ganglion of developing eu- and hypothyroid rats. *J. Autonomic Nerv. Syst.*, 36(1):33-38, 1991.

354. Cahill, A.L. and Perlman, R.L.: Phosphorylation of tyrosine hydroxylase in the superior cervical ganglion. *Biochim. Biophys. Acta*, 805:217-226, 1984.

355. Reymond, M.J., Speciale, S.G., and Porter, J.C.: Dopamine in plasma of lateral and medial hypophysial portal vessels: evidence for regional variation in the release of hypothalamic dopamine into hypophyseal portal blood. *Endocrinology*, 112:1958-1963, 1983.

356. Black, I.B.: The role of the thyroid in the growth and development of adrenergic neurons *in vivo*. *Neurology*, 24: 377, 1974.

357. Draves, D.J. and Timiras, P.S.: Thyroid hormone effects in neural (tumor) cell culture: differential effects on triiodothyronine nuclear receptors, Na⁺-K⁺-ATPase activity and intracellular electrolyte levels. In *Tissue Culture in Neurobiology*. Edited by E. Giacobini, A. Vernadakis, and A. Shahar, New York, Raven Press, 1980, pp.291-301.

358. Valcana, T. and Timiras, P.S.: Nuclear triiodothyronine receptors in the developing rat brain. *Mol. Cell. Endocrinol.*, 11:31-41, 1978.

359. Samuels, H.H., Stanley, F., and Shapiro, L.E.: Modulation of thyroid hormone nuclear receptor levels by 3,5,3'-triiodo-L-thyronine in GH₁ cells. *J. Biol. Chem.*, 252:6052-6060, 1977.

360. Samuels, H.H., Stanley, F., Casanova, J., and Shao, T.C.: Thyroid hormone receptor levels are influenced by the acetylation of chromatin associated proteins. *J. Biol. Chem.*, 255:2499-2508, 1980.

361. Rastogi, R.B. and Singhal, R.L.: The effect of thyroid hormone on serotonergic neurons: depletion of serotonin in discrete brain areas of developing hypothyroid rats. *Naunyn-Schmiedeberg's Arch. Pharmacol.*, 304(1):9-13,1978.

362. Mason, M., Mackin, J.L., Harrison, G.G., and Seubert, S.A.: *Nutrition and the Cell: The Inside Story*. Chicago, Year Book Medical Publishers, Inc., 1973.

363. Beisel, W.R.: *Fed. Proc.*, 39:3105, 1982.

364. Axelrod, A.E.: Immune processes in vitamin deficiency states. *Am. J. Clin. Nutr.*, 24(2):265-271, 1971.

365. Beisel, W.R.: Nutrition and infection. In *Nutritional Biochemistry and Metabolism: with Clinical Applications*, 2nd edition. Edited by M.C. Linder, New York, Elsevier, pp.507-542.

366. Linder, M.C.: Nutrition and metabolism of vitamins. In *Nutritional Biochemistry and Metabolism: with Clinical Applications*, 2nd edition. Edited by M.C. Linder, New York, Elsevier, pp.111-189.

367. Eisinger, J., Plantamura, A., and Ayavou, T.: Glycolysis

abnormalities in fibromyalgia. *J. Amer. Coll. Nutr.*, 13: 144-148, 1994.

368. Lefkowitz, R.J., Hoffman, B.B., and Taylor, P.: Neurohormonal transmission: the autonomic and somatic motor nervous systems. In *The Pharmacologic Basis of Therapeutics*, 8th edition. Edited by A.G. Gilman, T.W. Rall, A.S. Nies, and P. Taylor, New York, Pergamon Press, 1990, pp.84-121.

369. Mongeau, R., de Montigny, C., and Blier, P.: Electrophysiologic evidence for desensitization of α₂-adrenoceptors on serotonin terminals following long-term treatment with drugs increasing norepinephrine synaptic concentration. *Neuropsychopharmacology*, 10(1):41-51, 1994.

370. Rastogi, R.B. and Singhal, R.L.: Neonatal hypothyroidism: alteration in behavioral activity and metabolism of brain norepinephrine and dopamine. *Life Sci.*, 18:851-858, 1976.

371. Mooradin, A.D.: Metabolic fuel and amino acid transport into the brain in experimental hypothyroidism. *Acta Endocrinologica* (Copenh.), 122(2):156-162, 1990.

372. Ito, J.M., Valcana, T., and Timiras, P.S.: Effect of hypo- and hyperthyroidism on regional monoamine metabolism in the adult rat brain. *Neuroendocrinology*, 24:55-64, 1977.

373. Mongeau, R., de Montigny, C., and Blier, P.: Effects of long-term α₂ adrenergic antagonists and electroconvulsive treatments on the α₂-adrenoceptors modulating serotonin neurotransmission. *J. Pharmacol. Exp. Ther.*, 269(3): 1152-1159, 1994.

374. Kakahara, T., Uchimura, H., Hirano, M., Saito, M., and Ito, M.: Effects of gonadectomy and thyroidectomy on tyrosine hydroxylase activity in individual hypothalamic nuclei and lower brain stem catecholaminergic cell groups in the rat. *Brain Res.*, 117:351-356, 1976.

375. Schwark, W.W. and Keesey, R.R.: Cretinism: influence on rate limiting enzymes of amine synthesis in rat brain. *Life Sci.*, 19:1699-1704, 1976.

376. Vaccari, A., Valcana, T., and Timiras, P.S.: Effects of hypothyroidism on the enzymes for biogenic amines in the developing rat brain. *Pharmacol. Res. Commun.*, 9:763-780, 1977.

377. Rastogi, R.B. and Singhal, R.L.: Alterations in norepinephrine and tyrosine hydroxylase activity during experimental hypothyroidism in rats. *Brain Res.*, 81:253-266, 1974.

378. Katsurada, A., Iritani, N., Fukuda, H., Noguchi, T., and Tanaka, T.: Transcriptional and posttranscriptional regulation of malic enzyme synthesis by insulin and triiodothyronine. *Biochim. Biophys. Acta*, 950:113-117, 1988.

379. Safaei, R. and Timiras, P.S.: Thyroid hormone binding and regulation of adrenergic enzymes in two neuroblastoma cell lines. *J. Neurochem.*, 45(5):1405-1410, 1985.

380. Hoffman, B.B. and Lefkowitz, R.J.: Catecholamines and sympathomimetic drugs. In *The Pharmacologic Basis of Therapeutics*, 8th edition. Edited by A.G. Gilman, T.W. Rall, A.S. Nies, and P. Taylor, New York, Pergamon Press, 1990, pp.187-220.

381. Russell, I.J., Vipraio, G.A., Morgan, W.W., and Bowden, C.L.: Is there a metabolic basis for the fibrositis syndrome? *Am. J. Med.*, 81(3A):50-56, 1986.

382. Tilbe, K., Bell, D.A., and McCain, G.A.: Loss of diurnal variation in serum cortisol, growth hormone, and prolactin in patients with primary fibromyalgia. *Arthritis Rheum.*, 31:4, 1988.

383. Bennett, R.M., Clark, S.R., Burckhardt, C.S., and Cook, D.: IGF-1 assays and other GH tests in 500 fibromyalgia patients. (Abstract) *J. Musculoskel. Pain*, 3(Suppl.1):109, 1995.

384. Bennett, R.M., Clark, S.R., Burckhardt, C.S., and Walczyk, J.: A double-blind placebo controlled study of growth hormone therapy in fibromyalgia. (Abstract) *J. Musculoskel. Pain*, 3(Suppl.1):110, 1995.

385. Stratz, T., Schochat, T., Faber, L., Schweiger, C., and Müller, W.: Are there subgroups in fibromyalgia? (Abstract) *J. Musculoskel. Pain*, 3(Suppl.1):110, 1995.

386. Bennett, R.M., Clark, S.R., Campbell, S.M., and Burckhardt, C.S.: Low levels of somatomedin C in patients with the fibromyalgia syndrome: a possible link between sleep and muscle pain. *Arthritis Rheum.*, 35:1113-1116, 1992.

387. Nørregaard, J., Bülow, P.M., Volkman, H., Mehlsen, J., and Samsøe, B.D.: Somatomedin-C and procollagen aminoterminal peptide in fibromyalgia. *J. Musculoskel. Pain*, 3(4):33-40, 1995.

388. Hynes, R.C.: Adrenocorticotropic hormone: adrenocortical steroids and their synthetic analogs: inhibitors of the synthesis and actions of adrenocortical hormones. In *The Pharmacologic Basis of Therapeutics*, 8th edition. Edited by A.G. Gilman, T.W. Rall, A.S. Nies, and P. Taylor, New York, Pergamon Press, 1990, pp.1431-1462.

389. Baldessarini, R.J.: Treatment of depression by altering monoamine metabolism: precursors and metabolic inhibitors. *Psychopharmacol. Bull.*, 20:224-239, 1984.

390. Baldessarini, R.J.: Drugs and the treatment of psychiatric disorders. In *The Pharmacologic Basis of Therapeutics*, 8th edition. Edited by A.G. Gilman, T.W. Rall, A.S. Nies, and P. Taylor, New York, Pergamon Press, 1990, pp.383-435.

391. Karhunen, T., Tilgmann, C., Ulmanen, I., Julkunen, I., and Panula, P.: Distribution of catechol-*O*-methyltransferase enzyme in rat tissues. *J. Histochem. Cytochem.*, 42(8): 1079-1090, 1994.

392. Gripois, D., Klein, C., and Valens, M.: Influence of hypo- and hyperthyroidism on noradrenaline metabolism in brown adipose tissue of the developing rat. *Biol. Neonate*, 37(1-2):53-59, 1980.

393. Coulombe, P., Dussault, J.K., Lescault, A., and Walker, P.: Red blood cells catechol-*O*-methyl-transferase activity in thyroid dysfunction. *Canad. J. Physiol. Pharmacol.*, 55 (3):444-447, 1977.

394. Wills, C.: *Exons, Introns, and Talking Genes*. New York, Basic Books, 1991.

395. Marks, D.B.: *Biochemistry*. Baltimore, Williams & Wilkins, 1990.

396. Tkachenko, N.N., Potin, V.V., Beskrovnyi, S.V., and Nosova, L.G.: Hypothyroidism and hyperprolactinemia. *Akush. Ginekol.*, 10:40-43, 1989.

397. Baldessarini, R.J.: *Chemotherapy in Psychiatry: Principles and Practice*, 2nd edition. Cambridge, Harvard University Press, 1985.

398. Levine, M.A., Feldman, A.M., Robishaw, J.D., et al.: Influence of thyroid hormone status on expression of genes encoding G protein subunits in the rat heart. *J. Biol.*

Chem., 265(6):3553-3560, 1990.

399. Ewart, H.S. and Klip, A.: Hormonal regulation of the Na⁺/K⁺-ATPase: mechanisms underlying rapid and sustained changes in pump activity. *Am. J. Physiol.*, 269(Cell Physiol.38):C295-C311, 1995.

2.4

Thyroid Hormone Deficiency

The incidence of primary and especially central hypothyroidism among fibromyalgia patients far exceeds that in the general population. This chapter describes the different classifications of primary and central hypothyroidism, an overview of the various causes of each, and a survey of factors that may cause disruption of the thyroid system at multiple sites.

Much confusion in the thyroidology literature results from writers misusing two terms. They use the term hypothyroidism when referring to tissue hypometabolism and the term hyperthyroidism when referring to tissue thyrotoxicity. The terms hypothyroidism and hyperthyroidism refer respectively to thyroid hormone deficiency and excess due specifically to abnormal thyroid gland function. The terms tissue hypometabolism and hypermetabolism (or thyrotoxicity) refer to inadequate or excessive tissue stimulation by thyroid hormone.

Many patients' fibromyalgia symptoms are merely manifestations of hypothyroidism. When a patient has fibromyalgia symptoms, the clinician should suspect that hypothyroidism may be the underlying cause. Suspicion should be heightened if the clinician learns through a patient's history or examination that factors or conditions that are known to induce hypothyroidism are relevant to her case.

The factors and conditions included in this chapter are not exhaustive, but they are sufficient for the purposes of most clinicians who care for hypothyroid fibromyalgia patients. Nine factors are included that

may cause primary hypothyroidism by adversely affecting the function of the thyroid gland. These factors are autoimmune thyroid diseases, silent and subacute thyroiditis, antithyroid treatments, iodine deficiency or excess, use of lithium, thyroid gland trauma, use of bromide, growth hormone injections, and viral infections. Five factors are included that may induce central hypothyroidism by adversely affecting the hypothalamus or the pituitary gland. These factors are accidental and surgical trauma, radiotherapy, use of tricyclic and monoamine oxidase inhibiting antidepressants, use of exogenous dopamine, and excessive influence of endogenous adenosine. Factors that can disrupt the thyroid system at more than one site are also included: elevated glucocorticoids, chemical contaminants, and hemochromatosis.

To avoid confusion, it is critical to bear in mind that the terms hypothyroidism and hyperthyroidism refer to abnormalities in circulating levels of thyroid hormones *due to abnormal function of the thyroid gland itself.* Hypothyroidism is not synonymous with tissue hypometabolism, and hyperthyroidism is not synonymous with thyrotoxicosis. Hypo- and hyperthyroidism refer *solely* to thyroid hormone blood levels due to decreased and increased thyroid gland production.[104]

Hypothyroidism is the most common disorder related to thyroid hormones. It may result from any of a number of structural or functional abnormalities, all of which result in deficiency of circulating thyroid hormones. *Primary* or *thyroidal hypothyroidism* is decreased synthesis and secretion of thyroid hormones due to a disorder of the thyroid gland. *Central hypothyroidism* (also called *hypothyrotropic hypothyroidism*) is decreased thyroid gland synthesis and secretion of thyroid hormones because of decreased thyroid gland stimulation by thyroid stimulating hormone (TSH, or thyrotropin). Decreased TSH stimulation of an intrinsically normal gland may result from deficient synthesis or secretion of TSH by the anterior pituitary gland. In this case, the terms *pituitary hypothyroidism* or *secondary hypothyroidism* are appropriate. Deficient TSH secretion may also result from insufficient stimulation of the anterior pituitary gland because of a deficiency of the hypothalamic hormone, thyrotropin-releasing hormone (TRH). In this case, the terms *hypothalamic hypothyroidism* or *tertiary hypothyroidism* are proper.[235,p.919][236,pp.508-509][240,p.475]

In general, patients who abruptly develop hypothyroidism have more symptoms of worse severity than patients who develop it insidiously. For example, thyroidectomy can leave a patient severely symptomatic until he or she begins taking an adequate dosage of thyroid hormone. In most cases, the patient has overt hypothyroidism, defined as low serum T_4 and T_3 and high TSH levels due to low thyroid gland secretion. In contrast, the patient with autoimmune thyroid disease typically has subclinical hypothyroidism (defined as normal serum T_4 and T_3 and high TSH levels due to suboptimal thyroid gland secretion) for years or decades before the hypothyroidism becomes overt.[235,p.920] The subclinical hypothyroidism will continue as long as the thyroid gland is able to respond to increased TSH concentrations with increased thyroid hormone synthesis and secretion.[235][236] Braverman and Utiger wrote[235,p.919] that even in overt hypothyroidism, the severity of the clinical features varies widely. The condition will induce few signs and symptoms in some patients, and coma in others.

● THE INCIDENCE OF HYPOTHYROIDISM IN FIBROMYALGIA

A number of studies indicate a high incidence of hypothyroidism among fibromyalgia patients compared to the general population. Some researchers have attempted to identify hypothyroid patients (to

exclude them from their fibromyalgia studies) through testing with the T_4 and T_3 resin uptake blood tests.[36] Other researchers have included basal TSH measures.[66] The T_4 and T_3 resin uptake tests are no longer the preferable tests for identifying patients with abnormal thyroid function,[245,p.120] and the basal TSH level can identify only patients with primary (thyroidal) hypothyroidism. Even combining the T_4 and T_3 resin uptake with the basal TSH does not distinguish patients who may have thyroid hormone deficiency of pituitary or hypothalamic origin, termed central hypothyroidism. (See Chapter 4.2.)

PRIMARY HYPOTHYROIDISM AND FIBROMYALGIA

Five reports provide quantitative figures on the incidence of primary hypothyroidism among fibromyalgia patients. Shiroky and coworkers[243] reported that of 34 fibromyalgia patients, 4 (12%) had primary hypothyroidism. Eisinger and colleagues[244] reported that 6 of 62 (9.7%) patients had primary hypothyroidism. In my retrospective study of 38 consecutive fibromyalgia patients, test results for 4 patients (10.5%) were consistent with primary hypothyroidism.[237] Hershman wrote that the incidence of primary hypothyroidism has been reported to be 1% of the general adult population and 3% of geriatrics.[238,p.40] The incidence of primary hypothyroidism (4 patients) among my 38 patients is 10.5 times (10.5%/1%) the incidence in the general non-geriatric population, if the 1% estimate is accurate. In a second study of the thyroid status of 54 consecutive fibromyalgia patients,[242] my colleagues and I found that 8 patients (14.8%) had test results consistent with primary hypothyroidism. It is obvious from these studies that the incidence of primary hypothyroidism in fibromyalgia is relatively high.

CENTRAL HYPOTHYROIDISM AND FIBROMYALGIA

I found that 20 (52.6%) of 38 consecutive fibromyalgia patients had test results consistent with central hypothyroidism (suggesting hypothalamic or pituitary dysfunction).[237] Eleven patients had blunted TSH responses to TRH (<8.5 μU/mL). This is 28.9% of the 38 patients in the study, which is close to Ferraccioli's finding of blunted TSH responses in 5 of 24 patients (20.8%).[241] The incidence of central hypothyroidism has been reported to be only 0.00021% of the population.[238,p.40] According to this figure, central hypothyroidism is about 1/4,800 (0.00021%/1%) as frequent as primary hypothyroidism. The incidence of possible central hypothyroidism in my 38 patients was 250,476.19 times (52.6%/0.00021%) that in the general population. The incidence, therefore, of primary and central hypothyroidism in my 38 fibromyalgia patients was *exponentially* inversely proportional to incidences in the general population. In a second study of the thyroid status of 54 consecutive fibromyalgia patients,[242] test results were consistent with central hypothyroidism in 20 patients (37%). This is 176,190 times the incidence in the non-geriatric population at-large. (See Appendix B, paper titled "Thyroid Status of 38 Fibromyalgia Patients: Implications for the Etiology of Fibromyalgia," and abstract titled "Thyroid Status of Fibromyalgia Patients.")

AWARENESS BY CLINICIANS

Most cases of hypothyroidism escape recognition by clinicians. Ladenson pointed out that among primary care patients whose symptoms might be attributed to hypothyroidism, the diagnosis is established in only 1%-to-4% of cases.[268,p.1092] In attempting to explain why this diagnosis is made in so few cases, Ladenson, in chorus with Seshadri and coauthors, wrote that the clinical manifestations of hypothyroidism, while providing clues that a patient may have hypothyroidism, are too insensitive and nonspecific for a definitive diagnosis. He noted that even in some patients with overt biochemical hypothyroidism (low serum thyroid hormone and high TSH levels), symptoms and signs may be minimal or absent.[269] He gives numerous reasons for the subtle presentation of hypothyroidism.[268,p.1092] These include an insidious onset of thyroid gland failure, borderline hormone deficiencies, the passivity of many hypothyroid patients, and the common and nonspecific symptoms (such as fatigue and constipation) and signs (such as dry skin and weight gain). He also includes age- and gender-specific features of hypothyroidism such as growth retardation in children, menorrhagia in menstruating women, and dementia in old people. These features could be caused by many other conditions that clinicians pursue diagnostically while neglecting to consider hypothyroidism.

The clinician should be aware of the potential causes of hypothyroidism. In the sections below, I describe various conditions or factors that may cause primary hypothyroidism by damaging the thyroid gland, or may cause central hypothyroidism by impairing either the hypothalamus or the pituitary gland. After the clinician learns that one or more of these conditions or factors impinge on a patient, he should be attentive to the patient possibly having or developing hypothyroidism.

POLYMYALGIA-HYPOTHYROID INTRACTABILITY SYNDROME: EISINGER'S SYNDROME

In 1998, Prof. J. Eisinger of Toulon, France, described a syndrome not previously described in the medical literature. The descriptive name he gave the condition is "polymyalgia-hypothyroid intractability syndrome."[339] It is fitting that the condition should be designated "Eisinger's syndrome," in honor of the eminent researcher who first identified and described it, and documented its occurrence.

Four features characterize Eisinger's syndrome: (1) hypothyroidism with unsteady symptoms, (2) a poor response of symptoms to T$_4$, (3) a peculiar myofascial pain syndrome with multiple and unusual trigger points, and (4) a peculiar fibromyalgia syndrome with severe muscle pain and discrete mood disorders. Eisinger described the condition as rare and usually disabling. He wrote that the physical abnormalities of the myofascial pain syndrome are difficult to treat because they are diffuse. In addition, the biochemical abnormalities are additive—mitochondrial respiratory chain impairment and increased lipid peroxidation are associated with patients' hypothyroidism, and pentose pathway impairment, decreased nitric oxide production, and increased protein peroxidation are associated with their fibromyalgia.[339]

Eisinger wrote that balancing patients' thyroid status with T$_4$ is almost impossible and that some patients have clinical indications of both hypothyroidism (such as somnolence) and hyperthyroidism (such as palpitations). This suggests that different tissues respond differentially to exogenous thyroid hormone, some unaffected and others overstimulated. Patients usually have more than 6 tender points, but some have fewer than the 11 of 18 required by the ACR criteria for the diagnosis of fibromyalgia syndrome.

Eisinger wrote that treatment of the hypothyroidism remains the key problem. He recommended reducing the patient's T$_4$ dosage by a small amount and adding T$_3$ to the treatment regimen.[340] In his experience, the T$_3$ improves some clinical signs and biological abnormalities. Other treatment procedures he advised include supplementing with selenium or zinc (both favor the conversion of T_4 to T_3), and vitamin B_2.

After Eisinger described the syndrome to me, I realized in retrospect that some of my former fibromyalgia patients had the characteristic features of the syndrome. Because I had monitored some patients weekly for one year, I was aware that their status was unstable.[341] The prevalence of Eisinger's syndrome must yet be established.

● CAUSES OF PRIMARY HYPOTHYROIDISM

Several different conditions can impair thyroid gland function. The impairment results are elevated serum TSH levels, an exaggerated TSH response to injected TRH, and possibly low serum circulating levels of thyroid hormone.

AUTOIMMUNE THYROID DISEASES

Two forms of autoimmune thyroid disease are autoimmune thyroiditis and Graves' disease. These conditions have immunogenetic and clinical similarities and differences. The prototypical form of autoimmune thyroiditis is Hashimoto's thyroiditis. Hashimoto's is common but there are several variations of the prototype that have different features.[160,p.921]

Martin-du Pan studied 98 patients with Graves' disease and 95 patients with Hashimoto's thyroiditis. He found that 11% of Graves' patients and 6% of Hashimoto's patients developed the condition after exposure to stress factors. He also found that 25% of women of childbearing age developed Graves' disease and 10% developed Hashimoto's after a pregnancy.[337]

Patients with Graves' disease virtually always have thyroid-stimulating antibodies and infiltrative ophthalmopathy. By contrast, patients with Hashimoto's thyroiditis seldom do. There is a higher incidence of Sjögren's syndrome in Hashimoto's patients than in Graves' patients.[142]

Graves' and Hashimoto's result from separate specific defects in genes involved in immunoregulation.[160,p.922][166] Despite this, the two conditions are closely related genetically and immunologically. Both conditions tend to occur in the same families. Also, both conditions are likely to occur in the same pa-

tient's thyroid gland.[160,p.925] Hashimoto's thyroiditis, both with and without hypothyroidism, sometimes changes into Graves' disease and hyperthyroidism. Conversely, Graves' disease in some cases spontaneously changes to Hashimoto's thyroiditis and hypothyroidism.[141][142][160,p.925] The conditions share common features: Either may involve lymphocytic infiltration, increased levels of various immunoglobulins within the thyroid gland, thymic enlargement, and increased titers of thyroid autoantibodies.[142] These similarities warrant their being classified under the generic term "autoimmune thyroid disease."[160,p.921] Both disorders can result in hypothyroidism, and in susceptible individuals, the hypothyroidism manifests as fibromyalgia.

Autoimmune Thyroiditis

Autoimmune thyroiditis in some patients does not result in reduced thyroid hormone synthesis. Chronic autoimmune thyroiditis, however, is the most common disease that causes primary hypothyroidism.[235,p.919] Thyroid hormone deficiency is the main physiologic outcome of the autoimmune thyroiditis diseases.[164][171][174] Elevated TSH levels usually precede detectably low serum thyroid hormone levels. The pattern of elevated TSH and normal thyroid hormone levels due to impaired thyroid gland function is termed subclinical hypothyroidism.[160,p.927]

Antithyroid Antibodies. Virtually all Graves', Hashimoto's, and idiopathic hypothyroid patients have microsomal antibodies.[142][160,p.926][169] (Microsomes are small vesicles released from the endoplasmic reticulum of cell nuclei upon centrifuging.) Titers of microsomal antibodies are correlated with the histologic lesions of Hashimoto's thyroiditis.[163]

The enzyme thyroid peroxidase is the microsomal antigen.[168] It is located in the apical cytoplasm and plasma membrane of follicular cells.[169] Antibodies to thyroid peroxidase are complement-fixing antibodies. They exert cytotoxic effects in cultured thyroid cells[160,p.926] and can interfere with the enzymatic activity of thyroid peroxidase, thereby inducing thyroid dysfunction.[170] (See Chapter 2.1, section titled "Thyroid Hormone Production in the Thyroid Gland.") *Antibody levels usually decrease either when patients with autoimmune thyroiditis become hypothyroid[171] or they undergo treatment with T_4.[172][173]*

Clinical Features. The clinical features of autoimmune thyroiditis differ widely among patients. Some patients have no symptoms or signs.[177] Clinicians may inadvertently be alerted to a patient's autoimmune thyroiditis in different circumstances: upon seeing the results of thyroid function or thyroid antibody tests, during surgery or at biopsy, or upon observing an enlarged thyroid gland.[164][167][175][176] Rarely, a patient is hyperthyroid.[160,p.927] Other patients, who may or may not have goiters, are overtly hypothyroid.[164][171][175][176]

Forms of Autoimmune Thyroiditis. Several different forms of thyroiditis have a similar pathogenesis. Autoimmune thyroiditis is a generic term that subsumes these different forms. Most forms are "goitrous" (involving gland enlargement). At least one form, primary hypothyroidism, is "atrophic," meaning that the size of the thyroid gland decreases.[160,p.921]

Goitrous Autoimmune Thyroiditis. Histologically, the goitrous form of autoimmune thyroiditis involves inflammatory infiltrate. Follicular hypertrophy may occur: The follicular cells are tall and columnar, the follicular lumina are small, and the lumina contain little colloid. There are large numbers of lymphocytic and plasma cells and varying degrees of fibrosis.[160,p.923]

In 1912, Hashimoto described the form of autoimmune thyroiditis that is now considered the prototype and bears his name.[160,p.921] The thyroid glands of the patients Hashimoto described were diffusely infiltrated with lymphocytes and eosinophils; the glands were fibrotic and their follicular cells atrophied. The patients also had goiters;[161] in many, the thyroid glands were diffusely and symmetrically enlarged.[160,p.927][179] Clinicians continue to term the goitrous form of the condition Hashimoto's thyroiditis,[160,p.921] but it is also called chronic nonspecific thyroiditis, lymphocytic thyroiditis, or struma lymphomatosa.[153,p.608]

There are several variants of Hashimoto's thyroiditis. These include the chronic fibrous form, with predominant fibrosis and minimal lymphocytic infiltration; childhood and adolescent lymphocytic thyroiditis, with minimal fibrosis and lymphocyte infiltration; postpartum thyroiditis; and silent, painless thyroiditis.[160,p.921]

It appears that increased iodine intake in the last several generations has increased the incidence of autoimmune thyroiditis.[162] Thyroid autoantibodies indicate autoimmune thyroiditis.[165] Autoantibodies are found in some 15% of elderly women. In fact, autoimmune thyroiditis occurs most often in women.[153,p.608] In a study in Busselton, Western Australia, subclinical hypothyroidism (high serum TSH and normal thyroid hormone levels) was indicated in 59 (72%) of 82 individuals with persistently elevated thyroid microsomal antibodies, 18 (72%) of those with recently developed elevated antibodies, and 12 (23%) of those with transiently elevated antibodies.[163]

There are other forms of autoimmune thyroiditis that differ from Hashimoto's.[160,p.921] The clinical abnormalities range from no symptoms or signs to moderate hyperthyroidism to severe hypothyroidism. The pathological abnormalities range from a large goiter to atrophy of the gland. The gland may have sporadic groups of infiltrating lymphocytes or widespread chronic inflammation and fibrosis with loss of almost all follicular epithelium.[153,p.608]

Among the immune phenomena that occur in autoimmune thyroiditis are various types of circulating antithyroid antibodies, basement membrane changes of thyroid gland cells and *in situ* immune complex deposition, and expression of major histocompatibility complex antigens on thyroid cells.[151][152][154][155][156][157]

Atrophic Autoimmune Thyroiditis. The most common cause in the Western world of primary hypothyroidism is autoimmune thyroiditis during which the gland undergoes atrophy.[160,pp.921&930] Most adult hypothyroidism, except that induced by pituitary failure, radiation, or thyroidectomy, represents a form of autoimmune thyroiditis.[153,p.610] In many cases, clinicians determine that patients have autoimmune thyroiditis only after the patients consult them for symptoms that turn out to be due to hypothyroidism.[164][171][175][176] Patients with either goitrous or atrophic autoimmune thyroiditis may become hypothyroid, although thyroid hormone deficiency is more common in the atrophic form.[177]

Among patients with autoimmune thyroiditis, those with subclinical hypothyroidism outnumber those with overt hypothyroidism.[160,p.927] Only 10% of patients with goiters and elevated titers of thyroid autoantibodies develop hypothyroidism.[177] Others have unexplained remissions—with or without recurrences—of autoimmune thyroiditis, but do not become hypothyroid.[177][178] Some patients develop Graves' disease and become hyperthyroid.[142] Follicles are atrophied, and there are variable amounts of lymphocytes and fibrosis.[160,p.923]

Antibodies to TSH receptors on thyroid gland cell membranes block stimulation of adenylate cyclase activity, and this impedes the TSH-stimulated growth of thyroid cells. This may be the mechanism of atrophic thyroiditis that results in hypothyroidism.[167] But thyroid gland failure is more closely correlated with the presence of cytoplasmic antibodies than with thyroglobulin antibodies.[103,p.661]

Volpé wrote that when clinical and biochemical evidence indicate that a patient is hypothyroid and no other mechanism is obvious, the clinician should consider autoimmune thyroiditis. He wrote further that this is especially true when thyroid function test results of a middle-aged or elderly patient indicate subclinical hypothyroidism, and particularly when the patient is goitrous, regardless of the presence or absence of thyroid autoantibodies. A negative antibody test does not exclude the diagnosis, but a positive test confirms it. A positive test result makes a thyroid biopsy unnecessary.[160,p.930]

Hyperthyroid Variant of Autoimmune Thyroiditis. The hyperthyroid variant is similar to Graves' disease. In autoimmune thyroiditis, there is more cellular metaplasia than in Graves' disease. In Graves' disease, thyroid gland follicles are larger and contain more papillary structures than in autoimmune thyroiditis.[153,p.609] Otherwise, though, the gross and microscopic findings in the two conditions may be identical.[180] Hyperthyroidism can occur when Graves' disease and autoimmune thyroiditis are concurrent in the patient's thyroid gland.[79][80] Hyperthyroidism can also occur during the initial stages of Hashimoto's thyroiditis. Thyrotoxicosis may occur because inflammation of the gland causes the release of large amounts of preformed thyroid hormone.[160,p.928]

Extent of Involvement in Autoimmune Thyroiditis. The extent of involvement in autoimmune thyroiditis ranges from slight and focal to all-encompassing. Oertel and LiVolsi describe the variability: "In some glands, follicular epithelial hyperplasia is striking, and lymphocytic infiltration is minimal. In other examples, the inflammatory cells have replaced nearly all of the follicular epithelium, which can lead to confusion with lymphoma. Thus, a variety of changes occur, ranging from multifocal to diffuse; the amount of inflammatory infiltrate varies greatly; and the epithelium may be atrophic or hyperplastic, with oxyphilic cells or squamous cells. Combinations of these alterations lead to remarkably varied histologic patterns."[153,pp.609-610] The authors speculate that this variability is a product of the different types of antibodies assailing thyroid antigens and the population of lymphoid cells in the gland.

In classic Hashimoto's thyroiditis, the thyroid gland is enlarged, has widespread lymphoplasmacytic infiltrates, and extensive loss of colloid. Most of the epithelium disappears, and there is substantial fibrosis. In advanced cases, there may be little or no visible normal parenchyma. There are also infiltrates of lymphocytes, plasma cells, and macrophages.[153,pp.609-610] Oertel and LiVolsi wrote that in their experience, the thyroid gland of a Hashimoto's patient is fibrotic and small; it contains a few nests of abnormal epithelial cells and small scattered groups of lymphocytes and

plasma cells.[153,p.610] Stassi et al. found that infiltrating T lymphocytes are not directly involved in thyrocyte cell death during Hashimoto's thyroiditis. Instead, their findings suggest that autocrine/paracrine Fas-FasL interaction is a major mechanism in autoimmune thyrocyte destruction[115] (see section below titled "Treatment of Autoimmune Thyroiditis: Gene Therapy").

Treatment of Autoimmune Thyroiditis. In autoimmune thyroiditis, corticosteroids reduce the size of the enlarged thyroid gland and lower thyroid antibody titers.[181][182] Volpé wrote, however: "In view of the serious side effects of these and other immunosuppressive agents, and the ease with which autoimmune thyroiditis can be treated with thyroid hormone, any type of immunosuppressive therapy is unwarranted."[160,p.930]

Volpé[160,p.930] also wrote that all patients who are hypothyroid because of autoimmune thyroiditis should be treated with T_4.[164][171][176][179] He stipulated that patients with both overt and subclinical hypothyroidism should be treated with T_4. The patient should continue the treatment for life because when patients discontinue the treatment, hypothyroidism regularly recurs.[160,p.930] T_4 therapy usually reduces the size of a goiter, but the gland does not return to normal size in all cases.[179][183] Thyroid antibody titers typically decrease with T_4 therapy, especially in patients whose TSH levels were elevated before they began the therapy.[172][173]

Gene Therapy. Batteux et al. recently found that gene therapy inhibits lymphocytic infiltration of thyroid gland tissue in experimental autoimmune thyroiditis. The researchers obtained the effect by directly injecting DNA expression vectors encoding FasL (Fas-Fas ligand) into inflamed thyroid tissue. (Fas, APO-1/CD95, is a cell-surface receptor involved in cell death signaling. Germline mutations in the Fas gene are associated with conditions such as autoimmune lymphoproliferative syndrome; somatic Fas mutations are associated with multiple myeloma.[114]) In addition to inhibiting lymphocytic infiltration of the thyroid, the treatment caused the death of infiltrating T cells. The treatment also totally abolished the anti-thyroglobulin cytotoxic T cell response. The researchers wrote that their results show that FasL expression on thyrocytes may cure experimental autoimmune thyroiditis by causing the death of pathogenic autoreactive infiltrating T lymphocytes.[338]

Hypothyroidism Associated with Autoimmune Thyroiditis. Ladenson wrote that because autoimmune thyroiditis is the most common cause of primary hypothyroidism, indications of thyroiditis should prompt the clinician to order laboratory tests for possible hypothyroidism.[268,p.1092] Gordin and Lamberg reported, however, that only about 10% of patients who have autoantibodies to the thyroid gland ever develop overt thyroid dysfunction.[145] According to Volpé,[160,p.930] 10%-to-15% of patients with autoimmune thyroiditis become hypothyroid,[177] and some patients have unexplained remissions of their hypothyroidism or goiter.[142][178] "Thus," he wrote, "it is not clear whether T_4, if given, should be given indefinitely. For most patients, however, the most reasonable and practical solution is indefinite treatment, unless they are examined regularly by physicians aware of the vagaries of the natural history of the disorder." He continued, "Because therapy may at least limit further thyroid enlargement and because hypothyroidism, particularly in the elderly, may be subtle, easily overlooked, and dangerous, this approach seems to offer the greatest benefit to the most patients."[160,p.930]

Graves' Disease

In Graves' disease, an immunoglobulin G antibody to the TSH receptors on thyroid gland cell membranes acts as a thyroid gland stimulant; it is called thyroid-stimulating antibody. The antibody, as it binds to the TSH receptor, mimics TSH by activating adenylate cyclase and generating cAMP. It sustains these effects longer than does TSH. The antibody causes a primary diffuse hyperplasia of the gland[151][152] that is termed hyperplastic goiter. The hyperplasia results in hyperthyroidism with distinct thyrotoxicosis.[139,p.654] The hyperthyroid Graves' patient's TSH levels are usually suppressed.[142,p.73] If the patient also has Hashimoto's thyroiditis, however, the patient may not become hyperthyroid.[143][142] This condition is called hypothyroid Graves' disease.[143]

Patients with Graves' disease typically have pretibial myxedema. About 5% of patients also have thyroid acropachy, a thickening and clubbing of the digits.[149][150] Some 50% of patients also have infiltrative ophthalmopathy with protrusion of the eyes (exophthalmos),[144] stare, and eyelid retraction.[139,p.654] Preorbital edema due to impaired orbital venous drainage causes the ophthalmopathy, and swollen connective tissues and muscles behind the eye cause proptosis of the eye.[148,p.661]

Tests for TSH receptor antibodies are not essential to the diagnosis. Virtually all patients have elevated serum total and free T_4 levels and low TSH levels; these values indicate hyperthyroidism. Volpé wrote that if the patient has ophthalmopathy and a diffuse goiter, the clinician should consider Graves' disease to

be the cause. If these two signs are absent, he recommended a 24-hour radioactive iodine uptake or a thyroid radioisotope scan. These tests distinguish Graves' disease from other causes of hyperthyroidism.[139,p.655]

Hyperthyroidism in Graves' disease may follow a steady course of varying severity. The condition may occur as one isolated episode, or it may cease for varying periods and then resume.[139,p.654][146][147]

Hypothyroidism Associated with Graves' Disease. Graves' disease is of interest in regard to fibromyalgia because Graves' may culminate in hypothyroidism.[139,p.655] Of Graves' patients treated with antithyroid drugs and in remission, 10%-to-15% become hypothyroid 15-to-20 years later as a result of Hashimoto's thyroiditis.[140][141] Graves' disease and Hashimoto's thyroiditis, both of which appear to be induced genetically, sometimes occur in the same family, and one patient may have both diseases.[139,p.651] Graves' patients treated for thyrotoxicosis with thyroidectomy or ^{131}I therapy may develop early or late hypothyroidism.[268,p.1093] But even without these ablative therapies, Graves' disease may progress to hypothyroidism.[270]

Incidence of Systemic Autoimmune Disease Among Patients with Autoimmune Thyroid Diseases

Gaches et al. studied the incidence of autoimmune diseases among patients with autoimmune thyroid diseases. They included in a retrospective analysis 218 patients (202 women and 16 men) with autoimmune thyroid diseases treated between 1981 and 1993. The mean age at the time the autoimmune thyroid diseases were diagnosed was 49. One or more concomitant autoimmune diseases were associated with thyroid disease in 30 patients (13.7%). Lupus and Sjögren's syndrome were the most common accompanying autoimmune diseases. In 17 cases concomitant autoimmune diseases were diagnosed at the same time as the thyroid diseases. In 5 cases, the systemic diseases anteceded the thyroid disease by a mean of 8 years, and in 8 cases by a mean of 5 years. The incidence of systemic autoimmune diseases was higher in patients with thyroid disorders than in the population at-large. The investigators conjectured that there are probably common pathophysiological mechanisms in patients with both types of autoimmune diseases. They recommended that patients with only systemic autoimmune disease or with only autoimmune thyroid disease be reevaluated at intervals for possible development of the other type of disease.[113]

SILENT AND SUBACUTE THYROIDITIS

Silent thyroiditis and subacute thyroiditis refer to clinical syndromes that accompany various histopathological changes in the thyroid gland. Silent thyroiditis, which is painless, involves lymphatic thyroiditis with transient clinical manifestations of thyrotoxicosis. Postpartum thyroiditis is similar to silent thyroiditis except that it may involve transient thyrotoxicosis, transient or persistent hypothyroidism, or euthyroid goiter. The term subacute thyroiditis is used only to refer to granulomatous giant cell inflammation. Thyroid pain and tenderness are predominant in subacute thyroiditis.[180]

Silent Thyroiditis

Nikolai wrote that silent thyroiditis and subacute thyroiditis are most likely overlapping forms of thyroiditis provoked by different infectious, autoimmune, or other mechanisms. Onset occurs when some undetermined mechanism causes sudden inflammation. Damaged thyroid follicles release a large amount of preformed thyroid hormone.[184,p.710] (Other iodinated substances such as thyroglobulin also escape into the circulation.) This causes transient thyrotoxicosis that may reoccur several times in the same patient, lasting each time from 1-to-9 weeks.[184,p.714][185] Silent thyroiditis follows a time-limited course, from a few weeks-to-several months. About 40% of patients have transient hypothyroidism during recovery. This phase typically lasts from 4-to-16 weeks. For some patients, hypothyroidism persists indefinitely.[184,p.714]

Most patients seek care when they are in the thyrotoxic phase of the disease. A small percentage are euthyroid or hypothyroid. This is especially true of women in the postpartum period.[186][187] Thyroid function test results vary considerably, depending on the phase of the disease. Results reflect the pathological state of the thyroid gland.[185][188][189]

Diagnosis and Treatment. Diagnosis depends upon four factors: (1) mild-to-moderate thyrotoxicosis with elevated T_3 and T_4, (2) slight nontender thyroid gland enlargement (evident in 50%-to-60% of patients), (3) low ^{131}I uptake, and (4) no former use of iodine-containing medications or thyroid hormone. The finding of lymphocytic thyroiditis through fine-needle or core-needle biopsy of the thyroid gland confirms the diagnosis. This is not essential to the diagnosis, however.[184,p.716] Most patients' thyrotoxicosis is mild. Because of this, the use of a β-blocking drug is usually not necessary. However, the patient can use a β-blocker to stop bothersome symptoms, and with

proper precautions, an elderly patient should use a blocker if cardiac safety is of concern. If thyrotoxicosis is severe, an anti-inflammatory drug such as prednisone usually decreases the inflammation and serum T_3 and T_4 levels within 7-to-10 days.[190]

Hypothyroidism during the recovery phase is usually mild and typically lasts 4-to-10 weeks. The use of sufficient exogenous T_4 can relieve severe hypothyroid symptoms. Nikolai cautioned, however, that the dosage should be kept low enough not to decrease the serum TSH to normal. He wrote that continuing TSH secretion may accelerate recovery and enable the patient to slowly withdraw from the use of T_4.[184,p.718] "In the occasional patient who develops permanent hypothyroidism," Nikolai wrote, "the serum T_4 concentration falls and the TSH concentration rises when T_4 therapy is withdrawn. If hypothyroidism lasts for longer than six months, it is probably permanent, and no further attempts at withdrawal need be undertaken."[184,p.717] He also advised that the clinician monitor at 1-to-2 year intervals for goiter or thyroid failure. Some 50% of patients who have an episode of silent thyroiditis eventually have thyroid disease.[191]

Subacute Thyroiditis

Subacute thyroiditis is much less common than silent thyroiditis. Patients are most often between the ages of 20 and 60. It is rare in children and the elderly. The female/male ratio is between 3:1 and 6:1.[192] A variety of viruses are implicated in the etiology of subacute thyroiditis.[196] The absence of increased viral antibody titers in some cases suggests that other etiologic factors are involved. It is possible, though, that viruses cause the disease, but that researchers have not tested for the associated antibodies. Nevertheless, Nikolai[184,p.718] wrote that indirect yet strong evidence suggests that viral infections are the cause, as first proposed in 1952.[197]" There have been epidemics of this form of thyroiditis,[195] but the incidence is highest during the summer months[193][194] and is concurrent with summer enterovirus infections. The disease is often preceded by an upper respiratory infection. The prodromal phase may include muscle aches and pains, malaise, and fatigue.[184,p.718] Autoimmunity may play a role,[192][197][198][199][200] but none of the active thyroid autoantibodies appear to be involved.[184,p.719]

During subacute thyroiditis, the gland is edematous and enlarged. Follicular cells are extensively destroyed and colloid is extravasated. The thyroid tissues contain an inflammatory infiltrate of neutrophils, lymphocytes, histocytes, clusters of follicular cells, and multinucleated giant cells.[201][202][203] Follicles are regenerated in areas, and there is minimal residual fibrosis.[184,p.720]

Subacute thyroiditis typically lasts from 2-to-4 months, but it may persist for a year. When prolonged, pain and tenderness of the thyroid gland continue throughout the course of the disease. Thyrotoxicosis subsides early, however, lasting only 4-to-10 weeks in 50% of patients. Even though thyroid gland inflammation persists, colloid stores deplete during the acute phase, and the patient becomes euthyroid again. According to Nikolai, patients with more severe thyroiditis may have transient hypothyroidism that lasts 1-to-2 months. As the patient recovers, the follicles regenerate, the colloid accumulates, and the gland recovers normal function.[184,p.722] An occasional patient becomes permanently hypothyroid.[171][197] In contrast with silent thyroiditis, few patients with subacute thyroiditis have persistent or progressive thyroid disease.[190][205]

Diagnosis. Patients have neck pain, tenderness of the thyroid gland, and symptoms of inflammatory illness. They may or may not be thyrotoxic. About 50% of patients have had an upper respiratory tract infection that was followed in days or weeks by the symptoms of subacute thyroiditis. Patients usually report that they experienced abrupt malaise and fever spontaneously or after an upper respiratory infection. They complain of pain in the area of the thyroid gland on one or both sides that may radiate to the angle of the jaw and to the ipsilateral ear. Ear pain may be the only symptom. If the thyroid gland pain and tenderness are initially unilateral, they become bilateral within days or weeks. The pain may be localized to the throat or upper anterior chest and made worse by coughing, swallowing, or by rotating the neck or head. Some patients experience pain only when pressure is applied to the neck. Systemic symptoms may include malaise, myalgia, mild fever, and anorexia. It is possible that silent thyroiditis initiates fibromyalgia/chronic fatigue syndrome in some patients who report that a sore throat preceded the chronic illness. This would be especially likely in the patient left with some degree of hypothyroidism.

About 50% of patients experience a thyrotoxic phase. During this phase the patient may be nervous, tremulous, heat intolerant, and have tachycardia. The thyroid gland is usually firm or hard and is diffusely enlarged.[184,p.720][191][195][204]

During the acute phase, the spilling of T$_4$ and T$_3$ into the blood raises their serum levels and lowers the TSH level. As the colloid becomes depleted, the hormone levels decrease to normal.[206][207][208][209] In 20%-

to-30% of patients, however, thyroid hormone levels decrease further and are subnormal for a time before increasing to normal. After the acute phase, and when the thyroid hormone levels decrease toward normal, the TSH level increases. The TSH level may be elevated for 2-to-4 weeks while the thyroid hormone levels are subnormal. Hypothyroidism usually lasts 1-to-2 months. Some patients may be hypothyroid for longer times, and an occasional patient will be permanently hypothyroid.[184,p.723] During the acute phase, ^{131}I uptake is usually low, possibly due to the suppressed TSH secretion, and thyroid radioisotope scans show irregular tracer uptake.[211][212] The clinician should take care to avoid concluding that the hypothyroidism in the hypothyroid phase is permanent.[204] Over time, the distinction between transient and permanent hypothyroidism becomes obvious.[184,p.724]

Nikolai advised[184,p.723] the clinician to palpate the thyroid gland in all patients who have upper respiratory infections and complain of a sore throat or earache. Characteristically, the erythrocyte sedimentation rate is increased to above 100 mm/hr.[171][195][204] The leukocyte count may be normal or elevated to as much as 18,000/µL.[184,p.723] In the acute phase, some patients may have liver dysfunction.[210] An accurate diagnosis can be made by fine-needle aspiration biopsy in about 90% of cases.[184,p.723]

Treatment. Salicylates and other non-steroidal anti-inflammatory drugs may relieve mild symptoms.[213][214] Corticosteroids (such as prednisone) are more effective, work more rapidly, and provide partial or complete relief in 24-to-48 hours.[195][204] Because corticosteroids control thyrotoxicosis, β-adrenergic blocking drugs are not necessary in most cases. Nikolai recommended an initial dose of prednisone of 40-to-60 mg/d for roughly 1 week. After that, the dosage should be rapidly reduced with complete cessation in 4 weeks. He advised, "In the rare patient with a prolonged course with persistent neck pain and tenderness and malaise, near-total thyroidectomy or ablation of the thyroid with radioactive iodine may be justified."[184,p.724]

ANTITHYROID TREATMENTS

Typical hyperthyroid patients, most often those with Graves' disease, will undergo antithyroid treatments.[234,p.887] These treatments commonly convert patients from hyperthyroid to hypothyroid. This is of concern to those of us who care for fibromyalgia patients. The hypothyroidism, in many cases, is manifest as fibromyalgia. And in most cases, the patients are either undertreated or not treated at all with exogenous thyroid hormone. This is a product of erroneous conclusions within the current endocrinology paradigm. The patient is likely to remain hypometabolic and symptomatic until beginning thyroid hormone therapy. Without thyroid hormone therapy, the patient's quality of life is likely to deteriorate, and she is subject to developing diseases such as atherosclerosis that may result in heart attacks or strokes.

Antithyroid Drugs

Antithyroid drugs are the main form of treatment for the thyrotoxicity of Graves' disease. The drugs are sometimes used as secondary treatments for thyrotoxicity due to causes such as toxic nodular goiter.[234,p.888] Those drugs most commonly used are a family of compounds that share the thionamide grouping and inhibit organification of iodide.[291,p.324] Thyroid peroxidase catalyzes the oxidation and organification of iodine and the coupling of iodotyroxyl residues to produce iodothyronine. (See Chapter 2.1.) Thionamides inhibit these peroxidatic reactions.[291,p.325] These drugs include thiouracil and propylthiouracil. Goitrin is a compound from this family that is found in rutabaga, turnip, and cabbage.[292] Goitrin in milk was responsible for a particular goiter endemic to Finland.[290,p161]

The purpose of antithyroid drugs is to return the patient to a euthyroid state. The hope is an eventual remission of Graves' disease.[234,p.896] Some patients' Graves' disease undergoes remission after weeks-to-months of antithyroid drug use. Regardless, it is generally recommended that the patient continue the medication for 1-to-2 years.[293][294][295] Usually, the longer the drug is continued, the more likely the patient is to remain euthyroid after stopping use of the drug.[296][297]

A small goiter and mild biochemical hyperthyroidism are factors suggesting that remission will last longer than one year, which is considered long-term.[299] But the low predictability of any clinical finding makes it difficult to accurately forecast which patients will remain in remission after treatment.[234,p.896] An unfavorable outcome, nevertheless, is generally indicated by three factors: (1) persisting thyroid gland enlargement, (2) a continuing need for large doses of the antithyroid drug, and (3) T_3-predominant hyperthyroidism during treatment.

Cooper[300] recommended that the drug dosage gradually be lowered and eventually discontinued.[234] The clinician should monitor the patient clinically and order serial thyroid function tests. Relapses, if they occur, usually do so within 3-to-6 months. Research-

ers reported that hyperthyroidism reoccurred in 60%[301][302] and 91%[265][301] of patients within 5 years after treatment. Hirota et al. reported that of 45 Graves' patients who had discontinued thionamide drugs 10 years before, 2 (4.4%) had physical signs of mild hyperthyroidism. Four patients (8.9%) had T_3-toxicosis, and 3 (6.7%) had an elevated free thyroxine index and serum T_3 levels. Thirty-six (80%) of the patients were euthyroid.[305]

Hypothyroidism Associated with Thionamide Drug Use. Excessive thionamide drug dosages can impair thyroid function sufficiently to induce hypothyroidism. Cooper[234,p.896] pointed out that as thyrotoxicity decreases during antithyroid drug treatment, the dosage can repeatedly be lowered. If the clinician does not monitor the patient and properly lower the dosage, the patient may become hypothyroid. It is especially important to make sure the patient to be treated with thionamides has a sufficient iodine intake. Azizi [306] studied two groups of patients in Tehran, an iodine-deficient area, who were treated with the thionamide medication called methimazole. Within a month, 8 (44%) of a group of 18 patients and 7 (46%) of a group of 15 became hypothyroid.

Hypothyroidism may develop long after the patient undergoes treatment with thionamides. Ten years after ceasing thionamide use, 2 (4.4%) of 45 Graves' patients had subclinical hypothyroidism.[305] Of the 36 patients who were considered euthyroid at the end of the 10-year period, TRH stimulation tests showed hyporesponsiveness of the pituitary-thyroid axis in 3 patients, and hyperresponsiveness in 5 patients.[305] This result is consistent with central hypothyroidism. In another study of 102 Graves' patients treated with either propylthiouracil or carbimazole, 6 (5.9%) developed hypothyroidism at a mean of 3.5 years after ending the thionamide therapy.[307]

Cooper recommended long-term follow-ups after the patient stops taking a thionamide. Follow-up evaluations are advisable because relapses can occur at any time in the patient's life, or the patient may become hypothyroid.[234,p.898] Cooper[234,p.896] and others[298] have pointed out that prolonged courses of antithyroid medication use are safe, and the patient may prefer to take small daily doses of the medication for decades as an option to ablative therapies. The probability of ablative therapies making the patient hypothyroid is much higher than that of antithyroid drugs (see below). However, thyroidologists often recommend radioiodine treatment for most adult hyperthyroid patients if one or two courses of anti-thyroid drugs (each lasting from 1-to-2 years) do not bring about remission.[304]

Ablative Therapies

Graves' disease may result in hypothyroidism even when the patient is not treated with ablative therapies.[270] Hypothyroidism is even more likely, however, in the patient who undergoes treatments such as subtotal thyroidectomy and ¹³¹I therapy.[268,p.1093]

Thyroidectomy. Subtotal thyroidectomy is the oldest treatment for hyperthyroidism; it was the only form of treatment for many years. Cooper stated that today it is used only in three exceptional circumstances: (1) when a patient is allergic to or is not compliant in taking thionamides, (2) when a patient has a large goiter, or (3) when a patient prefers ablation over drug treatment but is apprehensive about radioiodine treatment.[234,p.904] Thyroidectomy is the preferable treatment for toxic adenoma in the fertile age groups and for hyperfunctional bulky goiters. Elderly patients, however, are at higher risk for post-surgical complications.[303]

In subtotal thyroidectomy, the surgeon removes most of the gland, but he leaves a few grams of the posterior part of each lobe.[259] Virtually no one today dies during this procedure.[259][260] Cooper cautioned,[234,pp.904-905] however, that serious complications can result even from carefully performed surgery. These include recurrent laryngeal nerve damage, hypoparathyroidism, post-operative bleeding, keloids, unsightly scars, and wound infection. The risk of these complications may be increasing with the availability of alternate therapies and the resulting decrease in the number of surgeons experienced in the procedure.[234,pp.904-905]

Hypothyroidism Associated with Subtotal Thyroidectomy.

During the first year after surgery, 10%-to-60% of patients become hypothyroid.[261][262][263] Each year following, 1%-to-3% of patients become hypothyroid.[261] Whether hypothyroidism ensues depends on the size of the remaining thyroid tissue and whether there are antithyroid antibodies.[264] About 5% of patients become hyperthyroid again.[259][260][265][266] Kalk et al.[234,p.905] reported that 43% of their patients became hyperthyroid again after 5 years.[267] Radioiodine treatment may be preferable if this occurs.

Radioiodine. Radioiodine therapy (especially as ¹³¹I) used to treat hyperthyroidism destroys thyroid gland tissue.[256] It is the treatment of choice for toxic adenoma in patients over 40 years old. It is especially preferred for elderly patients with hyperthyroidism because of the higher risks of thyroidectomy.[303] It is also the recommended treatment for Graves' disease patients whose hyperthyroidism fails to respond to thionamide drugs.[304] Radioiodine is also used to treat toxic diffuse goiter.[308]

Hypothyroidism Associated with Radioiodine Therapy.

Radioiodine therapy commonly induces primary hypothyroidism, and the hypothyroidism is usually permanent.[235,p.919] Williams[256,p.424] termed this "post-irradiation hypothyroidism." Cooper wrote,[234,p.902] "Hypothyroidism may be considered to be an inevitable consequence of radioiodine therapy rather than a side effect."

Reports of the incidence of post-irradiation hypothyroidism, however, vary considerably. According to early reports,[255][257] from 15%-to-78% of patients who had radioiodine therapy were hypothyroid 10 years later. The report of a large study[258] was that 20% of patients were hypothyroid after 1 year, 31% after 7 years, and 40% after 11 years. Other authors[246] reported that within the first year following therapy, 90% of patients were hypothyroid; an additional 2%-to-3% became hypothyroid each subsequent year.

A higher incidence of hypothyroidism among post-irradiation patients is associated with higher auto-antibody titers before treatment and with higher doses of ¹³¹I.[247][248] With lower dosages, 3% of patients were hypothyroid at 3 months, and 40% were hypothyroid at 1 year. With higher dosages, 36% were hypothyroid at 3 months and 91% at 1 year.[246] Von Hofe and co-workers[308] reported that at 3 months after treatment, 50% of patients were hypothyroid, and at 1 year, 69% were hypothyroid. The hypothyroidism may be associated with the transient increase in circulating antithyroid antibodies in some hyperthyroid patients following radioiodine treatment.[254] A few patients have a persisting increase in the antibodies.[255]

A third of patients may be transiently hypothyroid after radioiodine treatment.[252][253] Because of this, Cooper[234,p.902] recommended that unless hypothyroid symptoms are insufferable, the patient who becomes hypothyroid within the first 2 months after treatment should abstain from T_4 therapy for 1-to-2 months. This is especially true if there is a persisting goiter. If the hypothyroidism continues for 2 months, it is probably permanent. The patient should then begin taking exogenous T_4.

Cooper[234] stated that patients with nodular toxic goiter who start the use of thionamides soon after radioiodine therapy appear to reduce the rate of hypothyroidism.[249] However, this may also increase the rate of failure of the radioiodine treatment.[250][251] He recommended that if thionamides are to be used after radioiodine treatment to produce a faster relief from hyperthyroidism, the radioiodine dosage should probably be increased.[234,p.902]

IODINE DEFICIENCY OR EXCESS

Iodine deficiency is by far the most common factor that interferes with thyroid hormone biosynthesis.[235,p.919] Ingesting subthreshold amounts of iodine tends to increase TSH secretion and thyroid iodine uptake, decrease thyroxine synthesis, increase the ratio of T_3/T_4 secretion, increase the ratio of circulating T_3/T_4 concentrations, and induce goiter.

On the other hand, excess iodine ingestion can inhibit thyroid hormone synthesis by blocking biosynthetic enzymes in the thyroid gland. This is likely to result in decreased secretion of T_4, increased TSH levels, development of goiter, and if the iodine excess is chronic, hypothyroidism.[138] Amounts 50-to-1000 times more than the recommended minimum dietary allowance (which is 150-to-300 µg/d) induces clinical hypothyroidism.[285][286][287] Along the coastal regions of Japan, residents who consume large amounts of seaweed (which contains iodine) have a high incidence of goiter and hypothyroidism.[288] Braverman et al. argued that induction of goiter and hypothyroidism by iodine occurs in individuals who have an underlying thyroid disease such as Hashimoto's thyroiditis.[289]

Reinhardt evaluated the effect of small doses of iodine on thyroid function and thyroid antibody levels in euthyroid patients with Hashimoto's thyroiditis. The patients lived in an area of mild dietary iodine deficiency. Seven patients in the iodine-treated group developed subclinical hypothyroidism; 1 patient became hypothyroid. Three of the 7 patients who developed subclinical hypothyroidism became euthyroid again when they stopped taking iodine. One patient developed hyperthyroidism with an increased antibody titer but became euthyroid again after stopping the iodine. One control patient, not taking iodine, developed subclinical hypothyroidism. Four of the 8 patients who developed subclinical hypothyroidism had TSH concentrations above 3 mU/L. No change in thyroid function or antibody titers occured in 32 patients taking iodine. The researchers concluded that small amounts of supplementary iodine (250 µg) induced slight but significant changes in thyroid hormone function in predisposed patients.[112]

LITHIUM

The actions of lithium on thyroid function are similar to those of iodine.[234,p.900] The thyroid gland concentrates lithium,[274] probably after actively importing it. Lithium appears to block thyroid hormone release,[275][276][277] but it probably also inhibits hormone biosynthesis.[274][276] The inhibitory effects on the gland may diminish or cease with long-term use of lithium. Investigators compared the relative effectiveness of lithium and thionamides in the treatment of thyrotoxicosis in Graves' disease. Lithium was no more effective than thionamides, and its use is less desirable in that it is potentially more toxic.[278] It is useful in treating thyrotoxic storm in patients who are allergic to and cannot use iodine.[234,p.900]

Hypothyroidism Associated with Lithium Therapy

The use of lithium induces subclinical hypothyroidism in many patients.[280][281] Emerson and coworkers found that sometime during the course of lithium therapy, 30% of patients had mildly-to-moderately elevated TSH levels. Elevations occurred from 3 months-to-4 years after the patients started lithium treatment. In some patients, elevated TSH levels were not permanent. Most did not have low T_4 levels, which justifies the diagnosis of subclinical hypothyroidism.[281] Fauerholdt and Vendsborg wrote that about 3% of patients who take lithium salts for prolonged times form goiters, become hypothyroid, or both.[316]

Many patients also develop overt hypothyroidism during their use of lithium.[282][283] After 5 years of lithium use, 15% of patients developed hypothyroid symptoms and had low T_4 and high TSH levels.[284] They required T_4 therapy.

THYROID GLAND TRAUMA

Some musculoskeletal specialists contend that trauma to the thyroid gland during a whiplash injury can induce hypothyroidism. Sehnert and Croft studied 101 consecutive post-whiplash trauma patients. They found that the basal metabolic temperatures of 86.4% of the patients were below normal. Of these patients, 30% had abnormal laboratory thyroid function test results indicating hypothyroidism. Of the 13% of the patients whose temperatures were normal, 33% had abnormal laboratory test results. The researchers considered 30% of the 101 patients to have post-traumatic hypothyroidism. They concluded, "Whiplash seems to result in a form of hypothyroidism suggesting direct injury to central tissues."[336]

There are numerous ways by which the thyroid gland can be traumatized. Armstrong, Funk, and Rice reported that hemorrhage into cystic thyroid nodules occurs fairly often. In most cases, hemorrhage is slight and the only symptoms are pain and some neck swelling. Trauma occasionally causes massive hemorrhage. This can induce a rapidly expanding thyroid hematoma that can compromise passage of air through the airway.[215] Other researchers have reported similar findings.[216][217] Whiplashing the neck or traumatizing the chin on the dashboard of a car can vertically traction the larynx and trachea and cause laryngeal rupture.[219] In such cases, the laryngotracheal axis may kink and scar tissue may grow into the larynx. Stenosis of the airway can occur unless a straight dilator is installed as an internal splint. Thyroiditis has also been caused by trauma sustained from a seat belt.[218]

"Palpatory" thyroiditis is an iatrogenic traumatically-induced thyroid gland inflammation. Some thyroid gland specimens, such as those obtained from surgical resection, show occasional disorganized follicles with colloid breakdown, macrophages, and foreign-body giant cells.[153,pp.609-610] These microscopic findings appear to result from palpation of the thyroid gland by a clinician. The findings appear to constitute post-traumatic thyroiditis.[159]

After a life-threatening trauma, one patient had a traumatically-induced aneurysm of the inferior thyroid artery.[137] The aneurysm was found after hemodynamic instability prompted angiographical examination. The aneurysm was corrected by ligation and excision.

Some patients being treated for head or neck neoplasia develop hypothyroidism. In one study, T_4 levels became abnormally low in 10% of patients subsequent to treatment, and TSH levels became high in 15%. The authors conjectured that the hypothyroidism resulted from damage during surgery, from radiation therapy, or from a combination of both.[220]

In the War Hospital in Slavonski Brod, Croatia, between September 1, 1991, and December 31, 1992, 7,043 patients were treated.[136] Of these, 728 patients had combat head and neck injuries. Of the patients with penetrating neck injuries, vital structures were involved in 49 cases. Only 3 involved the thyroid gland. This suggests that external trauma during combat is not a common cause of thyroid gland injury.

Development of Fibromyalgia Following Neck Trauma

Buskila et al. assessed 102 patients with neck injury and 59 patients with leg fractures (control group) for nonarticular tenderness and the presence of fibromyalgia. None of the patients had a chronic pain syndrome prior to the trauma. Fibromyalgia developed at a mean of 3.2 months after the trauma. Of the patients with neck injury, 21.6% met the criteria for fibromyal-

gia. Only 1.7% of patients with lower extremity fractures met the criteria. The incidence of fibromyalgia among patients with neck injury was 13 times that of patients with lower extremity injury. The difference between the two groups was significant (P=0.001). Compared to the leg fracture patients with fibromyalgia, the 22 neck injury fibromyalgia patients had more fibromyalgia symptoms and their symptoms were more severe. They had more tenderness, more impaired physical functioning, and reported a lower quality of life than did patients without fibromyalgia.[335]

BROMIDE

Bromide has long been used as a sedative. Bromide use has been reported to induce hypothyroidism due to loss of iodine from the thyroid gland. In the one reported case, thyroid gland cells were hyperplastic, colloid was lost, and there were areas of papillary proliferation.[321] Van Gelderen et al., however, found no effect of sodium bromide use on the thyroid-binding globulin, T_4, free T_4, T_3, or TSH levels of healthy volunteers.[323] Also, Sangster and colleagues administered "acceptable" dosages of bromide to 21 healthy volunteers and found no changes in any thyroid function test, including the TRH stimulation test.[98]

In contrast to the results of these human studies, several studies with rats have shown significant endocrine effects of bromide. The difference may be the rats' unique reactions to this chemical or toxicity induced by the higher-end dosages used in rat studies. Vobecky and Babicky, for example, found that with increased bromide intake, the bromine concentration in the thyroid gland increased. At the same time, the iodine concentration of the gland decreased.[322]

Buchberger and coworkers studied the effects of bromide on the total and free T_4 and TSH levels in the blood and the thyroid hormone concentrations in the thyroid gland. They found typical indicators of hypothyroidism. They wrote, "The results of this study also indicate that bromide toxicity is dependent upon the state of the iodine supply, which should be taken into account for evaluation of acceptable daily intake values for bromide."[324]

Loeber and colleagues found that bromide decreased the amount of T_4 in the thyroid gland and serum and increased the serum TSH level. Spermatogenesis in the testes was decreased, as were testosterone and corticosterone in the serum. ACTH levels were also increased. Most of these effects were attained at the highest dosages of bromide given. The researchers concluded that bromide directly disturbs the function of the thyroid and adrenal glands and the testes. There were no obvious microscopic abnormalities in offspring. The investigators wrote that bromide appears to exert an inhibitory effect on the thyroid gland with a secondary increase in TSH secretion by the pituitary gland.[325]

Van Leeuwen and coworkers found that the most prominent effect of high-dose bromide in rats was reduction of thyroid hormone production and increased TSH levels. They also found decreased spermatogenesis by the testes, decreased secretory activity by the prostate, and a reduction in the number of corpora lutea in the ovaries. Follow-up for 3 generations showed decreased fertility that was reversed with withdrawal of bromide from the diet.[97]

GROWTH HORMONE INJECTIONS

Bennett et al. reported using growth hormone injections as a treatment for fibromyalgia. They concluded that impaired growth hormone secretion is a part of the fibromyalgia complex that can be treated with replacement therapy, and that the therapy provides relief for many patients with low somatomedin C levels.[317]

Injections of exogenous growth hormone may adversely affect patients in several ways. Antibodies to growth hormone have been reported in 30%-to-40% of children treated with injected somatrem (recombinant methionyl-growth hormone) and 7%-to-20% treated with somatropin (recombinant growth hormone).[319] These preparations, derived from recombinant DNA, are intramuscular injectables. The injections are minimally painful but may lead to local lipoatrophy.[320,p.1342] In addition, treatment with growth hormone inhibits the thyroid gland from taking up iodine,[318] possibly antagonizing formation of thyroid hormone.

Injected growth hormone may impede thyroid hormone metabolism.[63,p.E192] Some children treated with growth hormone develop hypothyroidism.[320,p.1342] As a result, if a fibromyalgia patient is hypothyroid, taking growth hormone may worsen the thyroid hormone deficiency. If a patient is not already hypothyroid, inhibition of iodine uptake by the gland may cause a thyroid hormone deficiency.

VIRAL INFECTION

I mention viral infection as a mechanism of hypo-

thyroidism only as a possibility for some cases without apparent cause. An example of this possibility is the thyroid hormone deficiency caused by infection of sheep with border disease virus. Anderson et al. inoculated pregnant sheep with the virus. After birth, staining showed sparse antibodies for the virus in the pituitary cells of the lambs and large numbers of antibodies in thyroid gland follicular epithelial cells.[76] This was consistent with other investigators' findings.[77] Infected cells were morphologically normal. TSH levels were normal, but T_3 and T_4 levels were significantly low in infected lambs. This study confirmed virus-induced hypothyroidism in sheep. Anderson et al.[76] noted that hypothyroidism has been documented to result from congenital rubella syndrome, the nonarbo togavirus infection of human beings.[78]

● CAUSES OF CENTRAL HYPOTHYROIDISM

A PRECAUTION

Braverman and Utiger cautioned that some of the causes of central hypothyroidism can be disabling and possibly fatal. They wrote, "For this reason, and because primary hypothyroidism may not be due to permanent thyroid destruction, an attempt should always be made to determine the cause of hypothyroidism in an individual patient."[235,p.919] They also wrote that although it may be difficult to identify the cause of hypothyroidism, it is possible to do so with a history, physical examination, and tests for thyroid autoantibodies.[235,p.920] At minimum, when evaluating a patient who has thyroid function test results consistent with hypothyroidism, the clinician should meticulously screen for clinical indications of hypothalamic or pituitary hormone abnormalities. Table 2.4.1 contains a list of factors and disorders associated with central hypothyroidism that Pinchera, Martino, and Faglia[227,p.969] provided. One or more of these factors or disorders may be responsible for a patient's central hypothyroidism.

ACCIDENTAL AND SURGICAL TRAUMA

The first case of documented hypothalamic hypothyroidism was reported in 1971. Pittman et al. attributed the responsible hypothalamic lesion to head trauma.[221] Subsequently, others have ascribed hypothalamic hypothyroidism to head injury. Some injuries were associated with prolonged coma[222][223][224] and others were not.[225]

Surgical therapy for pituitary tumors may result in hypothyroidism due to impaired TSH production.[226] This form of central hypothyroidism is subclassified as pituitary hypothyroidism. Pinchera et al. wrote that about 10% of patients who undergo radical tumor excision subsequently developed hypothyroidism. By contrast, patients who undergo selective excision of micro-adenomata rarely developed hypothyroidism as a result.[227,p.970]

RADIOTHERAPY

Hypothyroidism is in some cases a sequella to thyroid gland damage during surgery, radiation therapy, or a combination of both.[220] The hypothalamus, pituitary gland, and thyroid gland are often damaged during radiotherapy for tumors of the head or neck.[227,p.970] In patients irradiated for nasopharyngeal tumors, researchers believed that 8 of 15 developed hypothyroidism due to pituitary or hypothalamic lesions.[228] The same outcome resulted for 13 of 65 patients irradiated for carcinoma of the nasopharynx or paranasal sinuses.[229] When patients undergo conventional external radiotherapy for acromegaly or pituitary tumors, about 10% develop TSH deficiency and other features of pituitary insufficiency.[230][231][232] Of those treated with α-particle irradiation, up to 33% develop hypopituitarism with TSH deficiency.[233]

USE OF TRICYCLIC AND MONOAMINE OXIDASE (MAO) ANTIDEPRESSANTS

Riley and coworkers reported that administering fluoxetin (Prozac) to adult rats decreased the levels of TRH mRNA by 48%±4%.[109,p.254] They also found that the serotonin-reuptake inhibitor zimelidine decreased TRH mRNA by 69%±11%.[109,p253] These findings raise the possibility that Prozac and zimelidine may impair metabolism by inducing hypothalamic hypothyroidism.

Two antidepressants, imipramine and tranylcypromine, have been shown to profoundly decrease resting metabolic rate (17%-to-24%) and to increase body weight.[110] The antidepressant carbamazepine, while not producing "frank hypothyroidism," caused a significant fall in thyroid hormone levels.[111] The mean decrease in total T_4 was 1.78 µg/dL. The researchers

referred to this decrease of 23.7% as "robust."[111,p.783] The mean decrease in free T_4 was 0.27 µg/dL. Nine of 11 patients had a mean decrease in T_3 of 16 ng/dL, but this decrease did not reach significance. There was a 2.7% decrease in the resting metabolic rate (-0.84 kcal/m²/hr) which also did not reach significance. Clinicians should bear in mind, however, that significance refers to the difference between the means of treated and untreated patients. Some individuals within the treatment group might have had a substantial reduction in resting metabolic rate that was obscured by less marked or unchanged metabolic rates of others in the treated group. This is one of the shortcomings of group statistics studies: They do not reflect the true patterns of reaction of individuals. Instead, they bury the individual patterns in averaged figures. The researchers stated that they could not rule out the possibility of a significant subtle decrease in resting metabolic rate with a much larger sample size.[111,p.783]

There are questions of particular concern regarding patients who take antidepressants: Do the metabolism-slowing effects stop after the patients stop the antidepressant medication? And if so, does a longer and higher-dose exposure to tricyclics and MAOs render an individual hypometabolic even after ceasing the medication?[111,p.785] Herman and colleagues[111,p.785] found an inverse correlation between baseline resting metabolic rate and the number of months during the prior 5 years that depressed patients took carbamazepine. This suggests that repeated and lengthy use of tricyclic and MAO antidepressants may cause sustained hypometabolism.

USE OF EXOGENOUS DOPAMINE

Dopamine and dopamine-agonist drugs, acting through hypothalamic DA_2 (dopamine) receptors, stimulate TRH secretion by the rat hypothalamus.[82][83] The increased secretion of TRH increases TSH secretion. However, dopamine and dopamine-agonist drugs also stimulate release of somatostatin from the hypothalamus.[82][83] Administering somatostatin to humans has caused a number of effects that militate against increased TSH secretion after dopamine administration. Administering somatostatin (1) lowered the elevated TSH levels during untreated primary hypothyroidism,[84] (2) suppressed the TSH response to injected TRH,[85] (3) eliminated the nocturnal rise in TSH level,[86] and directly to the point, (4) blocked TSH release in subjects after researchers administrated dopamine agonist drugs.[81]

Table 2.4.1. Disorders associated with pituitary and hypothalamic (central) hypothyroidism*

Pituitary Disorders:

>   Aneurysm of internal carotid artery
>   Chronic lymphocytic hypophysitis
>   Genetic abnormality in TSH synthesis
>   Hemochromatosis
>   Histiocytosis (Hand-Schüller-Christian disease)
>   Iatrogenic disorders
>   Radiation therapy
>   Surgery
>   Idiopathic disorders
>   Infectious diseases
>   Pyogenic
>   Syphilis
>   Tuberculosis
>   Ischemic necrosis
>   Diabetes mellitus
>   Postpartum (Sheehan's syndrome)
>   Severe shock
>   Pituitary aplasia or hypoplasia
>   Sarcoidosis
>   Somatic joint dysfunction/upper cervical spinal
>   segments
>   Tumors
>   Caranipharyngiomas
>   Metastatic tumors
>   Pituitary adenomas (secreting and nonsecreting)

Hypothalamic Disorders:

>   Congenital malformation
>   Histiocytosis
>   Iatrogenic
>   Radiation therapy
>   Surgery
>   Ischemic necrosis
>   Idiopathic disorders
>   Sarcoidosis
>   Traumatic disorders
>   Tumors
>   Suprasellar spreading of pituitary adenomas
>   Craniopharyngiomas
>   Meningiomas, gliomas, and other primary tumors
>   Metastatic tumors

*After Pinchera, A., Martino, E., and Faglia, G.: Central hypothyroidism. In *Werner and Ingbar's The Thyroid: A Fundamental and Clinical Text*, 6th edition. Edited by L.E. Braverman and R.D. Utiger, New York, J.B. Lippincott Co., 1991.[227,p.969]

Scanlon pointed out that in humans it is well-established that dopamine inhibits release of TSH by the anterior pituitary thyrotrophs.[106,p.239] Dopamine seems poised to inhibit pituitary secretion of TSH: Its con-

centration in the hypophyseal portal blood is higher than in peripheral blood, and the concentration is high enough to effectively inhibit the thyrotrophs.[95][96] The inhibition is mediated by the binding of dopamine to anterior pituitary DA_2 receptors.[92] These receptors, upon binding to dopamine, decrease adenylate cyclase activity.[106,p.239]

TSH may specifically regulate its own secretion by induction of DA_2 receptors on thyrotroph cells.[93] Increased secretion of TSH increases the number (but not the affinity) of DA_2 receptors. In turn, binding of dopamine to the DA_2 receptors inhibits TSH secretion. This is indicated by the stronger inhibition of TSH secretion by dopamine in hypothyroid animals.[94]

Dopamine also suppresses TSH synthesis by inhibiting the genes for the two components of the TSH molecule: the α-subunit and TSH β-subunit. Dopamine most potently inhibits the genes in primary hypothyroid patients.[79][80] In cultured anterior pituitary cells from hypothyroid rats, dopamine reduced gene transcription with a 75% reduction in the levels of α-subunit and TSH β-subunit mRNAs.[91] (The α-subunit is also common to glycoprotein hormones other than TSH, such as luteinizing hormone, follicle-stimulating hormone, and chorionic gonadotropin. The β-subunit of each hormone provides the biologic specificity of the hormone.[87] α-Subunits and TSH β-subunits must be combined to exert biologic action.[106,p.230] Separate genes located on different chromosomes code for the two subunits:[89][90] The α-subunit is encoded on chromosome 6 and the TSH β-subunit on chromosome 1.[91])

The inhibition of TSH release by dopamine is greater in patients with mild or subclinical hypothyroidism than in either normal subjects or those with severe hypothyroidism.[81] Many fibromyalgia patients are mildly or subclinically hypothyroid, and these patients may be more prone than other individuals to inhibition of TSH secretion by exogenous dopamine.

ADENOSINE

Adenosine is a purine neurotransmitter. Administering adenosine into the cerebral ventricles of rats induced inhibition of TSH secretion and elevation of the prolactin level.[105] Because of this finding, Scanlon wrote that adenosine should be added to the growing list of chemicals that can influence TSH secretion but that do not have clear physiologic relevance.[106,p.241]

Adenosine has inhibitory effects on humans.[88] It is probably through inhibiting this inhibitory chemical that caffeine increases alertness and improves mood and cognitive function.[88] The stimulatory effect of caffeine may be mediated partly by freeing TSH of suppression by adenosine. It is possible that many people who perceive that caffeine benefits them may have hypometabolism due to an excessive influence of endogenous adenosine. If so, their health in general may be substantially improved by the intake of small-to-moderate amounts of caffeine at intervals throughout the day. I say this based on the presumption that the individual does not have adverse effects from caffeine. The patient should, of course, observe reasonable precautions (see Chapter 5.5).

● FACTORS THAT DISRUPT MULTIPLE STEPS OF THE THYROID SYSTEM

Elevated cortisol levels, environmental contaminants such as dioxins and PCBs, and the disease hemochromatosis can interfere with more than one step in, and thus disrupt, the thyroid system.

ELEVATED GLUCOCORTICOIDS

Thyroid function may be increased by acute stress. Thyroid function is temporarily suppressed, however, by elevated cortisol due to chronic stress or the use of exogenous cortisol.

Effects of Acute Stress on Thyroid Function

Reports of the effects of acute mental stress on thyroid hormone levels are confusing. An early study suggested that hormone levels were increased during acute stress. The investigators concluded this because the protein bound iodine was elevated in psychiatric patients under stress and in medical students while taking examinations.[121] Increases of the free thyroxine index were consistently found as acute psychiatric patients were being admitted (7%-to-18%).[123][124] Since acute stress has been shown to increase cortisol secretion (for example, emotional arousal prior to a gymnasium exercise program increased adrenal cortical activity[122][132]), an increase in cortisol secretion in these psychiatric patients could have inhibited T_4 to T_3 conversion, raising the T_4 level into the high-normal range and lowering the T_3 level into the low-normal range. Values, however, tended to become normal over time and as the patients were treated for their psychiatric conditions. Researchers have rarely found ab-

normal serum T_3 levels in psychiatric patients.[116,p.174]

Elevated Cortisol Due to Sustained Stress or the Use of Exogenous Cortisol

Brabant et al. wrote that cortisol does not play a primary role in regulating TSH secretion.[120] And Nicoloff et al. wrote that during normal physiology, cortisol does not markedly alter the overall circadian rhythms of TSH release, although cortisol does dampen the rhythms during stress. There is considerable evidence, however, that glucocorticoids exert a suppressive effect on the thyroid hormone system.[119]

Sufficiently high circulating cortisol levels suppress the thyroid hormone system in two ways: by suppressing TSH secretion by the anterior pituitary gland and by inhibiting conversion of T_4 to T_3. These effects may contribute to the decreases in serum T_3 during starvation, acute heat (due to high environmental temperature or febrile illness),[125][126] and non-thyroidal diseases.[116,p.173] It is important to realize, however, that these effects of elevated cortisol are *transient*. It is well-documented that the suppression reverses to normal within 1-to-3 weeks.[134] Nicoloff et al. described this as "escape" from the suppressive influence of cortisol. This is true even though circulating cortisol levels remain elevated due to continuing stress or because a patient continues to take exogenous cortisol.[119] (For documentation, see Chapter 2.5, section titled "Proposal of a Sustained Euthyroid Sick Syndrome Under the Expropriated Name 'Wilson's Syndrome.'")

Effects of Cortisol on TSH Secretion. Glucocorticoids suppress TSH secretion and blunt the TSH response to TRH.[129][130][131][134] The endocrine response to surgery is complex, but there is some typical interaction of the adrenal glands and the hypothalamic-pituitary-thyroid axis. The serum cortisol level undergoes a marked rise with its peak at night rather than the morning—the reverse of normal. There is a marked drop in serum T_3 and an increase in reverse T_3. The serum T_4 does not change. Immediately after surgery, the basal serum TSH level decreases sharply, and the normal nighttime surge in the serum TSH level disappears. About a week after surgery, these abnormal thyroid values return to normal.[117]

Wilbur and Utiger suggest that as well as suppressing TSH secretion, glucocorticoids also inhibit TRH secretion by the hypothalamus.[135] Taking high doses of cortisol (such as prednisone) tends to inhibit for a period of weeks TSH secretion induced by TRH. The magnitude of the effect of glucocorticoids is determined by the individual's endocrine status, the type of glucocorticoid used, the dose, and whether it is taken by mouth or injection.[127][128]

Inhibition of TSH secretion also occurs in patients with Cushing's syndrome,[119][127] a disorder resulting from increased adrenocortical secretion of cortisol. The normal nocturnal surge in TSH secretion does not occur in patients with primary adrenal cortisol-secreting tumors or ACTH-secreting pituitary adenomata. These findings indicate that increased cortisol levels suppress the nocturnal surge of TSH.[118,p.809][273] However, even in Cushing's syndrome patients, the suppression only lasts a few weeks (see above).

Decreased Conversion of T_4 to T_3 During Cortisol-Elevating Stresses. The rate of T_4 to T_3 conversion decreases during physical trauma, prolonged emotional arousal, sickness, or fasting. This results in decreased T_3 levels and increased rT_3 levels. The decreased conversion results from the elevated glucocorticoid levels typical of conditions such as trauma and emotional arousal.[116,pp.173&188-189] Glucocorticoids inhibit outer ring deiodination of T_4 in the peripheral tissues, and this increases the production of reverse T_3.[127][128] The serum T_3 level may be low compared to that of T_4.[116,p.188] Glucocorticoids suppress conversion of either endogenous or exogenous T_4.[133]

A low T_3 level due to the impaired conversion of T_4 to T_3 is not a form of hypothyroidism. The reason it is not is that the low T_3 level is not caused by reduced thyroid gland production of thyroid hormones. Instead, it is more useful to view the impaired T_4 to T_3 conversion as a mechanism of cellular resistance to thyroid hormone.

Clinical Hypometabolism Induced by Suppression of the Hypothalamic-Pituitary-Thyroid Axis by Elevated Cortisol Levels. Some authors have stated that although the TSH response to TRH injection is blunted in Cushing's syndrome[271] and during prolonged corticosteroid use,[272] clinical hypothyroidism (by which they mean the clinical syndrome resulting from inadequate thyroid hormone stimulation of tissues) does not occur. Braverman and Utiger pointed out that most T_3 production is extrathyroidal and that extrathyroidal production is impaired in "many" patients.[235,p.919] They also wrote that decreased T_3 production in these patients is not accompanied by recognizable features of hypothyroidism. There are good reasons to believe that this is not true (see Chapter 2.5, section titled "Do Low T_3 Levels Due to Impaired T_4 to T_3 Conversion in Nonthyroidal Illness Cause Features Typical of Hypothyroidism?").

Theoretically, whether decreased T_3 production generates symptoms of hypometabolism in any particular individual is determined by his or her tissue metabolic sufficiency beforehand. It is reasonable to expect symptoms to develop in at least one circumstance: when a small decrease in metabolic drive due to reduced T_3 availability is superimposed on tissue metabolic status that is barely above the threshold for symptom production. Thus, stress-mediated elevation of cortisol, by suppressing TSH secretion and blocking T_4 to T_3 conversion, may produce at least transient hypometabolism. If this metabolic slow-down compounds borderline metabolic sufficiency in the individual, symptoms of fibromyalgia may result.

Smythe conjectured that trauma could precipitate fibromyalgia,[99] and Wolfe reported that 24% of patients indicated that trauma caused their fibromyalgia.[100] Greenfield and colleagues found that 29 (23%) of 127 patients diagnosed as having primary fibromyalgia reported having trauma, surgery, or a medical illness before the onset of their fibromyalgia. (Of these 29 patients, 25 (86%) developed fibromyalgia following trauma or surgery. There is a high incidence of fibromyalgia in the hospital population.) These investigators classified this 23% as having "reactive" fibromyalgia. These patients had more disabling symptoms than patients whose fibromyalgia developed insidiously. As a result, they had an unemployment rate of 70%, a disability compensation rate of 34%, and a reduced activity rate of 35%.[101,p.680]

Greenfield speculated that the trauma or surgery that precipitated fibromyalgia in some of his patients may have done so by reducing physical activity. He derived this from the report by 45% of his reactive fibromyalgia patients that the trauma or surgery reduced their physical activity and that the reduced activity preceded the onset of fibromyalgia.[101,p.680] It may be, however, that the trauma, surgery, or illness increased cortisol output, and the elevated cortisol levels blocked TSH secretion and T_4 conversion to T_3. This proposition is supported by the finding that the use of prednisone worsened the status of fibromyalgia patients.[102]

ENVIRONMENTAL CONTAMINANTS

At least two classes of environmental contaminants pose potentially serious health problems among humans: polychlorinated dibenzo-*p*-dioxin and polychlorinated dibenzofuran (dioxins), and polychlorinated biphenyls (PCBs). The number of chlorine atoms in dioxins varies between 1 and 8. This variety results in possibly 75 different congeners (varieties of the same compound) of polychlorinated dibenzo-*p*-dioxin and 135 possible congeners of polychlorinated dibenzofuran. Different chlorine substitutions result in 209 possible congeners of PCB.[20,p.468]

Origin of the Problem of Dioxins and PCBs

Dioxins and PCBs are chemically and physically stable, and they have electrical insulating properties. Because of these features, dioxins and PCBs were commercially produced in the United States between 1930 and 1977. Mixtures of them were in wide industrial use, serving as coolant fluids in transformers and dielectric fluids in capacitors.[21] These same features are responsible for the problems with environmental contamination caused by these chemicals.[24] Production and use of these compounds were banned in the late 1970s as a response to their evident adverse health effects.[22][23] Since the early 1980s, there has been a general decline in PCB levels in environmental samples.[45,p.21]

Dioxins and PCBs are still used in significant amounts in older transformers and capacitors. The contaminants do not readily degrade after disposal or dissemination.[20,p.468] Because they are lipophilic, they bind mainly to lipids.[20] This permits them to accumulate and remain in biological organisms. The contaminants are nearly ubiquitous in our environment and are found abundantly in human and animal adipose tissue, milk, blood, and sediment.[24] They have, therefore, accumulated in the food chain. For human beings, the main sources of exposure to these toxic compounds are dairy products, meat, and fish.[20]

Dioxins and PCBs leave the body slowly. *The half-life in human beings is 6-to-10 years.*[25] At least theoretically, preventing the intake of more of these contaminants will eventually clear the body of them.

Transplacental transport exposes fetuses to small quantities of PCBs,[26] but breastfeeding transmits much higher quantities to infants. Human milk is especially polluted with dioxins in highly industrialized and densely populated countries, particularly Germany, Belgium, Sweden, Spain, the Netherlands, and the United Kingdom.[20,p.469] Infant formula contains very small amounts of these toxins. Accordingly, postnatal exposure of formula-fed infants is low.[45,p.21]

Some writers in the field of thyroidology have had a curiously reserved posture toward the possible relation of chemical contaminants to thyroid problems. Barsano, for example, wrote, "A large number of compounds other than drugs are known to interfere with thyroid hormone synthesis and secretion *in vitro*. Many of these are also goitrogenic in animals, but few

have been convincingly demonstrated to cause goiter or hypothyroidism in humans."[279,p.961] However, he cited three studies[309][310][311] showing that the concentration of organic pollutants (such as resorcinol) in the drinking water of Columbia and the state of Kentucky where shale and coal are abundant are positively correlated with a high incidence of thyroid disorders such as goiter. He also cited studies showing that people accidentally exposed to polybrominated biphenyls have low T_4 and high TSH levels.[312][313][314] But he stated that these are ". . . suggestive but not fully convincing of a significant polybrominated biphenyl-related antithyroid effect in humans."[279,p.961] There are many studies relating chemical pollutants to thyroid abnormalities. A surprising few of these, however, made their way into the 1996 edition of the major thyroidology reference text, *Werner's The Thyroid*.[315]

Adverse Effects in Human Beings

Dioxins and PCBs have a wide array of toxic effects in human beings.[30] These include body weight loss, atrophy of the thymus, teratogenicity, carcinogenicity, and toxicity of the liver and reproductive and immune systems.[27][28] The contaminants can also alter thyroid status and metabolism, as I describe in the sections below.

Inhibition of Thyroid Gland Activity. Numerous chemicals and pharmaceutical drugs lower thyroid hormone levels by adversely affecting thyroid gland activity. Perchlorate and thiocyanate, which are ionic inhibitors, suppress iodide uptake by the thyroid gland. They reduce synthesis of thyroid hormones by the gland.[1] Other chemicals, such as propylthiouracil (a thionamide), sulfonamides (aromatic amines), and hexylresorcinol (a polyhydric phenol), inhibit synthesis of thyroid hormones at various stages in the thyroid gland, and they are considered goitrogenic.[2,p.37] PCBs also inhibit thyroid gland synthesis and secretion of thyroid hormones.[3]

Increased Hepatic Degradation Rate of T_4. T_4 is degraded in the liver and excreted in the bile. The catabolic process is called glucuronidation.[12] The microsomal enzyme UDP-GT (uridine diphosphate-glucuronosyltransferase) catalyzes conversion of T_4 and glucuronic acid to T_4-glucuronide. This product is then excreted in the bile.[2,p.36] (Microsomes are particles contained in the endoplasmic reticulum of the cell nucleus.) The bile content of T_4-glucuronide was significantly increased after treatment with a number of UDP-GT inducers. These include PCBs,[8][13] polycyclic hydrocarbons,[14][15] TCDD,[7] phenobarbital,[4][15] and pregnenolone-16α-carbonitrile.[16] Microsomal enzyme inducers have also been shown to reduce circulating thyroid hormone levels. The inducers include phenobarbital,[4] 2,3,7,8-tetrachlorodibenzo-*p*-dioxin (TCDD),[5][6][7] PCBs, and polybrominated biphenyls.[8][9]

Barter and Klaassen found that phenobarbital and 3-methylcholanthrene moderately increased UDP-GT activity and lowered total and free T_4 levels. Pregnenolone-16α-carbonitrile had slightly stronger effects, and PCBs were the most potent in increasing enzyme activity and lowering T_4 levels. The researchers wrote that these chemicals represent a wide class that increases activity of UDP-GT and may reduce T_4. They also found that phenobarbital, PCBs, and pregnenolone-16α-carbonitrile reduced T_3 levels slightly. The reduction in T_3 levels, however, did not correlate with increased activity of UDP-GT, and the reduced levels were not related to glucuronidation of T_4. The reduced T_3 apparently resulted from some other extrathyroidal mechanism.[2,p.40]

In summary, a number of chemicals that induce microsomal enzymes increase the catabolism and excretion of T_4. The increased excretion decreases circulating T_4 levels.

As I describe in the following section, the decrease in circulating T_4 levels in turn increases TSH levels.[2][7][29][30][31][32] Plasma T_3 levels are typically less affected by dioxins and PCBs.[20,p.471] Effects of the contaminants on total T_3, total T_4, free T_4, and TSH are similar in rats, monkeys, and humans.[20,p.471]

Effects on the Thyroid Gland. When phenobarbital, PCBs, and other microsomal enzyme inducers reduce circulating levels of thyroid hormones, the pituitary thyrotrophs secrete more TSH. This feedback loop (see Chapter 2.1), under the influence of these chemicals, results in TSH stimulation of the thyroid gland.[8][10] When prolonged, the thyroid gland stimulation can induce hypertrophy, hyperplasia, and functional abnormalities in the gland.[4][17][18][19]

Phenobarbital promotes thyroid gland tumors.[11] The tumors do not appear to result from a direct toxic effect of phenobarbital on the thyroid gland. Instead, they appear to result from prolonged stimulation of the gland by elevated levels of TSH. The elevated TSH, in turn, results from the low T_4 level due to a phenobarbital-induced increase in the T_4-degrading enzyme UDP-glucuronosyl-transferase.[4][10]

Effects on Thyroid Hormone Transport Proteins. Structurally, dioxins and PCBs are markedly similar to T_4. They selectively bind to and occupy the T_4 binding pocket on transthyretin.[41][42][43][46] (Transthyretin is the most important thyroid hormone transport protein in rats.[34]) In binding to transthyretin, PCBs displace T_4 from the transport protein. The most important thyroid hormone carrier protein in humans, T_4-binding globulin, does not appear to be affected by dioxins and PCBs.[35] Competitive binding of dioxins and PCBs to transthyretin in humans, however, may contribute to a slight degree to the low plasma levels of total T_4. The lower levels would result from the rapid removal of the displaced, and therefore "free," T_4 from the circulation.[41,p.444]

Competitive binding of PCBs to transthyretin may also decrease the amount of T_4 that passes through the blood-brain barrier. T_4 is transported from the circulation into the cerebrospinal fluid by binding to transthyretin formed in the choroid plexus.[37] It is likely that the concentration of T_4 in the brain is lower than normal in fetal and neonatal rats with low plasma levels of total and free T_4 induced by PCBs. This is indicated by the increase of type II T_4 5'-deiodinase in the brains of the rats. This enzyme catalyzes conversion of T_4 to the metabolically active T_3 in the brain.[38] The activity of this enzyme serves to avert slight but dangerous changes in the concentration of T_3 in the brain. During a thyroid hormone deficiency, the conversion rate of T_4 to T_3 increases, and with thyroid hormone excess, the rate decreases. This occurs both in the brain and liver.

Dratman and coworkers measured the effects of chronic thyroid hormone deficiency and excess on brain iodothyronine economy and on the rate of intracranial conversion of T_3 from T_4. They found that after thyroidectomy, the rate of T_4 to T_3 conversion decreased in the liver and increased markedly in the brain. In hyperthyroidism, exactly the opposite direction of change occurred in brain and liver. They wrote, "The results demonstrate that despite extremes of thyroxine availability, brain thyroxine and triiodothyronine concentrations and brain triiodothyronine production and turnover rates are kept within narrow limits. Adjustments in the activity of both brain and liver help to maintain these relatively stable conditions." They concluded, "These responses suggest that brain iodothyronine homeostasis is important for the function of the whole organism. Because signs of nervous system dysfunction develop in hypothyroid and hyperthyroid individuals, it is possible that even relatively small deviations of brain iodocompound economy can produce significant changes in behavior and autonomic nervous system dysfunction."[63] If the amount of T_4 entering the brain is reduced because of competitive binding of PCBs to transthyretin, the protective system of increased activity of type II T_4 5'-

deiodinase may be taxed. If taxed excessively, the protective system may not be able to avert adverse effects on the brain, and in turn, the body as a whole.

I should also mention that during inadequate protein-calorie intake, transthyretin production undergoes a profound decrease. In malnutrition, the decrease may be related to the high tryptophan content of transthyretin. There is also an extremely reduced production of transthyretin in illness. These conditions could therefore lead to a deficiency in the amount of T_4 reaching the brain.[64,p.118]

One might expect that competitive binding to transthyretin, with displacement of T_4 by PCBs, would increase the peripheral metabolic rate by virtue of the resulting increase in free T_4. However, elevated TSH levels show that the pituitary is underexposed rather than overexposed to thyroid hormone. Patients exhibit some indication of hypermetabolic effects, such as hypotonicity and hyperreflexia. But they also have indications of hypometabolism such as elevated serum triglycerides and cholesterol.[24,p.239] Actually, the T_4 referred to in the literature as "free" is not free in the sense that it is displaced from transthyretin and can excessive stimulate cellular metabolism. Instead, the T_4 displaced from transthyretin merely shifts to what McKinney and Pedersen termed "nonspecifically protein bound hormone."[24,p.237] This means that T_4 binds to proteins not specific for transporting thyroid hormone. McKinney and Pedersen stated that T_4 bound to proteins not specific for thyroid hormone is biologically inactive.[24,p.237] As a result, the displaced T_4 is *less* available for conversion to T_3 in cells. Less T_3 is then available for binding to nuclear thyroid hormone receptors and exerting metabolic stimulatory effects.

Adverse Effects in the Fetus and Infant. Small quantities of the mother's thyroid hormones pass to the fetus through the placental barrier.[39] These hormones are important to early fetal development because the fetus does not produce its own thyroid hormones until the 12th week.[20,p.472] Adequate levels of T_4 (to be converted to T_3) are vital to normal brain development.[40] Porterfield[44] wrote that neurologic development in the fetus and neonate occurs in orderly sequences, and deficiencies or excesses of thyroid hormone can severely disturb the sequences. Such disturbed sequences can result in abnormalities of neurological development. At certain developmental stages, disturbances may cause irreversible neurological damage. Porterfield noted that the nature of the damage depends on the developmental period that is disturbed and the severity of the thyroid excess or deficiency.[44]

Adverse Developmental Effects of Thyroid Hor-

mone Deficiency and PCB Contamination. Potter et al. compared the effects on neonate lambs of thyroidectomy at 60 days of gestation to control neonate lambs. The thyroidectomized neonates had significantly lower mean body weight, brain weight, and lower brain DNA, RNA, and protein.[47] Thyroid hormone deficiency at birth caused marked impairment of rat brain differentiation.[54][55] Cell differentiation and synapse formation in the rat cerebellum was retarded in hypothyroidism.[60][61][62] Such effects occur with endemic goiter in humans[56,p.942] and represent a veritable medical and social scourge.[57][58][59] Endemic goiter, however, is due to an iodine deficiency, and this is probably seldom a problem in modern industrialized countries. The important question is whether the thyroid hormone deficiency resulting from contamination with dioxins and PCBs results in similar adverse effects.

McKinney and Pedersen point out that adverse human effects from PCBs may be largely limited to the initial growth phase as happens in hypothyroidism.[24,p.239] They reported the results of studies on the effects of transplacental exposure to PCBs in 912 neonates.[23] Neurologic and psychological tests showed that neonates of mothers with higher PCB levels in their breast milk had hypotonicity and hyperreflexia. Another study comparing clinical status with serum PCB levels revealed that elevated PCBs were associated with elevated serum triglycerides and cholesterol levels.[24,p.239] The elevated lipids probably resulted from inadequate thyroid hormone regulation of fat metabolism (see Chapter 4.3, section titled "Cholesterol, Triglycerides, and Low-Density Lipoproteins").

Jacobson and colleagues conducted two longitudinal studies of the effects of moderate and low exposure to PCBs in U.S. children. The 300 children included in the study were born in the early 1980s. The researchers tested them at birth, during infancy, and at 4 years after birth. The children made up two groups. One (the Michigan cohort) consisted of offspring of women who had eaten relatively large amounts of fish from Lake Michigan. At the time, Lake Michigan was the lake in the U.S. most contaminated with PCBs. The other group (the North Carolina cohort) was made up of offspring of breastfeeding mothers with PCB exposure levels tantamount to that in the population at-large. Testing involved the Bayley Scales (the most commonly used tests of infant development), the Mental Development Index (to assess attention, language, and fine motor coordination), and the Psychomotor Development Index (to assess gross motor function). The North Carolina cohort, at

6, 12, and 24 months, showed a significant relationship between prenatal PCB exposure and poor psychomotor performance. Effects were seen only in the most highly exposed infants. The main finding with the Michigan cohort was an association between prenatal PCB exposure and poor visual recognition memory at 7 months. Infants appeared normal clinically, but test results provided evidence of limited capacity for information processing. In the Michigan cohort, children with the highest exposure levels performed the worst on verbal and memory scales.[49][50]

Brouwer and coauthors commented on these studies. According to them, large quantities of PCBs are transferred to the infant after birth through breastfeeding. Nevertheless, results show that the vulnerability is greatest *in utero*. They conjectured that this is due to the greater sensitivity of cells undergoing mitosis to three factors: toxic substances, the absence of a blood-brain barrier, and different drug-metabolizing capabilities. They pointed out that testing showed the worst effects in children most heavily exposed through higher maternal levels of PCBs. This entailed the top 3%-to-5% in the general population sample from North Carolina, and 11% of the more heavily exposed fish-eating sample from Michigan.[45,p.21] Fein and colleagues found a lower birth weight among infants born to mothers who consumed larger amounts of Lake Michigan fish.[53] This result has also been found in regions where mothers consume relatively large amounts of fatty fish species such as salmon and herring.[52] (Recall that dioxins and PCBs are lipophilic and bind mainly to lipids.[20])

Koopman-Esseboom and coworkers studied 418 healthy Dutch Caucasian mother-infant pairs. Their purpose was in part to assess the effects of *in utero* and lactational PCB and dioxin exposure on thyroid status and neural development of young children.[51] Most infants had high TSH levels, and those with higher than average exposure also had low plasma total T_4 and free T_4 levels. Three months after birth, scores on the psychomotor scale were negatively correlated with prenatal PCB exposure: the higher the exposure, the lower the psychomotor score. Researchers found a significantly higher percentage of hypotonia with higher exposure levels of PCBs, and a tendency toward hypotonia with higher dioxin exposure levels. Brouwer et al., in reviewing the results, wrote that *in utero* and lactational exposures were "not related to a *serious* delay in neural development [italics mine]."[45,p.24] However, Koopman-Esseboom et al. found small changes in thyroid hormone levels. They suggested that even these small changes might ad-

versely influence the development of the fetus and infant.[20,p.472] Ahlborg et al. wrote that the 1992 level of exposure of Nordic populations (where consumption of locally-caught fatty fish was high) was within range for subtle adverse health effects in children *in utero* and possibly through breastfeeding.[52]

Possible Mechanism of Adverse Effects. Porterfield defined PCB and dioxin exposures as environmental insults to the fetus and neonate. The chemical structure of these two classes of pollutants is similar to that of thyroid hormones. This provides them with similar binding properties. As a result, problems arise from the pollutants' affinity for and binding to three types of molecules—the cytoplasmic Ah receptor (the "dioxin receptor"[24,p.232][48,p.79]), the nuclear thyroid hormone receptor, and the thyroid hormone transport protein transthyretin. *Depending on the congener and its dosage, PCBs and dioxins either decrease or mimic the biological action of thyroid hormones.*[44]

Either effect during critical stages of brain development can be disastrous for the fetus or neonate. Porterfield pointed out that children who were exposed to dioxins or PCBs in the uterus or during infancy may suffer from behavioral disorders that resemble those resulting from hypothyroidism *in utero* or as infants. He stated that the data suggest these abnormalities in dioxin- and PCB-exposed children can be partially or completely the result of abnormalities of thyroid hormone availability or action. "It is possible," he wrote, "that transient exposure of the mother to doses of toxins presently considered nontoxic to the mother could have an impact upon fetal or perinatal neurological development. If the toxins act via their effect on thyroid hormone action, it is possible that doses of toxins that would normally not alter fetal development could become deleterious if superimposed on a preexisting maternal or fetal thyroid disorder."[44]

Koopman-Esseboom and colleagues found that high levels of dioxins and PCBs were significantly correlated with lower plasma levels of total T_3 and total T_4 in mothers, and with high TSH levels in infants in the 2nd week and 3rd month after birth. The elevated TSH levels indicate compensation for low levels of thyroid hormones. Infants exposed to higher amounts of the pollutants also had lower plasma total and free T_4 levels in the 2nd week after birth.[20] The authors suggested that the small changes in thyroid hormone levels they found may adversely influence the development of the fetus and infant.[20,p.472]

Pluim et al. evaluated at 11 weeks after birth infants exposed to high levels of dioxins in human breast milk. The infants had higher mean plasma TSH levels than infants exposed to medium and low dioxin levels. In contrast to the results of the Koopman-Esseboom study, infants with high dioxin levels had high mean total T₄ levels at 1 and 11 weeks post-birth.[33]

Brouwer et al. studied developmental toxicity with dioxins and PCBs in experimental animals and human infants. After exposure *in utero* and during lactation, both animals and human beings had persistent neurobehavioral, reproductive, and endocrine abnormalities. The researchers reported that the lowest levels of the contaminants causing abnormalities were within the current range of background body levels. They suggested that the method now used to measure levels (the toxic equivalency factor) may underestimate the risk of neural developmental damage.[45]

Whether environmental contaminants play a role in thyroid hormone deficiency in fibromyalgia patients is yet to be determined. But considering the near ubiquitousness of PCBs and dioxins in the environment, their tendency to decrease plasma thyroid hormone levels, and their displacement of T₄ from transthyretin (perhaps lowering brain thyroid hormone concentration), their possible implication in fibromyalgia is worth pursuing.

Mixed Hypothyroid and Hyperthyroid Effects of Dioxins and PCBs. The clinical effects of dioxin and PCB exposure are likely to be typical of hypothyroidism.[24,p.232] McKinney and Pedersen pointed out,[42] however, that the overall toxic-biological effects of dioxins and PCBs are variably those of both hypothyroidism and hyperthyroidism. This is consistent with the finding of low thyroid hormone levels in many patients but high levels in others. Compared to nonexposed control subjects, for example, adults exposed to high levels of PCBs in food had elevated levels of T₃ and T₄ 16 years later.[20,p.471]

McKinney and coauthors proposed that the competitive binding of these pollutants to transthyretin provides a model for their binding to nuclear thyroid hormone receptors.[42] The researchers conjectured that hyperthyroid effects may result from the toxins attaching to thyroid hormone receptors and potently and persistently altering gene expression.[24,p.232][48] This might account for the initial "metabolic boost" found in studies of birds exposed to various chlorinated hydrocarbon insecticides.[107] It might also account for the initial stimulation of growth phase that precedes the inhibition of growth phase in tadpoles and rats exposed to the contaminants.[24,p.239]

Possible Dioxin- and PCB-Induced Pituitary Hypothyroidism. Transthyretin may transport dioxins and PCBs to the pituitary thyrotroph cells and release them there. It is possible that the pollutants bind to T₃ receptors on the TSH gene. The binding could then inhibit transcription for TSH mRNA. This might account for the low normal basal TSH levels in some fibromyalgia patients. It might also account for the blunted TSH response to TRH injection in some.[237][239][242]

Table 2.4.2 is a modified version of the table presented by Barsano. It lists the industrial and environmental chemicals shown to have goitrogenic or antithyroid effects in either humans or other animals.[279,p.962] I encourage interested readers to review the material on these chemicals in Barsano's chapter[279,p.961] and to read the comprehensive review edited by Gaitan.[290]

HEMOCHROMATOSIS

Hemochromatosis is a disease of iron metabolism in which iron accumulates in body tissues. When iron-overload reaches the stage where the tissue deposition is inducing injury and the patient has a total iron body load of greater than 15 gm, the condition is considered hemochromatosis. Primary hemochromatosis results from an autosomal recessive trait linked to the histocompatibility location on chromosome 6p.

Secondary hemochromatosis results from other diseases or disorders that increase the amount of iron ingested or retained in the body tissues. Patients usually have liver cirrhosis, bronze pigmentation of the skin, diabetes mellitus, and cardiomyopathy. It is common for patients to have pituitary failure. It is assumed that most such abnormalities result from the heavy deposit of iron in the parenchyma of tissues.[326,p.1146]

Primary Hypothyroidism

Iron usually accumulates in thyroid gland tissues.[328] In hemochromatosis of the neonate, which can rapidly progress to death, the thyroid gland is among the tissues with excess iron deposition.[330] When the thyroid gland is involved in hemochromatosis, hemosiderin accumulates in the follicular cells and connective tissues of the gland. The concentration of hemosiderin may be enough to discolor the tissues[153,p.613] and induce hypothyroidism.[279,p.958]

Some patients develop hemochromatosis due to multiple blood transfusions (a form of secondary hemochromatosis) and may subsequently become hypothyroid. Himoto and coworkers reported the case of an 11-year-old boy with refractory aplastic anemia who developed secondary hemochromatosis. By age 10, he

Table 2.4.2. Industrial and environmental chemicals shown to have goitrogenic or antithyroid effects in humans and other animals.*

Compounds

Flavonoids (Polyphenols)
　　Aglycons
　　C-ring fission metabolites (phloroglucinols and
　　　　phenolic acids)
　　Glycosides

Inorganic Atoms
　　Excess iodine
　　Lithium

Other Organoclorines
　　Dichlorodiphenyltrichloroethane (*p,p'*-DDT)
　　Dichlorodiphenyltrichloroethane (*p,p'*-DDT) and
　　　　dieldrin
　　2,3,7,8-Tetrachlorodibenzo-*p*-dioxin (TCDD)

Polyhydroxyphenols and Phenol Derivatives
　　2,4-Dinitrophenol
　　2-Methylresorcinol
　　5-Methylresorcinol (orcinol)
　　4-Chlororesorcinol
　　Phloroglucinol (1,3,5-trihydroxybenzene)
　　Pyrogallol (1,2,3-trihydroxybenzene)
　　Resorcinol (1,3-dihydroxybenzene)

**Polychlorinated (PCB) and Polybrominated (PBB)
Biphenyls**
　　PBBs and PBB oxides
　　PCBs (Aroclor)

Polycyclic Aromatic Hydrocarbons (PAH)
　　3,4-Benzpyrene (BaP)
　　3-Methylcolanthrene (MCA)
　　7,12-Dimethylbenzanthracene (DMBA)

Pyridines
　　Dihydroxypyridines

Sulfurated Organic Compounds
　　Disulfides (R-S-S-R)
　　Isothiocyanates
　　L-5-vinyl-2-thiooxazolidone (goitrin)
　　Thiocyanate

*Barsano, C.P.: Other forms of primary hypothyroidism. In *Werner's The Thyroid: A Fundamental and Clinical Text*, 5th edition. Edited by L.E. Braverman and R.D. Utiger, Philadelphia, J.B. Lippincott Co., 1991.[279, p. 962]

had received a total of 100 liters of blood through transfusions. For some reason, the use of iron-chelating agents in the transfused blood had been delayed. He was diagnosed with primary hypothyroidism at age 10 and hypoparathyroidism at age 11.[331] Shirota et al.[332] described a 56-year-old patient who developed secondary hemochromatosis after receiving a total of 20 liters of blood through regular dialysis. Thyroid function testing showed that he had developed primary hypothyroidism. MRI studies and histologic analysis showed that his thyroid gland was among the tissues that accumulated iron. The researchers pointed out that it is rare in hemochromatosis patients for iron deposition in the thyroid gland to cause primary hypothyroidism.

Oerter and coauthors[333] studied endocrine abnormalities in 17 hemochromatosis patients between the ages of 12 and 18. All 17 had at least one endocrine abnormality, and 12 had more than one. The most common abnormalities were of the hypothalamic-pituitary-gonadal axis and involved 14 children. Six had growth hormone abnormalities. Three had primary hypothyroidism.

Edwards et al. assessed the thyroid function of 49 patients who were homozygous for the hemochromatosis allele. Serum T_4 and TSH concentrations were measured. Thirty-four men were homozygous. Three of the 34 men were hypothyroid. They had T_4 levels less than 3.0 µg/dL and TSH levels above 40 µU/mL. One man was hyperthyroid; his T_4 level was 24 µg/dL. Fifteen women who were homozygous for the allele had normal thyroid function test results. The hypothyroid patients had elevated titers of antithyroid antibodies. One patient died and his non-goitrous thyroid gland was examined at autopsy. The histologic examination showed considerable iron deposition, extensive fibrosis, and minor infiltration of lymphocytes. The follicular epithelium that remained was atrophic and loaded with iron. The researchers conjectured that iron accumulation initiated a sequence of pathologic steps that resulted in hypothyroidism: injury of the follicular epithelium, release of thyroidal antigens from the damaged cells, stimulation of antithyroid antibodies by the antigens, inflammation of the gland, fibrosis, atrophy of the epithelium, and deficient thyroid hormone synthesis. They pointed out that men with hemochromatosis had more iron accumulation than women. They also noted that the prevalence of thyroid dysfunction in men with hemochromatosis is some 80 times that of men in the population at-large. The researchers stated that the reversal of the typical sex ration of thyroid dysfunction indicates that iron deposition plays a causative role in thyroid disease.[329]

Central Hypothyroidism

Iron can also accumulate in anterior pituitary cells and cause fibrosis and deficient function of the gland.[327] One result may be central (especially pituitary) hypothyroidism.[227,pp.969-970]

Hereditary Hemochromatosis, Hypothyroidism, and Fibromyalgia

Cindy Munn,[334]RN, contacted me to ask whether I was aware of a relationship between hereditary hemochromatosis (HH) and fibromyalgia. She pointed out that communications over the Internet indicate that there is considerable overlap between the symptoms of the two conditions. She also asked whether I had included ferritin and iron levels in my laboratory testing of fibromyalgia patients to identify those with iron overloads. I had included a ferritin level in the laboratory profile I ordered on some of my fibromyalgia patients, and I had ordered an iron level on all. By means of these tests, I had not identified a fibromyalgia patient who had a problem with iron metabolism.

Munn put me in contact with Cheryl Goodman, MPH, ACSW, a genetic social worker involved in the study of HH. She and her colleagues[108] reviewed the files of people who had been included in their study. They counted those who had thyroid problems and fibromyalgia. They had not, while assessing people during their study, asked specifically whether an individual had a thyroid disorder or fibromyalgia. Thus, when an individual's file indicated that he or she did, the information was unsolicited and anecdotal.

Goodman pointed out that when dealing with hemochromatosis due to mutations in the Hfe gene, there are 6 possible genotypes: CYS/CYS, CYS/-, -/-, CYS/HIS, HIS/HIS, and HIS/-. There were 1145 people in their study. Of these, 21 had reported thyroid problems and 21 had reported fibromyalgia. Only 2 patients had reported both thyroid problems and fibromyalgia. Neither of the 2 patients, however, had any of the hemochromatosis alleles. Their genotype was therefore -/-.

Goodman and her colleagues determined that 61.9% of the 40 people reporting either thyroid problems and/or fibromyalgia had at least one hemochromatosis allele. Of the hemochromatosis patients included in their study, 59% had at least one hemochromatosis allele. The researchers also found that 14% of patients reporting either thyroid problems or fibromyalgia had both copies of the mutant gene. Their genotypes are CYS/CYS, CYS/HIS, or HIS/HIS. Goodman wrote that these patients are at greatest risk for developing hemochromatosis because they have both alleles. Of the whole population of patients included in their study, 25% had both alleles.

Goodman noted that had a larger number of patients been included, it is doubtful whether those reporting thyroid problems and/or fibromyalgia would have had the same percentages with one and two mutant alleles. Having had only 21 patients reporting each clinical condition, the calculated percentages could be inaccurate due to the small sample size.

"In conclusion," Goodman wrote, "we can look at the charts and see that the resulting percentages in each genotypic group are somewhat similar, indicating that there is no difference in the HH incidence between people with thyroid problems or fibromyalgia and the patient population. Also, in the patient population, the percentage of patients with both alleles was slightly higher (25%). Based on this anecdotal evidence, with only a small group to study, more patients without any known or diagnosed thyroid problems were found to have a slightly higher incidence of developing hemochromatosis."

"Finally," she wrote, "the percentages in each genotypic group were quite similar when comparing patients with thyroid problems or fibromyalgia to people in the patient population. From this preliminary data, it does not appear as though there is a connection between developing thyroid problems or fibromyalgia and having HH. Further studies will have to be performed with a larger database in order to come to a more definitive conclusion."

Readers interested in HH can contact Cindy Munn's webpage. The Internet address is <http://www.zoomnet.net/~munsters/>. At this site, she tells of her family's plight with HH under the title "Are you tired all the time?" The Internet address of the American Hemochromatosis Society is <http://www.americanhs.org>.

REFERENCES

1. Haynes, R.C., Jr. and Murad, F.: Thyroid and antithyroid drugs. In *The Pharmacological Basis of Therapeutics*, 7th edition. Edited by A.G. Gilman, L.S. Goodman, T.W. Rall, and F. Murad, New York, MacMillan Co., 1985, pp.1389-1411.

2. Barter, R.A. and Klaassen, C.D.: UDP-glucuronosyltransferase inducers reduce thyroid hormone levels in rats by an extrathyroidal mechanism. *Toxicol. Appl. Pharm.*, 113: 36-42, 1992.

3. Collins, W.T., Jr., Capen, C.C., and Daily, R.E.: Effect of polychlorinated biphenyl (PCB) on the thyroid gland of rats. *Am. J. Pathol.*, 89:119-136, 1977.

4. McClain, R.M., Levin, A.A., Posch, R., and Downing, J.C.: The effect of phenobarbital on the metabolism and excretion of thyroxine in rats. *Toxicol. Appl. Pharmacol.*, 99:216-228, 1989.

5. Potter, C.L., Sipes, I.G., and Russell, D.H.: Hypothyroxinemia and hypothermia in rats in response to 2,3,7,8-

tetrachlorodibenzo-*p*-dioxin administration. *Toxicol. Appl. Pharmacol.*, 69:89-95, 1983.

6. Gorski, J.R. and Rozman, K.: Dose response and time course of hypothyroxinemia and hypoinsulinemia and characterization of insulin hypersensitivity in 2,3,7,8-tetrachlorodibenzo-*p*-dioxin (TCDD)-treated rats. *Toxicology*, 44:297-307, 1987.

7. Bastomsky, C.H.: Enhanced thyroxine metabolism and high uptake goiters in rats after a single dose of 2,3,7,8-tetrachlorodibenzo-*p*-dioxin. *Endocrinol.*, 101:292-296, 1977.

8. Bastomsky, C.H. and Murphy, P.V.N.: Enhanced *in vitro* hepatic glucuronidation of thyroxine in rats following cutaneous application or ingestion of polychlorinated biphenyls. *Can. J. Physiol. Pharmacol.*, 54:23-26, 1976.

9. Allen-Rowlands, C.F., Castracane, V.D., Hamilton, M.G., and Seifter, J.: Effect of polybrominated biphenyls (PBB) on pituitary-thyroid axis of the rat (41099). *Proc. Soc. Exp. Biol. Med.*, 166:506-514, 1981.

10. McClain, R.M., Posch, R.C., Bosakowski, T., and Armstrong, J.M.: Studies on the mode of action for thyroid gland tumor promotion in rats by phenobarbital. *Toxicol. Appl. Pharmacol.*, 94:254-265, 1988.

11. Hiasa, Y., Kitahori, Y., Ohshima, M., Fujita, T., Yuasa, T., Konishi, N., and Miyashiro, A.: Promoting effects of phenobarbital and barbital on the development of thyroid tumors in rats treated with *N*-bis (2-hydroxy-propyl) nitrosamine. *Carcinogenesis*, 3:1187-1190, 1982.

12. Taurog, A., Briggs, F.N., and Chaikoff, I.L.: I[131]-labeled L-thyroxine. II. Nature of the excretion product in bile. *J. Biol. Chem.*, 194:655-668, 1952.

13. Bastomsky, C.H.: Effects of polychlorinated biphenyl mixture (Arochlor 1254) and DDT on biliary thyroxine excretion in rats. *Endocrinol.*, 95:1150-1155, 1974.

14. Bastomsky, C.H. and Papapertou, P.D.: The effect of methylcholanthrene on biliary thyroxine excretion in normal and Gunn rats. *J. Endocrinol.*, 56:267-273, 1973.

15. Goldstein, J.A. and Taurog, A.: Enhanced biliary excretion of thyroxine glucuronide in rats pretreated with benzpyrene. *Biochem. Pharmacol.*, 11:1049-1065, 1968.

16. Japundzic, M.M., Bastomsky, C.H., and Japundzic, I.P.: Enhanced biliary thyroxine excretion in rats treated with pregnenolone-16α-carbonitrile. *Acta Endocrinol.*, 81:110-119, 1976.

17. Hill, R.N., Erdreich, L.S., Paynter, O.E., Roberts, P.A., Rosenthal, S.L., and Wilkinson, C.F.: Thyroid follicular cell carcinogenesis. *Fundam. Appl. Toxicol.*, 12:629-697, 1989.

18. Saunders, J.E., Eigenberg, D.A., Bracht, L.J., Wang, W.R., and VanZwieten, J.J.: Thyroid and liver trophic changes in rats secondary to liver microsomal enzyme induction caused by an experimental leukotriene antagonist (L-649,923). *Toxicol. Appl. Pharmacol.*, 95:378-387, 1988.

19. Comer, C.P., Chengelis, C.P., Levin, S., and Kotsonis, F.N.: Changes in thyroidal function and liver UDP-ucuronosyltransferase activity in rats following administration of a novel imidazole (SC-37211). *Toxicol. Appl. Pharmacol.*, 80:427-436, 1985.

20. Koopman-Esseboom, C., Morse, D.C., Weisglas-Kuperus, et al.: Effects of dioxins and polychlorinated biphenyls on thyroid hormone status of pregnant women and their infants. *Pediat. Res.*, 36(4):468-473, 1994.

21. De Voogt, P. and Brinkman, U.A.T.: Production, properties, and usage of polychlorinated biphenyls. In *Halogenated Biphenyls, Terphenyls, Naphthalenes, Dibenzodioxins, and Related Products*. Edited by R.D. Kimbrough and A.A. Jensen, Amsterdam, Elsevier, 1989, pp.3-45.

22. Kuratsune, M., Yoshimura, T., Matsuzaka, J., and Yamaguchi, A.: Epidemiological study on Yusho, a poisoning caused by ingestion of rice oil contaminated with a commercial brand of polychlorinated biphenyls. *Environ. Health Perspect.*, 1:119-128, 1972.

23. Rogan W.J., Gladen, B.C., Hung, K-L., et al.: Congenital poisoning by polychlorinated biphenyls and their contaminants in Taiwan. *Science*, 241:334-336, 1988.

24. McKinney, J.D. and Pedersen, L.G.: Do residue levels of polychlorinated biphenyls (PCBs) in human blood produce mild hypothyroidism? *J. Theor. Biol.*, 129:231-241, 1987.

25. Michalek, J.E., Tripathi, R.C., Caudill, S.P., and Pirkie, J.L.: Investigation of TCDD half-life heterogeneits in veterans of Operation Ranch Hand. *J. Toxicol. Environ. Health*, 25:20-28, 1992.

26. Schecter, A., Pëpke, O., and Ball, M.: Evidence for transplacental transfer of dioxins from mother to fetus: chlorinated dioxins and dibenzofuran levels in livers of stillborn infants. *Chemosphere*, 21:1017-1022, 1990.

27. Skene, S.A., Dewhurst, I.C., and Greenberg, M.: Polychlorinated dibenzo-*p*-dioxins and polychlorinated dibenzofurans—the risks to human health: a review. *Human Toxicol.*, 8:173-203, 1989.

28. Safe, S.: Polychlorinated biphenyls and polybrominated biphenyls (PBBs): biochemistry, toxicology, and mechanism of action. *Crit. Rev. Toxicol.*, 13:319-395, 1984.

29. Ness, D.K., Schantz, S.L., Moshtaghian, J., and Hanssen, L.G.: Effects of perinatal exposure to specific PCB congeners on thyroid hormone concentrations and thyroid histology in the rat. *Toxicol. Lett.*, 68:311-323, 1993.

30. Emmett, E.A., Maroni, M., Jefferys, J., Schmith, J., Levin, B.K., and Alvares, A.: Studies of transformer repair workers exposed to PCBs. II. Results of clinical laboratory investigations. *Am. J. Ind. Med.*, 14:47-62, 1988.

31. Brewster, D.W., Elwell, M.R., and Birnbaum, L.S.: Toxicity and disposition of 2,3,4,7,8-pentachlorodibenzofuran (4PeDCF) in the rhesus monkey (*Macaca mulatta*). *Toxicol. Appl. Pharmacol.*, 93:231-246, 1988.

32. Van den Berg, K.J., Zurcher, C., and Brouwer, A.: Effects of 3,4,3',4'-tetrachlorobiphenyl on thyroid function and histology in marmoset monkeys. *Toxicol. Appl. Pharmacol.*, 41:77-86, 1988.

33. Pluim, H.J., Koppe, J.G., Olie, K., et al.: Effects of dioxins on thyroid function in newborn babies. *Lancet*, 339:1303, 1992.

34. Brouwer, A. and Van den Berg, K.J.: Binding of a metabolite of 3,4,3',4'-tetrachlorobiphenyl to transthyretins reduces serum vitamin A transport by inhibiting the formation of the protein complex carrying both retinol and thyroxine. *Toxicol. Appl. Pharmacol.*, 85:301-312, 1986.

35. Lans, M.C., Spietz, C., Brouwer, A., and Koeman, J.H.: Different competition of thyroxine binding to transthyretin and thyroxine-binding globulin by hydroxy-PCBs,

PCDDs, and PCDFs. *Eur. J. Pharmacol.*, 270:129-136, 1994.

36. Kravitz, H.M., Katz, R.S., Helmke, N., Jeffriess, H., Bukovsky, J., and Fawcett, J.: Alprazolam and ibuprofen in the treatment of fibromyalgia: report of a double-blind placebo-controlled study. *J. Musculoskel. Pain*, 2(1):3-27, 1994.

37. Herbert, J., Wilcox, J.N., Pham, K-T.C., et al.: Transthyretin: a choroid plexus-specific transport protein in human brain. *Neurology*, 36:900-911, 1986.

38. Morse, D.C., Groen, D., Veerman, M., et al.: Interference of polychlorinated biphenyls in hepatic and brain thyroid hormone metabolism in fetal and neonatal rats. *Toxicol. Appl. Pharmacol.*, 122:27-33, 1993.

39. Vulsma, T., Gons, M.H., and De Vijider, J.J.M.: Maternal-fetal transfer of thyroxine in congenital hypothyroidism due to a total organification defect or thyroid agenesis. *N. Engl. J. Med.*, 321:13-16, 1989.

40. Porterfield, S.P. and Hendrich, C.E.: The role of thyroid hormones in prenatal and neonatal neurological development: current perspectives. *Endocr. Rev.*, 14:94-106, 1993.

41. Brouwer, A.: Inhibition of thyroid hormone transport in plasma of rats by polychlorinated biphenyls. *Arch. Toxicol.*, (Suppl.)13:440-445, 1989.

42. McKinney, J.D., Chae, K., Oatley, S.J., and Blake, C.C.: Molecular interactions of toxic chlorinated dibenzo-*p*-dioxins and dibenzofurans with thyroid binding prealbumin. *J. Med. Chem.*, 28:375-381,1985.

43. Pederson, L.G., Darden, T.A., Oatley, S.J., and McKinney, J.D.: A theoretical study of the binding of polychlorinated biphenyls (PCBs), dibenzodioxins, and dibenzofuran to human plasma prealbumin. *J. Med. Chem.*, 29:2451-2457, 1986.

44. Porterfield, S.P.: Vulnerability of the developing brain to thyroid abnormalities: environmental insults to the thyroid system. *Environ. Health Perspect.*, 102 (Suppl. 2):125-130, 1994.

45. Brouwer, A., Ahlborg, U.G., Van den Berg, M., et al.: Functional aspects of developmental toxicity of polyhalogenated aromatic hydrocarbons in experimental animals and human infants. *Euro. J. Pharmacol.*, 293(1):1-40, 1995.

46. Lans, M.C., Klasson-Wehler, E., Willemsen, M., Meussen, E., Safe, S., and Bouwer, A.: Structure-dependent, competitive interaction of hydroxy-polychlorobiphenyls, -dibenzo-*p*-dioxins and -dibenzo-furans with human transthyretin. *Chemico-Biological Interactions*, 88(1):7-21, 1993.

47. Potter, B.J., McIntosh, G.H., and Hetel, B.S.: The effect of iodine deficiency on fetal brain development in the sheep. In *Fetal Brain Disorders: Recent Approaches to the Problem of Mental Deficiency*. Edited by B.S. Hetzel and R.M. Smith, Amsterdam, Elsevier/North Holland Biomedical Press, 1981, p.119.

48. McKinney, J., Fannin, R., Jordan, K., Chae, U. Rickenbacher, U., and Pedersen, L.: Polychlorinated biphenyls and related compound interactions with specific binding sites for thyroxine in rat liver nuclear extract. *J. Med. Chem.*, 30:79-86, 1987.

49. Jacobson, J.L., Jacobson, S.W., and Humphrey, H.E.B.: Effects of *in utero* exposure to polychlorinated biphenyls and related contaminants on cognitive functioning in young children. *J. Pediatr.*, 116:38-45, 1990.

50. Jacobson, J.L., Jacobson, S.W., and Humphrey, H.E.B.: Effect of *in utero* exposure to PCBs and related compounds on growth and activity in children. *Neurotox. Teratol.*, 12:319, 1990.

51. Koopman-Esseboom, C.M., Huisman, N. Weisglas-Kuperus, C.G., et al.: PCB and dioxin levels in plasma and human milk of 418 Dutch women and their infants: predictive value of PCB congener levels in maternal plasma for fetal and infant's exposure to PCBs and dioxins. *Chemosphere*, 28:1721, 1994.

52. Ahlborg, U.G., Hanberg, A., and Kenne, K.: Risk assessment of polychlorinated biphenyls (PCB). Copenhagen, Nordic Council of Ministers Meeting, 26:1992.

53. Fein, G.G., Jacobson, S.W., Jacobson, P.M., Schwartz, P.M., and Dowler, J.K.: Prenatal exposure to polychlorinated biphenyls: effects on both size and gestational age. *J. Pediatr.*, 105:315, 1983.

54. Eayrs, J.R. and Taylor, S.M.: The effect of thyroid deficiency induced by methylthiouracil on the maturation of the central nervous system. *J. Anat.* (Lond.), 85:350, 1951.

55. Balazs, R., Kovacs, S., Cocks, W.A., Johnson, A.L., and Eayrs, J.T.: Effects of thyroid hormone on the biochemical maturation of rat brain: postnatal cell formation. *Brain Res.*, 25:555, 1971.

56. Delange, F.M.: Endemic cretinism. In *Werner and Ingbar's The Thyroid: A Fundamental and Clinical Text*, 6th edition. Edited by L.E. Braverman and R.D. Utiger, New York, J.B. Lippincott Co., 1991, pp.942-955.

57. Stanbury, J.B., Ermans, A.M., Hetzel, B.S., Pretell, E.A., and Querido, A.: Endemic goiter and cretinism: public health significance and prevention. *WHO Chron.*, 28:220, 1974.

58. Hetzel, B.S., Dunn, J.T., and Stanbury, J.B.: *The Prevention and Control of Iodine Deficiency Disorders*. Amsterdam, Elsevier, 1987.

59. Delange, F.: Endemic cretinism: an overview. In *Iodine and the Brain*. Edited by G.R. Delange, J. Robbins, and P.G. Condiffe, New York, Plenum Press, 1989, p.219.

60. Nicholson, J.L. and Altman, J.: The effects of early hypo- and hyperthyroidism on the development of rat cerebellar cortex. I. Cell proliferation and differentiation. *Brain Res.*, 44:13, 1972.

61. Nicholson, J.L. and Altman, J.: The effects of early hypo- and hyperthyroidism on the development of rat cerebellar cortex. II. Synaptogenesis in the molecular layer. *Brain Res.*, 44:25, 1972.

62. Clos, J. and Legrand, J.: Effects of thyroid deficiency on different cell populations of the cerebellum of the young rat. *Brain Res.*, 63:450, 1973.

63. Dratman, M.B., Crutchfield, F.L., Gordon, J.T., and Jennings, A.S.: Iodothyronine homeostasis in rat brain during hypo- and hyperthyroidism. *Am. J. Physiol.*, 245(2):E185-E193, 1983.

64. Robbins, J.: Thyroid hormone transport proteins and the physiology of hormone binding. In *Werner and Ingbar's The Thyroid: A Fundamental and Clinical Text*, 6th edition. Edited by L.E. Braverman and R.D. Utiger, New

York, J.B. Lippincott Co., 1991, pp.111-125.

65. Kohrle, J., Hesch, R.D., and Leonard, J.L.: Intracellular pathways of iodothyronine metabolism. In *Werner and Ingbar's The Thyroid: A Fundamental and Clinical Text*, 6th edition. Edited by L.E. Braverman and R.D. Utiger, New York, J.B. Lippincott Co., 1991, pp.144-189.

66. Jacobsen, S., Danneskiold-Samse,B., and Andersen, R.B.: Oral S-adenosylmethionine in primary fibromyalgia: double-blind clinical evaluation. *Scand. J. Rheum.*, 20:294-302, 1991.

67. Behne, D., Kyrıakopoulos, A., Meinhold, H., and Koehrle, J.: Identification of type I iodothyronine 5'-deiodinase as a selenoenzyme. *Biochem. Biophys. Res. Commun.*, 173:1143, 1990.

68. Berry, M.J., Banu, L., and Larsen, P.R.: Type I iodothyronine deiodinase is a selenocystein-containing enzyme. *Nature*, 349:438, 1991.

69. Adlkoferr, F., Schurek, H.J., and Sörje, N.: The renal clearance of thyroid hormones in the isolated rat kidney. *Horm. Metab. Res.*, 12:400, 1980.

70. Behne, D., Hilmert, H., Scheid, S., Gessner, H., and Elger, W.: Evidence for specific selenium target tissues and new biologically important selenoproteins. *Biochem. Biophys. Acta*, 966:12, 1988.

71. Behne, D., Scheid, S., Kyrakopoulos, A., and Hilmert, H.: Subcellular distribution of selenoproteins in the liver of the rat. *Biochem. Biophys. Acta*, 1033, 219, 1990.

72. Cody, V.: Thyroid hormone structure-function relationships. In *Werner and Ingbar's The Thyroid: A Fundamental and Clinical Text*, 6th edition. Edited by L.E. Braverman and R.D. Utiger, Philadelphia, J.B. Lippincott Co., 1991, pp.225-229.

73. Aufmkolk, M., Koehrle, J., Hesch, R.D., and Cody, V.: Inhibition of rat liver iodothyronine deiodinase: interactions of aurone with the iodothyronine deiodinase binding site. *J. Biol. Chem.*, 261:11623, 1986.

74. Koehrle, J., Fang, S.L., Yang, Y. , et al.: Rapid effects of the flavonoid EMD 21388 on serum thyroid hormone binding and thyrotropin regulation in the rat. *Endocrinol.*, 125:532, 1989.

75. Safran, M., Koehrle, J., Braverman, L.E., and Leonard, J.L.: Effect of biological alterations of type I 5'-deiodinase activity on affinity labeled membrane proteins in rat liver and kidney. *Endocrinol.*, 126:826, 1990.

76. Anderson, C.A., Higgins, R.J., Smith, M.E., and Osburn, B.I.: Border disease: virus-induced disease in thyroid hormone levels with associated hypomyelination. *Lab. Invest.*, 57(2):168-175, 1987.

77. Terpstra, C.: Detection of border disease antigen in tissues of affected sheep and in cell cultures by immunofluorescence. *Res. Vet. Sci.*, 25:350, 1978.

78. Hanid, T.K.: Hypothyroidism in congenital rubella. *Lancet*, 2:854, 1978.

79. Scanlon, M.F., Chan, V., Health, M., et al.: Dopaminergic control of thyrotropin, alpha-subunit and prolactin in euthyroidism and hypothyroidism: dissociated responses to dopamine receptor blockade with metoclopramide in euthyroid and hypothyroid subjects. *J. Clin. Endocrinol. Metab.*, 53:360, 1981.

80. Peters, J.R., Foord, S.M., Dieguez, C., and Scanlon, M.F.: TSH neuroregulation and alterations in disease states.

Clin. Endocrinol. Metab., 12:669, 1983.

81. Scanlon, M.F., Lewis, M., Weightman, D.R., Chan, V., and Hall, R.: The neuroregulation of human thyrotropin secretion. In *Frontiers in Neuroendocrinology*. Edited by L. Martini and W.F. Ganong, New York, Raven Press, 1980, p.333.

82. Lewis, B.M., Dieguez, C., Lewis, M.D., and Scanlon, M.F.: Dopamine stimulates release of thyrotropin-releasing hormone from perfused intact rat hypothalamus via hypothalamic D_2 receptors. *J. Endocrinol.*, 115:419, 1987.

83. Lewis, B.M., Dieguez, C., Ham, J., et al.: Effects of glucose on TRH, GHRH, somatostatin, and LHRH release from rat hypothalamus *in vitro*. *J. Neuroendocrinol.*, 1: 437, 1989.

84. Lucke, C., Hoffken, B., and Von Zur Muhien, A.: The effect of somatostatin on TSH levels in patients with primary hypothyroidism. *J. Clin. Endocrinol. Metab.*, 41: 1082, 1975.

85. Siler, T.M., Yen, S.S.C., Vale, W., and Guillemin, R.: Inhibition by somatostatin of the release of TSH induced in man by thyrotropin-releasing factor. *J. Clin. Endocrinol. Metab.*, 38:742, 1974.

86. Weeke, J. and Lauberg, P.: Diurnal TSH variations in hypothyroidism. *J. Clin. Endocrinol. Metab.*, 43:32, 1976.

87. Giudice, L.C. and Pierce, J.G.: Separation of functional and nonfunctional subunits of thyrotropin preparations by polyacrylamide gel electrophoresis. *Endocrinol.*, 101:776, 1977.

88. Erfurth, A. and Schmauss, M.: Perspectives on the therapy of neuropsychiatric diseases with adenosinergic substances. *Fortschritte der Neurologie-Psychiatrie*, 63(3):93-98, 1995.

89. Kourides, I.A., Barker, P.E., Gurr, J.A., Pravtcheva, D.A., and Ruddle, F.H.: Assignment of the genes for the alpha and beta subunits of thyrotropin to different mouse chromosomes. *Proc. Natl. Acad. Sci.*, 81:517, 1984.

90. Naylor, S.L., Chin, W.W., Goodman, H.M., Lalley, P.A., Grzeschik, K.H., and Sakagguchi, A.Y.: Chromosome assignment of genes coding the alpha and beta subunits of glycoprotein hormones in man and mouse. *Somatic Cell. Molec. Genet.*, 9:757, 1983.

91. Shupnik, M.A., Ridgway, E.C., and Chin, W.W.: Molecular biology of thyrotropin. *Endocr. Rev.*, 10:459, 1989.

92. Foord, S.M., Peters, J.R., Dieguez, C., Scanlon, M.F., and Hall, R.: Dopamine receptors on intact anterior pituitary cells in culture: functional association with the inhibition of prolactin and thyrotropin. *Endocrinol.*, 112:1567, 1983.

93. Foord, S.M., Peters, J.R., Dieguez, C., Shewring, A.G., Hall, R., and Scanlon, M.F.: TSH regulates thyrotroph responsiveness to dopamine *in vitro*. *Endocrinol.*, 118: 1319, 1985.

94. Foord, S.M., Peters, J.R., Dieguez, C., Jasani, B., Hall, R., and Scanlon, M.F.: Hypothyroid pituitary cells in culture: an analysis of TSH and PRL responses to dopamine and dopamine receptor binding. *Endocrinol.*, 115:407, 1984.

95. Ben-Jonathan, N., Oliver, C., Weiner, H.J., Mical, R.S., and Porter, J.C.: Dopamine in hypophyseal portal plasma of the rat during the estrous cycle and throughout pregnancy. *Endocrinol.*, 100:452, 1977.

96. Johnston, C.A., Gibbs, D.M., and Nigro-Vilar, A.: High

concentrations of epinephrine derived from a central source and of 5-hydroxyindole-3-acetic acid in hypophysial portal plasma. *Endocrinol.*, 113:819, 1983.

97. Van Leeuwen, F.X., den Tonkelaar, E.M., and van Logten, M.J.: Toxicity of sodium bromide in rats: effects on the endocrine system and reproduction. *Food Chem. Toxicol.*, 21(4):383-389, 1983.

98. Sangster, B., Krajnc, E.I., Loeber, J.G., Rauws, A.G., and van Logten, M.J.: Study of sodium bromide in human volunteers, with special emphasis on the endocrine system. *Human Toxicol.*, 1(4):393-402, 1982.

99. Smythe, H.A.: Nonarticular rheumatism. *Arthritis and Allied Conditions*, 10th edition. Edited by D.J. McCarty, Philadelphia, Lea & Febiger, 1985.

100. Wolfe, F.: The clinical syndrome of fibrositis. *Am. J. Med.*, 81(Suppl. 3A):7-14, 1986.

101. Greenfield, S., Fitzcharles, M.-A., and Esdaile, J.M.: Reactive fibromyalgia syndrome. *Arth. Rheumat.*, 35:678-681, 1992.

102. Clark, S., Tindall, E., and Bennett, R.: A double-blind crossover study of prednisone in the treatment of fibrositis (Abstr). *Arthritis Rheum.*, 27:S76,1984.

103. Evered, D.C., Ormston, B.J., Smith, P.A., Hall, R., and Bird, T.: Grades of hypothyroidism. *Brit. Med. J.*, 1:657-662, 1973.

104. Refetoff, S.: Written communication with J. Yellin, July 10, 1996.

105. Ondo, J.G., Walker, M.W., and Wheeler, D.D.: Central actions of adenosine on pituitary secretion of prolactin, luteinising hormone, and thyrotropin. *Neuroendocrinol.*, 49:654, 1989.

106. Scanlon, M.F.: Neuroendocrine control of thyrotropin secretion. In *Werner and Ingbar's The Thyroid: A Fundamental and Clinical Text*, 6th edition. Edited by L.E. Braverman and R.D. Utiger, New York, J.B. Lippincott Co., 1991, pp.230-256.

107. Jeffries, D.J.: *Organochlorine Insecticides*. Edited by F. Moriarty, New York, Academic Press, 1975, pp.131-230.

108. Goodman, C.: Personal communication, July 9, 1998.

109. Riley, L.A., Jonakait, G.M., and Hart, R.P.: Serotonin modulates the levels of mRNAs coding for thyrotropin-releasing hormone and preprotachykinin by different mechanisms in medullary raphe neurons. *Mol. Brain Res.*, 17:251-257, 1993.

110. Fernstrom, M., Epstein, L., Spiker, D., and Kupfer, D.: Resting metabolic rate is reduced in patients treated with antidepressants. *Biol. Psychiatry*, 20:688-692, 1985.

111. Herman, R., Obrzanek, E., Mikalauskas, K.M., Post, R.M., and Jimerson, D.C.: The effects of carbamazepine on resting metabolic rate and thyroid function in depressed patients. *Biol. Psychiatry*, 29:779-788, 1991.

112. Reinhardt, W., Luster, M., Rudorff, K.H., et al.: Effect of small doses of iodine on thyroid function in patients with Hashimoto's thyroiditis residing in an area of mild iodine deficiency. *Eur. J. Endocrinol.*, 139(1):23-28, 1998.

113. Gaches, F., Delaire, L., Nadalon, S., Loustaud-Ratti, V., and Vidal, E.: Frequency of autoimmune diseases in 218 patients with autoimmune thyroid pathologies. *Rev. Med. Interne.*, 19(3):173-179, 1998.

114. Gronbaek, K., Straten, P.T., Ralfkiaer, E., et al.: Somatic Fas mutations in non-Hodgkin's lymphoma: association

with extranodal disease and autoimmunity. *Blood*, 92(9): 3018-3024, 1998.

115. Stassi G, Todaro M, Bucchieri F, et al.: Fas/Fas ligand-driven T cell apoptosis as a consequence of ineffective thyroid immunoprivilege in Hashimoto's thyroiditis. *J. Immunol.*, 162(1):263-267, 1999.

116. DeGroot, L.J., Larsen, P.R., Refetoff, S., and Stanbury, J.B.: *The Thyroid and Its Diseases*, 5th edition. New York, John Wiley & Sons, 1984.

117. Bartalena, L., Martino, E., and Brandi, L.S.: Lack of nocturnal serum thyrotropin surge after surgery. *J. Clin. Endocrinol. Metab.*, 70:293, 1990.

118. Christy, N.P.: The adrenal cortex in thyrotoxicosis. In *Werner and Ingbar's The Thyroid: A Fundamental and Clinical Text*, 6th edition. Edited by L.E. Braverman and R.D. Utiger, Philadelphia, J.B. Lippincott Co., 1991, pp.806-815.

119. Nicoloff, J.T., Fisher, D.A., and Appleman, M.D.: The role of glucocorticoids in the regulation of thyroid function in man. *J. Clin. Invest.*, 49:1922, 1970.

120. Brabant, A., Brabant, G, and Schuermeyer, T.: The role of glucocorticoids in the regulation of thyrotropin. *Acta Endocrinol.* (Copenhagen), 121:95, 1989.

121. Tingley, J.O., Morris, A.W., Hill, S.R., and Pittman, J.A.: The acute thyroid response to emotional stress. *Ala. J. Med. Sci.*, 2:297, 1965.

122. Ulrich, A.C.: Measurement of stress evidenced by college women in situations involving competition. Ph.D. diss., University of Southern California, 1956.

123. Levy, R.P., Jensen, J.B., Laus, V.G., Agle, D.P., and Engel, I.M.: Serum thyroid hormone abnormalities in psychiatric disease. *Metabolism*, 30:1060, 1981.

124. Spratt, D.I., Pont, A., Miller, M.B., McDougall, I.R., Bayer, M.F., and McLaughlin, W.T.: Hyperthyroxinemia in patients with acute psychiatric disorders. *Am. J. Med.* 73:41, 1982.

125. Epstein, Y., Edassin, R., and Sack, J.: Serum 3,5,3'-triiodothyronine and 3,3',5'-triiodothyronine concentrations during acute heat load. *J. Clin. Endocrinol. Metab.*, 49: 677, 1979.

126. Ljunggren, J.-G., Kallner, G., and Tryselius, M.: The effect of body temperature on thyroid hormone levels in patients with nonthyroidal illness. *Acta Med. Scand.*, 202: 459, 1977.

127. Chopra, I.J., Williams, D.E., Orgiazzi, J., and Solomon, D.H.: Opposite effects of dexamethasone or serum concentration of 3,3',5'-triiodothyronine (reverse T_3) and 3,5,3'-triiodothyronine (T_3). *J. Clin. Endocrinol. Metab.*, 41:911, 1975.

128. Duick, D.W., Warren, D.W., Nicoloff, J.T., Otis, C.L., and Croxson, M.S.: Effect of a single dose of dexamethasone on the concentration of serum triiodothyronine in man. *J. Clin. Endocrinol. Metab.*, 39:1151, 1974.

129. Re, R.N., Kourides, I.A., Ridgway, E.C., Weintraub, B.D., and Maloof, F.: The effect of glucocorticoid administration on human pituitary secretion of thyrotropin and prolactin. *J. Clin. Endocrinol. Metab.*, 43:338, 1976.

130. Otsuki, M., Dakoda, M., and Baba, S.: Influence of glucocorticoids on TRH-induced TSH stimulation. *J. Clin. Endocrinol. Metab.*, 36:95, 1973.

131. Dussault, J.H.: The effect of dexamethasone on TSH and

prolactin secretion after TRH stimulation. *Can. Med. Assoc. J.*, 111:1195, 1974.

132. Renold, A.E., Quigley, T.B., Kenard, H.E., and Thorn, G.W.: Reaction of the adrenal cortex to physical and emotional stress in college oarsmen. *New Eng. J. Med.*, 244: 754-757, 1951.

133. Ingbar, S.H.: The effect of cortisone on the thyroidal and renal metabolism of iodine. *Endocrinol.*, 53:171, 1953.

134. Topliss, D.J., White, E.L., and Stockigt, J.R.: Significance of thyrotropin excess in untreated primary adrenal insufficiency. *J. Clin. Endocrinol. Metab.*, 50:52, 1980.

135. Wilber, J.F. and Utiger, R.D.: The effect of glucocorticoids on thyrotropin secretion. *J. Clin. Invest.*, 48:2096, 1969.

136. Prgomet, D., Danic, D., Milicic, D., and Leovic, D.: Management of war-related neck injuries during the war in Croatia: 1991-1992. *Eur. Arch. Oto-Rhino-Laryng.*, 253 (4-5):294-296, 1996.

137. Siegmeth, A., Gabler, C., Sandbach, G., and Vecsei, V.: Traumatic rupture of the inferior thyroid artery. *Unfallchirurg.*, 99(5):368-370, 1996.

138. Fisher, D.A.: Physiological variations in thyroid hormones: physiological and pathophysiological considerations. *Clin. Chem.*, 42(1):135-139, 1996.

139. Volpé, R.: Graves disease. In *Werner and Ingbar's The Thyroid: A Fundamental and Clinical Text*, 6th edition. Edited by L.E. Braverman and R.D. Utiger, New York, J.B. Lippincott Co., 1991, pp.648-657.

140. Tamai, H., Kasagi, K., Takaichi, Y., et al.: Development of spontaneous hypothyroidism in patients with Graves' disease treated with antithyroid drugs: clinical, immunological, and histological findings in 26 patients. *J. Clin. Endocrinol. Metab.*, 69:49, 1989.

141. Hirota, Y., Tamai, H., Hayashi, Y., et al.: Thyroid function and histology in forty-five patients with hyperthyroid Graves' disease in clinical remission more than ten years after thionamide drug treatment. *J. Clin. Endocrinol. Metab.*, 62:165, 1986.

142. Volpé, R.: Immunology of human thyroid disease. In *Autoimmunity in Endocrine Disease*. Edited by R. Volpé, Boca Raton, CRC, 1990, p.73.

143. Christie, J.H. and Morse, R.S.: Hypothyroid Graves' disease. *Am. J. Med.*, 62:291, 1971.

144. Volpé, R.: Graves' disease. In *Thyroid Function and Disease*. Edited by G.W. Burrow, J.H. Oppenheimer, and R. Volpé, Philadelphia, W.B. Saunders, 1989, pp.648-657.

145. Gordin, A. and Lamberg, B.A.: Natural course of symptomless autoimmune thyroiditis. *Lancet*, 2:1234, 1975.

146. Codaccioni, J.L., Oregiazzi, J., Blanc, P., Pugeat, M., Roulier, R., and Carayon, P.: Lasting remissions in patients treated for Graves' hyperthyroidism with propranolol alone. *J. Clin. Endocrinol. Metab.*, 67:656, 1988.

147. Mazzaferri, E.L., Reynolds, J.C., Young, R.L., Thomas, C.N., and Parisi, A.F.: Propranolol as primary therapy for thyrotoxicosis. *J.A.M.A.*, 136:50, 1976.

148. Gorman, C.A., Bahn, R.S., and Garrity, J.A.: Ophthalmopathy. In *Werner and Ingbar's The Thyroid: A Fundamental and Clinical Text*, 6th edition. Edited by L.E. Braverman and R.D. Utiger, New York, J.B. Lippincott Co., 1991, pp.657-676.

149. Thomas, H.M., Jr.: Acropachy: secondary subperiosteal new bone formation. *Arch. Intern. Med.*, 51:571, 1933.

150. Haydar, N.A.: Exophthalmos, digital clubbing and pretibial myxedema in thyroiditis (letter). *J. Clin. Endocrinol. Metab.*, 23:215, 1963.

151. Wick, M.R. and Sawyer, M.D.: Antigenic alterations in autoimmune thyroid diseases: observations and hypotheses. *Arch. Pathol. Lab. Med.*, 113:77, 1989.

152. DeGroot, L.J. and Quintans, J.: The causes of autoimmune thyroid disease. *Endocr. Rev.*, 10:537, 1989.

153. Oertel, J.E. and LiVolsi, V.A.: Pathology of thyroid diseases. In *Werner and Ingbar's The Thyroid: A Fundamental and Clinical Text*, 6th edition. Edited by L.E. Braverman and R.D. Utiger, New York, J.B. Lippincott Co., 1991, pp.601-644.

154. Aichinger, G., Fill, H., and Wick, G.: *In situ* immune complexes, lymphocyte subpopulations, and HLA-DR-positive epithelial cells in Hashimoto thyroiditis. *Lab. Invest.*, 52:132, 1985.

155. Yagi, Y.: Electron microscopic and immunohistochemical studies on Hashimoto's thyroiditis. *Acta Pathol. Japn.*, 31:611, 1981.

156. Katoh, R., Sugai, T., Ono, S., et al.: Mucoepidermoid carcinoma of the thyroid gland. *Cancer*, 65:2020, 1990.

157. Pfaltz, M. and Hedinger, C.E.: Abnormal basement membrane structures in autoimmune thyroid disease. *Lab. Invest.*, 55:531, 1986.

158. Fatourechi, V., McConahey, W.M., and Woolner, L.B.: Hyperthyroidism associated with histologic Hashimoto's thyroiditis. *Mayo Clin. Proc.*, 46:682, 1971.

159. Carney, J.A., Moore, S.B., Northcutt, R.C., Woolner, L.B., and Stillwell, G.K.: Palpation thyroiditis (multifocal granulomatous folliculitis). *Am. J. Clin. Pathol.*, 64:639, 1975.

160. Volpé, R.: Autoimmune thyroiditis. In *Thyroid Function and Disease*. Edited by G.W. Burrow, J.H. Oppenheimer, and R. Volpé, Philadelphia, W.B. Saunders, 1989, pp.921-933.

161. Hashimoto, H.: Zur kenntnis der lymphomatosen veranderung der schilddruse (struma lymphomatosal). *Arch. Klin. Chir.*, 97:21, 1912.

162. Beierwaltes, W.H.: Iodine and lymphocytic thyroiditis. *Bull. All-India Inst. Med. Sci.*, 3:145, 1969.

163. Hawkins, B.R., Cheah, P.S., Dawkins, R.L., et al.: Diagnostic significance of thyroid microsomal antibodies in randomly selected population. *Lancet*, 2(8203):1057-1059, 1980.

164. Fisher, D. and Beall, G.N.: Hashimoto's thyroiditis. *Pharmacol. Ther.*, 1:445, 1976.

165. Yoshida, H., Amino, N., Yagawa, K., et al.: Association of serum antithyroid antibodies with lymphocytic infiltration of the thyroid gland: a study of 70 autopsied cases. *J. Clin. Endocrinol. Metab.*, 46:459, 1978.

166. Todd, J.: A most intimate foe: how the immune system can betray the body it defends. *Science*, 30(2):20, 1990.

167. Cho, B.Y., Shong, Y.K., Lee, H.K., Koh, C.S., and Min, H.K.: Inhibition of thyrotropin-stimulated adenylate cyclase activation and growth of rat thyroid cells, FRTL5, by immunoglobulin G from patients with primary myxedema: comparison with activities of thyrotropin-binding inhibitory immunoglobulin. *Acta Endocrinol.*, 120:99, 1989.

168. Iitaka, M., Aguayo, J., Row, V.V., Ruf, J., Carayon, P., and Volpé, R.: Comparison of measurements of *in vitro* production of antithyroid microsomal antibody versus anti-thyroid peroxidase antibody. *Reg. Immunol.*, 1:106, 1988.

169. Pinchera, A., Fenzi, G.F., Bartalena, L., et al.: Thyroid antigens involved in autoimmune thyroid disorders. In *Autoimmunity in Thyroid Diseases*. Edited by E. Klein and F.A. Horster, Stuttgart, Schattauer, 1979, p.49.

170. Kohno, Y., Hiyama, Y., Shimojo, N., Nakajima, H., and Hosaya, T.: Autoantibodies to thyroid peroxidase in patients with chronic thyroiditis. *Clin. Exp. Immunol.*, 65: 534, 1986.

171. Bastenie, P.A. and Ermans, A.M.: Thyroiditis and thyroid function: clinical, morphological, and physiological studies. *International Series of Monographs on Pure and Applied Biology: Modern Trends in Physiological Sciences*, Vol. 36. Oxford, Pergamon Press, 1972, p.1.

172. Jannson, R., Karlsson, A., and Dahlberg, P.A.: Thyroxine, methimazole, and thyroid microsomal autoantibody titres in hypothyroid Hashimoto's thyroiditis. *Br. Med. J.*, 290: 11, 1985.

173. Trbojevic, B., Lalic, N., and Slijepcevic, D.: The effect of replacement therapy on thyroid antibody and serum thyrotropin concentrations in Hashimoto's thyroiditis. In *The Thyroid and Autoimmunity*. Edited by H.A. Drexhage and W.M. Wiersinga, Amsterdam, *Excerpta Medica*, 1986, p.113.

174. Volpé, R., Row, V.V., Webster, B.R., et al.: Studies of iodine metabolism in Hashimoto's thyroiditis. *J. Clin. Endocrinol. Metab.*, 25:593, 1965.

175. Greenberg, A.H., Czernichow, P., Hung, W., et al.: Juvenile chronic lymphocytic thyroiditis: clinical, laboratory, and histological correlations. *J. Clin. Endocrinol. Metab.*, 30:29, 1970.

176. LiVolsi, J.A. and LoGerfo, P.: *Thyroiditis*. Boca Raton, CRC Press, 1981, p.1.

177. Lamberg, B.A.: Aetiology of hypothyroidism. *Clin. Endocrinol. Metab.*, 8:3, 1979.

178. DePapendieck, L.R., Iorcansky, S., Rivarola, M.A., and Bergada, C.: Variations in the clinical, hormonal, and serological expressions of chronic lymphocytic thyroiditis in children and adolescents. *Clin. Endocrinol. Metab.*, 16: 19, 1982.

179. Doniach, D., Bottazzo, G.F., and Russell, P.C.G.: Goitrous autoimmune thyroiditis (Hashimoto's disease). *J. Clin. Endocrinol. Metab.*, 8:63, 1979.

180. Fatourechi, V., McConahey, W.M., and Woolner, L.: Hyperthyroidism associated with histologic Hashimoto's thyroiditis. *Mayo Clinic*, 46:682, 1971.

181. Ito, S., Tamura, T., and Mishikawa, M.: Effect of desiccated thyroid, prednisolone, and chloroquins on goiter and antibody titer in Hashimoto's thyroiditis. *Metabolism*, 7: 317, 1968.

182. Blizzard, R.M., Hung, W., Chandler, R.W., et al.: Hashimoto's thyroiditis: clinical and laboratory response to prolonged cortisone therapy. *N. Engl. J. Med.*, 267:1015, 1962.

183. Doniach, D.: Humoral and genetic aspects of thyroid autoimmunity. *Clin. Endocrinol. Metab.*, 4:267, 1979.

184. Nikolai, T.F.: Silent thyroiditis and subacute thyroiditis.

In *Werner and Ingbar's The Thyroid: A Fundamental and Clinical Text*, 6th edition. Edited by L.E. Braverman and R.D. Utiger, New York, J.B. Lippincott Co., 1991, pp.710-727.

185. Nikolai, T.F., Brosseau, J., Kettrick, M.A., Roberts, R., and Beltaos, E.: Lymphocytic thyroiditis with spontaneously resolving hyperthyroidism (silent thyroiditis). *Arch. Intern. Med.*, 140(4):478-482, 1980.

186. Nikolai, T.F., Turney, S., and Roberts, R.: Postpartum lymphocytic thyroiditis. *Arch. Intern. Med.*, 147:221, 1987.

187. Amino, N., Mori, H., Iwatani, Y., et al.: High prevalence of transient postpartum thyrotoxicosis and hypothyroidism. *N. Engl. J. Med.*, 306:849, 1982.

188. Woolf, P.D.: Transient painless thyroiditis with hyperthyroidism: a varient of lymphocytic thyroiditis. *Endocr. Rev.*, 4:411, 1980.

189. Yamamoto, M., Sakurada, T., Yoshida, K., et al.: Thyroid function and antimicrosomal antibody during the course of silent thyroiditis. *Endocrinol. Japan.*, 34:357, 1987.

190. Nikolai, T.F., Coombs, G.J., McKenzie, A.K., et al.: Treatment of lymphocytic thyroiditis with spontaneously resolving hyperthyroidism (silent thyroiditis). *Arch. Intern. Med.*, 142:2281, 1982.

191. Nikolai, T.F., Coombs, G.J., and McKenzie, A.K.: Lymphocytic thyroiditis with spontaneously resolving hyperthyroidism (silent thyroiditis) and subacute thyroiditis: long-term follow-up. *Arch. Intern. Med.*, 141:1455, 1981.

192. Volpé, R.: Subacute (de Quervain's) thyroiditis. *Clin. Endocrinol. Metab.*, 8:81, 1979.

193. Martino, E., Buratti, L., Bartalena, L., et al.: High prevalence of subacute thyroiditis during summer season in Italy. *J. Endocrinol. Invest.*, 10:321, 1987.

194. Saito, S., Sakurada, T., Yamamoto, M., et al.: Subacute thyroiditis: observations of 98 cases for the last 14 years. *Tohoku J. Exp. Med.*, 113:141, 1974.

195. Greene, J.N.: Subacute thyroiditis. *Am. J. Med.*, 51:97, 1971.

196. Fraser, R. and Harrison, R.J.: Subacute thyroiditis. *Lancet*, 1:382, 1952.

197. Volpé, R., Row, V.V., and Ezrin, C.: Circulating viral and thyroid antibodies in subacute thyroiditis. *J. Clin. Endocrinol. Metab.*, 27:1275, 1967.

198. Galluzzo, A., Giordano, C., Andronica, F., et al.: Leukocyte migration test in subacute thyroiditis: hypothetical role of cell-mediated immunity. *J. Clin. Endocrinol. Metab.*, 59:1038, 1980.

199. Chartier, B., Bandy, P., and Wall, J.R.: Fc receptor-bearing blood mononuclear cells in thyroid disorders: increased levels in patients with subacute thyroiditis. *J. Clin. Endocrinol. Metab.*, 51:1014, 1980.

200. Strakosch, C.R., Joyner, D., and Wall, J.R.: Thyroid stimulating antibodies in patients with subacute thyroiditis. *J. Clin. Endocrinol. Metab.*, 46:345, 1978.

201. Saunders, L.R., Moreno, A., Pittman, D.L., et al.: Painless giant cell thyroiditis diagnosed by fine needle aspiration and associated with intense thyroidal uptake of gallium. *Am. J. Med.*, 80:971, 1986.

202. Mizukami, Y., Michigishi, T., Kawato, M., et al.: Immunohistochemical and ultrastructural study of subacute thyroiditis with special references to multinucleated giant

cells. *Hum. Pathol.*, 18:929, 1987.

203. Jayaram, G., Marwaha, R.K., Gupta, R.K., et al.: Cytomorphologic aspects of thyroiditis: a study of 51 cases with functional, immunologic, and ultrasonographic data. *Acta Cytol.*, 31:687, 1987.

204. Volpé, R. and Johnston, M.: Subacute thyroiditis: a disease commonly mistaken for pharyngitis. *Can. Med. Assoc., J.*, 77:297, 1957.

205. Steinberg, F.U.: Subacute granulomatous thyroiditis: a review. *Ann. Intern. Med.*, 52:1014, 1960.

206. Gordin, A. and Lamberg, B.A.: Serum thyrotrophin response to thyrotrophin release hormone and the concentration of free thyroxine in subacute thyroiditis. *Acta Endocrinol.*, 74:111, 1973.

207. Larsen, P.R.: Serum triiodothyronine and thyrotrophin during hyperthyroid, hypothyroid, and recovery phases of subacute non-supprative thyroiditis. *Metabolism*, 23:467, 1974.

208. Weihl, A.C., Daniels, G.H., Ridgeway, E.D., et al.: Thyroid function tests during the early phase of subacute thyroiditis. *J. Clin. Endocrinol. Metab.*, 44:1107, 1977.

209. Staub, J.J.: TRH test in subacute thyroiditis. *Lancet*, 1: 868, 1975.

210. Babb, R.R.: Associations between diseases of the thyroid and the liver. *Am. J. Gastroenterol.*, 79:421, 1984.

211. Lewitus, W., Rechnic, J., and Lubin, E.: Sequential scanning of the thyroid as an aid in diagnosis of subacute thyroiditis. *Isr. J. Med. Sci.*, 3:847, 1967.

212. Hamburger, J.I., Kadian, G., and Rossin, H.W.: Subacute thyroiditis: evaluation depicted by serial ^{131}I scintigram. *J. Nucl. Med.*, 6:560, 1965.

213. Volpé, R.: Treatment of thyroiditis. *Mod. Treat.*, 6:474, 1969.

214. Van Herle, A.J., Vassart, G., and Dumont, J.E.: Control of thyroglobulin synthesis and secretion. *N. Engl. J. Med.*, 301:239, 1979.

215. Armstrong, W.B., Funk, G.F., and Rice, D.H.: Acute airway compromise secondary to traumatic thyroid hemorrhage. *Arch. Otolaryngology: Head and Neck Surgery*, 120(4):427-430, 1994.

216. Oertli, D. and Harder, F.: Complete traumatic transection of the thyroid gland. *Surgery*, 115(4):527-529, 1994.

217. Rupprecht, H., Rumenapf, G., Braig, H., and Flesch, R.: Acute bleeding caused by rupture of the thyroid gland following blunt neck trauma: case report. *J. Trauma*, 36 (3):408-409, 1994.

218. Leckie, R.G., Buckner, A.B., and Bornemann, M.: Seat belt-related thyroiditis documented with thyroid Tc-99m pertechnetate scans. *Clin. Nuclear Med.*, 17(11):859-860, 1992.

219. Schulze, W. and Kleinsasser, O.: Laryngeal ruptures. *HNO*, 25(4):117-121, 1977.

220. Cannon, C.R.: Hypothyroidism in head and neck cancer patients: experimental and clinical observations. *Laryngoscope*, 104(11 pt 2 Su 66):1-21, 1994.

221. Pittman, J.A., Jr., Haigler, E.D., Hershman, J.M., and Pittman, C.S.: Hypothalamic hypothyroidism. *N. Engl. J. Med.*, 285:844, 1971.

222. Rudman, D., Gleisher, A.S., Kutner, M.H., and Raggio, J.F.: Suprahypophysial hypogonadism and hypothyroidism during prolonged coma after head trauma. *J. Clin. Endocrinol. Metab.*, 45:747, 1977.

223. Kanade, A., Ruiz, A.E., Rornoyos, K., Wakabayashi, I., and Kastin, A.J.: Panhypopituitarism and anemia secondary to traumatic fracture of the sella turcica. *J. Endocrinol. Invest.*, 1:263, 1978.

224. Woolf, P.D. and Schalch, D.S.: Hypothyroidism secondary to hypothalamic insufficiency. *Ann. Intern. Med.*, 78: 88, 1973.

225. Valenta, L.J. and DeFeo, D.R.: Post-traumatic hypopituitarism due to a hypothalamic lesion. *Am. J. Med.*, 68:614, 1980.

226. Danial, P.M. and Prichard, M.M.L.: Studies of the hypothalamus and the pituitary gland with special reference to the effects of the transection of the pituitary stalk. *Acta Endocrinol.*, 80 (Suppl. 201):1, 1975.

227. Pinchera, A., Martino, E., and Faglia, G.: Central hypothyroidism. In *Werner and Ingbar's The Thyroid: A Fundamental and Clinical Text*, 6th edition. Edited by L.E. Braverman and R.D. Utiger, New York, J.B. Lippincott Co., 1991, pp.968-984.

228. Sawin, C.T. and McHugh, J.E.: Isolated lack of thyrotropin in man. *J. Clin. Endocrinol Metab.*, 26:955, 1966.

229. Samaan, N.A., Cangir, A., Maor, M.H., Sampiere, V.A., and Jesse, R.H.: Effect of irradiation on the hypothalamic, pituitary, and thyroid function in patients with tumors of the head and neck. In *Recent Advances in the Diagnosis and Treatent of Pituitary Tumors*. Edited by J.A. Linfoot, New York, Raven Press, 1979, p.148.

230. Sheline, G.E.: Radiation therapy of pituitary tumors. In *Hormone Secreting Pituitary Tumors*. Edited by V.J.R. Givens, Chicago, Year Book Medical Publilshers, 1982, p.121.

231. Samaan, N.A., Bakdams, M.M., Caderao, J.B., Cangir, A., Jesse, R.H., and Ballantyne, A.J.: Hypopituitarism after external irradiation: evidence for both hypothalamic and pituitary origin. *Ann. Intern. Med.*, 83:771, 1975.

232. Lawrence, A.M., Pinsky, S.M., and Goldfine, I.D.: Conventional radiation therapy in acromegaly: a review and reassessment. *Arch. Intern. Med.*, 128:369, 1971.

233. Linfoot, J.A.: Alpha particle pituitary irradiation in the primary and postsurgical management of pituitary microadenoma. In *Pituitary Microadenomas*. Edited by G. Faglia, M.A. Giovannelli, and R.M. MacLeod, New York, Academic Press, 1980, p.515.

234. Cooper, D.S.: Treatment of thyrotoxicosis. In *Werner and Ingbar's The Thyroid: A Fundamental and Clinical Text*, 6th edition. Edited by L.E. Braverman and R.D. Utiger, New York, J.B. Lippincott Co., 1991, pp.887-916.

235. Braverman, L.E. and Utiger, R.D.: Introduction to hypothyroidism. In *Werner and Ingbar's The Thyroid: A Fundamental and Clinical Text*, 6th edition. Edited by L.E. Braverman and R.D. Utiger, New York, J.B. Lippincott Co., 1991, pp.919-920.

236. Ingbar, S.H. and Woeber, K.A.: Diseases of the thyroid. In *Harrison's Principles of Internal Medicine*, 8th edition. Edited by G.W. Thorn, R.D. Adams, E. Braunwald, K.J. Isselbacher, and R.G. Petersdorf, New York, McGraw-Hill Book Co., 1977, pp.501-519.

237. Lowe, J.C.: Thyroid status of 38 fibromyalgia patients: implications for the etiology of fibromyalgia. *Clin. Bull. Myofascial Ther.*, 2(1):47-64, 1997.

238. Hershman, J.M.: Hypothalamic and pituitary hypothyroidism. In *Progress in the Diagnosis and Treatment of Hypothyroid Conditions*. Edited by P.A. Bastenie, M. Bonnyns, and L.VanHaelst, Amsterdam, *Excepta Medica*, 1980, pp.40-50.

239. Neeck, G. and Riedel, W.: Thyroid function in patients with fibromyalgia syndrome. *J. Rheum.*, 19:1120-1122, 1992.

240. Martin, J.B.: Hypothalamus and releasing hormones. In *Harrison's Principles of Internal Medicine*, 8ᵗʰ edition. Edited by G.W. Thorn, R.D. Adams, E. Braunwald, K.J. Isselbacher, and R.G. Petersdorf, New York, McGraw-Hill Book Co., 1977, pp.471-478.

241. Ferraccioli, G., Cavalieri, F., Salaffi, F., Fontana, S., Scita, F., Nolli, M., and Maestri, D.: Neuroendocrinologic findings in primary fibromyalgia (soft tissue chronic pain syndrome) and in other chronic rheumatic conditions (rheumatoid arthritis, low back pain). *J. Rheum.*, 17:869-873, 1990.

242. Lowe, J.C., Reichman, A.J., Honeyman, G.S., and Yellin, J.: Thyroid status of fibromyalgia patients. *Clin. Bull. Myofascial Ther.*, 3(1):69-70, 1997.

243. Shiroky, J.B., Cohen, M., Ballachey, M.L., and Neville, C.: Thyroid dysfunction in rheumatoid arthritis: a controlled prospective survey. *Ann. Rheumat. Dis.*, 52:454-456, 1993.

244. Eisinger, J., Arroyo, P., Calendini, C., Rinaldi, J.P., Combes, R., and Fontaine, G.: Anomalies biologiques au cours des fibromyalgies: III. Explorations endocriniennes. *Lyon Méditerranée Méd.*, 28:858-860, 1992.

245. Hamburger, J.I.: Use of modern thyroid tests in illustrative ambulatory patients. In *Diagnostic Methods in Clinical Thyroidology*. Edited by J.I. Hamburger, N.Y., Springer-Verlag, 1989, pp.111-123.

246. Cunnien, A.J., Hay, I.D., Gorman, C.A., Offord, K.P., and Scanion, P.W.: Radioiodine-induced hypothyroidism in Graves' disease: factors associated with the increasing incidence. *J. Nucl. Med.*, 23:978, 1982.

247. Lundell, G., Holm, L.E., Ljunggren, J.G., and Wasserman, J.: Incidence of hypothyroidism after ¹³¹I therapy for hyperthyroidism. *Acta Radiol.*, 20:225, 1981.

248. Lundell, G. and Holm, L.E.: Hypothyroidism after ¹³¹I therapy for hyperthyroidism in relation to immunologic parameters. *Acta Radiol. Oncol.*, 19:449, 1980.

249. Bliddal, H., Hansen, J.M., Rogwski, P., Johansen, K., Friis, T., and Siersbaek-Nielson, K.: ¹³¹I treatment of diffuse and nodular toxic goitre with or without antithyroid agents. *Acta Endocrinol.* (Copenh.), 99:517, 1982.

250. Vilkeniers, B., Vanhaelst, L., Cytryn, R., and Jonckheer, M.H.: Treatment of hyperthyroidism with radioiodine: adjunctive therapy with antithyroid drugs reconsidered. *Lancet*, 2:1127, 1988.

251. Steinbach, J.J., Donoghue, G.D., and Goldman, J.K.: Simultaneous treatment of toxic diffuse goiter with I-131 and antithyroid drugs: a prospective study. *J. Nucl. Med.*, 20:1263, 1979.

252. Connell, J.M., Hilditch, T.E., McCruden, D.C., and Alexander, W.D.: Transient hypothyroidism following radioiodine therapy for thyrotoxicosis. *Br. J. Radiol.*, 56:309, 1983.

253. Sawers, J.S.A., Toft, A.D., Irvine, W.J., Brown, N.S., and

Seth, J.: Transient hypothyroidism after iodine-131 treatment of thyrotoxicosis. *J. Clin. Endocrinol. Metab.*, 50:226, 1980.

254. Einhorn, J., Fagraeus, A., and Galinson, S.: Radiation of thyroid: experimental study in radiosensitivity of thyroid. *Radiology*, 29:40, 1937.

255. O'Gorman, P., Staffurth, J.S., and Ballentyne, M.R.: Antibody response to thyroid irradiation. *J. Clin. Endocrinol. Metab.*, 24:1072, 1964.

256. Williams, F.D.: Biologic effects of radiation on the thyroid. In *Werner's The Thyroid: A Fundamental and Clinical Text*, 6ᵗʰ edition. Edited by L.E. Braverman and R.D. Utiger, New York, J.B. Lippincott Co., 1991, pp.421-436.

257. Werner, S.C., Coelho, B., Quimby, E.H., and Day, R.McC.: Ten year results of I¹³¹ therapy of hyperthyroidism. *Bull. N.Y. Acad. Med.*, 33:783, 1957.

258. Dunn, J.T. and Chapman, E.M.: Rising incidence of hypothyroidism after radioactive-iodide therapy in thyrotoxicosis. *N. Engl. J. Med.*, 271:1037, 1964.

259. Klementschitsch, P., Shen, K., and Kaplan, E.L.: Reemergence of thyroidectomy as treatment for Graves' disease. *Surg. Clin. North Am.*, 59:35, 1979.

260. Maier, W.P., Derrick, B.M., Marks, A.D., Channick, B.J., Au, F.C., and Caswell, H.T.: Long-term follow-up of patients with Graves' disease treated by subtotal thyroidectomy. *Am. J. Surg.*, 147:267, 1984.

261. Hedley, A.J., Young, R.E., Jones, S.J., et al.: Late onset hypothyroidism after subtotal thyroidectomy for hyperthyroidism: implications for long-term follow-up. *Br. J. Surg.*, 70:740, 1983.

262. Toft, A.D., Irvine, W.J., Sinclair, I., McIntosh, D., Seth, J., and Cameron, E.H.D.: Thyroid function after surgical treatment of thyrotoxicosis. *N. Engl. J. Med.*, 298:643, 1978.

263. Lee, T.C., Coffey, R.J., Currier, B.M., Ma, X.P., and Canary, J.J.: Propranolol and thyroidectomy in the treatment of thyrotoxicosis. *Ann. Surg.*, 195:766, 1982.

264. Reid, D.J.: Hyperthyroidism and hypothyroidism complicating the treatment of thyrotoxicosis. *Br. J. Surg.*, 74:1060, 1987.

265. Sugrue, D., Drury, M.I., McEvoy, M., Heffernan, S.J., and O'Malley, E.: Long-term follow-up of hyperthyroid patients treated by subtotal thyroidectomy. *Br. J. Surg.*, 70:408, 1983.

266. Harada, T., Shimaoka, K., Arita, S., and Nakanisky, Y.: Follow-up evaluation of thyroid function after thyroidectomy for thyrotoxicosis. *World J. Surg.*, 8:444, 1984.

267. Kalk, W.J., Durbach, D., Kantor, S., and Levin, J.: Post-thyroidectomy thyrotoxicosis. *Lancet*, 1:291, 1978.

268. Ladenson, P.W.: Diagnosis of hypothyroidism. In *Werner's The Thyroid: A Fundamental and Clinical Text*, 5ᵗʰ edition. Edited by L.E. Braverman and R.D.Utiger, Philadelphia, J.B. Lippincott Co., 1991, pp.1092-1098.

269. Seshadri, M.S., Samuel, B.U., Kanagasabapathy, A.S., and Cherian, A.M.: Clinical scoring system for hypothyroidism: is it useful? *J. Gen. Intern. Med.*, 4:490, 1989.

270. Wood, L.C. and Ingbar, S.H.: Hypothyroidism as a late sequela in patients with Graves' disease treated with antithyroid drugs. *J. Clin. Invest.*, 64:1429, 1979.

271. Kuku, S.F., Child, D.F., Nader, S., and Fraser, T.R.: Thyrotropin and prolactin responsiveness to thyrotropin re-

leasing hormone in Cushing's disease. *Clin. Endocrinol.* (Oxf.), 4:437, 1975.

272. Otsuki, M., Dakoda, M., and Baba, S.: Influence of glucocorticoids on TRH-induced TSH response in man. *J. Clin. Endocrinol. Metab.*, 36:95, 1973.

273. Bartalena, L., Martino, E., Petrini, L., et al.: The nocturnal serum thyrotropin surge is abolished in patients with ACTH-dependent or ACTH-independent Cushing's syndrome. *J. Clin. Endocrinol. Metab.*, 72:1203, 1991.

274. Berens, S.C., Wolff, J., and Murphy, D.L.: Lithium concentration by the thyroid. *J. Endocrinol.*, 87:1085, 1970.

275. Berens, S.C., Bernstein, R.S., Robbins, J., and Wolff, J.: Antithyroid effects of lithium. *J. Clin. Invest.*, 49:1357, 1970.

276. Burrow, G., Burke, W.R., Himmehoch, J.M., Spencer, R.P., and Hershman, J.M.: Effect of lithium on thyroid function. *J. Clin. Endocrinol. Metab.*, 32:647, 1971.

277. Williams, J.A., Berens, S.C., and Wolff, J.: Thyroid secretion *in vitro*: inhibition of TSH and debutyryl cyclic-AMP stimulated ^{131}I release by Li. *Endocrinol.*, 88:1385, 1971.

278. Kristenson, O., Andersen, H.H., and Pallisgaard, G.: Lithium carbonate in the treatment of thyrotoxicosis. *Lancet*, 1:603, 1976.

279. Barsano, C.P.: Other forms of primary hypothyroidism. In *Werner's The Thyroid: A Fundamental and Clinical Text*, 5th edition. Edited by L.E. Braverman and R.D.Utiger, Philadelphia, J.B. Lippincott Co., 1991, pp.956-967.

280. Smigan, L., Wahlin, A., Jacobson, L, and von Knorring, L.: Lithium therapy and thyroid function tests: a prospective study. *Neuropsychobiology*, 11:39, 1984.

281. Emerson, C.H., Dyson, W.L., and Utiger, R.D.: Serum thyrotropin and thyroxine concentrations in patients receiving lithium carbonate. *J. Clin. Endocrinol. Metab.*, 36:338, 1973.

282. Schou, M.: Lithium prophylaxis: myths and realities. *Am. J. Psychiatry*, 146:573, 1989.

283. Clower, C.G.: Effects of lithium on thyroid function. (Letter) *Am. Psych.*, 146:1357, 1989.

284. Lindstedt, G., Nilsson, L.-A., Walinder, J., Skott, A., and Ohman, R.: On the prevalence, diagnosis, and management of lithium-induced hypothyroidism in psychiatric patients. *Br. J. Psychiatry*, 130:452, 1977.

285. Barsano, C.P.: Environmental factors altering thyroid function and their assessment. *Environ. Health Perspect.*, 38:71, 1981.

286. Wolff, J.: Iodide goiter and the pharmacologic effects of excess iodide. *Am. J. Med.*, 47:101, 1969.

287. Wagenakis, A.G., Downs, P., Braverman, L.E., Burger, A., and Ingbar, S.H.: Control of thyroid hormone secretion in normal subjects receiving iodides. *J. Clin. Invest.*, 52:528, 1973.

288. Suzuki, H., Higuchi, T., Sawa, K., Ohtaki, S., and Horiuchi, Y.: "Endemic Coast goitre" in Hokkaido, Japan. *Acta Endocrinol.*, 50:161, 1965.

289. Braverman, L.E., Vagenakis, A.G., Wang, C., Maloof, F, and Ingbar, S.H.: Studies on the pathogenesis of iodide myxedema. *Trans. Assoc. Am. Physicians*, 84:130, 1971.

290. Gaitan, E. (Editor): *Environmental Goitrogenesis*. Boca Raton, CRC Press, 1989.

291. Green, W.L.: Extrinsic and intrinsic variables: antithyroid compounds. In *Werner's The Thyroid: A Fundamental and Clinical Text*, 5th edition. Edited by L.E. Braverman and R.D.Utiger, Philadelphia, J.B. Lippincott Co., 1991, pp.322-335.

292. Greer, M.A.: Isolation from rutabaga seed of progoitrin, the percursor of the naturally occurring antithyroid compound, goitrin (L-1-5-vinyl-oxazolidinethione). *J. Am. Chem. Soc.*, 78:1260, 1956.

293. Greer, M.A., Kammer, H., and Bouma, D.J.: Short-term antithyroid drug therapy for the thyrotoxicosis of Graves' disease. *N. Engl. J. Med.*, 297:173, 1977.

294. Bouma, D.J., Kammer, H., and Greer, M.A.: Follow-up comparison of short-term versus 1 year antithyroid therapy for the thyrotoxicosis of Graves' disease. *J. Clin. Endocrinol. Metab.*, 55:1138, 1982.

295. Bing, R.F. and Rosenthal, F.D.: Early remission in thyrotoxicosis produced by short courses of treatment. *Acta Endocrinol.* (Copenh.), 100:221, 1982.

296. Allannic, H., Fauchet, R., Orgiazzi, et al.: Antithyroid drugs and Graves' disease: a prospective randomized evaluation of the efficacy of treatment duration. *J. Clin. Endocrinol. Metab.*, 70:675, 1990.

297. Tamai, H., Nakagawa, T., Fukino, O., et al.: Thionamide therapy in Graves' disease: relapse rate to duration of therapy. *Ann. Intern. Med.*, 92:488, 1980.

298. Slingerland, D.W. and Burrows, B.A.: Long-term antithyroid treatment in hyperthyroidism. *J.A.M.A.*, 242:2408, 1979.

299. Lauberg, P., Hansen, P.E.B., Iversen, E., Jansen, S.E., and Weeke, J.: Goitre size and outcome of medical treatment of Graves' disease. *Acta Endocrinol.* (Copenh.), 111:39, 1986.

300. Hershman, J.M., Givens, J.R., Cassidy, C.E., and Aswood, E.B.: Long-term outcome of hyperthyroidism treated with antithyroid drugs. *J. Clin. Endocrinol. Metab.*, 26:803, 1966.

301. Surgrue, D., McEvoy, M., Feely, J., and Drury, M.I.: Hyperthyroidism in the land of Graves': results of treatment by surgery, radio-iodine, and carbimazole in 837 cases. *Q. J. Med.*, 49:51, 1980.

302. Hedley, A.J., Young, R.E., Jones, S.J., Alexander, W.D., and Bewsher, P.D.: Antithyroid drugs in the treatment of hyperthyroidism of Graves' disease: long-term follow-up of 434 patients. *Clin. Endocrinol.* (Oxf.), 31:209, 1989.

303. Cramarossa, L., Astorre, P., and Ronchi, F.: Therapy of hyperthyroidism: indications, advantages, and disadvantages of treatment of the adult and the elderly. *Recent Prog. Med.*, 80(4):219-226, 1989.

304. Dunn, J.T.: Choice of therapy in young adults with hyperthyroidism of Graves' disease: a brief case-directed poll of fifty-four thyroidologists. *Ann. Intern. Med.*, 100:891, 1984.

305. Hirota, Y., Tamai, H., and Hayashi, Y., et al.: Thyroid function and histology in forty-five patients with hyperthyroid Graves' disease in clinical remission more than ten years after thionamide drug treatment. *J. Clin. Endocrinol. Metab.*, 62(1):165-169, 1986.

306. Azizi, F.: Environmental iodine intake affects the response to methimazole in patients with diffuse toxic goiter. *J. Clin. Endocrinol. Metab.*, 61(2):374-377, 1985.

307. Holm, L.E. and Alinder, I.: Relapses after thionamide

therapy for Graves' disease. *Acta Med. Scand.*, 211(6): 489-492, 1982.

308. Von Hofe, S.E., Dorfman, S.G., Carretta, R.F., and Young, R.L.: The increasing incidence of hypothyroidism within one year after radioiodine therapy for toxic diffuse goiter. *J. Nucl. Med.*, 19(2):180-184, 1978.

309. Jolley, R.L., Gaitan, E., Douglas, E.C., and Felker, L.K.: Identification of organic pollutants in drinking waters from areas with endemic thyroid disorders and potential pollutants of drinking water sources associated with coal processing areas. *Am. Chem. Soc. Environ. Chem.*, 26:59, 1986.

310. Gaitan, E.: Iodine-sufficient goiter and autoimmune thyroiditis: the Kentucky and Columbian experience. In *Frontiers in Thyroidology*, Vol.1. Edited by G. Medeiros-Neto and E. Gaitan, New York, Plenum Press, 1986, p.19.

311. Gaitan, E.: Endemic goiter in Western Columbia. *Ecol. Dis.*, 2:295, 1983.

312. Bahn, A.K., Mills, J.L., Snyder, P.J., et al.: Hypothyroidism in workers exposed to polybrominated biphenyls. *N. Engl. J. Med.*, 302:31, 1980.

313. Kreiss, K., Roberts, C., and Humphreys, H.E.B.: Serial PBB levels, PCB levels, and clinical chemistries in Michigan's PBB cohort. *Arch. Environ. Health*, 37:141, 1982.

314. Stross, J.K.: Hypothyroidism and polybrominated biphenyls. *N. Engl. J. Med.*, 302:1421, 1980.

315. *Werner's The Thyroid: A Fundamental and Clinical Text*, 7th edition. Edited by L.E. Braverman and R.D. Utiger, Philadelphia, Lippincott-Raven Publishers, 1996.

316. Fauerholdt, L. and Vendsborg, P.: Thyroid gland morphology after lithium treatment. *Acta Pathol. Microbiol. Immunol. Scand.* (A), 89:339, 1981.

317. Bennett, R.M., Clark, S.R., Burckhardt, C.S., and Walczyk, J.: A double-blind placebo-controlled study of growth hormone therapy in fibromyalgia (Abstr). *J. Musculoskel. Pain*, 3(Suppl. 1): 110, 1995.

318. Root, A.W., Bongiovanni, A.M., and Eberlein, W.R.: Inhibition of thyroidal radioiodine uptake by human growth hormone. *J. Pediatr.*, 76:422-429, 1970.

319. Marshak, D.R. and Liu, D.T. (Editors): *Banbury Report 29: Therapeutic Peptides and Proteins: Assessing the New Technologies.* New York, Cold Spring Harbor Laboratory, 1988.

320. Kuret, J.A. and Murad, F.: Adenohypophyseal hormones and related substances. In *The Pharmacologic Basis of Therapeutics*, 8th edition. Edited by A.G. Gilman, T.W. Rall, A.S. Nies, and P. Taylor, New York, Pergamon Press, 1990, pp.1334-1360.

321. Mizukami, Y., Funaki, N., Hashimoto, T., Kawato, M., Michigishi, T., and Matsubara, F.: Histologic features of the thyroid gland in a patient with bromide-induced hypothyroidism. *Am. J. Clin. Pathol.*, 89:802, 1988.

322. Vobecky, M. and Babicky, A.: Effect of enhanced bromide intake on the concentration ratio I/Br in rat thyroid gland. *Biol. Trace Elem. Res.*, 43-45:509-516, 1994.

323. Van Gelderen, C.E., Saavelkoul, T.J., Blom, J.L., van Dokkum, W., and Kroes, R.: The no-effect level of sodium bromide in healthy volunteers. *Human Experi. Toxicol.*, 12(1):9-14, 1993.

324. Buchberger, W., Holler, W., and Winsauer, K.: Effects of sodium bromide on the biosynthesis of thyroid hormones and brominated/iodinated thyronines. *J. Trace Elem. Electrol. Health Dis.*, 4(1):25-30, 1990.

325. Loeber, J.G., Franken, M.A., and van Leeuwen, F.X.: Effect of sodium bromide on endocrine parameters in the rat as studied by immunocytochemistry and radioimmunoassay. *Food Chem. Toxicol.*, 21(4):391-404, 1983.

326. *Merck Manual of Diagnosis and Therapy*, 16th edition. Edited by R. Berkow, A.J. Fletcher, and M.H. Beers, Rahway, Merck Research Laboratories, 1992.

327. Peillon F. and Racadot, J.: Histopathology of the hypophysis in six cases of hemochromatosis. *Ann. Endocrinol.* (Paris), 30(6):800-807, 1969.

328. MacDonald, R.A. and Mallory, G.K.: Hemochromatosis and hemosiderosis. *Arch. Intern. Med.*, 105:686, 1960.

329. Edwards, C.Q., Kelly, T.M., Ellwein, G., and Kushner, J.P.: Thyroid disease in hemochromatosis: increased incidence in homozygous men. *Arch. Intern. Med.*, 143(10): 1890-1893, 1983.

330. de Boissieu, D. and Badoual, J.: Perinatal hemochromatosis. *Pediatrie*, 46(2):141-145, 1991.

331. Himoto, Y., Kanzaki, S., Nomura, H., Araki, T., Takahashi, Y., and Seino, Y.: Hypothyroidism and hypoparathyroidism in an 11 year old boy with hemochromatosis secondary to aplastic anemia. *Acta Paediatr. Jpn.*, 37(4): 534-536, 1995.

332. Shirota, T., Shinoda, T., Aizawa, T., et al.: Primary hypothyroidism and multiple endocrine failure in association with hemochromatosis in a long-term hemodialysis patient. *Clin. Nephrol.*, 38(2):105-109, 1992.

333. Oerter, K.E., Kamp, G.A., Munson, P.J., Nienhuis, A.W., Cassorla, F.G., and Manasco, P.K.: Multiple hormone deficiencies in children with hemochromatosis. *J. Clin. Endocrinol. Metab.*, 76(2):357-361, 1993.

334. Munn, C.: Personal communication, April 21, 1998.

335. Buskila, D.; Neumann, L., Vaisberg, G., Alkalay, D., and Wolfe, F.: Increased rates of fibromyalgia following cervical spine injury. A controlled study of 161 cases of traumatic injury. *Arthritis Rheum.*, 40(3):446-452, 1997.

336. Sehnert, K.W. and Croft, A.C.: Basal metabolic temperature vs. laboratory assessment in "post-traumatic hypothyroidism." *J.M.P.T.*, 19(1):6-12, 1996.

337. Martin-du Pan, R.C.: Triggering role of emotional stress and childbirth: Unexpected occurrence of Graves' disease compared to 96 cases of Hashimoto thyroiditis and 97 cases of thyroid nodules. *Ann. Endocrinol.* (Paris), 59(2): 107-112, 1998.

338. Batteux, F., Tourneur, .L., Trebeden, H., Charreire, J., and Chiocchia, G.: Gene therapy of experimental autoimmune thyroiditis by *in vivo* administration of plasmid DNA coding for Fas ligand. *J. Immunol.*, 162(1):603-608, 1999.

339. Eisinger, J.: Place du syndrome polymyalgies-hypothyroidie instable dans le cadre des manifestations musculaires des hypothyroidiens traités. *Lyon Med. Med.*, 34 (5/6):5-7, 1998.

340. Eisinger, J.: Hypothyroidie et fibromyalgie: Indications d'une double hormonothérapie thyroidienne. *Lyon Med. Med.*, 35(2):37-40, 1999.

341. Lowe, J.C., Eichelberger, J., Manso, G., and Peterson, K.: Improvement in euthyroid fibromyalgia patients treated with T$_3$. *J. Myofascial Ther.*, 1(2):16-29, 1994.

2.5

Euthyroid Hypometabolism

As far back as the time of Galen (AD 130-to-200), medical writers have described symptoms that today are considered characteristic of hypothyroidism. These symptoms are also common to euthyroid hypometabolism—subnormal metabolism despite normal laboratory thyroid function test results. The symptoms are termed non-specific in that they are not specific to one disease but may be manifestations of different diseases. Some of the diseases are not necessarily related to inadequate thyroid hormone regulation of cell function. For example, some of the symptoms are common features of adrenal insufficiency, physical deconditioning, and B complex vitamin deficiencies. The non-specific symptoms are common to both hypothyroidism and euthyroid hypometabolism. Because of this, the symptoms in both of these conditions appear to be manifestations of inadequate thyroid hormone regulation of cell function.

Early in this century, some individuals with these symptoms were shown to have low basal metabolic rates (BMRs). According to the crude diagnostic methods of the day, most of the individuals appeared not to have diseases. Because of this, despite the non-specific symptoms, investigators concluded that the people were healthy. They also concluded that the low BMRs merely represented the low-normal end of the normal bell curve of human metabolic rates. The investigators denoted the putative phenomenon as "physiological hypometabolism." It was not possible to determine at that time which of the individuals included in these early studies had thyroid hormone deficiencies. Sensitive and reliable laboratory tests were not available until the 1970s. It is likely, however, that some of the individuals had either subclini-

cal or overt hypothyroidism, and that some had euthyroid hypometabolism due to partial cellular resistance to thyroid hormone.

The use of desiccated thyroid or T_4 relieved the non-specific symptoms and increased the low BMRs of some patients; others did not benefit from these forms of exogenous thyroid hormone. T_3 was discovered in 1952. Researchers soon found the use of T_3 relieved the non-specific symptoms and increased the low BMRs of patients who had failed to benefit from the use of desiccated thyroid and T_4.

In several studies published in the 1950s and 1960s, researchers described patients whose status improved with the use of T_3. These patients, as described by the authors of the studies, were remarkably similar to euthyroid fibromyalgia patients. The patients possibly would have met today's diagnostic criteria for fibromyalgia. This cannot be determined, however, because the authors of the studies did not report tenderness as a symptom. Unfortunately, the study of these patients ceased in the 1960s and did not commence again, to my knowledge, until my colleagues and I began to study euthyroid fibromyalgia patients in the late 1980s. The cessation of studies of these patients in the 1960s resulted from two factors. First, some physicians vigorously protested the advertising of T_3 as a general health elixir by two pharmaceutical companies. Second, researchers who conducted two studies in 1960 to assess the effectiveness of T_3 concluded that the hormone was not effective compared to placebos. This conclusion was erroneous for two reasons: Patients in the studies were not permitted to take T_3 long enough for the benefits to be clinically obvious, and a major statistical *error incorrectly indicated no significant difference between the groups taking T₃ and those taking placebos.*

During the first half of the 20ᵗʰ century, the only explanation for hypometabolism related to thyroid hormone was a deficiency of the hormone. In the 1950s, however, investigators proposed that some patients' cells had a subnormal response to thyroid hormone. This was the inception of the concept of partial cellular resistance to thyroid hormone as an explanation for hypometabolism. In 1981, Kaplan and co-workers reported the first carefully documented case of partial peripheral resistance to thyroid hormone. Peripheral resistance is a phenotype of thyroid hormone resistance in which the patient has normal thyroid function test results. Patients with the "non-specific" symptoms of metabolic insufficiency reported in the 1950s and 1960s and euthyroid fibromyalgia patients of today may be cases of this phenotype.

In 1967, Refetoff identified and described patients with a syndrome of resistance to thyroid hormone. This initiated studies to determine why some patients did not respond normally to their endogenous thyroid hormones. In 1988, Usala and colleagues established a tight linkage between thyroid hormone resistance and the c-erbAβ gene on chromosome 3. In 1990, Usala and his colleagues reported the identification of a mutation responsible for mutant T₃-receptors with low T₃-binding affinity. Most patients with mutant T₃-receptors have various clinical manifestations of inadequate DNA transcription regulation. Most mutant T₃-receptors regulate transcription properly when exposed to supraphysiologic dosages of T₃. At least theoretically, this phenomenon may explain why some patients with cellular resistance to thyroid hormone have therapeutic responses only to supraphysiologic dosages of T₃.

In the early 1970s, new and more reliable thyroid function laboratory tests were marketed. Requests for BMR testing decreased and insurance reimbursements for it ceased. So soon after the advent of the more reliable laboratory tests, instruments for measuring the BMR and technicians skilled at using the instruments became scarce. The predominant code of practice dictated that clinicians prescribe T₄ for patients who had non-specific symptoms and were hypothyroid according to the thyroid function tests. The code also dictated that clinicians refuse to prescribe T₃ for patients who had the symptoms but had normal thyroid function test results. Over time, this practice from the early 1970s crystalized into three rules: (1) the only mechanism through which the thyroid system can produce the

non-specific symptoms is a thyroid hormone deficiency, (2) normal laboratory test results conclusively rule out a thyroid hormone deficiency, and (3) only patients whose test results indicate a hormone deficiency should be treated with exogenous T₄. Underlying these rules is the belief that normal thyroid function test results are synonymous with normal tissue metabolism. Those who hold this belief overlook two phenomena for which there can be little doubt: (1) the responsiveness of tissues to thyroid hormone varies among individuals and among different tissues in the same individual, and (2) there is a multiplicity of potential faults in the regulation of cell function by normal concentrations of thyroid hormone.

A corollary to the belief that patients should only be treated with T₄ is that patients should only use dosages that maintain the basal TSH in the lower end of the normal range. The permitted dosage range is 0.05-to-0.15 mg, although some patients are permitted to use 0.2 mg. Before 1973, hypothyroid patients were customarily treated with dosages of T₄ between 0.2-to-0.4 mg or equivalent dosages of desiccated thyroid. The lower dosages allowed today are considered "replacement" dosages. This is the amount assumed to maintain exogenously the blood level of thyroid hormones and TSH maintained by a normal thyroid gland. The decision to use only these dosages is based on the theoretical concept of a "normal" range for thyroid function tests. Careful clinical observation indicates that this post-1970s dosage range probably leaves most hypothyroid patients hypometabolic. As a result, it is common today that many hypothyroid patients retain their non-specific symptoms. When hypothyroid fibromyalgia patients are given dosages in the former higher range as part of a full metabolic regimen, most recover from their non-specific symptoms. They then no longer meet the criteria for fibromyalgia. A recent study showed that the administration of exogenous T₄ to hypothyroid rats did not result in normal concentrations of T₄ and T₃ in most tissues. The researchers questioned the assumption that the use of T₄ alone in "replacement" dosages is effective in treating human hypothyroid patients.

In the 1990s, endocrinologists/thyroidologists came to argue that the only test needed to assess a patient's thyroid status and to make thyroid hormone dosage adjustments is the serum basal TSH level. Many of these practitioners now consider the patient's clinical status to be irrelevant to clinical decisions. These changes in the method of practice constitute the transition of the conventional endocrinologist/thyroidologist from medical clinician to laboratory technocrat. The extremist technocratic orientation of these practitioners has led to the development of highly specific and sensitive tests of the functional status of the pituitary-thyroid gland axis. Certainly, however, any value in these tests is more than offset by the incalculable suffering and premature deaths that have undoubtedly resulted from the extremism.

Regardless of this social and public health problem, the laboratory tests can be used to distinguish with a fair degree of reliability patients who have thyroid hormone deficiencies from those who do not. With patients who are hyperthyroid, as in Graves' disease, the tests are useful for the initial diagnosis and long-term monitoring. But with patients who are hypothyroid or euthyroid hypometabolic, the tests are useful only for initially establishing the patient's thyroid status. With these patients, adjustments in the dosage of exogenous thyroid hormone are best based on clinical judgment aided by the results of indirect tests of tissue metabolic status. Laboratory tests of thyroid function are of no value for the hypothyroid or euthyroid hypometabolic patient after the initial assessment of thyroid status.

In the late 1970s, investigators began observing, describing, and classifying patients with non-specific symptoms. The symptoms that were studied are the same as those of hypothyroid and euthyroid hypometabolic patients in reports scattered through the first half of the 20th century. Those whose predominant symptom was pain were diagnosed as having fibrositis, and after 1990, fibromyalgia. Since the mid-1980s, patients whose predominant non-specific symptom was fatigue have been diagnosed as having chronic fatigue syndrome.

In my experience, both these groups of patients typically have the same non-specific symptoms, signs, and physical exam results as patients with hypometabolism due to hypothyroidism. Yet many are not hypothyroid according to current laboratory test standards. Fibromyalgia and chronic fatigue syndrome investigators have failed to distinguish through laboratory testing the high percentage of these patients who have either primary or central hypothyroidism. My colleagues and I have determined that some 50% of fibromyalgia patients have test results consistent with either primary or central hypothyroidism. The failure of other investigators to recognize the hypothyroid status of a high percentage of these patients is based on the erroneous proposition that the basal TSH level and/or the measures of circulating thyroid hormones are sufficient to identify patients who are hypothyroid. As a result, fibromyalgia researchers have falsely concluded that hypothyroidism is rare among these patients. These researchers have largely ignored the possibility that fibromyalgia patients are hypometabolic.

When some fibromyalgia researchers and clinicians do use thyroid hormone as part of their treatment for fibromyalgia, they prescribe "replacement" dosages of T_4. Almost uniformly, patients do not benefit from these low dosages of T_4. The lack of benefit from the use of these dosages has apparently reinforced the researchers' and clinicians' belief that fibromyalgia is not related to thyroid hormone. As a result, acceptance by these fibromyalgia researchers and clinicians of the reigning endocrinology/thyroidology paradigm has diverted them from recognizing the pathophysiological process underlying fibromyalgia symptoms in many patients. The nature of this type of failure is inherent in a statement by Duesberg, "As often in the history of science, the biggest obstacle in finding the truth is not the difficulty in obtaining data, but the bias of the investigators on what data to chase and how to interpret them."

The definition of euthyroid hypometabolism is abnormally slow cellular metabolism despite normal thyroid function test results.[64] Plummer in 1917 was probably the first to write about patients with this condition.[53] Other writers between the 1930s and 1950s gave euthyroid hypometabolism several designations: "non-myxedematous hypometabolism,"[31] "low metabolism without myxedema,"[45] "hypometabolism without myxedema,"[46] "extrathyroidal hypometabolism,"[32,p.532] and "metabolic insufficiency."[29] [30][47] Despite normal laboratory test results (and presumably normal thyroid function), the typical euthyroid hypometabolic patient is clinically indistinguishable from the hypothyroid patient.

The non-specific symptoms of the euthyroid hypometabolic patient are features of a variety of diseases. In at least a subset of patients, however, the symptoms result from diminished responsiveness of the cells of specific tissues to thyroid hormone. The diminished responsiveness may result from a variety of faults in the action of thyroid hormone in cells. The most well-documented fault is the low affinity of T_3-receptors for T_3 due to point mutations in the c-erbAβ gene in chromosome 3. I subsume this fault with others under the classification of "partial cellular resistance to thyroid hormone." The reader should note that this term is distinct from "thyroid hormone resistance syndrome." According to recent convention, the term "hormone resistance syndrome" refers to defects at the site of action of different hormones. Because the main site of action of thyroid hormone is at genes where T_3-receptors are stationed, thyroid hormone resistance syndrome refers to defects at these nuclear sites. Thyroid hormone resistance syndromes, then, are forms of cellular resistance to thyroid hormone. "Cellular resistance to thyroid hormone" refers to the failure of normal concentrations of thyroid hormone (indicated by normal laboratory thyroid function test results) to properly regulate cell function, regardless of the particular mechanism at fault.

I will use the term euthyroid hypometabolism only in referring to patients studied after the early 1970s. This is because laboratory tests became available then that were specific and sensitive enough to distinguish with fair reliability patients who were hypothyroid from those who were euthyroid. We do not know whether hypometabolic patients studied before that time were hypothyroid or euthyroid.

For orientation, I will here emphasize one of the most important points in this chapter: Test results that indicate normal thyroid hormone levels and normal function of the pituitary-thyroid gland axis do not assure that the patient has normal or adequate tissue metabolism. Tissue responsiveness to thyroid hormone varies between individuals. Moreover, different tissues in the same individual vary in their responsiveness to thyroid hormone. Because of this, some individuals with normal circulating levels of thyroid hormone and TSH are nevertheless hypometabolic. The hypometabolism of some patients is severe enough to cause symptoms. In some, the hypometabolism is pathogenic. Thus, laboratory thyroid function test results tell us nothing of the metabolic status of a patient. In clinical practice today, metabolic status is best determined by indirect measures of tissue metabolism.

● CAUSES OF EUTHYROID HYPOMETABOLISM NOT DIRECTLY RELATED TO THYROID HORMONE

Hypometabolism is a clinical feature of several conditions that are not caused by inadequate thyroid hormone regulation of cell function: The hypometabolism that occurs in these conditions is independent of that caused by thyroid hormone deficiency or cellular resistance to the hormone. But because the hypometabolism that occurs in these conditions is independent of impaired thyroid gland function, the hypometabolism is properly classified as "euthyroid" hypometabolism.

Loss of muscle mass and adrenal insufficiency are two conditions in which hypometabolism can occur independently of thyroid gland function[29,p.124][45,p.895] They may be relevant to fibromyalgia. Also, Travell and Simons wrote that vitamin B_1 and folic acid deficiencies produce symptoms typical of hypometabolism.[2] It is understandable that a deficiency of these vitamins impairs metabolism considering the roles they play in cellular metabolic processes as synergists to thyroid hormone (see Chapter 2.2). Some authors have also reported that hypometabolism is a feature of depression and "psychoneurosis."[64,p.1053] I discuss this unlikely possibility below.

It is important to note that a patient with one of these conditions, say adrenal insufficiency, may concurrently have hypothyroidism or cellular resistance to thyroid hormone. If so, hypometabolism due to the inadequate thyroid hormone regulation of cell function will compound that due to the adrenal insufficiency. Some patients are likely to undergo treatment only for their thyroid hormone deficiency or resistance but not the adrenal insufficiency. In such a case, the hypometabolism due to the adrenal insufficiency will persist. Similarly, if the patient undergoes effective treatment only for the adrenal insufficiency, the portion of the hypometabolism caused by the inadequate thyroid hormone regulation of cell function will persist. All contributions to a patient's hypometabolism must be corrected, compensated for, or alleviated if the outcome for the patient is to be normal metabolism.

LOSS OF MUSCLE MASS

Any condition that results in loss of muscle mass will also decrease the resting metabolic rate[98][99][101][102][103] (see Chapters 3.4 and 5.5). The metabolic rate varies with the mass of metabolically active cells. Muscle cells are more metabolically active than fat cells,[98] so loss of muscle mass reduces the metabolic rate. A slowed metabolic rate occurs in many patients who become sedentary because of the fatigue and decreased motor drive associated with fibromyalgia. When the hypometabolism of deconditioning compounds that from inadequate thyroid hormone regulation of transcription, the symptoms are likely to be more severe.

ADRENAL INSUFFICIENCY

Disorders of the hypothalamic-pituitary-adrenal axis or primary damage to the adrenal cortices may result in adrenocortical insufficiency.[104,p.1051] A relative adrenal insufficiency has been reported in fibromyalgia patients.[106] A mild central adrenal insufficiency (decreased adrenocortical secretion due to hypothalamic or pituitary dysfunction) has been reported in chronic fatigue syndrome patients.[107] Griep and coauthors wrote that adrenal insufficiency in fibromyalgia patients might explain their reduced aerobic capacity and impaired muscle performance.[106] It is possible, however, that the adrenocortical abnormalities documented in some fibromyalgia patients are the manifestation of inadequate thyroid hormone regulation of peripheral and central nervous system cell function (see Chapter 3.5). In Addison's disease (primary adrenal insufficiency), the basal metabolic rate may decrease to -25% or -30% of normal.[115,p.578] Early symptoms of adrenal insufficiency during Addison's disease include weakness, fatigue, and orthostatic hypotension. When the adrenal insufficiency is the result of a primary adrenal disease, the patient may have increased pigmentation due to elevated ACTH and melanocyte stimulating hormone.[105][119] The increased pigmentation may be apparent as widespread tanning of exposed and unexposed parts of the body. Skin over body prominences, skin folds, scars, and extensor surfaces become especially pigmented. The patient may also have black freckles over the face, forehead, neck, and shoulders.[104,p.1051]

During environmental stress, the pituitary gland increases its secretion of ACTH. The ACTH in turn stimulates the adrenal cortices to secrete adrenocortical hormones.[104,p.2500] The increased circulating levels of adrenocortical hormones decreases pituitary secretion of ACTH. When primary adrenal insufficiency occurs, as during the exhaustion stage of the general adaptation syndrome,[108,p.229] ACTH levels are high (50 pg/mL or more). The high levels of ACTH continue until the circulating level of adrenocortical hormones suppresses pituitary secretion of ACTH. Basal PM levels of ACTH have been reported to be elevated in some chronic fatigue syndrome patients, and stimulation of ACTH release by corticotropin stimulating hormone has been reported to be exaggerated in some fibromyalgia patients (see Chapter 3.5). Because these patients typically do not have hyper-pigmentation,

however, it seems likely that any adrenocortical impairment they have is minor. This does not support a contention that these syndromes are manifestations of the exhaustion stage of the general adaptation syndrome. It is more likely that the low cortisol levels in fibromyalgia[106] and chronic fatigue syndrome[107] patients are largely a result of inadequate thyroid hormone regulation of central nervous system cells (see Chapter 3.5).

Adrenal insufficiency must be corrected if it is contributing to the hypometabolism of a fibromyalgia patient with inadequate thyroid hormone regulation of cell function. Otherwise, the benefits from metabolic rehabilitation involving the use of exogenous thyroid hormone will be compromised.

DEPRESSION AND B VITAMIN DEFICIENCY

I know of no evidence that hypometabolism is produced by depression, *per se*. Of course, many depressed individuals have low levels of physical activity. As a result, their muscles lose mass as part of the process of deconditioning. If an individual's ratio of lean-to-fat tissue decreases, his metabolic rate will decrease roughly proportionally (see Chapter 5.5). But the decrease in metabolic rate is secondary to, not primarily due to, the depression.

Depression may occur in patients who are deficient in vitamins B$_6$,[35] B$_{12}$,[36] or folic acid.[37] When evaluating a patient for symptoms of euthyroid hypometabolism, folic acid deficiency is an especially important consideration. Travell and Simons[2,p.132] wrote that patients with low normal (lowest quartile) or subnormal serum folic acid levels commonly have symptoms and signs typical of patients with thyroid gland hypofunction. These patients tire easily, sleep poorly, feel depressed and discouraged, frequently feel cold, and have low basal temperatures. Travell and Simons also wrote that these patients tend to have increased neuromuscular irritability and susceptibility to myofascial trigger points. Because nutritional insufficiencies and deficiencies are common in the U.S. (see Chapter 5.5), all patients should begin nutritional supplementation to relieve any associated symptoms.

Psychoneurosis. The concept that the symptoms characteristic of euthyroid hypometabolism result from abnormal psychological processes has no credible scientific corroboration. It should be completely abandoned (see Chapter 1.2).

● THYROID HORMONE-RELATED EUTHYROID HYPOMETABOLISM

In thyroid hormone-related euthyroid hypometabolism, the patient's thyroid gland produces a normal amount of thyroid hormones. Also, the patient's circulating concentration of thyroid hormones is normal. Nonetheless, the patient's cell metabolism, at least in some tissues, is subnormal for some reason related to thyroid hormone other than a deficient blood level. If the patient's cell metabolism is sufficiently subnormal to generate troublesome symptoms, the patient may seek clinical care. Symptoms are typically vague and suggest hypothyroidism.

From 1900 until the early 1970s, the hypometabolism of a patient who sought clinical care could be confirmed by a low basal metabolic rate (BMR). After the advent of laboratory thyroid function blood tests, however, instruments for measuring the BMR and technicians who could performed the test soon became inaccessible to practicing clinicians. Without access to the instruments and technicians, there was no longer a highly sensitive and reliable method of measuring a patient's basal metabolism.

According to measurements of BMR, some euthyroid hypometabolic patients' metabolism did not accelerate with desiccated thyroid, thyroglobulin, or synthetic T_4.[31,p.1355] Soon after the discovery of T_3 in 1952,[84][85] some clinicians found that the BMRs of these formerly treatment-resistant patients did accelerate when they used synthetic T_3.[31,p.1355] The patients responded with both increased BMRs and improvement or relief of their symptoms.

The failure of physiologic dosages of thyroid hormone to exert normal cellular effects in some euthyroid hypometabolic patients may result from faults at one or more cellular sites. Sonkin wrote of the possible mechanisms, "Abnormality in responsiveness or concentration of end organ receptors, antibodies against receptors, or abnormalities of intracellular carriers of thyroid hormones are intriguing possibilities."[43,p.162] Regardless of the fault, normal circulating levels of thyroid hormones may not result in these hormones exerting their normal transcription-regulating effects at the chromosomes. The net effect is what Jefferies in 1961 termed ". . . a deficiency of thyroid hormone activity at the tissue level . . . ."[48,p.583] The effects of such deficient activity are theoretically the same as those of a frank thyroid hormone deficiency. For example, the effects would include a cellular increase in the metabolism-inhibiting molecular products (α-adrenergic receptors, inhibitory G_i proteins, and phosphodiesterase) that are normally kept at lower levels by adequate transcription regulation by thyroid hormone.[114]

The reason it is believed that some patients' euthyroid hypometabolism is thyroid hormone-related is that these patients benefit from the use of exogenous thyroid hormone. They benefit in general as hypothyroid patients do from the exogenous hormone. However, euthyroid patients typically do not respond well to T_4. In my clinical and research experiences, "replacement" dosages of T_4 are thoroughly without benefit for the vast majority of euthyroid patients. Supraphysiologic dosages of T_3 can be effective if the dosages are properly adjusted (see Chapter 5.2).

Early in the 20th century, clinicians used a positive response to exogenous thyroid hormone as a criterion for the diagnosis of hypothyroidism.[60,p.373] That a patient's symptoms improve or are relieved by exogenous thyroid hormone, however, does not prove that the symptoms were related to thyroid hormone. It is possible that the exogenous hormone may override a symptom mechanism that is not related to thyroid hormone. But the positive response to thyroid hormone does raise the possibility that the symptoms were thyroid hormone-related. This justifies further investigation of the possibility.

NON-SPECIFIC SYMPTOMS AND SIGNS

Symptoms are the initial clues that a patient might be suffering from too little thyroid hormone regulation of cell function. Throughout the 20th century, clinically-oriented practitioners have valued symptoms as an index of the metabolic status of patients. The complete abandonment of an appreciation of the value of this index by many technocratic endocrinologists/thyroidologists does not diminish its importance. In fact, the ineffectiveness of these practitioners with hypothyroid patients is testimony to the cost of their technocratic orientation.

Greek physician and writer on medicine Claudius Galen lived between AD 130-to-200. As far back as then, medical writers have described patients with a variety of symptoms that today are known to be characteristic of the hypometabolism of hypothyroidism. The symptoms are varied. In 1942, Barnes wrote, "No single symptom has been found which would apply to every person with low metabolism. Some have fatigue, some have cutaneous disorders, some have dry skin, some have nervousness, some have menstrual difficulties, some have dry hair and some have other symptoms. But none of these signs could be considered reliable in all cases."[116,p.1072]

The same is true of the symptoms of hypometabolism, whether they occur in the hypothyroid or euthyroid hypometabolic patient. Table 2.5.1 displays the symptoms of euthyroid hypometabolism reported by different investigators.

From symptoms we can only conjecture about the underlying mechanism. Nevertheless, as Sonkin pointed out regarding the symptoms of these patients, "None of the complaints is specific, but a constellation of these symptoms should raise the question of impaired thyroid function."[62,p.47] The possibility of inadequate thyroid hormone regulation of cell function is made more likely, though not proven, when these patients' symptoms are improved or relieved subsequent to their beginning the use of exogenous thyroid hormone.

Table 2.5.2 is a list of hypothyroid signs and symptoms reported in two studies. Those in bold print are signs and symptoms of euthyroid hypometabolism reported by various authors. The terms writers have used to describe these signs and symptoms have not been uniform throughout this century. Because of this, I have in some cases taken liberties in considering what appears in the literature to be different but synonymous terms for the same signs and symptoms. Of the 54 symptoms and signs listed, at least 30 (56%) have been reported to occur in euthyroid hypometabolic patients.

Pursuit of Objective Confirmation That Non-specific Symptoms Are Thyroid-Related

It is clinicians' written descriptions of symptoms that suggest that patients have for centuries shared some discomforting, and in some cases debilitating, abnormality related to the thyroid system. Only late in this century, however, have we been able to determine with fair reliability which of these patients have hypothyroidism.

According to Werner, in 1603 Paracelsus described endemic cretinism in the Duchy of Salzburg,[76] and in 1871, Fagge[77] described sporadic cretinism.[75,p.4] In 1874, Gull described cretinism in adults.[11] This led to Ord's coining the term "myxedema" to describe hypothyroidism in 1878.[79] The term referred to the patients' tissue swelling. It was Ord who in 1888 first related myxedema to thyroid gland disease.[80] At that time, the diagnosis was based on

clinical observation. Gradually, the symptoms patients reported and the signs clinicians observed (such as cretinism, myxedema, a slow relaxation phase of the Achilles reflex, and drooping eyelids) became useful gauges of patient status within the armamentarium of clinical medicine. Today, as over the past hundred years, symptoms and signs are useful to those who practice clinical rather than technocratic medicine. Symptoms and signs are clues that a patient may be hypothyroid or euthyroid hypometabolic, and they can serve as indices of change during metabolic treatment.

Table 2.5.1. Symptoms of euthyroid hypometabolic patients listed by various writers.

WRITER	SYMPTOMS/SIGNS LISTED
Thompson & Thompson[44,p.495]	Headaches, dizziness, weakness, chronic fatigue, nervousness/low BMR.
Thurmon & Thompson[45,p.883-886]	Lack of endurance, marked nervousness, marked tendency to worry and emotional upset at slight provocation, cold sensitivity, numbness and tingling of extremities, constipation, headache, vague pains, dizziness, palpitation, dyspnea on exertion, delayed and scanty menstrual flow/low pulse rate.
Kurland, et al.[31]	Lethargy, easy fatigability, nervousness, irritability, emotional instability, cold sensitivity, headache, ill-defined skeletal pain, diminished sexual potency in men, menstrual irregularity in women.
Sonkin[43,p.157]	A variety of symptoms suggesting hypothyroidism/slow Achilles reflex.
Goldberg[64,p.1053-1054]	Anxiety states, irritability, mood swings, easy fatigability, lethargy, decreased libido, premenstrual tension, GI disturbances, scalp seborrhea or hair loss, palpitations, muscle and joint pains, shortness of breath /prolonged contraction phase of Achilles reflex, low BMR.

But symptoms and signs are not specific enough for a definitive diagnosis of hypothyroidism[71,p.1092] or thyroid hormone-related euthyroid hypometabolism. By "not specific enough," I mean that the symptoms and signs typical of inadequate thyroid hormone regulation of cell function may also be manifestations of underlying conditions that are independent of a pa-

Table 2.5.2. Symptoms and signs of hypothyroidism.*

SYMPTOMS AND SIGNS

Appetite poor **
Atrophic tongue
Basal metabolic rate low
Cardiac enlargement on x-ray
Cerebration slow
Choking sensation
Cholesterol high
Coarse skin
Cold skin, cold sensitivity
Constipation, disturbed bowel function
Cyanosis
Deafness
Decreased sweating
Depression
Dysphagia
Dyspnea
Edema of eyelids
Emotional instability, irritability, anxiety, restlessness
Exophthalmos ***
Face edematous
Fatigue, lethargy
Fineness of hair
Food intake reduced
Fundus oculi changes
Hair dry, hair loss, hair coarseness
Heat intolerance
Hoarseness
Infertility
Libido diminished, potency decreased
Loss of weight
Menstrual disturbances (dysmenorrhea)
Memory impaired
Nails brittle, nails broken
Nervousness
Pain, joints
Pain, muscle (headaches)
Pain, precordial
Pallor of skin
Pallor of lips
Palpitations
Paresthesias
Peripheral edema
Poor heart sounds
Poor vision
Reflex, Achilles, slow
Skin dry
Speech slow
Sparse eyebrows
Temperature, low
Thick tongue
Weakness
Weight gain

*From: a) *The Thyroid and Its Diseases*, by L.J. DeGroot, P.R. Larsen, S. Refetoff, and J.B. Stanbury, New York, John Wiley & Sons, 1984, pp.577-578. b) *Bedside Diagnostic Examination*, by R.L. DeGowin, and E.L. DeGowin, 3rd edition. New York, Macmillan Publishing Co., Inc., 1976. c) Lowe, J.C., et al.: Effectiveness and safety of T3 (triiodothyronine) therapy for euthyroid fibromyalgia: a double-blind placebo-controlled response-driven crossover study. *Clin. Bull. Myofascial Ther.*, 2(2/3)31-57, 1997.
**Those in bold represent signs and symptoms in euthyroid hypometabolic patients reported by various authors.
***Probably periorbital edema, p.989 in d) Smith, T.J.: Connective tissue in hypothyroidism. In *Werner's The Thyroid: A Fundamental and Clinical Text*, 6th edition. Edited by L.E. Braverman and R.D.Utiger, Philadelphia, J.B. Lippincott Co., 1991, pp.989-992.

tient's thyroid status (see section above, "Causes of Euthyroid Hypometabolism Not Directly Related to Thyroid Hormone"). The lack of specificity of the symptoms and signs and the desire for objective barometers of patient status were a stimulus to research. Clinicians and researchers began pursuing objective methods for determining whether patients had thyroid system abnormalities and to quantify the degree of abnormality. First came the basal metabolic rate, next the protein-bound iodine, and then the basal body temperature.

MEASURES OF METABOLISM AND LABORATORY TESTING OF THYROID FUNCTION

There is no direct measure of the effects of thyroid hormone on an individual patient's cell metabolism. Barnes wrote that an ideal test is not even possible: "What we ideally need to measure is the amount of thyroid hormone on the inside of each cell in the body where it controls the rate of oxidation of fuel burning with the cell. It is obvious, of course, why such a test is impossible. Since there are billions of cells in the body, billions of simultaneous analyses would have to be run and this can't be done even today with computers."[40,pp.16-17] Attempts have been made to find indirect methods of assessing the effects of thyroid hormone on cell metabolism. The two indirect methods most commonly used have been the basal metabolic rate (BMR) and the basal body temperature (BBT). Serum cholesterol level, the Achilles reflex, and pulse rate were once considered possible indicators. They were non-specific, however, in that other factors may also have influenced the outcome of these measures.[60,p.373][116,p.1072]

I want to emphasize that although measures such as the basal body temperature, serum cholesterol level, Achilles reflex, and pulse rate are not specific to thyroid status, they are useful indices of metabolic status related to thyroid hormone. This is especially true when the clinician uses several of the non-specific measures to assess patient status (see Chapter 4.3).

At the end of the 19th century, the basal metabolic rate (BMR) came into use. The BMR measures oxygen consumption at rest, which is considered equivalent to the metabolic rate of the body. Early in the 20th century, some clinicians also began using the basal body temperature (BBT). The BBT measures the body temperature at rest. Before these two measures, there was no fundamental way to assess whether an individual's cellular metabolism was normal or slow.

Before highly sensitive and reliable thyroid function laboratory tests were developed, clinicians had difficulty distinguishing between hypothyroid and euthyroid hypometabolic patients. Even with these tests, the distinction is not always certain. The earliest test in widespread use to assess the thyroid hormone level in the blood was the protein-bound iodine. Before its advent, clinicians had no way to determine whether a patient had normal circulating levels of thyroid hormones.

What Various Measures Do and Do Not Do

It is important to understand what the various measures do and do not do. Blood tests of thyroid function now show with a fair degree of accuracy when an individual is hypothyroid—that is, when the circulating thyroid hormone levels are low due to impaired synthesis and secretion of the hormones by the thyroid gland. Thyroid function tests are not, however, measures of cell metabolism. Conversely, the BMR and BBT are measures of cell metabolism (although the BBT is useful only with some patients), but they do not determine whether a patient's metabolic rate is related to her blood levels of thyroid hormone.

Measurement of the Basal Metabolic Rate (BMR)

At the end of the 19th century, the pioneer clinician Magnus-Levy showed that a nurse consumed more oxygen after she began taking thyroid substance as a treatment for obesity.[117][118] He termed the oxygen consumption at rest the basal metabolic rate (BMR). He showed that the BMRs of patients thought to be hypothyroid were low and those of patients thought to be hyperthyroid were high.

The normal range of the BMR is reported to be -15% to +5%.[2,p.145] The BMRs of patients with complete loss of thyroid gland function may fall to -35% or -45%. According to DeGroot et al., the BMRs of untreated hypothyroid patients usually decrease to between -35% and -45%, with an average of about -40%.[115,p.579] The BMRs of patients with complete absence of thyroid gland function are remarkably constant. BMRs differ less among hypothyroid patients than among normal individuals.

Conditions other than hypothyroidism may lower the BMR.[120,p.168] The condition most important to us in this chapter is peripheral resistance to thyroid hor-

mone.[10] In Addison's disease (primary adrenal insufficiency), the BMR may fall to -25% or -30%. In pituitary gland deficiency, it may drop to below -50%.[115,p.578] In a patient who fasted for 30 days, the BMR decreased by 30%.[121]

Some Researchers Designate Patients with Low Basal Metabolic Rates as "Healthy." Early in this century, some patients with the non-specific symptoms were shown to have low basal metabolic rates. It appears that if a patient with non-specific symptoms and a low metabolic rate had the swollen, doughy cutaneous appearance called myxedema, the researchers diagnosed hypothyroidism. If the patient did not have myxedema, despite having symptoms and a low metabolic rate, the researchers designated the patient as "healthy."[46,p.537][64,p.1053][81,pp.24-25]

The "Essential" Sign: Myxedema. Why was myxedema considered essential to the diagnosis of hypothyroidism in the early part of the 20th century? Kimball gave his opinion in 1933 as he worked to change the view of the medical profession that myxedema was essential to the diagnosis: ". . . Ord overemphasized the symptoms of myxedema when he analyzed the condition in 1874.[79] Sir William Gull first described the condition. Henceforth, Gull's disease became myxedema."[59,p.488] The general impression was that the patient with depressed thyroid gland function would invariably have obvious myxedema.

Kimball also attributed the erroneous view that all hypothyroid patients have myxedema in part to a paper by Boothby, Plummer and Wilson. The Mayo Clinic published the paper as a monograph in 1922.[59,p.488] At that time, there were no blood tests to measure thyroid hormone levels and from which to make inferences about hormone production by the thyroid gland. The diagnostic criterion for hypothyroidism at that time was a positive response (relief of symptoms and rise in the BMR) to desiccated thyroid by a person with a low BMR. In line with this criterion, Boothby, Plummer, Wilson, and other investigators[53] tried to differentiate hypothyroid from normal individuals. They did so by measuring each person's basal metabolic rate (BMR) and treating those with low BMRs with desiccated thyroid. They found that some people with low BMRs did not improve with desiccated thyroid. From this observation, they concluded that the BMR did not distinguish normal from hypothyroid individuals. Presumably, their assumption was that the non-specific symptoms of these patients were due to some condition not related to hypothyroidism or were not related to an underlying condition at all. Since some people they considered euthyroid had low BMRs, they could not conclude that a low BMR was diagnostic of hypo-thyroidism. In the end, they concluded that only the presence of myxedema distinguished which patients were hypothyroid. Their conclusions, combined with Ord's, initiated a misbelief within the medical profes-sion that proved difficult to dispel.

Table 2.5.3a. Percentages of hypothyroid patients in two studies with myxedematous swelling of different tissues, and the percentage of control subjects from one study with swelling of the same tissues.*

SYMPTOMS AND SIGNS	STUDY A % OF 77 CASES	STUDY B % OF 100 CASES	NORMAL CONTROL SUBJECTS
Edema of eyelids	90	86	28
Thick tongue	82	60	17
Edema of face	79	95	27
Peripheral edema	55	57	2
Exophthalmos[γ]	—[δ]	11	4

The Thyroid and Its Diseases, by L.J. DeGroot, P.R. Larsen, S. Refe-toff, and J.B. Stanbury, New York, John Wiley & Sons, 1984, pp.577-578.
[γ] Probably periorbital edema, p.989 in Smith, T.J. : Connective tissue in hypothyroidism. In *Werner's The Thyroid: A Fundamental and Clin-ical Text*, 6th edition. Edited by L.E. Braverman and R.D. Utiger, Phila-delphia, J.B. Lippincott Co., 1991, pp.989-992.
[δ]—Dash means not reported in the study.

Table 2.5.3a shows the percentage of hypothyroid patients in two studies who had myxedematous swel-ling or puffiness. The percentages for the patients are compared to the percentage of control subjects in one study who had swelling. It is understandable, consid-ering the high percentages in the hypothyroid patients, how early researchers mistakenly considered myx-edema diagnostic of hypothyroidism. It has been long established that not all hypothyroid patients have myx-edema. Nonetheless, some clinicians continued to use the term myxedema as a synonym for hypothyroid-ism.[74,p.762]

The Argument that Hypometabolism is Physio-logical and Not of Pathological Significance. Some researchers early in the 20th century argued that people with low BMRs represent the lower end of the normal bell curve for metabolic rates.[64,p.1053] Kirk and Kvor-ning wrote that low BMRs were not associated with pathology and referred to the phenomenon as "physio-logical hypometabolism."[81,pp.24-25]

Some clinicians and researchers continue to hold this view. Consider statements made by Linder in 1991: "As molecular biological research continues, the extremes of 'allowable' genetic differences for normal function will become ever clearer."[69,p.8] This is a seemingly benign statement. However, it expresses a philosophy of medical care perpetuated by the current endocrinology/thyroidology paradigm that has inflict-ed needless suffering and tragedy upon many hypo-metabolic individuals. Linder also wrote that genetic makeup may underlie ". . . metabolism differences among normal individuals." She wrote that indeed ". . . there is considerable 'biological variation' among individuals within the 'normal, healthy' population." She gave as an example people with different forms of hemoglobin. "Each of these will vary to some extent in its ability to bind oxygen under a variety of different physiological conditions, but will still allow overall 'normal' performance (not requiring medical inter-vention)."[69,p.8]

Linder's last stipulation exemplifies the implica-tion of the current endocrinology/thyroidology para-digm that hypometabolism is not a threat to health. Practitioners who subscribe to this implicit proposition neglect to consider the often debilitating non-specific symptoms of both euthyroid hypometabolic and hypo-thyroid patients. Many hypometabolic patients do not receive proper metabolism-accelerating treatment, and the human suffering that results is so great as to be in-calculable.

Thyroid Status of Patients with Low BMRs—Uncertain Prior to the 1970s. Specific and fairly reli-able thyroid function tests were not available until the 1970s. It is not possible to learn at this time which patients with low BMRs in pre-1970 studies actually had thyroid hormone deficiencies. Some patients may have been malnourished, folic acid-deficient, decondi-tioned, or anemic. Others may have been truly hypo-thyroid. While instruments for measuring the BMR were still available to clinicians, the protein-bound iodine and the radioactive iodine uptake became avail-able. These tests were not particularly useful: They were relatively insensitive, and their specificity was not certain because of the iodine contamination of patients' bodies. Conclusions about the percentages of patients who were hypothyroid and euthyroid based on the use of these tests are dubious.

Problems with the BMR. Barnes pointed out in a 1942 paper that unless the BMR is taken at a patient's home or in the hospital, it is not likely that the mea-surement will be accurate. Digestion and worry will prevent a true basal reading because they increase the metabolic rate. The activities of dressing and traveling to the facility where the BMR is to be measured will markedly increase the oxidative rate. This is true despite the patient resting for 30-to-60 minutes after arriving at the facility. Also, during the test the patient may not be able to relax, and this will keep the BMR higher than the basal value.[116,p.1072] In 1976, he also wrote, "And the test itself is anything but relaxing. A tight clothespin on the nose and a large rubber breathing tube stuffed in the mouth, or alternatively a tight mask over both the nose and mouth, do not make for calm and comfort."[40,p.17] He argued that instead of the BMR, the basal body temperature was the most reliable measure of metabolic status.[116]

Kimball also cautioned about errors in measuring the BMR. He wrote that a low BMR is more likely to be a correct reading than a high BMR. All errors tend to increase the reading or give a rate higher than the basal value.[59,p.495] In addition, Wharton explained that the calculation of the body surface area from height and weight, which is necessary for calculating the BMR, has an error of about 15%.[60,p.372]

Despite these problems, the BMR is potentially a valuable tool in diagnosing euthyroid hypometabolism and for adjusting thyroid hormone dosage for both hypothyroid and euthyroid hypometabolic patients. DeGroot and coauthors wrote that lowering of the BMR is the most reliable deviation from normal in hypothyroidism.[115,p.578] We can infer from this that increases in the BMR are a reliable index of increasing metabolism in response to the use of exogenous thyroid hormone, at least by the hypothyroid patient. Sonkin wrote that for the diagnosis and study of euthyroid hypometabolism, the BMR is essential.[62,p.59]

The BMR is not diagnostic of hypothyroidism, but when used in conjunction with laboratory tests of thyroid function, it could serve—were it available for practicing clinicians—as an almost indispensable clinical tool in the effort to obtain optimal cellular metabolism. Unfortunately, with the popularization among endocrinologists of the use of thyroid function tests, several medical organizations and Blue Cross/Blue Shield agreed to pronounce the BMR obsolete.[62,p.59] Insurance companies then began reimbursing for charges for the thyroid function tests and stopped reimbursing for BMRs.

Today, some BMR units cost around $25,000. This makes the purchase of a BMR unit economically impractical for most clinicians. This is especially true considering the dwindling income of clinicians due to managed care.

Measurement of the Basal Body Temperature (BBT)

As an historical figure in medicine, Broda Barnes

was a beacon of reason. He illuminated the failure of the current endocrinology/thyroidology paradigm to provide clinicians with methods to effectively identify and properly care for patients with thyroid hormone-related hypometabolism.

Barnes defined the basal body temperature (BBT) as the body temperature taken under conditions typically considered necessary for measuring the basal metabolic rate.[116,p.1072] He wrote that BBT was the most useful measure of the body's metabolic rate, and therefore it was the best method for identifying hypothyroidism.[40,p.36-50] He believed the BBT was more reliable than the BMR.[116] The BBT is not as vulnerable to false negatives as the BMR. When patients are not able to relax, the BBT may still show a subnormal temperature despite a BMR measurement above the true basal rate.[40,p.77] In addition, the BBT is inexpensive and convenient in that the patient can administer the test to herself. Barnes specified that before taking the BBT, the patient should have a good night's rest, no food for 12 hours, and no excitement or exercise.

Barnes wrote, "I certainly hold no brief for the basal temperature as the ultimate test. But until something better comes along, it can, I know, help many physicians to help patients."[40,p.137] He also wrote: "The basal temperature is not a perfect test for thyroid function. There are conditions other than hypothyroidism that may produce a low reading—for example, starvation, pituitary gland deficiency, or adrenal gland deficiency. But starvation is certainly not difficult to rule out—and some thyroid is frequently indicated, anyhow, for the other conditions."[40,p.46] And in light of these qualifications, he wrote, "More information often can be brought to the physician with only the aid of the ordinary thermometer than can be obtained with all other thyroid function tests combined."[40,p.46]

Based on his research and extensive use of the BBT, Barnes conjectured that 40% of the population has some degree of hypothyroidism. (He did not mention cellular resistance to thyroid hormone, but it appears likely that he included in his definition of hypothyroidism both thyroid hormone deficiency and cellular resistance to thyroid hormone.)

Problems with the BBT. Barnes wrote, "Very few patients with subnormal temperature fail to respond to thyroid therapy, both as to relief of symptoms and as to elevation in temperatures."[116,p.1073] In my clinical experience, however, in a considerable percentage of patients, increases in the BBT do not keep pace with other indices of metabolic change during thyroid hormone treatment. Because of this, for years I have used other indirect measures of metabolic status in lieu of the BBT.

Refetoff also found that the body temperature is not a reliable index of metabolic change. He hospitalized patients and measured various indices of metabolic status as he administered and increased the dosage of T_3. Simultaneously, he recorded changes in core temperature. To measure core temperature, he had patients swallow, at intervals, glass capsules that contained thermometers. Each capsule was equipped with a device that transmitted signals from the thermometer to a receiver that recorded the alimentary canal temperature during the day and night. Refetoff found that changes in temperature did not correlate well with other measures of metabolic status. For example, at high T_3 dosages, patients had negative nitrogen balance. This indicates protein catabolism and may have been a thyrotoxic effect. Temperatures in general, however, did not increase at rates or to levels that were proportional to this and other measures of metabolic status.[124]

Refetoff stated that the basal temperature is useful only with extreme changes in metabolism. According to him, in most humans whose hypothyroidism has been confirmed through other tests, there is no significant change in the basal temperature. And in laboratory animals, the basal temperature does not change unless the thyroid gland is totally ablated and the animal is left for a time with no thyroid hormones. He concluded from such findings that the body temperature is not a useful indicator of mild degrees of hypothyroidism. He also stated that there are many factors that affect the basal body temperature, so it is not a specific measure of metabolic status.[124]

Some clinicians have argued that increasing the body temperature with thyroid hormone is essential to activating enzymes that then normalize cell processes. Barnes cited Kleitman's observations that work efficiency parallels diurnal variations in body temperature.[116,p.1073][122] This may appear to imply that the health of the body and functional capacity depend upon an optimal body temperature. The higher body temperature during times of greater work efficiency is most likely a byproduct of the increased metabolism during these times. It is unlikely that the increased temperature is a *cause* of the increased work efficiency. In the early 1600s, Descartes expressed the same erroneous view as Barnes and Kleitman, writing that heat is the cause rather than the result of body motion.[123] Increases in body temperature with the use of exogenous thyroid hormone occur secondarily to the increased activity of various enzymes. For example, thyroid hormone controls the expression of sodium/

potassium-ATPase (Na^+/K^+-ATPase) through genomic action. Thyroid hormone increases the availability of Na^+/K^+-ATPase. Heat production is a *byproduct* of resulting increases in Na^+/K^+-ATPase activity, as a phosphate is cleaved from ATP molecules with the production of ADP (see Chapter 2.2, section titled "Thyroid Hormone and Membrane Na^+/K^+-ATPase Activity").

Laboratory Thyroid Function Tests

In 1888, Ord related what we now know as hypothyroidism signs and symptoms to disease of the thyroid gland.[80] After that advance in knowledge, there was a lengthy time before researchers developed tests for measuring levels of hormones of the pituitary-thyroid gland axis. Certainly, however, astute clinicians recognized that something was radically wrong with many patients who suffered from the symptoms and signs. Their recognition must have contributed to the pursuit of tests to determine the source of the signs and symptoms.

Clinicians were extremely limited in their understanding of the condition that afflicted their patients. Having no laboratory tests of thyroid function with established ranges of normal for thyroid hormones was only one of their limitations. TSH had not been discovered yet. They had no knowledge base for understanding why some patients with non-specific symptoms and low BMRs did not benefit from desiccated thyroid or T_4. Theorists would not originate the concept of cellular resistance to thyroid hormone for more than another half century. And even more time would pass before researchers would discover impaired conversion of T_4 to T_3. In light of such limitations, it would not be fair with hindsight to fault these early clinicians for false conclusions about the condition.

It is understandable that they believed the condition was rare.[12,p.246] Only after researchers developed blood tests for assessing the thyroid system did it become obvious that thyroid hormone deficiency was common, and in some areas, epidemic. It would also not be fair to fault the clinicians for an overly-simplistic line of reasoning—that when exogenous thyroid hormone relieved a patient's non-specific symptoms, it did so because the patient had a deficiency of the hormone. And if a patient failed to benefit from taking exogenous thyroid hormone, she must already have had a sufficient amount of the hormone and the symptoms were not due to a hormone deficiency.

The deduction the clinician made from this line of reasoning was this: Only a thyroid hormone deficiency can produce the symptoms and signs that are relieved by the patient's intake of exogenous thyroid hormone. Today, this deduction can no longer be logically or scientifically defended, yet it is the implicit proposition by which conventional endocrinologists/thyroidologists practice.

Late in the 19th century, the committee of the Clinical Society of London was appointed to study myxedema. In 1888, the committee reported, "the great majority of cases . . . have reached, when first recognized, a well advanced stage." They also stated hopefully, ". . . in the near future the disease may be detected in its beginnings."[63,p.1439] This last statement forecasted the development of laboratory thyroid function tests and documentation of degrees of hypothyroidism. Some 80 years would pass, however, before this would occur. In 1973, Evered and coauthors[125] published a study reporting their findings that hypothyroidism is a graded phenomenon. They reported that at the time, the most useful features defining an individual's grade of hypothyroidism were the clinical manifestations, the serum TSH, and the presence of circulating antibodies to the tissues of the thyroid gland. The three grades of hypothyroidism they used were normal status, subclinical hypothyroidism, and overt hypothyroidism.[125]

Earlier, in 1942, Barnes had noted that there was still considerable disagreement in the literature as to whether all patients with low metabolic rates were hypothyroid.[116,p.1072] The disagreements continued for at least two reasons. First, the BMR, which was in widespread use, is not a measure of thyroid hormone levels; second, reliable tests for thyroid hormone blood levels still were not available (until 1940, the only test of thyroid function was the BMR[40,p.135]). Concluding that the non-specific symptoms often relieved by exogenous thyroid hormone were due to hypothyroidism was an inference. The inference was based on the patients' low BMRs and peripheral indices such as a high serum cholesterol and a slow relaxation phase of the Achilles reflex, as well as the patients' positive responses to thyroid hormone use. Clinicians also depended on their judgment as to whether a particular patient's symptoms were likely, based on past experiences with other patients, to be relieved by exogenous thyroid hormone.

The earliest test of circulating thyroid hormone levels, and the one most often used before the 1970s, was the protein-bound iodine.[74,p.763] This test came into use about 1940.[40,p.136] The test is an estimate of the plasma level of thyroid hormones after the patient takes a dose of radioactive iodine 131I or 132I (measured

by a directional scintillation counter), and by inference, of thyroid hormone transport proteins. Patients usually take the iodine by mouth. The half-life of 131I is 8 days; that of 132I is 2-to-3 days. The range of normal is 11%-to-33%. In thyrotoxicosis, about 90% of values are above normal, and in hypothyroidism, about 80% are below normal.[74,pp.762,763] Later, clinicians began testing the rate of uptake of radioactive iodine (131I) by the thyroid gland. Both tests would eventually be considered relatively non-specific because of the already high iodine content of most patients' bodies.

Barnes wrote that after the protein-bound iodine came into use, other tests to measure thyroid function soon followed, and ". . . the era of the laboratory had begun."[40,p.136] He wrote of the irrational devotion of many physicians to laboratory tests such as the protein-bound iodine: "The result was a pendulum-like swing to an extreme. Many physicians came to look upon the results of laboratory tests as absolutes. If a patient was hypothyroid, the laboratory was the place to determine so. If laboratory tests failed to indicate hypothyroidism, it could not be present—no matter the patient's symptoms or even if a patient was already on thyroid therapy and benefitting from it. Willy-nilly, if the lab report came back negative for low thyroid function, the patient got no thyroid therapy, and if the patient was already on it he or she was taken off it."[40,pp.136-137] Barnes also noted that it was 1967 when Herbert Selenkow of Harvard began publicizing the pitfalls and unreliability of the protein-bound iodine. Barnes wrote that thyroid function tests are no substitute for ". . . a good physician's knowledge of what thyroid deficiency can bring about and his expert clinical impression of what it may be doing in the case of an individual patient."[40,pp.136-137]

Into the early 1970s, other clinicians tended to agree with Barnes about the value of indicators other than laboratory tests, such the patients' health history and symptoms and signs. In 1973,[73,p.52] Plankard recommended that clinicians use the symptoms, signs, and objective measures described in Table 2.5.3b to diagnose hypothyroidism. To my knowledge, this is one of the most comprehensive published protocols for the diagnosis of hypothyroidism. The two laboratory thyroid function tests he recommended (the protein-bound iodine and the 131I uptake by the thyroid gland) are less sensitive and specific than tests available today. But despite this, clinicians who used a multiple indicator method for diagnosis such as Plankard's were able to identify virtually all patients with hypometabolism, although the metabolism of some might not have been due to a thyroid hormone deficiency.

And if the clinicians used multiple indicators, they were certainly better able to manage cases than the technocratic endocrinologists/thyroidologists of today who use only the serum TSH (and possibly the free T_4) to diagnose and manage cases. The clinician using only the protocol these technocrats recommend will fail to identify most patients with central hypothyroidism and all those with thyroid hormone-related euthyroid hypometabolism.

Table 2.5.3b. The symptoms, signs, and objective measures Plankard recommended for clinicians to use in diagnosing hypothyroidism.

───────────────────

SYMPTOMS

(1) Cold sensitivity, even in warm weather.
(2) Worsening of symptoms during cold weather.
(3) Mental slowness, possible irritability, suspicion, delusions, and hallucinations.

SIGNS

(1) Slow pulse.
(2) Subnormal temperature.
(3) Increase in weight.
(4) Anemia.
(5) Decrease in basal metabolic rate (BMR), perhaps as much as 40% below normal.
(6) Raised cholesterol (normal = 154-to-260 mg/mL).
(7) Low ^{131}I uptake, thyroid gland (normal = 20%-to-50%).
(8) Low protein-bound iodine (normal = 3.5-to-8 μg/100 mL).
(9) Positive response to treatment with "thyroid."

───────────────────

Maclagan wrote in 1973 that the success of laboratory tests for assessing thyroid status "... has made metabolic procedures [such as the BMR] much less popular. However, the basal metabolic rate is still occasionally of value, as is the high blood-cholesterol of myxoedema, particularly as a check on the effects of treatment which may invalidate other tests."[74,p.764] The value of tests such as the serum cholesterol level and speed of the relaxation phase of the Achilles reflex for adjusting thyroid hormone dosage decreases because in most cases thyroid hormone treatment normalizes them. When normal, they do not reflect slight changes in metabolic status and their value for dosage adjustments diminishes. The BMR more sensitively measures subtle variations in metabolism. Maclagan also pointed out that when patients were seen who were

clinically thyrotoxic but had normal T_4 levels, the BMR could be useful.[74,p.764]

By the early 1970s, however, the BMR had come into disfavor. Soon after, instruments for measuring the BMR and technicians skilled at conducting the test were no longer available for the use of practicing clinicians. In a 1978 abstract submitted to the Endocrine Society, Sonkin wrote: "Sequential BMR and serum cholesterol measurements aid in the evaluation of therapeutic responses to thyroid hormones. The BMR, recently and inappropriately under pressure to be obsolete, remains a source of useful clinical information not currently available from other thyroid tests except serum cholesterol. It also remains a useful tool in the follow up of conventionally hypothyroid and thyrotoxic patients during and after treatment."[65] Fifteen years later, Sonkin wrote, "The test was useful in detecting thyroid dysfunction, and in following treatment with sequential measurements on the same patient, but had shortcomings as a single measurement because of its wide 'normal' range."[62,p.50]

The disappearance of the BMR from facilities available to practicing clinicians no doubt stemmed from the endocrinologists' interest in measuring the levels of circulating thyroid hormones. With tests that determined hormone levels, clinicians would not have to depend on inferences about the status of the patient's pituitary-thyroid gland axis from indirect measures such as the BMR. Theoretically, direct measures of thyroid hormone levels would enable the clinician to distinguish patients who had thyroid hormone deficiencies from those who did not. Many clinicians incorrectly assumed, though, that blood thyroid hormone levels—and later, the TSH level—are synonymous with tissue metabolic status. Their incorrect deduction was that if levels of circulating thyroid hormones and TSH are within the established normal reference range, metabolism in all tissues is also normal. They neglected to appreciate two critical facts: (1) there is variability in the responsiveness to thyroid hormone among individuals, and (2) there is variability in the responsiveness of different tissues in the same individual. The incorrect deduction has had a devastating impact on the quality and span of life of hypothyroid patients. Nevertheless, since 1973, the deduction has dictated many clinicians' decisions about their hypothyroid patients' dosages of T_4.[16][17][38,p.810]

The desire for more sensitive and specific measures of thyroid hormone levels led to the diagnosis of thyroid hormone abnormalities based on bioassays. As time passed, researchers developed increasingly specific tests for measuring serum thyroid hormone levels.[71,p.1092] By the late 1980s, the most often-ordered thyroid function tests were the T_4, T_3 uptake, and free thyroxine index (FTI).[172]

Advent of the TSH Assay. The doctrine that TSH stimulates T_4 secretion by the thyroid gland was in place by the 1930s.[19,p.305] In 1933, Kimball[59,p.492] wrote that recent studies had yielded a thyrotropin hormone that could be used to induce exophthalmos in normal animals. In 1949, Purves of New Zealand, one of the few who had measured TSH levels, visited Harvard. He reported that the hormone was elevated above normal in hypothyroidism.[57,p.44] As late as 1967, however, articles discussing common thyroid function tests did not mention the TSH.[20] The lack of mention was probably due to the lack of an established normal reference range for TSH blood levels. Investigators specified a range in the early 1970s, and authors began recommending the test.[21] In 1973, however, measurements of the TSH were ". . . only carried out in a few special centres . . . ."[74,p.763] The procedure used was to measure the amount of isotopically-labeled thyroid hormone released from an animal's thyroid gland after injecting the animal with the patient's serum or serum extract. Eventually, clinicians accepted that the TSH is usually high in hypothyroidism and low in hyperthyroidism.[74,p.763] Its increasing use in clinical practice contributed to researchers developing more sensitive TSH assays.

Sensitivity of TSH Assays. Today, second-generation TSH assays are sensitive and third-generation assays are even more so. The basal TSH and changes in endogenous TSH levels during the TRH stimulation test are reliable[71,p.1092] as long as various factors that alter the TSH level or the test procedure do not interfere. Even first-generation TSH assays were sensitive enough so that clinicians were able to classify patients as having subclinical or "incipient" hypothyroidism.[63,p.1442][65,p.661] The diagnosis of subclinical hypothyroidism is made when the TSH level is elevated, indicating hypofunction of the thyroid gland. The TSH level rises before other tests can detect decreased T_4 or T_3 levels. The elevated basal TSH is said to predict the eventual failure of thyroid function.

Abandonment of the Use of Hypothyroid Symptoms and Signs: Transition of the Conventional Endocrinologist/Thyroidologist from Medical Clinician to Laboratory Technocrat. It is noteworthy that TSH assays made it possible to establish definite criteria for the diagnosis of subclinical hypothyroidism. The criteria include a normal T_4 and T_3 level and an elevated TSH. Some investigators argue that an elevated TSH in the presence of a normal T_4 level indicates a failing thyroid gland and a high likelihood of future overt hypothyroidism.[22] Some investigators question whether the patient with a normal T_4 and elevated TSH should begin the use of exogenous thyroid hormone unless that patient has clinical symptoms of hypothyroidism.[21,p.608] Other investigators argue that the patient should begin treatment with T_4 strictly on the basis of laboratory test values indicating subclinical hypothyroidism. In 1987, endocrinologists/thyroidologists were still debating this issue.[12,p.246][23]

There is an irony in the history of endocrinology/thyroidology at that time. Beginning treatment with T_4 on the basis of laboratory values that prognosticate the future emergence of hypothyroid symptoms seems a liberal policy. Yet this very reliance on laboratory test values without consideration of patients' symptoms appears to have substantially contributed to an extremely conservative policy—denial of thyroid hormone treatment for patients with hypothyroid symptoms and signs because their laboratory test values do not corroborate their hypothyroidism. *Underlying this policy is the tacit belief of conventional endocrinologists/thyroidologists that all patients' tissues, and every tissue in each patient, are equally responsive to the same quantity of thyroid hormone.* As long as the conventional endocrinologist/thyroidologist holds this false belief, it will continue to reinforce his repudiation of any clinical value in patients' symptoms and signs and his extremist focus on laboratory test results. With this development, we witness the point of transition for the conventional endocrinologist/thyroidologist from medical clinician to laboratory technocrat.

Limitations of the TSH Test. There are at least two major limitations in a dependence on the TSH test. First, despite the contrary claims of writers such as Volpé,[96] the basal TSH (as well as the T_4 and free thyroxine index) may be normal in patients who have mild but symptomatic primary hypothyroidism.[62,p.48] In addition, my clinical and research experiences convince me that the basal TSH does not identify patients with central hypothyroidism (see Chapter 4.2, subsection titled "Basal TSH and Free T_4 Predict TSH Response to TRH in Euthyroid and Primary Hypothyroid Patients"). Moreover, even during the TRH stimulation test, post-injection TSH levels are normal in some patients with documented central hypothyroidism.[128]

Endocrinology/thyroidology laboratory technocrats generally ignore such limitations. Their mode of practice has resulted in legions of dissatisfied hypothyroid and euthyroid hypometabolic patients throughout the world.

One Diagnostic Step Forward: One Diagnostic

Step Backward. Modern laboratory thyroid function tests are reasonably reliable and readily accessible. They are a necessary tool for determining the probable functional status of a patient's pituitary-thyroid gland axis. On the other hand, with the virtual inaccessibility of units to measure the basal metabolic rate, we cannot so easily document the patient's metabolic status. Instead, we must form an impression from the use of indirect and non-specific peripheral indices such as the Achilles reflex, the basal body temperature, and symptoms lists. Thus, clinicians today can determine directly and with a high degree of probability whether a patient is euthyroid. But whether the patient is eumetabolic must remain far less definite, for euthyroid is *not* synonymous with eumetabolic. Clinicians are simply not able to accurately assess the patient with possible inadequate thyroid hormone regulation of cell function without methods for evaluating both the status of the pituitary-thyroid gland axis *and* the patient's metabolism. No net gain in quality patient care is inherent in having obtained one method at the cost of the other.

Laboratory Thyroid Function Testing Is of No Value in the Dosage Titration of Hypothyroid and Euthyroid Hypometabolic Patients

In 1986, Fraser and colleagues compared two methods of adjusting the T_4 of hypothyroid patients: thyroid function test results, and the clinical judgment of experienced clinicians. The laboratory tests used were the total T_4, total T_3, free T_4, free T_3, and basal TSH. Four clinicians experienced in the use of T_4 evaluated the patients clinically and used the Wayne index[39] (an assessment of patients' symptoms and signs) to classify the patients as euthyroid, hypothyroid, or hyperthyroid. (What the clinicians were actually assessing was whether the patients were clinically eumetabolic, hypometabolic, or hypermetabolic.) The clinicians' assessments of patients were determined not to be biased by subjecting the Wayne index scores to Kruskal-Wallis analysis of variance. The outcome showed that there was no significant difference in the median scores of the 4 clinicians. By contrast, tests of the total T_4, total T_3, free T_4, free T_3, and basal TSH were of *no* value in determining whether patients were taking enough, too much, or too little T_4. The researchers wrote, "These measurements are therefore of little, if any, value in monitoring patients receiving thyroxine replacement."[38]

The conclusion of Fraser et al.[38] in the above study is inherent in a statement by Stockigt in the 1996 edition of *Werner's The Thyroid*. He wrote, "In some situations (e.g., patients with ischemic heart disease

and hypothyroidism), the appropriate dose of T_4 should be based on clinical judgment rather than laboratory findings."[100,p.381] This was a concession that adjusting dosage by clinical indicators is superior to doing so on the basis of laboratory thyroid function test results. The implicit message in Stockigt's statement is that when adjusting the dosage of exogenous thyroid hormone is *really* important (as in avoiding exacerbation of ischemic heart disease), the patient's symptoms, signs, and physical exam results are more important than thyroid function test results. I consider adjusting the exogenous thyroid hormone dosage of all hypothyroid and euthyroid hypometabolic patients extremely important. The quality of their lives is at stake. And for some, the continuation of life by alleviating suicidal urges depends upon effective dosage adjustments. There is no justification for denying these patients the greater efficacy of care based on responsible clinical judgment rather than laboratory test values.

As conventional endocrinologists/thyroidologists are wont to do upon conceding that laboratory testing has limited value, Stockigt hedged: ". . . but there is justification for periodic serum TSH assessment to avoid subtle tissue effects of thyroid hormone excess or deficiency."[100,p.381] Notwithstanding this statement, it is indisputable that the TSH level does not assess the effects of thyroid hormone, subtle or otherwise, on any tissue other than the anterior pituitary. The TSH level is a measure of nothing more than the secretory activity of the anterior pituitary thyrotroph cells. The functional status of the thyroid gland can be inferred from the TSH level, but that is the extent of the value in measuring the TSH level during treatment with exogenous thyroid hormone.

DIAGNOSIS OF HYPOTHYROIDISM BY TREATMENT WITH THYROID HORMONE

After Sir William Gull first described myxedema in 1874, clinicians knew it was potentially fatal.[11] It was a great discovery, therefore, when Dr. George R. Murray (a physician in Newcastle, England) found that he could cure myxedema by giving patients thyroid substance. On April 13, 1891, he successfully treated his first patient, a hypothyroid woman, with a homemade thyroid extract. He macerated sheep thyroid tissue in glycerine and a weak phenol solution, and then he strained it through a "fine handkerchief." He injected her subcutaneously with this extract once or twice a week. Within 3 months, she had remarkably improved. She began the treatment in 1891 and continued until 1919, when she died at the age of 74.[14] Murray's presentation to the British Medical Association in July, 1891, and his published paper a few months later,[14] were the first reports of successful hormone therapy.[13,p.389] Since that time, incalculable numbers of patients' hypothyroid symptoms and signs have been relieved with oral thyroid hormone therapy.

Within a year, clinicians found that consuming thyroid tissue by mouth was also effective.[15] Sheep's thyroid tissue was distasteful, so patients "lightly fried" it or ate it with brandy or currant jelly. Within a few years, several companies supplied dried thyroid tissue as powder or tablets.[13,p.390] By 1916, attempts to standardize thyroid products led to the U.S.P. definition that a standard thyroid preparation contained 0.2% iodine.[13][112] By the 1940s, desiccated thyroid was established as a reliable product.[13,p.391] Desiccated thyroid is a mixture of T_3 and T_4 derived from pig thyroid tissue in the proportions found in the thyroid gland. By 1983, desiccated thyroid accounted for about 40% of the thyroid preparations sold in the U.S.A[89]

In 1915, Kendall reported that he had isolated a small amount of active crystalline substance from alkaline hydrolysates of a large amount of desiccated thyroid. He also reported that the material corrected hypothyroidism.[86] In 1919, Kendall and Osterberg synthesized the crystalline substance and named it thyroxine (T_4).[18] Harington in 1926[87] and Harington and Barger in 1927[88] determined the chemical structure of T_4. After these developments, some clinicians began using T_4 rather than desiccated thyroid to treat patients suspected of being hypothyroid.

Failure of Many Clinicians to Consider Hypothyroidism in Their Patients

Despite the availability of desiccated thyroid and T_4, many patients did not have the opportunity to use them because many clinicians did not believe the patients had a thyroid hormone deficiency.

The committee of the Clinical Society of London reported in 1888 that "the great majority of cases [of myxedema] . . . have reached, when first recognized, a well advanced stage," and ". . . in the near future the disease may be detected in its beginnings."[63,p.1439] We might infer from this that they regarded the condition as a graded phenomenon, possibly progressing along a continuum from incipient-to-severe. If so, many subsequent writers on the condition did not show this insight.

In the 1930s, writers of medical textbooks mentioned only distinct cretinism and myxedema as examples of hypothyroidism. They wrote little or nothing

about milder or unusual forms of the condition. As a result, Wharton wrote in 1939 that clinicians did not recognize as hypothyroid many patients who could benefit from thyroid hormone treatment. He said that mild or masked forms of hypothyroidism differ a great deal from cretinism and myxedema. To recognize it, the clinician must be constantly alert for its many and varied manifestations.[60,p.371]

In 1933, Kimball wrote of hypothyroidism, "In the practice of medicine today no more important condition is encountered or so often unrecognized as such, as hypothyroidism." He noted that many lecturers argued that hypothyroidism without myxedema (swelling or puffiness) did not exist. This is what his professors had taught him as a medical student 15 years before. He wrote, "Just why this teaching should persist now in the face of all the experimental evidence to the contrary is hard to understand."[59,p.488]

Kimball spent the next 10 years carrying out a clinical study of hypothyroid adults and children in the schools of Detroit and Cleveland. He observed and treated many patients continuously over this time.[59,p.488] Like other investigators, he found that *most* hypothyroid patients do not have the edematous swelling of myxedema. No longer, he concluded, should clinicians consider the term myxedema synonymous with hypothyroidism. If a clinician required patients to be myxedematous before considering them hypothyroid, he would miss most cases. Kimball concluded: "The differential diagnosis of a thyroid deficiency as being the underlying factor in any given condition is not so difficult; the real difficulty lies in the failure of the physician to consider it as a possibility in any given case."[59,p.495]

In 1957, Jackson wrote, "Hypothyroidism is the most frequent chronic affliction and at the same time the most often overlooked condition affecting persons residing in the Middle West." After treating thousands of hypothyroid patients over some 37 years, he also came to another conclusion. According to him, many clinicians failed to recognize hypothyroidism in many of their patients because they conducted BMR tests improperly.[61,p.121] The clinicians would not have patients rest prior to the tests to slow metabolism to a basal rate. The resulting measurements were higher than the patients' true BMRs. The clinicians would then conclude that the patients had normal BMRs and could not be hypothyroid.

Failure of Some Patients with Low BMRs to Benefit from Desiccated Thyroid or T_4. Before the BMR came into widespread use, a positive response to exogenous thyroid hormone served as a criterion for the diagnosis of hypothyroidism and for determining the proper dosage of thyroid hormone.[40,p.137][60,p.373] Some symptomatic patients with low BMRs, however, did not have a positive response to thyroid hormone. With the state of knowledge early in the 20th century, some clinicians decreed that these patients were not hypothyroid and did not need desiccated thyroid or T_4 therapy.

Winkler and coworkers, for example, described such patients in 1943. They wrote: "There are evidently a good many subjects who can tolerate two or three grains of oral thyroid daily, and some who can tolerate six or seven grains, without effect on the BMR. These patients had no other obvious clinical peculiarity in common, save possibly a tendency toward an initially low BMR. The BMR of myxedematous subjects, on the other hand, regularly increases by twenty-five or thirty per cent on two or three grains of thyroid daily, and shows no tendency to decline even after years of thyroid medication."[58] Some of Winkler's patients responded positively to T_4 injections but required much larger dosages than did "myxedematous" patients.[41] Lee in 1935[126] and Kirk and Kvorning in 1946[27] also described "hypothyroid" patients who did not show symptomatic or metabolic responses to desiccated thyroid, thyroglobulin, or thyroxine.

Recognition of Euthyroid Hypometabolism and the Advent of T_3

In retrospect, it is clear that the "hypothyroid" patients Wharton, Kimball, Jackson, and Barnes wrote about could have been either hypothyroid or euthyroid hypometabolic. We will never know, however, which classification any of their patients belonged to. Laboratory tests specific and sensitive enough to distinguish which patients had thyroid hormone deficiencies did not exist at the time; such tests were not available until the late 1970s.

In the 1950s, though, the discovery and use of T_3 led clinicians to make an important distinction. It was generally accepted among clinicians that a low BMR and characteristic symptoms indicated hypometabolism. An increase in the low BMR and relief of the symptoms through the use of desiccated thyroid or T_4 indicated that the hypometabolism had been the result of a thyroid hormone deficiency. Failure of the BMR to increase and symptoms to remit with the use of desiccated thyroid or T_4 suggested that the low BMR and symptoms were not due to a hormone deficiency. But then some clinicians found that patients unresponsive to desiccated thyroid and T_4 did respond to T_3. Why these patients responded to this form of thyroid hor-

mone and not to the others was up for conjecture. But the conclusion some clinicians reached was reasonable: Because the patients' low BMRs increased and their symptoms remitted with the use of T_3, their hypometabolism had been a result of insufficient thyroid hormone stimulation. The patients appeared to be euthyroid rather than hypothyroid, yet their hypometabolism appeared to be thyroid hormone-related. Clearly, they differed in some undetermined way from the other set of patients.

In 1952, two different research groups, one in England,[84][85] the other in France,[5][6] published reports of the discovery of T_3. Researchers had found the hormone in the thyroid gland and plasma. This ended a sort of short-term race by the two groups.[68,p.4] In a preliminary publication in 1951,[7,p.17] Gross and Pitt-Rivers of England reported finding that T_3 is a normal constituent of plasma in humans. They also isolated T_3 from the human thyroid gland and described its physiological activity. In 1952, they found that administering T_3 to hypothyroid rats reduced their goiters. In addition, they found that the hormone was an effective treatment for human hypothyroidism. The researchers wrote, ". . . from the above evidence it is suggested that triiodothyronine is the peripheral thyroid hormone and that thyroxine is its precursor." They acknowledged the simultaneous work of the French researchers who had identified radioactive T_3 and synthesized the molecule from diiodothyronine. Thyroxine or T_4 contains four iodine atoms and is accordingly named *tetra*-iodothyronine. In distinction, the T_3 compound contains three iodine atoms and is therefore suitably named *tri*-iodothyronine.

Researchers soon discovered that patients who failed to benefit from desiccated thyroid or T_4 improved or recovered from their non-specific symptoms with the use of T_3. In addition, their BMRs increased to normal values. As I noted in the previous section, investigators in 1935,[126] 1943,[58] and 1946[27] had described "hypothyroid" patients whose symptoms and BMRs did not improve with the use of desiccated thyroid, thyroglobulin, or thyroxine. Now, in the 1950s, such patients were the focus of study again, and researchers found that they benefitted from the use of T_3. These patients resemble the euthyroid fibromyalgia patients my research group and I have worked with since the late 1980s.[90][91][92][93][94][95][114][135][169] (Table 2.5.4 contains several researchers' lists of symptoms and signs of patients believed to have euthyroid hypometabolism.)

Therapeutic Responsiveness to T_3. When researchers in 1952 discovered T_3, they found that it had a potency far exceeding that of T_4. In July, 1955, the compound was made available for investigational use.[30,p.818] Several researchers soon found that it relieved the symptoms and signs and increased the BMRs of euthyroid hypometabolic patients.

In 1955, Freedberg, Kurland, and Hamolsky published a report of 2 patients with euthyroid hypometabolism. The patients' symptoms included aching of both knees, skin pallor, facial puffiness, feelings of dullness, and tiredness. Both had low BMRs and high cholesterol, and both failed to benefit from desiccated thyroid. The investigators reported that the patients' clinical and metabolic responses to T_3, or a combination of T_3 and T_4, were striking.[24]

After the 2 patients' BMRs had been normal for 3 weeks, each was taken off T_3 for 1 week and then started on a placebo that resembled the T_3 tablets they had taken before. The effects were dramatic. One complained of severe lethargy, fatigue, and puffiness of his eyes. His BMR promptly dropped. Within 3 weeks, his BMR had decreased from -5% and -10% to -23%. The other patient felt dull and fatigued and had pallor. His BMR dropped from -12% to -25%.[24,p.59]

Also in 1955, Kurland, Hamolsky, and Freedberg reported the cases of 4 patients who had low BMRs and were "resistant" to T_4: that is, their symptoms did not improve and their BMRs did not increase when taking the hormone. The patients' thyroid function tests were normal. The tests included the thyroidal ^{131}I uptake and turnover and serum levels of protein-bound iodine. Their serum cholesterol levels were also within normal limits. Their symptoms included lethargy, easy fatigue, nervousness, irritability, sensitivity to cold, headache, musculoskeletal pain, diminished sexual potency, and menstrual irregularities. Their BMRs were below -20%. Desiccated thyroid provided no sustained benefit, and some patients had thyrotoxic reactions to it. When given a combination of T_4 and T_3, or high doses of T_3 alone, their BMRs returned to normal levels. All patients' clinical status improved and their BMRs increased with the use of T_3 alone or a combination of T_3 and T_4.[31,p.1365]

Freedberg, Kurland, and Hamolsky wrote: "The dramatic relief of the clinical manifestations of myxedema [hypothyroidism] by the administration of desiccated thyroid is a striking example of the efficacy of hormone replacement therapy. Many patients are seen, however, with persistently low basal metabolic rates and with symptoms usually associated with thyroid deficiency (muscle or joint aching or stiffness, chronic fatigue, lethargy, facial or periorbital puffiness), in whom the administration of large doses of thyroid or

Table 2.5.4. Published symptoms and signs of patients thought to be euthyroid hypometabolic.*

WRITER	SYMPTOMS/SIGNS LISTED
Kurland[31] (1955)	Serum cholesterol levels were within normal limits. Symptoms included: lethargy, easy fatigue, nervousness, irritability, sensitivity to cold, headache, musculoskeletal pain, diminished sexual potency, and menstrual irregularities./ BMRs were below -20%.
Freedberg[24] (1955)	Aching in both knees, skin pallor, facial puffiness, a dull feeling, and tiredness./ Low BMRs and high cholesterol.
Tittle[47] (1956)	Chronic fatigue, muscle and joint aches, weight gain, disturbed bowel function, low body temperature.
Morton[29] (1957)	Obesity, infertility, salt and water imbalance, chronic fatigue (88%), "obesity" (75%), menstrual disturbances (67%); dry hair, dry skin, or brittle fingernails (57%); nervousness, irritability, depression, or mental apathy (51%); muscle aches and stiffness (47%); some had puffiness of the face.
Fields[30] (1957)	In school children of normal intelligence: poor grades, short attention span, poor concentration, "don't care" attitude, anxiety, restlessness, leanness, poor appetite, constipation.
Goldberg[64] (1961)	Anxiety states, irritability and mood swings, easy fatigability, lethargy, decreased libido, premenstrual tension, GI disturbances, scalp seborrhea or hair loss, palpitations, muscle and joint pains, shortness of breath./Prolonged contraction phase of Achilles reflex, low BMR.
Sonkin[43,p.157] (1985)	A variety of symptoms suggesting hypothyroidism./Slow Achilles reflex.
Lowe[90] (1997)	Normal thyroid function test results including TRH stimulation test, slow relaxation phase of Achilles reflex, chronic widespread pain, tender points, fatigue, stiffness, depression, cognitive dysfunction, anxiety, coldness, paresthesia, dry tissues, headaches, disturbed sleep, bowel disturbance, difficulty exercising, and other functional impairments.

*Some authors used alternate terms such as metabolic insufficiency. The term I use is euthyroid fibromyalgia. Not all the signs and symptoms listed by each author are (were) essential to the diagnosis. Some features merely support(ed) the diagnosis.

l-thyroxine does not elevate the basal metabolic rate or relieve the symptoms."[24,p.57] These authors also speculated, "We have considered the possibility that such patients are unable to utilize—that is, to absorb, convert to an active form, or metabolize—*l*-thyroxine."[24,p.57]

In 1957, Kurland et al. reported the results of a preliminary study of 12 euthyroid hypometabolic patients and 10 controls. Disappearance of radioactive T_4 from the patients' plasma was slower than from that of controls (8.3 days compared to 7.18 days). The researchers wrote that the study pointed to a possible abnormality of T_4 metabolism.[173,p.1371] This finding indicates that the liver clearance of T_4 was slowed in euthyroid hypometabolism, as it is in hypothyroidism.

Before long, a debate ensued as to whether or not the proposed condition, which the authors termed "nonmyxedematous hypometabolism," existed.[32] Those who argued that the condition was a fact tended to compromise that it was rare. In general, endocrinologists were skeptical. Some other practitioners were enthusiastic over the concept because of the relief T_3 gave their patients who had been chronically tired and resistant to T_4. Gynecologists and urologists were among the enthusiastic because of the benefits of T_3 for their patients with fertility problems.[1,p.652]

In 1954, Sonkin studied hypometabolic patients who were euthyroid according to laboratory test results. He scored their symptoms and signs.[62,pp.50-51] Table 2.5.5 shows the various complaints of his patients and the number of therapeutic responses for each complaint. Sonkin wrote,"Myofascial pain was the second most common complaint after fatigue. Of 63 patients with muscle pain, 46 (73%) had symptomatic improvement with thyroid therapy."[62,p.51]

In 1956, Tittle reported a study of 8 euthyroid hypometabolic patients; 5 were women and 3 were men. He assessed the effects of T_3 on their symptoms and BMRs, and he compared the results with those obtained from their prior treatment with desiccated thyroid. The patients had previously taken desiccated thyroid for a range of 6 months-to-5 years.[47,p.272] Despite this, they were all symptomatic and had low metabolism. The BMRs of the group ranged from -28% to -36%. The patients' serum protein-bound iodine and ^{131}I uptake were normal. Their cholesterol values ranged from 186 mg-to-240 mg/100 mL.[47,p.274]

Tittle had the patients take increasing amounts of T_3 until they reached a maximum of 50 µg-to-100 µg daily. Within 1-to-2 months, 6 of the 8 patients had improvement in symptoms. The treatment relieved their chronic fatigue and muscle and joint aches. They

lost weight, bowel function improved, and they had better thermal regulation. Their BMRs increased to -16% or higher. The average rise in BMR was 18%. Two of the 6 patients who improved showed signs of overstimulation with 75 µg of T_3. The signs subsided when their dosage was reduced to 37.5 µg daily. Two other patients did not tolerate T_3 well and Tittle discontinued their treatment. These latter 2 patients had also not tolerated desiccated thyroid well. Tittle wrote: "L-triiodothyronine [T_3] produced satisfactory symptomatic and physical improvement and elevation in basal metabolic rate. It is concluded, therefore, that L-triiodothyronine is a rapid and effective metabolic stimulant and therapeutic agent for treating metabolic insufficiency."[47,p.274]

In 1957, Joseph Morton wrote, "The syndrome of metabolic insufficiency (hypometabolic state) is perhaps one of the most common metabolic disorders seen in everyday practice." He also wrote that it may go unrecognized or misdiagnosed.[29,p.124] Morton studied the effects of T_3 on 51 patients with general metabolic insufficiency (Group 1) and 29 patients with "specific or localized metabolic disorders" (Group 2). Group 2 contained patients with obesity, infertility, salt and water imbalance, and menstrual disturbances. The predominant symptom of Group 1 was chronic fatigue (88%), and the predominant sign was obesity (75%). Patients also had menstrual disturbances (67%); dry hair, dry skin, or brittle fingernails (57%); nervousness, irritability, depression, or mental apathy (51%); muscle aches and stiffness (47%); and some had puffiness of the face.[29,p.125]

Morton's criteria for diagnosing metabolic insufficiency were: (1) low normal or subnormal BMR, (2) multiple coexistent signs and symptoms of deficient metabolism, and (3) normal thyroid gland function (indicated by protein-bound iodine and ^{131}I uptake tests).[29,p.128] (See Table 2.5.6.)

Morton reported that 46 (90%) of the 51 patients had good-to-excellent responses to T_3. Good meant a marked though incomplete response or remission of symptoms after more than 2 weeks; excellent meant complete remission of symptoms or a marked response in 1-to-2 weeks. The patients' most common and beneficial response was loss of fatigue. They had a sense of well-being and their muscle and joint aches and stiffness subsided or completely disappeared.[29,p.126]

Of this group, 36 patients had previously been treated with desiccated thyroid, thyroglobulin, or thyroxine. Only 3 (6% of the 51 patients) had good-to-excellent responses to these forms of thyroid hormone.

Of the 29 patients with localized hypometabolic

disorders, 25 (86%) had good-to-excellent responses to T₃. Twenty-one (72%) of the group had previously used other forms of thyroid hormone with poor results. Morton wrote that neither controls nor placebos were necessary in his study because he could use the patients' previous therapies for comparison.[29,p.126] He concluded that his results showed that T₃ is a highly effective and safe therapeutic agent for metabolic insufficiency.[29,p.128]

In a study published in 1957, Fields reported his treatment with T₃ of 100 children. He diagnosed 40 of the children as having metabolic insufficiency. This group consisted of 10 girls and 30 boys. They ranged in age from 1-to-17 years. None of the children were cretinoid or myxedematous. They were of normal intelligence. Nonetheless, many had poor school records, short attention spans, lack of ability to concentrate, and a "don't care" attitude. They were thin, had poor appetites, and were somewhat constipated. They showed moderate symptoms of anxiety and restlessness.[30,p.818]

For the children old enough to cooperate by lying still, BMRs were determined. The BMRs were low, ranging from -20% to -30%. The children's serum cholesterol averaged 290 mg/100 cc. Their protein-bound iodine levels were normal. Fluoroscopic exams showed that all the children were retarded in bone development. The average degree of retardation was 18 months.[30,p.818]

Fields considered that an excellent response to T₃ was relief of all or 90% of a patient's symptoms during treatment. A good response was relief of 70%-to-90% of symptoms. A fair response was relief of at least 50% of symptoms. Results were excellent in 22 children, good in 15, and fair in 3. Fields wrote that during treatment, the children's attitudes and behavior became normal. Each child's appetite and bowel function improved, and each gained an average of 2½ lbs. Cholesterol levels decreased, and BMRs increased to normal. During the 3-month treatment, the bone age of most of the children increased 6-to-9 months (about 100%-to-200% more than the growth typical of normal children of the same age). "The over-all responses," Fields wrote, "were most encouraging and dramatic."[30,pp.818-819]

In 1961, Goldberg reported a study of euthyroid hypometabolic patients. His paper is important because he produced more convincing laboratory data from this type of patient than did other investigators. He reported that he had identified 32 euthyroid hypometabolic patients among 500 patients he had screened. This was a 6.4% incidence. He pointed out,

Table 2.5.5. Complaints of euthyroid hypometabolic patients and the number of therapeutic responses to thyroid hormone therapy.*

COMPLAINT	TOTAL	POSITIVE RESPONSES
Fatigue	88	51
Myofascial pain	63	46
Weight gain	48	18
Dry skin	39	24
Depression	39	20
Thyroid nodules	24	7
Dysmenorrhea	20	5
Cold intolerance	17	13
Hair loss	14	3
Temporomandibular joint syndrome	7	3
Constipation	7	6
Swollen eyelids	6	3
Arthritis	5	1
Infertility	5	2
Hoarseness	4	1
Headache	4	3
Flushes	4	0
Fluid retention	3	1
Insomnia	3	1
Stiffness	2	0
Weakness	2	1
Nervousness	2	0
Bloating	2	2
Numbness	1	0
Nasal congestion	1	1
Anemia	1	0
Puffiness	1	1
Impotence	1	0
Menorrhagia	1	1

*Sonkin, L.S.: Myofascial pain due to metabolic disorders: diagnosis and treatment. In *Myofascial Pain and Fibromyalgia: Trigger Point Management.* Edited by E.S. Rachlin, St. Louis, Mosby, 1994, pp.45-60.

however, that this did not represent the incidence of euthyroid hypometabolism in the general population because the 500 patients he screened did not represent the population at-large. The patients were referred to him specifically for "psychoneurotic" and endocrine problems.[64,p.1054]

Goldberg used the following five criteria to diagnose euthyroid hypometabolic patients: (1) symptoms and appearance typical of hypothyroidism or "psychoneurosis," (2) normal protein-bound iodine level and normal rise in iodine level after 10 units of TSH, (3) low BMR and slowed Achilles reflex, (4) no response to placebos and equivocal or untoward response to desiccated thyroid, and (5) long-term objective and subjective improvement with T_3. I will address these seriatim. (See Table 2.5.6.)

(1) *Symptoms and appearance typical of hypothyroidism or "psychoneurosis."* Goldberg listed the ten most common symptoms of his hypometabolic patients: These were fatigue, irritability and mood swings, lethargy, decreased libido, premenstrual tension, gastrointestinal disturbances, scalp seborrhea or hair loss, palpitations, muscle and joint pains, and shortness of breath. Fourteen of his hypometabolic patients were overweight, and 4 were underweight.

Table 2.5.6. Different investigators' diagnostic criteria for euthyroid hypometabolism.

Morton[29,p.128] (1957)	1) low normal or subnormal BMR, 2) multiple coexistent signs and symptoms of deficient metabolism, and 3) normal thyroid gland function (indicated by protein-bound iodine and ^{131}I uptake tests).
Goldberg[64,p.1054] (1961)	1) Symptoms and appearance typical of hypothyroidism or psychoneurosis, 2) normal protein-bound iodine (PBI) level and normal rise after 10 units of TSH, 3) low BMR and slowed Achilles reflex, 4) no response to placebos and equivocal or untoward response to desiccated thyroid, and 5) long-term objective and subjective improvement with T_3.

It is instructive to note that Goldberg thought 2 of the underweight patients were hyperthyroid. Their BMRs, however, turned out to be -20%. They were clearly hypometabolic. These particular patients resemble euthyroid fibromyalgia patients with symptoms paradoxically similar to hyperthyroid symptoms (such as nervousness, anxiety, and excess body heat) that are relieved by the use of T_3. It is also not unusual for euthyroid fibromyalgia patients to have hypertension that is relieved by the use of T_3. When initially evaluated, some of these patients are taking β-adrenergic receptor blocking drugs such as propranolol. These medications may be contributing to the patients' hypometabolism. The patients must cease taking the medications because they nullify the β-adrenergic effects through which thyroid hormone accelerates metabolism (see Chapters 3.1, 4.3, and 5.2).

Goldberg described what he believed were four differences between the symptoms of hypothyroid and euthyroid hypometabolic patients: (a) hypometabolic patients usually complained of morning fatigue, while hypothyroid patients complained of late afternoon or early evening fatigue; (b) hypometabolic women had no or minimal menstrual flow, while hypothyroid women had varying menstrual flow; (c) hypometabolic patients had oily, seborrheic skin and scalp, as opposed to the dry, thick skin typical of hypothyroid patients; and (d) hypometabolic patients reported excess rather than minimal sweating.[64,p.1054]

(2) *Normal protein-bound iodine (PBI) level and normal rise in the PBI after 10 units of TSH.* According to Goldberg, a 1.5 μg rise in the PBI after a patient takes TSH indicates normal responsiveness of the thyroid gland to TSH. The patient whose PBI rises to this level after taking TSH is not likely to be hypothyroid. If the PBI fails to rise to 1.0 μg after taking TSH, the patient usually has hypothyroidism. The typical hypothyroid patient will permanently improve both objectively and subjectively with thyroid replacement.[49][64,p.1054]

Goldberg wrote that of the 500 patients he screened, he initially thought he had found 70 with euthyroid hypometabolism. Each of these patients had a normal PBI level and a normal elevation of the PBI after taking TSH. Each also had a sluggish Achilles reflex and a low BMR. He found later, however, that 38 of these patients had false-normal PBI levels due to iodine contamination from iodine-containing drugs and x-ray contrast media they had taken. The iodine contamination probably obscured inadequate PBI increases after the intake of TSH. Goldberg decided that these patients were actually hypothyroid. They responded to desiccated thyroid just as the euthyroid hypometabolic patients responded to T_3. (The 60 mg of desiccated thyroid the hypothyroid patients responded to was equivalent to 37 μg of T_3.) After excluding these 38 patients, this left 32 patients who were euthyroid hypometabolic. None of the euthyroid hypometabolic patients improved with the use of desiccated thyroid.

(3) *Low BMR and slowed Achilles reflex.* Goldberg wrote that a low BMR and slowed Achilles reflex indicate deficient end-organ metabolism. He wrote that the instrument he used to test patients' Achilles reflexes is over 94% accurate in distinguishing euthyroid hypometabolic and hypothyroid patients.[50] According to him, this measure is the most reliable objective criterion for screening for hypometabolic patients. Only about 50% of the patients' BMRs were low when they were tested the first time. Regarding this, he wrote, "The fact that the standard BMR procedure requires complete relaxation on the part of the patient, coupled with the fact that the typical 'hypometabolic' patient is a tense, anxious individual, often leads to a false elevation of the BMR, particularly if it is the first experience the patient has had with the BMR procedure."[64,p.1055]

Table 2.5.7 shows the BMRs, Achilles reflex speeds, and cholesterol values of Goldberg's 32 euthyroid hypometabolic patients. The table shows values before treatment and during treatment with a placebo, with desiccated thyroid, and with T_3.

(4) *No response to placebos and equivocal or untoward response to desiccated thyroid.* Goldberg put all patients through a 4-week placebo trial. Next, he started patients on 120 mg of desiccated thyroid. He increased the dosage by 60 mg biweekly until patients improved or showed intolerance. Fifteen patients had

toxic reactions to any more than 120 mg. They later tolerated an equivalent amount of T_3, however, and in some cases much higher dosages. Ten patients responded to desiccated thyroid, but only briefly—within 2-to-4 weeks, their symptoms and BMRs returned to pre-treatment levels.[64,p.1056]

(5) *Long-term objective and subjective improvement with T_3.* The criteria for improvement were: (a) relief of signs and symptoms, (b) return of a normal Achilles reflex, and (c) a rise of the BMR to normal levels. Treatment with T_3 was effective for all 32 euthyroid hypometabolic patients. The average effective daily dosage was between 100 μg and 125 μg. The range was 75 μg-to-150 μg. Goldberg examined patients every 2 weeks and adjusted their dosages according to the speed of their Achilles reflexes. (The optimum contraction phase of the reflex was 200 msec.)

Table 2.5.7. Pre- and post-treatment test values in 32 euthyroid hypometabolic patients.*

TEST	THERAPY			
	MEAN & (RANGE): NO THERAPY	PLACEBO	DESICCATED THYROID	T_3
BMR	-15% (-33%, +7%)	-17.5% (-37%, +5%)	-13% (-33%, +11%)	-5% (-14%, +18%)
Achilles reflex[λ]	255 (240-290)	255 (230-290)	250 (230-300)	200 (170-240)
Serum cholesterol	225 (180-350)	233 (160-370)	220 (165-360)	215 (140-345)

*After Goldberg, M.: Diagnosis of euthyroid hypometabolism. *Am. J. Obst. & Gynec.*, 81(5):1055, 1961.
[λ] Unit of measure is msec. Fewer msec indicate a more rapid reflex.

Falsely Crucial Studies. In 1958, Keating questioned whether there is a distinct clinical entity involving patients with low BMRs, lack of positive therapeutic responses to desiccated thyroid and T_4, but positive therapeutic responses to T_3. He recommended in an editorial that the controversy over metabolic insufficiency be settled by double-blind studies.[32] This was a time in medical research when investigators had just begun using double-blind studies. Unfortunately, studies then, even more so than now, were subject to serious methodological flaws. In 1960, soon after Keating's suggestion, two studies of the effectiveness

of T_3 were conducted. The statistical analyses of the results were crucially flawed. Sonkin wrote in 1994 that the conclusions from these studies ". . . appear to be flagrant examples of the β error, i.e., acceptance of a null hypothesis when it is, in fact, unproven."[62,p.49] The studies were also defective in ways other than statistical analyses. Patients participating in the studies did not continue treatment long enough, and it is questionable whether appropriate patients were included.

In the first study, 18 patients with fatigue and low BMRs were placed in three groups of 6 patients each. One group received T_4, another T_3, and the other a placebo. Dosages were increased gradually over a 2-week period.[133] Although some changes occurred within this short time, statistical tests did not detect a significant difference between the groups in symptom and BMR changes. In the second study, 19 subjects who had fatigue and moderately low BMRs were divided into a T_3 group and a control group and treated briefly. Again, no significant difference was detected between the responses of the two groups.[33] According to Sonkin, these poorly designed studies ultimately contributed to the "premature obsolescence of the BMR."[62,pp.49-50] In 1961, Jefferies commented on the studies.[48,p.582] He was not aware of the poor design of the studies and the faulty interpretation of the data. He wrote that the confusion over metabolic insufficiency was increased rather than dissipated by the studies showing that T_3 was ineffective in the treatment of the condition.

In 1962, two years after these studies were reported, Williams called for further studies.[132] Unfortunately, these were not done. Sonkin described the two original studies as poorly designed and irrelevant. He pointed out that the results conflict so much with reported clinical observations that the subject warrants further studies.[62,p.53] As far as I can determine, however, none were done between 1960 and 1995. That year, my research group and I began blinded efficacy studies of euthyroid fibromyalgia patients.[90][91][92]

Relevance of Studies in this Section to Euthyroid Fibromyalgia Patients. Some of the patients in the studies of euthyroid hypometabolism included in this section may have had hypothyroidism that was not detected with the crude laboratory measures available in the 1950s and 1960s. It is likely, however, that the patients who were reported to be resistant to desiccated thyroid, T_4, and thyroglobulin were not hypothyroid but were genuinely euthyroid hypometabolic and had partial cellular resistance to thyroid hormone. Some of the patients, of course, could have had both hypothyroidism and cellular resistance to thyroid hormone. (See Table 2.5.8 for a summary of the events in the investigation of forms of hypometabolism.)

In general, my experiences with euthyroid fibromyalgia patients in clinical and experimental settings are consistent with the reports I cite in this section. I have found that most fibromyalgia patients whose laboratory test results indicate hypothyroidism improve or recover with TSH-suppressive dosages of desiccated thyroid or T_4. Some of them do not, but virtually all of these patients respond when switched to T_3, as did a patient whose case I reported in 1995.[134] Fibromyalgia patients whose laboratory test results indicate

euthyroidism typically do not benefit from desiccated thyroid or T_4, even with TSH-suppressive dosages. Virtually all of them, however, improve or recover with T_3.

● **RESPONSES TO SIX CRITICISMS OF THE CONCEPT OF EUTHYROID HYPOMETABOLISM**

Most criticisms of the concept of euthyroid hypometabolism and its treatment were registered by two authors some 40 years ago. For the most part, their statements are outdated. It is important, however, to review the points they raised. Having participated in the sport of journal debating, I have learned that some critics of a concept will use to their advantage any weapon they can grab—notwithstanding its anachronistic status. To rebut such opportunists, familiarity with the old criticisms may serve well the clinician treating euthyroid hypometabolic patients today. This is especially true of the scientifically invalid criticism most often hurled forth by modern-day opponents: The patient's non-specific symptoms are features of one somatoform disorder or another. Early in this century, the term used was "psychoneurosis."

(1) SYMPTOMS OF EUTHYROID HYPOMETABOLISM AS MANIFESTATIONS OF "PSYCHONEUROSIS": A FALSIFIED CONCEPT

Keating of the Mayo Clinic critiqued the concept of euthyroid hypometabolism in 1958. He wrote that symptoms attributed to euthyroid hypometabolism are vague and non-specific. They ". . . obviously occur in a large proportion of patients, many of whom have anxiety tension states or psychoneurosis . . . ." He also wrote of such symptoms in hypothyroid patients: "Such symptoms as fatigability, nervousness, emotional instability, irritability or headaches in a patient who has frank myxedema frequently can be attributed to an associated psychoneurotic disturbance rather than to deficiency of thyroxine in itself. Furthermore, replacement therapy usually does not alleviate these complaints, even when the hypothyroid state is completely corrected."[32,p.532]

The opinion of Jefferies was similar to that of Keating. In 1961, Jefferies made this statement in the opening paragraph of his critique of euthyroid hypometabolism: "The similarity of the clinical picture to that of psychoneurosis is disturbing to the conscientious physician striving to reach a definitive diagnosis."[48,p.582]

The diagnosis of psychoneurosis as a cause of the non-specific symptoms characteristic of hypothyroidism completely lacks any scientific foundation. It is puzzling why critics of the diagnosis of euthyroid hypometabolism would offer in its place a subjective diagnosis with no scientific basis. One thing is clear, however: The concept, by any name, does not stand up to analysis by either traditional or critical rationalism. Because of this, the concept of psychoneurosis must be classified as a pseudo-scientific hypothesis. Clinicians should be held accountable for subjecting patients to misdiagnoses based on this concept (see Chapter 1.2).

(2) "HEALTHY" EUTHYROID HYPOMETABOLISM: DEFINING ABNORMAL AS NORMAL

In his 1956 editorial in *Lancet*, Keating quoted Means as saying, ". . . hypometabolism is sometimes seen in perfectly normal people, who have a low BMR just as others have a slow pulse-rate."[51,p.826] Keating wrote that discussions of euthyroid hypometabolism usually fail to take full account of extensive and careful observations recorded on the basal metabolic rate.[32,p.532] He pointed out that Boothby and Sandiford found metabolic rates lower than -15% in 1.2% of the 8,614 patients they studied.[53] Also, Means and Burgess found rates lower than -15% in 1.6% of their 1,000 patients.[54] This corresponds to the findings of others as well.[55][56] Thompson and Thompson wrote that there are healthy people whose metabolism is as low as -16% to -25%. According to them, "They differ in no apparent respect from healthy people with a standard normal metabolic rate."[44,pp.494-495] Sturgis mentioned a person he considered healthy whose metabolic rate was -22% to -25%.[82] And Wishart reported 3 cases of presumably healthy people whose metabolic rates were -16%, -21%, and -21%, respectively.[83]

Patients Deemed "Healthy" Despite Non-Specific Symptoms

According to Keating, "Many of these patients [those of Boothby and Sandiford [53]] were healthy; some had various menstrual irregularities; some had nasal conditions, such as rhinorrhea; and a substantial number (but by no means a majority) had a group of

Table 2.5.8. Events in the investigation of forms of hypometabolism.

RESEARCHERS AND DATES	EVENTS
Gull 1874	Describes myxedema in adults.
Ord 1878	Emphasizes myxedema.
Murray 1891	First to successfully treat hypothyroidism with thyroid extract.
Boothby 1922	Establishes range of BMR. Finds that some 1922 patients with symptoms but no myxedema have low BMRs.
Kimball 1933 & Wharton 1939	Demonstrate that most hypothyroid patients are not myxedematous.
Barnes 1940s	Establishes normal range of BBT. Demonstrates that the BBT can be a reliable test of patients' metabolic state.
Tittle, Morton, Fields, & Goldberg Mid-1950s to 1961	Demonstrate that some patients with hypothyroid-like symptoms, normal PBI, normal ^{131}I uptake, and low BMR do not respond to desiccated thyroid or T_4. Argue that some patients are euthyroid hypometabolic.
Refetoff 1967	Identifies patients with partial resistance to their endogenous thyroid hormones. They respond to T_3 but not T_4.
1970s	Serum TSH and thyroid hormone tests permit precise laboratory differentiation of hypothyroid from euthyroid hypometabolic patients.
Lowe 1990	Finds euthyroid hypometabolism is the common condition underlying euthyroid fibromyalgia.
Lowe 1996	Reports 10.5% of fibromyalgia patients have primary hypothyroidism, 52.6% have central hypothyroidism, and 36.8% are euthyroid.
Lowe 1996	Experimentally demonstrates that euthyroid fibromyalgia patients are "resistant" to thyroid hormone and improve or recover with metabolic therapy based on T_3.

symptoms analogous to those described as characteristic of "metabolic insufficiency."'[32,p.532] This is an important concession that contradicts Keating's own argument. He concedes that a substantial minority of patients with low BMRs had a group of symptoms analogous to those described as characteristic of "metabolic insufficiency."[32,p.532] Yet he considered these patients healthy. This foreshadowed the conclusion of many clinicians today that fibromyalgia and chronic fatigue syndrome patients are actually "healthy."

The pronouncement of "healthy" is not restricted to these patients, however. Many patients with disorders not yet accepted by the medical orthodoxy, but that reduce the quality of life and disable patients, are told emphatically by some clinicians that they are perfectly healthy. But when treated for hypoglycemia, systemic yeast infections, and other such conditions, many of these patients recover genuine health and well-being. Such experiences have contributed to the growing public disenchantment with conventional medicine and the increased use of alternative health care.

Possible Causes of Clinicians Pronouncing Patients Healthy Despite Non-specific Symptoms

There may be two causes for the tendency to pronounce that patients whose symptoms are non-specific are healthy: the hospital training of medical physicians, and the orthodoxy-driven erroneous conclusion that only symptoms with proven organic causes are worthy of medical care.

Hospital Training. The tendency of many medical physicians to pronounce patients with non-specific symptoms as healthy may be a result of the facilities in which they train. Medical physicians have their practical, hands-on training in hospitals. As a result, they may have little or no exposure to patients whose conditions do not warrant emergency room care or hospitalization. Such clinicians may be accustomed to ministering only or largely to patients with conditions such as broken arms, gun-shot wounds, seeping pustules, acute asthmatic episodes, cancerous tumors, and cardiac arrest. It is easy to comprehend their difficulty in changing mental set when in private practice they are confronted by the euthyroid hypometabolic patient. This patient is likely to complain of symptoms such as fatigue, depression, and diffuse aches and pains. Compared to patients the physician was trained to treat, the euthyroid hypometabolic patient may appear to have nothing to complain about. To appreciate the euthyroid hypometabolic patient's need for proper care, the physician must become reoriented. This reorientation must entail the physician's acceptance that many patients suffer from diseases that are far more subtle than those he encountered during his training.

Absence of Proven Pathology. Another reason some clinicians classify patients with non-specific

symptoms as healthy is that no pathogenic basis for the symptoms has been proven. However, there is no logical or scientific basis for concluding that the absence of a proven organic cause of symptoms means that the patient is healthy. This erroneous conclusion is undoubtedly rooted in social and political sensibilities. As Fredericks and Goodman wrote: "The weight of the consensus in medicine is formidable. It salutes a practitioner who uses the 'accepted form' of treatment even if this treatment does little or nothing for a patient; it condemns and may even punish a physician who uses an 'unaccepted form' of treatment, even if that treatment may help a patient. There is even a motto perpetuating this philosophy: Be not the first by whom the new are tried nor yet the last to lay the old aside!"[52,pp.44-45] Fredericks and Goodman were referring to treatment, but the same applies to diagnosis. Many members of the medical orthodoxy are oriented toward abject disease and trauma, and they tend to question and criticize those who attend to more subtle, borderline, or unfamiliar health problems, the diagnoses of which are uncertain.

The tendency for some clinicians and researchers to pronounce patients with non-specific symptoms "healthy" is well illustrated by two examples. Boothby and Sandiford (whom Keating referenced) plotted "the basal metabolic rates . . . obtained on 127 subjects whom we consider 'normal' because they had passed through a careful clinical examination without revealing any evidence of disease that could in any way affect their metabolism. The criticism that these subjects were practically all 'patients' and came for examination because they thought they were patients, or might be, is effectively offset by this careful negative examination."[53] Boothby and Sandiford made this statement in 1922. At that time, diagnostic technology was limited in the extreme. Because of the limits, these investigators could not possibly have ruled out all abnormalities related to metabolism in the subjects they studied.

Another example that illustrates the tendency to unjustly pronounce uncertain cases "healthy" is a study published in 1946. The study involved 308 hypometabolic patients in Denmark.[81] The investigators, Kirk and Kvorning, found that 199 patients in the study were hypometabolic due to one of four conditions: hypothyroidism, low levels of physical activity, inadequate nutrient intake, or hypogonadism. They were not certain of the cause of hypometabolism in the remaining 109 patients (roughly ⅓). These patients' BMRs were on the average 20% below normal. Kirk and Kvorning reported that most of the patients had reliable diagnoses, although the diseases they suffered from would not be expected to cause hypometabolism. In fact, a review of the list of diagnoses raises an interesting question: Rather than hypometabolism resulting from the conditions, was hypometabolism (due to inadequate thyroid hormone cell regulation) instead the underlying cause of some of the diagnosed conditions? The conditions included weakness and debility, constipation, hypertension, gallstones, eczema, myalgia, neurasthenia, and mental retardation due to faulty development. These are all clinical features that have been eliminated in some patients by the use of exogenous thyroid hormone.

Kirk and Kvorning wrote that in 21 of the hypometabolic individuals, ". . . there were no signs of disease at all, so these individuals must be regarded as healthy."[81,p.24] Fifty years later, it is a puzzle why logic and humility did not avert them from this conclusion. The decision that the people were healthy presumes that Kirk and Kvorning's diagnostic search was all-inclusive, infallible, and left no possible abnormalities unrevealed—presumptuous indeed for the time during which they collected their data, 1940-to-1942. Far more reasonable was Keating's 1956 statement that such signs and symptoms ". . . cannot be explained in terms of any known organic disorder."[51,p.826]

It is possible that no pathophysiology underlies the euthyroid hypometabolism of some patients. They may simply be on the slow end of the bell curve for metabolic rates. Still, if their metabolism is slow enough, their cells may not be able to meet increases in metabolic demand, as during exposure to severe cold, physical stresses such as intense exercise, or severe emotional arousal. During such times, the combination of the increased metabolic demand and their limited metabolic capacity may result in a metabolic crisis. The crisis may generate non-specific symptoms that physicians cannot relate to any demonstrable physical cause. Finding no documentable physical cause, some clinicians conclude that the patient is healthy. This means, of course, that no treatment is warranted. Nevertheless, any clinician is on precarious footing when he concludes that a symptomatic patient has *no* disease. This is true despite our latest technological advances. When a clinician has failed with all available diagnostic methods to identify a physical cause for a patient's symptoms, all he can correctly say is that he has not been able to find the cause. It is irrational for him to conclude further that the patient's symptoms do not *have* a physical cause. No matter what diagnostic procedures he has performed, this conclusion is never

scientifically justifiable.

(3) EUTHYROID HYPOMETABOLISM AS THE LOWER END OF THE NORMAL RANGE OF METABOLIC RATES: FROM PHYSIOLOGICAL TO PATHOGENIC HYPOMETABOLSIM

Goldberg wrote that hypometabolic individuals who do not have obvious disease may comprise the end-fraction of a normal distribution curve of BMRs.[64,p.1053] In a similar vein, Means believed that many perfectly normal people are hypometabolic; they have low BMRs just as others have slow pulse rates.[46,p.537] Kirk and Kvorning wrote that these people have "physiological hypometabolism"—their low basal metabolism is non-pathological. Kirk and Kvorning also wrote that the clinician may anticipate hypometabolism in patients and not regard it as a part of their primary diseases.[81,pp.24-25]

Kirk and Kvorning presented some evidence to support their argument that hypometabolic patients with no apparent diseases were merely part of a normal distribution curve. They entered the BMRs of 109 hypometabolic patients into a graph and compared this to a graph of the BMRs of 190 eumetabolic control subjects. They found that the hypometabolic patients' BMRs fell to the left of the curve, and those of the eumetabolic individuals fell in the middle. Hypermetabolic BMRs formed the right portion of the curve. The combined BMR values formed a normal distribution curve. We would expect, of course, that BMRs in the general population form a normal bell curve. However, that BMRs fall into a normal bell curve (as does most any other measurable human feature) in no way supports the contention that individuals with low (or high) BMRs are "normal" or "healthy" in the sense of the absence of aberrant physiology or pathology. Extreme BMRs may be associated with physiological dysfunction or even pathology, even though they form the wings of a normal bell curve of human features.

My clinical and research experiences indicate that fibromyalgia in most patients is a manifestation of inadequate thyroid hormone regulation of cell function in specific tissues. The inadequacy may result from a thyroid hormone deficiency or from partial cellular resistance to thyroid hormone. Patients with the latter problem are correctly termed euthyroid hypometabolic: The consequence of the inadequate thyroid hormone cell regulation is inhibition of metabolic processes that results in a general mental and physical slow-down. The organic consequences of this slow-down may indeed result in physiological dysfunction and eventual pathology.

Consider, for example, that many of these patients have elevated blood lipids that return to normal upon treatment with T_3. But if the patient is not treated with T_3, the long-term lipid elevation is likely to result in cardiovascular disease that may be lethal. In addition, the patient is typically fatigued and has low motor drive. These influence the patient to become generally hypokinetic, and the hypokinesis can compound the pathogenic effects of elevated blood lipids. I could follow several other such possibilities to their logical conclusions, but this example should clarify one point: "Physiological hypometabolism," which Kirk and Kvorning[81,pp.24-25] referred to, can lead to pathological hypometabolism.

(4) RARITY OF EUTHYROID HYPOMETABOLISM: FAILING TO SEE WHAT ONE DOES NOT LOOK FOR

According to Keating, Freedberg told him that he and Kurland had found only 15 euthyroid hypometabolic patients over a period of several years. Keating then commented, "The relative paucity of reports on 'metabolic insufficiency' from other centers perhaps might be interpreted as indicating that others also may have experienced difficulties in recognizing the condition."[32,p.534] The suggestion was that the condition was rare; otherwise, clinicians would have recognized and reported the condition in a higher percentage of patients. This criticism implies that most clinicians scrutinize their patients with minds as dispassionate, objective, and truth-ferreting as that of Star Trek's Mr. Spock. Had more than a few patients of these clinicians had euthyroid hypometabolism, they *certainly* would have recognized, documented, and reported it. Because they have not, the condition must therefore be rare.

For those who value truth, this would be the best of worlds. Unfortunately, perceptual mechanisms blind many clinicians to phenomena that are obvious to others. No other example of this is more relevant to the subject of this book than that of the typical practicing endocrinologist/thyroidologist today. He is blinded with satisfaction as he sees the mid-range TSH level in his patient's lab report. He looks straight at her to tell her the report shows that her thyroid hormone dosage is perfectly correct. But he completely fails to recognize that the woman sitting before him exhibits blatant,

classic signs of severe hypothyroidism. I am confident that if Keating were to ask such clinicians if patients taking replacement dosages of thyroid hormone (enough to keep the TSH within the middle of the normal reference range) are still clinically hypothyroid, he would hear a resounding "No." Perception is often conditioned so that clinicians do not see what is before them. Because of this, a paucity of reports of euthyroid hypometabolism is of no value in assessing its probable incidence.

The endocrinologist Sonkin has had clearer perception than most of his conventional colleagues. He wrote: "Patients are frequently encountered with a variety of symptoms suggesting hypothyroidism who in fact appear to be euthyroid when subjected to a battery of laboratory studies, including radioactive iodine uptake, blood thyroxine level, T_3-binding tests, and, more recently, pituitary thyroid-stimulating hormone (TSH) measurements. This condition is of great interest to the practitioner dealing with muscle problems since it may be a major cause of myofascial pain encountered in practice."[43,p.157] Barnes also described patients who appeared to be hypothyroid but had normal thyroid hormone blood tests. He estimated that 40% of the general population is afflicted with what he called hypothyroidism.[40,p.31] Many of this 40% with symptoms suggestive of hypothyroidism are most likely euthyroid hypometabolic.

Refetoff reported that the literature contains only one convincing case of a patient with peripheral resistance to thyroid hormone.[8,p.1304] I classify this patient as having thyroid hormone-related euthyroid hypometabolism. Kaplan, Swartz, and Larsen reported the case.[10] Refetoff pointed out that all the patient's hormone tests of thyroid function were normal. "It is possible," he wrote, "that many such patients remain undiagnosed because the clinical manifestations of apparent hypometabolism cannot be easily confirmed by specific tests measuring the action of thyroid hormone on peripheral tissues."[8,p.1304]

Other than the euthyroid fibromyalgia patients my coauthors and I have reported,[90][91][92] the case reported by Kaplan et al. is the only one in the medical literature that meets stringent definitional requirements. One study of mine indicated that 36.8%[94] of sequential fibromyalgia patients were euthyroid hypometabolic, and another by my research group indicated that 43.5% were in this same category.[95] These studies indicate that at least among fibromyalgia patients, euthyroid hypometabolism is anything but rare. The scarcity of reports of euthyroid hypometabolic patients in the medical literature is *not* testimony to its rarity. It is more likely that investigators' simply have not recognized the condition for what it is—or that those who have (as my experience attests) cannot get their observations published in conventional medical journals.

Among patients with symptoms that clinicians suspect are due to hypothyroidism, the diagnosis is established for only 1%-to-4%.[66][67] How many of the remaining 96%-to-99% of these patients actually have euthyroid hypometabolism? Its prevalence in the general population is a mystery. Fibromyalgia patients constitute a select population and may not reflect the incidence of euthyroid hypometabolism in the population at-large. I believe, however, that euthyroid fibromyalgia is only one clinical phenotype of euthyroid hypometabolism. I also suspect that euthyroid hypometabolism, manifest as other clinical phenotypes, is quite common in the population at-large.

(5) EUTHYROID HYPOMETABOLISM AS OCCULT HYPOTHYROIDISM: ANOTHER UNSETTLED ISSUE

In clinical practice, when the TRH stimulation test is performed, seldom is the subsequent increase in thyroid hormone levels assessed. In practice, therefore, we interpret the result of the TRH stimulation test without the benefit of knowing of changes in thyroid hormone levels. We assume that (1) a normal TSH response to a TRH injection is consistent with euthyroidism, and (2) an exaggerated TSH response is consistent with pituitary or hypothalamic dysfunction (the test does not allow us to distinguish between the two). There are, however, two possibilities for errors in diagnosis. First, the patient may have a normal or high-normal TSH response, yet have a slightly subnormal secretion of thyroid hormone by the thyroid gland. Without assessing the change in thyroid hormone levels before and after the TRH injection, we may incorrectly diagnose the patient's condition as euthyroidism rather than occult hypothyroidism.

Second, the patient's TSH response may be exaggerated not because of pituitary or hypothalamic dysfunction, but because of slightly subnormal thyroid gland secretion of thyroid hormones. (A subnormal thyroid hormone secretion, at least during the nocturnal TSH surge, may result in decreases in peak levels of circulating thyroid hormone. This may result in disinhibition of TSH synthesis and secretion and an increased TSH reserve in the anterior pituitary. A TRH injection may cause secretion of a sufficient amount of the reserve TSH to produce the exaggerated TSH res-

ponse during the test.) In this case, the problem is not that we may misdiagnose occult hypothyroidism as euthyroid hypometabolism. Instead, it is that we may misdiagnose occult primary hypothyroidism as central hypothyroidism.

Proper testing may shift some patients considered to be euthyroid or central hypothyroid to the classification of "occult" primary hypothyroid.[94][95] Up to this time, my research group has not addressed this diagnostic issue.

(6) NO EVIDENCE THAT THYROID HORMONES FAIL TO ACT AT THE CELLULAR LEVEL: A CRITICISM PROVEN FALSE

As well as I can determine, it was in the 1950s that authors first proposed the concept of cellular resistance to thyroid hormone—a weak or attenuated response of a patient's cells to normal concentrations of the hormone. The concept of thyroid hormone-related euthyroid hypometabolism implies that the pituitary-thyroid axis functions normally. Despite this, the cells of some tissues are hyporesponsive to normal concentrations of thyroid hormone. Reiss and Haigh suggested in 1954 that body tissues in general might be insensitive to thyroid hormones in euthyroid hypometabolic patients.[26] Means also referred to the concept in 1954.[57,p.48] In 1955, Freedberg, Kurland, and Hamolsky proposed that some patients' cells were partially insensitive to thyroid hormone.[31,p.1355] They reported that their nonmyxedematous hypometabolic patients were not able to use T_4—that is, ". . . to absorb, convert to an active form or metabolize it."[24,p.57] They also wrote, "Impaired permeability of the tissues of such patients to thyroxine but not to tri-iodothyronine is another possibility."[24,p.59]

Jefferies argued in 1961 that the premise of failed cellular action of thyroid hormones had not been tested.[48,p.583] At the time, this was true. But the conjectures of Reiss and Haigh, Means, and Freedberg, et al. in the 1950s have now been corroborated. As I wrote above, in the late 1980s the molecular defects were found that underlay some cases of partial cellular resistance to thyroid hormone described by a procession of authors through the 1970s, 1980s, and 1990s (see Chapter 2.6). Also, laboratory data have confirmed the partial cellular resistance to thyroid hormone in two groups of euthyroid fibromyalgia patients: those who have participated in studies by my research group, and other euthyroid fibromyalgia patients whom Honeyman-Lowe and I have treated in clinical practice. The pattern of thyroid function test results are the same for most of our euthyroid patients who no longer meet the criteria for fibromyalgia after undergoing metabolic rehabilitation including the use of T_3: The basal TSH, free T_4, and total T_4 are low, and the free T_3 is markedly elevated. This shows that the patients are not clearing the T_3 from their bodies at an accelerated rate; they are retaining it. The pattern of laboratory values is typical of patients who have what is termed "T_3-thyrotoxicosis," yet none of the tissues of our properly treated patients are thyrotoxic.

● **RESPONSES TO SIX CRITICISMS OF THE USE OF T_3 WITH EUTHYROID HYPOMETABOLIC PATIENTS**

(1) WARNING OF POTENTIAL DANGERS IN USING T_3 AS A TONIC: NO LONGER RELEVANT WITH REASONABLE PRECAUTIONS

In a 1956 editorial in *Lancet*,[51] Keating questioned the liberal use of T_3 as a tonic. He objected to use of the hormone as a tonic for physical and mental sluggishness, irritability, depression, nervousness, ". . . and similarly non-specific symptoms under the title 'metabolic insufficiency.'" He particularly criticized two pharmaceutical firms for promoting the use of therapeutic trials of T_3 without any evidence of hypometabolism such as low BMRs. The companies had apparently advertised that because hypometabolism may affect isolated tissues in patients, it may not markedly alter the BMR. So in the absence of objective signs or test results by which the clinician can identify the syndrome, the companies suggested that ". . . the diagnosis of metabolic insufficiency can be readily verified or discounted by a short therapeutic trial."[51]

Keating wrote, "What, in effect, this means is that patients complaining of almost any symptom which has no obvious cause should be given triiodothyronine to see whether they feel any better."[51,p.827] He argued that if the companies' advice were followed, we would have diagnostic confusion and serious harm would result from the inadvertent use of T_3 by individuals with severe coronary artery disease.

There was cause for extreme caution in the use of T_3 when Keating made the criticism in 1956. T_3 must be used cautiously by patients with cardiovascular abnormalities or adrenal insufficiency. Forty years ago, cardiac and adrenal status were more difficult to assess before prescribing a medication that might exacerbate cardiac abnormalities and adrenal insufficiency. In contrast, clinicians today can easily and accurately assess the likelihood of adverse cardiac or adrenal effects from a patient's use of T_3. From the standpoint of patient safety, then, this criticism is no longer appropriate, providing the clinician takes responsible precautionary measures. Disregard of precautions by some patients or their clinicians, however, is not a reason to discourage patients from undergoing a trial of T_3.

Virtually all prescription medications today have a lengthy list of potential adverse effects. In contrast, T_3 (most commonly used as the brand known as Cytomel) is without adverse effects when used properly. When pharmacists fill prescriptions for Cytomel, they usually provide patients with a print-out that contains the statement: "POSSIBLE SIDE EFFECTS: NO COMMON SIDE EFFECTS HAVE BEEN REPORTED with the proper use of this medicine. If you notice any unusual effects, contact your doctor, nurse, or pharmacist [quoted *verbatim et literatim*]."[129] Despite this notice, many physicians, including some endocrinologists/thyroidologists, misinform patients that T_3, in contrast to T_4, is likely to harm them in various ways.

But alas, T_3 *can* be used improperly. As a precaution, I encourage clinicians to be vigilant of euthyroid fibromyalgia patients who do not cooperate by using T_3 properly. Some patients find exercising repugnant and simply refuse to engage in it. Other patients will not take B complex vitamins. Interacting with thyroid hormone, exercise and supplemental nutrients are synergistic metabolism-regulators. Clinicians should convince patients that these measures are *essential* for obtaining and maintaining optimal metabolic status. Some patients, particularly those who do not like to exercise and take nutritional supplements, expect T_3 to relieve their symptoms. Yet the symptoms may be partly a product of inactivity and nutritional insufficiencies. Typically, such patients' symptoms improve somewhat with T_3. Without exercise and nutritional supplements, however, the patients remain symptomatic to some degree, and for some there is practically no improvement. Some of these patients state that they expect to improve further if they can progressively increase their T_3 dosage; some will increase it against the clinicians' advice. Many of these patients already have an increased probability of lifestyle-related cardiac abnormalities. Such abnormalities may be exacerbated by the increase in heart rate and contractile force induced by T_3. Use of supraphysiologic dosages of T_3 by these patients is potentially hazardous. Unless clinicians can motivate these patients to cooperate, it is to these patients' and their clinicians' advantage that the patients discontinue the use of T_3.

(2) NO CRITERIA FOR DETERMINING WHICH PATIENTS MAY BENEFIT FROM T_3: A FALSE COMPLAINT

Keating[51] argued that T_3 should not be prescribed *indiscriminately* as a tonic. The clinician should, of course, use specific criteria to predict which patients are likely to benefit from T_3. In fact, the authors of most studies of T_3 treatment for euthyroid hypometabolism provided clear-cut criteria. These included (1) a low BMR, (2) symptoms typical of hypothyroidism, and in some cases (3) failure to respond to desiccated thyroid hormone or T_4. These criteria are quite different from, ". . . patients complaining of almost any symptom which has no obvious cause . . . ."[51,p.827] My colleagues and I have also provided specific criteria for designating which fibromyalgia patients are likely to benefit from exogenous T_3[90][91][92] (see Chapter 4.3).

(3) EMPIRICAL USE OF T_3 "JUST TO SEE WHAT HAPPENS": CONSISTENT WITH THE COMMON PRACTICE OF EMPIRICAL MEDICINE

For a clinician to prescribe T_3 for "almost any symptom," just to see if it works is a liberal empirical use of T_3. This style of prescribing medications, however, is in fact common. And it is justified when the clinician has good reason to believe that the trial of medication is safe and may be effective. In the 1960s and 1970s, when other medicinal treatment measures failed, there was rampant use of hydrocortisone without a clear-cut rationale for its use in treating various diseases. This *ad libitum* use of hydrocortisone is not rare even today. During the 1970s and 1980s, Valium was prescribed this way, and today, antidepressant medications are taking their turn. Antidepressants have been lifesaving for many suicidal, depressed patients. Most often, however, these medications are undoubtedly prescribed just to see if they might relieve rel-

atively mild symptoms such as melancholy, other vaguely unpleasant moods, disturbed sleep, and pain. To criticize the empirical use of T_3 today would constitute a double standard in medical practice.

The diagnostic protocol I describe in this book can enable the clinician to predict fairly well which patients are likely to benefit from exogenous T_3 when used within the context of a more complete regimen for metabolic rehabilitation.

(4) T_3 AS A PLACEBO: A FALSIFIED VIEW

Keating argued that T_3 was probably a placebo and referred to the ". . . suggestibility of many patients."[32,p.533] He also wrote: "The practicing physician is, of course, often in a poor position from which to exercise critical judgment as to the relative efficacy of drugs in his patient. The patient consults a physician because he wishes to feel better, and the physician treats the patient with a sincere desire to oblige. Hence, the two together unconsciously conspire to produce a result pleasing to both."[32,p.534]

To suggest that a positive response of euthyroid hypometabolic patients to T_3 is a placebo reaction is to say that the patient would have responded just as well to tablets containing an inert substance rather than T_3. In most reported studies in the 1950s and 1960s, however, patients improved with T_3 *after they had failed to improve over a period of months or even years with desiccated thyroid or T_4.* This was true of one patient whose case I reported[134] and also of many other patients I have seen in clinical practice. Each patient was essentially his own control. The patient's lack of benefit from desiccated thyroid and T_4 (and in the case of my patients, other medications such as antidepressants) provided a baseline against which to plot the degree of benefit from T_3. To Keating's placebo hypothesis, the obvious reply is: Where was the placebo effect when the patient was taking desiccated thyroid or T_4? Why was T_3 the only form of thyroid hormone that caused a "placebo" response?

That improved status in euthyroid hypometabolic patients is not a placebo effect was made clear through the 1-to-5-year follow-up study Reichman, Yellin, and I recently conducted. Extensive statistical analyses showed that 9 euthyroid fibromyalgia patients treated with T_3 were significantly improved compared to 9 patients who did not use the hormone. We concluded, "The continuation of improved fibromyalgia status for 1-to-5 years effectively rules out a placebo effect as the mechanism of improvement."[93]

After implying a placebo effect, Keating[51] stated that investigators had to show unequivocally that patients benefit from T_3: ". . . and this would require," he wrote, "a rigorously controlled statistical study with the substitution of a placebo for the drug without the knowledge of either patient or observer."[51,p.826] Blinded studies of the effects of T_3 were certainly needed in 1956. Unfortunately, the first two studies in the 1960s were faulty and their conclusions are now known to be erroneous (see section above titled "Falsely Crucial Studies"). My research group has now provided the blinded studies Keating called for.[90][91][92] However, Keating's argument that only blinded studies could determine whether T_3 was a placebo is an early example of the extremist thinking that dominates many clinicians' thinking today. The absurd notion that discerning probable truth is utterly impossible except through blinded studies has largely canceled the use of common sense in medical practice. This is especially true in specialties such as endocrinology/thyroidology.

Consider the report by Goldberg in 1961. He showed that his patients had dramatic adverse reactions when he switched them from T_3 to a placebo.[64] His study was not double-blind; he and his patients were aware of the treatments the patients received. According to Keating's thinking, Goldberg's awareness alone could subtly but remarkably induce all 32 of his patients' BMRs to rise to normal, their Achilles reflexes to speed up to normal, their cholesterol levels to drop, and all their symptoms to evaporate. All other investigators who reported results similar to Goldberg's would also have had this uncanny power over hypometabolic patients. Paradoxically, some of these clinicians had previously used desiccated thyroid and T_4 without success with the same patients who responded positively to T_3. The putative placebo response was selective for T_3. This is certainly within the realm of possibility, but its probability is infinitesimally small. My statements are not an argument that blinded studies are not important. Instead, they are an argument that it is irrational and therefore unscientific to exclude other methods of investigation from the pursuit of truth.

(5) APPARENT RESISTANCE TO DESICCATED THYROID OR T_4 IN EUTHYROID HYPOMETABOLIC PATIENTS EXPLAINED BY PRACTICAL PHYSIOLOGICAL MECHANISMS: AN UNSETTLED ISSUE

Jefferies contended that patients diagnosed as having euthyroid hypometabolism are not resistant to desiccated thyroid or T_4; they just do not absorb these as well as T_3. He wrote that he had seen several hypothyroid patients with irregular, confusing responses to treatment with enteric-coated thyroid tablets. These patients' conditions "stabilized nicely when their medication was changed to ordinary, noncoated tablets." He then referred to a study by Winkler.[58] In this study, non-myxedematous patients with low BMRs failed to improve on doses of desiccated thyroid as high as 6 grains (0.4 gram) daily. Yet when Winkler injected some patients with large dosages of T_4 intravenously, their BMRs increased promptly. Jefferies concluded, "The relatively brisk response to intravenous thyroxine ruled out a defect in the use of thyroxine at the tissue level and suggested an impairment of absorption of desiccated thyroid as the cause of the resistance."[48,p.585]

This is not, however, what Winkler and his co-authors concluded. They wrote that deficient absorption could not be entirely eliminated as an explanation, but "there are weighty arguments against it." First, as far as he could determine, his patients had no other defect in absorption and no gastrointestinal lesions. Second, he was aware of no case in which a hypothyroid patient did not respond to oral desiccated thyroid or T_4 but did respond to injected thyroid. This suggested to him that malabsorption of desiccated thyroid and T_4 was not common. And third, failure to absorb desiccated thyroid or T_4 did not explain these patients' measurably reduced responses to injected T_4. He had to inject some patients with very large dosages of T_4 intravenously to increase their BMRs.[58,pp.542-543] Injections produced improvement in patient status, although not as much as in hypothyroid patients. Winkler and his coauthors wrote, the patients ". . . required much larger doses than do myxedematous subjects to produce a comparable rise in the BMR."[58,p.543] They tentatively concluded that the hormone is inactivated after absorption or injection. They conjectured that the amount of T_4 in the injection exceeded the rate at which the hormone was being inactivated, and this permitted the injected hormone to exert metabolic effects. Hormones being absorbed from the gastrointestinal tract, on the other hand, entered the circulation more slowly and were inactivated before being able to exert metabolic effects. Limited technology in the mid-1940s restricted Winkler and his coworkers to such speculations. A small percentage of my hypothyroid patients and most euthyroid hypometabolic fibromyalgia patients do not benefit from desiccated thyroid or T_4. It has been clear, however, from their elevated T_4 levels and their suppressed TSH levels that they have absorbed large amounts of T_4 with no clinical benefit. I do not believe that impaired conversion of T_4 to T_3 is the source of resistance to T_4 in these patients. In my laboratory testing of euthyroid hypometabolic fibromyalgia patients, I have not found test values that indicate impaired conversion. Yet when I have switched the typical patient who is apparently resistant to T_4 and desiccated thyroid to T_3, he or she significantly improves or recovers from fibromyalgia.[134][135] Unfortunately, sequencing of the nucleotides of the c-*erb*Aβ gene from my euthyroid patients has been too limited to determine whether mutations of this gene underlie the resistance of some euthyroid patients.

(6) LACK OF EVIDENCE THAT SOME PATIENTS RESPOND TO T_3 AFTER NOT RESPONDING TO T_4 OR DESICCATED THYROID: SIMPLY A FALSE CONCLUSION

Jefferies also argued that it could not be concluded that patients in most reports responded to T_3 after failing to respond to desiccated thyroid or T_4. He wrote that patients were not left on these latter supplements long enough for the supplements to exert their metabolic effects.[48,p.586] He was wrong about this. In Fields' study of 40 euthyroid hypometabolic and 60 hypothyroid children, 10 of the children had taken either desiccated thyroid, thyroglobulin, or T_4 for as long as 2 years with incomplete remission of symptoms.[30,p.818] Tittle included 10 patients in his study. "All the patients," he wrote, ". . . had been treated previously with 2-to-3 grains . . . of desiccated thyroid per day for as long as six months-to-five years."[47,p.272]

Many of my euthyroid fibromyalgia patients who recovered with metabolic rehabilitation involving the use of T_3 had taken desiccated thyroid or T_4 for years with no noticeable improvement. Some who had no thyrotoxicity to supraphysiologic dosages of T_3 had toxic reactions to more than 2 or 3 grains of desiccated thyroid. I reported the case of one central hypothyroid patient who had failed to respond to relatively high dosages of desiccated thyroid or T_4 despite her use of these agents for 6 years. She experienced a dramatic recovery with a physiologic dosage of T_3.[134] This case was reminiscent of those reported in the 1950s by Fields, Tittle, and others. Studies in the mid-to-late 1950s and my later clinical observations show that this criticism of Jefferies is not justified.

● PERSISTENT FAILURE TO CONVERT T_4 TO T_3 IN CELLS: A MECHANISM OF EUTHYROID HYPOMETABOLISM?

As early as 1955[24,p.57] and 1957,[78] investigators observed that some hypometabolic patients failed to benefit from T_4 or desiccated thyroid but benefitted from T_3. They speculated that the responsible mechanism was failure to convert the prohormone T_4 to the active thyroid hormone, T_3. In the 1950s, laboratory methods that could confirm the putative mechanism were not available. Documenting the phenomenon in individual patients has only been possible since the advent of more highly sensitive lab tests.[71,p.1092] Evidence for reduced activity of 5'-deiodinase (the enzyme that converts T_4 to T_3) in humans is not based on direct enzyme assessment but on kinetic studies using radiolabeled T_4 and T_3.[142,p.287] There are at least two documented conditions in which conversion of T_4 to T_3 fails to occur. In one condition, low T_3 sick syndrome, the conversion failure is temporary. In inherited 5'-deiodinase deficiency, the failure is permanent. I will discuss these after a brief review of T_4 to T_3 conversion. (For more extensive coverage, see Chapter 2.1, sections: "Deiodinases that Breakdown the Iodotyrosines (T_1 and T_2) and the Iodothyronines (T_3 and T_4)," and "Deiodinases that Convert T_4 to T_3 and Reverse-T_3.")

DISORDERS INVOLVING INHIBITION OF T_4 TO T_3 CONVERSION

Researchers differ in their opinions of the effects of T_4 to T_3 conversion. The difference depends upon whether the commentator believes that T_4 is or is not bioactive. Those who do not believe T_4 is bioactive contend that T_4 to T_3 conversion activates the inactive prohormone, T_4. I believe, in accord with Eisinger,[113][171] that the evidence indicates that T_4 has biological effects independent of T_3. Consistent with this position, I will say here that converting T_4 to T_3 increases many-fold the range of biological effects and the potency of thyroid hormone. The conversion, catalyzed by the enzymes termed deiodinases, constitutes critical steps in the cascade of changes in the iodothyronine molecules.[28,p.134] (See Chapter 2.1, section titled: "Deiodinases that Convert T_4 to T_3 and Reverse-T_3.")

Deiodination is the removal of an iodine atom from the thyroid hormone molecule. Removal of one iodine atom from T_4 (the 5'- atom) converts the molecule to T_3. Removal of one atom from T_3 converts the molecule to T_2. In turn, removal of one iodine atom from T_2 produces T_1. And removal of the single iodine atom from T_1 produces T_0.[139,p.147] Removal of the 5-atom of T_4 produces reverse-T_3 (rT_3). rT_3 appears to have no bioactivity.[28][139]

Euthyroid Sick Syndrome

Euthyroid sick syndrome, also termed low T_3 sick syndrome, is a form of euthyroid hypometabolism. The low T_3 level is not technically hypothyroidism. The term hypothyroidism refers to low production and release of thyroid hormones by the thyroid gland, and not to either a low T_3 or T_4 level. In euthyroid sick syndrome, the low T_3 level does not result from impaired thyroid gland production. Instead, it results from impaired conversion of T_4 to T_3, with an increase in the reverse-T_3 level.[111] The serum T_3 is low in many patients with nonthyroidal sickness, systemic illness, various chronic illnesses, anorexia nervosa, fasting, and other types of starvation.[70][72][111] That the serum T_3 level is low in different conditions means that the finding is "non-specific;" it is not specific to any particular disease. (Incidentally, as of 1991, the test for the serum T_3 level was also not considered sensitive: It was normal in about ⅓ of hypothyroid patients.[71,p.1095])

Presumably, the purpose of the low T_3 level is to slow metabolism for an adaptive purpose. For example, a low serum T_3 level would contribute to energy conservation and decrease glycolysis and gluconeogenesis during starvation.

Are Tissues Hypometabolic During Low T_3 Levels Due to Impaired T_4 to T_3 Conversion? Some thyroidologists believe the clinical features typical of hypothyroidism do not occur in euthyroid sick syndrome. In other words, they do not believe that a clinical syndrome of tissue hypometabolism occurs while the patient has low T_3 levels. For some patients, this is undoubtedly true; they do not appear to be hypometabolic. However, the symptoms of some nonthyroidal illness, such as nausea or pain, tend to dominate patients' perceptions. Such symptoms are likely to cloud their perception of more minor symptoms of hypometabolism. In addition, the onset of perceptual effects of inadequate thyroid hormone regulation of cell function can be gradual and insidious, and they can be subtle when full-blown.[71,p.1092] Moreover, the perceptual effects of hypometabolism due to inadequate thyroid hormone regulation can resemble those of chronic physical inactivity. Thus, the patient who is inactive because of non-thyroidal illness may interpret all such perceptions as due to physical inactivity, the non-thyroidal illness, or a combination of both. It is, therefore, more likely that the effects of a patient's hypometabolism will be perceptually obscure and not detected.

When failed T_4 to T_3 conversion is especially prolonged or severe, it is logical to expect that effects such as decreased gluconeogenesis would compound the patient's nonthyroidal illness. Some clinicians may misinterpret such effects as features of the nonthyroidal illness. Some patients with prolonged caloric deprivation, such as those with anorexia nervosa, have low serum T_3 levels and delayed tendon reflexes. It is possible that the delayed reflexes result from the impaired T_4 to T_3 conversion. In such cases, the mechanism of the delayed reflexes may be the same muscle effects that occur in hypothyroidism.[157] (See Chapter 4.3, section titled "Peripheral Indices of Metabolic Status: Achilles Reflex Time.")

Inherited 5'-Deiodinase Deficiency

In 1957, Hutchison et al. reported a single, isolated case of a child with cretinism who failed to benefit from "dry thyroid." Dry thyroid was a product that contained primarily T_4. (Cretinism is a clinical condition due to thyroid hormone deficiency in a child. The condition is characterized by dwarfism, physical deformity, and mental retardation.) The cretinism was completely reversed by the use of T_3. Hutchison and his coauthors conjectured that the child had "a deficiency in an enzyme concerned with the peripheral deiodination of T_4 to T_3."[78]

In 1980, when more sensitive thyroid function tests were available, Maxon et al. published a report of 8 of 13 family members who had elevated serum total T_4 levels but normal total T_3 levels. Their basal TSH levels and post-TRH stimulation levels were normal. The authors stated that the patients were euthyroid and did not have goiters. The patients did not have elevated thyroid hormone carrier proteins to account for the elevated T_4 levels.[136] In a second report on these patients in 1982, Maxon et al. confirmed the previous laboratory findings. In addition, however, they also found that the patients had elevated free T_4 levels. What is more, they found that in addition to the patients' normal total T_3 levels, their serum rT_3 levels were increased. There was also a slight increase in $3',5'$-T_2. This suggested a 5'-deiodinase deficiency[137] (see Chapter 2.1, section titled "Deiodinases that Convert T_4 to T_3 and Reverse-T_3").

Kleinhaus et al. reported a sporadic (single, isolated) case of an 11-year-old girl whom they believed had a general 5'-deiodinase defect. She had a high total T_4, free T_4, total rT_3, free rT_3 (3,3',5-T_3), and 3',5'-T_2. However, her 3,3'-T_2 was low. This pattern suggests a 5'-deiodinase but not 5-deiodinase deficiency. Such a deficiency was also indicated by another finding: 50 μg of T_3 suppressed her TSH level, but 200 μg of T_4 were required to do so. The investigators considered the deiodinase deficiency generalized because both type I and type II 5'-deiodinases were deficient.[138] Refetoff, Weiss, and Usala wrote in 1993 that the mechanism of these laboratory findings remains unknown.[131,p.388] It is not likely that the two forms of deiodinase are coded by the same mutant gene.

A 1-year-old boy treated by Jansen and coworkers had muscular hypotonia, constipation, and slow psychomotor development. The mother had toxemia during pregnancy. In addition, at delivery the boy had asphyxiation from umbilical cord strangulation. Thyroid function testing over 7.5 years showed elevated levels of serum free T_4, free T_3, and basal TSH. Also, the patient had a normal TSH response to injected TRH. But the serum total T_4, rT_3, and T_4-binding globulin were elevated. When the boy was 8.5 years old, 15 μg and 30 μg of exogenous T_3 were used to suppress his TSH, and total and free T_4 levels. Jansen and coauthors conjectured that the abnormal test results were due to an abnormality of membrane transport of T_4 or a deficit of 5'-deiodinase.[287] Refetoff and coauthors noted that the excess T_4-binding globulin could account for the elevated thyroid hormone.[131,p.389] However, this would not explain the elevated free T_4 levels.

Rösler and coauthors reported the cases of 6 women who probably had deficits of 5'-deiodinase. The women were members of 3 generations of the same family. They had high levels of basal TSH, T_3, and T_4, and they had increased radioactive iodine uptake by the thyroid gland. Their peripheral tissues responded normally to thyroid hormone. This was indicated by their hypermetabolism (BMRs ranging from +32% to +100%) and signs and symptoms of thyrotoxicosis. This pattern of findings fulfills the criteria for pituitary resistance to thyroid hormone (see Chapter 2.6). Physiologic dosages of T_3 (but not T_4) reduced to normal the TSH, total T_3, total T_4, and BMR; and eliminated symptoms and signs of thyrotoxicity. That the patients had a favorable response to physiologic dosages of T_3 was unusual; most patients with pituitary resistance require supraphysiologic dosages of T_3. In these pa-

tients, the physiologic dosages of T_3 apparently produced a brief increase in the serum T_3 levels, and this was sufficient to suppress TSH secretion. This decreased the synthesis and release of T_4. Conversion of T_4 to T_3 in peripheral tissues provided a continuous source of T_3. The authors speculated that the high TSH levels before T_3 treatment were maintained by a pituitary intracellular deficit of T_3, and this deficit enabled the TSH levels to remain abnormally high.[140] The T_3 deficit probably resulted from a deficiency of type II 5'-deiodinase. This enzyme is present in the pituitary but few peripheral tissues. This would have resulted in decreased conversion of T_4 to T_3 in the pituitary with disinhibition of TSH secretion.[140] These 6 patients did not have euthyroid hypometabolism resulting from failed conversion; they were hypermetabolic. But their cases illustrate the potential influence of a deiodinase deficiency.

PROPOSAL OF A SUSTAINED EUTHYROID SICK SYNDROME UNDER THE EXPROPRIATED NAME "WILSON'S SYNDROME"

Although the term "Wilson's syndrome" had been in use for many years,[158][159][160][161][162][163] in 1991 Dennis Wilson commandeered the name. He used it as the title of a book he authored[141] in which he described a hypothetical condition that he named after himself. The condition he hypothesized essentially would be a sustained euthyroid sick syndrome. He made the bold statement that T_4 to T_3 conversion ". . . is the most critical step in the thyroid hormone system because it is the step in which there is most often a problem."[141,p.34] He offered no objective evidence to support this assertion. The assertion conflicts with the extensive research findings that have accumulated since Utiger confirmed and reported T_4 to T_3 conversion in 1970.[20,p.10]

Using the usurped term, Wilson defined the supposed syndrome as: "The cluster of often debilitating symptoms especially brought on by significant physical or emotional stress that can persist even after the stress has passed, which responds characteristically to the special thyroid hormone treatment method recently developed (see this manual). It is characterized by a body temperature that runs on average below normal, and routine thyroid blood tests are often in the 'normal range.'"[144,p.206]

Wilson referred to a number of circumstances in

which T_4 to T_3 conversion decreases: periods of physical injury, chronic and acute illness, increased glucocorticoid levels during mental and emotional stresses, and fasting. In describing the problem with T_4 to T_3 conversion, Wilson wrote, "Wilson's Syndrome [sic] can be thought of as a survival mechanism that has gotten stuck." He wrote that under stress, the body makes less T_3 and more rT_3 and that the rT_3 ". . . can then start a vicious cycle by hogging the enzyme [referring to deiodinase]."[143,p.2]

Central to Wilson's proposal is the notion that rT_3 comes to secondarily inhibit T_4 to T_3 conversion, ". . . resulting in a sustained or persistent impairment and the associated symptoms." He cites two papers to support this idea. In the first, Schimmel and Utiger discussed the well-known decrease of T_3 and increase of rT_3 that occur in euthyroid sick syndrome.[145] When I obtained a copy of this paper, I could find nothing in it supporting the notion of the mechanism becoming "stuck" or otherwise persisting indefinitely. It is well documented that this adaptive change reverts to normal within 1-to-3 weeks. This reverting to normal occurs *even though* stress-induced cortisol remains elevated or *even though* a patient continues to take exogenous cortisol.[147][148][149]

In the other paper Wilson referenced,[146] the authors report finding higher rT_3 in elderly people than in younger ones. This report does not support Wilson's extrapolation that a sustained elevation in rT_3 occurs in younger people or in other conditions. The tendency toward a higher rT_3 in elderly people may be among other age-related changes that have no apparent implications for younger people.

Wilson also made several statements that were apparent attempts to justify his proposal of a sustained impairment of T_4 to T_3 conversion, particularly after fasting. He stated that: (1) during fasting, there is a decrease in T_4 to T_3 conversion, (2) fasting slows the metabolic rate, and (3) "sometimes fasting can result in a persistent slowing of the metabolism even after the starvation is over."[144,p.206] Each of these statements is true. It is a patent *non sequitur,* however, to conclude from this series of statements that a sustained decrease in T_4 to T_3 conversion accounts for persisting slow metabolism after fasting. After his statement "And sometimes fasting can result in a persistent slowing of the metabolism even after the starvation is over," Wilson cites three papers.[150][151][152] Presumably, these support his implied conclusion—that a sustained decrease in T_4 to T_3 conversion accounts for persisting slow metabolism after fasting. But in none of these studies, nor in other similar studies, did the researchers attribute the sustained slow metabolism after fasting to decreased T_4 to T_3 conversion.

In one of the studies Wilson cited, investigators determined how much subjects had to restrict their food intake to maintain lost weight. Obese women who had lost weight had to restrict their food intake 25% more than matched non-obese women to maintain the reduced weight.[152] In another study, the researchers found that when subjects lost 10% or more of their usual body weight, the total energy expenditure of previously obese subjects decreased more than that of subjects who had never been obese. When body weight was increased by 10% of usual weight, the energy expenditure of previously obese subjects increased, but less than that of subjects who had not been obese.[154] Findings such as these indicate that people with a history of obesity have a more profound decrease in metabolism after fasting. The responsible mechanisms involve peculiarities of adipocyte physiology[155] and genetics,[156] but not a sustained decrease in T_4 to T_3 conversion. Moreover, DeGroot and co-workers studied the mechanisms of reduced energy metabolism in overweight women 8 weeks after they began a slimming diet. The researchers determined that the reduced metabolism resulted from decreased physical activity, decreased body weight, and decreased thermogenesis related to caloric restriction. They wrote, "Measurements of physical activity indicated a reduction of spontaneous physical activity during slimming," and "There seems little reason to consider other adaptive mechanisms."[153]

There appears to be no evidence for the sustained decreased conversion mechanism that Wilson has proposed. The references he cited do not support the likelihood of such a mechanism. In addition, I have found no studies that would support his hypothesis, even after an extensive search of the research literature. Wilson presented no data from laboratory testing to support the occurrence of his putative mechanism. On the other hand, I conducted laboratory testing of euthyroid fibromyalgia patients. No patient had an elevated rT_3 or any pattern of test values that indicated impaired T_4 to T_3 conversion.

Wilson's hypothesis is fascinating to ponder and speculate about. Despite this, I find no reason to believe that what he has proposed actually occurs, particularly in euthyroid fibromyalgia patients. Some patients who have undergone the T_3 treatment Wilson recommended have reported that they improved. This I do not doubt. It is highly probable, though, that their improvement was mediated by T_3 affecting some mechanism other than the one Wilson hypothesized.

● DISCOVERY OF THYROID HORMONE RESISTANCE SYNDROMES

During the first half of the 20ᵗʰ century, symptoms relieved by the patient's use of exogenous thyroid hormone were thought to have been manifestations of a thyroid hormone deficiency. Why some patients' symptoms persisted, despite the use of exogenous thyroid hormone, was perplexing. One explanation was that the symptoms must be caused by some abnormality unrelated to thyroid hormone. But in the 1950s, some investigators proposed that some patients' cells were partially insensitive to thyroid hormone.[31,p.1355][57,p.48] This was the inception of the concept of cellular resistance to thyroid hormone—the weak or attenuated response of a patient's cells to normal concentrations of the hormone.

In 1967, Refetoff, Dewind, and DeGroot described a familial goiter that was caused by partial resistance of target tissues to the action of thyroid hormones.[3] In the involved family members, the peripheral tissues were resistant. In addition, as in all patients with general resistance to thyroid hormone, the pituitary gland was resistant. This resulted in elevated levels of serum TSH and thyroid hormones. This, in fact, is the pattern that resulted in Refetoff first identifying the condition.[3] The syndrome was considered rare for many years.[62,p.48] Writers of some textbooks wafted across the subject, typically with little more than, "Variations in peripheral tissue response have been reported but are believed to be rare."[110,p.746] But in the Winter 1991 *NIH Observer*, Weintraub stated, "Thyroid hormone resistance syndrome may affect thousands of unsuspecting Americans." [127]

Since Refetoff and his coauthors published their first paper on thyroid hormone resistance, progressively more investigators have reported both individual and familial cases of the phenomenon.[4] At this point, the existence of thyroid hormone resistance is well established. In fact, the condition has taken its place among the list of syndromes of primary hormone resistance.

Cellular resistance to thyroid hormone is partial, of course. Total resistance would be incompatible with life. It is noteworthy that supraphysiologic dosages of T_4 or T_3 are necessary to override cellular resistance. In general, supraphysiologic amounts of thyroid hormone induce cellular responses that physiologic amounts induce in normal cells.[8,p.1293]

Refetoff's identification of patients with a syndrome of thyroid hormone resistance prompted studies by other investigators. As indicated by the contents of Chapter 2.6, the study of patients who do not respond normally to their endogenous thyroid hormones is now a prolific research field. In 1988, Usala et al. determined the likelihood that general resistance (involving both pituitary and peripheral tissues) to thyroid hormone is linked to the c-*erb*Aβ gene on chromosome 3. This gene codes for the c-*erb*Aβ T_3-receptor.[164] In 1989[166] and 1990,[165] investigators reported point mutations (base changes in nucleotides) in this gene in members of two separate families with general resistance. Since then, researchers have identified mutations in many general resistance patients (see Chapter 2.6).

PARTIAL PERIPHERAL RESISTANCE TO THYROID HORMONE: A MECHANISM OF THYROID HORMONE-RELATED EUTHYROID HYPOMETABOLISM

The patient classified clinically as having peripheral resistance to thyroid hormone meets two criteria: his pituitary gland responds normally to thyroid hormone, but his peripheral tissues are hyporesponsive. The patient with this phenotype of resistance has normal circulating levels of thyroid hormone and TSH. But because the peripheral tissues are resistant and thyroid hormone levels are normal, the patient's peripheral tissues are hypometabolic. The symptoms that result are characteristic of those of hypothyroid patients.

In 1981, Kaplan and coworkers published extensive documentation of peripheral tissue resistance in one patient. The patient required 500 µg of T_3 to maintain normal tissue metabolism. In spite of this extraordinarily high intake, she had no indication of thyrotoxicity.[10] Usala and coworkers analyzed the T_3-binding domain of the c-*erb*Aβ gene in this patient and found normal nucleotide sequences.[167] This eliminates the possibility of mutations in this patient in the domains of the gene where most mutations have been identified in general resistance patients.

Euthyroid Fibromyalgia: A Clinical Phenotype of Peripheral Resistance to Thyroid Hormone

Until recently, Kaplan's patient was the only well-documented case of peripheral resistance in the medical literature. In 1989, I began exploring the possibility that euthyroid fibromyalgia is a clinical phenotype of peripheral resistance to thyroid hormone.[169] My clinical observations at that time suggested that this was the case. Unfortunately, my ability to reach firm conclusions was hampered. The problem was that my usual methods of assessing patient status in clinical practice were not quantitative and consistent enough. Nonetheless, my anecdotal observations were sufficiently convincing that I was not able to lay the subject aside despite many attempts to do so.

During the subsequent 5 years, I improved my method of systematically monitoring patients and keeping records of changes in their fibromyalgia status. In 1994[135] and 1995,[134] I published case reports involving these systematic observations. I reached the tentative conclusion from these open studies that these patients were clinically the same as the euthyroid hypometabolic patients described in published papers in the 1950s and 1960s. The evidence supporting the conclusion was (1) the non-specific symptoms of euthyroid fibromyalgia patients were the same as euthyroid hypometabolic patients; (2) the thyroid function test results of the patients were normal; (3) most patients had peripheral indices of inadequate thyroid hormone cell regulation such as sluggish Achilles reflexes, elevated cholesterol, low voltage ECGs, and low basal body temperature; (4) these peripheral indices normalized and the non-specific symptoms disappeared in most cases only when patients used supraphysiologic dosages of T_3; and (5) the supraphysiologic dosages did not cause target tissue thyrotoxicosis.

I have not measured the BMR of my fibromyalgia patients. Most have been deconditioned due to limited activity associated with fibromyalgia. Low BMRs were predictable because of the deconditioning. Sonkin performed BMRs of patients who appeared to be euthyroid hypometabolic, some of whom fit the clinical phenotype of euthyroid fibromyalgia. He found that the BMRs of some patients increased with thyroid hormone treatment. He wrote, "My series of therapeutic trials in symptomatic, chemically euthyroid patients who show no evidence of [hypothalamic-pituitary-thyroid] feedback and frequently respond to thyroid hormone, probably contain members of this putative population."[62,p.48] He also wrote, "This group of patients with symptomatic low metabolism responsive to thyroid probably reveals a population of patients with peripheral resistance to thyroid hormone that does not feed back to the [hypothalamic-pituitary-thyroid] axis, and is probably a result of one or more post-receptor defects in the cascade of biochemical reactions that translate hormonal action to the biological action of the cell."[62,p.53]

In 1996 and 1997, my colleagues and I conducted three rigorous double-blind placebo-controlled crossover studies with euthyroid fibromyalgia patients.[90][91][92] These studies confirmed the outcome of the previous open trials. We performed follow-up laboratory testing of the patients who participated in these studies. All were still taking supraphysiologic dosages of T_3. Their thyroid hormone and TSH levels were typical of those in patients said to have T_3-thyrotoxicosis due to the consumption of "excessive" amounts of T_3. The patients, however, were not thyrotoxic. This is clear from extensive serum and urinary biochemical tests, serial ECGs, and bone densitometry we obtained on each patient. All patients had low levels of TSH and total and free T_4, and all had high free T_3 levels. These values demonstrated that the patients were not merely clearing the exogenous T_3 at an accelerated rate. The T_3 levels were high, and presumably the high levels were overriding a mechanism of cellular resistance to thyroid hormone. These findings make it highly probable that our euthyroid fibromyalgia patients have cellular resistance to thyroid hormone. They appear in most respects to be modern examples of the euthyroid hypometabolic patients reported in the 1950s and 1960s to have benefitted from T_3 treatment. And they are similar to Kaplan's patient documented to have partial peripheral resistance to thyroid hormone.[10]

Some individuals appear to develop tolerance to large dosages of thyroid hormone.[50][168] Because of this, it has been suggested that T_3-receptors down-regulate in patients who are able to use supraphysiologic dosages of T_3 without thyrotoxicity.[131,p.383] This mechanism is considered a physiological adaptation to persistent exposure to high levels of thyroid hormone. An implication of this suggestion has been that although supraphysiologic dosages of thyroid hormone do not harm these patients, they also may not benefit them. In the case of most euthyroid fibromyalgia patients, experience shows that this is not the case. Many euthyroid fibromyalgia patients improve or recover from the condition when they use supraphysiologic dosages of exogenous T_3 within the context of a more comprehensive metabolic rehabilitation program. These patients no longer meet the ACR criteria for fibromyalgia, and most patients consider themselves improved or recovered. These results have largely been confirmed by other clinicians using the same or a similar treatment protocol. Garrison, a coauthor on two of our blinded studies, reported treating some 200 fibromyalgia patients with considerable success at the University of Texas Health Science Center.[97] Honeyman published a case history of the successful treatment of a hypothyroid fibromyalgia patient and a euthyroid fibromyalgia patient. Her paper is particularly useful for clinicians because she provides a detailed account of her use of metabolic therapy combined with the use of physical treatment.[170]

● RECOGNITION OF FIBROMYALGIA/ CHRONIC FATIGUE SYNDROME

In the late 1970s, investigators began observing, describing, and classifying patients with the non-specific symptoms typical of euthyroid hypometabolic patients. Patients whose predominant symptom was pain were diagnosed as having fibromyalgia; those whose predominant symptom was fatigue were diagnosed as having chronic fatigue syndrome. It is generally agreed at this time that these two conditions are the same or at least largely overlap. In my experience, these patients are indistinguishable from patients described in the 1950s and 1960s as having euthyroid hypometabolism. The clinical features of fibromyalgia/chronic fatigue syndrome and euthyroid hypometabolism are virtually the same. Also, fibromyalgia/chronic fatigue syndrome patients respond to metabolic therapy (centered around the use of T_3) exactly as euthyroid hypometabolic patients reportedly did in the 1950s and 1960s. And patients within these classifications respond to this treatment as patients with peripheral thyroid hormone resistance have.

MISBELIEFS ABOUT THE SERUM TSH THAT HAVE DIVERTED FIBROMYALGIA RESEARCHERS FROM AN UNDERSTANDING OF EUTHYROID FIBROMYALGIA

There is a high incidence of hypothyroidism among fibromyalgia patients. In virtually all cases of hypothyroid fibromyalgia, the symptoms of fibromyalgia are relieved when the patient undergoes metabolic rehabilitation involving three procedures: (1) the use of nutritional supplements, (2) exercise to tolerance, and (3) TSH-suppressive dosages of thyroid hormone. Some hypothyroid fibromyalgia patients improve or recover when the form of exogenous thyroid hormone is T_4 or desiccated thyroid. However, many do not improve or recover until they are switched to T_3. The hypothyroid patient I described in 1995 in a published

case history, who dramatically recovered after being switched to T_3, is typical of such patients[134] (see Appendix B).

The symptoms of most euthyroid fibromyalgia (euthyroid hypometabolic) patients are improved or relieved by supraphysiologic dosages of T_3—when used as part of a regimen that also includes the use of nutritional supplements and exercise to tolerance. It is my impression that virtually no fibromyalgia researcher or clinician operating within the rheumatologic paradigm of fibromyalgia is aware of the therapeutic potential of T_3 with these patients. With few exceptions, in my experience, such researchers and clinicians have rejected the possibility while vehemently refusing to consider the evidence in favor of it. The root of this psychosocial phenomenon appears to be the unquestioning acceptance of two false propositions perpetrated and maintained by modern conventional endocrinologists/thyroidologists.

The False Proposition that the Basal Serum TSH is Sufficient to Identify Primary Hypothyroid Patients

According to published papers, in most studies of fibromyalgia patients, investigators have attempted to identify and exclude hypothyroid patients. Most have used the basal TSH level to identify patients who were hypothyroid. By failing to use either the TRH stimulation test or the nocturnal TSH surge, they undoubtedly failed to identify two groups of patients with thyroid hormone deficiencies: (1) those with borderline primary hypothyroidism not revealed by a clearly elevated basal TSH, and (2) those with TRH stimulation test results consistent with central hypothyroidism. As a result, based on the findings of my research group,[94][95] perhaps all such fibromyalgia studies contained unidentified hypothyroid patients.

The failure of researchers and clinicians to recognize the high incidence of hypothyroidism among fibromyalgia patients results from one mistake: implicit trust in the judgment of endocrinologists that the basal TSH is sufficient to identify hypothyroid patients. Despite the claims of Volpé that the latest modern TSH assays invariably identify hypothyroid patients,[96] this proposition is patently false. I have had patients whose third-generation TSH levels were normal, yet they had extremely exaggerated TSH responses to TRH injections (which are consistent with both primary and central hypothyroidism). Invariably, these patients have completely recovered from fibromyalgia with TSH-suppressive dosages of T_4 (used as part of a regimen including dietary changes, nutritional supplements, and exercise to tolerance). In addition, the patients had no tissue thyrotoxicity from the use of exogenous thyroid hormone.

The False Proposition that the Basal Serum TSH is Sufficient to Properly Titrate the Dosage of T_4

An often expressed criticism directed to me is this: "If the fibromyalgia symptoms of a hypothyroid patient are manifestations of the patient's tissue hypometabolism, then replacement doses of thyroid hormone would certainly relieve the fibromyalgia symptoms. Thyroid hormone replacement does not relieve fibromyalgia symptoms. Therefore, fibromyalgia symptoms cannot be a manifestation of tissue hypometabolism caused by hypothyroidism."

It is easy to understand why a clinician would assert this criticism if we also know beforehand that he believes an erroneous endocrinology doctrine—that a basal TSH level within the normal reference range rules out inadequate thyroid hormone cell regulation. My impression is that clinicians who register the criticism have never permitted hypothyroid fibromyalgia patients under their care to use TSH-suppressive dosages of exogenous thyroid hormone. As a result, they have never witnessed the improvement or recovery that virtually always occurs when these patients use such dosages (as part of a complete regimen of metabolic rehabilitation). According to the clinicians' frame of reference, they have used exogenous thyroid hormone "properly" with hypothyroid fibromyalgia patients, yet they have not seen the improvement or recovery I have reported. In effect, their unquestioning subscription to the current endocrinology misbelief leaves them *non compos mentis* in regard to seeing a connection between inadequate thyroid hormone cell regulation and fibromyalgia.

In 1994, the medical director (a rheumatologist) of a Houston, Texas fibromyalgia support group made a preemptive response to my forthcoming presentation to the group. He wrote, "Clearly, if thyroid hormone replacement was the key, then no patient on thyroid medication would have fibromyalgia."[9] This is tantamount to arguing that if thirst were due to insufficient liquid intake, then no one who consumes liquid would be thirsty. Of course, thirst will persist if one consumes too little liquid; similarly, symptoms of hypometabolism will continue if the hypothyroid patient takes too little exogenous thyroid hormone. But the current endocrinology paradigm dictates that "enough" thyroid hormone is not the amount that relieves the patient's symptoms. Instead, it is an amount that keeps the basal TSH level within the normal reference range. According to this model, in adjusting liquid intake, a patient would be permitted to consume only enough liquid to keep the blood liquid content within a certain range despite the patient's pleas to be allowed to drink more to relieve his or her thirst.

The amount of exogenous thyroid hormone sufficient to keep the basal TSH within the normal reference range is termed the "replacement dosage."[16][17] The misbelief that such a dosage is enough thyroid hormone for *all* hypothyroid fibromyalgia patients has most likely been an obstacle to recovery for most of these patients. This erroneous belief is entrenched at high levels in the rheumatology fibromyalgia research community. This is illustrated by the recent rejection of a grant proposal my colleagues and I submitted to a funding organization. We had proposed a rigorously designed double-blind study of hypothyroid fibromyalgia patients. We were to compare the effects of replacement dosages with that of higher dosages of T_4. The proposal was rejected because the person assigned to review it (I later learned) was a prominent rheumatology fibromyalgia researcher. The damaging pronouncement was, "We find that replacement dosages of thyroid hormone do not benefit fibromyalgia patients." Because of this statement, our grant proposal was rejected.

This *illuminati* was correct—replacement dosages typically do not benefit hypothyroid fibromyalgia patients. We predicted in our grant proposal that our study would confirm this. In addition, we hypothesized that, in contrast, higher dosages *would* benefit the patients. But it appears that the reviewer did not bother to read far enough into the proposal to learn of this, and the decision-makers had the impression from his pronouncement that it was already established that exogenous thyroid hormone is of no benefit at all to fibromyalgia patients. "As often in the history of science," wrote Duesberg, "the biggest obstacle in finding the truth is not the difficulty in obtaining data, but the bias of the investigators on what data to chase and how to interpret them."[109,pp.409-410]

If rheumatology researchers have been looking through cloudy glasses regarding hypothyroid fibromyalgia patients, they wear a tight-fitting blindfold regarding euthyroid hypometabolic fibromyalgia patients. In two of their decision-making conferences on fibromyalgia, they have reached an implicit conclusion through a particular line of thinking. First, they erroneously believe that only an elevated basal TSH indicates hypothyroidism. Second, they note that only a small percentage of fibromyalgia patients have elevated TSH levels. Third, if hypothyroidism were the cause of all fibromyalgia, then all fibromyalgia patients would have elevated TSH levels. Thus, because most fibromyalgia patients do not have elevated TSH levels, hypothyroidism cannot be the cause of fibromyalgia. They also appear to believe that the only thyroid hormone-related problem that could produce symptoms of hypometabolism is a thyroid hormone deficiency; they completely ignore the phenomenon of cellular resistance to thyroid hormone. Moreover, they conclude that hypothyroidism is only a concomitant condition in a small percentage of fibromyalgia patients.

As a result of this line of reasoning, few members of the rheumatology fibromyalgia research clique have considered inadequate thyroid hormone cell regulation as a pathophysiological basis of fibromyalgia. (Prof. J.B. Eisinger, whose studies I reference throughout this book, is a highly notable exception. As I pointed out in a 1998 editorial in the *Clinical Bulletin of Myofascial Therapy*, "Eisinger's work, conducted in France, deserves the focused attention of all researchers and clinicians in the field. It should be clear to anyone who has scrutinized fibromyalgia patients that they suffer from metabolic impairment. In good science, such self-evident concepts serve as the postulates upon which forward-moving studies are based. Yet in this regard in the field of fibromyalgia, Eisinger's work almost stands alone. It is my view that his studies are the most important in the field. At a fundamental level, they are the most relevant to the self-evident nature of fibromyalgia."[130,p.1]) While most rheumatology researchers have paid little attention to the role of hypothyroidism in fibromyalgia, to my knowledge they have paid none to the role of euthyroid hypometabolism. They have implicitly exculpated inadequate thyroid hormone cell regulation from an etiological role in fibromyalgia. With this misbelief embedded in their common frame of reference, they presently wander aimlessly down alternate research paths that are impertinent to relieving fibromyalgia patients of their suffering.

● EUTHYROID HYPOMETABOLISM AND LABORATORY TESTS OF THYROID FUNCTION

The value of laboratory thyroid function tests for euthyroid fibromyalgia patients is in initially establishing the patients' euthyroid status. Unfortunately, once the patient's euthyroid status is established, few clinicians today will treat the patient. For treatment, most euthyroid fibromyalgia patients must seek the assistance of a prescribing clinician who rejects the current endocrinology/thyroidology paradigm. With the protocol I describe in this book, the clinician does not use thyroid function test results to disqualify euthyroid patients from the use of thyroid hormone. Instead, he uses the test results to determine with which form of thyroid hormone the patient would preferably begin treatment. Most patients who have any form of hypothyroidism would best begin with desiccated thyroid (or a combination of synthetic T_3 and T_4); those who are euthyroid should use T_3 (see Chapters 5.2, 5.3, and 5.4).

Clinicians should bear in mind what thyroid function test results provide: At best, they give information on the blood levels of TSH and thyroid hormones, and on the functional status of the pituitary-thyroid axis. *They do not in any way measure the metabolic status of tissues.* Thyroid function tests are of no value in identifying patients whose peripheral tissues are hypometabolic despite the patient's euthyroid status. In euthyroid patients, as with hypothyroid patients, hypometabolism may be a result of inadequate thyroid hormone regulation of transcription. Correction of the inadequacy will depend on a trial of thyroid hormone with the patient's dosage adjusted based on systematically monitored symptoms, signs, and peripheral indices (see Chapter 4.3). Dosage should *not* be titrated on the basis of thyroid function testing.

The pattern of values from the thyroid function tests is predictable for the euthyroid patient who uses supraphysiologic dosages of exogenous T_3. For most patients, the basal TSH and T_4 are low, and the free T_3 is elevated. This pattern alarms many clinicians, as they have been taught that such a pattern is synonymous with tissue thyrotoxicosis. However, short-term[90][91][92] and long-term[93] testing of our euthyroid fibromyalgia patients taking supraphysiologic dosages of T_3 and exhibiting the predictable test pattern have revealed no thyrotoxicity. Bone densitometry, serial ECGs, and serum and urine tests for biochemical evidence of toxicity in heart, muscle, liver, and bone indicate that these tissues of concern in our euthyroid fibromyalgia patients are resistant to thyroid hormone. In some patients at follow-up times ranging from 1-to-5 years, bone density was *higher* than age- and sex-matched individuals.

After establishing that the fibromyalgia patient is euthyroid, thyroid function tests are of no further benefit in the care of the patient. This means that after the patient begins using exogenous T$_3$, thyroid function tests are useless for determining the patient's safe and effective dosage. After the thyroid status is established, subjecting the patient or a third party payer to the cost of further thyroid function tests cannot be justified. It is necessary, of course, to know whether a particular T$_3$ dosage is adversely affecting a patient. Adverse tissue effects, however, can only be objectively determined through tests that specifically show thyrotoxicity of individual tissues (see Chapters 4.3 and 4.4).

It is scientifically indefensible to argue that thyroid function tests objectively demonstrate adverse tissue effects. At most, one can argue that a particular pattern of thyroid function test values is typical of patients who have tissue thyrotoxicity. But it is false to conclude in an individual case, based solely on the pattern of values, that the patient has tissue thyrotoxicosis.

CONCEPTUAL OBSTACLES TO EUTHYROID HYPOMETABOLIC PATIENTS RECEIVING PROPER TREATMENT

The concepts perpetrated and perpetuated by modern conventional endocrinology/thyroidology have created obstacles to the proper treatment of euthyroid hypometabolic patients.

Investigators began to consider euthyroid hypometabolism a clinical entity in the 1950s. (See Table 2.5.9 for the classification of the forms of hypometabolism.) Since then, it has been medical practitioners other than endocrinologists who have embraced the concept. These other practitioners have provided patients with relief through treatments derived from the concept. In 1960, Goldberg wrote, "Despite the preponderance of endocrinologists stating that they were still searching for their first *bona fide* case of euthyroid hypometabolism, or disparaging the entire matter as a commercial invention of the pharmaceutical houses, the controversy was kept alive by the enthusiasm of general practitioners who seemed to be getting favorable results with T$_3$ in several of their chronically tired, thyroid-resistant cases, and the gynecologists and urologists struggling with their infertility problems."[49,p.479]

Today, this circumstance in general has not changed. Sonkin—one of the few rational voices regarding euthyroid hypometabolism in the modern specialty of endocrinology/thyroidology—has commented on the circumstance. He attributed the problem with endocrinologists/thyroidologists to the current paradigm of their specialty.[62,p.49] According to this paradigm, symptomatic patients are permitted treatment with thyroid hormone only if thyroid function laboratory test results are indicative of hypothyroidism. In challenging the paradigm, Sonkin wrote that it contains three prevailing concepts: (1) the single cause of symptoms of thyroidal insufficiency is hypothyroidism, (2) patients with normal thyroid function test results should not be permitted to undergo therapeutic trials with thyroid hormone, and (3) patients should not be treated with thyroid hormone dosages that lower the TSH below "normal" levels.[62,p.53]

Because of the first two prevailing concepts Sonkin listed, euthyroid fibromyalgia patients are generally denied the opportunity to undergo a trial of thyroid hormone therapy. Regarding this, he wrote, "It seems reasonable, in the face of current evidence and uncertainty to give the patient the benefit of the doubt, and offer a therapeutic trial with thyroid, which is innocuous and frequently effective."[62,p.49]

As I indicated above, some euthyroid patients are permitted by other types of practitioners to undergo a trial of thyroid hormone. Because of the third concept Sonkin lists, however, most of these patients are not permitted to increase their thyroid hormone dosage enough. The dosage is kept low enough to avoid TSH suppression. With most patients, this effectively prevents the metabolic changes that are prerequisite to improved symptoms and signs. As a result, the patient remains symptomatic.

To effectively treat most euthyroid hypometabolic patients, the clinician must forswear the erroneous concepts of the current endocrinology/thyroidology paradigm. He must bear in mind the single most pertinent question in assessing endocrine function: "Does the target organ respond properly to the hormone in question?"[110,p.746] With the exception of the anterior pituitary, laboratory thyroid function tests cannot answer this question; only indirect measures of peripheral tissue metabolic status can (see Chapter 4.3).

● CONCLUSION

In this chapter, I have presented the historical development of the clinical concepts of both hypothyroidism and euthyroid hypometabolism. I have also considered the methods for diagnosing and treating these conditions. It should be clear from this overview that euthyroid hypometabolism is a genuine clinical phenomenon. As such, it is a condition worthy of the long-overdue attention of researchers.

Table 2.5.9. Classification of forms of hypometabolism.*

FORM OF HYPOMETABOLISM

Diagnostic features (not all features in every patient)	Overt hypothyroidism	Subclinical hypothyroidism	General resistance to thyroid hormone	Euthyroid hypometabolism[δ]
Non-specific & variable FMS-like clinical features	Yes	Yes	Varies	Yes
Adaptive changes in hypothalamic-pituitary axis	Elevation of serum TSH	Enhanced TSH response to TRH injection, basal TSH typically but not invariably slightly raised	Inappropriately high	None
Thyroid hormone levels	Low T_4 Low T_3	Normal	Inappropriately high levels typically	Normal
Basal metabolic rate (BMR)	Low	Low	Varies	Low
Basal body temperature (BBT)	Low	Low	Varies	Low
Response to desiccated thyroid or T_4	Positive to physiologic dosage[†]	Lowering of TSH with physiologic dosage	Positive in some cases; supraphysiologic dosage required	None
Response to T_3	Positive to physiologic dosage[†]	Lowering of TSH to physiologic dosage	Positive to supraphysiologic dosage	Positive to supraphysiologic dosage [‡]
Myofascial pain and trigger points	Yes	Yes	Varies	Yes

*Adapted from Evered, D.: Subclinical hypothyroidism. In *Werner's The Thyroid: A Fundamental and Clinical Text*, 5th edition. Edited by S.H. Ingbar and L.E. Braverman, Philadelphia, J.B. Lippincott Co., 1986, p.1440, and Sonkin, L.S.: Myofascial pain due to metabolic disorders: diagnosis and treatment. In *Myofascial Pain and Fibromyalgia: Trigger Point Management*. Edited by E.S. Rachlin, St. Louis, Mosby, 1994, pp.45-60.
[δ]Here I use the term euthyroid hypometabolism as synonymous with partial cellular resistance to thyroid hormone.
[†] Lowers TSH, raises blood thyroid hormone levels, relieves symptoms, and increases BMR.
[‡]Relieves symptoms and increases BMR.

For purposes of case management at this time, we are left with a question of practical concern to clinicians: Can we, with current technology, truly distinguish hypothyroidism from euthyroid hypometabolism? There are several components to my answer. First, we can, with a reasonable degree of accuracy, identify primary and central hypothyroid patients if—and *only* if—clinicians will use the proper thyroid function tests, and if they will interpret them properly (see Chapter 4.2). This would require that many clinicians abdicate their blind devotion to the idea that the TSH is the be-all and end-all in thyroid function testing, because it is not! It would also require that clinicians resume for diagnostic purposes the proper use of the TRH stimulation test or begin using the measures of the TSH nocturnal surge. If a clinician determines through proper thyroid function testing that the patient has normal TSH and thyroid hormone levels and that the pituitary-thyroid axis is functioning properly, does this mean that the patient is euthyroid? It does only if we assume that the ranges of normal that fluidly vary from laboratory-to-laboratory truly represent "normal."

This has yet to be convincingly established. In addition, no laboratory thyroid function test is 100% reliable. Some hypothyroid patients will not be identified through laboratory testing. Nonetheless, within the limits of this scientific uncertainty, yes—we can, with a fair degree of accuracy, determine which patients are, and which are not, hypothyroid.

Those who are not hypothyroid and are not hyperthyroid are euthyroid. Can we determine, however, whether some euthyroid patients are hypometabolic? We certainly cannot with any thyroid function test, including third generation TSH assays. Unfortunately, the BMR is for all practical purposes not available to most clinicians because of an agreement between medical organizations and Blue Cross/Blue Shield.[62,p.59] This leaves clinicians without a highly reliable method for assessing cellular metabolism. I say this because the basal body temperature is not sufficiently reliable, and it is specific only for the heat generating mechanisms of the body. A normal basal body temperature does not assure that a patient is eumetabolic, and a low basal body temperature does not assure that a patient is hypometabolic. An assessment is best based on a combination of indirect peripheral indices such as the basal body temperature, ECG voltage, Achilles reflex, pulse rate, cholesterol, and the five objective measures of fibromyalgia status (see Chapter 4.3).

Monitoring such indices through the course of metabolic rehabilitation can give a fairly accurate impression of changes in tissue metabolism. This protocol is far from ideal, but many euthyroid fibromyalgia patients (whom I consider euthyroid hypometabolic) have benefitted from it. At this time, the protocol is acceptable for purposes of case management.

REFERENCES

1. Willson, J.R., Beecham, C.T., and Carrington, E.R.: *Obstetrics and Gynecology*. Saint Louis, C.V. Mosby Co., 1975, p.652.
2. Travell, J.G. and Simons, D.G.: *Myofascial Pain and Dysfunction: The Trigger Point Manual*, Vol. 1. Baltimore, Williams and Wilkins, 1983.
3. Refetoff, S., Dewind, L.T., and DeGroot, L.J.: Familial syndrome combining deaf-mutism, stippled epiphyses, goiter and abnormally high PBI: possible target organ refractoriness to thyroid hormone. *J. Clin. Endocrinol. Metab.*, 27:279, 1967.
4. Refetoff, S.: Syndromes of thyroid hormone resistance. *Am. J. Physiol.*, 243:E88, 1982.
5. Roche, J., Lissitzky, S., and Michel, R.: Sur la présence de triiodothyronine dans la thyroglobuline. *Comptes Rendus de l'Acad. Sci.*, 10(234):1228-1230, 1952.
6. Roche, J., Lissitzky, S., and Michel, R.: Sur la triiodothyronine, produit itermédiaire de la transformation de diiodothyronine en thyroxine. *Comptes Rendus de l'Acad. Sci.*, 25(234):997-998, 1952.
7. Williams, E.D.: In memoriam to Rosalind Pitt-Rivers. *Prog. Thyroid Res.* Edited by A. Gordan, J. Gross, and G. Hennemann, Rotterdam, A.a.Balkema, 1991, pp.15-18.
8. Refetoff, S.: Thyroid hormone resistance syndromes. In *Werner's The Thyroid: A Fundamental and Clinical Text*, 5th edition. Edited by Sidney H. Ingbar and Lewis E. Braverman, Philadelphia, J.B. Lippincott Co., 1986, pp.1292-1307.
9. Rubin, R.: Primary versus secondary fibromyalgia. *The Fibromyalgia Connection: Newsletter of the Fibromyalgia Association of Houston, Inc.*, 1(5):2, 1994.
10. Kaplan, M.M., Swartz, S.L., and Larsen, P.R.: Partial peripheral resistance to thyroid hormones. *Am. J. Med.*, 70: 1115-1121, 1981.
11. Gull, W.W.: On a cretinoid state supervening in adult life in women. *Trans. Clin. Soc.* (Lond.), 7:180-185, 1874.
12. Cooper, D.S.: Subclinical hypothyroidism. *J.A.M.A.*, 258: 246-247, 1987.
13. Sawin, C.T.: The development and use of thyroid preparations. In *The Thyroid Gland: A Practical Clinical Treatise*. Edited by L. Van Middlesworth, Jr., Chicago, Year Book Medical Publishers, Inc., 1986, pp.389-403.
14. Murray, G.R.: Note on the treatment of myxoedema by hypodermic injections of an extract of the thyroid gland of a sheep. *Br. Med. J.*, 2:796, 1891.
15. MacKenzie, H.W.G.: A case of myxoedema treated with great benefit by feeding with fresh thyroid glands. *Br. Med. J.*, 2:940, 1892.
16. Stock, J.M., Surks, M.I., and Oppenheimer, J.H.: Replacement dosage of L-thyroxine in hypothyroidism. *N. Engl. J. Med.*, 290:529-533, 1974.
17. Evered, D., Young, E.T., Ornston, B.J., Menzies, R., Smith, P.A., and Hall, R.: Treatment of hypothyroidism: a reappraisal of thyroxine therapy. *Br. Med. J.*, iii:131-134, 1973.
18. Kendall, E.C. and Osterberg, A.E.: The chemical identification of thyroxin. *J. Biol. Chem.*, 40:265, 1919.
19. Reichlin, S.: Regulation of the hypothalamic-pituitary-thyroid axis. *Med. Clin. North Am.*, 62:305-312, 1978.
20. Braverman, L.E.: Sidney H. Ingbar remembered. In *Progress in Thyroid Research*. Edited by A. Gordan, J. Gross, and G. Hennemann, Rotterdam, A.a. Balkema, 1991, pp.9-13.
21. Vagenakis, A.G. and Braverman, L.E.: Thyroid function tests-which one? *Ann. Intern. Med.*, 84:607-608, 1976.
22. Toft, A.D., Irvine, W.J., and Seth, J.: Thyroid function in the long-term follow-up of patients treated with iodine-131 for thyrotoxicosis. *Lancet*, 2:576-578, 1975.
23. Tibaldi, J. and Barzel, U.S.: Thyroxine supplementation: method for the prevention of clinical hypothyroidism. *Am. J. Med.*, 79:241-244, 1985.
24. Freedberg, A.S., Kurland, G.S., and Hamolsky, M.W.: Effect of l-tri-iodothyronine alone and combined with l-thyroxine in nonmyxedematous hypometabolism. *New Engl. J. Med.*, 253:57-60, 1955.
25. Haines, S.F. and Mussey, R.D.: Certain menstrual disturbances associated with low basal metabolic rates with myx-

edema. *J.A.M.A.*, 105:557, 1935.

26. Reiss, M. and Haigh, C.P.: Various forms of hypothyroidism in mental disorder. *Proc. Roy. Soc. Med.*, 47:889, 1954.

27. Kirk, E. and Kvorning, S.A.: Hypometabolism: a clinical study of 308 consecutive cases. *Acta Med. Scandinav.*, Suppl.184:3-83, 1946.

28. Leonard, J.L. and Koehrle, J.: Intracellular pathways of iodothyronine metabolism. In *Werner and Ingbar's The Thyroid: A Fundamental and Clinical Text*, 7th edition. Edited by L.P. Braverman and R.D. Utiger, Philadelphia, Lippincott-Raven Publishers, 1996, pp.125-161.

29. Morton, J.H.: Sodium liothyronine in metabolic insufficiency syndrome and associated disorders. *J.A.M.A.*, 165:124-129, 1957.

30. Fields, E.M.: Treatment of metabolic insufficiency and hypothyroidism with sodium liothyronine. *J.A.M.A.*, 163:817, 1957.

31. Kurland, G.S., Hamolsky, M.W., and Freedberg, A.S.: Studies in non-myxedematous hypometabolism: I. The clinical syndrome and the effects of triiodothyronine, alone or combined with thyroxine. *J. Clin. Endocrinol.*, 15:1354, 1955.

32. Keating, F.R., Jr.: Editorial: Metabolic insufficiency. *J. Clin. Endocrinol.*, 18:531-537, 1958.

33. Sikkema, S.H.: Triiodothyronine in the diagnosis and treatment of hypothyroidism: failure to demonstrate the metabolic insufficiency syndrome. *J. Clin. Endocrinol.*, 20:546, 1960.

34. Milton, R.: *Alternative Science: Challenging the Myths of the Scientific Establishment*. Rochester, Park Street Press, 1996.

35. Sauberlich, H.E. and Canham, J.E.: Vitamin B_6. In *Modern Nutrition in Health and Disease*, 6th edition. Edited by R.S. Goodhart and M.E. Shils, Philadelphia, Lea & Febiger, 1980, pp.219-225.

36. Roe, D.A.: *Drug-induced Nutritional Deficiencies*. AVI Publishing, 1976, pp.72, 83, 120, 217.

37. Carney, M.W.P.: Psychiatric aspects of folate deficiency. In *Folic Acid in Neurology, Psychiatry, and Internal Medicine*. Edited by M.I. Botez and E.H. Reynolds, New York, Raven Press, 1979, pp.480-482.

38. Fraser, W.D., Biggart, E.M., O'Reilly, D. St. J., Gray, H.W., and McKillop, J.H.: Are biochemical tests of thyroid function of any value in monitoring patients receiving thyroxine replacement? *Br. Med. J.*, 293:808-810, 1986.

39. Wayne, E.J.: Clinical and metabolic studies in thyroid disease. *Br. Med. J.*, i:1-11. 78-90, 1960.

40. Barnes, B.O.: *Hypothyroidism: The Unsuspected Illness*. New York, Harper and Row, Publishers, 1976.

41. Winkler, A.W., Criscuolok, J., and Lavietes, P.H.: Quantitative relationship between basal metabolic rate and thyroid dosage in patients with true myxedema. *J. Clin. Invest.*, 22:531, 1943.

42. Andersen, B., Russell, I.J., Lewit, K., and McCain, G.A.: Panel discussion on management issues. *First International Symposium on Myofascial Pain and Fibromyalgia*, Minneapolis, May 10, 1989.

43. Sonkin, L.S.: Endocrine disorders and muscle dysfunction. In *Clinical Management of Head, Neck and TMJ Pain and Dysfunction*. Edited by B. Gelb, Philadelphia, W.B. Saunders Co., 1985, pp.137-170.

44. Thompson, W.O. and Thompson, P.K.: Low basal metabolism following thyrotoxicosis. II. Permanent type without myxedema. *J. Clin. Invest.*, 5:471,1928.

45. Thurman, F.M. and Thompson, W.O.: Low basal metabolism without myxedema. *Arch. Intern. Med.*, 46:879-897, 1930.

46. Means, J.H.: *The Thyroid and Its Diseases*, 2nd edition. Philadelphia, J.B. Lippincott Co., 1948.

47. Tittle, C.R.: Effects of 3,5,3' l-triiodothyronine in patients with metabolic insufficiency. *J.A.M.A.*, 162:271, 1956.

48. Jefferies, W.McK.: Occult hypothyroidism and "metabolic insufficiency." *J. Chron. Dis.*, 14:582-592, 1961.

49. Goldberg, M.: The case for euthyroid hypometabolism. *Am. J. Med. Sc.*, 240:479-493, 1960.

50. Danovski, T.S., Sarver, M.E, D'Ambrosia, R.D., and Moses, C.: Hydrocortisone and/or desiccated thyroid in physiologic dosage. X. Effects of thyroid hormone excesses on clinical status and thyroid indices. *Metabolism*, 13:702-716, 1964.

51. Keating, F.R.: Editorial: Triiodothyronine for "metabolic insufficiency." *Lancet*, Oct.20:826-827,1956.

52. Fredericks, C.: *Psycho-Nutrition*. New York, Crosset & Dunlap, 1976.

53. Boothby, W.M. and Sandiford, I.: Summary of the basal metabolism data on 8,614 subjects with especial reference to the normal standards for the estimation of the basal metabolic rate. *J. Biol. Chem.*, 54:783, 1922.

54. Means, J.H. and Burgess, H.W.: The basal metabolism in nontoxic goiter and in borderline thyroid cases: with particular reference to its bearing in differential diagnosis. *Arch. Int. Med.*, 30:507, 1922.

55. Haines, S.F. and Mussey, R.D.: Certain menstrual disturbances associated with low basal metabolic rates without myxedema. *J.A.M.A.*, 105:557, 1935.

56. Wishart, G.M.: Variability of basal metabolism. *Quart. J. Med.*, 20:193, 1927.

57. Means, J.H.: *Lectures on the Thyroid*. Cambridge, Harvard University Press, 1954.

58. Winkler, A.W., Lavietes, P.H., Robbins, C.L., and Man, E.B.: Tolerance to oral thyroid and reaction to intravenous thyroxine in subjects without myxedema. *J. Clin. Invest.*, 22:535-544, 1943.

59. Kimball, O.P.: Clinical hypothyroidism. *Kentucky Med. J.*, 31:488-495, 1933.

60. Wharton, G.K.: Unrecognized hypothyroidism. *Canadian Med. Assoc. J.*, 40:371-376, 1939.

61. Jackson, A.S.: Hypothyroidism. *J.A.M.A.*, 165:121-124, 1957.

62. Sonkin, L.S.: Myofascial pain due to metabolic disorders: diagnosis and treatment. In *Myofascial Pain and Fibromyalgia: Trigger Point Management*. Edited by E.S. Rachlin, St. Louis, Mosby, 1994, pp.45-60.

63. Evered, D.: Subclinical hypothyroidism. In *Werner's The Thyroid: A Fundamental and Clinical Text*, 5th edition. Edited by S.H. Ingbar and L.E. Braverman, Philadelphia, J.B. Lippincott Co., 1986, pp.1439-1444.

64. Goldberg, M.: Diagnosis of euthyroid hypometabolism. *Am. J. Obst. & Gynec.*, 81(5):1053-1058, May, 1961.

65. Sonkin, L.S.: Paired BMR and serum cholesterol measurements in therapeutic trials with thyroid hormones in

patients with normal levels of TSH and/or T_4, or PBI and symptoms suggesting thyroid deficiency (abstract 678). *Endocrine Society 60th Annual Meeting*, 1978.

66. Goldstein, B.J. and Muslin, A.I.: Use of a single thyroxine test to evaluate ambulatory patients for suspected hypothyroidism. *J. Gen Intern. Med.*, 2:20, 1987.

67. Schectman, J.M., Kallenberg, G.A., Shumacher, R.J., and Hirsh, R.P.: Yield of hypothyroidism in symptomatic primary care patients. *Arch. Intern. Med.*, 149:861, 1989.

68. Torresani, J.: In memoriam to professor Serge Lissitzky. *Progress Thyroid Research*. Edited by A. Gordan, J. Gross, and G. Hennemann, Rotterdam, A.a.Balkema, 1991, pp.3-8.

69. Linder, M.C.: Human nutrition in context. In *Nutritional Biochemistry and Metabolism: with Clinical Applications*, 2nd edition. Edited by M.C. Linder, New York, Elsevier, 1991.

70. Gooch, B.R., Isley, W.L., and Utiger, R.D.: Abnormalities in thyroid function tests in patients admitted to a medical service. *Arch. Intern. Med.*, 142:1801, 1982.

71. Ladenson, P.W.: Diagnosis of hypothyroidism. In *Werner's The Thyroid: A Fundamental and Clinical Text*, 6th edition. Edited by L.E. Braverman and R.D.Utiger, Philadelphia, J.B. Lippincott Co., 1991, pp.1092-1098.

72. Wartofsky, L. and Burman, K.D.: Alteration in thyroid function in patients with systemic illness: the "euthyroid" sick syndrome. *Endocr. Rev.*, 3:164, 1982.

73. Prankerd, T.A.J.: Anaemia. In *French's Index of Differential Diagnosis*, 10th edition. Edited by F.D. Hart, Chicago, Year Book Medical Publishers Inc., 1973, pp.28-62.

74. Maclagan, N.F.: Thyroid: tests of function. In *French's Index of Differential Diagnosis*, 10th edition. Edited by F.D. Hart, Chicago, Year Book Medical Publishers Inc., 1973, pp.762-764.

75. Werner, S.C.: History of the thyroid. In *Werner's The Thyroid: A Fundamental and Clinical Text*, 5th edition. Edited by S.H. Ingbar and L.E. Braverman, Philadelphia, J.B. Lippincott Co., 1986, pp.3-6.

76. Paracelsus. De generative stultorum: liber theophrasti. In *Omina Opera Tractatus I*, 1603.

77. Fagge, C.H.: On sporadic cretinism occurring in England. *Br. Med. J.*, 1:279, 1871.

78. Hutchison, J.H., Arneil, G.C., and McGerr, E.M.: Deficiency of an extrathyroid enzyme in sporadic cretinism. *Lancet*, 2:314-315, 1957.

79. Ord, W.M.: On myxoedema: a term proposed to be applied to an essential condition in the "cretinoid" affection occasionally observed in middle-aged women. *Med. Chir. Trans.*, 61:57, 1878.

80. Ord, W.M.: On myxoedema: a term proposed to be applied to an essential condition in the "cretinoid" affection occasionally observed in middle-aged women: report of the Myxoedema Commission of the Clinical Society of London. *Trans. Clin. Soc.* (Lond.), 13:15, 1888.

81. Kirk, E. and Kvorning, S.A.: *Hypometabolism: A Clinical Study of 308 Consecutive Cases*. Copenhagen, Einar Munksgaard, Publisher, 1946.

82. Sturgis, C.C.: A clinical study of myxedema with observations of the basal metabolism. *Med. Clin. of North Am.*, 5:1251, 1922.

83. Wishart, G.M.: The variability of basal metabolism. *Quart. J. Med.*, 20:193, 1927.

84. Gross, J. and Pitt-Rivers, R.: The identification of 3:5:3'-triiodothyronine in human plasma. *Lancet*, 1:439, 1952.

85. Gross, J. and Pitt-Rivers, R.: Triiodothyronine in relation to thyroid physiology. *Recent Prog. Horm. Res.*, 10:109, 1954.

86. Kendall, E.C.: The isolation in crystalline form of the compound containing iodine which occurs in the thyroid: its chemical nature and physiological activity. *Trans. Assoc. Am. Physician*, 30:420, 1915.

87. Harington, C.R.: Chemistry of thyroxine. I. Isolation of thyroxine from the thyroid gland. *Biochem. J.*, 20:293, 1926.

88. Harington, C.R. and Barger, G.: Chemistry of thyroxine. III. Constitution and synthesis of thyroxine. *Biochem. J.*, 21:169, 1927.

89. Sawin, C.T., Geller, A., Hershman, J.M., Castelli, W., and Bacharach, P.: The aging thyroid: the use of thyroid hormone in older persons. *J.A.M.A.*, 261:2653-2655, 1989.

90. Lowe, J.C., Garrison, R., Reichman, A.J., Yellin, J., Thompson, M., and Kaufman, D.: Effectiveness and safety of T_3 (triiodothyronine) therapy for euthyroid fibromyalgia: a double-blind placebo-controlled response-driven crossover study. *Clin. Bull. Myofascial Ther.*, 2(2/3):31-57, 1997.

91. Lowe, J.C., Reichman, A.J., and Yellin, J.: The process of change during T_3 treatment for euthyroid fibromyalgia: a double-blind placebo-controlled crossover study. *Clin. Bull. Myofascial Ther.*, 2(2/3):91-124, 1997.

92. Lowe, J.C., Garrison, R.L., Reichman, A.J., and Yellin, J.: Triiodothyronine (T_3) treatment of euthyroid fibromyalgia: a small-N replication of a double-blind placebo-controlled crossover study. *Clin. Bull. Myofascial Ther.*, 2(4):71-88, 1997.

93. Lowe, J.C., Reichman, A.J., and Yellin, J.: A case-control study of metabolic therapy for fibromyalgia: long-term follow-up comparison of treated and untreated patients (abstract). *Clin. Bull. Myofascial Ther.*, 3(1):23-24, 1998.

94. Lowe, J.C.: Thyroid status of 38 fibromyalgia patients: implications for the etiology of fibromyalgia. *Clin. Bull. Myofascial Ther.*, 2(1):47-64, 1997.

95. Lowe, J.C., Reichman, A.J., Honeyman, G.S., and Yellin, J.: Thyroid status of fibromyalgia patients. *Clin. Bull. Myofascial Ther.*, 3(1):45-48, 1998.

96. Volpé, R.: Misinformation on diagnosis and treatment. *Thyroid Foundation of Canada Thyrobulletin*, 19(2):10, 1998.

97. Garrison, R.L.: *First Congress on Defining a New Paradigm for the Healing Arts*. University of Texas: Houston Health Sciences Center, May 28-31, 1998, p.8.

98. Cunningham, J.J.: Body composition and resting metabolic rate: the myth of feminine metabolism. *Am. J. Clin. Nutri.*, 36(4):721-726, 1982.

99. Poelhman, E.T., Berke, E.M., Joseph, J.R., Gardner, A.W., Katzman-Rooks, S.M., and Goran, M.I.: Influence of aerobic capacity, body composition, and thyroid hormones on the age-related decline in resting metabolic rate. *Metab.: Clin. Experiment.*, 41(8):915-921, 1992.

100. Stockigt, J.R.: Serum thyrotropin and thyroid hormone measurements and assessment of thyroid hormone transport. In *Werner and Ingbar's The Thyroid: A Funda-

mental and Clinical Text, 7th edition. Edited by L.P. Braverman and R.D. Utiger, Philadelphia, Lippincott-Raven Publishers, 1996, pp.377-396.

101. Sanborn, C.F. and Jankowski, C.M.: Physiologic considerations for women in sports. *Clin. North Am.*, 13(2): 315-327, 1994.

102. Campbell, W.W., Crim, M.C., Young, V.R., and Evans, W.J.: Increased energy requirements and changes in body composition with resistance training in older adults. *Am. J. Clin. Nutri*, 60(2):167-175, 1994.

103. Broeder, C.E., Burrhus, K.A., Svanevik, L.S., and Wilmore, J.H.: The effects of either high-intensity resistance or endurance training on resting metabolic rate. *Am. J. Clin. Nutri.*, 55(4):802-810, 1992.

104. *The Merck Manual of Diagnosis and Therapy*, 15th edition. Edited by R. Berkow and A.J. Fletcher, Rahway, Merck, Sharp & Dohme Research Laboratories, 1987.

105. Krude, H,, Biebermann, H., Luck, W., Horn, R., Brabant, G., and Gruters, A.: Severe early-onset obesity, adrenal insufficiency and red hair pigmentation caused by POMC mutations in humans. *Nat. Genet.*, 1998 Jun;19(2):155-157, 1998.

106. Griep, E.N, Boersma, J.W., and Kloet, E.R.: Altered reactivity of the hypothalamic-pituitary-adrenal axis in the primary fibromyalgia syndrome. *J. Rheumat.*, 20(3):469-474, 1993.

107. Demitrack, M.A., Dale, J.K., Straus, S.E., Laue, L., and Listwak, S.J.: Evidence for impaired activation of the hypothalamic-pituitary-adrenal axis in patients with chronic fatigue syndrome. *J. Clin. Endocrinol. Metab.*, 73(6): 1224-1234, 1991.

108. Bloom, F.E. and Lazerson, A.: *Brain, Mind, and Behavior*, 2nd edition. New York, W.H. Freeman and Co., 1988.

109. Duesberg, Peter H.: *Inventing the AIDS Virus*. Washington, DC, Regnery Publishing, Inc., 1996.

110. Davidsohn, I. and Henry, J.B.: *Clinical Diagnosis by Laboratory Methods*, 15th edition. Philadelphia, W.B. Saunders, 1974.

111. Everts. M.E., de Jong, M., and Lim. C.F., et al.: Different regulation of thyroid hormone transport in liver and pituitary: its possible role in the maintenance of low T_3 production during nonthyroidal illness and fasting in man. *Thyroid*, 6(4):359-368, 1996.

112. *The Pharmacopeia of the United States of America*, 9th decennial revision. Philadelphia, P. Blakiston's Sons, 1916, p.443.

113. Eisinger, J.B.: Personal written communication, Aug., 1998.

114. Lowe, J.C., Cullum, M.E., Graf, L.H., and Yellin, J.: Mutations in the c-erbAβ_1 gene: do they underlie euthyroid fibromyalgia? *Med. Hypotheses*, 48(2):125-135, 1997.

115. DeGroot, L.J., Larsen, P.R., Refetoff, S., and Stanbury, J.B.: *The Thyroid and Its Diseases*, 5th edition. New York, John Wiley & Sons, Inc., 1984.

116. Barnes, B.: Basal temperature versus basal metabolism. *J.A.M.A.*, 119:1072-1074, 1942.

117. Magnus-Levy, A.: Ueber den respiratorischen Gaswechsel unter dem Einfluss der Thyreoidea sowie unter vreschiedenen pathologische. *Zustanden. Berl. Klin. Wochenschr.*, 32:650, 1895.

118. Magnus-Levy, A.: Energy metabolism in health and dis-ease. *J. Hist. Med.*, 2:307, 1947.

119. Hunt, G., Donatien, P.D., Lunec, J., Todd, C., Kyne, S., and Thody, A.J.: Cultured human melanocytes respond to MSH peptides and ACTH. *Pigment. Cell. Res.*, 7(4):217-221, 1994.

120. Tepperman, J. and Tepperman, H.M.: *Metabolic and Endocrine Physiology*, 5th edition. Chicago, Year Book Medical Publishers, Inc., 1987.

121. Du Bois, E.F.: *Basal Metabolism in Health and Disease.* Philadelphia, Lea & Febiger, 1927.

122. Kleitman, N.: *Sleep and Wakefulness.* Chicago, University of Chicago Press, 1939.

123. Descartes, R.: *Rules for the Direction of the Mind.* Translated by L.J. Lafleur, Indianapolis, Bobbs-Merrill Company, Inc., 1961.

124. Refetoff, S.: Personal communication, April 27, 1992.

125. Evered, D.C., Ormston, B.J., Smith, P.A., Hall, R., and Bird, T.: Grades of hypothyroidism. *Brit. Med. J.*, 1:657-662, 1973.

126. Lee, R.L.: Hypothyroidism: a common symptom. *Ann. Intern. Med.*, 9:712-716, 1935.

127. Weintraub, B.: Thyroid hormone resistance syndrome may affect thousands of unsuspecting Americans. *NIH Observer*, 1, Winter, 1991.

128. Thyrel® TRH (protirelin) product information. March 1994. Ferring Laboratories, Inc., 400 Rella Blvd., Suite 201, Suffern, NY 10901. Phone 914-368-7916, fax 914-368-1193.

129. Medi-Span, Inc.: Database Version 97.2. Data © 1997.

130. Lowe, J.C.: Editorial. *Clin. Bull. Myofascial Ther.*, 3(1): 1-2, 1998.

131. Refetoff, S., Weiss, R.E., and Usala, S.J.: The syndromes of resistance to thyroid hormone. *Endocrine Rev.*, 14(3): 348-399, 1993.

132. Williams, R.: Hypometabolism (metabolic insufficiency). In *Textbook of Endocrinology*, 3rd edition. Edited by R. Williams, Philadelphia, W.B. Saunders, 1962.

133. Levin, M.E.: "Metabolic insufficiency": a double blind study using triiodothyronine, thyroxine, and placebo: psychometric evaluation of the hypometabolic patient. *J. Clin. Endocrinol. Metab.*, 20:106, 1960.

134. Lowe, J.C.: T_3-induced recovery from fibromyalgia by a hypothyroid patient resistant to T_4 and desiccated thyroid. *J. Myofascial Ther.*, 1(4):26-31, 1995.

135. Lowe, J.C., Eichelberger, J., Manso, G., and Peterson, K.: Improvement in euthyroid fibromyalgia patients treated with T_3 (tri-iodothyronine). *J. Myofascial Ther.*, 1(2): 16-29, 1994.

136. Maxon, H.R., Burman, K.D., and Premachandra, B.N.: Euthyroid familial hyperthyroxinemia. *N. Engl. J. Med.*, 302:1263, 1980.

137. Maxon, H.R., Burman, K.D., Premachandra, B.N., Chen, I.-W., Burger, A., Levy, P., and Georges, L.P.: Familial elevation of total and free thyroxine in healthy, euthyroid subjects without detectable binding protein abnormalities. *Acta Endocrinol.* (Copenh.), 100:224-230, 1982.

138. Kleinhaus, N., Faber, J., Kahana, L., Schneer, J., and Scheinfeld, M.: Euthyroid hyperthyroxinemia due to a generalized 5'-deiodinase defect. *J. Clin. Endocrinol. Metab.*, 66:684-688, 1988.

139. Kohrle, J., Hesch, R.D., and Leonard, J.L.: Intracellular

pathways of iodothyronine metabolism. In *Werner and Ingbar's The Thyroid: A Fundamental and Clinical Text*, 6th edition. Edited by L.P. Braverman and R.D. Utiger, New York, J.B. Lippincott Co., 1991, pp.144-189.

140. Rösler, A., Litvin, Y., Hage, C., Gross, J., and Cerasi, E.: Familial hyperthyroidism due to inappropriate thyrotropin secretion successfully treated with triiodothyronine. *J. Clin. Endocrinol. Metab.*, 54:76-82, 1982.

141. Wilson, E.D.: *Wilson's Syndrome: The Miracle of Feeling Well*. Orlando, Cornerstone Publishing Co., 1991.

142. Nicoloff, J.T. and LoPresti, J.S.: Nonthyroidal illness. In *Werner and Ingbar's The Thyroid: A Fundamental and Clinical Text*, 7th edition. Edited by L.P. Braverman and R.D. Utiger, Philadelphia, Lippincott-Raven Publishers, 1996, pp.286-296.

143. Wilson's Syndrome Patient Instruction Sheet. Publisher and date not designated.

144. Wilson, E.D.: *Doctor's Manual for Wilson's Syndrome*, 2nd edition. Muskeegee Medical Publishing Co., 1995.

145. Schimmel, M. and Utiger, R.D.: Thyroidal and peripheral production of thyroid hormones: review of recent findings and their clinical implications. *Ann. Intern. Med.*, 87(6):760-768, 1977.

146. Szabolcs, I., Weber, M., Kovacs, Z., et al.: The possible reason for serum 3,3',5'-(reverse) triiodothyronine increase in old people. *Acta Med. Acad. Scient. Hung.*, 39(1-2):11-17, 1982.

147. Nicoloff, J.T., Fisher, D.A., and Appleman, M.D.: The role of glucocorticoids in the regulation of thyroid function in man. *J. Clin. Invest.*, 49:1922, 1970.

148. Alford, F.P., Baker, H.W.G., Burger, H.G., et al.: Temporal patterns of integrated plasma hormone levels during sleep and wakefulness. I. Thyroid-stimulating hormone, growth hormone and cortisol. *J. Clin. Endocrinol. Metab.*, 37:841, 1973.

149. Brabant, A., Brabant, G., Schuermeyer, T., et al.: The role of glucocorticoids in the regulation of thyrotropin. *Acta Endocrinol.* (Copenh), 121:95, 1989.

150. deBoer, J.O., van Es, A.J., Roovers, L.C., van Raaij, J.M., and Hautvast, J.G.: Adaptation of energy metabolism of overweight women to low-energy intake, studied with whole-body calorimeters. *Am. J. Clin. Nutri.*, 44(5):585-595, 1986.

151. Elliot, D.L., Goldberg, L., Kuehl, K.S., and Bennett, W.M.: Sustained depression of the resting metabolic rate after massive weight loss. *Am. J. Clin. Nutri.*, 49(1):93-96, 1989.

152. Leibel, R.L. and Hirsch, J.: Diminished energy requirements in reduced-obese patients. *Metab.: Clin. Experi.*, 33(2):164-170, 1984.

153. DeGroot, L.C., van Es, A.J., van Raaij, J.M., Vogt, J.E., and Hautvast, J.G.: Adaptation of energy metabolism of overweight women to alternating and continuous low energy intake. *Am. J. Clin. Nutri.*, 50(6):1314-1323, 1989.

154. Leibel, R.L., Rosenbaum, M., and Hirsch, J.: Changes in energy expenditure resulting from altered body weight. *New Engl. J. Med.*, 332(10):621-628, 1995.

155. Leibel, R.L. and Hirsch, J.: Metabolic characterization of obesity. *Ann. Intern. Med.*, 103(6):1000-1002, 1985.

156. Friedman, J.M., Leibel, R.L., Bahary, N., Siegel, D.A.,

and Truett, G.: Genetic analysis of complex disorders: molecular mapping of obesity genes in mice and humans. *Ann. N. Y. Acad. Sci.*, 630:100-115, 1991.

157. Croxson, M.S. and Ibbertson, H.K.: Low serum triiodothyronine (T_3) and hypothyroidism in anorexia nervosa. *J. Clin. Endocrinol. Metab.*, 44:167, 1977.

158. Rudin, C., Jenny, P.M., Fliegel, C.P., Ohnacker, H., and Heitz, P.U.: Zuelzer-Wilson's syndrome and absence of the enteric nervous system: two rare forms of anomalies of the enteric nervous system with identical clinical symptoms. *Zeitschrift fur Kinderchirurgie*, 41(5):287-292, 1986.

159. Weingartner, L.: D-penicillamine in various diseases in childhood. *Medizinische Klinik*, 74(26):1038-1042, 1979.

160. Gasbarrini, G., Miglio, F., Corazza, G.R., and Stefanini, G.F.: On the therapeutic combination of S-adenosylmethionine with D-penicillamine in Wilson's disease. *Minerva Medica*, 66(33):1600-1604, 1975.

161. Pawlak, J.: Copper metabolism disorders as an attempt at explaining analogous pathological mechanisms in Wilson's syndrome and severe cases of liver cirrhosis. *Wiadomosci Lekarskie*, 28(12):1041-1044, 1975.

162. Birau, N.C.: New aspects concerning the pathological histophysiology of Kimmelstiel-Wilson's syndrome. *Romanian Med. Rev.*, 14(1):10-17, 1970.

163. Yoshida, Y. and Sawada, S.: A case of diabetes mellitus associated with hypertension, nephrotic syndrome, and uremia (Kimmelstiel-Wilson's syndrome). *Japanese Arch. Intern. Med.*, 12(7):379-384, 1965.

164. Usala, S.J., Bale, A.E., Gesundheit, N., et al: Tight linkage between the syndrome of generalized thyroid hormone resistance and the human c-*erb*Aβ gene. *Mol. Endocrinol.*, 2:1217-1220, 1988.

165. Usala, S.J., Tennyson, G.E., Bale, A.E., et al.: A base mutation of the c-*erb*Aβ thyroid hormone receptor in a kindred with generalized thyroid hormone resistance: molecular heterogeneity in two other kindreds. *J. Clin. Invest.*, 85:93-100, 1990.

166. Skurai, A., Takeda, K., Ain, K., et al.: Generalized resistance to thyroid hormone associated with a mutation in the ligand-binding domain of the human thyroid hormone receptor β. *Proc. Natl. Acad. Sci.* (USA), 86:8977-8981, 1989.

167. Usala, S.J.: Molecular diagnosis and characterization of thyroid hormone resistance syndromes. *Thyroid*, 1:361-367, 1991.

168. Johnston, M.W., Squires, A.H., and Farquharson, R.F.: The effect of prolonged administration of thyroid. *Ann. Intern. Med.*, 35:1008-1022, 1951.

169. Lowe, J.C.: Results of an open trial of T_3 therapy with 77 euthyroid female fibromyalgia patients. *Clin. Bull. Myofascial Ther.*, 2(1):35-37, 1997.

170. Honeyman, G.S.: Metabolic therapy for hypothyroid and euthyroid fibromyalgia: two case reports. *Clin. Bull. Myofascial Ther.*, 2(4):19-49, 1997.

171. Eisinger, J.B.: Personal written communication, Sept., 1997.

172. DeGroot, L.J.: Abnormal thyroid function tests in euthyroid patients. In *Diagnostic Methods in Clinical Thyroidology*. Edited by J.I. Hamburger, New York, Springer-Verlag, 1989, pp.3-26.

173. Kurland, G.S., Bustos, J.G., Hamolsky, M.W., and Freedberg, A.S.: Studies in nonmyxedematous hypometabolism. II. Turnover of I[131]-labeled thyroxine after intravenous infusion. *J. Clin. Endocrinol. Metab.*, 17: 1365-1372, 1957.

2.6

Thyroid Hormone Resistance

Thyroid hormone action is determined not only by the availability of the hormone, but also by target organ sensitivity to it. In patients with thyroid hormone resistance syndromes, the responsiveness of different tissues to thyroid hormone is impaired to variable degrees. Some tissues are normally responsive, others may be hyporesponsive, and others hyperresponsive.

For clinical convenience, thyroid hormone resistance syndromes are divided into three forms: general, pituitary, and peripheral. In the general form, the pituitary and peripheral tissues are resistant. In the pituitary form, only pituitary tissue is resistant. In the peripheral form, the peripheral tissues, but not pituitary tissue, are resistant. Studies have shown that mutations in the c-erbAβ gene are the molecular mechanisms of general and pituitary resistance to thyroid hormone. The mutations cluster in the "hot spot" region of the gene. This region codes for the T_3-binding domain of the c-erbAβ thyroid hormone receptor. The mutation causes a substitution in the amino acid sequence in the T_3-binding domain, and results in low T_3-binding affinity of the receptor. The low affinity reduces the ability of the receptor to properly activate or repress transcription. Mutant c-erbAβ receptors bind normally to the DNA sequences termed T_3 response elements. These distinct sequences interact with normal T_3-receptors to control gene expression. When a normal T_3-receptor binds to a T_3 response element, transcription is either activated or repressed, depending on whether the gene is positively or negatively regulated by the T_3-bound receptor. Synthesis of

mRNA then increases or decreases accordingly.

Binding (to a T_3 response element) of a mutant c-erbAβ receptor not bound to T_3 (unliganded) fails to properly regulate transcription of the gene. Occupancy of DNA-binding sites by mutant receptors minimizes access of normal (wild type) receptors to the sites. The mutant receptor therefore prevents the normal c-erbAβ receptor from binding to DNA. Because the normal receptor cannot bind and properly regulate transcription of the target gene in question, it is said that the mutant inhibits the wild type receptor, a process called dominant-negative activity. Studies suggest that for the mutant receptor to inhibit normal receptors, it must form a heterodimer with an auxiliary protein (usually a retinoic X receptor). The heterodimer occupies the T_3 response element and blocks access of normal receptors.

The mutant c-erbAβ receptor fails to regulate transcription at low or normal T_3 concentrations. It becomes transcriptionally active, however, at high concentrations. In essence, high T_3 concentrations override the thyroid hormone resistance.

Recent studies show that individuals with different clinical symptoms and signs may share the same c-erbAβ gene mutation. The identical mutation has been found in some patients with general resistance and others with pituitary resistance. These data indicate that at least these two clinical forms of resistance to thyroid hormone are variable manifestations of a single type of genetic abnormality.

No molecular basis has been determined for peri-

pheral resistance because patients with this resistance phenotype have been the subject of only minimal study. There are several reasons for this. The patient with general or pituitary resistance is easily identified by laboratory thyroid test results. In peripheral resistance, thyroid function test results are normal, so the patient with this clinical phenotype is more difficult to identify. Identification must begin with recognition of signs and symptoms typical of hypothyroidism in a euthyroid patient. Many clinicians, due to the current paradigm in endocrinology, are not aware that inadequate thyroid hormone regulation of transcription can occur despite normal circulating levels of thyroid hormone. Also, due to the current excessive focus on laboratory tests and the virtual abandonment of clinical judgment, few clinicians are likely to recognize patients with possible peripheral resistance based on classic hypothyroid symptoms and signs. Consequently, other than patients identified by my fibromyalgia research group, only one such patient has come to the attention of researchers investigating thyroid hormone resistance syndromes. Even if a clinician suspects that a patient has peripheral resistance, the diagnostic tool that could verify hypometabolism, the BMR, is no longer readily available. Thus, while a clinician may suspect that a patient is hypometabolic due to peripheral cellular resistance, for all practical purposes, his hypothesis must remain unverified. Other tests that indicate deficient thyroid hormone action at the tissue level, such as urinary cortisol metabolites, are not readily available commercially, and they potentially demonstrate inadequate hormone action in only one specific tissue.

Nevertheless, it is probable that peripheral resistance to thyroid hormone is synonymous with thyroid-related euthyroid hypometabolism, which I describe in the previous chapter. Roughly 50% of fibromyalgia patients appear to have euthyroid hypometabolism. The euthyroid fibromyalgia patients my research team has investigated fit the profile of patients with peripheral resistance to thyroid hormone. Before beginning T_3 treatment, their thyroid function test results are normal, yet their clinical signs and symptoms are typical of hypothyroidism. They improve or recover from these signs and symptoms, and cease to meet the criteria for fibromyalgia, only with supraphysiologic dosages of T_3. The patients do not have the tissue thyrotoxicity expected from the use of such large dosages of T_3. The results of serum and urine biochemical tests, serial ECGs, and bone densitometry have been normal at short-term follow-up in all patients. Long-term follow-up (1-to-5 years) has also shown normal

safety test results in the limited number of patients tested at this time. The low serum TSH and total and free T_4, and the high free T_3 levels indicate that the absence of thyrotoxicity in these patients is not due to accelerated T_3 clearance. These data point to partial peripheral cellular resistance to thyroid hormone in our euthyroid fibromyalgia patients.

Garrison has proposed nomenclature for thyroid hormone deficiency and cellular resistance to thyroid hormone that is analogous to that used in diabetes. He proposes the term type I hypothyroidism as appropriate for thyroid hormone deficiency, and type II hypothyroidism as appropriate for subnormal responses of cells despite exposure to normal concentrations of thyroid hormone.

However, recently and by convention, hormone resistance has come to refer to a defect at the site of hormone action. In the case of thyroid hormone, this restricts the use of the term to failed action at the nucleus. This is an unfortunately specific use of the term "resistance." It requires the invention of other terms to refer to impaired responsiveness of cells to thyroid hormone not due to faulty action at the nucleus. I use the term "thyroid hormone resistance syndrome" in compliance with this convention. I use the term "cellular resistance to thyroid hormone" in a more general sense. I mean by this term a subnormal response of cells to thyroid hormone, regardless of the involved mechanism. Cellular resistance to thyroid hormone, then, subsumes such mechanisms as inadequate cellular influx of T_4 or T_3, excess cellular efflux of T_3, failed conversion of T_4 to T_3 due to inhibition of 5'-deiodinase by mercury, and failed T_3 action at the nucleus (thyroid hormone resistance syndrome).

Understanding euthyroid fibromyalgia requires an understanding that thyroid hormone action is determined not only by the availability of the hormone, but also by target tissue sensitivity to the hormone.[193] Failure of the cell to respond normally to thyroid hormone is variously termed cellular hyposensitivity, hyporesponsiveness, or resistance to thyroid hormone. Throughout this book, I use the term "cellular resistance to thyroid hormone" generally to refer to a failure of cells to respond normally to otherwise adequate amounts of thyroid hormone, regardless of the mechanism of the failure. Almost exclusively in the research literature today, however, the term "resistance" is used within the context of "thyroid hormone resistance syndrome."

Thyroid hormone resistance syndrome has been

described variously as a disorder in which body tissues are resistant to the effects of thyroid hormone,[57] a condition of impaired end-organ responsiveness to thyroid hormone,[150] hyposensitivity of target tissues to thyroid hormone,[152] and a syndrome of inherited tissue hyposensitivity to thyroid hormone.[56][148] (In that the condition occurs sporadically in some patients, it is not accurate to state that it is an inherited abnormality, although it is true that it is predominantly inherited.)

Refetoff, Weiss, and Usala wrote in 1993, "Recent studies, particularly those assisted by molecular biological techniques, have redefined the syndromes of hormone resistance, confining the term 'resistance' to those conditions caused by defects at the site of hormone action or the receptor level." They specify that thyroid hormone acts initially at the level of the nucleus.[3,p.349] In line with this designation, Hayashi and coauthors define resistance to thyroid hormone as "a dominantly inherited syndrome characterized by hyposensitivity to thyroid hormone caused by mutations in the thyroid hormone receptor-beta (TR beta) gene."[60] Others describe the condition as a rare disorder caused by mutations in the β thyroid hormone receptor (c-*erb*Aβ) gene.[61]

Researchers have now identified the molecular lesions responsible for some patients' partial resistance to their endogenous thyroid hormones. The lesions have been identified in patients with the general and pituitary forms of the condition, but not the peripheral form (see section on peripheral resistance later in this chapter). Structurally, the lesions are deleted or substituted bases within the c-*erb*Aβ gene, expressed as c-*erb*Aβ T_3-receptors with an amino acid deletion or substitution in the T_3-binding domain. Such deletions or substitutions constitute mutations.[125,p.72] Functionally, the lesions are impediments to T_3 action at the cellular level. The mutant receptors are unable to alter patterns of gene expression normally.[61] (For those interested in the state of knowledge of the molecular basis of thyroid hormone resistance syndromes, I recommend the excellent 1993 paper by Refetoff, Weiss, and Usala.[3] I have organized much of this chapter on the basis of their published reports, particularly their 1993 paper.)

For diagnostic and treatment purposes, researchers specify three classifications of thyroid hormone resistance syndrome. These forms essentially specify which of the patient's tissues are resistant to thyroid hormone. In the pituitary form, the pituitary is the only tissue that is resistant. In the general form, the pituitary and other tissues of the body are resistant. In the peripheral form, the pituitary is not resistant, but other body tissues are. These clinical distinctions are useful as a guide to the most appropriate treatment. However, recent studies indicate that at least general resistance and pituitary resistance are variable phenotypic manifestations of the same genetic abnormality. In most cases, the abnormality is a mutation in the c-*erb*Aβ gene. This is indicated by the same mutations underlying both general and pituitary resistance in different individuals, and by variable signs and symptoms in different individuals who have the same underlying mutation.[133][134][144][175][182][222] In one kindred (all relatives collectively), the same mutation is associated with general resistance in some members and pituitary resistance in others.[212] Nevertheless, some mutations are repeatedly identified in patients with the same form of resistance syndrome. For example, a point mutation at amino acid arginine 338-to-tryptophan (R338W) has been found in several patients with pituitary resistance, indicating that this mutation is associated with pituitary phenotypic expression.[222]

The three classifications of thyroid hormone resistance syndrome are dictated by our limited ability to assess the effects of thyroid hormone on body tissues other than the pituitary gland.[71,p.1032] We can easily and specifically measure the reaction of the pituitary gland as changing serum TSH levels. Some measures of thyroid hormone action on specific tissues other than the pituitary, such as urinary cortisol metabolites,[167] are being developed. But for practical purposes at this time, we cannot specifically measure the reactions of specific tissues other than the pituitary.

Because of the lack of specificity of measurements and for the purposes of classifying patients, all tissues other than the pituitary are termed *peripheral tissues*.[71,p.1032] The classifications, therefore, are based on our limited ability to assess the condition rather than on physiological differences in the way tissues other than the pituitary respond to thyroid hormones.

It is also important to emphasize, in the way of orientation, one more point about the three forms of thyroid hormone resistance syndrome. That is, they are not defined by an underlying molecular lesion unique to each form. The same molecular lesion will give rise to a different form of resistance syndrome, depending on the tissue that harbors it. Thus, any one lesion may cause any of the three forms of thyroid hormone resistance syndrome. The only requirement is that the lesion be present in the tissue(s) peculiar to each form of the syndrome. On the other hand, different molecular lesions can cause the same resistance syndrome in different patients. All that is necessary is that each type of lesion interfere with thyroid hormone expression in the tissues peculiar to that form of the syndrome. *The important point is that the form of the syndrome (general, pituitary, peripheral) tells us what tissue(s) are involved, not the nature of the underlying molecular lesion.*

Reviewing the available information on general resistance and pituitary resistance is informative. Most research into thyroid hormone resistance syndrome has focused on these two forms. To understand any form of thyroid hormone resistance syndrome, we must consider the information on these two forms. Peripheral resistance, however, is of greatest importance with regard to fibromyalgia. It is probable that thyroid hormone-related euthyroid hypometabolism, diagnosed as euthyroid fibromyalgia, is synonymous with peripheral resistance to thyroid hormone. This means that euthyroid fibromyalgia is a particular clinical phenotype of peripheral resistance. If this is true, the features of euthyroid fibromyalgia result from resistance of select tissues, the effects of which constitute the features of fibromyalgia.

Some writers have begun to describe peripheral resistance as a disorder in which the patient has the symptoms and signs of hypothyroidism, although the individual's thyroid function test results are normal. The writers have also begun to recommend more sophisticated diagnostic methods than thyroid function tests and that patients be allowed to undergo thyroid hormone treatment.[88] Our research group has acted in accord with this approach. The hypometabolism hypothesis of fibromyalgia is partly a result of this line of thought.

● THE THREE CLINICAL CLASSIFICATIONS OF THYROID HORMONE RESISTANCE

GENERAL RESISTANCE TO THYROID HORMONE (GENERAL RESISTANCE)

General resistance is the most commonly recognized form of thyroid hormone resistance. In general resistance, both the pituitary and other target tissues, such as the skeletal muscles, are partially resistant to thyroid hormone.[204]

The patient has either normal or elevated serum TSH level and elevated blood levels of T_3 and T_4. The TSH level can be suppressed only with a supraphysiologic dosage of thyroid hormone. Goiter is common in

patients with general resistance,[233] even though the TSH level may be normal. The goiter and elevated thyroid hormone levels conflict with the finding of a normal TSH level.[205] An explanation is provided by the recent finding that circulating TSH in patients with general resistance has enhanced bioactivity:[151] The TSH is more potent than normal in stimulating thyroid gland secretion of thyroid hormone. Normal amounts of TSH with enhanced bioactivity reaching the thyroid gland would result in secretion of amounts of thyroid hormone that are disproportionately high for the TSH level. The bioactivity of TSH returns to normal upon T_3 administration. Table 2.6.1 shows typical thyroid function test values for members of a family who have general resistance and members who do not.[150]

Despite high thyroid hormone levels, the patient typically does not have symptoms or signs characteristic of hyperthyroidism,[160] although some tissues in some patients may be hypermetabolic. The absence of hypermetabolism of peripheral tissues is due to the partial cellular resistance to thyroid hormone. When the patient's circulating thyroid hormone levels are normal, her tissues are hypometabolic. When circulating hormone levels are high, tissue metabolism normalizes. To remain eumetabolic, the patient must have a high blood level of thyroid hormone.

The general resistance patient's pituitary is also partially resistant to thyroid hormone. In non-resistant individuals, normal circulating levels of thyroid hormone regulate synthesis and secretion of TSH by the thyrotrophs. As a result, the circulating TSH is maintained within the normal range. If the circulating levels of thyroid hormone increase, upon passing some threshold point, the pituitary thyrotrophs are inhibited and TSH secretion decreases. Since the thyroid gland's secretion of thyroid hormones depends on exposure to TSH, the decreased TSH level results in decreased secretion of thyroid hormone. When the blood level of thyroid hormone drops below some threshold level, the thyrotrophs are disinhibited and the pituitary gland secretes more TSH.

In general resistance, the thyrotrophs are partially resistant to thyroid hormone. When the circulating thyroid hormone level is normal, TSH secretion continues as though the thyroid hormone level is too low. Accordingly, the thyrotrophs secrete an abnormally large amount of TSH which stimulates the thyroid gland to secrete abnormally large amounts of thyroid hormones. The high thyroid hormone level then inhibits the thyrotrophs, reducing their output of TSH. The pituitary thyrotrophs still respond during the TRH stimulation test with increased TSH secretion.[160] High dosages of T_3 are usually required to successfully suppress the TSH levels.[160]

The high circulating levels of thyroid hormone also override the resistance of the peripheral tissues, inducing a normal metabolic rate.[8] As a result of these mechanisms, the typical general resistance patient has normal metabolism[160] although her thyroid hormone levels are high and her TSH level is inappropriately high for her thyroid hormone level. Refetoff, Weiss, and Usala noted that all tissues other than the pituitary are at the mercy of the amount of thyroid hormone produced at the discretion of the thyrotrophs and that down-regulates TSH secretion.[3,p.349] *Clinicians should pay particular attention to this phenomenon—it illustrates the irrelevance of the metabolic status of all tissues except the pituitary thyrotrophs in regulating the circulating levels of thyroid hormone. As these authors stated, the peripheral tissues comply with the amount of thyroid hormone that down-regulates TSH secretion. But non-resistant pituitary thyrotrophs are more sensitive to thyroid hormone than are the peripheral tissues. Therefore, adjusting a peripheral resistance patient's exogenous thyroid hormone dosage according to the amount necessary to keep her TSH level in the middle of the range is likely to leave her peripheral tissues hypometabolic.*

In hyperthyroid patients, abnormally high thyroid hormone levels can be lowered through thyroid surgery, radioiodine treatment, or antithyroid drugs. Ideally, these measures relieve the patient's hyperthyroid symptoms and leave her euthyroid and eumetabolic. In contrast, with the general resistance patient, lowering the hormone levels into the normal range by such measures usually causes overt symptoms and signs of hypometabolism.[57][86][152][205][210] Hypometabolism occurs because high thyroid hormone levels are necessary to override the resistance of the peripheral tissues and maintain a eumetabolic state.[8]

General resistance patients are not likely to develop fibromyalgia because of the normal metabolism of their peripheral tissues. Lowering these patients' thyroid hormone levels with antithyroid treatment, however, would favor development of fibromyalgia in some patients. The patients who are susceptible are those with a high level of thyroid hormone resistance in the tissues selective for the generation of signs and symptoms of fibromyalgia.

Diagnostic Complications

Elevated TSH and thyroid hormone levels in general resistance patients can make the diagnosis of overlapping hypothyroidism complicated. Robinson and coauthors reported the case of a patient with general resistance who eventually developed symptomatic autoimmune hypothyroidism. The serum free T_4 level had decreased from its previous value, but it remained within the normal range. High dosages of T_4 were necessary to decrease the basal and TRH stimulated TSH to their prior mildly elevated levels. The authors noted that a high serum titer of antithyroid antibodies is of diagnostic value in such cases in which the basal TSH is initially elevated due to the resistance of the pituitary to thyroid hormone.[162]

Table 2.6.1. Mean thyroid function values typical of patients with general thyroid hormone resistance compared to values for family members not affected.*

TEST	AFFECTED FAMILY MEMBER	UNAFFECTED FAMILY MEMBER
Basal TSH	4.5 μU/L	2.4 μU/L
Free T_4 index	250	108
Total T_3	4.3 nmol/L	2.4 nmol/L

*Weiss, R.E., Chyna, B., Duell, P.B., Hayashi, Y., Sunthornthepvarakul, T., and Refetoff, S.: A new mutation (C446R) in the β thyroid hormone receptor gene of a family with resistance to thyroid hormone. *J. Clin. Endocrinol. Metab.*, 78(5):1253-1256, 1994.[150]

It is extremely important that clinicians recognize these patients' high TSH levels despite their elevated thyroid hormone levels. Failure to do so has often resulted in a correct diagnosis of hyperthyroidism but the incorrect use of antithyroid therapy.[57][152][205][210] By definition, the general resistance patient has hyperthyroidism: her thyroid hormone levels are elevated due to excess production by the thyroid gland. Most patients, however, do not have tissue thyrotoxicity. Antithyroid therapy leaves the patient hypometabolic. If the patient's TSH level is initially within the normal range, the elevated thyroid hormone levels are especially likely to result in a clinician recommending antithyroid therapy. This circumstance highlights the dangers of the current paradigm in endocrinology whereby the serum TSH and hormone levels are the sole basis for clinical decisions.

Watanabe and coauthors reported the case of a 21-year-old female with a condition they diagnosed as pituitary resistance to thyroid hormone. Her serum TSH, free T_3, and free T_4 levels were high. Her TSH level gradually decreased with T_3 administration in doses of 100 μg, 200 μg, and 400 μg/day. During her treatment, cranial CT and MRI imaging revealed a pituitary microadenoma. Upon histological examination of the surgical specimen, a TSH-secreting adenoma was found. The adenoma contained TSH cell cluster islets and an abnormally low number of TSH cells in the non-neoplastic regions of the pituitary tissue. When the adenoma cells were cultured, they secreted TSH spontaneously and when stimulated by TRH. T_3 exposure suppressed TRH-stimulated TSH secretion. One year following surgery, CT and MRI showed no residual pituitary tumor. However, the patient's TSH, free T_3, and free T_4 levels were still high. The TSH level was not responsive during the TRH stimulation test.[181] (Effective surgical or radiotherapeutic treatment of pituitary adenomas usually results in normal TSH levels within a week after the treatment, indicating a definitive cure.[223]) The hormone levels in this patient, despite the absence of a pituitary lesion, suggest pituitary resistance to thyroid hormone. This case illustrates the need for thoroughness in patient assessment.

PITUITARY RESISTANCE TO THYROID HORMONE (PITUITARY RESISTANCE)

In selective pituitary resistance, the peripheral tissues respond normally to thyroid hormone, but the thyrotrophs of the pituitary gland do not.[168][235][241] Normally, the c-*erb*Aβ receptor, when bound to T_3, represses transcription of TSH alpha subunits. Consequently, as thyroid hormone levels rise, TSH levels decline. In pituitary resistance, however, TSH levels increase above normal. The increase results from failure of mutant c-*erb*Aβ receptors to bind T_3 and repress transcription of TSH. The result is disinhibition of TSH alpha unit transcription and increased synthesis and secretion of TSH.[209][244] The elevated TSH induces the thyroid gland to secrete excess amounts of thyroid hormones. In response, the thyroid gland undergoes hypertrophy and forms a goiter. After the thyroid hormone levels rise high enough to override the resistance of the thyrotrophs, TSH secretion ceases to rise further but is maintained at the elevated level. The peripheral tissues are normally responsive to thyroid hormone, so the high thyroid hormone levels stimulate their metabolism excessively. The excess stimulation causes signs and symptoms of thyrotoxicosis,[159] such as heat intolerance, palpitations, and hand tremor.[194]

Exogenous T_4 suppresses TSH levels and relieves thyrotoxicosis in some pituitary resistant patients.[234] The dopamine agonist bromocriptine effectively inhib-

its excessive TSH secretion in pituitary resistance.[161] The T_3 analogues triac and triprop are more potent than T_3 in regulating transcription upon binding to mutant and normal c-*erb*Aβ$_1$ receptors. The greater potency of these drugs make them potentially useful in treating pituitary resistance.[192]

As in other forms of hyperthyroidism, the patient may experience muscle weakness. Some patients and clinicians mistake this weakness as a feature of fibromyalgia or chronic fatigue syndrome. In that fibromyalgia signs and symptoms arise from tissues with subnormal metabolism or other metabolic impairment, the patient with selective pituitary thyroid hormone resistance is essentially protected from fibromyalgia.

Patients diagnosed as having pituitary resistance have clinical features that overlap with those of general resistance. Some patients may have extreme pituitary resistance with only mild peripheral tissue resistance. The combined pituitary and peripheral involvement constitute general resistance. The patients elevated thyroid hormone levels would be expected to induce hypermetabolism in the least resistant peripheral tissues but maintain normal metabolism in more resistant tissues.

This possibility is indicated by at least two studies. Mixson and coworkers studied the first patient (L-F3) reported to have selective pituitary resistance to determine whether she had a mutation in the c-*erb*Aβ$_1$ gene. They found a cytosine-to-thymine substitution at base 1297 in codon 333. The base substitution caused a fourfold decrease in the affinity of the mutant c-*erb*Aβ$_1$ receptor for T_3. The nucleotide substitution at base 1297 was the same as in an unrelated patient (K-T3) whose diagnosis was general rather than pituitary resistance. This realization instigated a comparison of the two patients sharing the same mutation. The researchers found similar patterns of resistance in several tissues. Both patients had bone resistance, but only L-F3, diagnosed as pituitary resistant, had liver and neuromuscular resistance. The researchers concluded, "These findings suggest that apparent selective pituitary resistance and generalized resistance to thyroid hormone are not qualitatively different syndromes." Still, they emphasized that the clinical distinction between the two syndromes remains useful: patients with pituitary resistance have clinical and biochemical features of hyperthyroidism. It is important to identify them and treat them to lower serum thyroid hormone concentrations. Conversely, it is important to recognize general resistance to avoid the antithyroid therapies that lower thyroid hormone levels, leaving the patient hypometabolic for a time until thyroid gland goiter recurs.[175]

Sasaki and coworkers found a β gene mutation in a 30-year-old Japanese woman with pituitary resistance. The mutation was in one allele at nucleotide 1297, a cytosine-to-thymine substitution. The mutation resulted in substitution of tryptophan for arginine at the 333rd amino acid in the receptor. They noted that the same mutation, resulting in low T_3-binding affinity, has been reported in a general resistance patient. The researchers wrote that the presence of the same mutation in a patient with general resistance and another with pituitary resistance indicates that the syndrome of resistance represents a continuous spectrum of the same etiologic defect, resulting in variable tissue resistance.[59] Their view is shared by other researchers[59][175][182] and supported by the finding of a point mutation at the identical codon (H435L and H435Q) in the extreme carboxyl-terminus of the dimerization domain in one patient with general resistance and another with pituitary resistance. The mutation at codon 435 resulted in a histidine-to-leucine (CAT→CTT) substitution in the general resistance patient and a histidine-to-glycine (CAT→CAA) substitution in the pituitary resistance patient.[246]

PERIPHERAL TISSUE RESISTANCE TO THYROID HORMONE (PERIPHERAL RESISTANCE)

In peripheral resistance, the patient's serum levels of T_3, T_4, and TSH are within the normal range. Nonetheless, the patient exhibits peripheral signs and symptoms typical of thyroid hormone deficiency, and in most cases, clinical improvement is dependent on supraphysiologic dosages of T_3.[160] The patient's clinical profile, then, is that of thyroid hormone-related euthyroid hypometabolism.

In this form of resistance syndrome, the peripheral tissues are to some degree hyporesponsive to thyroid hormone. The pituitary gland is not resistant; and as a result, the pituitary and thyroid glands interact normally, maintaining circulating thyroid hormone levels within the normal range. The TRH stimulation test result is also normal in these patients. Normal levels of thyroid hormone, however, are not sufficient to override the resistance of the peripheral tissues. Consequently, the peripheral tissues are hypometabolic. Their metabolism accelerates to normal only when the thyroid hormone concentration within the cells is high enough to override the resistance.

It is instructive to contrast general resistance with peripheral resistance. In general resistance, both the peripheral tissues and pituitary gland are partially resistant to thyroid hormone.[169] Because of the pituitary resistance, the serum thyroid hormone blood level must become elevated before TSH secretion is suppressed. The elevated thyroid hormone levels override the resistance of the peripheral tissues, rendering them eumetabolic. Of 92 patients with general resistance, 81 (88%) had treatment (by physicians who did not understand the nature of the condition) to lower the circulating thyroid hormone levels.[3,p.363] Once the levels were lowered, the condition was no longer compensated, and the resistant peripheral tissues became hypometabolic. Many of these patients reported symptoms suggestive of hypothyroidism: fatigue, somnolence, cold intolerance, depression, weight gain, bradycardia, and reduced growth rate. Lowering of the thyroid hormone levels produced iatrogenically the hypometabolic symptoms of peripheral resistance. In the peripheral form of resistance syndrome, the normally responding pituitary imposes the same symptoms by keeping the thyroid hormone levels within the normal range. The lack of a compensatory elevation of the TSH, due to the normally responsive pituitary gland, leaves the thyroid hormone levels insufficiently elevated to override the resistance of the peripheral tissues. The peripheral tissues, as in the improperly treated general resistance patients, are left hypometabolic by the normal thyroid hormone levels, and the patient has symptoms typical of hypothyroidism.

The symptoms and signs of peripheral resistance in any one patient will depend on the peripheral tissues that are most highly resistant. A common phenotypic expression appears to be the nonspecific symptoms of patients with thyroid-related euthyroid hypometabolism. As I detailed in Chapter 2.5, numerous investigators published descriptions of these patients in the 1950s and 1960s. The euthyroid fibromyalgia patients studied by my research group appear to be modern counterparts who suffer from the same condition. The terms thyroid hormone-related euthyroid hypometabolism, peripheral thyroid hormone resistance syndrome, and euthyroid fibromyalgia are probably synonymous. As of 1994, researchers had identified more than 400 subjects with general resistance to thyroid hormone.[152][210] By contrast, prior to my research team reporting patients who have cellular resistance to thyroid hormone,[153][154][155] only one well-documented (and published) case of peripheral resistance had been reported.[81]

Clearly, the peripheral tissues of most of the euthyroid fibromyalgia patients my colleagues and I studied in three double-blind trials were resistant to thyroid hormone, although we do not know the mechanism of the resistance. The patients significantly improved or completely recovered from their fibromyalgia symptoms and signs and became "normal" according to five objective fibromyalgia measures. Supraphysiologic dosages of T_3 were required, but no patient had thyrotoxicity of any peripheral tissue. The patients were not clearing T_3 from their bodies too rapidly, as shown by their elevated free T_3 levels and low TSH and total and free T_4 values. These patients' pituitary glands were normally responsive, so they would be properly classified—if eventually shown to have molecular lesions at the level of the nucleus—as having peripheral thyroid hormone resistance syndrome.[153][154][155]

Difficulty Diagnosing Peripheral Resistance to Thyroid Hormone

The difficulty in diagnosing peripheral resistance is that thyroid function test results are normal and measures of peripheral tissue metabolic status are non-specific. Hopefully, markers that specifically indicate inadequate thyroid hormone action in peripheral tissues will become available. One such possibility is the measurement of the ratio of two urinary cortisol metabolites, tetrahydrocortisone (THE) and tetrahydrocortisol (THF). Taniyama, Honma, and Ban found that the THE/THF ratio was higher in hyperthyroidism (4.58 ± 1.49), and lower in hypothyroidism (1.31 ± 0.55) compared to controls (1.93 ± 0.35). They found a good correlation between the THE/THF ratio and serum thyroid hormone levels, especially in hypothyroidism. They concluded that the THE/THF ratio is a good biochemical indicator of deficient peripheral thyroid hormone action. They also found that in patients with general resistance the THE/THF ratio was low, despite the patients' elevated thyroid hormone levels. This low ratio indicates deficiency of thyroid hormone action in the resistant adrenal cortices despite elevated thyroid hormone levels in general resistance patients. The researchers concluded that the ratio of these cortisol metabolites is a good marker for peripheral thyroid hormone resistance. The ratio may be low in patients suspected of having peripheral resistance to thyroid hormone.[167]

● PATHOLOGY IN PATIENTS WITH THYROID HORMONE RESISTANCE

Little is known about tissue pathology in resistance patients because autopsy findings are not yet available.[3,p.357][71,p.1039] The tissue effects of thyroid hormone resistance vary between afflicted individuals. One patient may be free from an abnormality suffered by several others. Theoretically, the pathological effects depend on the tissues involved and the degree of the tissue resistance.

Striated muscle biopsied from one patient showed swollen mitochondria[35] typical of those found in thyrotoxicosis.[80] Fassbender reported swollen mitochondria in the earliest stage of damage in "fibrositic" muscle.[122,p.305]

Refetoff and coworkers stained the biopsied skin of a thyroid hormone resistant patient with toluidine blue dye. The biopsy showed extracellular metachromatic material (glycosaminoglycans or mucopolysaccharides) deposited in the upper layer of the dermis.[35] This material is typical of the myxedema of hypothyroidism. The material probably collected in the resistant patient because thyroid hormone failed to inhibit its synthesis by skin fibroblasts. When a hypothyroid patient takes a thyroid supplement, this material disappears. General resistance patients, however, did not respond in this way when taking thyroid supplements.[8,p.1296]

The studies cited in the paragraph above found pathophysiology typical of hyperthyroidism in one patient's muscle and pathophysiology typical of hypothyroidism in another patient's skin.[35] The seemingly paradoxical findings in resistance patients suggest that the sensitivity of various tissues to thyroid hormone is diverse in resistant patients. Some tissues are normally sensitive, others hyposensitive, and still others are hypersensitive. Such diversity prompted Sonkin to question the validity of the concept of *general* resistance to thyroid hormone.[62,p.48]

Kvetny and Bollerslev tested the effects of thyroid hormones on mononuclear blood cells from patients with thyroid hormone resistance. They reported that in patients with general resistance, results showed depressed thyroid hormone-stimulated glucose uptake. In other patients who had osteopetrosis, the mitochondria appeared to be insensitive to thyroid hormone-stimulated oxygen consumption.[178]

Some general resistance patients have normal thyroid glands,[35] but others have variable degrees of hyperplasia of the follicular epithelium.[78][86][87][117]

● MECHANISMS OF THYROID HORMONE RESISTANCE SYNDROMES

The discipline of clinical endocrinology was born in the mid-19th century. For some 75 years, the field developed as investigators pursued knowledge of two types of endocrine disorders: hormone deficiencies and hormone excesses. Virtually no one in the field investigated the mechanisms of action of hormones within target cells.

In 1937, however, researchers proposed that a third type of endocrine disorder exists—a defect in the ability of target cells to respond to hormones. Albright and his coauthors introduced this concept now called hormone resistance.[4][5] They described what they termed pseudo-hypoparathyroidism. They proposed that the mechanism of the seeming hypoparathyroidism was not due to a deficiency of parathyroid hormone. Instead, it resulted from a faulty response of target tissues to the hormone.

After Albright introduced the concept of hormone resistance and proposed that patients inherited the resistance, investigators began studies that eventually revealed the steps involved in hormone action. Through this pursuit, the investigators identified hormone receptors.[3,p.349] Recently, researchers' use of advanced techniques of molecular biology has led to a limited definition of syndromes of hormone resistance: conditions caused by defects at the site of hormone action or at the hormone's receptor.[3,p.349] This usage is unfortunate because there are other sites, both preceding and following the primary site of action of each hormone, where faults may result in the failure of a cell to respond to the hormone. Now, a different terminology is needed to refer to these other mechanisms of failed cellular response to a hormone.

Thus, while thyroid hormone resistance syndrome by convention now refers to failed action of thyroid hormone at its receptors, terms such as "cellular resistance to thyroid hormone" that employ the word "resistance" may be confused with thyroid hormone resistance syndrome. Clinicians interested in the study of impaired cellular responses to thyroid hormone must bear these distinctions in mind.

A few sporadic reports of resistance to thyroid hormones appeared prior to the mid-1960s.[2][5][41] In 1967, however, Refetoff and coauthors provided convincing evidence of thyroid hormone resistance.[1] Refetoff described two siblings who had deaf-mutism, delayed bone age, goiter, and elevated blood levels of protein-bound iodine. The children had normal metabolism. They had no apparent defects in thyroid hormone synthesis. They consumed an adequate amount of iodine in their diets and their thyroid glands took up the iodine in excess and bound it to form mainly T_4. The T_4 was secreted in excessive amounts. The patients' T_3 and T_4 molecules were normal structurally.[35] Excessive amounts of thyroid hormone penetrated the patients' peripheral tissue cells, and cells degraded the hormone through proper pathways. Although these patients obviously had resistance to thyroid hormone, no one knew the exact location of the responsible lesion. In 1990, the location of the lesion was found with the use of modern molecular biology laboratory techniques.

MOLECULAR BASIS OF GENERAL RESISTANCE SYNDROMES

Mutations in the c-erbAβ Gene: Mechanism of Most Cases of General Thyroid Hormone Resistance

The genetic basis of the general and pituitary forms of thyroid hormone resistance syndrome is now well understood. The resistance results from mutations in the β thyroid receptor gene (c-*erb*Aβ gene) that codes for synthesis of the β T_3-receptor (c-*erb*Aβ receptor). Researchers have found a diversity of mutations in that gene of general resistance patients. The diverse mutations result in a variety of clinical features in these patients. The cloned, synthesized, and tested mutant receptors have an impaired ability to bind T_3. The affinity of the receptor for T_3 varies between patients. In some patients, the affinity is reduced twofold. In other patients, the receptors have no detectable ability to bind T_3.[138,p.361]

In most cases, the gene harbors single mutations, but cloned receptors from some patients contain two mutations. Miyoshi reported two consecutive base substitutions (thymine-to-adenine and cytosine-to-adenine) in one patient.[240] In another patient, one of two mutations was "silent," causing no amino acid substitutions in the translater protein. But the other mutation caused histidine to substitute for arginine 438 in the receptor.[183] In contrast, Collingwood and coauthors described a novel leucine-to-valine mutation in codon 454 of the c-*erb*Aβ gene that resulted in normal T₃-binding affinity and normal formation of homo-dimers and heterodimers. Nevertheless, the ability of the receptor to activate transcription was markedly impaired.[215]

Cheng and coworkers examined eight naturally occurring mutated c-*erb*Aβ receptors derived from patients with general resistance. Compared to normal c-*erb*Aβ receptors, binding of T_3 and its analogues to the mutant receptors was reduced by as much as 97%. The order of binding affinities of normal receptors for thyroid hormone and its analogues was: T_3 > D-T_3 > L-T_4 > 3,5-diiodo-L-thyronine > 3,3',5'-triiodo-L-thyronine. Mutant receptors had practically the same order of reduced affinities for the thyroid hormone analogues. The degree of reduced binding affinity varied between mutant receptors. Cheng and coauthors wrote that this variety of reduced affinities suggests that different hormone analogues interplay with different specific mutated amino acid residues in the receptors.[156]

A mutant receptor fails to regulate transcription in the presence of physiological concentrations of T_3. It can regulate transcription only under the influence of supraphysiologic dosages.[163][179][242][245][248][249] Natural point mutations have been identified in the T_3-binding domain of one of the two alleles of the c-*erb*Aβ gene. No natural mutations have been found in the nucleotide regions that code for DNA-binding and dimerization (binding to auxiliary proteins, such as retinoid X receptors[185]).[146][217] The two T_3-binding domain regions with a strong propensity to mutations straddle the putative dimerization region.[210] Most mutations described so far have been clustered at exons 8 through 10. But other researchers have described mutations in exon 7 located close to or within the coding region for the hinge domain of the T_3-receptor that is essential to T_3-binding.[194][237][243]

The mutations identified so far are all clustered within restricted domains in the carboxyl-terminal region of the c-*erb*Aβ receptor gene. Groenhout and Dorin emphasized the critical role of the carboxyl-terminal region of the β receptor in mediating both positive and negative regulation of genes responsive to thyroid hormone.[149] In kindred G-H, who had an arginine-316-histidine mutation, the mutant β receptor had impaired DNA-binding properties.[133] In most kindreds, however, mutant receptors bind DNA normally. They also dimerize normally, but they do not bind T_3 or regulate transcription normally.[61] Bound to DNA and heterodimerized with auxiliary proteins such as

retinoic X receptors, mutant receptors constitute inactive complexes that neither activate nor repress gene transcription properly.[207] Hiramatsu and coworkers reported a novel mutation of one allele of the c-*erb*Aβ gene in two members of a Japanese family. The *in vitro* translation product of this gene, which had a significantly reduced T_3-affinity, had a new turn in its alpha helix structure.[208]

As of 1993, investigators had found sporadic occurrence of thyroid hormone resistance in only 14 families.[3,p.350][59][140][144] In 1995, Brucker-Davis and coworkers found that of 104 patients with resistance from 42 kindreds, inheritance was autosomal dominant in 22 families and sporadic in 14 families.[190] In the resistance patients studied, inheritance has been autosomal dominant except in one family in which it was recessive.[147][152][233] Frequency is about equal in both genders and the condition occurs in most races.[3,p.350]

Steps to the Discovery of Mutant T_3-Receptors

It is instructive to review the route investigators followed in discovering the mutations responsible for general resistance.

Defects at the Nuclear Receptor. Two types of measures led to discovery of the mutations causing general resistance: thyroid hormone binding to cell nuclei, and cell responses to thyroid hormone.[3, pp.374-377] These measures disclosed cellular hyposensitivity to thyroid hormone. Results of numerous studies of thyroid hormone binding to cell nuclei were inconsistent. The inconsistencies suggested that numerous defects might underlie thyroid hormone resistance syndrome, but nuclear receptors were the most likely site of putative lesions.[54]

Cell Responses to T_3 and Abnormal T_3-Binding to Cell Nuclei. In 1972, Oppenheimer demonstrated that liver and kidney contain sites that bind T_3. The sites were highly specific for T_3 and had a high T_3-binding affinity.[119] This discovery led researchers to describe the thyroid hormone receptor in theoretical terms.[115] After this, other investigators ran tests to determine whether the defect in general resistance was at the nuclear site where T_3 binds and acts.

Investigators have measured cell responses to T_3 in muscle, fibroblasts, and lymphocytes from resistance patients. In the first study of a general resistance patient in 1972, Refetoff et al. tested the response of striated muscle taken by biopsy to T_3.[35] The respiratory rate was initially similar to that found in thyrotoxic patients. The rate was labile, though, and as testing progressed, phosphorylation turned out to be low. Phosphorylation of proteins was also low in this patient's fibroblasts, as it was in other members of the patient's family who had general resistance.[84] The results were hard to interpret.

In one study, lymphocytes from one general resistance patient had a very low affinity for T_3.[37] Tests results in thirteen other laboratories, however, were not consistent with this finding.[3,p.374] Liewendahl[67] and colleagues[68] studied family members and sporadic individuals with mild thyroid hormone resistance. The researchers tested the patients' lymphocytes but found no defects in thyroid hormone binding to the nuclei. They suspected that the lymphocytes might harbor a defective step somewhere other than the presumed receptor. They also suggested that cells other than the lymphocytes from these patients might have defective thyroid hormone receptors.

Chait first found that fibroblasts had a diminished response to T_3 in general resistance patients. He cultured fibroblasts from three general resistance patients and found that the cells did not respond normally to T_3. They did not degrade low density lipoprotein as rapidly as fibroblasts from patients without general resistance. Despite this, the investigators were not able to find an abnormality of T_3-binding to the nuclei of the fibroblasts.[70] Refetoff could not reproduce these results in a subject from his original study, nor from general resistance patients from other families.[3,p.376]

Fibroblasts from patients with general resistance incorporated thymidine more slowly than fibroblasts from subjects without general resistance. The time for incorporation (the doubling-time) was 8-to-9 hours in general resistance patients. In subjects without general resistance, the time was 4-to-6 hours. The doubling-time in fibroblasts from general resistance patients reached normal (3-to-5 hours) only after exposure to a concentration of T_3 50 times that of the normal (physiological) free T_3.

Murata and coauthors cultured fibroblasts from six general resistance patients. In four of the patients neither T_3 nor T_4 normally inhibited the synthesis of glycosaminoglycans (mucopolysaccharides). Two of these four patients were siblings. The nuclei of fibroblasts from three of the four patients did not bind T_3 normally.[83] Refetoff wrote that such studies show that family members may share an identical defect, but that the site of the defect may vary from sites in patients from other families.[8,p.1295]

The diminished inhibitory effect of T_3 on skin fibroblasts' synthesis of fibronectin has been the most consistent physiological abnormality found in general resistance patients.[64][65] Refetoff stated that this test, measurement of the ability of T_3 to properly inhibit fibroblasts' fibronectin synthesis, is the only *in vitro* test of thyroid hormone resistance that offers promise.[3,p.377] (See Chapter 3.3 for more on fibronectin.)

Refetoff and coauthors reported that of 48 patients from 27 families with general resistance, only one-third had abnormal binding to their fibroblasts. Only one-half had abnormal binding to their mononuclear cell nuclei. Cells from one individual might show abnormal T_3-binding in one test but not in another.[3,p.375] The researchers proposed several reasons for these inconsistent findings of abnormal binding of thyroid hormone to cell nuclei. First, there was the variety of defects in thyroid hormone expression in cells that resulted in general resistance.[111][112][113] Second, normal values were not established for thyroid hormone binding to cell nuclei. In seven reports, for example, researchers used cells from only one-to-three normal subjects as the normal reference against which to measure abnormal values. This small N was insufficient to establish a normal range. Third, as Refetoff, Weiss, and Usala pointed out, the structure of the genes that code for T_3-receptors mitigates the effect of the mutation responsible for general resistance. They explain that mutations in general resistance typically involve only one of the four T_3-receptor alleles—specifically, one of the two thyroid hormone β (β-receptor) alleles. The three normal alleles (one β allele and two α alleles) are able to dictate the synthesis of an adequate number of thyroid hormone receptors. As a result, binding of T_3 in cell nuclei may be virtually normal during testing. They also noted that the contribution of a mutant c-*erb*Aβ receptor to the overall T_3-binding in cell nuclei may vary between different tissues. The contribution of the receptor to T_3-binding depends on the extent to which the normal β and α alleles express in T_3-receptor synthesis. If expression of the non-mutated alleles is sufficient, the quantity of normal receptors synthesized should allow enough T_3 to bind to properly regulate transcription.[3,p.375] Studies such as these led to the discovery of specific defects in the β T_3 gene and receptor in some patients.

Abnormal Binding of Thyroid Hormone to Nuclear Receptors. Three separate investigators showed that T_3-receptors of four patients from three unrelated families had *increased* maximum binding capacity for T_3. However, the receptors had low affinity for T_3.[37][67][72] In two other cases, affinity was normal but maximum binding capacity was slightly low.[67][73] Three of nine cases showed abnormal T_3-binding to the nuclei of fibroblasts.[37][38][74][75][76] Eight other cases showed no abnormalities in T_4-binding to nuclear receptors.[36][68][117] (T_4 has some binding affinity for

T_3-receptors, but far less than the affinity of T_3.[156]) Refetoff reiterated that these inconsistencies showed that general resistance was the result of a number of defects in thyroid hormone action and that nuclear receptor abnormality was only one of these.[8,p.1295]

Hot Spot Region of the c-*erb*Aβ gene: Location of Most Mutations in Thyroid Hormone Resistant Patients. In most cases, mutations occur in only one portion of the c-*erb*Aβ gene. This section codes for the polypeptide component of the receptor that binds T_3. This component is called the T_3-binding domain of the receptor; the mutated segment of the gene is called the T_3-binding domain of the gene. This portion of the gene is called a CpG island, or CpG dinucleotide.[142][144][237] C represents cytosine, G represents guanine, and p represents the phosphate linker. CpG islands are rich in the CpG dinucleotide and often indicate the presence of a gene. A large amount of CpG is usually found in the transcription initiation regions of genes. Statistically, CpG dinucleotides are underrepresented in DNA, and a large number of them are usually nonrandom.[143]

High Incidence of Mutations in Hot Spot Regions of the c-erbAβ Gene. In the part of the c-*erb*Aβ gene coded for the T_3-binding domain of the receptor, there are two "hot spots." These hot spots are regions where natural mutations tend to cluster.[231] These two regions sandwich the "cold spot" region. The cold spot region lacks the natural mutations that result in thyroid hormone resistance.

Hayashi and coworkers conducted a study to determine why mutations in the cold spot region do not cause thyroid hormone resistance. The researchers created 10 "artificial" mutations in the cold spot region, using the hot spot substitution rule of cytosine-to-thymine or guanine-to-adenine. Next, they compared the effects on cloned receptors of natural mutations in the hot spots and the artificial mutations in the cold spot. Natural mutations in the hot spots resulted in mild resistance to thyroid hormone with decreased T_3-binding affinity. In contrast, T_3-binding affinity was normal in six receptors from the gene with artificially-induced cold spot mutations. T_3-binding affinity of receptors coded by three of the artificial mutations was reduced, but the affinity was less reduced than for natural hot spot mutations. One receptor from an artificial mutation did not bind T_3 at all. The ability of all receptors from the naturally mutated genes (hot spots) to activate transcription was impaired, and they exhibited strong dominant-negative effects on normal thyroid hormone receptors. Receptors from artificially mutated genes had minimally impaired ability to activate transcription and weak or no dominant-negative effect on normal receptors. The one receptor from the artificially mutated gene that did not bind T_3 also did not activate transcription, but it had no dominant-negative activity. Thus, this cold spot region of the gene is relatively resistant to mutations. In addition, unlike the hot spot coding regions, the cold spot region does not appear to be critical for the binding of T_3 to the receptor.[142]

From these findings, Hayashi and coauthors concluded that natural mutations in the cold spot region of the c-*erb*Aβ receptor gene should remain covert and escape detection.[142] They would fail to manifest as thyroid hormone resistance because receptors coded by a naturally mutant cold spot region would only exhibit a slightly diminished affinity for T_3. Only a small increase in serum thyroid hormone levels is necessary to compensate for the lowered affinity. In a general resistance patient, expression of the mutant receptor would only slightly lower T_3-binding affinity in pituitary and peripheral cells. The TSH and thyroid hormone levels would rise slightly. The increased thyroid hormone level would inhibit further TSH secretion and maintain a eumetabolic state in the peripheral tissues. In a pituitary resistant patient, again only a slight increase in serum thyroid hormone levels would suppress TSH secretion, and the non-resistant peripheral tissues would be only slightly hypermetabolic. In a peripheral resistant patient, the pituitary-thyroid axis would function normally and maintain normal serum TSH and thyroid hormone levels. The peripheral tissues would be only slightly hypometabolic. The authors also pointed out that only in the homozygote would mutant receptors due to nucleotide substitutions in the cold spot region have a complete absence of T_3-binding, transcriptional activity, and dominant-negative effect.[142]

Researchers Discover Two c-*erb*A Genes That Code for Thyroid Hormone Receptors. Soon after Refetoff described thyroid hormone resistance syndrome, he and his colleagues proposed that the responsible defect was at the intracellular site where thyroid hormone exerted its effect.[35] They were not able to test this hypothesis, though, until Oppenheimer proposed the concept of the thyroid hormone receptor.[65] Their study employed mononuclear cells of a patient from a general resistance family. Testing showed markedly low T_3-binding affinity to the cell nuclei.[37] Other studies did not confirm this finding.

In 1986, two research groups contributed to the human genome project by identifying what they considered two different thyroid hormone receptor genes.

The genes coded for proteins that had a high affinity for thyroid hormone. The affinity of the proteins for thyroid hormone was similar to that of nuclear extracts in previous studies. This similarity led the researchers to consider that the proteins were receptors for thyroid hormone. Researchers have now isolated the two genes.[89][90]

Researchers mapped the two genes to human chromosomes 3 and 17.[49][63] Chromosome 3 contains the β gene; chromosome 17 contains the α gene. The α gene generates two mRNAs. They are designated c-*erb*Aα$_1$ RNA and c-*erb*Aα$_2$ RNA. c-*erb*Aα$_1$ RNA codes for a protein that binds T$_3$.[92] c-*erb*Aα$_2$ RNA codes for a protein similar to a thyroid hormone receptor, but the protein contains a carboxyl-terminus that renders it incapable of binding T$_3$. The protein is not a thyroid hormone receptor.[46,pp.210-211] The β gene also produces two mRNAs, c-*erb*Aβ$_1$ RNA and c-*erb*Aβ$_2$ RNA.[89][93] While both the c-*erb*Aβ$_1$ RNA and c-*erb*Aβ$_2$ RNA code for proteins that bind T$_3$, c-*erb*Aβ$_2$ RNA expresses mainly in the pituitary gland.[47]

How the c-erbA Genes Were Discovered. An interesting sequence of events led to the discovery of human thyroid hormone receptor genes. The two genes in humans are homologues of the viral oncogene *erb*-A. v-*erb*A is an avian retrovirus that carries the genetic code responsible for the development of the chicken disease erythroblastosis.[50][51] The v-*erb*A oncoprotein is a mutated version of a thyroid hormone receptor that is responsible for the arrest of differentiation in chicken erythroid cells. (In quail myoblasts v-*erb*A action does not interfere with T$_3$-induced mechanisms; instead, expression of the mutant oncoprotein results in a surprising increase in myoblast proliferation and myoblast terminal differentiation.[137]) The retroviral genome has two domains that must cooperate to fully express the virus: the v-*erb* B and the v-*erb*A genes. Researchers demonstrated that the homologue of the v-*erb*B gene codes for receptors for epidermal growth factor. The other gene, v-*erb*A, has a cellular homologue in humans in chromosome 17.[52]

Sequencing of the DNA nucleotides had shown a 50% structural homology between the steroid-binding region of the glucocorticoid receptor and the v-*erb*A protein.[53] Such findings led to the belief that the retroviruses derived some of their genes from their human hosts. This belief raised suspicion that the homologue of v-*erb*A in human cells might code for an unidentified steroid receptor.[53]

Two groups of researchers checked libraries of cloned DNA for homologues of v-*erb*A.[89][90] Each group found cDNAs in different libraries. They used

DNA polymerase (the enzyme that catalyzes a segment of DNA to transcribe its code—its nucleotide sequence—to mRNA) to synthesize the cDNAs *in vitro*. They allowed the resulting mRNAs to translate their code to proteins. The investigators found that steroid hormones did not bind to the proteins. They were aware, however, that the proteins corresponded to the estimated size of the T$_3$-receptor. When tested by exposing the protein to radioactive T$_3$ ([^{125}I]T$_3$), the protein and hormone bound with high specificity. T$_3$ and its analogues inhibited the binding, showing that these molecules had a higher affinity for the protein than did [^{125}I]T$_3$. The binding of the protein and T$_3$ closely resembled the binding of T$_3$ to nuclei and nuclear extracts.[45]

These findings provided firm evidence that the protein translated from the cDNA was a thyroid hormone receptor. The researchers concluded that a human cell homologue of the v-*erb*A gene coded the T$_3$-receptor in humans. They named this homologue the c-*erb*A gene.[90]

T$_3$-Receptor. The β gene in chromosome 3 transcribes its code to the two mRNAs, c-*erb*Aβ$_1$ and c-*erb*Aβ$_2$. Ribosomes in the cytoplasm then translate the mRNA codes to synthesize two isoforms of the β thyroid hormone receptor, β$_1$ and β$_2$. Similarly, the α gene in chromosome 17 transcribes its code to its two mRNAs, c-*erb*Aα$_1$ and c-*erb*Aα$_2$. Ribosomes then translate the codes of the mRNAs to synthesize the two isoforms of the α thyroid hormone receptor, α$_1$ and α$_2$.

Each T$_3$-receptor has three structural components. One component at its amino terminus, the DNA-binding domain (DBD), binds to DNA. The receptors that bind T$_3$, β$_1$, β$_2$, and α$_1$, do so at a second structural component called the T$_3$- (or ligand-) binding domain. Each of the three types of receptors bind to chromosomes proximal to specific sequences of DNA called T$_3$ (or thyroid hormone) response elements, or TREs.[3,pp.353-354] TREs reside in chromosomes near the location where transcription starts (termed transcription start points) in genes regulated by thyroid hormone.[3,p.383]

TREs consist of half-sites that have the consensus sequence AGGTCA. Their number, spacing (n), and orientation vary.[18][82][97] Half-sites may be oriented as direct repeats (AGGTCAnAGGTCA), a palindrome (AGGTCAnTGACCT), or an inverted palindrome (TGACCTnAGGTCA).[158] Refetoff and coauthors pointed out that typically, one half-site binds a single T$_3$-receptor molecule (monomer), and two half-sites bind two T$_3$-receptors (dimer), or one T$_3$-receptor and a nuclear cofactor termed a T_3-receptor-auxiliary-protein (TRAP).[3,p.384] Attachment of the T_3-receptor to the TRE is stabilized by a number of different TRAPs. Some TRAPs do not bind ligands. Others, such as retinoic X receptors, bind retinoic acid.

The retinoid X receptor is the main TRAP. This receptor is a member of a class of nuclear retinoic acid receptors each of which has α, β, and γ subtypes.[185] Like all other nuclear receptors, including the T_3-receptor, the retinoid X receptor has a DNA-binding domain, a ligand-binding domain, and a dimerization domain. This receptor form heterodimerizes with other receptors, such as the T_3-receptor, to form active transcription-inducing complexes. In a pattern analogous to that of a mutant T_3-receptor, the affinity of a mutant retinoid X receptor for its ligand (retinoic acid) is reduced. The mutant receptor binds normally to the retinoic acid response element of DNA, and the mutant exhibits dominant-negative inhibition of normal retinoid X receptors. It does so by binding to DNA without inducing transcription, and thereby competing with normal receptors for binding sites on the retinoic acid response element. (Mutant retinoic acid receptors, through their dominant-negative inhibition of normal receptors, may be involved in the etiology of neoplastic diseases such as acute promyelocytic leukemia.)

T_3-receptors located at TREs probably are not functional until thyroid hormone, largely T_3, attaches to the hormone binding domain of the receptor. The combination of the hormone and the receptor apparently induces a change in the conformation of the receptor. This change alters the rate of transcription of the target gene.[3,p.354]

At some genes, such as the rat growth hormone gene, binding of T_3 to a T_3-receptor accelerates transcription.[48] At such genes, binding of T_3 to the receptor has a *stimulatory* effect. At other genes, however, the effect of T_3 on transcription is *inhibitory*.[43] Refetoff, Weiss, and Usala pointed out[3,p.354] that when thyroid hormone is not present, the TRE has an effect opposite from that when thyroid hormone is present. If the combination of the liganded receptor and the TRE normally stimulates transcription, then the TRE in the absence of a liganded receptor is inhibitory. If the liganded receptor-TRE combination is normally inhibitory, then the TRE in the absence of the liganded receptor is stimulatory.[33][42][121,p.703] (See Section 3 for the clinical implications.)

Finding the Association Between General Resistance and the Mutant c-*erb*Aβ Receptor. In 1988, Bale, Usala, Weinberger, and McBride used the newly cloned human thyroid hormone receptors to search for

the defect in general resistance patients. They looked for a linkage between the syndrome and a single β allele in a large family. In sixteen family members, they found a linkage between the β site on chromosome 3 and general resistance.[94] According to Usala, analysis showed odds of 8000 to 1 that the observed linkage was due to chance.[95] This study and a subsequent one with another general resistance family suggested that the defects causing general resistance were mutations in the β gene of these two unrelated families.

The linkage between general resistance and the c-*erb*Aβ gene was present in multiple kindreds.[99] Establishing this linkage between c-*erb*Aβ and general resistance prompted the investigators to "sequence" the T_3-binding domain of the c-*erb*Aβ gene from affected members of family A.[101] Their aim was to compare to a normal reference sample the sequence of nucleotides in the gene (from family members) that codes for the component of the c-*erb*Aβ receptor that selectively binds the T_3 molecule.

First, they cloned part of the complementary DNA from fibroblasts that codes for the amino acid sequence of the T_3-binding domain of the thyroid hormone T_3-receptor.[31] At a certain DNA position (nucleotide position 1643), they found that one base, cytosine, was substituted for the appropriate one, adenine. They designated this gene "A-1643." This substitution altered the code for the sequence of amino acids in the polypeptide that makes up the binding domain of the T_3-receptor. As a result, in the amino acid sequence of the protein T_3-binding domain of the receptor, the amino acid histidine was substituted for proline. Usala pointed out that the normal amino acid sequence at the carboxyl-terminus in the β receptor may result in a unique conformation necessary for T_3-binding.[96,p.68] Substituting histidine for proline in the sequence, in these family members, may impede T_3-binding.

Next, Usala and his coworkers sequenced nucleotides from family A, including the suspected mutated gene. From the results, they concluded that the A-1643 gene was most likely the disease gene. Subsequently, they showed that the A-1643 gene, with its cytosine-to-adenine substitution, is possessed only by members of family A who have general resistance.[31] The investigators then screened seventeen members of family A, using parts of chromosomes (18 bases in length) containing the sections that would include the A-1643 gene. In seven family members who have general resistance, the A-1643 gene was present. The gene was not present in the ten members who did not have general resistance. The presence of gene A-1643 in individuals who had resistance and its absence in those who did not confirmed the link between general resistance and the c-erbAβ gene. The researchers published these results in 1991.[96,p.65]

The researchers had found that family members with general resistance had mutations, but members without resistance did not. In each family, only one of the two β alleles was mutated. This finding confirmed a dominant mode of inheritance.[3,p.354]

Sakurai and his coworkers found a different mutation in the c-erbAβ gene associated with general resistance in another family (family Mf). As in affected members of family A, the mutation involved a single nucleotide substitution in the β receptor coding region of chromosome 3: the nucleotide normally occupying the site was substituted with another nucleotide. In family A, the mutation resulted in short stature. But in family Mf, liver and heart cells were thyroid hormone resistant. Family members also had a history of learning disabilities, attention deficit, and hyperactivity.[24]

The mutation in family Mf involved a single substitution of cytosine for guanine at nucleotide position 1318. This substitution results in a change of arginine for glycine in the amino acid sequence of β T_3-receptors. When the investigators cloned these patients' DNA and produced protein from the relevant gene, the protein did not bind T_3.[24] The resistance was complete because the protein had *no* affinity for T_3.

In contrast, when Usala and his coworkers synthesized a receptor from the DNA of members of family A, the receptor had a diminished but measurable affinity for T_3.[25] Usala and Weintraub speculated about the difference between the T_3-binding affinity of receptors from families A and Mf. The difference was probably due, the researchers wrote, to the different protein structure of the T_3-receptors in the two families, dictated by their respective mutated genes.[96,p.68] Comparison of the data from family A and family Mf suggested that different substituted amino acids caused different degrees of impaired T_3-binding to the receptor. The mutant receptors in both families attached to non-mutated TREs on DNA.[23][24][25]

Usala and Weintraub wrote that the majority of patients with the inherited form of general resistance have mutations in one of the two c-erbAβ genes. Researchers can identify mutations by cloning and sequencing the T_3-binding domain of the gene.[96,p.68][98] They wrote that the tight linkage between general resistance and the c-erbAβ gene in various families with general resistance leaves no doubt that a genetic defect in the c-erbAβ thyroid hormone receptor is responsible for general resistance in multiple families.[96,p.71]

Thyroid Hormone Receptor Mutations and General Resistance. As of 1993, researchers had identified mutations in the β gene of 28 families with general resistance. They also found probable mutations in this gene in nine more families.[3,p.355] One family had a complete deletion of the β gene.[26] These family members are not able to synthesize β mRNA or c-erbAβ receptors. The paired nucleotides of the β receptor gene (alleles) completely lack T_3-binding and DNA-binding domains. Devoid of β receptors, thyroid hormone in these patients stimulates cells only by combining with their c-erbAα$_1$ receptors. Other members of the family who were missing only one of the paired β receptor genes were normal, with no thyroid hormone resistance.[35] On the other hand, in one homozygous member of another family (family S), both alleles dictated a single amino acid deletion in the T_3-binding domain of the β receptor.[136] In other members of family S, heterozygous members, only one of the alleles coded for this deletion. These patients also had general resistance but were less severely affected than the homozygous member.[35]

In 1993, Refetoff, Weiss, and Usala summarized gene analyses of general resistance patients.[3,p.355] (For additional details, I recommend reading the paper by these authors.) Of the 37 families with identified or putative mutations of the β gene, only one family has a complete deletion of the gene. The other 36 families have relatively minor mutations. One family had a deletion of three nucleotides, resulting in the loss of threonine-337. In two families, the addition of a single nucleotide in the gene produced a frame shift that changed the sequences of 14 (in one family) and of 8 (in another family) of the carboxyl-terminal amino acids and the addition of 2 terminal amino acids, leucine and aspartic acids. (A frameshift mutation involves an insertion or deletion of one or two bases in the coding region of a gene, changing the reading frame of the corresponding mRNA.[103,p.628])

In one family, a nucleotide substitution produced a *stop codon*. (A stop codon is a three nucleotide sequence within the mRNA nucleotide chain that signals cessation of synthesis of the protein at the ribosome. The three codons that code for termination of translation are UAG, UAA, and UGA.[103,p.637]) In this family, the stop codon resulted in a truncated receptor protein of 445 rather than 461 amino acids.

In the other 23 families, the only abnormalities were a single nucleotide substitution in the β gene from each family. Each nucleotide substitution caused substitution of a single amino acid in the β receptor. Identical mutations were found to be harbored by four pairs of unrelated families.

Except in the family whose β gene was deleted, all mutations were located within the T_3-binding domain of the receptor. The natural mutations cluster in two T_3-binding domain regions. These two regions straddle the putative dimerization binding region and DNA binding region.[19][20][21][22][179] Refetoff and coauthors suggested that this clustering may be of functional relevance.[3,p.355] The clustering may, for example, determine the degree of impaired T_3-binding.

At one point, it was believed that the degree of impaired T_3-binding did not correlate with the clinical severity of thyroid hormone resistance, judging from the large amounts of T_3 or T_4 needed to override resistance of the pituitary thyrotrophs in general resistance patients so that the patients maintain normal serum TSH levels).[3,p.355][56][210][219] In 1995, however, Refetoff and colleagues reported findings that revised this conclusion. They studied 124 resistant subjects representing 18 different β receptor mutations. Serum free T_4 levels correlated with the degree of T_3-binding impairment for 12 of the mutant receptors but not the other 6. The magnitude of elevated serum free T_4 at baseline correlated with the thyrotropin resistance shown by the incremental doses of T_3 necessary to properly suppress the TSH. The coauthors concluded that the clinical severity of thyroid hormone resistance can be predicted from the degree of impaired T_3-binding and potency of dominant-negative inhibition of mutant β receptors. They also concluded that the degree of peripheral tissue resistance and related clinical manifestations is restricted by putative environment and genetic factors that modify the effects of thyroid hormone.[225]

POSSIBLE MECHANISMS OF DOMINANT-NEGATIVE INHIBITION OF NORMAL THYROID HORMONE RECEPTORS BY MUTANT THYROID HORMONE RECEPTORS

The typical mutant c-*erb*Aβ$_1$ receptor is normal in that it binds DNA with high affinity. But it is abnormal in two functions: first, it binds T_3 with reduced affinity, <1% of that of normal receptors in some cases;[238] and second, it exhibits dominant-negative inhibition of normal c-*erb*Aβ and c-*erb*Aα$_2$ receptors.[219] The mechanism of this inhibition has been the subject of intense study, partly because it may help explain the variable phenotypic expression of thyroid hormone resistance syndrome.

Mutant c-*erb*Aβ receptors in families A, Mf, and D function as dominant-negative inhibitors. These mutants inhibit function of normal c-*erb*Aβ receptors (expressed from the one normal allele in heterozygotic patients) and the normal c-*erb*Aα receptors (expressed from two alleles).[133] This process impedes transcriptional regulation by the normal receptors.[104] Investigators have known of dominant-negative inhibition of normal c-*erb*Aβ receptors by mutant β receptors for some time,[23] but as of 1991, researchers did not know the mechanism of inhibition.[96,p.72]

Factors that Appear Critical to Dominant-Negative Inhibition

Point mutations have been identified in the T_3-binding domain on one of the two alleles of the c-*erb*Aβ gene, but not in the nucleotide regions that code for DNA-binding and dimerization (in the case of the T_3-receptors, binding to an auxiliary protein, such as the retinoid X receptor[185]). This indicates that DNA-binding and receptor dimerization are important for dominant-negative inhibition by mutant thyroid hormone receptors.[146]

Study of a woman with selective pituitary resistance indicated that arginine at codon 311 in the c-*erb*Aβ gene is also required for dominant-negative inhibition. This patient had markedly elevated serum free T_4 and total T_3, but inappropriately normal TSH, and was hyperthyroid. The patient had a single mutation, a guanine-to-adenine substitution at nucleotide 1,232 in one allele. The mutation altered codon 311 so that it coded for histidine rather than arginine. The patient's father and a half-sister harbored the same mutation but were clinically normal. The patient and her father had an equal expression of normal and mutant alleles. When the patient's receptors were cloned and tested, their T_3-binding affinity was significantly reduced. But in contrast to many other c-*erb*Aβ mutants found in general resistance patients, the mutant receptor from this patient did not inhibit normal receptors. The investigators reported that apparently, arginine at codon 311, which histidine had substituted for, is crucial to the structural integrity required for dominant-negative inhibition.[176]

Differential Interactions of Mutant β T_3-Receptors at Thyroid Response Elements

Zavacki and coworkers explored the hypothesis that the heterogeneous tissue-specific manifestations of general resistance result from differential interactions between the mutant β T_3-receptor on T_3 response elements (TREs) in different T_3-responsive genes.[163]

(TREs, remember, are distinct DNA sequences that interact with the T_3-receptor to control gene expression.[164,p.587] Interaction between the liganded T_3-receptor and a TRE increases or decreases the rate of mRNA synthesis, depending on whether the gene is activated or repressed by the liganded T_3-receptor.[165][166])

First, Zavacki tested the transcriptional activity of mutated c-*erb*Aβ and c-*erb*Aα receptors. Next, he measured the extent to which each mutant receptor inhibited corresponding normal c-*erb*Aβ and c-*erb*Aα receptors at four structurally distinct TREs. Transcriptional activity of the mutants was similarly reduced at all four TREs. The extent of reduction was T_3-dependent—the lower the T_3 concentration, the greater the reduction of activity; the higher the T_3 concentration, the less the reduction. The mutant c-*erb*Aα receptor characteristically had greater transcriptional activity. Nevertheless, the receptor continued to impede the normal c-*erb*Aα receptor even at a high T_3 concentration (500 nM). In general, dominant-negative inhibition of normal receptors by mutants was inversely correlated with the T_3 concentration. This correlation was expected because of the mutant receptors' decreased affinity for T_3. The concentration of T_3 that was sufficient to relieve the dominant-negative inhibition of normal receptors by mutant receptors at three of the different TREs did not do so at the fourth. The fourth continued to inhibit normal receptors. Also, mutant receptors varied in their dominant-negative inhibition at three of the four different TREs, based on the receptor isoform. The investigator concluded that in general resistance, both the distinct structure of the involved TRE and the isoform of the mutant c-*erb*A receptor determine the degree of dominant-negative inhibition of normal receptors.[163]

Interference with Access of Normal Receptors to Hormone Response Elements

Study of the mutant retinoic acid receptor, which also exhibits dominant-negative activity, suggests one possible mechanism of inhibitory activity by mutant thyroid hormone receptors.[139] The retinoic acid receptor is similar to the thyroid hormone receptor in structure and mode of action. The two types of receptors share many amino acids in their functionally important DNA-binding domains, ligand-binding domains, and sites where they interface when heterodiming. A sequence of steps is necessary for both types of normal receptors to function. Both receptors (1) dimerize with retinoid X receptors, (2) recognize their cognate hormone response elements, and (3) bind their respective ligands. When these three steps occur normally, each type of receptor properly regulates the target gene.

Recall that a mutation in the form of a single amino acid substitution in the ligand-binding domain of the c-*erb*Aβ receptor reduces its binding affinity for T_3. The mutation also confers dominant-negative phenotypicity to the receptor in that it inhibits normal T_3-receptors. Mutations in the c-*erb*Aβ receptor most commonly involve substitutions of amino acids also constitutive to the retinoic acid receptor. Saitou and coworkers mutated the ligand-binding domain of the retinoic acid receptor by substituting a single amino acid. The mutated receptor then had dominant-negative activity and suppressed the function of normal retinoic acid receptors when exposed to physiological concentrations of retinoic acid.[139] The mutated receptor exerts dominant-negative activity only when the receptor is structured so as to recognize its DNA-binding site, the retinoic acid response element[103,p.412] (tantamount to the DNA-binding site for the c-*erb*A receptor, the T_3 response element) in target genes. This requirement for dominant-negative activity indicates that the retinoic acid receptor must have intact dimeric-binding and DNA-binding sites. It appears that dominant-negative activity of the low ligand-binding affinity mutant results from its binding to the retinoic acid response element and blocking access by normal retinoic acid receptors.

The same appears to be true of the mutant c-*erb*Aβ receptor. Nagaya and Jameson tested the hypothesis that receptor dimerization is required for dominant-negative inhibition. They suspected that natural mutations do not occur in the dimerization domain (the cold spot region) of the β gene, a region that separates the two hot spot regions that code for T_3-binding and where natural mutations cluster. The researchers showed that two natural mutant c-*erb*Aβ receptors formed homodimers with other c-*erb*Aβ receptors and heterodimers with α retinoid X receptors. They induced an artificial mutation in the putative receptor dimerization domain of the gene. The resulting mutant c-*erb*Aβ receptors formed homodimers with other c-*erb*Aβ receptors, but they were impaired in forming heterodimers with α retinoid X receptors. The investigators then found that inducing the artificial dimerization mutation eliminated dominant-negative inhibition of normal c-*erb*Aβ receptors by the mutant c-*erb*Aβ receptors. They concluded that dominant-negative activity is dependent on formation of heterodimers that are transcriptionally inactive and block access of normal receptors to DNA.[179]

Mutations in the DNA-Binding Domain of the T₃-Receptor

In general, dominant-negative activity of the mutant T_3-receptor involves successful competition with the normal receptor for DNA binding. Also, binding of the mutant receptor to DNA is usually prerequisite to exertion of dominant-negative inhibition. Liu et al., however, reported an exception to this. They artificially induced a cysteine-73-serine substitution in the DNA-binding domain of an otherwise normal T_3-receptor. This substitution enabled the receptor to inhibit transcription induction by a normal α_1 T_3-receptor. Inhibition occurred regardless of the presence or absence of T_3 and on three different reporter genes containing TREs. The presence of the α_2 T_3-receptor variant (which because of its structure does not bind T_3 and normally inhibits c-erbAβ and c-erbAα_1 receptors) enhanced the dominant-negative inhibition by the T_3-receptor containing the mutant DNA-binding domain. (The dominant-negative effect did not occur at the α TSH luciferase reporter gene which the liganded T_3-receptor normally represses. With this gene, the mutant T_3-receptor exerted its normal negative regulatory effect. The mutant inhibited transcription of the TK-luciferase reporter gene linked with rat malic enzyme TRE.) The investigators concluded that the T_3-receptor with a mutated DNA-binding domain can have dominant-negative effects. They proposed that the mechanism may be similar to the inhibitory effect of the α_2 T_3-receptor variant that appears to involve interference with basal transcription factors. They also wrote that the clinical significance of the mutant is not clear, but that it is logical to expect that such mutants occur naturally.[218]

Structural Changes in TREs that Increase Binding to Dimers Containing Mutant β T₃-Receptors

Zavacki and colleagues reported that structural features of a TRE may favor dominant-negative inhibition by mutant c-erbA receptors. They found that structural features that favor potent binding of mutant T_3-receptor homodimers and mutant T_3-receptor/retinoid X receptor heterodimers heighten the sensitivity of the TRE to inhibition by the mutants. Two such TRE structural features are the everted palindromic conformation and the optimal T_3-receptor consensus octomer.[230] This finding indicates that both half-site orientation and TRE sequence can confer to a TRE sensitivity to dominant-negative inhibition by a mutant T_3-receptor.

Mutations of the c-erbAα Gene

Usala and colleagues established tight linkage between general resistance to thyroid hormone and the c-erbAβ gene. They pointed out, however, that future studies may show families in which the c-erbAβ gene and general resistance are not linked. In patients from these families, studies may show mutant T_3-receptors coded by the c-erbAα gene rather than the β gene.[95] No mutations have yet been identified in the c-erbAα gene.[177] It is the best candidate, however, as the source of general resistance not caused by a mutant c-erbAβ gene.[96,p.65]

Lee and Mahdavi induced substitution of two clusters of positively charged amino acids into the D domain of the c-erbAα_1 receptor. (The sequences lysine-134-arginine-lysine and arginine-188-arginine-lysine were substituted to the neutral residues TIT.) These mutant receptors then exhibited normal DNA-binding and normal T_3-binding but had no ability to activate or repress transcription. What is more, substituting either one of the amino acids converted the receptors into dominant antagonists of T_3-dependent receptors. The investigators noted the relevance of amino acid substitutions in the D domain to the function of the c-erbAα_1 receptor and suggested that it may have implications for general thyroid hormone resistance.[186]

The c-erbAα_2 receptor (a receptor variant that does not bind T_3) has been found to potentiate the dominant-negative inhibitory activity of mutant c-erbAβ receptors (but only within the context of a positively regulated reporter gene).[173] The c-erbAα_2 may therefore selectively increase the degree of dominant-negative activity at different target genes regulated by c-erbAβ receptors. Meier-Heusler and coworkers[193] found that in excessive concentrations, the c-erbAα_2 receptor partially displaces T_3-receptor/retinoic X receptor heterodimers from DNA. They concluded that the general dominant-negative inhibition by the c-erbAα_2 receptor results in part from competition with the T_3-receptor and its auxiliary proteins for DNA-binding.

Some investigators have proposed that expression of the normal c-erbAα gene (which would have to be the α_1 isoform, since the α_2 isoform does not bind T_3[173]) may increase as a compensation for the expression of a mutant c-erbAβ gene. The one family with homozygous deletion of the c-erbAβ gene, however, did not have an increase in expression of the α gene.[184]

The functions of the normal c-erbAα receptor have not been clearly defined yet, although it is known that the receptor forms heterodimers with retinoid X receptors to regulate transcription at TREs.[242] One function of the c-*erb*Aα$_2$ receptor, which does not bind T$_3$, is to competitively bind DNA and thereby inhibit the effects of T$_3$ bound to c-*erb*Aβ receptors.[260]

Note: The α$_1$ receptor is present in the testis only during certain developmental stages in the rat, and it is absent in the adult rat. The α$_1$ receptor is expressed only during fetal and prepubertal stages, and is found in fetal seminiferous cords and tubules. The c-*erb*Aβ receptor is absent in rat testis at all times. The testis of the adult rat does not respond to thyroid hormone as most other tissues do with an increase in oxygen consumption. High-affinity binding in the nuclei of rat testicular cells has not been demonstrated.[157]

● **VARIABLE MANIFESTATIONS OF THYROID HORMONE RESISTANCE**

What is known about the variable manifestations of thyroid hormone resistance has been derived largely from the study of general resistance. The effects of thyroid hormone resistance described in this section may result from molecular lesions common to all forms of thyroid hormone resistance syndrome.

VARIABLE CLINICAL FEATURES OF THYROID HORMONE RESISTANCE

Clinical features vary between general resistance patients. Some patients are normal, others have mild or moderate symptoms and signs, and still others have severe abnormalities.

Mutant c-*erb*Aβ receptors are associated with delayed bone growth and short stature in some families, such as family A.[221] Some affected members of this family have tachycardia. Their liver tissues and some brain regions are resistant, and their BMRs are low. In contrast, members of a second family, family D, have resistant heart tissues with bradycardia. Their livers are affected and their BMRs are low. They do not, however, have short stature. Affected members of both families A and D have low scores on IQ tests. Affected members of family A are hyperactive and have attention deficit. Some affected members of another family, family B, were hyperactive with attention deficit as children. Later, their school performance was normal. Also in family B, BMRs were low, and liver and heart were resistant to thyroid hormone.[96,p.60]

Hearing loss is a significant problem in thyroid hormone resistance patients.[236] There is an equal incidence of sensorineural deficits and conductive deficits. Conductive deficits appear to be related to frequent ear infections. In one study of 82 patients, 21% had hearing loss, 34% had abnormal tympanometry, 39% had abnormal acoustic reflexes, and 50% had cochlear dysfunction.[224]

Table 2.6.2 lists the clinical features that different investigators have reported in general resistance patients. In general resistance, both the pituitary and peripheral tissues are resistant. The pituitary resistance results in hypersecretion of TSH, which in turn, results in higher than normal levels of thyroid hormone. In most cases of general resistance, the elevated thyroid hormone levels compensate for the peripheral tissue resistance, and the individuals are eumetabolic with normal growth and development. Refetoff, Weiss, and Usala explain further:

> However, not infrequently, the compensation appears to be incomplete in spite of equally high thyroid hormone levels. More rarely, high endogenous thyroid hormone levels can produce toxic effects on peripheral tissues, an apparent state of overcompensation. Cases on the one extreme of the spectrum have produced hypothyroidism with typical cretinoid features, and on the other, thyrotoxicosis with extreme wasting, agitation, and tachycardia.[3,p.359]

The features listed in Table 2.6.2 occurred in some patients despite the compensation.[61] Some patients have features typical of both hypothyroidism and hyperthyroidism. An example is a single subject with a homozygous deletion of threonine-337[1] in the c-*erb*Aβ receptor (III2, F66). This individual's hypothyroid-like features included growth retardation, delayed skeletal maturation, hyperbilirubinemia, and hypofibrinogenemia. His thyrotoxic-like features included prominent stare, tachycardia, respiratory distress, poor weight gain, frequent stools, and hyperbilirubinemia.[3,p.359] Because of the variable tissue responsiveness, patients with general thyroid hormone resistance have no pathognomonic symptoms or signs and most often have heterogeneous clinical features.[3,p.359] In any one patient, some tissues may be hyporesponsive to thyroid hormone, others may be hyperresponsive, and others normally responsive. Such variability prompted Sonkin to question the validity of the concept of *generalized* resistance.[62,p.48] In contrast to general resistance patients, those with peripheral resistance to thyroid hormone largely have symptoms characteristic of hypothyroidism (see Chapter 2.5).

Attention Deficit Hyperactivity Disorder (ADHD) and Low Intelligence Level

ADHD is a neurodevelopmental abnormality. It is often found in children with general resistance to thyroid hormone, suggesting that thyroid abnormalities may be etiologically related to ADHD.[170][213] Refetoff, Weiss, and Usala[3,p.390] made reference to testimonials of improved behavior of children with ADHD from families 22 and 44 during their use of supraphysiologic doses of T_3.[74] But one child from family 54 did not benefit.[3,p.390]

Elia and coworkers evaluated boys with ADHD for evidence of general resistance to thyroid hormone. They tested 53 ADHD patients and 41 control subjects. They found no laboratory evidence of resistance. They concluded that resistance was rare, and that thyroid function should not be evaluated routinely in the nonfamilial form of ADHD.[55]

Weiss and colleagues found that among 277 ADHD children, fourteen children had abnormal thyroid function results: six had an elevated T_4 level but a normal free T_4 index (group 1); three had a high free T_4 index and a normal TSH level (group 2); five had a low free T_4 index and a normal TSH level (group 3). A detailed study of four of the children (from groups 1 and 2) did not demonstrate general resistance to thyroid hormone. Weiss and his coauthors wrote that although the prevalence of ADHD in those with general thyroid hormone resistance is reported to be 46%, they found no cases of general resistance among the 277 ADHD children they studied. However, the prevalence of abnormal thyroid function test results in the children they studied was higher (5.4%) than in the normal population (<1%).[170]

Similarly, Spencer and his colleagues found no cases of resistance in 132 ADHD children and adolescents. The researchers reported that the mildly abnormal thyroid function test results they found in a small minority of subjects were the same as those reported in the literature for normal children.[189]

Brucker-Davis and coworkers wrote that of 104 resistance patients studied at their facility, 60% had ADHD.[190] Weiss and coworkers wrote that 46%-to-50% of children with thyroid hormone resistance have ADHD. They studied sixteen members of a family, some of whom harbored the mutation R316H in the c-*erb*Aβ receptor gene. Three members had the R316H allele and had a mildly elevated free T_4 index and nonsuppressed TSH, suggesting general resistance. Blinded diagnostic interviews and psychometric testing indicated that two of the three patients with the mutant allele had ADHD. The other family member did not have resistance (thyroid function test results were normal) but also had ADHD. The three members had a lower mean IQ score than that of unaffected family members (77±5 compared to 93±7, p=0.006). Weiss and his coauthors concluded that their data do not support a linkage of ADHD with thyroid hormone resistance.[145] The data do, however, suggest that resistance is associated with lower IQ scores, and patients with lower IQ scores may be more likely to exhibit ADHD symptoms.

Usala and Weintraub reported low IQ test scores in thyroid hormone resistant members of families A and D. But only members of family A had ADHD.[96,p.60] According to Brucker-Davis and coworkers, 38% of their 104 resistance patients had IQs lower than 85, and 35% had speech impediments.[190] Stein and coworkers found that compared to ADHD children without thyroid hormone resistance, ADHD children with resistance had lower nonverbal intelligence and lower academic achievement. Mean nonverbal intelligence (as performance IQ) in resistant children was 85, compared to 99 in nonresistant children. Academic achievement in resistant children was >1-2 SD below the mean, compared to within 2 SD for nonresistant children. Stein and coauthors wrote that the weaker perceptual-organization ability and lower school achievement of resistant ADHD children suggest a more severe neurobehavioral impairment than in ADHD children without resistance.[239]

Leonard and colleagues studied 43 subjects (20 affected males and 23 affected females) with general resistance for developmental brain malformation. The researchers compared the results with 32 unaffected first degree relatives (18 unaffected males and 14 unaffected females). They used MRI brain scans to determine the volume of structures by 90 contiguous 2 mm-thick sagittal images. A blinded investigator examined contiguous images representing structures from a standard sagittal position lateral to the insula. In the bank of the Sylvian fissure (multimodal association cortex) and in Heschl's transverse gyri (primary auditory cortex), they found extra or missing gyri. They found an increased frequency of anomalous Sylvian fissures in the left hemisphere of males with resistance. Of males affected by thyroid hormone resistance, 70% had anomalies, compared to 30% of affected females and 28% of both unaffected males and females. In addition, affected males had a higher frequency of anomalous Sylvian fissures on the left combined with multiple Heschl's gyri in either hemisphere. The frequency was 50% compared with 9% in affected females, 6% in unaffected males, and 0% in unaffected females. Resistant subjects with these anomalies did not have a higher incidence of ADHD than resistant subjects without the anomalies. The researchers concluded that grossly observable cerebral anomalies of the left hemisphere are associated with abnormal thyroid hormone action in the male fetus during early brain development. These anomalies may have some relation to neurobehavioral abnormalities in general resistance males.[187]

Matochik and coworkers compared the ability of thirteen adult general resistance patients and normal subjects to perform a sustained attention task (a continuous auditory, discrimination task). The thirteen resistance patients were clearly impaired in this ability. Patients performed the task while undergoing positron emission tomography. This procedure showed higher metabolism during the task in both the right parietal cortex and the anterior cingulate gyrus in the patients. The increased metabolic activity in the cingulate gyrus may indicate a decreased signal-to-noise ratio for the neural processing. The authors concluded that mutations in the c-*erb*Aβ receptor gene are associated with attention deficit in adults.[227]

VARIABLE TISSUE RESPONSIVENESS IN THYROID HORMONE RESISTANCE SYNDROMES

Liewendahl[67] and colleagues[68] studied mildly affected family members and sporadic cases of general resistance. When they tested the patients' lymphocytes and found no defects in the lymphocyte nuclear receptors, they speculated as to the reason. They wrote that perhaps their laboratory techniques were not sensitive enough to illuminate the defect. On the other hand, maybe the defect causing hormone resistance was not in the nuclear receptors. It might be that some step of the post-receptor effector mechanism (chemical steps inside the inner cell membrane or the cytoplasm that mediate cellular reactions upon binding of a hormone to its receptor) might be faulty. Then again, the defect might be in cells other than lymphocytes.

Refetoff's conclusion after reviewing these studies is worthy of careful consideration. He first points out that the lymphocytes and fibroblasts used in some of the studies may not have been resistant to thyroid hormone, while other tissues of the patients may have been. Lymphocytes and fibroblasts, although convenient for study, may not be the resistant cells producing the patients' symptoms. He concluded:

Table 2.6.2. Clinical features of patients with general thyroid resistance syndromes.*

Adrenal insufficiency, primary**
Agitation
Attention deficit
Bone maturation, delayed
Early development, delayed
Congestive heart failure, refractory
Cretinoid appearance in infancy
Diarrhea in infants
Epiphyses, stippled**
Facial puffiness in adults
Failure to thrive
Fatigue
Fractures, multiple osteoporotic crush**
Goiter in children or adolescents***
Goiter, recalcitrant in adults after surgical ablation***
Growth retardation
Headaches**
Hearing defects (such as loss)
Hyperactivity
Hypotonia in infants
Infections, recurrent (ear, nose, and throat)**
Jaundice, congenital
Learning disabilities
Mental retardation
Myopathy typical of hypothyroidism
Nervousness
Nystagmus, congenital
Pain, chronic back**
Palpitations
Proptosis without ophthalmopathy**
Restlessness
Scaphocephaly**
School, difficulty adjusting to
Sleeplessness in children
Somnolence
Speech, delayed
Short stature
Syncope, recurrent**
Tachycardia
Tremulousness (most common thyrotoxic finding)
Variable features of hypo- and hyperthyroidism
   (a combination of both in some patients)
Weight loss in adults and children
Weight gain

*a) Refetoff, S., Weiss, R.E., and Usala, S.J.: The syndromes of resistance to thyroid hormone. *Endocrine Reviews*, 14:348-399, 1993.[3]
b) Kopp, P., Kitajima, K., and Jameson, J.L.: Syndrome of resistance to thyroid hormone: insights into thyroid hormone action. *Proc. Soc. Experim. Biol. Med.*, 211(1):49-61, 1996.[61]
c) Brucker-Davis, F., Skarulis, M.C., Grace, M.B., et al.: Genetic and clinical features of 42 kindreds with resistance to thyroid hormone: the National Institutes of Health prospective study. *Ann. Intern. Med.*, 123 (8):572-583, 1995.[190]
**Refetoff, Weiss, and Usala[3,p.359] stated that these features were related to a variety of apparently unrelated conditions in patients who sought medical care. With the possible exception of scaphocephaly and proptosis, however, the tagged features are common to thyroid hormone-related euthyroid hypometabolic patients (particularly in those with euthyroid fibromyalgia) and are often improved or relieved by proper metabolic treatment.
***Goiter is by far the most common finding in general resistance (85% in one study of 104 resistant patients[190]).

Consistent with the hypothesis of selective tissue involvement is the clinical impression of variable degrees of insensitivity, which are more pronounced in some peripheral tissues than in others, and which appear to follow a uniform pattern within each family, but show greater differences among affected members from unrelated families.[8, p.1295]

Refetoff's view is supported by an unusual case. Almost all general resistance patients have responded therapeutically to T_3. In one report, however, investigators wrote of a patient for whom T_4 was more potent than T_3 in overriding cell resistance and producing the appropriate tissue response.[116] The investigators were not certain why T_4 was more potent. But the fact that it was more effective highlights the variability of the possible defective mechanisms in thyroid hormone resistance.

The degree of resistance of different tissues within any particular patient varies. Moreover, different families have variable patterns of tissue resistance.[37] That is, the set of resistant tissues in one family may differ from that in another. Or the degree of resistance in one type of tissue may vary from family-to-family, one family affected severely, another only mildly.

Investigators have assessed the responsiveness of various tissues to T_3 in general resistance patients. The tested tissues include bone, brain, liver, heart, and pituitary. Investigators have also measured patients' basal metabolic rates. As shown in Table 2.6.3, Usala and Weintraub compared tissue responsiveness between families A, B and D.

The tissues involved in thyroid hormone resistance and the degree of resistance vary considerably among patients. There is wide variety between and within kindreds. The tissues involved among one group of 104 patients, in decreasing order, were the pituitary gland, the brain, bone, liver, and the heart.[190]

Refetoff, Weiss, and Usala correlated growth with mental function in resistant patients. Among the patients, more had mental dysfunction (59%) than growth retardation (26%). Abnormal mental function without growth retardation was common (37%), and growth retardation without mental dysfunction was rare (4%). (See Table 2.6.4.) The investigators noted that this latter percentage is similar to that for the general population. They concluded, "Thus, if functional deprivation of thyroid hormone were responsible for the observed abnormalities on growth and mental function, its consequences on the brain appears to be more important than that on bone."[3, p.361]

Patients with peripheral resistance may have similar variability in the resistance of tissues to thyroid hormones. Such variability could explain the diversity of clinical phenotypes such as hyperlipidemia, atypical depression, and fibromyalgia.

PUTATIVE FACTORS RESPONSIBLE FOR PHENOTYPIC VARIABILITY

The gene mutation *per se* does not account for the variability in clinical presentation between resistance patients. This is clear from the finding that patients from the same and different kindreds and with the general and pituitary forms of resistance have identical c-*erb*Aβ gene mutations.[133] The identical mutation occurs independently in unrelated families, and affected members of the families vary in their clinical features and the severity of their resistance according to their responses to exogenous T_3.[211] Within some kindreds harboring the same c-*erb*Aβ gene mutation, affected individuals have different clinical features and heterogeneous thyroid function test results, both before and after treatment with thyroid hormone.[140]

Similar translation products of mutant genes may not result in similar clinical manifestations in different patients. Truncation of part of the carboxyl-terminus of the c-*erb*Aβ receptor is an example. Taniyama and coworkers[216] reported the case of a 16-year-old eumetabolic male with mild general resistance who had a novel mutation in codon 449 in the end of exon 10 of the c-*erb*Aβ gene. When the researchers induced expression of the receptor protein coded by the mutant gene, the carboxyl-terminus was deficient of 13 amino acids. The patient's thyrotrophs and peripheral tissues responded well to exogenous T_3. The researchers contrasted the mildness of this patient's resistance to the severe resistance of two previously published cases. One of these cases had a 16-amino acid deficiency at the carboxyl-terminus; the other case had an 11-amino acid deficiency at the terminus. Truncation of amino acids in the carboxyl-terminus, therefore, does not result in uniform severity of resistance.

A number of investigators wrote that the variety of clinical manifestations indicate that general and pituitary resistance are variable manifestations of a single genetic entity. The investigators have also argued that factors other than c-*erb*Aβ gene mutations may account for the wide spectrum of phenotypes in thyroid hormone resistance patients.[134][141][144]

Lists of Possible Factors Causing Variability

In a recent review, Refetoff, Weiss, and Usala attributed variability in the clinical manifestations and laboratory findings in general resistance patients to several possible factors. Accounting for some variability could be different types of mutations, such as defects in different functional domains (the T_3-binding, DNA-binding, and auxiliary protein-binding domains) of the thyroid hormone receptor gene. Mutations in one or more of the three different T_3-binding isoforms of the receptor could also contribute. The level of expression of receptor isoforms in different tissues is another factor. Others include the interaction of the c-erbAβ gene with other nuclear factors and the effectiveness or ineffectiveness of various compensatory mechanisms.[3,p.349]

Chatterjee and Beck-Peccoz suggested that resistance in peripheral tissues may result from differences in the tissue distribution of α and β forms of the c-erbA receptor, variable dominant effects of the mutant receptors on different target genes, or other factors not directly related to the mutant receptor.[141]

Pohlenz and coauthors[191] and Takeda and Hashimoto[147] listed several factors that might account for variety in clinical phenotype: dominant-negative activity by heterodimerization of a mutant thyroid hormone receptor with a retinoid X receptor, and homodimerization of a mutant thyroid hormone receptor with a normal thyroid hormone receptor; variation in types of thyroid hormone response elements in different genes; and different thyroid hormone receptor isoforms and auxiliary proteins in different target tissues.

The findings of Meier-Heusler and coauthors indicate that three different mechanisms may modulate thyroid hormone action. First is increased binding of mutant α_1 and β_1 thyroid hormone receptors to specific TREs. Second is effective competition for limited amounts of retinoid X receptor by other heterodimers. (For example, they showed that human peroxisome proliferator-activated receptor completely inhibited DNA-binding by T_3-receptor/retinoid X receptor heterodimers. This result indicated that human peroxisome proliferator-activated receptor had a higher binding affinity for retinoid X receptor and constituted a potent competitor for intranuclear retinoid X receptors, resulting in formation of fewer T_3-receptor/retinoid X receptor heterodimers.) The third modulating mechanism is competition for binding to DNA and auxiliary proteins other than the retinoid X receptor. The investigators found, for instance, that c-erbAα_2 receptors only partially displaced T_3-receptor/retinoid

X receptor heterodimers from DNA. The partial displacement suggests that the c-erbAα_2 receptor, which has general dominant-negative inhibitory action at TREs, inhibits T_3-receptors by effectively competing for DNA-binding and for the auxiliary proteins that T_3-receptors must form heterodimers with to bind to DNA.[193]

Table 2.6.3. Responsiveness of various tissues in three families with general resistance.

	TISSUE RESPONSIVENESS*					
Family	Bone	Brain	Liver	Heart	Pituitary	Metabolism
A	R	SR	R	V	R	R
B	—	V	R	SR	R	R
C	—	SR	R	SR	R	R

*The following is the scale for tissue responsiveness: SR = severe resistance; R = resistance; V = variable resistance among family members; — = minimal or no resistance. Thyroid hormone action was determined by various measures peculiar to each tissue: Bone = adult height, bone age; Brain = intelligence quotient; Liver = sex hormone binding globulin, cholesterol; Heart = sleeping pulse, pulse wave arrival time; Pituitary = TSH; Metabolism = basal metabolic rate.

After Usala, S.J. and Weintraub, B.D.: Familial thyroid hormone resistance: clinical and molecular studies. In *Advances in Endocrinology and Metabolism*, Vol.2., New York, Mosby-Year Book, Inc., 1991.[96,p.61]

Relative Expression of Mutant and Normal Alleles

Bercu and coworkers found a variation between kindreds in the relative expression of normal and mutant alleles for the c-erbAβ_1 receptor. They compared the relative expression of mutated and normal alleles by measuring mutant and normal β_1 receptor mRNAs from fibroblasts of children of two different kindreds with general resistance. Children from kindred A had both delayed bone age and short stature. Bercu found that they overexpressed the mutant alleles. However, in children from kindred S, who had delayed bone age but normal growth curves, the level of normal β_1 receptor mRNAs was nearly twice as high as that for mutant mRNAs. The investigators wrote, "Relative expression of the c-erbAβ alleles thus appeared to be increased during this period of somatic growth. The relative overexpression of the normal allele [in kindred S] potentially counteracted the potent dominant-negative expression of the S [mutant] receptor during early childhood, ameliorating a deleterious effect on linear growth."[11]

Mixson and coworkers reported similar findings. They pointed out that heterogeneous phenotypic expression occurs not only between different kindreds, but also within the same kindred. They hypothesized that this variability was due to differing ratios of expression of mutant and normal thyroid hormone receptors in tissues. They found that in the A-H kindred, two members had equal amounts of normal and mutant mRNA levels for the c-*erb*Aβ_1 receptor. In two other members, at least 70% of the mRNA was mutant. Members with higher ratios of mutant-to-normal mRNA had considerably more bone resistance during their development. The authors proposed that differing ratios of mutant-to-normal receptors may be age- and growth-related. Differing ratios may also account for some phenotypic symptoms attenuating with age.[58]

Table 2.6.4. Correlation of growth retardation and mental dysfunction in patients with general resistance to thyroid hormone.*

Growth Retardation	Mental Dysfunction	Different Subjects	Families
Normal	Normal	26(37%)	13(31%)
Normal	Abnormal	26(37%)	21(50%)
Abnormal	Normal	3(4%)	3(7%)
Abnormal	Abnormal	15(21%)	10(24%)
Total		70	42[†]

*Refetoff, S., Weiss, R.E., and Usala, S.J.: The syndromes of resistance to thyroid hormone. *Endocrine Reviews*, 14:348-399, 1993.[3,p.362]
[†]According to Refetoff, et al., the number of families does not "sum up" because some members in the same families were "scored under different categories."

Klann and coworkers, however, found that the extreme mental and growth retardation in a severely affected homozygous mutant from a kindred with general resistance was not due to relative overexpression of the mutant allele.[174] Similarly, Hayashi and coworkers conducted a study to determine whether the lack of correlation between the severity of the clinical manifestations of thyroid hormone resistance and the functional impairment of the mutant receptor results from quantitative differences in expression of the normal or mutant β gene. They measured mutant and normal receptor mRNA in fibroblasts from heterozygous individuals with general resistance from two families.

The individuals varied in the severity of their clinical manifestations. Expression of both forms of mRNA were equal, indicating that quantitative differences in expression did not account for the variable manifestations. The investigators wrote that differences are more likely a result of variations in the interactions of the mutant and normal β receptors, α receptors, and nuclear stabilization factors.[184]

A study by Hayashi and coworkers showed that thyroid hormone resistance phenotype can be modified by thyroid hormone deficiency. In hypothyroid mice infected with mutated thyroid hormone receptors, T_3 treatment did not lower weight or serum cholesterol levels as expected. In addition, overexpression of normal c-*erb*Aβ receptors in hypothyroid mice further increased the elevated serum cholesterol. On the other hand, this overexpression of normal receptors potentiated the decrease in serum cholesterol when T_3 was administered. The study showed that at least *in vivo*, high levels of unliganded normal c-*erb*Aβ receptors can worsen the manifestations of hypothyroidism. The c-*erb*Aβ receptors bind to DNA, but with insufficient T_3 available to bind to the receptor, the receptor is not able to activate transcription regulation. With mutant c-*erb*Aβ receptors in the hypothyroid mice, supraphysiologic concentrations of T_3 would have been required to activate transcription regulation. This requirement was not met because of the T_3 deficiency associated with the hypothyroidism. Although T_3 was administered, the hypothyroidism probably increased the total amount of T_3 that would have been necessary to override the low binding T_3-affinity of the mutant receptors.[60]

Location of Mutations

The c-*erb*Aβ gene mutations found in general resistance patients are clustered in two regions, the distal and proximal regions of the T_3-binding domain. The mutant receptors are transcriptionally inactive and inhibit transcriptional activity of normal receptors. Nagaya et al. tested four mutant receptors from general resistance patients. Transcriptional activity of the mutant was correlated with its T_3-binding affinity. Two distal region mutants that displayed partial T_3-binding exhibited strong dominant-negative activity at low T_3 concentrations. At high T_3 concentrations, however, they were transcriptionally active. Two proximal region mutants did not bind T_3. They were 5-to-10 times less potent as inhibitors of normal receptors. The fact that they exhibited dominant-negative inhibition at all indicates that this activity is not correlated with T_3-binding. The investigators concluded from these findings that the location of mutations within the gene (distal or proximal) may influence the degree of dominant-negative activity, providing a potential basis for phenotypic variability in thyroid hormone resistance.[173]

Different Mutations Within the c-erbAβ Gene Have Divergently Different Effects on Dimerization

Hao and coworkers tested two different mutants. One was the S receptor (deletion of threonine-332). This receptor from a kindred with general resistance is a potent inhibitor of normal receptors. The researchers found that the S receptor augments homodimerization of the c-*erb*Aβ₁ receptor. The other receptor (from a patient with severe pituitary resistance with "compromised" dominant-negative inhibition) is coded by the mutant arginine-311-histidine gene. The mutant c-*erb*Aβ₁ receptor has severely impaired homodimerization and less severely impaired heterodimerization. The investigators wrote that these findings indicate that different mutations in the c-*erb*Aβ gene have divergent dimerization activities.[214]

In line with this view, Nomura and coworkers reported predominantly decreased formation of homodimers associated with mutations. They identified two mutations not previously reported in resistant patients. The mutations were situated close to the dimerization domain at codon 435 histidine (H435L and H435Q). The researchers also artificially created two additional mutations (H435R and H435E). The T_3-binding affinities of all four receptors were below detection, and the receptors were not able to induce transcription. Homodimer formation varied among the mutant receptors (especially at the DR4 TRE). With a basic amino acid at codon 435, the receptors formed homodimers normally, but when neutral and acidic amino acids were substituted, formation of homodimers decreased.[226]

Mutant Thyroid Hormone Receptors as Homodimers May Block Transcription of Some Genes

To regulate transcription, α and β T_3-receptors bind to specific T_3 response elements (TREs) in the promoter region of target genes.[188] High affinity binding of T_3-receptors to TREs requires heterodimerization with the retinoid X receptors.[195][196][197][198][199][200] The retinoid X receptors enhance transcriptional activity of T_3-receptors.[195][198][200][201] T_3-receptor/retinoid X receptor heterodimers function as repressors or as activators on TREs, respectively increasing or decreas-

ing transcription. In that T_3-receptors bind TREs with high affinity only as heterodimers, they differ from steroid hormone receptors. Steroid receptors function as ligand-dependent enhancers of transcription as homodimers.[188]

T_3-receptors activate transcription of some genes and repress transcription of other genes.[207] For example, the TREpal preferentially binds T_3-receptor/retinoid X receptor heterodimers.[202] On such TREs, heterodimers not activated by ligand can, through competitive binding to the TREs, repress otherwise ligand-activated heterodimers.[203]

Piedrafita and coworkers found that unliganded T_3-receptor/T_3-receptor homodimers (not bound to T_3), which form at a selective set of TREs,[208] block transcription.[188] A number of researchers failed to detect these homodimers in the absence of DNA, suggesting that the DNA binding sites catalyze formation of the homodimers.[195][196][199][200][208] Binding of T_3 to the T_3-receptor appears to prevent homodimers from forming on TREs. This prevents repression by homodimers, and possibly relieves repression by previously formed homodimers on the TREs, enabling transcription to proceed.[208] It is noteworthy that T_3-binding to the single normal T_3-receptor component of the heterodimer induces transcription. In contrast, binding of T_3 to the two T_3-receptors of the homodimer does not stimulate ligand-homodimer induced transcription. Transcriptional activity resumes with T_3 binding to the T_3-receptor/T_3-receptor homodimer probably because T_3-binding to the receptors of the homodimer causes them to detach from the TRE.

Piedrafita and coworkers analyzed c-*erb*Aβ receptor mutants from individuals with general resistance. The result was that the mutant receptors formed heterodimers and homodimers that exhibited normal binding to DNA. However, because of the low T_3-binding affinity of the mutant receptors, T_3 did not inhibit homodimer formation on TREs. Homodimers formed on the TREs as do homodimers composed of normal T_3-receptors in the absence of T_3, and transcription remains repressed.[188]

OTHER POSSIBLE MOLECULAR DEFECTS UNDERLYING GENERAL RESISTANCE TO THYROID HORMONE

Mutations in T_3-binding domain of the c-*erb*Aβ gene have been determined to be the molecular defect underlying most cases of general resistance to thyroid hormone. However, recent findings indicate that resistance may result from a variety of other molecular lesions. Lesions can potentially occur at any point in the action of thyroid hormone.

Mutant c-erbAβ₂ Receptors

Researchers have proposed that the mixed hyperthyroid-/hypothyroid-like symptoms of some resistant patients reflect the variable responsiveness of different tissues to T_3. The researchers have attributed this variable responsiveness of tissues to relative expression of the c-erbAβ₁ receptors and c-erbAα receptor variants in those tissues.[3] According to this view, in a resistant patient, tissues in which expression of the mutant c-erbAβ gene predominates would be more resistant to T_3 than tissues with a high expression of the c-erbAα gene.

Ng and coworkers wrote that their findings indicate a more complex scenario involving both c-erbAβ₁ and c-erbAβ₂ receptors. (The c-erbAβ₂ receptor has been largely neglected in studies of receptor function.) They found that both mutant c-erbAβ₁ and mutant c-erbAβ₂ receptors were totally ineffective in inducing transcription of reporters' nucleotide sequences carrying a palindromic or inverted repeat in fibroblasts and neuronal cells, even when exposed to high T_3 concentrations. Also, in both types of cells, both mutant c-erbAβ₁ and mutant c-erbAβ₂ receptors inhibited T_3-dependent transcription by normal T_3-receptors. The inhibition shows that both mutant c-erbAβ₁ and mutant c-erbAβ₂ receptors may impair transcription *in vivo*. The authors recommended that investigators reassess the conclusion that thyroid hormone resistance involves molecular lesions of only c-erbAβ₁ receptors. Mutant c-erbAβ genes may also mediate resistance through mutant c-erbAβ₂ receptors.[229]

Tissues differ in their relative expression of c-erbAβ₁ and c-erbAβ₂ receptors.[47][250][251][252][253][254] The receptors also differ in their DNA-binding properties. These findings suggest that the receptors may have a different range of activities in specific cells and at specific target genes. Expression of c-erbAβ₂ receptors is more restricted than that of c-erbAβ₁ receptors. β₂ receptors have been identified in anterior pituitary,[47][252] inner ear,[253][254] neuroretina,[251] and regions of the developing brain.[251][253] Hearing impairment, mental retardation, neuropsychological and psychiatric abnormalities, and loss of T_3-dependent suppression of the TSH gene in the thyrotrophs in general and pituitary resistance may involve mutations of one or both isoforms of the c-erbAβ receptor.[229]

Undetermined Abnormal Cofactors

Weiss and coauthors reported failure to find ab-

normalities in either the α or β T_3-receptor genes in a mother and her two children who had severe general resistance. Resistance of the thyrotrophs and peripheral tissues was so severe that therapeutic responses occurred only with 8-to-10 times normal replacement doses of T_4 and T_3. The defect occurred *de novo* in the mother and she transmitted it to her two children by unrelated fathers. An electrophoretic mobility shift assay of nuclear extract from cultured skin fibroblasts showed a strong band in addition to those seen in nuclear extract from normal individuals and patients with thyroid hormone resistance caused by substitution or deletion mutations of the β T_3-receptor gene. A similar additional band was seen in the nuclear extract from one of the children. The coauthors wrote that the etiology of thyroid hormone resistance is not confined to abnormalities in the β T_3-receptor gene: "An abnormal cofactor with a specific function in the regulation of thyroid hormone action is probably involved in the expression of the [thyroid hormone resistance] phenotype in this family."[220]

Increased Rate of Efflux of T₃ from Cells

Ribeiro and coworkers wrote that the intracellular concentration of free T_3 determines the rate and degree of T_3 occupancy of T_3-receptors. In turn, the occupancy determines the extent of T_3-regulated transcription. They reported that hepatoma cells can be made resistant to thyroid hormone by reducing the cellular content of thyroid hormone (by enhancing its efflux). Extrusion from cells was enhanced by a saturable, cold-sensitive mechanism. The researchers then used verapamil (a calcium channel blocker that inhibits mdr/P-glycoprotein function) to inhibit thyroid hormone efflux and thereby reverse the thyroid hormone resistance. They concluded from this that mdr/P-glycoprotein mediated thyroid hormone resistance in the hepatoma cells. They proposed that increased outward transport of thyroid hormone from the cell may be one mechanism of thyroid hormone resistance in the absence of T_3-receptor mutations. This mechanism might also account for the heterogeneity of response to thyroid hormone in different tissues in thyroid hormone resistance patients. Finally, the authors wrote that active thyroid hormone efflux may be a mechanism for physiological regulation of the cellular action of thyroid hormones.[232]

Altered DNA Sequences in Thyroid Hormone Response Elements (TREs)

Ikeda, Wilcox, and Chin pointed out that to regulate transcription T_3 forms a heterodimer with the retinoid X receptor on the TRE. They inquired, however, as to whether the T_3-receptor/retinoid X receptor heterodimer on a TRE is sufficient to induce transcription. They created several TRE mutations (DR4s, which are half-sites arranged as direct repeats with a nucleotide gap of four) that preferentially bound the T_3-receptor/retinoid X receptor heterodimer. They found that binding of T_3 to the heterodimer was not sufficient to activate transcription of the target gene. It is possible that different DNA sequences in specific TREs may alter T_3-mediated transcription by modulating the conformation of the liganded heterodimer.[228]

Absent or Mutant DNA-Binding Domain in the T_3-Receptor

Absence of the DNA-binding domain of the thyroid hormone receptor impairs its function. After introducing into a cell a mutant thyroid hormone receptor that lacked a DNA-binding region in its molecular structure, the investigators found that the function of the receptors was impaired.[21] Liu and colleagues [218] artificially-induced a cystine-73-serine substitution in the DNA-binding domain of a normal T_3-receptor. The receptor then inhibited transcription induction by the α_1 T_3-receptor.

OTHER DISORDERS ASSOCIATED WITH GENERAL RESISTANCE TO THYROID HORMONE

Refetoff, Weiss, and Usala cite four disorders reported to be associated with general resistance.[3,p.387]

Cytomegalovirus Infection

Hirano and colleagues studied an infant with congenital cytomegalovirus who had a clinical picture consistent with general resistance to thyroid hormone. At 3 weeks of age, the infant's serum total and free T_3 and T_4 were above normal despite a high TSH level of 154 µU/mL. She did not have the clinical syndrome of thyrotoxicosis. Only supraphysiologic doses of T_3 (16 µg/kg body weight) suppressed the high TSH to a normal level. While inherited general resistance is permanent, all thyroid function test results returned to normal in this case. The child had normal bone development, but she had mild psychomotor retardation, sensory hearing loss, and microcephaly.[255] Refetoff and coauthors surmised that the transient viremia caused a reduction in the concentration of T_3-receptors or a reduction of cofactors that resulted in general transient resistance to thyroid hormone.[3]

Autosomal Dominant Osteopetrosis

Bollerslev and Kvetny reported seven patients from three families who had autosomal dominant osteopetrosis. They had symmetric osteosclerosis and thickened calvarium vaults. Their mean total T_3 (123±12 ng/dL) was high compared to age-matched controls (94±5 ng/dL), but was within the normal range. No other thyroid function test result was abnormal. Mean maximum binding of T_3 to mononuclear blood cell nuclei was decreased (0.51±0.23 vs 1.8±0.4 fmol T_3/mg DNA), but there was a normal association constant.[256] Refetoff and coauthors stated that it is not clear that the patients had thyroid hormone resistance as reported by Bollerslev and Kvetny.[3]

Cystinosis

Patients with nephropathic cystinosis typically become hypothyroid because cystine crystals accumulate and destroy the thyroid gland parenchyma.[259] Bercu and colleagues reported resistance to thyroid hormone in twelve children with nephropathic cystinosis. The children had inappropriately high serum TSH levels, ranging from 4.5-to-132 µU/nL and exaggerated TSH responses to TRH injections. Only two children had elevated total T_4, total T_3, free T_4, and free T_3. Two had only elevated total T_4, four had only elevated total T_3, four had only elevated free T_4, and five had only elevated free T_3. The mean dosage of T_4 (6.2±1.2 µ/kg body weight) and T_3 (1.9±0.7 µ/kg body weight) necessary to suppress the high TSH levels was higher than that necessary for suppression in hypothyroid children.[257] Refetoff and coauthors noted that although Bercu reported that these patients had pituitary resistance, they appeared to have general resistance in that there was also evidence of peripheral tissue resistance: normal serum cholesterol, red blood cell sodium concentration, 24-hour urinary hydroxyproline, creatine excretion, and pulse rate during sleep. Refetoff and coauthors also wrote that the failure of T_3 secretion to increase after TRH stimulation indicates that the children had reduced thyroid hormone reserve, suggesting that they actually had compensated primary hypothyroidism.[3,p.387]

Childhood Blindness

Bellastella et al. described eight blind boys (ages 7-to-10 years). Blindness was induced before age 1 by sympathetic ophthalmia, ocular trauma, or retrolental fibroplasia. Compared to age- and sex-matched siblings, all had a high serum free T_4 (39±4.7 µg/mL vs 12.0±0.6 µg/mL) and free T_3 (14.0±1.3 µg/mL vs 4.7±0.2 µg/mL). The free T_4 and free T_3 levels were above the upper limit of the normal reference range. TSH levels were within the normal range, and all the blind boys were reported to be clinically euthyroid (probably meaning eumetabolic).[258] These clinical and laboratory findings indicate that the boys had general resistance to thyroid hormone.

● ARE MUTATIONS INSTRUMENTAL IN PERIPHERAL RESISTANCE TO THYROID HORMONE?

Thyroid researchers now consider hormone resistance syndromes to result from lesions at the site of hormone action.[3] If we define thyroid hormone resistance in this way, then there is no evidence at this time that patients who have peripheral cellular resistance to thyroid hormone (which exempts the pituitary gland) actually have thyroid hormone resistance. It is obvious from the available data, however, that in general, euthyroid fibromyalgia patients are hyporesponsive to thyroid hormone. Most require supraphysiologic dosages of T$_3$ before their symptoms of hypometabolism (fibromyalgia) are relieved.[153][154][155]

All general resistance patients are considered to have peripheral resistance, as both the pituitary and the peripheral tissues are resistant. Nonetheless, researchers have not yet identified a molecular lesion responsible for resistance to thyroid hormone in a patient with peripheral resistance only. Usala, one of the main investigators of general resistance, has stated that he is sure peripheral resistance is relatively common. He said that he and a colleague, D. Thomas, sequenced the c-erbAβ gene from one peripheral resistance patient and found no mutations.[132] In 1996, Prof. J. Torresani in Marseille, France, sequenced the c-erbAβ gene from two of my patients.[79] These patients had completely recovered from euthyroid fibromyalgia with supraphysiologic dosages of T$_3$ during a blinded study my colleagues and I conducted.[153] The sequenced genes from these patients were not mutated.

Refetoff, who first described thyroid hormone resistance syndromes, agrees that euthyroid hypometabolic patients are more common than is documented. He has observed euthyroid patients who take large doses (0.3 mg-to-0.4 mg) of synthetic T$_4$ but do not have tachycardia or other indications of excess thyroid hormone stimulation. He has found that some of these patients have negative nitrogen balance (greater excretion than intake of nitrogen). Because of this, he suspects they may have thyroid hormone resistance, but in

some cases, he speculates that the patients may be habituated to the T$_4$, therefore requiring progressively higher doses to maintain their subjective well-being.[85]

In 1928, Thompson and Thompson wrote of the mechanism of euthyroid hypometabolism, "It seems much more likely that the explanation lies in some other obscure pathology about which nothing is known at present."[44,p.495] Until investigators identify a specific molecular lesion in euthyroid hypometabolic patients,[27][29] there is no certainty of the nature of that "obscure pathology."

The patients with cellular resistance to thyroid hormone who come to the attention of clinicians have conditions severe enough to prompt the pursuit of professional assistance. Linus Pauling wrote: "It is harder to recognize a mild genetic disease than a serious one, but the mild genetic diseases may in the aggregate cause more suffering than the serious ones because so many more people suffer from them."[128,pp.114-115] This is true of most abnormal conditions, and recognition of this truth should motivate clinicians to remain vigilant for even subtle indications of hypometabolism that might be due to cellular resistance to thyroid hormone. My colleagues and I have found in blinded trials that euthyroid fibromyalgia patients typically improve or recover with metabolic therapy. When clinicians encounter such patients, the patients should be given an opportunity for possible relief through this form of treatment.

● "TYPE II HYPOTHYROIDISM": PROPOSED NOMENCLATURE FOR THYROID HORMONE RESISTANCE

Garrison recently recommended a change in nomenclature for thyroid hormone resistance.[262] He suggested that his proposed nomenclature could permit the creation of terms that meaningfully relate to one another. As he pointed out in the passage below, this could reduce the proliferation of terms for diagnostic classification.

> The issue of fibromyalgia requires an emphasis on precise use of language. Obviously, in classic hypothyroidism, insufficient thyroid hormone quantity leads to failure of that hormone to properly regulate gene transcription. However, when thyroid hormone is in normal supply, it can still fail to properly regulate gene transcription. One mechanism has been proven and several implied [see above and below in this chapter]. Mecha-

nisms for thyroid resistance may be diverse among patients, making nomenclature problematic.

Two types of nomenclature already exist for distinguishing between syndromes of endocrine deficiency and endocrine resistance. One of these, associated with parathyroid hormone resistance, is horrendous. The other, used in diabetes mellitus, is neatly organized and may be taken as a useful prototype.

Diabetes is currently separated into type I (insulin deficient) and type II (insulin resistant) categories. These categories are both theoretically and practically useful because proper classification is a good predictor of differential responsiveness to different treatments. Type I disease typically does better with insulin replacement therapy, whereas type II disease responds best to therapies directed to the mechanisms of resistance so that endogenous insulin can function with usual efficiency. Mixed disease is seen with both type I and type II elements. Finally, types of resistance are described in six general categories: reduced numbers of receptors; poor receptor affinity, whether genetic or acquired; post-receptor effects as are seen with glut-4 phosphorylation; oppositional effects of other biological pathways, such as from the stress hormones; absence of cofactor effects, as with hypothyroidism; and competitive inhibition as with insulin-antibody complexes and possibly placental lactogen. If this language were expanded to designate all disorders of production as type I endocrinopathies and disorders of utilization as type II endocrinopathies, most cases of fibromyalgia would reclassify as type II hypothyroidism. A few would be mixed type II/type I, and some would be type I hypothyroidism. Occasional cases of fibromyalgia would be found not to involve thyroid hormone. The various types of resistance to thyroid hormone could be classified in the same six categories listed above for type II diabetes.

This change in nomenclature would facilitate understanding fibromyalgia's relative position in the spectrum of known diseases. It may well be that the fibromyalgia-like syndromes such as chronic fatigue syndrome will be found to differ from fibromyalgia only in the mechanism of resistance. Just as importantly, good nomenclature will facilitate recognition of the importance of type II multiple endocrinopathy. This multiplicity can be seen in the occasional fibromyalgia patient who, in addition to being thyroid-resistant, may be, for example, insulin resistant, estrogen-resistant, or progesterone-resistant as well. Such patients may become less resistant to other hormones as the thyroid resistance clears, as in the case of restoration of normal glucose tolerance in the fibromyalgia patient effectively treated with thyroid hormone. Just as important, treatment of the other resistan-

ces may facilitate recovery from the thyroid resistance.

This entire question deserves more attention, as it seems likely that resistance to many or most hormones may engender other resistances. Multiple endocrine resistances have likewise been described in parathyroid hormone resistance. And it may be that insulin resistance in type II diabetes may be approachable much of the time by attacking other resistance.

Unplanned nomenclature, as typified by the classification of parathyroid hormone disorders, can lead to serious proliferation of idiosyncratic labels. Different endocrinology texts present diverse and even conflicting categories for these disorders, using words like "ineffective," "overwhelmed," and "inadequate" to describe varieties of resistance. Six of these involve, by various mechanisms, unavailability of vitamin D as a co-factor, whether because of deficiency or resistance. Four others use the tortuous terms "pseudohypoparathyroidism" and "pseudopseudohypoparathyroidism" to denote various kinds of receptor or post-receptor resistance. Recognition of the important multiple-resistance aspects of parathyroid hormone resistance is lost in these schematics.

As is apparent from the analogy to diabetes, appropriate therapy for thyroid hormone resistance would be directed in the future towards restoration of receptor sensitivity. Currently, however, properly titrating an effective dosage of T_3 for the thyroid hormone resistant fibromyalgia patient is the best available treatment.[262]

● **OTHER POSSIBLE MECHANISMS OF THYROID HORMONE RESISTANCE**

The general resistance patients Refetoff and his coworkers originally studied had no defect in: (1) the synthesis of normal thyroid hormone, (2) hormone binding in the plasma, (3) hormone penetration into the target cell, (4) conversion of T_4 to T_3, or (5) the rate of hormone breakdown.[3][35] The defect did not involve antibodies to T_3, although these have been demonstrated in some patients with acquired resistance to T_3.[6]

These exclusions led to the conclusion that the defect was either at the intracellular receptor or the post-receptor effector machinery.[7,p.276] Investigators later showed two abnormalities. First, receptors in the nuclei of peripheral lymphocytes from the two original general resistance patients bound less than one-tenth as much T_3 as do receptors in nuclei of normal individuals. Second, they showed that these T_3-receptors did not bind T_3 to the patients' lymphocyte chromatin.[66]

Table 2.6.5. Mechanisms of hormone resistance.[δ]

RESISTANCE TO ENDOGENOUS HORMONES ONLY:
(1) Incompletely synthesized or cleaved hormones
(2) Abnormal hormones

RESISTANCE TO ENDOGENOUS AND EXOGENOUS HORMONES:
(1) Physiologic antagonism
(2) Antibodies to hormones
(3) Antibodies to hormone receptors
(4) Absence of target cells
(5) Abnormal or absent receptors
(6) C-erbAβ gene mutations
(7) C-erbAα gene mutations[γ]
(8) Post-receptor-effector defects

[δ]After Verhoeven, G.F.M. and Wilson, J.D.: The syndromes of primary hormone resistance. *Metabolism*, 28(3):253-289, 1979.[7,p.254]
[γ]Verhoeven and Wilson did not include this defect in their list.

Finding these abnormalities aimed research toward T_3-receptors, and eventually toward the source of the receptor defect, the β gene that codes for the receptors. This discovery, and the identification of the mutation in many general resistance patients, did not eliminate the possibility that other molecular faults are instrumental in peripheral resistance to thyroid hormone. Refetoff wrote that inconsistent laboratory findings show that general resistance is the result of a number of defects in thyroid hormone action. Defects in nuclear receptors is only one of these.[8,p.1295] Peripheral resistance to thyroid hormone may also be caused by a variety of defects in thyroid hormone action. As I mentioned above, Usala and Darby[132] found no mutations in the β gene of the one peripheral resistance patient whose case is well-documented in the literature,[81] and Torresani did not find a mutation when sequencing the gene from two of my recovered patients.[79] One or more of these patients may have a mutation of the c-erbAα gene, which we did not sequence. However, they could have euthyroid hypometabolism due to a number of other mechanisms of cellular resistance to thyroid hormone. In fact, there may be a variety of molecular faults in any individual euthyroid hypometabolic patient. For this reason, I include in this section an outline of the possible defects researchers have investigated. This outline is in physiological sequence: it begins with defects in the thyroid gland and ends with the effects of thyroid hormones as they serve their cellular functions.

Table 2.6.5 lists a variety of causes of hormone resistance. A tissue may be resistant to thyroid hormone because of more than one defect. Any combination of defects may affect the pituitary, peripheral tissues, or both.

DEFECTS IN THE THYROID GLAND

Early investigators suspected that the defect in resistant patients was at the cellular level in the thyroid gland. Such defects would result in defective thyroid hormones incapable of adequately stimulating target cells. As of 1958, however, they had found no abnormalities in the gland itself. Patients' thyroid glands were normal in all important respects. The glands normally: (1) trapped iodine, (2) synthesized and released T_4 and T_3, (3) bound the hormone to proteins, and (4) responded to TSH. The researchers concluded that, evidently, the defect was outside the thyroid gland.[34]

DEFECTIVE THYROID HORMONES

Some patients are resistant to their endogenous hormones, but not to exogenous hormones. These patients may have hormones that are abnormal in some way. The molecular structure of the hormones, for example, may not be complete. Patients with abnormal endogenous hormones respond normally when they take exogenous hormones in roughly equivalent amounts. Patients with true hormone resistance, however, are insensitive to both endogenous and exogenous hormones. Many patients with euthyroid hypometabolism improve only with large doses of exogenous T_3, indicating that the defect is not abnormal molecular structure of endogenous thyroid hormones. Also, two studies showed that in the thyroid hormone resistance patients studied, endogenous T_3 and T_4 were authentic and stereochemically normal.[35][36]

DEFECTS AT THE CELLULAR LEVEL

Most defects in thyroid hormone resistance occur at the level of target cells,[7,p.254] and most studies of resistance have focused on these defects. Some of these studies have contributed to our knowledge of endocrinology by identifying some specific steps in the action of hormones in cells.

Verhoeven and Wilson arbitrarily divided disorders of hormone resistance into two types: (1) those involving hormones whose primary receptor mechanism is on the cell surface, and (2) those involving hormones whose receptors are intracellular. Protein hormones such as insulin bind to surface receptors, as do biogenic amines such as norepinephrine. Steroid hormones such as cortisol and estrogen bind to intracellular receptors.[7] Thyroid hormones bind to nuclear receptors and mitochondrial receptors, and also to surface receptors of cells such as fibroblasts.[7,p.254]

Free thyroid hormones, those not bound to carrier proteins in the plasma, passively diffuse into cells. Inside the cell, T_4 (H) undergoes conversion to T_3 (H'). This conversion "activates" the hormone. Some T_3, however, is formed from T_4 in other cells, leaves the converting cell, and is transported through the plasma to target cells. Steroids, in contrast to T_3, diffuse into the cell and combine with a specific receptor protein (R) in the cytoplasm of the cell. This forms a hormone-receptor complex (H'R'). This "activated" H'R' then passes from the cytoplasm into the nucleus. T_3 may bind minimally to proteins in the cytoplasm. For the most part, though, T_3 passes unbound from the cytoplasm into the nucleus. There it combines with a receptor protein to form H'R'. T_3, as part of this complex, then binds to chromatin (DNA attached to its base, a protein structure). One mechanism of resistance may involve the binding of T_3 to a protein in the cytoplasm, essentially causing the T_3 to be captured so that it is not available to enter the nucleus and bind to the nuclear T_3-receptor.

Upon combining with chromatin, the H'R' activates a series of reactions called post-receptor effector mechanisms. The minimum post-receptor effector mechanism is the formation of new messenger RNA (mRNA). The mRNA travels to and attaches to the ribosomes in the cytoplasm. There, it interacts with the ribosomes and transfer RNA to synthesize proteins.[7,p.267] The transfer RNA binds amino acids in the cytoplasm and transports them to the ribosomes where they bind in a sequence dictated by the sequences of bases of the mRNA. Transfer RNAs are specific for each individual amino acid.[91,p.162] (See Chapter 2.2.)

During this process, defects causing hormone resistance might occur at a minimum of five points: (1) conversion of T_4 to T_3, (2) formation and (3) activation of the T_3-receptor complex, (4) binding of the T_3-receptor complex to chromatin, and (5) various post-receptor effector mechanisms such as the process of translation.[7,p.267]

Defective Transport of T_4 Across Plasma Membranes

One study of general resistance patients found evidence of defective transport of T_4 across the plasma membrane of red blood cells.[36] Other studies, however, showed normal uptake of T_4 and T_3 by red and white blood cells and fibroblasts.[37][38][39]

Defects in the Conversion of T_4 to T_3

Several investigators have proposed that some hypothyroid and euthyroid hypometabolic patients are not able to deiodinate T_4 to T_3, the most metabolically active form of thyroid hormone. In 1957, Hutchison and Arneil reported the case of a cretinous girl who did not improve on desiccated thyroid. She became normal, though, in all respects, both physically and mentally, after beginning supplemental T_3. These authors proposed that because the girl did not improve with desiccated thyroid, which contains mostly T_4, and did improve with T_3, her cells did not effectively convert T_4 to T_3.[40]

Rosler and colleagues studied a hypermetabolic family whose pituitary resistance was apparently due to a reduced rate of conversion of T_4 to T_3 in the pituitary. In these family members, taking physiologic doses of T_3 in a single daily dose produced two effects. First, it caused intermittent elevations in their serum T_3 levels that effectively suppressed TSH secretion. Second, it relieved their hypermetabolism.[114]

Cooper and his associates reported that three patients with both pituitary and peripheral resistance responded to T_3. The investigators found normal binding of thyroid hormones to the nuclei of the patients' leukocytes. They wrote that because hormone receptors were normal in these patients' leukocytes, the defect was most likely at the post-receptor level. The investigators speculated, however, that conversion of T_4 to T_3 in these patients' thyroid glands or in their peripheral tissues was defective.[117,p.508] Cells other than the patients' circulating leukocytes, however, may have had defective receptors or too few receptors to effectively bind the hormone.

Refetoff wrote that a minor defect in T_3 generation is reasonable for two reasons. First, administering T_3 just above the physiologic level to general resistance patients from several families suppressed the secretion of TSH. This suppression suggested that the patients may be more sensitive to T_3 than T_4.[78][117][118] Second, other investigators found elevated T_4 and reverse T_3 in healthy, eumetabolic family members whose serum T_3 was normal. The elevated T_4 was not due to elevated binding protein. Generation of reverse T_3 is an alternate to T_3 production during deiodination of T_4. This laboratory picture is consistent with a primary abnormality in the deiodination of T_4 in peripheral tissues.[8,p.1294]

According to Refetoff, researchers have not used thyroid hormone resistant patients to carry out *in vivo* studies of the conversion of T_4 to T_3 outside the thyroid gland.[8] Schimmel and Utiger reported that the ratio of T_3 to T_4 in general resistance patients is similar to that of healthy euthyroid people (ranging from 0.010-to-0.025).[77] In an *in vitro* study of cultured fibroblasts from thyroid hormone resistant patients, T_3 formation by monodeiodination of T_4 was normal.[39] Refetoff found that general resistance patients converted T_4 to T_3 normally.[39]

Inhibition of T_4 to T_3 Conversion by Elevated Glucocorticoids. Another mechanism that may block thyroid hormone action is endogenous glucocorticoids. Glucocorticoids block T_4 to T_3 conversion, and they suppress TSH secretion by the pituitary thyrotrophs. *These effects reverse to normal within 1-to-3 weeks*, even though stress-induced cortisol remains elevated or even though a patient continues to take exogenous cortisol.[135][172][180]

Myofascial patients may have elevated levels of glucocorticoids.[9] Theoretically, these patients may generate a high enough glucocorticoid level to temporarily block the conversion of T_4 to T_3. About 30% of chronic fatigue syndrome patients have low, rather than high, cortisol levels.[32] To my knowledge, studies for thyroid hormone resistance have not been done on myofascial patients who have elevated blood levels of glucocorticoids.

I have observed patients who first injured a muscle, developed pain syndromes limited to one or a few muscles, and before recovering from these simple myofascial syndromes, developed what may be termed full-blown fibromyalgia. Goldenberg has also reported observing this sequence of events.[123] As time passes after the initial injury and the patient suffers neverending somatogenic stress in the form of myofascial pain, she develops insomnia, fatigue, gastrointestinal dysfunction, and depression. These are normal physiological and psychological sequelae to noxious myofascial stimulation.[107][108] Many of these patients are dramatically relieved of this syndrome partially or completely when treated with T_3, although T_4 seems to be of no benefit.[124] A possible explanation for these observations is that some patients' somatic stress is associated with elevated glucocorticoid levels that in turn inhibit TSH secretion and T_4 to T_3 conversion. A resulting low cellular concentration of T_3, in turn, may

produce and sustain the complex clinical syndrome from which the patient suffers. Based on available data, this condition should be time-limited in most patients. Most likely, however, these clinical symptoms are induced in patients already predisposed by either borderline thyroid hormone insufficiency or marginal cellular resistance to thyroid hormone.

Inhibition of T_4 to T_3 Conversion by Mercury. Studies of the effects of mercury on the thyroid system have produced mixed results. The mixed results may be a result of differences in the magnitude and chronicity of mercury exposure in study subjects.

Kawada et al. noted that both methylmercuric chloride and mercuric chloride caused a 50% inhibition of Na^+/K^+-ATPase in hog thyroid membranous tissue. In a 1980 study, they gave mice intraperitoneal injections of mercury (5 μg of mercurial per gram body weight daily for two consecutive days). At 4 and 24 hours, the uptake of ^{131}I by the thyroid gland was reduced. In addition, the production of radioactively labeled iodothyronines was reduced. (Iodothyronines are the thyroid hormones T_3 and T_4. These molecules are produced when the enzyme peroxidase catalyzes the coupling of T_1 and T_2 to form T_3 and T_4. See Chapter 2.1, subsection titled "Thyroid Hormone Production in the Thyroid Gland.") Iodotyrosine deiodinase was inhibited by mercury *in vitro* and *in vivo*. (Iodotyrosine deiodinases in the thyroid gland break down T_1 and T_2 that is not combined into T_3 and T_4. The breakdown frees iodide molecules. See Chapter 2.1, subsection titled "Enzymatic Breakdown of T_1, T_2, T_3, and T_4.") Four and 24 hours after administration of mercury, the serum bound ^{131}I-iodide had decreased. The investigators noted that the circulating T_4 levels, estimated by radioimmunoassay, were reduced. This result indicates that hormone secretion was acutely decreased by mercury.[106]

Langworth et al. reported that the mean basal serum TSH, T_3, and T_4 levels of dental personnel exposed to mercury vapor from dental amalgam did not differ from levels in an unexposed control group. The groups also did not differ in the mean TSH response to the injection of 25 μg of TRH. According to these findings, chronic, low-grade exposure to mercury vapor did not have a negative influence on the pituitary-thyroid axis.[247]

Erfurth et al. reported similar results. They noted that elementary mercury vapor results in an accumulation of mercury in the pituitary and thyroid glands. To determine whether the accumulation altered the function of the pituitary-thyroid axis, they compared the differences in urinary mercury concentration and thyroid indices of eleven workers and nine dentists. The mean urinary mercury of the workers was 26 nmol/mmol creatinine and of the dentists was 1.3 nmol/mmol creatinine. The basal serum levels of TSH and the TSH response to TRH injections did not differ between the eleven male workers and nine male dentists, despite the differences in their urinary mercury concentrations. There was also no association between urinary mercury levels and serum concentrations of free T_3 and free T_4.[102]

Emerson has indicated that some fibromyalgia patients have benefitted from removal of mercury amalgam dental fillings. As he suggested, chronic exposure due to high mercury uptake from dental amalgam fillings may inhibit 5'-deiodinase conversion of T_4 to T_3, creating a form of thyroid hormone resistance.[109]

Consistent with Emerson's view, the study results of Barregard et al. indicated that mercury may inhibit the activity of 5'-deiodinase. These researchers assessed the effects of occupational exposure to mercury vapor on the function of the thyroid system. They studied 41 workers exposed to chloralkali vapor for an average of 10 years and compared them with 41 age-matched controls. Chloralkali workers had a mean urinary mercury concentration of 27 µg/g (15 nmol/mmol) creatinine; the control group had a mean urinary concentration of 3.3 µg/g (1.9 nmol/mmol) creatinine. The workers had a mean blood level of 46 nmol/L; the mean blood level of the control group was 17 nmol/L. The mean TSH level was not associated with mercury exposure. However, the workers with the highest mercury exposure had a significantly higher mean serum free T_4 level and a high ratio of free T_4 to free T_3. The cumulative mercury exposure was inversely correlated with the serum free T_3. These results suggest that T_4 to T_3 conversion was impaired in the workers, possibly due to inhibition of 5'-deiodinase by mercury.[110]

The exposure of humans to mercury is widespread. Because of this, further studies should be carried out to explore the possible role of mercury in cellular resistance to thyroid hormone.

Note: In the Erfurth et al. mercury study, the researchers found that increased plasma levels of selenium were associated with increased basal serum levels of TSH.[102] The positive correlation of TSH and selenium levels is contrary to the finding of Hagmar et al. They studied the relationships between fish intake, selenium status, and thyroid hormone function in coastal fishermen and inland subjects from Latvia. The researchers found that the mean plasma selenium level in those with a high fish intake (21-to-50 fish meals per month) was 81% higher than in those with the lowest fish intake. Thyroid hormone levels were not correlated with fish intake, plasma selenium, or selenoprotein P levels. However, the mean serum TSH was inversely correlated with plasma selenium and selenoprotein P. The researchers concluded that (1) selenium from high fish consumption markedly increased all measures of selenium status, (2) selenium status did not alter T_3 and T_4 levels, but that (3) low selenium levels may be associated with increased TSH secretion.[105]

Mutant Thyroid Receptor Auxiliary Protein (TRAP)

Usala suggested sequencing a gene that codes for TRAP (a protein such as the retinoid X receptor[185]). This protein binds to the T_3-receptor and facilitates its function. If mutated, it would fail to facilitate the T_3-receptor and theoretically would give rise to thyroid hormone resistance.[132]

Mixed Hypothyroid and Hyperthyroid Effects of Dioxins and PCBs

McKinney and coauthors pointed out that the overall toxic biological effects of dioxins and PCBs are variably those of both hypothyroidism and hyperthyroidism. These authors proposed that the competitive binding of these pollutants to transthyretin provides a model for their binding to nuclear thyroid hormone receptors.[206] They conjectured that hyperthyroid effects may result from the toxins attaching to thyroid hormone receptors and potently and persistently altering gene expression.[171][261,p.232] The alterations would involve activation of genes normally activated by thyroid hormone and repression of genes normally repressed by the hormone. These alterations might account for the initial "metabolic boost" found in studies of birds exposed to various chlorinated hydrocarbon insecticides,[120] and the initial stimulation of the growth phase that precedes inhibition of growth phase in tadpoles and rats.[261,p.239] It could also possibly account for certain features of fibromyalgia that appear to resemble hyperthyroid characteristics (anxiety, nervousness, excess warmth, diarrhea) against a general background of hypometabolic features (lethargy, fatigue, low motor drive, depression). Such mixed metabolic effects have been found in some patients with general resistance to thyroid hormone. The effects might occur if dioxins or PCBs attach to T_3-receptors on the β- and α-adrenergic receptor genes and persistently activate transcription of mRNAs for the β-adrenergic receptor gene and repress mRNAs for the α-adrenergic receptor gene.

Possible Mechanism of Adverse Effects. Porterfield defines PCB and dioxin exposure as environmental insults to the fetus and neonate.[100] Because these two classes of pollutants and thyroid hormones have similar chemical structures, they also have similar binding properties. As a result, problems arise from the affinity for and binding of the pollutants to three types of molecules—the cytoplasmic Ah receptor (the "dioxin receptor"[171,p.79][261,p.232]), the nuclear thyroid hormone receptor, and the thyroid hormone transport protein, transthyretin. Depending on the congener and its dosage, PCBs and dioxins either decrease or mimic the biological action of thyroid hormones. Either effect during critical stages of brain development can harm a fetus or neonate.

Porterfield points out that children who were exposed to dioxins or PCBs in the uterus or during infancy may suffer from behavioral disorders that resemble those resulting from hypothyroidism *in utero* or in infancy. He stated that the data suggest that these abnormalities in dioxin- and PCB-exposed children can be partially or completely the result of abnormalities of thyroid hormone availability or action. "It is possible," he wrote, "that transient exposure of the mother to doses of toxins presently considered nontoxic to the mother could have an impact upon fetal or perinatal neurological development. If the toxins act via their effect on thyroid hormone action, it is possible that doses of toxins that would normally not alter fetal development, could become deleterious if superimposed on a preexisting maternal or fetal thyroid disorder."[100]

Post-Receptor Effector Defect: Genetically-Based Selective Resistance to Thyroid Hormones

Liewendahl[67] and colleagues[68] wrote that the defect causing thyroid hormone resistance might be a fault in the "post-receptor effector mechanism." Such a fault, for example, might be improper translation at the ribosomes.

Low Thyroid Hormone Receptor Density

In animals, reduced caloric intake,[126][127] uremia,[129][130] and other models of nonthyroidal illness reduce the density of T_3-receptors. DeGroot concluded that "a tenable hypothesis is that the changes represent a group of selective physiologic responses designed to . . . protect tissues from the catabolic effects of T_3 and T_4 during the illnesses."[131] It appears, then, that receptors can down-regulate for adaptive purposes. They may also down-regulate as a pathophysiologic process.

Guernsy and Moroshige have shown that ob/ob mice have a low density of nuclear T_3-receptors in liver and lung tissues. The mice have normal circulating levels of thyroid hormones and blunted end-organ responses to thyroid hormone. Probably as an adaptation, they have superefficient metabolism. They have low resting oxygen consumption. Since they cannot increase thermogenesis on exposure to cold, they inadequately adapt to cold.[10,p.324]

York and his group found a post-receptor effector mechanism defect in the ob/ob experimental mouse. The mouse has a selective resistance to thyroid hormone action. The specific defect is in the ability of the mouse to increase Na^+/K^+-ATPase in liver and kidney tissues in response to doses of T_3. The authors speculate that the mouse's Na^+/K^+-ATPase is structurally abnormal and has little or no activity. The result is that the mouse generates too little heat. Also, epinephrine in the mouse is not able to adequately induce fat breakdown, and the mouse is therefore obese. Thyroid action is otherwise normal in the mouse.[69]

Age-Related Decrease in Responsiveness to Thyroid Hormone

Some studies have shown an age-related decline in responsiveness to T_4 and T_3 in rats.[13][14][15][16] However, Gambert and colleagues found no age-related changes in T_3-receptors in human mononuclear cells.[12,p.350][17] Because of this finding, Gambert postulated that an undetermined alteration in post-receptor function must account for the age-related decline in responsiveness to thyroid hormone in rats.[12,p.350]

The range of possible defects is broad, and research may target multiple defects. Decreased numbers of thyroid hormone receptors can occur as in other hormone resistance syndromes. Individuals who have androgen resistance, for example, have an absence of androgen receptor protein in the cytoplasm of cells.[28,p.939] The defect in "resistance" may not be related directly to thyroid hormone or its receptors, although T_3 may override or compensate for the defect, increasing metabolism and improving symptoms.

Fibromyalgia patients may, for example, have energy deficits in cells because of a mutation in the genome of the mitochondria. German researchers reported a mutation of the mitochondrial genome of some fibromyalgia patients, but we cannot conclude from their data that the mutation is etiologically related to fibromyalgia.[30] Research that began in the 1950s showed that mitochondrial genes rather than nuclear genes control some mitochondrial features.[121,p.877] Several diseases result from mutations of mitochondrial genes. In these diseases, patients' mitochondrial structure and some enzyme activities are abnormal. Organ systems whose energy is dependent on mitochondrial activity, including the central nervous system and the skeletal muscles, are damaged.[121,p.879] Theoretically, T_3 could compensate for a mitochondrial gene mutation in fibromyalgia patients. A mitochondrial mutation would not account for all fibromyalgia symptoms and objective findings, however.

By analogy with pseudo-parathyroidism, some fibromyalgia patients may have defects of the G_s proteins of catecholamine-sensitive cells. G_s proteins are links in the chain of molecular steps that mediate cell stimulation by catecholamines. This defect impairs many cellular processes dependent on basal and surge levels of catecholamines. The result would be similar to pseudo-parathyroidism, a condition in which target organs have a blunted response to adequate levels of parathormone. The cause is a genetically-determined deficiency or functional inadequacy of G_s.[10,p.35]

Cooper, Bloom, and Roth conjecture that the local ionic environment of a receptor may desensitize it so that it does not respond normally to its chemical agonists such as hormones.[92,p.103] The first step in the desensitization of a receptor is uncoupling of the receptor from its G_s-adenyl cyclase complex. Uncoupling probably occurs when phosphate combines with the receptor molecule (receptor phosphorylation). The receptor is a substrate for most protein kinases, including cAMP-dependent kinase and C kinase. An adequate concentration of cAMP could activate kinases whose action is cAMP-dependent, and the kinases might stimulate phosphorylation of the β adrenergic receptor. Phosphorylation uncouples the receptor from its G_s protein.[92,p.254] Phosphorylation therefore impairs a receptor's ability to communicate with its G_s protein. If the receptor cannot combine with its G_s protein, adenylate cyclase will not be activated. As a result, the hormone attached to the receptor will have little or no effect on the target cell. Next, the receptor becomes sequestered in an endocytosed vesicle in the plasma membrane away from its G protein and adenyl cyclase. Vesicles containing the receptors are then processed by Golgi and recycled back to the plasma membrane, or phagocytosed and degraded by lysosomes. Resensitization involves either a Golgi package returning the receptor to the plasma membrane, or replacement in the membrane of phagocytosed receptors by new receptors synthesized in the cytoplasm of the cell.[10,pp.238-239]

Cooper, Bloom, and Roth also suggested that polymerization (clustering) of receptor subunits may occur. Also, depolymerization may inactivate receptors by changing them into an inactive structural form.[92,p.103]

Cooper, Bloom, and Roth wrote that investigators recently isolated the complimentary DNA clone that codes for synthesis of a protein that serves as a membrane transporter for norepinephrine. Its cDNA sequence predicts that it is constructed of 617 amino acids with 12-to-13 hydrophobic sections. Its function is dependent on sodium, and it is sensitive to pharmaceutical norepinephrine inhibitors. The researchers noted that its nucleotide sequence is strikingly similar to that of GABA (gamma aminobutyric acid) transporter protein. These investigators may have come upon a new family of genes that carry the code for transporters.[92,p.250]

Cooper et al. wrote that the availability of human cDNA that codes for norepinephrine transporter protein will be fortuitous, offering an opportunity to determine whether alterations in the corresponding genes play an etiological role in major depression or other affective disorders.[92,p.250] If so, some of the effects of this mechanism would overlap one effect of hypothyroidism and cellular resistance to thyroid hormone—impaired catecholamine regulation of cells due to a shift from α-adrenergic/β-adrenergic balance toward α-adrenergic dominance. Finding the gene coded for norepinephrine transporter protein has obvious implications for the study of fibromyalgia.

SUMMARY

Euthyroid fibromyalgia patients, despite normal thyroid function test results, appear to have hypometabolism of various tissues due to cellular resistance to thyroid hormone. Multiple mechanisms may interact to induce and sustain euthyroid fibromyalgia by rendering cells partially resistant to thyroid hormone. Regardless of the underlying mechanism, it is likely that in many cases, failed thyroid hormone expression mediates the signs and symptoms of euthyroid fibromyalgia.

REFERENCES

1. Refetoff, S., Dewind, L.T., and DeGroot, L.J.: Familial syndrome combining deaf-mutism, stippled epiphyses, goiter and abnormally high PBI: possible target organ refractoriness to thyroid hormone. *J. Clin. Endocrinol. Metab.*, 27:279, 1967.

2. Lasker, N.B. and Ryan, R.J.: Half-life of radiothyroxine in non-thyroidal hypometabolism. *J. Clin. Endocrinol.*,

18:538-539, 1958.

3. Refetoff, S., Weiss, R.E., and Usala, S.J.: The syndromes of resistance to thyroid hormone. *Endocr. Rev.*, 14:348-399, 1993.

4. Albright, F., Butler, A.M., and Bloomberg, E.: Rickets resistent to vitamin D therapy. *Am. J. Dis. Child.*, 54:531-547, 1937.

5. Albright, F., Burnett, C.H., Smith, P.G., and Parson, W.: Pseudohypoparathyroidism: an example of "Seabright-Bantam syndrome." *Endocrinology*, 30:922-932, 1942.

6. Ginsberg, J., Segal, D., Ehrlich, R.M., and Walfish, P.G.: Inappropriate triiodothyronine (T_3) and thyroxine (T_4) radioimmunoassay levels secondary to circulating thyroid hormone autoantibodies. *Clin. Endocrinol.*, 8:133-139, 1978.

7. Verhoeven, G.F.M. and Wilson, J.D.: The syndromes of primary hormone resistance. *Metabolism*, 28:(3)253-289, 1979.

8. Refetoff, S.: Thyroid hormone resistance syndromes. In *Werner's The Thyroid: A Fundamental and Clinical Text*, 5th edition. Edited by S.H. Ingbar and L.E. Braverman, Philadelphia, J.B. Lippincott Co., 1986, pp.1292-1307.

9. Lowe, J.C.: T_3 and chronic fatigue. *Dyn. Chiro.*, Dec. 19, 1990, p.9.

10. Tepperman, J. and Tepperman, H.M.: *Metabolic and Endocrine Physiology*, 5th edition. Chicago, Year Book Medical Publishers, Inc., 1987.

11. Bercu, B.B., Usala, S.J., Klann, R.C., et al.: Enhanced levels of wild-type versus mutant thyroid hormone receptor β_1 messenger RNA in fibroblasts from heterozygotes of kindred S with thyroid hormone resistance. *Thyroid*, 6 (3):189-194, 1996.

12. Gambert, S.R.: Environmental effects and physiologic variables. In *Werner and Ingbar's The Thyroid: A Fundamental and Clinical Text*, 6th edition. Edited by L.E. Braverman and R.D. Utiger, New York, J.B. Lippincott Co., 1991, pp.347-357.

13. Denkla, W.D.: Role of the pituitary and thyroid glands in the decline of minimal O_2 consumption with age. *J. Clin. Invest.*, 53:572, 1974.

14. Frolkis, V.V., Verzhakovskaya, N.V., and Valueva, G.V.: The thyroid and age. *Exp. Gerontol.*, 8:285, 1973.

15. Gambert, S.R.: Effect of age on basal and 3,5,3'triiodothyronine (T_3) stimulated human mononuclear cell sodium-potassium adenosine-triphosphatase (Na^+-K^+ ATPase) activity. *Horm. Metab. Res.*, 18(9):649-650, 1986.

16. Gambert, S.R., Ingbar, S.H., and Hagen, T.C.: Interaction of age and thyroid hormone status on Na^+-K^+ ATPase in rat renal cortex and liver. *Endocrinology*, 108(1):27-30, 1981.

17. Gambert, S.R. and Tsitouras, P.D.: Effect of age on nuclear triiodothyronine receptors in circulating human lymphocytes. *Age*, 6:76, 1983.

18. Forman, B.M., Casanova, J., Raaka, B.M., Ghysdael, J., and Samuels, H.H.: Half-site spacing and orientation determines whether thyroid hormone and retinoic acid receptors and related factors bind to DNA response elements as monomers, homodimers, or heterodimers. *Mol. Endocrinol.*, 6(3):429-442, 1992.

19. Darling, D.S., Beebe, J.S., Burnside, J., Winslow, E.R., and Chin, W.W.: 3,5,3'-triiodothyronine (T_3) receptor-

auxiliary protein (TRAP) binds DNA and forms heterodimers with the T_3 receptor. *Mol. Endocrinol.*, 5(1): 73-84, 1991.

20. Glass, C.K., Lipkin, S.M., Devary, O.V., and Rosenfeld, M.G.: Positive and negative regulation of gene transcription by a retinoic acid-thyroid hormone receptor heterodimer. *Cell*, 59:697-708, 1989.

21. Forman, B.M., Yang, C.R., Au, M., Casanova, J., Ghysdael, J., and Samuels, H.H.: A domain containing leucine zipper-like motifs mediate novel *in vivo* interactions between the thyroid hormone and retinoic acid receptors. *Mol. Endocrinol.*, 3:1610-1626, 1989.

22. O'Donnell, A.L., Rosen, E.D., Darling, D.S., and Koenig, R.J.: Thyroid hormone receptor mutations that interfere with transciptional activation also interfere with receptor interaction with a nuclear protein. *Mol. Endocrinol.*, 5:94-99, 1991.

23. Sakurai, A., Miyamoto, T., Refetoff, S., and DeGroot, L.J.: Dominant-negative transcriptional regulation by a mutant thyroid hormone receptor β in a family with generalized resistance to thyroid hormone. *Mol. Endocrinol.*, 4:1988-1994, 1990.

24. Sakurai, A., Takeda, K., Ain, K., et al.: Generalized resistance to thyroid hormone associated with a mutation in the ligand-binding domain of the human thyroid hormone receptor β. *Proc. Natl. Acad. Sci. (USA)*, 86:8977-8981, 1989.

25. Usala, S.J., Wondisford, F.E., Watson, T.L., Menke, J.B., and Weintraub, B.D.: Thyroid hormone and DNA binding properties of a mutant c-*erb*Aβ receptor associated with generalized thyroid hormone resistance. *Biochem. Biophys. Res. Commun.*, 171(2):575-580, 1990.

26. Takeda, K., Sakurai, A., DeGroot, L.J., and Refetoff, S.: Recessive inheritance of thyroid hormone resistance caused by complete deletion of the protein-coding region of the thyroid hormone receptor-β gene. *J. Clin. Endocrinol. Metab.*, 74(1):49-55, 1992.

27. Kirk, E. and Kvorning, S.A.: Hypometabolism: a clinical study of 308 consecutive cases. *Acta Med. Scand.*, 184 (Suppl.):3-83, 1946.

28. Horton, R.J.: Testicular steroid transport, metabolism and effects. In *Endocrinology and Metabolism*, 2nd edition. Edited by P. Felig, J.D. Baxter, A. Broadus, and L.A. Frohman, New York, McGraw-Hill Book Co., 1987, pp.937-942.

29. Kurland, G.S., Bustos, J.G., Hamolsky, M.W., and Freedberg, A.S.: Studies in nonmyxedematous hypometabolism: II. Turnover of I^{131}-labeled thyroxine after intravenous infusion. *J. Clin. Endocrinol. Metab.*, 17: 1365-1372, 1957.

30. Späth, M., Obermaier-Kusser, B., Fisher, P., and Pongratz, D.: Are point mutations or deletions of mitochondrial DNA of any significance for fibromyalgia? *J. Musculoskel. Pain*, 3(Suppl.1):116, 1995.

31. Usala, S.J., Tennyson, G.E., Bale, A.E., et al.: A base mutation of the c-*erb*Aβ thyroid hormone receptor in a kindred with generalized thyroid hormone resistance. Molecular heterogeneity in two other kindreds. *J. Clin. Invest.*, 85(1):93-100, 1990.

32. Straus, S.: Chronic fatigue syndrome. In *Mind-Body Interactions and Disease: Proceedings of a Conference on*

Stress, Immunity, and Health Sponsored by the National Institutes of Health. Edited by N.R.S. Hall, F. Altman, and S.J. Blumenthal, 1995, pp.95-104.

33. Damm, K., Thompson, C.C., and Evans, R.M.: Protein encoded by v-*erb*A functions as a thyroid hormone receptor antagonist. *Nature*, 339:593-597, 1989.

34. Lassiter, W.E. and Stanbury, J.B.: *J. Clin. Endocrinol.*, 18:903, 1958..

35. Refetoff, S., DeGroot, L.J., Benard, B., and DeWind, L.T.: Studies of a sibship with apparent hereditary resistance to the intracellular action of thyroid hormone. *Metabolism*, 21(8):723-756, 1972.

36. Wortsman, J., Premachandra, B.N., Williams, K., Burman, K.D., Hay, I.D., and Davis, P.J.: Familial resistance to thyroid hormone associated with decreased transport across the plasma membrane. *Ann. Intern. Med.*, 98:904-909, 1983.

37. Bernal, J., Refetoff, S., and DeGroot, L.J.: Abnormalities of triiodothyronine binding to lymphocyte and fibroblast nuclei from a patient with peripheral resistance to thyroid hormone action. *J. Clin. Endocrinol. Metab.*, 47(6):1266-1272, 1978.

38. Kaplowitz, P.B., D'Ercole, A.J., and Utiger, R.D.: Peripheral resistance to thyroid hormone in an infant. *J. Clin. Endocrinol. Metab.*, 53:958-963, 1981.

39. Refetoff, S., Matalon, R., and Bigazzi, M.: Metabolism of L-thyroxine (T_4) and L-triiodothyronine (T_3) by human fibroblasts in tissue culture: evidence for cellular binding proteins and conversion of T_4 to T_3. *Endocrinology*, 91: 934-947, 1972.

40. Hutchison, J.H. and Arneil, G.C.: Deficiency of an extrathyroid enzyme in sporadic cretinism. *Lancet*, 2:314-315, 1957.

41. Wiener, J.D. and Lindeboom, G.A.: Observations on an unusual case of myxoedema. *Acta Endocrinol.*, 39:439-456, 1962.

42. Brent, G.A., Dunn, M.K., Harney, J.W., Gulick, T., Larsen, P.R., and Moore, D.D.: Thyroid hormone aporeceptor represses T_3-inducible promoters and blocks activity of the retinoic acid receptor. *New Biol.*, 1:329-336, 1989.

43. Carr, F.E., Burnside, J., and Chin, W.W.: Thyroid hormones regulate rat thyrotropin β gene promotor activity expressed in GH3 cells. *Mol. Endocrinol.*, 3:709-716, 1989.

44. Thompson, W.O. and Thompson, P.K.: Low basal metabolism following thyrotoxicosis. II. Permanent type without myxedema. *J. Clin. Invest.*, 5:471,1928.

45. Koerner, D., Schwartz, H.L., and Surks, M.I.: Binding of selected iodothyronine analogues to receptor sites of isolated rat hepatic nuclei: high correlation between structural requirements for nuclear binding and biological activity. *J. Biol. Chem.*, 250:6417, 1975.

46. Oppenheimer, J.H.: Thyroid hormone action at the molecular level. In *Werner and Ingbar's The Thyroid: A Fundamental and Clinical Text,* 6th edition. Edited by L.E. Braverman and R.D. Utiger, Philadelphia, J.B. Lippincott Co., 1991, pp.204-223.

47. Hodin, R.A., Lazar, M.A., and Wintman, B.I.: Identification of a thyroid hormone receptor that is pituitary-specific. *Science*, 244:76-78, 1988.

48. Brent, G.A., Larsen, P.R., Harney, J.W., Koenig, R.J., and Moore, D.D.: Functional characteristics of the rat growth hormone promoter elements required for induction by thyroid hormone with and without a co-transfectant β type thyroid hormone receptor. *J. Biol. Chem.*, 264:178-182, 1989.

49. Naylor, S.L. and Bishop, D.T.: Report of the committee on the genetic constitution of chromosome 3 (HGM10). *Cytogenet. Cell Genet.*, 51:106-120, 1989.

50. Vennström, B.L. and Bishop, J.M.: Isolation and characterization of chicken DNA homologues to the putative oncogenes of avian erythroblastosis virus. *Cell*, 28:135, 1982.

51. Vennström, B.L., Fanshier, L., and Moscovici, C.: Molecular cloning of the avian erythroblastosis virus genome and recovery of oncogenic virus by transfection of chicken cells. *J. Virol.*, 36:575, 1980.

52. Spurr, N.K, Solomon, E., Jansson, M., et al.: Chromosomal localization of the human homologues to the oncogenes *erb*A and *erb*B. *EMBO J.*, 3(1):159-163, 1984.

53. Weinberger, C., Hollenberg, S.M., and Rosenfeld, M.G.: Domain structure of human glucocorticoid receptor and its relationship to the v-*erb* A oncogene product. *Nature*, 318:670, 1985.

54. Auchus, R.J. and Fuqua, S.A.: Clinical syndromes of hormone receptor mutations: hormone resistance and independence. *Semin. Cell Biol.*, 5(2):127-136, 1994.

55. Elia, J., Gulotta, C., Rose, S.R., Marin, G., and Rapoport, J.L.: Thyroid function and attention-deficit hyperactivity disorder. *J. Am. Acad. Child Adolesc. Psychiat.*, 33(2): 169-172, 1994.

56. Weiss, R.E., Marcocci, C., Bruno-Bossio, G., and Refetoff, S.: Multiple genetic factors in the heterogeneity of thyroid hormone resistance. *J. Clin. Endocrinol. Metab.*, 76(1):257-259, 1993.

57. McDermott, M.T. and Ridgway, E.C.: Thyroid hormone resistance syndromes. *Am. J. Med.*, 94(4):424-432, 1993.

58. Mixson, A.J., Hauser, P., Tennyson, G., Renault, J.C., Bodenner, D.L., and Weintraub, B.D.: Differential expression of mutant and normal β T_3 receptor alleles in kindreds with generalized resistance to thyroid hormone. *J. Clin. Invest.*, 91(5):2296-2300, 1993.

59. Sasaki, S., Nakamura, H., Tagami, T., et al.: Pituitary resistance to thyroid hormone associated with a base mutation in the hormone-binding domain of the human 3,5,3'-triiodothyronine receptor-beta. *J. Clin. Endocrinol. Metab.*, 76(5):1254-1258, 1993.

60. Hayashi, Y., Mangoura, D., and Refetoff, S.: A mouse model of resistance of a mutant thyroid hormone receptor. *Mol. Endocrinol.*, 10(1):100-106, 1996.

61. Kopp, P., Kitajima, K., and Jameson, J.L.: Syndrome of resistance to thyroid hormone: insights into thyroid hormone action. *Proc. Soc. Experim. Biol. Med.*, 211(1):49-61, 1996.

62. Sonkin, L.S.: Myofascial pain due to metabolic disorders: diagnosis and treatment. In *Myofascial Pain and Fibromyalgia: Trigger Point Management.* Edited by E.S. Rachlin, St. Louis, Mosby, 1994, pp.45-60.

63. Soloman, E. and Barker, D.F.: Report of the committee on the genetic constitution of chromosome 17 (HGM10). *Cytogenet. Cell Genet.*, 51:319-337, 1989.

64. Sobieszczyk, S. and Refetoff, S.: Abnormal response of

fibronectin messenger RNA to triiodothyronine in fibroblasts from patients with generalized resistance to thyroid hormone. *Endocrinology*, 121(Suppl.):T-24, 1988.

65. Ceccarelli, P., Refetoff, S., and Murata, Y.: Resistance to thyroid hormone diagnosed by the reduced response of fibroblasts to the triiodothyronine-induced suppression of fibronectin synthesis. *J. Clin. Endocrinol. Metab.*, 65: 242-246, 1987.

66. Bernal, J., DeGroot, I.J., and Refetoff, S.: Absent nuclear thyroid hormone receptors and failure of T_3-induced TRH suppression in the syndrome of peripheral resistance to thyroid hormone. In *Thyroid Research*. Edited by J. Robbins and L.E. Braverman, Amsterdam, *Excerpta Medica*, 1976, pp.316-319.

67. Liewendahl, K.: Triiodothyronine binding to lymphocytes from euthyroid subjects and a patient with peripheral resistance to thyroid hormone. *Acta Endocrinol.*, 83:64-70, 1976.

68. Liewendahl, K., Rosengard, S., and Lamberg, B.A.: Nuclear binding of triiodothyronine and thyroxine in lymphocytes from subjects with hyperthyroidism, hypothyroidism and resistance to thyroid hormones. *Clin. Chim. Acta*, 83(1-2):41-48, 1978.

69. York, D.A., Bray, G.A., and Yukimura, Y.: An enzymatic defect in the obese (ob/ob) mouse: loss of thyroid-induced sodium- and potassium-dependent adenosinetriphosphatase. *Proc. Natl. Acad. Sci.*, 75:477-481, 1978.

70. Chait, A., Kanter, R., Green, W., and Kenny, M.: Defective thyroid hormone action in fibroblasts cultured from subjects with the syndrome of resistance to thyroid hormone. *J. Clin. Endocrinol. Metab.*, 54:767-772, 1982.

71. Refetoff, S.: Resistance to thyroid hormone. In *Werner and Ingbar's The Thyroid: A Fundamental and Clinical Text*, 7th edition. Edited by L.P. Braverman and R.D. Utiger, Philadelphia, Lippincott-Raven Publishers, 1996, pp.1032-1048.

72. Daubresse, J.C., Dozin-van Roye, B., Denayer, P.H., and Devisscher, M.: Partial resistance to thyroid hormones: reduced affinity of lymphocyte nuclear receptors for T_3 in two siblings. In *Thyroid Research, Proceedings of the VI International Thyroid Congress*. Edited by J.R. Storkiot and S. Nagataki, *Aust. Acad. Sci.*, 1980, pp.295-298.

73. Maenpaa, J. and Liewendahl, K.: Peripheral insensitivity to thyroid hormones in a euthyroid girl with goitre. *Arch. Dis. Child.*, 55:207-212, 1980.

74. Bantle, J.P., Seeling, S., Mariash, C.N., Ulstrom, R.A., and Oppenheimer, J.H.: Resistance to thyroid hormones: a disorder frequently confused with Graves' disease. *Arch. Intern. Med.*, 142:1867-1871, 1982.

75. Chaussin, J.L., Binet, E., and Job, J.C.: Antibodies to human thyrotropin in the serum of certain hypopituitary dwarfs. *Rev. Europ. Studies Clin. Biol.*, 17:95-99, 1972.

76. Eil, C., Fein, H.G., and Smith, T.J.: Nuclear binding of ^{125}I-triiodothyronine in dispersed cultured skin fibroblasts from patients with resistance to thyroid hormone. *J. Clin. Endocrinol. Metab.*, 55:502-510, 1982.

77. Schimmel, M. and Utiger, R.: Thyroidal and peripheral production of thyroid hormones: review of recent findings and their clinical implications. *Ann. Intern. Med.*, 87:760-768, 1977.

78. Vandalem, J.L., Pirens, G., and Hennen, G.: Familial inappropriate TSH secretion: evidence suggesting a dissociated pituitary resistance to T_3 and T_4. *J. Endocrinol. Invest.*, 4:413-422, 1981.

79. Torresani, J.: Laboratoire de Biochimie Médicale, Faculté de Médecine, Université d'Aix-Marseille II, Marseille, France, 1996 (arranged by Prof. J. Eisinger, Centre Regional d'Exploration des Myalgies, Hospital G. Clemenceau, B.P. 1412-F, 83056, Toulon, France).

80. Hoch, F.L.: Thyrotoxicosis as a disease of mitochondria. *New Engl. J. Med.*, 266:446-454, 1962.

81. Kaplan, M.M., Swartz, S.L., and Larsen, P.R.: Partial peripheral resistance to thyroid hormone. *Am. J. Med.*, 70:1115-1121, 1981.

82. Umesono, K., Marakami, K.K., Thompson, C.C., and Evans, R.M.: Direct repeats as selective response elements for the thyroid hormone, retinoic acid, and vitamin D_3 receptors. *Cell*, 65:1255-1266, 1991.

83. Murata, Y., Refetoff, S., Horwitz, A.I., and Smith, T.J.: Hormonal regulation of glycosaminoglycan accumulation in fibroblasts from patients with resistance to thyroid hormone. *J. Clin. Endocrinol. Metab.*, 57:1233-1239, 1983.

84. Nakamura, H., Smith, T.J., Refetoff, S., Horwitz, A., and DeGroot, L.J.: T_3 effects on phosphorylation of endogenous proteins in rat liver cytosol and cultured human fibroblasts. (Abstract) *Endocrinology*, 109(Suppl.):T14, 1972.

85. Refetoff, S.: Personal communication. April 27, 1992.

86. Refetoff, S., Salazar, A., Smith, T.J., and Scherberg, N.H.: The consequences of inappropriate treatment due to failure to recognize the syndrome of pituitary and peripheral tissue resistance to thyroid hormone. *Metabolism*, 32:822, 1983.

87. Lamberg, B.A. and Liewendahl, K.: Thyroid hormone resistance. *Ann. Clin. Res.*, 12(5):243-253, 1980.

88. Rootwelt, K.: Hypothyroidism. Emphasis on clinical aspects or laboratory tests? Report about well known facts which, however, can be doubted. *Tidsskr. Nor. Laegeforen.*, 111(2):209-214, 1991.

89. Weinberger, C., Thompson, C.C., Ong, E.S., Lebo, R., Gruol, D.J., and Evans, R.M.: The c-erbA gene encodes a thyroid hormone receptor. *Nature*, 324:641-646, 1986.

90. Sap, J., Munoz, A., Damm, K., et al.: The c-erbA protein is a high-affinity receptor for thyroid hormone. *Nature*, 324:635-640, 1986.

91. BSCS Personnel: *Biological Science*. Boston, Houghton Mifflin Co., 1963.

92. Cooper, J.R., Bloom, F.E., and Roth, R.H.: *The Biochemical Basis of Neuropharmacology*, 6th edition. New York, Oxford University Press, 1991.

93. Drabkin, H., Kao, F.T., Hartz, J., et al.: Localization of human ERBA2 to the 3p22—3p24.1 region of chromosome 3 and variable deletion in small cell lung cancer. *Proc. Natl. Acad. Sci.* (USA), 85(23):9258-9262, 1988.

94. Bale, A.E., Usala, S.J., Weinberger, C., and McBride, O.W.: A cDNA probe from the hc-erbA β gene on chromosome 3 detects a high frequency RFLP. *Nucleic Acids Res.*, 16:7756, 1988.

95. Usala, S.J., Bale, A.E., Gesundheit, N., et al.: Tight linkage between the syndrome of generalized thyroid hormone resistance and the human c-erbA β gene. *Mol. Endocrinol.*, 2:1217-1220, 1988.

96. Usala, S.J. and Weintraub, B.D.: Familial thyroid hormone resistance: clinical and molecular studies. In *Advances in Endocrinology and Metabolism*, Vol. 2. New York, Mosby-Year Book, Inc., 1991, pp.59-76.

97. Brent, G.A., Harvey, J.W., Chen, Y., Warne, R.L., Moore, D.D., and Larsen, P.R.: Mutations of the rat growth hormone promoter which increase and decrease response to thyroid hormone define a consensus thyroid hormone response element. *Mol. Endocrinol.*, 3:1996-2004, 1989.

98. Usala, S.J., Menke, J.B., Watson, T.L., et al.: A new point mutation in the 3,5,3'-triiodothyronine-binding domain of the c-*erb*A β thyroid hormone receptor is tightly linked to generalized thyroid hormone resistance. *J. Clin. Endocrinol. Metab.*, 72(1):32-38, 1991.

99. Fein, H.G., Burman, K.D., Ojuh, Y.Y., et al.: Linkage between the syndrome of generalized thyroid hormone resistance (GTHR) and the human c-*erb*A β gene is present in multiple kindreds. (Abstract) *Endocrinology*, 122 (Suppl.):T-1, 1989.

100. Porterfield, S.P.: Vulnerability of the developing brain to thyroid abnormalities: environmental insults to the thyroid system. *Environ. Health Perspect.*, 102 (Suppl.2): 125-130, 1994.

101. Weintraub, B.D., Usala, S.J., Bale, A.E., et al.: Thyroid hormone resistance syndrome. In *Progress in Endocrinology*. Edited by H. Imura, Amsterdam, Elsevier Science Publishers BV, 1988, pp.797-802.

102. Erfurth, E.M., Schutz, A., Nilsson, A., Barregard, L., and Skerfving, S.: Normal pituitary hormone response to thyrotrophin and gonadotrophin releasing hormones in subjects exposed to elemental mercury vapor. *Brit. J. Ind. Med.*, 47(9):639-644, 1990.

103. Weaver, R.F. and Hedrick, P.W.: *Genetics*, 2nd edition. Dubuque, Wm. C. Brown Publishers, 1992.

104. Herskowitz, I.: Functional inactivation of genes by dominant-negative mutations. *Nature*, 329:219, 1987.

105. Hagmar, L., Persson-Moschos, M., Akesson, B., and Schutz, A.: Plasma levels of selenium, selenoprotein P and glutathione peroxidase and their correlations to fish intake and serum levels of thyrotropin and thyroid hormones: a study on Latvian fish consumers. *Eur. J. Clin. Nutr.*, 52(11):796-800, 1998.

106. Kawada, J., Nishida, M., Yoshimura, Y., and Mitani, K.: Effects of organic and inorganic mercurials on thyroidal functions. *J. Pharmacobiodyn.*, 3(3):149-159, 1980.

107. Lowe, J.C.: The myofascial genesis of unpleasant thoughts and emotions: its neural basis. *Dig. Chiro. Econ.*, 31(5):80, March/April, 1989.

108. Lowe, J.C.: The emotional effects of noxious myofascial stimulation. *Am. Chiropractor*, 22-24, January, 1989.

109. Emerson, S.: Personal communication. Nov. 11, 1998. Website: < http://www.teleport.com/~semerson/ fm.html#metals >

110. Barregard, L., Lindstedt, G., Schütz, A., and Sallsten, G.: Endocrine function in mercury exposed chloralkali workers. *Occup. Environm. Med.*, 51(8):536-540, 1994.

111. Lakka-Papadodima, E., Souvatzoglon, A., Pandos, P.G., Alivisatos, J., and Koutras, D.A.: Two cases of peripheral tissue resistance to thyroxine of different mechanisms. (Abstract) *Ann. Endocrinol.*(Paris), 38(Suppl):71A, 1977.

112. Menezes-Ferreira, M.M., Eil, C., Wortsman, J., and Weintraub, B.D.: Decreased nuclear uptake of [125I]tri-iodo-L-thyronine in fibroblasts from patients with peripheral thyroid hormone resistance. *J. Clin. Endocrinol. Metab.*, 59:1081-1087, 1984.

113. Eli, C., Fein, H.G., Smith, T.J., Furlanetto, R.W., Bourgeois, M., Sterling, M.W., and Weintraub, B.D.: Nuclear binding of [125I]triiodothyronine in dispersed cultured skin fibroblasts from patients with resistance to thyroid hormone. *J. Clin. Endocrinol. Metab.*, 55:502-510, 1982.

114. Rosler, A., Litvin, Y., and Hage, C.: Familial hyperthyroidism due to inappropriate thyrotropin secretion successfully treated with triiodothyronine. *J. Clin. Endocrinol. Metab.*, 54:76-82, 1982.

115. Tsai, J.S. and Samuels, H.H.: Thyroid hormone action: demonstration of putative nuclear receptors in human lymphocytes. *J. Clin. Endocrinol. Metab.*, 38(5):919-922, 1974.

116. Seif, F.J., Scherbaum, W., and Klingler, W.: Syndrome of elevated thyroid hormone and TSH blood levels: a case report. (Abstract) *Ann. Endocrinol.*(Paris), 87(215 Suppl.):81-82, 1978.

117. Cooper, D.S., Ladenson, P.W., Nisula, B.C., Dunn, J.F., Chapman, E.M., and Ridgway, E.C.: Familial thyroid hormone resistance. *Metabolism*, 31(5):504-509,1982.

118. Linde, R., Alexander, N., Island, D.P., and Rabin, D.: Familial insensitivity of the pituitary and periphery to thyroid hormone: a case report in two generations and a review of the literature. *Metabolism*, 31(5):510-513, 1982.

119. Oppenheimer, J.H., Koerner, D., Schwartz, H.I., and Surks, M.I.: Specific nuclear triiodothyronine binding sites in rat liver and kidney. *J. Clin. Endocrinol. Metab.*, 35:330-333, 1972.

120. Jeffries, D.J.: *Organochlorine Insecticides*. Edited by F. Moriarty, New York, Academic Press, 1975, pp.131-230.

121. Wolfe, S.L.: *Molecular and Cellular Biology*. Belmont, Wadsworth Publishing Co., 1993.

122. Fassbender, H.G.: *Pathology of Rheumatic Diseases*. New York, Springer-Verlag, 1975.

123. Bennett, R.M., Goldenberg, D.L., Simons, D.G., and Travell, J.G.: Panel discussion on definitions and diagnostic criteria for muscular pain syndromes. *First Iternational Symposium on Myofascial Pain and Fibromyalgia*, Minneapolis, May 8, 1989.

124. Lowe, J.C.: Results of an open trial of T3 therapy with 77 euthyroid female fibromyalgia patients. *Clin. Bull. Myofascial Ther.*, 2(1):35-37, 1997.

125. Shapiro, R.: *The Human Blueprint: The Race to Unlock the Secrets of Our Genetic Script.* New York, St. Martin's Press, 1991.

126. Burman, K.D., Lukes, Y., Wright, F.D., and Wartofsky, L.: Reduction in hepatic triiodothyronine binding capacity induced by fasting. *Endocrinology*, 101:1331, 1977.

128. Pauling, L.: *How to Live Longer and Feel Better.* New York, Avon Books, 1987.

127. Schussler, G.C.: Fasting decreases triiodothyronine receptor capacity. *Science*, 199:686, 1978.

129. Thompson, P., Jr., Burman, K.D., and Lukes, Y.G.: Uremia decreases nuclear 3,5,3'-triiodothyronine receptors in rats. *Endocrinology*, 107:1081, 1980.

130. Lim, V.S., Passo, C., and Murta, Y.: Reduced triiodothyronine content in liver but not pituitary of the uremic rat model: demonstration of changes compatible with thyroid hormone deficiency in liver only. *Endocrinology*, 114:280, 1984.

131. DeGroot, L.J., Coleoni, A.H., and Rue, P.A.: Reduced nuclear triiodothyronine receptors in starvation-induced hypothyroidism. *Biochem. Biophy. Res. Commun.*, 79:173, 1977.

132. Usala, S.J.: Personal communication. July 14, 1992.

133. Usala, S.J.: Resistance to thyroid hormone in children. *Curr. Opinion Pediat.*, 6(4):468-475, 1994.

134. Beck-Peccoz, P. and Chatterjee, V.K.: The variable clinical phenotype in thyroid hormone resistance syndrome. *Thyroid*, 4(2):225-232, 1994.

135. Nicoloff, J.T., Fisher, D.A., and Appleman, M.D.: The role of glucocorticoids in the regulation of thyroid function in man. *J. Clin. Invest.*, 49:1922, 1970.

136. Usala, S.J., Menke, J.B., Watson, T.L., et al.: A homozygous deletion in the c-*erb*A β thyroid hormone receptor gene in a patient with generalized thyroid hormone resistance: isolation and characterization of the mutant receptor. *Mol. Endocrinol.*, 5:327-335, 1991.

137. Cassar-Malek, I., Marchal, S., Altabef, M., Wrutniak, C., Samarut, J., and Cabello, G.: v-*erb*A stimulates quail myoblast differentiation in a T_3 independent, cell-specific manner. *Oncogene*, 9(8):2197-2206, 1994.

138. Usala, S.J.: Molecular diagnosis and characterization of thyroid hormone resistance syndromes. *Thyroid*, 1:361-367, 1991.

139. Saitou, M., Narumiya, S., and Kakizuka, A.: Alteration of a single amino acid residue in retinoic acid receptor causes dominant-negative phenotype. *J. Biol. Chem.*, 269(29):19101-19107, 1994.

140. Bartolone, L., Regalbuto, C., Benvenga, S., Filetti, S., Trimarchi, F., and Pontecorvi, A.: Three new mutations of thyroid hormone receptor-beta associated with resistance to thyroid hormone. *J. Clin. Endocrinol. Metab.*, 79(1):323-326, 1994.

141. Chatterjee, V.K. and Beck-Peccoz, P.: Hormone-nuclear receptor interactions in health and disease. Thyroid hormone resistance. *Baillieres Clin. Endocrinol. Metab.*, 8(2):267-283, 1994.

142. Hayashi, Y., Sunthornthepvarakul, T., and Refetoff, S.: Mutations of CpG dinucleotides located in the triiodothyronine (T_3)-binding domain of the thyroid hormone receptor (TR) beta gene that appears to be devoid of natural mutations may not be detected because they are unlikely to produce the clinical phenotype of resistance to thyroid hormone. *J. Clin. Invest.*, 94(2):607-615, 1994.

143. Yellin, T.: Personal communication. April 20, 1997.

144. Adams, M., Matthews, C., Collingwood, T.N., Tone, Y., Beck-Peccoz, P., and Chatterjee, K.K.: Genetic analysis of 29 kindreds with generalized and pituitary resistance to thyroid hormone: identification of 13 novel mutations in the β thyroid hormone receptor gene. *J. Clin. Invest.*, 94(2):506-515, 1994.

145. Weiss, R.E., Stein, M.A., Duck, S.C., et al.: Low intelligence but not attention deficit hyperactivity disorder is associated with resistance to thyroid hormone caused by mutation R316H in the β thyroid hormone receptor gene.

J. Clin. Endocrinol. Metab., 78(6):1525-1528, 1994.

146. Okamura, K. and Fujishima, M.: Point mutation of the β T_3 receptor gene and the syndrome of inappropriate secretion of TSH. *Japan. J. Clin. Med.*, 52(4):935-939, 1994.

147. Takeda, K. and Hashimoto, K.: Resistance to thyroid hormone. *Japan. J. Clin. Med.*, 52(4):922-928, 1994.

148. Sasaki, S. and Nakamura, H.: Diagnosis of thyroid hormone resistance by molecular biology. *Japan. J. Clin. Med.*, 52(4):929-934, 1994.

149. Groenhout, E.G. and Dorin, R.I.: Generalized thyroid hormone resistance due to a deletion of the carboxyl terminus of the c-*erb*A β receptor. *Mol. Cell. Endocrinol.*, 99(1):81-88, 1994.

150. Weiss, R.E., Chyna, B., Duell, P.B., Hayashi, Y., Sunthornthepvarakul, T., and Refetoff, S.: A new mutation (C446R) in the β thyroid hormone receptor gene of a family with resistance to thyroid hormone. *J. Clin. Endocrinol. Metab.*, 78(5):1253-1256, 1994.

151. Persani, L., Asteria, C., Tonacchera, M., et al.: Evidence for the secretion of thyrotropin with enhanced bioactivity in syndromes of thyroid hormone resistance. *J. Clin. Endocrinol. Metab.*, 78(5):1034-1039, 1994.

152. Refetoff, S.: Resistance to thyroid hormone and its molecular basis. *Acta Paediatri. Japon.*, 36(1):1-15, 1994.

153. Lowe, J.C., Garrison, R.L., Reichman, A.J., Yellin, J., Thompson, M., and Kaufman, D.: Effectiveness and safety of T_3 (triiodothyronine) therapy for euthyroid fibromyalgia: a double-blind placebo-controlled response-driven crossover study. *Clin. Bull. Myofascial Ther.*, 2(2/3):31-57, 1997.

154. Lowe, J.C., Reichman, A.J., and Yellin, J.: The process of change during T_3 treatment for euthyroid fibromyalgia: a double-blind placebo-controlled crossover study. *Clin. Bull. Myofascial Ther.*, 2(2/3):91-124, 1997.

155. Lowe, J.C., Garrison, R.L., Reichman, A., and Yellin, J.: Triiodothyronine (T_3) treatment of euthyroid fibromyalgia: a small-N replication of a double-blind placebo-controlled crossover study. *Clin. Bull. Myofascial Ther.*, 2(4):71-88, 1997.

156. Cheng, S.Y., Ransom, S.C., McPhie, P., Bhat, M.K., Mixson, A.J., and Weintraub, B.D.: Analysis of the binding of 3,3',5-triiodo-L-thyronine and its analogues to mutant human β_1 thyroid hormone receptors: a model of the hormone binding site. *Biochemistry*, 33(14):4319-4326, 1994.

157. Jannini, E.A., Dolci, S., Ulisse, S., and Nikodem, V.M.: Developmental regulation of the α_1 thyroid hormone receptor mRNA expression in the rat testis. *Mol. Endocrinol.*, 8(1):89-96, 1994.

158. Williams, G.R., Zavacki, A.M., Harney, J.W., and Brent, G.A.: Thyroid hormone receptor binds with unique properties to response elements that contain hexamer domains in an inverted palindrome arrangement. *Endocrinology*, 134(4):1888-1896, 1994.

159. Caron, P., Thalamas, C., Cogne, M., Calazel-Fournier, C., and Bayard, F.: Hyperthyroidism caused by inappropriate secretion of TSH. Apropos of 2 new cases. *Rev. Med. Interne.*, 14(10):990, 1993.

160. Mechain, C., Leger, A., Feldman, S, Kuttenn, F., and Mauvais-Jarvis, P.: Syndrome of resistance to thyroid hormones. *Presse Med.*, 22(37):1870-1875, 1993.

161. Ohzeki, T., Hanaki, K., Motozumi, H., et al.: Efficacy of bromocriptine administration for selective pituitary resistance to thyroid hormone. *Horm. Res.*, 39(5-6):229-234, 1993.

162. Robinson, D.B., Michaels, R.D., and Shakir, K.M.: Autoimmune hypothyroidism in a patient with generalized resistance to thyroid hormone. *South. Med. J.*, 86(12): 1395-1397, 1993.

163. Zavacki, A.M., Harney, J.W., Brent, G.A., and Larsen, P.R.: Dominant-negative inhibition by mutant thyroid hormone receptors is thyroid hormone response element and receptor isoform specific. *Mol. Endocrinol.*, 7(10): 1319-1330, 1993.

164. Pescovitz, O.H., Cutler, G.B., and Loriaux, D.L.: Synthesis and secretion of corticosteroids. In *Principles and Practice of Endocrinology and Metabolism.* Edited by K.L. Becker, J.P. Bilezinkian, and W.J. Bremner, et al., Philadelphia, J.B. Lippincott Co., 1990, pp.579-591.

165. Lavin, T.N.: In *Endocrinology,* 2nd edition. Edited by L.J. DeGroot, New York, Grune and Stratton, 1988, pp.562-573.

166. Oppenheimer, J.H.: The nuclear receptor-triiodothyronine complex: relationship to thyroid hormone distribution, metabolism, and biological action. In *Molecular Basis of Thyroid Hormone Action.* Edited by J.H. Oppenheimer and H.H. Samuels, New York, Academic Press, 1983, pp.1-35.

167. Taniyama, M., Honma, K., and Ban, Y.: Urinary cortisol metabolites in the assessment of peripheral thyroid hormone action: application for diagnosis of resistance to thyroid hormone. *Thyroid*, 3(3):229-233, 1993.

168. Ashizawa, K. and Nagataki, S.: Pituitary resistance to thyroid hormone. *Japan. J. Clin. Med.*, 51(10):2726-2730, 1993.

169. Refetoff, S.: Resistance to thyroid hormone. *Clin. Lab. Med.*, 13(3):563-581, 1993.

170. Weiss, R.E., Stein, M.A., Trommer, B., and Refetoff, S.: Attention-deficit hyperactivity disorder and thyroid function. *J. Pediatr.*, 123(4):539-545, 1993.

171. McKinney, J., Fannin, R., Jordan, S., Chae, K. Rickenbacher, U., and Pedersen, L.: Polychlorinated biphenyls and related compound interactions with specific binding sites for thyroxine in rat liver nuclear extracts. *J. Med. Chem.*, 30(1):79-86, 1987.

172. Brabant, A., Brabant, G., Schuermeyer, T., et al.: The role of glucocorticoids in the regulation of thyrotropin. *Acta Endocrinol.* (Copenh), 121:95, 1989.

173. Nagaya, T., Eberhardt, N.L., and Jameson, J.L.: Thyroid hormone resistance syndrome: correlation of dominant-negative activity and location of mutations. *J. Clin. Endocrin. Metab.*, 77(4):982-990, 1993.

174. Klann, R.C., Torres, B., Menke, J.B., Holbrook, C.T., Bercu, B.B., and Usala, S.J.: Competitive polymerase chain reaction quantitation of c-$erbA\beta_1$, c-$erbA\alpha_1$, and c-$erbA\alpha_2$ messenger ribonucleic acid levels in normal, heterozygous, and homozygous fibroblasts of kindred S with thyroid hormone resistance. *J. Clin. Endocrinol. Metab.*, 77(4):969-975, 1993.

175. Mixson, A.J., Renault, J.C., Ransom, S., Bodenner, D.L., and Weintraub, B.D.: Identification of a novel mutation in the gene encoding the beta-triiodothyronine receptor in a patient with apparent selective pituitary resistance to thyroid hormone. *Clin. Endocrinol*, 38(3):227-234, 1993.

176. Geffner, M.E., Su, F., Ross, N.S., et al.: An arginine to histidine mutation in codon 311 of the c-$erbA\beta$ gene results in a mutant thyroid hormone receptor that does not mediate a dominant negative phenotype. *J. Clin. Invest.*, 91(2):538-546, 1993.

177. Sakurai, A.: Genetic analysis of hormone resistance. *Japan. J. Clin. Pathol.*, 41(5):527-532, 1993.

178. Kvetny, J. and Bollerslev, J.: Relation between phenotype and intracellular thyroid hormone effect in patients with altered peripheral thyroid hormone sensitivity. *Clin. Endocrinol.*, 39(1):73-76, 1993.

179. Nagaya, T. and Jameson, J.L.: Thyroid hormone receptor dimerization is required for dominant-negative inhibition by mutations that cause thyroid hormone resistance. *J. Biol. Chem.*, 268(21):15766-15771, 1993.

180. Alford, F.P., Baker, H.W.G., Burger, H.G., et al.: Temporal patterns of integrated plasma hormone levels during sleep and wakefulness. I. Thyroid-stimulating hormone, growth hormone and cortisol. *J. Clin. Endocrinol. Metab.*, 37:841, 1973.

181. Watanabe, K., Kameya, T., Yamauchi, A., et al.: Thyrotropin-producing microadenoma associated with pituitary resistance to thyroid hormone. *J. Clin. Endocrinol. Metab.*, 76(4):1025-1030, 1993.

182. Yamashita, S. and Nagataki, S.: Thyroid hormone resistance. *Japan. J. Clin. Med.*, 51(Suppl.):83-91, 1993.

183. Sakurai, A., Miyamoto, T., Hughes, I.A., and DeGroot, L.J.: Characterization of a novel mutant human thyroid hormone β receptor in a family with hereditary thyroid hormone resistance. *Clin. Endocrinol.* (Oxf.), 38(1):29-38, 1993.

184. Hayashi, Y., Janssen, O.E., Weiss, R.E., Murata, Y., Seo, H., and Refetoff, S.: The relative expression of mutant and normal thyroid hormone receptor genes in patients with generalized resistance to thyroid hormone determined by estimation of their specific messenger ribonucleic acid products. *J. Clin. Endocrinol. Metab.*, 76(1): 64-69, 1993.

185. Pemrick, S.M., Lucas, D.A., and Grippo, J.F.: The retinoid receptors. *Leukemia*, 8(11):1797-1806, 1994.

186. Lee, Y. and Mahdavi, V.: The D domain of the α_1 thyroid hormone receptor specifies positive and negative transcriptional regulation functions. *J. Biol. Chem.*, 268(3): 2021-2028, 1993.

187. Leonard, C.M., Martinez, P., Weintraub, B.D., and Hauser, P.: Magnetic resonance imaging of cerebral anomalies in subjects with resistance to thyroid hormone. *Am. J. Med. Genetics*, 60(3):238-243, 1995.

188. Piedrafita, F.J., Bendik, I., Ortiz, M.A., and Pfahl, M.: Thyroid hormone receptor homodimers can function as ligand-sensitive repressors. *Mol. Endocrinol*, 9(5):563-578, 1995.

189. Spencer, T., Biederman, J., Wileens, T., Guite, J., and Harding, M.: ADHD and thyroid abnormalities: a research note. *J. Child Psychol. Psychia. Allied Discipl.*, 36 (5):879-885, 1995.

190. Brucker-Davis, F., Skarulis, M.C., Grace, M.B., et al.: Genetic and clinical features of 42 kindreds with resistance to thyroid hormone: the National Institutes of

Health prospective study. *Ann. Intern. Med.*, 123(8):572-583, 1995.

191. Pohlenz, J., Wirth, S., Winterpacht, A., Wemme, H., Zabel, B., and Schonberger, W.: Phenotypic variability in patients with generalized resistance to thyroid hormone. *J. Med. Genetics*, 32(5):393-395, 1995.

192. Takeda, T., Suzuki, S., Liu, R.T., and DeGroot, L.J.: Triiodothyroacetic acid has unique potential for therapy of resistance to thyroid hormone. *J. Clin. Endocrinol. Metab.*, 80(7):2033-2040, 1995.

193. Meier-Heusler, S.C., Zhu, X., Juge-Aubry, C., et al.: Modulation of thyroid hormone action by mutant thyroid hormone receptors, c-$erbA\alpha_2$ and peroxisome proliferation-activated receptor: evidence for different mechanisms of inhibition. *Mol. Cell. Endocrinol.*, 107(1):55-66, 1995.

194. Hidaka, Y., Tada, H., Kashiwai, T., et al.: A case of hyperthyroidism due to pituitary resistance to thyroid hormone. *Endocrine J.*, 41(4):339-349, 1994.

195. Zhang, X.K., Hoffmann, B., Tran, P.B., Graupner, G., and Pfahl, M.: Retinoid X receptor is an auxiliary protein for thyroid hormone and retinoic acid receptors. *Nature*, 355(6359):441-446, 1992.

196. Bugge, T.H., Pohl, J., Lonnoy, O., and Stunnenberg, H.G.: RXRα, a promiscuous partner of retinoic acid and thyroid hormone receptors. *EMBO J.*, 11:1409-1418, 1992.

197. Yu, V.C., Delsert, C., Andersen, B., et al.: RXRβ: a coregulator that enhances binding of retinoic acid, thyroid hormone, and vitamin D receptors to their cognate response elements. *Cell*, 67:1251-1266, 1991.

198. Marks, M.S., Hallenbeck, P.L., Nagata, T., et al.: H-2RIIBP (RXRβ) heterodimerization provides a mechanism for combinatorial diversity in the regulation of retinoic acid and thyroid hormone genes. *EMBO J.*, 11:1419-1435, 1992.

199. Leid, M., Kastner, P., Lyons, R., et al.: Purification, cloning, and RXR identity of the HeLa cell factor with which RAR or TR heterodimerizations bind target sequences efficiently. *Cell*, 68:377-395, 1992.

200. Kliewer, S.A., Umesonso, K., Mangelsdorf, D.J., and Evans, R.M.: Retinoid X receptor interacts with nuclear receptors in retinoic acid, thyroid hormone, and vitamin D_3 signaling. *Nature*, 355:446-449, 1992.

201. Herman, T., Hoffmann, B., Zhang, X.K., Tran, P., and Pfahl, M.: Heterodimeric receptor complexes determine 3,5,3'-triiodothyronine and retinoid signaling specificities. *Mol. Endocrinol.*, 6:1153-1162, 1992.

202. Zhang, X.K. and Pfahl, M.: Regulation of retinoid and thyroid hormone action through homodimeric and heterodimeric receptors. *Trends Endocrinol. Metab.*, 4:10-16, 1993.

203. Herman, T., Hoffmann, B., Piedrafita, F.J., Zhang, X.K., and Pfahl, M.: V-$erbA$ requires auxiliary proteins for dominant-negative activity. *Oncogene*, 8:55-65, 1993.

204. Harkonen, M.: Resistance to thyroid hormone. *Duodecim*, 110(21):2009-2011, 1994.

205. Westhoff, M.: Thyroid hormone resistance: rare cause of recurrence following goiter resection. *Deutsche Medizinische Wochenschrift*, 120(6):197, 1995.

206. McKinney, J.D., Chae, K., Oatley, S.J., and Blake, C.C.: Molecular interactions of toxic chlorinated dibenzo-*p*-dioxins and dibenzofurans with thyroxine binding prealbumin. *J. Med. Chem.*, 28(3):375-381, 1985.

207. Jameson, J.L.: Mechanisms by which thyroid hormone receptor mutations cause clinical syndromes of resistance to thyroid hormone. *Thyroid*, 4(4):485-492, 1994.

208. Hiramatsu, R., Abe, M., Morita, M., Noguchi, S., and Suzuki, T.: Generalized resistance to thyroid hormone: identification of a novel c-$erbA\beta$ thyroid hormone receptor variant (Leu450) in a Japanese family and analysis of its secondary structure by the Chou and Fasman method. *Japan. J. Human Genet.*, 39(4):365-377, 1994.

209. Collingwood, T.N., Adams, M., Tone, Y., and Chatterjee, V.K.: Spectrum of transcriptional, dimerization, and dominant-negative properties of twenty different mutant β thyroid hormone receptors in thyroid resistance syndrome. *Mol. Endocrinol.*, 8(9):1262-1277, 1994.

210. Refetoff, S.: Resistance to thyroid hormone: an historical overview. *Thyroid*, 4(3):345-349, 1994.

211. Refetoff, S., Weiss, R.E., Wing, J.R., Sarne, D., Chyna, B., and Hayashi, Y.: Resistance to thyroid hormone in subjects from two unrelated families is associated with a point mutation in the β thyroid hormone receptor gene resulting in the replacement of the normal proline 453 with serine. *Thyroid*, 4(3):249-254, 1994.

212. Chatterjee, V.K.: Resistance to thyroid hormone—an uncommon cause of thyroxine excess and inappropriate TSH secretion. *Acta Med. Austriaca*, 21(2):56-60, 1994.

213. Mala, E.: Hyperkinetic disorder—a new view? *Ceskoslovenska Psychiatr.*, 90(4):209-212, 1994.

214. Hao, E., Menke, J.B., Smith, A.M., et al.: Divergent dimerization properties of mutant β_1 thyroid hormone receptors are associated with different dominant-negative activities. *Mol. Endocrinol.*, 8(7):841-851, 1994.

215. Collingwood, T.N., Rajanayagam, O., Adams, M., et al.: A natural transactivation mutation in the β thyroid hormone receptor: impaired interaction with putative transcriptional mediators. *Proc. Nat. Acad. Sci* (U.S.), 94(1):248-253, 1997.

216. Taniyama, M., Kusano, S., Miyoshi, Y., et al.: Mild resistance to thyroid hormone with a truncated β thyroid hormone receptor. *Experi. Clin. Endocrinol. Diab.*, 104(4):339-343, 1996.

217. Weiss, R.E., Tunca, H., Gerstein, H.C., and Refetoff, S.: A new mutation in the β thyroid hormone receptor (TR) gene (V458A) in a family with resistance to thyroid hormone. *Thyroid*, 6(4):311-312, 1996.

218. Liu, R.T., Suzuki, S., Takeda, T., and DeGroot, L.J.: An artificial thyroid hormone receptor mutant without DNA binding can have dominant-negative effect. *Mol. Cell. Endocrinol.*, 120(1):85-93, 1996.

219. Ozata, M., Suzuki, S., Takeda, T., et al.: Functional analysis of a proline to serine mutation in codon 453 of the β_1 mutant thyroid hormone receptor gene. *J. Clin. Endocrinol. Metab.*, 80(11):3239-3245, 1995.

220. Weiss, R.E., Hayashi, Y., Nagaya, T., et al.: Dominant inheritance of resistance to thyroid hormone not linked to defects in the α or β thyroid hormone receptor genes may be due to a defective cofactor. *J. Clin. Endocrinol. Metab.*, 81(12):4196-4203, 1996.

221. Weiss, R.E. and Refetoff, S.: Effect of thyroid hormone on growth: lessons from the syndrome of resistance to

thyroid hormone. *Endocrinol. Metab. Clin. North Am.*, 25 (3):719-730, 1996.

222. Ando, S., Nakamura, H., Sasaki, S., et al.: Introducing a point mutation identified in a patient with pituitary resistance to thyroid hormone (Arg 338 to Trp) into other mutant thyroid hormone receptors weakens their dominant-negative activities. *J. Endocrinol.*, 151(2):293-300, 1996.

223. Beck-Peccoz, P., Persani, L., Mantovani, S., Cortelazzi, D., and Asteria, C.: Thyrotropin-secreting pituitary adenomas. *Metab. Clin. Experi.*, 45(8 Suppl.1):75-79, 1996.

224. Brucker-Davis, F., Skarulis, M.C., Pikus, A., Ishizawar, D., Mastroianni, M.A., Koby, M., and Weintraub, B.D.: Prevalence and mechanisms of hearing loss in patients with resistance to thyroid hormone. *J. Clin. Endocrinol. Metab.*, 81(8):2768-2772, 1996.

225. Hayashi, Y., Weiss, R.E., Sarne, D.H., et al.: Do clinical manifestations of resistance to thyroid hormone correlate with the functional alteration of the corresponding mutant β thyroid hormone receptors? *J. Clin. Endocrinol. Metab.*, 80(11):3246-3256, 1995.

226. Nomura, Y., Nagaya, T., Tsukaguchi, H., Takamatsu, J., and Seo, H.: Amino acid substitutions of thyroid hormone receptor-β at codon 435 with resistance to thyroid hormone selectively alter homodimer formation. *Endocrinology*, 137(10):4082-4086, 1996.

227. Matochik, J.A., Zametkin, A.J., Cohen, R.M., Hauser, P., and Weintraub, B.D.: Abnormalities in sustained attention and anterior cingulate metabolism in subjects with resistance to thyroid hormone. *Brain Res.*, 723(1-2):23-28, 1996.

228. Ikeda, M., Wilcox, E.C., and Chin, W.W.: Different DNA elements can modulate the conformation of thyroid hormone receptor heterodimer and its transcriptional activity. *J. Biol. Chem.*, 271(38):23096-23104, 1996.

229. Ng, L., Forrest, D., Haugen, B.R., Wood, W.M., and Curran, T.: N-terminal variants of β thyroid hormone receptor: differential function and potential contribution to syndrome of resistance to thyroid hormone. *Mol. Endocrinol.*, 9(9):1202-1213, 1995.

230. Zavacki, A.M., Harney, J.W., Brent, G.A., and Larsen, P.R.: Structural features of thyroid hormone response elements that increase susceptibility to inhibition by an RTH mutant thyroid hormone receptor. *Endocrinology*, 137(7):2833-2841, 1996.

231. Kijima, H., Kubo, M., Ishizuka, T., Kakinuma, M., and Koike, T.: A novel missense mutation in the β thyroid hormone receptor gene in a kindred with resistance to thyroid hormone. *Human Genet.*, 97(3):407-408, 1996.

232. Ribeiro, R.C.J., Cavalieri, R.R., Lomri, N., Rahmaoui, C.M., Baxter, J.D., and Scharschmidt, B.F.: Thyroid hormone export regulates cellular hormone content and response. *J. Biol. Chem.*, 271(29):17147-17151, 1996.

233. Forrest, D., Golarai, G., Connor, J., and Curran, T.: Genetic analysis of thyroid hormone receptors in development and disease. *Recent Prog. Horm. Res.*, 51:1-22, 1996.

234. Pohlenz, J. and Knobl, D.: Treatment of pituitary resistance to thyroid hormone (PRTH) in an 8-year-old boy. *Acta Paediatrica*, 85(3):387-390, 1996.

235. Forrest, D., Hanebuth, E., Smeyne, R.J., et al.: Recessive resistance to thyroid hormone in mice lacking β thyroid

hormone receptor: evidence for tissue-specific modulation of receptor function. *EMBO J.*, 15(12):3006-3015, 1996.

236. Forrest, D., Erway, L.C., Ng, L., Altschuler, R., and Curran, T.: Thyroid hormone receptor beta is essential for development of auditory function. *Nature Genetics*, 13(3): 354-357, 1996.

237. Pohlenz, J., Schonberger, W., Wemme, H., Winterpacht, A., Wirth, S., and Zabel, B.: New point mutation (R243W) in the hormone binding domain of the c-erbAβ₁ gene in a family with generalized resistance to thyroid hormone. *Human Mutat.*, 7(1):79-81, 1996.

238. Zhu, X.G., Yu, C.L., McPhie, P., Wong, R., and Cheng, S.Y.: Understanding the molecular mechanism of dominant-negative action of mutant β₁ thyroid hormone receptors: the important role of the wild-type/mutant receptor heterodimer. *Endocrinology*, 137(2):712-721, 1996.

239. Stein, M.A., Weiss, R.E., and Refetoff, S.: Neurocognitive characteristics of individuals with resistance to thyroid hormone: comparison with individuals with attention-deficit hyperactivity disorder. *J. Develop. Behav. Pediatr.*, 16(6):406-411, 1995.

240. Miyoshi, Y., Nakamura, H., Sasaki, S., et al.: Two consecutive nucleotide substitutions in the β T₃ receptor gene resulting in an 11-amino acid truncation in a patient with generalized resistance to thyroid hormone. *Mol. Cell. Endocrinol.*, 114(1-2):9-17, 1995.

241. Sasaki, S., Nakamura, H., Tagami, T., Miyoshi, Y., and Nakao, K.: Functional properties of a mutant β T₃ receptor (R338W) identified in a subject with pituitary resistance to thyroid hormone. *Mol. Cell. Endocrinol.*, 113 (1):109-117, 1995.

242. Piedrafita, F.J., Ortiz, M.A., and Pfahl, M.: β Thyroid hormone receptor mutants associated with generalized resistance to thyroid hormone show defects in their ligand-sensitive repression function. *Mol. Endocrinol.*, 9(11): 1533-1548, 1995.

243. Onigata, K., Yagi, H., Sakurai, A., et al.: A novel point mutation (R243Q) in exon 7 of the β c-erbA thyroid hormone receptor gene in a family with resistance to thyroid hormone. *Thyroid*, 5(5):355-358, 1995.

244. Kitajima, K., Nagaya, T., and Jameson, J.L.: Dominant-negative and DNA-binding properties of mutant thyroid hormone receptors that are defective in homodimerization but not heterodimerization. *Thyroid*, 5(5):343-353, 1995.

245. Grace, M.B., Buzard, G.S., and Weintraub, B.D.: Allele-specific associated polymorphism analysis: novel modification of SSCP for mutation detection in heterozygous alleles using the paradigm of resistance to thyroid hormone. *Human Mutat.*, 6(3): 232-242, 1995.

246. Tsukaguchi, H., Toshimasa, Y., Fujimoto, K., et al.: Three novel mutations of β thyroid hormone receptor gene in unrelated patients with resistance to thyroid hormone: two mutations of the same codon (H435L and H435Q) produce separate subtypes of resistance. *J. Clin. Endocrinol. Metab.*, 80(12):3613-3616, 1995.

247. Langworth, S., Rojdmark, S., and Akesson, A.: Normal pituitary hormone response to thyrotrophin releasing hormone in dental personnel exposed to mercury. *Swed. Dent. J.*, 14(2):101-103, 1990.

248. Nagaya, T., Madison, L.D., and Jameson, J.L.: Thyroid hormone receptor mutants that cause resistance to thyroid

hormone. *J. Biol. Chem.*, 267:13014-13019, 1992.

249. Meier, C.A., Dickstein, B.M., Ashizawa, K., et al.: Variable transcriptional activity and ligand binding of mutant β 1,3,5,3'-triiodothyronine receptors from four families with generalized resistance to thyroid hormone. *Mol. Endocrinol.*, 6:248-258, 1992.

250. Lechan, R.M., Qi, Y., Berrodin, T.J., et al.: Immunocytochemical delineation of thyroid hormone receptor β₂-like immunoreactivity in the rat central nervous system. *Endocinology*, 132:2461-2469, 1993.

251. Sjöberg, M., Vennström, B., and Forrest, D.: Thyroid hormone receptors in chick retinal development: differential expression for α and N-terminal variant β receptors. *Development*, 114:39-47, 1992.

252. Wood, W.M., Ocran, K.W., Gordon, D.F., and Ridgway, E.C.: Isolation and characterization of mouse complementary DNAs encoding α and β thyroid hormone receptors from thyrotroph cells: the mouse pituitary specific β₂ isoform differs at the amino terminus from the corresponding species from rat pituitary tumor cells. *Mol. Endocrinol.*, 5:1049-1061, 1991.

253. Bradley, D.J., Towle, H.C., and Young, W.S., III: Spatial and temporal expression of α- and β-thyroid hormone receptor mRNAs, including the β₂-subtype, in the developing mammalian nervous system. *J. Neurosci.*, 12(6): 2288-2302, 1992.

254. Bradley, D.J., Towle, H.C., and Young, W.S., III: α and β thyroid hormone receptor (TR) gene expression during auditory neurogenesis: evidence for TR isoform-specific transcriptional regulation *in vivo*. *Proc. Natl. Acad. Sci.* (USA), 91(2):439-443, 1994.

255. Hirano, T., Jogamoto, M., and Chin, I.: Syndrome of resistance to thyroid hormone in an infant with congenital cytomegalovirus infection. *Acta Paediatr. Japan*, 31(4): 504-508, 1989.

256. Bollerslev, J. and Kvetny, J.: Thyroid hormone resistance in blood monocyte cells and elevated serum T₃ in patients with autosomal dominant osteopetrosis. *Scand. J. Clin. Lab. Invest.*, 48(8):795-799, 1988.

257. Bercu, B.B., Orloff, S., and Schulman, J.D.: Pituitary resistance to thyroid hormone in cystinosis. *J. Clin. Endocrinol. Metab.*, 51:1262-1268, 1980.

258. Bellastella, A., Criscuolo, T., Sinisi, A.A., et al.: Plasma thyrotropin, thyroxine, triiodothyronine, free thyroxine, free triiodothyronine, and cortisol levels in blind prepubertal boys. *J. Endocrinol. Invest.*, 11:171-177, 1988.

259. Chan, A.M., Lynch, M.J.C., Baily, J.D., Ezerin, C., and Fraser, D.: Hypothyroidism in cystinosis: a clinical, endocrinologic, and histologic study involving sixteen patients with cystinosis. *Am. J. Med.*, 48:678-692, 1970.

260. Lazar, M.A., Hodin, R.A., and Chin, W.W.: Human carboxyl-terminal variant of α-type c-*erb*A inhibits transactivation by thyroid hormone receptors without binding thyroid. *Proc. Natl. Acad. Sci.*, 86:7771-7774, 1989.

261. McKinney, J.D. and Pedersen, L.G.: Do residue levels of polychlorinated biphenyls (PCBs) in human blood produce mild hypothyroidism? *J. Theor. Biol.*, 129:231-241, 1987.

262. Garrison, R.L.: Personal communication. February 4, 1999. < rgarrison@fpcm.med.uth.tmc.edu >

Section III

Interpretation of Fibromyalgia Symptoms and Objective Findings as Manifestations of Inadequate Thyroid Hormone Regulation

A. System Mechanisms

3.1

Adrenergic System

Overview of the Sympathetic-Catecholamine-Adrenoceptor System

The adrenergic system consists of three links: (1) sympathetic neurons, (2) catecholamine hormones, and (3) adrenergic receptors. The sympathetic nerves secrete the catecholamine hormones. The hormones include dopamine, norepinephrine, and epinephrine. Dopamine binds to dopamine receptors. Norepinephrine and epinephrine bind to α- and β-adrenergic receptors. The two types of adrenergic receptors occupy membranes of cells of most body tissues. α-Adrenergic receptors have a higher affinity for norepinephrine, and β-adrenergic receptors have a higher affinity for epinephrine. In general, binding of catecholamines to α-adrenergic receptors slows cell metabolism; binding to β-adrenergic receptors accelerates metabolism. In some tissues, such as the liver and some hypothalamic regions, liganded receptor types have the opposite effects on metabolism.

Thyroid Hormone Status and the Sympathetic-Catecholamine-Adrenoceptor Axis

Thyroid hormone potently regulates the adrenergic genes. In most tissues, binding of T_3 to T_3-receptors on β-adrenergic genes increases the genes' transcription, resulting in an increase in production of β-adrenergic receptors. Inadequate thyroid hormone regulation of β-adrenergic receptor genes decreases the genes' transcription, thus decreasing the production of β-adrenergic receptors. In most tissues, binding of T_3 to T_3-receptors on α-adrenergic genes decreases their transcription, resulting in decreased production of α-adrenergic receptors. Inadequate thyroid hormone regulation of the α-adrenergic receptor genes increases the genes' transcription, thus increasing the production of α-adrenergic receptors. These genomic effects of thyroid hormone are responsible for most of the metabolic and clinical features of hypothyroidism and hyperthyroidism. The effects are also responsible for most of the features of cellular resistance to thyroid hormone and the thyrotoxic effects of excessive thyroid hormone intake.

In hypothyroidism, the density of α-adrenergic receptors on cell membranes increases, and the density of β-adrenergic receptors decreases. In hyperthyroidism, the opposite occurs—the density of α-adrenergic receptors on cell membranes decreases, and the density of β-adrenergic receptors increases. As a result, overall, hypothyroid patients have α-adrenergic receptor dominance; consequently, their mental and physical processes are generally slowed. Hyperthyroid patients have β-adrenergic receptor dominance; as a result, their mental and physical processes are accelerated. The shift in the ratio of β- to α-adrenoceptors toward α-adrenoceptor dominance is a plausible mechanism for most of the symptoms and objective findings in fibromyalgia.

Abnormalities of the Sympathetic-Catecholamine-Adrenoceptor Axis in Fibromyalgia

In one study, the platelets of fibromyalgia patients had an increased density of α_2-adrenergic receptors. For an understanding of the underlying mechanism of fibromyalgia, this finding of an increased density of α_2-adrenergic receptors is the most important documented molecular abnormality.

The reported levels of catecholamines in fibromyalgia patients have been inconsistent, ranging from normal-to-elevated. Researchers found that breakdown products of dopamine and norepinephrine, but not serotonin, were significantly lower than in con-

341

trols. During exercise and other stresses, fibromyalgia patients were found to have a subnormal increase in norepinephrine and epinephrine levels; they also had subnormal increases in heart rate. At rest, however, sympathetic activity was normal in most cases. Fibromyalgia patients also have been found to have lower than normal levels of neuropeptide Y.

Inadequate Thyroid Hormone Regulation of Transcription May Mediate the Abnormalities of the Sympathetic-Catecholamine-Adrenoceptor System in Fibromyalgia

Inadequate thyroid hormone regulation of the sympathetic-catecholamine-adrenoceptor axis plausibly accounts for each of the abnormalities of the axis documented in fibromyalgia. Inadequate thyroid hormone regulation of the corticotropin-releasing hormone (CRH) gene may result in subnormal activation of the central sympathetic nervous system by corticotropin-releasing hormone.

Inadequate thyroid hormone regulation decreases the levels and activities of two enzymes critical to catecholamine production. Tyrosine hydroxylase is essential to the conversion of tyrosine to DOPA, the precursor of dopamine. Dopamine-β-hydroxylase is the enzyme critical to the conversion of dopamine to norepinephrine. Low levels and activity of these two enzymes adequately account for the low levels of the metabolites of dopamine and norepinephrine in the cerebrospinal fluid of fibromyalgia patients. In addition, hypothyroidism decreases β-adrenergic receptors in the striatum (the main locus of dopamine production); the decrease in β-adrenoceptors may contribute to low dopamine levels. The low dopamine levels can account for the low motor drive and in part for the fatigue of fibromyalgia patients. Low dopamine levels may also reduce systolic blood pressure (the pressure during heart contraction) and permit relative vasodilation.

Low central nervous system production of norepinephrine and an increase in α₂-adrenergic receptors in the central nervous system of fibromyalgia patients may be the molecular underpinnings of their cognitive dysfunction and depression. Moreover, subnormal activity of the enzymes in the nucleus of the solitary tract in the brain stem and in the paravertebral sympathetic ganglia may account for fibromyalgia patients' deficient secretion of norepinephrine and epinephrine during exercise. Blunted sympathetic responsiveness in fibromyalgia with a relative parasympathetic nervous system dominance might also explain the irritable bowel syndrome of some patients.

Inadequate thyroid hormone regulation of the adrenergic genes can account for several abnormalities of the sympathetic-catecholamine-adrenoceptor axis in fibromyalgia. The inadequate gene regulation can explain the increased density of α₂-adrenergic receptors on the platelets of fibromyalgia patients. Psychiatric researchers consider the platelet density of α₂-adrenergic receptors a reliable indicator of central nervous system density of the receptors. An increase of α₂-adrenergic receptors in the nucleus of the solitary tract of the brain stem and in the sympathetic ganglia can account in part for fibromyalgia patients' blunted sympathetic responses to stressors such as exercise. Accordingly, the increased receptor density can explain in part the subnormal increase in heart rate and in norepinephrine secretion during exercise.

An increase in the density of α₂-adrenergic receptors can also explain other features of fibromyalgia. Binding of catecholamines to α₂-receptors induces vasoconstriction, while also decreasing heart rate and force of contraction. These effects can explain the decreased brain and peripheral blood flow in fibromyalgia. Binding of catecholamines to α₂-adrenergic receptors on cell membranes can also account for the abnormalities of glucose breakdown (glycolysis) in fibromyalgia. α₂-Adrenergic receptors on serotonergic neurons inhibit their secretion of serotonin. The inhibition may explain the indicators of low peripheral serotonin levels. α₂-Adrenergic receptors also appear to decrease growth hormone secretion. This mechanism of inhibition may back up decreased growth hormone levels due to repressed transcription for growth hormone caused directly by inadequate thyroid hormone regulation of the growth hormone gene. The increase in α₂-adrenergic receptors may also explain fibromyalgia patients' anxiety, pain, and urinary frequency. An increase in α₂-adrenergic receptors or α₁-adrenergic receptors may result in disturbed sleep by altering synthesis and secretion of various hormones, neurotransmitters, and neuromodulators.

A line of evidence related to β-adrenergic receptors supports the hypothesis that most features of fibromyalgia are due to inadequate thyroid hormone regulation of the sympathetic-catecholamine-adrenoceptor axis. Activating β₂-adrenergic receptors in rat brain with salbutamol (a β-adrenergic receptor agonist) significantly increased serotonin levels in limbic forebrain, corpus striatum, and cerebral cortex. When fibromyalgia patients took salbutamol, the patients' fibromyalgia status improved, especially in measures of pain and exercise tolerance. In susceptible individuals, the use of β-adrenergic receptor blocking drugs *such as propranolol induce symptoms typical of fibromyalgia: slow heart rate (bradycardia), cold extremities, depression, fatigue, and sleep disturbances that might include insomnia and nightmares. Studies showed that fibromyalgia patients did not improve with the use of imipramine (a medication that increases the amount of norepinephrine in the synaptic clefts between noradrenergic nerves). Adverse effects motivated 35% of patients to stop taking imipramine. The adverse effects may have resulted from the increased norepinephrine binding to α_2-adrenergic receptors and inhibiting neuronal transmission.*

The low neuropeptide Y plasma levels in fibromyalgia patients cannot yet be interpreted in terms of inadequate thyroid hormone regulation. The reason is that no studies have been published in which researchers explored thyroid hormone regulation of neuropeptide Y in the peripheral circulation. However, neuropeptide Y is secreted with norepinephrine from sympathetic nerve terminals. Future studies may show that inadequate thyroid hormone regulation of sympathetic nerves diminishes neuropeptide Y synthesis and secretion.

Life for most human beings involves virtually relentless exposure to chemical, physical, physiological, and psychological disruptions of homeostatic balance. These disruptions constitute stress. Under normal circumstances, we adapt to stress and recover homeostatic balance through the activities of two major stress adaptation systems. One, the hypothalamic-pituitary-adrenocortical system, I cover in Chapter 3.5. The other, the sympathetic-catecholamine-adrenoceptor system, is the subject of this chapter.

My title for this chapter, the "Adrenergic System," may seem truncated. After all, the subject is the sympathetic-catecholamine-adrenoceptor axis—a system with multiple links. I chose this title for two reasons. First is its brevity. Second is the meaning of the term "adrenergic." Early investigators learned that a structure on top of each kidney secretes hormones that enable the organism to adapt to stress. They named the structures "adrenal" glands. This term is *apropos*: "ad" means "to," and "ren" is short for "renal" which means kidney. Thus, the adrenal glands are additions to the kidneys. Another synonym, "suprarenal" gland, means the gland atop the kidney. British researchers named the hormone secreted in greatest quantity by the adrenal glands "adrenaline." Later, researchers found that the adrenal gland also secretes a second hormone, "noradrenaline." Biochemists subsequently determined that adrenaline and noradrenaline are catecholamines. (A catecholamine is a pyrocatechol, a root chemical compound, with an alkylamine side chain. DOPA, norepinephrine, and epinephrine are the catecholamines I consider in this chapter.) The term researchers in the United States use for adrenaline is "epinephrine." For noradrenaline, they use "norepinephrine."

As researchers learned more about the sympathetic-catecholamine-adrenoceptor axis, they came to use the term "adrenergic" as an adjective to denote biochemical or physiological links in the axis. Thus, sympathetic nerves (the first link) secrete the "adrenergic hormones" epinephrine and norepinephrine. We use the terms "adrenergic neurons," "noradrenergic neurons," and "dopaminergic neurons" as synonyms for the nerves, depending on the catecholamine the nerves secrete. These hormones (the second link) affect cell metabolism by binding to proteins on cell membranes. We call the proteins (the third link), which are specific recipients of the hormones, "adrenergic receptors." Adrenergic receptors do not exclusively bind to either epinephrine or norepinephrine. We divide the receptors into two types, α-adrenergic receptors and β-adrenergic receptors. (For subtypes of these receptors, see section below titled "Adrenergic Receptors.") Each type binds both epinephrine and norepinephrine. However, α-adrenergic receptors have a higher affinity for (bind more readily to) norepinephrine, and β-adrenergic receptors have a higher affinity for epinephrine.

Researchers have reported abnormalities of each link of the axis in fibromyalgia patients. Inadequate thyroid hormone regulation of gene transcription can account for all of them.

● REVIEW OF THE SYMPATHETIC-CATECHOLAMINE-ADRENOCEPTOR AXIS

To understand the model of fibromyalgia I propose in this book, it is critical to have a general understanding of the sympathetic-catecholamine-adrenoceptor system.[112,pp.816-817][113,pp.243-251][114,pp.223-225] This first section is an overview of the system.

Function of the sympathetic-catecholamine-adrenoceptor axis involves four steps: (1) activation of sympathetic nerves, (2) secretion of the catecholamines norepinephrine and epinephrine, (3) binding of the catecholamines to adrenergic receptors, and (4) intracellular biochemical pathways that convert the catecholamine-adrenoceptor interaction into physiological responses. When the system functions normally, it aids homeostasis; when it dysfunctions, it permits physiological and psychological imbalances. When the dysfunction is sufficiently severe or prolonged, abject disease may result. This is the case, for example, with pheochromocytoma. The patient with this disease has a catecholamine-secreting tumor (typically benign) in an adrenal medulla. Laboratory testing makes obvious the abnormality underlying the patient's attacks of palpitation, headache, nausea, dyspnea, anxiety, pallor, sweating, and hypertension. On the other hand, testing available in commercial laboratories today does not initially enable the clinician to detect cellular resistance to thyroid hormone as a mechanism of patients' hypothyroid-like symptoms. For practical purposes, the underlying mechanism is invisible. As a result, due to a pseudoscientific presumption of conventional medicine, conventional clinicians are likely to falsely ascribe the patient's symptoms and signs to some psychogenic mechanism (see Chapter 1.2).

The sympathetic system is the component of the nervous system that sets in motion physiological processes that enable us to adapt rapidly to stimuli that signal the need for fast or vigorous activity. Several regions of the central nervous system mediate neural output of the autonomic nervous system, which includes both sympathetic and parasympathetic divisions. The regions include the cerebral cortex, hippocampus, entorrhinal cortex, and parts of the thalamus, basal ganglia, cerebellum, and the reticular formation of the brain stem. The autonomic activating influences of most of these are produced through the hypothalamus. The hypothalamus integrates neural input from other brain regions into coherent patterns of autonomic response. The hypothalamus influences autonomic function through projections to brain stem and spinal cord nuclei that act on preganglionic neurons. These projections alter functions such as heart rate, blood pressure, body temperature, and respiration.[165,pp.766-767] Stimulation of the lateral and posterior hypothalamus normally induces general sympathetic activation. The activation entails increases in heart rate and blood pressure. It also induces piloerection (erection of hair by contraction of the arrectores pilorum muscles), sweating, and pupil dilation. Stimulation of the anterior hypothalamus induces parasympathetic output.[158,p.143][165,pp.766-767]

The main autonomic coordinating center of the brain stem is the nucleus of the solitary tract. Afferent signals reach this nucleus from most organs and alter autonomic function. The structure receives input from viscera and the limbic system. Its main output is to the hypothalamus, limbic system, and other brain stem nuclei. Through signals it transmits to the hypothalamus, the nucleus influences hormonal secretions. Through signals it transmits to other brain stem nuclei, it alters autonomic preganglionic neuronal output to peripheral tissues. The nucleus mediates autonomic changes through sets of reflex circuits that interact with lower brain stem nuclei connected to autonomic motor neurons that control "effectors." (Charles Sherrington's term for a peripheral tissue that reacts to nerve signals: muscles react by contracting and glands react by secreting.) Also, the nucleus sends and receives input from other brain regions that integrate signals for complex autonomic control.[165,pp.767-768]

Sympathetic nerves conduct signals that cause their terminal axons to secrete norepinephrine into synapses in tissues. The norepinephrine binds to adrenergic receptors on the membranes of cells within the anatomic vicinity of its release. The epinephrine and norepinephrine secreted by the chromaffin cells (see subsection below titled "Locations of Catecholaminergic Neurons") of the adrenal medullae enter the blood. The circulation delivers the two catecholamines to tissues; there, the hormones influence cells upon binding to adrenergic receptors stationed on their membranes.

The medullae take part in sympathetic activity when signals reach them through a rich supply of fibers from the splanchnic and lumbar portions of the sympathetic chain. The medullae are therefore under direct control of the sympathetic nervous system. The medullae react by ejecting catecholamines into the bloodstream. About 80% of the ejection is epinephrine and 20% norepinephrine. (Except for some secretion in the brain, only the adrenal medullae secrete epinephrine.) The circulation then delivers the catecholamines to the tissues whose function the hormones will affect. The catecholamines released by the medullae reinforce the effects of norepinephrine released by sympathetic nerve endings in tissues.

The sympathetic nerves and the adrenal medullae release catecholamines when signaled by impulses reaching them from centers in the hypothalamus or brain stem. The sympathetic nerves and adrenal medullae may simultaneously activate. This occurs during strenuous exercise or exposure to extreme cold. They may also activate separately or to different degrees. Hypoglycemia, for instance, activates the adrenal medullae but inhibits the sympathetic nervous system.

After catecholamines are secreted, they set off reactions in cells by interacting with protein receptors embedded in the cells' plasma membranes. Because the receptors are specific for catecholamines, we call them adrenergic receptors. The membranes of most tissues and organs contain both α- and β-adrenergic receptors. Epinephrine has equal affinity for α- and β-adrenergic receptors. In most tissues, norepinephrine has greater affinity for α- than β-adrenergic receptors.[110,p.671] In reacting to norepinephrine and epinephrine, α- and β-adrenergic receptors mediate opposite or antagonistic responses. *The response of an organ to catecholamines depends on which type of receptor most densely populates its cell membranes.* This is important to an understanding of the role of inadequate thyroid hormone regulation of cell function in the etiology of many patients' fibromyalgia. Inadequate thyroid hormone regulation of the adrenergic receptor genes induces a predominance of α-adrenergic receptors on cell membranes. Overall, this type of adrenergic receptor, when bound to a catecholamine, initiates cellular effects that slow metabolic processes.

Overall, the β-adrenergic type, bound to a catecholamine, initiates cellular processes that accelerate metabolism and muster physiological processes that facilitate increased levels of activity. One physiological process is the mobilization of glucose and fatty acids—substances cells can oxidize to generate energy. For example, during psychological or physical stress, epinephrine stimulates the liver to break down glycogen and release its glucose molecules into the circulation. The release raises the blood glucose level. Also, epinephrine stimulates adipose tissue to release free fatty acids into the circulation. The glucose and fatty acids fuel the increased metabolic activities of cells during the stressful event.

In general, then, catecholamine/α-adrenoceptor interaction is inhibitory to mental and physical function; catecholamine/β-adrenoceptor interaction is excitatory. Some α-adrenoceptor-mediated functions, however, are excitatory. For example, catecholamine/α_2-adrenergic receptor interaction induces vasoconstriction. The constriction is an active contraction of the smooth muscle lining of blood vessels. The α_1- form of adrenergic receptor increases activity of the enzyme (type II T_4 5'-deiodinase) that converts T_4 to T_3 in brown fat.[219][220] In addition, the receptor mediates muscle contractions of the bladder (see Chapters 3.14 and 3.21), intestinal sphincters, and piloerector muscles.[110,p.671] Among the functions mediated by β-adrenergic receptors are vasodilation, acceleration of heart rate, fat breakdown, dilation of the bronchial tubes, and generation of body heat.[110,p.672]

Both α- and β-adrenergic receptors set off physiological responses by triggering chains of reactions in cell membranes and cytoplasm. The different biochemical reactions initiated by α- and β-adrenergic receptors transduce adrenergic receptor/catecholamine binding into physiological responses. The α_2-adrenergic receptor, for example, couples in the cell membrane to G_i (inhibitor G protein). This interaction reduces adenyl cyclase activity. Through subsequent biochemical reactions, the interaction diminishes physiological responses that would favor adaptation to stress. One such diminished response is secretion of norepinephrine by sympathetic neurons. The β_2-adrenergic receptor, upon binding to a catecholamine, activates adenylate cyclase in the cell membrane, generates cyclic adenosine monophosphate (cAMP) in the cytoplasm, and increases the intracellular concentration of Ca^{2+}. The increased calcium ion concentration activates kinases, and the activated kinases catalyze reactions in the cell that lead to adaptive physiological responses. Such responses include increased secretion of norepinephrine and increased glycolysis and ATP synthesis.[109,pp.244&252]

THYROID HORMONE AND THE ADRENERGIC SYSTEM

Most effects of thyroid hormone on the body are mediated by adrenergic receptors interacting with catecholamines. Thyroid hormone regulates transcription of the adrenergic genes. When thyroid hormone levels are sufficient and the hormone properly regulates transcription of the adrenergic genes, cell membranes have a normal balance of α- and β-adrenergic receptors. When thyroid hormone fails to properly regulate transcription of the adrenergic genes, α-adrenoceptor density on cell membranes increases, and β-adrenoceptor density decreases. Thus, the ratio of α-adrenergic receptors to β-adrenergic receptors increases, resulting in a predominance of α-adrenergic receptors on cell membranes. Because overall, α-adrenergic receptors impede metabolic process, a general slowdown of the individual results. I term this overall slowdown the α-adrenergic profile. Fibromyalgia patients exhibit this profile. In contrast to this profile, excessive exposure of the adrenergic genes to thyroid hormone induces a shift toward β-adrenergic dominance. The shift results in cellular hypermetabolism. If hypermetabolism generates symptoms, clinicians diagnose the individual as thyrotoxic. We may call thyrotoxicity a β-adrenergic profile, although β-adrenergic/catecholamine interaction does not mediate all features of thyrotoxicity.

Normally, sympathetic neurons and the adrenal

medullae secrete basal amounts of epinephrine and norepinephrine. The basal amounts of the catecholamines circulate through the body and modulate cell metabolism to accommodate the individual's varying biochemical and physiological needs. Basal amounts of catecholamines are sufficient to maintain normal sympathetic tone,[110,p.674] *but only if cell membranes contain a normal balance of α- and β-adrenergic receptors.* If cell membranes contain an excess of α-adrenoceptors, physiological features typical of hypothyroidism result. These features include reduced cardiac output, peripheral vasoconstriction, reduced blood flow, and decreased glycolysis. As I detail below, fibromyalgia patients exhibit these hypothyroid-like features. The finding of an increased density of α_2-adrenergic receptors on the platelets of fibromyalgia patients[91] suggests that the receptors mediate the hypothyroid-like features.

ANATOMY, PHYSIOLOGY, BIOCHEMISTRY, AND MOLECULAR BIOLOGY OF THE SYMPATHETIC-CATECHOLAMINE-ADRENOCEPTOR AXIS

Locations of Catecholaminergic Neurons

In the periphery, sympathetic nerve terminals and the chromaffin cells of the adrenal medullae contain catecholamines. The chromaffin cells are developmentally similar to sympathetic postganglionic neurons and secrete norepinephrine and epinephrine into the circulation.[158,p.142] In the central nervous system, several types of neurons contain and secrete catecholamines. The neurons may secrete one or more of the three main catecholamines: dopamine, norepinephrine, and epinephrine. (Throughout this chapter, for the most part, when I use the term catecholamines, I refer to norepinephrine and epinephrine, though dopamine is also a catecholamine.)

Adrenergic nerve cell bodies contain some 10-to-100 μg/g catecholamines. Their axons contain very little, but the varicosed regions of the nerve terminals contain very large amounts (1000-to-3000 μg/g). In both central and peripheral adrenergic neurons, vesicles store catecholamines in each nerve section until secreted.[109,p.259]

Dopaminergic System. Dopaminergic neurons (neurons that secrete dopamine) in the brain outnumber noradrenergic neurons by 3 or 4 to 1. Neuronal projections of the dopaminergic system are tightly organized topographically. We classify dopaminergic neurons into two major systems based on their efferent projections: (1) the mesostriatal system and (2) the mesolimbic and mesocortical systems.[157,p.697]

The mesostriatal dopaminergic system extends from the substantia nigra and ventral tegmentum to several striatal regions. This system mediates control of voluntary movement. Damage to this system results, for example, in the motor disorders of Parkinson's disease.[157,p.698]

The mesolimbic dopaminergic system projects from the ventral tegmentum to limbic areas, and the mesocortical system projects to cortical regions. Investigators believe these projections mediate cognition.[157,p.698]

There are also other dopaminergic cell groups. The diencephalon contains tuberohypophyseal, incertohypothalamic, and medullary periventricular dopaminergic neurons. Other neurons are present in the dorsal and ventrolateral preoptic regions and the hypothalamus. The olfactory bulb and the retina also contain dopaminergic neurons.[157,p.697]

Noradrenergic System. Two brain stem nuclei, the locus ceruleus and the lateral tegmental neurons, contain the cell bodies of noradrenergic neurons (neurons that secrete norepinephrine). The locus ceruleus is located in the rostral pontine central gray regions; the lateral tegmental neurons are widely dispersed in the medullary lateral pontine tegmentum.[157,p.696]

Projections of the dopaminergic system are highly organized. In contrast, the noradrenergic system has widespread projections through the central nervous system.[157,p.696] Some single neurons innervate wide areas of the brain.[229]

Locus Ceruleus. The locus ceruleus is a compact group of cells in the grey matter at the caudal end of the pons. It contains some 12,000 large noradrenergic neurons on each side of the brain stem. The axons project extensively and widely through the brain, and some descend through the spinal cord. Their terminals contain a great density of vesicles, as do the terminals of peripheral sympathetic nerves.[109,p.261] Axons from the cells bodies in the locus ceruleus form five main noradrenergic tracts. Three tracts ascend, mainly ipsilaterally, along pathways of blood vessels and bundles of nerves. They innervate all cortical areas, specific thalamic and hypothalamic nuclei, and the olfactory bulb. Specifically, these ascending tracts form a central tegmental tract, a central gray dorsal longitudinal fasciculus tract, and a ventral tegmental-medial forebrain bundle tract.[109,p.262] Most ascending projections terminate in the dorsal thalamus; a smaller proportion terminate in the hypothalamus.[157,p.696]

A fourth tract travels through the superior cerebellar peduncle and innervates the cortex of the cerebellum. A fifth tract descends into the midbrain and the spinal cord. Its axons travel in the ventral-lateral columns.

Noradrenergic axons from the locus ceruleus travel through the cortices of the cerebellum, hippocampus, and cerebrum; the axons pass up through the major myelinated tracts of the cortices and turn vertically toward the outer cortex. The axons then bend, forming T-shaped branches, and course parallel to the molecular layer of the cortical surface. At the cortical surface, the noradrenergic axon terminals form a complex network with other neuron terminals.[109,p.263]

Noradrenergic pathways in the central nervous system are for the most part efferent. For example, noradrenergic fibers that innervate the hypothalamus originate in the brain stem and travel mainly along two pathways that form part of the medial forebrain bundle. Fibers of the dorsal pathway originate in the locus ceruleus and reach out to other parts of the brain, such as the dorsal and paraventricular nuclei of the hypothalamus. Fibers of the ventral pathway originate in the ventral medulla and the nucleus of the solitary tract and provide most of the noradrenergic innervation of the hypothalamus.[123][124]

According to Cooper et al., in the cerebellum, hippocampus, and cerebral cortex, the major effect of activating noradrenergic neurons from the locus ceruleus is inhibition of spontaneous discharge of postsynaptic neurons. They wrote that postsynaptic neurons become hyperpolarized and their membrane resistance increases. They also wrote that the receptors of the postsynaptic target cells are the β-adrenoceptor form; they respond to norepinephrine with characteristic production of cAMP.[109,pp.263-264]

It is true that an increase in cAMP is an effect of norepinephrine/β-adrenergic receptor interaction (see subsection below titled "Post-Adrenergic Receptor Mechanisms in the Cell Membrane that Mediate Catecholamine-Adrenoceptor Signals"). However, the conclusion that β-adrenergic receptors mediate inhibition of spontaneous discharge of target cells conflicts with data suggesting that norepinephrine/β-adrenergic receptor interaction is excitatory to most brain cells. The inhibitory effect of noradrenergic neuron activation Cooper et al. describe is characteristic of norepinephrine/α-adrenergic receptor interaction. Role and Kelly wrote, ". . . norepinephrine activates α-adrenergic receptors, producing the opposite effect [from β-adrenergic receptors] on cellular excitability. In these cells, norepinephrine causes a slow hyperpolarization and a decrease in the rate of spontaneous

firing."[157,pp.696-697] Generally, norepinephrine/β-adrenergic interaction increases brain activity.[110,p.650] For example, binding of norepinephrine to β-adrenoceptors increases the excitability of the hippocampus cells that mediate recent memory.[164]

There are exceptions to the general rule that norepinephrine/β-adrenoceptor interaction has excitatory effects on brain cells. For example, in the paraventricular nucleus of the hypothalamus (which plays a major role in the neuroendocrine response to stress[123]), norepinephrine binds to α_1- and α_2-adrenergic receptors to induce secretion of corticotropin-releasing hormone (CRH).[119] This hormone stimulates pituitary section of ACTH, the hormone that in turn stimulates corticosteroid secretion by the adrenal cortices.

No brain function is associated with only one neurotransmitter. Thus, norepinephrine from the locus ceruleus generally wakes the brain, and serotonin induces sleep. Yet norepinephrine is not *the* transmitter for waking, and serotonin is not *the* transmitter for sleep. Each neurotransmitter is part of pathways that have several chemical relays involving other neurotransmitters or neuromodulators.[115,p.148]

Neural Input to the Locus Ceruleus. There are only two major afferent neural pathways to the locus ceruleus. These are from two brain stem nuclei: the nucleus paragigantocellularis and the nucleus hypoglossi prepositus. Role and Kelly noted that although the locus ceruleus provides broad efferent projections, afferent input to the structure is limited. Locus ceruleus neurons respond to novel afferent signals with a burst of norepinephrine secretion. These secretory bursts suggest that these neurons help the organism orient and attend to sudden contrasting or aversive stimuli.[157,p.696]

Activation of the Locus Ceruleus by Hypothalamic Corticotropin-Releasing Hormone. Hypothalamic cells secrete corticotropin-releasing hormone. The hormone stimulates the anterior pituitary gland to release ACTH, which in turn stimulates release of cortisol by the adrenal cortices. This series of hormones released by the hypothalamic-pituitary-adrenocortical axis constitutes one branch of the stress adaptation system. The other is the central locus ceruleus-norepinephrine system and its peripheral branch, the sympathetic nervous system.

These two systems are not independent of one another. Corticotropin-releasing hormone from the hypothalamus not only activates pituitary-adrenocortical components of the hypothalamic-pituitary-adrenocortical axis, it also stimulates the locus ceruleus-norepinephrine system and the central sources of the sympathetic nervous system.[148]

Lateral Tegmental Region. A large number of norepinephrine-secreting neurons are scattered about in the lateral and ventral tegmental regions.[157,p.696] Some authors state that the fibers projecting from the lateral tegmental region intermingle complexly with those projecting from the locus ceruleus.[109,p.264] Others contend that overlap is minimal. They explain that locus ceruleus neurons provide the major noradrenergic input to the neocortex, and in contrast, neurons from the lateral tegmentum provide the major input to the brain stem and spinal cord.[157,p.696]

Norepinephrine-secreting neurons from the more anterior tegmental area send axons to the forebrain and the diencephalon. The physiological effects of this noradrenergic pathway have not been established; however, it may innervate basal forebrain structures such as the amygdala and septum. Noradrenergic neurons of the more posterior tegmental area send fibers to the midbrain and spinal cord.[109,p.264]

Noradrenergic fibers from the lateral tegmentum facilitate integration of the autonomic nervous system. From the tegmentum, the neurons project to three sites: (1) the intermediolateral horn cells of the spinal cord, the origin of sympathetic preganglionic neurons; (2) the nucleus of the solitary tract, the major coordinating center for autonomic function in the brain stem;[165,p.767] and (3) the dorsal motor nucleus of the vagus nerve. Activating cells of the lateral tegmentum profoundly decrease heart rate, blood pressure, and mean arterial pressure.[157,p.697]

Storage of Norepinephrine in Neurons. Most of the norepinephrine in sympathetic nerve terminals and adrenal medullary chromaffin cells is housed in specialized vesicles. The vesicles limit the diffusion of norepinephrine out of the neurons and protect it from breakdown by the enzyme monoamine oxidase.[109,p.239] Presumably, the same is true of norepinephrine-containing neurons in the central nervous system. A vesicle contains about four ATP molecules for every molecule of norepinephrine. At physiological pH, norepinephrine is a cation (positively charged ion). The phosphate groups of ATP are anions (negatively charged ions). Due to their opposite charges, the phosphate groups of ATP form a salt link with norepinephrine, and this binds the neurotransmitter inside the vesicles. This binding to ATP, and perhaps a similar binding to protein, keeps norepinephrine out of the free state that would cause osmotic breakdown of the vesicle.[929,p.238]

The vesicle has a limiting membrane. The membrane holds within the vesicle a high volume of catecholamines and ATP, a protein that aids storage, and the enzyme dopamine-β-hydroxylase. The vesicle stores norepinephrine until nerve conduction commands its release. The membrane also protects the norepinephrine from lysis by monoamine oxidase, which also is present inside the neuronal terminal, outside the vesicle, particularly in mitochondria. The vesicle takes in dopamine as well and shields it from breakdown by monoamine oxidase. Inside the vesicle, however, dopamine-β-hydroxylase oxidizes dopamine to norepinephrine.[109,pp.238-240]

Release of Norepinephrine from Neuronal Vesicles. How norepinephrine is released from central nervous system neurons or from peripheral sympathetic neurons is not completely clear. Catecholamine secretion in the adrenal medullae is better understood. When a preganglionic sympathetic nerve conducts signals to an adrenal medulla, the terminal of the nerve releases acetylcholine.[158,p.142] This transmitter combines with proteins in the plasma membrane of the chromaffin cells. The protein changes shape and makes the membrane more permeable to calcium and other ions. Calcium ions flow into the cell and initiate a complex series of chemical reactions that mobilize catecholamines. The cells then secrete the catecholamines by exocytosis.[109,p.242]

Several factors modulate the release of catecholamines from nerve endings. First, once a neuron releases catecholamines into a synapse, some of the catecholamines bind to autoreceptors on the presynaptic ending of the neuron that released the catecholamines. An autoreceptor is a receptor on a presynaptic neuron that modulates release of the chemical transmitter the neuron secretes. The autoreceptor may regulate secretion by the neuron by binding to the transmitter secreted by the neuron or to transmitters secreted by closely adjacent neurons.[109,p.34] An example relevant to this chapter is the α_2-adrenergic autoreceptor. Upon binding to norepinephrine, this autoreceptor inhibits further norepinephrine secretion by the presynaptic neuron it occupies. High concentrations of norepinephrine inhibit further release, and low concentrations increase release.

Epinephrine System. Epinephrine-secreting nerve cell bodies lie in three central nervous system locations. Two of these are intermingled with norepinephrine-secreting neurons. One of these two locations is in the lateral tegmental region. The other is in the dorsal medulla. The axons of the nerve cell bodies in these two regions ascend to and enter the hypothalamus. The other location of epinephrine-secreting neurons is the midbrain. Axons of these nerve cells innervate the visceral efferents and afferents. A main site of innervation is the dorsal motor nucleus of the vagus nerve.

Epinephrine-secreting axons innervate cells in the locus ceruleus and the periventricular regions of the fourth ventricle. The axons also innervate the lateral horn cells of the spinal cord. Researchers have a limited understanding of the function of epinephrine-secreting neurons in the central nervous system. The neurons may inhibit neural impulses in the locus ceruleus, and they may take part in controlling blood pressure and neurohormonal secretions.[109,p.265]

Substances that Modulate Catecholamine Release

Substances that may take part in modulating catecholamine release are prostaglandins, amines that affect blood vessels, angiotensin II, and acetylcholine.[109,pp.242-243]

THE CATECHOLAMINES: DOPAMINE, NOREPINEPHRINE, AND EPINEPHRINE

The catecholamines are a group of compounds that include dopamine, epinephrine, and norepinephrine. Dopamine is the precursor of norepinephrine, and norepinephrine is the precursor of epinephrine.

Central Nervous System Locations of the Three Catecholamines

Dopamine. Although dopamine is the precursor of norepinephrine, its distribution in the brain is different from that of norepinephrine. This suggests that dopamine serves roles other than conversion to norepinephrine.

Dopamine makes up more than 50% of brain catecholamines. Its highest levels are in the neostriatum. This structure consists of the caudate nucleus and putamen (the major input nuclei for the basal ganglia),[163,p.648] the tuberculum olfactorum, and the nucleus accumbens. The nucleus accumbens, part of the limbic system, receives extensive dopaminergic input. Stimulation of the nucleus accumbens is reinforcing, and cocaine appears to induce euphoria by heightening the action of dopamine at the accumbens.[162,p.759] The carotid body and superior cervical ganglia also concentrate dopamine.[109,pp.223-224] Puymirat et al. wrote that most catecholamine cells in the hypothalamus are dopaminergic neurons.[120,pp.444-445] When visualized by au-

toradiography, catecholamine neurons in rat fetus hypothalamic tissue consisted almost exclusively of dopamine neurons. Inhibiting uptake of radioactive dopamine by the specific dopamine uptake inhibitor benztropin showed the predominance of dopaminergic neurons. Researchers also found a predominance of dopaminergic neurons in fetal mouse hypothalamus.[121] A specific norepinephrine uptake inhibitor did not reveal noradrenergic neurons. This finding concurs with data showing that most of the norepinephrine in rat hypothalamus originates from nerve terminals in anatomical sites other than the hypothalamus.[122]

Norepinephrine. Peripheral postganglionic sympathetic nerves secrete norepinephrine.[158,p142] This means that peripherally, norepinephrine is secreted at any site innervated by sympathetic nerves. The highest concentration of norepinephrine in nerves is in the varicosities of the terminals. Sympathetic nerves innervate diffuse areas in peripheral tissues. The terminal branches off a nerve may extend 10-to-20 cm and contain several thousand norepinephrine-containing varicosities.[109,pp.220-221]

Norepinephrine is a normal brain constituent, but its distribution in the brain is not uniform. Its highest concentrations are in central nervous system structures associated with regulation of the sympathetic nervous system, such as the hypothalamus. Although nerve terminals secrete norepinephrine in these brain areas, the neurotransmitter originates in cells bodies located in the locus ceruleus and lateral tegmentum. In these two locations, clusters of nerve cell bodies in gray matter concentrate norepinephrine.[109,p.223]

Epinephrine. The central nervous system contains little epinephrine, perhaps only 5%-to-17% as much as its norepinephrine concentration.[109,p.224] The pituitary portal blood contains a higher concentration of epinephrine (and dopamine) than does the peripheral blood. (The portal blood delivers substances from the hypothalamus to the posterior pituitary gland.) The concentration of epinephrine in the portal blood is high enough to act physiologically on the pituitary thyrotroph cells.[132][133]

Synthesis of Catecholamines

Catecholamines are synthesized from the amino acid tyrosine. Tyrosine is derived from dietary phenylalanine through the action of the enzyme phenylalanine hydroxylase. Both phenylalanine and tyrosine are present in their free forms in the brain. Of all the tyrosine used for synthesis of endogenous compounds, however, less than 2% is converted to catecholamines.[109,pp.225-226]

Tyrosine circulates in the blood until an active transport system takes it into the brain or into sympathetic neurons in peripheral tissues. After entering a peripheral neuron, enzymes chemically transform tyrosine solely into norepinephrine. In the central nervous system, enzymes transform tyrosine into norepinephrine, epinephrine, or dopamine. The form tyrosine takes depends upon the predominant abundance of one of two enzymes, phenylethanolamine-N-methyl transferase and dopamine-β-hydroxylase[109,pp.224-225] (see below).

Heuther et al. gave healthy young men infusions of L-tryptophan, the amino acid precursor of serotonin.[217] The infusions caused a depletion of other neutral amino acids. Measurements showed a dose-dependent decrease in the ratio of plasma tyrosine to the sum of the plasma concentrations of the other large neutral amino acids. Because of these findings, the investigators speculated that two factors account for some central nervous system effects of L-tryptophan administration: (1) the L-tryptophan-stimulated production of serotonin and (2) a simultaneous decrease in the availability of tryrosine for catecholamine synthesis.

Tyrosine Hydroxylase. Tyrosine hydroxylase is the first enzyme in the biochemical pathway for synthesis of norepinephrine.[170,p.187] The enzyme is also the rate-limiting step in the synthesis of the catecholamines (dopamine, norepinephrine, and epinephrine) from DOPA.

The enzyme tyrosine hydroxylase catalyzes conversion of the amino acid tyrosine to DOPA. DOPA is then converted to dopamine and in turn to norepinephrine. Tyrosine hydroxylase is present only in the brain, adrenal medullae, the superior cervical ganglion, and all sympathetic fibers that innervate other tissues. Activity of the enzyme requires the presence of iron ions. The enzyme is highly specific for and oxidizes naturally formed L-tyrosine and, to a lesser degree, L-phenylalanine. The action of tyrosine hydroxylase is the chemical step that limits the rate of norepinephrine synthesis in both the peripheral and central nervous systems. It is also the rate-limiting enzyme for dopamine synthesis in the central nervous system.[109,p.225]

Competitive binding by some chemicals blocks the conversion of tyrosine by tyrosine hydroxylase. A methylated tyrosine, for example, blocks the conversion. Clinicians have used methylated tyrosine to inhibit catecholamine synthesis in patients with the catecholamine-secreting tumor pheochromocytoma.[109,pp.228-229] (A pheochromocytoma is a catechol-amine-producing tumor of the adrenal medullae). Clinicians may also use the chemicals to block catecholamine synthesis in patients with malignant hypertension. (Malignant hypertension is a rapidly escalating hypertension that severely damages blood vessels and may cause death.)[109,pp.228-229]

Dihydroxyphenylalanine Decarboxylase. The second enzyme that catalyzes synthesis of catecholamines is dihydroxyphenylalanine decarboxylase. This enzyme converts DOPA to dopamine. Dopamine is next converted to norepinephrine.[109,p.227] Because 3,4-dihydroxyphenylalanine is the complete term for DOPA, researchers also call the enzyme DOPA-decarboxylase. The enzyme removes carboxyl (COOH) groups from L-DOPA. DOPA-decarboxylase is highly active in the synthesis of norepinephrine. The enzyme requires vitamin B_6 (pyridoxal phosphate) as a cofactor. Vitamin B_6 deficiency reduces the activity of DOPA-decarboxylase. This does not critically reduce the levels of catecholamines in tissues. It has been shown, however, to impede recovery of complete adrenal stores of catecholamines after the administration of insulin depletes them.[109,p.230]

Dopamine-β-Hydroxylase. Dopamine is converted to norepinephrine in the brain, tissues with sympathetic innervation, sympathetic ganglia, and the adrenal medullae. The enzyme responsible for the conversion is dopamine-β-hydroxylase. Adrenergic neurons store the enzyme. The precise location of storage is the membrane of the granules that store amines such as dopamine. Chemically blocking this enzyme selectively reduces the amount of norepinephrine in the brain.[125]

Dopamine-β-hydroxylase contains copper and requires molecular oxygen and vitamin C as cofactors. Compounds that chelate copper can inhibit the enzyme. The inhibition leads to reduced norepinephrine synthesis in the brain and elevated dopamine levels.[109,pp.231-232] The drug reserpine produces behavioral depression by blocking access of dopamine to the site on dopamine-β-hydroxylase where it is converted to norepinephrine.[109,p.237]

Phenylethanolamine-*N*-Methyl Transferase. The enzyme phenylethanolamine-*N*-methyl transferase methylates norepinephrine. The methylation converts norepinephrine to epinephrine. The highest rate of conversion occurs in the adrenal medulla, but conversion also occurs at a lower rate in the heart and brain.[109,p.232]

Regulation of Norepinephrine Synthesis

When sympathetic nerves fire, they release norepinephrine from their endings to transmit nerve signals across synapses. The more the nerves fire, the more norepinephrine they release. The concentration of norepinephrine in a sympathetic nerve ending, however, stays fairly constant despite high levels of sympathetic activity. Some norepinephrine is lost during synaptic transmission by two means: dissipation from the local region where the catecholamine is released, and enzymatic decomposition. A mechanism obviously must exist that replenishes stores in the nerve terminal. Studies show that electrical stimulation of sympathetic nerves increases the amount of norepinephrine in the tissues innervated by the nerves. Electrical stimulation also increases the activity of the enzyme that controls the rate of norepinephrine synthesis. The amount of this enzyme, tyrosine hydroxylase, does not increase, but its level of activity does.[109,p.233]

In turn, norepinephrine acts as a feedback inhibitor of tyrosine hydroxylase. Norepinephrine inhibits tyrosine hydroxylase by binding to the protein component of the enzyme (apoenzyme). When norepinephrine binds to the apoenzyme, it competitively blocks the binding of a cofactor called pteridine. The cofactor is essentially an activator of the enzyme. So, when the cofactor is not able to bind to the apoenzyme, activity of the enzyme decreases. When a sympathetic nerve is firing slowly, norepinephrine concentration in the nerve terminal increases. The increase happens because tyrosine hydroxylase—free from the inhibiting effect of norepinephrine—becomes more active.

Conversely, when the sympathetic nerve fires frequently, the nerve terminal releases more norepinephrine; more of the neurotransmitter dissipates from the region, or enzymes break down more. As a result, the amount of norepinephrine in the nerve terminal decreases. Pteridine is then free to bind to the apoenzyme component of tyrosine hydroxylase, activating it. The increased enzymatic activity synthesizes norepinephrine to replace that depleted by the nerve firing.

Norepinephrine therefore controls its own synthesis through a negative feedback inhibition. This mechanism operates both in peripheral sympathetic nerves and the brain. Researchers have shown this by administering inhibitors of monoamine oxidase, the enzyme that breaks down norepinephrine, and recording the resulting reduction in norepinephrine production.[109,p.234]

Inhibition by norepinephrine, however, is not the sole mechanism that regulates synthesis of tyrosine hydroxylase. The frequency of depolarization of sympathetic nerves also plays a regulating role. Frequent neuronal firing, for example, allosterically activates

tyrosine hydroxylase. Researchers call these alterations "allosteric changes."[117,pp.326-327] (See Glossary: "Allosteric change.") Allosteric activation means that the rate of discharge of the sympathetic nerves changes the structural conformation of the tyrosine hydroxylase. The changed structure increases the affinity of tyrosine hydroxylase for its cofactor pteridine. Increased affinity means the two bind to one another more readily. The change also decreases the enzyme's affinity for its inhibitors, norepinephrine and dopamine. So, increased signal conduction may disinhibit the enzyme so that it increases its synthesis of norepinephrine. How impulse flow causes these effects is not clear, but researchers know that the binding of phosphorous to the enzyme (phosphorylation) increases its activity. Other enzymes called kinases catalyze phosphorylation of the enzyme. These enzymes include C-kinase, cAMP-dependent protein kinase, and calcium/calmodulin-dependent kinase. Some researchers believe that calcium/calmodulin kinase is the main phosphorylating enzyme.[109,p.235]

In summary, the enzyme tyrosine hydroxylase catalyzes the conversion of the amino acid tyrosine to DOPA. Tyrosine attaches to an active site on the enzyme and undergoes conversion to DOPA. The active site is receptive to tyrosine when the cofactor pteridine is attached to the allosteric site. When the allosteric site binds to pteridine, the active site binds any available tyrosine and converts it to DOPA. If norepinephrine or dopamine is present in significant concentrations, however, one of them binds to the allosteric site on the enzyme. The binding allosterically changes the conformation of the active site so that it binds tyrosine poorly, if at all. Tyrosine to DOPA conversion then slows or stops. This occurs when a sympathetic nerve fires rapidly and releases a large amount of norepinephrine in the local region of tyrosine hydroxylase. The large quantity of norepinephrine displaces pteridine from the allosteric site on the enzyme. Norepinephrine then replaces pteridine by binding to the site. The replacement changes the molecular shape of the molecule so that it slows or ceases its catalytic conversion of tyrosine to DOPA. The ultimate result is reduced norepinephrine synthesis. Norepinephrine thus engages in a self-regulatory loop. A critical component of the loop is the allosteric alteration in the rate-limiting enzyme responsible for norepinephrine synthesis.

Metabolic Degradation of Catecholamines

The most important enzymes that metabolically degrade catecholamines are monoamine oxidase and catechol-*O*-methyltransferase. Monoamine oxidase degrades epinephrine and norepinephrine to their aldehyde forms. The enzyme aldehyde dehydrogenase then oxidizes the aldehydes to their acid forms. In the brain, the enzyme aldehyde reductase reduces the aldehyde form of norepinephrine to alcohol or glycol (a dihydric alcohol).[109,p.244]

Monoamine oxidase resides mainly in the outer membrane of mitochondria. The enzyme may contain a compound that resembles vitamin B_2 (riboflavin). Monoamine oxidase is more abundant outside neurons, but it is the enzyme inside neurons that metabolizes catecholamines. Monoamine oxidase has two forms. Type A catabolizes norepinephrine and serotonin; type B catabolizes β-phenylalanine and benzydamine. Either enzyme type can metabolize dopamine, tyramine, and tryptamine. Catecholamines that are outside their protective vesicles are susceptible to breakdown by the enzyme.[109,p.245]

The other enzyme, catechol-*O*-methyltransferase, is present in cytoplasm in both the central nervous system and tissues with sympathetic innervation. The enzyme stimulates transfer of methyl groups from *S*-adenosylmethionine to the *m*-hydroxyl group of catecholamines. Researchers have tested S-adenosyl-methionine as a fibromyalgia medication and found it ineffective. (See Chapter 5.1, subsection titled "Nonsteroidal Anti-inflammatory Drugs (NSAIDs): S-adenosylmethionine.") Catechol-*O*-methyltransferase requires *S*-adenosylmethionine and magnesium ions to function. Theoretically, chemically blocking the enzyme at sympathetic nerve terminals should increase the lifespan of released catecholamines. Accordingly, the prolonged presence of catecholamines in the synaptic cleft should prolong activity of the postsynaptic nerve. However, in peripheral tissues, activation of postsynaptic nerves by catecholamines released from presynaptic nerves (the adrenergic response to nerve stimulation) is prolonged only slightly. This suggests that catechol-*O*-methyltransferase only weakly inactivates catecholamines after their release. Diffusion and particularly neuronal reuptake, rather than enzymatic breakdown, must account for a good proportion of elimination of catecholamines from the synaptic cleft.

Monoamine oxidase may break down catecholamines more weakly than does catechol-*O*-methyltransferase. Blocking the activity of monoamine oxidase may not prolong the postsynaptic nerve response at all. The two enzymes may be more potent in the central nervous system.[109,p.247]

Uptake of Catecholamines after Release

When researchers experimentally stimulate postganglionic nerves at intensities typical of normal physiological function, the nerves release norepinephrine into the synaptic cleft. The route of exit of norepinephrine from the cleft was once a subject of debate. Now it is clear that most of the neurotransmitter is not "washed away" into the circulation; nor is it completely broken down by monoamine oxidase or catechol-*O*-methyltransferase. When researchers use pharmaceutic agents to block these two norepinephrine-catabolizing enzymes, norepinephrine does not "puddle" in the synapse. Instead, the sympathetic nerve that released the norepinephrine takes it back up. When a small dose of norepinephrine is injected into a vein, some 40%-to-60% is catabolized by monoamine oxidase and catechol-*O*-methyltransferase. Rapid neuronal reuptake removes the remainder. The uptake is proportional to the density of sympathetic nerves in the tissue.

Once heart, spleen, artery, and vein take up radioactive norepinephrine, stimulating their sympathetic nerves causes them to release the labeled norepinephrine. The nerves of the tissue take up labeled norepinephrine by active membrane transport. Uptake is sodium-dependent. Blocking sodium and potassium-activated ATPase impedes uptake. A transport protein is probably involved.[929,pp.247-249]

Reuptake Blockers

Inhibition of Monoamine Oxidase. A diverse group of drugs blocks oxidative deamination of various biogenic amines, including norepinephrine. The drugs do so by inhibiting the action of monoamine oxidase. Inhibitors of monoamine oxidase increase tissue levels of amines such as norepinephrine, and some clinicians use them for treating depression. However, Cooper, Bloom, and Roth noted the lack of correlation between monoamine oxidase inhibition and therapeutic changes in depressed patients. The drugs also inhibit other enzymes that may have therapeutic as well as adverse effects.[109,p.257]

Inhibition of Storage. Several compounds block storage of monoamines. The dried roots of Rauwolfia serpentina are the source of most of these drugs. Serpentine and reserpine are examples. The drugs block monoamine storage (1) by impeding uptake of the amines into storage vesicles or (2) by interfering with amine binding inside the vesicles. By blocking storage, the drugs cause release of the amines from the vesicles inside the nerve terminals where monoamine oxidase degrades them.[109,p.257] Effects of the drugs include decreased blood pressure and tranquilization.

Calcium-Channel Blockers. Calcium ions are necessary for catecholamine release from nerve terminals; reducing the calcium level in nerve terminals decreases catecholamine release.[109,pp.257-258] Verapamil is a calcium-channel blocking medication currently marketed to correct arrhythmias. It blocks α-adrenergic activity but has no β-blocking ability.[118,p.869]

Inhibiting Reuptake. Several drugs inhibit reuptake of norepinephrine by both central and peripheral nerve endings. These include cocaine, desipramine, and some other tricyclic antidepressants. These drugs augment impulse transmission to adrenergic receptors on postsynaptic neurons by making more norepinephrine available in the synapse.[109,p.258]

Table 3.1.1 lists four commonly prescribed antidepressant drugs and the neurotransmitters whose reuptake they inhibit. Amitriptyline inhibits only serotonin reuptake, and desipramine inhibits only norepinephrine. Nortriptyline and imipramine, however, block reuptake of both neurotransmitters.[106,p.241] The drugs have different effects because of differences in their molecular structure. Nortriptyline is the demethylated metabolite of amitriptyline, and desipramine is the major metabolite of imipramine.[959,p.407]

ADRENERGIC RECEPTORS

Adrenergic receptors are proteins stationed on cell membranes. Norepinephrine, epinephrine, and adrenergic drugs bind to the receptors. We say that the binding "activates" the receptors. The activation alters the function of the cells. The chemicals that bind to adrenoceptors reach the receptors by one or both of two ways. First, the terminals of postganglionic fibers of the sympathetic nervous system release norepinephrine near the cells. Second, circulating blood delivers norepinephrine, epinephrine, and adrenergic drugs to the cells.

Two main types of adrenergic receptors occupy cell membranes and bind catecholamines—α- and β-adrenergic receptors. α-Adrenergic receptors are important to the understanding of fibromyalgia caused by hypothyroidism or cellular resistance to thyroid hormone. α-Adrenergic receptor dominance in fibromyalgia—suggested by an increased density of α_2-adrenoceptors on the platelets of some patients[91]—may mediate most of the features of fibromyalgia.

In the late 1980s, investigators classified three subtypes of α_2-adrenoceptor: α_{2A}-, α_{2B}-, and α_{2C}-adrenoceptors. Researchers have not yet learned the distinct roles of the subtypes.[194]

Transcription of the α_{1B}-adrenergic receptor gene produces multiple α_{1B}-adrenergic receptor mRNAs; the mRNAs are distributed in a tissue-specific fashion. Multiple α_{1B}-adrenergic receptor mRNAs may play a role, yet undetermined, in regulating α_{1B}-adrenergic receptor responsiveness in different tissues. Interactions of catecholamines with α_{1B}-adrenergic receptors on the surfaces of different types of cells mediate physiologic and pathologic functions.[195]

Investigators have intensely studied the β_1- and β_2-adrenoceptor subtypes of adrenergic receptors.[199] More recently, researchers have investigated the β_3-adrenoceptor subtype. A Trp→Arg mutation at amino acid position 64 in the human β_3-adrenergic receptor gene is associated with morbid obesity. Individuals with the mutation tend to gain mass, have early-onset diabetes, insulin resistance, and an increased waist to hip ratio.[196] These abnormalities may result in part from the failure of catecholamines to induce a sufficient maximum cAMP accumulation in cells that express the mutant β_3-adrenergic receptor.[197] The mutation is not harmful in individuals who are not obese. Also, the mutation is apparently not the main determinant of obesity in populations of people who consume the low fat/low energy diet typical of the Japanese.[198]

Table 3.1.1. Inhibitory effects of tricyclic antidepressant drugs on reuptake of neurotransmitters.*

DRUG	NEUROTRANSMITTER	
	Serotonin	Norepinephrine
Amitriptyline	++++	0
Nortriptyline	++	++
Imipramine	+++	++
Desipramine	0	++++

*Adapted from Tepperman, J. and Tepperman, H.M.: *Metabolic and Endocrine Physiology*, 5th edition. Chicago, Year Book Medical Publishers, Inc., 1987.[106,p.241]

In adipose tissue, β_3-adrenergic receptors are regulated in part by thyroid hormone. Adipose tissue in the epididymides of hypothyroid rats contained low levels of β_3-adrenoceptor mRNA. Twelve hours after researchers administered T_3, β_3-adrenoceptor mRNA increased 147%. In response to T_3, an increase in the lipolytic (fat decomposing) response to a specific β_3-adrenergic agonist paralleled the increase in β_3-adrenergic receptor mRNA. This parallel is important in relation to how much leptin (the obese gene product) mutant individuals have. Hypothyroid male rats had markedly elevated leptin mRNA levels. Administering T$_3$ to the rats for 8 hours decreased leptin mRNA by 40%. This reduction in leptin mRNA correlated with a 50% reduction in circulating leptin level at 24 hours.[203] El Hadri et al. found that T$_3$ did not significantly alter the transcription rate of the β$_3$-adrenoceptor gene. However, the hormone increased by 36% the half-life of β$_3$-adrenoceptor mRNA. The researchers concluded that T$_3$ exerts a post-transcriptional effect on β$_3$-adrenoceptor expression in fat cells.[204] An increase in β$_3$-adrenoceptor number correlated with β$_3$-adrenoceptor coupling to the adenylate cyclase system. Tissue site variations in the expression and function of β- and α$_2$-adrenoceptors in adipose tissue may be partly instrumental in regional obesity.[188]

Types of Adrenergic Receptors that Mediate Catecholamine Release

α$_2$-Adrenoceptors on presynaptic nerves inhibit release of norepinephrine from presynaptic adrenergic nerves; chemical blockade of α$_2$-adrenoceptors increases norepinephrine release.[109,p.258] The receptors may inhibit norepinephrine release by several possible mechanisms. The receptors, upon binding catecholamines, may (1) reduce calcium ion flow through membrane calcium channels, (2) impede impulse conduction over nerve terminal varicosities, (3) increase polarization of the neuron by favoring potassium flow into the cell, and (4) decrease cAMP and calcium ion concentrations in the cell by blocking adenyl cyclase. Opiate, dopamine, and muscarinic receptors, like α$_2$-adrenoceptors, inhibit the release of catecholamines.[109,p.243]

β$_2$-Autoreceptors induce norepinephrine release by stimulating adenyl cyclase. The stimulation increases intracellular cAMP, and in turn, cAMP increases the calcium ion concentration in the nerve cell. Chemical blockade of β$_2$-autoreceptors inhibits norepinephrine release.[109,p.258]

Nicotinic and angiotensin II receptors, upon binding to their ligands, excite catecholamine release. A β-adrenergic receptor agonist, for example, may activate a postsynaptic β$_2$-receptor in a blood vessel wall. The activation causes synthesis and release of angiotensin II. Angiotensin II passes back across the synapse and stimulates angiotensin II receptors that provoke norepinephrine release.[109,p.243]

By α$_2$-adrenergic receptors decreasing norepinephrine release, and by β$_2$-adrenergic receptors increasing its release, a balance of these receptors provides fine adjustments of norepinephrine release at synapses.

Epinephrine has a higher affinity than norepinephrine for β$_2$-adrenergic receptors. When a small amount of epinephrine is released at the synapse, it activates β$_2$-receptors and increases the release of norepinephrine. When norepinephrine release increases, however, the norepinephrine activates α$_2$-receptors reducing norepinephrine release.[109,pp.243-244]

The E series of prostaglandins is present in tissues that have sympathetic innervation. These chemicals limit the calcium ion concentration in the neuron that is necessary for release of norepinephrine. Through this mechanism, E series prostaglandins strongly inhibit the release of norepinephrine provoked by neural signals. Blocking local tissue production of prostaglandins increases norepinephrine release. The blocking also potentiates the cellular effects of norepinephrine following nerve stimulation.[109,p.244]

Nature of the Adrenergic Receptor Molecule

Adrenergic receptors are compounds composed of carbohydrates and proteins (glycoproteins) and are all about the same size. Whether the different types of adrenergic receptors are actually one interconvertible molecule or distinctly different molecules has been a subject of debate.

Hypothesis of One Generic Interconvertible Adrenergic Macromolecule. Some researchers once argued that all adrenergic receptors were one interconvertible macromolecule. The conformation of the molecule presumably alternately changed from the α- to the β-type, depending on the concentration of thyroid hormone the molecule was exposed to.[68][107] According to this hypothesis, adrenergic receptors are not static molecular entities.

Kunos et al. removed the thyroid glands of rats. Six-to-ten weeks later, the investigators tested the left atria of the rats' hearts for β- and α-adrenergic responsiveness. The atria exhibited greater α-adrenoceptor responsiveness. Kunos et al. allowed that the shift toward α-adrenoceptor responsiveness could have resulted from (1) a change in α-adrenoceptor sensitivity or (2) an increase in the number of α-adrenoceptors from a pool of receptors different from that of β-adrenoceptors. On the other hand, the change in balance could have resulted from one type of adrenergic receptor—a single macromolecule—shifting its structure (an allosteroic change) in response to inadequate exposure of atrial cells to thyroid hormone.[68]

Kunos favored the latter explanation by analogy with other studies of β- and α-adrenoceptors. In the other studies, the balance of α- and β-adrenergic responsiveness of heart tissue was systematically changed by exposing the hearts to lower temperatures. α-Adrenoceptor dominance occurred at lower temperatures and β-adrenoceptor dominance at warmer ones. After finding this temperature-related difference, investigators alkylated the receptors when the hearts were exposed to lower temperatures. Alkylating locks the receptors in the structural form that produces α-responsiveness. When the researchers exposed the alkylated receptors to warmth, the receptors did not respond as β-adrenoceptors. This outcome suggested that alkylating a single macromolecule that constitutes the generic adrenergic receptor locks it into one shape. Afterward, its molecular shape resists change, even when exposed to temperatures that would normally change it to the alternate form. If there were two distinctly different populations of receptors (α and β macromolecules), alkylating the α molecule would not block β-adrenoceptor responsiveness when the environment is warmed. The β-adrenoceptor would, according to the model, be dormant at cold temperatures but would activate at warm temperatures despite locking α-adrenoceptors by alkylation. But since alkylating the receptor molecule during cold exposure prevented further β-adrenoceptor responsiveness, regardless of the temperature, it seemed likely that the α- and β-adrenoceptor is one and the same. The studies by Kunos et al. suggested that exposure to thyroid hormone changes the three dimensional shape of the generic adrenoceptor molecule. Researchers were to learn later, however, that adrenergic receptor types are distinctly different molecules.

Different Adrenergic Receptor Types are Distinctly Different Molecules that are Products of Separate Genes. Tepperman and Tepperman wrote that α- and β-adrenergic receptors have unique glycoprotein compositions, and the distinctly different composition suggests that the receptors are products of separate genes.[106,p.238] Thyroid hormone binds to T_3-receptors at the thyroid hormone response elements of the genes. Upon binding, T_3 potently regulates expression of the genes (see next section).

Inadequate Thyroid Hormone Regulation of Adrenergic Gene Transcription

In a variety of physiological and pathological conditions, functional expression of α-adrenoceptors and β-adrenoceptors is inversely regulated.[68][69][70][71][72] In general, alterations in mRNA levels for the two receptor types correlate with changes in cell adrenoceptor density and reactivity.[71][72][73][74][75][76][77][78][79][80] Hypothyroidism reduces the density of β-adrenergic receptors on cell membranes and reduces β-adrenoceptor-mediated cellular responsiveness in most tissues.[71][72][73][74][75][76][80][81] Increases in α_{1B}-adrenoceptor mRNA in heart tissue of hypothyroid rats correlate with decreases in inotropic and chronotropic heart responsiveness mediated by α_{1B}-adrenoceptors.[71][74][80] α_2-Adrenergic receptor antagonists increase heart rate and force of contraction by relieving inhibition of norepinephrine secretion by presynaptic α_2-adrenergic receptors.[223][224][225][226] Moreover, selective α_2-adrenoceptor agonists decrease heart rate by inhibiting norepinephrine release from presynaptic neurons.[227][228] Conversely, administering thyroid hormone increases β-adrenoceptor mRNA and the membranous population of β-adrenoceptors.[82][84][85][186] At the same time, the hormone decreases α-adrenoceptor density in most tissues.[75][80][83]

Both α- and β-adrenoceptor genes contain thyroid hormone response elements. Binding of T_3 to T_3-receptors on these response elements activates transcription of the β-adrenergic receptor gene and represses transcription of the α-adrenergic receptor gene. When T_3 is not bound to T_3-receptors on the response elements, as during hypothyroidism, the transcription pattern reverses—transcription of the α-adrenergic receptor gene activates, and transcription of the β-adrenergic receptor gene represses. (In the liver, however, this relationship is reversed.)[86][199]

Researchers do not know the factors that determine expression of different subtypes of adrenergic receptors in different tissues. In many tissue cells, such as cardiac muscle cells, T_3 controls expression of β_1-adrenoceptors. T_3 does not, however, control expression of these receptors in other tissue cells such as the C6 glioma cells in the brain. The cell-specific absence of T_3 regulation may result in part from a low expression of T_3-receptors in these cells. However, studies suggest that high expression of the c-*erb*Aα_2 splice variant that inhibits T_3 genomic action is not an instrumental factor.[202]

Exposure of cultured ventricular muscle cell to T_3 is illustrative.[82] Within 24 hours, exposure to T_3 increased the number of β_1-adrenergic receptors per cell by 2.1±0.3-fold. β_2-Adrenergic receptor mRNA levels in the muscle cells were unaffected by T_3. Nevertheless, the rat β_2-adrenoceptor gene (present in the genome of the muscle cell) contains a thyroid hormone response element,[200] and the receptor expresses in response to T_3 in some tissues. The researchers concluded that in rat muscle cells, T_3 regulates the cardiac β-adrenergic receptor/adenylate cyclase system by controlling the transcription rate of the β_1-adrenergic receptor gene. This regulation involves nuclear T_3-receptors—ventricular cells contain nuclear T_3-receptors and mRNAs of c-*erb*A genes that encode T_3-binding proteins. The mechanism is not known, but transcription regulation of the β_1-adrenoceptor gene is exerted in a tissue-specific manner.

Biochemical Factors Other than T_3 that Augment α-Adrenergic Responsiveness and Decrease β-Adrenergic Responsiveness of Cells in Hypothyroidism

α-Adrenergic receptor dominance in hypothyroidism results from repression of β-adrenoceptor gene transcription and activation of α-adrenergic gene transcription due to the thyroid hormone deficiency.[86][199] In addition, evidence suggests that four other biochemical alterations facilitate decreased β-adrenoceptor responsiveness and increased α-adrenergic responsiveness. The four alterations are: (1) reduced coupling of β-adrenergic receptors to adenylate cyclase by increased expression of inhibitor G proteins (G_i);[214][215][221] (2) decreased expression of stimulatory G proteins (G_s);[222] (3) increased sensitivity to the inhibitory effects of adenosine due to increased G_i; and (4) increased production of phosphodiesterase, the cytoplasmic enzyme that decomposes cAMP after it is produced by β-adrenergic receptor/G_s/adenylate cyclase interaction in the cell membrane. (See Chapter 3.11, section titled "Fatigue Due to Increased Production of Three Inhibitory Molecules in Hypothyroidism" and Chapter 2.3, section titled "Molecular Byproducts of Thyroid Hormone-Regulated Transcription: Relevance to Fibromyalgia.")

Factors Other than Thyroid Hormone that Regulate Adrenergic Receptors

Several factors other than thyroid hormone regulate production of adrenergic receptors or alter their function. Various factors potently influence β-adrenoceptors. Insulin, estrogens, and androgens also regulate the receptors. Nutritional factors, diabetes, autonomic neuropathy, and β-blocking agents alter the function of the receptors. α-Adrenergic receptors are less responsive to these influences. (There are two exceptions: (1) during infancy when there are marked developmental alterations in the function of α_2-adrenoceptors, and (2) during fasting when there is a decrease in expression of the receptors.) β-Adrenoceptor responsiveness decreases after exposure to agonists, but this does not seem to be true of α_2-adrenoceptors. Some tissue cells have substantial adrenoceptor reserves; this is especially true of fat cells. Some 50% of β- and α_2-adrenoceptors in fat cells are spare receptors.[188]

Estrogen. Karakanias et al. found that in ovariectomized rats, administering estradiol for 48 hours decreased frontal cortex α_2-adrenoceptor density. The reduction correlated with a 50% reduction in mRNA levels encoding the predominant $\alpha_{2A/D}$-adrenoceptor subtype expressed in cortex. Levels of mRNA and receptor density did not change in the preoptic area of the hypothalamus. The authors pointed out that the study provided the first evidence that estradiol regulates expression of postsynaptic α_2-adrenoceptors in female rat frontal cortex. The reduction in $\alpha_{2A/D}$-adrenoceptor density may be a molecular substrate for modulation of cognitive function by estradiol.[189] It is possible that the emotional and cognitive upswing that occurs between day 4 and day 7 of the menstrual period[212,p.127] results from the renewed secretion of estrogen and the down-regulation of α_2-adrenergic receptors in the brain. We would expect these changes to increase neuronal metabolic processes (see Chapter 3.6).

Cyclic-AMP. Cyclic-AMP (cAMP) partly regulates expression of β_1-,[190] β_2-,[220] α_{1A}-,[193] and α_{1B}-adrenergic receptors.[192] Researchers have found cAMP response elements on the β_1-adrenoceptor gene[190] and the α_{1B}-adrenoceptor gene.[192]

Glucocorticoids. The β_1-adrenoceptor gene has glucocorticoid regulatory elements.[199] Collins et al. found that 3.1 kb of the nucleotide sequence from the 5'-flanking region of the human β_1-adrenergic receptor gene contains thyroid hormone, glucocorticoid hormone, and cAMP transcriptional response elements. These hormone response elements provide physiological evidence that thyroid hormone, glucocorticoid hormone, and cAMP regulate expression of β_1-adrenoceptors.[190]

The β_2-adrenergic receptor also contains a glucocorticoid-response element.[200] Malbon and Hadcock identified a glucocorticoid response element in the 5'-noncoding region of the hamster β_2-adrenergic receptor gene. These are obligate for glucocorticoid regulation of β_2-adrenoceptor mRNA transcription. The researchers reported that incubation of wild-type Chinese hamster ovary cells with dexamethasone, a potent glucocorticoid, elevated both β_2-adrenoceptor mRNA levels and β_2-adrenergic receptor number.[191]

Gao et al. reported that the 5'-flanking region of the rat liver α_{1B}-adrenoceptor gene contains three transcriptional response elements—one for cAMP, glucocorticoid hormone, and thyroid hormone. Investigators compared the rat α_{1B}-adrenergic receptor gene sequence to that of the cloned human α-$_{1B}$-adrenergic receptor gene. The overall structure of the human gene was highly conserved; that is, it was similar to that of the rat gene. However, the 5'-flanking region had notable differences. The α-$_{1B}$-adrenergic receptor gene is involved in mediating processes in diseases such as myocardial hypertrophy and benign prostatic hyperplasia.[192]

POST-ADRENERGIC RECEPTOR MECHANISMS IN THE CELL MEMBRANE THAT MEDIATE CATECHOLAMINE-ADRENOCEPTOR SIGNALS

Early observations indicated that thyroid hormone interacted with catecholamines and adrenergic receptors to affect cell function. Epinephrine is a physiological stimulant. Administering it to humans or laboratory animals increases pulse rate, blood pressure, and basal metabolic rate. Exposure to excessive amounts of thyroid hormone increases the magnitude of the stimulating effects of epinephrine.[104][126] β-Adrenergic receptor blocking drugs inhibit symptoms such as a rapid heart rate, hypertension, and elevated basal metabolic rate when they occur in hyperthyroid or anxious subjects.[127] The inhibiting effects of the drugs show that β-adrenergic receptors mediate the symptoms.

Hyperthyroid humans have normal amounts of cAMP in their urine. When given epinephrine, however, the cAMP in their urine increases.[210]

In 1984, DeGroot et al. reviewed studies indicating an interaction of thyroid hormone with the adrenergic system.[108,p.75] Some but not all studies showed that thyrotoxic animals have increased adenylate cyclase activity.[96][97][98] Making rats hypothyroid with propylthiouracil reduced the density of β-adrenergic receptors in their myocardial tissues. Treating the rats with large amounts of T_4 increased β-adrenoceptor density.[74][97] Mature red blood cells from hypothyroid turkeys had fewer β-adrenergic receptors. Thus, production of cAMP was abnormally low when researchers exposed the turkey cells to the β-adrenergic receptor agonist isoproterenol.[100] Immature red blood cells in hypothyroid rats had a reduced amount of β-adrenergic receptors and reduced coupling of the receptors to adenylate cyclase. A lowered concentration of GTP-binding nucleotide (see below in this section) caused the reduced coupling.[101] Some researchers found increases of β-adrenergic receptors on lymphocytes in thyrotoxic humans,[102] although others

did not find β-receptor increases.[103]

These observations led to the speculations about how thyroid hormone increased cellular responsiveness to catecholamines. One view was that thyroid hormone increased catecholamine secretion so that more was available to drive the metabolism of cells. However, studies showed that the catecholamine content of tissues did not increase after T_4 treatment; neither did the urinary content of catecholamine breakdown products.[61][128] These study results led to an alternative hypothesis: that thyroid hormone exerts many of its effects by modulating the sensitivity of cells to normal concentrations of catecholamines.[97]

DeGroot et al. listed four possible mechanisms by which thyroid hormone alters adrenergic response: (1) an increase in the number of adrenergic receptors on the plasma membrane of cells, (2) an increase in the adrenergic receptor's affinity for catecholamines, (3) activation of adenylate cyclase, or (4) an increased metabolism of or response to cAMP inside the cell.[108,p.75] Later studies showed that thyroid hormone regulates transcription of the adrenergic genes, thereby controlling the density of β-adrenergic receptors on cell membranes (see section above titled "Inadequate Thyroid Hormone Regulation of Adrenergic Gene Transcription"). Further research has elucidated the biochemical mechanisms by which thyroid hormone/catecholamine/adrenoceptor interaction affects the cell.

G Proteins

Part of the adrenergic receptor faces outward from the plasma membrane, and part faces inward to the cytoplasm. It is the outward facing part that binds epinephrine and norepinephrine. Once the hormone binds, the inward facing part of the receptor reacts. It recognizes and interacts with a specific transducing protein dissolved in the plasma membrane. The protein is loosely affiliated with the adrenergic receptor.[106,p.238]

There are two types of transducing proteins. We call them G proteins (G for short). The G proteins are guanine nucleotide-binding regulatory proteins. When a catecholamine binds to an adrenergic receptor, G splits into subunits. The largest subunit promptly binds to a regulatory protein, GTP-binding nucleotide (abbreviated as GTP for guanosine triphosphate). The G protein subunit is GTP-dependent. GTP activates G and enables it to exert its effect inside the cell.[109,pp.252-253] There are two types of G: a stimulating form (G_s) and an inhibitory form (G_i). The type of G that takes part depends on the type of adrenergic receptor that binds the catecholamine.

When a catecholamine binds to a β-adrenergic

receptor, a complex interaction involving G_s increases fuel metabolism inside the cell. Intially, the binding of a catecholamine to a β-adrenergic receptor activates a G_s by replacing the guanine diphosphate (GDP) bound to G_s with guanine triphosphase (GTP). The γ and β subunits of G_s separate from the α subunit. The α subunit then moves to adenylate cyclase and activates it. Adenylate cyclase then catalyzes the conversion of ATP to 3',5'-cyclic AMP (cAMP).[231,p.763]

There are at least two subtypes of β-adrenoceptor, $β_1$ and $β_2$. Both subtypes activate G_s to stimulate adenyl cyclase. The β-adrenoceptors cause G_s to split. The split releases the subunit of the G protein that combines with GTP and then activates the enzyme adenyl cyclase. Adenyl cyclase converts ATP to cAMP. In the cytoplasm, cAMP stimulates various protein kinases, and these enzymes set into motion a cascade of cellular reactions.[109,p.252]

There are at least two subtypes of α-adrenoceptors, $α_1$ and $α_2$. The membranes of presynaptic norepinephrine-secreting neurons contain $α_2$-adrenoceptors. The receptors inhibit release of norepinephrine. The receptors are linked in the cell membrane to the inhibitory G protein, G_i. When a catecholamine binds to an $α_2$-adrenoceptor, G_i splits from its subunits. One of the subunits, when activated by GTP, inhibits G_s from splitting from its protein. As a result, the subunit of G_s that potentially can activate adenyl cyclase stays locked within G_s. With adenyl cyclase at a standstill, cAMP production decreases, and the cascade of biochemical reactions in the cell slows or halts.[106,p.238]

With $β_1$-, $β_2$-, and $α_2$-adrenoceptor, GTP is a central figure in mediating the effects of catecholamines. GTP activates both G_s and G_i, causing G_s to stimulate the enzyme adenyl cyclase and G_i to inhibit it.[106,p.35]

Unlike the two β-adrenoceptors and the $α_2$-adrenoceptor, the $α_1$-adrenoceptor does not, upon binding a catecholamine, activate adenyl cyclase. (The β-adrenoceptors affect the enzyme positively and the $α_2$-adrenoceptor affects it negatively.) Instead, the $α_1$-adrenergic receptor causes mobilization of calcium ions in the cell. In the cell membrane, the $α_1$-adrenergic receptor activates phospholipase C.[109,p.253] Phospholipase C splits phospholipids in the membrane into second messengers. Through a series of reactions, these messengers move into the cytoplasm and mobilize calcium ions from mitochondria and the endoplasmic reticulum.[110,p.815]

Dynamics of Catecholamines in Synapses

Alterations in Synaptic Activity. Blocking secretion of norepinephrine by presynaptic noradrenergic nerves increases the sensitivity of postsynaptic nerves to test doses of norepinephrine. In addition, an absence of norepinephrine at a postsynaptic nerve increases the number of noradrenergic receptors on the nerve membrane. The absence of norepinephrine also increases the affinity of adrenergic receptors on the postsynaptic nerve for norepinephrine. This upregulation of adrenergic receptors occurs in the brain and the peripheral sympathetic system.[109,p.253]

Increasing the amount of norepinephrine in the synapse (by administering a tricyclic antidepressant drug or a monoamine oxidase inhibitor) renders the postsynaptic neuron hyposensitive to test doses of norepinephrine. Adrenergic receptors on the postsynaptic neuron downregulate. Cooper, Bloom, and Roth described the increases or decreases in the sensitivity of postsynaptic nerves to norepinephrine as compensatory responses to varying levels of synaptic transmitter substance.[109,p.253] In this sense, the changes in postsynaptic neuron responsiveness are a plastic quality of the nervous system—the quality helps maintain homeostatic balance between structural and functional components.

When investigators destroy noradrenergic neurons in the brain and the peripheral sympathetic system, the count of $α_1$- and $α_2$-adrenergic receptors increase. When they destroy noradrenergic neurons in the cerebral cortex, the count of $β_1$-adrenoceptors increases. *Chronic use of tricyclic antidepressants increases the amount of norepinephrine in synapses. As a result, the density of $β_1$-adrenoceptors in the cerebral cortex decreases.* These changes show that adrenergic neurons innervate $β_1$-adrenoceptors in the cortex.[109,p.253] Destroying norepinephrine neurons in the cortex, however, does not decrease the count of $β_2$-adrenoceptors. The lack of change in $β_2$-adrenoceptors results from their low affinity for norepinephrine. They have a higher affinity for epinephrine, and epinephrine content in the brain is low.

THYROID STATUS AND THE SYMPATHETIC-CATECHOLAMINE-ADRENOCEPTOR AXIS

Goetsch, in 1918, was the first to point out the interaction of thyroid hormone and the sympathetic nervous system.[36] Since then, many physiological studies have confirmed the relationship.[37] Thyroid hormone and the sympathetic nervous system interact in coordinated fashion for adaptation. In the positive direction, interaction occurs when cells need metabolic substrates such as glucose for energy release. In a negative direction, conditions such as starvation and severe illness result in decreases in sympathetic drive, thyroid gland secretion of thyroid hormone, and conversion of T_4 to T_3.

Internal cues (such as perceived threats) and external cues (such as substantial environmental temperature changes) rapidly activate the sympathetic nervous system; the system enables prompt adjustments to the cues. Thyroid hormone provides a positive gain in the capacity of most tissues to respond to the catecholamines released by adrenergic neurons.[55,p.661] Thyroid hormone potentiates sympathetic activity mainly by increasing β-adrenergic receptor density and adenyl cyclase activity.[201]

Changes in Catecholamine Secretion in Altered Thyroid States

A paradox in severe hypothyroidism is the increase in norepinephrine levels in some patients despite an increased density of α-adrenergic receptors. Inadequate thyroid hormone regulation of the adrenoceptor genes results in an increase in α-adrenoceptors and a decrease in β-adrenoceptors. Presynaptic $β_2$-autoreceptors induce noradrenergic neurons to release norepinephrine,[109,p.243] and we would expect a decreased density of the receptors to reduce norepinephrine levels. $α_2$-Adrenergic autoreceptors decrease secretion of norepinephrine by noradrenergic neurons (see section above titled "Types of Adrenergic Receptors that Mediate Catecholamine Release"). The increased density of $α_2$-adrenergic autoreceptors in hypothyroidism should decrease norepinephrine secretion. Why severely hypothyroid individuals may have increased peripheral norepinephrine levels is not clear.

In hypothyroidism, the α- and β-adrenoceptor balance on cell membranes shifts to relative α-adrenergic receptor dominance. The general consequence of this shift is a slowing of cellular functions. When the shift reaches some threshold, the peripheral sympathetic nervous system compensates by increased activity.[35,p.934] The increase in sympathetic activity appears to compensate for the slowing of metabolism due to the thyroid hormone deficiency. Sympathetic compensatory activity increases the metabolic rate and body heat.[35,p.904] The increased sympathetic activity of the hypothyroid patient may increase her plasma concentration and urinary excretion of norepinephrine.[30][43][56][57] The increases result from increased norepinephrine secretion by noradrenergic neurons.[58][59] The patient with prolonged or severe hypothyroidism is especially likely to have increased norepinephrine secretion. Thyroid hormone deficiency

significantly increases the turnover rate of norepinephrine, which is a measure of sympathetic activity. Treatment with thyroid hormone reduces the turnover rate in animals.[62][63][64][65]

Thyroid hormone deficiency or excess apparently does not alter secretion of epinephrine by the adrenal medullae. The epinephrine level is usually normal.[30][60] In thyrotoxicosis, plasma concentrations and urinary excretion of epinephrine are normal or low.[30][61] Although peripheral norepinephrine levels may be high in prolonged or severe hypothyroidism, most hypothyroid patients have normal urinary excretion of both norepinephrine and epinephrine.[32]

ADRENERGIC EFFECTS OF INADEQUATE THYROID HORMONE REGULATION OF ADRENERGIC GENE TRANSCRIPTION

In a variety of physiological and pathological conditions, the functional expression of α-adrenoceptors and β-adrenoceptors is inversely regulated.[68][69][70][71][72] In general, alterations in mRNA levels for these two receptor types correlate with changes in cell adrenoceptor density and reactivity.[71][72][73][74][75][76][77][78][79][80] In general, hypothyroidism reduces β-adrenoceptor density and reactivity[71][72][73][74][75][76][80][81] and increases α-adrenoceptor density and reactivity in most tissues.[71][74][80] Conversely, administration of thyroid hormone increases β-adrenoceptor mRNA and the membranous population of β-adrenoceptors[82,p.15867][84,p.539][85] and decreases α-adrenoceptor density in most tissues.[75][80][83]

On the chromosomes, T_3 binds to the ligand-binding domain of the T_3-receptors. The receptors reside on genes at nucleotide sequences termed thyroid hormone response elements. When T_3 binds to T_3-receptors on the response elements, transcription regulation begins. Transcription regulation by T_3/T_3-receptor binding is stimulatory to some target genes; a well-studied example is the growth hormone gene.[87] Transcription regulation by T_3 is inhibitory to other genes such as the pituitary TSH gene.[88] When T_3 is absent from the genes, the unliganded T_3-receptor attached to the response element has the opposite transcriptional effect from that of a liganded (T_3-bound) T_3-receptor on the element. If T_3/T_3-receptor binding activates transcription, absence of binding represses it; if T_3/T_3-receptor binding represses transcription, absence of binding activates it.[89][90] (See Chapter 2.3, section: "Nuclear T_3-Receptors.")

Both α- and β-adrenoceptor genes have thyroid

hormone response elements.[86,p.1118] T_3/T_3-receptor binding to the response elements has opposite effects at the two types of genes. In most tissues, T_3/T_3-receptor binding activates the β-adrenoceptor gene and represses the α-adrenoceptor gene. Absence of T_3/T_3-receptor binding represses the β-adrenoceptor gene and activates the α-adrenoceptor gene. Activation of the β-adrenoceptor gene (by T_3/T_3-receptor binding) increases the levels of β-adrenoceptor mRNA and the density of β-adrenoceptors on cell membranes. Activation of the α-adrenoceptor gene (by absence of T_3/T_3-receptor binding) increases levels of α-adrenoceptor mRNA and the density of α-adrenergic receptors on cell membranes.[86,p.1117]

Interaction of the Sympathetic-Catecholamine-Adrenoceptor System and Thyroid Hormone

The sympathetic-catecholamine-adrenoceptor system and thyroid hormone interact to maintain homeostasis. The sympathetic-catecholamine-adrenoceptor system allows rapid adjustments when needed, and thyroid hormones "sensitize" adrenergic receptors so that they respond more readily to catecholamines. "Sensitize" is a figurative term in that thyroid hormone increases the number of β-adrenergic receptors, and the receptors mediate stimulation of cells by catecholamines. To early researchers, the heightened excitatory response of cells to catecholamines after a patient began taking thyroid hormone appeared to sensitize adrenergic receptors. When metabolic demand increases over time, as during prolonged cold exposure, the sympathetic-catecholamine-adrenoceptor system and the thyroid system interact to adjust the metabolic rate to meet the individual's needs. When metabolic demand is low, as during fasting or starvation, both systems act independently to slow metabolism. The sympathetic-catecholamine-adrenoceptor system reduces blood and tissue levels of catecholamines, the thyroid gland releases fewer hormones, and T_4 to T_3 conversion decreases.

When too few thyroid hormones are available to adequately maintain homeostasis, the sympathetic-catecholamine-adrenoceptor system tends to compensate. Sympathetic nerves, for example, increase their output of norepinephrine, at least in severe hypothyroidism. The increased amounts of norepinephrine bind to α-adrenergic receptors, which are also increased in hypothyroidism. The binding constricts blood vessels in the skin and preserves the diminished body heat.

● ABNORMALITIES OF THE SYMPATHETIC-CATECHOLAMINE-ADRENOCEPTOR AXIS IN FIBROMYALGIA

Researchers have reported several abnormalities of the sympathetic-catecholamine-adrenoceptor axis in some fibromyalgia patients. The abnormalities include an increase in $α_2$-adrenergic receptors, low cerebrospinal fluid concentrations of norepinephrine and dopamine metabolites, and low sympathetically-induced physiological responsiveness.

INCREASED DENSITY OF $α_2$-ADRENERGIC RECEPTORS ON PLATELETS OF FIBROMYALGIA PATIENTS

One research group found an increase in the density of $α_2$-adrenoceptors on platelets from fibromyalgia patients.[91] To elucidate the underlying pathophysiology of fibromyalgia, this is perhaps the most important objectively documented abnormality reported to date. After reviewing the available evidence, Wirz-Justice wrote that $α_2$-adrenergic receptor binding in platelets and the central nervous system is similar. He also wrote, "this homogeneous preparation of human cells is an increasingly important tool in studying mechanisms in pathophysiology."[17] The increased density of $α_2$-adrenergic receptors on fibromyalgia patients' platelets may indicate a similar increased density on the membranes of central nervous system cells. If so, the increased density provides a plausible mechanism for most symptoms and objective findings of fibromyalgia.

LOW CEREBROSPINAL FLUID LEVELS OF NOREPINEPHRINE AND DOPAMINE METABOLITES IN FIBROMYALGIA PATIENTS

In one study of fibromyalgia patients, investigators measured the breakdown products in the cerebrospinal fluid of three central nervous system neurotransmitters: serotonin, dopamine, and norepinephrine.[54] (The latter two neurotransmitters are catecholamines.) The measured metabolite of serotonin is 5-hydroxyindoleacetic acid (5-HIAA), of dopamine is 3-methoxy-4-hydroxyphenethylene glycol (MHPG), and of norepinephrine is homovanillic acid (HVA). Concentrations of norepinephrine and dopamine were lower in the cerebrospinal fluid of fibromyalgia patients than in rheumatoid arthritis patients and control subjects. The low levels of MHPG and HVA were statistically significant. The concentration of 5-HIAA in fibromyalgia patients' cerebrospinal fluid did not statistically differ from that of arthritis patients and control subjects. (See Table 3.1.2.)

NORMAL-TO-ELEVATED PERIPHERAL NOREPINEPHRINE LEVELS IN FIBROMYALGIA PATIENTS AT REST

Investigators measured the epinephrine and norepinephrine urinary excretion in untreated fibromyalgia patients and normal controls.[31][33][34,p.151] The patients' epinephrine excretion before treatment was almost identical to that of the controls. The investigators found that 4 of 20 patients (20%) had much higher norepinephrine excretion. Their norepinephrine secretion was more than two standard deviations above the mean of control subjects' secretion. The means of fibromyalgia and control groups overlapped, but the means were not significantly different. Caffeine intake was the only factor that significantly correlated with increased norepinephrine secretion in fibromyalgia patients.[31][33][34,p.151] Results of tests of fibromyalgia patients' 24-hour urinary excretion of epinephrine and norepinephrine have been inconsistent.[31][33] Russell et al. wrote, however, ". . . evidence is now available that suggests an increased production of catecholamines in fibrositis syndrome."[31]

LOW PERIPHERAL INCREASE IN NOREPINEPHRINE AND EPINEPHRINE SECRETION DURING EXERCISE

Mengshoel also reported no rise in blood norepinephrine concentrations during exercise in fibromyalgia patients compared with a many-fold rise in healthy subjects.[152] In response to the exercise, fibromyalgia patients had lower serum levels of epinephrine and norepinephrine. They also had low creatine kinase, myoglobin, and cortisol. The researchers concluded that their fibromyalgia patients had disturbed sympathetic activity.[134]

SUBNORMAL SYMPATHETIC RESPONSE TO EXERCISE IN FIBROMYALGIA PATIENTS

Some researchers have hypothesized that fibromyalgia/chronic fatigue syndrome patients have exaggerated sympathetic nervous system responsiveness. Sendrowski et al., for example, recently referred to ". . . the sympathetic hypersensitivity condition called fibromyalgia syndrome . . . ." They conducted a study to determine whether chronic fatigue syndrome patients had "denervation hypersensitivity of the sympathetic system." Twenty-nine chronic fatigue syndrome patients and 33 normal subjects took part in the study. The investigators used a standardized supersensitivity test in which they instilled patients eyes with two drops of 1.0% phenylephrine (an α_1-adrenergic receptor agonist). They measured pupil size by a pupil gauge and flash photography. Their criterion for sympathetic denervation hypersensitivity was pupillary dilation in response to the stimulus of greater than 2.5 mm. All patients and normals had a small but statistically significant increase in pupil size (a mean of 0.931 mm in patients and 0.788 mm in normals). The increase in pupil size is the normal reaction to binding of a catecholamine analog to α_1-adrenoceptor receptors. The overlap in the change in pupil size in the two groups was substantial but not significant (t=0.83, p=0.42, dF=60). When the investigators applied 1.0% topical phenylephrine, patients and normal subjects responded the same. The researchers were not able to distinguish patients from normals by a hypersensitive sympathetic reaction. The study results suggest that chronic fatigue syndrome patients do not have a denervation hypersensitivity of the pupil.[149]

The hypothesis of Sendrowski et al. that fibromyalgia is a sympathetic hypersensitivity condition[149] brings to mind a common assumption of early fibromyalgia researchers. They suspected that patients' muscle symptoms and objective abnormalities such as impaired microcirculation resulted from excessive muscle sympathetic nerve activity. The suspicion was contradicted by findings of Elam et al. They found that at rest, sympathetic activity in fibromyalgia patients was no different from that in normal controls. They found that in 8 fibromyalgia patients and 8 normal controls, basal (at rest) sympathetic nerve discharge (measured by intraneuronal recordings of peroneal nerve activity), heart rate, and blood pressure were similar. Also, in 4 or 5 [sic] of 6 patients, sympathetic activity increased normally in response to various stressors. However, in 4 or 5 [sic] of 6 patients, the increase in sympathetic activity was slightly less than in normal controls. In addition, in 1 or 2 [sic] patients, sympathetic activity actually decreased to a slight-to-marked degree.[150,p.372]

Similarly, van Derderen et al. reported evidence

of subnormal sympathetic activity in fibromyalgia patients when performing exhaustive exercise. Lower-than-normal heart rates and increases in norepinephrine secretion indicated subnormal activity.[134]

LOW NEUROPEPTIDE Y LEVELS IN FIBROMYALGIA

Crofford et al.[137] and Clauw[138] reported that fibromyalgia patients had lower plasma levels of neuropeptide Y than controls. Clauw reported that fibromyalgia patients had lower neuropeptide Y levels after 30 minutes on a tilt table.[138]

● INADEQUATE THYROID HORMONE REGULATION OF TRANSCRIPTION MAY MEDIATE SYMPATHETIC-CATECHOLAMINE-ADRENOCEPTOR AXIS ABNORMALITIES IN FIBROMYALGIA

The reported effects of inadequate thyroid hormone regulation of transcription in hypothyroidism suggest that such inadequate regulation can account for most of the abnormalities of the sympathetic-catecholamine-adrenoceptor axis in fibromyalgia. Subnormal sympathetic responsiveness in fibromyalgia may result from two main effects of inadequate regulation of gene transcription: (1) decreased corticotropin-releasing hormone secretion and (2) a shift in the ratio of β- to α-adrenergic receptors on cell membranes, with a predominance of α-adrenoceptors. The symptoms and objective findings in fibromyalgia that can be explained by one of these mechanisms is likely to be equally well explained by the other. This may be true in some cases of cellular resistance to thyroid hormone in which the corticotropin-releasing hormone gene and the adrenergic genes are involved. It is likely to be true in most cases of hypothyroidism because most tissues are subjected to the thyroid hormone deficiency.

SUBNORMAL SECRETION OF CORTICOTROPIN-RELEASING HORMONE

Some investigators have reported evidence consistent with decreased hypothalamic corticotropin-releasing hormone in fibromyalgia patients. Hypothalamic corticotropin-releasing hormone activates

pituitary-adrenocortical components of the hypothalamic-pituitary-adrenocortical axis. Thyroid hormone regulates corticotropin-releasing hormone levels through controlling its transcription (see Chapter 3.5). When thyroid hormone regulation of corticotropin-releasing hormone transcription is inadequate, as in hypothyroidism, secretion of corticotropin-releasing hormone is deficient. The deficient secretion results in hypothalamic-pituitary-adrenocortical axis dysfunction.

Corticotropin-releasing hormone also stimulates the locus ceruleus-norepinephrine system and the central sympathetic system.[148] Deficiency of corticotropin-releasing hormone due to inadequate thyroid hormone regulation of corticotropin-releasing hormone gene transcription may result in subnormal activation of the locus ceruleus-norepinephrine system and the central sympathetic system. The subnormal activation may in part account for the findings indicative of subnormal sympathetic activity in fibromyalgia patients: blunted sympathetic response to exercise[150][151][152] and low cerebrospinal fluid concentrations of norepinephrine and dopamine metabolites.[54]

HIGH RATIO OF α- TO β-ADRENERGIC RECEPTORS ON CELL MEMBRANES

Increased α₂-Adrenoceptors on the Platelets of Fibromyalgia Patients

The increased density of α_2-adrenoceptors on the platelets of fibromyalgia patients[91] may be the most important indicator of the underlying pathophysiological mechanism in most fibromyalgia patients—inadequate thyroid hormone regulation of cell function, particularly of the adrenoceptor genes.

The activity level of a patient's sympathetic nervous system (specifically, her secretion of norepinephrine) may vary with her degree of inadequate thyroid hormone regulation of cell function. When a patient's hypothyroidism is mild or of recent onset, she is likely to have normal plasma and urinary norepinephrine levels. When her hypothyroidism is severe or of long duration, her norepinephrine levels may be elevated (see subsection above titled "Changes in Catecholamine Secretion in Altered Thyroid States"). The effects of her increased norepinephrine secretion (viewed as increased sympathetic nervous system activity) are determined by the ratio of β- to α-adrenergic receptors occupying cell membranes and binding the norepinephrine.

The cellular and physiological responses to the release of norepinephrine by sympathetic nerves depend on the type of adrenergic receptor that predominates on the cell membranes of target cells. Binding of norepinephrine to α-adrenergic receptors reduces blood flow and slows or halts cell metabolism. Binding of catecholamines, especially epinephrine, to β-adrenergic receptors increases blood flow and increases cell metabolism. Understanding these ligand/receptor relationships makes it clear that inadequate thyroid hormone regulation of adrenergic gene transcription can account for most features of fibromyalgia.

Two studies by Bengtsson et al. strongly support the possibility that fibromyalgia patients have increased α_2-adrenergic receptors in peripheral tissues in addition to those on their platelets.[49][179] In one study, the researchers used two techniques to induce sympathetic ganglion blocks in fibromyalgia patients. As a result, the blocks diminished the patients' fibromyalgic pain.[49] The results indicate that the blocks reduced norepinephrine secretion in peripheral tissues, stopped norepinephrine/α_2-adrenergic receptor binding, permitted blood vessels to dilate, and relieved ischemic pain. (See subsection below titled "Pain.")

α-Adrenergic Dominance

The pathological potential of a physiological process is often best elucidated by considering it in the extreme. The effects of extreme α-adrenergic dominance are exemplified by the arterial insufficiency (by vasoconstriction) induced in some patients by the drug cafergot, a combination of caffeine and ergotamine tartrate, often used to treat migraine. Some patients may have a hypersensitivity to the combined ingredients and the dosage may be excessive. It can induce symptoms of peripheral vascular insufficiency. Wells et al. wrote that the clinician should suspect iatrogenic ergotism in patients with ischemic symptoms while taking cafergot. Ishemia may progress to necrosis and gangrene.[29]

The ischemic symptoms may result from interactions of prostaglandins, calcium, and serotonin, and from activation of α-adrenergic receptors. Through these mechanisms, cafergot induces vasoconstriction of both arteries and veins. For the patient with iatrogenic ergotism, discontinuing caffeine may be all that is necessary to relieve the symptoms. Prazosin, an α-adrenergic receptor antagonist, is used in emergency circumstances to relieve acute vascular insufficiency.

The potential adverse effects of fibromyalgia due to inadequate thyroid hormone regulation of transcription, with a relative increase in α-adrenergic receptors, is obvious from the contraindications to the use of cafergot. These include renal or hepatic failure, peripheral vascular disease, hypertension, ischemic heart disease, and Raynaud's phenomenon.[29] The vascular effects of fibromyalgia due to inadequate thyroid hormone regulation of adrenoceptor gene transcription can be predicted to be similar to the ischemic effects of cafergot.

β-Adrenergic Receptors

Induction of Fibromyalgia-Like Symptoms by a β-Adrenergic Receptor Blocker. The β-blocking drug propranolol is often prescribed for thyrotoxic patients. Most of the clinical benefit from use of this drug, especially at lower dosages, derives from β_1-adrenoceptor blockade.[55,p.665] This is indicated by the results of studies of the levels of cAMP[66] and selective β_1-adrenoceptor antagonists.[67]

Peripheral adverse effects to β-blocking drugs may include bradycardia and cold extremities, and central nervous system effects may include fatigue, disturbed sleep (such as insomnia and nightmares), and depression.[161,pp.238-239] Such adverse effects from β-blocking drugs in susceptible patients illustrates an important potential of a decreased ratio of functional β- to α-adrenergic receptors on cell membranes: Induction of symptoms typical of fibromyalgia.

Therapeutic Response of Fibromyalgia Patients to a β-Adrenergic Agonist. Eisinger treated fibromyalgia patients with a β_2-adrenergic receptor agonist, salbutamol (8-12 mg/d, per os). The researchers reported that the agonist improved the status of 7 of 10 patients. The symptoms especially improved were muscle pain and exercise tolerance.[218] It is likely that the agonist forcibly activates the relatively few β-adrenergic receptors on patients' cell membranes. The effect would mimic the effects of norepinephrine-β-adrenergic receptor interaction.

A study by Hallberg et al. suggests two mechanisms by which Eisinger's fibromyalgia patients improved with the use of salbutamol. Hallberg et al. administered the β_2-adrenergic receptor agonist salbutamol to rats twice per day for 14 days. The treatment significantly increased serotonin levels in the limbic forebrain, corpus striatum, and cerebral cortex. The levels of tryptophan, the amino acid from which cells synthesize serotonin, were not increased. As a result, the investigators concluded that salbutamol increased the rate of tryptophan hydroxylation in the rats' brains. Salbutamol-activation of β_2-adrenergic receptors also significantly increased norepinephrine levels and use in the rat brains. The investigators concluded that the activation of noradrenergic and serotonergic systems in the brain by the β_2-adrenergic receptor agonist salbutamol explains the antidepressant effects of the agonist.[151] A shift toward decreased β_2-adrenergic receptor density in the brain (due to inadequate thyroid hormone regulation of β-adrenergic gene transcription) may in part explain the low levels of the norepinephrine metabolite in the cerebrospinal fluid of fibromyalgia patients.

Contrasting the study by Eisinger et al. with another by Wysenbeek (see next section) is informative. The two reports considered together support the proposition that inadequate regulation of adrenergic gene transcription mediates some features of fibromyalgia. Support is inherent in the improved fibromyalgia status from activating β-adrenoceptors with salbutamol despite a low ratio of β- to α-adrenergic receptors. Support is also inherent in the failure of medicinally-increased norepinephrine to improve fibromyalgia status, presumably because of the patients' decreased β-adrenoceptor/α-adrenoceptor ratio.

Table 3.1.2. Cerebrospinal fluid, plasma, serum, or urine levels of neurotransmitters or their metabolites in fibromyalgia patients.

NEUROTRANSMITTER	METABOLITE	SAMPLE SOURCE	LEVEL
Serotonin	5-hydroxyindoleacetic acid (5-HIAA)	5-HIAA in cerebrospinal fluid	Normal*
Dopamine	3-methoxy-4-hydroxyphenethylene glycol (MHPG)	MHPG in cerebrospinal fluid	Low*
Norepinephrine	homovanillic acid (HVA)	HVA in cerebrospinal fluid	Low*
Norepinephrine		Serum (during exercise)	Low[†‡]
Epinephrine		Serum (during exercise)	Low[†]
Norepinephrine		Urine	Normal or elevated[γ]
Epinephrine		Urine	Normal[γ]
Neuropeptide Y		Plasma	Low[δλ]

* Russell, I.J., Vaeroy, M., Jabors, M., and Nyberg, F.: Cerebrospinal fluid biogenic metabolites in fibromyalgia/fibrositis syndrome and rheumatoid arthritis. *Arthritis Rheum.*, 35:550-556, 1992.[54]
†van Denderen J.C., Boersma, J.W., Zeinstra, P., Hollander, A.P., and van Neerbos, B.R.: Physiological effects of exhaustive physical exercise in primary fibromyalgia syndrome (PFS): is PFS a disorder of neuroendocrine reactivity? *Scand. J. Rheumatol.*, 21:35-37, 1992.[134]
‡ Mengshoel, A.M.: Effect of physical exercise in fibromyalgia. *Tidsskr Nor Laegeforen*, 116:746-748, 1996.[152]
γ Russell, I.J.: Neurohormonal aspects of fibromyalgia syndrome. *Rheum. Dis. Clin. North Am.*, 15:149-168, 1989.[34]
δ Crofford, L.J., Pillemer, S.R., Kalogeras, K.T., et al.: Hypothalamic-pituitary-adrenal axis perturbations in patients with fibromyalgia. *Arthritis Rheum.*, 37:1583-1592, 1994.[137]
λ Clauw, D.J., Sabol, M., Radulovic, D., et al.: Serum neuropeptides in patients with both fibromyalgia (FM) and chronic fatigue syndrome (CFS). *J. Musculoskel. Pain*, 3(Suppl.1):79, 1995.[138]

Blunted Response to Norepinephrine-Increasing Medication. Wysenbeek et al. administered the drug imipramine to fibromyalgia patients. Imipramine essentially makes more norepinephrine available at synapses.[38,p.47][45] Typically, the additional norepinephrine has stimulatory, antidepressive effects on central nervous system neurons. The increased norepinephrine also facilitates stage 4 sleep.[48,p.407] Imipramine, however, had no effect on fibromyalgia patients' signs or symptoms. Nineteen of the 20 patients stopped therapy because of no response (70%), adverse effects (35%), or a combination of both.[46] Unfortunately, the study had no control subjects, and it is not certain that the researchers' conclusions were accurate. But the report that 70% of the fibromyalgia patients failed to respond suggests that the patients did not have a sufficient concentration of β-adrenergic receptors to bind the norepinephrine and increase neuronal metabolism. In addition, adverse effects in 35% of patients suggest that the increased norepinephrine interacted instead with α-adrenergic receptors, slowing metabolism and increasing symptom intensity. This is presumably the main mechanism by which exercise worsens fibromyalgia status—increased levels of exercise-induced catecholamines interacting with a high density of α-adrenergic receptors in cell membranes (see Chapter 3.4).

Subnormal Sympathetic Response to Stress in Hypothyroid and Fibromyalgia Patients

The subnormal responsiveness of the sympathetic nervous system in fibromyalgia may result in part from insufficient hypothalamic secretion of corticotropin-releasing hormone. It may also result from inhibited sympathetic ganglionic neural transmission due to an increase in α-adrenergic receptors and a decrease in β-adrenergic receptors (see section immediately below). Inhibition of the sympathetic ganglia reduces sympathetic flow to peripheral tissue. Exercise in normal individuals above 50%-to-60% VO$_2$ max increases catecholamine secretion.[22,p.204][23][24][25][26][27] The reduced sympathetic outflow in fibromyalgia patients may account in part for their subnormal norepinephrine secretion and cardiorespiratory response during exercise. (See Chapter 3.4, subsection titled "Increased Catecholamine Secretion During Exercise.")

Inhibition of Sympathetic Ganglionic Neural Transmission by an Increased α$_2$-Adrenergic Receptor Density on Ganglion Cells. Binding of catecholamines to β-adrenergic receptors in the sympathetic ganglia increases sympathetic ganglionic transmission. Binding of catecholamines to α-adrenergic receptors in the ganglia has the opposite effect: inhibition of transmission. Researchers more often record inhibition rather than facilitation of transmission.[10]

α-Adrenergic receptors inhibit transmission through two mechanisms: (1) blocking of acetylcholine release from preganglionic cholinergic sympathetic neurons (presynaptically),[234] and (2) hyperpolarization of postganglionic noradrenergic neurons (postsynaptically).[160] In some species such as the rabbit, rat, and guinea pig, inhibition of transmission is clearly presynaptically-mediated. Depressed excitability of postsynaptic nerves occurred even when the nerves were not hyperpolarized.[235,pp.99-100] However, binding of α-adrenergic receptors to catecholamines on postsynaptic neurons hyperpolarized them. Inhibition of the postsynaptic neurons by α-adrenergic receptors was associated with an increase in potassium conductance.[237] α$_2$-Adrenergic receptors are the inhi-

biting receptor subtype on both presynaptic[236] and postsynaptic neurons.[206][211] Use of the α$_2$-adrenergic receptor agonist clonidine hyperpolarized sympathetic ganglionic cells.[160]

Reduction in Sympathetic Outflow to Peripheral Tissues by Activation of Central α-Adrenergic Receptors. Studies showed that activating α$_2$-adrenergic receptors in the ventrolateral medulla of the brain stem reduced sympathetic outflow to peripheral tissues. The reduction lowered arterial blood pressure and induced bradycardia.[50,pp.120-122] Also, activation of α$_2$-adrenergic receptors in the solitary tract nucleus in the medulla (see Glossary and section above titled "Review of the Sympathetic-Catecholamine-Adrenoceptor Axis") has an antihypertensive effect.[180]

Norepinephrine Levels in Fibromyalgia Patients at Rest. Investigators have studied the catecholamine levels in the blood and urine of hypothyroid and fibromyalgia patients. The levels reported have been inconsistent.

Hypothyroid patients usually have normal epinephrine levels. The norepinephrine excretion, especially by those with severe or prolonged hypothyroidism, tends to be high.[30][56][57] However, there is considerable variability in findings among patients with abnormal thyroid status.[55,p.664][62][63]

Fibromyalgia patients had normal urinary excretion of epinephrine. Norepinephrine excretion was normal for 80%; it was significantly elevated in 20%.[31][33][34,p.151] The findings for fibromyalgia patients overlapped those of control subjects.[31][33][34,p.151] These findings are consistent with those of hypothyroid patients.

As Russell et al. commented, ". . . evidence is now available that suggests an increased production of catecholamines in fibrositis syndrome."[31] The patient with prolonged or severe hypothyroidism is also likely to have increased norepinephrine secretion.

Low Increase in Norepinephrine and Epinephrine Secretion During Exercise. Norepinephrine and epinephrine secretion during stresses such as exercise are measures of sympathetic nervous system function. The abnormally low norepinephrine secretion in fibromyalgia patients during exercise may result from two mechanisms that are secondary to inadequate thyroid hormone regulation of gene transcription: (1) blunted central sympathetic nervous system activation due to reduced corticotropin-releasing hormone, and (2) impeded sympathetic outflow due to an increase in α$_2$-adrenergic receptors in the brain stem and sympathetic ganglia. Activation of α$_2$-adrenergic receptors inhibits norepinephrine secretion by sympathetic nerves, and blockade of the receptors increases norepinephrine secretion. Conversely, β_2-autoreceptors induce norepinephrine secretion, and blockade of these receptors inhibits norepinephrine release.[109,p.258]

Low Production of Catecholamine-Inducing Enzymes Due to Inadequate Thyroid Hormone Regulation During Fetal Development and Infancy.

Thyroid hormone regulates tyrosine hydroxylase (the enzyme that converts tyrosine to DOPA, which is then converted to dopamine) and dopamine-β-hydroxylase (the enzyme that converts dopamine to norepinephrine) at the transcriptional level in some cells, at least during development. One group of such cells is the post-synaptic noradrenergic neurons of the superior cervical ganglion. Researchers found that thyroid hormone regulates transcription for dopamine-β-hydroxylase in developing rats.[208,p.37] Depriving young and adult rats of thyroid hormone or administering the hormone to them did not change sympathetic ganglion synthesis of dopamine-β-hydroxylase. But rats made hypothyroid in infancy had markedly lower basal tyrosine hydroxylase and dopamine-β-hydroxylase activity. Perhaps more important, rats made hypothyroid at birth showed no evidence of induction of the enzyme at any age. (See Chapter 2.3, subsection titled "Effect of Thyroid Status on Tyrosine and Dopamine-β-Hydroxylase Induction in the Superior Cervical Ganglion.") De Lonlay et al. wrote, "Indeed, there may be a 'critical period' during development when the action of thyroid hormone is particularly important for the complete functional organization of the superior cervical ganglion."[208,p.37]

This finding shows that at one or more developmental stages in rats, adequate exposure to thyroid hormone is essential for inducing the enzyme dopamine-β-hydroxylase. We would expect that low availability or activity of the enzyme would decrease the conversion of dopamine to norepinephrine. As a result, when stresses prompt activation of the sympathetic ganglia, too little norepinephrine would be available to provide normal secretion. The organism would thus have an inadequate sympathetic response to stress.

This finding raises an interesting question. Do some humans have inadequate thyroid hormone regulation of transcription for the two enzymes during some critical developmental stage? If so, does a subsequent deficient induction of these catecholamine-inducing enzymes in the superior cervical ganglion predispose humans to subnormal sympathetic nervous system responses to stress? If so, we can anticipate several essentially sympatholytic features: low norepinephrine secretion during exercise, low neuropeptide

Y levels, low cerebral and peripheral blood flow, slow and weak heart contractions, and low blood pressure. These sympatholytic features of inadequate thyroid hormone regulation of gene transcription are, of course, documented features of fibromyalgia.

Possible Stress-Induced Consequences of Subnormal Catecholamine Production.

A putative low production of enzymes critical to catecholamine production can have serious stress-induced consequences. An increase in the production and secretion of catecholamines is essential for adapting well to stress. During stresses in normal humans (such as immobilization stress,[1] cold exposure,[2] insulin hypoglycemia[3][4] injection of nerve growth factor,[5] or injection of reserpine[6][7][8][9]), tyrosine hydroxylase activity and dopamine-β-hydroxylase activity increase. As a result of catalytic activities of the enzymes, catecholamine secretion in peripheral tissues increases. Through this effect, increases in the activities of the enzymes help the organism adapt to the stress.

Subnormal thyroid hormone regulation of transcription for the enzymes during some critical development period may render some humans unable to normally adapt to stress. During stresses, these individuals may have a subnormal increase in tyrosine hydroxylase and dopamine-β-hydroxylase activity. Consequently, they will also have a subnormal production of DOPA, dopamine, norepinephrine, and epinephrine. Without enough production and secretion of these hormones, the individuals may not have a sufficient amount of the hormones to adapt to the stresses. Affected individuals who already have borderline sufficient metabolism may undergo a metabolic crisis during increased metabolic demand. This may occur during stresses such as surgery, accidental trauma, or severe viral infection. The metabolic slow-down may be worsened by stress-induced elevation of the adrenal cortical hormone cortisol. Cortisol can transiently impede metabolic capacity by its anti-thyroid system effects. (See Chapter 3.5, section titled "A Putative Etiological and Exacerbating Role for Increased Cortisol Levels: Stress-Related Cortisol Elevation May Precipitate Fibromyalgia by Slowing Already Marginally Adequate Metabolism in Fibromyalgia-Related Tissues.") The symptoms of the metabolic crisis may worsen debilitation from surgery, accidental trauma, or infection. Debility may impose prolonged physical inactivity on the individual so that she quickly loses lean tissue mass. The lean tissue loss may reduce her basal metabolism enough to induce symptoms of hypometabolism. This set of factors may explain in part why some people develop fibromyalgia following stresses.

Low Central Nervous System Dopamine Metabolite Levels. In one study, researchers found low levels of the dopamine metabolite MHPG in the cerebrospinal fluid of fibromyalgia patients.[54] The low level may reflect low synthesis of dopamine in the patients' central nervous systems. Low dopamine production in fibromyalgia patients could cause low motor drive that they perceive as fatigue or weakness (see Chapters 3.4 and 3.11). The low levels might also contribute to patients' depressed mood by reduced dopaminergic stimulation of the nucleus accumbens of the limbic system[162,p.759] (see Chapter 3.10). Moreover, low dopamine levels in fibromyalgia patients may lower systolic blood pressure and permit relative vasodilation. This is suggested by the finding that low doses of dopamine increase systolic blood pressure, and high doses cause vasoconstriction. These effects of dopamine are probably mediated by binding of dopamine to both D_1-dopaminergic receptors and β_1-adrenergic receptors.[99,pp.280-281]

Thyroid Hormone Regulation of Tyrosine Hydroxylase and Dopamine Synthesis. Thyroid hormone increases dopamine production in the hypothalamus. Thyroid hormone deficiency decreases dopamine synthesis in the striatum (where dopamine is the main catecholamine produced) and the hypothalamus. An increase in the activity of tyrosine hydroxylase increases conversion of tyrosine to DOPA. In turn, DOPA is sequentially converted to dopamine and norepinephrine. In hypothyroidism, DOPA accumulates at a reduced rate, and in hyperthyroidism, DOPA accumulates at an exaggerated rate. In some tissues, such as the superior sympathetic ganglion, hypothyroidism inhibits production of tyrosine hydroxylase, possibly at the transcriptional level.[208,p.37]

Investigators found that in cultured, immature cells called neuroblastomas, hypothyroidism decreased the activity of tyrosine hydroxylase. This reflected a decreased rate of protein synthesis, a possible genomic effect. Subjecting neuroblastoma to thyroid hormone increased the activity of the enzyme; the higher the exposure to thyroid hormone, the greater the increase in activity of the enzyme. Enzyme activity was dose-dependent and correlated with the percentage of nuclear T_3-receptor sites occupied by the hormone. The researchers concluded that through binding to nuclear T_3-receptors, thyroid hormone directly affects the activity of tyrosine hydroxylase in cultured, immature neurons. The effect is not consistent, however, in all brain regions. In some brain regions, thyroid hormone decreased tyrosine hydroxylase activity and thyroid hormone deficiency increased it.[207,p.1409] (See Chapter

2.3, subsection titled "Effects of T_3 on Catecholamine Enzymes in Cultured Neuroblastoma Cells.")

Thyroid Hormone Regulation of β-Adrenergic Receptors in the Striatum. The decrease in dopamine production in the striatum in hypothyroidism may result in part from a decrease in β-adrenergic receptors. Atterwill et al. found that inducing hypothyroidism in rats caused a 12% reduction in β-adrenergic receptors in the striatum. Administering T_3 caused an 18% increase in the receptors. The investigators noted the possible significance to low dopamine production in the striatum.[116]

Neuropeptide Y. The lower neuropeptide Y plasma levels in some fibromyalgia patients[137][138] may be a sympathetic nervous system consequence of inadequate thyroid hormone cell regulation. (See section below titled: "Low Neuropeptide Y Levels in Fibromyalgia.")

Neuropeptide Y secretion during stress, like norepinephrine and epinephrine secretion, is a measure of sympathetic nervous system function. In the hypothalamus, the peptide increases secretion of corticotropin-releasing hormone (CRH).[140] If the low plasma levels are accompanied by low central nervous system secretion, this may contribute to the apparent suboptimal CRH secretion in fibromyalgia patients. Neuropeptide Y acts in conjunction with CRH to stimulate ACTH secretion by the pituitary gland.[141] In the adrenal cortex, neuropeptide Y has an effect similar to that of ACTH in stimulating glucocorticoid secretion.[142]

Neuropeptide Y (NPY) is synthesized, stored, and secreted along with norepinephrine in sympathetic nerve terminals.[146] The peptide is widely distributed throughout the body and has vasoconstrictive properties. When exogenous NPY is applied intranasally, it produces a long-lasting nasal vasoconstriction without cardiovascular effects.[147]

Neuropeptide Y secretion is augmented by increased sympathetic nerve impulse frequency,[144] and plasma levels are assumed to be proportional to the secretory activity of sympathetic nerves and the adrenal medullae. Thus, intense exercise[136] or, for example, heart failure[146] increases NPY secretion.

As Crofford has noted, it is not known whether plasma levels of neuropeptide Y correspond to concentrations in any brain region.[139,p.190] She proposed that low NYP levels in fibromyalgia may represent subnormal function or depletion of the sympathetic stress axis.[139,p.190] This is consistent with the view of Sun et al.[145] that plasma neuropeptide Y is a useful marker of sympathetic nervous system activity, possibly a more sensitive one than epinephrine and norepinephrine levels. For example, Sun et al.[145] found that aortic occlusion caused a significant increase in neuropeptide Y but not in catecholamines. Others argue, however, that norepinephrine is a more sensitive index, at least for sympathetic neural responses that regulate the systemic circulation.[146]

Hashimoto et al. found that patients with major depressive disorder had lower plasma levels of neuropeptide Y than normal controls.[143]

IMPAIRED SYMPATHETIC NERVOUS SYSTEM FUNCTION DUE TO INADEQUATE THYROID HORMONE REGULATION OF CELL FUNCTION: PHYSIOLOGICAL EFFECTS

Most of the objective findings in fibromyalgia patients could result from a shift to predominance of α_2-adrenoceptors on cell membranes due to inadequate thyroid hormone regulation of adrenergic gene transcription. Fibromyalgia patients have increased α_2-adrenoceptors on platelets.[91]

Bradycardia and Low Blood Pressure

When catecholamines bind to β-adrenergic receptors on heart cells, heart rate and contractile force increase. The receptors are especially dense in the sinoatrial node, and the left ventricle contains the highest density of β-adrenergic receptors in the heart.[205,pp.235-238] A reduction in the density of these receptors during inadequate thyroid hormone regulation of adrenergic gene transcription can account for the reduced cardiovascular response to exercise in hypothyroidism and fibromyalgia. Valente et al. found that thyroidectomy produced a more intense bradycardia than sympathectomy. Treatment with T_3 relieved the bradycardia caused either by thyroidectomy or sympathectomy. The investigators suggested that the direct effect of the thyroid hormone on heart rate results from an early enhancement of β-adrenoceptors.[187]

A factor possibly contributing to the bradycardia and low blood pressure of some fibromyalgia patients is reduced sympathetic outflow to the cardiovascular system from the sympathetic ganglia, with increased parasympathetic outflow. Stimulation of central nervous system α_2-adrenergic receptors induces these effects.[131][156] Investigators found that stimulation of α_2-adrenergic receptors in the ventrolateral medulla reduced sympathetic outflow to peripheral tissues, reduced arterial blood pressure, and induced bradycardia.[50,pp.120-122] Both central and peripheral admin-

istration of α_2-adrenergic receptor agonists, such as norepinephrine and the drug clonidine, induce hypotension and bradycardia.[159]

Blunted Cardiac Response to Stress

The shift toward α-adrenergic predominance can also impede cardiac response to catecholamines released during stress. This can account for the impaired cardiac response to exercise found in some fibromyalgia patients. Activation of α_2-adrenergic receptors hyperpolarizes and decreases neural firing of the sympathetic postganglionic cells. The hyperpolarization decreases the outflow of sympathetic signals to peripheral tissues. The hyperpolarization could also result in failure of the cardiorespiratory system to meet the demands for increased oxygen delivery to exercising muscles in fibromyalgia patients.

Altered Cardiac Cyclic-AMP Response to Catecholamines Due to the Decrease in β-Adrenergic Receptors from Inadequate Thyroid Hormone Regulation of the β-Adrenoceptor Gene. Burack et al. reported that exercise intolerance in hypothyroid patients results mainly from cardiac limitation due to impaired ability to increase stroke volume and cardiac output. During exercise, patients had low oxygen consumption. Their arterial lactate levels increased more than normal.[209] The cardiac limitation is partly explained by the decrease in β-adrenergic receptors on cardiac membranes.

Guttler et al. measured urinary cyclic-AMP excretion in euthyroid, hyperthyroid, and hypothyroid individuals. Urinary excretion of cyclic-AMP in normal individuals is increased by the binding of catecholamines to β-adrenergic receptors at cell membranes. The investigators found no significant difference between the three groups when at rest (comparable to the similar finding for fibromyalgia patients). Infusions of epinephrine over a 2-hour period increased excretion of cyclic-AMP in euthyroid men; excretion increased even more in hyperthyroid men. Hypothyroid men, however, did not have a significant increase in excretion. Cardiovascular responses to the epinephrine infusions were greatest in hyperthyroid men and were virtually absent in hypothyroid men.[210]

Muscle Sympathetic Nerve Activity

Elam et al. studied intraneural recordings of peroneal nerve activity in fibromyalgia patients. They found a tendency toward lower sympathetic muscle activity when subjected to stressors than in controls.[150] The low level of sympathetic nerve activity can be explained by an increase in α_2-adrenergic receptors in the sympathetic ganglia, a related hyperpolarization of the ganglia, and consequent reduced activity of the postganglionic sympathetic nerves innervating muscle. (See subsection above titled "Inhibition of Sympathetic Ganglionic Neural Transmission by an Increased α_2-Adrenergic Receptor Density on Ganglion Cells.")

Also, an increase in the density of α_2-adrenergic autoreceptors on sympathetic nerve terminals in muscle could explain any decrease in norepinephrine secretion during stress. Elam et al., however, did not measure secretion of the neurotransmitter. Nonetheless, from lowered sympathetic nerve activity, we would expect a subnormal secretion of norepinephrine. If the patient's blood vessels and muscle cells have a lower than normal β-adrenergic receptor density and a higher than normal α-adrenergic density, any secreted norepinephrine—even a subnormal amount—would induce vasoconstriction and decrease cellular metabolism. The decreased blood flow and metabolism would predispose the patient to suboptimal muscle function and muscle-related symptoms.

Some researchers have reported increased muscle sympathetic nerve activity in hypothyroid patients. Matsukawa et al. measured muscle sympathetic nerve activity in hyperthyroid and hypothyroid patients and compared the results with normal controls. Hyperthyroid patients tended to have less muscle sympathetic activity than normal controls. In contrast, hypothyroid patients had significantly greater muscle sympathetic nerve activity than controls. All subjects had a significant, negative correlation between serum levels of free T_3 or free T_4 and muscle sympathetic nerve activity. There was a significant positive correlation between serum TSH levels and muscle sympathetic nerve activity. The researchers wrote that their results suggest an inverse relationship between thyroid function and muscle sympathetic nerve activity.[63]

Such increased muscle sympathetic nerve activity may account in part for the increased circulating and urinary levels of norepinephrine in severe or prolonged hypothyroidism (see section above titled "Changes in Catecholamine Secretion in Altered Thyroid States"). However, I do not know the severity or chronicity of hypothyroidism of patients in the study by Matsukawa et al.

Pending further study, we must suspend judgment on a possible difference in muscle sympathetic nerve activity in fibromyalgia and hypothyroid patients. The conflicting results (lower than normal activity in fibromyalgia patients and higher than normal activity in hypothyroid patients) are moot for several reasons.

First, inadequate thyroid hormone regulation of cell function tends to be tissue specific: The tissues affected vary to some degree between patients, resulting in variable clinical phenotypes within the same diagnostic category such as fibromyalgia. *Thus, while some hypothyroid and fibromyalgia patients will have low muscle sympathetic activity, others may have normal activity, and others may have high activity. This reflects tissue variability—only in some patients is the peripheral sympathetic nervous system inhibited by the effects of inadequate thyroid hormone cell regulation.* A close inspection of the data reported by Elam et al.[150] shows this to be true of the 8 fibromyalgia patients they studied. In 4 or 5 [sic] of 6 patients, stressors increased muscle sympathetic activity, although slightly less than in normal controls. But in 1 or 2 [sic] of the 6 patients, muscle sympathetic activity in response to stressors was slightly-to-markedly decreased.[150] Thus, the low mean obscured the normal activity in more of the fibromyalgia patients.

In addition, the study by Elam et al.[150] may have contained too few patients to document sympathetic muscle activity in fibromyalgia patients at-large. Elam et al. included only 6 fibromyalgia patients and 6 controls in their study.[150] In attempting to establish the features of a clinical condition, larger numbers of subjects in studies are preferable. This is especially true when a finding, such as that of Elam et al., conflicts with predictions of a highly productive hypothesis such as the one I posit in this book. Considering this qualification, the finding of low muscle sympathetic activity in the Elam et al. study may have resulted from selection bias; the result of another study with a larger number of patients may differ from that of the study by Elam et al. Thus, the mean tendency reported by Elam et al., and even the variability that their detailed data show, may not accurately represent the unknown mean and variability of muscle sympathetic activity of fibromyalgia patients in general. As a result, we must consider their conclusion tentative.[150] A larger study may, however, show reduced muscle sympathetic activity in fibromyalgia patients. If so, this will be one way in which fibromyalgia patients differ from hypothyroid patients. The difference may constitute a challenge to the adequacy of the hypothesis of the etiology of fibromyalgia that I present in this book.

Blood Flow

Klemp et al. used injected ^{133}xenon to measure local blood flow through a large tissue volume in fibromyalgia patients. They found no abnormality.[154] Lund, Bengtsson, and Thorborg,[155] however, using a more sensitive method, found low oxygenation of the trapezius and brachioradialis muscles of fibromyalgia patients. They speculated that the low oxygenation was due to structural and function changes affecting the microvessels in tender points. They also found low oxygen pressure in the patients' subcutaneous tissues although the tissues were not hypoxic. The reduced oxygen pressure could be a result of an increase in α-adrenergic receptors and a decrease in β-adrenergic receptors on the blood vessels of muscle due to inadequate thyroid hormone regulation of the adrenergic receptor genes. This altered ratio of the adrenoceptors would, upon catecholamine binding, induce muscle vasoconstriction—the ". . . neuro-effector mechanism . . ." of ". . . sympathetically-mediated muscle ischemia . . ." allowed for by Elam et al.[150,p.375]

The possibility that this mechanism is operative in fibromyalgia is strongly supported by a study by Bengtsson et al. They used two techniques to induce sympathetic ganglion blocks in fibromyalgia patients. The blocks diminished the patients' fibromyalgic pain.[49] The results indicate that the blocks reduced norepinephrine secretion in peripheral tissues, stopped norepinephrine/α_2-adrenergic receptor binding, and permitted blood vessels to dilate. (See section below titled "Pain.")

Circulation through hypothyroid skeletal muscle is decreased because the density of β-receptors on muscle blood vessels is reduced.[84] The smooth muscle of blood vessels that supply skeletal muscles has both β_2- and α-adrenergic receptors. The adrenergic receptors on the blood vessels of the skin are almost exclusively the α- type. When catecholamines bind to α-adrenergic receptors, the blood vessels constrict. Binding of catecholamines to β_2-receptors abolishes the vasoconstriction induced by α-adrenergic receptor stimulation.[48,p.190] In other words, the blood vessels in skeletal muscle dilate only in reversing the constriction induced by catecholamine binding to α-adrenergic receptors.[48,p.199] Norepinephrine has little effect on β_2-adrenergic receptors, but is a potent activator of α-adrenergic receptors. The number of β-adrenergic receptors is decreased in hypothyroidism and the density of α-adrenergic receptors is increased. As a result, the release of catecholamines reduces blood flow through both skeletal muscle and skin.[48,p.199] Precisely the same mechanism may account for reduced blood flow in fibromyalgia (see Chapter 3.2).

Abnormal Glycolysis in Fibromyalgia

Eisinger et al. found that fibromyalgia patients had glycolysis impairment (which is similar to the finding

in hypothyroid patients). The researchers also found that fibromyalgia patients had low red blood cell ATP concentrations.[130][218]

These abnormalities may result from the shift from a balance of α- and β-adrenergic receptors on cell membranes to a predominance of α-adrenergic receptors. Inadequate thyroid hormone regulation of the β-adrenergic receptor genes results in a decreased β-adrenoceptor density on cell membranes. The inadequacy also results in reduced glycogenolysis (which is mediated by β_2-adrenoceptors).[110,p.671] Binding of catecholamines to β-adrenergic receptors increases energy production through activation of glycogenolysis and glycogenesis; binding of catecholamines to α-adrenergic receptors decreases energy production by inactivating the two cytoplasmic pathways. (See Chapter 2.2, section titled "Energy Processes in the Cytoplasm.")

Molecular Changes during Hypothyroidism that Impede β-Adrenergic Responsiveness of Cells. Adequate thyroid hormone regulation potently maintains four molecular conditions: a proper ratio of β- to α-adrenergic receptors, a proper ratio of stimulatory (G_s) to inhibitory (G_i) G proteins, normal levels of phosphodiesterase, and normal responsiveness to the inhibitory molecule adenosine. In hypothyroidism, the density of β-adrenergic receptors on cell membranes decreases, the content of G_i in cell membranes increases, phosphodiesterase levels increase, and cell responsiveness to adenosine increases. (See section above titled "Biochemical Factors Other than T_3 that Augment α-Adrenergic Responsiveness and Decrease β-Adrenergic Responsiveness of Cells in Hypothyroidism.") Thus, inadequate thyroid hormone regulation results in four molecular changes that impede the activation of fuel metabolism in cells. Because of these changes, hypothyroid patients have a diminished ability to muster the cell processes necessary to adapt well to stress.

Growth Hormone

Thyroid hormone potently regulates transcription of the growth hormone gene. The hormone positively regulates the gene. When thyroid hormone binds to a T_3-receptor on the gene, transcription increases. Absence of the hormone at the gene stops transcription and results in low growth hormone levels. Thyroid hormone also regulates the production of growth hormone-releasing hormone by hypothalamic cells. Growth hormone-releasing hormone controls growth hormone secretion by the anterior pituitary. Thus, in addition to directly regulating the growth hormone gene, thyroid hormone indirectly regulates growth hormone secretion by regulating production of growth hormone-releasing hormone. Moreover, thyroid hormone increases: somatomedin C levels, production of somatomedin C receptors, and somatomedin-binding proteins that transport somatomedins through the circulation. For the most part, thyroid hormone increases somatomedin production by regulating pituitary production of growth hormone. However, thyroid hormone also appears to have direct effects on somatomedin production. In hypothyroidism, for example, somatomedin C levels may be low despite normal growth hormone production (see Chapter 3.12).

In some hypothalamic cells, inadequate thyroid hormone regulation of transcription of the adrenergic genes increases production of α-adrenergic receptors and decreases production of β-adrenergic receptors. This is true of the cells that synthesize and secrete growth hormone-releasing hormone. The binding of ligands to α_2-adrenergic receptors usually increases growth hormone secretion. However, Bennett et al. reported that in fibromyalgia patients, the growth hormone response to clonidine (α_2-adrenoceptor agonist) was blunted.[135] Inadequate thyroid hormone regulation of the α-adrenergic receptor gene in fibromyalgia patients may account for the increased density of α_2-adrenergic receptors on their platelets.[91] Conversely, inadequate regulation of the α-adrenergic receptor gene in hypothalamic cells may lower the density of α_2-adrenergic receptors on these cells' membranes. The result would be a decreased production of growth hormone-releasing hormone and, in turn, low growth hormone production by the pituitary—even when pituitary secretion of growth hormone is provoked by clonidine. Thus, inadequate thyroid hormone regulation of hypothalamic cells may indirectly decrease growth hormone secretion via a decreased density of α_2-adrenergic receptors. (See Chapter 3.12, section titled "Thyroid Hormone, Adrenergic Receptor Type, and Regulation of Growth Hormone-Releasing Factor and Growth Hormone Secretion.")

Serotonin

α_2-Adrenoceptors located presynaptically on serotonergic nerve terminals inhibit secretion of serotonin.[92] Inhibition occurs when the receptors bind to norepinephrine secreted by noradrenergic neurons in the neighborhood of the serotonergic neurons.[95] Studies have shown α_2-adrenergic receptor inhibition of serotonin secretion in neocortex from humans,[95] hippocampus[93] and solitary tract nuclei from rats,[94] and cerebral cortex from rats and rabbits.[94] The finding

that α_2-adrenoceptors inhibit serotonin secretion is important in relation to fibromyalgia. In view of this finding, the increased density of α_2-adrenoceptors on the platelets of fibromyalgia patients[91] makes a conjecture plausible: that inadequate thyroid hormone regulation of α_2-adrenergic receptor gene transcription is responsible for the low peripheral serotonin levels in fibromyalgia.

Serotonin Levels and the β_2-Adrenergic Receptor Agonist Salbutamol. That inadequate regulation of the adrenergic genes is responsible for peripheral low serotonin levels in fibromyalgia is supported by other findings. Hallberg et al. administered the β_2-adrenergic receptor agonist salbutamol to rats twice per day for 14 days. As a result, serotonin levels significantly increased in limbic forebrain, corpus striatum, and cerebral cortex. The levels of tryptophan, the amino acid from which cells synthesize serotonin, were not affected. The results indicate that the *in vivo* rate of tryptophan hydroxylation in the brain was increased by salbutamol-activated β_2-adrenergic receptors.[151] β_2-adrenergic receptor activation may also increase serotonin levels in the periphery. If so, low peripheral serotonin levels in fibromyalgia may result from a shift toward increased α_2-adrenergic receptors and decreased β_2-adrenergic receptors due to inadequate thyroid hormone regulation of adrenergic gene transcription.

Serotonin Metabolism in Mature Rat Brain Is Critically Dependent on Thyroid Hormone Adequacy During Early Life: Implications for Fibromyalgia. I described in a section above studies showing that the ability of adult rats to increase production of two catecholamine-increasing enzymes (tyrosine hydroxylase and dopamine-β-hydroxylase) during stress depends on the rats having had normal exposure to thyroid hormone during a critical time in their development. Inadequate exposure to thyroid hormone during that critical time presumably impaired the ability of the rats to adapt to stress with sufficient catecholamine synthesis and secretion. (See subsection above titled "Low Production of Catecholamine-Inducing Enzymes Due to Inadequate Thyroid Hormone Regulation During Fetal Development and Infancy.")

A similar phenomenon occurs with serotonin metabolism: Hypothyroidism in neonatal rats resulted in abnormal serotonin metabolism in adulthood.[11][177][178] Rastogi and Singhal induced hypothyroidism in 1-day-old rats.[11] Subsequently, the mid-brains of the rats had a low level of tryptophan hydroxylase. This enzyme hydroxylates tryptophan to 5-hydroxytryptophan, the stage preceding formation of serotonin.[109,p.262] Serotonin levels were reduced in the cerebellum by 22%, the mid-brain by 29%, and the striatum by 31%. The serotonin metabolite 5-hydroxyindoleacetic acid was significantly decreased in the cerebellum, mid-brain, and striatum. When the researchers administered T_3 5 days after the beginning of thyroid hormone deficiency and continued for 25 days, tryptophan hydroxylase activity and tryptophan and serotonin levels returned to normal values. The concentration of 5-hydroxyindoleacetic acid also increased.

When the researchers postponed T_3 administration until the rats reached adulthood, none of the serotonin-related abnormalities improved. Rastogi and Singhal wrote: "Our data demonstrate that deficiency of thyroid hormone in early life disrupts the normal upsurge of 5-hydroxytryptamine [serotonin] metabolism in brain. A critical period exists in early life of rats during which thyroid hormone must be present for the optimal development of 5-hydroxytryptamine metabolizing systems in maturing brain."[11] This finding raises an interesting question: Does suboptimal thyroid status in susceptible humans at a critical early stage in life predispose them to the adverse effects of low serotonin levels, such as depression, hypersensitivity to pain, and disturbed sleep? I know of no evidence that provides an answer to this question.

Norepinephrine

α_2-Adrenergic receptor activation inhibits norepinephrine secretion in the central nervous system. Activation of α_2-adrenergic receptors on neurons increases membrane potassium conductance. The increase hyperpolarizes the nerves,[50,p.119] reducing their spontaneous neural firing rate.[53] Researchers have shown this effect in norepinephrine-secreting neurons of the locus ceruleus in the brain stem. α_2-Adrenergic receptor agonists hyperpolarize the neurons, and receptor antagonists reduce polarization.[52]

Autoreceptors are stationed in and modulate norepinephrine secretion by locus ceruleus neurons. The autoreceptors are presynaptic α_2-adrenergic receptors on the cell bodies of the neurons.[50,p.120] When stimulated, locus ceruleus neurons secrete norepinephrine locally and through their axons in widespread parts of the brain. Locally secreted norepinephrine binds to presynaptic α_2-adrenergic receptors. The binding hyperpolarizes the neurons and reduces their excitability and secretion of norepinephrine.[52] A predominance of α_2-adrenergic receptors on locus ceruleus neurons due to inadequate thyroid hormone regulation of adrenergic gene transcription may account for the low concentration of the metabolite of norepinephrine

in fibromyalgia patients' cerebrospinal fluid. (See section above titled "Low Cerebrospinal Fluid Levels of Norepinephrine and Dopamine Metabolites in Fibromyalgia Patients.") Moreover, an increase of α_2-adrenergic receptors in the nucleus of the solitary tract can account in part for decreased central sympathetic drive in fibromyalgia patients. (See subsection above titled "Reduction in Sympathetic Outflow to Peripheral Tissues by Activation of Central α-Adrenergic Receptors.") Similarly, an increase in the density of the receptors in the sympathetic ganglia may explain subnormal norepinephrine secretion in the periphery of patients. (See subsection above titled "Inhibition of Sympathetic Ganglionic Neural Transmission by an Increased α_2-Adrenergic Receptor Density on Ganglion Cells," and section below titled "Pain.")

Through a more complicated change in adrenergic receptor type during inadequate thyroid hormone regulation of adrenergic receptor genes, hypothalamic secretion of corticotropin-releasing hormone may decrease as β-adrenergic receptors increase. (In some cells of the hypothalamus, inadequate thyroid hormone regulation increases β- and decreases α-adrenergic receptor density.) Since stimulation of CRH secretion by norepinephrine is mediated primarily by α-adrenoceptors, an increase in β-adrenergic receptor density in the hypothalamus is likely to result in dysregulation of the hypothalamic-pituitary-adrenocortical axis, and it may decrease central activation of the sympathetic nervous system. (See Chapter 3.5, section titled "Control of CRH Secretion," and subsections above titled "Activation of the Locus Ceruleus by Hypothalamic Corticotropin-Releasing Hormone" and "Locus Ceruleus.")

Low Neuropeptide Y Levels in Fibromyalgia

I have not found published studies on the possible regulation of peripheral circulating neuropeptide Y (NPY) levels by thyroid hormone. Therefore, at this time, I am not able to interpret low plasma NPY levels in fibromyalgia in terms of inadequate thyroid hormone regulation of cell function.[137][138] However, as Clauw et al. speculated, low plasma NPY levels in fibromyalgia patients indicate diminished sympathetic function and may contribute to some fibromyalgia symptoms.[138] Diminished sympathetic function is consistent with the predicted effects of α_2-adrenergic receptor dominance in fibromyalgia patients that I proposed above (see subsection titled "Inhibition of Sympathetic Ganglionic Neural Transmission by an Increased α_2-Adrenergic Receptor Density on Ganglion Cells").

IMPAIRED SYMPATHETIC NERVOUS SYSTEM FUNCTION: CLINICAL CONSEQUENCES

Impaired sympathetic nervous system function due to inadequate thyroid hormone regulation of cell function (mainly inadequate regulation of gene transcription) may result in several clinical conditions that we consider features of fibromyalgia.

Pain

The results of a study by Bengtsson et al.[49] provide strong evidence that an increase in the density of α_2-adrenergic receptors on sympathetic ganglion neurons can account for some features of fibromyalgic pain. The investigators used two techniques to block the outflow of sympathetic nerve signals from sympathetic ganglia. The first was a stellate ganglion block. In this procedure, an investigator injected a sufficient amount of local anesthetic through the neck into the tissue area of the stellate ganglion. In most patients, this ganglion is made up of a fusion of the first thoracic sympathetic ganglion and the lower of the three cervical ganglia. Clinicians use stellate ganglion blocks to relieve vascular insufficiency and pain as features of a wide variety of conditions. Relief occurs because the block reduces norepinephrine secretion by the postganglionic sympathetic neurons that travel from the ganglia to peripheral tissues of the head, neck, and upper extremities.[185,pp.773&775] The blocking procedure enables blood vessels to dilate by stopping the norepinephrine/α_2-adrenergic receptor binding that sustains vasoconstriction in peripheral tissues. With this procedure, however, some of the vasodilation and pain relief occur because the anesthetic also blocks acetylcholine secretion by preganglionic fibers in the glanglia.

Bengtsson et al. also used another procedure—injections of guanethidine to block patients' sympathetic ganglia.[49] Injecting guanethidine intravenously does not block acetylcholine release by preganglionic sympathetic neurons; instead, the procedure exclusively blocks secretion of norepinephrine by postganglionic nerves.[153,p.754] Thus, the vasodilation and pain relief result specifically from reduced norepinephrine secretion from postganglionic sympathetic neurons that innervate the peripheral tissues. Reduced norepinephrine secretion decreases the norepinephrine/α_2-adrenergic receptor binding that maintains vasoconstriction; consequently, blood vessels dilate.

This study by Bengtsson et al.[49] lends support to the hypothesis that α-adrenergic receptor dominance is a mechanism of fibromyalgia symptoms and signs.

Fifteen minutes after stellate ganglion block by injection in 8 fibromyalgia patients, pain decreased and the number of tender points decreased. Maximum results occurred at 4 hours. Using a visual analog scale, patients reported that their pain at rest decreased from 29.2 to 2.8 mm. The number of tender points decreased from an average value of 7.6 to 3.1. When patients were given an intravenous regional sympathetic blockade with guanethidine, the number of tender points decreased, although pain at rest did not significantly decrease. Chemical blockade of the sympathetic ganglion reduces norepinephrine secretion. Relief of symptoms under such conditions indicates that the symptoms were mediated by norepinephrine interaction with α-adrenergic receptors.

Apparently, one mechanism by which sympathetic blockade, regardless of the technique employed, relieves pain is by relieving ischemia.[185,p.779] Raynaud's-like symptoms, such as cold fingers, are a feature of fibromyalgia. For more than 50 years, clinicians have surgically disrupted sympathetic innervation of the extremities as a treatment for Raynaud's phenomenon.[184] It is likely that the mechanism of reduced fibromyalgic pain in the study by Bengtsson et al. is the same as that from sympathetic blockade—relief of vasoconstriction induced by norepinephrine/α_2-adrenergic receptor binding. In fibromyalgia, it is also likely that the vasoconstriction ultimately is the result of inadequate thyroid hormone regulation of adrenergic gene transcription.

Activating α_2-adrenergic receptors in the dorsal horns of the spinal cord with agonists such as norepinephrine and clonidine inhibits nociception.[182] Clinicians have administered clonidine, an α_2-adrenergic receptor agonist, within the subdural space of the spinal cord to relieve cancer patients' pain.[183] Inhibition of nociceptive processing by activation of α_2-adrenergic receptors is a local effect that occurs when agonists are administered intrathecally.[181] The local effect apparently is not sufficient to override at least two nociceptive effects of inadequate thyroid hormone regulation of transcription of different genes: high substance P and low serotonin levels. While an increased density of α_2-adrenergic receptors is an effect of inadequate regulation by thyroid hormone, the net effect of the inadequacy appears to be increased pain perception. (See Chapter 3.15.) I would predict that (all other factors held constant) patients with normal thyroid hormone regulation of transcription would obtain pain relief from intrathecal administration of clonidine, but fibromyalgia patients whose central nervous systems have high substance P and low serotonin levels would not.

Worsening of Fibromyalgia Status with Stresses such as Exercise

Data in the section above titled "Blunted Cardiac Response to Stress" indicate that the response of target cells to catecholamines is diminished when thyroid hormone inadequately regulates transcription of the adrenergic genes. This finding may in part explain the worsening of fibromyalgia symptoms in patients who exercise enough to induce substantial catecholamine secretion (see Chapter 3.4, section titled "Exercise Intolerance: Worsening of Fibromyalgia Status During Exercise and Other Stresses"). Norepinephrine released during stresses such as exercise will bind predominantly to α-adrenergic receptors on blood vessel and muscle cell membranes. The binding will reduce muscle blood flow (see section above titled "Blood Flow") and inhibit the very metabolic adaptation of cells that is needed to meet the demands imposed by the stress-activated sympathetic nervous system. The decreased blood flow and metabolism would induce a metabolic crisis that would worsen the patient's fibromyalgia status.

Low Motor Drive, Low Fitness Level, and Exercise Intolerance

Fibromyalgia patients commonly report a lethargy and disinclination to mobilize themselves (see Chapter 3.4, section titled "Thyroid Hormone Regulation of Dopamine Levels and Motor Drive"). This symptom may result from the reduced dopamine synthesis and secretion due to inadequate thyroid hormone regulation of dopaminergic cells (see section above titled "Low Cerebrospinal Fluid Levels of Norepinephrine and Dopamine Metabolites in Fibromyalgia Patients"). The lack of motor drive may overlap with depression in patients with behavioral suppression (see next section).

Depression and Cognitive Dysfunction

Fibromyalgia patients have anxiety, depression, and cognitive dysfunction (see Chapter 3.10). These psychological abnormalities may be understood by consideration of the catecholamine hypothesis of affective disorders.

The catecholamines epinephrine and norepinephrine have marked effects on the nervous system. Norepinephrine-secreting neurons in the central nervous system mediate learning, memory, reinforcement, sleep-wake cycles, anxiety-related pain sensitivity, and affective disorders. Some writers have proposed that

the most important roles of norepinephrine are regulation of cerebral blood flow and cerebral metabolism. These roles are important in that studies have shown decreased regional brain blood flow in fibromyalgia patients (see Chapter 3.2). Reduced blood flow and metabolism of central nervous system neurons can substantially affect mood and cognition.

Cooper, Bloom, and Roth wrote that the major function of noradrenergic neurons projecting from the locus ceruleus is to regulate the brain's global orientation to visceral and exogenous stimuli. Rat studies have shown that the locus ceruleus responds to an array of innocuous sensory stimuli. The level of "behavioral vigilance" determines the responsiveness of the rat's locus ceruleus to such stimuli. Exogenous sensory stimuli that "surprise" rats increase noradrenergic neuronal activity in the locus ceruleus. Behaviors that mediate a tonic, vegetative state decrease locus ceruleus neuronal activity.[109,p.276]

The catecholamine hypothesis of affective disorders posits that a deficiency of catecholamines, particularly norepinephrine, produces depression. The hypothesis attributes mania to an excess of catecholamines.[109,p.278][232] Considerable evidence supports the hypothesis.

Many norepinephrine-releasing neurons of the locus ceruleus project to the limbic system (a brain structure involved in emotion and motivation), the thalamus, and cerebral cortex. Also, many serotonin-secreting neurons of the midline raphe nuclei of the lower pons and medulla send fibers to the limbic system. Drugs such as reserpine that block norepinephrine and serotonin release cause depression. Tricyclic antidepressant drugs and monoamine oxidase inhibitors relieve depression in many people; they do so by sustaining the life-span of norepinephrine and serotonin at synapses and potentiating their excitatory effects. As Guyton wrote, "It is presumed that the norepinephrine system especially and perhaps the serotonin system as well normally function to provide motor drive to the limbic system to increase a person's sense of well-being, to create happiness, contentment, good appetite, appropriate sex drive, and psychomotor balance, although too much of a good thing can cause mania."[110,p.665] Guyton also noted that the hypothalamic centers that mediate pleasure and reward receive many norepinephrine-secreting nerve endings. I cannot overemphasize, however, that *the responses of tissues to secreted norepinephrine are dictated by the adrenergic receptor type that predominates on the cell membranes of the tissues.* We can accurately predict the effects of secreted norepinephrine only by considering the adrenergic receptor type that predominates. This is true because in most tissues, the interaction of norepinephrine with α- and β-adrenergic receptors has opposite effects. Thyroid hormone potently regulates the adrenergic genes and controls the ratio of β- to α-adrenergic receptor density on cell membranes. By doing so, thyroid hormone also potently regulates the effects of norepinephrine on cells. Some individuals' affective disorders result from inadequate thyroid hormone regulation of the adrenergic genes. The inadequate regulation results in decreased responsiveness of central nervous system tissues to catecholamines.[233] The decreased responsiveness appears to result from the increase in α-adrenergic receptor density on neurons. (See Chapter 3.10.)

We can apply an extension of the catecholamine hypothesis of affective disorders to fibromyalgia patients. The application posits that α-adrenergic receptor predominance on central nervous system neuronal membranes mediates the patients' psychological abnormalities. When brain stem locus ceruleus neurons are stimulated, they secrete norepinephrine. A high density of α₂-adrenergic receptors on the noradrenergic neurons (due to inadequate thyroid hormone regulation of adrenergic gene transcription) hyperpolarizes them and reduces their excitability.[52] Predictable effects of these molecular changes include slowing of cognitive function and dampening of emotion. Patients' depression is thus not primarily due to stress or a psychogenic mechanism—instead, it is the psychological manifestation of a molecularly-based physiological process.

Two findings support the possibility that this molecular mechanism contributes to the psychological abnormalities of fibromyalgia: (1) an increased density of α₂-adrenergic receptors on the platelets of some fibromyalgia patients,[91] and (2) the significantly low concentration of homovanillic acid, the breakdown product of norepinephrine, in the cerebrospinal fluid of other patients.[54] (See Chapter 3.10.)

Anxiety

Activation of α₂-adrenergic receptors hyperpolarizes and decreases neural firing of the sympathetic postganglionic cells. The hyperpolarization decreases the outflow of sympathetic signals to peripheral tissues. (See subsection above titled "Inhibition of Sympathetic Ganglionic Neural Transmission by an Increased α₂-Adrenergic Receptor Density on Ganglion Cells.") The hyperpolarization is similar to the "relative refractory period" rather than the "absolute refractory period" of nerve fibers. Two factors cause

a relative refractory period: (1) an inactive state of some sodium channels (keeping sodium outside neurons), and (2) wide-open potassium channels (enabling potassium to accumulate inside the neuronal membrane). These ion changes hyperpolarize nerve fibers, rendering them more resistant than normal to stimulation. Only strong stimuli can cause the fibers to begin conducting action potentials.[110,p.64]

The requirement for a strong stimulus to activate the sympathetic system may account in part for physiological cues that the patient perceives as anxiety (see Chapter 3.10, section titled "Perceptual or Cognitive Set as a Possible Cause of Anxiety in Fibromyalgia Patients"). The sympathetic system may be inactive until a sufficiently strong stimulus activates it. When the system is activated, the patient may experience a sympathetic surge. With her apprehensions associated with fibromyalgia, she may interpret the surge as anxiety.

Irritable Bowel Syndrome

Gervais Tougas wrote that besides immune and endocrine mechanisms, neural pathways enable communication along the brain-gut axis. The sympathetic and parasympathetic branches of the autonomic nervous system are important neural pathways in regulating the homeostasis of gut function. Many researchers have found that different disorders of autonomic nervous system function are relevant to subgroups of patients who have functional bowel disorders. Patients whose disorders involve slowed gastrointestinal motility generally have two autonomic abnormalities: (1) decreased parasympathetic (vagal/cholinergic activity) nervous system outflow and (2) increased sympathetic outflow. Patients with symptoms associated with increased motility usually have either (1) increased parasympathetic outflow or (2) decreased sympathetic outflow. Gervais Tougas wrote that autonomic dysfunction may account for the common gastrointestinal complaints of fibromyalgia and chronic fatigue syndrome patients.[166] The autonomic imbalance that underlies diarrhea-like irritable bowel syndrome in fibromyalgia, as suggested by Gervais Tougas' review, may be the same as underlies bradycardia and hypotension (see section above titled "Bradycardia and Low Blood Pressure"). The underlying molecular mechanism may be an increase in central nervous system α₂-adrenergic receptors due to inadequate thyroid hormone regulation of the α-adrenergic genes. Central nervous system α₂-adrenergic receptors can both reduce sympathetic outflow and increase parasympathetic nervous system outflow.[131][156]

Altered Sleep Patterns

Prange and his coworkers pointed out three points of similarity between hypothyroid and depressed patients. Hypothyroid and depressed patients tend to have: (1) a diminished response to infused norepinephrine,[40][41] (2) a high urine level of catecholamines and their metabolites,[42][43] and (3) altered sleep patterns.[44] Fibromyalgia patients are similar to hypothyroid and depressed patients by virtue of the same three points of similarity. (See Table 3.1.3.)

The disturbed sleep pattern of fibromyalgia patients is similar to that of hypothyroid patients[44][47][174] This similarity may be a result of the same underlying process—inadequate thyroid hormone regulation of cell function. Several findings support this possibility.

Table 3.1.3. Similarities between depressed, hypothyroid, and fibromyalgic patients.

PATIENT TYPE:	DEPRESSED	HYPOTHYROID	FIBROMYALGIC
Blunted response to NE*	Yes	Yes	Yes
High NE* urinary excretion	Yes	Yes†	Yes
Altered sleep pattern	Yes	Yes	Yes

*(NE = norepinephrine)
†Studies indicate that NE is elevated in severe or prolonged hypothyroidism.

First, central nervous system norepinephrine plays a role in the regulation of the sleep-wake cycle.[109,p.276] Researchers found that fibromyalgia patients' cerebrospinal fluid levels of the metabolite of norepinephrine were significantly low.[54] Based on this finding, low central nervous system levels of norepinephrine may be involved in dysregulation of sleep in fibromyalgia patients. However, a more important factor may be a decreased density of β-adrenergic receptors and an increased density of α-adrenergic receptors in patients' brains. Relevant to this possibility is a study by Hilakivi. He found that in cats, a low level of β-adrenergic receptor activity, especially when combined with a high level of α$_2$-adrenoceptor activity, facilitated production of "drowsy waking."[167] Even a low level of norepinephrine interacting with a low ratio of β- to α-adrenergic receptors would be likely to produce the effect reported by Hilakivi.

Second, α$_2$-adrenergic receptors on serotonergic neurons inhibit serotonin synthesis and secretion.[18][19][92] Serotonin is involved in sleep induction and maintenance of slow wave sleep.[105][129] Studies have not shown that fibromyalgia patients have low central nervous system levels. In one study, patients' cerebrospinal fluid levels of the serotonin metabolite were not significantly low.[54] However, if some patients do have a low central nervous system serotonin level, the low level may contribute to their sleep disturbance. The responsible factor may be an increase in α$_2$-adrenergic receptors on serotonergic neurons due to inadequate regulation of the α$_2$-adrenoceptor gene.

Third, increased histamine secretion heightens alertness[20] and can interfere with sleep.[21] Histamine probably induces arousal and pain perception that interfere with sleep. Lin et al. found that administering an agent that inhibited the histamine-synthesizing enzyme decreased wakefulness and increased slow wave sleep.[21] Although study results are inconsistent,[172] binding of catecholamines to α$_2$-adrenergic receptors on mast cells may increase histamine secretion.[173] Prazosin, an α$_1$-adrenergic receptor antagonist, when inhaled, reduced the severity of post-exercise bronchoconstriction in asthmatic children. This finding indicates that α$_1$-adrenergic receptors facilitate the release of histamine from mast cells.[171] Thyroid hormone treatment of rats significantly decreased the density of α$_{1A}$- and α$_{1B}$-adrenergic receptors in heart tissue; the treatment increased the density of α$_{1D}$-adrenoceptors.[168] Sabria et al. found that treating rats up to 5 days old with thyroid hormone or TSH decreased the number of mast cells and the levels of histamine in the rats' brains. Treating them with an antithyroid chemical that rendered them hypothyroid increased both the number of mast cells and histamine levels.[169] This finding of increased mast cells in hypothyroid rats corresponds to the higher mean number of mast cells in skin biopsies of fibromyalgia patients compared to healthy subjects and rheumatoid arthritis patients.[15] Thus, inadequate thyroid hormone regulation of the α-adrenergic genes may result in sleep interference from increased histamine secretion from mast cells. (See Chapter 3.18.)

Fourth, thyroid hormone is a powerful positive regulator of transcription of the growth hormone gene (see Chapter 3.12). In addition, α$_2$-adrenergic receptors (increased during inadequate thyroid hormone regulation of the α$_2$-adrenoceptor gene) inhibit growth hormone secretion.[135] In turn, growth hormone deficiency appears to disrupt sleep.[28][175][176] (See Chapter 3.18.)

Urinary Frequency

Inadequate thyroid hormone regulation of adrenergic gene transcription can cause abnormalities in the function of the hypothalamic-pituitary-kidney-bladder axis. One or more of these abnormalities may account for increased urgency and frequency among fibromyalgia patients. The main abnormality may be a shift toward an increased α-adrenoceptor density on cell membranes and a shift toward decreased density of β-adrenoceptors on the membranes.

Increased α_2-adrenoceptor activity is associated with decreased pituitary secretion of vasopressin (a hormone that causes contraction of the smooth muscle of blood vessels). Also, increased numbers of α_2-adrenergic receptors on the renal tubules decrease the count of vasopressin receptors on the tubules. This decrease in vasopressin receptors renders the kidneys partially resistant to vasopressin. The resistance impedes the water-retaining effect of vasopressin and increases kidney excretion of water in the urine. In addition, subnormal sympathetic drive in the fibromyalgia patient might impede renal vasoconstriction. The subnormal vasoconstriction might allow excessive loss of water in the urine.

The urinary urgency and frequency of some fibromyalgia patients may result partly from α-adrenergic receptor dominance in the bladder. α-Adrenergic receptors induce increased tone or frank contraction of the muscle coat of the bladder wall. β-Adrenergic receptors relax the muscle lining of the bladder. A decrease in β-adrenergic receptor density in the bladder wall, and a shift toward α-adrenergic dominance, increases the muscle tone of the bladder muscle wall and can cause it to contract. Increased α-adrenergic receptor density at the trigone (the base of the bladder) increases its tone. The resulting total increase in tone of the bladder musculature would decrease its capacity for filling. The decreased filling capacity would lower the threshold for the urination reflex that induces urgency. The urination reflex is regulated at the level of the brain stem; α_1-adrenergic receptors facilitate the reflex. It is plausible, then, that a shift toward α-adrenergic receptor dominance (sustained by inadequate thyroid hormone regulation of transcription of the adrenoceptor genes) underlies urinary urgency and frequency in fibromyalgia.

Finally, a patient may have subnormal sympathetic innervation and increased parasympathetic innervation of the ureters (the tubes that conduct urine from the kidneys to the bladder). Increased peristalsis (contraction of the muscle lining) of the ureters would result. The increase in peristalsis would cause more rapid filling of the contracted low-capacity bladder, contributing to urgency and frequency. (See Chapter 3.21.)

REFERENCES

1. Kvetnansky, R., Gewirtz, G.P., Weise, V.K., and Kopin, I.J.: Enhanced synthesis of adrenal dopamine-β-hydroxylase induced by repeated immobilization in rats. *Mol. Pharmacol.*, 7:81-86, 1971.
2. Thoenen, H.: Induction of tyrosine hydroxylase in peripheral and central adrenergic neurones by cold-exposure of rats. *Nature*, 228(274):861-862, 1970.
3. Viveros, O.H., Arqueros, L., Connett, R.J., and Kirshner, N.: Mechanism of secretion of catecholamines from the adrenal medulla. IV. The fate of the storage vesicles following insulin and reserpine administration. *Mol. Pharmacol.*, 5:69-82, 1969.
4. Patrick, R.L. and Kirshner, N.: Effect of stimulation on the levels of tyrosine hydroxylase, dopamine-β-hydroxylase, and catecholamines in intact and denervated rat adrenal glands. *Mol. Pharmacol.*, 7:87-96, 1971.
5. Otten, U., Schwab, M., Gagnon, C., and Thoenen, H.: Selective induction of tyrosine hydroxylase and dopamine-β-hydroxylase by nerve growth factor: comparison of adult and newborn rats. *Brain Res.*, 133:291-303, 1977.
6. Carmichael, S.W.: *The Adrenal Medulla, Vol. 1: Annual Research Reviews*, Montreal, Eden Press, 1979.
7. Gagnon, C., Otten, U., and Thoenen, H.: Increased synthesis of dopamine-β-hydroxylase in cultured rat adrenal medullae after *in vivo* administration of reserpine. *J. Neurochem.*, 27:259-265, 1987.
8. Joh, T.H., Geghman, C., and Reis, D.: Immunochemical demonstration of increased accumulation of tyrosine hydroxylase protein in sympathetic ganglia and adrenal medulla elicited by reserpine. *Proc. Natl. Acad. Sci. (USA)*, 70:2767-2771, 1973.
9. Ungar, A. and Phillips, J.H.: Regulation of the adrenal medulla. *Physiol. Rev.*, 63:787-843, 1983.
10. Volle, R.L.: Pharmacology of ganglionic transmission. In *Handbook of Pharmacology*, Vol. 53. Edited by D.A. Kharkevich, Berlin, Springer-Verlag, 1980, pp.385-410.
11. Rastogi, R.B. and Singhal, R.L.: The effect of thyroid hormone on serotonergic neurons: depletion of serotonin in discrete brain areas of developing hypothyroid rats. *Naunyn-Schiedeberg's Arch. Pharmacol.*, 304(1):9-13, 1978.
12. Cahill, A.L. and Perlman, R.L.: Phosphorylation of tyrosine hydroxylase in the superior cervical ganglion. *Biochem. Biophys. Acta*, 805:217-226, 1984.
13. Reymond, M.J., Speciale, S.G., and Porter, J.C.: Dopamine in plasma of lateral and medial hypophysial portal vessels: evidence for regional variation in the release of hypothalamic dopamine into hypophyseal portal blood. *Endocrinology*, 112:1958-1963, 1983.
14. Wang, P.S., Gonzales, H.A., Reymond, M.J., and Porter, J.C.L: Mass and in situ molar activity of tyrosine hydroxylase in the median eminence. *Neuroendocrinology*, 49:659-663, 1989.
15. Enestrom, S., Bengtsson, A., and Frodin, T.: Dermal IgG deposits and increase of mast cells in patients with fibromyalgia: relevant findings or epiphenomena? *Scand. J.*

Rheumatol., 26(4):308-313, 1997.

16. Black, I.B.: The role of the thyroid in the growth and development of adrenergic neurons *in vivo. Neurology*, 24: 377, 1974.

17. Wirz-Justice, A.: Platelet research in psychiatry. *Experientia*, 44(2):145-152, 1988.

18. Aslanian, V. and Renaud, B.: Changes in serotonin metabolism in the rat raphe magnus and cardiovascular modifications following systemic administration of clonidine and other central α_2-agonists: an *in vivo* voltammetry study. *Neuropharmacology*, 28:387, 1989.

19. Svensson, T.H., Bunney, B.S., and Aghajanian, G.K.: Inhibition of both noradrenergic and serotonergic neurons in brain by the α-adrenergic agonist clonidine. *Brain Res.*, 92:291, 1975.

20. Nicholson, A.N., Pascoe, P.A., Turner, C., et al.: Sedation and histamine H_1-receptor antagonism: studies in man with the enantiomers of chlorpheniramine and dimethindene. *Brit. J. Pharmacol.*, 104(1):270-276, 1991.

21. Lin, J.S., Sakai, K., and Jouvet, M.: Hypothalamo-preoptic histaminergic projections in sleep-wake control in the cat. *Eur. J. Neurosci.*, 6(4):618-625, 1994.

22. deVries, H.A.: *Physiology of Exercise*, 4th edition. Dubuque, Wm. C. Brown Publishers, 1986.

23. Galbo, H., Holst, J.J., and Christensen, N.J.: Glucogon and plasma catecholamine responses to graded and prolonged exercise in man. *J. Appl. Physiol.*, 38:70-76, 1975.

24. Haggendal, J., Hartley, L.H., and Saltin, B.: Arterial noradrenaline concentration during exercise in relation to the relative work levels. *Scand. J. Clin. Lab. Invest.*, 26:337-342, 1970.

25. Von Euler, U.S.: Sympatho-adrenal activity in physical exercise. *Med. Sci. Sports*, 6(3):165-173, 1974.

26. Howley, E.T.: The effect of different intensities of exercise on the excretion of epinephrine and norepinephrine. *Med. Sci. Sports*, 8:219-222, 1976.

27. Bannister, E.W. and Griffiths, J.: Blood levels of adrenergic amines during exercise. *J. Appl. Physiol.*, 33:674-676, 1972.

28. Davidson, J.R., Moldofsky, H., and Lue, F.A.: Growth hormone and cortisol secretion in relation to sleep and wakefulness. *J. Psychiat. Neurosci.*, 16(2):96-102, 1991.

29. Wells, K.E., Steed, D.L., Zajko, A.B., and Webster, M.W.: Recognition and treatment of arterial insufficiency from cafergot. *J. Vascular Surg.*, 4(1):8-15, 1986.

30. Christiansen, C.J.: Increased levels of plasma noradrenaline in hypothyroidism. *J. Clin. Endocrinol.*, 35:359, 1972.

31. Russell, I.J., Vipraio, G.A., and Morgan, W.W.: Is there a metabolic basis for the fibrositis syndrome? *Amer. J. Med.*, 81(3A):50-56, 1986.

32. Lee, W.Y., Morimoto, P.K., Bronsky, D., and Waldstein, S.S.: Studies of thyroid and sympathetic nervous system interrelationships: I. the blepharoptosis of myxedema. *J. Clin. Endocrinol. Metab.*, 21:1402, 1961.

33. Russell, I.J., Vipraio, G.A., Morgan, W.W., et al.: Catecholamine excretion in fibromyalgia syndrome. Unpublished material, 1988.

34. Russell, I.J.: Neurohormonal aspects of fibromyalgia syndrome. *Rheum. Dis. Clin. North Amer.*, 15:149-168, 1989.

35. Landsberg, L.: Catecholamines and the sympathoadrenal system. In *The Thyroid*, 4th edition. Edited by S.C. Werner and S.H. Ingbar, New York, Harper and Row Publishers, 1987.

36. Goetsch, E.: New methods in the diagnosis of thyroid disorders: pathological and clinical. *NY State Med. J.*, 18: 257, 1918.

37. Harrison, T.S.: Adrenal medullary and thyroid relationships. *Physiol. Rev.*, 44:161, 1964.

38. Prange, A.J., Wilson, I.C., Rabon, A.M., and Lipton, M.A.: Enhancement of imipramine antidepressant activity by thyroid hormone. *Am. J. Psychiat.*, 126:39-51, 1969.

39. Clark, G.T., Rugh, J.D., and Handelman, S.L.: Nocturnal masseter muscle activity and urinary catecholamine levels in bruxers. *J. Dent. Res.*, 59(10):1571-1576, 1980.

40. Prange, A.J., Jr., Lipton, M.A., and Love, G.N.: The effects of thyroid status on the toxicity of imipramine and the toxicity of drugs with common actions in the mouse. In *Proceedings of the Third International Congress on Chemotherapy*. Edited by H.P. Kuemmerle and P. Preziosi, Stuttgart, Georg Thieme Verlag, 1964, pp.341-344.

41. Prange, A.J., Jr., McCurdy, R.L., and Cochrane, C.M.: The systolic blood pressure response of depressed patients to infused norepinephrine. *J. Psychiat. Res.*, 5:1-13, 1967.

42. Bunney, W.E., Jr., Davis, J.M., Weil-Malherbe, H., and Smith, E.R.B.: Biochemical changes in psychotic depression: high norepinephrine levels in psychotic vs. neurotic depression. *Arch. Gen. Psychiat.*, 16:448-460, 1967.

43. Wiswell, J.G., Hurwitz, G.E. Coronban, A., Bing, O.H.L., and Child, D.L.: Urinary catecholamines and their metabolites in hyperthyroidism and hypothyroidism. *J. Endocrinol.*, 23:1102-1105, 1963.

44. Kales, A., Heuser, G., Jacobsen, A., Kales, J.D., Hanley, J., Zweizig, J.R., and Paulson, M.J.: All night sleep studies in hypothyroidism patients, before and after treatment. *J. Clin. Endocrinol.*, 27:1593-1599, 1967.

45. Glowinski, J. and Axelrod, J.: Inhibition of uptake of titrated noradrenaline in the intact rat brain by imipramine and structurally related compounds. *Nature*, 204:1318-1319, 1964.

46. Wysenbeek, A.J., Nor, F., Lurie, Y., and Weinburger, A.: Imipramine for the treatment of fibrositis: a therapeutic trial. *Ann. Rheum. Dis.*, 44:752-753, 1985.

47. Moldofsky, H.: The contribution of sleep-wake physiology to fibromyalgia. In *Advances in Pain Research and Therapy*, Vol.17. Edited by J.R. Fricton and E.A. Awad, New York, Raven Press, Ltd., 1990, pp.227-240.

48. Gilman, A.G., Rall, T.W., Nies, A.S., and Taylor, P. (Editors): *The Pharmacological Basis of Therapeutics*, 8th edition. New York, Pergamon Press, 1990.

49. Bengtsson, H. and Bengtsson, M.: Regional sympathetic blockade in primary fibromyalgia. *Pain*, 33(2):161-167, 1988.

50. Nichols, A.J. and Ruffolo, R.R., Jr.: Functions mediated by α-adrenoceptors. In α-*Adrenoceptors: Molecular Biology, Biochemistry and Pharmacology*. Basel, Karger, 1991, pp.113-179.

51. Dashwood, M.R., Gilbey, M.P., and Spyer, K.M.: The localization of adrenoceptors and opiate receptors in regions of the cat nervous system involved in cardiovascular control. *Neuroscience*, 15:537-551, 1985.

52. Williams, J.T., Surprenant, A.-M., and North, R.A.: Inhi-

bitory synaptic transmission mediated by catecholamines. VI. Adrenergic neuron electrophysiology and behavior. In *Epinephrine in the Central Nervous System.* Edited by P. Stolk, E. U'Prichard, and J. Fuxe, New York, Oxford University Press, 1988, pp.252-258.

53. Simson, P.E., Cierpial, M.A., Heyneman, L.E., and Weiss, J.M.: Pertussis toxin blocks the effects of α_2-agonists and antagonists on locus ceruleus activity *in vivo. Neurosci. Lett.,* 89:361-366, 1988.

54. Russell, I.J., Vaeroy, M., Jabors, M., and Nyberg, F.: Cerebrospinal fluid biogenic metabolites in fibromyalgia/fibrositis syndrome and rheumatoid arthritis. *Arthritis Rheum.,* 35:550-556, 1992.

55. Silva, J.E.: Catecholamines and the sympathoadrenal system in thyrotoxicosis. In *Werner and Ingbar's The Thyroid: A Fundamental and Clinical Text,* 7th edition. Edited by L.P. Braverman and R.D. Utiger, Philadelphia, Lippincott-Raven Publishers, 1996, pp.661-670.

56. Coulombe, P., Dussault, J.H., and Walker, P.: Plasma catecholamine concentrations in hyperthyroidism and hypothyroidism. *Metabolism,* 25:973, 1976.

57. Manhem, P., Bramnert, M., Hallengren, B., Lecerof, H., and Werner, R.: Increased arterial and venous plasma noradrenaline levels in patients with primary hypothyroidism during hypothyroid as compared to euthyroid state. *J. Endocrinol. Invest.,* 15(10):763-765, 1992.

58. Polikar, R., Kennedy, B., Ziegler, M., et al.: Plasma norepinephrine kinetics, dopamine-β-hydroxylase, and chromogranin-A, in hypothyroid patients before and following replacement therapy. *J. Clin. Endocrinol. Metab.,* 70:277, 1990.

59. Coulombe, P. and Dussault, J.H.: Catecholamine metabolism in thyroid disease. I. Norepinephrine secretion rate in hypothyroidism and hyperthyroidism. *J. Clin. Endocrinol. Metab.,* 44:1185, 1977.

60. Coulombe, P., Dussault, J.H., Letarte, J., and Simard, S.J.: Catecholamine metabolism in thyroid disease. I. Epinephrine secretion rate in hypothyroidism and hyperthyroidism. *J. Clin. Endocrinol. Metab.,* 42:125, 1976.

61. Bayless, R.I.S. and Edwards, O.M.: Urinary secretion of free catecholamines in Graves' disease. *Endocrinology,* 49:167, 1971.

62. Gross, G. and Lues, I.: Thyroid-dependent alterations of myocardial adrenoceptors and adrenoceptor-mediated responses in the rat. *Naunyn-Schmiedeberg's Arch. Pharmacol.,* 329:427, 1985.

63. Matsukawa, T., Mano, T., Gotoh, E., et al.: Altered muscle sympathetic nerve activity in hyperthyroidism and hypothyroidism. *J. Auton. Nerv. Syst.,* 42:171, 1993.

64. Lansberg, L. and Axelrod, J.: Influence of pituitary, thyroid, and adrenal hormones on norepinephrine turnover and metabolism in the rat heart. *Circ. Res.,* 22:559, 1968.

65. Tu, T. and Nash, C.W.: The influence of prolonged hyper- and hypothyroid states on the noradrenaline content of rat tissues and the accumulation of efflux rates of titrated noradrenaline. *Can. J. Physiol. Pharmacol.,* 53:74, 1975.

66. Guttler, R.B., Croxson, M.S., DeQuattro, V.L., Warren, D.W., Otis, C.L., and Nicoloff, J.T.: Effects of thyroid hormone on plasma adenosine 3',5'-monophosphate production in man. *Metabolism,* 26(10):1155-1162, 1977.

67. Tsai, J.S. and Chen, A.: Effect of L-triiodothyronine on (-) ^{3}H-dihydroalprenolol binding and cyclic AMP response to (-) adrenaline in cultured heart cells. *Nature,* 275(5676): 138-140, 1978.

68. Kunos, G., Vermes-Kunos, I., and Nickerson, M.: Effects of thyroid state on adrenoceptor properties. *Nature,* 250: 779-781, 1974.

69. Kunos, G. and Ishac, E.J.N.: Mechanism of inverse regulation of α_1- and β-adrenergic receptors. *Biochem. Pharmacol.,* 36:1185-1191, 1987.

70. Ishac, E.J.N., Lazar-Wesley, E., and Kunos, G.: Rapid inverse changes in α_{1B}- and β_2-adrenergic receptors and gene transcripts in acutely isolated rat liver cells. *J. Cell. Physiol.,* 152:79-86, 1992.

71. Kunos, G.: Thyroid hormone-dependent interconversion of myocardial α- and β-adrenoceptors in the rat. *Brit. J. Pharmacol.,* 59:177-189, 1977.

72. Kupfer, L.E., Bilezikian, J.P., and Robinson, R.B.: Regulation of α- and β-adrenergic receptors by triiodothyronine in cultured rat myocardial cells. *Naunyn- Schmiedeberg's Arch Pharmacol.,* 334:275-281, 1986.

73. Kunos, G.: Modulation of adrenergic reactivity and adrenoceptors by thyroid hormone. In *Adrenoceptors and Catecholamine Action,* Part A. Edited by G. Kunos, New York, John Wiley & Sons, 1981, pp.297-333.

74. Williams, L.T., Lefkowitz, R.J., Watanabe, A.M., Hathaway, D.R., and Besch, H.R., Jr.: Thyroid hormone regulation of β-adrenergic receptor number. *J. Biol. Chem.,* 252: 2787-2789, 1977.

75. Sharma, V.K. and Banerjee, S.P.: α-Adrenergic receptor in rat heart. *J. Biol. Chem.,* 253:5277-5279, 1978.

76. Ishac, E.J.N., Pennefather, J.N., and Handberg, G.M.: Effect of changes in thyroid state on atrial α- and β-adrenoceptors, adenylate cyclase activity, and catecholamine levels in the rat. *J. Cardiovasc. Pharmacol.,* 5:396-405, 1983.

77. Preiksaitis, H.G. and Kunos, G.: Adrenoceptor-mediated activation of liver glycogen phosphorylase: effects of thyroid state. *Life Sci.,* 24(1):35-41, 1979.

78. Malbon, C.C.: Liver cell adenylate cyclase and β-adrenergic receptors: increased β-adrenergic receptor number and responsiveness in the hypothyroid rat. *J. Biol. Chem.,* 255:8692-8699, 1980.

79. Preiksaitis, H.G., Kan, W.H., and Kunos, G.: Decreased α_1-adrenoceptor responsiveness and density in the hypothyroid rat. *J. Biol. Chem.,* 257:4320-4326, 1982.

80. Kunos, G., Mucci, L., and O'Regan, S.: The influence of hormonal and neuronal factors on rat heart adrenoceptors. *Brit. J. Pharmacol.,* 71:371-386, 1980.

81. Baker, S.P.: Effects of thyroid status on β-adrenoreceptors and muscarinic receptors in the rat lung. *J. Autonom. Pharmacol.,* 1:269-277, 1981.

82. Bahouth, S.W.: Thyroid hormone transcriptionally regulates the β_1-adrenergic receptor gene in cultured ventricular myocytes. *J. Biol. Chem.,* 266(24):15863-15869, 1991.

83. Williams, L.T. and Lefkowitz, R.J.: Thyroid hormone regulation of α-adrenergic receptors: studies in rat myocardium. *J. Cardiovasc. Pharmacol.,* 1:181-189, 1979.

84. Sharma, V.K. and Banerjee, S.P.: β-adrenergic receptors in rat skeletal muscle: effects of thyroidectomy. *Biochim. Biophys. Acta,* 539:538-542, 1978.

85. Mason, G.A., Bondy, S.C., Nemeroff, C.B., Walker, C.H.,

and Prange, A.J., Jr.: The effects of thyroid state on β-adrenergic and serotonergic receptors in rat brain. *Psychoneuroendocrinology*, 12(4):261-270, 1987.

86. Lazar-Wesley, E., Hadcock, J.R., Malbon, C.C., Kunos, G., and Ishac, J.N.: Tissue-specific regulation of α_{2B}, β_1, and β_2-adrenergic receptor mRNAs by thyroid state in the rat. *Endocrinology*, 129(2):1116-1118, 1991.

87. Brent, G.A., Larsen, P.R., Harney, J.W., Koening, R.J., and Moore, D.D.: Functional characterization of the rat growth hormone promoter elements required for induction by thyroid hormone with and without a co-transfectant β type thyroid hormone receptor. *J. Biol. Chem.*, 264:178-182, 1989.

88. Carr, F.E., Burnside, J., and Chin, W.W.: Thyroid hormones regulate rat thyrotropin β gene promoter activity expressed in GH3 cells. *Mol. Endocrinol.*, 3:709-716, 1989.

89. Brent, G.A., Dunn, M.K., Harney, J.W., Gulick, T., Larsen, P.R., and Moore, D.D.: Thyroid hormone aporeceptor represses T_3-inducible promoters and blocks activity of the retinoic acid receptor. *New Biol.*, 1:329-336, 1989.

90. Damm, K., Thompson, C.C., and Evans, R.M.: Protein encoded by v-*erbA* functions as a thyroid-hormone receptor antagonist. *Nature*, 339:593-597, 1989.

91. Bennett, R.M., Clark, S.R., Campbell, S.M., et al.: Symptoms of Raynaud's syndrome in patients with fibromyalgia: a study utilizing the Nielsen test, digital photoplethysmography and measurements of platelet α_2-adrenergic receptors. *Arthritis Rheum.*, 34:264-269, 1991.

92. Frankhyzen, A. and Muller, A.: *In vitro* studies on the inhibition of serotonin release through α-adrenoreceptor activity in various regions of the rat CNS. *Abstract of the 5th Catecholamine Symposium*, 1983, p.137.

93. Benkirane, S., Arbilla, S., and Langer, S.Z.: Newly synthesized noradrenaline mediates the α_2-adrenoceptor inhibition of [3H]5-hydroxytryptamine release induced by β-phenylethylamine in rat hippocampal slices. *Eur. J. Pharm.*, 131(2-3):189-198, 1986.

94. Yang, J., Bao, J., and Su, D.F.: Effects of serotonin and norepinephrine on neuronal discharges of the nucleus tractus solitarii in medullary slices. *Acta Pharm. Sinica*, 13(1):42-44, 1992.

95. Trendelenburg, A.U., Trendelenburg, M., Starke, K., and Limberger, N.: Release-inhibiting α_2-adrenoceptor at serotonergic axons in rat and rabbit brain cortex: evidence for pharmacological identity with α_2-autoreceptors. *Naunyn-Schmiedeberg's Arch. Pharm.*, 349(1):25-33, 1994.

96. Sobel, B.E., Dempsey, P.J., and Cooper, T.: Normal myocardial adenyl cyclase activity in hyperthyroid cats. *Proc. Soc. Exp. Biol. Med.*, 132:6, 1969.

97. Ciaraldi, T. and Marinetti, G.V.: Thyroxine and propylthiouracil effects *in vivo* on α and β receptors in rat heart. *Biochem. Biophys. Res. Commun.*, 74:984, 1977.

98. Tse, J., Wrenn, R.W., and Kuo, J.F.: Thyroxine-induced changes in characteristics and activities of β-adrenergic receptors and adenosine 3',5'-monophosphate systems in the heart may be related to reputed catecholamine supersensitivity in hyperthyroidism. *Endocrinol.*, 107:6, 1980.

99. Theoharides, T.C. and Munsat, T.L.: Autonomic nervous system. In *Pharmacology*. Edited by T.C. Theoharides, Boston, Little, Brown and Company, 1992, pp.240-288.

100. Furukawa, H., Loeb, J.N., and Bilezikian, J.P.: β-Adrenergic receptors and isoproterenol-stimulated potassium transport in erythrocytes from normal and hypothyroid turkeys. *J. Clin. Invest.*, 66:1057, 1980.

101. Stiles, G.L., Stadel, J.M., Delean, A., and Lefkowitz, R.J.: Hypothyroidism modulates β-adrenergic receptor-adenylate cyclase interactions in rat reticulocytes. *J. Clin. Invest.*, 68:1450, 1981.

102. Ginsberg, A.M., Clutter, W.E., Shah, S.D., and Cryer, P.E.: Triiodothyronine-induced thyrotoxicosis increases mononuclear leukocyte β-adrenergic receptor density in man. *J. Clin. Invest.*, 67:1785, 1981.

103. Williams, R.S., Guthrow, C.E., and Lefkowitz, R.J.: β-Adrenergic receptors of human lymphocytes are unaltered by hyperthyroidism. *J. Clin. Endocrinol. Metab.*, 48:503, 1979.

104. Zwillich, C.W., Matthay, M., Potts, D.E., Alder, R., Hofeldt, F., and Weil, J.V.: Thyrotoxicosis: comparison of effects of thyroid ablation and β-adrenergic blockade on metabolic rate and ventilatory control. *J. Clin. Endocrinol. Metab.*, 46:491, 1978.

105. Morgane, P.J.: Serotonin: twenty years later—monoamine theory of sleep: the role of serotonin: a review. *Psychopharmacol. Bull.*, 17:13-17, 1981.

106. Tepperman, J. and Tepperman, H.M.: *Metabolic and Endocrine Physiology*, 5th edition. Chicago, Year Book Medical Publishers, Inc., 1987.

107. Oppenheimer, J.H. and Samuels, H.H.: *Molecular Basis of Thyroid Hormone Action*. New York, Academic Press, Inc., 1983.

108. DeGroot, L.J., Larsen, P.R., Refetoff, S., and Stanbury, J.B.: *The Thyroid and Its Diseases*, 5th edition. New York, John Wiley & Sons, Inc., 1984.

109. Cooper, J.R., Bloom, F.E., and Roth, R.H.: *The Biochemical Basis of Neuropharmacology*, 6th edition. New York, Oxford University Press, 1991.

110. Guyton, A.C.: *Textbook of Medical Physiology*, 8th edition. Philadelphia, W.B. Saunders Co., 1991.

111. Baldessarini, R.J.: Drugs and the treatment of psychiatric disorders. In *The Pharmacological Basis of Therapeutics*, 8th edition. Edited by A.G. Gilman, T.W. Rall, A.S. Nies, and P. Taylor, New York, Pergamon Press, 1990, pp.383-435.

112. Silva, J.E. and Landsberg, L.: Catecholamines and the sympathoadrenal system in thyrotoxicosis. In *Werner and Ingbar's The Thyroid: A Fundamental and Clinical Text*, 6th edition. Edited by L.E. Braverman and R.D. Utiger, Philadelphia, J.B. Lippincott Co., 1991, pp.816-827.

113. Hoag, J.M.: Disorders of the adrenal gland. In *Osteopathic Medicine*. Edited by J.M. Hoag, W.V. Cole, and S.G. Bradford, New York, McGraw-Hill Book Co., Inc., 1969, pp.243-251.

114. Janig, W.: The autonomic nervous system. *Fundamentals of Neurophysiology*. Edited by R.F. Schmidt, New York, Springer-Verlag, 1985, pp.216-269.

115. Changeux, J.-P.: *Neuronal Man: The Biology of Mind*. New York, Oxford University Press, 1985.

116. Atterwill, C.K., Bunn, S., Atkinson, D., Smith, S.L., and Heal, D.: Effects of thyroid status on presynaptic α_2-adrenoceptor function and β-adrenoceptor binding in the rat brain. *J. Neural Transm.*, 59(1):43-55, 1984.

117. Baum, S.J.: *Introduction to Organic and Biological Chemistry.* New York, The Macmillan Co., 1970.

118. Bigger, J.T. and Hoffman, B.F.: Antiarrhythmic drugs. In *The Pharmacological Basis of Therapeutics*, 8th edition. Edited by A.G. Gilman, T.W. Rall, A.S. Nies, and P. Taylor, New York, Pergamon Press, 1990, pp.840-873.

119. Calogero, A.E., Gallucci, W.T., Chrousos, G.P., and Gold, P.W.: Catecholamine effects upon rat hypothalamic corticotropin-releasing hormone secretion *in vitro. J. Clin. Invest.*, 82(3):839-846, 1988.

120. Puymirat, J., Luo, M., and Dussault, J.H.: Immunocytochemical localization of thyroid hormone nuclear receptors in cultured hypothalamic dopaminergic neurons. *Neuroscience*, 30(2):443-449, 1989.

121. Puymirat, J., Barret, A., Picart, R., et al.: Triiodothyronine enhances the morphological maturation of dopaminergic neurons from fetal mouse hypothalamus cultured in serum-free medium. *Neuroscience*, 10:801-810, 1983.

122. Brownstein, M., Palkovits, M., Tappaz, M., Saavedra, J., and Kizer, J.: Effects of surgical isolation of the hypothalamus on its neurotransmitter content. *Brain Res.*, 117:282-295, 1976.

123. Swanson, L.W., Sawchenko, P.E., and Lind, R.W.: Regulation of multiple peptides in CRF parvocellular neurosecretory neurons: implications for the stress response. *Prog. Brain Res.*, 68:169-190, 1986.

124. Nieuwenhuys, R., Geeraedts, L.M.G., and Veening, J.G.: The medial forebrain bundle of the rat. I. General introduction. *J. Comp. Neurol.*, 206(1):49-81, 1982.

125. Mogilnicka, E., Szmigielski, A., and Niewiadomska, A.: The effect of α, α'-dipyridyl on noradrenaline, dopamine, and 5-hydroxytryptamine levels and on dopamine-β-hydroxylase activity in brain. *Pol. J. Pharmacol. Pharm.*, 27:619-624, 1975.

126. Murray, J.F., and Kelly, J.J., Jr.: The relation of thyroid hormone level to epinephrine response: a diagnostic test. *Ann. Intern. Med.*, 51:309, 1959.

127. Turner, P., Granville-Grossman, K.L., and Smart, J.V.: Effect of adrenergic receptor blockade on the tachycardia of thyrotoxicosis and anxiety state. *Lancet*, 2:1316, 1965.

128. Goodkind, M.J., Fram, D.H., and Roberts, M.: Effect of thyroid hormone on myocardial catecholamine content of the guinea pig. *Amer. J. Physiol.*, 201:1049, 1961.

129. Chase, T.N. and Murphy, D.L.: Serotonin and central nervous system function. *Ann. Rev. Pharmacol.*, 13:181-197, 1973.

130. Eisinger, J., Plantamura, A., and Ayavou, T.: Glycolysis abnormalities in fibromyalgia. *J. Amer. Coll. Nutr.*, 13:144-148, 1994.

131. Kobinger, W.: Central α-adrenergic system as targets for antihypertensive drugs. *Rev. Physiol. Biochem. Pharmacol.*, 81:39-100, 1978.

132. Ben-Jonathan, N., Oliver, C., Weiner, H.J., Mical, R.S., and Porter, J.C.: Dopamine in hypophyseal portal plasma of the rat during the estrous cycle and throughout pregnancy. *Endocrinology*, 100:452, 1977.

133. Johnston, C.A., Gibbs, D.M., and Nigro-Vilar, A.: High concentrations of epinephrine derived from a central source and of 5-hydroxyindole-3-acetic acid in hypophysial portal plasma. *Endocrinology*, 113:819, 1983.

134. van Denderen, J.C., Boersma, J.W., Zeinstra, P., Hollander, A.P., and van Neerbos, B.R.: Physiological effects of exhaustive physical exercise in primary fibromyalgia syndrome (PFS): is PFS a disorder of neuroendocrine reactivity? *Scand. J. Rheumatol.*, 21:35-37, 1992.

135. Bennett, R.., Clark, S.R., Burckhardt, C.S., and Cook, D.: IGF-1 assays and other GH tests in 500 fibromyalgia patients. *J. Musculoskel. Pain*, 3(Suppl.):109, 1995.

136. Lundberg, J.M., Franco-Cereceda, A., Lacroix, J.-S., and Pernow, J.: Neuropeptide Y and sympathetic neurotransmission. *Ann. N.Y. Acad. Sci.*, 611:166-174, 1990.

137. Crofford, L.J., Pillemer, S.R., Kalogeras, K.T., et al.: Hypothalamic-pituitary-adrenal axis perturbations in patients with fibromyalgia. *Arthritis Rheum.*, 37:1583-1592, 1994.

138. Clauw, D.J., Sabol, M., Radulovic, D., et al.: Serum neuropeptides in patients with both fibromyalgia (FM) and chronic fatigue syndrome (CFS). *J. Musculoskel. Pain*, 3 (Suppl.1):79, 1995.

139. Crofford, L.J.: The hypothalamic-pituitary-adrenal axis in the fibromyalgia syndrome. *J. Musculoskel. Pain*, 4(1/2): 181-200, 1996.

140. Haas, D.A. and George, S.R.: Neuropeptide Y administration acutely increases hypothalamic corticotropin-releasing factor immunoreactivity: lack of effect in other rat brain regions. *Life Sci.*, 41:2725-2731, 1987.

141. Koening, J.I.: Regulation of the hypothalamo-pituitary axis by neuropeptide Y. *Ann. N.Y. Acad. Sci.*, 611:317-328, 1990.

142. Kamilaris, T.C., Calogero, A.E., and Johnson, E.O.: Effect of neuropeptide Y on hypothalamic-pituitary-adrenal function in the rat. *19th Annual Meeting of the Society for Neuroscience*, Phoenix, AZ, 1989.

143. Hashimoto, H., Onishi, H., Koide, S., Kai, T., and Yamagami, S.: Plasma neuropeptide Y in patients with major depressive disorder. *Neurosci. Lett.*, 216(1):57-60, 1996.

144. Kennedy, B., Shen, G.H., and Ziegler, M.G.: Neuropeptide Y-mediated pressor responses following high-frequency stimulation of the rat sympathetic nervous system. *J. Pharmacol. Exper. Thera.*, 281(1):291-296, 1997.

145. Sun, L.S., Du, F., Schechter, W.S., Quaegebeur, J.M., and Vulliemoz, Y.: Plasma neuropeptide Y and catecholamines in pediatric patients undergoing cardiac operations. *J. Thorac. Cardiovasc. Surg.*, 113(2):278-284, 1997.

146. Morris, M.J., Cox, H.S., Lambert, G.W., et al.: Region-specific neuropeptide Y overflows at rest and during sympathetic activation in humans. *Hypertension*, 29:137-143, 1997.

147. Lacroix, J.S., Ricchetti, A.P., Morel, D., et al.: Intranasal administration of neuropeptide Y in man: systemic absorption and functional effects. *Brit. J. Pharmacol.*, 118(8): 2079-2084, 1996.

148. Calogero, A.E., Bernardini, R., Gold, P.W., and Chrousos, G.P.: Regulation of rat hypothalamic corticotropin-releasing hormone secretion *in vitro*: potential clinical implications. *Adv. Experi. Med. Biol.*, 245:167-181, 1988.

149. Sendrowski, D.P., Buker, E.A., and Gee, S.S.: An investigation of sympathetic hypersensitivity in chronic fatigue syndrome. *Optomet. Vis. Sci.*, 74(8):660-663, 1997.

150. Elam, M., Johansson, G., and Wallin, B.G.: Do patients with primary fibromyalgia have an altered muscle sympathetic nerve activity? *Pain*, 48:371-375, 1992.

151. Hallberg, H., Almgren, O., and Svensson, T.H.: Increased

brain serotonergic and noradrenergic activity by the β₂-agonist salbutamol: a putative antidepressant drug. *Psychopharmacology*, 73:201-204, 1981.

152. Mengshoel, A.M.: Effect of physical exercise in fibromyalgia. *Tidsskr Nor Laegeforen*, 116:746-748, 1996.

153. Hannington-Kiff, J.G.: Pharmacological target blocks in painful dystrophic limbs. In *Textbook of Pain*, 2ⁿᵈ edition. Edited by P.D. Wall and R. Melzack, Edinburgh, Churchill Livingstone, 1989, pp.754-766.

154. Klemp, P., Nielsen, H.V., Korsgard, J., and Crone, P.: Blood flow in fibromyotic muscles. *Scand. J. Rehabil. Med.*, 14(2):81-82, 1982.

155. Lund, N., Bengtsson, A., and Thorborg, P.: Muscle tissue oxygen pressure in primary fibromyalgia *Scand. J. Rheumatol.*, 15:165-173, 1986.

156. Connor, H.E., Drew, G.M., and Finch, L.: Clonidine-induced potentiation of reflex vagal bradycardia in anesthetized cats. *J. Pharm. Pharmacol.*, 34:22-26, 1982.

157. Role, L.W. and Kelly, J.P.: The brain stem: cranial nerve nuclei and the monoaminergic systems. In *Principles of Neural Science*, 3ʳᵈ edition. Edited by E.R. Kandel, J.H. Schwartz, and T.M. Jessell, Norwalk, Appleton & Lange, 1991, pp.683-699.

158. Berne, R.M. and Levy, M.N.: *Principles of Physiology*, St. Louis, C.V. Mosby Co., 1990.

159. Head, G.A. and Burke, S.: Importance of central noradrenergic and serotonergic pathways in the cardiovascular actions of rilmenidine and clonidine. *J. Cardiovasc. Pharmacol.*, 18(6):819-826, 1991.

160. Brown, D.A. and Caulfield, M.P.: Hyperpolarizing α₂-adrenoceptors in rat sympathetic ganglia. *Br. J. Pharmacol.*, 65:435-445, 1979.

161. Hoffman, B.B. and Lefkowitz, R.J.: Adrenergic receptor antagonists. In *Goodman and Gilman's The Pharmacological Basis of Therapeutics*, 8ᵗʰ edition. New York, Pergamon Press, 1990, pp.221-243.

162. Kupfermann, I.: Hypothalamus and limbic system: motivation. In *Principles of Neural Science*, 3ʳᵈ edition. Edited by E.R. Kandel, J.H. Schwartz, and T.M. Jessell, Norwalk, Appleton & Lange,1991, pp.750-760.

163. Côté, L. and Crutcher, M.D.: The basal ganglia. In *Principles of Neural Science*, 3ʳᵈ edition. Edited by E.R. Kandel, J.H. Schwartz, and T.M. Jessell, Norwalk, Appleton & Lange,1991, pp.647-659.

164. Nicoll, R.A.: The coupling of neurotransmitter receptors to ion channels in the brain. *Science*, 241:545-551, 1988.

165. Dodd, J. and Role, L.W.: The autonomic nervous system. In *Principles of Neural Science*, 3ʳᵈ edition. Edited by E.R. Kandel, J.H. Schwartz, and T.M. Jessell, Norwalk, Appleton & Lange, 1991, pp.761-775.

166. Gervais Tougas, G.: The autonomic nervous system in functional bowel disorders. *Can. J. Gastroenterol.*, 13 (Suppl.A):15A-17A, 1999.

167. Hilakivi, I.: The role of β- and α-adrenoceptors in the regulation of the stages of the sleep-waking cycle in the cat. *Brain Res.*, 277:109-118, 1983.

168. Han, C., Yu, G., Zhang, Y., Xu, K., Qu, P., and Dong, E.: Alterations of α₁-adrenoceptor subtypes in the hearts of thyroxine-treated rats. *Eur. J. Pharmacol.*, 294(2-3):533-539, 1995.

169. Sabria, J., Ferrer, I., Toledo, A., Sentis, M., and Blanco, I.:

Effects of altered thyroid function on histamine levels and mast cell number in neonatal rat brain. *J. Pharmacol. Exp. Ther.*, 240(2):612-616, 1987.

170. Schwartz, J.H. and Kandel, E.R.: Synaptic transmission mediated by second messengers. In *Principles of Neural Science*, 3ʳᵈ edition. Edited by E.R. Kandel, J.H. Schwartz, and T.M. Jessell, Norwalk, Appleton & Lange, 1991, pp.173-193.

171. Barnes, P.J., Wilson, N.M., and Vickers, H.: Prazosin, an α₁-adrenoceptor antagonist, partially inhibits exercise-induced asthma. *J. Allergy Clin. Immunol.*, 68(6):411-415, 1981.

172. Phillips, M.J., Barnes, P.J., and Gold, W.M.: Characterization of purified dog mastocytoma cells: autonomic membrane receptors and pharmacologic modulation of histamine release. *Am. Rev. Respir. Dis.*, 132(5):1019-1026, 1985.

173. Moroni, F., Fantozzi, R., Masini, E., and Mannaioni, P.F.: The modulation of histamine release by α-adrenoceptors: evidences in murine neoplastic mast cells. *Agents Actions*, 7(1):57-61, 1977.

174. Hayashi, M., Saisho, S., Suzuki, H., Shimozawa, K., and Iwakawa, Y.: Sleep disturbance in children with congenital and acquired hypothyroidism. *No To Hattatsu. Brain Dev.*, 20:294-300, 1988.

175. Hayashi, M., Saisho, S., Suzuki, H., Shimozawa, K., and Iwakawa, Y.: Sleep disturbance in children with growth hormone deficiency. *No To Hattatsu. Brain Dev.*, 14:170-174, 1992.

176. Asrom, C. and Lindholm, J.: Growth hormone-deficient young adults have decreased deep sleep. *Neuroendocrinology*, 51(1):82-84, 1990.

177. Savard, P., Merand, Y., Di Paolo, T., and Dupont, A.: Effect of neonatal hypothyroidism on the serotonin system of the rat brain. *Brain Res.*, 292(1):99-108, 1984.

178. Rastogi, R.B. and Singhal, R.L.: Influence of neonatal and adult hyperthyroidism on behavior and biosynthetic capacity for norepinephrine, dopamine, and 5-hydroxytryptamine in rat brain. *J. Pharma. Exper. Therap.*, 198(3):609-618, 1976.

179. Backman, E., Bengtsson, A., Bengtsson, M., Lennmarken, C., and Henriksson, K.G.: Skeletal muscle function in primary fibromyalgia: effect of regional sympathetic blockade with guanethidine. *Acta Neurol. Scand.*, 77:187-191, 1988.

180. Reis, D.J., Joh, M.A., Nathan, B., et al. (Editors): *Nervous System and Hypertension*. New York, Wiley-Flammarion, 1979, pp.147-164.

181. Headley, P.M., Duggan, A.W., and Griersmith, B.T.: Selective reduction by noradrenaline and 5-hydroxytryptamine of nociceptive responses of cat dorsal horn neurons. *Brain Res.*, 145:185-189, 1978.

182. Howe, J.R., Wang, J.Y., and Yaksh, T.L.: Selective antagonism of the antinociceptive effect of intrathecally applied α-adrenergic agonists by intrathecal prazosin and intrathecal yohimbine. *J. Pharmacol. Exp. Ther.*, 224(3):552-558, 1983.

183. Coombs, D.W., Saunders, R., Gaylor, M., LaChance, D., and Jensen, L.: Clinical trial of intrathecal clonidine for cancer pain. *J. Region. Anesth.*, 9:34-35, 1984.

184. Gillespie, J.A.: Sympathectomy. *Brit. J. Hosp. Med.*, 14:

418-428, 1975.

185. Verrill, P.: Sympathetic ganglion lesions. In *Textbook of Pain*, 2nd edition. Edited by P.D. Wall and R. Melzack, Edinburgh, Churchhill Livingstone, 1989, pp.773-783.

186. Moalic, J.M., Bourgeois, F., Mansier, P., et al.: β_1-adrenergic receptor and α-G_s mRNAs in rat heart as a function of mechanical load and thyroxine intoxication. *Cardiovasc. Res.*, 27(2):231-237, 1993.

187. Valente, M., De Santo, C., de Martino Rosaroll, P., Di Maio, V., Di Meo, S., and De Leo, T.: The direct effect of the thyroid hormone on cardiac chronotropism. *Arch. Int. Physiol. Biochim.*, 97(6):431-440, 1989.

188. Arner, P.: Adrenergic receptor function in fat cells. *Amer. J. Clin. Nutri.*, 55(1 Suppl.):228S-236S, 1992.

189. Karakanias, G.B., Li, C.S., and Etgen, A.M.: Estradiol reduction of α_2-adrenoceptor binding in female rat cortex is correlated with decreases in $\alpha_{2A/D}$-adrenoceptor m RNA. *Neuroscience*, 81(3):593-597, 1997.

190. Collins, S., Ostrowski, J., and Lefkowitz, R.J.: Cloning and sequence analysis of the human β_1-adrenergic receptor 5'-flanking promoter region. *Biochim. Biophys. Acta*, 1172(1-2):171-174, 1993.

191. Malbon, C.C. and Hadcock, J.R.: Evidence that glucocorticoid response elements in the 5'-noncoding region of the hamster β_2-adrenergic receptor gene are obligate for glucocorticoid regulation of receptor mRNA levels. *Biochem. Biophys. Res. Comm.*, 154(2):676-681, 1988.

192. Gao, B. and Kunos, G.: Isolation and characterization of the gene encoding the rat α-$_{1B}$-adrenergic receptor. *Gene*, 131(2):243-247, 1993.

193. Razik, M.A., Lee, K., Price, R.R., et al.: Transcriptional regulation of the human α_{1A}-adrenergic receptor gene: characterization of the 5'-regulatory and promoter region. *J. Biol. Chem.*, 272(45):28237-28246, 1997.

194. Macdonald, E., Kobilka, B.K., and Scheinin, M.: Gene targeting: homing in on α_2-adrenoceptor-subtype function. *Trends Pharmacol. Sci.*, 18(6):211-219, 1997.

195. Jones, S.M., Deng, C.L., MacLeod, V., and Cornett, L.E.: Evidence for alternative splicing in hepatic α_{1B}-adrenergic receptor gene expression. *J. Recept. Signal Transduct. Res.*, (6):815-832, 1997.

196. Clement, K., Vaisse, C., Manning, B.S., et al.: Genetic variation in the β_3-adrenergic receptor and an increased capacity to gain weight in patients with morbid obesity. *N. Engl. J. Med.*, 333(6):352-354, 1995.

197. Pietrirouxel, F., Manning, B.S., Gros, J., and Strosberg, A.D.: The biochemical effect of the naturally-occurring Trp64-Arg mutation on human β_3-adrenoceptor activity. *Eur. J. Biochem.*, 247(3):1174-1179, 1997.

198. Yuan, X.H., Yamada, K., Koyama, K., et al.: β_3-adrenergic receptor gene polymorphism is not a major genetic determinant of obesity and diabetes in Japanese general population. *Diabetes Res. Clin. Pract.*, 37(1):1-7, 1997.

199. Padbury, J.F., Tseng, Y.T., and Waschek, J.A.: Transcription initiation is localized to a TATAless region in the ovine β_1-adrenergic receptor gene. *Biochem. Biophys. Res. Comm.*, 211(1):254-261, 1995.

200. Jiang, L. and Kunos G.: Sequence of the 5' regulatory domain of the gene encoding the rat β_2-adrenergic receptor. *Gene*, 163(2):331-332, 1995.

201. Silva, J.E.: Thyroid hormone control of thermogenesis and energy balance. *Thyroid*, 5(6):481-492, 1995.

202. Lopez-Barahona, M., Iglesias, T., Garcia-Higuera, I., et al.: Post-transcriptional induction of β_1-adrenergic receptor by retinoic acid, but not triiodothyronine, in C6 glioma cells expressing thyroid hormone receptors. *Eur. J. Endocrinol.*, 135(6):709-715, 1996.

203. Fain, J.N., Coronel, E.C., Beauchamp, M.J., and Bahouth, S.W.: Expression of leptin and β_3-adrenergic receptors in rat adipose tissue in altered thyroid states. *Biochem. J.*, 322(Pt.1):145-150, 1997.

204. el Hadri, K., Pairault, J., and Feve, B.: Triiodothyronine regulates β_3-adrenoceptor expression in 3T$_3$-F442A differentiating adipocytes. *Eur. J. Biochem.*, 239(2):519-525, 1996.

205. Venter, J.C.: β-Adrenoceptors, adenylate cyclase, and the adrenergic control of cardiac contractility. In *Adrenoceptors and Catecholamine Action*, Part A. Edited by G. Kunos, New York, John Wiley & Sons, 1981, pp.213-245.

206. Starke, K.: Regulation of noradrenaline release by presynaptic receptor systems. *Rev. Physiol. Biochem. Pharmacol.*, 77:1-124, 1977.

207. Safaei, R. and Timiras, P.S.: Thyroid hormone binding and regulation of adrenergic enzymes in two neuroblastoma cell lines. *J. Neurochem.*, 45(5):1405-1410, 1985.

208. de Lonlay, A., Blouquit, M.F., Valens, M., Chami, N., Edwards, D.A., and Gripois, D.: Tyrosine hydroxylase and dopamine β-hydroxylase inductions evoked by reserpine in the superior cervical ganglion of developing eu- and hypothyroid rats. *J. Autonomic Nerv. Syst.*, 36:33-38, 1991.

209. Burack, R., Edwards, R.H.T., Green, M., et al.: The response to exercise before and after treatment in myxedema with thyroxine. *J. Pharm. Exp. Ther.*, 176:212, 1971.

210. Guttler, R.B., Shaw, J.W., Otis, C.L., and Nicoloff, J.T.: Epinephrine-induced alterations in urinary cyclic AMP in hyper- and hypothyroidism. *J. Clin. Endocrinol. Metab.*, 41(4):707-711, 1975.

211. Langer, S.Z.: Presynaptic regulation of catecholamine release. *Biochem. Pharmacol.*, 23(13):1793-1800, 1974.

212. Pert, C.: *Molecules of Emotion*. New York, Scribner, 1997.

213. Milligan, G., Spiegel, A.M., Unson, C.G., and Saggerson, E.D.: Chemically induced hypothyroidism produces elevated amounts of the α subunit of the inhibitory guanine nucleotide binding protein (G_i) and the β subunit common to all G-proteins. *Biochem. J.*, 247:223-227, 1987.

214. Rapiejko, P.J., Watkins, D.C., Ros, M., and Malbon, C.C.: Thyroid hormones regulate G-protein β-subunit mRNA expression *in vivo*. *J. Biol. Chem.*, 264:16183-16189, 1989.

215. Ros, M., Northup, J.K., and Malbon, C.C.: Steady-state levels of G-proteins and β-adrenergic receptors in rat fat cells. *J. Biol. Chem.*, 263:4362-4368, 1988.

216. Goswami, A. and Rosenberg, I.N.: Effects of thyroid status on membrane-bound low K_m cyclic nucleotide phosphodiesterase activity in rat adipocytes. *J. Biol. Chem.*, 260:82-85, 1985.

217. Heuther, G., Hajak, G., Reimer, A., et al.: The metabolic fate of infused L-tryptophan in men: possible clinical implications of the accumulation of circulating tryptophan and tryptophan metabolites. *Psychopharmacology*, 109(4):

422-432, 1992.

218. Eisinger, J., Dupond, J.L., and Cozzone, P.J.: Anomalies de la glycolyse au cours des fibromyalgies: étude biologique et thérapeutique. *Lyon Méd. Méd.*, 27:2180-2181, 1996.

219. Silva, J.E. and Larsen, P.R.: Adrenergic activation of triiodothyronine production in brown adipose tissue. *Nature*, 305:712, 1983.

220. Silva, J.E. and Larsen, P.R.: Hormonal regulation of iodothyronine 5'deiodinase in rat brown adipose tissue. *Amer. J. Physiol.*, 251:E639, 1986.

221. Levey, G.S.: Catecholamine-thyroid hormone interactions and the cardiovascular manifestations of hyperthyroidism. *Amer. J. Med.*, 88:642, 1990.

222. Ransnas, L., Hammond, H.K., and Insel, P.A.: Increased G_s in myocardial membranes from hyperthyroid pigs. (Abstract) *Clin. Res.*, 36:552A, 1988.

223. Benfey, B.G. and Varma, D.R.: Stimulation of the heart of the spinal dog by phynoxybenzamine. *Nature*, 191:919-920, 1961.

224. Benfey, B.G. and Varma, D.R.: Studies on the cardiovascular actions of antisympathomimetic drugs. *Intern. J. Neuropharmacol.*, 1:9-12, 1962.

225. Starke, K., Montel, H., and Schumann, H.J.: Influence of cocaine and phenoxybenzamine on noradrenaline uptake and release. *Naunyn-Schmiedeberg's Arch. Pharmacol.*, 270:210-214, 1971.

226. Starke, K., Montel, H., and Wagner, J.: Effect of phentolamine on noradrenaline uptake and release. *Naunyn-Schmiedeberg's Arch. Pharmacol.*, 271(2):181-192, 1971.

227. Starke, K.: α-Sympathomimetic inhibition of adrenergic and cholinergic transmission in the rabbit heart. *Naunyn-Schmiedeberg's Arch. Pharmacol.*, 274:18-45, 1972.

228. Starke, K.: Influence of extracellular noradrenaline on the stimulation-evoked secretion of noradrenaline from sympathetic nerves: evidence for an α-receptor mediated feedback inhibition of noradrenaline release. *Naunyn-Schmiedeberg's Arch. Pharmacol.*, 275:11-23, 1972.

229. McQueen, J.L.: Classical transmitters and neuromodulators. *Basic Clin. Aspects Neurosci.*, 2:7-16, 1978.

230. Lehninger, A.L.: *Biochemistry: The Molecular Basis of Cell Structure and Function,* 2nd edition. New York, Worth Publishers, Inc., 1975.

231. Lehninger, A.L., Nelson, D.L., and Cox, M.M.: *Principles of Biochemistry*, 2nd edition. New York, Worth Publishers, 1993.

232. Shildkraut, J.J.: The catecholamine hypothesis of affective disorders: a review of supporting evidence. *Am. J. Psychiat.*, 122:509-522, 1965.

233. Whybrow, P.C. and Prange, A.J., Jr.: A hypothesis of thyroid-catecholamine-receptor interaction. Its relevance to affective illness. *Arch. Gen. Psychiatry*, 38(1):106-113, 1981.

234. Paton, W.D.M. and Thompson, J.W.: Abstract. *XIX International Physiology Congress*, 1953, pp.664-665.

235. Brown, D.A. and Caulfield, M.P.: Adrenoceptors in ganglia. In *Adrenoceptors and Catecholamine Action*, Part A. Edited by G. Kunos, New York, John Wiley & Sons, 1981, pp.99-115.

236. Caulfield, M.P.: *Pharmacological Characteristics of Catecholamine Receptors in Rat Sympathetic Ganglia.* PhD thesis, University of London, 1978.

237. Ivanov, A.Y. and Skok, V.I.: Slow inhibitory postsynaptic potentials and hyperpolarization evoked by noradrenaline in the neurones of mammalian sympathetic ganglion. *J. Auton. Nerv. Syst.*, 1(3):255-263, 1980.

3.2

BLOOD PRESSURE AND CIRCULATION

Throughout this book, the term "peripheral" refers to structures and functions outside the central nervous system. These structures and functions are distinct from "central" ones, that is, those within the central nervous system. This convention continues in this chapter. In addition, however, the term "peripheral" is also used to distinguish structures and functions outside the kidneys. For example, "peripheral vascular resistance" is distinct from both "central vascular resistance" and "kidney vascular resistance." Hence, the term "peripheral" refers to structures and functions outside both the CNS and kidneys.

Normal Tissue Circulation

Individual tissues regulate their own blood flow based on their specific need for nutrients. This is true of both central, peripheral, and kidney tissues. The sympathetic nervous system, however, regulates general systemic blood flow. A general discharge of the sympathetic system shifts the balance of blood flow from visceral structures and the skin to the skeletal muscles and brain.

Normal Blood Pressure

Three physiological systems maintain normal blood pressure: (1) stretch receptors in the aorta and arteries of the upper body interacting with the autonomic nervous system, (2) regulation of body fluid content by the kidney, and (3) the renin-angiotensin-aldosterone system. The stretch receptors and autonomic nervous system correct rapid, acute changes in blood pressure. The body fluid-kidney system and the renin-angiotensin-aldosterone system help correct rapid changes in blood pressure. However, these systems exert corrective action far more slowly than do the stretch receptors and autonomic nervous system. The renin-angiotensin-aldosterone system regulates blood pressure over the long term.

Cardiovascular Effects of Hypothyroidism

Hypothyroidism substantially reduces cardiovascular function. Hypothyroid patients have decreased cardiac output, peripheral tissue circulation time, circulating blood volume, velocity of blood flow, pulse rate, pulse pressure, and respiratory capacity. In the arteries of many tissues, including skeletal muscle, large arteries such as the aorta, the mesentery, and the brain, resistance to blood flow is increased. Patients typically have low blood pressure, although some have high blood pressure. Blood flow is reduced in peripheral and cerebral tissues. These changes are appropriate to the reduced tissue metabolic rate in hypothyroidism and cellular resistance to thyroid hormone. Inadequate regulation by thyroid hormone directly affects the heart and blood vessels. However, an increased density of α-adrenergic receptors and a decreased density of β-adrenergic receptors on cell membranes mediate most effects of inadequate regulation by thyroid hormone.

Cardiovascular Effects of Hyperthyroidism

Excessive thyroid hormone stimulation has cardiovascular effects largely opposite from those of hypothyroidism. In hyperthyroidism, systemic vascular resistance is lower than normal, the heart rate is rapid, and cardiac stroke volume is increased. The rapid *heart rate and larger stroke volume increase the amount of blood projected through tissues. The reduced vascular resistance increases blood flow in peripheral and cerebral tissues. These changes are proper in view of the increased metabolic rate and increased requirement of tissues for nutrients. Excessive regulation by thyroid hormone directly affects the heart and blood vessels. However, a decreased density of α-adrenergic receptors and an increased density of β-adrenergic receptors on cell membranes mediate most effects of excessive thyroid hormone regulation.*

Blood Flow and Blood Pressure in Fibromyalgia

Some researchers reported finding no decrease in peripheral blood flow in fibromyalgia patients. However, using more sensitive techniques, other researchers found decreased oxygenation of subcutaneous tissues and the trapezius and brachioradialis muscles. Several studies have shown reduced brain blood flow, and other studies suggest reduced blood flow in some peripheral tissues. A subset of fibromyalgia patients have chronic hypotension and/or orthostatic or postural hypotension.

Model of Reduced Blood Flow and Abnormal Blood Pressure in Fibromyalgia

The reduced circulation and blood pressure in a subset of fibromyalgia patients virtually duplicate the findings in a subset of hypothyroid and thyroid hormone resistant patients.

Reduced Blood Flow. *Three factors related to inadequate regulation by thyroid hormone plausibly explain the reduced blood flow through the brain and peripheral tissues in fibromyalgia: (1) an increase in α-adrenergic receptors and a decrease in β-adrenergic receptors on arterioles, (2) reduced release of the vasodilator nitric oxide by nerve endings, and (3) an increased calcium ion concentration in the smooth muscle cells lining arterioles. Hypothyroid rats and humans have a marked reduction in cerebral blood flow. The reduced cerebral blood flow in fibromyalgia and chronic fatigue syndrome patients is likely a result of hypothyroidism and/or cellular resistance to thyroid hormone.*

Hypotension. *At least four mechanisms may be involved in fibromyalgia patients' hypotension. These mechanisms may prevent a normal adaptation to hypotension long term and/or to the abrupt fall in arterial pressure when the patient assumes an upright posture from recumbency. First is a high density of α$_2$-adrenergic receptors on sympathetic nerve cell bodies*

in three structures: (1) the nucleus of the solitary tract in the brain stem, (2) the paravertebral sympathetic ganglia, and (3) the dorsal vagal nucleus. The first two structures contain sympathetic nerve cell bodies and the third, the parasympathetic nerve cell bodies. The high density of α$_2$-adrenergic receptors inhibits the sympathetic nerve cells and activates the parasympathetic nerve cells. The resulting diminished sympathetic innervation and increased parasympathetic innervation of the heart causes a subnormal heart rate and decreased stroke volume (decreased cardiac output).

The second possible mechanism of hypotension is subnormal innervation of the kidneys due to the high density of α$_2$-adrenergic receptors in the nucleus of the solitary tract and the sympathetic ganglia. The subnormal sympathetic innervation results in dilation of the kidney arterioles with an undue loss of salt and water in the urine. Normally, when blood pressure falls, sympathetic signals induce the kidney arterioles to constrict. The result is retention of more water in the blood. The retention contributes to an increase of plasma volume which helps raise the blood pressure. However, kidney vasoconstriction may not occur when sympathetic innervation is subnormal, and this important contributor to recovery of a normal blood pressure may fail. The subnormal sympathetic innervation of the kidney arterioles, with excess water loss, may also lead to urinary frequency.

Moreover, subnormal sympathetic innervation of the afferent arterioles of the kidneys results in subnormal renin release when blood pressure is too low. The subnormal renin release by the kidneys results in a failure of the renin-angiotensin-aldosterone system to increase salt and water retention in the blood. Consequently, plasma volume and blood pressure may remain too low. The subnormal renin release may be reinforced by an increased density of α$_1$-adrenergic receptors on the juxtaglomerular cells of the kidney afferent arterioles. These receptors inhibit the release of renin, blocking renin release in response to low blood pressure.

The third possible mechanism of hypotension is an increased density of α$_2$-adrenergic receptors in the dorsal vagal nucleus. The high density of α$_2$-adrenergic receptors increases parasympathetic innervation of the heart. Increased parasympathetic innervation reduces the heart rate and stroke volume. When cardiac output is decreased enough, vasovagal type symptoms result, often including fainting. Researchers have recently described vasovagal type symptoms in fibromyalgia and chronic fatigue syndrome patients.

Terms to describe the symptoms are orthostatic intolerance, orthostatic hypotension, orthostatic tachycardia, neurogenic hypotension, and postural hypotension.

A fourth possible mechanism is tissue hypometabolism. An increased density of α-adrenergic receptors and a decreased density of β-adrenergic receptors on cell membranes in hypothyroidism and/or thyroid hormone resistance strongly contribute to cell hypometabolism. The hypometabolism reduces the need of tissues for oxygen and other nutrients. The reduced need diminishes activity of the autoregulatory mechanism for dilating local arterioles and increasing local blood flow. The result is an increase in vasoconstrictive tone of arterioles with an increase in vascular resistance. The increased resistance to blood flow combined with subnormal cardiac output reduces cerebral and peripheral blood flow.

In addition, two other effects of deficient regulation by thyroid hormone may intensify the vasoconstriction: (1) reduced release of the vasodilator nitric oxide by nerve endings and (2) increased calcium ion concentration in the smooth muscle cells lining the arterioles. Further, reduced sympathetic innervation of the veins permits them to dilate slightly. Venous dilation and reduced blood flow of blood from the arteries to the veins may result in venous hypotension. With venous hypotension, too little blood returns to the heart. The reduced venous return contributes to subnormal stroke volume and cardiac output.

For a more thorough description of the possible mechanisms involved in reduced circulation and hypotension in fibromyalgia, see the section below titled "Model of Reduced Blood Flow and Hypotension in Fibromyalgia."

A small percentage of fibromyalgia patients, as with a few hypothyroid patients, have high blood pressure. This may result from conditions unrelated to the patients' thyroid status. Commonly, the hypertension is related to lifestyle factors that override the blood pressure-lowering mechanisms of hypothyroidism or resistance to thyroid hormone. The fibromyalgia symptoms of many such patients are exacerbated by β-adrenergic receptor blockers such as propranolol prescribed to decrease the hypertension.

Reduced blood flow, especially reduced brain blood flow, and low blood pressure are features of fibromyalgia for many patients. Blood flow is the quantity of blood that passes any point in the circulation during a given time. Two factors determine the flow through the vessel: (1) the difference in pressure between the two ends of the vessel, which forces the blood through the vessel; and (2) resistance to the movement of the blood through the vessel.[66,pp.152-153] The state of contraction of the smooth muscle lining of the arterioles determines their resistance to blood flow. The arterioles are largely smooth muscles and function as the major site of resistance to blood flow.[139,p.267]

Blood pressure, also called arteriotony, is the tension of the blood within the arteries. For the most part, two factors determine blood pressure: (1) the force of contraction of the left ventricle, which forces blood into the aorta, and (2) the resistance of the arteries, arterioles, and capillaries to the flow of blood. Other factors contribute to blood pressure. These include the elasticity of the arterial walls and the volume and viscosity of the blood.

Adequate and inadequate thyroid hormone regulation of cell function potently affect the force of contraction of the heart and the resistance of arterioles to the flow of blood. Thyroid hormone has direct effects on the heart muscle and blood vessels. The hormone also profoundly affects the cardiovascular system by interacting with the sympathetic and parasympathetic divisions of the autonomic nervous system and by affecting kidney function. Adequate thyroid hormone regulation increases contractility and shortens the relaxation time of the heart muscle (myocardium), sensitizes the myocardium to the sympathetic nervous system, and decreases resistance to blood flow in arteries.[81] During inadequate thyroid hormone regulation of the cardiovascular system, the force of contraction of the myocardium decreases, relaxation time of the left ventricle is prolonged, the myocardium becomes desensitized to the sympathetic nervous system, and vascular resistance increases.

Hypothyroidism is associated with decreased heart rate, aortic pressure, pressure within the left ventricle, total blood volume, and cardiac output.[115] A minority of hypothyroid patients have high blood pressure.

Blood pressure may be normal in hyperthyroid patients. Usually, however, they have a rapid heart rate and increased heart stroke volume (the volume of blood pumped out of the left ventricle in a single beat). The pressure of the left ventricle is usually elevated.[115]

Several other factors may profoundly influence blood pressure. These include adiposity, stress-related high circulating catecholamine levels, sodium chloride intake, and fluid intake.

● MECHANISMS THAT NORMALLY REGULATE CIRCULATION AND CONTROL BLOOD PRESSURE

In this section, I describe five physiological systems that normally maintain a constant circulation and blood pressure. These systems usually operate to maintain blood flow and blood pressure at levels sufficient to enable the individual to function normally and survive. One system, termed "autoregulation of blood flow" adjusts local circulation so that the blood delivers the quantity of nutrients needed to meet the metabolic needs of the local tissues. Two of the systems, the "baroreceptors" and the "central nervous system ischemic response," act to correct acute, rapid changes in blood pressure. The other two systems, the "kidney-body fluid-blood pressure system" and the "renin-angiotensin-aldosterone system" maintain normal blood pressure long term.

BLOOD FLOW TO INDIVIDUAL TISSUES: AUTOREGULATION OF BLOOD FLOW

Adjustments to the blood flow to the various tissues of the body are largely controlled by local tissue mechanisms. Each tissue controls its blood flow according to its metabolic needs. The greater the metabolic needs of a tissue, the greater its blood flow. The lower the metabolic needs, the further local blood flow is reduced.[66,p.185] Autoregulation controls blood flow to both peripheral and cerebral tissues. Autoregulation normally keeps the cerebral blood flow from increasing more than slightly during exercise.[139,p.634]

The metabolic hypothesis of autoregulation of blood flow states this: When the oxygen supply to a tissue does not meet its requirement for oxygen, the tissue releases vasodilator metabolites. The metabolites dilate local arterioles, increasing blood flow through the capillary bed. When the blood flow meets the oxygen requirement of the tissue, the release of vasodilator metabolites decreases and local blood flow diminishes.[139,pp.277-278] If the oxygen requirement of the tissue decreases because metabolism slows, as during hypothyroidism, the release of vasodilator metabolites decreases, permitting local vasoconstriction and reduced blood flow.

The local tissue requirement for oxygen is not the only factor that regulates local blood flow. During in-

adequate thyroid hormone regulation of the adrenergic genes, the density of α-adrenergic receptors on arterioles increases and the density of β-adrenergic receptors decreases. This change in adrenergic receptors causes a sustained increase in vasoconstrictive tone. Conversely, blockade of α-adrenergic receptors enables epinephrine to induce vasodilation upon binding to β-adrenergic receptors on arterioles.[40] (See section below titled "Role of Adrenergic Receptors in Vascular Resistance and Blood Flow in Hypothyroidism.") Also, thyroid hormone stimulates release of the vasodilator nitric oxide from sympathetic nerve endings near arterioles, and the hormone increases the activity of Ca^{2+}-ATPase within the smooth muscle cells of arterioles. Both effects dilate the arterioles and increase blood flow. (See the section below titled "Effects of Thyroid Hormone on Blood Vessels.")

RAPID CORRECTION OF CHANGES IN BLOOD PRESSURE

The nervous system controls changes in the overall rate of circulation and acute changes in blood pressure. The nervous system responds powerfully within seconds-to-minutes to changes in blood pressure, acting to recover a normal level. The two main systems for correcting acute changes in blood pressure are the baroreceptors in the peripheral arteries and the aorta, and the central nervous system ischemic response system. The renin-angiotensin-aldosterone system also contributes to correct acute changes in blood pressure (see section below titled "Renin-Angiotensin System" and the subsection titled "Angiotensin and Aldosterone"). However, the nervous system acts faster by far to correct blood pressure changes.

Effects of Standing Up on the Cardiovascular System: Orthostasis

Passive Effects. When the human stands up from a lying position, gravity causes some 600 ml of blood to shift into veins below the level of the heart. The veins accommodate the increased blood volume. Usually, about 75% of the total blood volume is below the heart level and contained in veins, which are 20-to-30 times more expansive than arteries. At first, the valves of the veins prevent the blood from pooling in the lower extremities. This function of the valves is protective, for sufficient pooling would cause cerebral ischemia and fainting. Patients with damaged and ineffective valves are likely to faint. Even when the valves have normal integrity, standing causes continued filling of the veins, increasing the intravenous pressure. The pressure eventually widens the veins, opening the valves. Opening of the valves creates a continuous orthostatic column between the heart and feet. The resulting pooling of blood in the lower extremities decreases the amount of blood in the thorax. Filling pressure of the ventricles falls close to zero, and stroke volume decreases by some 40%. This passive hydrostatic pooling in the distensible veins causes cardiovascular changes. Reflexes are quickly initiated that enable the cardiovascular system to recover normal function.[139,pp.622-624]

Reflex Adaptations. Normally, roughly 3 minutes after a human assumes an upright posture from a lying position, the cardiopulmonary, aortic, and carotid pulse pressures decline. Decreases occur in the right atrial mean pressure, stroke volume, cardiac output, and central blood volume. Blood flow also decreases through the kidneys, other viscera, and the skeletal muscles. On the other hand, the heart rate and total peripheral vascular resistance increase. The accelerated heart rate does not usually compensate for the decreased stroke volume, so the net cardiac output briefly remains low. Nonetheless, total peripheral vascular resistance increases enough to maintain the mean arterial pressure. The diastolic pressure may increase slightly due to the increased total peripheral vascular resistance, and the systolic pressure may decrease slightly because of the decreased stroke volume. After about 8 minutes, increases occur in the right atrial mean pressure, stroke volume, cardiac output, and central blood volume. In addition, blood flow increases through the kidneys, other viscera, and the skeletal muscles. At the same time, the heart rate and total peripheral vascular resistance decrease. The diastolic pressure may decrease slightly due to the decreased total peripheral vascular resistance, and the systolic pressure may increase slightly because of the increased stroke volume. Again, the mean arterial pressure remains normal.[139,pp.623-624]

Baroreceptors

The baroreceptors are stretch receptors in the carotid sinuses, the aorta, and other arteries. The baroreceptor reflex system of arteries is a powerful and rapidly acting mechanism for the control of arterial pressure.[150]

Increasing Blood Pressure. When blood pressure rises, as during strenuous exercise, several nervous system changes rapidly occur. First, stretch receptors (called baroreceptors) in large arteries in the neck and thorax begin generating nerve signals. The main baroreceptors are in the sinuses of the carotid arteries and the arch of the aorta. Nerve fibers transmit the signals from the baroreceptors to the medulla of the brain stem. In the medulla, the signals reach the nucleus of the solitary tract. From there, secondary nerve signals inhibit sympathetic nerves in the vasoconstrictor center of the medulla. The inhibition dramatically decreases the flow of sympathetic nerve signals to the arterioles and veins of peripheral parts of the body.[134] The decrease of sympathetic signals reduces resistance to blood flow from the arterioles to the capillary beds, and decreased signals reduce the return of blood to the heart through the veins. A decrease in sympathetic nerve signals to the heart reduces the heart rate and stroke volume. In addition, baroreceptor signals reflexly increase parasympathetic nerve signals (through the vagus nerves) to the heart, further reducing heart rate and stroke volume. (The reader may appreciate the potent effect of increased parasympathetic signals by considering vasovagal syncope. The term "vasovagal" refers to action of the vagal nerve on blood vessels, and "syncope" is fainting. Fainting involves an abrupt drop in blood pressure with "cerebral anemia" followed by a loss of consciousness. Vasovagal syncope is a sudden fall in blood pressure, slowing of the pulse rate, and possibly convulsions. Researchers believe the condition results from sudden stimulation of the vagus nerves mediated by the baroreceptors. Two circulatory phenomena occur in most vasovagal syncope patients—systemic arterial vasodilation and bradycardia. A third phenomenon, cerebrovascular constriction, occurs in some patients, but its contribution to the fainting is less well established.[149]) The combined effect of decreased sympathetic signals and increased parasympathetic signals during a rise in blood pressure is reduced cardiac output. The two nervous system changes lower blood pressure toward normal.[66,pp.198-201]

Sympathetic involvement in peripheral vasodilation or vasoconstriction is more complex than mere regulation via the baroreceptors. Henriksen studied local sympathetic innervation of human skeletal muscle, skin, and subcutaneous tissues of the arms and legs. He reported that besides the sympathetic reflexes regulated by spinal and supraspinal centers, the innervated tissues have local sympathetic nerves. Each nerve conducts sympathetic signals from a vein to an arteriole. Increased pressure within the vein of about 25 mm Hg activates the nerve. The signals induce constriction of the arteriole.[134] Constriction of the arteriole reduces blood flow through the capillary bed, reducing the entry of blood into the venules and veins. These local sympathetic nerves likely contribute to adaptive decreases and increases of arterial pressure.

Decreasing Blood Pressure. When blood pressure decreases, the nervous system rapidly responds to bring the pressure back to normal. First, the decreased pressure in the carotid arteries and aorta shorten the baroreceptors. The shortening ceases the flow of nerve signals from the receptors. The reduction of signals reaching the brain stem increases the transmission of sympathetic nerve signals to the heart and blood vessels. The sympathetic signals increase heart rate and stroke volume and induce constriction of the arterioles. The signals also cause a slight constriction of veins. The venous constriction increases the delivery of venous blood to the heart.

Simultaneously, the signals reaching the brain stem decrease the flow of parasympathetic signals to the heart and blood vessels through the vagus nerves. The decrease of parasympathetic signals increases heart rate and stoke volume.

The combined effect of the increased sympathetic innervation and decreased parasympathetic innervation is to raise the blood pressure back to normal by inducing vasoconstriction and increasing cardiac output.[66,p.198-201]

A sufficient decrease of pressure in veins is likely to reduce activity of the local sympathetic fibers that transmit signals from veins to arterioles. The decrease of signals results in dilation of the arterioles.[134] Dilation of the arterioles increases blood flow through the capillary bed, enabling more blood to enter the venules and veins. The increased flow of blood into the venous system increases intravenous pressure.

Normal function of the baroreceptors, the brain stem centers, and the sympathetic nervous system is critical to rapidly correcting a fall in blood pressure when someone gets upright after sitting or lying. If the nervous system does not act quickly to reverse the fall in arterial pressure, fainting may result from reduced blood flow to the head. In many fibromyalgia and chronic fatigue syndrome patients, the system for correcting a fall in blood pressure is faulty (see section below titled "Hypotension in Fibromyalgia"). As a result, they have chronic hypotension and/or orthostatic hypotension. The hypotension is plausibly explained by faults in the blood pressure regulating systems that occur in many hypothyroid and thyroid hormone resistant patients. (See section below titled "Model of Reduced Blood Flow and Hypotension in Fibromyalgia.")

Central Nervous System Ischemic Response

When the circulation is so slow that the CO_2 in the vasomotor center in the brain stem rises above a threshold concentration, the CO_2 strongly stimulates the sympathetic nervous system. The increase of sympathetic nerve transmission throughout the body raises the blood pressure and accelerates blood flow through the lungs. The increased pulmonary blood flow accelerates the exchange of CO_2 for oxygen. A rise in the concentrations of acidic substances such as lactic acid may also activate the sympathetic nervous system. Loosely considered, this mechanism is part of the central nervous system ischemic response system. Strictly, though, the ischemic system involves activation of the sympathetic nervous system with an increase in blood pressure triggered by ischemia of the cerebrum.[66,p.202]

Cerebral blood vessels have properties that protect the brain from deficient circulation. Normally, cerebral vessels can change their own diameter. When the systemic blood pressure rises, cerebral vessels constrict, and when systemic blood pressure falls, cerebral vessels dilate. Also, when the arterial CO_2 level rises, cerebral arterioles dilate and brain blood flow increases. When the arterial CO_2 level falls, cerebral blood vessels constrict and blood flow through the brain decreases.[82,p.1044] This dynamic flow-regulating feature of cerebral blood vessels normally ensures a constant blood supply to the brain.

According to Guyton, ischemia of the cerebrum is one of the most powerful stimulants of sympathetic nervous system activity. Sympathetic activity does not increase, however, until the arterial pressure falls to 60 mm Hg or lower. Thus, the ischemic system does not regulate blood pressure under normal circumstances. Guyton described the ischemic system as a "last ditch" mechanism when a decrease in blood flow to the brain reaches a potentially lethal level. The system is critically important because nerve cells of the brain can survive a loss of nutrients for only 3-to-10 minutes. Subsequently, their metabolism completely ceases. This, of course, is neuronal cell death.[66,p.202]

LONG-TERM CONTROL OF BLOOD PRESSURE

The baroreceptors in arteries and the aorta do not play an important role in maintaining blood pressure over the long term. Over a few days, the baroreceptors adjust to any sustained level of blood pressure. Accordingly, if low or high blood pressure continues, the baroreceptors reset and act to keep the pressure fairly constant at the low or high level.

Also, reactions of the sympathetic nervous system to acute changes in blood pressure are short-lived. With a sudden fall in blood pressure, increased sympathetic discharge helps raise the pressure to normal. In one sense, however, sympathetic nervous system activity contributes to long-term blood pressure status. Chronically increased sympathetic nervous system tone may contribute to high blood pressure. This is evident from the finding that regular cardiovascular exercise can lower blood pressure by reducing sympathetic nervous system tone.[148] Conversely, progressive physical deconditioning can increase sympathetic nervous system tone with an associated increase in blood pressure. Overall, however, physiologists classify the sympathetic nervous system as a mechanism for adapting to acute blood pressure changes.

Long-term regulation of blood pressure mainly involves the kidneys. Over days, weeks, and months, the kidneys respond to increases in arterial pressure and interact with several substances to maintain normal body fluid levels and blood pressure. These kidney functions are the most important mechanism for keeping the blood pressure constant over the long term.

Kidney-Body Fluid System

Normally, the kidneys sensitively respond to changes in arterial blood pressure by altering salt and water excretion.[135] When the blood pressure rises, salt and water excretion increases. The increased excretion involves accelerated glomerular filtration and reduced reabsorption of salt and water back into the blood from the kidney tubules.[130] An increase in arterial pressure of only a few mm Hg can double the kidney excretion of salt and water. (This is true only if the individual does not have organic kidney disease or an excess of aldosterone, the hormone that stimulates reabsorption of salt and water from the kidney tubules. Those who do may not properly excrete salt and water, and may develop hypertension.[132][135]) The excretion of salt is roughly equal to that of water.

Long-term changes in arterial pressure result from an alteration of one or both of two factors: (1) an increase or decrease in the intake of salt and water, and/or (2) an increase or decrease in the excretion rate of salt and water by the kidneys. If the amount of water in the extracellular fluids markedly increases, both cardiac output and arterial pressure increase. The kidneys potently react by eliminating large amounts of salt and

water. The increased salt and water excretion reduce plasma volume and lower cardiac output and arterial pressure back to normal. If the amount of water in the extracellular fluids markedly decreases, both cardiac output and arterial pressure decrease. The kidneys react by decreasing the excretion of salt and water. As a result, plasma volume increases and cardiac output and arterial pressure return to normal. The kidneys usually return the arterial pressure to normal within hours or days.[66,pp.205-208]

The kidneys are highly effective in adjusting the long-term arterial pressure level, even when cardiac output and/or peripheral vascular resistance are abnormal. This is true during hyperthyroidism and hypothyroidism. Most hyperthyroid patients have increased cardiac output. The increased output results from three factors: (1) direct stimulation of heart muscle cells by thyroid hormone, (2) an increase in the density of β-adrenergic receptors on heart muscle cells, and (3) increased sympathetic innervation. However, peripheral resistance of arterioles is decreased due to an increased density of β-adrenergic receptors on arterioles. When the excretion of salt and water by the kidneys is normal in hyperthyroidism, increased cardiac output compensates for the decreased peripheral vascular resistance. The compensation results in normal arterial pressure.

In contrast to hyperthyroid patients, most hypothyroid patients have decreased cardiac output. The decrease results from three factors: (1) subnormal direct stimulation of heart muscle cells by thyroid hormone, (2) a decrease in the density of β-adrenergic receptors on the muscle cells, and (3) decreased sympathetic innervation of the heart. However, peripheral resistance of arterioles is heightened due to a decreased density of β-adrenergic receptors and an increased density of α-adrenergic receptors on the arterioles. When salt and water excretion by the kidneys is normal in the hypothyroid patient, the decreased cardiac output compensates for the increased peripheral vascular resistance. The compensation results in normal arterial pressure.[66,p.208]

When an individual ingests a large amount of water and the kidney-body fluid system is functioning normally, arterial pressure remains normal. The kidneys easily excrete large amounts of water. But the kidneys do not excrete salt as easily, and a high salt intake usually results in an accumulation in the body. Due to the accumulation, a high salt intake usually raises the arterial pressure.[66,p.209] The salt accumulates in the body and stimulates the thirst center, inducing the person to increase liquid intake. As a result, the extracellular body fluid content increases. The increased osmolality of the blood stimulates hypothalamic-posterior pituitary secretion of vasopressin (antidiuretic hormone). Vasopressin stimulates the reabsorption of water from the kidney tubules. The consequent increased water content of the blood raises plasma volume. The raised volume increases the return of venous blood to the heart and stimulates increased cardiac output. The increased output increases the blood flow to tissues, and the increased flow activates local tissue mechanisms to induce vasoconstriction. The combination of vasoconstriction and increased cardiac output raises arterial pressure.[66,p.209]

The reverse circumstance (from high salt intake described in the previous paragraph), low salt intake and resulting low arterial pressure, has recently become an issue. Over the past several decades, at the behest of medical organizations and health care providers, many people have decreased their salt ingestion to avoid or correct hypertension. In general, reduced salt intake appears to have accomplished the objective without adverse effects.[132] But as with most human interventions that are generally beneficial, this one has adversely affected some individuals. Low salt intake by some fibromyalgia and chronic fatigue syndrome patients seems to result in low blood pressure. The low pressure may be chronic, or it may manifest as neurogenic, orthostatic, or postural hypotension (see the section below titled "Hypotension in Fibromyalgia"). Understanding these patients' hypotension requires knowledge of the mechanism I presented above for the rapid control of a fall in blood pressure. However, understanding also requires knowledge of how low salt ingestion contributes to low arterial pressure.

With low salt intake, the salt concentration in the blood may decrease to such a low level that activity of the thirst center decreases. With decreased thirst, the person consumes less water. The reduced intake of salt and water decreases the extracellular fluid content of the body. The decreased salt level of the circulating blood may create low osmolality. The low osmolality would in turn reduce hypothalamic-posterior pituitary secretion of vasopressin. The decreased vasopressin level would reduce the reabsorption of water from the kidney tubules. The reduced reabsorption of water would decrease extracellular fluid volume and the plasma volume. The decreased plasma volume would reduce the return of blood to the heart, resulting in decreased cardiac output. Decreased cardiac output reduces blood flow to tissues. In response to the reduced blood flow, the local blood flow-regulating mechanism of the tissues would dilate blood vessels to increase the supply of nutrients reaching the tissues. Vasodilation in the tissues while cardiac output is low further reduces arterial pressure. The arterial pressure may be so low in some patients that they become dizzy and faint if they do not sit or lie down.

Low salt intake, with low cardiac output, low arterial pressure, and local tissue vasodilation, may account for a finding of Grassi et al. After studying transcapillary permeability in the nail fold capillaries of fibromyalgia patients, the researchers speculated that the patients had low capillary flow and/or capillary bed hypotension.[129] The hypotension may have resulted from hypotension due to low salt intake, despite vasoconstriction from an increase in α-adrenergic receptors on arterioles.

When increased peripheral vascular resistance accompanies increased vascular resistance in the kidneys, arterial pressure rises. Conversely, when decreased peripheral vascular resistance accompanies decreased resistance of the kidney arterioles, arterial pressure falls. The reduced vascular resistance in the kidneys is mainly responsible for the fall in blood pressure.[66,p.208] Similarly, in hypertension, substantial evidence points to a primary role of increased vasoconstriction in the kidneys. The increase in resistance of the kidney arterioles initially results from heightened tone of kidney arterioles. Eventually, the increased resistance becomes irreversible. The irreversibility results from structural changes. An overgrowth and contraction of the interstitial connective tissues with hardening of the kidneys causes the structural changes. This pathological process is called nephrosclerosis.[135]

Fine adjustments to this kidney-body fluid system are managed by the renin-angiotensin mechanism (see section immediately below).

Renin-Angiotensin System

The renin-angiotensin system is a potent regulator of arterial pressure. The system activates to correct acute changes in blood pressure,[131] but it also serves to powerfully regulate arterial pressure over the long term.[153]

As a feedback mechanism, the renin-angiotensin system normally keeps arterial pressure near normal despite a high salt intake. Renin secretion decreases or ceases when blood pressure is high, and renin secretion begins or increases when blood pressure is low.

Renin is an enzyme that the afferent arterioles of the kidneys secrete when the arterial pressure becomes too low. A reaction of the sympathetic nervous system to the low pressure can induce renin secretion through sympathetic fibers to the kidney arterioles.[146] Renin is formed and stored as prorenin in the smooth muscle cells of the arterioles. When the arterial pressure falls, prorenin splits and releases renin. Some renin remains in the kidneys to influence them, but most enters the systemic circulation. While circulating in the blood, renin acts on a globulin called angiotensinogen. When acted upon by renin, angiotensinogen releases angiotensin I. Angiotensin I is a weak vasoconstrictor that has little effect on raising the low blood pressure. (The term "angio" means blood or lymph vessel. The term "tensin" refers to tension, as when the smooth muscle cells lining arterioles contract.) Each renin molecule circulates in the blood for 30-to-60 minutes. As it circulates, it converts angiotensinogen to angiotensin I.[66,p.211] This short time circulating in the blood for each renin molecule ensures a timely offset of the hypotension-relieving effects of the vasoconstrictors renin generates.

Angiotensin I circulates to the small blood vessels of the lungs where, within seconds, angiotensin converting enzyme catalyzes its conversion to angiotensin II.[87,p.785] (Inhibitors of angiotensin converting enzyme are important anti-hypertensive medications. See the section below titled "β-Adrenergic Receptor Blockers and Other Anti-Hypertensive Medications.") Angiotensin II is a powerful vasoconstrictor.[153] After 1 or 2 minutes, various enzymes classified as angiotensinase decompose angiotensin II. Before angiotensinase decomposes angiotensin II, however, angiotensin II exerts two main effects that raise blood pressure.

One way angiotensin II raises blood pressure is by powerfully inducing peripheral vasoconstriction. Angiotensin II induces extreme constriction of arterioles, increasing peripheral resistance and raising blood pressure. It also induces a milder constriction of veins. The venous constriction facilitates return of blood to the heart. The increased venous return helps increase the force with which the heart sends blood into the arteries against the higher vascular resistance.[66,p.212]

A second way angiotensin II raises arterial pressure is by reducing the excretion of salt and water by the kidneys. The main site of action of angiotensin II in the kidneys is the efferent arterioles.[151] The reduced excretion increases the salt and water content of the blood and increases extracellular fluid volume. Under this influence, the arterial pressure increases over hours or days. Guyton wrote that the long-term effect of angiotensin II in the kidneys is more powerful than

its induction of peripheral vasoconstriction. He also wrote that about 20 minutes is needed for the renin-angiotensin system to fully activate and induce vasoconstriction. This is a longer time than required for the baroreceptors and sympathetic nervous system to react and raise blood pressure. Nevertheless, the slower-acting renin-angiotensin system can be lifesaving in conditions such as circulatory shock.[66,p.212]

Physiologists have long studied angiotensin I and II. However, it appears that several other angiotensins take part in the central and peripheral effects of the renin-angiotensin system. For example, angiotensin-(1-7) binds to receptors in the periphery and on central sites involved in the control of arterial pressure. Peripherally angiotensin-(1-7) exerts a potent antidiuretic effect on water-loaded rats. Injection of angiotensin-(1-7) into the dorsomedial or ventrolateral medulla of the brain stem produces cardiovascular effects comparable to those of angiotensin II. Angiotensin-(1-7) also strongly stimulates the release of vasopressin and prostaglandin. It also provokes neuronal activity in the hypothalamus and medulla.[147]

According to Dzau, some blood vessel walls other than those of the afferent kidney arterioles contain a renin-angiotensin system. He wrote that this system induces constriction of arterioles and it may affect compliance of the large conduit arteries.[131]

Angiotensin and Aldosterone. Besides angiotensin directly inducing the kidneys to reduce salt and water excretion, it also indirectly potentiates this effect by stimulating the adrenal cortices to secrete the hormone aldosterone. In fact, angiotensin is among the most potent stimuli for aldosterone release. Aldosterone stimulates the reabsorption of salt and water from the kidney tubules. The increased absorption raises the salt concentration of the extracellular fluids. The increased salt concentration increases the extracellular fluid volume, and the increased volume raises blood pressure over the long term.[66,p.213]

Angiotensin, Sympathetic Nervous System Discharge, and Vasopressin. Angiotensin exerts a direct effect in the central nervous system that increases sympathetic nervous system discharge and vasopressin secretion. The sympathetic discharge increases vasoconstriction, and the vasopressin increases reabsorption of water from the kidney tubules. This effect of angiotensin is integrated at the level of the AV3V brain region. In addition, sensory signals from the kidneys, by a complex route to the forebrain, can induce sympathetic discharge.[133]

● CIRCULATION AND BLOOD PRESSURE IN FIBROMYALGIA

Studies have shown that fibromyalgia patients have reduced blood flow through both the brain and the peripheral tissues.

DECREASED BRAIN BLOOD FLOW IN FIBROMYALGIA

In studies using SPECT (see Glossary), regional cerebral blood flow of fibromyalgia patients was lower than normal. In one study, researchers found that fibromyalgia patients with moderate-to-severe headaches had reduced blood brain flow. The most common finding was reduced blood flow through the frontal lobes. Of the 100 patients in the study, 97 had asymmetries in blood perfusion of the cerebrum. Twenty-one patients had reduced blood flow through the right frontal lobe, and 23 patients had reduced flow through the left frontal lobe. Some patients also had reduced blood flow through the temporal lobes. The left temporal lobe was involved more than the right.[4]

Other investigators used SPECT to examine the brains of 10 patients with severe fibromyalgia.[5] They inspected the thalamus, cortex, and caudate nuclei. Blood flow through the thalamus was normal. Cerebral blood flow was significantly lower than controls. Flow through the caudate heads was significantly lower than normal. Flow was 2-to-3 standard deviations below normal. The investigators wrote, "The low caudate activity may reflect decreased excitatory input from the thalamus, a structure important in pain perception and discrimination. The low caudate activity supports the hypothesis that [fibromyalgia] may result from a primary dysregulation within the limbic system."

San Pedro et al. conducted a study to detect any relation between pain states and blood perfusion of the caudate, thalamus, and anterior cingulate. They tested a father and daughter who had restless leg syndrome and induced pain by restricting their mobility. During increasing pain, SPECT showed that regional cerebral blood flow in the father was 13% below normal in the caudate nuclei. Also with increasing pain, blood flow was 7% above normal in the thalamus and 6.6% in the anterior cingulate. During increased pain, SPECT showed that regional cerebral blood flow in the daughter was 12% below normal in the caudate and 1.2% above normal in the anterior cingulate. San Pedro et al. concluded, "The study supports the association between pain and decreased regional cerebral blood flow

of the caudate nucleus as reported in fibromyalgia syndrome."[72]

Goldstein et al. found that the brain SPECT images of fibromyalgia patients were virtually identical to those of chronic fatigue syndrome patients. The location of decreased regional cerebral blood flow was the same in both groups. They compared the blood flow of chronic fatigue syndrome patients who did not meet the tender point criterion for fibromyalgia and fibromyalgia/chronic fatigue syndrome patients who did meet the criterion. Those who did had more severely decreased blood flow.[68][69,p.52] Goldstein reported that SPECT scans of chronic fatigue syndrome patients revealed reduced brain blood flow that in some cases was in the ischemic range.[83,p.177] He also wrote that PET scans, which show regions of reduced metabolism, indicated hypometabolism in various limbic structures: the medial frontal lobes, the hippocampus, amygdala, cingulate gyrus, anterior caudate nucleus, superior colliculus, and parietal lobe areas. He wrote that in some cases, PET scans show the premotor cortex and the anterior cerebellum to be hypometabolic.[83,p.117] On the basis of neuropsychological testing, he proposed that one of the conditions chronic fatigue syndrome patients have is "metabolic encephalopathy."[83,p.118] This description resembles that given by investigators of a patient with subclinical hypothyroidism[70] (see section below titled "Reduced Cerebral Blood Flow in Hypothyroidism").

Streeten and Bell measured the red blood cell mass and plasma volume of patients with severe chronic fatigue syndrome. Of the 19 patients, 15 were females and 4 were males. They found a red cell mass below the normal range in 14 of the 15 females (93.8%) and 2 of the 4 males (50%). The plasma volume was below normal in 10 of the 19 patients (52.6%), and the total blood volume was subnormal in 12 (63.2%). The researchers speculated that the low red blood cell mass in a high percentage of chronic fatigue syndrome patients might contribute to their symptoms by reducing the amount of oxygen delivered to the brain by the blood. They noted that the red blood cell mass is also significantly low in patients with orthostatic hypotension who do not have fibromyalgia or chronic fatigue syndrome. Some fibromyalgia and chronic fatigue syndrome patients have orthostatic hypotension.[116]

PERIPHERAL BLOOD FLOW IN FIBROMYALGIA

Fassbender and Wegner proposed that hypoxia is

an essential causative factor in fibromyalgia.[24] Fassbender wrote, "We have postulated that a local vascular disturbance is responsible for both a muscular and a connective tissue lesion. In muscle, this leads to degeneration of small foci of the parenchyma and may show features of necrosis. Fibrous tissue, on the other hand, may respond by a proliferation of cells."[21,p.310]

Lund, Bengtsson, and Thorborg found low oxygenation of the trapezius and brachioradialis muscles of fibromyalgia patients. The researchers speculated that the low oxygenation was due to structural and functional changes affecting the microvessels in tender points. They also found low oxygen pressure in the patients' subcutaneous tissues, although the tissues were not hypoxic. They wrote that the low oxygen pressure suggests that tissues other than the skeletal muscles are involved in fibromyalgia.[22] (They wrote this in 1986 when some researchers suspected that fibromyalgia was primarily a skeletal muscle disorder.) However, Klemp et al. used a technique ([133]xenon injection) that measures local blood flow through a larger tissue volume. They found no abnormality, but because the technique is not as sensitive as that used by Lund and his group, the results were not conclusive.[23]

Bengtsson, Henriksson, and Larsson suggested that a mechanism of hypoxia in fibromyalgia tissue is swollen endothelial cells of capillaries protruding into the capillary lumen (reported by Fassbender[21]). They wrote that the swelling may cause intravascular obstruction of the capillaries and that the obstruction reduces blood flow.[35,p.820] Gidlöf et al. found swollen capillary endothelial cells in samples taken from the quadriceps muscle of fibromyalgia patients after 150 minutes of induced ischemia.[34] The ischemia may cause an energy crisis in the capillary endothelial cells, with contractures of the actomyosin and an increase in intracellular organelles. Both changes could alter the shape of the cells from flat to spherical. The spherical form would protrude into the capillary lumen.

Some studies have shown that ischemia causes metabolic changes. The changes include decreased ATP and phosphocreatine and an increase in AMP and creatine.[25][26][27] These are changes also found in muscles of both fibromyalgia and hypothyroid patients. Researchers suggest that elevated lactate in hypothyroid (thyroidectomized) dogs may be due to reduced blood flow.[28] But some patients with ischemia have increased lactate and pyruvate levels.[26][27]

Bengtsson et al. did not find an increase in lactate in fibromyalgia patients. They explained that the patients' circulation was adequate to clear lactate.[35,p.820] Eisinger also found an increase in blood pyruvic acid

levels in fibromyalgia patients. The patients' lactate production during forearm ischemic exercise testing was normal-to-decreased. The experimentally-induced ischemia reduced the oxygen supply to the exercising muscles. The reduced oxygen supply should have increased lactate production, but pyruvate-to-lactate conversion did not increase. Conversion occurred at a normal rather than increased rate probably because of the low lactate dehydrogenase levels Eisinger found. Hypoxia may contribute to such biochemical abnormalities in fibromyalgia. However, an increased density of α-adrenergic receptors on skeletal muscle cells and arterioles can account for hypoxia and the biochemical abnormalities. (See Chapter 2.2, subsection titled "Lactate Dehydrogenase in Fibromyalgia and in Hypothyroidism," and the subsection titled "Glycolysis." Also see Chapter 3.1, the section titled "High Ratio of α- to β-Adrenergic Receptors on Cell Membranes," and the section titled "Abnormal Glycolysis in Fibromyalgia.")

For descriptions of additional studies of peripheral blood flow in fibromyalgia, see Chapter 3.4, section titled "Subnormal Circulation."

BLOOD ABNORMALITIES IN FIBROMYALGIA

Hypercoagulability in Fibromyalgia Patients. Berg et al. included 21 female patients (9 with chronic fatigue syndrome and 12 with fibromyalgia) in a study in which investigators used four laboratory tests for hypercoagulation. They reported that in one test, 19 of 21 patients (90%) had abnormal values; in a second test, results were abnormal for 15 of 18 patients (83%); in a third, results were abnormal for 14 of 21 patients (67%); and in a fourth, 11 of 21 patients (52%) had abnormal results. The researchers wrote that their test results prove the truth of their hypothesis that a subgroup of chronic fatigue syndrome/fibromyalgia patients have a hypercoagulable state. They wrote that their results showed thrombin (IIa) generation in these patients, and in addition, two thirds of the patients had platelet activation. They wrote, "A hypercoagulable state exists in a subset of CFS/FM patients. New sensitive coagulation assays . . . allow detection of low grade thrombin generation, platelet activation, and prove a hypercoagulable condition exists. The size of the subset (small, medium, or large number of CFS/FM patients) remains unanswered."[137]

Berg et al. treated patients with heparin, which they reported downregulates the hypercoagulable state. They also reported that low-dose coumadin therapy prevents most patients' symptoms from reappearing. They reported that most of the patients had moderate-to-excellent results and remained symptom-free. Of the 21 patients, they wrote, only 1 had minimal symptom improvement. They wrote that the treatment may not relieve symptoms for 1-to-3 months. The researchers also stated that 2 patients required an additional week of heparin therapy after they converted to the use of coumadin.[137] (See section below titled "Blood Changes in Hypothyroidism.")

HYPOTENSION IN FIBROMYALGIA

A subset of both fibromyalgia[136][159][160] and chronic fatigue syndrome[136][162][163][165][166][167][168][169][170][171][172][173][174][175][176] patients have neurally mediated hypotension. Grassi et al. proposed that abnormal microvascular dynamics in fibromyalgia patients are induced by low capillary flow and/or capillary bed hypotension.[129]

In one study, 12 of 20 fibromyalgia patients (60%) had an abnormal response to the head-up tilt test. The investigators defined an abnormal response as (1) fainting or pre-fainting with a drop in systolic blood pressure of at least 25 mm Hg and (2) no increase in heart rate. Of 18 fibromyaliga patients who tolerated the upright tilt for more than 10 minutes, all reported the onset of widespread pain. The investigators concluded that fibromyalgia is strongly associated with neurally mediated hypotension.[175] Many of my fibromyalgia patients have been hypotensive, with systolic/diastolic pressures in some cases as low as 90/58. Most of these patients have had chronic hypotension. A smaller number have reported orthostatic hypotension, especially upon quickly changing from a recumbent to a standing posture. Some patients, a small percentage, have been hypertensive.

A symptom characteristic of low blood pressure is malaise. In fact, many clinicians consider malaise a signal that a patient's dosage of anti-hypertensive medications is excessive, causing episodes of hypotension.[154] Rowe wrote that over the past 50 years, researchers and clinicians have considered chronic fatigue a prominent symptom of several overlapping syndromes of orthostatic intolerance. (Orthostatic intolerance is a decrease in heart rate and blood pressure upon assuming an upright posture, as in the head-up tilt test, and associated symptoms.) The overlapping syndromes Rowe listed are neurally mediated (or vasovagal) hypotension, delayed orthostatic hypotension, postural orthostatic tachycardia syndrome, and idio-

pathic hypovolemia. Rowe and Calkins also wrote that considerable evidence supports a relationship between hypotension and both idiopathic chronic fatigue and chronic fatigue syndrome.[169] Some have proposed that chronic hypotension is the underlying mechanism of chronic fatigue syndrome.[163]

Most patients with hypotension have symptoms other than fatigue. In one study, all 50 patients with orthostatic intolerance had at least four symptoms within the first 45 minutes of assuming an upright posture. Of the 50 patients, 82% had fatigue, 78% had lightheadedness, 70% had pain other than headache, and 62% had nausea. The mean time to the onset of hypotension was 39 minutes.[126] In another study, 25 of 26 chronic fatigue syndrome patients experienced severe orthostatic symptoms. Seven of 25 patients fainted, 15 of 25 had orthostatic tachycardia with hypotension, 3 of 25 had orthostatic tachycardia without significant hypotension, and 18 of 25 had cold and blue extremities (acrocyanosis) and edema.[166] Schondorf et al. reported that of 75 patients with chronic fatigue syndrome, 30 (40%) had orthostatic intolerance during the head-up tilt test. Sixteen of the 30 patients (53%) exhibited neurally-mediated fainting alone, 7 patients (23%) had tachycardia, and 6 patients (20%) had both tachycardia and fainting.[165]

According to Rowe, researchers now recognize neurally mediated hypotension as the most common mechanism of orthostatic intolerance in chronic fatigue syndrome patients. Some patients faint. Rowe also wrote that postural orthostatic tachycardia syndrome is common among these patients.[127] Postural orthostatic tachycardia syndrome is a rapid heart rate with hypotension upon assuming an upright posture.

Some authors have described neurally mediated hypotension in fibromyalgia and chronic fatigue syndrome as an abnormal vasovagal response to the upright posture.[160][161] The abnormal vasovagal response resembles "vasovagal syncopy." Vasovagal syncope is fainting due to excessive parasympathetic innervation of the heart via the vagus nerves. Blood pressure promptly falls, "cerebral anemia" follows, and the individual loses consciousness. (For a more detailed description, see the subsection above under "Baroreceptors" titled "Increasing Blood Pressure.")

Stewart et al. described orthostatic tachycardia syndrome (heart rate over 100 upon assuming an upright posture) in chronic fatigue syndrome patients. During the head-up tilt test, all 25 chronic fatigue syndrome patients (100%) in the study experienced severe orthostatic symptoms. Two of the 25 fainted and 16 of 23 had early orthostatic tachycardia. Of the 16 tachycardic patients, 13 had low blood pressure. Of 23 patients, 7 experienced delayed orthostatic tachycardia, and 6 of the 7 patients were hypotensive. Eighteen of 25 patients had edema and cold and blue hands.[161]

LaManca et al. defined a positive head-up tilt test as (1) a drop in systolic blood pressure of >25 mmHg without a concurrent increase in heart rate and/or (2) the occurrence of pre-fainting symptoms. Of 12 chronic fatigue syndrome patients they tested, 11 had positive results. The patients with positive test results had higher baseline heart rates and smaller stroke volumes. During the last 4 minutes before being returned to a reclining posture, the patients who had positive test results had higher heart rates, lower pulse pressures, and lower pulsatile-systolic areas. The researchers wrote that patients who have positive test results have a cardiovascular profile that differs from those of patients with negative results and control subjects. Also, during the test, the profile of patients with positive results is maintained.[164]

● CIRCULATION AND BLOOD PRESSURE IN HYPOTHYROIDISM

The reduced blood flow found in studies of fibromyalgia and chronic fatigue syndrome patients is virtually the same as that found in studies of hypothyroid patients. Inadequate thyroid hormone regulation of cell function accounts well for the reduced blood flow in both the central nervous system and the peripheral tissues of fibromyalgia.

PERIPHERAL BLOOD FLOW IN HYPOTHYROIDISM

Decreased local tissue metabolism during inadequate thyroid hormone regulation of cell function results in decreased circulation to those tissues This is true of both the cerebrum and peripheral tissues. (See section above titled "Blood Flow to Individual Tissues.") Each tissue locally regulates its own blood flow so as to fill its unique metabolic needs. At rest, for example, skeletal muscles have a very low rate of circulation, but during vigorous exercise, the circulation may increase 20-fold. This occurs because the metabolic rate of muscle may increase 50-fold during exercise.[66,p.185] Hence, in hypothyroid and thyroid hor-

mone resistant patients, both at rest and during exercise, skeletal muscle circulation can be expected to be low.

Most hypothyroid patients have reduced cardiovascular function. Thyroid hormone has direct effects on the heart muscle, and subnormal heart function directly reflects deficient thyroid hormone exposure. Reduced cardiovascular function, however, is also mediated by a decrease in β-adrenergic receptors and an increase in α-adrenergic receptors. These changes in the numbers of the two types of adrenergic receptors result from inadequate thyroid hormone regulation of the adrenergic genes.

Effects of Thyroid Hormone on Blood Vessels

Exposure of arterioles to thyroid hormone relaxes them, decreasing vascular resistance. Deficient exposure of arterioles to the hormone constricts them, increasing vascular resistance.

Researchers have reported that administering T_3 to animals causes a rapid decrease in systemic vascular resistance. The decrease results from T_3-induced relaxation of the smooth muscle cells that line the arterioles. The relaxation results from two effects of T_3 on the muscle cells, one direct and the other indirect. Within the smooth muscle cells of arterioles, T_3 reduces the cytoplasmic calcium concentration by increasing the activity of Ca^{2+}-ATPase. This enzyme catalyzes the transport of calcium from the cytoplasm to the sarcoplasmic reticulum. This effect of thyroid hormone is direct. The indirect vasodilating effect of thyroid hormone is mediated by the vasodilator nitric oxide. T_3 increases secretion of nitric oxide by sympathetic nerve terminals near arterioles. The released nitric oxide then dilates the arterioles.

These two effects of T_3 occur before changes in heart rate or cardiac contractility.[57] However, as systemic vascular resistance decreases in response to thyroid hormone, blood pressure drops. The drop in pressure causes a reduction of nerve signals from baroreceptors to the brain stem. Brain stem centers respond by increasing the heart rate and stroke volume. Thus, cardiac output increases.[58,p.610]

During a thyroid hormone deficiency, we can expect the reverse effects—increased systemic peripheral vascular resistance (due to an increase in calcium concentration of the cytoplasm of vascular smooth muscle cells and decreased nitric oxide secretion) and decreased cardiac output. Increased vascular resistance with decreased cardiac output decreases blood flow.

Reduced Cardiovascular Function in Hypothyroidism

Hypothyroidism substantially reduces peripheral circulation. Studies of hypothyroid patients show that they typically have decreased cardiac output,[30][81] circulating blood volume,[31] velocity of blood flow, heart rate, pulse pressure, and respiratory capacity.[32] The peripheral circulation is also slowed.[29,p.318][33][63][64] The arm-to-lung and arm-to-tongue circulation time is prolonged.[3,p.169] Also, the distribution of tissue blood flow varies from normal. For example, skin blood flow markedly decreases and commonly causes cold skin.[63][64]

When thyroid hormone therapy increases patients' metabolic rates, their peripheral blood flow increases. Stewart and Evans, for example, wrote: "At a time when the basal metabolic rate was low in the untreated subjects, the peripheral blood flow was also decreased. During the progressive rise in basal metabolic rate with administration of thyroid, there were successive and parallel increases in peripheral blood flow."[33,p.817] Stewart and his coworkers found that when the metabolic rate was low, cardiac output per minute decreased and the velocity of blood flow (from tongue to arm) slowed.[30,p.237] "The circulation rate," they wrote, "is slowed to such an extent that it is inadequate even to the decreased tissue requirements for oxygen."[30,pp.247-248]

Klein et al. wrote that hypothyroidism is associated with elevated cholesterol which increases the risk of atherosclerosis. As the main cardiovascular complications of hypothyroidism, they listed angina pectoris, atrioventricular block, and pericarditis, and diastolic hypertension in some patients. They cautioned that even mild hypothyroidism might be associated with an increased risk of such complications.[81]

Role of Adrenergic Receptors in Vascular Resistance and Blood Flow in Hypothyroidism

Park et al. found that increasing concentrations of both T_4 and T_3 produced vasodilation in rat skeletal muscle resistance arteries. T_3 was more potent than T_4. They wrote that the modest vasodilatory effect accounts for the cardiovascular actions of thyroid hormone when administered to patients during cardiac surgery.[51] Zwaveling et al.[53] tested the direct relaxant effects of thyroid hormones on mesenteric resistance vessels. Both the L- and D-isomers of T_4 and T_3 induced blood vessel relaxation, but the T_4 isomers were more potent.

In hypothyroidism, the reduced density of β-adrenergic receptors on blood vessels decreases circulation.[39] The increased density of α-adrenergic receptors on blood vessels contributes to the decreased circulation. The smooth muscle of blood vessels that supply skeletal muscles has both $β_2$- and α-adrenergic receptors. In contrast, the smooth muscle of the blood vessels of the skin has α-adrenergic receptors almost exclusively. Stimulation of α-adrenergic receptors causes the smooth muscle of blood vessels to contract. The contraction reduces blood through the vessels. Stimulation of $β_2$-adrenergic receptors on blood vessels abolishes the vasoconstriction induced by stimulation of α-adrenergic receptors.[38,p.190] In other words, the blood vessels in skeletal muscles do not dilate except in reversing the constriction induced by α-adrenergic receptors.[38,p.199] Administering T_3 reduces the resistance of peripheral blood vessels. However, administering the α-adrenergic receptor stimulant phenylephrine prevents the reduction in resistance otherwise induced by T_3.[54] This shows that α-adrenergic dominance increases peripheral vascular resistance. The increased resistance decreases tissue blood flow.

Norepinephrine has little effect on $β_2$-adrenergic receptors, but it is a potent activator of α-adrenergic receptors. Because the number of β-adrenergic receptors is decreased in hypothyroidism and norepinephrine levels may be increased, α-adrenergic function dominates. As a result, blood flow through both the skeletal muscle and skin is reduced.[38,p.199]

A combined population of $α_1$- and $α_2$-adrenergic receptors mediates the constriction of arteries. The receptors reside on the vascular side of the junctions of sympathetic nerves and blood vessels.[20,p.131] When researchers administered catecholamines at the junctions, the catecholamines traveled some distance from the nerve/vessel junctions and acted as pressors, inducing vasoconstriction. However, administering $α_1$- and $α_2$-adrenergic receptor blockers first mitigated or blocked the vasoconstriction induced by the catecholamine. Inducing the release of norepinephrine by stimulating sympathetic nerves also induced vasoconstriction. But first administering an $α_1$-adrenergic receptor blocker diminished the vasoconstriction induced by norepinephrine release. The investigators reached two conclusions from these observations: (1) α-adrenergic receptors at the junction of sympathetic nerves and arteries are of the $α_1$-subtype, and (2) the receptors located away from the junction are of the $α_2$-subtype.[12] Other studies support these conclusions.[13][14][15]

$α_1$-Adrenergic receptors maintain vascular tone by

interacting with endogenous norepinephrine released by sympathetic nerves at the junctions of sympathetic nerves and blood vessels. α_2-Adrenergic receptors are located some distance from the junction of sympathetic nerve and blood vessels. Since norepinephrine is released from sympathetic nerve terminals, the catecholamine must travel some distance before binding to and activating α_2-adrenergic receptors.[20,p.132] The norepinephrine reuptake pump on sympathetic nerve terminals is efficient and keeps the amount of norepinephrine in the synapses low. The pump also minimizes diffusion of norepinephrine toward the distant α_2-adrenergic receptors.[13] During stress, however, the amount of norepinephrine secreted by nerve endings may be great enough to exceed the capacity of the reuptake pump. The residual may reach α_2-adrenergic receptors and activate them.

Langer and Shepperson suggested that rather than responding to norepinephrine secreted by distant sympathetic nerve endings, α_2-adrenergic receptors bind epinephrine delivered by the circulation. Normally, the level of circulating norepinephrine is well below that necessary to produce physiological effects.[14] During stress, however, norepinephrine levels may rise high enough to reach and activate α_2-adrenergic receptors stationed on blood vessels.[16] When circulating catecholamine levels are high enough, the catecholamines activate α_2-adrenergic receptors. The receptor activation constricts blood vessels, increasing total peripheral vascular resistance. Activation of the receptors by chronically high catecholamine levels may contribute to pathophysiological states such as hypertension and congestive heart failure.[17][18][19]

The exacerbation of fibromyalgia status after cognitive activation stress and vigorous exercise[69,p.67] may also be explained by high catecholamine levels interacting with an increased density of α_2-adrenergic receptors on cell membranes. Bennett et al. reported an increased count of α_2-adrenergic receptors on the platelets of fibromyalgia patients.[67] Patients are likely to have an increased density of the receptors on the cell membranes of other tissues. During emotional stress and exercise, the amount of norepinephrine secreted by sympathetic nerves at the junctions of nerves and blood vessels may exceed the amount the reuptake pump can recover. This would leave residual norepinephrine to spread to distant α_2-adrenergic receptors on blood vessels. In addition, an increased amount of the epinephrine delivered by blood vessels would reach the receptors. Activation of α_2-adrenergic receptors slows metabolic processes in cells that are essential for adapting to stresses. For a time after the increased lev-

els of catecholamines bind to the α_2-adrenergic receptors on cell membranes, the patient may undergo a metabolic crisis with a severe worsening of fibromyalgia symptoms.

Treatment with Thyroid Hormone. Fibromyalgia patients improve with thyroid hormone therapy as a component of a more comprehensive regimen of metabolic rehabilitation. This is true of both hypothyroid and thyroid hormone resistant fibromyalgia patients. Honeyman-Lowe, Garrison, and I have found this in extensive independent clinical experience, and our clinical experience has been confirmed in systematic open trials,[73][74][75] a 1-to-5 year follow-up,[76] and several blinded studies.[77][78][79] Observations of patients suggest that their improvement is based partly on increased blood flow. This is evident in patients whose previous cold intolerance and cold skin become normal with metabolic rehabilitation involving thyroid hormone therapy. Reports by other researchers support this view. For example, Gledhill et al. studied 9 patients with Raynaud's phenomenon. Somatic neuropathy was indicated in 8 of the patients by clinical evidence and 9 patients by electrophysiological evidence. They used 3 measures of heart rate and 2 measures of blood pressure (a total of 45 measures for the group of 9 patients). The patients' use of T_3 improved their autonomic function. Before treatment, 24 of the 45 measures (53%) were abnormal, and after treatment, 5 of 40 tests (12.5%) were abnormal. The investigators conjectured that the T_3 corrected autonomic dysfunction in the patients by increasing blood flow to ischemic peripheral nerves or by directly acting on the autonomic system. Evidence I present in this chapter suggests that T_3 could have acted through both proposed mechanisms to improve blood supply and provide clinical improvement in the patients' symptoms, heart rate, and blood pressure.

Blood Changes in Hypothyroidism

Some changes in blood measures of chronic fatigue syndrome patients match those of hypothyroid patients. At least one measured change reportedly found in fibromyalgia/chronic fatigue syndrome patients does not match.

Similar Blood Findings Between Patients with Chronic Fatigue Syndrome and Hypothyroidism. The low red cell mass, plasma volume, and total blood volume Streeten and Bell found in chronic fatigue syndrome patients[116] can be explained by inadequate thyroid hormone regulation of red blood cell formation (erythropoiesis) and cardiovascular function.

Thyrotoxic patients have an increase in red blood

cell production, red cell mass, and plasma volume.[117,p.786] In contrast, about a third or more of hypothyroid patients are anemic,[118][119][120] and a quarter of the patients have reduced red cell mass.[121,pp.1023-1024] They also have low plasma volume[121,p.1023] and low total blood volume.[115] These blood-related findings in hypothyroidism match those in chronic fatigue syndrome patients reported by Streeten and Bell.[116]

The decreased red cell mass and the anemia in hypothyroidism appear to result from a reduction in erythropoietin levels. Erythropoietin (also termed erythropoietic hormone or hematopoietin) is a protein that increases red cell production by bone marrow. Erythropoietin production increases when the oxygen requirement of tissues increases. This occurs during thyrotoxicosis. The increase in erythropoietin results in an increase in circulating red blood cells which delivers more oxygen to the hypermetabolic tissues. During hypothyroidism, the metabolic rate of tissues decreases, and their oxygen requirement correspondingly decreases. As a result, erythropoietin levels decrease, and in turn, red cell production decreases.[122][123][124] The rate of red cell production may be reduced enough to result in anemia.[120] The anemia may be obscured by low plasma volume.[121,p.1023]

Bleeding Time, Brusing, and Decreased Coagulability in Hypothyroidism. Hypothyroid patients may have a decrease in platelet adhesiveness, an increase in bleeding time, and easy bruising.[125][121,p.1023][138]

Zeigler et al. reported the case of a hypothyroid patient who had profuse bleeding following a tooth extraction. She had a prolonged aspirin bleeding time and reduced retention of platelets on glass beads. They subsequently studied 12 other hypothyroid patients who were taking no medications. Following the ingestion of aspirin, most patients had a subnormal thrombin-induced platelet serotonin release. They wrote that the effects of aspirin on bleeding in these patients might account for the easy bruising and menorrhagia in hypothyroid patients.[138]

Masunaga et al. reported that in hypothyroid patients, administering collagen induced an increase in platelet aggregation.[142] However, more researchers have reported a decrease in platelet aggregation in untreated hypothyroidism. O'Regan and Fong reported that hypothyroid rats had subnormal platelet aggregation.[144] Sjoberg et al. also reported that hypothyroidism in rats resulted in decreased platelet aggregation. They found that administering T$_4$ to 23-week-old hypothyroid rats for 28 days relieved the decreased aggregation and caused a rapid increase in platelet

count.[140]

As in rats, hypothyroidism in humans reduces platelet aggregation. Lazurova et al., for example, tested platelet aggregation in 10 controls and 17 primary hypothyroid patients before and after T$_4$ therapy. Before treatment, hypothyroid patients had reduced aggregation compared to controls. Of the 17 hypothyroid patients, 11 (65%) had reduced aggregation. After treatment, aggregation increased in 7 of the 11 patients (63%). Reduced aggregation continued in 4 patients. It is possible that aggregation would also have increased in these 4 patients with one of two conditions: (1) adjusting T$_4$ dosages according to peripheral indices rather than thyroid function test results, or (2) treating with desiccated thyroid or T$_3$ alone rather than T$_4$.[141]

Edson et al. reported that 12 of 16 hypothyroid patients had low platelet adhesiveness (measured as platelet retention in a glass bead column). In one other patient, adhesiveness was borderline normal. Treatment with T$_4$ increased platelet adhesiveness in 6 patients. The researchers concluded that patients with untreated hypothyroidism have coagulation factor deficiencies.[145]

Myrup et al. noted reports of a bleeding tendency in hypothyroidism that is similar to that in von Willebrand's disease. (Synonyms for von Willebrand's are "angiohemophilia" and "vascular hemophilia"; von Willebrand's is a hemorrhagic disease. Patients have normal blood clot retraction, but their bleeding time is prolonged. They bleed mainly from mucous membranes. Their platelet counts are usually normal, but the platelets may be structurally defective.) The investigators tested 10 hyperthyroid patients and 9 hypothyroid patients. Patients with untreated hypothyroidism had a prolonged bleeding time, although they had a shortened maximum time to platelet agglutination. Myrup et al. concluded that diminished arrest of bleeding (hemostasis) is a general feature of hypothyroidism, but hemostasis usually becomes normal after T$_4$ treatment.[143]

The Hypothesis of Hypercoagulability in Fibromyalgia. Berg et al. reported that fibromyalgia patients have hypercoagulable state[137] (see subsection above titled "Hypercoagulability in Fibromyalgia Patients"). The report appears inconsistent with the hypothesis that inadequate thyroid hormone regulation of cell function underlies most patients' fibromyalgia. Several methodological problems raise doubt that we can extrapolate the findings in their patients to fibromyalgia patients in general.

The first methodological problem is that Berg et

al. did not describe in their report the method the researchers used to identify fibromyalgia patients for inclusion in the study. The only indication of selection criteria was the statement that some of the immune-mediated symptoms included "headache, pelvic pain, and fatigue." Without selection criteria, we cannot be sure that 12 of the patients in the study reported to have fibromyalgia met any generally-accepted criteria for the condition. Second, although most patients in the study had abnormal test results, we do not know that these results were related to the symptoms of "headache, pelvic pain, and fatigue." This uncertainty relates to a third methodological problem: The researchers did not report any objective methods for assessing patients' initial fibromyalgia status, their post-treatment status, and any quantitative difference between the two. Without such assessment methods, the researchers' and/or patients' expectations may have influenced their judgment of post-treatment improvement.

In addition to these methodological problems, I doubt on theoretical grounds that a significant percentage of fibromyalgia patients at-large have hypercoagulation. My reason for this conjecture is another conjecture—that most fibromyalgia patients have either thyroid hormone deficiency or cellular resistance to thyroid hormone. If this is true, a significant percentage of fibromyalgia patients are likely to have blood abnormalities that conflict with the hypercoagulation hypothesis. A significant percentage of fibromyalgia patients are likely to have abnormalities of blood measures similar to those described in the beginning to this subsection (see subsection immediately above titled "Bleeding Time, Brusing, and Decreased Coagulability in Hypothyroidism").

Finally, I am aware of no plausible mechanism by which hypercoagulation would underlie most of the well-documented symptoms and objective findings in fibromyalgia that I have included in Section III of this book.

Cardiovascular Effects of Hyperthyroidism

Excessive thyroid hormone stimulation has cardiovascular effects that are largely opposite from those of hypothyroidism. These effects of hyperthyroidism in part show the impact on cardiovascular function of an increased density of β-adrenergic receptors and a decreased density of α-adrenergic receptors. In thyrotoxicosis, systemic vascular resistance is lower than normal.[55][56]

Hyperthyroidism usually increases contractile strength of the heart muscle, increases cardiac output, and reduces systemic vascular resistance.[81] Hyperthyroid patients have a rapid heart rate and increased stroke volume. The more rapid heart rate and larger stroke volume increase the amount of blood projected through the tissues. It is commonly believed that in hyperthyroidism, despite an increased cardiac output, blood flow remains constant in the liver and cerebrum but blood flow increases in coronary arteries, skin, and skeletal muscles.[59][60][61]

Administering T_3 causes a more rapid reduction in resistance to blood flow than does hyperthyroidism. The rapidly reduced resistance probably results from local tissue formation of lactic acid or a direct vasodilatory action of T_3 on the smooth muscle of blood vessels.[58,p.609] Administering T_3 causes a decrease in coronary artery resistance and increases coronary blood flow.[62] Administering T_3 to animals also causes a rapid reduction of systemic vascular resistance. The reduction of resistance to blood flow occurs before the increase in heart rate or force of contraction.[57] The reduced resistance increases blood flow in many organs. The increased flow provides for the increased need for oxygen and metabolic substrates.

Some thyrotoxic patients are at risk for "high output" cardiac decompensation. Their thyrotoxicosis may trigger arrhythmias. Even patients with mild or subclinical hyperthyroidism may develop complications.[81]

Reduced Cerebral Blood Flow

Three factors related to inadequate regulation by thyroid hormone plausibly explain the reduced brain blood flow of fibromyalgia patients. The first factor is inadequate thyroid hormone regulation of transcription of the adrenergic genes. The inadequate regulation would result in an increase in the density of α-adrenergic receptors and a decrease in the density of β-adrenergic receptors on cerebral arterioles. Activation of the α-adrenergic receptors would induce cerebral vasoconstriction. Activation of β-adrenergic receptors causes dilation of arterioles. The low density of β-adrenergic receptors would result in a failure of dilation to counterbalance the vasoconstriction induced by the high density of α-adrenergic receptors. The vasoconstriction would militate against the autoregulatory mechanism for increasing local blood flow when the circulation fails to deliver enough nutrients to meet the need of brain tissue (see section above titled "Blood Flow to Individual Tissues: Autoregulation of Blood Flow").

The second factor related to inadequate regulation

by thyroid hormone is reduced secretion by nerve terminals of the vasodilator nitric oxide. The third factor is an increase of calcium ions in the cytoplasm of the smooth muscle cells that line the arterioles. The increased calcium concentration results in a sustained vasocontriction of the arterioles. I discuss these two mechanisms in the subsection below titled "Nitric Oxide and Thyroid Hormone."

Normally, cerebral blood flow increases in response to an elevated carbon dioxide blood level[36] or a low oxygen blood level.[37] The increased blood flow serves a compensatory function—it reduces the carbon dioxide concentration and raises the oxygen concentration. However, whether the cerebral blood flow increases appropriately in response to a high carbon dioxide or low oxygen level critically depends on the three factors I discussed in the two paragraphs above. If thyroid hormone is not properly regulating the adrenergic genes, not stimulating nitric oxide release, and not keeping the arteriolar muscle cell calcium concentration low enough, blood flow will not increase sufficiently to meet even the reduced nutrient needs of hypometabolic brain cells. (See the subsection below titled "α-Adrenergic Receptors on Cerebral Arteries," the subsection titled "Vasodilation in the Cerebral Cortex is Mediated in Part by Nitric Oxide," and the subsection titled "Reduced Nitric Oxide Availability and Increased α_2-Adrenergic Activity: Combined Inhibiting Effect on Hypoxia-Induced Vasodilation in the Cerebral Cortex.")

The superior sympathetic ganglion may also contribute to the reduced flow, but for the most part, this source of sympathetic stimulation functions only to raise blood pressure during severe cerebral ischemia (see the section above titled "Central Nervous System Ischemic Response"). However, if the three factors discussed above induce cerebral ischemia or near-ischemia, the superior cervical sympathetic ganglia may activate. If so, the catecholamines the sympathetic nerve endings secrete in the brain will bind to the high density of α-adrenergic receptors on cerebral arterioles and may induce more severe vasoconstriction. In fact, increased sympathetic innervation of cerebral arterioles containing a high density of α-adrenergic receptors may partly explain the exacerbation of fibromyalgia symptoms by strenuous exercise.

In one study, the mean level of the metabolite of norepinephrine in the cerebrospinal fluid of fibromyalgia patients was low.[101] The reduced norepinephrine level may result from an increased density of α_2-adrenergic receptors on noradrenergic nerve endings in the central nervous system. These presynaptic receptors inhibit norepinephrine release by the nerve endings. (See Chapter 3.1, subsection titled "Release of Norepinephrine from Neuronal Vesicles" and the section titled "Types of Adrenergic Receptors that Mediate Catecholamine Release.") The reduced norepinephrine secretion might minimize vasoconstriction of cerebral arterioles, but a predominance of α-adrenergic receptors on the vessels would result in a tonic vasoconstriction (see Glossary) even with subnormal exposure to norepinephrine.

High Brain Requirement for Blood Flow and Oxygen. An extreme reduction of cerebral blood flow and oxygen supply can impair the function of brain cells. If the reduced blood flow and oxygen supply are extreme enough, brain cells die. Brain cells are more vulnerable to damage from reduced blood flow than are cells of other body tissues. The greater vulnerability of brain cells is due to their higher metabolic rate. Because brain cells have a higher metabolic rate than peripheral tissue cells, their requirement for metabolic substrates, such as oxygen and energy-yielding nutrients, is higher than the requirements of other body cells.

The brain makes up only about 2% of body weight. Despite this, the brain receives some 15% of cardiac output, and it consumes about 20% of the body's oxygen at rest.[1,pp.282-284][82,p.1044] In relation to the size of the rest of body, the percentage of the body's oxygen supply consumed by brain cells is disproportionately high. The general metabolic rate of gray matter is roughly 4 times that of white matter.[66,p.681] (Gray matter consists mostly of cell bodies of neurons, and white matter consists mostly of the myelinated tracts of nerve fibers.) The gray cerebral cortex consumes about 8 times the oxygen consumed by the white matter below the cortex.[1,pp282-284] These findings suggest that gray matter of the brain (the nerve cell bodies) is more vulnerable to a reduced oxygen supply when cerebral blood flow is subnormal. This is consistent with the high incidence of cognitive dysfunction among fibromyalgia patients (see Chapter 3.10).

Reduced Cerebral Blood Flow in Hypothyroidism. Each individual tissue in the body adjusts its blood flow through local mechanisms to meet its metabolic requirements.[66,p.185] In hypothyroidism and thyroid hormone resistance, tissue metabolism is subnormal. The lower metabolic rate diminishes local circulation in each tissue according to its individual metabolic rate. In hypothyroidism, blood flow through the kidneys and cerebrum decreases, but the reduction in blood flow is more modest than in most peripheral tissues.[2][63][64] That reduction in blood flow is more modest in the brain is consistent with the brain's higher metabolic rate than that of peripheral tissues (see the subsection immediately above titled "High Brain Requirement for Blood Flow and Oxygen").

In sufficiently severe hypothyroidism, however, arteriolar resistance to blood flow in the brain may markedly increase. As a result, cerebral blood flow will substantially decrease. A study by Lefauconnier et al. showed the potential magnitude of the reduction in brain blood flow in hypothyroid rats. The researchers chemically induced hypothyroidism in rats the 1st day after their birth. At the 16th day after birth, cerebral blood flow in the rats was 50% lower than normal. Blood flow was lowest in the cerebellum. The brain plasma volume was 30% below normal.[113]

The reduced brain blood flow in hypothyroidism decreases the delivery of oxygen and glucose to cerebral tissues by blood vessels. As a result, the cells' consumption of oxygen and other metabolic substrates decreases.[2][3,p.170] In some patients, the decreased quantity of nutrients that reach brain cells through the diminished blood flow may be sufficient to meet the metabolic needs of the hypometabolic cells. Hypometabolic cells have a reduced requirement for nutrients. However, in some hypothyroid patients, the density of α-adrenergic receptors on cerebral blood vessels may be greatly increased (see subsection below titled "α-Adrenergic Receptors on Cerebral Arteries"). If the α-adrenergic receptor density is high enough, vasoconstriction is likely to be severe, resulting in extremely reduced blood flow. In turn, the vascular delivery of nutrients to the hypometabolic brain cells may fall short of meeting even their reduced needs. The nutrient deficit can have profoundly adverse effects on brain cells, even though the reduction in blood flow is more modest in the brain than in most other tissues. The adverse effects may occur despite the strong homeostatic mechanisms that work to maintain normal brain function.[2][63][64]

Several reports show the potential adverse effects of reduced brain blood flow in hypothyroid humans.[70] Kinuya and colleagues reported the case of a 69-year-old man with hypothyroid dementia. The hypothyroidism and the dementia were caused by radioactive iodine therapy and an overdose of methimazole (a drug that inhibits the synthesis of thyroid hormones in the thyroid gland). A SPECT scan showed that the hypothyroid patient had diffuse subnormal blood perfusion of the brain. The blood flow was 25%-to-26% below normal. When therapeutic efforts returned the patient's TSH and thyroid hormone levels to normal, his hypothyroid dementia disappeared and a SPECT scan showed normal blood perfusion of his brain. Kinuya et al. wrote that this was the first report in which brain imaging with SPECT showed reversible subnormal brain blood flow associated with hypothyroid dementia.[112] Tanaka et al. reported the case of a hypothyroid patient with cerebellar ataxia. Blood flow through the patient's cerebellum and the rate of oxygen metabolism within it were subnormal.[114]

Forchetti et al. reported the case of a 59-year-old woman with encephalopathy due to *subclinical* hypothyroidism—the mildest of laboratory-confirmed thyroid hormone deficiencies. Her SPECT scan revealed global subnormal blood perfusion of her brain. Forchetti et al. found that the woman had autoimmune thyroiditis and rapidly progressive dementia. The clinicians diagnosed Hashimoto's encephalopathy based on three findings: (1) an elevated TSH, (2) an abnormal EEG, and (3) clinical improvement and normalization of her SPECT scan after she began thyroid hormone replacement therapy. Forchette et al. suggested that the low blood perfusion of her brain was the mechanism of the encephalopathy.[70] This case appears to represent a severe selective involvement of the brain in thyroid hormone deficiency. Apparently, the woman lacked the tightly regulated homeostatic mechanisms that normally provide some protection of the brain during hypothyroidism. (The description of this patient's encephalopathy resembles that given by Goldstein of chronic fatigue syndrome patients based on neuropsychological testing. See the section above titled "Decreased Brain Blood Flow in Fibromyalgia.")

Reduced Cerebral Blood Flow in Fibromyalgia. In fibromyalgia patients who have hypothyroidism and/or cellular resistance to thyroid hormone, reduced cerebral blood flow is likely to result from the same mechanisms as in other hypothyroid patients (see the section above titled "Reduced Cerebral Blood Flow" and the subsection above titled "Reduced Cerebral Blood Flow in Hypothyroidism").

α-Adrenergic Receptors on Cerebral Arteries. Memory problems and other cognitive disturbances may accompany reduced cerebral blood flow.[82,p.1047] It is highly probable that the reduced cerebral blood flow of fibromyalgia/chronic fatigue syndrome patients is a major contribution to their cognitive dysfunction (see Chapter 3.10).

As I described in the section above titled "Reduced Cerebral Blood Flow," cerebral arterioles normally change their diameter to protect the brain from deficient circulation. In response to a rise in systemic blood pressure, cerebral arterioles constrict; in response to a fall in system pressure, the arteries dilate. These arterial adjustments normally assure a constant flow of blood to the cerebrum. Also, a rise in arterial carbon dioxide levels causes the cerebral arterioles to dilate, resulting in an increase of blood flow through the brain. A fall in arterial carbon dioxide levels normally causes cerebral blood vessels to constrict, resulting in decreased blood flow through the brain.[82,p.1044] (See section above titled "The Central Nervous System Ischemic Response.")

In view of these protective mechanisms, the reduced cerebral blood flow of fibromyalgia patients must involve underlying abnormalities that potently resist the protective mechanisms. An increased density of α-adrenergic receptors on cerebral arterioles is one likely mechanism. α_2-Adrenergic receptor agonists, upon binding to α_2-adrenergic receptors, induce vasoconstriction. Administering α_2-adrenergic receptor blockers prevents vasoconstriction in response to norepinephrine.[20,pp.139-140]

Cerebral blood vessels have widespread sympathetic innervation.[8] Compared to peripheral vessels, however, cerebral vessels exhibit a minimal response to α-adrenergic receptor-mediated sympathetic nerve stimulation.[9] The lower-magnitude response may be due to lower density of α-adrenergic receptors on cerebral vessels or a lower sensitivity of the receptors to catecholamines.[10] Another explanation may be that the high metabolic rate of brain tissue produces metabolic products that strongly sustain cerebral vasodilation. Regardless, the sympathetic nervous system does modulate cerebral blood flow through the mediation of α-adrenergic receptors.[11]

Researchers have found binding sites for blockers of both α_1-adrenergic receptors (prazosin) and α_2-adrenergic receptors (yohimbine) in human and monkey cerebral arteries. α_2-Adrenergic receptor binding sites have been identified in dog and cow cerebral arteries. A predominance of α_2-adrenergic receptor binding sites has been found in cats. The regulatory role of α-adrenergic receptors in cerebral arterial circulation may decrease as vascular diameter decreases. For example, the reactivity of the vertebral and carotid arteries of the rat to norepinephrine decreases markedly just proximal to the transit of the vessels into the subarachnoid space.[6] Because of this, the arteries most extensively regulated by adrenergic receptors may be the large ones such as the basilar and middle cerebral arteries.[7] Constriction of these larger arteries rather than lower caliber arteries might result in more severely reduced brain blood flow in response to the binding of norepinephrine to α-adrenergic receptors.

Vasodilation in the Choroid Plexuses is Mediated in Part by α-Adrenergic Receptors. Williams et al. assessed the response of blood flow through the choroid plexuses (see Glossary) of rats during elevated carbon dioxide blood levels (hypercapnia). The researchers induced high arterial carbon dioxide levels by having the rats breathe a mixture of 5%-to-8% carbon dioxide in air. In rats with high arterial carbon dioxide, blood flow in the cerebral cortex increased by 67%. Blood flow in the choroid plexuses was similar in three groups of rats: those with (1) normal carbon dioxide levels, (2) elevated carbon dioxide levels, and (3) normal carbon dioxide levels and simultaneous treatment with phentolamine (an α_1- and α_2-adrenergic receptor blocker). However, in rats that received the α-adrenergic receptor blocker and were then subjected to high carbon dioxide levels, blood flow increased by 26% in the choroid plexuses of the lateral, third, and fourth ventricles. This result suggests that activation of α-adrenergic receptors prevents an increase in blood flow through the choroid plexuses in response to high carbon dioxide levels. But when the receptors are blocked, elevated carbon dioxide levels increase the flow of blood to the plexuses.[36] These results suggest that the normal function of α-adrenergic receptors in the choroid plexuses is to maintain a relative degree of vasoconstriction, even in the presence of levels of carbon dioxide that otherwise would cause vasodilation.

Vasodilation in the Cerebral Cortex is Mediated in Part by α_2-Adrenergic Receptors. A question of interest regarding fibromyalgia is whether treatment with an α-adrenergic receptor agonist decreases blood flow through the choroid plexuses. If so, this would suggest that an increased density of α-adrenoceptors due to inadequate thyroid hormone transcription regulation of the α-adrenoceptor gene might account for reduced blood flow in some fibromyalgia patients.

McPherson et al. tested the effects of α-adrenergic receptor stimulation on cerebral blood flow.[37] They measured changes in cerebral blood flow in dogs with normal blood oxygen levels after treatment with an α_2-adrenergic receptor agonist (dexmedetomidine). Administering the agonist reduced cerebral blood flow to 54±8 mL-1 x 100 g-1. When hypoxia was induced, cerebral blood flow increased to 97±14 mL min-1 x 100 g-1. In control dogs not treated with the α_2-adrenoceptor agonist, hypoxia increased cerebral blood flow from 83±4 to 210±30 mL min-1 x 100 g-1 in one trial, and in another from 88±7 to 205±27 mL min-1 x 100 g-1. The investigators concluded that when blood oxygen levels are normal, the α_2-adrenoceptor agonist decreased cerebral O_2 transport (cerebral blood flow x arterial O_2 content). They noted, however, that during hypoxia, the increase in cerebral blood flow, despite treatment with the α_2-adrenoceptor agonist, was sufficient to maintain oxygen levels within the normal range for cerebral blood flow.

Implications for Fibromyalgia. It is reasonable to expect that the reduced cerebral blood flow in fibromyalgia patients results from a (1) predominance of α-adrenergic receptors on cerebral arterioles due to inadequate thyroid hormone regulation of transcription of the adrenergic genes, in combination with (2) subnormal nitric oxide release, and (3) excessive calcium in arteriolar smooth muscle cells. These same putative vasoconstrictive factors also make it reasonable to expect that the resulting low brain blood perfusion will persist despite the use of vasodilating medications. Persistence of low perfusion due to a predominance of α-adrenergic receptors on cerebral arteries might account for a report by Goldstein. According to him, medications that increase cerebral blood flow lessen the severity of patients' symptoms but do not reliably improve symptoms.[83,p.116] It is likely that a predominance of α-adrenergic receptors on cerebral arteries due to inadequate thyroid hormone regulation of the adrenergic genes (if the inadequate regulation persists) would outlast the beneficial effects of blood flow-increasing medications. α-Adrenergic receptor-induced vasoconstriction might also account for Goldstein's report that the α_2-adrenergic receptor blocker yohimbine improved the status of some of his patients.[69,p.63] It may explain his report that β-blockers,[83,p.241] including propranolol,[83,242] were of no benefit to his patients.

Goldstein wrote that he and Day found that after exercise, chronic fatigue syndrome patients did not have the expected elevations of cortisol, catecholamines, and growth hormone. He also wrote, "most surprising of all, core temperature did not change, and sometimes even went down!"[69,p.88] These findings, however—including the failure of body temperature to rise, and even to decline—are directly predictable from α-adrenergic dominance on cell membranes due to inadequate thyroid hormone regulation of the adrenergic genes. During exercise of sufficient intensity, more catecholamines are released. As more catecholamines reach cells and bind to α-adrenergic receptors on their membranes, energy metabolism within the cells will decrease. The inhibited metabolism would prevent the rise in temperature that normally occurs when catecholamines bind to β-adrenergic receptors on cell membranes during exercise (see Chapter 3.4, section titled "Impaired Aerobic and Anaerobic Metabolism in Fibromyalgia: Possible Effect of Increased

α- and Decreased β-Adrenergic Receptors"). The reduced regional cerebral blood flow in fibromyalgia/chronic fatigue syndrome patients during the stresses of exercise and cognitive activation[69,p.67] is also predictable largely from an increase in catecholamine binding to a predominance of α-adrenergic receptors on blood vessels.

Low Nitric Oxide Levels in Fibromyalgia. Eisinger reported low levels of the vasodilator nitric oxide in fibromyalgia patients.[157][158] In one study, the mean plasma nitric oxide level of 7 control subjects was 26 ± 11 µmol/mL. In comparison, the mean level in 14 female fibromyalgia patients was only 12 ± 9 µmol/mL.[157] In another study by Eisinger, 28 fibromyalgia patients had a mean plasma nitric oxide level that was significantly below normal values.[158] Low nitric oxide levels can reduce tissue blood flow.

Nitric Oxide and Thyroid Hormone. Low nitric oxide levels in fibromyalgia may result from impaired sympathetic nervous system activity secondary to inadequate thyroid hormone regulation of the adrenergic genes. Increased nitric oxide secretion occurs with higher levels of sympathetic nerve activity. Nitric oxide secretion increases during increased sympathetic nerve activity.[48] Fibromyalgia patients have a tendency toward low muscle sympathetic nerve activity[52] and a blunted sympathetic nervous system response to exercise.[44][45] The blunted sympathetic nervous system activity may cause low nitric oxide levels. The low sympathetic nervous system activity may result from inhibition by α_2-adrenergic receptors due to inadequate thyroid hormone regulation of α-adrenergic genes (see the subsection below titled "Inhibition of Central Centers for Activation of the Sympathetic Nervous System,"and Chapter 3.1).

In addition, reduced exposure of sympathetic nerve endings to thyroid hormone may reduce the release of nitric oxide.[50][51][53] The reduced nitric oxide production due to too little exposure of sympathetic nerves to thyroid hormone may contribute to low nitric oxide levels resulting from blunted sympathetic activity. (See Chapter 3.4, subsection titled "Low Nitric Oxide Levels in Fibromyalgia: Possibly Due to Impaired Sympathetic Function Secondary to Inadequate Thyroid Hormone Regulation.")

At least three isoforms of the enzyme nitric oxide synthase generate nitric oxide. The endothelial isoform is found in vascular endothelial cells. This isoform plays a role in the thyroid hormone-induced relaxation of the smooth muscle lining of arterioles.[50]

Thyroid hormone relaxes vascular smooth muscle by inhibiting Ca^{2+}-induced vascular contractions. (By activating membrane Ca^{2+}-ATPase through a non-genomic effect, thyroid hormone increases Ca^{2+} efflux from cells. The reduced cytoplasmic concentration of Ca^{2+} favors muscle relaxation. See Chapter 2.2, subsection titled "Thyroid Hormone, Membrane Ca^{2+}-ATPase Activity, and the Cell Content of Calcium.") Incubation with a nitric oxide inhibitor impaired the vascular relaxant effect of thyroid hormone. This finding suggests that thyroid hormone increases production of endothelium-derived nitric oxide. The investigators concluded that thyroid hormone indirectly relaxes vascular smooth muscle by stimulating nitric oxide production by the endothelium. They also concluded that thyroid hormone directly relaxes the muscle through increasing calcium flux. Thyroid hormone induced this direct effect, however, only at supraphysiologic concentrations of thyroid hormone (about 100 times basal levels). Because supraphysiologic doses were necessary, the investigators concluded that the direct effect on mesenteric vascular smooth muscle cells is not relevant under physiological conditions.[53]

Park et al. concluded that thyroid hormone has a "modest" vasodilating effect. When they induced vasodilation with isoproterenol (a β-adrenergic receptor stimulant), the resulting vasodilation (56%±6%) exceeded that induced by T_3 (36%±9%) and T_4 (24%±6%).[51] When thyroid hormone inadequately regulates transcription of the β- and α-adrenergic receptor genes, α-adrenergic receptors predominate on cell membranes, overriding β-isoform mediated functions. When vascular smooth muscle is affected, vasoconstriction results. If inadequate thyroid hormone regulation also disinhibits Ca^{2+}-induced vascular contractions, vasoconstriction induced α-adrenergic receptor dominance may be enhanced.

Vasodilation in the Cerebral Cortex is Mediated in Part by Nitric Oxide. McPherson et al. conducted a study to learn whether an inhibitor of nitric oxide synthase (the enzyme that increases the synthesis of nitric oxide) would diminish cerebral blood flow in response to hypoxia. They administered a nitric oxide synthase inhibitor (N omega-nitro-L-arginine methyl ester) to dogs. In dogs with normal blood oxygen levels, administering the synthase inhibitor reduced cerebral blood flow (52±2 mL min-1 x 100 g-1). Blood flow in control dogs not given the inhibitor was 83±4 mL min-1 x 100 g-1. In control dogs, hypoxia increased cerebral blood flow from 83±4 to 210±30 mL min-1 x 100 g-1 in one trial, and in another trial from 88±7 to205±27 mL min-1 x 100 g-1. In dogs pretreated with the synthase inhibitor, hypoxia increased

cerebral blood flow only to 177±13 mL min-1 x 100 g-1.[37] Thus, inhibition of nitric oxide production reduced vasodilation in response to low oxygen levels.

Reduced Nitric Oxide Availability and Increased $α_2$-Adrenergic Activity: Combined Inhibiting Effect on Hypoxia-Induced Vasodilation in the Cerebral Cortex. McPherson et al. administered to dogs both the nitric oxide synthase inhibitor and an $α_2$-adrenergic receptor agonist. As shown in Table 3.2.1, when oxygen levels were normal, the combination of the two agents caused the greatest reduction in cerebral blood flow. When oxygen levels were low, the $α_2$-adrenergic receptor agonist caused the greatest reduction in flow.[37]

Each of the two agents reduced cerebral blood flow when blood oxygen levels were normal. The agents also impeded the increase in blood flow in response to hypoxia.[37] I know of no studies of the effects of the nitric oxide inhibitors and α-agonists on cerebral blood flow in humans. It is possible that the effects could be stronger, accounting for the virtual cerebral ischemia in some fibromyalgia and chronic fatigue syndrome patients revealed by SPECT scans.[83,p.177] If $α_2$-adrenoceptor dominance and reduced nitric oxide production are responsible for the reduced brain blood flow in some fibromyalgia patients, the reduced blood flow through the cerebrum may be sufficient to cause some patients' cognitive dysfunction (see Chapter 3.10).

Role of the Superior Cervical Sympathetic Ganglion. Goldstein wrote that the superior cervical ganglion is "the major mediator of cerebral vasoconstriction."[83,p.244] One might assume, if this were true, that deficient neural output of the superior cervical sympathetic ganglion due to inhibition from α-adrenergic receptors would increase cerebral blood flow. However, this is highly unlikely. The superior cervical ganglion innervates both the large superficial cerebral arteries and the smaller arteries that penetrate into brain tissue. However, neither severing nor mildly-to-moderately stimulating the sympathetic nerve fibers induce a significant change in cerebral blood flow. Guyton explained that one reason sympathetic stimulation from the ganglion does not normally regulate cerebral blood flow is that the local brain blood flow autoregulatory mechanism is powerful. It normally completely compensates for sympathetic stimulation. This is not to say, however, that sympathetic stimulation from the ganglion never affects cerebral blood flow; it does under extreme circumstances. For example, when the local autoregulatory mechanism is not able to compensate, as during extreme arterial hypertension during vigorous exercise, the sympathetic nerves from the superior cervical ganglion stimulate large and moderately sized cerebral arteries to constrict. The vasoconstriction prevents the high arterial pressure from reaching the small arteries of the cerebrum.[66,p.680] Part of the reason that strenuous physical activity worsens fibromyalgia symptoms may be the powerful vasoconstriction caused by superior cervical ganglion stimulation of the cerebral arteries containing a predominance of α-adrenergic receptors. However, under non-stressful conditions, an increase of α-adrenergic receptors and reduced nitric oxide release are enough to explain fibromyalgia patients' reduced cerebral blood flow.

Another reason the superior cervical sympathetic ganglia may not serve a greater regulatory role in cerebral blood flow in fibromyalgia patients is a predominance of α_2-adrenergic receptors on the nerve cell bodies in the sympathetic ganglia. The receptors raise their threshold for activation of ganglion cells. As a result, signal outflow from the sympathetic ganglia to the cerebral blood vessels may be subnormal even during severe ischemia.

For the model I propose for reduced blood flow in fibromyalgia, see the section below titled "Model of Reduced Blood Flow and Hypotension in Fibromyalgia."

HYPOTENSION IN HYPOTHYROIDISM

Low blood pressure is divided into two types: chronic constitutional hypotension and hypotension resulting from faulty cardiovascular adjustment mechanisms during changes in posture.[163] The latter condition is referred to as orthostatic hypotension or orthostatic intolerance. Low blood pressure, whether chronic or only orthostatic, is not a disease itself.[163] Instead, it is a consequence of faulty physiological regulatory systems. In the section below, I have included the mechanisms by which thyroid hormone deficiency may cause faults in the regulatory systems that normally control blood pressure (see section titled "Mechanisms of Hypotension in Hypothyroidism").

Inadequate thyroid hormone regulation of gene transcription in hypothyroidism plausibly accounts for both chronic and orthostatic hypotension in fibromyalgia patients. In my clinical experience, the cardiovascular abnormalities of hypothyroid and euthyroid hypometabolic fibromyalgia patients are indistinguishable.

Most hypothyroid patients have either normal or low blood pressure, but some patients' blood pressure is high. The same is true among fibromyalgia patients. What we must ask ourselves in trying to understand either hypotension or hypertension in hypothyroidism or resistance to thyroid hormone is this: What components of the blood pressure regulation systems do inadequate thyroid hormone regulation impair so that the arterial pressure is too low or high? The starting point for understanding this is a familiarity with the regulating mechanisms. I described them in the above section titled "Mechanisms that Normally Regulate Circulation and Control Blood Pressure."

Table 3.2.1. Cerebral blood flow during normal and low blood oxygen levels in four groups of dogs: normal controls, those pretreated with an α_2-adrenergic stimulant, those pretreated with a nitric oxide synthase inhibitor, and those pretreated with a combination of the α_2-adrenergic stimulant and the nitric oxide synthase inhibitor.

CEREBRAL BLOOD FLOW DURING NORMAL AND LOW BLOOD OXYGEN LEVELS		
CONDITION	NORMAL O₂ LEVEL	LOW O₂ LEVEL
Control group	83±4*	210±30
α_2-adrenergic stimulation	54±8	97±14
NO† synthase blockade	52±2	177±13
α_2-adrenergic stimulation + NO synthase blockade	37±3	106±18

*Units: mL min-1 x 100 g-1   †NO=nitric oxide

Hypothyroid Hypotension

Hypothyroid laboratory rats usually have low arterial blood pressure and heart rate.[183][184] Food deprivation also lowers the blood pressure and heart rate of rats but not as much as hypothyroidism does.[183] In extreme hypothyroidism, total body water and extracellular fluid volume increase. However, the blood fluid volume decreases. The reduced blood volume contributes to hypotension.[186,p.872] Compared to control surgery patients, hypothyroid patients have roughly twice the incidence of hypotension during surgery (30% vs 61%).[185] Tachycardia often accompanies hypotension in hypothyroidism,[187] although some patients develop bradycardia.[188] Thyroid hormone replacement improves or relieves the hypotension.[186,p.872] Orthostatic hypotension is a feature of some patients' hypothyroidism.[182]

Sabio et al. found that low blood pressure in hypothyroidism resulted partly from decreased sensitivity to chemicals that normally induce vasoconstriction of the large arteries. In contrast, the aorta of hyperthyroid rats was normally responsive to vasoconstricting chemicals.[71]

Mechanisms of Hypotension in Hypothyroidism

Several possible mechanisms of hypotension in fibromyalgia are related to hypothyroidism or cellular resistance to thyroid hormone. The mechanisms involve inadequate thyroid hormone regulation of the adrenergic genes, the smooth muscle lining of blood vessels, renin and vasopressin secretion, and fibroblast function. In addition, low salt and/or fluid intake, venous pooling, and excessive catecholamine secretion, and the use of antidepressant medications may contribute to the hypotension.

Adrenergic Receptors. Two changes in adrenergic receptors contribute to hypotension in hypothyroidism and cellular resistance to thyroid hormone: (1) a decreased density of β-adrenergic receptors on heart cells and blood vessels, and (2) an increased density of α-adrenergic receptors on blood vessels and cells within the central nervous system nuclei that regulate sympathetic and parasympathetic nervous system activity.

Decreased β-Adrenergic Receptors. As I detailed in Chapter 3.1, inadequate thyroid hormone regulation of the β-adrenergic genes results in a decreased density of these receptors on cell membranes. Dodd and Role wrote that norepinephrine released from post-ganglionic sympathetic nerves binds to β-adrenergic receptors on heart cells. The binding increases the heart rate and force of heart contraction. These effects of norepinephrine are potently reinforced by epinephrine released into the circulation by the adrenal medullae.[177,p.770] When the β-adrenergic receptor count on heart cells is low, decreased heart rate and stroke volume occur during sympathetic stimulation. These effects compound the decreased cardiac output from sympathetic nerve stimulation during hypothyroidism or cellular resistance to thyroid hormone.

Increased α-Adrenergic Receptors. The increase in the density of α₂-adrenergic receptors on the platelets of fibromyalgia patients[67] suggests that they, like hypothyroid and thyroid hormone resistant patients, have inadequate thyroid hormone regulation of the adrenergic genes (see Chapter 3.1). An increased density of α-adrenergic receptors on cells of sympathetic centers in the central nervous system and the paravertebral sympathetic ganglia can cause hypotension.

According to Head and Burke, both central and peripheral administration of α₂-adrenergic receptor agonists, such as norepinephrine and the drug clonidine, induce hypotension and bradycardia.[189] These effects are mediated in part by an increase in prejunctional α₂-adrenoceptor activity in the sympathetic ganglia. The use of clonidine as an α₂-adrenergic receptor agonist has shown that increased α₂-adrenoceptor activity hyperpolarizes sympathetic ganglionic cells.[65][203] One result is subnormal activation of the sympathetic nervous system in response to a fall in blood pressure.

Kooner et al. wrote that clonidine is a presynaptic and postsynaptic α₂-adrenoceptor agonist that lowered blood pressure in normal subjects. The fall in blood pressure after clonidine infusion was accompanied by a reduction in cardiac output (decreased heart rate and stroke volume). Also, the blood vessels of the skin of the subjects' fingers dilated. Plasma norepinephrine levels after clonidine infusion fell substantially in the subjects. Clonidine exerts these sympatholytic effects largely at the supraspinal level and requires intact descending sympathetic nerve pathways. According to Kooner et al., compared to the central nervous system effects, clonidine has only minor effects on spinal preganglionic nerves or peripheral presynaptic α₂-adrenoceptors.[181]

In high doses, the α₂-adrenergic receptor agonist clonidine induces hypotension.[84] When researchers administered α₂-adrenergic receptor agonists (clonidine and rilmenidine) centrally (intracisternally) to rabbits, blood pressure and heart rate decreased by as much as 24%. When administered peripherally, doses of these drugs 25-to-30 times higher were needed to induce substantially decrease blood pressure and heart rate. Hypotension and bradycardia occurred in about 8 minutes after researchers administered the agonists. Chemically destroying central noradrenergic nerve pathways reduced the magnitude of hypotension and bradycardia in response to the two α₂-adrenergic receptor agonists. The reduced magnitude of hypotension and bradycardia suggests that both norepinephrine and α₂-adrenergic receptors were instrumental in the cardiovascular effects of the drugs. The maximum reduction of bradycardia in response to the drugs occurred after 2 weeks with some recovery by 8 weeks. The maximum reduction of hypotension in response to the agonists occurred at 8 weeks. Interestingly, destruction of central serotonergic neurons also attenuated the hypotension and bradycardia induced by rilmenidine and clonidine. The attenuation may have resulted from an indirect effect of serotonin on α₂-adrenergic receptors. Onset of this effect was slower than that from destruction of noradrenergic pathways, reaching maximum in 8 weeks.[189]

The main indication for treatment with selective α_1-adrenergic receptor blocking drugs is vascular hypertension. Adverse effects of the blockers result from excessive vasodilatation. For this reason, α_1-adrenergic blockers are contraindicated for patients who have cardiac or renal failure, a prior history of cerebrovascular incidents, or a tendency toward hypotension.[179] Prazosin is a commonly prescribed anti-hypertensive drug. It lowers peripheral vascular resistance by selectively blocking α_1-adrenergic receptors on the smooth muscle of arterioles.[180] Doxazosin is a long-acting α_1-adrenergic receptor blocker. It is structurally related to prazosin and terazosin. It induces an anti-hypertensive effect by reducing smooth muscle tone of peripheral vascular beds. The reduction in muscle tone decreases total peripheral resistance without a significant effect on heart rate or cardiac output.[178]

α_1-Adrenergic Receptor Inhibition of Renin Secretion. DeLorenzo et al. found that 22 of 78 chronic fatigue syndrome patients had orthostatic hypotension during the head-up tilt test. Eight weeks of salt therapy resulted in a normal follow-up test for 12 of the patients. These 12 patients had normal plasma renin levels. Ten patients still had orthostatic hypotension, despite the salt therapy. These 10 patients had significantly reduced plasma renin levels. The investigators concluded that an abnormal function of the renin-angiotensin-aldosterone system may explain the mechanism underlying orthostatic hypotension and an abnormal response to anti-hypotension treatment.[173]

Some fibromyalgia patients may have orthostatic intolerance due to deficient renin release. When the arterial blood pressure falls beyond a threshold point, the juxtaglomerular cells of the kidney release renin. Renin passes into the blood and causes the release of angiotensin I from a plasma protein, angiotensinogen. Angiotensin I induces mild vasoconstriction. Within seconds, angiotensin I splits to release angiotensin II, a powerful vasoconstrictor. Angiotensin II elevates arterial blood pressure, and to a lesser degree, elevates venous pressure. As the arterial pressure elevates, peripheral resistance increases. Simultaneously, as the venous pressure increases, more blood returns to the heart. The increased return of blood to the heart enables the heart to pump against the increasing pressure. Angiotensin II also reduces the excretion of both salt and water by the kidneys. The reduced excretion increases extracellular fluid volume and helps elevate arterial pressure.[66,pp.211-212][139,p.421] The reduced excre-

tion also keeps urine from accumulating in excess. However, binding of α_1-adrenergic receptors to catecholamines in the juxtaglomerular cells inhibits renin release.[65,p.43] Inhibiting the release of renin may allow the arterial blood pressure to remain low, leaving the patient hypotensive. A predominance of α_1-adrenergic receptors on the juxtaglomerular cells can result from inadequate thyroid hormone regulation of transcription of the adrenergic genes. This mechanism is likely to contribute to hypothyroid hypotension in some patients.

Inhibition of Central Centers for Activation of the Sympathetic Nervous System. Stewart et al. studied children who had chronic fatigue syndrome and neurally mediated hypotension. During the head-up test, heart rate variability was markedly depressed. They wrote that sympathetic nervous system and vagal (parasympathetic nervous system) balance did not properly shift. As a result, during the test, the children had too little sympathetic stimulation of heart rate and excessive parasympathetic stimulation. Also during the test, heart rate variability during fainting was blunted. Stewart et al. concluded that overall, the data suggest autonomic impairment in patients with chronic fatigue syndrome.[168] The deficient sympathetic innervation and excess vagal innervation of the heart may result from inadequate thyroid hormone transcription regulation of the adrenergic genes.

An increase in the density of α-adrenergic receptors on sympathetic nerve cells in the central nervous system and the paravertebral sympathetic ganglia can strongly contribute to hypotension. The nucleus of the solitary tract is one site of action of α_2-adrenergic receptor agonists.[194] Stimulation of α_2-adrenergic receptors in the ventrolateral medulla reduces sympathetic outflow to peripheral parts of the body with reduced arterial blood pressure and bradycardia.[190][191][192][193] Microinjections of the α_2-adrenergic receptor agonist clonidine into the lateral reticular nucleus in the ventrolateral medulla have an anti-hypertensive effect.[195] Since the nucleus is accessible from the ventral surface of the medulla, it serves as a site for the effective local application of α_2-adrenergic receptor agonists.[195][196][197][198] Inhibition of sympathetic nerve cell bodies in these centers inhibits sympathetic nervous system discharge in response to baroreceptor activation during a fall in blood pressure. The inhibited discharge results in a failure of the heart rate and stroke volume to increase in response to a fall in blood pressure.

The sympathetic nerve endings that innervated the heart have presynaptic α_2-adrenergic receptors. Activation of these receptors makes a minor contribution to the low blood pressure and bradycardia that is more potently induced by central α_2-adrenergic activation.[199][200][201][202]

α_2-Adrenergic receptor activation also increases parasympathetic nervous system activity.[20,p.122] α_2-Adrenergic receptors occupy cells in the dorsal vagal nucleus.[204] Activating the receptors with clonidine increases vagal outflow to the periphery.[164] The increase of parasympathetic signals to the heart through the vagus nerves slows the heart rate and decreases stroke volume. The net effect is decreased cardiac output. When extreme enough, these effects resemble the vasovagal phenomenon in which blood pressure drops and the patient experiences fainting or near-fainting. (See subsection above titled "Decreasing Blood Pressure.")

Thyroid hormone regulates gene transcription for corticotropin-releasing hormone (CRH). In hypothyroidism, secretion of CRH by hypothalamic cells is reduced. (See Chapter 3.1, section titled "Subnormal Secretion of Corticotropin-Releasing Hormone.") CRH normally stimulates the locus ceruleus in the brain stem to secrete norepinephrine. CRH also stimulates the central sympathetic system. Deficient secretion of CRH (due to inadequate thyroid hormone regulation of CRH gene transcription) may result in subnormal activation of locus ceruleus cells, resulting in the low norepinephrine levels in the cerebrospinal fluid of fibromyalgia patients.[101] Deficient CRH might also result in subnormal activation of the central sympathetic system. The subnormal activation may contribute to the inadequate sympathetic nervous system response to a drop in blood pressure in fibromyalgia patients.

Inhibition of the sympathetic nervous system due to α-adrenergic receptor-mediated inhibition of brain stem centers and the paravertebral sympathetic ganglia may reduce sympathetic innervation of the kidney arterioles. As a result, the arterioles may not properly constrict when the blood pressure falls. Consequently, too little salt and water would be retained in the blood to increase plasma volume and contribute to a recovery of normal blood pressure. This failure to adapt to a fall in blood pressure would be reinforced by an α-adrenergic receptor inhibition of renin release by the kidney afferent arterioles. In two ways, subnormal renin secretion would contribute to a failure to adapt to an acute fall in blood pressure:[146] (1) angiotensin II would not form and constrict peripheral and kidney blood arterioles, and (2) aldosterone secretion would not increase and stimulate reabsorption of salt and water from the kidney tubules. (See subsection above titled "α_1-Adrenergic Receptor Inhibition of Renin Secretion.") Without constriction of kidney arterioles and exposure of the tubules to aldosterone, circulating salt and water concentrations would remain low. As a result, plasma volume would remain low and fail to counteract the low arterial pressure.

Excessive Connective Tissue Elasticity, Hypermobility, and Orthostatic Intolerance. Rowe et al. described 11 chronic fatigue syndrome patients with orthostatic intolerance who also met the criteria for Ehlers-Danlos syndrome. All the patients responded to orthostatic stress with either postural tachycardia or neurally mediated hypotension. Of the 11 patients, 6 had hypermobility typical of Ehlers-Danlos (see Glossary). Rowe et al. hypothesized that the patients with both orthostatic intolerance and Ehlers-Danlos have excessive elasticity of connective tissues. The hyperelastic connective tissues would permit excessive distension of veins in response to ordinary hydrostatic pressures. The excessive distension would allow more venous pooling than normal. The hemodynamic consequences of the excessive pooling would be hypotension and lightheadedness. The investigators advised clinicians to examine patients with orthostatic intolerance syndromes for inordinately elastic connective tissues and hypermobility.[176]

Hypermobility suggests decreased connective tissue restriction of joint motion, possibly due to collagen and elastic fiber abnormalities. Both abnormalities can result from inadequate thyroid hormone inhibition of fibroblast activity. I detailed the possible mechanisms in Chapter 3.3. (In Chapter 3.3, see the sections titled "Mitral Valve Prolapse" and "Articular Hypermobility" under the section titled "Connective Tissue Abnormalities in Fibromyalgia" and the section titled "Possible Relation of Connective Tissue Abnormalities in Fibromyalgia to Inadequate Thyroid Hormone Regulation of Connective Tissue.") If hyper-elastic connective tissues are involved in orthostatic intolerance in some fibromyalgia/chronic fatigue syndrome patients, inadequate thyroid hormone regulation of fibroblasts may be the underlying mechanism.

Low Salt and/or Fluid Intake, Venous Pooling, and Excessive Catecholamine Secretion. For several decades, health care practitioners have advised the public to restrict salt intake as a method for preventing hypertension. It is possible that this preventive effort has contributed to hypotension and orthostatic intolerance in some individuals.

Calkins and Rowe reported that in uncontrolled studies, treatment intended to correct neurally mediated hypotension improved the hypotensive status of

⅔ of chronic fatigue syndrome patients.[162]

Rowe described the empiric treatment to help control the symptoms of neurally mediated hypotension and orthostatic tachycardia in chronic fatigue syndrome patients. Rowe wrote that neurally mediated hypotension and other orthostatic intolerance syndrome appear to involve three classes of events: (1) conditions that cause inordinate venous pooling (these may include prolonged quiet sitting or standing, increased histamine secretion, or the use of vasodilating medications); (2) low blood volume, possibly due to too little salt and/or fluid intake, the use of diuretics, or high environmental heat; and (3) excess catecholamine secretion, possibly due to the use of adrenergic agonist medications. The empiric treatment appears to work through preventing or providing some degree of correction for these mechanisms. The treatment involves three methods. He advised that patients avoid the three events. To reduce venous pooling, he recommended the use of compression stockings and an abdominal binder. For this purpose, he also recommended activities that increase muscle activity of the legs and raise blood pressure: standing in a crossed leg position, squatting, sitting in a knee-chest position or with the knees higher than the hips, bending forward, or resting a foot on a chair while standing. To increase blood volume, he recommended increased salt ingestion and consumption of at least 2 liters of fluids each day. He also noted that exercise to tolerance may increase plasma and red cell volume. To avoid excessive catecholamines, he recommended that asthma patients use a glucocorticoid inhaler rather than using adrenergic agonists that may activate the vasovagal reflex. As oral agents that may help, he listed fludrocortisone, which expands blood volume, but always with supplemental potassium.[127]

Rowe cautioned that researchers have not conducted controlled studies to learn whether the therapy does more harm than good.[127] Honeyman-Lowe has successfully used the therapy described by Rowe with fibromyalgia patients undergoing metabolic rehabilitation.[128]

Antidepressant Medications. Conventional clinicians often prescribed amitriptyline and other antidepressant medications for fibromyalgia patients (see Chapter 5.1). Besides being ineffective in the treatment of fibromyalgia, amitriptyline may cause adverse effects. Bryson and Wilde wrote that patients using amitriptyline commonly report dry mouth and sedation. These antimuscarinic effects tend to occur even at the low dosages of amitriptyline prescribed to control pain. Also among the potential adverse effects are orthostatic hypotension and tachycardia.[49] Other medical writers have also reported anticholinergic effects and orthostatic hypotension.[46][47]

For the model I propose for hypotension in fibromyalgia, see the section below titled "Model of Reduced Blood Flow and Hypotension in Fibromyalgia."

Hypertension in Hypothyroidism

Hypertension is defined as a systolic or diastolic pressure of 140/90 or higher. Hypertension, is defined as mild when the diastolic pressure is from 90-to-104 mm Hg, moderate when 105-to-114, and severe when over 115. Benign hypertension is the main risk factor for stroke, congestive heart failure, and coronary heart disease. Hypertension is the most common cardiovascular disease in the United States.[87,p.784] More hypothyroid patients have low blood pressure than high blood pressure. Nonetheless, because hypertension is so common, it should not be surprising that some hypothyroid patients, like some fibromyalgia patients, are hypertensive (see section above titled "Hypotension in Hypothyroidism").

Klein et al. listed the potential complications of hypothyroidism as angina pectoris, atrioventricular block, pericarditis, and diastolic hypertension. They wrote that even mild hypothyroidism might be associated with an increased risk of these complications.[81] In older age groups, hypertension is more common in hypothyroid patients than in euthyroid control subjects. Correcting the thyroid hormone deficiency relieves the hypertension in most hypothyroid patients without other therapeutic measures. Most hypothyroid patients share the same hemodynamic status: reduced cardiac output and increased peripheral vascular resistance. This pattern results largely from an increase in the density of α-adrenergic receptors on the cells of the heart and blood vessels.[45]

By contrast, in hyperthyroidism, patients have increased cardiac output and decreased peripheral vascular resistance. However, diastolic hypertension is not common in hyperthyroidism. Systolic hypertension is common in hyperthyroidism, although the prevalence is higher in younger than in older patients. Relieving the hyperthyroidism usually decreases the systolic hypertension without other therapeutic interventions.[45]

In patients using exogenous thyroid hormone, the therapeutic aim should be to achieve an intermediate state in which cardiac output and peripheral resistance are normal.

Hypothyroid Hypertension

Some researchers have reported finding no association between hypothyroidism and hypertension.[98][110] Many other researchers, however, have found an association.[90][91][92][93][94][95][96][97][99][100][102][103][104][105][106][107][108][109][111] They generally refer to the condition as "hypothyroid hypertension" or hypertension secondary to hypothyroidism. Numerous researchers have also reported that replacement dosages of T_4 have lowered the blood pressure of most hypertensive hypothyroid patients.[90][93][94][97][102][103][104] [105][106][107][108] The exact mechanism(s) of hypertension in hypothyroidism is not certain. Researchers have implicated one or more of three possible mechanisms: (1) increased α-adrenergic receptors on systemic arteries, (2) an uncharacteristic hyperactivity of the sympathetic nervous system resulting in elevated catecholamine levels, and (3) dysfunction of the renin-angiotensin-aldosterone system.[90][108] These mechanisms would mainly increase peripheral vascular resistance but would also increase cardiac output.

The use of desiccated thyroid or T_3 alone will most likely increase the therapeutic success rate. I have found that the use of T_3 has lowered the blood pressure of some euthyroid fibromyalgia patients. In most hypothyroid patients who are hypertensive, it is the diastolic pressure that is elevated.[95][104][108] Of 688 consecutive hypertensive patients referred by other clinicians, Streeten et al. found that 25 (3.6%) were hypothyroid. These patients' ceased taking anti-hypertensive medications and normalized their circulating TSH levels and T_4 levels by the use of T_4. As a result, diastolic pressures decreased below 90 mm Hg in 8 patients (32%).[104] In another study, Streeten et al. reported treating 40 thyrotoxic patients with radioiodine to relieve their hyperthyroidism. The treatment significantly increased the diastolic blood pressure to more than 90 mm Hg in 16 (40%). Treatment with T_4 returned the patients' circulating TSH and thyroid hormone levels to within the normal range. As a result, the patients' systolic and diastolic pressures declined. Moreover, the diastolic pressures of 9 of the 16 patients (56%) decreased below 90 mm Hg.[104] Two conditions would likely have increased the percentage of patients whose diastolic pressures became normal: (1) the use of T_3 or desiccated thyroid rather than T_4, and (2) titration of the patients' T_4 dosages by peripheral indicators rather than circulating T_4 and TSH levels.

Makolkin et al. cautioned clinicians not to miss the diagnosis of primary hypothyroidism because of "its running under the mask of myocardiodystrophy, coronary heart disease, bacterial and allergic myocar-

ditis, and arterial hypertension."[100] Several researchers reported that the mean blood pressure of older patients is higher, whether they are hypothyroid or not. Anderson found that increased age and concomitant atherosclerosis are likely to increase the incidence of hypothyroid hypertension.[111] Saito and Saruta found that in older age groups, hypertension is more common in hypothyroid patients than in euthyroid control subjects.[90] Also, older patients' hypertension is less responsive to the correction of hypothyroidism.[102][110][111] Streeten et al. emphasized the importance of age to prognosis. They found that a smaller percentage of patients over age 40 recovered normal blood pressure after being treated for conditions, including hypothyroidism, that caused secondary hypertension. They emphasized the importance of treating patients at the youngest possible age.[102]

Hypertension from Excess Thyroid Hormone Stimulation

Some thyrotoxic patients develop elevated systolic pressure. Rarely, an elevated systolic pressure may be the only sign of thyrotoxicity. However, the perceptive clinician is likely to identify other signs and symptoms of thyrotoxicity. Signs of thyrotoxicity might include hyperactivity, hyperreflexia, muscle weakness, stare and eyelid retraction, tachycardia or cardiac arrhythmias, tremor, and warm, moist, smooth skin. Symptoms of thyrotoxicity may include appetite change (typically an increase), fatigue, heat intolerance, hyperactivity, irritability, increased perspiration, menstrual disturbances, nervousness, palpations, tremor, weakness, and weight change (usually a decrease).[86,p.646]

Lifestyle as the Underlying Factor in Hypertension

Some hypothyroid patients have hypertension related to lifestyle factors that override the blood pressure-lowering tendency of hypothyroidism. Epidemiological studies suggest that variations in blood pressure in the population are based on genetic factors and environmental factors to the same magnitude.[152][155][156] Despite the role of genetic factors, in many patients, perhaps most, hypertension is underlain by factors within the patients' control through non-medicinal methods. For some 70% of patients with high blood pressure, the hypertension is mild and asymptomatic. If making lifestyle changes can lower blood pressure to normal, the wise patient will make this choice and incorporate the changes into her way of life. As Gerber and Nies wrote, "All drugs have side effects. If minor alterations of normal activity or diet can reduce blood pressure to a satisfactory level, the complications of drug therapy can be avoided. In addition, non-pharmacological methods to lower blood pressure allow the patient to participate actively in the management of his or her disease." Gerber and Nies listed the non-drug methods patients can use to lower blood pressure: ceasing to smoke cigarettes, reducing body weight, restricting sodium intake, increasing potassium intake, reducing heavy alcohol consumption, engaging in regular physical exercise, and using relaxation techniques.[87,pp.807-808]

Before deciding that lifestyle factors are the exclusive cause of a patient's hypertension, clinicians should rule out medical conditions that may cause secondary hypertension. Among these are primary aldosteronism, kidney-vascular hypertension, Cushing's syndrome, and hypothyroidism.[102] Clinicians should also rule out peripheral resistance to thyroid hormone.

β-Adrenergic Receptor Blockers and Other Anti-Hypertensive Medications

β-Adrenergic receptor blockers such as propranolol prescribed to decrease hypertension exacerbate some patients' fibromyalgia symptoms. Some patients have the dilemma of stopping the β-blockers so that fibromyalgia symptoms improve, but at the same time risking a return of hypertension that the β-blockers have presumably decreased. For some patients, the hypertension may originally have been an idiosyncratic function of hypothyroidism or cellular resistance to thyroid hormone (see section above titled "Hypothyroid Hypertension"). In this case, stopping the β-blockers and effectively treating the hypothyroidism or resistance to thyroid hormone are proper.

Probably in most cases, however, hypertension is related to lifestyle factors. If these patients stop using the β-blockers so that their fibromyalgia will improve, they must simultaneously change the responsible lifestyle factors; otherwise, their hypertension will soon resume. It is clear from our extensive experience with metabolic rehabilitation that the lifestyle changes that are likely to relieve hypertension without the use of β-blockers are also essential for the improvement of fibromyalgia. This is true whether the patient's metabolic rehabilitation does or does not include the use of exogenous thyroid hormone. The use of thyroid hormone without the lifestyle changes may be dangerous for the patient: For some such patients, a dosage of thyroid hormone that contributes to marked improvement will increase the risk of adverse cardiovascular effects. In my experience, some patients who decline to make the needed lifestyle changes nevertheless feel

some benefit from the use of thyroid hormone. They subsequently want to augment the improvement by progressively increasing their thyroid hormone dosages. But increasing the dosage trying to achieve a level of improvement that only lifestyle changes can provide increases the chances of inducing a catastrophic cardiovascular consequence. Clinicians should carefully consider whether patients who will not make the lifestyle changes should use thyroid hormone. Hypertension is more imminently dangerous and potentially fatal than is fibromyalgia. Because of this, the patient who will not make the lifestyle changes might best continue the β-blockers, despite the obvious adverse effects on fibromyalgia status.

Anti-hypertensive medications are available for regulating blood pressure without the use of β-blockers. Researchers developed the early anti-hypertensive drugs after learning that bilateral excision of the thoracic sympathetic nervous system chain reduced blood pressure. However, adverse effects resulted from both the surgical procedure and medications that inhibited sympathetic nervous system activity.[87,p.789] Researchers have developed safer medications that affect the sympathetic-catecholamine-adrenoceptor axis. But most of these medications are likely to worsen features of fibromyalgia mediated by deficient sympathetic nervous system activation. If inadequate thyroid hormone regulation of the sympathetic nervous system is a mechanism of some features of fibromyalgia, the use of anti-hypertensive medications is contraindicated. This is true of clonidine, guanabenz, and guanfacine. These medications stimulate α_2-adrenergic receptors in the brain stem and sympathetic ganglia. The stimulation reduces the outflow of sympathetic signals to the periphery.[85]

If lifestyle changes as a part of metabolic rehabilitation (after the patient ceases to use β-blocking medication) do not relieve the hypertension, the clinician may prescribe a medication that is an alternative to β-blockers and α_2-agonists. Prescribing clinicians may choose one or more medications from the list of diuretics, vasodilators, calcium channel blockers, and angiotensin converting enzyme inhibitors.[87,p.785] Studies have shown that calcium channel blockers and inhibitors of angiotensin converting enzyme can be effective "first-line" anti-hypertensive therapy.[87,p.809] One or more of these medications may regulate blood pressure until the complete regimen of metabolic rehabilitation eliminates the mechanism of hypertension. However, if a patient's hypertension is lifestyle related, using the medications chronically *in lieu of* the lifestyle changes is imprudent—for hypertension is only one of many medical disorders likely to result from a failure to make the changes.

Compound Effects of Hypothyroidism and Hypertension

For patients with severe, uncontrolled hypertension, hypothyroidism may for a time provide some protection from strokes and congestive heart failure. The deficient sympathetic discharge that usually occurs in hypothyroidism might prevent peaks in arterial blood pressure that are potentially lethal to some patients. Nevertheless, maintaining hypothyroidism is not a wise strategy for avoiding dangerous exacerbations or complications of hypertension. In hypothyroidism, inadequate thyroid hormone regulation of lipid metabolism strongly contributes to the progression of coronary artery disease and atherosclerosis.[89] Systolic hypertension appears to contribute to the progression of atherosclerosis.[88] In addition, atherosclerosis can worsen hypertension. In fact, elevation of the systolic pressure is an end-stage of atherosclerosis, resulting in a bounding pulse and a substantial increase in the pulse pressure (the difference between the systolic and diastolic pressures).[66,p.164] Therefore, complications from hypothyroidism and hypertension are likely to compound one another.

● MODEL OF REDUCED BLOOD FLOW AND HYPOTENSION IN FIBROMYALGIA

The subnormal circulation and hypotension of a subset of fibromyalgia patients are likely to be the result of hypothyroidism or cellular resistance to thyroid hormone. In hypothyroidism and resistance to thyroid hormone, subnormal circulation and hypotension result from one or more of the effects of inadequate thyroid hormone regulation of cell function or of transcription. I describe these effects in the sections below on reduced blood flow and hypotension. Decreased circulation and hypotension in fibromyalgia and chronic fatigue syndrome are virtually indistinguishable from that in hypothyroidism.

REDUCED BLOOD FLOW

In fibromyalgia patients with hypothyroidism or cellular resistance to thyroid hormone, three main factors can account for reduced blood flow: (1) an increased density of α-adrenergic receptors and a decreased density of β-adrenergic receptors on cell membranes, (2) subnormal direct effects of thyroid hormone on blood vessels, and (3) subnormal tissue metabolism due to inadequate thyroid hormone regulation of cellular metabolic processes. I will describe these factors seriatim.

(1) Reduced thyroid hormone regulation of the adrenergic genes results in an increased density of α-adrenergic receptors and a decrease in the density of β-adrenergic receptors on cell membranes. The results of several studies suggest that fibromyalgia patients have a decrease in β-adrenergic receptors and an increase in α-adrenergic receptors (see Chapter 3.1, section titled "High Ratio of α- to β-Adrenergic Receptors on Cell Membranes").

An increase of α-adrenergic receptors and a decrease of β-adrenergic receptors on the smooth muscle cells of arterioles result in increased vasoconstrictive tone. The vasoconstriction increases resistance to blood flow through the vessels. (See section above titled "Peripheral Blood Flow in Hypothyroidism.")

Were cardiac output normal, blood flow might remain close to normal despite the arterial vasoconstriction—a sufficiently rapid heart rate and stroke volume would propel blood through arteries at a near normal rate, although left ventricular hypertrophy might develop due to the resistance to blood flow. However, in many hypothyroid and thyroid hormone resistant patients, cardiac output is subnormal. The cause of the subnormal output is inadequate thyroid hormone regulation of transcription of the adrenergic genes. The main effect of the inadequate regulation is a high density of α_2-adrenergic receptors on 1) the dorsal vagal nucleus[164] and 2) sympathetic nerve cell bodies within the nucleus of the solitary tract and the paravertebral sympathetic ganglia (see Chapter 3.1, subsection titled "Inhibition of Sympathetic Ganglionic Neural Transmission by an Increased α_2-Adrenergic Receptor Density on Ganglion Cells," and the subsection titled "Reduction in Sympathetic Outflow to Peripheral Tissues by Activation of Central α-Adrenergic Receptors").

The increased vagal (parasympathetic) innervation and decreased sympathetic innervation lower cardiac output. In some patients, the heart rate slows to the level of bradycardia.[38,pp.191,199][81][164] The reduced heart rate and stroke volume result in low blood pressure. The hypotension occurs despite vasoconstriction and vascular resistance due to the increased density of α_1- and α_2-adrenergic receptors on arterioles.

In addition, an increased count of presynaptic α_2-

adrenergic receptors on sympathetic nerve endings in cardiac tissues inhibits the release of norepinephrine. The reduced release of norepinephrine next to heart muscle cells contributes, albeit to a small degree, to the low heart rate and stroke volume. (See subsection above titled "Inhibition of Central Centers for Activation of the Sympathetic Nervous System.") Further, a reduced β-adrenergic receptor density on heart cells reduces the responsiveness of the heart muscle cells to the reduced amounts of norepinephrine released (see subsection above titled "Decreased β-Adrenergic Receptors").

Decreased corticotropin-releasing hormone (CRH) secretion during hypothyroidism and resistance to thyroid hormone may augment subnormal sympathetic nervous system innervation of the heart. CRH is a sympathetic nervous system activation within the central nervous system. Deficient CRH secretion attenuates responsiveness of the sympathetic nervous system to stimulation. The attenuation would contribute to low cardiac output. (See Chapter 3.1, section titled "Subnormal Sympathetic Response to Stresses in Hypothyroid and Fibromyalgia Patients,"and the subsection titled "Bradycardia and Low Blood Pressure.")

Inadequate thyroid hormone regulation of transcription of the adrenergic genes is likely to increase the density of α_2-adrenergic receptors on nerve cell bodies within the dorsal vagal nucleus. Activation of the receptors increases the flow of parasympathetic nerve signals to the heart. The increase in signals reduces heart rate and stroke volume, compounding the decreased cardiac output from diminished sympathetic nerve signals to the heart.

Decreased sympathetic nerve signals to blood vessels reduces the release of norepinephrine next to them. The reduced norepinephrine release is not likely to diminish the vasoconstrictive tone induced by α-adrenergic receptors on blood vessels. In individuals with normal thyroid hormone levels and normal cellular responsiveness to the hormone, sympathetic signals induce norepinephrine secretion. The norepinephrine binds to both α- and β-adrenergic receptors on blood vessels. The binding to β-adrenergic receptors induces vasodilation that counteracts the vasoconstriction resulting from noepinephrine binding to α-adrenergic receptors. The net effect is reduced vascular resistance and increased blood flow. In hypothyroid and thyroid hormone resistant patients, this β-adrenergic receptor-mediated vasodilating effect is subnormal or absent due to the reduced density of β-adrenergic receptors on the vessels.

In individuals with normal thyroid hormone regu-lation of the sympathetic nervous system, sympathetic nerve endings secrete nitric oxide, a potent vasodilator that lowers resistance to blood flow. A reduction in signals reaching sympathetic nerve endings reduces nitric oxide secretion. In addition, decreased exposure of nerve terminals to thyroid hormone decreases their release of nitric oxide. Decreased secretion of the vasodilator would contribute to sustained vasoconstriction (see section above titled "Effects of Thyroid Hormone on Blood Vessels").

More intense vasoconstriction would probably occur when strong stimulation activates sympathetic ganglia hyperpolarized by a high density of α_2-adrenergic receptors (see Chapter 3.1, section titled "Anxiety"). Such strong stimulation might occur, for example, during strenuous exercise. This could account in part for the worsening of fibromyalgia status after a patient engages in exercise that is beyond her tolerance.

An increase in α_1-adrenergic receptors in the arterioles just proximal to the kidney glomeruli inhibits renin release (see subsection above titled "α_1-Adrenergic Receptor Inhibition of Renin Secretion"). In normal individuals, renin release sets into motion reactions that lead to the formation of angiotensin II, a powerful vasoconstrictor. When blood pressure falls, renin secretion increases, and angiotensin II forms and induces vasoconstriction. Constriction of peripheral arterioles increases arterial pressure and slightly increases venous pressure. Vasoconstriction of the kidney blood vessels decreases water and salt excretion. The gain in water and salt in the peripheral circulation increases plasma volume. The rise of plasma volume and the slight venous constriction increase the return of venous blood to the heart, enabling the heart to work against the increased peripheral resistance. Angiotensin II also stimulates the secretion of aldosterone by the adrenal cortices. Aldosterone induces the kidneys to reabsorb salt and water, further increasing plasma volume. Thus, a normally responsive renin-angiotensin-aldosterone system is critical to normalizing circulation that is reduced due to α-adrenergic receptor-induced arteriolar constriction. But when inadequate thyroid hormone regulation of transcription of the adrenergic genes increases the density of α_1-adrenergic receptors in the afferent arterioles of the kidneys, the renin-angiotensin-aldosterone system is not likely to respond normally to reduced arterial pressure. As a result, plasma volume will remain low. Consequently, the heart will not compensate for the reduced blood flow caused by α-adrenergic receptor-induced vasoconstriction and increased vascular resistance.

(2) Thyroid hormone relaxes the smooth muscle lining of blood vessels, and inadequate thyroid hormone exposure to the muscle may result in vasoconstriction (see section above titled "Effects of Thyroid Hormone on Blood Vessels"). Too little exposure of blood vessels to thyroid hormone, or failure of the normal amounts of thyroid hormone to exert proper action, can cause vasoconstriction in two ways. The first is reduced activity of the enzyme Ca^{2+}-ATPase. Reduced activity of the enzyme permits an excess of calcium to accumulate in the smooth muscle cells of blood vessels. The excess calcium induces tonic vasoconstriction with increased resistance to blood flow. The second way is subnormal stimulation of nitric oxide release by thyroid hormone. Nitric oxide is a potent vasodilator. When its secretion is subnormal, as during inadequate thyroid hormone stimulation of its synthesis and secretion, the smooth muscle lining of blood vessels maintains constriction.

(3) Local flow-regulating factors powerfully control blood flow to each tissue. These factors induce vasodilation when the metabolic needs of the cells of the tissue increase. The local factors permit vasoconstriction when the metabolic needs are low. During hypothyroidism or resistance to thyroid hormone, cell metabolism is subnormal in many, perhaps most, tissues. As a result, local flow-regulating mechanisms permit vasoconstriction to occur. This locally dictated vasoconstriction compounds the vasoconstriction induced by a high density of α-adrenergic receptors and a low density of β-adrenergic receptors on arterioles. The resulting vasoconstriction causes a high resistance to blood flow.

Low plasma volume due to a loss of water and salt in the urine may contribute to reduced blood flow. The loss of water and salt would result from two sources: 1) an increase of α_2-adrenergic receptors on the kidney afferent arterioles and 2) an increase in α_2-adrenergic receptors in the cervical sympathetic ganglia. The increase in α_2-adrenergic receptors in the afferent arterioles would inhibit renin secretion. The decreased renin secretion would have two effects, both of which would permit water and salt excretion—failure of angiotensin II to form and failure of angiotensin II to stimulate aldosterone secretion. The increase of α_2-adrenergic receptors within the cervical sympathetic ganglia might result in diminished vasopressin production by hypothalamic cells. Normally, when corticotropin-releasing hormone secretion by hypothalamic cells is subnormal, as during hypothyroidism, hypothalamic cells increase their production of arginine-vasopressin. This hor-

mone then compensates for the failure of corticotropin-releasing hormone to stimulate ACTH secretion by the pituitary. The vasopressin also inhibits water and salt excretion in the kidneys. Production of vasopressin, however, is partially dependent on stimulation of hypothalamic cells by sympathetic signals from the superior cervical ganglia. When sympathetic innervation of the hypothalamic cells is diminished due to α_2-adrenergic receptor inhibition of sympathetic ganglion cells, vasopressin secretion may be subnormal. The subnormal secretion may contribute to a loss of water and salt in the urine, contributing to reduced blood volume and reduced blood flow. The subnormal secretion might also cause urinary frequency. (See Chapter 3.1, section titled "Urinary Frequency," and Chapter 3.21.)

HYPOTENSION

Many fibromyalgia patients with hypothyroidism or cellular resistance to thyroid hormone have orthostatic hypotension. Other fibromyalgia patients have both chronic hypotension and orthostatic hypotension.

Orthostatic Intolerance

The orthostatic intolerance in fibromyalgia patients appears to be the same as that in hypothyroid and thyroid hormone resistant patients. In patients with inadequate thyroid hormone regulation of cell function, three phenomena described in the above section plausibly explain orthostatic intolerance during the head-up tilt test: (1) imbalanced autonomic nervous system regulation of cardiovascular function, (2) subnormal renin secretion, and (3) in some, subnormal secretion of vasopressin. As a result of these phenomena, the cardiovascular system would fail to normally adjust to assumption of an upright posture.

When someone assumes an erect posture, blood pressure falls. Normally, the fall in pressure inactivates the baroreceptors in the major upper body arteries. As a result, nerve signals from the baroreceptors to the brain stem decrease or cease. The decrease or cessation stimulates the flow of sympathetic nerve signals to the heart and blood vessels. The sympathetic signals accelerate the heart rate, increase stroke volume, and induce constriction of the arterioles. These peripheral effects rapidly raise the blood pressure back to normal. The decreased signals from the baroreceptors also decrease the flow of parasympathetic nerve signals to the heart by the vagus nerves. The decreased parasympathetic innervation contributes to the increased cardiac

In the patient with inadequate thyroid hormone regulation of the adrenergic genes, however, these blood pressure-correcting mechanisms are faulty. The increased density of α_2-adrenergic receptors within the nucleus of the solitary tract and paravertebral sympathetic ganglia cause a blunted response of the sympathetic nervous system. Also, an increased density of α_2-adrenergic receptors within the dorsal vagal nucleus enables parasympathetic signals to continue flowing to the heart. As a result, the fall in blood pressure is sustained long enough for symptoms associated with hypotension to occur. The patient's reduced cerebral blood flow may be so extreme that she faints.

In some patients, sympathetic activation is sufficient to cause tachycardia. However, stroke volume remains insufficient to project enough blood into the circulation to counteract arterial hypotension. In addition, in some patients, renin release is subnormal. With subnormal renin release, angiotensin II does not form and the adrenal cortices do not secrete aldosterone into the blood. As a result, salt and water continue to be excreted in the urine rather than being retained in the blood to increase plasma volume. The failure of plasma volume to increase contributes to continuation of the low blood pressure.

In addition, vasopressin secretion is subnormal. In these patients, the subnormal vasopressin secretion contributes to the failure to increase plasma volume through restriction of salt and water excretion. Moreover, whereas normal sympathetic innervation of the kidneys stimulates salt and water reabsorption, subnormal innervation allows salt and water excretion to continue apace.[139,p.440]

As a result of these faulty adaptations to the acute fall in blood pressure, and despite peripheral α-adrenergic receptor-induced vasoconstriction, hypotension may be sustained and severe enough to constitute orthostatic intolerance.

Chronic Hypotension

Chronic hypotension in fibromyalgia patients is likely to involve the same faulty adaptations to an abrupt fall in blood pressure as in patients who only have orthostatic hypotension. However, patients with chronic hypotension may have a predominant selective involvement of the renin-angiotensin-aldosterone system. The selective failure of this system could result mainly from inhibition of renin release by a high density of α_1-adrenergic receptors in the afferent arterioles of the kidneys. An increased density of α_2-adrenergic receptors in the nucleus of the solitary tract and the

paravertebral sympathetic ganglia, and an increased density of the receptors in the dorsal vagal nucleus, would reinforce the chronic hypotension primarily underlain by the blunted renin-angiotensin-aldosterone system.

REFERENCES

1. Schmidt, R.F.: Integrative functions of the central nervous system. *Fundamentals of Neurophysiology*, 3rd edition. New York, Springer-Verlag, 1985, pp.270-316.
2. Scheinberg, P., Stead, E.A., Jr., Brannon, E.S., and Warren, J.V.: Correlative observations on cerebral metabolism and cardiac output in myxedema. *J. Clin. Invest.*, 29: 1139, 1950.
3. Tepperman, J. and Tepperman, H.M.: *Metabolic and Endocrine Physiology*, 5th edition. Chicago, Year Book Medical Publishers, Inc., 1987.
4. Romano, T. and Govindan, S.: Brain SPECT findings in fibromyalgia patients with headache. *Arthritis Rheum.*, 36:R23, 1993.
5. Mountz, J.M., Bradley, L., Modell, J.G., Triana, M., Alexander, R., and Mountz, J.D.: Limbic system dysregulation in fibromyalgia measured by regional cerebral blood flow. *Arthritis Rheum.*, 36:R23, 1993.
6. Bevan, J.A.: Sites of transition between functional systemic and cerebral arteries of rabbits occur at embryological junctional sites. *Science*, 204:635-637, 1979.
7. Bevan, J.A., Bevan, R.D., and Laher, I.: Role of α-adrenoceptors in vascular control. *Clin. Sci.*, 68(Suppl.10):83s-88s, 1985.
8. Duckles, S.P.: Functional activity of the noradrenergic innervation of large cerebral arteries. *Br. J. Pharmacol.*, 69: 193-199, 1980.
9. McCalden, D.A.: Sympathetic control of the cerebral circulation. *J. Autonom. Pharmacol.*, 1:421-431, 1981.
10. Bevan, J.A.: Autonomic pharmacologist's guide to the cerebral circulation. *Trends Pharmacol. Sci.*, 5:234-236, 1984.
11. Rosendorff, C., Mitchell, G., Scriven, D.R.L., and Shapiro, C.: Evidence for a dual innervation affecting local blood flow in the hypothalamus of the conscious rabbit. *Circ. Res.*, 38:140-145, 1976.
12. Yamaguchi, I. and Kopin, I.J.: Differential inhibition of α_1- and α_2-adrenoceptors mediated pressor responses in pithed rat. *J. Pharmacol. Exp. Ther.*, 214:275-281, 1980.
13. Langer, S.Z. and Shepperson, N.B.: Recent developments in vascular smooth muscle pharmacology: the post-synaptic α_2-adrenoceptor. *TiPS*, 1982.
14. Langer, S.Z. and Shepperson, N.B.: Postjunctional α_1- and α_2-adrenoceptors: preferential innervation of α_1-adrenoceptors and the role of neuronal uptake. *J. Cardiovasc. Pharmacol.*, 4:S8-S13, 1982.
15. Wilffert, B., Timmermans, P.B.M.W.M., and van Zwieten, P.A.: Extrasynaptic location of α_2- and noninnervated β_2- adrenoceptors in the vascular system of the pithed normotensive rat. *J. Pharmacol. Exp. Ther.*, 221:762-768, 1982.
16. Clutter, W.E., Bier, D.M., Shah, S.D., and Cryer, P.E.:

Epinephrine plasma metabolic clearance rates and physiologic thresholds for metabolic and hemodynamic actions in man. *J. Clin. Invest.*, 66:94-101, 1980.

17. Bolli, P., Erne, P., Block, L.H., Ji, B.H., Kiowski, W., and Bühler, F.R.: Adrenaline induces vasoconstriction through post-junctional α_2-adrenoceptors and this response is enhanced in patients with essential hypertension. *J. Hypertens.*, 2(Suppl.3):115-118, 1984.

18. de Moraes, S., Bento, A.C., and de Lima, W.T.: Responsiveness to epinephrine in adult spontaneously hypertensive rat tail artery: preferential mediation by post-junctional α_2-adrenoceptors. *J. Cardiovasc. Pharmacol.*, 11:473-477, 1988.

19. Jie, K., van Brummelen, P., Vermey, P., Timmermans, P.B.M.W.M., and van Zwieten, P.A.: α_1- and α_2-Adrenoceptor mediated vasoconstriction in the forearm of normotensive and hypertensive subjects. *J. Cardiovasc. Pharmacol.*, 8:190-196, 1986.

20. Nichols, A.J. and Ruffolo, R.R., Jr.: Functions mediated by α-adrenoceptors. In *α-Adrenoceptors: Molecular Biology, Biochemistry and Pharmacology*. Basel, Karger, 1991, pp.113-179.

21. Fassbender, H.G.: *Pathology of Rheumatic Diseases*. New York, Springer-Verlag, 1975.

22. Lund, N., Bengtsson, A., and Thorborg, P.: Muscle tissue oxygen pressure in primary fibromyalgia. *Scand. J. Rheumatol.*, 15:165-173, 1986.

23. Klemp, P., Nielsen, H.V., Korsgard, J., and Crone, P.: Blood flow in fibromyotic muscles. *Scand. J. Rehab. Med.*, 14:81, 1982.

24. Fassbender, H.G. and Wegner, K.: Morphologie und pathogenese des weichteilrheumatismus. *Z. Rheumaforschg.*, 32:355, 1973.

25. Harris, R.C., Hultman, E., Kaijser, L., and Nordesjo, L.-O.: The effect of circulatory occlusion on isometric exercise capacity and energy metabolism of the quadriceps muscle in man. *Scand. J. Clin. Lab. Invest.*, 35:87-97,1975.

26. Larsson, J. and Hultman, E.: The effect of long term occlusion on energy metabolism of the human quadriceps muscle. *Scand. J. Clin. Lab. Invest.*, 39:257-264, 1979.

27. Bergstrom, J., Bostrom, H., Furst, P., Hultman, E., and Vinnars, E.: Preliminary studies of energy-rich phosphagens in muscle from severely ill patients. *Crit. Care Med.*, 4:197-204, 1976.

28. Kruk, B., Brzezinska, Z., Kaciuba-Uscilko, H., and Nazar, K.: Thyroid hormones and muscle metabolism in dogs. *Horm. Metabol. Res.*, 20:620-623, 1988.

29. Du Bois, E.F.: *Basal Metabolism in Health and Disease*. Philadelphia, Lea & Febiger, 1936.

30. Stewart, H.J., Deitrick, J.E., and Crane, N.F.: Studies of the circulation in patients suffering from spontaneous myxedema. *J. Clin. Invest.*, 17:237-248, 1938.

31. Gibson, J.G., II and Harris, W.H.: Clinical studies of the blood volume: II. Hyperthyroidism and myxedema. *J. Clin. Invest.*, 18:65, 1939.

32. Blumgart, H.L., Gargill, S.L., and Gilligan, D.R.: Studies in velocity of blood flow: XIV. The circulation in myxedema with a comparison of the velocity of blood flow in myxedema and thyrotoxicosis. *J. Clin. Invest.*, 9:91, 1930.

33. Stewart, H.J. and Evans, W.F.: Peripheral blood flow in myxedema. *Arch. Intern. Med.*, 69:808-821, 1942.

34. Gidlöf, A., Hammersen, F., Larsson, J., Lewis, D.H., and Liljedahl, S.O.: Is capillary endothelium in human skeletal muscle an ischemic shock tissue? *Symposium on Induced Skeletal Muscle Ischemia in Man.* Linköping, Sweden, November 6-7, 1980, pp.361-365.

35. Bengtsson, A., Henriksson, K.G., and Larsson, J.: Reduced high-energy phosphate levels in the painful muscles of patients with primary fibromyalgia. *Arthritis Rheum.*, 29:817-821, 1986.

36. Williams, J.L., Jones, S.C., Page, R.B., and Bryan, R.M., Jr.: Vascular responses of the choroid plexus during hypercapnia in rats. *Am. J. Physiol.*, 260:R1066-R1070, 1991.

37. McPherson, R.W., Koehler, R.C., and Traystman, R.J.: Hypoxia, α_2-adrenergic, and nitric oxide-dependent interactions on canine cerebral blood flow. *Am. J. Physiol.*, 266:H476-H482, 1994.

38. Hoffman, B.B. and Lefkowitz, R.J.: Catecholamines and sympathomimetic drugs. In *The Pharmacological Basis of Therapeutics*, 8th edition. Edited by A.G. Gilman, T.W. Rall, A.S. Nies, and P. Taylor, New York, Pergamon Press, 1990.

39. Sharma, V.K. and Banerjee, S.P.: β-Adrenergic receptors in rat skeletal muscle: effects of thyroidectomy. *Biochim. Biophys. Acta*, 539:538, 1978.

40. Hamilton, T.C.: Involvement of the adrenal glands in the hypotensive response to bromocriptine in spontaneously hypertensive rats. *Br. J. Pharmacol.*, 72(3):419-425, 1981.

41. Ceccatelli, S., Giardino, L., and Calza, L.: Response of hypothalamic peptide mRNAs to thyroidectomy. *Neuroendocrinology*, 56(5):694-703, 1992.

42. Cooper, J.R., Bloom, F.E., and Roth, R.H.: *The Biochemical Basis of Neuropharmacology*, 6th edition. New York, Oxford University Press, 1991.

43. Russell, I.J. Neurohormonal hypothesis: abnormal laboratory findings related to pain and fatigue in fibromyalgia. *J. Musculoskel. Pain*, 3(2):59-65, 1995.

44. van Denderen, J.C., Boersma, J.W., Zeinstra, P., Hollander, A.P., and van Neerbos, B.R.: Physiological effects of exhaustive physical exercise in primary fibromyalgia syndrome (PFS): is PFS a disorder of neuroendocrine reactivity? *Scand. J. Rheumat.*, 21:35-37, 1992.

45. Mengshoel, A.M.: Effect of physical exercise in fibromyalgia. *Tidsskr Nor Laegeforen*, 116:746-748, 1996.

46. Le Feuvre, C., Baubion, N., Berdah, J., Heulin, A., and Vacheron, A.: Drug-induced cardiovascular complications. *Ann. de Med. Intern.*, 140(7):597-599, 1989.

47. Jenike, M.A.: Treatment of affective illness in the elderly with drugs and electroconvulsive therapy. *J. Geratric Psychiat.*, 22(1):77-112, 1989.

48. Skarphedinsson, J.O., Elam, M., Jungersten, L., and Wallin, B.G.: Sympathetic nerve traffic correlates with the release of nitric oxide in humans: implications for blood pressure control. *J. Physiol.*, 501(Pt.3):671-675, 1997.

49. Bryson, H.M. and Wilde, M.I.: Amitriptyline. A review of its pharmacological properties and therapeutic use in chronic pain states. *Drugs Aging*, 8(6):459-476, 1996.

50. Colin, I.M., Kopp, P., Zbaren, J., Haberli, A., Grizzle, W.E., and Jameson, J.L.: Expression of nitric oxide syn-

thase III in human thyroid follicular cells: evidence for increased expression in hyperthyroidism. *Eur. J. Endocrinol.*, 136(6):649-655, 1997.

51. Park, K.W., Dai, H.B., Ojamaa, K., Lowenstein, E., Klein, I., and Selke, F.W.: The direct vasomotor effect of thyroid hormones on rat skeletal muscle resistance arteries. *Anesth. Analg.*, 85(4):734-738, 1997.

52. Elam, M., Johansson, G., and Wallin, B.G.: Do patients with primary fibromyalgia have an altered muscle sympathetic nerve activity? *Pain*, 48:371-375, 1992.

53. Zwaveling, J., Pfafferdorf, M., and van Zwieten, P.A.: The direct effects of thyroid hormones on rat mesenteric resistance arteries. *Fundamen. Clin. Pharmacol.*, 11(1): 41-46, 1997.

54. Ojamaa, K., Balkman, C., and Klein, I.: Acute effects of triiodothyronine on arterial smooth muscle cells. *Ann. Thorac. Surg.*, 56:S61, 1993.

55. Graettinger, J.S., Muenster, J.J., Selverstone, L.A., and Campbell, J.A.: A correlation of clinical and hemodynamic studies in patients with hyperthyroidism with and without heart failure. *J. Clin. Invest.*, 19:1316, 1959.

56. Anthonsen, P., Holst, E., and Thomsen, A.A.: Determination of cardiac output and other hemodynamic data in patients with hyper- and hypothyroidism, using dye dilution technique. *Scand. J. Clin. Lab. Invest.*, 12:472, 1960.

57. Kapitola, J. and Vilimovska, D.: Inhibition of the early circulatory effects of triiodothyronine in rats by propranolol. *Physiol. Bohemoslov.*, 30:347, 1981.

58. Klein, I. and Levey, G.S.: The cardiovascular system in thyrotoxicosis. In *Werner and Ingbar's The Thyroid: A Fundamental and Clinical Text*, 7th edition. Edited by L.P. Braverman and R.D. Utiger, Philadelphia, Lippincott-Raven Publishers, 1996, pp.607-615.

59. Kontos, H.A., Shapiro, W., Mauch, H.P. Jr., et al.: Mechanisms of certain abnormalities of the circulation to the limbs in thyrotoxicosis. *J. Clin. Invest.*, 44:947, 1965.

60. Myers, J.D., Brannon, E.S., and Holland, B.C.: Correlative study of the cardiac output and hepatic circulation in hyperthyroidism. *J. Clin. Invest.*, 29:1069, 1950.

61. Sokoloff, L., Wechsler, R.L., Balls, K., Mangold, R., and Kety, S.S.: Cerebral blood flow and oxygen consumption in hyperthyroidism before and after treatment. *J. Clin. Invest.*, 32:202, 1953.

62. Klemperer, J.D., Zelano, J., Helm, R.E., et al.: Triiodothyronine improves left ventricular function without oxygen wasting effects after global hypothermic ischemia. *J. Thorac. Cardiovas. Surg.*, 109(3):457-465, 1995.

63. Amidi, M., Leon, D.F., DeGroot, L.J., Kroetz, F.W., and Leonard, J.H.J.: Effect of the thyroid state on myocardial contractility and ventricular ejection rate in man. *Circulation*, 38:229, 1968.

64. Stewart, J.H. and Evans, W.F.: Peripheral blood flow in myxedema. *Arch. Intern. Med.*, 69:808, 1942.

65. Bilezikian, J.P.: Defining the role of adrenergic receptors in human physiology. In *Adrenergic Receptors in Man*. Edited by P.A. Insel, New York, Marcel Dekker, Inc., 1987, pp.37-67.

66. Guyton, A.C.: *Textbook of Medical Physiology*, 8th edition. Philadelphia, W.B. Saunders Co., 1991.

67. Bennett, R.M., Clark, S.R., Campbell, S.M., et al.: Symptoms of Raynaud's syndrome in patients with fi-

bromyalgia. A study utilizing the Nielsen test, digital photoplethysmography and measurements of platelet α_2-adrenergic receptors. *Arthritis Rheum.*, 34(3):264-269, 1991.

68. Goldstein, J.A., Mena, I., and Yunus, M.B.: Regional cerebral blood flow by SPECT in chronic fatigue syndrome with and without fibromyalgia syndrome. *Arthritis Rheum.*, 39(9/Suppl.):205, 1993.

69. Goldstein, J.A.: *Betrayal by the Brain*. New York, Haworth Medical Press, 1996.

70. Forchetti, C.M., Katsamakis, G., and Garron, D.C.: Autoimmune thyroiditis and a rapidly progressive dementia: global hypoperfusion on SPECT scanning suggests a possible mechanism. *Neurology*, 49(2):623-626, 1997.

71. Sabio, J.M., Rodriguez-Maresca, M., Luna, J.D., Garcia, A., del Rio, C., and Vargas, F.: Vascular reactivity to vasoconstrictors in aorta and renal vasculature of hyperthyroid and hypothyroid rats. *Pharmacol.*, 49(4):257-264, 1994.

72. San Pedro, E.C., Mountz, J.M., Mountz, J.D., Liu, H.G., Katholi, C.R., and Deutsch, G.: Familial painful restless legs syndrome correlates with pain dependent variation of blood flow to the caudate, thalamus, and anterior cingulate gyrus. *J. Rheumatol.*, 25(11):2270-2275, 1998.

73. Lowe, J.C., Eichelberger, J., Manso, G., and Peterson, K.: Improvement in euthyroid fibromyalgia patients treated with T3 (triiodothyronine). *J. Myofascial Ther.*,1(2):16-29, 1994.

74. Lowe, J.C.: T3-induced recovery from fibromyalgia by a hypothyroid patient resistant to T4 and desiccated thyroid. *J. Myofascial Ther.*, 1(4):26-31, 1995.

75. Lowe, J.C.: Results of an open trial of T3 therapy with 77 euthyroid female fibromyalgia patients. *Clin. Bull. Myofascial Ther.*, 2(1):35-37, 1997.

76. Lowe, J.C., Reichman, A.J., and Yellin, J.: A case-control study of metabolic therapy for fibromyalgia: long-term follow-up comparison of treated and untreated patients. *Clin. Bull. Myofascial Ther.*, 3(1): 23-24, 1998.

77. Lowe, J.C., Garrison, R.L., Reichman, A.J., Yellin, J., Thompson, M., and Kaufman, D.: Effectiveness and safety of T3 (triiodothyronine) therapy for euthyroid fibromyalgia: a double-blind placebo-controlled response-driven crossover study. *Clin. Bull. Myofascial Ther.*, 2 (2/3):31-58, 1997.

78. Lowe, J.C., Reichman, A.J., and Yellin, J.: The process of change during T3 treatment for euthyroid fibromyalgia: a double-blind placebo-controlled crossover study. *Clin. Bull. Myofascial Ther.*, 2(2/3):91-124, 1997.

79. Lowe, J.C., Garrison, R.L., Reichman, A.J., and Yellin, J.: Triiodothyronine (T3) Treatment of euthyroid fibromyalgia: a small-N replication of a double-blind placebo-controlled crossover study. *Clin. Bull. Myofascial Ther.*, 2(4):71-88, 1997.

80. Gledhill, R.F., Dessein, P.H., and van der Merwe, C.A.: Treatment of Raynaud's phenomenon with triiodothyronine corrects co-existent autonomic dysfunction: preliminary findings. *Postgrad. Med. J.*, 68(798):263-267, 1992.

81. Klein, M., Pascal, V., Aubert, V., Weryha, G., Danchin, N., and Leclere, J.: Heart and thyroid. *Ann. Endocrinol.* (Paris), 56(5):473-486, 1995.

82. Brust, J.C.M.: Cerebral circulation: stroke. In *Principles*

of Neural Science, 3rd edition. Edited by E.R. Kandel, J.H. Schwartz, and T.M. Jessell, Norwalk, Appleton & Lange, 1991, pp.1041-1049.

83. Goldstein, J.A.: *Chronic Fatigue Syndrome: The Limbic Hypothesis.* Binghamton, Haworth Medical Press, 1993.

84. Arnstein, A.F.T., Cai, J.X., and Goldman-Rakic, P.S.: The α_2-adrenergic agonist guanfacine improves memory in aged monkeys without sedative or hypotensive effects. *J. Neurosci.,* 8:4287-4298, 1988.

85. Langer, S.Z., Cavero, I., and Massingham, R.: Recent developments in noradrenergic neurotransmission and its relevance to the mechanism of action of certain antihypertensive agents. *Hypertension,* 2:372-382, 1980.

86. Braverman, L.E. and Utiger, R.D.: Introduction to thyrotoxicosis. In *The Thyroid: A Fundamental and Clinical Text,* 6th edition. Edited by L.E. Braverman and R.D. Utiger, Philadelphia, J.B. Lippincott Co., 1991, p.646.

87. Gerber, J.G. and Nies, A.S.: Antihypertensive agonists and the drug therapy of hypertension. In *Goodman and Gilman's The Pharmacological Basis of Therapeutics,* 8th edition. New York, Pergamon Press, 1990, pp.784-813.

88. Sutton-Tyrrell, K., Kuller, L.H., and Wolfson, S.K., Jr.: Causes, implications, and treatment of systolic hypertension. *Curr. Opin. Nephrol. Hypertens.,* 3(3):264-270, 1994.

89. Mohr-Kahaly, S., Kahaly, G., and Meyer, J.: Cardiovascular effects of thyroid hormones. Hypothyroidism leads to atherosclerosis and cardiac disease. *Z. Kardiol.,* 85 (Suppl.6):219-231, 1996.

90. Saito, I. and Saruta, T.: Hypertension in thyroid disorders. *Endocrinol. Metab. Clin. North Amer.,* 23(2):379-386, 1994.

91. Bramnert, M., Hallengren, B., Lecerof, H., Werner, R., and Manhem, P.: Decreased blood pressure response to infused noradrenaline in normotensive as compared to hypertensive patients with primary hypothyroidism. *Clin. Endocrinol.* (Oxf), 40(3):317-321, 1994.

92. Machado, C., Bhasin, S., Nona, W., and Steinman, R.T.: Hypothyroid cardiac tamponade presenting with severe systemic hypertension. *Clin. Cardiol.,* 16(6):513-516, 1993.

93. Gasiorowski, W. and Plazinska, M.T.: Arterial hypertension associated with hyper and hypothyroidism. *Pol. Tyg. Lek.,* 47(44-45):1009-1010, 1992.

94. Garg, P.K., Singh, V., Saigal, R., and Mathur, U.S.: Vasculitis: a complication of hypothyroidism. *J. Assoc. Physicians India,* 38(2):182-183, 1990.

95. Ponte, E. and Ursu, H.I.: Overt and subclinical hypothyroidism and atherosclerotic arteriopathy of the lower limbs (clinical and subclinical). *Rom. J. Endocrinol.,* 31 (1-2):71-79, 1993.

96. Egart, F.M., Kamalov, K.G., Vasil'eva, E.V., Bobrovskaia, T.A., Dobracheva, A.D., and Kolesnikova, G.S.: Atypical clinical variants of hypothyrosis. *Probl. Endokrinol.* (Mosk), 37(5):4-7, 1991.

97. Adogu, A.A., Njepuome, N., Anyiam, C.A., and Abegowe, C.U.: Primary hypothyroidism with secondary hypertension: a case report. *East Afr. Med. J.,* 69(3):165-166, 1992.

98. Bergus, G.R., Mold, J.W., Barton, E.D., and Randall, C.S.:The lack of association between hypertension and

hypothyroidism in a primary care setting. *J. Hum. Hypertens.,*13(4):231-235, 1999.

99. Chentsova, O.B., Kalinin, A.P., and Guzei, L.A.: Glaucoma and symptomatic hypertension in hypothyroidism. *Oftalmol. Zh.,* 33(1):20-23, 1978.

100. Makolkin, V.I., Starovoitova, S.P., and Shchedrina, I.S.: Therapeutic "masks" of primary hypothyroidism. *Ter. Arkh.,* 68(1):49-52, 1996.

101. Russell, I.J., Vaeroy, M., Jabors, M., and Nyberg, F.: Cerebrospinal fluid biogenic metabolites in fibromyalgia/fibrositis syndrome in rheumatoid arthritis. *Arthritis Rheum.,* 35:550-556, 1992.

102. Streeten, D.H., Anderson, G.H., Jr., and Wagner, S.: Effect of age on response of secondary hypertension to specific treatment. *Amer. J. Hypertens.,* 3(5 Pt.1):360-365, 1990.

103. Bing, R.F., Briggs, R.S., Burden, A.C., Russell, G.I., Swales, J.D., and Thurston, H.: Reversible hypertension and hypothyroidism. *Clin. Endocrinol.* (Oxf), 13(4):339-342, 1980.

104. Streeten, D.H., Anderson, G.H., Jr., Howland, T., Chiang, R., and Smulyan, H.: Effects of thyroid function on blood pressure: recognition of hypothyroid hypertension. *Hypertension,* 11(1):78-83, 1988.

105. Starkova, N.T., Egart, F.M., Atamanova, T.M., and Nazarov, A.N.: Pathogenesis and treatment of arterial hypertension in hypothyroidism patients. *Klin. Med.* (Mosk), 64(8):27-30, 1986.

106. Richards, A.M., Nicholls, M.G., Espiner, E.A., Ikram, H., Turner, J.G., and Brownlie, B.E.: Hypertension in hypothyroidism: arterial pressure and hormone relationships. *Clin. Exp. Hypertens.,* 7(11):1499-1514, 1985.

107. Saito, I., Ito, K., and Saruta, T.: Hypothyroidism as a cause of hypertension. *Hypertension,* 5(1):112-115, 1983.

108. Fletcher, A.K. and Weetman, A.P.: Hypertension and hypothyroidism. *J. Hum. Hypertens.,* 12(2):79-82, 1998.

109. Okamura, K., Inoue, K., Shiroozu, A., et al.: Primary hypothyroidism as a possible cause of hypertension from long-term follow-up studies of patients with Graves' disease. *Nippon Naibunpi Gakkai Zasshi,* 56(6):767-775, 1980.

110. Endo, T., Komiya, I., Tsukui, T., et al.: Re-evaluation of a possible high incidence of hypertension in hypothyroid patients. *Amer. Heart J.,* 98(6):684-688, 1979.

111. Anderson, G.H., Jr., Blakeman, N., and Streeten, D.H.: The effect of age on prevalence of secondary forms of hypertension in 4429 consecutively referred patients. *J. Hypertens.,* 12(5):609-615, 1994.

112. Kinuya, S., Michigishi, T., Tonami, N., Aburano, T., Tsuji, S., and Hashimoto, T.: Reversible cerebral hypoperfusion observed with Tc-99m HMPAO SPECT in reversible dementia caused by hypothyroidism. *Clin. Nucl. Med.,* 24(9):666-668, 1999.

113. Lefauconnier, J.M., Lacombe, P., and Bernard, G.: Cerebral blood flow and blood-brain influx of some neutral amino acids in control and hypothyroid 16-day-old rats. *J. Cereb. Blood. Flow Metab.,* 5(2):318-326, 1985.

114. Tanaka, M., Kawarabayashi, T., Okamoto, K., Morimatsu, M., and Hirai, S.: Reduction of cerebellar blood flow and metabolic rate of oxygen in a case of hypothyroidism presenting cerebellar ataxia. *Rinsho Shinkeigaku,* 27(10):

1262-1265, 1987.

115. Gay, R.G., Raya, T.E., Lancaster, L.D., Lee, R.W., Morkin, E., and Goldman, S.: Effects of thyroid state on venous compliance and left ventricular performance in rats. *Amer. J. Physiol.*, 254(1 Pt.2):H81-H88, 1988.

116. Streeten, D. and Bell, D.: Circulating blood volume in chronic fatigue syndrome. *J. Chron. Fatig. Synd.*, 4(1):3-11, 1998.

117. Ansell, J.E.: The blood in thyrotoxicosis. In *Werner's The Thyroid: A Fundamental and Clinical Text*, 6th edition. Edited by L.E. Braverman and R.D. Utiger, Philadelphia, J.B. Lippincott Co., 1991, pp.785-792.

118. Tudhope, G.R. and Wilson, G.M.: Anemia in hypothyroidism. *Q.J. Med.*, 29:513, 1960.

119. Horton, L., Coburn, R.J., England, J.M., and Hinesworth, R.L.: The hematology of hypothyroidism. *Q.J. Med.*, 45:101, 1975.

120. Green S.T. and Ng, J.P.: Hypothyroidism and anemia. *Biomed. Pharmacother.*, 40:326, 1986.

121. Ansell, J.E.: The blood in hypothyroidism. In *Werner's The Thyroid: A Fundamental and Clinical Text*, 6th edition. Edited by L.E. Braverman and R.D. Utiger, Philadelphia, J.B. Lippincott Co., 1991, pp.1022-1026.

122. Das, K.C., Mukherjee, M., Sarkar, T.K., Dash, R.J., and Rastogi, G.K.: Erythropoiesis and erythropoietin in hypo and hyperthyroidism. *J. Clin. Endocrinol. Metab.*, 40:211, 1975.

123. Muldowney, F.P., Crooks, J., and Wayne, E.J.: The total red cell mass in thyrotoxicosis and myxedema. *Clin. Sci.*, 16:309, 1957.

124. Axelrod, A.R. and Berman, L.: The bone marrow in hyperthyroidism and hypothyroidism. *Blood*, 6:436, 1951.

125. Hymes, K., Blum, M., Lackner, H., and Karpatkin, S.: Easy bruising, thrombocytopenia, and elevated platelet immunoglobulin G in Graves' disease and Hashimoto's thyroiditis. *Ann. Intern. Med.*, 94:27, 1981.

126. Rowe, P.C.: Neurally mediated hypotension and chronic fatigue syndrome. Abstracts presented at the Sydney 1998 CFS Conference.

127. Rowe, P.C.: New clinical insights in the treatment of chronic fatigue syndrome. Abstracts presented at the Sydney 1998 CFS Conference.

128. Honeyman-Lowe, G.: Personal communication, September, 1999.

129. Grassi, W., Core, P., Carlino, G., Salaffi, F., and Cervini, C.: Capillary permeability in fibromyalgia. *J. Rheumatol.*, 21(7):1328-1331, 1994.

130. Hall, J.E., Guyton, A.C., Coleman, T.G., Mizelle, H.L., and Woods, L.L.: Regulation of arterial pressure: role of pressure natriuresis and diuresis. *Fed. Proc.*, 45(13):2897-2903, 1986.

131. Dzau, V.J.: Vascular angiotensin pathways: a new therapeutic target. *J. Cardiovasc. Pharmacol.*, 10(Suppl.7):S9-S16, 1987.

132. Haddy, F.J.: Dietary sodium and potassium in the genesis, therapy, and prevention of hypertension. *J. Amer. Coll. Nutr.*, 6(3):261-270, 1987.

133. Brody, M.J.: Central nervous system and mechanisms of hypertension. *Clin. Physiol. Biochem.*, 6(3-4):230-239, 1988.

134. Henriksen, O.: Sympathetic reflex control of blood flow in human peripheral tissues. *Acta Physiol. Scand. Suppl.*, 603:33-39, 1991.

135. Ruilope, L.M., Lahera, V., Rodicio, J.L., and Carlos Romero, J.: Are renal hemodynamics a key factor in the development and maintenance of arterial hypertension in humans? *Hypertension*, 23(1):3-9, 1994.

136. Schloeffel, R.: Case presentation (abstract). 1999 Sydney ME/CFS Conference, November 27, 1999.

137. Berg, D., Berg, L.H., and Couvaras, J.: Is CFS/FM due to an undefined hypercoagulable state brought on by immune activation of coagulation? Does adding anticoagulant therapy improve CFS/FM patient symptoms? Abstract presented at the Sydney ME/CFS Conference, November 27, 1999.

138. Zeigler, Z.R., Hasiba, U., Lewis, J.H., Vagnucci, A.H., West, V.A., and Bezek, E.A.: Hemostatic defects in response to aspirin challenge in hypothyroidism. *Amer. J. Hematol.*, 23(4):391-399, 1986.

139. Berne, R.M. and Levy, M.N.: *Principles of Physiology*. St. Louis, C.V. Mosby Co., 1990.

140. Sjoberg, R.J., Kidd, G.S., Swanson, E.W., O'Barr, T.P., Corby, D.G., and Hofeldt, F.D.: Effects of hypothyroidism and short-term aging on whole blood thromboxane and arterial prostacyclin synthesis. *J. Lab. Clin. Med.*, 110(5):576-582, 1987.

141. Lazurova, I., Lazur, J., Mosanska, M., Trejbal, D., Trejbalova, L., and Zemberova, E.: Changes in thrombocyte aggregation in primary hypothyroidism. *Vnitr. Lek.*, 44(7):383-386, 1998.

142. Masunaga, R., Nagasaka, A., Nakai, J., et al.: Alteration of platelet aggregation in patients with thyroid disorders. *Metabolism*, 46(10):1128-1131, 1997.

143. Myrup, B., Bregengard, C., and Faber, J.: Primary haemostasis in thyroid disease. *J. Intern. Med.*, 238(1):59-63, 1995.

144. O'Regan, S. and Fong, J.S.: Platelet hypoaggregability in hypothyroid rats. *Proc. Soc. Exp. Biol. Med.*, 158(4):575-577, 1978.

145. Edson, J.R., Fecher, D.R., and Doe, R.P.: Low platelet adhesiveness and other hemostatic abnormalities in hypothyroidism. *Ann. Intern. Med.*, 82(3):342-346, 1975.

146. DiBona, G.F.: Neural control of renal function in health and disease. *Clin. Auton. Res.*, 4(1-2):69-74, 1994.

147. Santos, R.A. and Campagnole-Santos, M.J.: Central and peripheral actions of angiotensin-(1-7). *Braz. J. Med. Biol. Res.*, 27(4):1033-1047, 1994.

148. Krieger, E.M., Brum, P.C., and Negrao, C.E.: Role of arterial baroreceptor function on cardiovascular adjustments to acute and chronic dynamic exercise. *Biol. Res.*, 31(3):273-279, 1998.

149. Benditt, D.G., Fabian, W., Iskos, D., and Lurie, K.G.: Review article: heart rate and blood pressure control in vasovagal syncope. *J. Interv. Card. Electrophysiol.*, 2(1):25-32, 1998.

150. Irigoyen, M.C. and Krieger, E.M.: Baroreflex control of sympathetic activity in experimental hypertension. *Braz. J. Med. Biol. Res.*, 31(9):1213-1220, 1998.

151. Brands, M.W. and Granger, J.P.: Control of renal function and blood pressure by angiotensin II: implications for diabetic glomerular injury. *Miner Electrolyte Metab.*, 24(6):371-380, 1998.

152. Ferrari, P.: Molecular genetics of hypertension in the human. *Ther. Umsch.*, 56(1):5-11, 1999.

153. Jagadeesh, G.: Angiotensin II receptors-antagonists, molecular biology, and signal transduction. *Indian J. Exp. Biol.*, 36(12):1171-1194, 1998.

154. Belmin, J.: Current aspects of arterial hypertension: hypertension in the aged. *Presse Med.*, 28(16):862-869, 1999.

155. Kornitzer, M., Dramaix, M., and De Backer, G.: Epidemiology of risk factors for hypertension: implications for prevention and therapy. *Drugs,* 57(5):695-712, 1999.

156. Ambler, S.K. and Brown, R.D.: Genetic determinants of blood pressure regulation. *J. Cardiovasc. Nurs.*, 13(4):59-77, 1999.

157. Ayavou, T., Marie, P.A., Pouly, E., Zakarian, H., and Eisinger, J.: Oxyde nitrique et fibromyalgie. *Lyon Med. Med.*, 27:2194-2196, 1996.

158. Eisinger, J., Gandolfo, C., Zakarian, H., and Ayavou, T.: Reactive oxygen species: antioxidant status and fibromyalgia. *J. Musculoskel. Pain,* 5:5-11, 1997.

159. Bennett, R.: Fibromyalgia, chronic fatigue syndrome, and myofascial pain. *Curr. Opin. Rheumatol.*, 10(2):95-103, 1998.

160. Wilke, W.S., Fouad-Tarazi, F.M., Cash, J.M., and Calabrese, L.H.: The connection between chronic fatigue syndrome and neurally mediated hypotension. *Cleve. Clin. J. Med.*, 65(5):261-266, 1998.

161. Stewart, J.M., Gewitz, M.H., Weldon, A., and Munoz, J.: Patterns of orthostatic intolerance: the orthostatic tachycardia syndrome and adolescent chronic fatigue. *J. Pediatr.*, 135(2 Pt.1):218-225, 1999.

162. Calkins, H. and Rowe, P.C.: Relationship between chronic fatigue syndrome and neurally mediated hypotension. *Cardiol. Rev.*, 6(3):125-134, 1998.

163. Owens, P.E. and O'Brien, E.T.: Hypotension: a forgotten illness? *Blood Press. Monit.*, 2(1):3-14, 1997.

164. Connor, H.E., Drew, G.M., and Finch, L.: Clonidine-induced potentiation of reflex vagal bradycardia in anesthetized cats. *J. Pharm. Pharmacol.*, 34:22-26, 1982.

165. Schondorf, R., Benoit, J., Wein, T., and Phaneuf, D.: Orthostatic intolerance in the chronic fatigue syndrome. *J. Auton. Nerv. Syst.*, 75(2-3):192-201, 1999.

166. Stewart, J.M., Gewitz, M.H., Weldon, A., Arlievsky, N., Li, K., and Munoz, J.: Orthostatic intolerance in adolescent chronic fatigue syndrome. *Pediatrics,* 103(1):116-121, 1999.

167. Low, P.A.: Autonomic neuropathies. *Curr. Opin. Neurol.*, 11(5):531-537, 1998.

168. Stewart, J., Weldon, A., Arlievsky, N., Li, K., and Munoz, J.: Neurally mediated hypotension and autonomic dysfunction measured by heart rate variability during head-up tilt testing in children with chronic fatigue syndrome. *Clin. Auton. Res.*, 8(4):221-230, 1998.

169. Rowe, P.C. and Calkins, H.: Neurally mediated hypotension and chronic fatigue syndrome. *Amer. J. Med.*, 105 (3A):15S-21S, 1998.

170. Peroutka, S.J.: Chronic fatigue disorders: an inappropriate response to arginine vasopressin? *Med. Hypotheses,* 50 (6):521-523, 1998.

171. Smit, A.A., Bolweg, N.M., Lenders, J.W., and Wieling, W.: No strong evidence of disturbed regulation of blood pressure in chronic fatigue syndrome. *Ned. Tijdschr. Geneeskd.*, 142(12):625-628, 1998.

172. Streeten, D.H. and Anderson, G.H., Jr.: The role of delayed orthostatic hypotension in the pathogenesis of chronic fatigue. *Clin. Auton. Res.*, 8(2):119-124, 1998.

173. De Lorenzo, F., Hargreaves, J., and Kakkar, V.V.: Pathogenesis and management of delayed orthostatic hypotension in patients with chronic fatigue syndrome. *Clin. Auton. Res.*, 7(4):185-190, 1997.

174. van de Luit, L., van der Meulen, J., Cleophas, T.J., and Zwinderman, A.H.: Amplified amplitudes of circadian rhythms and nighttime hypotension in patients with chronic fatigue syndrome: improvement by inopamil but not by melatonin. *Angiology,* 49(11):903-908, 1998.

175. Bou-Holaigah, I., Calkins, H., Flynn, J.A., Tunin, C., Chang, H.C., Kan, J.S., and Rowe, P.C.: Provocation of hypotension and pain during upright tilt table testing in adults with fibromyalgia. *Clin. Exp. Rheumatol.*, 15(3): 239-246, 1997.

176. Rowe, P.C., Barron, D.F., Calkins, H., Maumenee, I.H., Tong, P.Y., and Geraghty, M.T.: Orthostatic intolerance and chronic fatigue syndrome associated with Ehlers-Danlos syndrome. *J. Pediatr.*, 135(4):494-499, 1999.

177. Dodd, J. and Role, L.W.: The autonomic nervous system. In *Principles of Neural Science*, 3rd edition. Edited by E.R. Kandel, J.H. Schwartz, and T.M. Jessell, Norwalk, Appleton & Lange, 1991, pp.761-775.

178. Fulton, B., Wagstaff, A.J., and Sorkin, E.M.: Doxazosin: an update of its clinical pharmacology and therapeutic applications in hypertension and benign prostatic hyperplasia. *Drugs,* 49(2):295-320, 1995.

179. Stockamp, K.: Therapy of benign prostatic hyperplasia with α receptor blockers. *Urologe Ausgabe A.*, 34(1):3-8, 1995.

180. Dwyer, P.L. and Teele, J.S.: Prazosin: a neglected cause of genuine stress incontinence. *Obst. Gyn.*, 79(1):117-121, 1992.

181. Kooner, J.S., Birch, R., Frankel, H.L., Peart, W.S., and Mathias, C.J.: Hemodynamic and neurohormonal effects of clonidine in patients with preganglionic and postganglionic sympathetic lesions: evidence for a central sympatholytic action. *Circulation,* 84(1):75-83, 1991.

182. Lambert, M., Thissen, J.P., Doyen, C., Col, J., and Coche, E.: Orthostatic hypotension associated with hypothyroidism. *Acta Clin. Belg.*, 39(1):48-50, 1984.

183. Delia, A.J. and Thompson, E.B.: A time-course study of hypothyroidism-induced hypotension: its relation to food deprivation. *Arch. Int. Pharmacodyn. Ther.*, 296:210-223, 1988.

184. Thompson, E.B. and Lum, L.: A time-course study of hypothyroidism-induced hypotension: its relation to hypothermia. *Arch. Int. Pharmacodyn. Ther.*, 283:141-152, 1986.

185. Ladenson, P.W., Levin, A.A., Ridgway, E.C., and Daniels, G.H.: Complications of surgery in hypothyroid patients. *Am. J. Med.*, 77(2):261-266, 1984.

186. Wartofsky, L.: Myxedema coma. In *Werner and Ingbar's The Thyroid: A Fundamental and Clinical Text*, 7th edition. Edited by L.P. Braverman and R.D. Utiger, Philadelphia, Lippincott-Raven Publishers, 1996, pp.871-877.

187. Ragaller, M., Quintel, M., Bender, H.J., and Albrecht,

D.M.: Myxedema coma as a rare postoperative complication. *Anaesthesist*, 42(3):179-183, 1993.

188. Abouganem, D., Taylor, A.L., Donna, E., and Baum, G.L.: Extreme bradycardia during sleep apnea caused by myxedema. *Arch. Intern. Med.*, 147(8):1497-1499, 1987.

189. Head, G.A. and Burke, S.: Importance of central noradrenergic and serotonergic pathways in the cardiovascular actions of rilmenidine and clonidine. *J. Cardiovasc. Pharmacol.*, 18(6):819-826, 1991.

190. Kobinger, W.: Central α-adrenergic systems as targets for antihypertensive drugs. *Rev. Physiol. Biochem. Pharmacol.*, 81:39-100, 1978.

191. Kobinger, W.: Centrally induced reduction in sympathetic tone, a postsynaptic α-adrenoceptor stimulating action of imidazolidines. *Eur. J. Pharmacol.*, 40:311-320, 1976.

192. van Zwieten, P.A., Thoolen, M.J.M.C., and Timmermans, P.B.M.W.M.: The pharmacology of centrally acting antihypertensive drugs. *Br. J. Clin. Pharmacol.*, 15:455S-462S, 1983.

193. Roffolo, R.R., Jr.: α-Adrenoceptors. In *Monographs in Neural Science*, Vol. 10. Edited by J. Cohen, Basel, Karger, 1984.

194. Schmitt, H.: Action des sympathomimétiques sur les structures nerveuses. *Actual. Pharmacol.*, 24:93-131, 1971.

195. Gillis, R.A., Gatti, P.J., and Quest, J.A.: Mechanism of the antihypertensive effect of α₂-agonists. *J. Cardiovasc. Pharmacol.*, 7(Suppl.8):S38-S44, 1985.

196. Bousquet, P. and Guertzenstein, P.G.: Localization of the central cardiovascular action of clonidine. *Br. J. Pharmacol.*, 49:573-579, 1973.

197. Scholtysik, G., Lauener, H., Eichenberger, E., Burki, H., Salzmann, R., Muller-Schweinitzer, E., and Waite, R.: Pharmacological actions of the antihypertensive agent N-amidino-2-(2,6-dichlorophenyl) acetamide hydrochloride (BS 100-141). *Arzneimittel Forsch*, 25:1483-1491, 1975.

198. Srimal, R.C., Gulati, K., and Dhawan, B.N.: On the mechanism of the central hypotensive action of clonidine. *Can. J. Physiol. Pharmacol.*, 55:1007-1014, 1977.

199. Walland, A.: Inhibition of a somato-sympathetic reflex via peripheral presynaptic α-adrenoceptors. *Eur. J. Pharmacol.*, 47:211-221, 1978.

200. Drew, G.M.: Effects of α-adrenoceptor agonists and antagonists on pre- and postsynaptically located α-adrenoceptors. *Eur. J. Pharmacol.*, 36:313-320, 1976.

201. Miso, Y. and Kubo, T.: Central and peripheral cardiovascular responses of rats to guanabenz and clonidine. *Jap. J. Pharmacol.*, 40:87-119, 1982.

202. de Jonge, A., van den Berg, G., Qian, J.Q., Wilffert, B., Thoolen, M.J.M.C., and Timmermans, P.B.M.W.M.: Inhibitory effect of α₁-adrenoceptor stimulation on cardiac sympathetic neurotransmission in pithed normotensive rats. *J. Pharmacol. Exp. Ther.*, 236:500-504, 1986.

203. Brown, D.A. and Caulfield, M.P.: Hyperpolarizing α₂-adrenoceptors in rat sympathetic ganglia. *Br. J. Pharmacol.*, 65:435-445, 1979.

204. Dashwood, M.R., Gilbey, M.P., and Spyer, K.M.: The localization of adrenoceptors and opiate receptors in regions of the cat nervous system involved in cardiovascular control. *Neuroscience*, 15:537-551, 1985.

3.3

Connective Tissue

Some fibromyalgia patients have biochemical and histological connective tissue abnormalities. Clinically, these may manifest as mitral valve prolapse, articular hypermobility, or a higher-than-average susceptibility to musculoskeletal injury.

Important components of what is termed loose connective tissue are its amorphous, gel-like ground substance and several constituents embedded in it. (Loose connective tissue, which is a normal tissue form, should be distinguished from abnormally lax ligaments—or ligamentous laxity—which result in joint hypermobility.) Of special significance are the fibroblast cells. These cells synthesize, secrete, and maintain all the major constituents of the extracellular matrix. Among the other constituents are water-binding proteoglycans (protein-glycogen molecules), high-tensile strength collagen, and fibronectin and elastin fibers. Fascia is the continuous, loose connective tissue that spans the body and provides a strong yet semi-elastic matrix and support for the other organs.

Many fibromyalgia and hypothyroid patients have low levels of hydroxyproline, a marker of collagen turnover. (Both collagen and elastin contain hydroxyproline, but collagen contains more.) Biochemical markers indicate that both groups of patients have decreased collagen cross-binding in their connective tissues. These markers are pyridinoline, an indicator of connective tissue disease, and deoxypyridinoline, an indicator of bone degradation.

Both groups of patients also have high levels of hyaluronic acid. The high water-binding capacity of this connective tissue compound is the chief determinant of the viscosity and permeability of connective tissue. Hyaluronic acid's binding of excess water in connective tissues plausibly explains the myxedematous swelling of the skin of some hypothyroid and fibromyalgia patients. The high hyaluronic acid levels indicate lack of normal inhibition of fibroblasts by thyroid hormone.

One researcher has reported a high incidence of mitral valve prolapse in fibromyalgia. The prolapse is possibly related to loosening of connective tissue in fibromyalgia patients, as it appears that prolapse of the valve is a manifestation of connective tissue abnormalities of the heart. Some researchers have reported mitral valve prolapse in hypothyroidism, but hyperthyroidism is the thyroid disorder most associated with prolapse of the valve. Connective tissues affected by hyperthyroidism become myxedematous as in hypothyroidism. The mechanism in hyperthyroidism appears to be autoimmune. In contrast, in hypothyroidism and resistance to thyroid hormone, myxedema results from inadequate thyroid hormone inhibition of fibroblast activity.

One study found a high incidence of articular hypermobility in fibromyalgia patients. Another reported hypermobility in hypothyroid patients who also had rheumatic signs and symptoms. Hypermobility suggests decreased connective tissue restriction of joint motion, possibly due to collagen and elastin fiber abnormalities. Both abnormalities can result from inadequate thyroid hormone inhibition of fibroblast activity.

It is plausible that inadequate thyroid hormone regulation underlies the connective tissue abnormalities found in some fibromyalgia patients. The abnormalities would be the same as those that occur in some patients with hypothyroidism or resistance to thyroid hormone. The main direct effect of inadequate thyroid hormone regulation on connective tissues is dysregulation of fibroblasts. The dysregulation would produce the biochemical and histological connective tissue abnormalities found in some fibromyalgia patients.

According to these documented abnormalities, these patients probably also have decreased collagen deposition, decreased collagen cross-binding, and increased water-binding in their connective tissues. These would result in weakened connective tissues, which can explain the joint hypermobility and mitral valve prolapse in some patients. It would also explain some patients' general or localized non-pitting edema that fails to subside during recumbency.

Inadequate thyroid hormone regulation of fibroblasts can cause any one or a combination of the above effects, which can account for the variability of connective tissue findings in fibromyalgia patients. Some patients may have weakened connective tissues and edema, some may have weakened connective tissues but no edema, and some may have edematous swelling but normal connective tissue strength. And still others, whose connective tissues are not affected by thyroid hormone inadequacy, may have fibromyalgia symptoms related only to other tissues that are affected by the thyroid hormone inadequacy.

Inadequate thyroid hormone regulation can also potentially affect connective tissues indirectly. First, the inadequacy may lower motor drive and cause a disinclination to engage in physical activities that would condition connective tissues. As a result, the thickness and strength of connective tissues would decrease. Second, thyroid hormone inadequacy can decrease the time a patient spends in stages 3 and 4 sleep. The reduced time in these sleep stages may result in decreased growth hormone secretion. In turn, low growth hormone secretion can cause subnormal protein synthesis, decreased connective tissue strength, increased susceptibility to micro-trauma, and delayed healing of exercise-induced injury. Third, inadequate thyroid hormone regulation of transcription of the growth hormone gene decreases growth hormone synthesis and secretion.

In patients who are physically inactive due to inadequate thyroid hormone regulation, connective tissues are likely to decrease in density and strength. In addition, the inadequate thyroid hormone regulation of connective tissue fibroblasts is likely to decrease collagen synthesis and cross-binding. These patients would be expected to become relatively hypermobile with subnormal joint stability. A higher incidence of mechanical injuries of joints with physical activity would suggest this. However, the low level of physical activity by those with inadequate thyroid hormone regulation may minimize the incidence of such injuries. The low incidence of injuries due to low activity levels may account for the dearth of published reports

on both articular hypermobility and injuries among fibromyalgia and hypothyroid patients.

Fascia, like other loose connective tissue, is dynamic. It adapts structurally and functionally to conditions such as immobility, repetitive work loading, or resolved inflammation. As fascia adapts, its water content decreases, its collagen content increases, collagen fibers move closer together, and cross-binding increases. Though this process is normally adaptive, it can progress to pathophysiological extremes. Clinically, the process can lead to musculoskeletal symptoms such as pain from ischemia and myofascial trigger points. (These symptoms would tend to occur less in patients whose connective tissues have inadequate thyroid hormone regulation, and more in patients whose connective tissues have adequate regulation—though other of their fibromyalgia-related tissues may not have adequate thyroid hormone regulation.)

Fascia thins and weakens during prolonged abstention from resistance-type physical activities, loss of stages 3 and 4 sleep, or low growth hormone secretion. All these may be the result of inadequate thyroid hormone regulation of cells.

The connective tissue abnormalities that occur in hypothyroidism also tend to occur in fibromyalgia. The similarity of the connective tissue abnormalities in these two conditions—in view of the almost uniform similarity of other features between the two—favors the proposition that the connective tissue abnormalities in fibromyalgia are caused by inadequate thyroid hormone regulation. The most likely mechanism is inadequate thyroid hormone regulation of fibroblast cells of the ground substance of connective tissues.

● OVERVIEW OF CONNECTIVE TISSUE

ANATOMY AND HISTOLOGY

The connective tissues are a diverse tissue group and serve various purposes in the body. They provide structure, serve as packing substance, provide insulation, and are one medium for defense of the body.[97,p.53] This chapter focuses on loose connective tissue, which is the prototypical form of connective tissue. (*Loose* connective tissue, which is a normal tissue form, should be distinguished from the abnormally lax ligaments—or ligamentous laxity—that result in joint hypermobility.) All other forms of connective tissue are variations. The constituents of connective tissue relevant to this chapter are ground substance, proteoglycans, collagen and elastin fibers, and fibroblast cells.

Ground Substance

The fibers and cells of connective tissue are inlaid in the ground substance. This is an amorphous, transparent gel that constitutes the matrix of connective tissue. The viscosity of ground substance varies in different forms of connective tissue and even in loose connective tissue at different times and under different conditions.

Proteoglycans

Ground substance contains proteoglycans. These are made up of proteins and complex hexosamine-containing carbohydrates called glycosaminoglycans,[97,p.69] mucopolysaccharides, and mucin.[104] The proteoglycan filaments are extremely thin, coiled molecules that are difficult to see even with the aid of electron microscopy. Their placement forms a fine mat network.[52,p.173]

The proteoglycan molecule consists of a protein core. Glycosaminoglycan side chains project off the protein core and give the molecule a "bottle brush" appearance. Proteoglycans and long chain carbohydrates bind large amounts of water, creating the gelatinous material of ground substance. Tissue levels of proteoglycans are elevated in some fibromyalgia, hypothyroid, and thyroid hormone resistant patients. The diminished inhibitory effect of T_3 on skin fibroblasts' synthesis of one proteoglycan, fibronectin, is the most common physiological abnormality found in patients with general resistance to thyroid hormone (see section and subsection below: "Possible Relation of Connective Tissue Abnormalities in Fibromyalgia to Inadequate Thyroid Hormone Regulation of Connective Tissue: Proteoglycan Accumulation").

The main proteoglycan that binds water in loose connective tissue is hyaluronic acid. Some 98% of proteoglycans are hyaluronic acid (the other 2% consist of protein).[52,p.173] Hyaluronic acid's high water-binding power is the chief determinant of the viscosity and permeability of connective tissue. Water bound to hyaluronic acid provides a vehicle for the transport of nutrients, gases, and metabolites between the circulating blood and cells.[97,p.54] Levels of hyaluronic acid are elevated in some fibromyalgia and hypothyroid

patients (see section and subsection below: "Possible Relation of Connective Tissue Abnormalities in Fibromyalgia to Inadequate Thyroid Hormone Regulation of Connective Tissue: Elevated Serum Hyaluronic Acid").

Collagen and Elastin Fibers, and Fibronectin

Collagen is a fibrous, insoluble connective tissue protein. About a third of body proteins are collagen. In the ground substance, collagen fibers and proteoglycan filaments are the two most abundant solid constituents. The collagen molecule is flexible but has high tensile strength. The length of collagen fibers varies, but most extend long distances in the ground substance[52,p.173] and they branch extensively.[97,p.54] Collagen has a higher content of the amino acid hydroxyproline than do elastin fibers. Hydroxyproline serves as a marker of collagen turnover, and is low in some fibromyalgia and hypothyroid patients. (See sections and subsections below: "Possible Relation of Connective Tissue Abnormalities in Fibromyalgia to Inadequate Thyroid Hormone Regulation of Connective Tissue: Changes in Connective Tissue Fibers: Decreased Hydroxyproline Levels.")

Collagen fibers form cross-links or cross-bindings with adjacent collagen. These links contribute to the semi-elastic yet stabilizing capacity of connective tissues. Biochemical markers indicate reduced collagen cross-binding in some fibromyalgia and hypothyroid patients. (See sections and subsections below: "Connective Tissue Abnormalities in Fibromyalgia: Decreased Collagen Cross-Binding" and "Possible Relation of Connective Tissue Abnormalities in Fibromyalgia to Inadequate Thyroid Hormone Regulation of Connective Tissue: Decreased Collagen Cross-Binding in Hypothyroidism.")

Elastin fibers enable connective tissue to stretch considerable distances and then resume its original shape after the distorting force ceases. Elastin fibers are smaller than collagen fibers. They are made up of an amorphous component with bundles of microfibrils embedded around it. Elastin fibers contain less hydroxyproline than does collagen.[97,p.54]

Fibronectin is a cell surface protein that attaches cells to underlying tissue and adjacent cells. Fibronectin binds to the fibronectin cell surface receptors, and a single cell may have as many as 500,000 receptors.[47,p.739] The network fibronectin forms with collagen, elastin, and proteoglycans makes up the connective tissue extracellular matrix.

Fibroblast and Mast Cells

Any cell from which connective tissue develops is considered a fibroblast. Fibroblasts are not the only connective tissue cells, but they are the most prevalent. They synthesize, secrete, and maintain all the major constituents of the extracellular matrix.[53,p.62]

Thyroid hormone inhibits excess secretion of proteoglycans by fibroblasts. In inadequate thyroid hormone regulation of fibroblasts (either due to hypothyroidism or thyroid hormone resistance due to mutant T_3-receptors), the cells secrete excessive amounts of proteoglycans. Some fibromyalgia patients have elevated tissue levels of proteoglycans (see section and subsection below: "Possible Relation of Connective Tissue Abnormalities in Fibromyalgia to Inadequate Thyroid Hormone Regulation of Connective Tissue: Proteoglycan Accumulation").

The mast cells of loose connective tissue are important as a component of the immune system. They secrete heparin, an anticoagulant, and histamine, a compound that induces vasodilation and increases the permeability of capillaries and venules.[97,pp.55-56] During inadequate thyroid hormone regulation of the adrenergic genes, an increased density of α-adrenergic receptors on mast cells may cause the cells to secrete excess histamine. This may give rise to increased allergy tendencies or chemical sensitivities syndrome. In addition, increased histamine secretion may interfere with sleep by heightening awareness and pain perception (see Chapter 3.1, section titled "Altered Sleep Patterns" and Chapter 3.18).

Fascia

Fascia is the semiflexible fibrous membrane of connective tissue that binds together the various components of the body. Pockets in the fascia contain the various body organs. One of these is the skeletal muscles, which fascia covers, supports, and separates.

Fascia is a dynamic tissue. It increases in density and relative rigidity during chronic repetitive muscle stresses, immobility, or resolution of inflammation. Various types of manual therapies and systematic stretching can, in many cases, restore normal or near-normal fascial elasticity.[66][67][69][71] (See section below: "Adaptive and Pathophysiological Processes of Fascia.")

● CONNECTIVE TISSUE ABNORMALITIES IN FIBROMYALGIA

BIOCHEMICAL AND HISTOLOGICAL ABNORMALITIES IN FIBROMYALGIA

Researchers have reported several biochemical and histological connective tissue abnormalities in fibromyalgia patients. I have listed some of these in Tables 3.3.1 and 3.3.2.

Proteoglycan Accumulation

Brendstrup et al.,[16] Awad,[2][20] and others[17][18][19][51,p.132] have found increased proteoglycans in biopsy samples from fibromyalgia patients.

Elevated Serum Hyaluronic Acid

Yaron et al. measured the serum levels of hyaluronic acid in 42 female fibromyalgia patients. The researchers compared the results with measures of serum hyaluronic acid from 27 female rheumatoid arthritis patients and 36 healthy female controls matched for age. The fibromyalgia patients had significantly higher serum levels. The mean level in healthy controls was 41±8.7 μg/L, in rheumatoid arthritis patients was 113±15.9 μg/L, and in fibromyalgia patients was 420±26 μg/L. Yaron et al. concluded that the elevated hyaluronic acid level of fibromyalgia patients is a biochemical abnormality that may serve as a laboratory marker for diagnosing the condition.[55]

Changes in Connective Tissue Fibers

Researchers have reported biochemical abnormalities in collagen, collagen cross-binding, and in elastin in some fibromyalgia patients.

Decreased Hydroxyproline Levels: Indication of Changes in Collagen. Sprott et al. measured urinary hydroxyproline levels in 39 fibromyalgia patients. The levels were significantly lower than in healthy controls.[56] The lower hydroxyproline levels suggest impaired collagen turnover in connective tissues in these fibromyalgia patients.

Decreased Collagen Cross-Binding. Sprott and coauthors conducted their study to learn whether abnormal collagen metabolism characterizes fibromyalgia. They took skin biopsy samples from the trapezii muscles of 8 patients. They also obtained urine samples from 39 patients and 55 control subjects, and they collected serum from 22 patients and 17 controls. The researchers performed analyses for two products of lysyl oxidase-mediated cross-binding in collagen. One product was pyridinoline, an indicator of connective tissue disease. The other was deoxypyridinoline, an indicator of bone degradation. They found low ratios of pyridinoline to deoxypyridinoline in the urine and serum. This suggests decreased levels of collagen cross-binding. They concluded that fibromyalgia patients had decreased collagen cross-binding.[56]

Sprott and colleagues also found highly ordered "cuffs" of collagen around the terminal nerve fibers in biopsy tissue samples from all 8 patients with fibromyalgia. Such "cuffs" were not present in control skin samples. The investigators suggested that the decrease in collagen cross-binding may contribute to remodeling of the extracellular matrix and deposition of collagen around nerve fibers. It is possible, as they wrote, that deposition of collagen around nerve fibers can lower the pain threshold at the tender points.[56] As the contents of this chapter attest, I concur with their view that the study of altered metabolism in collagen and other connective tissue constituents in fibromyalgia patients may help clarify the pathogenesis of the condition.

Elastin Fibers Connecting Muscle Fibers. Danneskiold-Samsøe et al. performed microscopic exams of muscle from normal and "fibrositis" patients. The researchers reported finding muscle fibers connected by an abnormal network of reticular or elastic fibers.[46]

STRUCTURAL/FUNCTIONAL ABNORMALITIES

Mitral Valve Prolapse

Pelligrino et al. reported that according to echocardiography, 75% of his fibromyalgia patients had mitral valve prolapse, and 33% had myxedematous degeneration (mucous connective tissue tumors).[39] Goldman reported that fibromyalgia patients have an increased incidence of both joint hypermobility (see next section) and mitral valve prolapse. He speculated that in fibromyalgia, the hypermobility and prolapse are part of a more generalized connective tissue abnormality.[32] (Klemp et al. did not find mitral valve prolapse in hypermobile ballet dancers,[36] but other researchers have documented the association.[37][38])

Articular Hypermobility

Goldman tested 210 fibromyalgia patients and found that 136 (65%) had joint hypermobility of the upper and/or lower extremities. Of the 136 hypermobile patients, 133 were women. He proposed that hypermobile patients are more at risk for sports-related and other injuries, depending on which of their joints are hypermobile.[32] His view is in line with the finding of Klemp et al. that injuries were significantly more common in hypermobile ballet dancers than in controls. The researchers wrote that they regard hypermobility as a liability to the ballet dancer.[36] Goldman also speculated that injuries associated with hypermobility may influence the development of fibromyalgia.[32,p.1195]

● POSSIBLE RELATION OF CONNECTIVE TISSUE ABNORMALITIES IN FIBROMYALGIA TO INADEQUATE THYROID HORMONE REGULATION OF CONNECTIVE TISSUE

BIOCHEMICAL AND HISTOLOGICAL ABNORMALITIES

Table 3.3.1 contains a list of the biochemical and histological connective tissue abnormalities reported in hypothyroidism and fibromyalgia.

Proteoglycan Accumulation

Inadequate thyroid hormone inhibition of fibroblasts causes edematous swelling of connective tissues in some patients.[50,p.854] The swelling, termed myxedema, results from accumulation of excess ground substance glycosaminoglycans[4][5][6][7][8][9][10][11][12] and fibronectin.[13][14]

Clinicians call the swelling edema. Edema may be responsible for pain when it causes compression of mechanoreceptors (types C and A delta fibers). This may occur because of the limited ability of fascia to expand and accommodate increasing fluid pressure. The increasing pressure inside tissues may mount sufficiently to activate the mechanoreceptors. Edema may form in aponeuroses, ligaments, tendons, and the fascia of skeletal muscles. Edema in some ligaments causes clinical conditions. For example, in hypothyroidism, myxedema of the flexor retinaculum (the ligament that surrounds the wrist) may compress the medial nerve and cause carpal tunnel syndrome with abnormal sensations of the hands. (See Chapter 3.16, sections titled: "Carpal Tunnel Syndrome: A Mononeuropathy in Fibromyalgia" and "Carpal Tunnel Syndrome in Hypothyroidism: A Mononeuropathy.") The tissues of the heart and intestinal tract may also become myxedematous.[37] Myxedema of the heart may cause slow heart rate, and myxedema of the intestinal tract may cause constipation.[50,p.854]

Conversely, exposure of fibroblasts to sufficient amounts of T_3 inhibits secretion of ground substance constituents[11]—if the T_3-receptors in the fibroblasts have normal ligand affinity. T_3 exerts this inhibitory effect on glycosaminoglycans by decreasing synthesis rather than by increasing degradation.[12] Administering supraphysiologic amounts of T_3 does not, however, excessively inhibit secretion of the major glycosaminoglycan, hyaluronic acid.[47,p.737]

Investigators have found accumulated glycosaminoglycans [4][13][15] and fibronectin [13] in the skin of patients with thyroid hormone resistance. The diminished inhibitory effect of T_3 on skin fibroblasts' synthesis of fibronectin has been the most consistent physiological abnormality found in patients with general resistance to thyroid hormone.[13][14][43][45]

In the early 1970s,[20] and again in the late 1980s and early 1990s,[1][2,p.253] Awad tried to interest researchers in the myxedematous connective tissue changes he found in biopsies of "fibrositic nodules." This was to little avail, however.[21] The tissue changes he found were similar to or the same as those found in hypothyroidism. In Table 3.3.1, I have compared his biopsy findings[2] to those reported in the hypothyroidism literature.[3,pp.147-151] Pelligrino et al. found that 33% of fibromyalgia patients had myxedematous degeneration; researchers refer to the degeneration as "mucous connective tissue tumors."[39]

Brendstrup et al.,[16] Awad,[2][20] and others[17][18][19][51,p.132] reported finding increased proteoglycans in biopsy samples from fibromyalgia patients. Moreover, when Brendstrup took a biopsy sample from "fibrositic" muscle, he also took a control sample of "normal" muscle from the fibrositis patient. Of the 12 control samples, he found some evidence of increased proteoglycan material (metachromatic staining) in 3 samples, an increased number of nuclei in 3, and a few lymphocytes around blood vessels in 1 sample. These findings may indicate that some patients had mild and more widespread inadequate thyroid hormone inhibition of fibroblasts than merely at "fibrositic" loci.

Thyroid researchers conjectured that some complaints of hypothyroid patients (transient pain, stiffness, and cramps in the muscles) are due to the separation of muscle fibers by "mucoedema."[22,p.571] Similarly, Awad argued that some muscle symptoms of fibromyalgia patients are due to separation of the

muscle fibers by the proteoglycans he found in biopsies.[1] The proteoglycan accumulation constitutes "a space-occupying lesion that produces a mass effect."[2,p.257] Beyond some threshold, accumulating myxedematous material will compress vascular channels and impede blood flow. By compressing vessels, the material impairs oxygen flow and compromises the supply of energy-yielding nutrients to muscle fibers.[2,p.257] The decreased blood flow may also reduce exposure of fibroblasts to T_3 enough to further disinhibit their secretion of proteoglycan. This might intensify the myxedema in the local areas. Awad concurred that this is possible.[21]

In addition, inadequate thyroid hormone regulation of fibroblasts may result in impaired blood flow through arterioles and capillaries due to an accumulation of a glycosominoglycan called glycocalyx. Glycocalyx has molecular sieving properties and constitutes a selective barrier to the movement of macromolecules from the plasma in the lumen to the endothelial surface of the vessels. The glycocalyx also impedes the flow of red blood cells farther downstream in the lumen of the vessels.[112]

In the fibromyalgia patients I have seen with myxedematous-appearing skin, the edema has been nonpitting and has not dispersed when the patients were recumbent. These are indicators that the edema was due to increased proteoglycan content of their ground substance. In most patients, the edema has been bilaterally localized to the area just above the clavicles, the upper arms, anterior legs, or the back. Fewer patients have had the generalized edema typical of that in longstanding or severe inadequate thyroid hormone inhibition of fibroblasts.[98,p.989] In all cases I have observed, the tissue puffiness has disappeared after the patients began taking exogenous thyroid hormone of various dosages. This is consistent with disappearance of myxedema in the connective tissues of the hypothyroid patient after she attains eumetabolic status.[98,p.990] (Some differences in reported findings in these two types of patients may be due to variations in the sensitivity of techniques used to examine biopsy samples.)

Elevated Serum Hyaluronic Acid

Yaron et al. measured the serum levels of hyaluronic acid in 42 female fibromyalgia patients. They found that the levels were significantly higher than in rheumatoid arthritis patients and healthy control subjects.[55] This finding is consistent with high hyaluronic acid levels during inadequate thyroid hormone inhibition of fibroblasts.

Regulation of Fibroblast Activity by Thyroid

Hormone. In 1950, Asboe-Hansen reasoned that high levels of TSH in hypothyroidism stimulate the mast cells of the amorphous ground substance to increase their output of hyaluronic acid.[5,p.227] Later studies, however, showed that the increased output of hyaluronic acid is not due to elevated TSH; instead, a deficiency of thyroid hormones causes increased output of the hyaluronic acid, and the cells that synthesize and secrete the substance are fibroblasts rather than mast cells.

That thyroid hormones regulate fibroblast secretion of hyaluronic acid was made clear through systematic testing. When a patient takes exogenous thyroid hormones, excess hyaluronic acid secretion begins to reverse within 2-to-3 weeks.[7] When a patient with pituitary hypothyroidism (deficient thyroid hormone output secondary to inadequate TSH secretion by the pituitary) receives exogenous TSH, the thyroid gland increases secretion of thyroid hormones and excess hyaluronic acid secretion reverses. But when the thyroid gland itself is impaired and cannot respond to injected TSH, excess hyaluronic acid secretion persists. This phenomenon was confirmed in the skin[8][9] and heart muscles[10] of myxedematous rats, and more recently, in the skin and various other tissues of humans (see subsection below: "Increased Tissue Hyaluronic Acid in Hypothyroidism").

In 1987, Kohn wrote that in hypothyroidism, the net content of glycosaminoglycans in the tissues does not significantly increase. In fact, he wrote that the rat skin content of one form of glycosaminoglycan, chondroitin sulfate, decreases.[50,p.855] (Chondroitan sulfate is a sulfur-containing mucopolysaccharide present among ground substance materials in the extracellular matrix of connective tissue.) This was reported in 1962 by Schiller et al. They found that hypothyroid rats had a decreased turnover rate of chondroitan sulfate although the skin concentration was low. The presumed cause was that chondroitin sulfate degrades at a normal rate, but synthesizes more slowly.[9] This would leave a net decrease in tissue content. However, in 1981, Smith et al. reported that as they deprived cultured fibroblasts of T_3, the fibroblasts secreted chondroitin sulfate at 2.1 times the normal rate.[11] The discrepancy in these two findings is yet unexplained.

Consistent with reports more recent than 1987, Kohn wrote that in hypothyroidism the content of hyaluronic acid increases about 150%. He noted that hyaluronic acid synthesizes more slowly than it normally would, but it degrades even more slowly, leaving a net increase in tissue content.[50,p.855] (See next section.) This excess hydrophilic hyaluronic acid increases the water-binding capacity of the ground substance. As a result, the tissues retain excess fluid. This produces edema-based puffiness that is most common in severe hypothyroidism. Adequate dosages of T_3[13][43][45] eliminate the edema. T_4 has the same effect if the patient's cells are able to deiodinate T_4 to T_3[50,p.855] and are not resistant to thyroid hormone.

Recent Studies of Hyaluronic Acid and Hypothyroidism. Hyaluronic acid is the most prevalent glycosaminoglycan in normal skin. Matsuoka et al. found that hyaluronic acid is also the most prevalent water-binding substance in the highly glycosaminoglycan-infiltrated myxedematous skin of hypothyroid patients.[75] Smith and coauthors grew human skin fibroblasts in culture media. They exposed the fibroblasts to T_3 in some cultures, and they deprived fibroblasts of the hormone in other cultures. Then they compared the hyaluronic acid levels in the two groups of cultures. In the cultures in which fibroblasts were deprived of T_3, hyaluronic acid content had increased 2.8-fold. (Chondroitin sulfate, a sulfated glycosaminoglycan, increased 2.1-fold.)[11] It appears that depriving fibroblasts of thyroid hormone increases hyaluronic acid synthesis by increasing the activity of the enzyme hyaluronate synthetase.[98,p.991] Smith et al. also found that adding T_3 to the T_3-deprived fibroblasts reduced the accumulation of hyaluronic acid. The reduced levels were almost the same as in cultures where fibroblasts were never deprived of T_3.[11] These laboratory findings indicate that T_3 decreases hyaluronic acid secretion by human skin fibroblasts. It probably does so by inhibiting activity of hyaluronate synthetase.[98,p.991]

In a similar study, Shishiba et al. incubated fibroblasts in media deficient of thyroid hormone. Synthesis of all species of proteoglycans increased by 85%. The net synthesis of hyaluronic acid increased by roughly 50%. The deficit of thyroid hormone in the media did not affect the rate of proteoglycan breakdown.[76]

The *in vitro* findings of Smith et al. are consistent with other researchers' *in vivo* findings.[11] Studies have shown that hypothyroid patients have elevated serum levels of hyaluronic acid, as do some fibromyalgia patients. Faber et al. measured the serum levels of hyaluronic acid during hypothyroidism and hyperthyroidism. Twenty-three hypothyroid patients had a significant mean elevation in hyaluronic acid levels. Sixteen of the patients underwent treatment with T_4, and their mean level of hyaluronic acid decreased to normal (71 ± 50 ng/mL before treatment and 41 ± 20 ng/mL after treatment, $P < 0.02$). The researchers concluded that fibroblast secretion of hyaluronic acid increases during hypothyroidism and decreases with thyroid hormone replacement.[73]

Increased Tissue Hyaluronic Acid in Hypothyroidism. Savage and Sipple pointed out that the bone marrow ground substance of hypothyroid patients tends to become replaced by hyaluronic acid-rich mucopolysaccharides. They called the process gelatinous transformation. Histologically, the process is similar to skin myxedema. They noted that visceral myxedema may occur through the same mechanism.[77]

McDaniel and Besada wrote that an increase in hyaluronic acid may cause primary open-angle glaucoma in hypothyroidism. In hypothyroidism, hyaluronic acid accumulation within the trabecular meshwork of the eye may cause an increase in outflow resistance and increased pressure within the eyeball. The pressure increase may be reversible with the use of thyroid hormone. The researchers described a hypothyroid patient whose intraocular pressure varied inversely with the use or discontinuation of thyroid hormone therapy.[72]

Table 3.3.1. Connective tissue abnormalities in fibromyalgia*† and hypothyroidism‡

CHANGES	FIBROMYALGIA	HYPOTHYROIDISM
Increase in proteoglycans	+	+
Increased interstitial nuclei (possibly sarcolemmal nuclei)	+	+
Distended interstices from proteoglycan accumulation	+	+
Increased mast cells	+	-
Extravasated blood between muscle fibers	+	-
Large clusters of blood platelets	+	-
Capillary endothelial changes	+	-
Lymphocytic infiltration (evidence of inflammation)	+	+
Basophilia of fibers	-	+

*Awad, E.A.: Pathological changes in fibromyalgia. *First International Symposium on Myofascial Pain and Fibromyalgia.* Minneapolis, Minnesota, May 9, 1989.
†Awad, E.A.: Histopathological changes in fibrositis. In *Advances in Pain Research and Therapy*, Vol. 17. Edited by J.R. Fricton and E.A. Awad, New York, Raven Press, Ltd., 1990, pp.249-258.
‡Ramsay, I.: *Thyroid Disease and Muscle Dysfunction.* Chicago, Year Book Medical Publishers, Inc., 1974, pp.147-151.

Hyaluronic acid is a component of synovial fluid. An increased concentration of hyaluronic acid—with a resulting increase in synovial water content—may account for the findings reported by Dorwart and Schumacher. They studied 12 severely hypothyroid patients who had rheumatic signs and symptoms. They found synovial effusions in 8 patients. The effusions in 7 patients were extremely viscous; effusions in 6 of the 7 patients contained calcium pyrophosphate crystals. Each patient complained of generalized stiffness. The patients had thickened flexor tendon sheaths, joint laxity, and popliteal cysts. Needle biopsy of the thick synovium specimens from 5 patients revealed only mild inflammation. Dorwart and Schumacher speculated that hypothyroidism was the cause of the musculoskeletal problems.[80]

Myxedema in Hyperthyroidism. A hundred years ago, clinicians used the presence of myxedema as the diagnostic indicator that a patient needed to use exogenous thyroid hormone (see Chapter 2.5). Later, researchers established that myxedematous tissues contain high levels of glycosaminoglycans, especially hyaluronic acid. The association of glycosaminoglycan infiltration and myxedema with hypothyroidism may cause confusion when the clinician reads that hyperthyroidism is also associated with glycosaminoglycan infiltration.[26] But localized myxedema does occur in some patients who are hyperthyroid due to Graves' disease,[75][78] and in other conditions such as scleromyxedema and scleredema.[75]

Some researchers debate whether the myxedema in Graves' patients results from a localized accumulation of glycosaminoglycans. Smith stated that such accumulation does occur.[44,p.678] Peacey et al. noted that a previous study had shown an increase in glycosaminoglycan eosition in the forearm skin of Graves' patients who did not have pretibial myxedema. Peacey and his group tried to confirm the presence of subclinical dermopathy in the forearm tissues of Graves' patients. They studied the forearms of 16 Graves' patients. However, they found no evidence of either widespread activated fibroblasts or of increased glycosaminoglycan deposition in the skin. They did find HLA-DR expression by fibroblast-like cells in the skin. HLA stands for human leukocyte antigen. These antigens are controlled by genes at three loci (HLA-A, HLA-B, and HLA-C) on chromosome 6. Specific antigen types are associated with specific diseases. The HLA-DR expression suggests activation of these cells in Graves' dermopathy specimens.[104]

Kriss wrote that studies show pretibial myxedema to be an autoimmune condition; it is a complication not only of "primary myxedema" (probably referring to primary hypothyroidism) but also of Hashimoto's thyroiditis and Graves' disease. According to Kriss, the most likely mechanism is stimulation by antithyroid antibodies of skin target cells, probably fibro-blasts. The stimulated cells secrete excessive amounts of glycosaminoglycans, especially hyaluronic acid. Other sites such as the skin over the radial aspect of the forearm (the thumb side) may also be infiltrated. Why these sites and not others are involved is unknown. The infiltration may last for months or years and then spontaneously subside.[78] Smith reviewed the data on the etiology of localized myxedema in Graves' disease. He pointed out that most of these patients have thyroid-stimulating antibodies. However, he wrote that the association of immunoglobulins, long-acting thyroid stimulator, and fibroblast-stimulating factor with localized myxedema has been inconsistent.[44,pp.678-679]

Changes in Connective Tissue Fibers

Biochemical changes suggesting abnormalities in collagen and elastin fibers in fibromyalgia are consistent with those reported during inadequate thyroid hormone regulation of fibroblast function.

Decreased Hydroxyproline Levels. Sprott et al. found that mean hydroxyproline levels were low in 8 fibromyalgia patients. The low levels indicate impaired collagen turnover. Levels were significantly lower than in healthy controls.[56]

Kaplan et al. reported that a patient with thyroid hormone resistance had low urinary hydroxyproline. She was hypometabolic and had a markedly subnormal oxygen consumption rate when taking 50-to-100 μg of T_3 daily. Her oxygen consumption did not increase much above predicted normal values despite high serum T_3 concentrations. Her low levels of urinary hydroxyproline increased to normal with higher (supraphysiologic) T_3 doses. She was normal according to most indices only with a daily dosage of 500 μg per day.[65]

Foscolo et al. studied urinary excretion of hydroxyproline in patients with adult onset idiopathic myxedema. The 13 untreated hypothyroid patients included 11 women and 2 men. They ranged in age from 24-to-64 years. Compared to healthy controls, these patients had a significantly lower urinary excretion of hydroxyproline (4.45±0.41 ng/mL vs 7.76±0.55 ng/mL, p < 0.001). The researchers wrote that the low hydroxyproline indicated reduced osteoclastic bone resorption.[63]

Elevated hydroxyproline is typically found in hyperthyroid patients.[57][58][59] (Preemptively, I should emphasize that, as Faber and others have reported, increased levels of such biochemical markers of collagen turnover in bone are not correlated with significant loss of bone density, osteoporosis, or fracture risk.[58] For evidence for this conclusion, see Chapter 4.4, section titled "Bone.") Bijlsma et al. found that when 4 hyperthyroid patients became eumetabolic with treatment, their urinary hydroxyproline/creatinine ratio decreased (69.9±12 vs 20.7±2.4 μmol/mmol, P < 0.01). Conversely, when hypothyroid patients became eumetabolic with treatment, their urinary hydroxyproline/creatinine ratio increased (15.9±4.3 vs 25.3±3.2 μmol/mmol, P < 0.05).[64] This study highlights the association between hypothyroidism and low hydroxyproline levels.

Indications of Changes in Collagen. The decrease in hydroxyproline in fibromyalgia patients suggests a reduction in collagen turnover in connective tissues. In addition, Jensen reported low serum levels of procollagen III, a collagen precursor, in 16 fibromyalgia patients who had disturbed sleep.[42] Both these findings are consistent with the reduced levels of procollagen III in hypothyroidism that increase to normal levels during thyroid hormone therapy.

Nørregaard et al. found that in 43 fibromyalgia patients, procollagen aminoterminal peptide was 12% lower than in normal men (P<0.01). It is important to note that in these fibromyalgia patients, the mean somatomedin-C levels were not lower than those of controls. Forty-one of the somatomedin-C values for the fibromyalgia patients were inside the 95% confidence interval.[41] This suggests that low growth hormone levels, with secondary low somatomedin C levels, were not responsible for underactivity of fibroblasts and consequent low procollagen levels. Instead, inadequate thyroid hormone regulation of fibroblasts may have been responsible.

Faber et al. measured serum levels of procollagen III N-peptide (a collagen precursor) to learn whether they changed during hyperthyroidism and hypothyroidism. Two-thirds of 28 hyperthyroid patients had elevated serum levels of the collagen precursor. Levels decreased to normal when the patients became eumetabolic. Hypothyroid patients had reduced serum levels of the collagen precursor. In the 16 patients who underwent T_4 treatment, levels increased significantly.[73] Serum levels of procollagen III were therefore positively correlated with adequate thyroid hormone levels. This indicates that during inadequate thyroid hormone regulation of fibroblasts, the amount of collagen in patients' tissues tends to decrease. This finding is compatible with the reduced hydroxyproline levels in some fibromyalgia patients.

Decreased Collagen Cross-Binding in Hypothyroidism. Sprott et al. reported finding low ratios of pyridinoline to deoxypyridinoline in the urine and serum of fibromyalgia patients. This suggests decreased levels of collagen cross-binding in some fibromyalgia patients. The researchers speculated that decreased cross-binding could lower the pain threshold at tender points.[56]

Kriss wrote that biopsies show evidence of damage to collagen in the skin of hypothyroid and other patients who have myxedema and increased levels of hyaluronic acid[78] (see section above, "Increased Tissue Hyaluronic Acid in Hypothyroidism").

Nakamura et al. found that hypothyroid patients had low urinary excretion of both pyridinoline and deoxypyridinoline. The researchers measured pyridinium cross-links in 8 hypothyroid patients before and after treatment with T_4. The aim was to see whether bone resorption was reduced in hypothyroidism and whether it increased with T_4 treatment. Initially, TSH levels were elevated (268.1 ± 87.7 µU/L). Patients were treated with 100 µg (0.1 mg) T_4 daily. The researchers assayed for the excretion of both products of urinary pyridinium cross-binding, pyridinoline and deoxypyridinoline, before and after T_4 treatment. Concentrations of both compounds were low in untreated hypothyroid patients. Levels increased gradually as thyroid hormone status improved from hypothyroidism to eumetabolism. One month after treatment, TSH levels were still as high as 74.4 ± 44.5 µU/L. At that time, urinary deoxypyridinoline excretion had increased by 2.6 times the pretreatment level. By the time the TSH levels of these patients decreased below 10 µU/L, the levels of both compounds had increased significantly: pyridinoline by 3.8 times pretreatment values, and deoxypyridinoline by 3.3 times. The investigators wrote that this was the first evidence that (1) urinary excretion of the products of pyridinium cross-linking are reduced in hypothyroidism, and (2) excretion of the products becomes normal after patients begin using physiologic dosages of thyroid hormone.[61]

The low urinary excretion of the two compounds, pyridinoline and deoxypyridinoline, in hypothyroid patients is the reverse of urinary excretion and serum levels in hyperthyroid patients. Nagasaka et al., for example, reported that urinary deoxypyridinoline and the serum pyridinoline (the cross-linked telopeptide domain of type I collagen) are elevated in hyperthyroidism. Before therapy, urinary deoxypyridinoline was elevated by +553%, and serum pyridinoline was elevated by +396%. Concentrations of each compound decreased to within the normal range during the second month of treatment.[62]

Langdahl et al. used another measure of collagen cross-links in 33 patients who had undergone surgery to correct hyperthyroidism. The patients had surgery 6 years before but had not used exogenous thyroid hormone. The researchers compared these results with 27 other patients who had undergone the same surgery, but who had taken T_4 over the 6 subsequent years. According to the investigators, all patients were eumetabolic. Patients taking T_4 had higher serum T_4 and serum free T_4-index levels than patients not taking T_4. The two groups did not differ in serum T_3 levels and the serum free T_3-index. The patients not taking T_4 had TSH levels within the normal range but higher than control levels. Urinary excretion of collagen cross-link products was normal. However, serum cross-linked carboxy-terminal telopeptide of type I collagen (ICTP) was decreased by 11% in untreated patients.[60]

Elastin Fibers Connecting Muscle Fibers. Danneskiold-Samsøe and coauthors reported muscle fibers connected by a network of reticular or elastic fibers in fibromyalgia patients. Normal muscle does not contain such a network. The researchers stated that the network of elastic fibers connected muscle cells and formed constricting bands around them. They called these "rubber-band structures."[46]

Danneskiold-Samsøe and colleagues proposed that in these patients, when one muscle cell contracts, it pulls other muscle cells connected to it by the abnormal elastic network. This causes a passive sideways stretch or pull. When adjacent muscle cells contract, they too exert a pull on other cells, creating a cascade of passive movement. The movement is painful and exhausting. The exhaustion, according to the researchers, accounts for muscle weakness in fibromyalgia patients. Danneskiold-Samsøe, et al. stated that these findings may indicate the nature of fibromyalgia.[46] They published their findings in 1982, an extremely early date for availability of objective data on fibromyalgia. In 2000, it is clear that such a mechanism could not account for the other objectively verified abnormalities in fibromyalgia. All other abnormalities and the "rubber-band structures" are best explained as features of another underlying pathophysiological process—inadequate thyroid hormone regulation of cell function.

Kriss wrote that biopsies show evidence of damage to elastin fibers in the skin of hypothyroid patients and others with increased hyaluronic acid and myxedema[78] (see section above titled, "Increased Tissue Hyaluronic Acid in Hypothyroidism").

Matsuoka and colleagues studied the elastin fiber constituent of skin as a possible source of decreased elasticity in myxedema. They found that elastin fiber concentration was significantly lower than normal in hypothyroid pretibial myxedema. The low elastin fiber concentration was due to the glycosaminoglycan infiltration. Ultrastructural examination of myxedematous skin revealed wide variations in the diameter of elastin fibers, as well as decreased numbers of microfibrils. The researchers wrote that hypothyroid pretibial myxedema is consistently associated with quantitative and qualitative defects of dermal elastin fibers.[103]

These studies indicate that elastin, as well as other connective tissue constituents, responds dynamically to deficient and excessive amounts of thyroid hormone. The abnormalities of elastin fibers in hypothyroidism are not entirely consistent with Danneskiold-Samsøe's report of an abnormal network of reticular or elastic fibers in fibromyalgia patients.[46] The hypothyroidism studies do show, however, that inadequate thyroid hormone regulation of fibroblasts (which synthesize, secrete, and maintain all the major constituents of the extracellular matrix[53,p.62]) can induce abnormalities of elastin. We must wait for additional studies to decide whether this mechanism generates in some fibromyalgia patients the abnormalities reported by Danneskiold-Samsøe.

Excess Mobility of Connective Tissue: Weakened Fascia. It may be, however, that the presence of an elastic fiber network in fibromyalgia patients is a result of weakened fascia. A patient's weakened fascia may permit unusually extensive movement of the endomysium and perimysium that ensheathe the muscle fibers and fascicles. (The endomysium is the thin fascial sheath that invests each muscle fiber; the perimysium, which is continuous with the endomysium, invests each bundle of muscle fibers. The fascial tissues are composed mostly of reticular fibers, but the tissues also contain the other constituents of loose connective tissue.) Extensive movement in turn may cause biochemical precursors to precipitate into elastin fibers. For example, immobile scar tissue does not contain newly formed elastin. Movement, however, can induce the appearance of elastin in scars.[48] Elastin is scanty in the fetal lung. After birth, when respiration ensues, the rhythmic mechanical stress causes elastin to accumulate in the pulmonary alveoli, the pleura, the myocardium and pericardium.

Keech removed the collagen from connective tissue and reduced the remaining contents to powder. When she subjected the powder to movement, such as scraping it off the sides of a test-tube, it formed a structureless gel. More movement converted the gel into a solid "rubber ball." Keech wrote that the mass "consisted entirely of elastin-like material in various stages of formation and exhibiting an underlying fibrous structure."[49,p.509] The more extensive the manipulation, the more complete was the conversion to fibrous structures typical of elastin.[49,p.510] Such excess mobility of connective tissue matrix due to abnormally low fascial tone may induce formation of the elastin network Danneskiold-Samsøe found in fibromyalgia patients' tissues.

Glucocorticoids. The process described in the section above may be more advanced in fibromyalgia patients who have taken supraphysiologic dosages of exogenous glucocorticoids. King and Carter-Su, for example, showed that supraphysiologic dosages of dexamethasone, administered for 24 hours, inhibited growth hormone from eliciting several early cellular events in fibroblasts. Glucocorticoids interfere with growth hormone cellular action by reducing the number of growth hormone receptors on fibroblast cell membranes.[109] The decrease in growth hormone receptors results in reduced binding of growth hormone to the cell. (See sections below: "Physical Deconditioning" and "Low Growth Hormone Secretion.")

By impeding collagen synthesis, glucocorticoids impair wound healing.[101] Hydrocortisone reduced synthesis of type I and type III collagen in smooth muscle cells of the ureters, serving as an anti-fibrotic agent.[102] Dexamethasone can disrupt the connective tissue filamentous cage-like structures around nascent lipid droplets. The mechanism of disruption by the glucocorticoid is expression of filaments with a carboxyl-terminal deletion.[99]

Haapasaari et al. reported that in skin treated topically with a corticosteroid, collagen synthesis was inhibited and down-regulated. A treatment period of 3 days decreased collagen synthesis. Synthesis did not increase during 1 corticoid-free week. During a 2-week corticoid-free period, synthesis increased to about 50% of the level seen in the non-treated skin.[100] This finding indicates that collagen synthesis does not completely normalize in human skin even during corticoid-free periods of up to 2 weeks. The thinning of skin that usually accompanies the use of topical glucocorticoids (as in the treatment of psoriasis) results, then, from inhibition of fibroblasts by the glucocorticoids.

STRUCTURAL/FUNCTIONAL ABNORMALITIES

Mitral Valve Prolapse

That some fibromyalgia patients have lax connective tissues is indicated by a higher than normal incidence of joint hypermobility (see next section) and mitral valve prolapse. Several researchers have reported mitral valve prolapse in fibromyalgia.[37][38][39] Goldman[32] conjectured that both the hypermobility and valve prolapse are part of a more generalized connective tissue abnormality in these patients.

Patients with Marfan syndrome, Ehlers-Danlos syndrome, and osteogenesis imperfecta have excessively elastic connective tissues and hyperflexible joints. They also have a higher prevalence of mitral valve prolapse than the general population.[96][98] The higher prevalence in these conditions suggests that mitral valve prolapse is a manifestation of abnormalities of the connective tissues of the heart valves.[84,p.765] Moreover, hyperflexible joints in other tissues are associated with a high prevalence of prolapse of the mitral valve.[92][93][94][95] The association of lax connective tissues with mitral valve prolapse raises the question as to whether mitral valve prolapse in some fibromyalgia patients results from influences that could loosen their connective tissues. One such influence is low growth hormone and/or somatomedin-C levels due to inadequate thyroid hormone regulation of the growth hormone gene (see Chapter 3.12). Low growth hormone may cause subnormal fibroblast activity (see Figure 3.3.1).

Studies of Laron's syndrome patients help elucidate the effects of inadequate growth hormone on fibroblasts. In Laron's syndrome, patients have a congenital growth hormone insensitivity due to dysfunctional growth hormone receptors. Freeth et al. found that the effects of growth hormone on fibroblasts in Laron's syndrome children is subnormal compared to normal control subjects. Cultured fibroblasts from affected children either do not respond to growth hormone or have reduced responses. These researchers believed that the growth hormone insensitivity in some children is caused by growth hormone receptor mutations, and in others, by dysfunctional growth hormone signaling.[108] In another study, Freeth et al. found that growth hormone activates some signaling pathways in skin fibroblasts. The hormone, for example, induced rapid tyrosine phosphorylation of proteins.[107]

I am not certain that low growth hormone and somatomedin C levels due to inadequate thyroid hormone regulation of the growth hormone gene result in laxity of the tendinous attachments of the mitral valve with consequent prolapse. At this time, there are too few studies of valve prolapse in hypothyroidism to give an impression of the likelihood of this mechanism.

In one study, procollagen aminoterminal peptide levels were low in fibromyalgia patients compared to normal controls. The patients' somatomedin-C levels, however, were not low. This finding decreases the likelihood that the low procollagen levels were due to low growth hormone and somatomedin-C levels.[41] It is more likely that instead, the low levels were a result of inadequate thyroid hormone regulation of fibroblasts.

A few authors have indicated an association of mitral valve prolapse with hypothyroidism. Paggi et al. described a 35-year-old woman with a congenital "sub-hyoid ectopy of the thyroid gland." She had clinical symptoms of hypothyroidism, myxedematous cardiopathy, and mitral valve prolapse. They reported that the cardiomyopathy resolved with thyroid hormone therapy.[87] Ardura et al. reported a pediatric case of hypothyroidism associated with mitral valve prolapse syndrome, with rupture of cordae tendinae. A sister of the patient died, presumably with a complication of mitral valve prolapse associated with hypothyroidism.[88]

However, Brauman et al. reported mitral valve prolapse in only 6% of patients with nongoitrous hypothyroidism. The incidence in normal controls was 5.2%. In the normal population, the incidence range is wide.[83] Kahaly et al. reported that 238 of 2410 normal controls (9.9%) had prolapse.[82] Marks et al. found that 4 of 50 controls (8%) had prolapse.[81] Others have reported a range from 6% to more than 20% in the presumably normal population.[89][90][91] The incidence of prolapse in hypothyroidism reported by the Brauman et al. study[83] is therefore well within the incidence range for normal control subjects.

More studies are available on valve prolapse in hyperthyroidism. These point to autoimmunity as the underlying pathology. Early study results showing a high incidence of prolapse among hyperthyroid patients raised the possibility of an association between excessive thyroid hormone levels and prolapse. But more definitive studies indicated that the valve prolapse is associated with the autoimmune process in some hyperthyroid patients, rather than with thyrotoxicosis.

Alvarado et al. also found that thyroid function test results did not correlate with prolapse in Graves' disease. The researchers studied three groups: hyperthyroid Graves' patients ($T_4 > 11.5$ μg/100 mL), euthyroid Graves' patients ($T_4 < 11.5$ μg/100 mL), and healthy controls. The incidence of prolapse was similar between hyperthyroid (31%) and euthyroid (25%) Graves' patients, but was higher than in controls (5%). The researchers concluded that prolapse is not associated with thyroid status, although Graves' patients have a higher incidence than normal controls.[86] This finding raises the possibility that another factor is responsible in these patients, most likely the autoimmune process.

Kahaly et al. assessed the prevalence of mitral valve prolapse in 60 patients with Graves' disease. The investigators compared the results with the prevalence in 20 patients with toxic nodular goiter, which is not an autoimmune disease. Thirty-six of 60 Graves' patients (60%) had prolapse, compared to 2 of 20 toxic nodular goiter patients (10%). The incidence in controls was 9.9%. Thyroid function test results were not correlated with incidence or intensity of prolapse. The researchers concluded that thyroid test results were virtually the same between the two groups. The difference between the hyperthyroid groups was the autoimmunity of the Graves' patients. Kahaly and coauthors concluded that mitral valve prolapse in Graves' patients is probably associated with the autoimmune process.[82]

This view is again supported by the finding of a high incidence of mitral valve prolapse in Graves' disease regardless of whether patients are thyrotoxic or eumetabolic.[83] Marks et al. found mitral valve prolapse in 31 of 75 patients (41%) with chronic lymphocytic thyroiditis. The researchers found no correlation, however, between the prevalence of mitral valve prolapse and the presence of hypothyroidism, serum antithyroid antibodies, or the duration of chronic lymphocytic thyroiditis.[81] Brauman et al. found that 16.09% of 87 patients with autoimmune chronic lymphocytic thyroiditis had mitral valve prolapse. The incidence was significantly increased compared to controls. Brauman et al. concluded that prolapse is significantly increased (P < 0.02) in patients with autoimmune disorders of the thyroid gland.[83] However, Blumberg et al. found that of 23 patients (ranging in age from 5-to-20 years) with juvenile autoimmune thyroiditis, only 1 patient (4.3%) had cardiac echo and Doppler evidence of mitral valve prolapse. The investigators concluded that the incidence of prolapse in such patients is probably not increased above that of healthy controls.[111]

Articular Hypermobility

Goldman reported that 65% of the fibromyalgia patients he studied had hypermobile joints. Most hypermobile patients were women.[32] This result is consistent with the report that women are more hyper-

mobile than men.[34]

In the general population of people with hypermobility, the joints that are hypermobile vary between individuals. Most articular hypermobility appears to be on the nondominant side.[33] Some people are more hypermobile in the upper extremities and others in the lower extremities. Other people have a more generalized joint laxity[34] and they tend to have joint and muscle pain.[35] Goldman reported that fibromyalgia patients have joint hypermobility of the upper or lower extremities. He noted that hypermobile individuals are more likely to be injured in sports activities, and he surmised that this could lead to the development of fibromyalgia.[32,p.1195]

Dorwart and Schumacher studied 12 severely hypothyroid patients who had rheumatic signs and symptoms. In 8 patients, the researchers found synovial effusions which may have resulted from increased levels of the water-binding compound hyaluronic acid in the fluid. All patients complained of generalized stiffness, and their flexor tendon sheaths were thickened. However, they had joint laxity, indicating loosening of the articular connective tissue supports. This possibly resulted from decreased collagen synthesis and cross-binding. The investigators hypothesized that hypothyroidism was the cause of these articular findings.[80]

It is also likely that the joints of physically inactive fibromyalgia patients (especially those who do little resistance-type activity) become more mobile as connective tissues progressively lose tone. Studies have shown that endurance exercises do not increase the tone of connective tissues as much as resistance exercises do. Investigators sectioned the gastrocnemius muscles of rats' legs. Absence of the gastrocnemius muscles subjected the plantaris muscles to more resistance activity. As a result, the plantaris muscles underwent compensatory hypertrophy. Also, attaching a weight to the wings of chickens, which increased resistance during use of the wings, increased the total collagen content of the wing muscles.[24,p.63] This does not mean necessarily that a lack of resistance activities will always result in hypermobility due to lax connective tissues. But this is a likely outcome for individuals whose connective tissues have genetically-determined greater elasticity. Hypermobility may occur among such individuals who are disinclined to exercise or who have exercise intolerance due to untreated or undertreated hypothyroidism or cellular resistance to thyroid hormone (see Chapter 3.4).

● A MODEL OF CONNECTIVE TISSUE ABNORMALITIES IN FIBROMYALGIA

In hypothyroidism and cellular resistance to thyroid hormone, connective tissue may lose tone and become more extensible; mitral valve prolapse and articular hypermobility may be the clinical outcome. Inadequate thyroid hormone regulation may induce these changes by several mechanisms. One mechanism is the low physical activity level of the patient. For several reasons, inadequate thyroid hormone regulation can render the patient disinclined to engage in enough physical activity to maintain physical conditioning. Other mechanisms include low growth hormone and/or somatomedin C secretion, decreased collagen synthesis and cross-binding, and increased connective tissue myxedema due to increased binding of water in the ground substance by excessive hyaluronic acid accumulation (see Figure 3.3.1).

PHYSICAL DECONDITIONING

In some patients, connective tissues may not be directly affected by inadequate thyroid hormone regulation. These patients would most likely not have myxedema. But if as a feature of their inadequate thyroid hormone regulation they are disinclined to engage in sufficient physical activity, one result might be that their connective tissues would have a decreased content of collagen fibers.

In 1989, Bennett posited a deconditioning hypothesis of fibromyalgia.[40,pp.187-188] At the time, he lacked the benefit of later evidence of growth hormone deficiencies in some patients. His hypothesis asserted that fibromyalgia pain resulted from micro-trauma to muscle. I will include connective tissues here because, as I have noted elsewhere,[70][71] injury to muscle seldom occurs without damage to its fascial sheaths. At the time, Bennett's hypothesis was instructive. It focused attention on inadequate physical activity by fibromyalgia patients, examining its possible but unlikely role as the cause of fibromyalgia as opposed to a precipitating or compounding factor.

Many fibromyalgia patients have difficulty engaging in conditioning-level physical activities (see Chapter 3.4). It is reasonable to expect that the consequent lessening of connective tissue strength in these patients renders them more susceptible to micro-trauma. The state of an individual's physical conditioning determines the level of mechanical stress necessary to induce micro-trauma, as well as the severity of the resulting symptoms.[85][110] One reason for this is that resistance exercises increase both the density of muscle myofibrils and the thickness of connective tissues.[24] The connective tissues that thicken with resistance exercises include: ligaments, tendons, junctions between tendons and bone and ligaments and bone, joint cartilage, and the fascial sheaths within muscle (epimysium, perimysium and endomysium).[24][25] The two training effects—an increase in myofibrils and a thickening of connective tissues—increase myofascial resistance to trauma. As a result, individuals who engage in sufficient resistance exercises can perform intense, repetitive, or prolonged activities with few adverse results.

The differential effects of exercise in deconditioned and conditioned men were reported in a study by Evans et al. Exercise by deconditioned men participating in the study produced evidence of harmful effects: intense muscle soreness and impaired locomotion 1-to-2 days after eccentric exercise; and increases in CK, interleukin-1, proteolysis-induced factor, and urinary 3-methylhistidine. These effects were absent or significantly less severe in conditioned runners.[27] The effects of training on connective tissues are further portrayed by a comparison of wild hares with caged laboratory rabbits. Wild hares can sustain a running load possibly 50-to-100 times greater than that sustained by caged rabbits. Wild hares' hip joints tend to show fewer degenerative changes. Staff wrote that in many ways, the lifestyle of modern man is more like that of the caged rabbit than of the wild hare.[28,pp.371-372] In view of such data, it seems likely that the joint hypermobility of some fibromyalgia patients results in part from detraining—from thinning of their connective tissues due to deconditioning.[32,p.1194] The deconditioning would most severely impact the patient with hypermobility due to (1) inherited higher-end connective tissue elasticity and (2) inadequate thyroid hormone regulation of fibroblasts.

Bennett conjectured that persistent and debilitating pain in some patients after they exercised was caused by sleep deprivation and poor physical fitness. These complementary and additive influences can reduce connective tissue tone and impair tissue repair.[40,p.188] Failure to sleep restoratively would leave the patient more fatigued, and the fatigue would decrease her inclination to exercise. In turn, an additional decrease in physical activity would tend to further reduce the amount of stage 4 non-REM slow wave sleep she gets, causing more fatigue. The patient's poor physical conditioning would in turn predispose her to more injury from exercise-induced muscle micro-trauma. Any associated pain would interfere even more with sleep and heighten the disinclination to exercise.

Bennett also noted that secretion of growth hormone depends on adequate slow wave sleep (mainly in stage 4) and the stress of exercise. Insufficient slow wave sleep and relative inactivity may result in subnormal secretion of growth hormone. The low growth hormone secretion in turn can cause suboptimal protein synthesis, decreased connective tissue strength, increased susceptibility to micro-trauma, and delayed healing of exercise-induced injury.[40]

Bennett wrote in summary: "The stimulus for the development of fibromyalgia syndrome is hypothesized to be any condition that leads to a continuation of slow wave sleep disturbance and reduced physical activity."[40,p.188] It is clear that inadequate thyroid hormone regulation can do both. In addition, inadequate thyroid hormone regulation also provides a plausible answer to the question: *Why are some individuals with deconditioned myofascia prone to develop fibromyalgia while others are not?* The susceptibility of some can be explained by numerous effects of inadequate thyroid hormone regulation. Bennett himself wafted over one highly probable effect. First he noted that those destined to develop fibromyalgia may be at the lower end of the VO$_2$ max distribution curve on an inherited basis. This would make them less inclined to enjoy exercise. He then proposed that these people "have a genetically predetermined *abnormality of the central controls of adrenergic activity*, making them less able to deal with stress, as well as exposing them to depressive illness and primary Raynaud's phenomenon [italics mine]."[40,p.188] The lower-end VO$_2$ max (see Chapter 3.4), low stress tolerance, depression (see Chapter 3.10), and Raynaud's (see Chapter 3.9) can indeed be attributed to altered adrenergic activity—all due to inadequate thyroid hormone transcription regulation of α- and β-adrenergic receptor genes. And, inadequate thyroid hormone regulation can feasibly account for other factors that directly or indirectly adversely impact the connective tissues: low growth hormone secretion (see Chapter 3.12), disinclination to exercise because of low motor drive (see Chapter 3.4), and reduced strength of connective tissues due to a decrease in collagen content and cross-binding (see section above titled "Changes in Connective Tissue Fibers").

Increased amounts of collagen in the ground substance, and increased collagen cross-binding, contribute substantially to the stability and tensile strength of connective tissues. By decreasing these, inadequate

thyroid hormone regulation may weaken connective tissues and increase susceptibility to mechanical injury. Moreover, loss of muscle and connective tissue strength favors the slumping, flexed posture that some believe induce the predictable tender points in fibromyalgia patients.[23] The progressively-flexing posture can cause changes in the myofascial tissues, the spine, and joints that contribute to the fibromyalgia patient's pain (see Chapter 3.11).

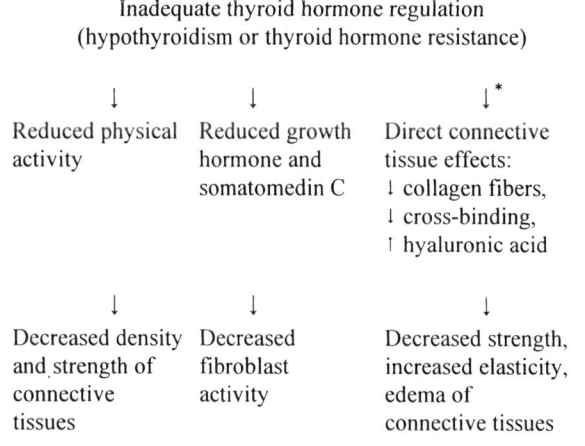

Figure 3.3.1. Pathways through which inadequate thyroid hormone regulation may affect the connective tissues.
*This pathway predominates during inadequate thyroid hormone regulation.

LOW GROWTH HORMONE SECRETION

Several factors can reduce growth hormone secretion. As I touched on in the above section, two factors are inadequate physical activity and insufficient stage 4 non-REM sleep. As I describe in Chapter 3.12, however, thyroid hormone potently regulates the growth hormone gene, and inadequate thyroid hormone regulation of this gene's transcription reduces growth hormone synthesis and secretion. Any one or combination of these three factors can lead to inadequate growth hormone regulation of fibroblasts, with resulting diminished strength of connective tissues. Inadequate thyroid hormone regulation is the most probable primary mechanism in reduced growth hormone secretion, compounded secondarily by the other two factors (both of which can be accounted for by inadequate thyroid hormone regulation).

Reduced Physical Activity
Growth hormone blood levels increase with ex-

ercise of moderate intensity[30][31] and decrease with inadequate physical activity.[29,p.267] As I describe in Chapter 3.4, inadequate thyroid hormone regulation can reduce dopamine levels in the brain. This can lower motor drive and motor activity, and it can leave an individual disinclined to engage in anything other than minimal physical activity. The reduced physical activity may secondarily lower the circulating levels of growth hormone. The reduced growth hormone levels may contribute to the connective tissue abnormalities in fibromyalgia.

Inadequate Stage 3 and Stage 4 (Deep) Sleep

Growth hormone secretion increases during stages 3 and 4 sleep.[30][31] Conversely, growth hormone levels decrease with loss of stages 3 or 4 sleep.[29,p.267]

Kales et al. found that hypothyroid patients had deficient stage 3 and stage 4 sleep. The deficit was relieved by thyroid hormone therapy.[79] Wilke, Sheeler, and Makarowski reported that most of their hypothyroid fibromyalgia patients, before starting thyroid replacement therapy, complained of "poor, interrupted" or "restless" sleep. With treatment, however, both their muscle pain and sleep disturbance disappeared simultaneously. The authors wrote, "*It is tempting for us to postulate that hypothyroidism in our patients impaired stage IV sleep, which then resulted in myalgias typical of the fibrositis syndrome* [again, italics are mine]."[74] (See Chapter 3.18.)

Inadequate Thyroid Hormone Regulation Can Cause Reduced Physical Activity, Inadequate Deep Sleep, and Low Growth Hormone Secretion

Inadequate thyroid hormone regulation can plausibly account for reduced physical activity, loss of deep sleep, and low growth hormone secretion in some fibromyalgia patients. The inadequacy of thyroid hormone regulation can cause a disinclination to exercise as well as exercise intolerance (see Chapter 3.4); it is associated with insufficient stages 3 and 4 sleep (see Chapter 3.18); and because thyroid hormone potently regulates the growth hormone gene, it can reduce growth hormone levels and, in turn, levels of somatomedin C. Inadequate thyroid hormone regulation is the interlinking mechanism that can most comprehensively account for all these documented abnormalities of fibromyalgia.

POSSIBLE EXPLANATION FOR VARIABLE PHENOTYPES AMONG FIBROMYALGIA PATIENTS

The fibroblasts in different tissues appear to respond differentially to different growth factors. Haase et al. found that responses of fibroblasts to growth factors varied, depending on the anatomical location within the periodontium. Somatomedin C (insulin-like growth factor), but not growth hormone, stimulated mitosis (somatic cell division) by periodontal and gingival ligament fibroblasts. However, periodontal fibroblasts were more responsive. Altered expression of matrix proteoglycan mRNA accompanied the mitosis. Some proteoglycan mRNAs decreased and others increased.[106] The results of this study suggest that differential tissue responsiveness of fibroblasts to different growth factors, such as growth hormone and somatomedin C, may account for the variable connective tissue findings in fibromyalgia patients. A greater deficiency of one growth factor than another may partially account for different phenotypes of fibromyalgia: some patients have joint hypermobility and mitral valve prolapse; others do not.

LOW GLUCOCORTICOID LEVELS

Glucocorticoids can mimic T_3-inhibition of fibroblasts. When a fibromyalgia patient has low cortisol secretion[47,p.738] (see Chapter 3.5), the inadequacy may have some disinhibiting effect on fibroblasts, increasing their hyaluronic acid secretion. (See subsection above titled "Glucocorticoids.") It would be interesting to determine whether there is correspondence between biochemical and histological connective tissue abnormalities, myxedema, and low glucocorticoid levels in fibromyalgia patients. Nevertheless, considering the bulk of available evidence, biochemical and histological abnormalities and myxedema in fibromyalgia patients are more likely to be associated with inadequate thyroid hormone inhibition of fibroblasts. In addition, while inadequate thyroid hormone regulation can feasibly account for decreased glucocorticoid secretion and low serum cortisol levels, the reverse is not likely.

ADAPTIVE AND PATHOPHYSIOLOGICAL PROCESSES OF FASCIA

Fascia is a dynamic tissue that adapts structurally and functionally to changing conditions. Because of this, fascia is as important to pain management as are muscles fibers. The conditions that induce dynamic adaptation of fascia are prolonged immobility, repetitive work load, and resolution of inflammation. Adaptation involves increased collagen deposition, collagen cross-binding, and a roughly concentric inward coiling of the collagen fibers. The involved area may become a fibrous adhesion that restricts normal myofascial mobility. The adhesion may lead to the need for clinical care because of resulting limitation of musculoskeletal mobility and the local compression of blood vessels and nerves.[54][69][105]

Healthy Fascia

In healthy, non-fibrotic fascia, collagen fibers are cross-linked to a degree that stabilizes interfaces at necessary loci. This occurs at anatomical sites that are relatively immobile and that are subjected to repetitive work loads. Cross-links are minimized at sites that are highly mobile, such as anatomical sites involved in frequent stretching movements. At these sites, fascial sheets are able to slide past one another or otherwise distort with sufficient flexibility and expansibility. When the tissue spaces collect an abnormally high content of fluid (as occurs during sodium retention or during myxedema), fascial tissue adapts: the distance between collagen fibers increases and elastin fibers stretch to permit the expansion required by the high fluid content.

Abnormal Fascia

When the ground substance contains an overabundance of collagen fibers that have cross-bound and coiled in on themselves (as would happen in chronic overload and immobility of fascial tissues), fascia is less able to adapt. This inelastic fascial meshwork is relatively unyielding and expands poorly. When fluid is retained, tremendous tension may mount inside the tissue spaces. As the tension mounts, veins and lymphatics may collapse. This results in the retention of metabolites that lower the thresholds of mechanoreceptors, such as those of type C nerve fibers. When the receptors are subjected to relatively slight degrees of mechanical pressure, the metabolites lower the threshold for noxious signal transmission. And at some threshold point, the mechanoreceptors will begin reacting to the intramuscular pressure much as they respond to a palpating digit that compresses them. The nerves will conduct noxious signals into the central nervous system and stimulate referred pain.[70,pp.36-37][71]

Immobility. When fascia is relatively immobile, water content of the ground substance decreases. This permits its collagen fibers to more closely approximate one another and to knit together with cross-bindings.[67] We would expect this to occur, for example, when someone habitually holds her neck in hyperextension, keeping the upper cervical myofascia relatively immobile. Also, when the fascia is not stretched sufficiently, as in this posture, its helical collagen fibers tend to coil in on themselves and shorten.[68] As a result, the fascia progressively contracts and compresses whatever is contained within it, including blood vessels and mechanoreceptors.[69] Under these conditions, fascia becomes a shrinking, pain-producing straightjacket of fibrotic flesh.

Repetitive Work Load. When a muscle is subjected to high-frequency work overload (the "stretch-hypertrophy rule"), fibroblasts in the muscle's investing fascia become more active and deposit more collagen fibers.[66] If the work overload is chronic, progressively more collagen deposits in the fascia. If the tissues are relatively immobile (as, for example, the erector muscles of the upper thoracic paraspinal region), the immobility reduces water-binding in the fascia. This enables the collecting collagen fibers to move more closely toward one another. When some threshold decreased distance is reached, cross-linking increases between the fibers.[67] This reinforces tensile strength and reduces expansibility of the myofascia. With increased intensity of this process, intra-myofascial pressure can mount sufficiently to impede circulation, and the patient may experience chronic, ischemic pain.

Resolved Inflammation. Inflammation of fascial tissue heals partly through the accumulation of type III collagen. The fibers are inlaid in the ground substance in a seemingly erratic pattern, resembling the arrangement of thousands of tooth picks dropped onto the floor. This arrangement is ideal for closing any traumatically-induced breach in the inflamed tissue. The collagen fibers form cross-links and then shorten through coiling. The coiling gradually pulls together the underlying tissues in a roughly concentric direction. The process stabilizes the tissues. The resulting adhesion (scar tissue) is less elastic than normal myofascial tissue and has a lower threshold than normal tissue for traumatic disruption. Treatments such as ultrasound and manual cross-frictioning, when expertly used, can increase the elasticity of the adhesion.[71]

Variable Tendency Toward Pathophysiological Fascia Among Fibromyalgia Patients. Immobility, repetitive work load, and resolution of inflammation are common in patients with musculoskeletal pain. These three potentially pathophysiological processes

Table 3.3.2. A comparison of markers of connective tissue abnormalities in fibromyalgia and hypothyroidism.

ABNORMALITY	FIBROMYALGIA	HYPOTHYROIDISM
Tissue proteoglycans* (water-binders)	High	High
Serum hyaluronic acid (water-binders)	High	High
Procollagen III (collagen precursor)	Low	Low
Hydroxyproline (collagen constituent)	Low	Low
Serum & urine pyridinoline and deoxypyridinoline (measures of collagen cross-binding)	Low	Low
Mitral valve prolapse	High incidence	Normal incidence, but sporadic cases[†]
Articular hypermobility	High incidence	Some reports

*Also found in thyroid hormone resistance patients.
[†]The lower incidence may result from detection and treatment of hypothyroidism.

are particularly common in patients with pain due to myofascial trigger points, including many fibromyalgia patients. But these processes depend on a sufficient ability to generate new collagen fibers that form cross-links. Some fibromyalgia patients with hypothyroidism or cellular resistance to thyroid hormone have a diminished ability to do so. This is evident from the diminished cross-linking and decreased numbers of collagen fibers in their connective tissues. These patients may be less susceptible to clinical disorders that develop from the fibrous adhesions that sometimes result from the three processes. However, variable tissue responsiveness to thyroid hormone ensures that some patients will have normal connective tissue structure and function. These patients may be as prone as individuals without fibromyalgia to clinical problems from fibrous adhesions.

MYXEDEMA AS A POSSIBLE SOURCE OF MYOFASCIAL TRIGGER POINT PAIN

As the hyaluronic acid content increases in connective tissues, they have a greater water-binding capacity. As I have pointed out in previous publications,[69][71] when the retained fluid causes a myofascial tissue to swell beyond its ability to expand, pressure inside the tissue's interstitial spaces increases. The extensibility of a region of fascial tissue may be reduced by factors that increase collagen inlaying and cross-linking, such as those I mention in the above section (prolonged immobility, repetitive mechanical stress, or resolved inflammation). As the pressure mounts from increased water-binding, it can exceed the threshold for mechanical compression of the local type C and A delta nerve receptors. The involved nerve fibers may then begin conducting afferent signals to the central nervous system, causing pain perception, sympathetically-induced vasoconstriction, and alpha motor neuron-mediated skeletal muscle contractions.

This process may mechanically activate latent trigger points. For illustration, consider latent trigger points in the small caliber muscles of the upper cervical area. When the muscles and their tendinous attachments have acquired adhesions due to repetitive biomechanical stress, their fascial latticework has a limited ability to expand. Edema of the minimally expandable tissue will create high internal pressure. This mechanical pressure will increase irritability of latent trigger points and, at some threshold, stimulate them to actively refer pain—in most cases to the head. (Clinicians often misinterpret such myofascial headaches as migraines.[54])

Further, the swelling may compress arteries and

veins coursing through the myxedematous fascia of the region. This can cause deficient entry of energy-yielding nutrients and deficient exit of metabolic wastes. Theoretically, this vascular impairment may contribute to the formation, maintenance, and activation of trigger points.

I have treated some fibromyalgia patients who had intermittent headaches mediated by the mechanism I describe above. In most cases, the headaches accompanied edema associated with their menstrual periods. My impression, however, is that the incidence of pain in fibromyalgia patients due to this mechanism is moderate. In fact, I would expect some patients with inadequate thyroid hormone regulation of fibroblasts (by virtue of their reduced ground substance collagen content and collagen cross-linking) to be consequently protected to some degree from pain due to this mechanism. Thus, the fascial component of the myofascial tissues may not be a major source for the headaches that are so problematic for some female fibromyalgia patients during their menstrual periods. Trigger points housed in the muscles may be a more common source.

A more potent factor related to the occurrence or worsening of headaches and general pain may be an increase in α_2-adrenergic receptors associated with the decrease of estrogen secretion between ovulation and the beginning of the menstrual period. The pain would possibly be worst just following ovulation and immediately before the onset of the period when estrogen secretion is typically lowest (see Chapter 3.6).

REFERENCES

1. Awad, E.A.: Pathological changes in fibromyalgia. *First International Symposium on Myofascial Pain and Fibromyalgia.* Minneapolis, Minnesota, May 9, 1989.
2. Awad, E.A.: Histopathological changes in fibrositis. In *Advances in Pain Research and Therapy*, Vol. 17. Edited by J.R. Fricton and E.A. Awad, New York, Raven Press, Ltd., 1990, pp.249-258.
3. Ramsay, I.: *Thyroid Disease and Muscle Dysfunction.* Chicago, Year Book Medical Publishers, Inc., 1974.
4. Murata, Y., Refetoff, S., Horwitz, A.L., and Smith, T.J.: Hormonal regulation of glycosaminoglycan accumulation in fibroblasts from patients with resistance to thyroid hormone. *J. Clin. Endocrinol. Metab.*, 57:1233, 1983.
5. Asboe-Hansen, G.: The variability in the hyaluronic acid content of the dermal connective tissue under the influence of thyroid hormone. *Acta Dermato-Venereologica*, 30:221-229, 1950.
6. Kohn, L.D.: Connective tissue. In *The Thyroid*, 4th edition. Edited by S.C. Werner and S.H. Ingbar, New York, Harper and Row Publishers, 1987.
7. Gabrilove, J.L. and Ludwig, A.W.: The histogenesis of myxedema. *J. Clin. Endocrinol. Metab.*, 17:925, 1957.
8. Schiller, S.: Mucopolysaccharides in relation to growth and thyroid hormones. *J. Chronic Dis.*, 16:291, 1962.
9. Schiller, S., Slover, G.A., and Dorfman, A.: Effect of thyroid gland on metabolism of acid mucopolysaccharide in skin. *Biochem. Biophys. Acta*, 58:27, 1962.
10. Von Knorring, J.: Changes in myocardial acid mucopolysaccharides in experimental hyper- and hypothyroidism in the rat. *Scand. J. Clin. Lab. Invest.*, [Suppl]19(95):57, 1967.
11. Smith, T.J., Horwitz, A.L., and Refetoff, S.: The effect of thyroid hormone on glycosaminoglycan accumulation in human fibroblasts. *Endocrinology*, 108(6):2397-2399, 1981.
12. Smith, T.J., Murata, Y., Horwitz, A.L., Philipson, L., and Refetoff, S.: Regulation of glycosaminoglycan accumulation by thyroid hormone *in vitro*. *J. Clin. Invest.*, 70: 1066, 1982.
13. Ceccarelli, P., Refetoff, S., and Murata, Y.: Resistance to thyroid hormone diagnosed by the reduced response of fibroblasts to the triiodothyronine-induced supression of fibronectin synthesis. *J. Clin. Endocrinol. Metab.*, 65: 242-246, 1987.
14. Murata, Y., Ceccarelli, P., Refetoff, S., Horwitz, A.L., and Matsui, N.: Thyroid hormone inhibits fibronectin synthesis by cultured human skin fibroblasts. *J. Clin. Endocrinol. Metab.*, 64:334, 1987.
15. Refetoff, S., Degroot, L.J., Benard, B., and Dewind, L.T.: Studies of a sibship with apparent hereditary resistance to the intracellular action of thyroid hormones. *Metabolism*, 21:723-756, 1972.
16. Brendstrup, P., Jespersen, K., and Asboe-Hansen, G.: Morphological and chemical connective tissue changes in fibrositis muscles. *Ann. Rheum. Dis.*, 16:438-440, 1957.
17. Stockman, R.: The causes, pathology, and treatment of chronic rheumatism. *Edinburgh Med. J.*, 15:107-116, 1904.
18. Glogowski, G. and Wallroff, J.: Ein beitrag zur klinik und histologie der muskelharten (myogelosen). *Ztschr. Orthop.*, 80:237-268, 1951.
19. Miehlke, K., Schulze, G., and Eger, W.: Klinische und experimentelle untersuchungen zum fibrositissyndrom. *Z. Rheumaforsch*, 19:310-330, 1960.
20. Awad, E.A.: Interstitial myofibrositis: hypothesis of the mechanism. *Arch. Phy. Med. Rehabil.*, 54:449-453, 1973.
21. Awad, E.A.: Personal communication. April 6, 1992.
22. DeGroot, L.J., Larsen, P.R., Refetoff, S., and Stanbury, J.B.: *The Thyroid and Its Diseases*, 5th edition. New York, John Wiley & Sons, Inc., 1984.
23. Hiemeyer, K., Lutz, R., and Menninger, H.: Dependence of tender points upon posture: a key to the understanding of fibromyalgia syndrome. *J. Manual Med.*, 5:169-174, 1990.
24. Fleck, S.J. and Falkel, J.E.: Value of resistance training for the reduction of sports injuries. *Sports Med.*, 3:61-68, 1986.
25. Laurent, G.J., Sparrow, M.P., Bates, P.C., and Millward, D.J.: Collagen content and turnover in cardiac and skeletal muscles of the adult fowl and the changes during

stretch-induced growth. *Biochemistry J.*, 176:419-427, 1978.

26. Shishiba, Y., Takeuchi, Y., Yokoi, N., Ozawa, Y., and Shimizu, T.: Thyroid hormone excess stimulates the synthesis of proteoglycan in human skin fibroblasts in culture. *Acta Endocrinol.*, 123(5):541-549, 1990.

27. Evans, W.J., Meredith, J.G., Cannon, J.G., et al.: Metabolic changes following eccentric exercise in trained and untrained men. *J. Appl. Phys.*, 61:1864-1868, 1986.

28. Staff, P.H.: Clinical consideration in referred muscle pain and tenderness: connective tissue reactions. *Eup. J. Appl. Physiol.*, 57:369-372, 1988.

29. Frohman, L.A.: Diseases of the anterior pituitary. In *Endocrinology and Metabolism*, 2nd edition. Edited by P. Felig, J.D. Baxter, A. Broadus, and L.A. Frohman, New York, McGraw-Hill Book Co., 1987, pp.247-337.

30. Hartley, L.H.: Growth hormone and catecholamine response to exercise in relation to physical training. *Med. Sci. Sports*, 7:34-36, 1975.

31. Karagiorgos, A., Garcia, J.F., and Brooks, G.A.: Growth hormone response to continuous and intermittent exercise. *J. Appl. Physiol.*, 11:302-307, 1979.

32. Goldman, J.A.: Hypermobility and deconditioning: important links to fibromyalgia/fibrositis. *Southern Med. J.*, 84:1192-1196, 1991.

33. Beighton, P., Soloman, L., and Soskolne, C.L.: Articular mobility in an African population. *Ann. Rheum. Dis.*, 32:413-418, 1973.

34. Larsson, L.G, Baum, J., and Mudholkar, G.S.: Hypermobility: features and differential incidence between sexes. *Arthritis Rheumatol.* 30:1426-1430, 1987.

35. Kirk, J.A., Ansell, B.M., and Bywaters, E.G.L.: The hypermobility syndrome: musculoskeletal complaints associated with generalized joint hypermobility. *Ann. Rheum. Dis.*, 26:419-425, 1967.

36. Klemp, P., Stevens, J.E., and Isaacs, S.: A hypermobility study in ballet dancers. *J. Rheumatol.*, 11:692-696, 1984.

37. Pitcher, D. and Grahame, R.: Mitral valve prolapse and joint hypermobility: evidence for a systemic connective tissue abnormality? *Ann. Rheum. Dis.*, 41:352-354, 1982.

38. Grahame, R., Edwards, J.C., Pitcher, D., et al.: A clinical and echocardiographic study of patients with the hypermobility syndrome. *Ann. Rheum. Dis.*, 40:541-546, 1981.

39. Pelligrino, M.J., Fossen, D.V., Gordon, C., et al.: Prevalence of mitral value prolapse in primary fibromyalgia: a pilot investigation. *Arch. Phys. Med. Rehabil.*, 70:541-543, 1989.

40. Bennett, R.M.: Beyond fibromyalgia: ideas on etiology and treatment. *J. Rheumatol.*, 16(Suppl.19):185-191, 1989.

41. Nørregaard, J., Volkman, H., and Danneskiold-Samsøe, B.: Somatomedin-C and procollagen aminoterminal peptide in fibromyalgia. *J. Musculoskel. Pain*, 3(Suppl.1):104, 1995.

42. Jensen, L.T., Jacobsen, S., and Hørsley-Petersen, K.: Serum procollagen type III aminoterminal peptide in primary fibromyalgia. *Br. J. Rheumatol.*, 27(6):496, 1988.

43. Sobieszczyk, S. and Refetoff, S.: Abnormal response of fibronectin messenger RNA to triiodothyronine in fibroblasts from patients with generalized resistance to thyroid hormone. *Endocrinology*, 121(Suppl.):T-24, 1988.

44. Smith, T.J.: Localized myxedema and thyroid acropachy. In *Werner and Ingbar's The Thyroid: A Fundamental and Clinical Text*, 6th edition. Edited by L.E. Braverman and R.D. Utiger, Philadelphia, J.B. Lippincott Co., 1991, pp.676-681.

45. Chait, A., Kanter, R., Green, W., and Kenny, M.: Defective thyroid hormone action in fibroblasts cultured from subjects with the syndrome of resistance to thyroid hormone. *J. Clin. Endocrinol. Metab.*, 54:767-772, 1982.

46. Danneskiold-Samsøe, B., Christiansen, E., Lund, B., and Bach-Andersen, R.: Regional muscle tension and pain (fibrositis). *Scand. J. Rehab. Med.*, 15:17-20, 1982.

47. Smith, T.J.: Connective tissue in thyrotoxicosis. In *Werner and Ingbar's The Thyroid: A Fundamental and Clinical Text*, 6th edition. Edited by L.E. Braverman and R.D. Utiger, Philadelphia, J.B. Lippincott Co., 1991, pp.734-743.

48. Bunting, C.H.: *Arch. Path.*, 28:306, 1939.

49. Keech, M.K.: The effect of mechanical factors on connective tissue *in vitro*. 81:505-510, 1961.

50. Kohn, L.D.: Connective tissue. In *The Thyroid*, 4th edition. Edited by S.C. Werner and S.H. Ingbar, New York, Harper and Row Publishers, 1987, pp.851-855.

51. Sockman, R.: *Rheumatism and Arthritis*. Edinburgh, W. Green and Son Ltd., 1920.

52. Guyton, A.C.: *Textbook of Medical Physiology*, 8th edition. Philadelphia, W.B. Saunders Co., 1991.

53. Pausen, D.F.: *Basic Histology*. Norwalk, Appleton & Lange, 1990.

54. Lowe, J.C.: Fascia and premenstrual headaches. *Mass. Ther. J.*, 30(2):21-24, 1991.

55. Yaron, I., Buskila, D., Shirazi, I., Neumann, L., Elkayam, O., Paran, D., and Yaron, M.: Elevated levels of hyaluronic acid in the sera of women with fibromyalgia. *J. Rheumatol.*, 24(11):2221-2224, 1997.

56. Sprott, H., Müller, A., and Heine, H.: Collagen crosslinks in fibromyalgia. *Arthritis Rheumat.*, 40(8):1450-1454, 1997.

57. Popelier, M., Jollivet, B., Fouquet, B., et al.: Phosphorus-calcium metabolism in hyperthyroidism. *Presse Med.*, 19(15):705-708, 1990.

58. Faber, J., Overgaard, K., Jarlov, A.E., and Christiansen, C.: Bone metabolism in premenopausal women with nontoxic goiter and reduced serum thyrotropin levels. *Thyroidology*, 6(1):27-32, 1994.

59. Krakauer, J.C. and Kleerekoper, M.: Borderline-low serum thyrotropin level is correlated with increased fasting urinary hydroxyproline excretion. *Arch. Intern. Med.*, 152(2):360-364, 1992.

60. Langdahl, B.L., Loft, A.G., Eriksen, E.F., Mosekilde, L., and Charles, P.: Bone mass, bone turnover, calcium homeostasis, and body composition in surgically and radioiodine-treated former hyperthyroid patients. *Thyroid*, 6(3):169-175, 1996.

61. Nakamura, H., Mori, T., Genma R., et al.: Urinary excretion of pyridinoline and deoxypyridinoline measured by immunoassay in hypothyroidism. *Clin. Endocrinol.*, 44(4):447-451, 1996.

62. Nagasaka, S., Sugimoto, H., Nakamura, T., et al: Antithyroid therapy improves bony manifestations and bone metabolic markers in patients with Graves' thyrotoxico-

sis. *Clin. Endocrinol.*, 47(2):215-221, 1997.

63. Foscolo, G., Roiter, I., De Menis, E., Da Rin, G., Legovini, P., and Conte, N.: Bone metabolism in primary hypothyroidism in the adult. *Minerva Endocrinol.*, 16(1): 7-10, 1991.

64. Bijlsma, J.W., Duursma, S.A., Roelofs, J.M., and der Kinderen, P.J.: Thyroid function and bone turnover. *Acta Endocrinol.* (Copenh), 104(1):42-49, 1983.

65. Kaplan, M.M., Swartz, S.L., and Larsen, P.R.: Partial peripheral resistance to thyroid hormone. *Amer. J. Med.*, 70(5):1115-1121, 1981.

66. Chamberlain, G.J.: Cyriax's friction massage: a review. *J. Orthopaeic. Sports Physi. Ther.*, 4(1):20, 1982.

67. Akeson, W.H., Amiel, D., and LaViolette, D.: The connective tissue response to immobility: an accelerated aging response? *Experi. Geront.*, 3:289-301, 1968.

68. Guyton, A.C.: Personal communication, Oct. 9, 1990.

69. Lowe, J.C.: Hypertonic fascia. *Dyn. Chiro.*, 8:28, 1990.

70. Lowe, J.C.: *Spasm.* Houston, McDowell Publishing Co., 1983.

71. Lowe, J.C.: *The Purpose and Practice of Myofascial Therapy* (audio album). Houston, McDowell Publishing Co., 1989, tape 1.

72. McDaniel, D. and Besada, E.: Hypothyroidism: a possible etiology of open-angle glaucoma. *J. Amer. Optometric Assoc.*, 67(2):109-114, 1996.

73. Faber, J., Horslev-Petersen, K., Perrild, H., and Lorenzen, I.: Different effects of thyroid disease on serum levels of procollagen III N-peptide and hyaluronic acid. *J. Clin. Endocrinol. Metab.*, 71(4):1016-1021, 1990.

74. Wilke, W.S., Sheeler, L.R., and Makarowski, W.S.: Hypothyroidism with presenting symptoms of fibrositis. *J. Rheum.*, 8:627-630, 1981.

75. Matsuoka, L.Y., Wortsman, J., Carlisle, K.S., Kupchella, C.K., and Dietrich, J.G.: The acquired cutaneous mucinoses. *Arch. Intern. Med.*, 144(10):1974-1980, 1984.

76. Shishiba, Y., Yanagishita, M., and Hascall, V.C.: Effect of thyroid hormone deficiency on proteoglycan synthesis by human skin fibroblast cultures. *Connect. Tiss. Res.*, 17(2):119-135, 1988.

77. Savage, R.A. and Sipple, C.: Marrow myxedema. Gelatinous transformation of marrow ground substance in a patient with severe hypothyroidism. *Arch. Path. Lab. Med.*, 111(4):375-377, 1987.

78. Kriss, J.P.: Pathogenesis and treatment of pretibial myxedema. *Endocrinol. Metab. Clinics North Amer.*, 16(2): 409-415, 1987.

79. Kales, A., Heuser, G., and Jacobson, A.: All night sleep studies in hypothyroid patients, before and after treatment. *J. Clin. Endocrinology*, 27:1593-1599, 1967.

80. Dorwart, B.B. and Schumacher, H.R.: Joint effusions, chondrocalcinosis and other rheumatic manifestations in hypothyroidism. A clinicopathologic study. *Amer. J. Med.*, 59(6):780-790, 1975.

81. Marks, A.D., Channick, B.J., Adlin, E.V., Kessler, R.K., Braitman, L.E., and Denenberg, B.S.: Chronic thyroiditis and mitral valve prolapse. *Ann. Intern. Med.*, 102(4): 479-483, 1985.

82. Kahaly, G., Erbel, R., Mohr-Kahaly, S., Zenker, G., von Olshausen, K., Krause, U., and Beyer, J.: Basedow's disease and mitral valve prolapse. *Dtsch. Med. Wochen-*

schr., 112(7):248-253, 1987.

83. Brauman, A., Rosenberg, T., Gilboa, Y., Algom, M., Fuchs, L., and Schlesinger, Z.: Prevalence of mitral valve prolapse in chronic lymphocytic thyroiditis and nongoitrous hypothyroidism. *Cardiology*, 75(4):269-273, 1988.

84. Dillman, W.H.: The cardiovascular system in thyrotoxicosis. In *Werner and Ingbar's The Thyroid: A Fundamental and Clinical Text*, 6th edition. Edited by L.E. Braverman and R.D. Utiger, Philadelphia, J.B. Lippincott Co., 1991, pp.759-770.

85. Newham, K.J., Mills, K.R., Quigley, B.M., and Edwards, R.H.T.: Muscle pain and tenderness after exercise. *Austr. J. Sports Med. Exerc. Sci.*, 14:129-131, 1982.

86. Alvarado, A., Ribeiro, J.P., Freitas, F.M., and Gross, J.L.: Lack of association between thyroid function and mitral valve prolapse in Graves' disease. *Braz. J. Med. Biol. Res.*, 23(2):133-139, 1990.

87. Paggi, A., Coppotelli, L., Astarita, C., and Sacchi, I.: Congenital thyroid abnormality (subhyoid ectopy) associated with mitral valve prolapse. *Minerva Med.*, 73(19): 1305-1310, 1982.

88. Ardura, J., de Nicolas, R., and Sanchez-Villares, E.: Mitral prolapse syndrome and hypothyroidism. *An. Esp. Pediatr.*, 11(11):789-794, 1978.

89. Markiewicz, W., Stoner, J., London, E., Hunt, S.A., and Popp, R.L.: Mitral valve prolapse in one hundred presumably healthy females. *Circulation*, 53:464, 1976.

90. Devereux, R.B., Kramer-Fox, R., and Kligfield, P.: Mitral valve prolapse: causes, clinical manifestations, and management. *Ann. Intern. Med.*, 111:305, 1989.

91. Jeresaty, R.M.: Mitral valve prolapse-click syndrome. *Prog. Cardiovasc. Dis.*, 15:623, 1973.

92. Child, A.: Increased prevalence of mitral valve prolapse associated with an elevated skin type III/III+I collagen ratio in joint hypermobility syndrome. *Agents Actions Suppl.*, 18:125-129, 1986.

93. Rajapakse, C.N.: Joint mobility and mitral valve prolapse in an Arab population. *Br. J. Rheumatol.*, 26(6):442-444, 1987.

94. Ondrasik, M.: Joint hypermobility in primary mitral valve prolapse patients. *Clin. Rheumatol.*, 7(1):69-73, 1988.

95. Suzuki, K.: Four boys with multiple floppy valves involving all cardiac valves and hyperextensive joints. *J. Cardiol. Suppl.*, 25:161-172, 1991.

96. Dolan, A.L.: Clinical and echocardiographic survey of the Ehlers-Danlos syndrome. *Br. J. Rheumatol.*, 36(4): 459-462, 1997.

97. Krause, W.J. and Cutts, J.H.: *Concise Textbook of Histology*, 2nd edition. Baltimore, Williams and Wilkins, 1986.

98. Smith, T.J.: Connective tissue in hypothyroidism. In *Werner and Ingbar's The Thyroid: A Fundamental and Clinical Text*, 6th edition. Edited by L.E. Braverman and R.D. Utiger, Philadelphia, J.B. Lippincott Co., 1991, pp.989-992.

99. Lieber, J.G. and Evans, R.M.: Disruption of the vimentin intermediate filament system during adipose conversion of 3T3-L1 cells inhibits lipid droplet accumulation. *J. Cell. Sci.*, 109(Pt 13):3047-3058, 1996.

100. Haapasaari, K.M., Risteli, J., and Oikarinen, A.: Recovery of human skin collagen synthesis after short-term

topical corticosteroid treatment and comparison between young and old subjects. *Br. J. Dermatol.*, 135(1):65-69, 1996.

101. Bitar, M.S.: Glucocorticoid dynamics and impaired wound healing in diabetes mellitus. *Amer. J. Pathol.*, 152 (2):547-554, 1998.

102. Wolf, J.S., Jr., Soble, J.J., Ratliff, T.L., and Clayman, R.V.: Ureteral cell cultures II: collagen production and response to pharmacologic agents. *J. Urol.*, 156(6):2067-2072, 1996.

103. Matsuoka, L.Y., Wortsman, J., Uitto, J., Hashimoto, K., Kupchella, C.E., Eng, A.M., and Dietrich, J.E.: Altered skin elastic fibers in hypothyroid myxedema and pretibial myxedema. *Arch. Intern. Med.*, 145(1):117-121, 1985.

104. Peacey, S.R., Flemming, L., Messenger, A., and Weetman, A.P.: Is Graves' dermopathy a generalized disorder? *Thyroid*, 6(1):41-45, 1996.

105. Lowe, J. C.: When fibrosis complicates trigger points. *J. Nat. Assoc. Trigger Point Myotherap.*, 3:7-8, 1990.

106. Haase, H.R., Clarkson, R.W., Waters, M.J., and Bartold, P.M.: Growth factor modulation of mitogenic responses and proteoglycan synthesis by human periodontal fibroblasts. *J. Cell. Physiol.*, 174(3):353-361, 1998.

107. Freeth, J.S., Silva, C.M., Whatmore, A.J., and Clayton, P.E.: Activation of the signal transducers and activators of transcription signaling pathway by growth hormone (GH) in skin fibroblasts from normal and GH binding protein-positive Laron Syndrome children. *Endocrinology*, 139(1):20-28, 1998.

108. Freeth, J.S., Ayling, R.M., Whatmore, A.J., Towner, P., Price, D.A., Norman, M.R., and Clayton, P.E.: Human skin fibroblasts as a model of growth hormone (GH) action in GH receptor-positive Laron's syndrome. *Endocrinology*, 138(1):55-61, 1997.

109. King, A.P. and Carter-Su, C.: Dexamethasone-induced antagonism of growth hormone (GH) action by down-regulation of GH binding in 3T3-F442A fibroblasts. *Endocrinology*, 136(11):4796-4803, 1995.

110. Komi, P.V. and Buskirk, E.R.: Effect of eccentric and concentric muscle conditioning on tension and electrical activity of human muscle. *Ergonomics*, 15:417-434, 1972.

111. Blumberg, D., Rutkowski, M., Sklar, C., Reggiardo, D., Friedman, D., and David, R.: Juvenile autoimmune thyroiditis and mitral valve prolapse. *Pediatr. Cardiol.*, 13 (2):89-91, 1992.

112. Henry, C.B. and Duling, B.R.: Permeation of the luminal capillary glycocalyx is determined by hyaluronan. *Am. J. Physiol.*, 277(2 Pt.2):H508-H514, 1999.

3.4

Fitness and Exercise Intolerance

Most fibromyalgia patients have low fitness levels and are intolerant of exercise. Compared to normal individuals, low levels of exercise worsen the patients' signs and symptoms for a time. This intolerance of exercise limits their physical activities, resulting in progressively declining levels of fitness. However, exercise intolerance is clearly not the sole factor accounting for the patients' low fitness levels. Moreover, their exercise intolerance is not simply a distaste for strenuous physical activity or laziness.

Some patients exercise despite their fibromyalgia symptoms. They appear to have normal or near-normal fitness levels, but they still have fibromyalgia. Other patients exercise at various levels of intensity, but they do not benefit as normal individuals do from proportional levels of exercise. Many other patients' pain and fatigue are too intense for them to exercise. Still other patients, aside from their pain and fatigue, have an overwhelming disinclination to engage in physical activities. They lack the drive to take part even in most low-level household activities. They simply cannot engage in exercise sufficient to provide conditioning.

Deconditioning Hypotheses

A low level of physical activity is not the cause of most patients' fibromyalgia. Instead, the low levels of activity, imposed by fibromyalgia symptoms and/or their underlying mechanism(s), compound and complicate the patients' fibromyalgia.

However, some researchers have asserted that chronic fatigue syndrome (and by extension, fibromyalgia) is simply the adverse effects of the deconditioning of individuals who choose not to engage in physical activity. This hypothesis accurately applies only to a very small percentage of fibromyalgia patients. For these rare fibromyalgia patients, low physical fitness is the main factor maintaining their fibromyalgia symptoms. When they begin physical fitness training, their fibromyalgia improves or is relieved with only few other therapeutic interventions. The outcome is most favorable for such individuals when they also abandon the conventional "American diet" for a more wholesome one and begin using a wide array of nutritional supplements.

Ample evidence, however, falsifies the speculation that volitional low physical activity levels underlie most patients' fibromyalgia. In some cases, the speculation reflects the researchers' prejudice against and prejorative mindset toward fibromyalgia/chronic fatigue syndrome patients. This deconditioning hypothesis has not led to a better understanding of fibromyalgia and has provided patients with no therapeutic benefits. It has instead generated burdensome psychosocial consequences for many fibromyalgia patients, and it has intensified the distress from which many already suffer.

Most fibromyalgia patients do not merely choose to be physically inactive. At the time of onset of their fibromyalgia, some were physically active and had physical fitness levels proportional to their levels of activity. The severity of some patients' fibromyalgia symptoms, and symptom exacerbations following exercise, force some patients to stop their exercise regimens. Among this latter subset of fibromyalgia patients are many who were athletes when they de-

veloped fibromyalgia. After developing fibromyalgia, their ability to exercise abruptly or gradually diminished. Accordingly, their physical fitness levels declined. Some patients, at the cost of considerable discomfort, continue to engage in vigorous physical activity. Yet they continue to suffer from fibromyalgia despite the activity. What is more, systematic, professionally-guided fitness training provides patients only modest improvement at best. These findings make it clear that exercise does not protect some individuals from developing fibromyalgia, and exercise does not relieve most patients' fibromyalgia.

A more humane conjecture regarding deconditioning in fibromyalgia is that some patients have deficiencies of growth hormone and somatomedin C. (Somatomedin C is an anabolic hormone synthesized in the liver and kidneys under the influence of growth hormone. It stimulates the synthesis of DNA, RNA, and proteins, incorporation of sulfur into mucopolysaccharides, and growth and repair of bone, cartilage, and other connective tissues.) This hypothesis is reasonable only if it stipulates that some features of some patients' fibromyalgia result from deficiencies of these two hormones. This stipulation is necessary because growth hormone and somatomedin C deficiencies can account for only a few of the multiple documented features of fibromyalgia. For example, deficiencies of growth hormone and somatomedin C can account for subnormal conditioning effects from exercise and subnormal tissue repair.

At least three findings, however, falsify the hypothesis that growth hormone and somatomedin C deficiencies underlie fibromyalgia, per se. *First, in growth hormone deficiency, the use of glucose for energy increases. But increased glucose use is inconsistent with the impaired glycolysis Eisinger et al. have documented in fibromyalgia. Second, in a growth hormone deficiency, cellular glycogen deposition decreases, but biopsies of tissues from fibromyalgia patients show increased glycogen deposition. Third, while growth hormone treatment of some fibromyalgia patients has provided modest improvements, patients have not recovered with this form of treatment. It is likely that the improvements with growth hormone therapy are limited to the few features of fibromyalgia that result from mild growth hormone and somatomedin C insufficiencies. It is also likely that the mild growth hormone and somatomedin C deficiencies in some fibromyalgia patients result from inadequate thyroid hormone regulation of transcription of the growth hormone and somatomedin C genes (see Chapter 3.12).*

The Inadequate Thyroid Hormone Regulation Hypothesis

The hypothesis that most patients' fibromyalgia results from inadequate thyroid hormone regulation of cell function provides a plausible mechanism for the low fitness levels and exercise intolerance of fibromyalgia patients. The low fitness levels and exercise intolerance of hypothyroid patients substantially overlap those of fibromyalgia patients. Inadequate thyroid hormone regulation of various body systems can account for low fitness levels and exercise intolerance.

Dopamine Secreting Neurons. *Some researchers have described impaired central nervous system activation of the motor system of fibromyalgia patients. Other researchers reported low levels of the metabolite of dopamine (3-methoxy-4-hydroxyphenethylene) in the cerebrospinal fluid of fibromyalgia patients. Thyroid hormone is a regulator of dopamine secretion. Dopamine is a hormone that mediates motor drive and motor activity. Hypothyroid animals have low motor drive and low levels of physical activity. The disinclination of many fibromyalgia patients to engage in exercise may result from subnormal dopamine levels. The subnormal levels may result from inadequate thyroid hormone regulation of dopamine synthesizing and secreting neurons in the basal ganglia of the brain. Subnormal dopamine levels may contribute to the heightened perception of weakness and fatigue of some fibromyalgia patients. Impaired cardiopulmonary and circulatory function with reduced delivery of energy-yielding nutrients to muscle cells, due to inadequate regulation by thyroid hormone, may contribute to the perception of weakness.*

Subnormal Oxidative Metabolism. *Physical exercise normally increases the activity of oxidative enzymes in the mitochondria. The increase raises the individual's capacity for oxidative metabolism during exercise. Thyroid hormone regulates the transcription of some enzymes that catalyze oxidative reactions, and it regulates the activity of others. Inadequate thyroid hormone regulation of the enzymes can limit the ability of the patient to benefit from physical exercise by imposing a low ceiling on the increase in enzyme activity in response to exercise. Thus, low physical fitness levels in hypothyroid or thyroid hormone resistant fibromyalgia patients may be underlain partly by subnormal activity of some oxidative enzymes.*

Subnormal Respiratory Drive. *Respiratory (ventilatory) drive is the output of the central nervous system respiratory centers in response to physiological stimuli as during exercise. Respiratory drive largely dictates respiration. At rest or during exercise, respir-*

ation normally ensures adequate amounts of oxygen for normal cellular function.

Many patients with untreated hypothyroidism usually have low respiratory drive. The low respiratory drive of patients with severe untreated hypothyroidism increases their carbon dioxide levels. In one study, hypothyroid women with the highest TSH levels had the most severe decreases in respiratory drive. Respiratory drive increases when patients use exogenous thyroid hormone.

Some degree of exercise intolerance in hypothyroid and/or thyroid hormone resistant fibromyalgia patients may be due to low respiratory drive. Some authors have described fibromyalgia patients with chronic, severe, episodic dyspnea. (Dyspnea is "shortness of breath," subjective difficulty or distress in breathing. Dyspnea occurs during strenuous exercise.) Some fibromyalgia patients also have subnormal chest expansion. Subnormal chest expansion during respiration can cause dyspnea, especially when the individual tries to exercise. Low chest expansion may be part of the effect of low respiratory drive caused by inadequate thyroid hormone regulation of CNS centers.

Increased α-Adrenergic Receptors and Decreased β-Adrenergic Receptors. Inadequate thyroid hormone regulation of transcription of the adrenergic genes may be the strongest contribution to fibromyalgia patients' low fitness levels and exercise intolerance. The inadequate transcription regulation increases the density of α-adrenergic receptors and decreases the density of β-adrenergic receptors on cell membranes. In one study, researchers found an increased density of α_2-adrenergic receptors on the platelets of fibromyalgia patients. Other studies support the hypothesis that an increase of α-adrenergic receptors and a decrease of β-adrenergic receptors mediate features of fibromyalgia (see Chapter 3.1, "High Ratio of α- to β-Adrenergic Receptors on Cell Membranes").

The altered ratio of α- to β-adrenergic receptors can cause subnormal sympathetic nervous system activity and excessive parasympathetic activity. It can also impair aerobic and anaerobic metabolism, decreasing the capacity of the fibromyalgia patient to exercise at high enough intensities to acquire physical conditioning.

Sympathetic and Parasympathetic Nervous System Activity. An increase of α_2-adrenergic receptors on sympathetic nerve cell bodies in the nucleus of the solitary tract and the paravertebral sympathetic ganglia inhibits activity of sympathetic nerves. In addition, an increase of α_2-adrenergic receptors on the dorsal

vagal nucleus results in excessive parasympathetic activity. Sympathetic inhibition and parasympathetic facilitation will have a combined impairing effect on adaptation to exercise.

Also, inadequate thyroid hormone regulation of hypothalamic corticotropin-releasing hormone (CRH) in fibromyalgia patients may also contribute to subnormal sympathetic nervous system activity. CRH stimulates the brain stem locus ceruleus-norepinephrine system and the central sympathetic nervous system (see Chapter 3.5). When CRH is deficient, central activation of the sympathetic nervous system may be subnormal. This additional source of subnormal sympathetic activity may contribute to impaired adaptation to exercise.

The subnormal sympathetic activity and excessive parasympathetic activity would render the patient exercise intolerant by causing subnormal heart rate and cardiac output during exercise. Some researchers have reported that fibromyalgia patients have lower than normal heart rates during exercise. The reduced heart rates and cardiac output may result in deficient delivery of oxygen and other nutrients to muscle cells during exercise. This may account in part for fibromyalgia patients in one study reaching the anaerobic threshold at lower heart rates than in healthy control subjects. An oxygen deficiency during exercise can place an undue demand on anaerobic metabolism in affected patients. An excessive demand can cause a crisis in energy metabolism that transiently worsens the patient's fibromyalgia status.

Aerobic and Anaerobic Metabolism. During exercise, "aerobic" and "anaerobic" metabolism provide energy for cellular processes such as muscle contraction. Aerobic metabolism is what physiologists call energy-providing metabolic processes that require oxygen, and they call energy-providing processes that proceed without oxygen anaerobic metabolism.

When exercise begins, a time is required for the heart, lungs, and arteries (the "cardiorespiratory" or "cardiopulmonary" system) to accelerate oxygen delivery to muscle cells and catch up to the exertion-increased need of the cells for oxygen. Also, during intense enough exercise, too little oxygen reaches muscles to meet their requirement. The deficient delivery of oxygen during intense exercise occurs because each individual's cardiorespiratory system has a limited capacity for providing oxygen to exercising muscle cells. Cardiorespiratory capacity is lower in deconditioned individuals and higher in conditioned ones.

Also, with intense enough exercise, the individual

will exceed her aerobic capacity. This essentially means that the cardiorespiratory system will deliver too little oxygen for aerobic metabolism to continue providing energy for cell processes. At that time, anaerobic metabolism begins providing energy. Normally, anaerobic metabolism provides energy until the individual decreases the intensity so that the delivery of oxygen to muscle cells is sufficient to enable aerobic metabolism to again provide energy.

However, inadequate thyroid hormone regulation in fibromyalgia patients with hypothyroidism or resistance to thyroid hormone may limit both the capacity for aerobic and anaerobic metabolism. Inadequate regulation may impede aerobic metabolism in at least two ways: (1) subnormal delivery of oxygen and energy-yielding nutrients such as glucose through arteries to muscle cells, and (2) decreased oxidative enzymes in the mitochondria. These impediments are likely to result in subnormal aerobic power (low VO_2 max).

Inadequate thyroid hormone regulation is also likely to impair anaerobic metabolism in at least three ways: (1) decreased stored ATP and creatine phosphate to release energy, (2) impaired release of glucose from glycogen molecules, and (3) impaired glycolysis.

Conditioning mainly involves two changes: increased competence of the cardiorespiratory system in delivering oxygen to cells for aerobic metabolism, and increased capacity for both aerobic and anaerobic metabolism. But inadequate thyroid hormone regulation is likely to limit these conditioning effects in most fibromyalgia patients with hypothyroidism and/or thyroid hormone resistance. A patient's subnormal capacities for aerobic and anaerobic metabolism may result in even mild exercise exceeding both capacities and inducing an energy metabolism crisis. The crisis may worsen the patient's fibromyalgia status for days or weeks.

These effects are similar to those that occur in chronically sedentary people. First consider the effects of regular conditioning exercises: cardiorespiratory efficiency improves, more oxygen reaches cells through the circulation, and aerobic and anaerobic capacities increase. As conditioning increases, higher intensities of exercise are needed to exceed aerobic capacity. Also, once anaerobic metabolism is invoked by more intense exercise, the person can sustain anaerobic exercise longer due to three benefits of conditioning—increased ATP and creatine phosphate, more efficient glycolysis, and more oxygen bound to myoglobin within muscle cells. The effects of decon-

ditioning are the reverse of those just described that result from conditioning through exercise. As the patients conditioning declines, progressively lower levels of exertion exceed the ability of aerobic metabolism to provide energy. Also progressively, anaerobic metabolism comes to be induced by lower levels of exercise. Yet anaerobic metabolism becomes less able to provide energy.

Inadequate regulation by thyroid hormone may also induce these effects characteristic of deconditioning due to a lack of exercise. The patient with inadequate regulation by thyroid hormone may have these effects even if she continues to exercise. If the patient is unable to exercise, the deconditioning from her low activity level will compound the effect from inadequate thyroid hormone regulation. The combined effect results in exercise intolerance and low levels of physical fitness.

In patients with hypothyroidism and/or thyroid hormone resistance, subnormal respiratory drive (see above, "Subnormal Respiratory Drive") may further limit oxygen delivery to muscle cells during exercise. A deficient oxygen supply reduces the metabolic rate of muscle cells. The reduction from this source would compound the reduced metabolic rate from inadequate thyroid hormone regulation of cellular process. So, low respiratory drive is likely to compound the patient's exercise intolerance and low fitness levels.

Summary

The combination of all these potential results of inadequate regulation by thyroid hormone—decreased motor and respiratory drive, low sympathetic activity, excess parasympathetic activity, and subnormal aerobic and anaerobic capacity—may render the fibromyalgia patient unable to benefit from exercise or unable to engage in it. The patient will experience metabolic distress during mild-to-moderate exercise or during ordinary daily activities. Consequently, she will descend though a spiral of exercise intolerance, decreasing fitness, and worsening fibromyalgia status.

Moldofsky and Scarisbrick wrote that as far back as the 12th century, Maimonides had remarked that sedentary people tend to develop musculoskeletal symptoms [7,p.43]. Maimonides wrote, "If one leads a sedentary life and does not take exercise, neglects the calls of nature, or is constipated—even if he eats wholesome food and takes care of himself in accordance with medical rules—he will, throughout his life, be subject to aches and pains and his strength will fail him."[123]

Maimonides' observation is true of people today—those with low physical fitness levels have lower metabolic rates, and they are more prone than physically fit individuals to develop fibromyalgia. However, if an individual who exercises regularly has inadequate thyroid hormone regulation of cell function, her metabolism will remain subnormal despite regular exercise. Thus, the individual whose fibromyalgia is underlain by hypothyroidism or cellular resistance to thyroid hormone will have subnormal metabolism despite exercising. Inadequate thyroid hormone regulation of cell function prevents many fibromyalgia patients from exercising, and it imposes on those who can exercise a low ceiling on the capacity for improved fitness. This mechanism renders many patients exercise intolerant and physically unfit. Although patients who can exercise may be more tolerant of their fibromyalgia signs and symptoms, exercise is not likely to relieve the signs and symptoms.

● LOW FITNESS LEVEL AND EXERCISE INTOLERANCE IN FIBROMYALGIA

LOW FITNESS LEVELS

Bennett et al. found that fibromyalgia patients have low aerobic fitness.[1] He has attributed the symptoms of fibromyalgia to the patients' low fitness levels.[1]

Jacobsen and his coworkers found in several studies that fibromyalgia patients' maximum voluntary muscle strength and endurance were low.[9][10][11] They also found that patients' maximum power output (exertion) was lower than that of controls.[12,p.160]

Klug et al. reported that fibromyalgia patients failed to achieve full physical fitness with exercise.[2,p.35] On the other hand, Wigers et al. found that aerobic exercise had some positive short-term effects on fibromyalgia patients, but ". . . effects on symptom severity are few, if any, in the longer term."[59,p.83] Exercise can improve the physical fitness of some fibromyalgia patients, but it does not significantly improve their pain. Mengshoel compared the effects of a 20-week exercise program with 18 fibromyalgia patients and 17 patients who did not exercise. He reported that the exercise group had a modest improvement in strength, but no improvement in pain or coping.[112] "In the long run," Mengshoel wrote, "fibromyalgia pa-

tients who exercise report less symptoms than sedentary patients do. Thus, exercise should be aimed at preventing physical inactivity and improving patients' physical fitness."[17]

Natvig, Bruusgaard, and Eriksen sent questionnaires to 588 female members of a local fibromyalgia association in Oslo, Norway. Eighty other fibromyalgia patients not members of the group filled out the questionnaires, as did 918 women who did not have fibromyalgia. Through the questionnaires, patients provided self-reports of the levels of physical leisure activity and physical fitness. According to the self-reports, the patients had higher levels of leisure activity than did the non-patients. This finding held even when the researchers controlled for factors such as employment status and work load. The researchers found a weak correlation between high physical leisure activity and high physical fitness levels. However, healthy women of the general population were able to engage in heavier physical activities than were fibromyalgia patients.[139]

EXERCISE INTOLERANCE

Many fibromyalgia patients report that their symptoms, particularly pain,[15][17] worsen following exercise. Mechtouf, Collard, and Eisinger reported that strenuous exercise aggravated the pain of 68 of 80 female fibromyalgia patients (85%); strenuous exercise aggravated the depression of 40 of the women (50%).[122]

Wigers et al. reported that some patients improved significantly with aerobic exercise and no longer met the criteria for fibromyalgia. However, 9 of 16 of their patients (56%) either did not improve or were worse after the 14 weeks of exercise.[59,p.83] Mengshoel also noted that exercise may exacerbate fibromyalgia patients' pain. He wrote in a 1996 review: "Exercise has been used in the treatment of fibromyalgia. Training has shown little benefit as regards pain, but has improved the physical fitness of the patients. Since pain may be exacerbated by physical activity, many patients become physically inactive, with possible development of reduced physical fitness."[17] Verstappen et al. pointed out that patients formerly active in sports performed better in fitness tests than did "always sedentary" patients. They also noted, however, that fibromyalgia patients tend to avoid physical exercise because of the muscle soreness it provokes.[15]

These reports of exercise intolerance are consistent with my experience with fibromyalgia patients not treated, or not treated effectively, with metabolic rehabilitation. For most, exercise worsens their pain and other symptoms. As a result, many avoid exercise and over time their fitness levels decline. Correspondingly, they also become progressively less tolerant of vigorous physical activity.

OBJECTIVE FIBROMYALGIA FINDINGS THAT MAY ACCOUNT FOR PATIENTS' LOW FITNESS LEVELS AND EXERCISE INTOLERANCE

Subnormal Measure of Energy Metabolism

Studies have shown reduced high-energy phosphate levels (ATP and creatine phosphate) in the muscles of fibromyalgia patients[95][96][158] and low ATP levels in their red blood cells.[91][171]

At least one study has shown a low increase in circulating creatine kinase levels in fibromyalgia patients after they exercised. Nørregaard et al. found that fibromyalgia patients who performed a stepwise incremental maximal bicycle ergometer test did not have creatine kinase levels that differed from that of controls.[153] However, the results of van Dederen et al. were different. They had 10 fibromyalgia patients and 10 healthy controls perform exhaustive physical exercise. The exercise involved a bicycle ergometer test and a step test. During both exercises, the mean maximum workload of fibromyalgia patients was lower than that of the control subjects. In response to the exercise, the mean serum level of creatine kinase did not rise as much in patients as in controls.[5] (For an explanation of creatine kinase, see section below titled "Low Stress-Induced Increase in Creatine Kinase Levels.")

Maximum Oxygen Uptake (VO₂ Max)

Simms et al. reported that the VO_2 max and maximum voluntary contraction of the upper trapezius and tibialis anterior muscles of 13 fibromyalgia patients was similar to that of 13 healthy controls.[128] (VO_2 max is the abbreviation for rate of oxygen usage during maximum aerobic metabolism.[20, p.946])

Sietsema et al. pointed out that some researchers have reported that some patients have low VO_2 max. They measured the pattern of VO_2 max in patients subjected to graded exercise. The patients exercised on an upright bicycle ergometer. The researchers measured respiratory gas exchange and grading of pain with a visual analog scale. Patients had higher pain levels

than controls after graded exercise. Three measures did not differ between patients and controls: 1) VO_2 max, 2) onset of anaerobic metabolism measured as respiratory gas exchange, and 3) the relationship between VO_2 max and work rate through the range of work rates. The researchers concluded that although patients reported more pain, measurements did not reveal abnormalities in the overall rate or pattern of oxygen use during muscle exercise.[129]

Bennett assessed the aerobic fitness of 25 female fibromyalgia patients. The patients exercised to exhaustion on an electronically braked bicycle ergometer. Based on their VO_2 max, in comparison with published standards, 80% of the patients were not physically fit. The researchers suggested that the etiology of fibromyalgia may involve detraining.[1]

Lower Central Nervous System Dopamine Levels

In one study, investigators measured the levels of the metabolites of serotonin, norepinephrine, and dopamine in the fibromyalgia patients' cerebrospinal fluids. The metabolite of dopamine, 3-methoxy-4-hydroxyphenethylene glycol, and that of norepinephrine, homovanillic acid, were significantly lower than those of patients with rheumatoid arthritis and normal controls (Table 3.4.1). The metabolite of serotonin, 5-hydroxyindole acetic acid, was not significantly lower than in normal controls.[60]

Deficient Hypothalamic Secretion of Corticotropin-Releasing Hormone (CRH)

Documented abnormalities in the function of the hypothalamic-pituitary-adrenocortical axis in fibromyalgia patients point to deficient secretion of CRH (see Chapter 3.5).

Catecholamine Levels

Results of tests of fibromyalgia patients' 24-hour urinary excretion of epinephrine and norepinephrine have been inconsistent. Caffeine use correlated with the elevated norepinephrine levels in 20% of fibromyalgia patients studied. (See Chapter 3.1, section titled "Normal to Elevated Peripheral Norepinephrine Levels in Fibromyalgia Patients at Rest.")

Yunus et al. measured plasma and urinary catecholamines in 30 fibromyalgia patients and 30 healthy controls. They found no significant difference.[126]

In a double blind study of the clinical effects of cyclobenzaprine, Hamaty et al. found that 7 fibromyalgia patients had normal-to-very high norepinephrine plasma levels and continuously low-to-normal epinephrine levels. The researchers reported that their fibromyalgia patients had a neurotransmitter plasma profile similar to that of other patients with chronic pain conditions. An exception, however, was fibromyalgia patients' low circulating epinephrine levels.[125]

Disturbed Sympathetic Function: Lower Stress-Induced Secretion of Epinephrine and Norepinephrine

Vaeroy et al. subjected fibromyalgia patients to two conditions: an auditory stimulus of 80 dB, 1000 Hz for 2 seconds and a cold pressor test at 10° C and 4° C (50° F and 39.2° F). (A "pressor" is a stimulus that induces vasoconstriction and resistance to blood flow.) The researchers reported that vasoconstriction in response to the stimuli was less in fibromyalgia patients than in controls. They wrote that this finding conflicts with the report that fibromyalgia patients have Raynaud's phenomenon.[127] However, a subset of fibromyalgia patients have Raynaud's symptoms. Frodin et al. reported that of 10 fibromyalgia patients, 7 had normal nail fold capillary structure and blood flow. However, 3 patients with a history of Raynaud's phenomenon, had sluggish capillary flow that correlated with subnormal skin temperature.[130] Similarly, Qiao et al. reported that compared to 29 healthy controls, 27 fibromyalgia patients had increased skin electrical conductance and less vasoconstriction during acoustic stimulation and a cold pressor test. They wrote that these results suggest that the patients had increased cholinergic (parasympathetic nervous system) activity and decreased adrenergic (sympathetic nervous system) activity.[131]

Lapossy et al. tested the vascular responses to cold applications in 50 fibromyalgia patients. Vasospasm in response to cold occurred in 38% of fibromyalgia patients. Vasospasms occurred in only 20% of 50 low back pain patients and 8% of 50 healthy controls. The responses between the groups were statistically significant.[132]

Adler et al. induced hypoglycemia in fibromyalgic premenopausal women and normal controls. In the fibromyalgia patients, urine tests showed significantly reduced ACTH and epinephrine responses to hypoglycemia. The responses were about 30% below the responses for control subjects. The two groups did not differ in norepinephrine, prolactin, cortisol, and dehydroepiandrosterone (DHEA) responses to hypoglycemia. The fibormyalgia patients' low epinephrine

response to hypoglycemia correlated (P=0.01) inversely with overall health status, determined by the Fibromyalgia Impact Questionnaire. Adler et al. concluded that the fibromyalgia patients had impaired activation of the hypothalamic-pituitary portion of the hypothalamic-pituitary-adrenal axis. The impairment results in a low ACTH response. The patients also had impaired activation of the sympathetic nervous system-adrenal medulla axis. This results in subnormal epinephrine secretion in response to hypoglycemia.[124]

Table 3.4.1. The breakdown products of the two neurotransmitters found to be low in the cerebrospinal fluid of fibromyalgia patients.

NEUROTRANSMITTER	METABOLITE
Dopamine	3-methoxy-4-hydroxyphenethylene glycol
Norepinephrine	homovanillic acid

Mengshoel also reported that during exercise, the circulating norepinephrine level of fibromyalgia patients did not rise. In contrast, the levels of healthy subjects underwent a many-fold rise.[17]

Van Dederen et al. had 10 fibromyalgia patients and 10 healthy controls perform exhaustive physical exercise. The exercise involved a bicycle ergometer test and a steptest. The mean maximum workload of fibromyalgia patients was lower than that of control subjects. In response to the exercise, the patients also had lower serum levels of creatine kinase, myoglobin, cortisol, epinephrine, and norepinephrine. When subjected to the same workload as control subjects, the patients had lower heart rates. The investigators noted that the lower heart rates of fibromyalgia patients during both exercises was "a striking finding." They wrote that the patients' lower norepinephrine and epinephrine levels and slower heart rates suggest disturbed reactivity of two systems—the sympathetic nervous system and the hypothalamic-pituitary-adrenal axis.[5,p.37]

Lower Muscle Sympathetic Activity

Elam et al. stimulated sympathetic nervous system activity of muscle by mental stress, contraction of the jaw muscles, static handgrip, and post-contraction ischemia. They found a tendency toward low muscle sympathetic activity.[50]

Increased α₂-Adrenoceptors on the Platelets of Fibromyalgia Patients, and Positive Therapeutic Responses to a β-Adrenoceptor Agonist (Salbutamol)

Several studies support the conjecture that fibromyalgia patients have an increased density of α-adrenergic receptors and a decreased density of β-adrenergic receptors on cell membranes (see Chapter 3.1, the section titled "High Ratio of α- to β-Adrenergic Receptors on Cell Membranes"). This alteration in the normal balance of adrenergic receptor types on cell membranes probably plays a prominent role in fibromyalgia patients' exercise intolerance and low fitness levels.

Subnormal Circulation

Several researchers have found reduced brain blood flow during SPECT scans (see Chapter 3.2, section titled "Decreased Brain Blood Flow in Fibromyalgia").

Based on studies available before 1989, Henriksson wrote that the most likely cause of pain in fibromyalgia is hypoxia. He sited four findings that support this conclusion: (1) a pathological distribution of tissue oxygen pressure in painful muscles of fibromyalgia patients, (2) muscle stiffness in most patients, (3) reduced concentrations of high-energy phosphates, and (4) ragged red fibers typically found in mitochondrial disorders. He concluded that long-standing hypoxia can explain muscle structural and biochemical abnormalities.[136][138] Bengtsson and Henriksson wrote that three phenomena can account for fibromyalgia patients' muscle pain, fatigue, and stiffness: (1) disturbed micro-circulation, (2) mitochondrial damage, and (3) a low concentration of high-energy phosphates in the muscles of patients. They proposed that abnormal motor nerve patterns induced by hypoxia cause these three phenomena.[137] According to Caro, studies suggest that the tissue changes in fibromyalgia may be consistent with altered micro-vascular permeability and blood flow, tissue hypoxia, and chronic muscle spasm.[135]

Fassbender and Wegner proposed that hypoxia due to a local vascular disturbance is responsible for the muscle lesions in fibromyalgia patients.[106] It is not clear whether they were referring to patients with fibromyalgia or myofascial trigger points. Klemp et al. used ¹³³xenon injections that measure local blood flow through a large tissue volume. They found no abnormality.[108] Lund, Bengtsson and Thorborg, using a more sensitive method, found abnormal oxygenation of the trapezius and brachioradialis muscles of fibromyalgia patients. They speculated that the low oxygenation was due to structural and function changes affecting the microvessels in tender points. They also found low oxygen partial pressure in the patients' subcutaneous tissues, although the tissues were not hypoxic.[107] Bennett et al. measured ¹³³xenon clearance to assess the blood flow in muscles of 16 fibromyalgia patients during exercise. Compared to the result in 16 sedentary control subjects, patients had reduced clearance.[1]

Bjelle et al. noted that studies have shown unevenly distributed low oxygen pressure in the skeletal muscles of fibromyalgia patients. They wrote that muscle hypoxia sensitizes nociceptors and result in hyperalgesia with a diffuse pain distribution.[134]

Bruckle et al. reported that measurements with polarographic needle probes in fibromyalgic erector spinae muscles showed an elevated total mean tissue oxygen pressure. The total mean pressure was higher than in control subjects. They found no evidence of small hypoxic areas in the muscles. They wrote that an increase in local blood flow or disturbance of oxygen use by muscle cells might underlie the elevated pressure. They wrote finally that they found no evidence of hypoxia or hypoxia-related pain in fibromyalgic muscle.[90]

A study by Bengtsson et al. strongly supports the possibility that fibromyalgia patients have increased α₂-adrenergic receptors in peripheral tissues as well as on their platelets. The researchers used two techniques to induce sympathetic ganglion blocks in fibromyalgia patients. The blocks diminished the patients' fibromyalgic pain. This result suggests that the blocks reduced norepinephrine secretion in peripheral tissues, stopped norepinephrine/α₂-adrenergic receptor binding, permitted arterioles to dilate, and relieved ischemic pain. (See Chapter 3.1, subsection "Pain.")

For additional descriptions of studies of peripheral blood flow in fibromyalgia, see Chapter 3.2, section titled "Peripheral Blood Flow in Fibromyalgia."

Nonspecific Muscle Changes

In a summary paper on muscle pathology in fibromyalgia, Simms noted that early studies suggested abnormalities in the skeletal muscles of fibromyalgia patients. Later studies, he went on, have not confirmed muscle metabolic abnormalities. He wrote, "More recent studies of morphology have shown only nonspecific or mild changes, perhaps consistent with subtle metabolic abnormalities, especially at tender point sites."[133]

● PROBLEMS WITH THE HYPOTHESIS THAT FIBROMYALGIA IS THE MANIFESTATION OF LOW FITNESS LEVELS

Bennett and his colleagues conjectured in the late 1980s that physical deconditioning played an important role in the etiology of fibromyalgia.[1] Based on the data available then, this was a reasonable hypothesis. In fact, physical deconditioning apparently is the most instrumental factor in a minority of patients' fibromyalgia.

Tragically, Steven Straus has implied that this is generally true of chronic fatigue syndrome patients. Straus, in an address to the American College of Rheumatology, blamed patients for at least some of their problem. As Hillary Johnson wrote, "A significant portion of the symptomatology of the disease, he commented, was a result of 'poor sleep hygiene' and failure to exercise." For this and other such statements, the audience roundly applauded Straus, and Johnson wrote that at least one audience member shouted, "'Hear, hear!'"[145,p.685] Actually, Straus' suggestion that exercise and improved sleep hygiene accounts for a significant portion of the symptoms of chronic fatigue syndrome—and by extension, fibromyalgia—was nonsensical. The suggestion appears to reflect an insensitivity to the plight of the patients he was charged with helping through the resources of the National Institutes of Health. That suggestion was not far afield from Straus' pseudo-scientific accusation of a psychiatric basis for chronic fatigue syndrome. (For descriptions of the conduct of this representative of the National Institutes of Health and its adverse effects on chronic fatigue syndrome patients, I strongly recommend Johnson's book *Osler's Web*.[145])

The hypothesis that fibromyalgia results largely or solely from deconditioning suffers from several problems.

LOW HEART RATES UNDER PHYSICAL LOADS

Were it true that fibromyalgia symptoms are the result of low fitness levels, fibromyalgia patients would have high heart rates under physical loads. The deconditioned individual has a higher resting heart rate and a higher heart rate at any work load.[146,p.124] The lower resting heart rate results from a decrease in va-

gal (parasympathetic) nerve stimulation.[147] The higher heart rate during exercise results from high-level sympathetic nerve stimulation.[148]

Van Denderen et al., however, found that the opposite was true of fibromyalgia patients who engaged in exhaustive physical exercise—the patients' heart rates were subnormal. The researchers commented that the low mean heart rate was "a striking finding."[5,p.37] They suggested that the low heart rates of fibromyalgia patients resulted from subnormal sympathetic activity. This fits in with the hypothesis that inadequate thyroid hormone regulation of the adrenergic genes in fibromyalgia results in α-adrenergic receptor dominance in select tissues. α_2-Adrenergic receptors hyperpolarize the sympathetic nerve cell bodies in the nucleus of the solitary tract and in the chain of paravertebral sympathetic ganglia. The hyperpolarization inhibits sympathetic nerve activity. Since increased sympathetic activity is required for normally adapting to vigorous physical exercise, the patients have low heart rates for increased work loads during exercise. As a result, as in the study by van Denderen et al., fibromyalgia patients have low heart rates, although their low level of physical fitness would predict high heart rates.[5]

In addition, an increase in α_2-adrenergic receptors in the dorsal vagal nucleus would increase the flow of parasympathetic nerve signals to the heart through the vagus nerves. The increased vagal signals would cause a low resting heart rate. In my clinical experience, this finding is common among fibromyalgia patients—uncharacteristically low resting heart rates for the patients' low cardiovascular fitness levels.

For descriptions of the effects of α_2-adrenergic receptor dominance on the sympathetic and parasympathetic divisions of the autonomic nervous system, see Chapter 3.2, subsection titled "Inhibition of Central Centers for Activation of the Sympathetic Nervous System."

EXERCISE PROVIDES ONLY MINIMAL IMPROVEMENT FOR SOME FIBROMYALGIA PATIENTS

Some authors contend that general physical activity is important in preventing fibromyalgia.[6,p.680][7] Others have argued that increased physical activity is an effective treatment.[7][8] These arguments are misleading, however, because their authors do not properly qualify them. Many individuals develop and continue to suffer from fibromyalgia despite remaining highly active physically. For most patients, exercise provides only minimal improvement in fibromyalgia status. Exercise does not improve the status of others, and it worsens the fibromyalgia status of many. If fibromyalgia were due merely to low aerobic fitness levels, we could expect that increasing the patients' fitness levels would eliminate their fibromyalgia. Aerobic and resistance training *to tolerance* improve the fibromyalgia status of some patients. However, the improvements are typically minimal. Physical training clearly is not a reliable path to improvement, and training alone provides recovery only in rare cases. (See Chapter 5.1, section titled "Exercise.")

I caution the reader, however, not to conclude that fibromyalgia status has no relation to physical fitness levels. A relationship definitely exists. Fibromyalgia status is likely to worsen as physical fitness levels decline. For few patients is a low physical fitness level the main factor underlying symptoms and signs that result in a diagnosis of fibromyalgia. It appears to me that borderline metabolic sufficiency predisposes many individuals to fibromyalgia, and a progressive decline in the level of physical fitness precipitates the onset of symptoms and signs severe enough to lead to a diagnosis of fibromyalgia. (For a more complete description of this process, see Chapter 3.5, subsection titled "Putative Etiologic Role of Decreased Physical Activity.")

● POSSIBLE RELATION OF LOW FITNESS LEVELS AND EXERCISE INTOLERANCE IN FIBROMYALGIA TO INADEQUATE THYROID HORMONE REGULATION OF CELL FUNCTION

Clark stated that women with fibromyalgia not engaging in regular aerobic activities was "unacceptable," since endurance exercises are important to reducing physical limitations associated with fibromyalgia.[42,p.195] I agree with her in that without physical exercise to tolerance, few patients' fibromyalgia status improves, despite improving their diet and nutrition and using exogenous thyroid hormone.

Some fibromyalgia patients use extraordinary will power to exercise, and they do so despite discomforts associated with their fibromyalgia. I believe, however, that other patients are strongly disinclined to exercise for one or more of four reasons. First, some patients have just never learned how to exercise, and they have never experienced its positive effects. Second, some

patients are simply unwilling to go to the inconvenience. Third, many patients appear to have decreased central motor drive and consequent low locomotor activity. And fourth, many patients have found that exercise exacerbates their fibromyalgia symptoms. These latter patients typically are apprehensive of experiencing exacerbations again.

LOW FITNESS LEVELS ASSOCIATED WITH INADEQUATE THYROID HORMONE REGULATION OF CELL FUNCTION

Fibromyalgia patients' low fitness levels occur partly because of their exercise intolerance. Because many of them tolerate exercise poorly, they decline to engage in it. In addition, some effects of inadequate regulation of thyroid hormone of cell function render patients disinclined to exercise. Progressively, their low physical activity levels cause their physical fitness levels to decline. However, for patients whose fibromyalgia is secondary to hypothyroidism or thyroid hormone resistance, low fitness levels are in part the result of physiological consequences of inadequate thyroid hormone regulation of various body systems.

In the section above titled "Low Fitness Levels," I describe the study by Natvig et al. They had 668 women with fibromyalgia and 918 women without fibromyalgia to complete a questionnaire. The responses were self-reports of the levels of physical leisure activity and physical fitness. The responses suggested that the patients had higher levels of leisure activity than did the non-patients. The researchers found a weak correlation between high physical leisure activity levels and high physical fitness levels. However, healthy women in the general population could engage in heavier physical activities than could fibromyalgia patients.[139]

As Bennett noted regarding the results of this study, "As this study was based on self-reports, it is possible that the fibromyalgia patients in this study were overstating their level of physical leisure activity, as they may have been 'programmed' that this is an important aspect of management." He also speculated, however, that the results suggest that reduced physical fitness in fibromyalgia patients is not related to reduced levels of physical leisure activities.[140] The material I have included in this section supports this latter possibility—fibromyalgia patients may be able to engage in leisure activities, yet their doing so does not translate into a level of condition that enables them to engage in more strenuous activities that would increase their levels of physical fitness. This is entirely possible, considering the limitations on exercise tolerance and achievable levels of physical fitness imposed by inadequate thyroid hormone regulation of cell function. Patients are likely to tolerate well physical activities that do not invoke the release of catecholamines. But activities that invoke catecholamine release may worsen fibromyalgia status so severely that some patients feel little inclination to again embark on bouts of vigorous physical activity. Hence, some effects of inadequate thyroid hormone regulation of cell function impose a ceiling on how much activity some fibromyalgia can engage in without severe adverse effects. This ceiling imposes a limit to the level of physical activity a patient can tolerate. The ceiling also restricts the level of physical fitness a patient can achieve through physical activity.

Several effects of inadequate thyroid hormone regulation of cell function in fibromyalgia can account for both low motor drive and symptom exacerbation with exercise. Comparisons with patients who have hypothyroidism, the prototypical form of hypometabolism, are informative. Hypothyroid patients typically complain of "fatigue and exercise intolerance."[24,p.994] The thyroidologist Ingbar wrote that these subjective sensations of hypothyroid patients may arise from several phenomena. These include limited pulmonary reserve, limited cardiac reserve, decreased muscle strength, and increased fatigability.[24,p.994] Below, I discuss these factors and others as they may relate to fibromyalgia patients' subnormal physical fitness levels.

Disinclination Toward Physical Activity in Fibromyalgia and Hypothyroidism

Bäckman et al. concluded from studies of fibromyalgia patients' skeletal muscle function that their lower-than-normal muscle strength resulted from impaired central activation of motor units.[114] In view of this conclusion, Bengtsson et al. remarked, ". . . it seems possible for patients with fibromyalgia to perform the same amount of work as healthy controls if a considerable amount of pain is accepted."[113,p.78]

The implication of this remark is that apprehension of pain reduces the central activation of motor units, causes volitional low activity levels, and results in lower test scores for muscle strength. Certainly, anticipation of pain from physical exertion contributes to some patients' disinclination to exert themselves. Several research groups have written that fear of and avoidance of physical activities contribute to the de-

velopment and maintenance of chronic musculoskeletal pain and disability.[141][142][143][144]

However, another and possibly more potent influence on the disinclination to engage in physical activity is impaired centrally-mediated motor drive. This is predictable from the hypothesis of inadequate thyroid hormone regulation of transcription in central dopaminergic neurons. Impaired motor drive may also explain study results reported by Elert et al.[115] They assessed fibromyalgia patients' perception of fatigue. On average, healthy control subjects did not perceive maximum fatigue after 100 muscle contractions. In contrast, fibromyalgia patients reached maximum perception of fatigue after 20-to-30 contractions. Despite the perception, the patients continued with the test until they completed 100 contractions. This outcome suggests that the patients' muscles were not weak *per se* and that the perception of fatigue was centrally-mediated. The perception of fatigue was disproportional to the actual work capability of the patients' muscles. (See Chapter 3.11, section titled "Decreased Dopamine and Low Locomotor Drive and Motor Activity in Hypothyroidism.")

Impaired Motor Drive and Decreased Motor Activity in Hypothyroidism

Many fibromyalgia patients report that they simply cannot muster the will to exercise; in fact, some report having no will to move about even for leisure activities. Many patients have too little drive to activate themselves to move about their living domains, and exercise is out of the question for them. My questioning of these patients and the forthright answers of many have lead me to a belief—that most have centrally-mediated subnormal motor drive. The subnormal drive militates against their efforts to engage in physical activities except through an extreme mustering of will power. Their lack of drive, to me, explains at least in part three research findings: fibromyalgia patients' low maximum voluntary muscle strength, their low endurance,[9][10][11] and their low maximum power output (exertion).[12,p.160] The finding of a low mean level of the breakdown product of dopamine (3-methoxy-4-hydroxyphenethylene) in the cerebrospinal fluid of fibromyalgia patients[60] makes feasible the hypothesis of low centrally-mediated motor drive. Low dopamine levels would account at least in part for the low drive.

Thyroid Hormone Regulation of Dopamine Levels and Motor Drive

Berne and Levy wrote that one mechanism which may initiate the close match between blood flow and metabolism during exercise is centrally-generated neural activity. The central command activates both the cardiovascular system and the skeletal muscle motor system, and it heightens the perception of effort. The command signals may arise from motor neurons in the spinal cord, motor cortex, cerebellum, and the basal ganglia.[160,p.642] It is likely that normal dopamine secretion by neurons in the basal ganglia is part of the central command, providing the motor drive for the individual to exert herself. Anything that impairs these cells' synthesis and secretion of dopamine may decrease motor drive, leaving the individual disinclined to exert herself. Inadequate thyroid hormone regulation of dopaminergic cells may provide such impairment.

Whether or not thyroid hormone could be responsible for the low dopamine metabolite levels in fibromyalgia patients is not an easy question to answer. One reason is that, depending on the region of the brain studied, researchers have reported that hypothyroidism increased,[63][64][65][66][72,p.585] decreased,[67][68] or left unchanged[69] the levels of catecholamines, including dopamine. Dopamine synthesizing and secreting neurons have nuclear T_3-receptors.[61] Thyroid hormone activates gene transcription for dopamine by binding to T_3-receptors. This is a direct genomic action. Moreover, thyroid hormone regulates the rate of synthesis of dopamine by controlling the activity of tyrosine hydroxylase, the rate-limiting enzyme in catecholamine synthesis.[62]

Decreased Dopamine in Hypothyroidism Lowers Locomotor Drive and Activity. Locomotor activity is the tendency to move or rate of movement. Dopaminergic neurons in the meso-limbic and nigro-striatal pathways control locomotor activity.[76][77][78][79][80][81][82][83] Hypothyroidism decreases catecholamine synthesis in the striatum, where dopamine is the main catecholamine.[70][71] Hypothyroidism decreases the locomotor activity of young rats.[75] Also, reduced synthesis of dopamine in the striatum accounts for impaired locomotor activity of developing hypothyroid rats.[70] Inadequate thyroid hormone regulation of dopamine synthesis, due to hypothyroidism or thyroid hormone resistance, may explain low motor drive and locomotor activity of fibromyalgia patients.

Modulation of the Effect of Decreased Dopamine on Locomotor Activity by α_2-Adrenergic Receptors. Lowered motor drive or locomotor activity caused by reduced dopamine production may be compounded by a concurrently increased population of α_2-adrenergic receptors on cell membranes. Both the reduced dopamine levels and the increase in α_2-ad-

renergic receptors can result from inadequate T_3 regulation of transcription. The α_2-adrenoceptor agonist clonidine inhibited both normal[84][85][86] and amphetamine-driven[87] locomotor activity.

Whether or not this compounding effect occurs, however, may depend on the isoform of α-adrenergic receptor increased by inadequate T_3 regulation. While α_2-adrenergic receptor agonists inhibited motor activity, α_1-adrenergic receptor agonists (phenylephrine and methoxamine) increased locomotor activity.[84][88][89] The finding of increased α_2-adrenoceptors on the platelets of fibromyalgia patients[45] raises the possibility that inadequate thyroid hormone transcription regulation is instrumental in the low motor drive and locomotor activity of these patients.

Low Dopamine Levels Due to Inadequate Thyroid Hormone Transcription Regulation in Dopaminergic Neurons May Decrease Growth Hormone Secretion. Low growth hormone levels, with secondarily low somatomedin C levels, in fibromyalgia may contribute to patients' low fitness levels. The low levels of the two hormones may impair tissue repair and reduce connective tissue tone in patients.[18,p.188] (See Chapter 3.3.)

Dopamine stimulates growth hormone secretion.[73][74] This phenomenon raises a possibility relevant to findings in fibromyalgia patients: that low dopamine levels, resulting from inadequate thyroid hormone regulation of dopamine synthesis and release, may contribute to low growth hormone and somatomedin C levels. Of course, thyroid hormone potently controls growth hormone gene transcription. Inadequate thyroid hormone regulation of the growth hormone gene may be directly responsible for low growth hormone and somatomedin C levels in fibromyalgia (see Chapter 3.12).

For more detailed information on the effects of thyroid hormone on dopaminergic neurons, see Chapter 2.3, the sections titled "Norepinephrine" and "Dopamine."

Perception of Weakness in Hypothyroidism Possibly Due to Diminished Cardiopulmonary and Circulatory Function

In fibromyalgia patients with inadequate thyroid hormone regulation of transcription, due either to hypothyroidism or thyroid hormone resistance, the perception of weakness may contribute to a disinclination to engage in physical activity.

In hypothyroidism, skeletal muscle is essentially an under-fueled contractile machine. Due to this, when hypothyroidism is severe enough, muscles are measurably weak. At least two other factors, however, contribute to the muscle weakness. One factor is diminished cardiopulmonary and circulatory function. Diminished circulation reduces the amounts of energy-yielding substrates that reach muscle cells. The other factor is a central perception of weakness. Tepperman and Tepperman wrote, "The perception of weakness must be at least as complicated as the perception of hunger, satiety, thirst or similar sensations, and although thyroid hormone availability or lack may have effects on the perception of the sensation of fatigue, we cannot describe these at present."[111,p.169]

Subnormal Capacity for Exercise-Induced Increased Oxidative Metabolism

Physical conditioning can increase by 40% the activity of oxidative enzymes in skeletal muscles. The increased enzyme activity does not usually contribute to an increase in VO_2 max, which may increase by only 15%. However, the increased enzyme activity may enable the physically conditioned individual to increase her capacity for heavy, prolonged exercise by as much as 300%. The increased activity of oxidative enzymes in the conditioned individual allows more of the pyruvate formed during glycolysis to be oxidized in the mitochondria to carbon dioxide and water. Also, physical conditioning mobilizes free fatty acids. These can then be oxidized to enter the citric acid cycle as acetyl-CoA through β-oxidation. The increased use of free fatty acids spares muscle glycogen to some degree.[160,p.642] It also provides more substrate for glycolysis in that the glycerol from the breakdown of fatty acids enters the glycolytic pathway in the cytoplasm of cells. (See Chapter 2.2, subsection titled "Fatty Acid Oxidation.")

In patients whose fibromyalgia is due to hypothyroidism or thyroid hormone resistance, the production of oxidative enzymes may be subnormal. The subnormal production may limit the patients' capacity to increase oxidative metabolism through physical training. Thyroid hormone may not directly affect the activity of the citric acid cycle. However, the hormone may influence the cycle by regulating the availability of citric acid cycle intermediates. In part, thyroid hormone does so by regulating the availability or activity of various enzymes. I will give three examples. (For a more complete description, see Chapter 2.2.)

In liver and adipose, thyroid hormone deficiency decreases the activity of different enzymes that either precede or take part in the citric acid cycle. For exam-

ple, pyruvate dehydrogenase catabolizes the oxidative decarboxylation of pyruvate, but in hypothyroidism, the activity of this enzyme in peripheral tissues may be reduced by a third.

In hypothyroid rats, activity of the enzyme pyruvate carboxylase in the liver was reduced by two-thirds. Pyruvate carboxylase thus plays a critical role in maintaining proper levels of citric acid cycle intermediates. Pyruvate is converted to oxaloacetate whenever citric acid cycle intermediates are deficient. This conversion catalyzed by pyruvate carboxylase is considered a "filling up" enzymatic reaction that replenishes a citric acid cycle intermediate.

Also, through genomic action, thyroid hormone regulates malic acid, an enzyme that takes part in the citric acid cycles. Malate is derived from foods and from synthesis in the citric acid cycle. Malate is an intermediate in the citric acid cycle. Oxidation of malate to oxaloacetate is another "filling up" enzymatic reaction. When citric acid cycle intermediates are deficient, malate dehydrogenase (malic enzyme) catalyzes the oxidation of malate to oxaloacetate. The conversion replenishes the available supply of oxaloacetate. The reaction also occurs in the opposite direction, with malate dehydrogenase catalyzing reduction of oxaloacetate to malate. (See Chapter 2.2, subsection titled "Citric Acid Cycle.")

Such findings suggest that a subnormal level or activity of oxidative enzymes in the mitochondria of hypothyroid or thyroid hormone resistant fibromyalgia patients may limit their capacity to further increase the activity of these oxidative enzymes through physical conditioning. Thus, inadequate thyroid hormone regulation of oxidative metabolism may be the primary condition underlying their low fitness levels.

Other studies show that inadequate thyroid hormone regulation of glycolysis reduces its rate. The reduced rate may limit the fibromyalgia patient's capacity for anaerobic metabolism. (See section below titled "Impaired Aerobic and Anaerobic Metabolism in Fibromyalgia: Possible Effect of Increased α- and Decreased β-Adrenergic Receptors.")

EXERCISE INTOLERANCE: WORSENING OF FIBROMYALGIA STATUS DURING EXERCISE (AND OTHER STRESSES)

Increased α-Adrenergic Receptors and Decreased β-Adrenergic Receptors

The single most important means by which inadequate thyroid hormone regulation of body function results in exercise intolerance is through its effects on adrenergic receptor types. Overall, inadequate thyroid hormone regulation of the adrenergic genes increases the density of α-adrenergic receptors and decreases the density of β-adrenergic receptors on cells membranes (see Chapter 3.1, section titled "Inadequate Thyroid Hormone Regulation of Adrenergic Gene Transcription"), including the membranes of skeletal muscle cells.[109] A number of studies give reason to believe that fibromyalgia patients have this pattern of adrenergic receptor types (see Chapter 3.1, section titled "High Ratio of α- to β-Adrenergic Receptors on Cell Membranes"). An increase of α-adrenergic receptors and a decrease of β-adrenergic receptors would interfere at several sites with normal physiological adaptation to exercise.

Decreased Cyclic-AMP Formation in Hypothyroidism. A study by Guttler et al. showed the effects on cyclic-AMP production during inadequate thyroid hormone regulation of gene transcription for adrenergic receptors. (Cyclic-AMP is a nucleotide within the cell membrane. Catecholamines, upon binding to β-adrenergic receptors on cell membranes, stimulate the formation of cyclic-AMP within the cell. Cyclic-AMP then stimulates a cascade of reactions that accelerate metabolism.) The purpose of the study by Guttler et al. was to measure the rate of urinary cyclic-AMP excretion in euthyroid, hyperthyroid, and hypothyroid men. They found no significant difference in the urinary excretion of cyclic-AMP between the three groups of men when at rest (when not ambulating). When given infusions of epinephrine over a 2-hour period, hyperthyroid and euthyroid men excreted more cyclic-AMP than hypothyroid men. Hyperthyroid men excreted more than euthyroid men. Hypothyroid men did not have a significant increase in cyclic-AMP excretion.[48]

Blunted Cardiovascular Responses in Hypothyroidism. Guttler et al. also evaluated cardiovascular system responses to the epinephrine infusions. The responses were greatest in hyperthyroid men. Responses were virtually absent in hypothyroid men. These differences reflect the difference in β-adrenergic receptor cell membrane density in hyperthyroid and hypothyroid individuals. The greater β-adrenergic receptor density in hyperthyroid men resulted in an increased excretion of cyclic-AMP and stronger cardiovascular responses. Two findings indicate a blunting of biochemical and physiological adaptations in hypothyroid men to epinephrine as a biochemical mediator of stress: (1) the lack of a significant increase in their urinary excretion of cyclic-AMP when infused with

epinephrine, and (2) their lack of a cardiovascular response to the infusions.

Activation of Intracellular Energy Metabolism. It is interesting that Guttler et al. (see the two subsections immediately above) found in "ambulating" hyperthyroid men, a slight, significant increase in the 24-hour urinary cyclic-AMP excretion. They wrote that the increase may have resulted from the exaggerated stimulation by endogenous catecholamines secreted in response to ambulation.[48] Ambulation, and especially more vigorous activity, induces catecholamine secretion, and the increased catecholamines stimulate muscle blood flow. When β-adrenergic receptor density on cell membranes is normal, catecholamines bind to these, induce an increase in cyclic-AMP formation, and through reactions triggered by the cyclic-AMP, induce the conversion of glycogen to glucose. The glucose is then degraded to provide energy to meet the increased energy needs for ambulation or other activities. Also, triglycerides in adipose tissue are hydrolyzed and the liberated fatty acids are then used to generate energy.[47,p.27] If a fibromyalgia patient has more α-adrenergic receptors than β-adrenergic receptors, then increased catecholamine secretion does not stimulate glycogenolysis, glycolysis, and lipolysis, and the patient is not able to normally adapt to the increased energy demand of activity—as reflected in the blunted response to epinephrine in the hypothyroid men in the Guttler et al. study.[48] (See the section below titled "Impaired Aerobic and Anaerobic Metabolism in Fibromyalgia: Possible Effect of Increased α- and Decreased β-Adrenergic Receptors.")

When I tracked patients' fibromyalgia status for a year,[49] I found that during times of physical or psychological stress, patients' status deteriorated to a significant degree. This phenomenon may be explained by intensification of diminished blood flow and slowed energy metabolism due to an increase in the density of α_2-adrenergic receptors and a decreased density of β-adrenergic receptors on blood vessels and cell membranes.

Sympathetic and Parasympathetic Nerve Cell Bodies. An increased density of α_2-adrenergic receptors on sympathetic and parasympathetic nerve cell bodies is likely to cause subnormal sympathetic nervous system activity and exaggerated parasympathetic activity. The altered autonomic nervous system function impairs adaptation of the cardiovascular system to the physiological demands of exercise. (See the next section, "Hyperpolarization of Sympathetic Neurons and Facilitation of Parasympathetic Neurons by an Increased Density of α_2-Adrenergic Receptors." Also, see the section below titled "Deficient Hypothalamic Secretion of Corticotropin-Releasing Hormone (CRH) in Fibromyalgia: Possible Impaired Activation of the Locus Ceruleus-Norepinephrine System and the Central Sympathetic System.")

Hyperpolarization of Sympathetic Neurons and Facilitation of Parasympathetic Neurons by an Increased Density of α_2-Adrenergic Receptors. Normally, when someone begins exercising, a substantial fall in arterial blood pressure does not occur. Baroreceptor reflexes prevent a substantial fall in pressure by inducing two effects that increase the heart rate and stroke volume: (1) reduced parasympathetic (vagus) nerve stimulation of the heart, and (2) increased sympathetic nerve stimulation.[160,p.624] However, an increased density of α_2-adrenergic receptors on sympathetic neurons hyperpolarizes them, making them resistant to activation. An increased density of the receptors on parasympathetic neurons facilitates their activation. As a result, the baroreceptor reflexes fail to increase the heart rate and stroke volume. Therefore, when the fibromyalgia patient engages in exercise of mild-to-moderate intensity, her cardiorespiratory system fails to respond properly. Hence, the system fails to meet the demand for increased oxygen delivery to the working muscles. Subnormal sympathetic activity due to the increase of α_2-adrenergic receptors in the nucleus of the solitary tract and the sympathetic ganglia may be reinforced by resistance to central nervous system sympathetic activation by another mechanism—reduced secretion of corticotropin-releasing hormone due to inadequate regulation by thyroid hormone (see the section below titled "Deficient Hypothalamic Secretion of Corticotropin-Releasing Hormone (CRH) in Fibromyalgia: Possible Impaired Activation of the Locus Ceruleus-Norepinephrine System and the Central Sympathetic System").

Both central and peripheral administration of α_2-adrenergic receptor agonists, such as norepinephrine and the drug clonidine, induce hypotension and bradycardia.[103] This effect is mediated in part by an increase in prejunctional α_2-adrenoceptor activity in the nucleus of the solitary tract and the paravertebral sympathetic ganglia (see Chapter 3.2, section titled "Inhibition of Central Centers for Activation of the Sympathetic Nervous System"). Activation of α_2-adrenergic receptors by clonidine hyperpolarized sympathetic ganglionic cells.[104]

The hyperpolarization is similar to the "relative refractory period" of nerve fibers rather than an "absolute refractory period." An absolute refractory period is the time following an action potential during which

a second action potential cannot be initiated, not even by strong stimuli. Following the absolute refractory period, a briefer relative refractory period follows. During the relative refractory period, the voltage-activated sodium channels are in an inactive state. The inactive state blocks further entry of sodium ions (Na^+, positive ions) into the neuronal cells. In addition, potassium channels remain wide open, and an excess of potassium ions (K^+, positive ions) flow out of the cell. The efflux of potassium ions temporarily leaves the inside of the cell in extreme negativity (hyperpolarization). Hyperpolarization renders the cell more resistant than normal to initiation of action potentials. As a result, stimuli of mild-to-moderate intensity cannot initiate action potentials. Similarly, an increased density of α_2-adrenergic receptors on sympathetic nerve cell bodies makes the cells more resistant to activation. An increased density of the receptors may account for a finding of Elam et al. They reported that when at rest, fibromyalgia patients had normal muscle sympathetic nerve activity. However, their muscle sympathetic innervation was subnormal during mild stimulation—mental stress, post-contraction ischemia, contraction of the jaw muscles, and static handgrip.[50]

While stimuli of mild-to-moderate intensity cannot initiate action potentials during hyperpolarization, sufficiently strong stimuli can.[20,p.64] This can adversely affect patients (see the next section: "Sympathetic Neuronal Activation by Strong Stimuli").

An increased density of α_2-adrenergic receptors on parasympathetic (vagal) neurons within the dorsal vagal nucleus facilitates the transmission of signals through the vagal nerves to the heart. (See Chapter 3.2, section titled "Inhibition of Central Centers for Activation of the Sympathetic Nervous System.") These vagal signals cause persistence of a slow heart rate and low stroke volume. Normally, when exercise begins, blood pressure falls slightly due to muscle metabolite-induced vasodilation. During this time, parasympathetic nervous system innervation of the heart rapidly diminishes. This occurs before an increase in sympathetic innervation. The offset of parasympathetic innervation causes the heart rate to increase within 1-to-2 beats. Up to a heart rate of about 100, the offset of parasympathetic innervation accounts for the increase in the heart rate. Above roughly 100 beats per minute, further increases in heart rate occur because of increased sympathetic innervation.[160,pp.624&628]

The combination of subnormal sympathetic innervation and persistent parasympathetic innervation can account for some fibromyalgia patients' lower heart rates during exercise.[5,p.37] The combination can also account for the blunted sympathetic nervous system responsiveness and parasympathetic nervous system dominance when fibromyalgia patients exercise (see Chapter 3.1, section titled "Subnormal Sympathetic Response to Stresses in Hypothyroid and Fibromyalgia Patients," and the section titled "Impaired Sympathetic Nervous System Function Due to Inadequate Thyroid Hormone Regulation of Cell Function: Physiological Effects").

Sympathetic Neuronal Activation by Strong Stimuli. Intensely strenuous exercise by fibromyalgia patients may provide the strong stimulation that overcomes the resistance of sympathetic nerve cell bodies to activation. This is tantamount to a strong stimulus overriding a relative refractory period in sympathetic neurons that I described above in this section. The result would be a sudden sympathetic nervous system discharge that the patient perceives as anxiety or panic (See Chapter 3.10). In addition, the increased norepinephrine and epinephrine secreted during sudden intense sympathetic nervous system activation bind to predominant α-adrenergic receptors on arterioles and muscle cell membranes. The result will be intense vasoconstriction and diminished energy metabolism within the muscle cells. In individuals with a normal count of both α- and β-adrenergic receptors on muscle arterioles, local dilation of the arterioles by vasodilating metabolites from local muscle cells effectively opposes the vasoconstriction induced by norepinephrine binding to α-adrenergic receptors on the arterioles.[160,p.636] However, the increased density of α-adrenergic receptors and the decreased density of β-adrenergic receptors on arterioles permit a far more potent vasoconstriction in response to norepinephrine binding to α-adrenergic receptors. (Conversely, when α-adrenergic receptors are chemically blocked, binding of epinephrine to β-adrenergic receptors on blood vessels strongly dilates them.[164]) Strong vasoconstriction upon sympathetic nervous system activation would critically reduce both muscle and cerebral blood flow during intense exercise. This can account for the severely reduced cerebral blood flow in some fibromyalgia patients (see Chapter 3.2, section titled "Reduced Cerebral Blood Flow"). The diminished energy metabolism may cause an intracellular metabolic crisis (see section below titled "Impaired Aerobic and Anaerobic Metabolism in Fibromyalgia: Possible Effect of Increased α- and Decreased β-Adrenergic Receptors"). Both the reduced blood flow and slowed energy metabolism would worsen fibromyalgia status.

Subnormal Catecholamine Secretion. Studies of catecholamine levels in fibromyalgia and hypothyroid patients at rest have given variable results. The variable results for the two groups largely overlap.

Fibromyalgia patients have subnormal norepinephrine secretion during exercise. (See Chapter 3.1, subsection titled "Norepinephrine Levels in Fibromyalgia Patients at Rest," and the subsection titled "Low Increase in Norepinephrine and Epinephrine Secretion during Exercise.") Yunus et al. reported that the plasma and urinary norepinephrine and epinephrine levels of fibromyalgia patients at rest were no different from that of controls.[126] During 5 months of treatment with cyclobenzaprine, fibromyalgia patients had normal-to-very high norepinephrine levels and low-to-normal epinephrine levels.[125]

Van Denderen reported that during exhaustive exercise, the norepinephrine and epinephrine levels of fibromyalgia patients were significantly lower than those of controls.[5] During insulin-induced hypoglycemia, fibromyalgia patients had about 30% lower rise in epinephrine than did control subjects.[124]

The low norepinephrine and epinephrine levels in fibromyalgia patients during stressors such as hypoglycemia or exercise suggest subnormal sympathetic reactivity at two sites: (1) sympathetic nerve endings, which secrete norepinephrine in tissues, and (2) the adrenal medullae, which secrete into the circulating blood a catecholamine ratio of about 80% epinephrine to 20% norepinephrine, although the ratio can vary under different physiological conditions. Compared to norepinephrine secreted directly into tissues, deficient adrenal gland secretion of catecholamines may have a greater overall dampening effect on fibromyalgia patients' ability to sustain exercise. This is possible because norepinephrine and epinephrine, secreted into the circulation by the adrenal medullae, clear slowly from the blood. As a result, the effects of these circulating hormones last 5-to-10 times longer than norepinephrine secreted directly into the tissues.[20,p.673]

Inadequate regulation by thyroid hormone can account for subnormal catecholamine secretion in two ways. First, thyroid hormone regulates enzymes involved in catecholamine synthesis, and inadequate thyroid hormone regulation decreases production of these enzymes (see Chapter 3.1, subsection titled "Low Production of Catecholamine-Inducing Enzymes Due to Inadequate Thyroid Hormone Regulation During Development"). Second, inadequate thyroid hormone regulation of transcription of the adrenergic genes increases the density of α_2-adrenergic receptors on presynaptic membranes of sympathetic nerve endings. The α_2-adrenergic receptors inhibit norepinephrine release from the nerve endings. Presynaptic β_2-adrenergic receptors induce norepinephrine release from sympathetic nerve endings,[116,p.243] but inadequate thyroid hormone regulation of the adrenergic genes decreases the density of β-adrenergic receptors on neuronal cell membranes. The result of this change in adrenergic receptor types is subnormal secretion of norepinephrine from sympathetic neurons. This may account for the failure of levels of norepinephrine to normally increase in fibromyalgia patients during exercise.

Studies show that activation of a normal count of β_2-adrenergic receptors in the adrenal glands stimulates adrenal secretion of epinephrine and norepinephrine. A decrease in the density of β_2-adrenergic receptors reduces adrenal gland catecholamine secretion. β_2-Adrenergic receptors on the outer surface of sympathetic nerve endings (termed presynaptic β_2-adrenergic receptors) in the adrenal medullae enhance norepinephrine and epinephrine secretion in response to electrical nerve stimulation. In other tissues, the receptors activate the release of norepinephrine from sympathetic nerve endings. However, in these other tissues, norepinephrine does not stimulate the receptors to activate norepinephrine release. Instead, epinephrine secreted by the adrenal medullae activates the receptors. The epinephrine either reaches the receptors through the circulation, or it reaches them after being taken up by sympathetic nerve endings and then secreted along with norepinephrine. It then stimulates the β_2-adrenergic receptors to augment norepinephrine release.[168] This is an example of a positive feedback loop—increases in epinephrine release stimulate further norepinephrine release.

Strenuous exercise normally increases both norepinephrine and epinephrine levels in the bloodstream. However, when rats were give a β_2-adrenergic receptor blocker before strenuous exercise, the increase in their norepinephrine and epinephrine levels were markedly subnormal. Intravenous infusion of a β_2-adrenergic receptor agonist caused a normal rise in the norepinephrine level during exercise. Infusion of epinephrine also caused a normal rise in the norepinephrine levels, showing that epinephrine stimulates β_2-adrenergic receptors to increase norepinephrine secretion. Injecting the selective α_2-adrenergic receptor blocker yohimbine along with a β_2-adrenergic receptor agonist caused an enormous rise in plasma norepinephrine levels during exercise. This showed that α_2-adrenergic receptors inhibit the adrenal gland release of norepinephrine.[169]

Koganei et al. reported that activation of β_2-adren-

ergic receptors in the adrenal medullae of anesthetized dogs increased the adrenal secretion of catecholamines.[166] Foucart et al. reported that same result.[170] On the other hand, activation of β_1-adrenergic receptors inhibited the catecholamine release caused by β_2-adrenergic receptor activation.[166] Foucart et al. reported that administering a β_2-adrenergic receptor blocker significantly decreased the release of adrenal catecholamines during electrical stimulation of the splanchnic nerves.[167]

Cardiac Function. deVries emphasized that when an individual uses large muscle masses during exercise, as in running, cardiac output limits aerobic power.[13,p.189] Van Dederen et al. had 10 fibromyalgia patients and 10 healthy controls perform exhaustive physical exercise, using a bicycle ergometer test and a step test. They wrote that the lower heart rates of fibromyalgia patients during both exercises were "a striking finding."[5,p.37] This suggests that cardiac output may impose a narrow limit on aerobic power in fibromyalgia patients. In turn, the low cardiac output may be partly a function of depressed sympathetic drive due to inadequate thyroid hormone transcription regulation of the adrenergic genes.

Similarly, Burack et al. reported that hypothyroid patients' exercise intolerance results mainly from cardiac limitation—an impaired ability to increase stroke volume and cardiac output. During exercise, hypothyroid patients had low oxygen consumption and work loads. Their arterial lactate levels increased above normal levels. Some hypothyroid patients also have an abnormal distribution of blood flow during exercise.[29]

Visuri et al. measured the sympathetic responses of 17 fibromyalgic males to several conditions that stimulate sympathetic responses: deep breathing, repetitive hand gripping, orthostasis, and the Valsalva maneuver. They had more than a 10 mm Hg rise in diastolic blood pressure.[162] Bennett commented that the results reported by Visuri et al. suggest enhanced sympathetic arousal in fibormyalgia patients.[163] The results of Visuri et al. may have resulted from the inadvertent selection of a subset of fibromyalgia patients whose sympathetic nervous systems were excessively responsive to stimulation.

When the sympathetic nerves in the heart secrete norepinephrine, the neurotransmitter normally binds to β-adrenergic receptors on the cells in the sinoatrial node. The sinoatrial node is a group of specialized cardiac muscle fibers. The group of fibers acts as the "pacemaker" of the heart conduction system. Most of the increase in heart rate during exercise results from the offset of parasympathetic innervation of the heart through the vagal nerves. When the heart rate nears or reaches 100, norepinephrine appears in the blood, showing that the sympathetic nervous system has activated. As the norepinephrine level rises in the blood, the heart rate increases beyond 100. The increase in heart rate results mainly from the binding of norepinephrine to β-adrenergic receptors in the sinoatrial node. A reduced count of β-adrenergic receptors on cells in the sinoatrial node, due to inadequate thyroid hormone regulation of the adrenergic genes, limits the capacity of the heart rate to rise substantially. Even if sympathetic nerve fibers to the heart continued to release norepinephrine near the sinoatrial node, too few β-adrenergic receptors on sinoatrial node cells nullify the neurotransmitters' ability to increase the heart rate.[160,p.628]

Norepinephrine is released by sympathetic nerve endings in the heart, and epinephrine (and a small amount of norepinephrine) reaches the heart through the circulation after being released from the adrenal medullae. In heart cells, these catecholamines bind to β_1-adrenergic receptors. If the heart cells have a normal count of the receptors, binding of norepinephrine and epinephrine to a normal density of β_1-adrenergic receptors causes powerful inotropic effects—that is, the binding potently increases contractility of the heart muscle. However, if inadequate thyroid hormone regulation of transcription of the adrenergic genes has reduced the density of β_1-adrenergic receptors on heart cells, the catecholamines will cause only a subnormal increase in heart contractility.

A reduced density of β-adrenergic receptors on heart cell membranes will compound the low heart rate and force of contraction that result from the subnormal sympathetic innervation and exaggerated parasympathetic innervation I described above (see subsection titled "Sympathetic and Parasympathetic Nerve Cell Bodies").

Deficient Hypothalamic Secretion of Corticotropin-Releasing Hormone (CRH) in Fibromyalgia: Possible Impaired Activation of the Locus Ceruleus-Norepinephrine System and the Central Sympathetic System

Documented abnormalities in the function of the hypothalamic-pituitary-adrenocortical axis in fibromyalgia patients point to deficient secretion of CRH (see Chapter 3.5). Thyroid hormone regulates CRH gene transcription. A deficiency of thyroid hormone or resistance of CRH-synthesizing hypothalamic cells to thyroid hormone may account for the CRH deficiency in some fibromyalgia patients. Hypothyroidism mar-

kedly reduces hypothalamic CRH gene expression: when thyroid hormone is deficient, CRH mRNA decreases; when thyroid hormone levels are adequate, CRH mRNA increases.

Hypothalamic CRH, which activates the pituitary-adrenocortical components of the hypothalamic-pituitary-adrenal axis, also stimulates the locus ceruleus-norepinephrine system and the central sympathetic system.[30] When thyroid hormone regulation of CRH transcription is inadequate, as in hypothyroidism, CRH is deficient, resulting in HPA axis dysfunction. In addition, however, CRH deficiency may result in subnormal activation of the locus ceruleus-norepinephrine system and the central sympathetic system. This may in part account for the depressed sympathetic nervous system response to exercise by fibromyalgia patients, with low increases in serum epinephrine and norepinephrine.[5] This mechanism would also account for the low increase in cortisol during exercise reported by van Dederen et al.[5]

Subnormal activation of the central sympathetic system due to low CRH secretion is likely to reinforce other mechanisms that impede sympathetic nervous system activation in fibromyalgia patients (see the subsection above titled "Hyperpolorization of Sympathetic Neurons and Facilitation of Parasympathetic Neurons by an Increased Density of α_2-Adrenergic Receptors").

Deficient Delivery of Oxygen to Muscle During Exercise

Decreased sympathetic nervous system innervation of muscles while fibromyalgia patients exercise may impair function of the muscle. The impaired function might be difficult to detect but sufficient to for the patient to perceive.

Simms wrote that recent studies have not shown distinct muscle metabolic abnormalities in fibromyalgia patients. He wrote, "Recent studies of morphology have shown only nonspecific or mild changes, perhaps consistent with subtle metabolic abnormalities, especially at tender point sites."[133] This is consistent with the characteristic but nonspecific and inconsistent abnormalities revealed by pathologic studies of skeletal muscle from patients with hypothyroid myopathy.[56]

Henriksson wrote: "In metabolic myopathies, with deficiency in enzymes necessary for sufficient adenosine triphosphate (ATP) production, muscle activity causes pain. From this perspective, studies on the regulation of intramuscular microcirculation and studies of muscle energy metabolism are of interest for understanding muscle pain. In the vast majority of patients with chronic muscle pain, there is, however, neither a primary metabolic myopathy nor any major disturbance in blood circulation. This does not exclude that there are changes in the muscle that could excite and sensitize intramuscular nociceptors and give rise to localized pain."[161,p.103]

The main change in muscle underling subtle muscle dysfunction may be circulation insufficient to provide the increased oxygen and nutrients needed during exercise. And pain due to insufficient ATP production may occur even during rest. An early study and a recent one have shown decreased production of ATP and creatine phosphate in muscle of fibromyalgia patients.[96][158] In 1986, Bengtsson et al. found low ATP and phosphocreatine concentrations in tender points in fibromyalgia patients' trapezius muscles at rest.[96] In 1998, Park et al. reported finding low ATP and phosphocreatine concentrations in fibromyalgia patients' quadriceps muscles at rest.[158] Inadequate thyroid hormone regulation of muscle cell metabolism can account for subnormal ATP production.

Also, the effects of inadequate thyroid hormone regulation on the sympathetic and parasympathetic branches of the autonomic nervous system can contribute to reduced energy metabolism in muscle. The decreased sympathetic innervation and increased parasympathetic innervation can cause subnormal cardiac output by decreasing heart rate and stroke volume. The decreased cardiac output results in a lower propulsion of blood through the arteries.

In addition, inadequate thyroid hormone regulation of the adrenergic genes increases the density of α-adrenergic receptors and decreases the density of β-adrenergic receptors on arterioles. The result is increased vasoconstriction, increased vascular resistance, and decreased blood flow to tissues.

Moreover, three other factors resulting from inadequate regulation by thyroid hormone can contribute to reduced blood flow to muscles: (1) decreased release of vasodilator metabolites from muscle cells, (2) decreased thyroid hormone-induced relaxation of the smooth muscle lining of blood vessels, and (3) decreased production of the vasodilator nitric oxide. Inadequate thyroid hormone regulation of muscle cell function reduces the metabolic rate of the cells. The decreased metabolic rate reduces the oxygen requirement of the cells, which reduces their release of vasodilating metabolites. The reduced release of the metabolites provides little opposition to vasoconstriction caused by an increase of α-adrenergic receptors on arterioles, deficient thyroid hormone-induced arteriolar relaxation, and subnormal nitric oxide secretion.

(For a description of the blood vessel relaxing effect of thyroid hormone, and thyroid hormone-induced production of nitric oxide, see Chapter 3.2, subsection titled "Nitric Oxide and Thyroid Hormone.") The following section describes the nitric oxide phenomenon.

Low Nitric Oxide Levels in Fibromyalgia: Possibly Due to Impaired Sympathetic Function Secondary to Inadequate Thyroid Hormone Regulation. The secretion of the vasodilator nitric oxide is coupled to the intensity of sympathetic nerve activity. Skarphedinsson et al. found that in normotensive, resting men, the intensity of muscle sympathetic nerve activity was positively correlated with plasma nitrate concentrations. (Plasma nitrate is a measure of nitric oxide release.) Higher sympathetic activity was correlated with greater nitric oxide release. The researchers proposed that nitric oxide, as a circulating vasodilator, counteracts vasoconstriction induced by sympathetic nerve traffic. They noted that the degree of increased sympathetic nerve activity varies between individuals. They suggested that with different degrees of nerve activity, nitric oxide release varies, and the variable release accounts for individual differences in vasoconstriction in nerves, muscle, the heart, and the kidneys. They also proposed that the failure of blood pressure to rise with increased sympathetic activities is due to a simultaneous increase in nitric oxide release.[32]

Low secretion of nitric oxide in fibromyalgia may be a result of low sympathetic activity. Eisinger found evidence of low peripheral nitric oxide levels in fibromyalgia patients.[33] The low nitric oxide levels may contribute to patients' vasoconstriction and reduced muscle and brain blood flow. The low nitric oxide level may be tied to fibromyalgia patients' blunted sympathetic response during exercise [5][17] and their tendency toward low muscle sympathetic activity.[50] The resulting vasoconstriction may contribute to subtle muscle dysfunction and pain.

Relation of Thyroid Hormone to Nitric Oxide Levels. As I explained in the two sections immediately above, low CRH secretion and inhibition of sympathetic nerve cell bodies in the nucleus of the solitary tract and the paravertebral sympathetic ganglia—all due to inadequate thyroid hormone regulation of cell function—inhibit sympathetic nervous system activation, unless provoked by strong stimuli. The reduced sympathetic nervous system activity may decrease nitric oxide production. In addition, however, reduced exposure of the endothelial cells of arteries to thyroid hormone may reduce endothelial vascular production of low nitric oxide.[34][35][105] The reduced production may contribute to the low nitric oxide levels resulting from the blunted sympathetic activity.

An advantage of fibromyalgia patients engaging in mild to moderate exercise, as Eisinger noted,[33] is that exercise increases nitric oxide production.[31] However, fibromyalgia patients who have hypothyroidism or thyroid hormone resistance may have a limited capacity for nitric oxide production without the use of large enough dosages of exogenous thyroid hormone. (See Chapter 3.2, subsection titled "Low Nitric Oxide Levels in Fibromyalgia.")

Metabolic Crisis in Fibromyalgia Patients During and Following Exercise

At least three mechanisms related to thyroid hormone may worsen fibromyalgia patients' symptoms during and after exercise: (1) increased catecholamine secretion, (2) binding of the catecholamines to the α-adrenergic receptors that predominate on cell membranes, and (3) a resulting critical slowdown of metabolism. The crisis may result from the slowdown of cell metabolism while muscle work during exercise increases metabolic demand. The crisis will result in transient worsening of patients' fibromyalgia status.

Increased Catecholamine Secretion During Exercise. During exercise at a high enough intensity, norepinephrine and epinephrine secretion increase.[39][40] deVries wrote that the effects of exercise on norepinephrine are well defined.[13,p.204] Exercise up to 50%-to-60% of VO_2 max causes only a small rise in norepinephrine levels. With heavier vigorous exercise, norepinephrine levels rise exponentially.[117][118][119][120] Howley found that at 49% of VO_2 max, norepinephrine excretion increased slightly. At 82% of VO_2 max, however, norepinephrine excretion increased 5-fold.[120] Berne and Levy wrote that when the heart rate during exercise reaches about 100 beats per minute, norepinephrine released from sympathetic nerves begins to appear in the circulating blood. When the heart rate rises above 100, the norepinephrine level in the blood rises sharply.[160,p.628]

Epinephrine increases less during exercise than does norepinephrine. However, despite the different magnitude in the rise of the two catecholamines, they increase in parallel.[121]

According to deVries, mild exercise, with a lack of catecholamine secretion, has a relaxing effect. But the effect of strenuous exercise, with catecholamine secretion, differs: "We see the importance of endocrine effects in allowing (if not to some extent causing) the 'tranquilizer' effect of exercise of low intensity, while heavy or exhausting exercise becomes an excitatory stressor."[13,p.204]

deVries also wrote that all investigators have reported that the catecholamine response to exercise diminishes with training.[13,p.204] The diminished response is important for endurance exercise. The lower heart rate and blood pressure from extensive training reduce myocardial O_2 uptake at any work load. The reduced O_2 uptake is important to the training regimen in health and disease.[13,p.205]

However, low catecholamine release in some fibromyalgia patients during exercise to exhaustion is not due to a physical training effect. Instead, it is most likely due to inhibited sympathetic nerve activity by a high density of α_2-adrenergic receptors on sympathetic neurons. In these patients, during exercise that is strenuous for them, sympathetic nerves are not likely to secrete normal amounts of norepinephrine into the tissues. Also, the adrenal medullae are not likely to secrete normal amounts of norepinephrine and epinephrine into the bloodstream.

Even in these fibromyalgia patients, some norepinephrine and epinephrine will be secreted. Still, the catecholamines are not likely to appropriately increase heart rate, cardiac output, and muscle cell metabolism. The catecholamines will bind predominantly to α_2-adrenergic receptors on cell membranes. The binding will then blunt energy metabolism. Hence, rather than the much needed increase in energy metabolism to meet the heightened energy demands from intense muscle work, muscle cells will be abruptly deprived of energy.

Impaired Aerobic and Anaerobic Metabolism in Fibromyalgia: Possible Effect of Increased α- and Decreased β-Adrenergic Receptors. Aerobic and anaerobic metabolism normally provide the energy needed for individuals to adapt physiologically to the stress of exercise.[13,pp.219-220] However, most fibromyalgia patients with hypothyroidism and/or thyroid hormone resistance are likely to have impairments during various steps in both aerobic and anaerobic metabolism. The expected result is the low fitness levels and exercise intolerance that are typical of fibromyalgia.

The conversion of pyruvate and fatty acids to acetyl Co-A and the production of ATP in the citric acid cycle in mitochondria require oxygen. Because oxygen is required, the transfer of energy within this system is called aerobic metabolism.[20,p.756] Release of glucose from glycogen and the production of ATP and pyruvate from glucose molecules do not require oxygen. These steps are therefore features of anaerobic metabolism. Both aerobic and anaerobic metabolism are critical to adaptation to exercise, and impairment of either can render the individual exercise intolerant.

Aerobic Metabolism. The glucose components of glycogen molecules are converted to pyruvate under anaerobic conditions, and the pyruvate is completely broken down to CO_2 and H_2O[13,p.219] in the mitochondria under aerobic conditions. In the presence of sufficient O_2, pyruvate, as the end product of glycolysis, is converted to acetyl-CoA. The aceytl-CoA combines with oxaloacetic acid to form citric acid which takes part in the citric acid cycle.[20,p.748] Although Eisinger's laboratory investigations did not show mitochondrial respiratory chain abnormalities in fibromyalgia patients,[33] further investigation is likely to show abnormalities that closely overlap those of hypothyroid patients.

The metabolic pathways that provide energy through aerobic metabolism to meet the increased need of muscles during exercise depend on a normal ability of the heart, lungs, and blood vessels (the cardiorespiratory system) to deliver enough O_2 to the cells. However, in hypothyroid and thyroid hormone resistant fibromyalgia patients, the cardiorespiratory system may have a low capacity for providing oxygen to muscle. First, inadequate thyroid hormone regulation of the adrenergic genes increases the density of α-adrenergic receptors and decreases the density of β-adrenergic receptors on various cells. The results are a subnormal heart rate and stroke volume (subnormal cardiac output), and increased resistance to blood flow due to vasoconstriction. Thus, blood flow to exercising muscle may be subnormal. In addition, respiration may be subnormal in hypothyroid and thyroid hormone resistant patients. Hence, the reduced flow of blood to exercising muscle may be insufficiently oxygenated. Subnormal oxygen delivery to muscle cells reinforces fibromyalgia patients' exercise intolerance by contributing to their low aerobic metabolic capacity. (See section below titled "Ventilatory (Respiratory) Drive in Hypothyroidism.")

Exercise physiologists in the past believed that maximum O_2 consumption (called "aerobic power," or VO_2 max) was a product mainly of blood O_2 transport. The also held that aerobic power was a product of cardiac output and hemoglobin level, which determine blood transport,[21] and O_2 consumption of the ventilatory muscles.[22] More recent evidence indicates that endurance in exercise may be determined mainly by the ability of muscles to use O_2 rather than the ability of blood to deliver it.[23] However, deVries emphasized that when large muscle masses are used in exercise, as in running, aerobic power is to a great degree limited by cardiac output.[13,p.189] Many fibromyalgia patients

apparently have subnormal cardiac output. The subnormal output seems to result from deficient sympathetic innervation and excessive parasympathetic innervation of the heart. The deficient sympathetic innervation and excessive parasympathetic innervation probably result from inadequate thyroid hormone regulation of the adrenergic genes. Patients' decreased cardiac output may result in too little delivery of oxygen to muscle during exercise, contributing to exercise intolerance (see Chapter 3.2, section titled "Mechanisms of Hypotension in Hypothyroidism").

(See section above titled "Subnormal Capacity for Exercise-Induced Increased Oxidative Metabolism.")

Anaerobic Metabolism and Glycolysis. As exercise intensity progressively increases, an intensity is reached when the heart, lungs, and blood vessels are not able to provide enough oxygen to cells for aerobic metabolism to proceed in providing energy. At this point, the O_2 supply fails to satisfy the increasing need of working cells for O_2. Physiologists call the degree of failure to meet the increased need an "oxygen (O_2) deficit." Patients with low aerobic metabolic capacity due to inadequate thyroid hormone regulation of oxidative enzymes (see section above titled "Subnormal Capacity for Exercise-Induced Increased Oxidative Metabolism") will enter anaerobic metabolism at a lower intensity of exercise. That this occurs in fibromyalgia patients is supported by a study by Nørregaard et al. They had 15 female fibromyalgia patients and 15 age- and sex-matched controls perform a stepwise incremental maximal bicycle ergometer test. Fibromyalgia patients reached an estimated anaerobic threshold at a heart rate of 124 per minute. Control subjects reached anaerobic threshold at a heart rate of 140 beats per minute. This statistically significant difference showed that fibromyalgia patients reached anaerobic metabolism with less exertion.[153]

The ability of muscle cells to continue functioning during the exercise-induced oxygen deficit depends on several energy sources not dependent on the deliver of O_2 to cells by the cardiorespiratory system. These sources are mainly: 1) O_2 bound to myoglobin in muscle, 2) cleaving ATP and creatine phosphate, and 3) glycolysis (the anaerobic degradation of glycogen to lactic acid). In other words, when exercise temporarily induces a metabolic need for more O_2 than the cardiorespiratory system can provide, the individual contracts an "oxygen debt," and from that point on, muscle energy needs are normally met by the three sources above. For the most part, muscle energy needs are met by the anaerobic metabolic process called glycolysis.[13,p.219]

Eisinger et al. were the first to conjecture that fibromyalgia patients suffer from a crisis in energy metabolism. The specific impaired pathway they proposed was glycolysis. They urged clinicians to treat fibromyalgia patients with metabolic therapy rather than analgesics.[91]

Along with other regulatory factors, thyroid hormone regulates the rate of glycolytic activity. The hormone does so partly by regulating the availability of and activity of various enzymes. It also regulates the release of glucose from glycogen (glycogenolysis) by regulating transcription of the adrenergic genes, indirectly providing a normal ratio of α- and β-adrenergic receptors on cell membranes. A normal density of β-adrenergic receptors and their binding to epinephrine and norepinephrine on muscle cell membranes is necessary for the conversion of glycogen to glucose. Catecholamine binding to β-adrenergic receptors is therefore essential for mobilizing glycogen so that energy can be derived from its glucose molecules. β-Adrenergic receptors also increase fuel metabolism from the breakdown of fat.[41,p.763]

When transcription regulation of the genes by thyroid hormone is inadequate, the result is an increased density of α-adrenergic receptors and a decreased density of β-adrenergic receptors on cell membranes (see Chapter 3.1, the section titled "High Ratio of α- to β-Adrenergic Receptors on Cell Membranes"). This change in the density of the two types of adrenergic receptors on cell membranes results in subnormal glycogenolysis and slowed energy metabolism. (See subsection above titled "Activation of Intracellular Energy Metabolism.")

What is more, during exercise, the sudden binding of catecholamines to the high density of α-adrenergic receptors on cell membranes blunts energy production. (See Chapter 2.2, subsection titled "Glycogenolysis.") Abruptly, cAMP formation decreases inside the cell. The decrease is followed by slowing of a cascade of chemical reactions that result in reduced release of glucose from glycogen molecules. The decrease can account for the increased glycogen deposits found in the muscles of both hypothyroiod[36][37] and fibromyalgic[99][100][101] patients. In turn, ATP production decreases and energy metabolism slows. When this α-adrenergic receptor-mediated slowing occurs upon catecholamine release during exercise, when the energy demands of muscle are heightened, the result is a crisis of energy metabolism.

In liver and adipose, thyroid hormone deficiency decreases the activity of enzymes of the glycolytic and pentose phosphate pathways. These effects are part of the diminished responsiveness of tissues in hypothyroidism to the rapidly-acting hormones epinephrine, glucagon, and insulin (despite normal circulating levels of insulin). (See Chapter 2.2, subsection titled "Citric Acid Cycle.") During 11 days in a culture absent of thyroid hormone, the glucose depletion rate in neonatal rat heart cells decreased by 32%. The decrease indicates reduced glycolytic activity. (See Chapter 2.2, subsection titled "Glycolysis.") Such findings as these show that too little regulation by thyroid hormone limits glycolysis and the capacity for anaerobic metabolism.

Eisinger et al. reported glycolysis abnormalities in 40% of fibromyalgia patients.[46] One abnormality reported by Eisinger et al. is an increase in the blood pyruvate levels and an increased pyruvate-to-lactate ratio in fibromyalgia patients during the forearm ischemic exercise test.[102] Nørregaard et al. also found low lactate production in fibromyalgia patients. They had 15 female fibromyalgia patients and 15 age- and sex-matched controls perform a stepwise incremental maximal bicycle ergometer test. The patients' maximal lactate concentration during the test was 4.2 mmol l-1 (3.5-5.6). The control subjects' concentration was 4.9 mmol l-1 (3.9-5.9). Thus, the patients' lactate production was lower.[153] According to Eisinger, the increased pyruvate-to-lactate ratio in fibromyalgia patients, like several other abnormalities, is similar in fibromyalgia and hypothyroid patients.[97][172] Indeed, other researchers have reported similar abnormalities in hypothyroidism.[93][94] The reduced oxygen supply should have increased lactate production, but pyruvate-to-lactate conversion did not appear to increase. It occurred at the normal rather than the expected increased rate during the test. The cause for this altered ratio may have been low lactate dehydrogenase levels (see Chapter 2.2, subsection titled "Lactate Formed from Pyruvate in Contracting Muscle: Converted into Glucose by the Liver"). Eisinger et al. reported that in fibromyalgia patients, the muscle isoenzyme lactate dehydrogenase was 23% lower than in control subjects. The investigators reported that the level of the isoenzyme was also lower in hypothyroid patients.[91][102]

The subnormal availability of energy in the muscles of some fibromyalgia patients probably contributes to the patients' fatigue. The fatigue is likely to render them disinclined to exercise and contributes to exercise intolerance. According to Sahlin et al., energy supply limits performance during high-intensity exercise. The muscle glycogen content before exercise begins largely determines performance during moderate intensity exercise.[19] Impaired glycolysis due to inadequate thyroid hormone regulation of muscle cell function probably provides an effect similar to a glycogen deficiency, limiting exercise performance.

Inadequate thyroid hormone regulation of oxidative enzymes in mitochondria also may limit the patient's capacity for aerobic metabolism (see section above titled "Subnormal Capacity for Exercise-Induced Increased Oxidative Metabolism").

Low ATP and Creatine Phosphate Levels in Fibromyalgia. Impaired glycolysis in fibromyalgia patients limits their anaerobic metabolism, and subnormal activity of oxidative enzymes limits their aerobic metabolism. The expected net effect is deficient ATP production and subnormal energy metabolism. Studies have shown reduced high-energy phosphate levels (ATP and creatine phosphate) in the muscles of fibromyalgia patients[95][96][158] (see section above titled "Deficient Delivery of Oxygen to Muscle During Exercise") and low ATP levels in their red blood cells.[91][171] Eisinger wrote that these findings in fibromyalgia patients are similar to those in hypothyroid patients.[91][92] Subnormal ATP and creatine phosphate levels in fibromyalgia patients undoubtedly contribute to their low fitness levels and exercise intolerance.

The potential impact of reduced ATP levels on the ability to exercise in fibromyalgia may be appreciated by considering Hocachka's report of the normally-maintained homeostasis of ATP concentrations in muscle cells. He wrote that normally, skeletal and cardiac muscle undergo substantial changes in ATP turnover during large changes in muscle work. In skeletal muscles, the changes can exceed 100-fold. Within muscle, ATP concentration is almost universally "homeostatic." ATP is the most precisely regulated intermediate of cellular metabolism. Even with large rates of turnover of ATP, no change in ATP concentrations can usually be detected. This is true even when the turnover of ATP increases or decreases by two or more orders of magnitude. The only other intermediate in aerobic energy metabolism that is homeostatically controlled, at least during muscle work, is oxygen. To illustrate, over large changes in work, a 1-to-1 relationship is found between oxygen delivery and metabolic rate.[159]

Low Stress-Induced Increase in Creatine Kinase Levels. Nørregaard et al. reported that plasma creatine kinase levels were similar between fibromyalgia patients and controls after they all performed a stepwise incremental maximal bicycle ergometer test.[153] However, van Dederen et al. reported that after exhaustive physical exercise, circulating creatine kinase did not rise as much in fibromyalgia patients as in control subjects.[5] A subnormal rise in creatine kinase levels following exhaustive exercise suggests that the fibromyalgia patients had a muscle cell deficit of phosphocreatine. The phosphocreatine molecule has a high-energy phosphate bond. This compound is normally 3-to-8 times more abundant than ATP in cells.

Creatine kinase is an enzyme that catalyzes the transfer of phosphate from phosphocreatine to ADP, forming creatine and ATP. The creatine kinase is important for muscle contraction. When ATP is abundant, much of its energy is transferred and stored as phosphocreatine. Then, when ATP levels fall with muscle contractions during exercise (which takes only a second or two), energy is rapidly transferred back from phosphocreatine to ATP molecules. Recovery of the energy as ATP is critical because phosphocreatine cannot serve the vital function ATP does. ATP is a coupling agent that stores energy from foods and transfers it to the mechanisms of cells, such as muscle contractile filaments, that require energy to function. Creatine kinase is essential for reconstituting ATP from phosphocreatine.[20,p.790]

Physiologists have widely used plasma creatine kinase activity as a marker for muscle damage during exercise.[3] In normal individuals, elevated circulating levels of creatine kinase accompanies post-exercise soreness.[4] Creatine kinase is usually elevated for a few days after exercise.[16] Patients with exercise-induced enzymatic myopathies such as McArdle's disease usually have increased creatine kinase levels.[110]

Clinical Effects of an Exercise-Induced Metabolic Crisis. Energy deprivation may cause symptoms in several ways. First, energy deprivation within muscle cells may cause energy-deficiency contractures, with severe shortening of the contractile filaments. The contractures may activate trigger points, causing the referral of pain or other types of paresthesia. (See Chapter 3.16, section titled "Trigger Points as a Source of Paresthesia.")

In addition, a high density of α-adrenergic receptors on arterioles is likely to induce vasoconstriction and severely decrease blood flow. Goldstein reported reduced regional cerebral blood flow in fibromyalgia/chronic fatigue syndrome patients during the stresses of exercise and cognitive activation[166,p.67] In the brain, the decreased blood flow may be severe, as revealed by SPECT scans. An acute, severely reduced brain blood flow may cause extreme cognitive dysfunction and fatigue for several days to a week or more. (See Chapter 3.2, section titled "Decreased Brain Blood Flow in Fibromyalgia," and the section titled "Reduced Cerebral Blood Flow.")

In peripheral tissues, the reduced blood flow may reach an ischemic level, sensitizing and exciting myofascial nociceptors, and inducing ischemic type pain.[161,p.103][165] (See the section above titled "Subnormal Circulation," and the section titled "Deficient Delivery of Oxygen to Muscle During Exercise.")

Ventilatory (Respiratory) Drive in Hypothyroidism

Ventilatory or respiratory drive describes the net output of the respiratory centers in response to physiological stimuli.[24,p.995] Ventilatory drive largely dictates ventilatory activity (respiration).

Low ventilatory drive accounts for the old reports that patients in myxedema coma retained CO_2.[25] Researchers have found low ventilatory drive in hypothyroid patients during two types of tests: (1) those that increase the blood carbon dioxide level (hypercapnia), and (2) those that maintain normal carbon dioxide but reduce oxygen levels (isocapneic hypoxia).[24,p.995] Ladenson et al. reported that 34% of 38 hypothyroid patients had low ventilatory drive. The incidence was highest among hypothyroid women who had the highest TSH levels.[28] Hypothyroid patients' diminished respiratory responses improved after they began using thyroid hormone.[26][27] In one study, ventilatory drive became normal within a week after patients began thyroid hormone therapy.[28]

Some degree of exercise intolerance in fibromyalgia patients with hypothyroidism and/or thyroid hormone resistance may be due to low ventilatory drive. Weiss et al. described 2 patients with chronic, severe, episodic dyspnea. (Dyspnea is subjective difficulty or distress in breathing. It is also described as shortness of breath. Dyspnea may occur in heart and/or lung diseases, but it also normally occurs with extremely strenuous physical activity.) The patients had undergone prolonged, extensive, and invasive evaluations without a resulting diagnosis. Eventually, both patients received a diagnosis of fibromyalgia. Weiss et al. wrote that clinicians rarely include fibromyalgia in the differential diagnosis of dyspnea.[150] The subnormal chest expansion in fibromyalgia that Ozgocmen reported[151] may explain the dyspnea of the patients that Weiss et al. described. Their dyspnea may have resulted from subnormal ventilatory drive associated with hypothyroidism or thyroid hormone resistance.

A low level of oxygen in the arteries normally increases respiration.[13,p.161] Hornbein et al. wrote that sudden mild hypoxia increases respiration.[152] If fibromyalgia patients have subnormal ventilatory drive,

their respiration may not increase sufficiently during exercise to meet the heightened demand of their muscles for oxygen. The main resulting symptom would be dyspnea. The result of dyspnea may be a diminished oxygen supply to muscle cells during exercise. According to Richardson, exercise during hypoxia reduces VO_2 max, and the oxygen supply to muscle cells limits their maximal respiratory rate.[157] Thus, decreased ventilatory drive may contribute to fibromyalgia patients' exercise intolerance by contributing to their low aerobic metabolic capacity.

Possibly Subnormal Anaerobic Metabolism Related to Low Myoglobin in Fibromyalgia Patients

During the O_2 deficit at the beginning of exercise, several energy sources independent of the transport and delivery of O_2 by the cardiorespiratory system make body function possible. One of these sources is O_2 bound to muscle myoglobin.[13,p.219] According to Richardson, the oxygen pressure of myoglobin is an indicator of oxygen transport and cellular respiration rate.[157] Hochachka wrote that in working muscles, myoglobin buffers oxygen concentrations at stable and constant values at work rates up to the aerobic maximum.[159]

Myoglobin is an iron-containing protein similar to hemoglobin in red blood cells. It is particularly abundant in slow (red) muscle fibers. It binds oxygen and stores it in muscle until intracellular oxidative processes require it. It rapidly transports the oxygen to the mitochondria where oxidative metabolism occurs. The reddish color of slow muscle is due to its high myoglobin content. The whitish color of fast (white) muscle is due to its low myoglobin content.[20,p.75]

Myoglobin has a fairly high molecular weight and the pores of muscle capillaries are minimally permeable to the protein. The permeability of capillaries to myoglobin is only 0.03 that of water.[20,p.172] Urinary myoglobin levels can increase due to ischemic constrictions of muscle, crush injuries, or deep thermal or electrical burns of muscle. When urinary myoglobin levels are extremely high due to severe muscle damage, kidney tubular necrosis may occur if treatment is not prompt and accurate.[149,p.1505] Increased circulating levels of myoglobin in hypothyroidism are not of this magnitude.

The oxygen content of blood appears to be the stimulus to increased myoglobin levels. Terrados et al. found that myoglobin content decreased when legs were trained under a barometric pressure equivalent to that of sea level (normobaroic) conditions. Myoglobin levels increased in legs trained under a barometric pressure below that of sea level (hypobaric) conditions. They concluded that myoglobin increases with decreased oxygen blood content.[57] In another study, Terrados et al. studied the effect of physical training on muscle metabolism at a moderate altitude where oxygen pressure is lower. They found that training at a moderate altitude increase subjects' mean myoglobin level. They concluded that hypoxia is a stimulus that increases myoglobin levels.[98]

Myoglobin is synthesized in muscle cells rather than in hemopoietic tissues such as bone marrow. The intracellular localization of myoglobin mRNA in the skeletal muscles of normal subjects was mainly on the A-bands of the myofibrils where ribosomes predominantly reside. However, the mRNA was also located at the cytoskeletal filaments in the intermyofibrillar space, intermyofibrillar spaces, perinuclear space, and the I-bands. The A-band may be related to the regulation of myoglobin synthesis in skeletal muscle cells. Apparently, myoglobin synthesis is not related to erythropoietin which decreases the erythrocyte count in hypothyroidism.[58]

Myoglobin Levels in Hypothyroidism. Roti et al. found that hypothyroid patients had elevated mean muscle myoglobin levels and hyperthyroid patients had decreased levels. Levels were inversely related to T_3 and T_4 levels.[54] Kasai[55] and Karlsson et al.[53] reported the same findings. Drouet reported a mean elevated myoglobin level in hypothyroid patients with distinct hypothyroid myopathy,[56] suggesting myoglobin leak from damaged muscle cell membranes.

Whether hypothyroid patients have elevated myoglobin levels, and how high the myoglobin levels become, are related to the severity of hypothyroidism.[53] Consistent with this view was the finding of Staub et al. that serum myoglobin levels did not become elevated in hypothyroid patients until their TSH levels exceeded 12 µU/mL. This was also the TSH level at which patients' Achilles reflex time became significantly slow.[51]

Martino et al. found that in patients with short-term hypothyroidism, myoglobin levels were higher than in controls, but not as high as in patients with long-term hypothyroidism. In long-term hypothyroidism, myoglobin levels inversely correlated with serum thyroid hormone levels, but this was not true in short-term hypothyroidism. The investigators concluded that the duration and severity of hypothyroidism are impor-

tant in determining whether the serum myoglobin level rises.[52]

Karlsson et al. found that when hypothyroid patients' thyroid hormone levels returned to normal, the elevated myoglobin levels decreased to normal.[53] Martino et al. reported that with T_4 therapy, serum myoglobin levels became normal faster than did the serum TSH. Also, less T_4 was needed to normalize myoglobin levels than to normalize TSH secretion.[52]

Myoglobin in Fibromyalgia Patients. Van Dederen et al. found that during exercises, 10 fibromyalgia patients had a lower increase in myoglobin than did 10 healthy control subjects. If this is consistent with lower levels of muscle myoglobin, the lower levels would decrease oxygen transport to mitochondria. The decrease would contribute to the putative energy crisis during anaerobic metabolism.[5]

However, myoglobin may be normal in most fibromyalgia patients. Bengtsson et al. found that 55 fibromyalgia patients had normal myoglobin levels.[154] Nørregaard et al. had 15 female fibromyalgia patients and 15 age- and sex-matched controls perform a stepwise incremental maximal bicycle ergometer test. The patients' myoglobin concentrations were normal.[153]

Danneskiold-Samsøe et al. found that plasma myoglobin concentrations were increased after massage in women with regional muscle pain and tension. The increase peaked 3 hours after the massage. When therapists massaged muscles that were not tense and painful, myoglobin levels did not increase.[156] In another study of 26 women with myofascial pain, Danneskiold-Samsøe et al. found that myoglobin increased after massage. A positive correlation was found between the increase in the myoglobin level and the degree of muscle pain and tension. The authors wrote, "The observed increase in myoglobin in plasma after massage indicates a leak of myoglobin from the muscle fibres in 21 patients, whose myofascial pain seemed to be linked with a muscle fibre disease."[155] In fibromyalgia patients, increased plasma myoglobin levels after massage or other soft tissue manipulation might result from increased friability of muscle cell membranes due to subnormal cortisol secretion. Cortisol is a membrane stabilizer. When cell exposure to cortisol is subnormal, cell membranes may be more easily disrupted. Cell membrane disruption would enable intracellular substances such as myoglobin to escape into the blood, increasing circulating levels. (See Chapter 5.1, section titled "Soft Tissue Manipulation.")

Patients Most Prone to Develop Fibromyalgia Appear to be Those with Marginally Adequate Metabolism of Fibromyalgia-Related Tissues: A Predisposing Factor for Fibromyalgia

Greenfield reported that trauma, surgery, or illness appeared to precipitate fibromyalgia in 23% of his fibromyalgia group. He surmised that some of his patients developed fibromyalgia because of reduced physical activity following the surgery, trauma, or illness. He arrived at this tentative explanation from the reports by 45% of his reactive fibromyalgia patients that trauma or surgery reduced their physical activity, and that the reduced activity preceded the onset of fibromyalgia. The reduced activity levels persisted after the patients recovered from the precipitating event. Only 10% of his reactive fibromyalgia patients resumed normal activity levels. The question that must be addressed, however, is why all individuals who become sedentary following trauma do not develop fibromyalgia. Obviously, some other factor is at play. It is reasonable to consider that patients who develop fibromyalgia from the metabolism-slowing influence of inactivity are predisposed by previously marginally adequate metabolism of the tissues that give rise to fibromyalgia symptoms and signs.

Bunt wrote that physical training appeared to increase the sensitivity of cells to thyroid hormone.[14,p.337] An apparent decrease in the sensitivity of cells to thyroid hormone occurs without physical training and with a decline in physical fitness levels. Thus, the inability of fibromyalgia patients to engage in physical activity may amplify features of fibromyalgia underlain by too little thyroid hormone regulation.

INCREASED EXERCISE TOLERANCE DUE TO A THYROID HORMONE-INDUCED β-ADRENERGIC DOMINANCE

Many fibromyalgia patients do not exercise because it worsens their symptoms after they do so. At the beginning of metabolic rehabilitation, we advise these patients to exercise well below tolerance until their status improves. Most patients find that after beginning the use of thyroid hormone as a part of their rehabilitation regimen, they cease to feel a strong disinclination to exercise. Some report feeling a strong inclination to do so. Upon exercising, they may experience such common effects as post-exercise soreness. However, they remark that this soreness is different from the exacerbation of their fibromyalgia symptoms that they experienced before beginning metabolic therapy.

Presumably, the substantial increase in physical activity level and improved tolerance of exercise by some patients I have carefully monitored[43] were due mainly to a decrease of α-adrenergic receptors and an increase of β-adrenergic receptors on cell membranes.[44] This possibility is supported by two findings: 1) increased $α_2$-adrenoceptors on the platelets of fibromyalgia patients,[45] and 2) increased exercise tolerance and improvement in muscle pain of 7 of 10 patients taking the β-adrenergic agonist salbutamol (8- to 12 mg per day).[46] These improvements in fibromyalgia status may have resulted from an increased metabolic rate enabled by the β-adrenergic agonist,[38] increased blood flow, and a higher capacity for anaerobic metabolism.

Exercise During the Use of Thyroid Hormone: A Requirement for Optimal Metabolic Improvement

Without exogenous thyroid hormone, many fibromyalgia patients have neither the motor drive nor the metabolic capacity to exercise. Thyroid hormone increases the patients' metabolic capacity to exercise. The hormone provides metabolic capacity, but the patient must exercise to capitalize on the increased capacity. Even when most fibromyalgia patients are taking sufficient amounts of thyroid hormone, exercise is indispensable to their improvement or recovery.

REFERENCES

1. Bennett, R.M., Clark, S.R., Goldberg, L., Nelson, D., Bonafede, R.P., Porter, J., and Specht, D.: Aerobic fitness in the fibrositis syndrome: a controlled study of respiratory gas exchange and ^{133}xenon clearance from exercising muscle. *Arthritis Rheumat.*, 32:454-460, 1989.
2. Klug, G.A., McAuley, E., and Clark, S.: Factors influencing the development and maintenance of aerobic fitness: lessons applicable to the fibrositis syndrome. *J. Rheumatol.*, 16(Suppl.19):30-39, 1989.
3. Kuipers, H.: Exercise-induced muscle damage. *Int. J. Sports Med.*, 15(3):132-135, 1994.
4. Miles, M.P. and Clarkson, P.M.: Exercise-induced muscle pain, soreness, and cramps. *J. Sports Med. Phys. Fitness,* 34(3):203-216, 1994.
5. van Denderen, J.C., Boersma, J.W., Zeinstra, P., Hollander, A.P., and van Neerbos, B.R.: Physiological effects of exhaustive physical exercise in primary fibromyalgia syndrome (PFS): is PFS a disorder of neuroendocrine reactivity? *Scand. J. Rheumat.*, 21:35-37, 1992.
6. Greenfield, S., Fitzcharles, M.-A., and Esdaile, J.M.: Reactive fibromyalgia syndrome. *Arth. Rheumat.*, 35:678-681, 1992.

7. Moldofsky, H. and Scarisbrick, P.: Induction of neurasthenic musculoskeletal pain syndrome by selective sleep stage deprivation. *Psychosom. Med.*, 38:35-44, 1976.

8. McCain, G.A., Bell, D.A., Mai, F.M., and Halliday, P.D.: A controlled study of the effects of a supervised cardiovascular fitness training program on the manifestations of primary fibromyalgia. *Arthritis Rheum.*, 31:1135-1141, 1988.

9. Jacobsen, S. and Danneskiold-Samsøe, B.: Interrelations between clinical parameters and muscle function in patients with primary fibromyalgia. *Clin. Exp. Rheumatol.*, 7: 493-498, 1989.

10. Jacobsen, S. and Danneskiold-Samsøe,, B.: Isometric and isokinetic muscle strength in patients with fibrositis syndrome. *Scand. J. Rheumatol.*, 16:61-65, 1987.

11. Jacobsen, S. and Danneskiold-Samsøe,, B.: Dynamic muscular endurance in primary fibromyalgia syndrome compared with chronic myofascial pain syndrome. *Arch. Phys. Med. Rehabil.*, 73(2):170-173, 1992.

12. Jacobsen, S., Jensen, K.E., Thomsen, C., Danneskiold-Samsøe, B., and Henriksen, O.: 31P magnetic resonance spectroscopy of skeletal muscle in patients with fibromyalgia. *J. Rheumatol.*, 19:160-163, 1992.

13. deVries, H.A.: *Physiology of Exercise*, 4th edition. Dubuque, Wm. C. Brown, Publishers, 1986.

14. Bunt, J.C.: Hormonal alterations due to exercise. *Sports Med.*, 3:331-345, 1986.

15. Verstappen, F.T.J., van Santen-Hoeufft, H.M.S., van Sloun, S., Bolwijn, P.H., and van der Linden, S.: Fitness characteristics of female patients with fibromyalgia. *J. Musculoskel. Pain*, 3(3):45-58, 1995.

16. Pedersen, B.K., Ostrowski, K., Rohde, T., and Bruunsgaard, H.: The cytokine response to strenuous exercise. *Can. J. Physiol. Pharmacol.*, 76(5):505-511, 1998.

17. Mengshoel, A.M.: Effect of physical exercise in fibromyalgia. *Tidsskr Nor Laegeforen*, 116:746-748, 1996.

18. Bennett, R.M.: Beyond fibromyalgia: ideas on etiology and treatment. *J. Rheumatol.*, 16(Suppl.19):185-191, 1989.

19. Sahlin, K., Tonkonogi, M., and Soderlund, K.: Energy supply and muscle fatigue in humans. *Acta Physiol. Scand.*, 162(3):261-266, 1998.

20. Guyton, A.C.: *Textbook of Medical Physiology*, 8th edition. Philadelphia, W.B. Saunders Co., 1991.

21. Shepard, R.J.: The validity of the oxygen conductance equation. *Int. Z. Anew. Physiol.*, 28:61-75, 1969.

22. Martin, B.J. and Steger, J.M.: Ventilatory endurance in athletes and non-athletes. *Med. Sci. Sports Exer.*, 13:21-26, 1981.

23. Miller, A.T., Jr.: Influence of oxygen administration on cardiovascular function during exercise and recovery. *J. Appl. Physiol.*, 5:165-168, 1952.

24. Ingbar, D.H.: The respiratory system in hypothyroidism. In *Werner and Ingbar's The Thyroid: A Fundamental and Clinical Text*, 6th edition. Edited by L.E. Braverman and R.D. Utiger, Philadelphia, J.B. Lippincott Co., 1991, pp.993-1001.

25. Nordqvist, P., Dhuner, K.G., Stenberg, K., et al.: Myxedema coma and CO_2 retention. *Acta Med. Scand.*, 166: 189, 1960.

26. Weg, J.G., Calverly, J.R., and Johnson, C.: Hypothyroidism and alveolar hypoventilation. *Arch. Intern. Med.*, 115: 302, 1965.

27. Massumi, R.A. and Winnacker, J.L.: Severe depression of the respiratory center in myxedema. *Am. Rev. Respir. Dis.*, 127:504, 1983.

28. Ladenson, P.W., Goldenheim, P.D., and Ridgway, E.C.: Prediction and reversal of blunted ventilatory responsiveness in patients with hypothyroidism. *Am. J. Med.*, 84:877, 1988.

29. Burack, R., Edwards, R.H.T., Green, M., et al.: The response to exercise before and after treatment in myxedema with thyroxine. *J. Pharm. Exp. Ther.*, 176:212, 1971.

30. Calogero, A.E., Bernardini, R., Gold, P.W., and Chrousos, G.P.: Regulation of rat hypothalamic corticotropin-releasing hormone secretion *in vitro*: potential clinical implications. *Adv. Experi. Med. Biol.*, 245:167-181, 1988.

31. Bode-Boger, S.M., Boger, R.H., Schroder, E.P., and Frolich, J.C.: Exercise increases systemic nitric oxide production in men. *J. Cardiovas. Risk*, 1(2):173-178, 1994.

32. Skarphedinsson, J.O., Elam, M., Jungersten, L., and Wallin, B.G.: Sympathetic nerve traffic correlates with the release of nitric oxide in humans: implications for blood pressure control. *J. Physiol.*, 501(Pt.3):671-675, 1997.

33. Eisinger, J.: Metabolic abnormalities in fibromyalgia. *Clin. Bull. Myofascial Ther.*, 3(1):3-21, 1998.

34. Colin, I.M., Kopp, P., Zbaren, J., Haberli, A., Grizzle, W.E., and Jameson, J.L.: Expression of nitric oxide synthase III in human thyroid follicular cells: evidence for increased expression in hyperthyroidism. *Eur. J. Endocrinol.*, 136(6):649-655, 1997.

35. Park, K.W., Dai, H.B., Ojamaa, K., Lowenstein, E., Klein, I., and Selke, F.W.: The direct vasomotor effect of thyroid hormones on rat skeletal muscle resistance arteries. *Anesth. Analg.*, 85(4):734-738, 1997.

36. Ramsay, I.: *Thyroid Disease and Muscle Dysfunction*. Chicago, Year Book Medical Publishers, Inc., 1974, pp.147-151.

37. Rodolico, C., Toscano, A., Benvenga, S., et al.: Myopathy as the persistently isolated symptomatology of primary autoimmune hypothyroidism. *Thyroid*, 8(11):1033-1038, 1998.

38. Cawthorne, M.A., Sennitt, M.V., Arch, J.R., and Smith, S.A.: BRL 35135, a potent and selective atypical β-adrenoceptor agonist. *Am. J. Clin. Nutri.*, 55(1 Suppl.):252S-257S, 1992.

39. Poehlman, E.T., Toth, M.J., and Fonong, T.: Exercise, substrate utilization, and energy requirements in the elderly. *Intern. J. Obesity Related Metab. Disord.*, 19(Suppl.4): S93-S96, 1995.

40. Herring, J.L., Mole, P.A., Meredith, C.N., and Stern, J.S.: Effect of suspending exercise training on resting metabolic rate in women. *Med. Sci. Sport Exer.*, 24(1):59-65, 1992.

41. Lehninger, A.L. and Nelson, D.L.: *Principles of Biochemistry*, 2nd edition. New York, Worth Publishers, 1993.

42. Clark, S.R.: Fitness characteristics and perceived exertion in women with fibromyalgia. *J. Musculoskel. Pain*, 1:191-197, 1993.

43. Lowe, J.C.: T_3-induced recovery from fibromyalgia by a hypothyroid patient resistant to T_4 and desiccated thyroid. *J. Myofascial Ther.*, 1(4):26-31, 1995.

44. Lowe, J.C., Cullum, M.E., Graf, L.H., Jr., and Yellin, J.: Mutations in the c-erbAβ₁ gene: do they underlie euthyroid

fibromyalgia. *Med. Hypoth.*, 48(2):125-135, 1997.

45. Bennett, R.M., Clark, S.R., Campbell, S.M., et al.: Symptoms of Raynaud's syndrome in patients with fibromyalgia: a study utilizing the Nielsen test, digital photoplethysmography and measurements of platelet α_2-adrenergic receptors. *Arthritis Rheum.*, 34:264-269, 1991.

46. Eisinger, J., Dupond, J.L., and Cozzone, P.J.: Anomalies de la glycolyse au cours des fibromyalgies: étude biologique et thérapeutique. *Lyon Méditerranée Méd.*, 27:2180-2181, 1996.

47. Linder, M.C.: Nutrition and metabolism in carbohydrates. In *Nutritional Biochemistry and Metabolism with Clinical Applications*, 2nd edition. Edited by M.C. Linder, New York, Elsevier, 1991.

48. Guttler, R.B., Shaw, J.W., Otis, C.L., and Nicoloff, J.T.: Epinephrine-induced alterations in urinary cyclic AMP in hyper- and hypothyroidism. *J. Clin. Endocrinol. Metab.*, 41(4):707-711, 1975.

49. Lowe, J.C., Eichelberger, J., Manso, G., and Peterson, K.: Improvement in euthyroid fibromyalgia patients treated with T_3 (tri-iodothyronine). *J. Myofas. Ther.*, 1(2):16-29, 1994.

50. Elam, M., Johansson, G., and Wallin, B.G.: Do patients with primary fibromyalgia have an altered muscle sympathetic nerve activity? *Pain*, 48:371-375, 1992.

51. Staub, J.J., Althaus, B.U., Engler, H., et al.: Spectrum of subclinical and overt hypothyroidism: effect on thyrotropin, prolactin, and thyroid reserve, and metabolic impact on peripheral target tissues. *Amer. J. Med.*, 92(6):631-642, 1992.

52. Martino, E., Sardano, G., Vaudagna, G., et al.: Serum myoglobin in primary hypothyroidism and effect of L-thyroxine therapy. *J. Nuclear Med.*, 23(12):1088-1092, 1982.

53. Karlsson, F.A., Dahlberg, P.A., Venge, P., and Roxin, L.E.: Serum myoglobin in thyroid disease. *Acta Endocrinol.*, 94(2):184-187, 1980.

54. Roti, E., Bandini, P., Robuschi, G., et al.: Serum concentrations of myoglobin, creatine kinase, lactate dehydrogenase and cardiac isoenzymes in euthyroid, hypothyroid and hyperthyroid subjects. *Ricerca in Clinica e in Laboratorio*, 10(4):609-617, 1980.

55. Kasai, K.: Serum myoglobin level in altered thyroid states. *J. Clin. Endocrinol. Metab.*, 48(1):1-4, 1979.

56. Drouet, A. and Valance, J.: Hypothyroid hypertrophic myopathy in adults related to chronic lymphocytic thyroiditis: A case. *Rev. Med. Interne*, 14(9):864-868, 1993.

57. Terrados, N., Jansson, E., Sylven, C., and Kaijser, L.: Is hypoxia a stimulus for synthesis of oxidative enzymes and myoglobin?. *J. Appl. Physiol.*, 68(6):2369-2372, 1990.

58. Mitsui, T., Kawai, H., Naruo, T., and Saito, S.: Ultrastructural localization of myoglobin mRNA in human skeletal muscle. *Histochemistry*, 101(2):99-104, 1994.

59. Wigers, S.H., Stiles, T.C., and Vogel, P.A.: Effects of aerobic exercise versus stress management treatment in fibromyalgia. *Scand. J. Rheumatol.*, 25:77-86, 1996.

60. Russell, I.J., Vaeroy, M., Jabors, M., and Nyberg, F.: Cerebrospinal fluid biogenic metabolites in fibromyalgia/fibrositis syndrome in rheumatoid arthritis. *Arthritis Rheuma.*, 35:550-556, 1992.

61. Puymirat, J., Luo, M., and Dussault, J.H.: Immunocytochemical localization of thyroid hormone nuclear receptors in cultured hypothalamic dopaminergic neurons. *Neuroscience*, 30(2):443-449, 1989.

62. Levitt, M., Spector, S., Sjoerdsma, A., and Udenfriend, S.: *J. Pharmacol. Exp. Ther.*, 148:1-8, 1965.

63. Prange, A.J., Meek, J.L., and Lipton, M.A.: Catecholamines diminished rate of synthesis in rat brain and heart after thyroxine pretreatment. *Life Sci.*, 9:901-907, 1970.

64. Singhal, R.L., Rastogi, R.B., and Hedina, P.D.: Brain biogenic amines and altered thyroid function. *Life Sci.*, 17:1617-1626, 1975.

65. Jacoby, J.H., Mueller, G., and Wurtman, R.J.: Thyroid state and brain monoamine metabolism. *Endocrinology*, 97:1332-1335, 1975.

66. Rastogi, R.B. and Singhal, R.L.: Neonatal hyperthyroidism: alterations in behavioural activity and the metabolism of brain norepinephrine and dopamine. *Life Sci.*, 18(8):851-857, 1976.

67. Engstrom, G., Svensson, T.H., and Waldeck, B.: Thyroxine and brain catecholamines: increased transmitter synthesis and increased receptor sensitivity. *Brain Res.*, 77(3):471-483, 1974.

68. Ito, J.M., Valcana, T., and Timiras, P.S.: Effect of hypo- and hyperthyroidism on regional monoamine metabolism in the adult rat brain. *Neuroendocrinology*, 24:55-64, 1977.

69. Lipton, M.A., Prange, A.J., Dairman, W., and Udenfriend, S.: Increased rate of norepinephrine biosynthesis in hypothyroid rats. *Proc. Fed. Am. Soc. Exp. Biol.*, 27:399, 1968.

70. Diarra, A., Lefauconnier, J.M., Valens, M., Georges, P., and Gripois, D.: Tyrosine content, influx, and accumulation rate, and catecholamine biosynthesis measured *in vivo*, in the central nervous system and in peripheral organs of young rats: influence of neonatal hypo- and hyperthyroidism. *Arch. Intern. Physiologie Biochem.*, 97:317-332, 1989.

71. Bertler, A. and Rosengren, E.: *Experientia*, 15:10-11, 1959.

72. Feek, C.M., Sawers, J.S.A., Brown, N.S., Seth, J., Irvine, W.J., and Toft, A.D.: Influence of thyroid status on dopaminergic inhibition of thyrotropin and prolactin secretion: evidence for an additional feedback mechanism in the control of thyroid hormone secretion. *J. Clin. Endocrinol. Metab.*, 51(3):585-589, 1980.

73. Tuomisto, J. and Männisto, P.: Neurotransmitter regulation of anterior pituitary hormones. *Pharmacol. Rev.*, 37:249-332, 1985.

74. Ericksson, E. and Modigh, K.: Depression, α_2-receptors, and sex hormones: neuroendocrine studies in the rat. In *Frontiers in Biochemical and Pharmacological Research in Depression*. Edited by E. Usdin, M. Äsberg, L. Bertilsson, and F. Sjögvist, New York, Raven Press, 1984, pp.161-178.

75. Rastogi, R.B., Lapierre, Y., and Singhal, R.L.: Evidence for the role of brain biogenic amines in depressed motor activity seen in chemically thyroidectomized rats. *J. Neurochem.*, 26(3):443-449, 1976.

76. Heffner, T.G. and Seiden, L.S.: Synthesis of catecholamines from [3H]tyrosine in brain during the performance of operant behavior. *Brain Res.*, 183(2):403-419, 1980.

77. Plaznik, A. and Kostowski, W.: The interrelationship between brain noradrenergic and dopaminergic neuronal

systems in regulating animal behavior: possible clinical implications. *Psychopharmacol. Bull.*, 19(1):5-11, 1983.

78. Creese, I. and Iversen, S.D.: The pharmacological and anatomical substrates of the amphetamine response in the rat. *Brain Res.*, 83:419-436, 1975.

79. Jackson, D.M., Anden, N.-E., and Dahlstrom, A.: A functional effect of dopamine in the nucleus accumbens and in some other dopamine-rich parts of the rat brain. *Psychopharmacology*, 45:139-149, 1975.

80. Kelly, P.H., Seviour, P.W., and Iversen, S.D.: Amphetamine and apomorphine responses in the rat following 6-OHDA lesions of the nucleus accumbens septi and corpus striatum. *Brain Res.*, 94:507,1975.

81. Pijnenburg, A.J.J., Honig, W.M.M., and Van Rossum, J.M.: Effects of antagonists upon locomotor stimulation induced by injection of dopamine and noradrenaline into the nucleus accumbens of nialamide-pretreated rats. *Psychopharmacology*, 41:175-180, 1975.

82. Costall, B., Marsden, C.D., Maylor, R.J., and Pycock, C.J.: Stereotyped behavior patterns and hyperactivity induced by amphetamine and apomorphine after discrete 6-hydroxy-dopamine lesions of extrapyramidal and mesolimbic nuclei. *Brain Res.*, 123:89-111, 1977.

83. Makanjuola, R.O.A., Dow, R.C., and Ashcroft, G.W.: Behavioural responses to stereotactically controlled injections of monoamine neurotransmitters into the accumbens and caudate-putamen nuclei. *Psychopharmacology*, 71:227-235, 1980.

84. Clineschmidt, B.V., Flataker, L.M., Faison, E., and Holmes, R.: An *in vivo* model for investigating α_1- and α_2-receptors in the CNS: studies with mianserin. *Arch. Int. Pharmacodyn. Ther.*, 242(1):59-76, 1979.

85. Delini-Stula, A., Baumann, P., and Buch, O.: Depression of exploratory activity by clonidine in rats as a model for the detection of relative pre- and postsynaptic central noradrenergic receptor selectivity of α-adrenolytic drugs. *Naunyn Schmiedeberg's Arch. Pharmacol.*, 307:115-122, 1979.

86. Drew, G.M., Gower, A.J., and Marriott, A.S.: α_2-Adrenoceptors mediate clonidine-induced sedation in the rat. *Br. J. Pharmacol.*, 67(1):133-141, 1979.

87. Mueller, K. and Nyhan, W.I.: Modulation of the behavioral effects of amphetamine in rats by clonidine. *Eur. J. Pharmacol.*, 83:339-342, 1982.

88. Pifl, Ch.F. and Hornykiewicz, O.: α-Noradrenergic involvement in locomotor activity. *Naunyn Schmiedeberg's Arch. Pharmacol.*, 330(Suppl.):R71, 1985.

89. Dickinson, S.L., Gadie, B., and Tulloch, I.F.: α_1- and α_2-Adrenoreceptor antagonists differentially influence locomotor and stereotyped behavior induced by *d*-amphetamine and apomorphine in the rat. *Psychopharmacology*, 96:521-527, 1988.

90. Bruckle, W., Suckfull, M., Fleckenstein, W., Weiss, C., and Muller, W.: Tissue pO_2 measurement in taut back musculature. *Z. Rheumatol.*, 49(4):208-216, 1990.

91. Eisinger, J., Plantamura, A., and Ayavou, T.: Glycolysis abnormalities in fibromyalgia. *J. Am. Coll. Nutr.*, 13:144-148, 1994.

92. Mathur, A.K., Gatter, R.A., and Bank, W.J.: Abnormal P NMR spectroscopy of painful muscles of patients with fibromyalgia. *Arthritis Rheum.*, 31:523, 1988.

93. Kaminsky, P., Robin-Lherbier, B., and Brunotte, F.: Energetic metabolism in hypothyroidism skeletal muscles, as studied by phosphorus magnetic resonance spectroscopy. *J. Clin. Endocrinol. Metab.*, 74:124-129, 1992.

94. Schwark, W.S., Singhal, R.L., and Ling, G.H.: Glyceraldehyde phosphate dehydrogenase activity in developing brain during experimental cretinism. *Biochim. Biophys. Acta*, 273:308-317, 1972.

95. Yunus, M.B., Masi, A., and Calabro, J.: Primary fibromyalgia (fibrositis): clinical study of 50 patients with matched normal controls. *Semin. Arthritis Rheum.*, 11: 151-170, 1981.

96. Bengtsson, A., Henriksson, K.G., and Larsson, J.: Reduced high-energy phosphate levels in the painful muscles of patients with primary fibromyalgia. *Arthritis Rheum.*, 29:817-821, 1986.

97. Valen, P.A., Flory, W., Pauwel, M., et al.: Forearm ischemic testing and plasma ATP degradation products in primary fibromyalgia. *Arthritis Rheum.*, 31:115, 1988.

98. Terrados, N.: Altitude training and muscular metabolism. *Int. J. Sports Med.*, 13(Suppl.1):S206-S209, 1992.

99. Kalyan-Raman, U.P., Kalyan-Raman, K., Yunus, M.B. and Masi, A.T.: Muscle pathology in primary fibromyalgia syndrome: a light microscopic, histological and ultrastructural study. *J. Rheumatol.*, 11:808-813, 1984.

100. Awad, E.A.: Pathological changes in fibromyalgia. *First International Symposium on Myofascial Pain and Fibromyalgia*. Minneapolis, Minnesota, May 9, 1989.

101. Awad, E.A.: Histopathological changes in fibrositis. In *Advances in Pain Research and Therapy*, Vol.17. Edited by J.R. Fricton and E.A. Awad, New York, Raven Press, Ltd., 1990, pp.249-258.

102. Eisinger, J., Mechtouf, K., Plantamura, A., et al.: Anomalies biologiques au cours des fibromyalgies: I. lactacidemie et pyruvicemie. *Lyon Méditerranée Med.*, 28: 851-854, 1992.

103. Head, G.A. and Burke, S.: Importance of central noradrenergic and serotonergic pathways in the cardiovascular actions of rilmenidine and clonidine. *J. Cardiovasc. Pharmacol.*, 18(6):819-826, 1991.

104. Brown, D.A. and Caulfield, M.P.: Hyperpolarizing α_2-adrenoceptors in rat sympathetic ganglia. *Br. J. Pharmacol.*, 65:435-445, 1979.

105. Zwaveling, J., Pfafferdorf, M., and van Zwieten, P.A.: The direct effects of thyroid hormones on rat mesenteric resistance arteries. *Fundamen. Clin. Pharmacol.*, 11(1): 41-46, 1997.

106. Fassbender, H.G. and Wegner, K.: Morphologie und pathogenese des weichteilrheumatismus. *Z. Rheumaforschg.*, 32:355, 1973.

107. Lund, N., Bengtsson, A., and Thorborg, P.: Muscle tissue oxygen pressure in primary fibromyalgia. *Scand. J. Rheumatol.*, 15:165-173, 1986.

108. Klemp, P., Nielsen, H.V., Korsgard, J., and Crone, P.: Blood flow in fibromyotic muscles. *Scand. J. Rehab. Med.*, 14:81, 1982.

109. Sharma, V.K. and Banerjee, S.P.: β-Adrenergic receptors in rat skeletal muscle: effects of thyroidectomy. *Biochim. Biophys. Acta*, 539(4):538-542, 1978.

110. Dupond, J.L., de Wazieres, B., Monnier, G., Closs, F., and Desmurs, H.: Silent exercise-induced enzymatic my-

opathies at rest in adults: a cause of confusion with fibromyalgia. *Presse Med.*, 21(21):974-978, 1992.

111. Tepperman, J. and Tepperman, H.M.: *Metabolic and Endocrine Physiology*, 5th edition. Chicago, Year Book Medical Publishers, Inc., 1987.

112. Mengshoel, A.M., Komnates, H.B., and Förre, O.: The effects of 20 weeks of physical fitness training in female patients with fibromyalgia. *Clin. Exp. Rheumatol.*, 10: 345-349, 1992.

113. Bengtsson, A., Bäckman, E., Lindblom, B., and Skogh, T.: Long term follow-up of fibromyalgia patients: clinical symptoms, muscular function, laboratory tests: an eight year comparison study. *J. Musculoskel. Pain*, 2(2):67-80, 1994.

114. Bäckman, E., Bengtsson, A., Bengtsson, M., Lenmarken, C., and Henriksson, K.G.: Skeletal muscle function in primary fibromyalgia: effect of regional sympathetic blockade with guanethidine. *Acta Neurol. Scand.*, 77:187-191, 1988.

115. Elert, I.E., Rantapää-Dahlqvist, S.B., Henriksson-Larsen, K., and Gerdle, B.: Increased EMG-activity during short pauses in patients with fibromyalgia. *Scand. J. Rheumatol.*, 18:321-323, 1989.

116. Cooper, J.R., Bloom, F.E., and Roth, R.H.: *The Biochemical Basis of Neuropharmacology*, 6th edition. New York, Oxford University Press, 1991.

117. Galbo, H., Holst, J.J., and Christensen, N.J.: Glucagon and plasma catecholamine responses to graded and prolonged exercise in man. *J. Appl. Physiol.*, 38:70-76, 1975.

118. Haggendal, J., Hartley, L.H., and Saltin, B.: Arterial noradrenaline concentration during exercise in relation to the relative work levels. *Scand. J. Clin. Lab. Invest.*, 26:337-342, 1970.

119. von Euler, U.S.: Sympatho-adrenal activity in physical exercise. *Med. Sci. Sports*, 6:165-173, 1974.

120. Howley, E.T.: The effect of different intensities of exercise on the excretion of epinephrine and norepinephrine. *Med. Sci. Sports*, 8:219-222, 1976.

121. Bannister, E.W. and Griffiths, J.: Blood levels of adrenergic amines during exercise. *J. Appl. Physiol.*, 33:674-676, 1972.

122. Mechtouf, K., Collard, O., and Eisinger, J.: Depression and pain evolution in fibromyalgia. *Z. Rheumatol*, 56: 378, 1997.

123. Maimonides, M.: Mishneh Torah. In *The Book of Knowledge*. Edited by M. Hyamson, Boys Town Jerusalem Publishers, 1962.

124. Adler, G.K., Kinsley, B.T., Hurwitz, S., Mossey, C.J., and Goldenberg, D.L.: Reduced hypothalamic-pituitary and sympathoadrenal responses to hypoglycemia in women with fibromyalgia syndrome. *Amer. J. Med.*, 106(5):534-543, 1999.

125. Hamaty, D., Valentine, J.L., Howard, R., Howard, C.W., Wakefield, V., and Patten, M.S.: The plasma endorphin, prostaglandin and catecholamine profile of patients with fibrositis treated with cyclobenzaprine and placebo: a 5-month study. *J. Rheumatol.*, 19(Suppl.):164-168, 1989.

126. Yunus, M.B., Dailey, J.W., Aldag, J.C., Masi, A.T., and Jobe, P.C.: Plasma and urinary catecholamines in primary fibromyalgia: a controlled study. *J. Rheumatol.*, 19(1): 95-97, 1992.

127. Vaeroy, H., Qiao, Z.G., Morkrid, L., and Forre, O.: Altered sympathetic nervous system response in patients with fibromyalgia (fibrositis syndrome). *J. Rheumatol.*, 16(11):1460-1465, 1989.

128. Simms, R.W., Roy, S.H., Hrovat, M., et al.: Lack of association between fibromyalgia syndrome and abnormalities in muscle energy metabolism. *Arthritis Rheum.*, 37(6): 794-800, 1994.

129. Sietsema, K.E., Cooper, D.M., Caro, X., Leibling, M.R., and Louie, J.S.: Oxygen uptake during exercise in patients with primary fibromyalgia syndrome. *J. Rheumatol.*, 20(5):860-865, 1993.

130. Frodin, T., Bengtsson, A., and Skogh, M.: Nail fold capillaroscopy findings in patients with primary fibromyalgia. *Clin. Rheumatol.*, 7(3):384-388, 1988.

131. Qiao, Z.G., Vaeroy, H., and Morkrid, L.: Electrodermal and microcirculatory activity in patients with fibromyalgia during baseline, acoustic stimulation and cold pressor tests. *J Rheumatol.*, 18(9):1383-1389, 1991.

132. Lapossy, E., Gasser, P., Hrycaj, P., Dubler, B., Samborski, W., and Muller, W.: Cold-induced vasospasm in patients with fibromyalgia and chronic low back pain in comparison to healthy subjects. *Clin. Rheumatol.*, 13(3): 442-445, 1994.

133. Simms, R.W.: Is there muscle pathology in fibromyalgia syndrome? *Rheum. Dis. Clin. North Amer.*, 22(2):245-266, 1996.

134. Bjelle, A., Bengtsson, A., Henriksson, K.G., Idstrom, J.P., Torebjork, E., and Thornell, L.E.: Fibromyalgia—a new name for a syndrome with diffuse muscular disorders. *Lakartidningen*, 86(7):528-530, 1989.

135. Caro, X.J.: New concepts in primary fibrositis syndrome. *Compr. Ther.*, 15(5):14-22, 1989.

136. Henriksson, K.G.: Muscle pain in neuromuscular disorders and primary fibromyalgia. *Neurologija*, 38(3):213-221, 1989.

137. Bengtsson, A. and Henriksson, K.G.: The muscle in fibromyalgia: a review of Swedish studies. *J. Rheumatol.*, 19 (Suppl.):144-149, 1989.

138. Henriksson, K.G.: Muscle pain in neuromuscular disorders and primary fibromyalgia. *Eur. J. Appl. Physiol.*, 57 (3):348-352, 1988.

139. Natvig, B., Bruusgaard. D., and Eriksen, W.: Physical leisure activity level and physical fitness among women with fibromyalgia. *Scand. J. Rheumatol.*, 27(5):337-341, 1998.

140. Bennett, R.M.: Fibromyalgia review. *J. Musculoskel. Pain*, 7(3):83-101, 1999.

141. Klennerman, L., Slade, P.D., Stanley, I.M., et al.: The prediction of chronicity in patients with an acute attack of low back pain in a general practice setting. *Spine*, 20:478-484, 1995.

142. Hasenbring, M., Marienfeld, G., Kuhlendahi, D., and Soyka, D.: Risk factors of chronicity in lumbar disc patients. *Spine*, 19:2759-2765, 1994.

143. Potter, R.G. and Jones, M.J.: The evolution of chronic pain among patients with musculoskeletal problems: a pilot study in primary care. *Brit. J. Gen. Prac.*, 42:462-464, 1992.

144. Growley, D. and Kendall, N.A.S.: Development and initial validation of a questionnaire for measuring fear-avoidance associated with pain: the fear-avoidance of

pain scale. *J. Musculoskel. Pain,* 7(3):3-19, 1999.

145. Johnson, H.: *Osler's Web.* New York, Penguin Books, 1996.

146. deVries, H.A.: *Physiology of Exercise,* 4th edition. Dubuque, Wm. C. Brown Publishers, 1986.

147. Katona, P.G., McLean, M., Dighton, D.H., and Guz, A.: Sympathetic and parasympathetic cardiac control in athletes and non-athletes at rest. *J. Appl. Physiol.,* 52:1652-1657, 1982.

148. Frick, M.H., Elovainio, R.O., and Somer, T.: The mechanism of bradycardia evoked by physical training. *Cardiologia,* 51:46-54, 1967.

149. *The Merck Manual of Diagnosis and Therapy,* 16th edition. Edited by R. Berkow, A.J. Fletcher, and M.H. Beers, Rahway, Merck Research Laboratories, 1992.

150. Weiss, D.J., Kreck, T., and Albert, R.K.: Dyspnea resulting from fibromyalgia. *Chest,* 113(1):246-249, 1998.

151. Ozgocmen, S.: Reduced chest expansion in primary fibromyalgia syndrome. *Yonsei Med. J.,* 40(1):90-91, 1999.

152. Horbein, T.F., Roos, A., and Griffo, Z.J.: Transient effect of sudden mild hypoxia on respiration. *J. Appl. Physiol.,* 16:11-14, 1961.

153. Nørregaard, J., Bulow, P.M., Mehlsen, J., and Danneskiold-Samsøe,, B.: Biochemical changes in relation to a maximal exercise test in patients with fibromyalgia. *Clin. Physiol.,* 14(2):159-167, 1994.

154. Bengtsson, A., Henriksson, K.G., Jorfeldt, L., Kagedal, B., Lennmarken, C., and Lindstrom, F.: Primary fibromyalgia: a clinical and laboratory study of 55 patients. *Scand. J. Rheumatol.,* 15(3):340-347, 1986.

155. Danneskiold-Samsøe, B., Christiansen, E., and Bach Andersen, R.: Myofascial pain and the role of myoglobin. *Scand. J. Rheumatol.,* 15(2):174-178, 1986.

156. Danneskiold-Samsøe,, B., Christiansen, E., Lund, B., and Andersen, R.B.: Regional muscle tension and pain ("fibrositis"): effect of massage on myoglobin in plasma. *Scand. J. Rehabil. Med.,* 15(1):17-20, 1983.

157. Richardson, R.S.: Oxygen transport: air to muscle cell. *Med. Sci. Sports Exerc.,* 30(1):53-59, 1998.

158. Park, J.H., Phothimat, P., Oates, C.O., Hernanz-Schulman, M., and Olsen, N.J.: Use of P-31 magnetic resonance spectroscopy to detect metabolic abnormalities in muscles of patients with fibromyalgia. *Arthritis Rheum.,* 41(3):406-413, 1998.

159. Hochachka, P.W.: Two research paths for probing the roles of oxygen in metabolic regulation. *Braz. J. Med. Biol. Res.,* 32(6):661-672, 1999.

160. Berne, R.M. and Levy, M.N.: *Principles of Physiology.* St. Louis, C.V. Mosby Company, 1990.

161. Henrikson, K.G.: Muscle activity and chronic muscle pain. *J. Musculoskel. Pain,* 7(1/2):101-109, 1999.

162. Visuri,T., Lindholm, H., Lindqvist, A., Dahlström, S., and Viljanen, A.: Cardiovascular functional disorder in primary fibromyalgia: a noninvasive study in 17 young men. *Arthritis Care Res.,* 5(4):210-215, 1992.

163. Bennett, R.M.: Exercise and exercise testing in fibromyalgia patients: lessons learned and suggestions for future studies. *J. Musculoskel. Pain,* 2(3):143-152, 1994.

164. Hamilton, T.C.: Involvement of the adrenal glands in the hypotensive response to bromocriptine in spontaneously hypertensive rats. *Br. J. Pharmacol.,* 72(3):419-425, 1981.

165. Mense, S.: Nociception from skeletal muscle in relation to clinical muscle pain: review article. *Pain,* 54:241-289, 1993.

166. Goldstein, J.A.: *Betrayal by the Brain.* New York, Haworth Medical Press, 1996.

166. Koganei, H., Kimura, T., and Satoh, S.: Effects of β- adrenoceptor agonists and antagonists on adrenal catecholamine release in response to splanchnic nerve stimulation in anesthetized dogs: role of β_1- and β_2-adrenoceptors. *J. Pharmacol. Exp. Ther.,* 273(3):1337-1344, 1995.

167. Foucart, S., de Champlain, J., and Nadeau, R.: Modulation by β-adrenoceptors and angiotensin II receptors of splanchnic nerve evoked catecholamine release from the adrenal medulla. *Can. J. Physiol. Pharmacol.,* 69(1):1-7, 1991.

168. Nedergaard, O.A. and Abrahamsen, J.: Modulation of noradrenaline release by activation of presynaptic β-adrenoceptors in the cardiovascular system. *Ann. N.Y. Acad. Sci.,* 604:528-544, 1990.

169. Scheurink, A.J., Steffens, A.B., Bouritius, H., Dreteler, G.H., Bruntink, R., Remie, R., and Zaagsma, J.: Adrenal and sympathetic catecholamines in exercising rats. *Amer. J. Physiol.,* 256(1 Pt.2):R155-R160, 1989.

170. Foucart, S., Nadeau, R., and de Champlain, J.: Local modulation of adrenal catecholamine release by β_2-adrenoceptors in the anaesthetized dog. *Naunyn Schmiedeberg's Arch. Pharmacol.,* 337(1):29-34, 1988.

171. Eisinger, J., Clairet, D., Zakarian, H., and Ayavou, T.: ATP érythrocytaire et apparel locomoteur: action de la calcitonine. *Lyon Méditerranée Med.,* 26:326-328, 1990.

172. Eisinger, J.: Personal written communication. April 17, 1996.

7

3.5

Hypothalamic-Pituitary-Adrenal Axis

Hypothalamic-Pituitary-Adrenal (HPA) Axis Physiology

The HPA axis is one of the two major stress adaptation systems. The axis is highly sensitive. Activation of the axis is part of the overall physiological arousal often set off by mild stimuli.

The apparent relation of fibromyalgia status to episodes of stress warrants study of the abnormalities of the axis in fibromyalgia. Stress may immediately precede the onset of fibromyalgia. In addition, fibromyalgia status often worsens during times of stress, and many patients report that they often perceive high levels of stress.

In response to stressful physical, physiological, chemical, mechanical, or psychological stimuli, hypothalamic cells secrete corticotropin releasing hormone (CRH) and arginine-vasopressin (AVP), the two hormones that most powerfully regulate adrenocorticotropin hormone (ACTH) secretion. CRH and AVP stimulate pituitary corticotroph cells to secrete ACTH. In turn, ACTH stimulates cells of the adrenal cortices to secrete glucocorticoids, especially cortisol.

Increased cortisol levels in response to ACTH feed back to hypothalamic and anterior pituitary cells, decreasing secretion of CRH and ACTH. A decreased cortisol level disinhibits hypothalamic and pituitary cells, consequently increasing secretion of CRH and ACTH. When functioning normally, this feedback circuit increases or decreases activity of the axis to meet the needs of the individual for adapting to the stresses of life.

HPA Abnormalities in Fibromyalgia

Several abnormalities of the HPA axis occur in a subset of fibromyalgia patients. The abnormalities include possible (although undocumented) deficient CRH secretion; a trend toward increased AVP secretion; an exaggerated ACTH response to injected CRH and insulin-induced hypoglycemia; a blunted cortisol response to ACTH; a subnormal increase in plasma cortisol after exercise; normal peak morning levels of cortisol but abnormally elevated evening levels (an absence of the normal nighttime cortisol "trough"); and a low 24-hour urine free cortisol level.

A subset of chronic fatigue syndrome patients have several of the same HPA abnormalities as fibromyalgia patients. These abnormalities include a low 24-hour urinary free cortisol level and a low maximum cortisol response to ACTH. These indices of low cortisol secretion resemble adrenal atrophy secondary to CRH deficiency. Three findings in a subset of chronic fatigue syndrome patients differ from those in fibromyalgia patients: elevated evening basal ACTH levels, low evening plasma cortisol levels, and blunted ACTH responses to injected CRH.

Similarities of Clinical Features of Adrenal Insufficiency and Fibromyalgia

Some features of the clinical syndrome resulting from adrenal insufficiency overlap features of fibromyalgia. Patients with adrenal insufficiency may have a low BMR, muscle contractures and pain, low blood pressure, postural hypotension, weakness, lethargy, *and fatigue.*

The clinician may be able to distinguish these symptoms and signs as features of adrenal insufficiency by laboratory testing. A normal or high basal cortisol level suggests normal hypothalamic-pituitary-adrenocortical function. However, an inadequate increase in plasma cortisol 30 minutes following an ACTH injection indicates insufficient adrenal reserve. The patient may also have low serum sodium and elevated serum potassium levels. The patient with a low basal cortisol level is likely to have an abnormally low rise of the cortisol level during the ACTH stimulation test.

The clinician must bear in mind that inadequate thyroid hormone regulation of gene transcription for CRH results in decreased CRH secretion. Reduced CRH secretion, by reducing ACTH secretion, can result in atrophy of the adrenal cortex. In addition, inadequate thyroid hormone regulation of cells of the adrenal cortex (those of the zona fasciculata-reticularis) reduce cortisol synthesis and secretion. Thus, although laboratory testing shows deficient secretion of cortisol, inadequate thyroid hormone regulation (due either to hypothyroidism or cellular resistance to thyroid hormone) may be the underlying cause. Exogenous cortisol can alleviate clinical features of cortisol deficiency even when caused by inadequate thyroid hormone regulation of adrenocortical cells. However, other clinical features of inadequate thyroid hormone regulation of cell function not due to the cortisol deficiency will continue apace.

Putative Role of Inadequate Thyroid Hormone Regulation of Cell Function

A plausible hypothesis is that the HPA abnormalities in fibromyalgia result from inadequate thyroid hormone regulation of the HPA axis. Inadequate thyroid hormone regulation of two components of the axis, CRH- and cortisol-synthesizing cells, can account for the HPA abnormalities of fibromyalgia. The axis abnormalities impair the ability of the HPA axis to facilitate adaptation to chronic stress. The impairment may compound fibromyalgia symptoms and signs caused by inadequate thyroid hormone regulation of tissues other than those of the HPA axis.

Inadequate thyroid hormone regulation of the axis as a mechanism of HPA abnormalities in fibromyalgia patients is plausible: HPA axis abnormalities in a subset of hypothyroid humans and laboratory animals closely resemble those of fibromyalgia patients. Overall, fibromyalgia patients have depressed HPA activity, as do hypothyroid patients.

Thyroid hormone activates transcription for CRH mRNA. In hypothyroidism, CRH production is subnormal. For two reasons, subnormal CRH secretion does not necessarily result in low production of ACTH: (1) hypothalamic secretion of AVP may increase in compensation for low CRH secretion, and (2) low CRH and suboptimal basal ACTH secretion decrease cortisol secretion by the adrenal cortices. Increased AVP stimulates the corticotrophs to increase synthesis of ACTH, and low circulating cortisol levels disinhibit the pituitary corticotrophs, increasing their production of ACTH. Thus, the possible increase in AVP and the documented subnormal cortisol production in fibromyalgia patients—both of which may result from inadequate thyroid hormone regulation of cell function—may account for the patients' exaggerated ACTH response to injected CRH. Hypothyroid laboratory animals and humans have the same pattern of deficient cortisol secretion and exaggerated ACTH response to CRH.

In hypothyroidism, CRH secretion may be subnormal due to inhibited neural output of the sympathetic superior cervical ganglion. An increase in α_2-adrenergic receptors in the sympathetic ganglia in hypothyroidism results in inhibition of both pre- and post-ganglionic sympathetic neurons. Reduced sympathetic drive is the result of this adrenergically-mediated blockade of the sympathetic ganglia. In the periphery, one result of the diminished sympathetic drive is a subnormal cardiovascular response to stressors such as exercise. This occurs in both hypothyroidism and fibromyalgia. In the central nervous system, a result is decreased secretion of CRH, as appears to occur in fibromyalgia. A predictable result is exaggerated ACTH secretion and deficient cortisol secretion during stress.

Researchers found that blockade of the superior cervical sympathetic ganglion diminished AVP secretion. In some fibromyalgia patients, an increase in α_2-adrenergic receptors on superior cervical ganglion cells may impair neural flow from the ganglion to the hypothalamus. If so, in these patients, the exaggerated ACTH response to injected CRH may not result from increased AVP secretion as a compensation for reduced CRH secretion. Instead, the exaggerated ACTH response may occur solely by another mechanism—high ACTH reserve in the pituitary corticotrophs due to disinhibition of the corticotrophs resulting from subnormal circulating cortisol levels.

The high mean level of AVP in some fibromyalgia patients in one study may have resulted from copious secretion of AVP. The AVP secretion of 5 of 12 patients was greater than two standard deviations above the value of control subjects. It is possible that in these 5 patients, AVP secretion was not inhibited by α_2-adrenergic receptor-mediated inhibition of the superior cervical sympathetic ganglia.

If the liver is selectively involved in hypothyroidism, the cortisol clearance rate from the liver may be reduced. A reduced clearance rate will increase the plasma cortisol level despite low cortisol secretion by the adrenal cortices. In some hypothyroid patients, adrenocortical output is normal or near normal, but a low hepatic clearance rate results in elevated basal plasma cortisol levels. A reduced liver clearance rate may account for two findings in fibromyalgia patients: the abnormally elevated evening cortisol level (absence of the pm cortisol "trough") and the low 24-hour urinary free cortisol level.

The Stress Hypothesis of Fibromyalgia

Some researchers have speculated that the HPA abnormalities identified in a subset of fibromyalgia patients result from chronic stress. Some have also conjectured that the HPA abnormalities mediate some features of fibromyalgia. The hypothesis that stress plays a role in fibromyalgia has merit. Fibromyalgia patients are subjected to chronic stressors: continuous pain, loss of functional abilities, the precarious prognosis of fibromyalgia, failed treatments, and accusations that their condition is psychogenic. Such stressors exacerbate many fibromyalgia patients' status. In normal individuals, stressors upregulate activity of the HPA axis. But in some fibromyalgia patients, as in some hypothyroid patients, normal upregulation does not occur. Instead, inadequate thyroid hormone regulation of gene transcription in CRH- and cortisol-secreting cells hinder the axis from serving its normal role in stress adaptation. In these patients, HPA axis dysfunction is not the underlying cause of fibromyalgia but may contribute to the patient's symptoms. During stress, the HPA axis dysfunction would compound the symptoms and signs of fibromyalgia that persist even during non-stressful times.

It is not likely, however, that a cortisol deficiency is a principle causative factor in fibromyalgia. First, a cortisol deficiency would increase the use of glucose, increase glycolysis, and reduce glycogen stores. But studies have shown glycolysis impairment in fibromyalgia and an increase in tissue glycogen deposition. If a cortisol deficiency were a causative factor in fibromyalgia, treatment with glucocorticoids would be expected to relieve fibromyalgia symptoms. In one study, though, the use of prednisone worsened fibro-

myalgia patients' status. In another report, polymyalgia rheumatica patients taking glucocorticoid medication developed fibromyalgia. Moreover, several studies have shown that glucocorticoid treatment benefits chronic fatigue syndrome patients minimally at best.

Some may argue that inadequate thyroid hormone regulation of cell function in fibromyalgia may itself result from stress. According to this model, increased cortisol secretion during stress-induced activation of the HPA axis suppresses TSH secretion and T_4 to T_3 conversion. The resulting inadequate T_3 regulation of CRH- and cortisol-secreting cells produces the HPA axis abnormalities in fibromyalgia—reduced CRH and cortisol secretion, and augmented ACTH secretion due to the low cortisol level. This model posits that the starting point of the HPA abnormalities is stress, not a failure of thyroid hormone to properly regulate the axis. Inadequate thyroid hormone regulation of the axis is merely a mediator of the axis-disrupting effects of stress. An implication of the model is that stress relief is necessary to alleviate the HPA abnormalities. This model fails on several counts. First, published studies and clinical experience show that anti-stress treatments for fibromyalgia are largely ineffective. Second, the anti-thyroid effects of elevated cortisol during stress would not sustain HPA axis abnormalities. The anti-thyroid effects of elevated cortisol are short-lived, lasting no more than a few weeks. After this time, the thyroid system "escapes" the anti-thyroid effects, even if cortisol levels remain elevated. Following the escape, T_3 levels return to normal. At that time, CRH and cortisol secretion would return to normal. After secretion became normal, patients would no longer have low CRH and cortisol secretion and exaggerated ACTH responses to CRH or stress. Third, the low T_3 level resulting from the stress-induced cortisol increase would reduce CRH secretion. The reduced CRH secretion would reduce cortisol secretion toward normal. The reduced cortisol level would relieve the anti-thyroid effects and, in turn, alleviate the axis abnormalities mediated by the low T_3 level.

Stress may, however, precipitate fibromyalgia symptoms in the individual who—before undergoing the stress—had only marginally adequate metabolism in fibromyalgia-related tissues due to mild hypothyroidism or cellular resistance to thyroid hormone. The patient's elevated cortisol level during stress, by lowering her T_3 level, would further reduce her barely adequate metabolism. If the reduction in metabolism is sufficient, symptoms of hypometabolism (fibromyal-

gia) will occur. This mechanism is supported by two reports. Again, in one study, use of prednisone worsened the status of fibromyalgia patients. In another report, the author noted that treatment of polymyalgia rheumatica patients with glucocorticoid medication resulted in some of the patients developing fibromyalgia.

Symptoms of hypometabolism such as pain and fatigue, if severe enough, may keep the patient from engaging in enough physical activity to maintain normal muscle mass. A loss of muscle mass will further lower her metabolism. The reduced metabolism from the lost muscle mass, imposed on her already marginally adequate metabolism, may be sufficient to keep her symptomatic even after her thyroid system escapes the suppressive effects of the elevated cortisol. In this model, the patient's long-standing, merely marginally adequate metabolism is the most fundamental underlying factor leading to continuing fibromyalgia (hypometabolism) symptoms. Her previous borderline metabolic status is the starting point of the process leading to chronic fibromyalgia. Her metabolism, already slowed due to lost muscle mass, slows further during the transient low T_3 levels caused by stress-induced elevated cortisol levels. The stress and elevated cortisol only contribute to the additional reduction of the patient's metabolic rate and her chronic fibromyalgia.

Under normal conditions, we recover from chemical, mechanical, or psychological disruptions of homeostatic balance—which we term "stress"—through two major stress-adaptation systems. One, the sympathetic-adrenergic system, I discuss in Chapter 3.1. The other, the hypothalamic-pituitary-adrenal (HPA) axis, is the subject of this chapter.

Study of the abnormalities of these systems may elucidate the nature of the relation of fibromyalgia status to stress. Many fibromyalgia patients have reported that their illness began with an episode of stress.[94][98] Others have reported a high level of perceived stress,[99] and still others have reported that their fibromyalgia status worsens during times of stress.[100] In one study, no difference was found in major life stress between fibromyalgia and rheumatoid arthritis patients.[99] However, fibromyalgia patients had higher "daily hassles" according to the "Hassles" scale. In another study, fibromyalgia patients had more psychological and life stress than rheumatoid arthritis patients.[74]

I monitored the status of some fibromyalgia patients for up to 10 years, graphing their scores on objective fibromyalgia measures. This process showed that intense physical or psychological stress worsened the patients' fibromyalgia status according to the graphed scores. (This was true even for patients who had formerly improved or recovered from fibromyalgia with metabolic rehabilitation. Patients resumed their improved or recovered status after the stresses ended.) The worsening or resumption of fibromyalgia symptoms during times of intense stress may result from transient suppression of the thyroid system by a stress-induced elevation of cortisol (see section below titled "High Cortisol Transiently Suppresses the Thyroid System").

● **OVERVIEW OF THE HYPOTHALAMIC-PITUITARY-ADRENAL (HPA) AXIS**

Physical, physiological, chemical, and psychological stimuli that disrupt homeostasis induce physiological and behavioral responses that correct the disruption. (Some sources of stress that researchers have studied are social isolation in mice,[46] hypoglycemia,[48] exercise,[49] and intravenous angiotensin II and ether.[50]) Two main systems take part in restoring homeostasis. One is the central locus ceruleus-norepinephrine system and its peripheral branch, the sympathetic nervous system, which I cover in Chapter 3.1. The other is the central hypothalamic corticotropin-releasing hormone system and its peripheral branch, the pituitary-adrenocortical axis. These two systems coordinate the stress response, allowing the organism to recover homeostatic balance, adapt, and increase its chances of survival.[147] The stress response of these two systems is closely integrated with other central and peripheral systems involved in the regulation of physiology and behavior, and with axes associated with reproduction, growth, and immunity.[134]

In this chapter, I consider abnormalities of the HPA axis-stress response system in fibromyalgia. The axis includes four links: (1) release of corticotropin-releasing hormone (CRH) and arginine-vasopressin (AVP) by hypothalamic cells, (2) CRH and AVP stimulated release of adrenocorticotropin hormone (ACTH) by pituitary corticotroph cells, (3) ACTH stimulated release of glucocorticoids (mainly cortisol) from the adrenal cortices, and (4) inhibition of the hypothalamic CRH-synthesizing cells and pituitary corticotrophs by glucocorticoids.[47][135] The glucocorticoids, especially cortisol, inhibit glucose use by cells. At the same time, glucocorticoids mobilize fats and proteins. Cells ultimately use the fatty acids from the fats and the amino acids from the proteins for energy.[2,pp.846-848]

CORTICOTROPIN-RELEASING HORMONE (CRH)

In response to stress, cells of the paraventricular nucleus of the hypothalamus secrete the peptide corticotropin-releasing hormone (CRH) into the primary capillary plexus of the hypothalamic-pituitary portal system. (The portal system consists of blood vessels that transmit hypothalamic releasing hormones from the hypothalamus to the anterior pituitary.) CRH travels through the portal system to the anterior pituitary gland, where it stimulates corticotroph cells to secrete adrenocorticotropin hormone (ACTH).

Most stimuli that cause high ACTH secretion initiate the process in the basal regions of the brain, especially the hypothalamus. Hypothalamic cells release CRH to stimulate ACTH secretion by the pituitary gland.[2,p.850] ACTH in turn provokes release of glucocorticoids from the adrenal cortex. Glucocorticoids (mainly cortisol in man) inhibit CRH neurons in the hypothalamus. ACTH and cortisol are therefore successive links in a negative feedback mechanism that regulates hypothalamic CRH release. In addition to this regulatory mechanism, CRH release varies throughout the day, and extreme stress perturbs its regulation.[82,pp.141-142]

Upon attaching to receptors on pituitary cells, CRH stimulates ACTH secretion by activating the cAMP "second messenger." CRH is the major stimulant to ACTH release, but it is not the only one. Arginine-vasopressin (AVP) and serotonin also stimulate ACTH release, but they are apparently synergists to CRH that potentiate its effects on ACTH release.[82,p.142] In prolonged stress, CRH secretion may diminish and AVP secretion may increase to continue ACTH secretion. Infusion of CRH for 48 hours caused a 40% decrease in anterior pituitary CRH receptor concentration. Concomitantly infusing AVP in chronically stressed rats significantly decreased the reduction of pituitary CRH receptors from 62% to 43%.[109]

Control of CRH Secretion

Many factors contribute to the complex mechanisms that control secretion of CRH by the hypothalamus. These factors help regulate CRH gene expression in the cells of the paraventricular nucleus of the hypothalamus.[78] The factors include neural input to the hypothalamus from the limbic system, lower brain stem, and spinal cord; release of modifying chemicals by local glial cells; interleukins; osmotic and metabolic factors such as glucose; feedback involving glucocorticoids, proopiomelanocortin (POMC)-related peptides (from which ACTH is derived), and other hypothalamic hormones;[110,p.138] and thyroid hormone (see subsection below titled "Thyroid Hormone Status and the HPA Axis").

Many ascending and descending neural pathways converge on the hypothalamus and contribute to the release of CRH. Especially influential are nerve fibers that originate in the brain stem, raphe nucleus, hippocampus, and amygdala. Nerve fibers from the cerebral cortex and within the hypothalamus itself are also important.[110,p.138] Mental stress involves neural transmission from the upregulated limbic system (particularly the hippocampus and amygdala) to the posterior medial hypothalamus. This stress-induced transmission increases CRH secretion. The CRH then promptly increases pituitary secretion of ACTH. Nociceptive signals (as from a broken leg) ascend the spinal cord and brain stem. The signals then pass to the perifornical region of the hypothalamus, to the hypothalamic paraventricular nucleus, and finally to the median eminence of the hypothalamus. The signals stimulate the median eminence (at the inferior aspect of the hypothalamus) to release CRH into the hypothalamic-pituitary portal system. After the portal system delivers it to the anterior pituitary gland, CRH stimulates the release of ACTH.[2,p.850]

Cholinergic and serotonergic neural pathways stimulate the release of CRH into the portal circulation. On the other hand, γ-aminobutyric acid (GABAergic) neural pathways potently inhibit CRH release into the portal system.[111] These three pathways (the cholinergic, serotonergic, and GABAergic) are involved in stress-provoked CRH secretion. In addition, serotonin is important to the circadian rhythm of HPA activity.[112] Both acetylcholine and serotonin are involved in the secretion of CRH and AVP.[111][113]

Opioid secreting neurons strongly contribute to the regulation of CRH secretion. Opioids tonically inhibit ACTH secretion. In the hypothalamus, k-opioid receptors mediate the inhibition. Apparently, these receptors decrease CRH and AVP release by inhibiting catecholaminergic neurons that stimulate CRH and AVP secretion.[116]

Interaction of norepinephrine with α-adrenergic

receptors strongly stimulates ACTH secretion. During stress, terminals of norepinephrine-secreting neurons in the hypothalamus (the cell bodies of which reside in the locus ceruleus of the brain stem) secrete norepinephrine. The norepinephrine binds to α_1- and α_2-adrenergic receptors and induces release of CRH. Norepinephrine interaction with β-adrenergic receptors weakly stimulates secretion of CRH.[114]

In most tissues, the density of α-adrenergic receptors increases with inadequate thyroid hormone regulation of transcription of the gene that codes for the receptor. And in most tissues, α-adrenergic receptors inhibit metabolism. In some tissues, however, such as liver and some hypothalamic cells, inadequate thyroid hormone regulation of the α_2-adrenergic receptor gene decreases production of the receptors. Conversely, adequate regulation of the gene by the hormone increases production of the receptors. Moreover, in the cells of these tissues, α-adrenergic receptors stimulate metabolic processes.[145,pp.315-316] (See Chapter 3.12, section titled "Thyroid Hormone, Adrenergic Receptor Type, and Regulation of Growth Hormone-Releasing Factor and Growth Hormone Secretion," and Chapter 3.1, subsection titled "Inadequate Thyroid Hormone Regulation of Adrenergic Gene Transcription.") The decrease in CRH in hypothyroidism suggests that inadequate thyroid hormone regulation of the α_2-adrenoceptor gene in paraventricular nuclei decreases production of α_2-adrenergic receptors. Conversely, the increase in CRH in thyrotoxicosis suggests that adequate thyroid hormone regulation of the gene increases production of the receptors. These findings indicate that thyroid hormone regulation of the adrenergic gene contributes to the hormones regulation of CRH secretion. In addition, the decrease in CRH mRNA in hypothyroidism suggests that thyroid hormone regulates the CRH gene. (See subsection below titled "Thyroid Hormone Status and the HPA Axis: CRH.") Thus, thyroid hormone may regulate CRH synthesis and secretion by two routes.

Stimulation of CRH secretion by norepinephrine is mediated primarily by α_1-adrenoceptors.[111][114][146] The subpopulation of hypothalamic cells that secrete CRH also contain AVP. The cells are located in a catecholamine-rich area of the paraventricular nucleus. An α_1-adrenoceptor agonist (methoxamine) caused significant depletion of vesicles from axons containing CRH and AVP.[146] The depletion suggests that the α_1-adrenoceptor agonist selectively activates the CRH- and AVP-secreting neurons, causing them to release their content of the two hormones. The neurons were within the blood-brain barrier and thus not in the pitui-

tary. In another study,[114] exposing the neurons to methoxamine caused elevations of plasma ACTH and cortisol. The researchers concluded, "Stimulation of central α_1-adrenergic mechanisms results in secretion of ACTH in man, presumably by increased release of a corticotropin-releasing factor." These results point to α_1-adrenoceptor activation of CRH secretion.

Administering epinephrine to the cerebral ventricles facilitated CRH secretion. Interaction of the epinephrine with α_1-and β-adrenoceptors facilitated secretion.[111] Epinephrine caused release of CRH only at high concentrations. Administering only an α_2-adrenoceptor antagonist (idazoxan) did not affect ACTH and cortisol secretion.[115] But administering the antagonist with the opioid antagonist naloxone, which stimulates ACTH secretion, increased ACTH secretion. This finding suggests that under some conditions of ACTH secretion, α_2-adrenergic receptors exert a permissive effect on secretion. Catecholamine binding to α_1- and β-adrenergic receptors, and to α_2-adrenoceptors under limited circumstances, stimulated rather than inhibited the release of CRH.[79] Under normal conditions, then, it appears that catecholamine-adrenergic receptor interaction stimulates secretion of CRH, and, in turn, the CRH stimulates secretion of ACTH.[42][71]

Other stimulatory transmitters include neuropeptide Y, angiotensin II, atrial natriuretic factor, and vasoactive intestinal peptide.[110,p.140] The pituitary pro-opiomelanocortin (POMC)-derived peptides ACTH and β-endorphin strongly inhibit hypothalamic CRH secretion.[117][118] These peptides do not cross the brain-blood barrier, so they probably exert their effects through the median eminence.[110,p.143]

ARGININE-VASOPRESSIN (AVP)

AVP is a hormone that functions as an auxiliary to CRH in stimulating the pituitary corticotrophs to release ACTH. Hypothalamic cells called supraoptic nuclei synthesize AVP. AVP is then transported down the hypothalamic-pituitary nerve tract to nerve endings in the posterior pituitary gland. When nerve impulses pass down the tracts from the supraoptic nuclei, AVP is released from the nerve endings and enters the adjacent capillaries.[2,p.828][108]

The parvocellular neurons in the paraventricular nucleus that contain CRH also contain AVP. Both hormones are released together from the median eminence. AVP strongly potentiates CRH-stimulated release of ACTH from the pituitary gland. This potentiation indicates that the two hormones are synergists.[36,p.418][37,p.743]

Repeated stress leads to plastic changes in hypothalamic CRH neurons: AVP stores increase and the two hormones "colocalize" in CRH nerve terminals.[104] Angelucci and Scaccianoce repeatedly administered CRH to the pituitary, a test that is presumably equivalent to chronic or repetitive stress. They reported that the pituitary became unresponsive to CRH 15 minutes after the first dose. During this time, the response of the adrenal cortices to AVP increased. The increased adrenocortical response suggests that AVP enables repeated activation of the pituitary-adrenocortical axis. However, glucocorticoids released during previous stressors blocked activation of the HPA axis. Cold stress (4°-to-6° C for 90 minutes) suppressed responsiveness of the HPA axis to a subsequent psychic stressor but not to a somatic one.[144]

AVP has different effects on TSH secretion depending on whether the hormone acts in the hypothalamus or the pituitary. In the hypothalamus, AVP indirectly inhibits pituitary secretion of TSH.[140] When present in the pituitary, however, AVP induces a specific and dose-related release of TSH with a potency equaling that of TRH.[140][143] Researchers found that AVP increased the synthesis and secretion of thyroid hormones by the thyroid gland.[148] Besides increasing TSH and T_4 levels, AVP increased thyroid gland weight. These findings suggest that AVP potently stimulates thyroid gland function, and that the pituitary gland mediates the stimulation.[149] Some hypothyroid patients have elevated AVP levels. The elevation may be a compensatory increase due to low CRH levels caused by thyroid hormone deficiency.

ADRENOCORTICOTROPIN HORMONE (ACTH)

The primary role of ACTH is to stimulate the synthesis and release of steroid hormones by the adrenal cortices. The adrenocortical steroid hormones are the glucocorticoids, mineralocorticoids, and weak androgens.

Plasma levels of ACTH vary during the day. Levels generally peak from 6am-to-8am, decline late in the day, and reach their lowest levels around midnight. Ordinarily, secretory bursts of ACTH occur during the day, especially in response to stress. Plasma levels of cortisol closely follow those of ACTH, although the correlation is not exact.[83] Bloom and Lazerson wrote that the early morning secretion of ACTH and cortisol

ready the body for the activities of the coming day. In nocturnal animals, cortisol levels peak in the early evening, preparing them for night activities.[80,p.178]

Increased cortisol secretion during early morning hours and during stress results from more frequent and higher volume bursts of ACTH secretion. The bursts probably result from heightened central nervous system stimulation that overrides the normal negative feedback effects of cortisol on the hypothalamus and pituitary.[84,p.590]

During stress, the increased glucocorticoid level decreases TSH secretion but does not significantly disrupt the rhythm of TSH secretion.[64] In contrast, stress disrupts the diurnal rhythm of ACTH secretion; increased secretion occurs within minutes.[2,p.850] In fact, the most trivial stimuli provoke ACTH secretion.[90,p.807] After a stressful event, the ACTH level peaks within a few minutes and plasma cortisol peaks some 30 minutes later. A stay in a hospital is stressful to many patients and may increase ACTH and cortisol levels. The secretion of cortisol is greater in anxious hospitalized patients than in controls. Anxious patients have higher plasma cortisol levels and increased urinary excretion of cortisol.[41][55] The clinician should consider these effects of stress on cortisol levels when evaluating a hospitalized fibromyalgia patient for HPA function.[82,p.142]

Neural pathways from the hypothalamus that regulate pituitary secretions conduct information concerning the circadian periodicity, environmental conditions, physical and psychological activities, and osmotic and metabolic status.[110,p.138] Adrenergic and noradrenergic pathways that originate in the brain stem[119] and cervical sympathetic plexus[120] terminate in the hypothalamic median eminence. Neurons of these pathways may contribute to the regulation of ACTH secretion by secreting norepinephrine into the portal circulation.[121] This possibility is controversial, however.[110,p.137]

Substances other than CRH and AVP that stimulate ACTH release include epinephrine, norepinephrine, oxytocin, angiotensin II, and vasoactive intestinal peptide. In response to hypothalamic extracts, substance P inhibited ACTH secretion *in vitro* and *in vivo*.[69]

CORTISOL

The adrenal cortices secrete glucocorticoids in response to ACTH. Cortisol, also called hydrocortisone, is the most abundantly secreted glucocorticoid. It is by far the most potent naturally synthesized glucocorticoid.[2,p.846] The blood transports glucocorticoids both as free steroids and bound to corticosteroid-binding globulin (also called transcortin). Inside cells, glucocorticoids significantly influence intermediary metabolism. One important metabolic role is to promote the deposition of glycogen in the liver. A role for glucocorticoids that is crucial to human health is their anti-inflammatory effect. Glucocorticoids are catabolized chiefly in the liver, but they are also catabolized in the kidneys, connective tissues, fibroblasts, and muscle. The half-time for hepatic clearance of cortisol is 80-to-120 minutes. When radioactively labeled cortisol is injected, some 90% is excreted in the urine.[70,p.210]

Mechanisms of Action

The actions of the glucocorticoids, like those of thyroid hormones, are virtually ubiquitous in the body. Cortisol potently inhibits secretion of CRH by the hypothalamus. Through inhibiting CRH secretion, cortisol indirectly inhibits ACTH secretion by the pituitary gland. However, cortisol also directly inhibits pituitary secretion of ACTH. Cortisol thereby tightly regulates activity of the HPA axis.[2,p.851] Most cells contain cortisol receptors that have a high affinity for the hormone. These receptors mediate the cellular effects of the hormone,[90,p.806] and only cells with receptors respond to cortisol.

Glucocorticoids diffuse through cell membranes. After entering a cell, the hormones travel to receptors which are located either in the cytoplasm or the nucleus, depending on the steroid hormone involved. After the hormone and a receptor bind, the hormone-receptor complex attaches to a specific DNA sequence, usually one situated at the 5'-flanking region of the hormone responsive gene.[87] The attachment activates or represses gene transcription, depending on the target gene. Activation of transcription increases mRNA and protein synthesis.[84,p.587]

One type of steroid hormone may bind with more than one type of steroid receptor, but the hormone usually has a higher affinity for one type of receptor than for the others. Cortisol has a high affinity for glucocorticoid receptors and a weak affinity for mineralocorticoid receptors. Because of its tight binding to the glucocorticoid receptor, cortisol has stronger glucocorticoid activity than mineralocorticoid activity. The role of steroid hormones in the cell, like that of thyroid hormones, is to regulate the expression of various genes. Glucocorticoids regulate different genes in different types of cells. In liver cells, for instance, glucocorticoids exert metabolic effects, and in lymphoid cells they mainly exert anti-inflammatory effects.

Glucocorticoids also play roles in cells other than controlling gene expression. One important non-genomic role is stabilization of lysosomal membranes. Stabilizing the membranes prevents the release of lysosomal enzymes within cells.[84,p.587] This membrane stabilizing role is critically important to the survival of the cells. Lysosomal enzymes, upon escaping from the membranes within cells that contain them, decompose the organic compounds that make up the structure of the cells; cell "death" results. A low circulating level of this hormonal membrane stabilizer in some fibromyalgia patients may explain the release of myoglobin from their skeletal muscles when therapists massaged "fibrositic" nodules in the muscles.[76][77] The investigators did not report the cortisol levels of the patients who had increased myoglobin levels following massage.

Presumably, low cortisol levels would leave patients' cell membranes, including the sarcolemmal membranes of the noduled muscles, friable—that is, the membranes would rupture easily when mechanically distorted by manual manipulation. The rupturing would enable myoglobin to escape. This theoretical effect of a low cortisol level in the general circulation might be intensified by reduced circulation at the site of the tender nodule. The nodule may consist of a circumscribed locus of myofascial tissue severely shortened by contracture of the muscle fibers. If so, the heightened pressure within the locus may compress arteries and arterioles. Sufficient compression would reduce the amount of blood constituents such as cortisol that the vessels deliver to the muscle cells. Reduced delivery of cortisol to the muscle cells due to the vascular compression would compound the inadequate exposure of cells to cortisol due to the low levels in the general circulation. The compounding of inadequate exposure of cells to cortisol would possibly worsen the friability of the muscle cell membranes.

Stress Hormone

Cortisol is responsible for roughly 95% of glucocorticoid activity. (A small but important amount of glucocorticoid activity is due to corticosterone,[2,p.846] the only other glucocorticoid secreted in significant amounts.[81,p.520]) Cortisol functions as a stress hormone. The cortisol level increases within minutes during stress. Secretion can increase 20-fold.[2,p.850] By inducing various physiological effects, cortisol increases the individual's chances of survival. The adrenocortical hormone potentiates the activating effects of catecholamines. The catecholamines in turn aid survival by providing energy. The increased energy enables increased cardiac output and work capacity of skeletal muscles. Cortisol also increases energy availability by mobilizing free fatty acids from adipose tissue and proteins from most cells of the body. Enzymes in the liver promptly deaminate amino acids, converting them to substrates for conversion to glucose.[84,p.589] Glucocorticoids, especially cortisol, are the most potent promoters of gluconeogenesis—conversion of glycerol and amino acids into glucose when normal amounts of carbohydrates do not meet the energy needs of cells.[2,p.752]

Suppression of ACTH Secretion

Cortisol and its synthetic glucocorticoid analogues such as prednisone and dexamethasone suppress ACTH secretion. Glucocorticoids suppress ACTH secretion in two phases. "Fast feedback" suppression occurs within minutes, probably by glucocorticoids acting at pituitary corticotroph cell membranes. "Delayed feedback" suppression occurs hours-to-days later, probably due to the effects of glucocorticoids at the chromosomal level in cell nuclei.[82,p.143]

Effects on Thyroid Function

Cortisol impedes the release of TSH by the pituitary thyrotrophs in response to TRH. Cortisol also inhibits the conversion of T_4 to T_3, resulting in an increase in reverse T_3. (See Chaper 2.5, section titled "Proposal of a Sustained Euthyroid Sick Syndrome Under the Expropriated Name "Wilson's Syndrome."") Cortisol also reduces both thyroid binding globulin and thyroid-binding prealbumin. According to Pescovitz et al., decreases in these transport proteins result in low-normal total T_4 and free T_4 levels but without clinical manifestations of hypothyroidism.[84,p.589]

Effects on Calcium

Glucocorticoids tend to reduce serum calcium by two means: reduction of intestinal absorption of calcium and decreased renal reabsorption of calcium and phosphorus. The serum calcium level typically does not drop below normal, however, because the parathyroid glands increase their secretion of parathyroid hormone. Parathyroid hormone mobilizes calcium from bone. It also increases intestinal absorption and renal tubular reabsorption of calcium. Parathyroid hormone action at these three sites sustains normal serum calcium levels.[85]

One of the most important long-term effects of high levels of glucocorticoids is osteoporosis. The steroids increase the number of osteoclasts, and the increased number accelerates the rate of osteolysis. Also, an elevated level of parathyroid hormone increases osteoclastic activity to maintain a normal serum calcium level. The increased osteoclastic activity intensifies the loss of calcium from bone and increases the tendency toward osteoporosis.[86]

Effects on Carbohydrate, Lipid, and Protein Metabolism

Glucocorticoids activate enzymes that have glucose-regulating effects.[88] In the liver, various enzymes stimulate the conversion of triglycerides to fatty acids and glycerol and break down proteins to amino acids. Other enzymes convert the glycerol and amino acids to glucose—a process called gluconeogenesis. This promotion of glucose availability is vital for life and justifies the term "*gluco*corticoids" for these hormones.[89]

When a person is not stressed during the day, her glucocorticoid secretion varies little.[84,pp.587-588] With increased stress, however, glucocorticoid secretion increases. The increased secretion is reflected in substantial metabolic effects on carbohydrates, lipids, and proteins.

Glucocorticoids exert these effects through two mechanisms. First, they activate gene transcription in liver cells. The activation increases production of many enzymes that take part in converting amino acids to glucose in the liver. Second, glucocorticoids mobilize amino acids from tissues other than the liver, especially muscle. As a result, more amino acids are available in the plasma to enter the liver and undergo gluconeogenesis.

These mechanisms cause an increase in the amount of glycogen stored in liver cells. Under normal non-stress circumstances, glucocorticoids work with insulin to induce glycogen deposition and storage in the liver. Stored glycogen can provide glucose reserves for long periods without food consumption. Both insulin and glucocorticoids stimulate the enzyme glycogen synthetase, thereby stimulating glucose storage and inhibiting glycogen breakdown.[84,p.588] Glycogen synthetase catalyzes the linking of glucose molecules to starch chains. As part of the glycogen, glucose is stored in muscle and other cells. As a part of the stress response, catecholamines bind to β-adrenergic receptors on liver cell membranes and start a cascade of cellular reactions that release glucose from the glycogen.

Decreased Glycolysis. Glucocorticoids cause a moderate decrease in glycolysis, reducing the use of glucose in cells. This may result from inhibition of oxidation of nicotinamide-adenine dinucleotide (NADH). Oxidation of NADH is required for rapid glycolysis.[2,p.847]

Lipid Metabolism. Triglycerides are the main storage form of lipids in the body. Triglycerides are formed of free fatty acids combined with glycerol through ester bonds. Glucocorticoids decrease the synthesis of glycerol molecules and therefore the formation of triglycerides. In this way, glucocorticoids mobilize free fatty acids from adipose tissue, increasing the fatty acids' plasma concentration and availability to cells for energy use.[2,p.759] Glycerol can undergo conversion to glucose through gluconeogenesis, and the fatty acids enter the citric acid cycle in mitochondria after being converted to acetyl-CoA.[2,pp.752&756]

Also, glucocorticoids inhibit insulin, so that fewer glucose molecules enter fat cells. The reduction of glucose in fat cells decreases intracellular levels of a glucose-derived substance called α-glycerophosphate. α-Glycerophosphate is necessary for the deposition and maintenance of triglycerides in adipose cells. When glucocorticoids reduce the concentration of α-glycerophosphate in fat cells, free fatty acids are liberated.[2,p.847]

Glucocorticoids favor the lipid-catabolizing effect of epinephrine.[84,p.588] This effect increases the concentration of free fatty acids in the plasma and their availability for energy use. Cortisol increases oxidation of free fatty acids within the cell. Through this mechanism, during times of stress (such as during starvation), cells shift from the use of glucose to the use of fatty acids for energy.[2,p.847]

Protein Metabolism. Glucocorticoids impede amino acid transport into tissues other than the liver.[2,p.847][84,p.588] Glucocorticoids also induce protein catabolism in most tissues of the body, including fat, bone, lymphoid, skeletal muscle, and connective tissue. In skeletal muscle, protein catabolism involves type 2 (white, fast twitch) "glycolytic" fibers more than type 1 (red, slow twitch) fibers. Heart muscle, the diaphragm, and especially the liver are, for the most part, spared from protein catabolism. The release of amino acids from tissues increases plasma amino acid levels. Upon being transported into the liver, the amino acids are available for gluconeogenesis.[2,p.847][84,p.588]

Glucocorticoids also decrease RNA production in cells.[2,p.847][84,p.588] Protein transport into liver cells increases, and an increase occurs in the synthesis of liver enzymes necessary for protein synthesis. Thus, the protein content of the liver increases, and the plasma levels of proteins produced by the liver increase.[2,p.847]

● ABNORMALITIES OF THE HYPOTHALAMIC-PITUITARY-ADRENAL AXIS IN FIBROMYALGIA

STRESS SYSTEM DYSFUNCTION: A HYPOTHESIS OF THE PATHOGENESIS OF FIBROMYALGIA

In a series of papers, Demitrack and Crofford presented data showing abnormalities of the hypothalamic-pituitary-adrenal axis in fibromyalgia and chronic fatigue syndrome patients.[92][93][94][95][96][128] These researchers hypothesized that the abnormalities are related to the pathogenesis of fibromyalgia.

Hypothalamic-Pituitary-Adrenal Axis Abnormalities in Fibromyalgia

Dexamethasone Suppression Test. In the dexamethasone suppression test, the clinician injects 1 mg of dexamethasone (a synthetic glucocorticoid 30 times more potent than cortisol[2,p.843]) at 11pm, and the serum cortisol level is measured the next day at 4pm and 11pm.[170][171] Cortisol levels are suppressed in a normal test result. Cortisol levels are not suppressed in roughly 50% of depressed patients, suggesting limbic-dienchephalic dysfunction.[44,p.1517] Dexamethasone does not suppress cortisol levels in patients with Cushing's syndrome, a condition of excessive cortisol synthesis and secretion by the adrenal cortices.

In one study, dexamethasone failed to suppress cortisol levels in only 4% of 22 fibromyalgia patients.[8] In another, dexamethasone failed to suppress cortisol levels in 28.7% of 20 patients.[9]

Cortisol. Griep et al.[97] and Crofford et al.[93] reported a blunted cortisol response to ACTH in fibromyalgia patients. The blunted cortisol response is consistent with the lower increase in plasma cortisol in fibromyalgia patients after exercise.[101] McCain and Tilbe reported a reduced 24-hour urine free cortisol.[67] Crofford et al. found cortisol binding globulin levels to be normal in fibromyalgia patients.[93]

Altered Circadian Cortisol Rhythm. Evidence suggests a disordered circadian plasma cortisol rhythm in fibromyalgia patients. Normally, the cortisol level is highest early in the morning, lower in the evening, and lowest about midnight. Crofford et al.[93] and McCain and Tilbe[67] reported loss of this diurnal variation in cortisol in fibromyalgia patients. The patients had normal peak morning levels of cortisol, but the levels were abnormally elevated in the evening. We can view the elevated evening levels as an absence of the normal pm cortisol "trough."

Tilbe et al. found abnormalities in the diurnal variation of the serum cortisol level in 10 of 20 patients (50%) who had fibromyalgia for fewer than 2 years. In patients whose fibromyalgia had begun more than 2 years before, the percentage with abnormalities was 70%.[9]

ACTH Response. Griep et al. tested fibromyalgia patients for changes in the secretion of ACTH in response to insulin-induced hypoglycemia and injected CRH. Both stimuli induced exaggerated ACTH secretion.[97] In that CRH directly stimulates the pituitary corticotroph cells, the exaggerated ACTH response to injected CRH suggests that the corticotrophs had a high reserve of ACTH. A high reserve could result from a lack of inhibition of the corticotrophs due to subnormal cortisol levels. Two findings suggest this mechanism: the low 24-hour urinary free cortisol levels and the low maximum cortisol response to ACTH found in some fibromyalgia patients (see section above titled "Hypothalamic-Pituitary-Adrenal Axis Abnormalities in Fibromyalgia: Cortisol").

Insulin-induced hypoglycemia activates the whole HPA axis by provoking a hypothalamic response to the low blood sugar level. Thus, the exaggerated ACTH response to insulin-induced hypoglycemia in the patients of Griep et al. suggests one of two possible phenomena. First, the CRH-secreting cells of the hypothalamus may have been normally responsive. Second, the CRH-secreting cells may not have been normally responsive, but AVP from the hypothalamus adequately stimulated the corticotrophs to synthesize and secrete ACTH. In addition, the patients' low cortisol levels may have disinhibited the corticotrophs so that they produced a high reserve of ACTH in response to the AVP. It is highly likely that this latter mechanism at least contributed to the exaggerated ACTH response. The report by Griep et al. suggests that their patients had a blunted mean cortisol response to insulin-induced hypoglycemia and injected CRH.

The results reported by Griep et al. are similar to those reported by Demitrack et al.[92] and Crofford et al.[93] Crofford et al. administered CRH in the evening. At that time, the fibromyalgia patients had abnormally elevated cortisol levels. The difference between the ACTH responses of patients and controls was not statistically significant. However, patients had a nonsignificant mean elevation of basal and CRH-stimulated ACTH levels despite the elevated cortisol levels.

Arginine-Vasopressin (AVP)

Researchers found that during prolonged stress or insufficient CRH secretion, AVP assumes a more prominent role in regulating ACTH secretion.[103][104][105] Crofford et al. found a trend toward increased AVP secretion following postural change (from reclining to vertical position) in fibromyalgia patients. The increase in 5 of 12 patients was greater than two standard deviations above that of control patients.[93] Crofford wrote that during chronic HPA axis activation, AVP becomes increasingly active in stimulating ACTH secretion.[95,p.189] She cited studies in which investigators subjected rats to chronic experimental stress—chemically-induced polyarthritis or blocked bile flow due to surgically-induced bile duct obstruction.[102][106][107] The stress resulted in reduced CRH mRNA, decreased secretion of CRH, loss of the circadian rhythm of ACTH and corticosterone, and substantially increased AVP secretion.

Hauger and Aquilera wrote that the physiological regulation of ACTH secretion largely depends on the interaction of CRH and AVP in the pituitary corticotrophs. They found that infusing CRH for 48 hours caused a 40% decrease in CRH receptors in the anterior pituitary gland. Simultaneously infusing AVP potentiated the anti-receptor effect of CRH, further decreasing the CRH receptor count. The researchers concluded that activation of the parvicellular (but not the magnocellular) vasopressin-secreting neurons enhanced the down-regulation of pituitary CRH receptors by CRH. The enhanced down regulation of the receptors with the infusion of AVP suggests a critical role for parvicellular AVP in the control of corticotroph function.[109] Aguilera added that sensitivity to feedback inhibition from glucocorticoids is also critical to the regulation of ACTH secretion in chronic stress. During chronic stress, the normal inhibitory effect of elevated plasma levels of glucocorticoids on ACTH secretion is mitigated. The mitigation involves changes in glucocorticoid receptors with transcription factors induced by CRH and AVP.[38] Crofford surmised that the increased AVP secretion during chronic stress in fibromyalgia patients is compensatory for the reduced CRH secretion.[95,p.189]

Similar HPA Axis Abnormalities in Chronic Fatigue Syndrome

HPA axis abnormalities in chronic fatigue syndrome are similar to those in fibromyalgia.[92][102] In one study, basal cortisol levels were normal in chronic fatigue syndrome patients.[179] Like fibromyalgia patients, however, chronic fatigue syndrome patients had low 24-hour urinary free cortisol levels.[94] Their evening basal ACTH levels were high. However, their mean ACTH response to CRH was blunted,[179] while that of fibromyalgia patients was exaggerated. The maximum cortisol response to ACTH in chronic fatigue syndrome patients was low, as in fibromyalgia patients. The low cortisol response resembles adrenal atrophy secondary to CRH deficiency.[94]

We cannot be certain, however, that the two groups of patients really differ. One problem in learning the features of newly-researched diseases, such as fibromyalgia and chronic fatigue syndrome, is the inclusion of too few patients in studies. The purpose of these "descriptive" studies is to clarify the characteristics of patients with the diseases. Then, having learned their distinguishing characteristics, we can describe them accurately. Including large numbers of patients in these studies is important; including only small numbers of patients may result in findings that are skewed and not truly representative of the entire populations of patients. Feasibly, the differences in the reported HPA features of fibromyalgia and chronic fatigue syndrome will fade as researchers test larger percentages of the two patient populations.

(Preemptively, I qualify that large numbers of patients are *not* needed for other study purposes. For example, as my colleague John Gedye observes, NASA finds it sufficient to use only one subject, John Glenn, to initially discern effects of space flight on the elderly human male. Similarly, researchers often use single subjects in studies to learn dose-response curves for medications. Also, large numbers of study subjects are not necessary to show the effectiveness of a treatment for a disease *if the treatment is highly effective.* We must include large numbers of patients only if the intention is to detect an extremely mild treatment effect. I mention these exceptions to the need for large numbers of study subjects because of a common problem—the mistaken belief of many clinicians, journal editors, and journal and committee peer-reviewers that large numbers of patients are necessary in *all* studies, regardless of differing purposes of the studies.)

CRITIQUE OF THE GLUCOCORTICOID DEFICIENCY HYPOTHESIS OF FIBROMYALGIA

Some 90% of cortisol is excreted in the urine.[70,p.210] In view of this, reduced 24-hour urinary concentrations of cortisol in fibromyalgia patients suggest deficient production of cortisol by the adrenal cortices (see subsection above titled "Hypothalamic-Pituitary-Adrenal Axis Abnormalities in Fibromyalgia:

Cortisol"). Demitrack and Crofford recently suggested that a relative glucocorticoid deficiency contributes to the symptoms of fibromyalgia.[94,p.69]

However, a cortisol deficiency in fibromyalgia appears inconsistent with Eisinger's finding of impaired glycolysis in fibromyalgia.[43][153][168] Cortisol moderately decreases glucose use by cells. In fact, some researchers hold a teleological view of glucocorticoids—that glucocorticoids evolved to protect functions of the cerebral cortex of the brain that depend on glucose. The hormones serve this protective role by stimulating the formation of glucose, reducing its use in peripheral tissues, and promoting the storage of glucose as glycogen.[169,p.1438] Cortisol may decrease the use of glucose mainly by inhibiting oxidation of NADH. Oxidation of NADH is necessary for rapid glycolysis, and inhibition by cortisol of the oxidation may impede glycolysis.[2,p.846] Increased oxidation of NADH due to a cortisol deficiency may enable glycolysis to proceed rapidly. (See Chapter 2.2, subsection titled "Lactate Formed from Pyruvate in Contracting Muscle: Converted into Glucose by the Liver.") This liberating effect of subnormal cortisol levels on glycolysis seems contrary to the impaired glycolysis in fibromyalgia reported by Eisinger.

That a subnormal cortisol level is not a principle etiologic factor in fibromyalgia is further suggested by a microscopic and histologic muscle tissue finding of Awad[172][173] and Kalyan-Raman et al.[174] These researchers found increased glycogen deposition in the tissues of fibromyalgia patients. This finding is similar to the increased glycogen deposition in hypothyroid patients.[175] Increased glycogen deposition in fibromyalgia is contrary to the depletion of carbohydrate stores in patients with cortisol deficiency.[176] (For example, when consuming food *ad libitum*, an animal without adrenal cortices has no carbohydrate abnormalities; its plasma glucose level remains normal and its liver continues to store glycogen. But a short period of fasting promptly depletes the animal's carbohydrate reserves. The glycogen concentration diminishes in the animal's liver and less dramatically in its muscles, and the animal becomes hypoglycemic.[169,p.1438])

An additional weakness in the glucocorticoid deficiency hypothesis of fibromyalgia and chronic fatigue syndrome is the results of treatment of the patients with glucocorticoids: Glucocorticoids worsened or initiated fibromyalgia symptoms. In one study, prednisone exacerbated patients' fibromyalgia status.[12] Also, some patients taking glucocorticoids as a treatment for polymyalgia rheumatica developed fibromyalgia during the treatment.[13,p.14] (See subsection below titled "Exacerbation and Induction of Fibromyalgia by Exogenous Corticosteroids.") In addition, several studies have shown that treatment with hydrocortisone provided only slight symptom improvement in chronic fatigue syndrome patients.[177][178] In another study, researchers evaluated the benefits to chronic fatigue syndrome patients of treatment with low-dose fludrocortisone (a synthetic mineralocorticoid). The researchers reported that the treatment was of no benefit to the patients.[141] The likely explanation for these results is that the exogenous glucocorticoids slowed metabolism by inhibiting TSH secretion and T_4 to T_3 conversion (see section below titled "High Cortisol Transiently Suppresses the Thyroid System").

That a cortisol deficiency is a primary causative factor in fibromyalgia is not likely. This conclusion is indicated by four findings: (1) the inconsistency of a cortisol deficiency with the impaired glycolysis in fibromyalgia, (2) the finding of increased glycogen deposition in fibromyalgia patients' tissues, (3) induction of fibromyalgia or exacerbation of fibromyalgia symptoms by exogenous glucocorticoids, and (4) the minimal benefits from the use of glucocorticoids by chronic fatigue syndrome patients. Despite the conclusion, however, the similarities in the clinical features of cortisol deficiency and fibromyalgia warrant scrutiny (see next section).

If a patient has a cortisol deficiency due to inadequate thyroid hormone regulation of the HPA axis, the deficiency may contribute features to the patient's fibromyalgia. Metabolic rehabilitation involving thyroid hormone should relieve the cortisol-related features as it does other features not related to the cortisol deficiency. However, a patient may have a cortisol deficiency because of a primary condition of the adrenal cortices unrelated to the patient's fibromyalgia. The use of exogenous thyroid hormone by this patient is likely to increase the metabolism of cortisol and provoke symptoms of cortisol deficiency. The clinician must be prepared to recognize symptoms related to the cortisol deficiency so that he can promptly treat the patient for it. (See Chapter 5.2, section titled "Adrenal Insufficiency.")

Similar Features of Fibromyalgia and Glucocorticoid Deficiency

Some features of adrenal insufficiency can lead to a diagnosis of fibromyalgia. The features include an onset of symptoms precipitated by stress, a low basal metabolic rate (BMR), muscle pain and contractures, arthralgias, low blood pressure, postural hypotension, weakness, chronic lethargy and fatigue, postexercise

fatigue, exacerbation of allergic responses, feverishness, adenopathy, disturbed sleep, and disturbed mood.

Demitrack and Crofford noted that the debilitating fatigue of fibromyalgia especially overlaps with that of glucocorticoid deficiency. They wrote that CRH serves as a principal stimulus to the hypothalamic-pituitary-adrenal axis. In addition, though, it is a behavior-driving neurohormone. Administering it to the central nervous system of nonhuman primates and other animals induced signs of physiological and behavioral arousal. "Hence," they wrote, "a relative or absolute deficiency of hypothalamic corticotropin releasing hormone could contribute to the profound lethargy and fatigue that are inherent characteristics of these 'atypical' depressive syndromes, fibromyalgia, and/or chronic fatigue syndrome, either through direct effects upon the central nervous system or indirectly by causing glucocorticoid deficiency."[94,p.69]

Fibromyalgia patients are clearly hypometabolic. Similarly, in Addison's disease (frank adrenal insufficiency), the BMR may fall to -25% or -30%. In pituitary gland deficiency, it may drop to below -50%.[24,p.578] The severely low BMR in pituitary gland deficiency possibly results from a combined metabolism-slowing effect of thyroid hormone deficiency and cortisol deficiency.

Differentiating Glucocorticoid Deficiency as the Source of Fibromyalgia Symptoms

One group of rheumatologists reported that muscle pain and contractures were the initial complaints of 5 patients with Addison's disease.[53] Indeed, muscle pain, spasm, or muscle contractures may be the first indications of insidiously developing primary adrenal insufficiency. These effects probably result from low serum sodium and elevated serum potassium.[52] Such values in the SMAC or ACP of a patient with pain should prompt the clinician to explore the possibility of adrenal insufficiency. Sonkin wrote that the clinician can confirm adrenal insufficiency by several findings: pigmentation of skin and mucous membranes, low blood pressure, postural hypotension, cachexia, weakness, electrolyte abnormalities, high serum ACTH, and a subnormal or absent rise of the serum cortisol 1 hour after an injection of synthetic ACTH. He also wrote that male patients often have a eunuchoid appearance, thin facial hair, sallowness, poor muscle development, weakness, low libido, testicular atrophy, and possibly a high-pitched voice.[54,p.57]

Hyperpigmentation is absent, however, in adrenal insufficiency secondary to pituitary tumor, infarction, or hemorrhage. As in primary adrenal insufficiency, the patient may have muscle pain, stiffness, and spasm due to low levels of sodium ions in the circulation (hyponatremia).[54,p.57]

Thyroid Hormone Status and the Chronic Stress of Fibromyalgia

Demitrack and Crofford noted that low cortisol levels increase the likelihood of inflammatory disease.[94,p.69] In inflammatory disease due either to withdrawal of cortisol medication or surgical removal of the adrenal glands, the autoimmune thyroiditis of some patients may be exacerbated.[122] The exacerbation may account in part for the patients experiencing symptoms of myalgia, arthralgia, and muscle weakness.[123] It is possible, then, that severe enough adrenal insufficiency may precede thyroiditis and subsequent hypothyroidism. The hypothyroidism may manifest as fibromyalgia signs and symptoms. My colleagues and I[124][125] and other researchers[126][127] found that between 10% and 14% of fibromyalgia patients had primary hypothyroidism. Considering this, even if adrenal insufficiency increases autoimmune thyroiditis in some fibromyalgia patients, resulting in hypothyroidism, this mechanism would probably not occur in more than about 14% of patients. That leaves 86% of fibromyalgia patients free from this putative HPA or adrenal mechanism. If the hypothesis I present in this book is true, and accordingly fibromyalgia is most often a manifestation of inadequate thyroid hormone regulation of fibromyalgia-related tissues, then adrenal insufficiency would induce the inadequate thyroid hormone regulation in only a small percentage of patients.

In response to my initial report of a high incidence of primary and central hypothyroidism in fibromyalgia,[124] Bennett wrote to me in 1996, "I suspect the central hypothyroidism you described . . . is a chronic stress response to long-term pain and its consequences."[56] Riedel et al. reiterated this conjecture in a 1998 paper. Among other hormonal abnormalities in fibromyalgia, they surmised that the blunted TSH response to TRH and low basal levels of T_3 result from a central nervous system adjustment to chronic pain and stress. These researchers proposed a putative mechanism for the blunted TSH response to TRH and the low T_3 levels in fibromyalgia patients: stress-induced secretion of CRH increases hypothalamic secretion of somatostatin, and the somatostatin in turn inhibits TSH secretion.[164]

This putative mechanism is unlikely for several reasons. First, in one study of fibromyalgia patients' thyroid status, of those who had laboratory results con-

sistent with central hypothyroidism, 45% had exaggerated rather than blunted TSH responses to TRH.[124] Results from a second study by my colleagues and I were consistent with this result.[125] Second, to my knowledge, Riedel et al. did not confirm elevated somatostatin levels in fibromyalgia patients. Third, increased secretion of CRH, which Riedel et al. wrote stimulates somatostatin secretion, is contrary to Demitrack's and Crofford's proposals that low CRH secretion is instrumental in the HPA axis abnormalities in fibromyalgia (see section above titled "Hypothalamic-Pituitary-Adrenal Axis Abnormalities in Fibromyalgia"). Fourth, if central hypothyroidism were a result of prolonged stress in fibromyalgia patients, the patients would benefit from anti-stress treatments rather than metabolic rehabilitation involving the use of exogenous thyroid hormone. But the available data do not support the proposition that prolonged stress is the cause of the central hypothyroidism: studies of anti-stress treatments for fibromyalgia have shown that the treatments benefit fibromyalgia patients minimally at best,[58][59][60][61][62][63] and I know of no patient who has markedly improved or recovered from fibromyalgia through even prolonged anti-stress therapies. Fifth, the measures of elevated cortisol that Riedel et al. reported are not likely to account for the low TSH and T_3 levels in fibromyalgia patients. Reduced conversion of T_4 to T_3 and suppression of TSH due to elevated cortisol are transient anti-thyroid effects, lasting only a few weeks even when cortisol levels remain elevated.[64][65][66][90][132,p.843] In addition, the report by Riedel et al. of elevated cortisol in fibromyalgia patients conflicts with the reports of other researchers.[57,p.101][67][94] If the other reports are accurate, even a transient anti-thyroid effect in fibromyalgia patients is unlikely.

It is therefore unlikely that stress is the underlying cause of the abnormal thyroid status of fibromyalgia patients. Despite this, elevated cortisol levels may precipitate the tissue hypometabolism that underlies fibromyalgia. Careful scrutiny of patients' histories and other medical records suggests that some individuals had marginal metabolic sufficiency long before developing fibromyalgia (see subsection below titled "Stress-Related Cortisol Elevation May Precipitate Fibromyalgia by Slowing Already Marginally Adequate Metabolism in Fibromyalgia-Related Tissues"). Presumably, the marginally adequate metabolic rate of these patients was not so low as to produce persistent or intense symptoms and signs of hypometabolism. The patients either had no symptoms or only mild, intermittent symptoms. In these patients, further metabolic slow-down due to a slight, temporary decrease in

T_3 levels[136] from cortisol elevation during stress may have precipitated their fibromyalgia symptoms and signs. (See section below titled "High Cortisol Transiently Suppresses the Thyroid System.") This mechanism might explain the proposal of Crofford that in women, postnatal stress may cause dysfunction of the hypothalamic-pituitary-adrenal stress system, and the dysfunction may leave the women vulnerable to developing fibromyalgia.[95,p.193] Of course, most women with postnatal stress do not develop fibromyalgia. In some women, however, who already have marginally adequate metabolism in fibromyalgia-related tissues, elevated cortisol levels associated with postnatal stress may slow their metabolism sufficiently more to generate symptoms of hypometabolism. Clinicians may then diagnose the symptoms as fibromyalgia.

Conclusions

If adrenal insufficiency mediates the features of a patient's fibromyalgia, the patient should recover from fibromyalgia when the use of exogenous cortisol corrects the insufficiency. In this case, we can consider the patient's fibromyalgia a clinical phenotype of adrenal insufficiency—meaning, of course, that the symptoms and signs diagnosed as fibromyalgia are merely manifestations of the deficiency of cortisol. (For the proper protocol for diagnosing adrenal insufficiency see Chapter 5.2, section titled "Adrenal Insufficiency.") However, not all fibromyalgia patients have abnormalities of the HPA axis. In addition, abnormalities of the HPA axis do not provide a plausible explanation for a number of features of fibromyalgia. These features include the exaggerated TSH responses to TRH in some patients. Inadequate thyroid hormone regulation of cell function more cogently accounts for all the features of fibromyalgia, including the HPA axis abnormalities.

A PUTATIVE ETIOLOGICAL AND EXACERBATING ROLE FOR INCREASED CORTISOL LEVELS

Stress-Related Cortisol Elevation May Precipitate Fibromyalgia by Slowing Already Marginally Adequate Metabolism in Fibromyalgia-Related Tissues

From my communications with fibromyalgia patients, I learned that many had the same, albeit milder, symptoms and signs of hypometabolism typical of fibromyalgia for many years before some acute physical or psychological stress precipitated full-blown fibro-

myalgia. The conclusion is compelling that marginally sufficient metabolism—at least in some tissues—predisposed these patients to fibromyalgia. Occasionally through the years, the marginally sufficient metabolism gave rise to fibromyalgia-like symptoms and signs upon the occurrence of some metabolism-slowing event. Such events include physical trauma; psychological stress; deconditioning from periods of physical inactivity; dieting; and abstention from the use of nutritional supplements, particularly B complex vitamins. It is my suspicion that in some patients, the HPA axis is normal until some inciting stress slows metabolism by increasing cortisol levels,[11] or until some other factors further slow metabolism. Then, the patient with marginally sufficient metabolism in fibromyalgia-related tissues develops distinct symptoms of hypometabolism.

High Cortisol Transiently Suppresses the Thyroid System

Cortisol inhibits TSH secretion.[10][17][22] The resulting decreased TSH level reduces thyroid hormone secretion by the thyroid gland. Cortisol also inhibits T_4 to T_3 conversion, reducing the circulating T_3 level.[1][68] Through these two anti-thyroid effects, increased cortisol levels during stress may reduce the metabolic rate of tissues. The reduction may be sufficient to result in symptoms of hypometabolism.[11]

Investigators have debated whether patients are hypometabolic during transient impairment of T_4 to T_3 conversion. However, a study of fasting individuals suggests that hypometabolism does occur. During fasting, if the metabolic rate were to remain normal, tissue proteins would be mobilized from virtually all tissues to produce glucose through gluconeogenesis. As a result, the individual would undergo protein loss. Decreased conversion of T_4 to T_3 minimizes protein loss during fasting. The reduced T_3 level slows the metabolic rate. The reduced metabolic rate reduces the glucose requirement of tissues, and the reduced requirement for glucose minimizes how much protein the body must mobilize for glucose production. So despite the reduced food intake, the individual may not lose much tissue protein. However, if the individual's metabolic rate increases during fasting because she takes exogenous T_3, more protein loss occurs.[136] This finding suggests that reduced T_4 to T_3 conversion spares tissue proteins during fasting by decreasing the metabolic rate. Thus, reduced T_3 levels during fasting appear to decrease the metabolic rate and may cause transient tissue hypometabolism.

Two factors appear to facilitate a patient's developing symptoms of hypometabolism in the above scenario: (1) marginal metabolic adequacy in fibromyalgia-related tissues slowing further from the reduced T_3 level; and (2) the individual interpreting events in her life (such as her fibromyalgia prognosis) as threatening, thereby potentiating ACTH and cortisol secretion and further slowing metabolism. The individual with a substantial metabolic safety margin may not develop symptoms of hypometabolism during times of stress. However, the individual with marginally adequate metabolism may easily develop symptoms.

Exacerbation and Induction of Fibromyalgia by Exogenous Corticosteroids. Two reports suggest that the use of exogenous glucocorticoids may induce or worsen fibromyalgia. Supraphysiologic levels of glucocorticoids may interfere with the secretion of TSH and conversion of T_4 to T_3. The interference may induce fibromyalgia symptoms through inadequate metabolic drive, or the interference might worsen fibromyalgia through worsening metabolic insufficiency. A study by Clark et al. supports the latter possibility. They reported that when fibromyalgia patients were treated with prednisone (a glucocorticoid), their condition actually worsened somewhat.[12]

A report by Yunus suggests that the use of glucocorticoids may induce fibromyalgia. He studied polymyalgia rheumatica (PMR) patients who developed fibromyalgia when treated with glucocorticoids. He wrote, "We have encountered cases of typical PMR with greatly increased ESR [erythrocyte sedimentation rate] who responded satisfactorily to a low-dose corticosteroid preparation, only to develop features of FMS at a later date. Fatigue disproportional to disease activity of PMR, increased number of tender points, a lack of satisfactory response to an increased dose of the corticosteroid preparation, and a normal (or modestly increased) ESR are indicative of a diagnosis of concomitant FMS."[13,p.14]

Trauma (Stress)-Precipitated Fibromyalgia. A patient's cortisol level may rise subsequent to the trauma that precipitates her fibromyalgia or during subsequent periods of emotional distress. Smythe conjectured that trauma could precipitate fibromyalgia,[19] and Wolfe wrote that 24% of patients reported that trauma caused their fibromyalgia.[20] A study by Greenfield et al. illustrates this. They found that 29 of 127 patients (23%) diagnosed as having primary fibromyalgia reported having trauma, surgery, or a medical illness (all of which most likely upregulate the HPA axis in normal individuals) before the onset of their fibromyalgia. Of these 29 patients, 25 developed fibromyalgia following trauma or surgery. The population

of hospital patients has a high incidence of fibromyalgia. Greenfield et al. classified the 23% of patients with pre-fibromyalgic trauma as having "reactive" fibromyalgia. These patients had more disabling symptoms than patients with fibromyalgia not associated with trauma. As a result, the traumatized patients had an unemployment rate of 70%, disability compensation rate of 34%, and reduced rate of physical activity of 35%.[18,p.680]

Putative Etiologic Role of Decreased Physical Activity. Greenfield et al. speculated that the trauma or surgery that precipitated fibromyalgia in some of their patients may have done so by reducing physical activity. They concluded this from the report by 45% of his reactive fibromyalgia patients that the trauma or surgery reduced their physical activity, and that the reduced activity preceded the onset of fibromyalgia.[18,p.680] Inactivity following stress-activated cortisol increase could well contribute to the development of fibromyalgia in individuals with marginally sufficient metabolism in fibromyalgia-related tissues. This would occur because decreased physical activity further reduces their metabolic rate (see Chapter 5.5, sections titled "Effects of Aerobic Exercise on Resting Metabolic Rate" and "Resistance Training"). This reduction may cause their metabolic rate to cross the threshold into the critically low range where symptoms and signs of fibromyalgia can occur.

If this mechanism is instrumental in some patients developing fibromyalgia, we must ask a question that leads back to the hypothesis I propose in this book—why does physical inactivity induce symptoms and signs of hypometabolism (fibromyalgia) in some individuals but not others? The most plausible answer is that individuals who develop symptoms and signs are predisposed by too small a safety margin of tissue metabolic sufficiency.

Myofascial Lesions as Stress Stimuli. The metabolic rate of patients with myofascial pain may be slowed in a similar way: by being predisposed by too small a safety margin of tissue metabolic sufficiency. Noxious signals from myofascial trigger points are transmitted into the central nervous system through types C and A delta nerve fibers. In the brainstem, collateral branches of these fibers stimulate the reticular activating system (RAS). Stimulation of the reticular system gives rise to intense generalized physical and mental arousal. The signals may also be transmitted to the thalamus and then relayed to the hypothalamus, producing mass discharge of the sympathetic nervous system. This activation of the RAS and discharge of the sympathetic nervous system constitute intense stress of myofascial origin.[2][3][4]

An important component of this type of stress response is the secretion of increased amounts of stress hormones. Patients with pain of myofascial origin had higher than normal glucocorticoid secretion[6][7] and increased urine levels of adrenaline and noradrenaline.[5] These endocrine findings would be far more likely found in patients with multiple myofascial pain syndromes.[137] The stress-induced increased output of endogenous glucocorticoids may be sufficient to transiently inhibit TSH secretion and the conversion of T_4 to T_3. This in turn may impair the patient's energy metabolism enough in various tissues to produce the complex of symptoms termed fibromyalgia, and these symptoms are likely to lead to a diagnosis of fibromyalgia. When an increased glucocorticoid level transiently impairs T_4 to T_3 conversion during stress, rT_3 is elevated while the free T_3 is low or low-normal. The 24-hour urinary cortisol is high. The clinician should find this pattern of laboratory test values before concluding that inhibited T_4 to T_3 conversion is instrumental in the patient's condition. The pattern is likely to be found only early during the patient's stress experience, as elevated cortisol levels impair T_4 to T_3 conversion for only a few weeks.

Other Anti-Thyroid Effects of Elevated Cortisol from Acute Stress

Elevated Glucocorticoids May Increase the Rate of Hepatic Clearance of T_4 from the Body. An elevated glucocorticoid level may hasten the liver's clearance of T_4 from the patient's body. The increased rate of clearance decreases the amount of T_4 available for conversion to T_3. Testing showed that glucocorticoids caused a small increase of the T_4 disappearance rate from the plasma. Wiener and Lindeboom wrote that after administering 20 mg per day of prednisone to a patient with "impaired peripheral utilization" of thyroid hormones, the disappearance rate of T_4 increased from 4.6% to 11.4%. They judged this rate of increase a significant change. The clearance rate of T_4 is also increased by the intake of Tegretol®, dioxins, and PCBs[21, pp.452-453] (see Chapter 2.4).

Elevated Cortisol May Lower Thyroid Binding Globulin Levels. Elevated glucocorticoid levels decrease the level of thyroid binding globulin (TBG) by speeding its hepatic clearance.[23] A patient's blood profile may show low-normal T_3, low-normal T_4, high-normal or high T_3 uptake, and low-normal or normal TSH.[24,pp.188-189] The clinician may refer to increased T_3 uptake and conclude that the patient is euthyroid or slightly hyperthyroid, although the patient may actual-

ly be hypometabolic due to decreases in TSH secretion and T_4 to T_3 conversion. An elevated rT_3 would indicate that the high cortisol level is blocking deiodination of T_4 to T_3. However, if a patient with elevated cortisol actually has primary hypothyroidism, her rT_3 may be low rather than high.[24,p.188] Even so, making the diagnosis of true hypothyroidism in patients using glucocorticoids is difficult and perhaps impossible.[24,p.189]

● INADEQUATE THYROID HORMONE REGULATION OF TRANSCRIPTION MAY MEDIATE THE ABNORMALITIES OF THE HYPOTHALAMIC-PITUITARY-ADRENAL AXIS IN FIBROMYALGIA

Fibromyalgia researchers have largely ignored the role of thyroid hormone in the regulation of the HPA axis. The basis of this mistake is the researchers' subscription to the false propositions of the current endocrinology paradigm regarding the use of TSH levels in the diagnosis and treatment of hypothyroidism (see Chapters 2.5 and 5.3). Nonetheless, inadequate thyroid hormone regulation of cell function can account for the abnormalities of the HPA axis found in some fibromyalgia patients.

INADEQUATE THYROID HORMONE REGULATION OF CRH AND CORTISOL SECRETION IN FIBROMYALGIA

Fibromyalgia patients have a precarious prognosis, and they are often distressed over failed treatments and accusations that their condition is psychogenic. These experiences for most patients constitute adverse stimuli (stressors) that are likely to increase activity of the HPA axis. When patients experience such stressors chronically, upregulation of the HPA axis would be expected. The decreased CRH response to insulin-induced hypoglycemia is consistent with chronic stress-induced activation of the axis, and so are elevated AVP levels. But subnormal cortisol secretion due to stress is not consistent with the finding in fibromyalgia patients of normal ACTH secretion. Normal ACTH would be maintained by increased AVP secretion compensating for reduced CRH secretion. However, inadequate thyroid hormone regulation of both the hypothalamic CRH- and AVP-secreting cells and of the adrenal cortices provides a plausible explanation for fibromyalgia patients' exaggerated ACTH secretion and their subnormal cortisol secretion.

When thyroid hormone regulation of CRH-synthesizing hypothalamic cells is inadequate, CRH secretion decreases. We would expect the synthesis and secretion of ACTH by the pituitary corticotrophs to be subnormal as a result of the decreased CRH secretion (see next section: "Effects of Thyroid Hormone Deficiency on the Hypothalamic-Pituitary-Adrenal Axis"). However, in hypothyroidism (and in fibromyalgia), hypothalamic cells secrete more AVP to compensate for the reduced CRH secretion. In response to AVP, ACTH secretion may be normal. In fibromyalgia, however, ACTH in response to injected CRH or insulin-induced hypoglycemia is exaggerated. The exaggerated response suggests that the pituitary corticotrophs have a reserve of ACTH. This is an unexpected result of normal ACTH synthesis and secretion maintained by AVP in compensation for reduced CRH. The most likely explanation for the exaggerated ACTH response is subnormal secretion and circulating levels of cortisol caused by other factors. The most probable other factor is inadequate regulation by thyroid hormone of the cortices of the adrenal gland. Cortisol normally inhibits pituitary ACTH-synthesizing corticotroph cells. When cortisol secretion is subnormal, as in some hypothyroid patients, the corticotrophs are disinhibited and increase their production of ACTH. The increased synthesis causes an increased reserve of ACTH in the cells. The increased reserve is detected as an exaggerated ACTH response to injected CRH or to insulin-induced hypoglycemia.

EFFECTS OF THYROID HORMONE DEFICIENCY ON THE HYPOTHALAMIC-PITUITARY-ADRENAL AXIS

The material in this section highlights the similarities between the HPA abnormalities in fibromyalgia and those in hypothyroidism (the archetypal form of inadequate thyroid hormone regulation of cell function). Table 3.5.1 displays the documented HPA axis abnormalities in hypothyroid patients compared to those in fibromyalgia and chronic fatigue syndrome patients. We must keep in mind that such comparisons are based on limited data from the study of fibromyalgia and chronic fatigue syndrome. Some differences or similarities between these conditions may be due to sampling error and differences in assessment techniques. Future studies should gradually disclose the

true degree of overlap between these two diagnostic groups.

Thyroid Hormone Status and the HPA Axis

In view of the evidence that thyroid status profoundly influences the HPA axis, it is puzzling that so many researchers have ignored the association. An example is the review by Grossman et al. of the factors that regulate the secretion of CRH. As factors that inhibit CRH synthesis and secretion, they list GABA, substance P (see Chapter 3.19), atrial natriuretic peptide, opioid peptides, and precursors of nitric oxide; as factors that stimulate CRH production and release, they list noradrenaline, acetylcholine, serotonin, neuropeptide Y, and interleukins 1 and 6. They fail altogether to mention the potent and omnipresent stimulatory influence of thyroid hormone, and they fail to list the inhibitory influence of inadequate exposure of hypothalamic cells to thyroid hormone.[91] The same neglect is obvious in the fibromyalgia literature where HPA abnormalities are explored. Demitrack and Crofford, for example, propose six possible causes of the HPA abnormalities in fibromyalgia and chronic fatigue syndrome: a primary adrenocortical defect, altered pituitary sensitivity, altered hypothalamic drive, disruption of neural or biochemical suprahypothalamic influences, altered circadian rhythm, and increased sensitivity to negative feedback by glucocorticoids.[94,p.71] They do not mention thyroid status.

Below, I review the literature bearing on the relation of thyroid status to the function of the HPA axis. The studies show that adequate or inadequate exposure of HPA axis cells to thyroid hormone profoundly affects the axis.

CRH. Crofford conjectured that the decreased responsiveness of the adrenal cortex in fibromyalgia patients could be due to impaired function of the adrenal cortex itself. The evidence I present in the section below on cortisol, however, suggests that inadequate thyroid hormone regulation is the most likely candidate for impaired adrenocortical function.

Crofford also proposed an alternative cause for decreased responsiveness of the adrenal cortex: "in the context of chronic overstimulation . . ." she wrote, the cause might be a CRH deficiency.[95] Demitrack et al. made a similar speculation: that the low maximum adrenocortical response to ACTH is compatible with secondary adrenal atrophy and that this suggests CRH insufficiency.[92] However, secondary adrenal atrophy due to a deficiency of CRH may be incompatible with Crofford's finding of increased AVP in fibromyalgia patients. If the increased AVP maintains normal

ACTH secretion, the normal ACTH secretion would in turn maintain normal cortisol secretion—that is, if the adrenal cortices are capable of normal responsiveness to ACTH. Inadequate thyroid hormone regulation of CRH- and AVP-secreting cells and the adrenal cortices is a highly plausible mechanism for the decreased CRH, increased AVP, exaggerated ACTH, and subnormal cortisol in fibromyalgia. Exactly the same pattern occurs in hypothyroidism. (See section below titled "ACTH.") However, if decreased CRH secretion is instrumental in subnormal cortisol secretion in fibromyalgia, inadequate thyroid hormone regulation of CRH-secreting hypothalamic cells is the most likely mechanism.

In one study, response of the HPA axis to insulin-induced hypoglycemia was normal-to-slightly decreased in mild hypothyroidism.[130] In progressively more severe hypothyroidism, the HPA axis was markedly less responsive.[131] Kamilaris et al. tested the response of the HPA axis to induced hypocortisolemia in hypothyroid patients. The researchers lowered cortisol levels with the drug metyrapone. They found increased sensitivity of the pituitary corticotrophs to CRH, but a decreased ACTH response to lower plasma cortisol levels. They concluded, in accord with other researchers, that hypothyroid patients have reduced HPA axis responsiveness to both low cortisol levels and to induced hypoglycemia. They wrote that the results suggest that the secretion of hypothalamic CRH and other ACTH secretagogues are decreased in hypothyroidism.[129]

Several studies have documented thyroid hormone regulation of the CRH transcript. When thyroid hormone levels are adequate, CRH mRNA increases;[25,p.1577] when thyroid hormone is deficient, CRH mRNA decreases.[25][29][30] Ceccatelli and colleagues induced hypothyroidism in rats by surgical ablation of the thyroid gland. At 28 and 50 days after surgery, the hypothalamic paraventricular nuclei of the rats contained a significantly decreased quantity of CRH mRNA. Administering T_4 increased mRNA levels.[30] Similarly, Shi et al. used propylthiouracil to chemically induce hypothyroidism in rats. The hypothyroidism caused a significant decrease in transcription of the CRH gene in the paraventricular nuclei of the rats.

Shi et al. also found a decrease in pituitary pro-opiomelanocortin (POMC).[25] (POMC is the precursor to eight peptide hormones, each produced through an alternate cleavage pathway. ACTH is one of the cleavage products.[26,pp.682-683][27,p.1351][28,p.486]) The decreased POMC most likely resulted from decreased secretion of CRH. The decrease in POMC found by Shi et al.

was reversed by treatment with T_3.

Shi et al. also found that hypothyroidism decreased circulating corticosterone.[25,p.1580] Decreased POMC in hypothyroidism, with a consequent decrease in its cleaved product, ACTH, caused decreased cortisol levels. In contrast, increased POMC in thyrotoxicosis[32][33][34] caused increased ACTH activity and increased circulating cortisol.[35]

The effects of thyroid hormone on the HPA axis reported by Shi et al. were not secondary to reduced levels of circulating corticosterone. The investigators concluded this because hypothyroidism decreased CRH transcription even when adrenalectomized rats received replacement doses of corticosterone. (Administering high doses of corticosterone or removing the adrenal glands did not affect the pituitary-thyroid gland axis.)[25]

Shi et al. wrote, "We conclude that circulating levels of thyroid hormones have a major effect on the central regulation of the hypothalamic-pituitary-adrenal axis."[25,p.1577] Thus, they argued that ". . . hypothyroidism causes a highly significant depression of the activity of the hypothalamic-pituitary-adrenal axis."[25,p.1579]

Indirect Effects of Inadequate Thyroid Hormone Regulation. I mentioned above that thyroid hormone directly effects the HPA axis. Thyroid hormone also has indirect effects on the axis. Thyroid hormone exerts its main indirect effect by regulation of the adrenergic system (see Chapter 3.1).

One anatomic site where thyroid hormone regulates the adrenergic system is the norepinephrine-secreting neurons in the brain stem. The axons of these neurons ascend to higher brain centers and secrete norepinephrine.[36,p.261] Thyroid hormone significantly impacts catecholamine-secreting neurons that project from the brain stem to the hypothalamic paraventricular nucleus.[39] Activation of these neurons increases the hypothalamic levels of CRH mRNA in response to stress.[40][42]

Szafarczyk and coworkers found that disruption of the catecholamine innervation of the paraventricular nucleus alone reduced CRH levels in the hypothalamic-pituitary portal vessels. (The portal vessels are the blood vessels through which hormone releasing factors travel from the hypothalamus to the anterior pituitary gland.) Disrupting catecholamine innervation reduced CRH levels by 57%. In addition, the disrupted innervation reduced plasma levels of ACTH by 35%. The lesion did not impair stress-induced ACTH release.[42] The failure of the lesion of the paraventricular nucleus to more completely suppress ACTH secretion suggests that other noradrenergic pathways (such as the ventral noradrenergic ascending bundle) also play a role in stress-induced activation of the HPA axis.[42]

Another indirect effect of thyroid hormone is regulation of serotonin secretion through the adrenergic system. During inadequate thyroid hormone regulation of transcription of the α_2-adrenergic receptor gene in serotonergic neurons, the density of α_2-adrenergic receptors on serotonergic neuronal membranes increases. The receptors, upon binding to catecholamines, inhibit the synthesis and secretion of serotonin by the neurons. (See Chapter 3.1, subsection titled "Serotonin.") Serotonin is important to the circadian rhythm of HPA activity[112] and is involved in the secretion of CRH and AVP.[111][113] By decreasing serotonin secretion via an increased density of the inhibitory α_2-adrenergic receptors on serotonergic neurons, inadequate thyroid hormone regulation of the α_2-adrenergic receptor gene may indirectly diminish the regulatory impact of serotonin on the HPA axis.

Still another mechanism through which inadequate thyroid hormone regulation of the α_2-adrenergic receptor gene may reduce CRH secretion is inhibition of superior cervical sympathetic ganglion function. In hypothyroidism, both CRH and AVP secretion may be subnormal due to inhibited function of the superior cervical sympathetic ganglia. The sympathetic afferent fibers originating in the superior cervical sympathetic ganglion terminate in the median eminence of the hypothalamus.[120] In hypothyroidism, the density of α_2-adrenergic receptors on sympathetic ganglion cells increases. These receptors inhibit both pre- and post-ganglionic sympathetic neurons. This adrenergically-mediated blockade of the sympathetic ganglia reduces sympathetic nervous system drive. As a result, neural output from the sympathetic ganglia is diminished. In the periphery, one result is a subnormal cardiovascular response to stressors such as exercise, as happens in fibromyalgia patients. (See Chapter 3.1, subsection titled "Inhibition of Sympathetic Ganglionic Neural Transmission by an Increased α_2-Adrenergic Receptor Density on Ganglion Cells.") Inhibition of the superior cervical ganglion impacts structures in the central nervous system. One effect is decreased secretion of both CRH (as appears to occur in fibromyalgia) and AVP. Decreased secretion of CRH and AVP occurred following superior cervical ganglionectomy.[154] Impaired superior cervical sympathetic ganglion function by chemical blockade from α_2-adrenergic receptors may be similar to surgical blockade by ganglionectomy.

AVP. Demitrack and Crofford wrote that their preliminary data indicated increased AVP levels in fibromyalgia patients.[94,p.71] Crofford et al. found a trend toward increased AVP secretion following postural change in fibromyalgia patients. The increase in 5 of 12 patients (41%) was greater than two standard deviations above the highest value for a control patient.[93] Crofford noted that AVP becomes increasingly active in stimulating ACTH secretion when the HPA axis is chronically stimulated.[95,p.189] She also cited studies showing that when rats are subjected to chronic stress (through polyarthritis or surgically-induced cholestasis), they produce less CRH mRNA, secrete less CRH, lose the circadian rhythm of ACTH and corticosterone release, and secrete much more AVP.[102][106][107]

Salomez-Granier et al. reported that of 22 patients with untreated hypothyroidism, 4 (18%) had elevated AVP levels.[161] Others have also reported finding elevated AVP levels in hypothyroidism.[138][139][140][142][158][160] However, others reported both high and normal levels[155][160] and others, low levels.[157][159] In the hypothyroid rat, vasoactive intestinal peptide (VIP) and VIP mRNA increase in the parvocellular and magnocellular neurons and the hypothalamic paraventricular nucleus. In that VIP stimulates AVP secretion, increases in VIP may mediate increased AVP secretion in hypothyroidism.[156] Low or even normal AVP levels in hypothyroid patients may result from suppressed hypothalamic secretion due to impaired superior cervical sympathetic ganglion function. Impairment of the ganglion in hypothyroidism results from hyperpolarization of pre- and post-ganglia cells by an increased density of α_2-adrenergic receptors on the cells (see section above "Indirect Effects of Inadequate Thyroid Hormone Regulation"). Elevated AVP levels in hypothyroid patients return to normal upon treatment with exogenous thyroid hormone.[138][142]

By suppressing the thyroid system, acute stress may decrease CRH and increase AVP secretion. Acute stress increases circulating cortisol levels. The elevated cortisol decreases TSH secretion and blocks T_4 to T_3 conversion. The resulting low levels of T_3 may decrease CRH production and increase production of AVP. However, the thyroid system escapes from the suppressive effects of cortisol within a few weeks; the system escapes even if cortisol levels remain elevated. So this mechanism might account for decreased CRH levels and increased AVP levels only transiently. (See Chapter 2.5, section titled "Proposal of a Sustained Euthyroid Sick Syndrome Under the Expropriated Name 'Wilson's Syndrome.'")

Table 3.5.1. Comparison of HPA abnormalities in fibromyalgia, chronic fatigue syndrome,* and hypothyroidism.

		FIBROMYALGIA	CHRONIC FATIGUE SYNDROME	HYPOTHYROIDISM
Hypothalamus	● Insulin-induced hypoglycemia	Impaired ?	?	?
	● CSF CRH, ACTH	Reduced ?	Reduced ?	?
	● CRH mRNA	?	Reduced	Reduced
	● Arginine-vasopressin	Elevated	Elevated	Elevated
	● Diurnal rhythm	Blunted	?	?
Pituitary	● Basal pm ACTH	Normal	Elevated	?
	● ACTH response to CRH	Exaggerated	Blunted	Exaggerated
	● POMC (precursor to ACTH)	?	?	Reduced (secondary to decreased CRH)
Adrenocortices	● Basal blood cortisol	Elevated in pm	Reduced	Low-to-elevated. Elevated with slowed liver clearance Reduced when POMC low
	● Cortisol secretion	Low	Low	Low
	● Liver cortisol clearance	?	?	Reduced
	● Corticosterone	?	?	Reduced when CRH & POMC low
	● Corticosterone response to ACTH	?	?	Blunted
	● 24-hr urinary cortisol	Reduced	Reduced	Increased with slowed liver clearance
	● Cortisol response to ACTH	Blunted	↑ sensitivity ↓ capacity	? ?
	● Cortisol response to CRH	Blunted	Normal	?
Cortisol binding globulin		Normal	?	?

*Modified from: Demitrack, M.A. and Crofford, L.J.: Hypothalamic-pituitary-adrenal axis dysregulation in fibromyalgia and chronic fatigue syndrome: an overview and hypothesis. *J. Musculoskel. Pain*, 3(2):67-73, 1995.[94,p.70]

ACTH. In the last few years, several investigators have reported exaggerated ACTH secretion in laboratory animals and humans with overt[155][162][163] and subclinical hypothyroidism.[165] This finding is consistent with the reports of exaggerated ACTH responses to insulin-induced hypoglycemia and injected CRH in fibromyalgia patients (see subsection above titled "Hypothalamic-Pituitary-Adrenal Axis Abnormalities in Fibromyalgia: ACTH Response").

Sànchez-Franco et al. reported that ACTH and corticosterone levels decreased in hypothyroid rats and increased in hyperthyroid rats. They concluded,

"These data give support to the important role of thyroid hormones in ACTH regulation and, therefore, in the adaptation to stress."[34] Similarly, Martino et al. wrote that in patients with primary or central hypothyroidism, pituitary hormones other than TSH are commonly deficient. They recommended specific basal and stimulation tests, such as the CRH stimulation test, to identify deficiencies. They noted that the thyroid hormone deficiency may be the cause of deficiencies of other pituitary hormones.[51,p.787] For example, ACTH (and in turn, cortisol) may be deficient. Thyroid hormone therapy may restore ACTH (and cortisol) levels to normal.[152]

In 1987, Kamilaris et al. reported results that contradict the reports of Sànchez-Franco et al. and Martino et al. of reduced ACTH secretion in hypothyroidism. Kamilaris and colleagues reported an exaggerated ACTH response to intravenous CRH in short-duration hypothyroidism. They concluded that hypothyroidism increased pituitary corticotroph sensitivity to CRH. At the same time, however, the ACTH response to hypocortisolemia (induced by metyrapone, a drug that suppresses adrenocortical secretion) was decreased.[129]

In 1991, Kamilaris et al. reported more definitive results. In this study, they assessed the plasma ACTH and corticosterone responses to CRH in two groups of rats: (1) hypothyroid rats at 7, 15, and 60 days after thyroidectomy and (2) rats made thyrotoxic with excessive amounts of T_4. The investigators' purpose was to learn the time-dependent effects of altered thyroid status on the function of the HPA axis. They found that after becoming hypothyroid, the rats initially had a decrease in cerebrospinal fluid levels of corticosterone, a decrease in weight of the adrenal gland, and an increase in the ACTH response to CRH. These findings were consistent with those they reported in 1987. But they also reported a decreased corticosterone response to ACTH released in response to CRH. This is similar to the reduced cortisol response of fibromyalgia patients.[93][97] As the rats' hypothyroidism continued, cerebrospinal fluid levels of corticosterone fell progressively, and the ACTH response to CRH progressively increased. In rats made thyrotoxic by T_4 treatment, the findings were generally the converse of those in hypothyroidism. The investigators wrote that their data did not reveal the precise HPA axis location principally affected by altered thyroid status. "However," they concluded, "these data are most compatible with a subtle hypothyroid-induced centrally mediated adrenal insufficiency and a subtle hyperthyroid-induced centrally mediated hypercortisolism. These data also suggest that alterations in HPA axis function in states of disturbed thyroid function become somewhat more pronounced as the duration of thyroid dysfunction increases."[133] The increased incidence of altered HPA axis function in longer duration hypothyroidism may be similar to the finding of Tilbe et al. regarding fibromyalgia patients. The researchers found that the diurnal variation of the serum cortisol level was abnormal in 10 of 20 patients (50%) who had fibromyalgia for fewer than 2 years. But in patients whose fibromyalgia had begun more than 2 years before, the percentage with abnormalities was 70%.[9]

Cortisol. Demitrack and Crofford wrote that decreased secretion of the adrenal cortices is a common feature of fibromyalgia and chronic fatigue syndrome. They suggested that the decreased adrenocortical reserve occurs late in the course of the syndromes, probably developing from chronic overstimulation of the adrenal cortices.[94,pp.71-72]

When the adrenal cortices are involved in hypothyroidism, they secrete a subnormal amount of glucocorticoids. The circulating cortisol levels in hypothyroid patients, however, are not solely a matter of how much the adrenal cortices secrete. The cortisol level is also influenced by the rate at which the liver clears cortisol.

Cortisol Levels in Hypothyroidism. Cortisol levels vary considerably among hypothyroid patients. Studies show that in hypothyroidism, secretion of adrenocortical hormones, their blood levels, hepatic clearance, and urinary excretion may be normal, low, or high. Some researchers have found normal cortisol levels in hypothyroidism,[15][31] and others have found elevated 24-hour urinary cortisol levels.[14]

However, some researchers have reported that thyroid hormone deficiency caused low adrenocortical secretion.[34][72][73][75] Other researchers reported low plasma cortisol levels, low urinary cortisol excretion,[16,p.137][150] and subnormal secretion of corticosterone in response to ACTH administration.[151] Hellman et al. wrote that in hypothyroidism, the rate of cortisol secretion and metabolism can decrease by 50%.[45]

Lo et al. chemically (propylthiouracil) induced hypothyroidism in rats. Then they measured the effects on corticosterone secretion *in vivo* and *in vitro*. Basal secretion and ACTH-stimulated secretion of corticosterone by the zona fasciculata-reticularis cells of the adrenal cortices were reduced. (The zona fasciculata-reticularis is the inner layer of cells of the adrenal cortex. It is located beneath the zona glomerulosa, the outer layer of cells of the cortex just beneath the outer capsule. The reticularis cells secrete cortisol, corticosterone, and dehydroepiandrosterone or DHEA.) Accordingly, the basal and ACTH-stimulated plasma levels of corticosterone in the hypothyroid rats were low. ACTH-stimulated levels of cAMP within cells of the adrenal cortices were low. Also, the activity of three enzymes (β-hydroxysteroid dehydrogenase, 21 β-hydroxylase, and 11 β-hydroxylase) was inhibited. Lo et al. concluded that propylthiouracil nullifies both basal and ACTH-stimulated adrenal steroid hormone production; it does so by attenuating the activity of 11 β-hydroxylase and cAMP production in zona fasciculata-reticularis cells.[166][167]

Variations in the severity and duration of hypothyroidism may partially account for variations in cortisol measures among patients. Noting that hypothyroid patients have subtle abnormalities of HPA function, Dluhy wrote that the severity of the abnormalities correlates with the severity and duration of thyroid hormone deficiency. The relevance of the severity and duration of hypothyroidism is evident in studies of the responses of the adrenal cortices to exogenous ACTH in patients. The response of the adrenal cortices in patients with mild hypothyroidism may be normal or blunted.[132,p.841] Patients with more severe hypothyroidism are more likely to have blunted responses.[130][131] In fibromyalgia patients, the responses of the adrenal cortices to ACTH may differ, depending on the severity or longevity of a patient's inadequate thyroid hormone regulation of adrenocortical function. In one study, a higher percentage of patients with longer-term fibromyalgia had abnormalities of the diurnal variation in cortisol levels.[9]

A contribution to adrenocortical insufficiency in prolonged or severe fibromyalgia may be inadequate compensation of CRH deficiency by AVP. To some degree, AVP compensates for deficient CRH. The compensation sustains ACTH secretion by the pituitary and, in turn, cortisol secretion by the adrenal cortices. However, during prolonged or severe CRH deficiency due to inadequate thyroid hormone regulation of CRH-synthesizing cells, increases in AVP secretion may not be sufficient to compensate for the reduced CRH. Failure of AVP secretion to compensate may occur when the patient has inadequate transcription regulation of the adrenergic receptor genes. The inadequate gene regulation increases the density of α_2-adrenergic receptors on the membranes of the superior cervical sympathetic ganglion cells. An increased density of these receptors on the cells reduces neural flow from the sympathetic ganglia. If the superior cervical sympathetic ganglion is involved, sympathetic innervation of the hypothalamus may be reduced. Consequently, both CRH and AVP secretion may be subnormal (see section above titled "Indirect Effects of Inadequate Thyroid Hormone Regulation"). Low cortisol secretion and resulting exaggerated ACTH secretion may then result.

Reduced Liver Clearance Rate. After cortisol is injected intravenously in some hypothyroid patients, it disappears from the plasma at a slower rate than in euthyroid subjects.[15] The slower rate occurs because of slowed clearance by the liver.[132,p.841] The slowed removal maintains a higher plasma level than when thyroid hormone normally stimulates liver cells.[16,p.137]

Decreased thyroid hormone stimulation of liver cells results in reduced activity of two enzymes (delta4-steroid reductase and 11-β-hydroxysteroid dehydrogenase) that catabolize cortisol.[132,p.841] Reduced activity of the enzymes slows the removal of cortisol from the plasma and clearance of the hormone from the liver.[14] If the blood level of cortisol is normal, normal amounts of cortisol will probably reach the peripheral tissues. The normal exposure should permit normal peripheral tissue responses to cortisol during stress.[132,p.841]

The clinician should bear in mind the relation of liver clearance to the rate of cortisol secretion by the adrenal cortices. Selective involvement of the liver and/or the adrenal cortices can result in different circulating levels of cortisol (see Table 3.5.2). If the liver clearance of cortisol is normal and secretion of cortisol by the adrenal cortices is normal, the circulating cortisol level is likely to be normal. If the liver clearance of cortisol is slowed and secretion of cortisol by the adrenal cortices is decreased, the circulating cortisol level is likely to be normal. If the liver clearance of cortisol is normal and secretion by the adrenal cortices is decreased, the circulating cortisol level is likely to be low. If the liver clearance of cortisol is slowed and the secretion of cortisol by the adrenal cortices is normal, the circulating cortisol level is likely to be elevated.

Slowed liver clearance of cortisol due to inadequate thyroid hormone regulation of liver cells may contribute to the elevated basal pm cortisol levels in some fibromyalgia patients.[67][93] Other factors may also be involved (see next section).

● A MODEL FOR THE HPA ABNORMALITIES IN FIBROMYALGIA

Inadequate thyroid hormone regulation of CRH- and cortisol-secreting cells is sufficient to explain the HPA abnormalities in fibromyalgia. Some hypothyroid patients have the same pattern of laboratory values that some fibromyalgia patients have: decreased CRH, increased AVP, subnormal cortisol, and an exaggerated ACTH response to stimulation. Some investigators have proposed that this pattern of values in fibromyalgia patients results from chronic stress. However, chronic stress does not plausibly account for most of the symptoms and objectively verified abnormalities in fibromyalgia covered in Section III of this book. Especially noteworthy is fibromyalgia patients' impaired glycolysis and increased glycogen deposition. Subnormal cortisol secretion is expected to produce the opposite—increased glycolysis and decreased glycogen deposition. While these findings are contrary to subnormal cortisol levels due to chronic stress, they are consistent with inadequate thyroid hormone regulation of cell function. This putative thyroid hormone-related mechanism plausibly explains both the glycolytic abnormalities and the subnormal cortisol levels.

Table 3.5.2. Different expected levels of circulating cortisol in relation to involvement of the liver and/or the adrenal cortices in thyroid hormone deficiency.

LIVER CLEARANCE OF CORTISOL	ADRENAL SECRETION OF CORTISOL	CIRCULATING CORTISOL LEVEL
↓	↓	normal
normal	↓	↓
↓	normal	↑

Elevated cortisol levels during stress may precipitate fibromyalgia in individuals made susceptible by marginally adequate metabolism in fibromyalgia-related tissues. In normal individuals, increased cortisol levels during stress decrease TSH secretion. The reduced TSH decreases thyroid hormone secretion by the thyroid gland. Increased cortisol levels also decrease the conversion of T_4 to T_3. Both "anti-thyroid" effects decrease circulating T_3 levels. However, the effects last only a few weeks at most. The tissues of most individuals have a metabolic safety margin: The tissue metabolic rate is sufficient to allow some degree of reduction during low T_3 levels without symptoms of hypometabolism developing.

In other individuals, the metabolic rate is marginally sufficient. A small decrease in metabolism when T_3 levels are low results in symptoms of hypometabolism, and clinicians are likely to diagnose the symptoms as fibromyalgia. While experiencing the symptoms, these individuals may become less physically active. If their reduced activity decreases their muscle mass, their metabolism will slow even more. The further slowing of metabolism is likely to increase the intensity of their symptoms.

Within one-to-several weeks, the transient suppression of TSH secretion and decrease of T_4 to T_3 conversion will subside. If the individuals are able to begin exercising again, their metabolism will increase, and their symptoms may completely resolve. But the loss of muscle mass from the reduced physical activity may sustain the reduced metabolism and perpetuate the fibromyalgia symptoms. If the symptoms (such as fatigue and widespread aches and pains) are severe enough, they may prevent the individual from becoming active again. As a result, a progressive loss of muscle mass will further worsen the fibromyalgia. The patient finds herself caught in a downward spiral of progressively worsening symptoms and loss of ability to engage in physical activities.

REFERENCES

1. *Physician's Desk Reference*, 44th edition. Oradell, Medical Economics Co., Inc., 1990, p.715.
2. Guyton, A.C.: *Textbook of Medical Physiology*, 8th edition. W.B. Saunders Co., 1991.
3. Lowe, J.C.: The myofascial genesis of unpleasant thoughts and emotions: its neural basis. *Dig. Chiro. Econ.*, 31(5):80, March/April, 1989.
4. Lowe, J.C.: The emotional effects of noxious myofascial stimulation. *Am. Chiropractor*, 22-24, January, 1989.
5. Russell, I.J.: Is there a metabolic basis for the fibrositis syndrome? *Am. J. Med.*, 81(3A):50:29, 1986.
6. Evaskus, D.S. and Laskin, D.M.: A biochemical measure of stress in patients with myofascial pain-dysfunction syndrome. *J. Dent. Res.*, 51:1464-1466, 1972.
7. Ferraccioli, G., Cavalieri, F., Salaffi, F., Fontana, S., Scita, F., Nolli, M., and Maestri, D.: Neuroendocrinologic findings in primary fibromyalgia (soft tissue chronic pain syndrome) and in other chronic rheumatic conditions (rheumatoid arthritis, low back pain). *J. Rheumatol.*, 17: 869-873, 1990.
8. Hudson, J.I., Pliner, L.F., Hudson, M.S., Goldenberg, D.L., and Melby, J.C.: The dexamethasone suppression test in fibrositis. *Biol. Psychiatry*, 19:1489-1493, 1984.
9. Tilbe, K., Bell, D.A., and McCain, G.A.: Loss of diurnal variation in serum cortisol, growth hormone and prolactin in patients with primary fibromyalgia. *Arthritis Rheumatol.*, 31:S99, 1988.
10. Otsuki, M., Dakoda, M., and Baba, S.: Influence of glucocorticoids on TRH-induced TSH stimulation. *J. Clin. Endocrinol. Metab.*, 36:95, 1973.
11. Lowe, J.C.: T_3 and chronic fatigue. *Dyn. Chiro.*, 9, December 19, 1990.
12. Clark, S., Tindall, E., and Bennett, R.: A double-blind crossover study of prednisone in the treatment of fibrositis (Abstract). *Arthritis Rheumatol.*, 27:S76,1984.
13. Yunus, M.B.: Fibromyalgia syndrome and myofascial pain syndrome: clinical features, laboratory tests, diagnosis, and pathophysiologic mechanisms. In *Myofascial Pain and Fibromyalgia: Trigger Point Management.* Edi-

ted by E.S. Rachlin, St. Louis, Mosby, 1994, pp.3-29.

14. Iranmanish, A., Lizarralde, G., Johnson, M.L., and Veldhuis, J.D.: Dynamics of 24-hour endogenous cortisol secretion and clearance in primary hypothyroidism assessed before and after partial thyroid hormone replacement. *J. Clin. Endocrinol. Metab.*, 70:155, 1990.

15. Peterson, R.E.: The influence of the thyroid on adrenal cortical function. *J. Clin. Invest.*, 37:736, 1958.

16. Peterson, R.E.: Metabolism of adrenal cortical steroids. In *The Human Adrenal Cortex*. Edited by N.P. Christy, New York, Harper and Row, 1971.

17. Re, R.N., Kourides, I.A., Ridgway, E.C., Weintraub, B.D., and Maloof, F.: The effect of glucocorticoid administration on human pituitary secretion of thyrotropin and prolactin. *J. Clin. Endocrinol. Metab.*, 43:338, 1976.

18. Greenfield, S., Fitzcharles, M.-A., and Esdaile, J.M.: Reactive fibromyalgia syndrome. *Arthritis Rheum.*, 35:678-681, 1992.

19. Smythe, H.A.: Nonarticular rheumatism. *Arthritis and Allied Conditions*, 10th edition. Edited by D.J. McCarty, Philadelphia, Lea & Febiger, 1985.

20. Wolfe, F.: The clinical syndrome of fibrositis. *Am. J. Med.*, 81(Suppl.3A):7-14, 1986.

21. Wiener, J.D. and Lindeboom, G.A.: Observations on an unusual case of myxoedema. *Acta Endocrinol.*, 39:439-456, 1962.

22. Bartalena, L., Martino, E., and Brandi, L.S.: Lack of nocturnal serum thyrotropin surge after surgery. *J. Clin. Endocrinol. Metab.*, 70:293, 1990.

23. Oppenheimer, J.H. and Werner, S.C.: Effect of prednisone on thyroxine-binding proteins. *J. Clin. Endocrinol. Metab.*, 26:715, 1966.

24. DeGroot, L.J., Larsen, P.R., Refetoff, S., and Stanbury, J.B.: *The Thyroid and Its Diseases*, 5th edition. New York, John Wiley & Sons, 1984.

25. Shi, Z-X., Levy, A., and Lightman, S.L.: Thyroid hormone-mediated regulation of corticotropin-releasing hormone messenger ribonucleic acid in the rat. *Endocrinology*, 134(3):1577-1580, 1994.

26. Wolfe, S.L.: *Molecular and Cellular Biology*. Belmont, Wadsworth Publishing Co., 1993.

27. Kuret, J.A. and Murad, F.: Adenohypophyseal hormones and related substances. In *The Pharmacologic Basis of Therapeutics*, 8th edition. Edited by A.G. Gilman, T.W. Rall, A.S. Nies, and P. Taylor, New York, Pergamon Press, 1990, pp.1334-1360.

28. Jaffe, J.H. and Martin, W.R.: Opioid analgesics and antagonists. In *The Pharmacologic Basis of Therapeutics*, 8th edition. Edited by A.G. Gilman, T.W. Rall, A.S. Nies, and P. Taylor, New York, Pergamon Press, 1990, pp.485-521.

29. Zoeller, R.T. and Rudeen, P.K.: Ethanol blocks the cold-induced increases in thyrotropin-releasing hormone mRNA in paraventricular nuclei, but not the cold-induced increase in thyrotropin. *Mol. Brain Res.*, 13:321-330, 1992.

30. Ceccatelli, S., Giardino, L., and Calzá, L.: Response of hypothalamic peptide mRNAs to thyroidectomy. *Neuroendocrinology*, 56:694-703, 1992.

31. Brien, T.G.: The adrenocortical status of patients with thyroid disease. *Clin. Endocrinol.* (Oxf.), 5(1):97-99, 1976.

32. Gallagher, T.F., Helmann, L., Finkelstein, J., et al.: Hyperthyroidism and cortisol secretion in man. *J. Clin. Endocrinol. Metab.*, 34:919-927, 1972.

33. Bigos, R., Ridgeway, E.C., Kourides, A., and Maloof, F.: Spectrum of pituitary alterations with mild and severe thyroid impairment. *J. Clin. Endocrinol. Metab.*, 2:317-325, 1978.

34. Sánchez-Franco, F., Fernández, L., Fernández, G., and Cacicedo, L.: Thyroid hormone action on ACTH secretion. *Horm. Metab. Res.*, 21:550-552, 1989.

35. Hilton, J.G., Black, W.C., Athos, W., McHugh, B., and Westermann, C.D.: Increased ACTH-like activity in plasma of patients with thyrotoxicosis. *J. Clin. Endocrinol. Metab.*, 22:900-905, 1962.

36. Cooper, J.R., Bloom, F.E., and Roth, R.H.: *The Biochemical Basis of Neuropharmacology*, 6th edition. New York, Oxford University Press, 1991.

37. Kupfermann, I.: Hypothalamus and limbic system: peptidergic neurons, homeostasis, and emotional behavior. In *Principles of Neural Science*, 3rd edition. Edited by E.R. Kandel, J.H. Schwartz, and T.M. Jessell, Norwalk, Appleton & Lange, pp.735-749.

38. Aguilera, G.: Regulation of pituitary ACTH secretion during chronic stress. *Frontiers in Neuroendocrinology*, 15(4):321-350, 1994.

39. Andersson, K. and Eneroth, P.: Thyroidectomy and central catecholamine neurons of the male rat: evidence for the existence of an inhibitory dopaminergic mechanism in the external layer of the paraventricular hypothalamic nucleus for the regulation of TSH secretion. *Neuroendocrinology*, 45:14-27, 1987.

40. Harbuz, M.S. and Lightman, S.L.: Stress and the hypothalamo-pituitary-adrenal axis: acute, chronic, and immunological activation. *J. Endocrinol.*, 134(3):327-339, 1992.

41. Bliss, E.L., Migeon, C.J., Branch, C.H.H., and Samuels, L.T.: Reaction of the adrenal cortex to emotional stress. *Psychosom. Med.*, 18:56, 1956.

42. Szafarczyk, A., Guillaume, V., Conte-Devolx, B., et al.: Central catecholaminergic system stimulates secretion of CRH at different sites. *Am. J. Physiol.*, 255(4 Pt.1):E463-E468, 1988.

43. Eisinger, J., Plantamura, A., and Ayavou, T.: Glycolysis abnormalities in fibromyalgia. *J. Amer. Coll. Nutri.*, 13:144-148, 1994.

44. *Merck Manual of Diagnosis and Therapy*, 15th edition. Edited by R. Berkow and A.J. Fletcher, Rahway, Merck, Sharp & Dohme Research Laboratories, 1987.

45. Hellman, L., Bardlow, H.L., Zumoff, B., and Gallagher, T.F.: The influence of thyroid hormone on hydrocortisone production and metabolism. *J. Clin. Endocrinol. Metab.*, 21:1231, 1961.

46. Murakami, K., Akana, S., Dallman, M.F., and Ganong, W.F.: Correlation between the stress-induced transient increases in corticotropin-releasing hormone content of the median eminence of the hypothalamus and adrenocorticotropic hormone secretion. *Neuroendocrinology*, 49(3):233-241, 1989.

47. Calogero, A.E., Bernardini, R., Gold, P.W., and Chrousos, G.P.: Regulation of rat hypothalamic corticotropin-releasing hormone secretion *in vitro*: potential clinical

implications. *Adv. Exper. Med. Biol.*, 245:167-181, 1988.

48. Watabe, T., Tanaka, K., Kumagae, M., et al.: Hormonal responses to insulin-induced hypoglycemia in man. *J. Clin. Endocrinol. Metab.*, 65(6):1187-1191, 1987.

49. Smoak, B., Deuster, P., Rabin, D., and Chrousos, G.: Corticotropin-releasing hormone is not the sole factor mediating exercise-induced adrenocorticotropin release in humans. *J. Clin. Endocrinol. Metab.*, 73(2):302-306, 1991.

50. Ojima, K., Maatsumoto, K., Tohda, M., and Watanabe, H.: Hyperactivity of central noradrenergic and CRF systems is involved in social isolation-induced decrease in pentobarbital sleep. *Brain Res.*, 684(1):87-94, 1995.

51. Martino, E., Bartalena, L., Faglia, G., and Pinchera, A.: Central hypothyroidism. In *Werner and Ingbar's The Thyroid: A Fundamental and Clinical Text*, 7th edition. Edited by L.P. Braverman and R.D. Utiger, Philadelphia, Lippincott-Raven Publishers, 1996, pp.779-791.

52. Blandford, R.L., Samanta, A.C., Burden, A.C., et al.: Muscle contractures associated with glucocorticoid deficiency. *Br. Med. J.*, 291:127, 1985.

53. Shapiro, M.S., Trebich, C., Shilo, L., et al.: Myalgias and muscle contracture as the presenting signs of Addison's disease. *Postgrad. Med.*, 64:222, 1988.

54. Sonkin, L.S.: Myofascial pain due to metabolic disorders: diagnosis and treatment. In *Myofascial Pain and Fibromyalgia: Trigger Point Management*. Edited by E.S. Rachlin, St. Louis, Mosby, 1994, pp.45-60.

55. Weiner, S., Dorman, D., Persky, H., et al.: Effect on anxiety of increasing the plasma hydrocortisone level. *Psychosom. Med.*, 25:69-77, 1963.

56. Bennett, R.M.: Personal written communication with J.C. Lowe, February 27, 1996.

57. Straus, S.: Chronic fatigue syndrome. In *Mind-Body Interactions and Disease: Proceedings of a Conference on Stress, Immunity, and Health Sponsored by the National Institutes of Health*. Edited by N.R.S. Hall, F. Altman, and S.J. Blumenthal, Whitten Publishers, 1995, pp.95-104.

58. Ferraccioli, G., Chirelli, L., and Scita, F.: EMG-biofeedback training in fibromyalgia syndrome. *J. Rheumatol.*, 14:820-825, 1987.

59. Molina, E., Cecchettin, M., and Fontana, S.: Failure of EMG-biofeedback after sham biofeedback training in fibromyalgia. *Fed. Proc.*, 46:A1357, 1987.

60. Walco, G.A. and Ilowite, N.T.: Cognitive-behavioral intervention for juvenile primary fibromyalgia syndrome. *J. Rheumatol.*, 19:1617-1619, 1992.

61. Nielson, W.R., Walker, C., and McCain, G.A.: Cognitive behavioral treatment of fibromyalgia syndrome: preliminary findings. *J. Rheumatol.*, 19:98-103, 1992.

62. Haanen, H.C., Hoenderdos, H.T., van Romunde, L.K., et al.: Controlled trial of hypnotherapy in the treatment of refractory fibromyalgia. *J. Rheumatol.*, 18(1):72-75, 1991.

63. Kaplan, K.H., Goldenberg, D.L., and Galvin-Nadeau, M.: The impact of a meditation-based stress reduction program on fibromyalgia. *Gen. Hosp. Psychiatry*, 15:284-289, 1993.

64. Nicoloff, J.T., Fisher, D.A., and Appleman, M.D.: The role of glucocorticoids in the regulation of thyroid function in man. *J. Clin. Invest.*, 49:1922, 1970.

65. Alford, F.P., Baker, H.W.G., Burger, H.G., et al.: Temporal patterns of integrated plasma hormone levels during sleep and wakefulness. I. Thyroid-stimulating hormone, growth hormone and cortisol. *J. Clin. Endocrinol. Metab.*, 37:841, 1973.

66. Brabant, A., Brabant, G., Schuermeyer, T., et al.: The role of glucocorticoids in the regulation of thyrotropin. *Acta Endocrinol. (Copenh.)*, 121:95, 1989.

67. McCain, G.A. and Tilbe, K.S.: Diurnal hormone variation in fibromyalgia syndrome: a comparison with rheumatoid arthritis. *J. Rheumatol.*, 16(Suppl):154-157, 1989.

68. Chopra, I.J., Williams, D.E., Orgiazzi, J., and Solomon, D.H.: Opposite effects of dexamethasone or serum concentration of 3,3',5'-triiodothyronine (reverse T_3) and 3,5,3'-triiodothyronine (T_3). *J. Clin. Endocrinol. Metab.*, 41:911, 1975.

69. Jones, M.T., Gillham, B., Holmes, M.C., Hodges, J.R., and Buckingham, J.C.: Influence of substance P on hypothalamo-pituitary-adrenocortical activity in the rat. *J. Endocrinol.*, 76(1):183-184, 1978.

70. Brownie, A.C.: The metabolism of adrenal cortical steroids. In *The Adrenal Gland*, 2nd edition. Edited by V.H.T. James, New York, Raven Press, Inc., 1992, pp.209-224.

71. Nagasaka, T.: Adrenocortical hormone rhythm in blood and metabolism of the hypothalamic biogenic amines in rats. *Hokkaido J. Med. Science*, 63(5):811-926, 1988.

72. Levin, M.E. and Daughaday, W.H.: The influence of the thyroid on adrenocortical function. *J. Clin. Endocrinol. Metab.*, 15:1499-1511, 1955.

73. Harvard, C.W.H., Saldanha, U.F., Bird, R., and Gardner, R.: Adrenal function in hypothyroidism. *Brit. Med. J.*, 1:337-339, 1970.

74. Uveges, J.M., Parker, J.C., Smarr, K.L., et al.: Psychological symptoms in primary fibromyalgia syndrome: relationship to pain, life stress, and sleep disturbance. *Arthritis Rheum.*, 33:1279-1283, 1990.

75. Linquette, M., Lefebre, J., Racapot, A., and Cappoen, J.P.: Taux de production et concentration plasmatique mayeure du cortisol dans l'hyperthyrodie. *Ann. d'Endocrinologie*, 37:331-345, 1976.

76. Danneskiold-Samsöe, B., Christiansen, E., Lund, B., and Bach-Andersen, R.: Regional muscle tension and pain (fibrositis). *Scand. J. Rehab. Med.*, 15:17-20, 1982.

77. Danneskiold-Samsöe, B., Christiansen, E., and Bach-Andersen, R.: Myofascial pain and the role of myoglobin. *Scand. J. Rehab. Med.*, 15:174-178, 1986.

78. Young, W.S.: Regulation of gene expression in the hypothalamus: hybridization histochemical studies. *Ciba Foundation Symposium*, 168:127-138, 1992.

79. Calogero, A.E., Gallucci, W.T., Chrousos, G.P., and Gold, P.W.: Catecholamine effects upon rat hypothalamic corticotropin-releasing hormone secretion *in vitro*. *J. Clin. Invest.*, 82(3):839-846, 1988.

80. Bloom, F.E. and Lazerson, A.: *Brain, Mind, and Behavior*, 2nd edition. New York, W.H. Freeman and Co., 1988.

81. Baxter, J.D. and Tyrrell, J.B.: The adrenal cortex. In *Endocrinology and Metabolism*, 2nd edition. Edited by P. Felig, J.D. Baxter, A. Broadus, and L.A. Frohman, New York, McGraw-Hill Book Co., 1987, pp.511-650.

82. Kendall, J.W. and Allen, R.G.: Adrenocorticotropin and

related peptides, and their disorders. In *Principles and Practice of Endocrinology and Metabolism*. Edited by K.L. Becker, J.P. Bilezinkian, W.J. Bremner, et al., Philadelphia, J.B. Lippincott Co., 1990, pp.140-144.

83. Krieger, D.T.: Rhythms of ACTH and corticosteroid secretion in health and disease and their experimental modification. *J. Steroid Biochem.*, 6:785, 1975.

84. Pescovitz, O.H., Cutler, G.B., and Loriaux, D.L.: Synthesis and secretion of corticosteroids. In *Principles and Practice of Endocrinology and Metabolism*. Edited by K.L. Becker, J.P. Bilezinkian, W.J. Bremner, et al., Philadelphia, J.B. Lippincott Co., 1990, pp.579-591.

85. Hahn, T.J., Halstead, L.R., and Baran, D.T.: Effects of short term glucocorticoid administration on intestinal absorption and circulating vitamin D metabolite concentrations in man. *J. Clin. Invest.*, 64:655, 1979.

86. Hahn, T.J., Halstead, L.R., and Teitelbaum, S.L.: Altered mineral metabolism in glucocorticoid-induced osteopenia. *J. Clin. Invest.*, 64:655, 1979.

87. Morris, D.J.: The metabolism and mechanism of action of aldosterone. *Endocr. Rev.*, 2:234, 1981.

88. Baxter, J.D. and Forsham, P.H.: Tissue effects of glucocorticoids. *Am. J. Med.*, 53:573, 1972.

89. Baxter, J.D.: Glucocorticoid hormone action. *Pharmacol. Therap.*, 2:605, 1976.

90. Christy, N.P.: The adrenal cortex in thyrotoxicosis. In *Werner and Ingbar's The Thyroid: A Fundamental and Clinical Text*, 6th edition. Edited by L.E. Braverman and R.D. Utiger, Philadelphia, J.B. Lippincott Co., 1991, pp.806-815.

91. Grossman, A., Costa, A., Navarra, P., and Tsagarakis, S.: The regulation of hypothalamic corticotropin-releasing factor release: *in vitro* studies. *Ciba Foundation Symposium*, 172:129-143, 1993.

92. Demitrack, M.A., Dale, J.K., Straus, S.E., et al.: Evidence for impaired activation of the hypothalamic-pituitary-adrenal axis in patients with chronic fatigue syndrome. *J. Clin. Endocrinol. Metab.*, 73:1224-1234, 1991.

93. Crofford, L.J., Pillemer, S.R., Kalogeras, K.T., et al.: Hypothalamic-pituitary-adrenal axis perturbations in patients with fibromyalgia. *Arthritis Rheum.*, 37:1583-1592, 1994.

94. Demitrack, M.A. and Crofford, L.J.: Hypothalamic-pituitary-adrenal axis dysregulation in fibromyalgia and chronic fatigue syndrome: an overview and hypothesis. *J. Musculoskel. Pain*, 3(2):67-73, 1995.

95. Crofford, L.J.: The hypothalamic-pituitary-adrenal axis in the fibromyalgia syndrome. *J. Musculoskel. Pain*, 4(1/2): 181-200, 1996.

96. Crofford, L.J., Engleberg, N.C., and Demitrack, M.A.: Neurohormonal perturbations in fibromyalgia. *Baillieres Clin. Rheumatol.*, 10:365-378, 1996.

97. Griep, E.N., Boersma, J.W., and deKloet, E.R.: Altered reactivity of the hypothalamic-pituitary-adrenal axis in the primary fibromyalgia syndrome. *J. Rheumatol.*, 20:469-474, 1993.

98. Crofford, L.J.: Neuroendocrine aspects of fibromyalgia. *J. Musculoskel. Pain*, 2(3):125-132, 1994.

99. Dailey, P.A., Bishop, G.D., Russell, I.J., and Fletcher, E.M.: Psychological stress and the fibrositis/fibromyalgia syndrome. *J. Rheumatol.*, 17:1380-1385, 1990.

100. Yunus, M.B., Masi, A.T., Calabro, J.J., Miller, K.A., and

Feigenbaum, S.L.: Primary fibromyalgia (fibrositis): clinical study of 50 patients with matched normal controls. *Semin. Arthritis Rheum.*, 11:151-171, 1981.

101. van Denderen J.C., Boersma, J.W., Zeinstra, P., Hollander, A.P., and van Neerbos, B.R.: Physiological effects of exhaustive physical exercise in primary fibromyalgia syndrome (PFS): is PFS a disorder of neuroendocrine reactivity? *Scan. J. Rheumatol.*, 21:35-37, 1992.

102. Harbuz, M.S., Rees, R.G., Eckland, D., Jessop, D.S., Brewerton, D., and Lightman, S.L.: Paradoxical responses of hypothalamic corticotropin-releasing factor (CRF) messenger ribonucleic acid (mRNA) and CRF-41 peptide and adenohypophyseal proopiomelanocortin mRNA during chronic inflammatory stress. *Endocrinology*, 130(3):1394-1400, 1992.

103. Hashimoto, K., Suemaru, S., Takao, T., Sugawara, M., Makino, S., and Ota, Z.: Corticotropin-releasing hormone and pituitary-adrenocortical responses in chronically stressed rats. *Regulatory Peptides*, 23:117-126, 1988.

104. de Goeij, D.C.E., Kvetnansky, R., Whitnall, M.H., Jezova, D., Berkenbosch, F., and Tilders, F.J.H.: Repeated stress-induced activation of corticotropin-releasing factor neurons enhances vasopressin stores and colocalization with corticotropin-releasing factor in the median eminence of rats. *Neuroendocrinology*, 53(2):150-159, 1991.

105. Scaccionoce, S., Muscolo, L.A.A., Cigliana, G., Navarra, D., Nicolai, R., and Angelucci, L.: Evidence for a specific role of vasopressin in sustaining pituitary-adrenocortical stress response in the rat. *Endocrinology*, 128:3138-3143, 1991.

106. Swain, M.G., Patchev, V., Vergalla, J., Chrousos, G., and Jones, E.A.: Suppression of hypothalamic-pituitary-adrenal axis responsiveness to stress in a rat model of acute cholestasis. *J. Clin. Invest.*, 91(5):1903-1908, 1993.

107. Sarlis, N.J., Dhowdrey, H.S., Stephanou, A., and Lightman, S.L.: Chronic activation of the hypothalamic-pituitary-adrenal axis and loss of circadian rhythm during adjuvant-induced arthritis in the rat. *Endocrinology*, 130: 1775-1779, 1992.

108. Mitchell, D.H. and Owens, B.: Replacement therapy: arginine vasopressin (AVP), growth hormone (GH), cortisol, thyroxine, testosterone, and estrogen. *J. Neurosci. Nursing*, 28(3):140-152, 1996.

109. Hauger, R.L. and Aguilera, G.: Regulation of pituitary corticotropin-releasing hormone (CRH) receptors by CRH: interaction with vasopressin. *Endocrinology*, 133 (4):1708-1714, 1993.

110. Buckingham, J.C., Smith, T., and Loxley, H.D.: The control of ACTH secretion. In *The Adrenal Gland*, 2nd edition. Edited by V.H.T. James, New York, Raven Press, Inc., 1992, pp.131-158.

111. Plotsky, P.M., Otto, S., and Sutton, S.: Neurotransmitter modulation of corticotropin releasing factor secretion into the hypophyseal-portal circulation. *Life Sci.*, 41:1311-1317, 1987.

112. Krieger, D.T. and Rizzo, F.: Serotonin mediation of circadian periodicity of plasma 17-hydroxycorticosteroids. *Am. J. Physiol.*, 217:1703-1707, 1969.

113. Hillhouse, E.W. and Milton, N.G.N.: Effect of acetylcholine and 5-hydroxytryptamine on the secretion of corticotropin-releasing factor-41 and arginine vasopressin

from the rat hypothalamus *in vitro. J. Endocrinol.*, 122: 713-718, 1989.

114. al-Damluji, S., Perry, L., Tomlin, S., et al.: Alpha-adrenergic stimulation of corticotropin secretion by a specific central mechanism in man. *Neuroendocrinology*, 45(1): 68-76, 1987.

115. al-Damluji, S., Bouloux, P., White, A., and Besser, G.M.: The role of α_2-adrenoceptors in the control of ACTH secretion; interaction with the opioid system. *Neuroendocrinology*, 51(1):76-81, 1990.

116. Grossman, A. and Besser, G.M.: Opiates control ACTH through a noradrenergic mechanism. *Clin. Endocrinol.* (Oxf.), 17:287-290, 1982.

117. Buckingham, J.C.: Stimulation and inhibition of corticotropin releasing factor secretion by β-endorphin. *Neuroendocrinology*, 42:148-152, 1986.

118. Motta, M., Fraschim, F., Piva, F., and Martini, L.: Hypothalamic and extrahypothalamic mechanisms controlling adrenocorticotrophin secretion. *Mem. Soc. Endocr.*, 17:3-18, 1968.

119. Palkovits, M.: Catecholamines in the hypothalamus: an anatomical review. *Neuroendocrinology*, 33:123-128, 1981.

120. Gallardo, E., Chiocchio, S.R., and Tramezzani, J.H.: Sympathetic innervation of the median eminence. *Brain Res.*, 290:333-335, 1984.

121. Gibbs, D.M.: Hypothalamic epinephrine is released into hypophysial portal blood during stress. *Brain Res.*, 335 (2):360-364, 1985.

122. Takasu, N., Komiya, I., Nagasawa, Y., Asawa, T., and Yamada, T.: Exacerbation of autoimmune thyroid dysfunction after unilateral adrenalectomy in patients with Cushing's syndrome due to an adrenocortical adenoma. *N. Engl. J. Med.*, 322(24):1708-1712, 1990.

123. Dixon, R.B. and Christy, N.P.: On the various forms of corticosteroid withdrawal syndrome. *Am. J. Med.*, 68(2): 224-230, 1980.

124. Lowe, J.C.: Thyroid status of 38 fibromyalgia patients: implications for the etiology of fibromyalgia, *Clin. Bull. Myofascial Ther.*, 2(1):47-64, 1997.

125. Lowe, J.C., Reichman, A.J., Honeyman, G.S., and Yellin, J.: Thyroid status of fibromyalgia patients (Abstract). *Clin. Bull. Myofascial Ther.*, 3(1):69-70, 1998.

126. Shiroky, J.B., Cohen, M., Ballachey, M.L., and Neville, C.: Thyroid dysfunction in rheumatoid arthritis: a controlled prospective survey. *Ann. Rheumat. Dis.*, 52:454-456, 1993.

127. Eisinger, J., Arroyo, P., Calendini, C., Rinaldi, J.P., Combes, R., and Fontaine, G.: Anomalies biologiques au cours des fibromyalgies: III. Explorations endocriniennes. *Lyon Méditerranée Méd.*, 28:858-860, 1992.

128. Crofford, L.J. and Demitrack, M.A.: Evidence that abnormalities of central neurohormonal systems are key to understanding fibromyalgia and chronic fatigue syndrome. *Rheum. Dis. Clin. N. Am.*, 22(2):267-284, 1996.

129. Kamilaris, T.C., DeBold, C.R., Pavlou, S.N., et al.: Effect of altered thyroid hormone levels on hypothalamic-pituitary-adrenal function. *J. Clin. Endocrinol. Metab.*, 65: 994-999, 1987.

130. Ridgway, E.C., McCammon, J.A., Benotti, J., and Maloof, F.: Acute metabolic responses in myxedema to large doses of intravenous L-thyroxine. *Ann. Intern. Med.*, 77(4):549-555, 1972.

131. Bigos, S.T., Ridgway, E.C., Kourides, I.A., and Maloof, F.: Spectrum of pituitary alterations with mild and severe thyroid impairment. *J. Clin. Endocrinol. Metab.*, 46:317, 1978.

132. Dluhy, R.G.: The adrenal cortex in hypothyroidism. In *Werner and Ingbar's The Thyroid: A Fundamental and Clinical Text*, 7ᵗʰ edition. Edited by L.P. Braverman and R.D. Utiger, Philadelphia, Lippincott-Raven Publishers, 1996, pp.841-844.

133. Kamilaris, T.C., DeBold, C.R., Johnson, E.O., et al.: Effects of short and long duration hypothyroidism and hyperthyroidism on the plasma adrenocorticotropin and corticosterone responses to ovine corticotropin-releasing hormone in rats. *Endocrinology*, 128(5):2567-2576, 1991.

134. Johnson, E.O., Kamilaris, T.C., Chrousos, G.P., and Gold, P.W.: Mechanisms of stress: a dynamic overview of hormonal and behavioral homeostasis. *Neurosci. Biobehavioral Rev.*, 16(2):115-130, 1992.

135. Iranmanesh, A., Lizarralde, G., and Veldhuis, J.D.: Coordinate activation of the corticotropic axis by insulin-induced hypoglycemia: simultaneous estimates of β-endorphin, adrenocorticotropin and cortisol secretion and disappearance in normal men. *Acta Endocrinol.*, 128(6): 521-528, 1993.

136. Molitch, M.E. and Hou, S.H.: Neuroendocrine alterations in systemic disease. *Clin. Endocrinol Metab.*, 12(3):825-851, 1983.

137. Lowe, J.C.: Globalization of a myofascial pain syndrome. *Dyn. Chiro.*, March 14, 1990, p.18.

138. Waters, A.K.: Increased vasopressin excretion in patients with hypothyroidism. *Acta Endocrinol.*, 88(2):285-290, 1978.

139. Laczi, F., Janaky, T., Ivanyi, T., Julesz, J., and Laszlo, F.A.: Osmoregulation of arginine-8-vasopressin secretion in primary hypothyroidism and in Addison's disease. *Acta Endocrinol.*, 114(3):389-395, 1987.

140. Lumpkin, M.D., Samson, W.K., and McCann, S.M.: Arginine vasopressin as a thyrotropin-releasing hormone. *Science*, 235(4792):1070-1073, 1987.

141. Peterson, P.K., Pheley, A., Schroeppel, J., et al.: A preliminary placebo-controlled crossover trial of fludrocortisone for chronic fatigue syndrome. *Arch. Intern. Med.*, 158(8):908-914, 1998.

142. Arnaout, M.A., Awidi, A.S., el-Najdawi, A.M., Khateeb, M.S., and Ajlouni, K.M.: Arginine-vasopressin and endothelium-associated proteins in thyroid disease. *Acta Endocrinol.*, 126(5):399-403, 1992.

143. Childs, G.V.: Structure-function correlates in the corticotropes of the anterior pituitary. *Front. Neuroendocrinol.*, 13(3):271-317, 1992.

144. Angelucci, L. and Scaccianoce, S.: Mechanisms in the control of stress responsiveness. *Annali del Istituto Superiore di Sanita*, 26(1):75-78, 1990.

145. Kunos, G.: Modulation of adrenergic reactivity and adrenoceptors by thyroid hormones. In *Adrenoceptors and Catecholamine Action*, Part A. Edited by G. Kunos, New York, John Wiley & Sons, 1981, pp.297-333.

146. Whitnall, M.H., Kiss, A., and Aguilera, G.: Contrasting effects of central α_1-adrenoreceptor activation on stress-

responsive and stress-nonresponsive subpopulations of corticotropin-releasing hormone neurosecretory cells in the rat. *Neuroendocrinology*, 58(1):42-48, 1993.

147. Chrousos, G.P. and Gold, P.W.: The concepts of stress and stress system disorders: overview of physical and behavioral homeostatis. *J.A.M.A.*, 267(9):1244-1254, 1992.

148. Ditiateva, G.V., Krasnovskaia, I.A., and Skopicheva, V.I.: Effect of arginine-vasopressin on the rat thyroid gland *in vitro*. *Biulleten Eksperimentalnoi Biologii i Meditsiny*, 110(10):423-425, 1990.

149. Malendowicz, L.K. and Miskowiak, B.: Effects of prolonged administration of neurotensin, arginine-vasopressin, NPY, and bombesin on blood TSH, T₃, and T₄ levels in the rat. *In Vivo*, 4(4):259-261, 1990.

150. Velardo, A., Pantaleoni, M., Zizzo, G., et al.: Isolated adrenocorticotropic hormone deficiency secondary to hypothalamic deficit of corticotropin releasing hormone. *J. Endocrinol. Invest.*, 15(1):53-57, 1992.

151. Meserve, L.A. and Leathem, J.H.: Development of hypothalamic-pituitary-adrenal response to stress in rats made hypothyroid by exposure to thiouracil from conception. *J. Endocrinol.*, 90(3):403-409, 1981.

152. Meserve, L.A. and Russ, E.V.: Long-term hypothyroidism and hypothalamus-pituitary-adrenal (HPA) response in adult mice. *Ohio J. Sci.*, 97(1):10-13, 1997.

153. Eisinger, J.: Metabolic abnormalities in fibromyalgia. *Clin. Bull. Myofascial Ther.*, 3(1):3-21, 1998.

154. Cardinali, D.P. and Stern, J.E.: Peripheral neuroendocrinology of the cervical sympathetic autonomic nervous system. *Braz. J. Med. Biol. Res.*, 27(3):573-599, 1994.

155. Tohei, A., Watanabe, G., and Taya, K.: Hypersecretion of corticotrophin-releasing hormone and arginine vasopressin in hypothyroid male rats as estimated with push-pull perfusion. *J. Endocrinol.*, 156(2):395-400, 1998.

156. Toni, R., Mosca, S., Ruggeri, F., et al.: Effect of hypothyroidism on vasoactive intestinal polypeptide-immunoreactive neurons in forebrain-neurohypophysial nuclei of the rat brain. *Brain Res.*, 682(1-2):101-115, 1995.

157. Ota, K., Kimura, T., Sakurada, T., et al.: Effects of an acute water load on plasma ANP and AVP, and renal water handling in hypothyroidism: comparison of before and after L-thyroxine treatment. *Endocr. J.*, 41(1):99-105, 1994.

158. Laczi, F., Julesz, J., Janaki, T., Ivanyi, T., Boda, K., and Laszlo, F.: Regulation of vasopressin release in primary hypothyroidism and Addison's disease as well as in central diabetes insipidus. *Orv. Hetil.*, 131(22):1175-1180, 1990.

159. Iwasaki, Y., Oiso, Y., Yamauchi, K., Takatsuki, K., Kondo, K., Hasegawa, H., and Tomita, A.: Osmoregulation of plasma vasopressin in myxedema. *J. Clin. Endocrinol. Metab.*, 70(2):534-539, 1990.

160. Archambeaud-Mouveroux, F., Dejax, C., Jadaud, J.M., Vincent, D., Laroumagne, G., Hessel, L., and Laubie, B.: Myxedema coma with hypervasopressinism: two cases. *Ann. Med. Intern.* (Paris), 138(2):114-118, 1987.

161. Salomez-Granier, F., Lefebvre, J., Racadot, A., Dewailly, D., and Linquette, M.: Antidiuretic hormone levels (arginine-vasopressin) in cases of peripheral hypothyroidism. 26 cases. *Presse Med.*, 12(16):1001-1004, 1983.

162. Tohei, A., Watanabe, G., and Taya, K.: Effects of thyroidectomy or thiouracil treatment on copulatory behavior in

adult male rats. *J. Vet. Med. Sci.*, 60(3):281-285, 1998.

163. Tohei, A., Imai, A., Watanabe, G., and Taya, K.: Influence of thiouracil-induced hypothyroidism on adrenal and gonadal functions in adult female rats. *J. Vet. Med. Sci.*, 60 (4):439-446, 1998.

164. Riedel, W., Layka, H., and Neeck, G.: Secretory pattern of GH, TSH, thyroid hormones, ACTH, cortisol, FSH, and LH in patients with fibromyalgia syndrome following systematic injection of the relevant hypothalamic-releasing hormones. *Z. Rheumatol.*, 57(Suppl.2):81-87, 1998.

165. Koshiyama, H., Ito, M., Yoshinami, N., et al.: Two cases of asymptomatic adrenocortical insufficiency with autoimmune thyroid disease. *Endocr. J.*, 41(4):373-378, 1994.

166. Lo, M.J., Wang, S.W., Kau, M.M., et al.: Pharmacological effects of propylthiouracil on corticosterone secretion in male rats. *J. Investig. Med.*, 46(9):444-452, 1998.

167. Lo, M.J., Kau, M.M., Chen, Y.H., et al.: Acute effects of thyroid hormones on the production of adrenal cAMP and corticosterone in male rats. *Am. J. Physiol.*, 274(2 Pt.1): E238-E245, 1998.

168. Eisinger, J., Dupond, J.L., and Cozzone, P.J.: Anomalies de la glycolyse au cours des fibromyalgies: etude biologiques et thérapeutique. *Lyon Méditerranée Méd.* 32: 2180-2181, 1996.

169. Haynes, R.C., Jr.: Adrenocorticotropic hormone; adrenocortical steroids and their synthetic analogs; inhibitors of the synthesis and actions of adrenocortical hormones. In Goodman and Gilman's *The Pharmacological Basis of Therapeutics*, 8ᵗʰ edition. Edited by A.G. Goodman, T.W. Rall, A.S. Nies, and P. Taylor, New York, Pergamon Press, 1990, pp.1431-1462.

170. Duick, D.W., Warren, D.W., Nicoloff, J.T., Otis, C.L., and Croxson, M.S.: Effect of a single dose of dexamethasone on the concentration of serum triiodothyronine in man. *J. Clin. Endocrinol. Metab.*, 39:1151, 1974.

171. Dussault, J.H.: The effect of dexamethasone on TSH and prolactin secretion after TRH stimulation. *Can. Med. Assoc. J.*, 111:1195, 1974.

172. Awad, E.A.: Pathological changes in fibromyalgia. *First International Symposium on Myofascial Pain and Fibromyalgia*. Minneapolis, Minnesota, May 9, 1989.

173. Awad, E.A.: Histopathological changes in fibrositis. In *Advances in Pain Research and Therapy*, Vol.17. Edited by J.R. Fricton and E.A. Awad, New York, Raven Press, Ltd., 1990, pp.249-258.

174. Kalyan-Raman, U.P., Kalyan-Raman, K., Yunus, M.B., et al.: Muscle pathology in primary fibromyalgia syndrome: a light microscopic, histologic and ultrastructure study. *J. Rheumatol.*, 11:808-814, 1984.

175. Ramsay, I.: *Thyroid Disease and Muscle Dysfunction*. Chicago, Year Book Medical Publishers, Inc., 1974, pp.147-151.

176. Cori, C.F. and Cori, G.T.: The fate of sugar in the animal body. VII. The carbohydrate metabolism of adrenalectomized rats and mice. *J. Biol. Chem.*, 74:473-494, 1927.

177. McKenzie, R., O'Fallon, A., Dale, J., et al.: Low-dose hydrocortisone for treatment of chronic fatigue syndrome: a randomized controlled trial. *J.A.M.A.*, 280(12):1061-1066, 1998.

178. Cleare, A.J., Heap, E., Malhi, G.S., Wessely, S., O'Keane, V., and Miell, J.: Low-dose hydrocortisone in chronic fa-

tigue syndrome: a randomised crossover trial. *Lancet*, 353 (9151):455-458, 1999.

179. Scott, L.V., Medbak, S., and Dinan, T.G.: The low dose ACTH test in chronic fatigue syndrome and in health. *Clin. Endocrinol.* (Oxf.), 48(6):733-737, 1998.

3.6

Sex Hormones: Hypothalamic-Pituitary-Gonadal Axis

Normal Function of the Hypothalamic-Pituitary-Gonadal Axis

The hypothalamic-pituitary-gonadal (HPG) axis and the hormones secreted by the three structures of the axis regulate sexual functions of the female and male. The hypothalamus secretes gonadotropin-releasing hormone (GnRH). GnRH stimulates anterior pituitary cells called gonadotrophs to secrete follicle stimulating hormone (FSH) and luteinizing hormone (LH). In the male's testicles, FSH stimulates production of sperm and LH stimulates production of testosterone.

An understanding of the menstrual cycle is necessary to appreciate the roles of FSH and LH in the female. Menstruation is the cyclic shedding and discharge of the endometrial mucosal lining of the uterus. Menstruation occurs during the first 4-to-7 days of the follicular phase of the monthly cycle. The follicular phase lasts a total of about 14 days and ends when ovulation occurs. During the follicular phase, an ovum matures in an ovarian follicle. When the ovum extrudes from the follicle, the follicle becomes the corpus luteum. If pregnancy does not occur, after another 14 days or so, the corpus luteum degenerates, and menstrual bleeding begins.

During the follicular phase of the cycle, FSH stimulates ovarian follicles. The stimulation influences a dominant follicle to mature. As the follicle matures, the granulosa cells that line its wall secrete some progesterone and larger amounts of estrogen. Thyroid hormone and other factors augment the stimulating effects of FSH on the follicles. The estrogen stimulates the endometrial lining of the uterus to develop, with proliferation of its glands and vascular system. Appropriately, these changes are termed the proliferative phase of endometrial development.

The rise in the estrogen level during the follicular phase causes a surge in the secretion of GnRH. A surge of LH secretion immediately follows the surge in GnRH secretion. The LH level peaks just before ovulation. The increased LH acts on the granulosa cells of the follicle, converting them to luteal cells that secrete large amounts of estrogen and even larger amounts of progesterone. Increased circulating levels of estrogen and progesterone suppress secretion of FSH and LH by pituitary gonadotrophs. Circulating levels of FSH and LH decrease and toward the end of the luteal phase descend to their lowest levels. The large amounts of progesterone during the luteal phase stimulate changes in the endometrium that prepare it to support and nourish a fertilized embryo. These changes constitute the secretory phase of endometrial development.

If pregnancy does not occur, in some 14 days after ovulation (about the 28th day since the previous onset of menstruation), the luteal phase of the cycle ends. The corpus luteum undergoes changes that end its secretion of progesterone and estrogen. Without further sex hormone stimulation, the endometrium degenerates and sheds, causing the bloody discharge known

509

as menstruation. The drop in the circulating levels of estrogen and progesterone disinhibits the pituitary gonadotrophs. As a result, they begin secreting FSH and LH, initiating development of other ovarian follicles.

If pregnancy does occur, the corpus luteum does not degenerate but continues to secrete progesterone. The progesterone sustains the endometrium in a condition favorable to survival of the embryo. After the placenta develops, it secretes the hormones necessary to maintain pregnancy, and the corpus luteum then degenerates.

Sex-Related Findings in Fibromyalgia

Researchers have conducted few studies on the relation of sex to fibromyalgia. This is surprising in view of two commonly acknowledged sex-related findings: (1) most fibromyalgia patients are women, and (2) the onset or exacerbations of fibromyalgia often occur during sex-related events for women—menarche, childbirth, premenstrual time, peri-menopause, and menopause.

Men and women with fibromyalgia complain of subnormal libido and reduced sexual activity, and men complain of impotence. Patients often attribute these symptoms to their pain and low level of well-being.

Women with fibromyalgia have a higher frequency of dysmenorrhea and PMS (premenstrual syndrome) than other women. Fibromyalgic women were reported to have elevated basal FSH levels and low basal estrogen levels. In response to injections of GnRH, patients' pituitary secretion of LH was blunted. In another study, premenopausal fibromyalgic women had significantly lower testosterone levels, and post-menopausal fibromyalgic women had levels that were just short of being significantly low. Pregnancy had negative effects on fibromyalgia patients and resulted in increased functional impairment and disability in the postpartum period.

Possible Relation of Sex-Related Findings to Thyroid Hormone

Several studies have shown that fibromyalgic patients have either hypothyroidism or cellular resistance to thyroid hormone. Thyroid hormone is not considered a sex hormone, but thyroid hormone status potently regulates the HPG axis. A relation between hypothyroidism and/or thyroid hormone resistance and sex-related abnormalities in fibromyalgia patients is highly probable. Several possible mechanisms may account for the high prevalence of females with fibromyalgia: (1) the lower metabolic rate of women, (2) a higher incidence of hypothyroidism among females, (3) thyroid hormone-lowering effects of estrogen, and (4) greater susceptibility to injury due to lower androgen levels than men.

During the luteal phase of the menstrual cycle, females have an increased density of α_2-adrenergic receptors. The degree of increased receptor density correlated with the severity of luteal phase anxiety and depression in patients with premenstrual dysphoric syndrome. Also, estrogen deficiency caused a 50% increase in the density of α_2-adrenergic receptors in the frontal region of the cerebral cortex. The increased density of the receptors may cause cognitive dysfunction and possibly depression in estrogen deficient women. In that α_2-adrenergic receptors are generally inhibitory, reducing metabolism, reduced density of the receptors suggests a molecular mechanism of some symptoms and signs associated with low estrogen levels, especially during the luteal phase of the cycle. Fibromyalgia patients had an increased density of α_2-adrenergic receptors on their platelets. During hypothyroidism and cellular resistance to thyroid hormone, inadequate thyroid hormone regulation of the adrenergic genes increases the density of α-adrenergic receptors on cell membranes. In hypothyroid and thyroid hormone resistant women, symptoms of hypometabolism resulting from an increased density of α_2-adrenergic receptors on cell membranes are likely to be exacerbated by an additional increase in α_2-adrenergic receptor density when estrogen levels decrease during the menstrual cycle. In women whose fibromyalgia is underlain by hypothyroidism and/or thyroid hormone resistance, low estrogen levels during the late luteal phase or during peri-menopause or menopause may induce or severely worsen their symptoms.

The low libido of fibromyalgia patients may result from low testosterone levels due to subnormal pituitary LH secretion and/or reduced responsiveness of gonadal interstitial cells to LH.

Dysmenorrhea in fibromyalgia may result from a combination of unbalanced endometrial stimulation and excessive activity of the uterine muscle, both of which can result from inadequate thyroid hormone regulation of the ovaries. Low FSH and a subnormal LH response to GnRH may be explained by inadequate thyroid hormone regulation of the HPG axis, the same findings having been reported in hypothyroid humans and rats.

The worsening of fibromyalgia symptoms during the premenstrual time and peri-menopause may result from inadequate thyroid hormone regulation of the function of the ovaries. Optimal amounts of thyroid hormone are needed for FSH to properly stimulate the granulosa cells of the ovarian follicles. During inadequate thyroid hormone regulation of the ovaries, the granulosa cells do not mature. As a result, estrogen and progesterone production are impaired. Also, thyroid hormone is necessary for the normal production of pregnenolone, the precursor of progesterone. Thyroid hormone is also necessary for normal activity of the enzyme that converts pregnenolone to progesterone. Inadequate thyroid hormone regulation can result in a progesterone deficiency. Deficient progesterone can mediate physical and psychological effects characteristic of PMS. The low basal estrogen levels of some fibromyalgia patients may result from reduced ovarian secretion of estrone and estradiol due to inadequate thyroid hormone facilitation of FSH-stimulation of ovarian granulosa cells.

Adequate thyroid hormone exposure to the granulosa cells of the ovaries is necessary for the cells to properly differentiate, for sufficient numbers of LH and hCG receptors to appear on the cells, and for the cells' production of estrogen and progesterone. For ovulation to occur normally, and for the follicle to convert to a corpus luteum, LH must bind to the granulosa cells. LH can do so only if the cells contain enough LH receptors, which is partly dependent on sufficient exposure to thyroid hormone. If the corpus luteum does not form properly, the follicular granulosa cells will not convert to progesterone-secreting luteal cells, and the patient may have a progesterone deficit during the luteal phase of the menstrual cycle. Low TRH secretion in fibromyalgia patients with hypothalamic hypothyroidism may also reduce LH secretion.

Many women with fibromyalgia complain of infertility and/or difficulties carrying fetuses to term. Hypothyroidism causes infertility in many women. It causes the pregnancies of some to end with spontaneous abortion in the first trimester, stillbirth, or premature birth. Also, hypothyroidism is a risk factor for the development of gestational diabetes and preeclampsia.

Thyroid Hormone Therapy

Restoring the premenopausal sex hormone status of some fibromyalgic women may free them from their symptoms. One experienced clinician who observed the responses of fibromyalgic women to cyclic estrogen and progesterone therapy noted that patients improved. However, he qualified that the therapy was not a cure of the fibromyalgia. Instead, patients typically continued to have partially controlled chronic pain. More patients are likely to improve with other

therapeutic procedures in addition to sex hormone therapy, including exercise to tolerance, adoption of a wholesome diet and the use of a wide array of nutritional supplements. However, most patients do not markedly improve or recover from their fibromyalgia symptoms—including exacerbations during the premenstrual time, peri-menopause, or menopause—until they undergo metabolic rehabilitation involving the use of exogenous thyroid hormone.

Many female fibromyalgia patients report that their symptoms began during their peri-menopausal years or about the time of menopause. Many other female patients report that their fibromyalgia symptoms worsen during the premenstrual time, a week or so before their periods begin. Despite these common reports of female patients, fibromyalgia researchers have conducted precious few studies that explore possible relationships between the female menstrual cycle and fibromyalgia. The paucity of studies may be a result of the failure of the rheumatology fibromyalgia paradigm—a failure to provide a plausible explanation for the phenomena commonly reported by female fibromyalgia patients. Because the rheumatology model of fibromyalgia provides no reasonable explanation, the model has failed to provide testable propositions to work with. In contrast, the hypothesis I posit in this book—that most patients' fibromyalgia is a clinical expression of inadequate thyroid hormone regulation of cell function—provides a highly tenable explanation for the female patients' reports. Accordingly, in this chapter, I present evidence showing that inadequate thyroid hormone regulation of the HPG axis may render a woman susceptible to the onset or exacerbation of fibromyalgia symptoms during her premenstrual time, peri-menopause, or menopause. I also provide information on the possible impact of inadequate thyroid hormone regulation of the hypothalamic-pituitary-gonadal axis on male fibromyalgia patients. First, however, a review of the axis is in order.

● **SEXUAL ABNORMALITIES IN HYPOTHYROIDISM AND RESISTANCE TO THYROID HORMONE**

Guyton wrote that for normal sexual function, thyroid hormone secretion must be close to normal.[78, p 836] When the thyroid gland secretes too little thyroid hormone, which by definition is hypothyroidism, the HPG axis is one of many body systems that is likely to malfunction. Researchers have long known of adverse effects of hypothyroidism such as diminished sex drive, heavy or prolonged menstrual bleeding, and painful or difficult menstruation.[207][288] However, as shown by studies I cite in this chapter, thyroid hormone deficiency can adversely affect sexual function in many other ways.

Some researchers have reported that women with euthyroid hypometabolism (thyroid hormone resistance) also suffer adverse sexual effects, such as PMS, abnormal menstruation, and decreased sex drive.[209][287] My extensive clinical experience with euthyroid fibromyalgia patients confirms their reports. Thus, for normal sexual function, it is necessary, as Guyton wrote,[78,p.836] that thyroid hormone secretion is normal. But equally essential, sufficient amounts of thyroid hormone must reach HPG cells, enter them, and exert normal regulatory actions within them. If the thyroid gland secretes normal amounts of thyroid hormone, but normal amounts fail to properly regulate the function of HPG axis cells, the sexual abnormalities that result will be virtually the same as those that occur in hypothyroidism.

In my clinical and research experiences, when sexual abnormalities result from hypothyroidism and/or thyroid hormone resistance, the patients' use of the proper form and dosage of thyroid hormone corrects the abnormalities. In some cases, of course, other therapeutic interventions are also necessary. However, the other interventions are not likely to correct the sexual abnormalities unless the patient also undergoes proper thyroid hormone therapy.

● HYPOTHALAMIC-PITUITARY-GONADAL (HPG) AXIS

The HPG axis and the hormones secreted by the different components of the axis regulate sexual function. The same three classes of sex-related hormones—estrogens, progesterone, and androgens—regulate sexual function in males and females. However, the levels of the hormones differ in males and females. Also, the effects of the hormones differ in males and females, dictated by differences in structures and functions peculiar to each sex. Release of the sex hormones by the gonads is regulated by two pituitary hormones called gonadotropins—follicle stimulating hormone and luteinizing hormone. In turn, the pitui-

tary release of the gonadotropins is regulated by the hypothalamic hormone gonadotropin-releasing hormone.

GONADOTROPIN-RELEASING HORMONE (GnRH)

One hypothalamic hormone, GnRH, stimulates the release of the two pituitary hormones (gonadotropins) that regulate the function of the gonads. Hypothalamic neurons located mainly in the arcuate nuclei synthesize GnRH. The neuronal terminals in the median eminence then release GnRH in pulses into the portal blood veins. The veins transport the hormone to the anterior pituitary gland.

In the anterior pituitary gland, GnRH acts on a population of heterogenous cells called gonadotrophs that contain GnRH receptors. Most gonadotrophs contain both follicle stimulating hormone and luteinizing hormone. Some gonadotrophs, however, contain only one or the other of the gonadotropins. In response to GnRH, the gonadotrophs secrete follicle stimulating hormone and luteinizing hormone. In the absence of GnRH, the gonadotrophs secrete virtually no gonadotropins. The gonadotrophs secrete follicle stimulating hormone at a rate that varies only slightly with the pulses of GnRH. In contrast, the pituitary cells secrete luteinizing hormone in a pattern that more closely matches the pulsatile secretions of GnRH. Because of the closer match between GnRH and luteinizing hormone secretion, some physiologists refer to GnRH as luteinizing hormone-releasing hormone.[78,p.894][228,p.581][229][301]

Several central and peripheral factors modulate the activity of the neurons that produce and release GnRH. Factors that stimulate GnRH release include norepinephrine and neuropeptide Y. Factors that inhibit the neurons include dopamine, β-endorphin, and interleukin-1. 17β-Estradiol may stimulate or inhibit the neurons.[228,p.581][297]

The substantial increase in the circulating estrogen level during the follicular phase of the menstrual cycle appears to trigger a surge in GnRH release (see Figures 3.6.1, 3.6.2, and 3.6.3). The estrogen probably does not act directly on the GnRH secreting neurons in the hypothalamus. Researchers have not found estrogen receptors on the GnRH neurons. The brain stem may be the site where estrogen acts to stimulate GnRH release. Estrogen may stimulate noradrenergic neurons in the brain stem that release norepinephrine from their terminals in the hypothalamus. Two findings suggest this: (1) the rate-limiting enzyme in norepinephrine synthesis, tyrosine hydroxylase, increases when estrogen levels increase in the follicular phase, and (2) norepinephrine levels surge at the time when GnRH levels peak just before ovulation.[297]

GONADOTROPINS

A gonadotropin is a hormone that stimulates the growth and function of the gonads—ovaries in the female and testicles in the male. The two gonadotropins secreted by the anterior pituitary gland are follicle stimulating hormone (FSH) and luteinizing hormone (LH). Both FSH and LH exert effects in females and males, but the effects differ in the two sexes. Each gonadotropin exerts specific effects on different histological components of the gonads.

Pituitary secretion of the gonadotropins is stimulated by GnRH and regulated by estradiol, progesterone, and testosterone. The three steroid hormones bind to their receptors in pituitary gonadotroph cells. Then, the hormone-receptor complexes enter the nuclei and bind to regulatory elements of genes. This genomic action accounts for the slow alteration in the secretion of FSH and LH. More rapid changes in gonadotropin secretion are regulated non-genomically by a variety of other hormonally active steroids that have only recently been discovered.[299]

Follicle Stimulating Hormone (FSH)

The anterior pituitary gland secretes FSH. In the female, the hormone stimulates the maturing of follicles in the ovaries. In the male, FSH stimulates production of sperm cells in the Sertoli cells of the seminiferous tubules of the testicles.

Luteinizing Hormone (LH)

LH is also termed "interstitial cell-stimulating hormone" because it stimulates cells in the interstitial tissues of the ovaries and the testicles. In the female, the hormone stimulates the formation of the corpus luteum from the Graafian follicle after the follicle releases an ovum during ovulation. In the female, LH also stimulates secretion of progesterone by the corpus luteum.

In the male, LH stimulates testosterone production by the interstitial cells of the testicles called Leydig's cells. These testosterone synthesizing and secreting cells reside in the interstitial tissues between the seminiferous tubules of the testicles that secrete testosterone. The corresponding interstitial cells in females are derived from the theca interna of atretic follicles of the ovary. These follicular cells, which form a layer just outside the wall of granulosa cells, produce mainly two androgens, testosterone and androstenedione. However, the granulosa cells convert most of these androgens to female sex hormones.[78,p.903][228,p.595]

SEX HORMONES

The three classes of sex hormones are the estrogens, progesterone, and androgens. Estrogens and progesterone travel through the circulation bound to either albumin or specific estrogen- and progesterone-binding globulins. The hormones loosely bind to the proteins and easily release from them and enter cells within 30 minutes or so after their secretion.[78,p.905]

Estrogens and progesterone pass freely into cells. In the cytoplasm, they bind to receptors. The hormone-receptor complexes then enter the cell nuclei and interact with specific DNA sequences. The interaction initiates transcription which increases protein synthesis in tissues such as the breasts, uterus, bone, and some fatty tissue areas.[78,p.907]

Testosterone and dihydrotestosterone circulate bound to sex steroid-binding globulin. A minority of the two hormones circulates bound to albumin.[228,p.595]

Estrogens

An estrogen is any natural or synthetic hormone that exerts the growth and maturation and feminizing effects characteristic of endogenous estradiol. Estrogens are produced in the ovaries, testicles, the placenta, and the adrenal cortex. They are also produced by a variety of plants. The main estrogens are estradiol and estrone. Estriol is the metabolc product of estradiol and estrone. Estradiol has 12 times the estrogenic potency of estrone and 80 times that of estriol.[78,p.904]

Estrogens are also called "estrins." The term estrin derives from the production of "estrus" by the hormone. The term estrus comes from the Greek word meaning "mad desire." The term refers to the time during the sexual cycle when a female animal is willing, judged by physiological changes and behavior, to engage in sexual intercourse.

The ovaries are the main source of estrogens in the female, and the testicles are the main source in the male. The adrenal cortex and the placenta also synthesize estrogens. After the ovaries secrete estradiol, the liver converts it to estrone and estriol. After the testicles secrete testosterone, some of it is converted to estrogen in fatty tissues, the liver, skeletal muscles, and hair follicles.

In the fertile years of the woman, during the follicular phase of the menstrual cycle, FSH from the pituitary gland stimulates the ovaries to secrete more estrogen. As a result, the circulating estrogen level rises during the follicular phase. (See Figures 3.6.2 and 3.6.3.)

Before ovulation, the ovarian follicle synthesizes small quantities of progesterone. After ovulation, the follicle becomes the corpus luteum and synthesizes and secretes large amounts of progesterone (see section below titled "Progestins and Progesterone").

In women who menstruate, most of the circulating estrogen is estradiol secreted by the ovaries. In postmenopausal women, however, most circulating estrogen is estrone. The estrone is derived from the conversion of androstenedione in peripheral tissues. The androstenedione is secreted by the adrenal glands and then converted to estrone in subcutaneous fat, hair follicles, and breast tissue. In that the estrone is derived from the conversion of androstenedione, the adrenal glands are the main source of estrogens in postmenopausal women.[33,p.568] In the premenopausal woman, estrone accounts for less than 4% of the circulating estrogen.

Estrogen is excreted in the urine after liver cells conjugate it with sulfur or glucoronic acid.[228,p.608]

Actions of Estrogens. These natural, endogenous estrogens produce female secondary sexual characteristics. During the follicular phase of the menstrual cycle, estrogens stimulate growth of the glands, vascular system, and layers of the endometrial lining in the uterus. The hormones also stimulate the smooth muscle (the myometrium) of the uterus.[30,p.135] Estrogens also stimulate the growth and maturation of bones. By some unknown mechanism, estrogen inhibits bone absorption. No estrogen receptors on bone have been identified. The effects of estrogen on bone may be indirect through mechanisms such as potentiation of the release of calcitonin, a hormone that stimulates bone formation.[30,p.150]

In women using oral contraceptives or oral estrogen replacement therapy, the synthetic estrogens may increase the levels of circulation thyroid hormone transport proteins. Elevated levels of endogenous estrogen may have the same effect in pregnant women. The estrogens inhibit the breakdown of the transport proteins,[30,p.150] and as a result, the patient's total T_4 is usually elevated. (See Chapter 4.2, section titled "Estrogens.") Estrogens enter the central nervous system and exert effects that influence mental functions, emotions, and overt behaviors (see section below titled "Premenstrual Syndrome (PMS)").

Progestins and Progesterone

Progesterone is a natural, endogenous hormone that plays an essential role in the menstrual cycle and pregnancy. The word "gestation" is synonymous with pregnancy, and the term progesterone means pro-gestation hormone—that is, progesterone *promotes gestation*. The term "progestins" refers to the classification of synthetic chemicals that exert effects in the body similar to those of progesterone. The term "progestogen" is a synonym for progestin. Progestins are designed to mimic the effects of progesterone. However, while progesterone is an orthomolecular substance (see Glossary), progestins are not. The chemical structures of progestins are different from that of progesterone, and the different structures account for the adverse effects progestins typically have on women (see section below titled "Glucose Intolerance and Low-Dose Oral Contraceptive Use," and the section below titled "Progesterone Replacement Therapy ").

During the female sex cycle, the corpus luteum secretes progesterone. The corpus luteum forms from the Graafian follicle after it extrudes the ovum at midcycle. During the first or follicular phase of the menstrual cycle, estrogen induces the endometrial lining of the uterus to thicken and to become highly vascularized. During the subsequent luteal phase of the cycle, the progesterone secreted by the corpus luteum sustains the estrogen-induced, thick, secretory endometrium. Sustaining the endometrium in this estrogen-induced state is critical. Only a blood- and nutrient-rich endometrium, maintained by progesterone, can support and nourish the ovum, should it become fertilized by a sperm cell as it approaches the uterus through a fallopian tube.

Progesterone promotes the survival and development of the embryo during pregnancy. The placenta secretes progesterone, estrogen, and gonadotrophins. These hormones enable the uterus to maintain pregnancy until term.

Synthetic progestins are hormones derived from progesterone or nortestosterone. The main prescribed synthetic progestin is medroxy-progesterone acetate (Provera). The structures of synthetic progestins differ slightly from that of natural, endogenous progesterone. Synthetic progestins are therefore not orthomolecular compounds (see Glossary); they are chemicals alien to animals. As with most synthetic and non-orthomolecular compounds, progestins have an array of adverse effects in women. Nonetheless, they exert the same uterine effects as natural, endogenous progesterone and yam- or soybean-derived progesterone.

Progestins diffuse into cells, bind to cytoplasmic

receptors, and upon entering the cell nuclei, activate transcription of genes coded for various proteins. The resulting synthesized proteins regulate various physiologic functions. For example, acting through the genome, progesterone modifies the uterine epithelium during the second half of the menstrual cycle, preparing it for implantation of the blastocyst.[30,pp.136-137] Progesterone induces salt loss through the kidneys, probably by inhibiting the salt-retaining adrenal hormone aldosterone.[30,p.150]

During the follicular phase of the female cycle, the ovaries secrete about 50% of circulating progesterone and the adrenal glands secrete the other 50%. During the luteal phase, virtually all progesterone is derived from the corpus luteum. Progesterone is excreted in the urine after it is reduced to pregnanediol.[228,p.608]

Androgens

The term androgen refers to hormones that produce male secondary sexual characteristics. The main androgens in humans are testosterone, dihydrotestosterone, and androstenedione. Testosterone is the most potent of the endogenous androgens. Testosterone is mainly a prohormone. Most androgen effects occur after testosterone is reduced in peripheral tissues to dihydrotestosterone.[228,p.959] Nonetheless, testosterone and dihydrotestosterone produce most of the androgenic effects in the human body.[30,p.137][33,p.568] The principal hormone produced by the testicles is testosterone. The testicles also produce a very small amount of dihydrotestosterone and estrogen.[30,p.109] The testicles produce about 20% of the estradiol and 25% of the dihydrotestosterone in the general circulation.[34,p.158][35]

The testicles produce testosterone in response to LH binding to LH receptors. LH receptors are stationed in Leydig cells embedded in the interstitial tissues of the lobules of the testicles. The LH-receptor complex causes production of cAMP inside the cells, and the cAMP sets into motion the intracellular events that increase testosterone production.[30,p.109] Testosterone levels are lower during the evening. Throughout the day, however, levels of the hormone pulse in close relation to the pulsatile release of LH by the pituitary gonadotrophs.[228,p.959]

Peripheral, nonendocrine tissues produce some testosterone. Nonendocrine tissues produce testosterone from at least three adrenal products: (1) androstenedione, (2) DHEA (dehydroepiandrosterone or prasterone), and (3) DHEA-S (sulfated DHEA). These precursors have only minimal androgen-like effects on cells before being converted to testoster-

one.[30,p.137][33,p.568]

In the prostate and skin, the enzyme 5-α-reductase converts testosterone to dihydrotestosterone. Dihydrotestosterone then undergoes 3-α-reduction to androstanediol.[36,p.939] The major source of circulating estrogens in males is estradiol derived from the conversion of small amounts of testosterone in peripheral tissues.[36,p.939]

In men, the adrenal glands contribute only about 5% of the plasma testosterone.[32] Women synthesize only a small amount of testosterone, and about two thirds of this derives from the adrenal product androstenedione. (Androstenediol is a steroid metabolite that differs from androstanediol by a double bond within its structure between the 5th and 6th carbon atoms). Testosterone produced in the adrenal glands is responsible for most androgenic activity in women. The role of androgen in women is not clear, but the hormone appears to influence sex drive and the growth of pubic and axillary hair.

Proteins transport both testosterone and estrogen in the blood. The liver synthesizes the transport proteins. Testosterone and estrogen are inactive when they are bound to transport proteins.[30,p.109] Most testosterone is excreted in the urine after being oxidized at the 17-position.[228,p.595]

Actions of Androgens. Testosterone crosses cell membranes freely. In the cytoplasm near the nuclear membrane, the hormone is converted by the enzyme 5-α-reductase to dihydrotestosterone. The enzyme also converts androstenedione to dihydrotestosterone. Dihydrotestosterone binds to an androgen receptor.[37][38] The androgen receptor binds either testosterone or dihydrotestosterone, but it has a higher affinity for dihydrotestosterone.[36,p.939] The hormone-androgen receptor complex, bound to specific chromosomal sites, stimulates transcription of genes that code for proteins.[36,p.940][30,pp.116-117]

The secondary sex characteristics induced by androgens in some male animals are far more colorful than those of human males. Charles Darwin pointed this out and sited examples such as deer antlers, rooster heads, and peacock feathers. When administered in studies, androgens increased nitrogen, potassium, and phosphorus retention. It also increased total skeletal muscle mass.[30,p.116][240] Pharmacologic dosages of androgens increased the lean body mass in normal men,[242] and the dosages increased the size of muscles of men undergoing athletic training.[243] Castrated men have a smaller muscle mass than other men until they receive androgen replacement therapy. Muscle mass and strength increase in women who use exogenous androgens.[30]

Increased protein synthesis stimulated by androgen increases the thickness of connective tissues and muscles. The increased thickness provides protection against musculoskeletal injuries. This anabolic effect renders males less prone to musculoskeletal injuries and provides a higher capacity for the repair of injured tissues. Because of their lower androgen levels, women have less dense connective tissues and lower muscle mass. As a result, they are more susceptibility to musculoskeletal injuries and have a lower capacity for tissue repair. If a female fibromyalgia patient also has low growth hormone and/or somatomedin C levels due to inadequate thyroid hormone regulation of genes that code for these hormones, she is likely to be even more vulnerable to tissue injury and less capable of tissue repair (see Chapter 3.12).

The recent use of androgens by athletes has publicized the anabolic or tissue-building effects of these hormones.[30,pp.115-116] My observations of men using anabolic steroids have convinced me that the hormones can generate intense behavioral tendencies such as aggressiveness and pugnacity. These observations have caused me to question the wisdom of permitting males to hold the reigns of political or military power without first determining that their behavioral tendencies are free from undue influence by high androgen levels or high tissue sensitivity to normal levels of the hormones.

Androgens enter the central nervous system and exert effects that influence mental functions, emotions, and overt behaviors (see section below titled "Premenstrual Syndrome (PMS)").

The generally lower muscle mass of women, due to lower androgen activity in their bodies, accounts partly for their lower metabolic rate compared to that of men. However, factors other than muscle mass play a role (see the subsection below titled "Role of Gender Differences in Women's Lower Metabolic Rate").

Sex Steroid Receptors

Unlike hormones such as norepinephrine and epinephrine, steroid hormones such as estradiol and progesterone do not bind to receptors on the surfaces of cells. Instead, like thyroid hormone, they bind to receptors in the cytoplasm of cells. Before exerting most of its cellular effects, T_3 travels to cell nuclei and binds to T_3-receptors attached to chromosomes. In contrast, steroid hormones bind to receptors in the cytoplasm of cells. After the steroid hormones and receptors bind, the hormone-receptor complexes enter cell nuclei and bind to chromosomes. Binding of the hormone-receptor complexes to specific sites on DNA strands activates transcription. The resulting mRNAs are then translated into specific proteins that control cell functions.[78,p.814][103,p.244][296][298][302][303]

Berne and Levy wrote that few spare estrogen and progesterone receptors are available. Because of this, how responsive a tissue is to the hormones is proportional to the concentration of estrogen and progesterone receptors in the cell. Through receptor recruitment, estradiol or progesterone receptors can bolster or inhibit the action of the other type of receptors. For example, estradiol increases the density of both estrogen and progesterone receptors in the uterus during the follicular phase of the cycle when the endometrium is proliferating. On the other hand, progesterone reduces the density of estrogen receptors in the endometrium during the luteal phase when the endometrium is in the secretory phase.[228,p.608] Also, binding of progesterone to subtypes A and B progesterone receptors can inhibit estradiol-induced estrogen receptor activity.[302]

Estrogen receptors have a high affinity for many substances other than endogenous estrogens. The range of substances the receptors will bind to is so wide that some researchers refer to them as "promiscuous." The feature is both advantageous and disadvantageous. For example, the receptors bind an array of natural plant estrogens that women can use to their advantage during peri-menopause and menopause (see section below titled "Estrogen Replacement Therapy"). On the other hand, estrogen receptors bind many man-made chemical contaminants. According to McLachlan, "In endocrinology textbooks, one still finds flat assertions that receptors are highly discriminating about chemical structure and will bind only to their intended hormone or a very closely related compound. Although theory holds true in a general way, reality is proving considerably messier and unpredictable, not only in the case of the estrogen receptor but with other hormone receptors as well." A variety of man-made chemicals that are ubiquitous in our environment can bind to estrogen receptors. The effects are hard to predict because they vary, depending on the sex of the contaminated individual, whether the person is a child or adult, and whether a woman is pre- or post-menopausal. Some chemicals preferentially bind to estrogen receptors and activate them, regardless of circulating endogenous estrogen levels. Others bind to the receptors and keep them inactive, again, regardless of circulating endogenous estrogen levels.[87,pp.71&79]

● THE MENSTRUAL CYCLE

Menstruation begins in most females between the ages of 11 and 15. The ability to reproduce begins after FSH and LH secretion increases from low childhood levels.[228,p.608] During the reproductive years, females have menstrual cycles at roughly 1-month intervals. Each cycle has three sequential phases—the follicular, ovulatory, and luteal.

THREE PHASES OF THE MENSTRUAL CYCLE

Division of the menstrual cycle into three phases is based on the events in the development of each monthly ovum. Normally, during the different phases, the production and circulating levels of FSH, LH, estrogen, and progesterone vary in characteristic ways. The length of a normal menstrual cycle ranges from 21-to-35 days. Variations in the length of the cycle depend mostly on differences in the time span of the follicular phase.[228,p.602]

The main regulators of the phases of the menstrual cycle are GnRH, FSH and LH. In response to these gonadotropins, cells of the ovary release variable amounts of estrogen, progesterone, and testosterone.[228,p.602][313] These sex hormones regulate the function of tissues involved in sexual functions and alter the levels of GnRH, FSH, and LH. Figures 3.6.1, 3.6.2, and 3.6.3 show the approximate normal plasma levels of GnRH, FSH, LH, estrogen, and progesterone throughout the menstrual cycle.

Follicular Phase of the Menstrual Cycle

Menstruation. The follicular phase, which varies in length, starts when menstrual bleeding begins.[228,p.602] Menstruation is the cyclic shedding and discharge of the mucous membrane of the endometrium of the uterus that occurs about every 4 weeks. That menstruation occurs every 4 weeks is implied by the term "menses," a synonym for menstruation that derives from the Latin term for "monthly." Menstruation occurs during the early part of the follicular phase, normally lasting about 4-to-7 days.

FSH and LH Levels. Circulating levels of FSH and LH are at their lowest levels just before the beginning of the follicular phase. The level of FSH is slightly higher than that of LH. One day before menstruation begins, the FSH level begins rising, and it continues to rise during the first half of the follicular phase. During the second half of the follicular phase,

the FSH level declines somewhat, and the LH level rises. By the end of the follicular phase, the LH level has increased enough so that it is considerably higher than the FSH level.

During the first 6-to-8 days of the follicular phase, FSH stimulates progressively increased estradiol secretion by the follicle's granulosa cells. The granulosa cells form the granular layer that lines the wall of the follicle. The circulating estradiol level correspondingly rises. About midway through the follicular phase, estradiol secretion steeply increases, and the circulating estradiol level peaks just before the onset of ovulation. The high circulating estradiol level inhibits FSH release by pituitary gonadotroph cells. As a result, the circulating FSH level decreases during the second half of the follicular phase.

Granulosa and Thecal Cell Changes in the Follicular Phase. Within the first 2 or 3 days after menstruation begins, the FSH level increases moderately and the LH level increases slightly. These hormones, especially FSH, hasten the growth of several ovarian follicles. Initially, more granulosa cells (which form the granular layers of the wall of the follicle) are produced, and more layers of granulosa cells form in the follicles.

Other cells that arise from the interstitial tissues of the ovary aggregate outside the granulosa cells.[306] These other cells separate into two layers. The outer layer, the "theca externa," becomes the connective tissue capsule of the developing follicle. The capsule contains an extensive network of blood vessels. The internal layer, the "theca interna," is made up of cells that secrete a slightly different combination of sex hormones than do the granulosa cells.

During the follicular phase, the granulosa cells secrete a fluid that contains a high concentration of estradiol.[308][311] The estradiol in the fluid is an element critical to the maturing of the follicle. The fluid accumulates in the follicle, forming a cavity the walls of which are made up of layers of granulosa cells and the two thecal layers. Then the granulosa and thecal cells multiply, accelerate their rates of secretion, and the follicle grows. Estradiol secreted into the follicle by the granulosa cells increases the density of FSH cells on the granulosa cells, augmenting their responsiveness to FSH.[310] FSH and estrogen stimulate an increase in LH receptors on the granulosa cells. With the appearance of LH receptors, LH acts in concert with FSH to markedly increase secretions within the follicle. LH and increasing amounts of estradiol from the follicle stimulate reproduction of the thecal cells and increase their rate of secretion.

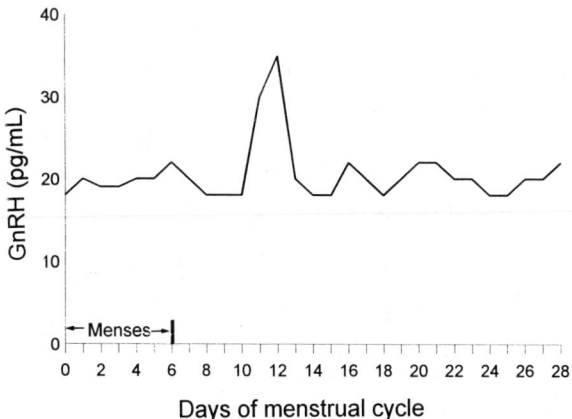

Figure 3.6.1. Approximate plasma levels of gonadotropin-releasing hormone during the normal female menstrual cycle.

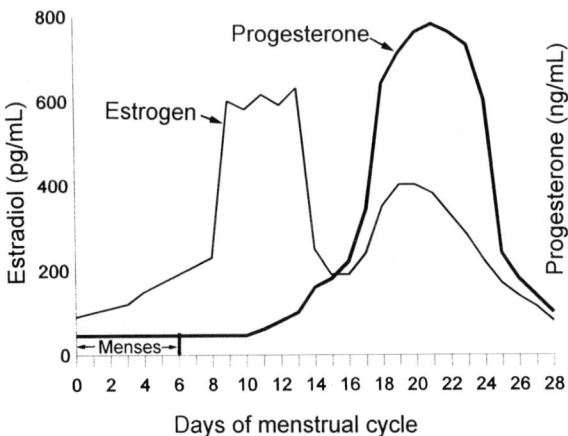

Figure 3.6.2. Approximate plasma levels of estradiol and progesterone during the normal female menstrual cycle.

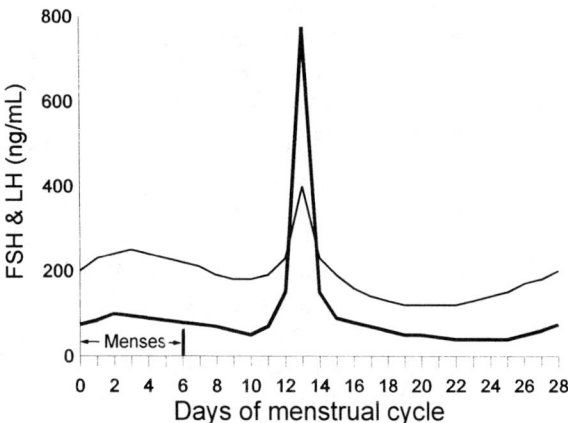

Figure 3.6.3. Approximate plasma levels of FSH and LH during the normal female menstrual cycle.

LH plays an important role in the second half of the follicular phase. In the follicles undergoing development, the granulosa and thecal cells exchange steroid hormones. LH stimulates the thecal cells to produce greater amounts of testosterone.[309] The testosterone diffuses to granulosa cells where the enzyme aromatase catalyzes their conversion to estradiol. In addition, LH stimulates the granulosa cells to secrete more progesterone. The progesterone diffuses to the thecal cells where it is converted to testosterone. The testosterone then diffuses back to the granulosa cells for conversion to estradiol.

After 7 days or so, all but one developing follicle become atretic. One follicle, the dominant one, continues to develop. The follicle that survives as the dominant one probably has more FSH receptors and a higher rate of aromatase activity. Both the higher density of receptors and the higher rate of enzymatic activity enable the follicle to produce estradiol more effectively than the other follicles that become atretic.[314]

The dominant follicle secretes a large amount of estrogen. The estrogen further increases the density of FSH receptors on the granulosa and thecal cells, further increasing their responsiveness to FSH. The increased number of cells provides even larger amounts of estrogen which further increase the density of FSH receptors. Moreover, the FSH and increased amounts of estradiol stimulate an even further increased density of LH receptors of granulosa and thecal cells.[307]

Eventually, in the latter part of the follicular phase, the follicle comes to secrete so much estradiol that the circulating level rises high enough to inhibit the pituitary gonadotroph cells. As a result, the circulating levels of FSH and LH diminish somewhat. Now, all follicles except the dominant one cease to grow. The dominant follicle continues to grow for two reasons: (1) its high estradiol content, and (2) its high density of FSH and LH receptors render it highly responsive to the somewhat reduced FSH and LH levels.[78,pp.901-902][228,p.603]

Uterine Changes in the Follicular Phase. The uterus is a muscular organ that encloses a cavity lined with a mucous membrane called the endometrium. After menstruation, the endometrium is thin, contains few glands, and a fertilized ovum cannot implant in it. In the follicular phase, after menstruation ends, increased estradiol secreted by the granulosa cells of the follicle induces the proliferative phase of endometrial development. The endometrium thickens 3- to 5-fold.[305] The glands of the membrane become more tortuous and its arteries elongate. In addition, the metabolism of glucose, lipids, and amino acids increases in cells of the membrane.[304] The increased estradiol also decreases the viscous nature of the mucous of the cervix, the opening to the uterus. The more watery consistency of the mucous makes it easier for sperm to enter the uterine cavity.

Ovulatory Phase of the Menstrual Cycle

The ovulatory phase occurs when the ovarian follicle expels the ovum. This phase lasts only 1-to-3 days. At the beginning of the ovulatory phase, the LH level sharply peaks, and to a far lesser degree, the FSH level also peaks. Two events in the late follicular phase immediately precede these peaks: (1) a "saw-tooth" peak of estradiol levels and (2) increased pulsatile releases of GnRH.[228,p.602][313] The estradiol peak indirectly stimulates GnRH release, and the increased GnRH stimulates a slightly increased release of FSH and a dramatically increased release of LH.

After the follicle expels the ovum, LH also stimulates the granulosa cells to quickly change into luteal cells. The luteal cells secrete small amounts of "inhibin," a nonsteroidal hormone that inhibits the pituitary gonadotrophs, especially their secretion of FSH.[78,pp.903&909][312] Because of the previously elevated estradiol level and the presence of inhibin in the circulating blood, the pituitary gonadotrophs sharply decrease their secretion of FSH and LH during the ovulatory phase of the menstrual cycle.

Ovulation may not occur because various influences disrupt the normal pattern of FSH and LH release by the pituitary. Such influences include stress, emotional disturbance, calorie deprivation, and regular strenuous physical exercise. These appear to override the influence of estradiol and progesterone on the normal pituitary secretion of FSH and LH. Hypothyroidism is particularly disruptive of ovulation.[228,p.605]

Uterine Changes in the Ovulatory Phase. During the ovulatory phase, progesterone secretion begins to increase. Increased exposure of the endometrium to the higher concentration of progesterone induces changes characteristic of the secretory phase of endometrial development. The rapid growth of the endometrium induced by estradiol ceases. Endometrial glands become more complex and store more glycogen.[228,p.606]

Luteal Phase of the Menstrual Cycle

The luteal phase, the third and final phase of the menstrual cycle, lasts 13-to-14 days. It ends when menstrual bleeding begins. During the luteal phase, the markedly reduced FSH and LH levels remain low.

They reach their lowest levels toward the end of the luteal phase, just before the beginning of menstruation. The sustained low FSH and LH levels result from gonadotroph cell inhibition by a high estradiol level and an even higher progesterone level. The high levels of estradiol and progesterone result from copious secretion of the hormones by the corpus luteum. Corpus luteum secretion of progesterone is 10 times that during other phases.[228,p.603] (See Figures 3.6.2 and 3.6.3.)

If pregnancy occurs, human chorionic gonadotropin (hCG—the placental equivalent of LH) secreted by the placenta sustains the corpus luteum (see section below titled "Pregnancy"). If pregnancy does not occur, in the late luteal phase, the corpus luteum begins to degenerate about the 8th day after ovulation. By the 14th day after ovulation, it completely ceases to secrete progesterone and estradiol. The corpus luteum begins to degenerate without exposure to hCG because the high estradiol, progesterone levels, reinforced by inhibin, have inhibited the pituitary gonadotrophs. The gonadotrophs have reduced their secretion of FSH and LH. If the LH level decreases early, the corpus luteum will, within 4-to-8 days, pass through a process of proliferation, enlargement, and secretion, and then degeneration. If LH levels are high enough for a longer time, the corpus luteum will continue functioning for 12 days. But the reduced FSH and LH levels, induced by elevated progesterone, estradiol, and inhibin levels, cause the corpus luteum to degenerate by the 12th day after ovulation, which is the 26th day of the menstrual cycle. Lysis of the corpus luteum is mediated mainly by prostaglandins.

As the corpus luteum degenerates, its secretion of progesterone and estradiol diminishes. By the 12th day after ovulation, about 2 days before menstruation, the levels of estradiol and progesterone are at their lowest during the cycle. At this time, circulating progesterone and estradiol levels fall low enough to disinhibit the pituitary gonadotrophs. Freed from sex hormone inhibition, the gonadotrophs begin secreting FSH, beginning the next follicular phase. The suddenly reduced circulating levels of estradiol and progesterone, especially that of progesterone, induce menstrual bleeding.[78,p.907][228,p.605]

Luteinization and the Corpus Luteum. Luteinization is the formation of a corpus luteum within a ruptured ovarian follicle shortly after ovulation. LH stimulates the conversion of granulosa cells to luteal cells. The cells enlarge to about twice the size of their precursor granulosa cells, and the entire mass of cells constitutes the corpus luteum. Luteinization occurs within a couple of hours after ovulation. If ovulation does not occur, then luteinization seldom occurs.

The corpus luteum is a small yellow body, its yellow color due to the high lipid content of its luteal cells. When initially formed, the corpus luteum develops an endoplasmic reticulum that produces large amounts of estradiol and even larger amounts of progesterone (see Figure 3.6.2). The corpus luteum also develops an extensive network of blood vessels. Its blood content increases and the network of vessels provides the luteal cells with LH and the cholesterol that is essential to progesterone synthesis.

If a sperm fertilizes the ovum, the corpus luteum continues to secrete progesterone. The progesterone sustains the endometrium in a condition favorable for continued pregnancy. The hormone also inhibits contractions of the uterus. If a sperm does not fertilize the ovum, the corpus luteum promptly stops its secretion of progesterone. The level of the hormone abruptly declines, initiating the onset of menstruation.[103,p.247]

Uterine Changes in the Luteal Phase. The corpus luteum secretes both estradiol and progesterone during the luteal phase. The estradiol causes endometrial cells to continue proliferating to a slight degree. The progesterone causes swelling and secretion, giving rise to the designation "secretory phase." During the secretory phase, vacuoles of stored glycogen migrate from the base toward the surface of the endometrium, and the glands markedly increase their rate of secretion. With the vacuoles closer to the surface, the fertilized ovum has easier access to the glycogen they contain. The endometrial stroma accumulates fluid and the arteries further elongate and coil. With these changes, the endometrium is better able to receive, implant, and nourish a fertilized ovum. Also, the high progesterone level causes the mucous of the cervix to thicken again, making it more difficult for sperm to enter the uterine cavity.[228,p.606]

If pregnancy does not occur, no placental progesterone is available to sustain the corpus luteum. Degeneration of the corpus luteum precipitously reduces progesterone and estradiol levels. The reduced levels result in spasms of the endometrial arteries. The spasms critically reduce blood flow to the superficial endometrium and cause tissue death. The superficial cells and clotted blood then shed, providing the bloody discharge of menstruation.[228,p.606]

PREGNANCY

If pregnancy occurs—that is, if a sperm fertilizes the ovum in the fallopian tube—the zygote develops into a blastocyst. Within 3 days, the blastocyst traverses the fallopian tube. Within another 2 or 3 days, the blastocyst implants in the endometrial lining of the uterus.

Whether or not the blastocyst implants depends upon events that occur only in the presence of sufficient concentrations of progesterone. The events include alternate contractions of the blastocyst and the release of substances in uterine secretions that help dissolve the outer layer of the ovum (the zona pellucida).

For the pregnancy to continue, the ovum must be nourished by "decidual cells." These are enlarged stroma cells of the uterus that have accumulated glycogen and lipid. Continual exposure of the stroma cells to progesterone and estrogen quickly alters the entire stroma into a layer of decidual cells. Until arteries and veins form between the mother and fetus, the decidual cells provide nutrients to the developing embryo.[228,p.610]

Placenta

When the placenta forms, it serves several functions on behalf of the fetus: arterial supply of oxygen and nutrients, venous elimination of metabolic wastes and carbon dioxide, and regulation of fluid volume. In addition, the placenta is an endocrine gland. It synthesizes and secretes protein and steroid hormones that regulate the metabolism of both the fetus and mother. Among the hormones produced by the placenta are human hCG, progesterone, and estrogens.[228,pp.610-611]

Human Chorionic Gonadotropin (hCG). During the first trimester, hCG stimulates the ovaries to secrete estrogen and progesterone. In the second and third trimesters, hCG does not serve this purpose because the placenta secretes estrogen and progesterone. Within 9 days of conception, hCG is measurable in the mother's plasma and urine. The outer cells of the placenta (called synctiotrophoblast cells) secrete hCG. Synthesis and production of the hormone increases when the placenta is exposed to GnRH secreted by adjacent placental cells. The level of hCG in the plasma rapidly increases and reaches a peak at 9-to-12 weeks of gestation. The level then declines slightly and remains stable throughout pregnancy.

If pregnancy does not occur, the corpus luteum degenerates. But if pregnancy does occur, hCG maintains the corpus luteum. The corpus luteum responds to hCG as it does to LH with the secretion of progesterone and estradiol. Between 6 and 12 weeks of gestation, the placenta synthesizes adequate amounts of progesterone and estrogens. At this time, hCG secretion decreases and the corpus luteum regresses.[78,p.903][228,p.611]

The adrenal glands of the fetus are dependent on hCG stimulation for production of sulfated DHEA (DHEA-S).[228,p.611] Fetal DHEA-S is necessary for the production of estrogen by the placenta (see subsection below in this section titled "Placenta and Estrogens").

Placenta and Progesterone. At 6 weeks of gestation, the placenta begins producing progesterone, mainly from maternal cholesterol. By 12 weeks, placental production increases enough that further production by the corpus luteum is not necessary. By the time of delivery, the placental production of progesterone is some 10 times the maximum produced by the corpus luteum.[228,p.611]

Progesterone is necessary for the fertilized ovum to implant, and the hormone is essential to the nourishment of the implanted ovum. Without enough progesterone, glycogen- and lipid-containing stromal cells are not converted to the decidual cells that nourish the embryo. In addition, progesterone also sustains the lining of decidual cells. The hormone also passes to the fetus where it serves as a substrate in the fetal adrenal cortices for the synthesis of aldosterone and cortisol.

Progesterone stimulates the synthesis of prolactin by the uterine lining. Prolactin inhibits the mother's immune system from forming antibodies to fetal antigens. The prolactin inhibition prevents rejection of the fetus. Also, progesterone prevents premature expulsion of the fetus by reducing uterine muscle contractions. The hormone stimulates development of the breasts, increases the capacity of the breasts to secrete milk, and increases the mother's respiration so that she efficiently eliminates the increased quantity of carbon dioxide associated with pregnancy.

Placenta and Estrogens. Throughout pregnancy, the levels of estradiol, estrone, and estriol steadily increase. The estrogens augment growth of the uterine muscles and stimulate relaxation of the pelvic ligaments so that they accommodate the expanding uterus.[228,p.611] The corpus luteum secretes the hormone relaxin, and its level reaches a peak in the first trimester. This hormone facilitates the relaxation of the uterine muscle and expansion of the pelvis.[228,p.612]

The corpus luteum initially provides the pregnant woman's estrogens. By the 18th or 20th week of gestation, however, the placenta has taken over estrogen production. To synthesize estrogens, placental cells must acquire an androgen precursor, DHEA-S produced by the adrenal glands of the mother and fetus. The placental cells remove the sulfate and convert the DHEA to estradiol and estrone. Estriol is also derived from DHEA-S but only after the liver of the fetus 16-hydroxylates DHEA-S, converting it to 16-OH-DHEA.[228,p.611]

PERI-MENOPAUSE AND MENOPAUSE

Menopause, the end of the female's capacity for reproduction, usually occurs between the ages of 50 and 60. Menstruation usually ends at about age 50.[319] Before this, between the ages of 40 and 50, menstrual cycles become irregular and ovulation occurs only during some cycles. This time is considered peri-menopause.

Peri-Menopause

The age of onset and the duration of peri-menopause vary considerably.[324] The peri-menopausal period, which may take years, is the transition to menopause. When the reproductive years are coming to an end, most women do not move from a time of regular menstruation to an abrupt cessation of menses. Instead, they go through peri-menopause, the transition into menopause that takes years. During peri-menopause, menstrual periods are irregular. The length of the menstrual cycle and the level of discomfort women experience in association with menses change. Hormonal levels usually fluctuate more in the extreme, precipitating symptoms.[325] The conventional view is that declining estrogen levels are the basis of health risks associated with peri-menopause, such as osteoporosis. The American College of Obstetricians and Gynecologists states that "preventive care, life style modification, and early diagnosis and intervention can play a valuable role in maintaining patients' overall health and quality of life."[326][327] In practice, however, the conventional medical approach involves prescriptions for estrogen replacement therapy with synthetic estrogen. Fortunately, other options are now available for women (see section below titled "Hormone Replacement Therapy").

For several years before menopause, the woman ovulates less often than during most of her reproductive years, and menstuation occurs at variable intervals. She also has decreased menstrual flow caused by two factors: (1) irregular peaks in estrogen levels, and (2) too little progesterone secretion during the luteal phase of the cycle. Her ovarian follicles become progressively less sensitive to FSH and LH, and accordingly, the levels of these hormones undergo a compensatory elevation.[228,p.608]

The peri-menopausal woman with diminished

menstrual blood flow may have an increase in menstrual cycle length, increased plasma FSH levels, and decreased plasma estradiol levels. She may also have decreased bone density[318] if she does not engage in physical exercise and does not maintain dietary and nutritional habits that militate against loss of bone density.

The variations in FSH and estradiol levels in peri-menopausal women in their 40s make these two hormones unreliable indicators of menopausal status. This is true even of women who are continuing to cycle regularly. These women are likely to have lower inhibin-B levels. Early in peri-menopause, when cycle irregularity first becomes obvious, the first hormonal change is a decline of inhibin-B levels early in the follicular phase. In late peri-menopause, levels of inhibin-A and estradiol also decline, inhibin-B levels remain low, and FSH remains elevated.[319]

Many patients have few or no symptoms when estrogen levels first begin to decline during early peri-menopause. But most women eventually experience symptoms as final ovarian failure approaches.[324] During peri-menopause, women may experience a variety of symptoms and physiological phenomena: depression, multiple discomforts that affect the patient's whole physical and psychologic self, hot flashes; cold sweats; joint, head, and neck pains; decreasing bone mass; changes in the urinary and genital tracts; infertility; irregular uterine bleeding; thinning skin; cognitive dysfunction, and psychosexual dysfunction.[322][323][324][327][329]

Some women are not aware that symptoms they are experiencing are due to peri-menopause. Cook wrote that an empathetic approach can be effective in educating these woman about the multiple body systems involved in peri-menopause and the various symptoms that can result. The approach can also help in counseling them to take up lifestyle changes that can promote health during this time of life.[317][322] (See section below titled "Hormone Replacement Therapy.")

Menopause

With menopause, all ovarian follicles disappear. As a result, the ovaries cease secreting estrogen. As long as a few follicles survive, the ovaries continue to secrete small amounts of estrogen. But as the last follicles become atretic, ovarian secretion of estrogen completely ends.[319]

The reduced estrogen and inhibin levels release the pituitary gonadotroph cells from inhibition. The release increases gonadotropin secretion—the plasma levels of FSH and LH rise 4-to-10 times higher than their levels during the follicular phase in the reproductive years. FSH levels remain continuously high, and higher than LH levels. After menopause, the cycle of FSH and LH secretion ceases, but pulsatile gonadotropin secretion continues.[228,p.608]

The woman with an estrogen deficiency during menopause has several physiological effects: thinning of the vaginal epithelium and loss of vaginal secretions, reduced breast mass, increased rate of bone loss, thinning of the skin, hot flushes, emotional lability, dyspnea, irritability, fatigue, anxiety, and an increased incidence of coronary artery disease.[78,p.911][228,p.608][315][316][317] According to Guyton, menopausal symptoms are severe enough to justify treatment.[78,p.911]

Matthews et al. found that menopausal women did not have an increased incidence of depression. However, peri-menopausal women who became postmenopausal had decreased levels of high-density lipoprotein and gradually increased levels of low-density lipoproteins. The women reported a decrease in symptoms. The researchers concluded that during mid-life, women have an increase of cardiovascular risk factors and a temporary increase in symptoms.[329]

● SEX-RELATED FINDINGS IN FIBROMYALGIA

Unfortunately, researchers have conducted few studies to learn the possible relation of fibromyalgia to sex hormone status. This is odd considering the two most commonly reported sex-related findings among fibromyalgia patients: (1) a much higher percentage of women in the population of fibromyalgia patients, and (2) the onset or worsening of fibromyalgia symptoms in the premenstrual time, during peri-menopause, or during menopause. Considering these common reports, it is odd that more studies have not been done on the possible relation of fibromyalgia to sex hormone status.

SEX-RELATED SYMPTOMS OF FIBROMYALGIA PATIENTS

Wolfe reported that some 40.6% of female fibromyalgia patients report a history of dysmenorrhea.[152] Some writers list PMS as a common symptom of fibromyalgia.[332,p.14]

Men with chronic fatigue syndrome have reported

a loss of sex drive, decreased sexual activity, and impotence.[349,pp.59,137,203] In clinical practice, female fibromyalgia patients report a loss of libido, often attributing the loss to their pain and general discomfort.

HIGHER INCIDENCE OF
FIBROMYALGIA AMONG FEMALES

Several studies have shown that most fibromyalgia patients are women. Guler et al. reported that among fibromyalgia patients, the female to male ratio is 5 to 1.[79] In a German town, researchers examined 541 citizens for fibromyalgia, and 10 met the criteria. Of the 10, 8 were females.[12,p.8] Of the general population in a town in eastern Denmark, 6% had fibromyalgia. All the people who meet the 1990 ACR criteria for fibromyalgia were women.[13,p.8] A study in England of patients from general medical practices found that 13.2% had chronic widespread pain. Widespread pain was twice as common in women as in men.[14,p.8] Campbell studied 596 patients from a general medical clinic. Seven percent possibly had fibromyalgia and 5.7% definitely did. Of the patients with possible fibromyalgia, 71.4% were females. Of those who definitely had fibromyalgia, 72.7% were female.[17] Felson wrote that clinical experience shows that 75%-to-95% of fibromyalgia patients are women.[18,p.8]

In one study, more patients with osteoarthritis who also had fibromyalgia were women. Of 105 male osteoarthritis patients, 42 (40%) met the criteria for fibromyalgia. In contrast, of 257 female osteoarthritis patients, 142 (55%) met the criteria for fibromyalgia.[15,p.11] In another study, more patients with rheumatoid arthritis who also had fibromyalgia were women. Of 52 males with rheumatoid arthritis, 12 (23%) had fibromyalgia. Of 102 females with rheumatoid arthritis, 37 (38%) had fibromyalgia.[16,p.11] For consideration of factors that may be responsible for the higher incidence of females among fibromyalgia patients, see section below titled "Factors Possibly Responsible for the Higher Incidence of Fibromyalgia Among Females."

ONSET AND EXACERBATIONS OF
FIBROMYALGIA IN RELATION TO
FEMALE SEX HORMONE CHANGES

Of 26 fibromyalgia patients, 19 (73%) reported that their symptoms worsened during the premenstrual time.[260]

The onset of many women's fibromyalgia is about the time of the onset of menopause.[76] Waxman and Zatzkis wrote that fibromyalgia is often associated with decreased ovarian function and often mimics an exaggerated menopausal state. They found the mean age at which 100 female patients received a diagnosis of fibromyalgia was 48. Patients ranged in age from 24-to-70. On average, patients had experienced fibromyalgia symptoms for 2 years before receiving the diagnosis. Menopause developed in 65 women before they received the diagnosis of fibromyalgia and in 3 after they received the diagnosis. Of the 65 women who developed menopause before fibromyalgia, 14 had undergone natural menopause, 21 had undergone surgery to remove both ovaries and fallopian tubes, and 30 had an abdominal hysterectomy and/or removal of one ovary and its fallopian tube. (A total of 51 women developed fibromyalgia after surgically-induced menopause.) The authors wrote that 49 of the women had reached menopause by age 50, and 36 of the 65 women were not using estrogen therapy when they developed fibromyalgia. They also noted that 24 of the 65 women received a diagnosis of fibromyalgia within 5 years of the onset of menopause, and the remaining 41 patients developed fibromyalgia up to 11 years after menopause. They also found that fibromyalgia patients aged 24-to-45 were prematurely menopausal, either due to surgery or natural processes.[77]

Anderberg et al. wrote that for most female patients, fibromyalgia begins after one or more childbirths, during middle age, or during the peri-menopausal time when estrogen and progesterone levels are decreasing. Some women's fibromyalgia symptoms begin at the time of the first menstrual period, and others' symptoms begin with delivery of a child.[333,pp.6-7]

Anderberg et al. studied changes in 15 different symptoms during the menstrual cycles of 16 premenopausal fibromyalgia patients and 15 healthy control subjects. Fibromyalgia patients had more severe symptoms than controls during the luteal phase and the premenstrual time. Patients had more fatigue, distress, depression, and sensitivity to pain. Of the 15 fibromyalgia patients, 7 (44%) also met the criteria for premenstrual dysphoric disorder. This is much higher than the 10% of women in the general population who have severe premenstrual dysphoric disorder.[336][337] However, fibromyalgia patients, both those with and without premenstrual dysphoric disorder, were more depressed and pain sensitive during the luteal phase and about the time of menstruation. The researchers concluded that during the premenstrual time, when estrogen and progesterone levels were declining, premenopausal fibromyalgia patients had more numerous and more severe symptoms than did healthy control subjects.[333,pp.6-7]

In another study, Anderberg et al. found that post-menopausal fibromyalgia patients had worse psychological status than premenopausal fibromyalgia patients. The post-menopausal fibromyalgia patients also had significantly worse psychological and physical status than post-menopausal healthy control subjects. Compared to premenopausal fibromyalgia patients, post-menopausal fibromyalgia patients had more psychological symptoms (compared during the time of the premenstrual patients' ovulatory phase, days 12-to-17 of their cycle), but the two groups did not differ regarding physical symptoms such as pain. The investigators noted that the post-menopausal patients' worse psychological status may have been related to their lower estrogen levels during this time. They wrote that during the ovulatory phase in premenopausal patients, estrogen levels are elevated (although the levels actually decline precipitously throughout this phase) while progesterone levels are comparatively low (progesterone levels gradually elevate throughout the phase). Their statement implies a positive role for estrogen, which is certainly possible. Around the time of their menstruation, premenopausal women did not differ psychologically from post-menopausal women. This premenopausal group may have had better psychological status on average were it not for the 44% of the women in the group who had premenstrual dysphoric disorder. Post-menopausal healthy control subjects had significantly better psychological status than all fibromyalgia patients. However, the psychological status of the healthy control subjects was especially better than that of post-menopausal fibromyalgia patients. About the time of the premenopausal patients' premenstrual time, they and post-menopausal patients had more stress-related symptoms (anxiety, stiffness, and headache) than did healthy post-menopausal women.[334]

PREGNANCY AND FIBROMYALGIA

Ostensen et al. interviewed 26 patients to learn the relation of fibromyalgia to pregnancy. The women had a total of 40 pregnancies while they had been fibromyalgic. All the women except one described their fibromyalgia symptoms as worse during pregnancy. They reported that their symptoms were worst during the last trimester. Six months after 37 of the 40 pregnancies, patients reported that their symptoms changed: 4 patients' symptoms improved, and 33 patients' symp-

toms worsened. The worsened symptoms resulted in 14 patients taking prolonged sick leave. The worst postpartum symptoms were anxiety and depression. The patients' fibromyalgia apparently did not adversely affect the mother or the neonate. The severity of the patients' fibromyalgia symptoms did not appear to be influenced by hormonal alterations associated with abortion, use of oral contraceptives, or breast feeding. The researchers wrote they compared the 26 patients who had borne their children after they had become fibromyalgic with 18 patients who had all their children before they developed fibromyalgia. They result showed that pregnancy had negative effects on the fibromyalgia patients and resulted in increased functional impairment and disability in the postpartum period.[260]

LEVELS OF FSH, ESTROGEN, GNRH, AND LH

Riedel et al. reported finding that 16 fibromyalgia patients had elevated basal FSH levels and low basal estrogen levels. When 6 patients were given GnRH injections, the patients had significantly blunted pituitary LH responses. They also found that the patients had low T_3 levels and blunted TSH responses to TRH. The investigators speculated that elevated CRH could have inhibited hypothalamic GnRH secretion and ovarian estrogen secretion. However, although they measured CRH levels, they did not report finding that it was low.[331] In addition, there is reason to believe that CRH secretion in fibromyalgia patients is low rather than high (see Chapter 3.5, section titled "Hypothalamic-Pituitary-Adrenal Axis Abnormalities in Fibromyalgia," and section titled "Thyroid Hormone Status and the HPA Axis").

ANDROGEN LEVELS IN FIBROMYALGIC WOMEN

Dessein et al. studied 57 consecutive female fibromyalgia patients and compared the results with 114 normal controls. They found that premenopausal women had significantly low testosterone levels, and post-menopausal women had lower levels that were short of statistical significance. Testosterone levels were correlated with levels of physical functioning—that is, women with lower testosterone levels had lower levels of physical functioning. The researchers concluded that they had found deficient adrenal secretion of androgens in fibromyalgic women.[330]

● INADEQUATE THYROID HORMONE REGULATION OF THE FEMALE HPG AXIS

Adequate thyroid hormone regulation of the HPG axis is essential to the normal function of the axis components and secretion of the hormones peculiar to each. Adequate thyroid hormone regulation is therefore indirectly responsible for normal function of the tissues that are dependent on HPG axis hormones. Inadequate thyroid hormone regulation of the HPG axis results in abnormalities that can plausibly account for the sex-related abnormalities of fibromyalgia patients.

SEX-RELATED ABNORMALITIES OF HYPOTHYROID FEMALES

In the female, inadequate thyroid hormone regulation of the HPG axis, during hypothyroidism and/or thyroid hormone resistance, can have variable adverse effects on female sex-related functions. In 1933, Kimball wrote: "The chronic type of hypothyroidism is practically always seen because of some condition secondary to low thyroid activity. The majority of my patients have come because of symptoms of hypogonadism. The complaint of the women is some abnormality of the menstrual cycle. You soon learn, however, of associated symptoms such as fatigue, lack of energy, or spells of drowsiness of which they are ashamed, and frequently nervousness. We have seen practically every type of amenorrhea and dysmenorrhea which was eventually proven to be secondary to hypothyroidism and relieved by adequate thyroid therapy." He also stated, "Dysmenorrhea due to primary hypothyroidism may simulate any and every form of menstrual disorder."[206,p.493] Many other medical writers have echoed Kimball's early statements.[124][125][126][127][128][150][151] For example, Maruo et al. wrote, "It is clinically evident that women suffering from thyroid disorders are associated with frequent occurrence of menstrual disturbances and impaired fertility, and these abnormalities are improved by thyroid hormone therapy."[86,p.1233] Similarly, Thomas and Reid wrote that thyroid disorders, which may develop insidiously, are implicated in a broad spectrum of reproductive disorders ranging from abnormal sexual development to menstrual irregularities and infertility.

POSSIBLE MECHANISMS OF SEX-RELATED ABNORMALITIES IN FIBROMYALGIA

Several possible mechanisms can account for the high prevalence of females with fibromyalgia: (1) the lower metabolic rate of women, (2) a higher incidence of hypothyroidism among females, (3) thyroid hormone-lowering effects of estrogen, and (4) greater susceptibility to injury due to lower androgen levels than men (see section below titled "Factors Possibly Responsible for the Higher Incidence of Fibromyalgia Among Females").

The low libido of fibromyalgia patients may result from low testosterone levels (see section below titled "Reduced Sex Drive"). Dysmenorrhea in fibromyalgia may result from a combination of unbalanced endometrial stimulation and excessive activity of the uterine muscle. The same mechanism may account for the excessive menstrual bleeding that leads to a high frequency of hysterectomies among fibromyalgia patients (see section below titled "Mechanisms of Menstrual Abnormalities in Hypothyroidism"). Inadequate thyroid hormone regulation of the HPG axis may explain low FSH and the subnormal LH response to GnRH (see section below titled "Thyroid Hormone, FSH, and LH"). However, Wortsman et al. found that men with primary hypothyroidism had blunted LH responses to GnRH and low T$_3$ levels.[195] The same pattern was found in hypothyroid rats[321] (see section below titled "Effects of Hypothyroidism on Male Sex Hormones").

The worse symptoms of fibromyalgic women during the premenstrual time and peri-menopause may result from inadequate thyroid hormone regulation of the function of the ovaries. Optimal amounts of thyroid hormone are needed for FSH to properly stimulate the granulosa cells of the ovarian follicles. Also, thyroid hormone is necessary for the normal production of estrogen and progesterone by the cells of the follicles of the ovaries. Thyroid hormone is required for the normal production of pregnenolone, the precursor of progesterone, and for normal activity of the enzyme that converts pregnenolone to progesterone. In addition, the low basal estrogen levels of some fibromyalgia patients[331] may result from reduced ovarian secretion of estrone and estradiol due to inadequate thyroid hormone facilitation of FSH-stimulation of ovarian granulosa cells (see section below titled "Estrogen Production in Granulosa Cells").

Without sufficient exposure of the granulosa cells of the ovaries to thyroid hormone, three critical problems develop that can account for some of fibromyalgic women's sex-related problems: incomplete differentiation of the granulosa cells, too few LH and hCG receptors in the cells, and subnormal production of estrogen and progesterone. For ovulation to occur normally, and for the follicle to convert to a corpus luteum, LH must bind to the granulosa cells. LH can do so only if the cells contain enough LH receptors, which is partly dependent on sufficient exposure to thyroid hormone. If the corpus luteum does not form properly, the follicular granulosa cells will not convert to progesterone-secreting luteal cells, and the patient will have a progesterone deficiency during the luteal phase of the menstrual cycle. The progesterone deficiency may be worsened by low pituitary secretion of LH secondary to low hypothalamic TRH secretion in fibromyalgia patients with hypothalamic hypothyroidism. (See section below titled "Luteinization.")

Many women with fibromyalgia complain of infertility and/or difficulties carrying fetuses to term. Hypothyroidism causes infertility in many women. It causes the pregnancies of some to end with spontaneous abortion in the first trimester, stillbirths, or premature birth. Also, hypothyroidism is a risk factor for the development of gestational diabetes and pre-eclampsia.

REDUCED SEX DRIVE

Many hypothyroid women have markedly reduced or absent libido.[78,p.836] This is also true of many female patients with fibromyalgia. Most such patients attribute their low libido to distractions by their other symptoms, especially pain and fatigue. However, the finding of low testosterone levels in fibromyalgia patients[330] raises the possibility that the loss of libido is hormonally based (see section above titled "Androgen Levels in Fibromyalgic Women").

The woman's sex desire usually reaches a peak in the time just before ovulation, probably because of the elevated estrogen level.[78,p.911] However, the woman's sex drive is partially dependent on testosterone. Basson, for example, wrote that testosterone is an important metabolic and sex hormone produced by the ovaries, and reduced ovarian testosterone at menopause is associated in some women with a loss of sex desire and sexual response. He noted that estrogen deficiency can also impair libido and sex response, but estrogen replacement does not improve and may worsen sexual symptoms from an androgen deficiency.[343] Sarrel reported that with menopausal women, therapy with both estrogen and androgens provides results su-

perior to those of estrogen alone. He wrote that the use of both hormones more effectively relieved poor concentration, depression, and fatigue, and low libido, and inability to reach orgasm.[344][345] Riley reported the case of a woman who had a lifelong absence of sex drive. Testing showed she had a low level of 5-dehydrotestosterone. After she began applying to her vulva a gel containing dehydrotestosterone, she developed sex drive and began experiencing sexual arousal.[346]

MENSTRUAL DISTURBANCES

In many hypothyroid women, the length of the menstrual cycle and the amount of bleeding become abnormal.[199][213][214] The changes may seem paradoxical. Some hypothyroid women have a total lack of menstrual bleeding (amenorrhea),[207,p.568][215][216][217][218] but most have excessive bleeding (menorrhagia).[137][207,p.568][219] Others have a high frequency of bleeding (polymenorrhea). Some hypothyroid women have episodes of amenorrhea interspersed with periods of heavy vaginal bleeding.[222]

DeGroot et al. wrote, "Menorrhagia is sufficiently impressive in ordinary myxedema so that in several cases that have come to our attention, patients have actually had dilatation and curettage or hysterectomy for it, the diagnosis of myxedema having been missed."[207,p.568] Such patients have been far from rare in my clinical practice. The high incidence of such women in my practice may be due to the unusually high incidence of hysterectomies among fibromyalgia patients,[289] probably due to menorrhagia. Most of the patients in my practice had willingly undergone hysterectomies because their menstrual bleeding was so profuse that it was problematic for them. Before their hysterectomies, their hypothyroidism was either unrecognized by clinicians or undertreated with T4. When they finally underwent metabolic rehabilitation including the use of the proper form and dosage of thyroid hormone, other symptoms and signs that existed when they had menorrhagia disappeared. The menorrhagia of such women is probably estrogen breakthrough bleeding secondary to failure to ovulate (anovulation).[137]

Even mild hypothyroidism may cause menorrhagia. Wilansky and Greisman studied 67 "apparently euthyroid" menorrhagic women. Fifteen of the 67 women (22%) had a mean basal TSH level that at the time was considered only slightly elevated, 5.9±0.76 μU/mL. In comparison, the mean level for the other 52 women was 2.4±0.24 μU/mL. The 15 women with elevated basal TSH levels also had a lower mean serum T_4 level than did the other women (85±4.2 vs 105±3.0 nmol/L). During TRH stimulation tests, the 15 patients also had exaggerated TSH responses, suggesting hypothyroidism. Wilansky and Greisman considered the 15 women to have "early and potential" hypothyroidism. With T_4 treatment, the patients' menorrhagia disappeared within 3-to-6 months. It had not recurred during a 1-to-3 year follow-up.[190]

In one study, 16 of 18 (91%) classically hypothyroid patients reported dysmenorrhea.[208,p.19] In another study of 77 cases of hypothyroidism, 18% of female patients reported dysmenorrhea, and among the premenopausal patients, 32% also reported menorrhagia.[207,pp.577-578]

Several writers have report menstrual disturbances as a symptom of euthyroid hypometabolism.[209][210][211] Menstrual disturbance has been a symptom of most of my female fibromyalgia patients.

In contrast to the menstrual disturbances in hypothyroid women, thyrotoxic women typically have scanty or infrequent menstrual flow (oligomenorrhea), or they have total amenorrhea.[78,p.836]

Mechanisms of Menstrual Abnormalities in Hypothyroidism

Menstrual abnormalities during hypothyroidism and/or thyroid hormone resistance may result from at least two mechanisms: excessive endometrial stimulation and increased muscle activity of the uterine muscle.

Increased FSH Secretion, Increased Estrogen, and Excessive Endometrial Stimulation. DeGroot et al. wrote that alterations of estrogen levels in hypothyroid women are the result of thyroid hormone deprivation on the production, metabolic pathways, and serum transport of the hormone.[207,p.568] Some researchers believe there is an overlap between the excessive production of TSH in hypothyroidism and the gonadotropins. Thus, when the hypothyroid woman's pituitary gland increases its secretion of TSH, it also increases its secretion of gonadotropins. The increased gonadotropins may cause early ovarian secretion of estrogen. The estrogen would cause endometrial overstimulation and bleeding. If the prolactin level is elevated, the patient may have galactorrhea.[347,p.1052]

Ruh et al. reported that uterine tissue from hypothyroid rats had an increased uptake and retention of estrogen.[355] Despite this finding, Gardner et al. found that hypothyroid rats had diminished uterine responses to estradiol, with low web weight, dry weight, protein content, RNA content, and thymidine incorporation in-

to uterine DNA.[356] The latter finding suggests that in hypothyroidism, estrogen may be taken up by the uterus more readily, but the effects of the estrogen may be subnormal.

Proliferative Endometrium and Urinary Progesterone Metabolite. Amenorrhea interspersed with menorrhea in some hypothyroid women corresponds to the proliferative endometrium found upon endometrial biopsy.[199] The proliferative endometrium is usually accompanied by low urinary concentration of pregnanetriol, a urinary metabolite of progesterone. The proliferative endometrium and low urinary pregnanetriol concentration suggest subnormal LH release and consequent failure of ovulation.[199] Fibromyalgia patients were found to have low LH responses to injected GnRH. It is interesting that they also had low FSH and estrogen levels. A subnormal LH level might cause the patient not to ovulate and for luteinization to fail. But low estrogen levels would also be expected to cause subnormal proliferation of the endometrium. Without sufficient proliferation, they would not have breakthrough bleeding. (See section above titled "Levels of FSH, Estrogen, GnRH, and LH.")

Excessive Contractions of the Myometrium. Pain associated with menstruation may result in part from abnormal contractions of the uterine muscle, the myometrium.[219] Two mechanisms may underlie the abnormal contractions—an increased density of α-adrenergic receptors and subnormal progesterone levels.

The rabbit uterus has both α_1- and α_2-adrenergic receptors. Activation of only the α_1-adrenergic receptors has been shown to produce smooth muscle contraction.[221,p.159] It is possible that some degree of pain associated with menstrual periods, a feature of dysmenorrhea in fibromyalgic women, results from an increase density of these receptors due to inadequate thyroid hormone transcription of the adrenergic genes (see Chapter 3.1).

As Berne and Levy wrote, "Progesterone quiets uterine muscle activity." In fact, progesterone-induced relaxation of the myometrium during pregnancy prevents premature expulsion of the fetus.[228,p.611] When progesterone is deficient, uterine muscle activity may be markedly increased.

It is possible, then, that the fibromyalgia patient may have pain-inducing contractions of the uterine muscle at menstruation for two reasons: (1) increased myometrial hypertonicity due to increased α-adrenergic receptors in the uterine muscle, and (2) a failure of the myometrium to relax properly during the luteal phase due to deficient progesterone. As a result, the uterine muscle may be hypertonic throughout the luteal phase and primed to contract painfully toward the end of the phase just before menstruation when the progesterone level reaches its lowest level during the cycle.

THYROID HORMONE STATUS AND FEMALE SEXUAL DEVELOPMENT

Longcope wrote that hypothyroidism during fetal life apparently does not impair development of the reproductive tract.[347,p.1052] However, hypothyroidism before puberty usually results in short stature and delayed sexual maturity.[134] Some girls with juvenile hypothyroidism experience precocious menstruation, a milky discharge from the nipples (galactorrhea), and enlargement of the selle turcica due to pituitary enlargement.[135][136] The possible mechanism underlying these abnormalities is overlap in pituitary production of the TSH (in response to low circulating thyroid hormone levels) and gonadotropins. If gonadotropin secretion increases with that of TSH, the increased gonadotropins reaching the ovaries are expected to have two main effects: (1) direct stimulation of the ovaries, causing precocious ovarian estrogen secretion, and (2) indirectly through the estrogen secretion, endometrial stimulation with vaginal bleeding. Prolactin is usually elevated in hypothyroid patients, and elevated prolactin would account for the girls' nipple discharge. Thyroid hormone therapy quickly relieves this syndrome.[135][136]

THYROID HORMONE, FSH, AND LH

During the normal mid-cycle surge of LH and FSH, LH secretion increases 6- to 10-fold; FSH secretion increases 2- to 3-fold. The mid-cycle surge of LH is essential to ovulation.[207,p.569]

The results of studies of gonadotropin levels in hypothyroidism have been inconsistent. According to some investigators, most hypothyroid women have normal serum FSH and LH levels, but their mid-cycle surges of the two hormones are subnormal.[207,p.569] Others researchers have reported that while the LH surge is subnormal, FSH and LH levels are persistently elevated.[220][78,p.902] When researchers tested at prolonged times after thyroidectomy of female rats, basal plasma LH and FSH levels were lower than normal,[224] the LH surge was subnormal,[225] and the number of ovulations was decreased.[226][227] Urinary gonadotropin levels in hypothyroidism may be normal or low.[207,p.569]

Mattheij et al. measured the effects of short-term hypothyroidism on rats' estrous cyclicity and the levels of LH, progesterone, and prolactin. They noted that the lower number of ovulations of hypothyroid rats reported by some researchers[226][227] was thought to result from the lower LH surge.[225] However, they found that the rate of ovulation was reduced even when a spontaneous or induced LH surge on the preceding day was higher than in control rats. They wrote that this suggests that thyroid hormone deficiency reduces the number of ovarian follicles that can ovulate. Their suggestion was confirmed by the finding of a decreased number of healthy, large follicles in the ovaries of hypothyroid rats. The ovaries contained more large atretic follicles (see Atresia in the Glossary). When the investigators suddenly stopped the T_3 treatment of hypothyroid rats, progesterone production within corpora lutea was high. However, follicles destined for the next ovulation were smaller than normal and were not able to ovulate. Administering GnRH to the rats did not induce progesterone secretion and did not increase estradiol secretion. Mattheij et al. wrote that the development of growing follicles into healthy, mature Graafian follicles depends on the follicles producing and secreting steroid hormones. Otherwise, the growing follicles undergo atresia. They conjectured that the increased numbers of atretic follicles in the rats they studied resulted from impaired steroid hormone production within the follicles due to hypothyroidism.[84]

The findings of Mattheij et al.[84] suggest that although gonadotropin levels may be abnormal in hypothyroidism, ovarian hormone secretion is a more fundamental problem (see section below).

THYROID HORMONE AND THE OVARY

Early *in vivo* studies documented a relationship between patients' thyroid status and their ovarian function. Thyroidectomy of rabbits halted the maturation of ovarian follicles. Compared to normal rabbits, thyroidectomized rabbits required far greater amounts of gonadotropins to stimulate conversion of a corpus luteum from a ruptured ovarian follicle (see subsection above titled "Luteinization and the Corpus Luteum," and section below titled "Luteinization").[129] In rats,[130] rabbits,[131] and humans,[132] treatment with drugs (such as thiouracil) that suppress thyroid gland production of thyroid hormone halted the development of ovarian follicles and caused atrophy of the ovaries.

Granulosa Cells

Differentiation of Granulosa Cells. FSH is the primary regulator of granulosa cell differentiation. Thyroid hormone is one of several amplifiers of the FSH-mediated differentiation.[83]

Maruo et al. studied the effects of thyroid hormone on ovarian function at the cellular level. They found that thyroid hormone exerted profound effects on the structure of immature granulosa cells. Combined exposure of the cells to T_3 and FSH induced an epitheloid cell structure typical of differentiated granulosa cells. T_3 or FSH alone was incapable of inducing this effect. This outcome suggests that T_3 and FSH act synergistically to induce granulosa cell differentiation.[86,pp.1237-1238][237][239]

FSH normally increases the density of LH receptors[138][139] and hCG receptors on granulosa cells.[140] [141] Maruo et al. found that the combination of T_3 and FSH greatly augmented the increased density of the two types of receptors on granulosa cells. T_3 selectively augmented FSH induction of the two receptor types in immature granulosa cells. The combination of T_3 and FSH increased the density of the receptors in small but not medium and large sized follicles.[86,p.1238]

Maruo et al. noted that the induction of LH and hCG receptors on granulosa cells is critical for the functional differentiation of granulosa cells. Because thyroid hormone acts synergistically with FSH to increase the density of the receptors, the thyroid hormone takes part in the functional differentiation of immature granulosa cells.[86,p.1238]

Thyroid Hormone and T_3-Receptors in Human Granulosa Cells. In 1987, Wakim, Ramani, and Rao reported that T_3 enhanced gonadotropin- and insulin-stimulation luteinization and progesterone secretion by cultured pig granulosa cells. They speculated that the effects of T_3 are direct and mediated by binding of T_3 to T_3-receptors in the cells. To test this hypothesis, they obtained granulosa cells from pig ovarian follicles. They found that T_3 had a higher binding affinity to sites in the nuclei than did T_4, and T_4 had a higher binding affinity than reverse-T_3. They also found that neither gonadotropins, prostaglandins, epidermal growth factor, nor insulin competed with radioactive T_3 (^{125}I-T_3) for binding to the sites. It was obvious from these findings that pig granulosa cells contain nuclear binding sites with characteristics expected of T_3-receptors. It was also likely that binding of T_3 to these receptors mediated the action of T_3 on granulosa cells.[145]

The first report of T_3 and T_4 in fluid from human ovarian follicles was by Wakim et al. published in 1993. They also reported that the use of three different specific antibodies against T_3 receptors also revealed the receptors in the nuclei of granulosa cells.[144] In 1994, Wakim et al. tested for mRNAs for α and β T_3-receptors in human granulosa cells. The cells were taken from the ovarian follicles of normally cycling women before ovulation occurred. The investigators reported positive staining for probes for both types of T_3-receptors. Ovarian stromal cells were also positive for both receptor types. They reported that the finding of α and β T_3-receptors in the granulosa cells and ovarian stroma makes it conceivable that thyroid hormone plays a direct role in regulating human ovarian physiology.[146] Also in 1994, Wakim et al. reported finding both α_1 and β_1 T_3-receptors in human granulosa cells.[147]

Maruo et al. had already determined in 1992 that T_3-receptors are expressed in granulosa cells early during maturation of ovarian follicles, at least in pig granulosa cells.[148]

Thyroid Hormone-Induced Increases in Granulosa Cell Secretion of Progesterone and Estrogen. Biswas et al.[143] and Maruo et al.[86] reported that thyroid hormone increased sex hormone production by cultured animal granulosa cells. Wakim et al. reported that thyroid hormone had the same effect on cultured human granulosa cells.[85] Apparently, insulin must be present for thyroid hormone to increase sex hormone production in granulosa cells.[86][133]

The thyroid hormone-induced increases in sex hormone production probably account for a report by Maruo et al. They found that when subclinically hypothyroid women underwent thyroid hormone replacement therapy, they had a higher success rate with ovulation induction by clomiphene citrate.[83] (Clomiphene citrate is an analogue of a nonsteroid estrogen. Clomiphene is a pituitary gonadotropin stimulant, and clinicians use it to induce ovulation. It competes with estrogen for cell binding in the hypothalamus, blocking the estrogen inhibition of GnRH secretion. The increased GnRH secretion induced by clomiphene enables continued secretion of FSH and especially LH. These gonadotropins then induce ovulation.) It is possible that the use of exogenous thyroid hormone in amounts that exceed replacement dosages might lead to normal ovulation without the need to simultaneously use clomiphene.

Progesterone Production in Granulosa Cells. Compared to immature granulosa cells exposed to FSH alone, those exposed to T_3 and FSH secreted significantly more progesterone and estrogen.[86,p.1238] FSH increases the production of progesterone in granulosa cells in two ways: by stimulating (1) synthesis of pregnenolone, and (2) activity of 3β-hydroxysteroid dehydrogenase. Thyroid hormone is involved in both pregnenolone production and 3β-hydroxysteroid dehydrogenase activity.

Pregnenolone is a sterol derived from cholesterol. It is synthesized in mitochondria and serves as the precursor of all other female sex hormones, including progesterone. The enzyme 3β-hydroxysteroid dehydrogenase (also called 3β-ol-dehydrogenase[228,p.580]) catalyzes the conversion of pregnenolone to progesterone.[142] Deficient T_3 may reduce progesterone levels by reducing the production of pregnenolone. Deficient exposure of rat adrenal cortex mitochondria to T_3 profoundly reduced biochemical reactions involved in the synthesis of pregnenolone. Apparently, the limiting step in pregnenolone synthesis was slowed because deficient T_3 inhibited the reaction that transfers energy from NADH to NADP.[231] Maruo et al. reported that an optimal concentration of T_3 appeared to augment the FSH-induced conversion of pregnenolone to progesterone by increasing the activity of 3β-hydroxysteroid dehydrogenase.[86,p.1239]

Exposing granulosa cells to FSH and LH increases their production of progesterone. However, exposing the cells to FSH, LH, and T_4 augments the increased progesterone production. Wakim et al. obtained human female granulosa cells by aspirating ovarian follicles. The follicles were pre-ovulatory—that is, they had not yet released their ova. The researchers exposed the granulosa cells from the follicles to one of two conditions: (1) the presence of FSH and LH, or (2) the presence of FSH, LH, and T_4. Cells exposed to FSH, LH, and T_4 secreted 1.29-to-1.51 times the progesterone as cells exposed only to FSH and LH.[85]

Goldman et al. studied the direct effects of T_3 on human luteinized granulosa cells (also termed luteal cells). They found that T_3 alone stimulated proliferation of the cells.[151] During pregnancy, hCG, secreted by placental cells, serves its major purpose of preventing involution of the corpus luteum and increasing luteal cell secretion of estrogen and progesterone.[78,p.919] A critical step in the stimulation of sex hormone synthesis in luteal cells by hCG is an increase in the concentration of cAMP within the cells. Goldman et al. found that exposing luteal cells to T_3 markedly increased their hCG-induced accumulation of cAMP. T_3 did so by preventing cAMP breakdown by inhibiting the cytoplasmic enzyme phosphodiesterase.[151]

Bandyopadhyay et al. reported that T_3 bound to the nuclear material of granulosa cells, induced a 2.5-fold increase in mRNA, caused a 2-fold increase in protein synthesis in the cells, and greatly increased the cells' release of progesterone. Next, after purifying the protein induced by T_3, they found that adding it to granulosa cells increased their release of progesterone. They concluded that the T_3-induced protein is a mediator of the T_3-stimulated release of progesterone by granulosa cells.[232]

Estrogen Production in Granulosa Cells. Studies show that thyroid hormone augments FSH-stimulated estrogen secretion by granulosa cells. Maruo et al. reported that FSH alone increased granulosa cell secretion of estrone after exposing the cells to the substrate androstenedione. Androstenedione is the precursor of estrogen produced in the adrenal glands (see section above titled "Estrogens"). The researchers exposed granulosa cells to androstenedione, and androgen that can be converted to estrone. After this preexposure, they exposed the cells to both T_3 and FSH. As a result, the cells significantly increased the secretion of estrone. Maruo et al. concluded that an optimal concentration of T_3 enhances the FSH-stimulated enzyme activity that increases estrone secretion.[86,p.1239]

Wakim et al. subjected granulosa cells from preovulatory human ovarian follicles to one of two conditions: exposure to FSH and LH, or exposure to FSH, LH, and T_4. Granulosa cells exposed to FSH, LH, and T_4 secreted 1.18-to-1.37 times the estradiol as cells exposed only to FSH and LH.[85]

Effective Doses of Thyroid Hormone. Maruo et al. wrote that the doses of thyroid hormone needed to effectively augment FSH-induced increases in progesterone and estrone secretion were equivalent to the physiologic range of circulating thyroid hormone levels in human plasma.[86,p.1239] This finding from a rat study cannot be extrapolated to all humans for one important reason—many humans, especially fibromyalgia patients, have partial cellular resistance to thyroid hormone. In these individuals, the granulosa cells of the ovarian follicles may be among the cells selectively involved in thyroid hormone resistance. If so, preferably, the source of the resistance can be identified and corrected. If not, then the individual's granulosa cells are likely to function normally only when exposed to supraphysiologic dosages of T_3. This approach must be carefully considered on an individual basis. While supraphysiologic dosages of T_3 may override the resistance of the granulosa cells and induced normal function, the same dosages may overstimulate other cells that are normally responsive to T_3 or less resistant to it than the granulosa cells.

In addition, *many* hypothyroid patients do not

have thyroid hormone resistance, but they nevertheless do not benefit enough or at all from the use of replacement dosages of T_4. These patients may not have normal ovarian function until they use a combination of T_4 and T_3 or T_3 alone. (See Chapter 5.3, section titled "Mandates of the Conventional Medical Hypothyroidism Paradigm," and particularly the section titled "The Patient Should Only be Permitted to Use Replacement Dosages of Thyroid Hormone," and the section titled "Hypothyroid Patients Should be Permitted to Use Only T_4.")

Luteinization

A high surge of LH and a lesser surge of FSH are necessary for ovulation. In turn, ovulation and LH are necessary to quickly change the estrogen-secreting granulosa cells of the dominant ovarian follicle more into progesterone-secreting lutein cells. At the same time, LH stimulates the theca cells to secrete androstenedione and testosterone which then serve as precursors for the luteal cells to convert into estrogens.[78,p.903] These changes at the time of ovulation, for which LH is essential, are called luteinization—formation of a corpus luteum from a ruptured ovarian follicle (see subsection above titled "Luteinization and the Corpus Luteum").

Thyroid hormone is also important for normal luteinization. Maruo et al. found that in the presence of FSH, T_3 stimulated several effects in immature pig granulosa cells: differentiation of granulosa cells, increased density of LH and hCG receptors on granulosa cells, and increased estrone and progesterone production. T_3 was effective only within an optimal dosage range. When the investigators administered FSH alone to the cells (without T_3), LH and hCG receptor density decreased, progesterone secretion decreased, and the cells underwent fibrous changes. They wrote that their finding that T_3 and FSH act synergistically to regulate the structure and function of immature granulosa cells may explain an *in vivo* observation—"ovarian follicles of thyroidectomized animals failed to mature and required much greater amounts of gonadotropic hormone to produce luteinization than did normal animals." The conclusion of Maruo et al. is worth quoting: "It is highly possible that the optimal concentration of thyroid hormone plays a physiological role in amplifying FSH-stimulated morphological luteinization, LH/hCG receptor induction, and ovarian steroid production in immature granulosa cells *in vivo*. Hence, the frequent occurrence of decreased gonadal function seen during the states of hypo- and hyperthyroidism may represent a direct consequence of in-

adequate thyroid hormone availability at the granulosa cell level, followed by a diminished responsiveness to FSH."[86,p.1240]

Channing et al. found that *in vitro*, a combination of insulin and thyroid hormone increased luteinization of pig granulosa cells. Thyroid hormone and insulin increased both LH- and FSH-induced luteinization and spontaneous luteinization.[133]

Thyroid Hormone and Luteal Phase Defect. In luteal phase defect, maturing of the endometrium is delayed.[83][236] The most characteristic finding is decreased levels of circulating progesterone. The women are infertile or have habitual first-trimester abortions.[234] The defect can result from ovarian abnormalities during the follicular phase.[149][233] One such abnormality is inadequate thyroid hormone regulation of granulosa cells.

Maruo et al. studied four women with "luteal phase defect." Each woman had a short luteal phase during the menstrual cycle. The phase lasted fewer than 10 days (the normal length is 14 days) based on body temperature or the time from the LH surge to the first day of menstrual flow. The women also had low progesterone levels during the luteal phase. Compared to normal control subjects, these patients had lower circulating thyroid hormone levels and higher TSH levels, but the differences from control subjects were not statistically significant. The use of clomiphene (which induces ovulation) alone did not relieve the luteal defects. However, despite the lack of significantly lower thyroid hormone levels, the combined use clomiphene and exogenous thyroid hormone "remarkably improved" the short luteal phase and low progesterone levels of the women. Maruo et al. concluded that the use of thyroid hormone is "of great value" for the treatment of luteal phase defect associated with subclinically low thyroid hormone levels. They wrote that thyroid hormone therapy can successfully relieve deficient luteal function and failure to ovulate (anovulation).[83]

TRH and LH Secretion. Colon et al. found that TRH stimulated gonadotroph secretion of LH but not FSH. TRH stimulated LH secretion in both the early follicular phase and the mid-luteal phases of the menstrual cycle in normal women. The researchers wrote that TRH may take part in the complex interplay of variables that control gonadotropin secretion in women.[230] This finding raises the possibility that inadequate TRH stimulation of pituitary cells due to hypothalamic hypothyroidism may contribute to subnormal LH secretion in fibromyalgia patients. My colleagues and I have found laboratory test results consistent with central hypothyroidism in many fibromyalgia patients, some of whom may have had hypothalamic hypothyroidism (see Appendix B, paper titled "Thyroid Status of 38 Fibromyalgia Patients: Implications for the Etiology of Fibromyalgia," and paper titled "Thyroid Status of Fibromyalgia Patients"). Low LH secretion can cause anovulation (see above section).

THYROID HORMONE AND PREGNANCY

Infertility

Clinicians have long recognized impaired fertility as a consequence of hypothyroidism.[137][150][151][168][188][199] Women with mild hypothyroidism may ovulate and conceive. However, their pregnancies often end with spontaneous abortion in the first trimester, stillbirths, or premature birth.[137][168][347,p.1052] The fertility of rats decreases a few weeks after thyroidectomy, and the rats who become pregnant have decreased litter numbers.[198]

Davis et al. reported that pregnancy was rare in hypothyroid women,[168] but as Longcope noted, this is difficult to document.[347,p.1052] Gerhard et al. found that spontaneous conception was more frequent in euthyroid (16%) than in hypothyroid (6%) women. They concluded that subclinical hypothyroidism plays a role in infertility.[295]

Tkachenko et al. performed complete endocrine workups on 14 patients with primary hypothyroidism. They found that all had anovulatory infertility. Eight of the 14 patients had elevated prolactin levels. The researchers wrote: "It is shown that hyperprolactinemia, developing in cases of primary hypothyroidism, is associated with impaired dopaminergic inhibition of pituitary lactotropics. Substitution thyroid therapy resulted in the recovery of the normal ovulatory cycle in all but one patient with secondary pituitary microprolactinoma, and 8 patients became pregnant. It is believed that damaged dopaminergic regulation of hypothalamic luliberin (RH) secretion is a direct cause of ovarian dysfunction associated with primary hypothyroidism."[27]

Burrow[169] and Nikolai et al.[170] reported that *low* doses of T_4 did not benefit euthyroid women with PMS, premenstrual syndrome, and infertility. I do not doubt these reports. Small amounts of T_4 often suppress euthyroid patients' TSH levels and in turn decrease thyroid gland secretion of both T_4 and T_3. In my clinical experience, these patients usually experience symptoms of hypometabolism (usually worsening of their fibromyalgia symptoms) after beginning the use of small dosages of T_4. I would therefore expect that among euthyroid women taking small dosages of T_4, menstrual disturbances, PMS, and difficulty conceiving would not improve but would worsen. However, among my female euthyroid fibromyalgia patients, high enough dosages of T_3 have often improved or completely relieved menstrual disturbances, PMS, and infertility without adverse effects.

Miscarriage, Spontaneous Abortion, and Adverse Effects on Pregnant Hypothyroid Women

Miscarriage is a spontaneous expulsion of the embryo or of the fetus before the middle of the second trimester, that is, before 18 weeks of pregnancy. (A human "embryo" is the product of conception during the 2nd and 8th weeks of development. Many people use the term "fetus" to mean the unborn young in the uterus between conception and birth. More specifically, however, the human fetus is the developing young from the 8th week after conception until the moment of birth.) Abortion refers to giving birth to an embryo or fetus before the stage of viability. Viability usually occurs at 20 weeks of gestation, just after the middle of the second trimester. Abortion differs from premature birth. While abortion occurs before the stage of viability, the premature infant is born after the stage of viability but before the 37th week. (A term infant has a gestational age of 259 completed days or 37 completed weeks.)

Emerson wrote that maternal hypothyroidism may adversely affect the development and survival of the progeny.[175,p.1268] Hypothyroid pregnant women are susceptible to spontaneous miscarriage and/or fetal malformations.[188] According to one report, the miscarriage rate was almost double that of euthyroid women.[181] In one study, researchers found that the outcome of pregnancy correlated with the severity of the woman's hypothyroidism—the more severe the patient, the worse the probable outcome.[182] Hypothyroid women whose pregnancies persist into the third trimester are predisposed to placental separation or detachment (abruption), preeclampsia, and adverse perinatal outcome.[183][184][185]

Maruo et al. assessed the possible role of thyroid hormone in sustaining early pregnancy. They measured the serum levels of TSH, thyroid hormone, and T_4-binding globulin of 32 patients who had a clinical diagnosis of "threatened abortion." The researchers compared the hormone and globulin levels to favorable and unfavorable outcomes of pregnancy. Compared to women who did not abort, women who subsequently did abort had lower serum levels of T_4, T_3, free T_4 and free T_3 at the onset of clinical signs of threatened abortion. Also, at the onset of clinical signs of threatened abortion, serum T_4 and T_3 levels were significantly higher in women who did not subsequently abort. These findings suggest that higher serum thyroid hormone levels help maintain early pregnancy. The findings also suggest that lower thyroid hormone levels are associated with an unfavorable outcome of threatened abortion.[163]

Winikoff and Malinek described the thyroid test profile typical of pregnant women. The profile consists of elevated total T_4 and T_4-binding globulin levels, a lowered T_3 uptake, and normal free T_4 level. (This is predictable from the elevated thyroxine binding globulin due to elevated estrogen levels. See Chapter 4.2, section titled "Estrogens," and Table 4.2.5.) In a study they conducted, normal pregnant women reached this typical test profile by 7-to-8 weeks. But women who habitually aborted reached the profile at 14-to-15 weeks. Most women who miscarried never reached the profile. The researchers had 4 women who previously aborted use exogenous T_4 through 6 pregnancies. During these pregnancies, the women developed normal test profiles and successfully carried their pregnancies to term.[164]

Montoro et al. wrote that infants of hypothyroid mothers may nonetheless be normal. The reason they gave is that the infants' hypothalamic-pituitary-thyroid axis develops independently from the mother's and provides sufficient fetal thyroid hormone levels.[183] This is not always the case, however.

Vojvodic et al. reported that hypothyroidism is a risk factor for the development of gestational diabetes and preeclampsia. Hypothyroid pregnant women had a significantly higher incidence of both conditions. The investigators reported that 83.9% of hypothyroid women delivered their babies, but 12.8% of these were delivered before term. The other 16.1% of women had spontaneous abortions. Stillbirths occurred in 4.2% of cases. One infant was born with hydrocephalus. Vojvodic et al. wrote, "In the authors' opinion, it is necessary to achieve a normal metabolic state before pregnancy which should be maintained with substitutional therapy during the whole pregnancy."[187]

Leung et al. studied the perinatal outcome of the pregnancies of 68 hypothyroid women. They reported that gestational hypertension (eclampsia, preeclampsia, and pregnancy-induced hypertension) was significantly more common in overt and subclinical hypothyroid patients than in the general population. Gestational hypertension occurred in 22% of overtly hypothyroid women, 15% of subclinical hypothyroid women, and 7.6% of euthyroid women. Moreover, of women who remained hypothyroid until delivery, 36% of the overt hypothyroid and 25% of the subclinical hypothyroid women developed gestational hypertension. Low birth weight of the neonates of overt and subclinical hypothyroid women resulted from premature delivery due to gestational hypertension. The only adverse fetal or neonatal outcomes were one stillbirth and one case of clubfeet. The authors wrote that normalizing the results of hypothyroid patients' thyroid function tests may prevent gestational hypertension and its complications.[189]

Ross et al. compared the free T_4 and T_4-binding globulin levels of two groups of pregnant women: (1) 8 women who later had spontaneous abortions between 8 and 20 weeks of pregnancy, and (2) 32 women who had successful pregnancy outcomes. The free T_4 levels between the two groups did not differ. The researchers wrote that this outcome suggests that impaired thyroid function of the mother plays no role in the unsuccessful outcome of pregnancy. (This conclusion is inconsistent with the findings of other researchers. See the next subsection, titled "Effect of Thyroid Hormone on the Placenta and Early Pregnancy.") However, at 5.2 weeks (range of 0-to-13 weeks), T_4-binding globulin levels were lower in the women who later aborted. Ross et al. concluded that serum T_4-binding globulin levels might serve as a minor predictor of pregnancy outcome.[162] Skjoldebrand et al. came to a similar conclusion. They evaluated several laboratory thyroid function test values in 144 apparently healthy, euthyroid pregnant women who had miscarriages. The tests included a T_4-binding globulin, T_4-binding prealbumin, T_4, free T_4, T_3, and TSH. They compared the values with those of 228 women who had normal pregnancies. Women who miscarried had significantly lower values of T_4-binding globulin. The researchers concluded that a significantly lower value of T_4-binding globulin was most predictive of an unfavorable outcome of pregnancy.[160]

Effect of Thyroid Hormone on the Placenta and Early Pregnancy. The placenta is the organ though which the developing child receives nourishment from the mother. The membrane that encloses the embryo is attached to the margin of the placenta. Nutrients, oxygen, and antibodies pass from the mother to the child through the two umbilical arteries. The arteries originate from the uterine arteries and longitudinally traverse the placenta. Metabolic wastes pass from the fetal blood to the maternal blood through the umbilical vein that traverses the placenta. Maternal and fetal blood do not mix.[78,pp.917-919][228,p.610]

The placenta is an endocrine organ. It produces estrogen, progesterone, and hCG. One type of pregnancy test is designed to detect hCG in the urine. The presence of hCG determines pregnancy. Estrogen and progesterone secreted by the placenta during pregnancy help maintain pregnancy. Optimal exposure of placental trophoblast cells (see below) to thyroid hormone helps maintain early pregnancy. Thyroid hormone stimulates placental production of hCG, estrogen, and progesterone.[78,pp.917-919][228,p.610]

Thyroid Hormone and Hormone Production by Placental Trophoblast Cells. Maruo et al. investigated the direct effects of T_3 and T_4 on the function of trophoblast cells (see Glossary) in cultured early and term human placentas. Adding T_3 or T_4 to placental tissues caused a maximum daily increase in the production of progesterone, 17β-estradiol, hCGα, hCGβ, hCG, and human placental lactogen. (The term "lactogen" refers to the synthesis or secretion of milk. Lactogen secreted by the human placenta is structurally similar to growth hormone. It induces mild effects similar to those of growth hormone and prolactin.) Increased production of progesterone and 17β-estradiol by thyroid hormone was further increased when the placental tissues were exposed to testosterone or pregnenolone. The increased production suggests that thyroid hormone intensifies the enzymatic activities of 3β-hydroxysteroid dehydrogenase and aromatase in the placenta. (3β-Hydroxysteroid dehydrogenase catalyzes the conversion of pregnenolone to progesterone,[142] and aromatase converts testosterone to estradiol.[228,p.580]) Higher or lower doses of thyroid hormone produced weaker stimulatory effects. Maruo et al. concluded that spontaneous abortion in early pregnancy by hypothyroid women may be a result of too little exposure of placental trophoblasts to thyroid hormone. The subnormal exposure reduces estradiol and progesterone production and secretion by the trophoblasts.[159]

Matsuo et al. studied the direct effects of T_3 on the production of hormones by cultured human early and term placentas. Administering an optimal dose of T_3 stimulated the daily secretion of estradiol and progesterone. The T_3 stimulated estradiol and progesterone production by increasing the activity of the enzymes 3β-hydroxysteroid dehydrogenase and aromatase. T_3 also increased hCGα and hCGβ and human placental lactogen. Excessive amounts of T_3 inhibited estradiol and progesterone secretion. Matsuo et al. wrote that optimal exposure of early placentas to thyroid hor-

mone acts as a biological amplifier of the endocrine function of trophoblast cells of the placenta. They pointed out, however, that term placental tissues did not respond to the addition of graded doses of T_3 with increased hormone production. They wrote, as did Maruo et al.,[159] that during maternal hypothyroidism, spontaneous abortion may occur in early pregnancy, resulting from inadequate direct thyroid hormone regulation of trophoblast cells.[156]

La Marca et al. reported that women who miscarried had significantly lower hCG levels than women who did not abort. The free T_3 was normal in women who miscarried, their free T_4 levels were lower and their TSH levels were higher. In women who miscarried, the plasma levels of hCG and thyroid hormones correlated. The researchers concluded that in women with threatened abortion, low hCG and free T_4 levels and a high TSH level suggest a negative pregnancy outcome.[155]

Mochizuki and Maruo reported that in early placental tissue, an optimal dose of thyroid hormone stimulated the production of progesterone, estradiol, hCG, and human placental lactogen. Compared to women who had favorable pregnancy outcomes, women who aborted had lower levels of total T_4 and T_3 and free T_4 and T_3. Mochizuki and Maruo wrote that their findings suggest a role for thyroid hormone in maintaining early pregnancy.[157]

Mochizuki et al. investigated the effects of epidermal growth factor and T_3 on early human placenta during pregnancy. They found that in 4-to-5 week old placentas, epidermal growth factor stimulated secretion of hCG and human placental lactogen. Adding T_3 increased the secretion of epidermal growth factor by placental cells. It thus appears that T_3 may increase secretion of hCG and human placental lactogen at least partly by increasing the placenta secretion of epidermal growth factor.[154] Normal secretion of epidermal growth factor is important during pregnancy. It contributes to fetal growth by regulating the supply of glucose through the placenta.[204] The growth factor also stimulates some trophoblast cells (cytotrophoblasts) and inhibits apoptosis.[205] (The term "apoptosis" is from the Greek word for "falling off." It is a process by which single cells are deleted from a tissue by fragmenting into membrane-bound particles that are then phagocytized. Some researchers believe the process is a feature of genetically programmed cell death.)

Effects of Maternal Hypothyroidism on Progeny. The fetuses of pregnant hypothyroid rats were found to have subnormal organ weights. Organ weights were lower in the fetuses of pregnant rats that were hypothyroid during the second rather than the first half of gestation.[200] Fetuses of pregnant thyroidectomized sheep had slowed brain and body growth. By term, brain growth had reached normal, but body weight was subnormal.[201] Thyroidectomized guinea pigs had a low percentage of live births.[202]

The offspring of women who are hypothyroid during their pregnancies may have lasting adverse effects. Greenman et al. compared the infants of women who had severe hypothyroidism during pregnancy with those of women who had mild hypothyroidism. Infants of severely hypothyroid mothers had a higher incidence of mental and motor retardation.[184] This is consistent with the finding of mental and developmental abnormalities among children of women who were hypothyroid during their pregnancies.[196][197]

Thyroid Therapy During Pregnancy. Longcope advised that when a woman's hypothyroidism is diagnosed during pregnancy, she should immediately begin treatment with T_4. He wrote that beginning the T_4 therapy may increase the chances of a normal pregnancy.[347,p.1053]

Some thyroid hormone crosses the placenta, at least during late pregnancy. Valsma et al. wrote that this is evident from the fact that neonates who subsequently have severe hypothyroidism have no evidence of the condition at birth. This suggests a placental transfer of thyroid hormone from the mother to the fetus. They concluded from rat studies that substantial amounts of T_4 are transferred from the mother to the fetus during late gestation.[171]

Based on their studies, Sack et al. agreed that some T_4 is transferred from the mother to the fetus. However, they also concluded that too little T_4 is transferred to suppress fetal levels of TSH and to prevent intrauterine hypothyroidism in congenitally hypothyroid infants who have organification defects.[172] It is possible that the development of the fetus depends partially on maternal thyroid hormone reaching it through the placenta, and severe enough maternal hypothyroidism may impair fetal development in some way.

Longcope recommended that the clinician occasionally monitor the TSH level during the patient's pregnancy to insure that the T_4 dosage remains adequate. He wrote that the TSH is probably the best indicator of changes in thyroid function.[347,p.1053] Of course, measures of thyroid hormone levels are also important in a thorough assessment of thyroid status. But I vigorously disagree that the TSH alone or the TSH and thyroid hormone levels are adequate for evaluating the adequacy of thyroid hormone regulation of tissue metabolic status. The clinician should bear in

mind that "thyroid status" refers only to the status of the hypothalamus-pituitary-thyroid gland axis. As I have expounded in different chapters of this book, to focus on thyroid status alone is to neglect the most fundamentally important question in the treatment of the hypothyroid patient—Is the form and dosage of thyroid hormone the patient is using exerting adequate tissue metabolic effects? The clinician cannot find the answer to this question by measuring the circulating TSH and/or thyroid hormone levels. He can find the answer only by assessing the response of various tissues to the therapy. (See Chapter 5.3, section titled "Mandates of the Conventional Medical Hypothyroidism Paradigm.")

Conventional clinicians have a double standard for assessing the effects of understimulation and those of overstimulation by thyroid hormone. For example, clinicians are advised to determine fetal overstimulation by thyroid hormone according to tissue responses typical of thyrotoxicosis,[175] such as tachycardia. But the same approach is not generally advised for determining fetal understimulation by thyroid hormone. Instead, the clinician is advised to infer possible understimulation from laboratory thyroid function test results that indicate hypothyroidism.

Clinicians are often concerned that the mother's exogenous thyroid hormone may adversely affect the embryo or fetus. Over the past 30 years, conventional thyroidologists have exaggerated the potential adverse effects of amounts of thyroid hormone larger than replacement dosages. Because of this, clinicians often ask pregnant hypothyroid women to reduce their thyroid hormone dosages as a safety measure. However, for some women, compliance with this recommendation may be responsible for adverse effects on the developing embryo, fetus, or the neonate.

Longcope wrote that hypothyroid women who begin using exogenous thyroid hormone before pregnancy should continue to do so throughout pregnancy.[347,p.1053] Utiger,[173] Mandel et al.,[174] and McDougall and Maclin[186] wrote that many hypothyroid women may need to increase their dosages of thyroid hormone during pregnancy. Mandel et al. studied 12 women with primary hypothyroidism before, during, and after pregnancy. The mean TSH level increased from 2.0 ± 0.5 μU/mL before pregnancy to 13.5 ± 3.3 μU/mL during pregnancy. The mean serum T_4 level decreased from 111.0 ± 5.8 nmol/L before pregnancy to 86.5 ± 5.2 nmol/L during pregnancy (normal range is 64-to-142 nmol/L). Nine of the 12 patients increased their thyroid hormone dosages due to their elevated TSH levels. Mandel et al. concluded:

"Our results indicate that the need for thyroxine increases in many women with primary hypothyroidism when they are pregnant, as reflected by an increase in serum thyrotropin concentrations. Although the effects of this modest level of hypothyroidism are not known, we think it prudent to monitor thyroid function throughout gestation and after delivery and to adjust the thyroxine dose to maintain a normal serum thyrotropin level."[174]

McDougall and Maclin reported that to maintain a normal TSH level during pregnancy, 20 women with primary hypothyroidism had to increase their T_4 dosages by an average of 36 µg (0.036 mg). However, among the women, there was substantial variation in the increased dosages required during pregnancy.[186] Thyrotoxicosis of the mother predisposes to miscarriage,[176] and congenital malformations may result from maternal thyrotoxicosis.[177] Obviously, the mother should not be overstimulated with thyroid hormone. However, whether she is overstimulated or understimulated can only be determined by measures of tissue metabolic status and not by the results of thyroid function laboratory tests.

The clinician can monitor the response of the fetus to maternal thyroid hormone intake in several ways. For example, he can monitor the fetal heart rate. The fetal heart rate should be about 140 beats per minute.[180] The thyrotoxic fetus will most likely have tachycardia. A fetal heart rate over 160 beats per minute after 22 weeks of gestation suggests cardiac overstimulation of the fetus by thyroid hormone.[179,p.1238] The clinician can order ultrasonography of the fetal thyroid gland size.[175,p.1272] If the clinician includes TSH, free T_4 and free T_3 tests in the evaluation of the newborn, he should keep in mind that values are higher in normal neonates than in normal adults.[180,pp.1214-1216] The clinician caring for the pregnant hypothyroid woman should study the literature relevant to the effects of exogenous thyroid hormone on the embryo, fetus, and neonate. Doing so may increase the chances of making case management decisions that insure normal fetal development.

● **SPECIAL CONSIDERATIONS: ORAL CONTRACEPTIVES, PREMENSTRUAL SYNDROME, MENOPAUSE, AND HORMONE REPLACEMENT THERAPY**

The use of oral contraceptives, the experience of peri-menopause, menopause, and the use of estrogen replacement therapy have implications for the fibromyalgia status of women.

ORAL CONTRACEPTIVES AND MYOFASCIAL PAIN

Oral contraceptives contain female sex steroids that prevent pregnancy. Diabetic-like effects—elevated blood glucose and insulin levels—appear to mediate some adverse effects in a subset of women who use oral contraceptives.

As a pain management specialist, oral contraceptives have commanded my attention as an iatrogenic source of pain for some women. I have reported in several publications that some women using oral contraceptives experience recurrent episodes of acute, severe, treatment-resistant myofascial pain.[24][25][93] In my clinical experience, patients' pain is most often regional and usually involves the small caliber muscles of the neck and upper thorax. The fibromyalgia patient often attributes these episodes of acute treatment-resistant pain associated with oral contraceptives to "flares," acute exacerbations expressed as severe regional pain. However, stopping use of the contraceptives usually has two effects: it enables the patients to benefit from specific myofascial therapy as most other patients do, and it ends recurrences of the regional pain.

Some of my patients have had similar acute treatment-resistant myofascial pain during episodes of hypoglycemia.[90][93] Travell and Simons have also described this phenomenon[95,pp.147-148][96,pp.219-220] Myofascial pain resulting from hypoglycemia due to the patient failing to eat at regular enough intervals is highly resistant to myofascial therapy that typically stops acute myofascial pain in most other patients. This hypoglycemia-based, treatment-resistant pain dramatically subsides within 30-to-60 minutes after I have the patient ingest one or two bananas or slices of bread. After this time, specific myofascial therapy usually relieves any residual pain. (Honeyman-Lowe and I have described elsewhere a highly effective treatment protocol for myofascial pain.[10][11][89][90][91][92] This protocol, when expertly used, promptly and effectively relieves the myofascial pain of most patients who do not have treatment resistance due to underlying factors such as hypothyroidism and hypoglycemia. Myofascial trigger points are the most common source of musculoskeletal pain,[98][99][100] although many clinicians—even pain management and musculoskeletal specialists—are not aware of this.[97][101] Yet expertly applied myofascial therapy promptly and dramatically relieves most patients' pain caused by myofascial trigger points.) Eating may also reduce the severity of myofascial pain associated with oral contraceptive use. The relief is usually not complete, however, and it lasts only briefly. The recurrences completely cease only after the patients stop using the contraceptives.

In clinical practice, I have advised my patients who had recurrent, severe myofascial pain while using oral contraceptives to discuss the relation with their gynecologists.[24] Some of these specialists have open-mindedly considered a possible relation and have been cooperative. Others, however, have dogmatically denied any relation between the two. Yet when these patients stop using oral contraceptives, their recurrent episodes of pain cease. Mendelsohn wrote to women: "Problems with oral contraceptives were predictable because of the way they affect the body. Don't expect to hear this from your doctor, because the Pill wouldn't have many takers if women were told that it alters hormonal balance to create a physiological dysfunction. The desired result is to interfere with a natural process—ovulation—by causing the body to malfunction." He also wrote, "Doctors continue to prescribe oral contraceptives despite repeated instances of adverse effects that they see in their patients and an abundance of evidence in the scientific journals that they are responsible for a host of ills and countless deaths."[13,p.120]

I am aware of no controlled studies of the relation of myofascial pain to oral contraceptive use. Nonetheless, I am certain that other clinicians who look for the relation I describe here will identify it in some women who use oral contraceptives. It is important that clinicians remain vigilant for adverse effects of oral contraceptives on patients. Skouby et al. wrote that the metabolic effects of oral contraceptives differ from adverse reactions to other drugs, which typically have an acute onset. The adverse effects of oral contraceptives are insidious, and both patients and clinicians can easily overlook the relation between the two.[65,p.347] The adverse metabolic effects Skouby et al. referred to involve problems with glucose metabolism. Some patients' impaired glucose metabolism, as during episodes of hypoglycemia, selectively involves skeletal muscles. The resulting energy deficiency muscle contractures may form or activate myofascial trigger points that refer pain. Skouby et al. wrote that even "discrete changes in glucose metabolism may promote development of coronary heart disease."[65,p.347] Similarly, a mild impairment of glucose metabolism in

some patients produces severe referral of pain from myofascial trigger points.

Skouby et al. wrote that glucose tolerance decreases in women as they age. Because of this, the authors recommended caution with women over age 35 using oral contraceptives. "In young women," they wrote, "there is no reason to believe that the modern types of combined low-dose contraceptives will have any influence on glucose metabolism that will result in any clinical problem."[65,p.347] I vehemently disagree with this reassurance. Most women I have treated for myofascial pain associated with oral contraceptives use have been in their 20s or early 30s. Also, they used combined low-dose contraceptives. These patients did not have other obvious health problems such diabetes. This suggests that age-related physiological deterioration did not underlay their adverse reactions to oral contraceptives. Hence, myofascial pain occurs even in some young, apparently healthy women who use low-dose oral contraceptives. I have no idea what the incidence may be of myofascial pain syndromes associated with oral contraceptive use.

Glucose Intolerance and High-Dose Oral Contraceptive Use

In one study, high-dose oral contraceptive users had higher serum glucose levels in the 1-hour glucose tolerance test. Glucose intolerance (see Glossary) was more severe in women who were older, obese, or had a family history of diabetes. Glucose intolerance was reversed when women stopped their use of contraceptives.[39] Other researchers found a 20% impairment of glucose tolerance in women using high-dose oral contraceptives. Women had impaired tolerance no matter how long they had used the contraceptives. Glucose tolerance test results returned to normal 1-to-2 months after the women stopped using oral contraceptives.[44] This study and others[40][41][42][43] led Gaspard and Lefedvre to reach a preliminary conclusion: High-dose oral contraceptives can chronically raise blood glucose and insulin levels and increase the incidence of impaired glucose tolerance. They pointed out that these abnormalities are likely to occur in "a predisposed population" and are probably reversible.[45,p.336]

Glucose Intolerance and Low-Dose Oral Contraceptive Use

Low-dose oral contraceptives were developed with the aim of reducing the disease risks that are increased by high-dose oral contraceptives. It is worth emphasizing, however, that some investigators have admitted that they do not expect problem-free use of contraceptives, regardless of the dosage level. Gaspard and Lefebvre, for example, wrote: "If most of the impact on carbohydrate metabolism in OC [oral contraceptive] users is related to the dose and potency of the progestin content, adaptation of low-dose OC formulation is mandatory *in view of reducing carbohydrate alterations to a minimum*, because chronic abnormalities can lead to increased cardiovascular morbidity and mortality."[45,p.336] And they wrote further: "Certainly in that regard, the new OCs with overall reduced levels of estrogen and progestin, with particular emphasis on reducing the most potent progestins such as levonorgestrel and other gonanes, *should be suited better to exerting only a minor impact on carbohydrate metabolism and thereby partly on potential atherogenicity* [italics mine]."[45,p.337] Such admissions should sensitize the clinician to the possibility that low-dose oral contraceptives may adversely affect women who use them.

Low-dose contraceptives contain low doses of both estrogens and progestins. Many studies have been published, and in most, the researchers have used repeated, standardized oral glucose loads to evaluate the effects of low-dose contraceptives on carbohydrate metabolism. Usually, researchers administered the tests before participating women began using contraceptives, and then again at 3-to-12-month intervals[45,p.340] In spite of "worrisome shortcomings" of methodology, Gaspard and Lefebvre wrote that most of these studies show slight decreases in glucose tolerance. Only rarely did the intolerance progress to impaired glucose intolerance. Typically, the insulin response mildly increased when women in the studies ingested glucose. The researchers interpreted the increase as a reflection of increased cell resistance to insulin, possibly at some post-receptor step.[45,p.340]

Godsland et al. do not dismiss "worrisome shortcomings" as easily as do Gaspard and Lefebvre. In discussing methodological problems in studies of low-dose oral contraceptives, they wrote, "it is not sufficient to conclude, on the basis of 10 or 20 patient studies, that if no changes in the glucose response during the oral glucose tolerance test occurred outside the normal range, there were no important effects on carbohydrate metabolism." Doubting the favorable conclusions of some studies, they also wrote, "The magnitude of the effects on glucose and insulin levels reported in many studies that claim no effect of low-dose oral contraceptives on carbohydrate metabolism must raise questions about the power of their design."[62,p.351]

Godsland et al. also complained that no studies

had assessed the wide range of low-dose contraceptives being marketed. They conducted a study of 1127 women taking either of 5 monophasic- or 2-triphasic-combined estrogen-progestin contraceptives and two progestin-only contraceptives.[63,pp.287-298] In the group taking the combined contraceptives, there was a significant elevation in the glucose and insulin responses during the oral glucose tolerance test. Also, they found that progestins had effects on the glucose and insulin responses. "The higher progestogen dose," they wrote, "had the greatest impact in every case." The concluded that even with the use of low-dose oral contraceptives, the adverse effects on carbohydrate metabolism is still an issue.[62,p.352]

Gaspard and Lefebvre wrote that a better understanding of the mechanism of decreased glucose tolerance in oral contraceptive users is mandatory. They stated that a better understanding may lead to oral contraceptives with a softer impact on carbohydrate metabolism. The softer impact is needed because chronically elevated blood glucose and insulin levels, even of moderate levels, promote cardiovascular disease.[45,p.341] This warning is justified. Admonishment is also warranted in relation to chronic, widespread, treatment-resistant myofascial pain. For some of my female patients, recurrent myofascial pain has been severe and debilitating until they stopped using low-dose oral contraceptives.

Adverse Effects of Synthetic Estrogens and Progestins

The most commonly used oral contraceptives contain combinations of both estrogen and progestin. The estrogens in the contraceptives are usually ethinyl estradiol and mestranol. The progestins may be norethindrone or norgestrel. Progestin capsules implanted subcutaneously in the upper arm usually contain levonorgestrel. The estrogens in contraceptives suppress ovulation. The progestins prevent implantation of the ovum in the endometrium and render the cervical mucous impenetrable to sperm.[103,p.248]

Synthetic Estrogens. Most of the natural estrogens are rapidly metabolized by microsomal enzymes during their first pass in the circulation through the liver. Because of this, they are not administered orally as medications. Instead, clinicians may give esters of estradiol intramuscularly. A far smaller percentage of these esters are metabolized during the first pass through the liver. Ethinyl estradiol and mestranol are taken orally, are fat soluble, and are stored in fat tissues from which they escape only slowly. Synthesized nonsteroidal compounds with estrogenic activity are used clinically. These include diethylstilbestrol, quin-estrol, and chlorotranisene.[103,pp.243-244]

The use of synthetic estrogens over the long term may adversely affect glucose regulation, although not to the degree likely from the use of progestins (see subsection immediately below titled "Synthetic Pro-gestins"). One group reported that long-term use of the estrogenic compounds ethinyl estradiol and mestranol did not significantly affect blood glucose or insulin during the oral glucose tolerance test.[59] The women included in the study had taken estrogen for no longer than 6 months. The same group later reported that after 2 years of use of the estrogen compound mestranol (80 mg), oral glucose tolerance tests revealed small in-creases in serum glucose and insulin levels.[58]

Synthetic Progestins. Harvey and Champe wrote that natural progesterone has low bioavailability be-cause it is rapidly metabolized during the first pass in the circulation through the liver. Because of this, syn-thetic progestins, including medroxyprogesterone ace-tate, norethindrone, hydroxyprogesterone acetate, and norgestrel, are used in medications such as contracep-tives. These are used, they explained, because they are not rapidly inactivated in the first pass through the liver.[103,p.247] Lee proposed that the slow metabolism of synthetic progestins accounts for some of their po-tential for adverse effects. He wrote, "their activity is prolonged, creating reactions in the body that are not consistent with natural progesterone." He also wrote that the chemical alterations of progesterone or nor-testerone to produce synthetic progestins—which make them patentable and therefore commercially profitable—"undoubtedly explains the alarming array of listed warnings, contraindications, precautions, and adverse reactions to progestins, all of which are uncharacteristic of natural progesterone."[102,pp.88-89] Despite the array of adverse effects associated with synthetic progestins in oral contraceptives, new ones continue to be developed.[104]

The potential for problems in the use of synthetic progestins was shown in a 1986 rat study by Thomas et al. After the researchers removed the ovaries of vir-gin rats, the rats' food intake remained the same. How-ever, their activity levels and T_3 levels decreased. As a result, the rats lost weight. Also, their insulin levels were greatly reduced. After beginning estrogen re-placement, the rats' activity levels increased and they regained their lost weight. Insulin levels and T_3 levels also normalized, but T_4 and glucose levels remained low. Giving the rats both estrogen and progestin re-placement increased their weight and raised their T_3 and T_4 levels to normal. However, despite having low-er than normal body weight, the rats had high glucose and insulin levels. Thomas et al. wrote this finding indicated insulin resistance. They wrote that the study results had important implications for the role of progestins in disturbances of glucose regulation and energy balance.[203]

Studies reviewed by two separate investigators suggest that several forms of progestins (progesterone, 17-acetoxy-progesterone derivatives, and 19-nor-tes-tosterone-derived compounds) increased both glucose and insulin levels after either oral or intravenous doses of glucose. Elevations occurred even when the proges-tins were given alone and in small doses.[60][61,pp.395-410] Gaspard and Lefebvre wrote that the progestin com-ponent of oral contraceptives is primarily responsible for abnormal carbohydrate metabolism. They also concluded that among the progestins, derivatives of 19-nor-testosterone are more pernicious than 17-ace-toxy-progesterone derivatives. Among the 19-nor-progestins, the gonane group such as norgestrel was more abnormality-provoking than the estrane com-pounds.[45,p.340]

Gaspard and Lefebvre also commented that most progestins contained in oral contraceptives are derived from 19-nor-testosterone. These progestins have the greatest potential for inducing glucose intolerance. According to Gaspard and Lefebvre, they "have the potential to decrease glucose tolerance and increase insulin resistance by mechanisms still largely un-known. In some studies the use of standard dose [oral contraceptives] containing high levels of these proges-tins has been associated not only with biochemical alterations in the carbohydrate metabolism previous-ly described but also with a trend to increasing the incidence of [impaired glucose tolerance] and even progression to overt [diabetes mellitus], which is sometimes not reversible, despite discontinuation of the OCs."[45,p.340] Perlman et al. reported that some women taking oral contraceptives that contained the progestin developed impaired glucose tolerance, and others developed diabetes mellitus. They wrote that compared to estrane progestins, norgestrel progestins cause a slightly higher incidence of impaired glucose tolerance and diabetes.[41]

Norplant, the progestin levonorgestrel, contained in 6 flexible silicone rubber tubes that are implanted in the woman's upper arm, causes at least minor altera-tions of glucose metabolism.[110]

Health Risks of Oral Contraceptive Use

Oral contraceptives can potentially cause a wide array of adverse health effects. Some medical writers describe these and caution against them. Other writers, however, suggest that the potential adverse effects have been exaggerated and that the risks are worth taking for the potential benefits from use of the medications.

Reassurances of Safety of Oral Contraceptives. Many medical writers trivialize the potential perniciousness of oral contraceptives. Instead, they focus attention on "a broad range of noncontraceptive health benefits" of the medications.[105] Fuchs et al. wrote, "Women are poorly informed about oral contraceptive use, and are largely unaware of the important long-term non-contraceptive benefits."[107] And Jones wrote, "Probably even more women would use the pill if they had more accurate information regarding the higher failure rates with barrier methods (especially the condom), if misperceptions about OC safety were put to rest, and if greater awareness of the noncontraceptive health benefits of OC could be achieved."[108] Similarly, Tyrer recently wrote, "Almost 40 years after its introduction, the pill's [sic] contraceptive efficacy is proven, its improved safety has been established, and the focus has shifted from *supposed* health risks to documented and real health benefits [italics mine]."[105] In the same vein, Davis and Wysocki recently wrote, "Myths and misperceptions continue to influence women's opinions about oral contraceptives (OC), despite the immense body of evidence regarding OC safety and efficacy. Patient opinions about OC failure rates and health risks are often far from proven fact, and the health benefits of OC are too often unrecognized." They advised, "Because successful OC use requires an informed patient, effective communication between clinicians and their patients is needed to correct misinformation, relieve unnecessary fears, and increase OC use."[106]

Potential Adverse Effects of Oral Contraceptives. Recurrent, acute, severe myofascial pain is only one potential health risk of oral contraceptive use. As Mendelsohn forthrightly explained in *MalePractice: How Doctors Manipulate Women*, the worst of the health risks is death.[94] Lee has explained many of the other adverse effects of both synthetic progestins and estrogen. I strongly recommend his book *What Your Doctor May Not Tell You About Menopause*.[102] Some other health risks, that may or may not lead to premature death, are associated with elevated glucose and insulin levels. A comparison with other conditions involving elevated glucose and insulin levels suggests that the use of oral contraceptives may increase the risks for several conditions: hypertension, abnormal blood patterns of lipid-conjugated proteins (dyslipo-

proteinemia, with high low-density lipoproteins and low high-density lipoproteins), glucose intolerance, obesity, and coronary artery disease.[46][47][48][74,p.285]

The major adverse effects of synthetic estrogens are nausea and vomiting, breast tenderness, endometrial hyperplasia, postmenopausal bleeding, hyperpigmentation, migraine headaches, hypertension, edema due to sodium retention, facilitation of estrogen-dependent neoplasms, cholestasis, and gallbadder disease. The major adverse effects of synthetic progestins are weight gain, edema, depression, thrombophlebitis, and pulmonary embolism.[103,pp.246-247]

In 1999, Sherif described the potential adverse effects of low-dose oral contraceptives: "Major risks are cardiovascular. Preliminary data from nonrandomized studies suggest that oral contraceptives containing third-generation progestins are associated with increased risk of venous thromboembolism, particularly in carriers of the coagulation factor V Leiden mutation. The risk of arterial thrombosis, such as myocardial infarction or stroke, may be directly related to estrogen dose, particularly in women who have hypertension, smoke, or are >35 years old." Sherif also wrote that it is contraceptive users who are older than 30 and who smoke more than 25 cigarettes per day who "have a higher estimated mortality rate than that of pregnant women." This statement logically means that more of these users die, but death with oral contraceptive use is not restricted to them. Considering this, Sherif continued, "the benefits of oral contraceptives appear to outweigh their risks."[109] Perhaps for contraceptive purposes, this may be. But in that natural alternatives to synthetic female sex hormones are available for hormone replacement therapy, and the natural alternatives can be used virtually without risks, the synthetic hormones seem a risky option indeed. (See subsection below titled "Phramaceutical vs Natural Sex Hormones.")

Panay and Studd, in 1997, described "progestogen intolerance" as one of the main causes of women not complying with their progestin treatment regimens. They wrote, "Progestogens have a variety of effects apart from the one for which their use was intended, that of secretory transformation of the endometrium. Endometrial effects vary between individuals and between different progestogens, leading to bleeding problems. Symptoms of fluid retention are produced by the sodium-retaining effect on the renin-aldosterone system. The nor-testosterone-derived progestogens can have adverse effects on skin, lipids, vasculature and insulin resistance. Negative mood effects are produced by most progestogens due to the effect on neurotransmitters via central nervous system progesterone receptors."[111]

An elevated blood glucose level during the 2-hour glucose tolerance test reveals glucose intolerance. In glucose intolerance, the fasting blood glucose level is usually normal, but the glucose level after meals is abnormally elevated.[48,p.292] Glucose intolerance is associated with a 2-fold increase in death from cardiovascular disease.[50][51]

Elevated blood insulin levels (hyperinsulinemia) are also associated with a 2-fold increase in the rate of death from heart disease. This holds true whether insulin levels are elevated during fasting, at 1 or 2 hours during the oral glucose tolerance test, at any blood glucose level, and despite the absence of other risk factors for cardiovascular disease.[52][53][54,pp.143-148] Studies of patients with diabetes mellitus who are not insulin-dependent showed that elevated blood insulin levels may cause a pathological proliferation of the smooth muscle cells in blood vessels.[55] Also, elevated insulin blood levels increase production of very low-density lipoproteins. In addition, the elevated levels decrease high-density lipoprotein cholesterol, especially the HDL_2 cholesterol subfraction. The latter is considered the "heart-protective" fraction,[56][57] and its reduction leads to dangerous cardiovascular consequences. Gaspard and Lefebvre wrote that these findings may explain the increased risk for cardiovascular disease associated with hyperinsulinemia in oral contraceptive users.[45,p.337]

Mechanisms of Glucose Abnormalities Associated with Oral Contraceptive Use

Glucose abnormalities during oral contraceptive use are of particular concern to me because they appear to underlie the pain associated with some women's use of oral contraceptives.

Those who have speculated on the mechanism by which oral contraceptive constituents cause elevated glucose and insulin levels have cited the literature on other conditions that share these blood patterns. To consider the mechanism by which the contraceptives may cause myofascial pain, we must also look at the data from this other literature.

Beck-Nielsen et al. indicate that keeping glucose levels within homeostatic limits after a meal depends on two factors—normal insulin secretion and insulin action. When one of these factors is faulty, the other tends to compensate for it. The compensation keeps glucose levels within normal limits even when one factor is excessive or deficient. For example, when cells are partially resistant to insulin, insulin secretion

increases to compensate for the deficient cellular action of insulin.[48,p.292] Spellacy et al. were appealing to this model when they wrote that in their patients taking high-dose oral contraceptives, elevated insulin levels suggest peripheral cellular resistance to insulin. The resistance, by impeding insulin action, resulted in increased insulin secretion to maintain glucose homeostasis.[49,p.562] Skouby et al. agreed with this mechanism, although they surmised that slowed clearance of insulin from the circulation by the liver may also play a role in elevated circulating insulin levels.[65,p.343] However, Godsland et al. measured C-peptide concentrations in response to combination oral contraceptives. C-peptide is a 30 amino acid chain binding the A and B chains of insulin in proinsulin (the single chain precursor of insulin). Conversion of proinsulin to insulin removes the C-peptide. Godsland et al. wrote that their results suggested a relative difference in insulin responses, showing that the increased insulin levels in the women were due to increased pancreatic secretion.[62,p.352]

Insulin Resistance in Oral Contraceptive Users. When I refer to "insulin resistance," I am referring to deceased sensitivity or responsiveness of cells to insulin. Resistance increases circulating insulin and glucose levels, and it decreases glucose entry into cells. Studies suggest that estrogens protect against and progestins contribute to insulin resistance.

Estrogen and Insulin Resistance. Hulman et al. made rats insulin resistant by feeding them a high sucrose diet. Subsequent estrogen withdrawal caused insulin levels to elevate during both fasting and glucose intake. The insulin elevation with estrogen withdrawal suggests that estrogen provides some protection against the induction of insulin resistance by a high sucrose intake.[120]

Many post-menopausal women have insulin resistance, and estrogen replacement decreases the resistance.[113] Brussaard et al. found that estrogen replacement increased insulin sensitivity (decreased insulin resistance) in the livers of post-menopausal women with non-insulin-dependent diabetes mellitus.[112]

Too high a dosage of estrogen, however, may diminish the degree of estrogen-induced improvement in insulin resistance. For 3 months, Wu, Bi, and Wang had post-menopausal women use two different dosages of ethinyl estradiol, 0.05 mg and 0.025 mg. Both dosages decreased the levels of fasting plasma glucose and insulin. Insulin sensitivity increased significantly. However, Wu, Bi, and Wang wrote that the outcome indicated that 0.025 mg is a more appropriate dosage because women using 0.05 mg underwent a deterioration of glucose tolerance.[119]

Progestin and Insulin Resistance. Several studies have shown increased insulin resistance and carbohydrate abnormalities with oral contraceptive use.[45][48][49][121][122] Progestins derived from nor-testosterone increase insulin resistance.[111]

Colcurci et al. reported that women treated with estrogen alone had a lower insulin response during an oral glucose loading test. The lower insulin response suggests greater insulin sensitivity. This effect was more evident in women who used transdermic 17β-estradiol treatment than in those who took conjugated equine estrogens orally. Adding a progestin (medroxy-progestogen) to the estrogens diminished the increase in insulin sensitivity induced by estrogens.[114]

Kimmerle et al. tested the effects of low-dose vs. high-dose combination estrogen-progestin on insulin sensitivity in post-menopausal nondiabetic women. The preparation contained both 17β-estradiol and nor-ethisterone acetate. They reported that 3 months continuous use of a low-dose preparation, consisting of 1 mg estradiol and 0.5 mg norethisterone, did not change insulin sensitivity in postmenopausal women. But the use of a high-dose preparation, containing 2 mg estradiol and 1 mg norethisterone, caused a modest decrease in insulin sensitivity (an increase in insulin resistance).[117]

Raudaskoski et al. reported that transdermal estradiol improved insulin sensitivity by 22% in healthy postmenopausal women. However, combining intra-uterine levonorgestrel (a progestin) to transdermal estradiol minimzed this benefit, providing only a small 3.6% increase in insulin tolerance. The researchers wrote, however, that the combination therapy did not induce frank insulin resistance.[116]

Increased Insulin Resistance in the Luteal Phase of the Menstrual Cycle. Escalante et al. tested for variations in insulin resistance during the menstrual cycles of 12 healthy regularly menstruating women. The women had normal fasting glucose levels of < 100 μg/dL, and they had no family history of diabetes mellitus. The researchers tested for insulin sensitivity, glucose effectiveness, and the acute insulin response to glucose during intravenous glucose tolerance tests. The mean sensitivity to insulin decreased (insulin resistance increased) during the cycle. Mean insulin sensitivity was higher (insulin resistance was lower) during the follicular phase (5.03±0.72), and insulin sensitivity decreased (resistance increased) during the luteal phase (2.22±0.45). Glucose effectiveness did not differ in the follicular and luteal phases. The mean ac-

ute insulin response to glucose was 276.4±27.8 AIRg mU/mL in the follicular phase. In the luteal phase, when the women had decreased insulin sensitivity (increased insulin resistance), the mean acute insulin response to glucose was adaptively increased to 304.4 +/- 51.1 AIRg mU/mL. This increase of 28 AIRg mU/mL, however, was not statistically significant.[118]

The slight increase in insulin resistance during the luteal phase, the third phase of the menstrual cycle, may result from the decreased secretion of endogenous estrogen. This observation may indicate that in susceptible women, energy deficiency muscle contractures and activation of treatment-resistant myofascial trigger points are more likely to occur during the luteal phase of the menstrual cycle. If so, the association would allow us to predict that the patients' myofascial pain will subside at the end of the luteal phase when estrogen secretion begins anew, decreasing insulin resistance and possibly relieving energy deficiency contractures.

Adverse Effects of Elevated Insulin Due to Cellular Resistance to Insulin. In individuals with glucose intolerance due to cellular resistance to insulin, insulin levels may be elevated during the fasting state and after meals. If as a result, the ability of the beta cells of the pancreas to synthesize and secrete insulin becomes impaired, diabetes mellitus results.[48,p.292] In the meantime, however, chronically elevated insulin levels due to insulin resistance serve as a major common denominator of at least three clinical conditions: dyslipoproteinemia, arterial hypertension, and obesity.[48,p.293]

For some women, the progestin constituent of contraceptives may cause insulin resistance and result in impaired glucose metabolism in skeletal muscle cells.

During insulin resistance, three putative mechanisms may decrease muscle cell energy metabolism: (1) increased triglyceride synthesis, (2) reduced density and activity of insulin receptors, and (3) decreased glycogen synthetase activity.

Increased Triglyceride Synthesis. In genetically obese mice, the skeletal muscles are insulin resistant. Elevated blood glucose following a meal is not adequately disposed of by their skeletal muscles. Thus, the beta cells of the pancreas are stimulated to continue releasing insulin. Elevated insulin levels are associated with increases in the activity of two enzymes that increase fat formation: glucose-6-phosphate dehydrogenase and malic enzyme 3-hydrooxyacyl-CoA. (There is no change in the activity of the glycolytic enzymes phosphofructokinase, hexokinase, pyruvate kinase, and alpha-glycerophosphate.)[66] Increased activity of the enzymes results in accelerated synthesis of triglycerides, cholesterol, and phospholipids. Consequently, adipose tissue progressively accumulates.[48,p.293] Insulin resistant patients usually have high levels of very low-density lipoproteins and low levels of high-density lipoproteins.[64]

This fat-storing abnormality is important to some patients' treatment resistance myofascial pain syndromes. Muscle cells are dependent on a steady flow of free fatty acids for energy metabolism between meals. When the activity of fat synthesizing enzymes increases during insulin resistance, fewer free fatty acids are mobilized to fuel muscle cell activity between meals. An energy deficit may occur in muscles cells, resulting in energy deficient contractures and activation of pain-referring trigger points.

Decreased Density and Activity of Insulin Receptors. De Pirro et al. proposed that oral contraceptives reduce the number and binding affinity of insulin receptors on cell membranes.[123] In a condition called syndrome X, there appears to be a genetic defect that causes resistance of skeletal muscle cells to insulin.[67,p.565] The insulin receptor may be the defective locus. Researchers have found reduced numbers of insulin receptors in skeletal muscle cell membranes in obese subjects, only some of whom are diabetic. A kinase makes up the β component of the receptor, and it mediates the insulin signal across the cell membrane once insulin binds to the α component of the receptor.[30,p.263] This kinase is impaired in syndrome X patients.[68] Changes in diet alter the decreased density of insulin receptors on cell membranes and the decreased kinase activity.[69] This suggests that they are responsible for insulin resistance in the patients, and the resistance involves desensitization due to excess exposure of cell membranes to insulin.

Decreased Glycogen Synthetase Activity. Beck-Nielsen et al. suggested that the main defect in glucose processing of insulin resistant patients is inside cells. The defect may involve the anaerobic pathway of glycogen synthesis. They wrote that the key enzyme in glycogen synthesis is glycogen synthetase.[48,p.294] This enzyme enables the cell to store glucose molecules as glycogen so that the glucose can later be released for ATP synthesis. If glucose is not effectively stored as glycogen, too little glucose may be available for ATP production. In lean individuals with normal glucose tolerance, insulin stimulates a several-fold increase in the activity of glycogen synthetase. In obese individuals, the ability of insulin to increase activity of the enzyme is much weaker. In obese diabetic patients, the enzyme is completely resistant to insulin.[70] Beck-Nielsen et al. speculated that oral contraceptives

impair the ability of insulin to activate glycogen synthetase in muscle cells.[48,pp.294-295] Progestins bind to receptors in the cell nucleus[31,p.98] and affect gene transcription.[30,p.23] It is possible that changes in glycogen synthetase and/or insulin receptors may be genomic effects of the progestins.

It is possible that in some women, the progestin component of contraceptives, by inducing insulin resistance, impedes muscle cell metabolism by one of more of these mechanisms—decreasing the availability of free fatty acids, reducing the density and activity of insulin receptors on cell membranes, and reducing the activity of glycogen synthetase. In susceptible women, the energy deficiency might induce and sustain myofascial pain syndromes. I am speculating, of course, about these possible mechanisms. But whatever the mechanisms may be, I am certain of the clinical phenomena that result from them—oral contraceptive use by some women results in episodes of acute, severe, treatment-resistant myofascial pain, and the episodes cease to occur when the women stop using the contraceptives. Fibromyalgic women who have deficient muscle energy metabolism due to inadequate thyroid hormone regulation of muscle cell metabolism may be even more susceptible than most women to his iatrogenic source of myofascial pain.

PREMENSTRUAL SYNDROME (PMS)

R.T. Frank first described PMS in 1931.[252] The condition is a variety of physical, cognitive, emotional, and behavioral symptoms that some women experience during the perimenstrual time. The symptoms usually begin 7-to-10 days before menstruation, and relief usually occurs within a few hours to a day or so after the onset of menstruation.[81] Hence, PMS symptoms occur during the last half of the luteal phase of the cycle, which lasts 13-to-14 days and during the earliest part of the follicular phase. (See section above titled "Luteal Phase of the Menstrual Cycle.")

PMS Symptoms and Their Prevalence

Medical writers have attributed more than 150 symptoms to PMS.[246] Prominent somatic symptoms include bloating (water retention), breast swelling and pain, bowel disturbances, skin disorders, increased weight, pelvic pain, unstable blood sugar, and headaches. Psychological symptoms include irritability, aggressiveness, depression, anxiety, panic attacks, poor concentration, mood swings, diminished sense of well-being, crying, tension, lethargy, sleep disturbance, altered appetite, loss of sex drive, craving for sweets and caffeine, morning sluggishness, low metabolism, and symptoms of hypothyroidism despite normal thyroid hormone levels.[81][102,pp.135-136[251][278]

Most researchers have reported that 30%-to-40% of women experience PMS.[247][248][249] Other researchers, however, have reported a prevalence of 92%.[250] PMS is most common among women who work outside the home, have had more children, are alcoholics, or have had hypertensive disorders (toxemia) during pregnancies.[81]

Factors Possibly Underlying PMS

Researchers have proposed several possible causative factors: progesterone deficiency, hypothyroidism, prolactin excess, abnormalities of the renin-angiotensin system, vasopressin excess, excess prostaglandins, decreased osmotic pressure of the blood, vitamin deficiencies, ovarian infection, yeast overgrowth, and psychosocial factors.[81] Other common associated factors are endometriosis, chronic pelvic inflammatory disease, and benign smooth muscle growths in the uterus (leiomyoma uteri).[245] Learning the causes of PMS is a formidable challenge, partly because usually, multiple factors are involved.[102,p.234] Many researchers recognized that PMS, like peri-menopausal and menopausal symptoms, are worse in women who do not exercise, have poor nutrition, and are subjected to intense and relentless stress. My task here is not to explore all the contributions but to consider those most likely to interact with inadequate thyroid hormone regulation of the HPG axis.

Array of Possible Hormonal Underpinnings of PMS. Studies conducted to identify hormonal abnormalities associated with PMS have given inconsistent results. Consequently, no hormone abnormalities are reliably associated with PMS. Based on the available studies, it is exceedingly difficult to draw conclusions about the possible mechanisms of PMS that are not contradicted by other study results. This outcome does not prove, as some researchers might assume, that PMS is unrelated to alterations of estrogen, progesterone, and/or thyroid hormone levels. Instead, the variable results may mean that PMS is a *heterogenous* condition, as Lurie and Borenstein have defined it.[81,p.220] PMS is probably heterogenous in that altered levels of multiple hormones, and variations in the responsiveness of different tissues, cause a variety of overlapping symptoms in different women. Some women's symptoms may be caused by low estrogen levels, some by estrogen dominance, others by low progesterone levels, and still others by various combi-

nations of these. Other women's symptoms are caused mainly by inadequate thyroid hormone regulation of the HPG axis. Other patients' symptoms may result from abrupt changes in estrogen and/or progesterone levels. This is suggested by reports that women experience symptoms at times when their hormone levels vary—during PMS, after childbirth, peri-menopause, and menopause[278] (see section below titled "Peri-Menopause and Menopause"). Some women may be highly sensitive to changes in estrogen and/or progesterone levels—so much so that the women experience symptoms when their estrogen and/or progesterone levels vary within their respective ranges of normal.

Some medical writers such as Arpels have hypothesized that the symptoms of PMS, postpartum period, peri-menopause, and menopause result from a fall in estrogen levels below that required of the brain.[278] Others such as Hargrove, Lee, and Laux contend that the symptoms result from low progesterone levels.[102][276] Studies have not reliably shown abnormal levels of estradiol, progesterone, or LH in women with PMS.[277] Despite the failure of studies to show a consistent hormone imbalance, evidence suggests a link between various PMS symptoms and altered hormone levels. For example, women are more susceptible to depression than men. Their susceptibility to depression is greatest at times when estrogen and progesterone levels rapidly fluctuate. For example, many women become deeply depressed before their menstrual periods start, after giving birth, and during the transition to menopause.[277]

Estrogen Deficiency as a Factor in PMS. Estrogen, like progesterone, exerts potent effects on brain function. Estrogen passes the blood-brain barrier and binds to receptors in brain cells. The onset of the effects of the estrogen-receptor complexes are generally delayed and have prolonged duration. However, both rapid and delayed actions of estrogen can alter the electrical properties of nerve membranes and thus their firing patterns. In brain cells, estradiol mainly exerts excitatory effects, whether the effects are rapid or delayed.[300] Rosie et al. described several effects of estrogen on central nervous system neurotransmitters: increased dopamine$_2$ receptors and serotonin$_{2A}$ receptors, and increased arginine vasopressin secretion.[281]

Rosie et al. referred to estrogen as "Nature's psycho-protectant." They wrote that by acting on monoamine and neuropeptide transmitter mechanisms in the brain, estrogen exerts profound effects on mood, mental state, and memory. Estrogen stimulates an increase in dopamine$_2$ (D$_2$) receptors in the striatum. It also stimulates transcription of the arginine vasopressin

(AVP) gene in the stria terminalis of rats. It stimulates a 100-fold increase in AVP mRNA and a massive increase in AVP peptide in the projections from the stria terminalis to the lateral septum and lateral habenula. AVP within this system enhances and/or maintains "social" or "olfactory" memory. According to Rosie et al., estrogen thus provides a powerful model for correlating transcriptional control of neuropeptide gene expression with behavior. In addition, estrogen also stimulates an increase in the density of serotonin$_{2A}$ receptors (5-HT$_{2A}$) in anterior frontal, cingulate, and primary olfactory cortices and in the nucleus accumbens. These areas of the brain are concerned with the control of mood, mental state, cognition, emotion and behavior. (Serotonin, interacting with 5-HT$_{2A}$ receptors in the central grey matter, may, through increasing the intensity of an aversive stimulus needed to induce flight or escape, improve clinical conditions such as chronic anxiety, panic states, and pain disorders.[290]) Rosie et al. speculate that the estrogen-induced increase in 5-HT$_{2A}$ receptors may explain why estrogen gives some women relief from depression as a PMS symptom.[281] Some medical writers appear to reason that a reduction of serotonin receptors in the brain from low estrogen levels explains why antidepressant medications are useful with some women who have depression related to PMS and menopause.[291][292] Estrogen improves the sense of well-being of post-menopausal women including those made menopausal by surgery.[339][340][341][342]

Anderberg et al. reported that premenstrual fibromyalgia patients had better psychological status than post-menopausal fibromyalgia patients during the premenopausal women's ovulatory phase. They defined this phase as the 12th through the 17th day of the menstrual cycle; ovulation is expected to occur on the 14th day of the cycle. They appeared to argue that this shows that estrogen and not progesterone underlay the better psychological status of the premenopausal women.[334,pp.32-33] They cited reports that estrogen replacement therapy had improved both the physical and mental status of post-menopausal women who had diminished well-being.[339][340][341][342] Concerning a previous study they conducted, they wrote,[333] "Premenopausal FMS patients have been found to have relief of the pain during the ovulatory phase when estrogen is raised without influence from progesterone."[334,p.33]

The likelihood that some patients' PMS is underlain by estrogen deficiency is supported by the finding that some women have an increased density of α$_2$-adrenergic receptors on cell membranes during the luteal phase of the cycle. The increased density results from

reduced estradiol levels, although the receptor density increases further when thyroid hormone inadequately regulates transcription of the adrenergic genes. Activation of the receptors by catecholamines impedes metabolic processes and gives rise to hypothyroid-like symptoms. (See subsection below titled "α$_2$-Adrenergic Receptor Density in the Luteal Phase of the Menstrual Cycle.")

Estrogen Dominance. Seippel and Backstrom found that the severity of premenstrual symptoms was worse in women who had higher luteal phase levels of estradiol and LH.[362] Redei and Freeman found that in PMS patients, estradiol and progesterone levels were both consistently higher throughout the cycle, but the levels were short of significance. Patients with more severe PMS symptoms had significantly higher estradiol levels from the follicular to the early luteal phase.[363] Wang et al. found that PMS patients had significantly higher estradiol and lower progesterone levels. The worst PMS symptoms occurred in cycles with higher luteal phase estradiol. The researchers wrote that their results suggest a relation between the hormones and the severity of distressing PMS symptoms.[365]

Some researchers have reported that high progesterone levels appear to be associated with PMS symptoms. However, in most studies, estrogen levels were also high and may have accounted for the PMS symptoms. (See subsection below titled "Dubious Association of Elevated Progesterone with PMS.")

Guyton pointed out that in the liver, estrogen is conjugated and sulfated. About a fifth of the conjugated estrogen is excreted in the bile, and the rest is excreted in the urine. The liver converts the strong estrogens estradiol and estrone to the weak estriol. Guyton wrote, "Therefore, diminished liver function *increases* the activity of estrogens in the body, sometimes causing *hyperestrinism* [italics his]."[78,p.905] Sluggish liver function, of course, typically accompanies inadequate thyroid hormone stimulation due to hypothyroidism. Thus, hypothyroidism might be the underlying cause of some women's estrogen dominance.

Progesterone Deficiency as a Factor in PMS. Progesterone, like estrogen, strongly influences brain function. Progesterone passes the blood-brain barrier and binds to progesterone receptors in brain cells. The effects of the progesterone-receptor complexes on cell function are generally delayed compared to the effect of other hormones such as norepinephrine, yet the effects are prolonged when they occur. Nonetheless, both rapid and delayed actions of progesterone can alter the electrical properties and firing patterns of nerve membranes. In brain cells, progesterone mainly exerts inhibitory effects, and usually the effects are rapid compared to those of estrogen.[300] Progesterone has sedative, hypnotic, and anesthetic effects on the central nervous system.[81,p.221][254][279] One progesterone metabolite is a gamma amino butyric acid-A receptor agonist that has anxiety relieving effects.[338] These known effects of progesterone suggest that a decrease of the hormone produces the dysphoria, irritability, aggressiveness, and anxiety that occur in the late luteal phase.[81,p.221] Also, progesterone inhibits the action of aldosterone in the distal kidney tubules, resulting in a net increase of sodium and water excretion.[255] A deficiency of progesterone is expected to cause sodium and water retention. Moreover, oral natural progesterone therapy, when combined with proper diet and exercise, is an effective PMS treatment for many women.[256][257]

Because progesterone is soporific, deficient progesterone levels may result in inadequate sleep. Lee et al. found no differences in various sleep stages between the menstrual cycle phases. However, women who had unpleasant emotional symptoms during the premenstrual time had significantly less slow-wave (delta) sleep during both the follicular and luteal phases compared to asymptomatic subjects.[286] Deficient slow-wave sleep is also associated with hypothyroidism (see Chapter 3.18). It is possible that a combination of deficient progesterone and inadequate thyroid hormone regulation of the sleep cycle can worsen slow-wave sleep deprivation and thereby amplify PMS symptoms.

Some studies have shown low progesterone levels in PMS patients. Hargrove and Abraham studied 137 premenopausal PMS patients. The patients' major complaints were bleeding, pain, and/or infertility. On average, during the middle of the luteal phase, the women had significantly decreased progesterone levels and elevated 17β-estradiol levels.[245] Wang et al. found that PMS patients had significantly higher estradiol and lower progesterone levels. The researchers wrote that their results suggest a relation between the hormones and the severity of distressing PMS symptoms.[365]

Lee has proposed a cogent and convincing hypothesis of PMS. He wrote that PMS results from a progesterone deficiency due to anovulatory cycles and adrenal exhaustion. He conjectured that the main cause of anovulatory cycles is xenoestrogens (see subsection below titled "Effects of Xenoestrogens"). He also proposed that due to the extremely stressful lifestyle of most women today, the ovaries shut down in

favor of survival. (This possibility is supported by studies showing that adverse environmental conditions inhibit ovulation.[357][358]) They stop ovulating, and as a result, no corpus luteum is formed. When a corpus luteum does not form, the ovaries produce no progesterone. The only source of progesterone then is the adrenal cortices. However, due to poor diet, the woman's adrenal cortices may lack enough of the nutrients that serve as substrates for the production of adrenal steroid hormones. Moreover, the woman's stressful lifestyle burdens the adrenal cortices with chronic, excessive activity. Thus, the resources of the adrenal cortices are invested in manufacturing hormones that enable the woman to adapt to the stress, such as cortisol and aldosterone, rather than sex hormones. Adrenal conversion of androgens to progesterone slows to a rate too low to provide the woman with sufficient amounts of progesterone. Because of the lack of progesterone production by a corpus luteum and the failure of the adrenal glands to compensate, the woman becomes progesterone deficient. By virtue of her low progesterone levels, she has estrogen dominance—that is, unopposed estrogenic effects on the body. Progesterone normally balances the effects of estrogen, but when progesterone is deficient, the effects of estrogen are not properly modulated. Estrogen dominance is normal during a week or so of the follicular phase of the cycle, but during the luteal phase, progesterone is normally dominant. But progesterone deficiency during the luteal phase exposes the woman to unoppposed estrogen effects throughout this 14-day phase of the cycle. Adverse effects may occur, including fatigue, depression, diminished sex desire, weight gain, water retention, headaches, and mood swings.[102,pp.130-149]

Lee's proposed mechanism is highly plausible, and it dovetails with the model of fibromyalgia I propose in this book. First, as Lee wrote, increased estrogen levels impede the thyroid system[102,pp.145-149] (see section below titled "Increased Estrogen Levels May Lower Circulating Thyroid Hormone Levels and Inhibit T$_4$ to T$_3$ Conversion"). As a result, during estrogen dominance, symptoms caused by the dominance and/or progesterone deficiency may be complicated by symptoms of inadequate thyroid hormone regulation of cell function.

Second, I believe that at least in fibromyalgia patients, inadequate thyroid hormone regulation of the HPG axis, particularly the ovaries, is a common mechanism of failure to ovulate and failed luteinization (see section above titled "Luteinization"). Anovulatory cycles are common among primary hypothyroid patients and corrected by the use of exogenous thyroid hormone.[27] As Lee has described,[102] when luteinization fails, a corpus luteum does not form, and the woman has low progesterone levels during the luteal phase of the menstrual cycle. Thus, low progesterone levels may be mainly responsible for their PMS symptoms. If so, improvement or relief of fibromyalgia patients' PMS symptoms with the use of the proper form and dosage of exogenous thyroid hormone, as we have found, suggests that the thyroid hormone normalized ovulation and luteinization. In addition, the thyroid hormone might increase the production of pregnenolone in the adrenal cortices, making more available for conversion to progesterone. Moreover, thyroid hormone might augment the FSH-induced conversion of pregnenolone to progesterone by increasing the activity of 3β-hydroxysteroid dehydrogenase (see section above titled "Progesterone Production in Granulosa Cells"). The use of thyroid hormone has not been completely successful with all female fibromyalgia patients, however, and I suspect that the poor outcome in some cases resulted from my failure to include proper progesterone therapy as part of their treatment regimen.

Dubious Association of Elevated Progesterone with PMS. Seippel and Backstrom wrote that the presence of a corpus luteum is necessary for PMS symptoms to occur.[362] Redei and Freeman wrote that PMS patients had significantly elevated progesterone levels along the entire menstrual cycle, and the levels correlated with PMS symptoms. The increased progesterone levels preceded the PMS symptoms by 5-to-7 days. They wrote, "These preliminary results provide support for the hypothesis that the presence of progesterone at early luteal phase levels is required for PMS symptoms to occur." It should be noted, however, that these patients' estradiol levels were also elevated.[363] Hammarback et al. studied 18 PMS patients through two consecutive menstrual cycles. More severe PMS symptoms occurred in cycles when both luteal phase estradiol and progesterone levels were high. However, high luteal phase estradiol levels were related to worse symptoms. The researchers wrote that their results contradict the hypothesis that progesterone deficiency plays a role in the etiology of PMS.[364] We should note that while progesterone levels were not low, estradiol levels were high. This supports Lee's contention that estrogen dominance is the source of many women's symptoms.[102]

Inadequate Thyroid Hormone Regulation in PMS

Inadequate thyroid hormone regulation of the HPG axis is the main factor underlying some patients' PMS, and the clinician should consider hypothyroidism and cellular resistance to thyroid hormone as possible factors underlying PMS. In addition to clinical experience, several PMS studies support this view.

Schmidt et al. reported the case of a woman with autoimmune thyroiditis whose initial diagnosis was "menstrual-related mood disorder." Thyroid hormone therapy eliminated the mood disorder. The authors wrote that the successful outcome highlights the importance of assessing the thyroid status of women with a diagnosis of menstrual-related mood disorder.[258]

Roy-Byrne et al studied the TSH responses to injected TRH stimulation in PMS patients and normal controls. In both patients and controls, mean basal TSH levels and mean maximum increases in TSH in response to TRH were the same in all phases of the menstrual cycle. However, 7 of the 10 patients had significantly greater variability in TSH responses to TRH: 3 had blunted and 4 had exaggerated TSH responses. This outcome is consistent with incipient central hypothyroidism in the 7 of 10 patients.[259]

Girdler et al. found that mean thyroid hormone levels during the follicular and luteal phases did not differ between 15 PMS patients and 15 normal controls. However, PMS patients had significantly greater variations in the values of the TSH, T_3 uptake, total T_4, and the free T_4 index. In addition, PMS patients had significantly higher reverse-T_3 levels during the luteal phase of the cycle. (This suggests that T_4 to T_3 conversion was impaired during this phase in PMS patients.) The investigators wrote that these findings indicate that a subset of PMS patients have thyroid axis abnormalities that contribute to their PMS.[266]

Schmidt et al. found that PMS patients had a high incidence of abnormalities during the TRH stimulation test. Of the women tested, basal thyroid function test values suggested that 10.5% had either grade I or II hypothyroidism or hyperthyroidism, and (13%) had elevated thyroid auto-antibody titers. In addition, 30% of the patients, all with normal basal TSH levels, had abnormal responses to injected TRH. Twice as many patients had exaggerated TSH responses than had blunted TSH responses. These NIH researchers then treated 30 PMS patients with T_4 replacement in a double-blind placebo controlled design. They concluded from the results that T_4 was not superior to a placebo in the treatment of PMS. They wrote, "L-T_4 supplementation appears to have no place in the routine management of PMS."[267] This poor treatment outcome was predictable, of course, in that T_4 replacement typically has a poor outcome, whether it is used in studies or clinical practice. T_4 alone, compared to desiccated thyroid or T_3 alone, is highly ineffective, and replacement dosages are woefully inadequate in relieving inadequate thyroid hormone regulation of cell function. As my clinical experience has shown, had the researchers used sufficiently high dosages of desiccated thyroid or T_3, their results would have been different—most or all features of PMS caused by inadequate thyroid hormone regulation of the HPG axis would have been alleviated.

α_2-Adrenergic Receptor Density in the Luteal Phase of the Menstrual Cycle. α_2-Adrenergic receptors are inhibitory in general. Binding of the receptor to catecholamines on cell membranes inhibits cell energy metabolism and other processes. Most of the metabolism slowing effects of hypothyroidism are mediated by a shift toward α_2 adrenergic receptor dominance on cell membranes. (See Chapter 3.1, section titled "Inadequate Thyroid Hormone Regulation of Adrenergic Gene Transcription.")

Several researchers, which I cite below, have reported increases in α_2-adrenergic receptors associated with the luteal phase of the menstrual cycle, and the increased receptors are associated with more severe PMS symptoms. This is an important finding because fibromyalgia patients were found to have an increased density of α_2-adrenergic receptors on their platelets.[361]

The increased density of α_2-adrenergic receptors appears to be a response to reduced estradiol levels. That the increase in the density of the receptors is related to reduced estradiol levels may mean that symptoms mediated by the increased receptor density do not occur during estrogen dominance but do so in estrogen deficiency. Regardless, an increased density of α_2-adrenergic receptors on cell membranes is likely to be associated with symptoms. These symptoms are likely to be accentuated by simultaneous inadequate thyroid hormone regulation of the adrenergic gene transcription. The inadequate thyroid hormone regulation potently increases the density of α_2-adrenergic receptors on cell membranes. Thus, an estrogen deficiency combined with hypothyroidism or resistance to thyroid hormone may produce more severe symptoms related to increased α_2-adrenergic receptors than either condition alone.

Jones studied variations in α_2-adrenergic receptor binding in human platelets during the menstrual cycle. They found that females had cyclic variations in the number of α_2-adrenergic receptors that coincided with

their menstrual cycles. The density was highest at the onset of menstruation. The density of α_2-adrenergic receptors at the middle of the cycle, at ovulation, was only 74%-to-79% of the highest value during the entire cycle. The density increased from lowest to the highest through the luteal phase.[360]

Gurguis et al. studied α_2-adrenergic receptors in women with premenstrual dysphoric disorder, a condition characterized by anxiety and depression. They found that a high α_2-adrenergic receptor density during the follicular phase predicted more severe luteal symptoms in patients with dysphoric disorder. During the luteal phase, α_2-adrenergic receptor density correlated positively with symptom severity in patients.[359]

Amplifying of Estradiol-Induced Cerebral Cortex Inhibition by Inadequate Thyroid Hormone Regulation of Adrenergic Gene Transcription. An important finding was recently reported by Karakanias et al. The finding provides an explanation of how some features of PMS may be caused by an interaction of low estrogen levels with thyroid hormone deficiency or cellular resistance to thyroid hormone.

Karakanias et al. found that administering estradiol for 48 hours to rats whose ovaries were removed caused a 50% reduction in the concentration of $\alpha_{2A/D}$-adrenoceptor mRNA in the frontal region of the cerebral cortex. The reduced concentration of $\alpha_{2A/D}$-adrenoceptor mRNA was accompanied by reduced density of cortical α_2-adrenergic receptors. The researchers noted that the result provides the first evidence that estradiol regulates the expression of postsynaptic α_2-adrenergic receptors in female rat frontal cortex. The finding suggests that the density of $\alpha_{2A/D}$-adrenergic receptors increases in the cortex when estrogen levels are low, as during the luteal phase of the menstrual cycle. Karakanias et al. wrote that this is evidence of a molecular substrate for the changes in cognitive function during decreases and increases of estradiol.[284]

Sustained α_2-adrenergic receptor dominance in a woman's brain due to inadequate thyroid hormone transcription regulation of the adrenergic genes is likely to cause cognitive impairment and depression (see Chapters 3.1 and 3.10). The cognitive dysfunction and depression may result from the inhibition of norepinephrine secretion by α_2-adrenergic receptors.[221,pp.123-124] In such women, the reduced level of estrogen during the luteal phase of the cycle may compound the α-adrenergic receptor dominance, worsening her cognitive dysfunction and depression. A rise in the estrogen level during the follicular phase of the cycle would reduce or relieve these adverse effects mediated by α-adrenergic receptors in the cortex. The relief of the adverse effects might be followed by the "emotional upswing occurring between days five and seven" of the menstrual cycle, referred to by Candace Pert.[285,p.127] Pert asked whether the upswing could be caused by an endorphin release. But it is possible that the upswing results from a reduction in the density of α-adrenergic receptors in the cortex due to increased levels of estrogen.

Abnormal Responses to Normal Hormone Levels

The failure to find a consistent hormonal pattern that typifies PMS has prompted some researchers to look elsewhere for the source of the women's symptoms. Lurie and Borenstein wrote that it is convenient to agree with Merriam et al.:[81,p.222] PMS may result from abnormal responses to normal hormone levels.[253]

Redmond wrote that despite the low mood, depression, and irritability that commonly occur in the late luteal-early menstrual phase, women with PMS and those without it do not differ in circulating hormone levels during their cycles. Instead, they may differ in their brain response to hormones. He noted that estrogen and progesterone receptors exist in the brain and change during the cycle.[280] Exactly what could account for the different brain responses is not clear. One factor that can alter cell responsiveness to estrogen is xenoestrogens. The prefix "xeno" means strange or foreign, and xenoestrogens refer to chemical substances alien to the body that exert estrogenic effects on cells.

Effects of Xenoestrogens. In Chapter 2.4, I described in detail the thyroid system abnormalities potentially caused by dioxins, PCBs, and similar man-made chemical contaminants (see section titled "Environmental Contaminants"). The reproductive system is among the body systems that these contaminants may disrupt.[353][354]

Some contaminants are estrogen mimics, that is, they bind to estrogen receptors. Upon binding to the receptors, the mimics may activate cell processes normally activated by the binding of endogenous estrogen to estrogen receptors. Activation of estrogen-driven cell processes by the mimics can contribute to estrogen dominance.[87,pp.71&79] Dominance might occur even in the menopausal woman whose endogenous estrogen production is minimal and who consumes little or no phytoestrogens. Still, due to a high enough body level of estrogen mimics, she may be estrogen dominant. Treating such a woman with synthetic estrogen is like-

ly to be less than successful, and adding tranquilizers and antidepressants to her medication regimen, which is now common practice in conventional medicine, is to miss entirely the proper therapeutic target. If the tranquilizers and antidepressants provide some relief, the woman may be ill served by it. The xenoestrogens may insidiously induce life-threatening pathology while during the process, the medications make the associated symptoms tolerable.

Rather than activating cell processes, estrogen mimics may bind with a higher affinity than endogenous estrogen to estrogen receptors and inhibit the cell processes. In this case, the mimics function as estrogen blockers.[87,pp.71&79] The clinician may consider the resulting symptoms from this estrogen blockade as due to an estrogen deficiency, and as a result may prescribe synthetic estrogen or increase the woman's current dosage. The only result is likely to be excessive exposure of cells normally responsive to estrogen with possible production of estrogen dominance symptoms.

Deciding what possible roles these estrogen mimics play in the symptoms of PMS, peri-menopause, and menopause is exceedingly difficult. Unfortunately, probably most clinical decisions about female sex hormone replacement therapy are based on the clinician's unquestioning acceptance of the myth that estrogen deficiency is the cause of most or all female sex-related health problems. Making treatment decisions based on this myth may be a serious disservice to the treated woman. Lee contended, for example, that xenoestrogens are likely to be the main cause of anovulatory cycles.[102,p.111] Anovulatory cycles result in low progesterone levels during the luteal phase of the cycle and relative estrogen dominance. If xenoestrogens are the main cause, or even a common cause, then prescribing estrogen is precisely the wrong treatment choice. Probably the best we can do at this stage of investigation is to educate patients about the potential complications caused by these contaminants and encourage and motivate them to free themselves from them, to the extent that this is possible.

Evaluation

Lurie and Borenstein wrote that the diagnosis of PMS is based on establishing a relationship between the symptoms and the luteal phase of the menstrual cycle. They wisely cautioned, however—although PMS occurs cyclically, all that cycles is not PMS; not all premenstrual changes may be PMS; and PMS may be more than one condition.[81]

Evaluating the patient for PMS first requires a monthly diary to establish a relationship between the symptoms and the luteal phase of the cycle. Also, the clinician should examine the patient and order biochemical tests to rule out other disorders that might account for the symptoms.[81][283] The clinician can best determine the woman's hormonal status by ordering tests for estrogen, progesterone, testosterone, FSH, LH, and DHEA levels. He should also order thyroid function tests, possibly including a TRH stimulation test and thyroid antibodies. Only ordering tests for FSH and estrogen levels, based on the assumption that only an estrogen deficiency can be of concern, will not provide sufficient information for accurate conclusions about a patient's condition. Progesterone levels must be included. As Lee wrote, "Since progesterone levels are rarely measured, most doctors are unaware that their menstruating patients may be progesterone deficient in progesterone. Adding estrogen and tranquilizers will not solve their problems."[102,p.112]

PERI-MENOPAUSE AND MENOPAUSE

The symptoms women report during peri-menopause and menopause are virtually the same as some women report during PMS and after childbirth: depression, sleep disturbance, irritability, anxiety, panic, memory and cognitive dysfunction, and a decreased sense of well-being.[278][282] Luax and Conrad wrote that the woman with PMS has a hormonal imbalance, and she is also likely to experience menopausal symptoms.[276,p.98] The conventional view is that an estrogen deficiency, due to loss of ovarian follicles, is the cause of the symptoms of peri-menopause and menopause.

The view that an estrogen deficiency is solely responsible for the symptoms of peri-menopause and menopause is, with an extremely high degree of probability, wrong. Progesterone, like the estrogens, normally helps regulate numerous peripheral and central nervous system functions (see section above titled "Progesterone Deficiency as a Factor in PMS"). Thus, it is predictable that a subnormal level or absence of progesterone will have adverse effects on the woman.

Of course, estrogen and progesterone production by the ovaries diminishes at intervals during peri-menopause and ceases after menopause. However, the adrenal glands and some peripheral tissues interact to provide a lower quantity of the hormones than the ovaries previously did. These small amounts, supplemented by estrogens from plant foods and natural progesterone applied through the skin, provide many women with enough of the sex hormones to keep them free from deficiency symptoms—provided, of course,

that they exercise regularly, eat a wholesome diet, and take nutritional supplements (see section below titled "Hormone Replacement Therapy"). However, for the woman with hypothyroidism or thyroid hormone resistance, estrogen and progesterone supplementation and the lifestyle practices I mentioned are likely to provide relief only under one condition—that she also takes a high enough dosage of the proper form of exogenous thyroid hormone (see next section, titled "Thyroid Hormone, Peri-menopause, and Menopause").

Thyroid Hormone, Peri-Menopause, and Menopause

The American Association of Clinical Endocrinologists announced in 1999 that an undiagnosed thyroid disorder may actually underlie symptoms (such as fatigue, forgetfulness, depression, and mood swings) thought to be caused by menopause.[235] Studies support this report. For example, Ballinger et al. measured hormone levels in 85 peri-menopausal women. All the women completed the General Health Questionnaire and 48 of them had standardized psychiatric interviews. Women who had clinical depression had significantly higher TSH levels and lower T_3 levels.[238]

Surgical Menopause and Traumatic Onset of Fibromyalgia. Waxman and Zatzkis wrote that the rapid hormone changes associated with menopause may initiate fibromyalgia. They speculated, however, that the physical and mental stress of gynecological surgery may also precipitate fibromyalgia.[77] This is a reasonable speculation in that fibromyalgia may develop following other stresses, such as falls, automobile accidents, emotionally traumatic experiences, and other types of surgery. (See Chapter 3.5, section titled "A Putative Etiological and Exacerbating Role for Increased Cortisol Levels.")

(Unfortunately, I must pause here to make a parenthetical statement. Waxman and Zatzkis, after their reasonable observation that I cited in the previous paragraph, go on to make a highly nonsensical conjecture. Their conjecture was based on the assumption that "Most investigators consider these patients [fibromyalgic women] to be highly anxious and variably depressed and to have personality abnormalities ranging from hysteria to hypochondriasis." They tried to explain fibromyalgic women's pain as "a somatized expression of the anxiety-depression state of these patients."[77,pp.166-167] It is unfortunate that the authors of this otherwise good report ended it with pseudo-scientific psychosilliness. I recommend their paper with the qualification that patients and clinician ignore the authors psychologizing and first read Chapter 1.2 of this book.)

I suspect that a variety of "changes" in the average woman's life may act as stressors that may precipitate fibromyalgia. As Anderderg et al. wrote, the "changes" include first menstrual period, one or more childbirths, middle age, and peri-menopausal time when estrogen and progesterone levels are decreasing.[333,pp.6-7] Menopause, whether spontaneously or surgically induced, is a major stimulus to the onset of fibromyalgia.[77] For some women, probably those in extremely poor physical condition and suffering from nutritional deficiencies, the hormonal changes during the peri-menstrual time of the month may be a sufficiently severe stressor to initiate fibromyalgia. These precipitators may initiate fibromyalgia in women predisposed by marginally sufficient metabolism. For many, the marginally sufficient metabolism is due to undertreated or undiagnosed and untreated hypothyroidism and/or thyroid hormone resistance.

HORMONE REPLACEMENT THERAPY

A need for hormone replacement therapy may be peculiar to the last 100 years. As Seligmann et al. wrote in 1992: "A century ago, few women lived very long after their ovaries stopped functioning. Today most women have another 30 years—almost one third of their lives—yet to live after the age of 50, and they are determined to make the best of them."[244,p.71] Samsioe added, "Women can nowadays expect to live one-third of their lives in a potential hormonal deficiency state."[328] Some females, to avoid the potential deficiency, will require hormone replacement therapy at the onset of menopause and some males may require replacement after the onset of andropause.

In 1991, Dhar and Murphy wrote of the numerous theories of the cause of PMS and the variety of available treatments, noting that these attest to our ignorance of the exact nature of PMS. The hypothalamic-pituitary-ovarian axis is obviously involved in PMS, but the exact mechanism of the symptoms remains elusive. They wrote: "Progestin in the presence of estrogen appears to be essential. Excess estrogen may aggravate the condition. The popular theory of progesterone deficiency has not been supported by double blind trials of progesterone in various forms versus placebo. Because of the important placebo effect in this condition, double blind trials are essential in the assessment of any form of treatment."[293] If Dhar and Murphy intended to imply that treatment with estrogen (as opposed to progesterone) has been

adequately tested, they erred.[277] In fact, no matter which school of thought the treating clinician belongs to, his belief about the cause is theoretical and his choice of treatment empirical.

Severino and Moline recently wrote that because of the uncertain source of the symptoms, treatment consists of the management of specific symptoms, preferably based on symptom ratings.[283] The same is true of similar symptoms experienced by women during the postpartum time, peri-menopause, and menopause. Treatment is empirical, and the aim should be to *safely* alleviate the suffering of the women. The qualification of "safely" means that the synthetic estrogens and progestins used as first line treatments by mainstream medical clinicians should be the last resort, used only when no other methods have proven effective. (See section above titled "Oral Contraceptives and Myofascial Pain," and the subsection titled "Potential Adverse Effects of Oral Contraceptives.")

My judgment is that the best approach is the holistic one that has recently become popular—exercise to tolerance, antistress techniques, psychological and spiritual methods consistent with one's value system, wholesome diet, nutritional supplementation, avoidance of environmental contaminants (especially xenoestrogens), and when needed, increased dietary phytoestrogens, transdermal natural progesterone, and the proper form and dosage of thyroid hormone.

My main intention in this chapter is to establish that inadequate thyroid hormone regulation of the HPG axis can potentially underlie the female health problems of fibromyalgic woman. However, inadequate thyroid hormone regulation of the axis is certainly not the only hormonal-based contribution to the health problems peculiar to female fibromyalgia patients. The estrogens, progesterone, and the androgens exert potent effects on the psychological and physical status of women, and these hormones are almost certain to interact with inadequate thyroid hormone regulation to cause female related health problems. As Lee wrote, "Though each hormone is unique, hormone balance involves a complex harmonious blend of all hormones. I tend to think of hormones as instruments in an orchestra—the harmony we seek is the proper contribution of all the instruments together not only in pitch but also in volume and rhythm. The same is true of sex hormones and thyroid hormone."[102,p.145]

Overall, my view of the interaction of thyroid hormone and the sex hormones concurs with Lee's, and I believe we should keep his view in mind when individualizing treatment strategies for patients. However, I want to emphasize that I do not believe that our therapeutic aim should be predetermined blood levels of the involved hormones. That our therapeutic target for all women would best be the hormone blood levels of some statistically "normal" woman is an unverified hypothesis. It is a hypothesis that is most likely false. Instead, our clinical aim should be satisfactory scores on measures indicating that we have safely attained normal tissue effects and have relieved the suffering of treated women. The protocol should be fashioned after that I describe in Chapter 5.2.

Phramaceutical vs Natural Sex Hormones

Lurie and Borenstein wrote that properly managing PMS symptoms requires education, reassurance, and drug therapy.[81] It is my belief that the education of women should be about the comparative adverse effects of pharmaceutical sex hormones. Reassurance should come from the advice that they can probably live a fairly symptom-free life by using natural sex hormones. For most women, pharmaceutical sex hormones can improve or relieve the symptoms associated with PMS, peri-menopause, and menopause. At the same time, though, pharmaceutical hormones are likely to cause other health problems—the effects of which range from mild annoyance to death. Usually, natural sex hormones, used in combination with other health-inducing practices, effectively relieve the symptoms of PMS, peri-menopause, and menopause. As a bonus, the use of natural hormones does not carry the risks associated with pharmaceutical alternatives.

Some medical writers recognize the adverse effects of progestins, although they may not distinguish between synthetic progestins and natural progesterone. Mortola wrote: "Substantial evidence indicates that the pathophysiology of PMS is dependent on cyclic progesterone changes which, after a time delay, influence central neurotransmitter systems and peripheral tissues. Because of the myriad of neurotransmitter changes induced by progesterone, the most comprehensive treatment of the complex array of symptoms in severe PMS may require pharmacologic agents *that reduce circulating progesterone levels* [italics mine]." He also recommends that PMS patients be treated with gonadotrophin-releasing hormone, estrogen, and progestins.[292]

Similarly, Tiemstra and Patel wrote that some clinicians recommend progesterone therapy but that their recommendations are based on anecdotal evidence. Tiemstra and Patel state that controlled studies have shown progesterone to be ineffective. They wrote, "Estrogen is clearly effective in relieving symptoms of PMS, *whereas progesterone is ineffective and might even worsen symptoms* [italics mine]." They wrote further, "Combination oral contraceptives are effective, undoubtedly as a result of the estrogen component. While little comparative data exist to guide choice of an oral contraceptive, maximizing the relative estrogenic potency of the oral contraceptive seems logical."[275]

Confusion often results from medical writers' use of some words, such as progestins and progesterone, as synonyms when in fact they are not. Passages such as those in the two preceding paragraphs can leave readers with the impression that progesterone has adverse effects when it is actually synthetic progestins that do. Indeed, progestins, such as Provera, appear to worsen the PMS, peri-menopausal, and menopausal symptoms of most women who use them. (See section titled "Oral Contraceptives and Myofascial Pain," and the subsection titled "Synthetic Progestins.") But adverse effects from progestins is not a good reason for women to avoid the use of natural progesterone. Natural progesterone is an orthomolecular substance (see Glossary) which has a chemical structure different from the structures of synthesized progestins.

Laux, a naturopathic physician, and Conrad, his coauthor, wrote: "It has been estimated that as many as one-half of all women on the Premarin/Provera regimen stop after a year, unable to tolerate the side effects. Two-thirds of all women stop the Provera (frequently without telling their doctors) and continue to take just Premarin, foregoing the more difficult side effects of Provera, which can mimic the worst of PMS symptoms, such as bloating, irritability, and depression."[276,pp.8-9] Cabot wrote that fewer than 50% of women who start the use of sex hormone replacement therapy continue for more than a few months, mainly because of the annoying adverse effects.[294,p.75] Nachtigall, a reproductive endocrinologist, noted that most women do not stay on hormone replacement therapy (conventional medications such as Premarin and Provera) longer than 9 months. Utian, a gynecologist, surmised, "That's probably because doctors don't explain the long-term benefits, and they don't make themselves available to answer women's questions and concerns."[244,p.81] I have witnessed first hand the severe adverse effects of synthetic progestins on my pain patients, and I have listened to patients' descriptions of the noxious effects of Provera in particular. Based on these experiences, I doubt that doctors explaining the presumed long-term benefits of pharmaceutic sex hormones, particularly progestins, is likely to dissolve resistance of most women to tolerating the noxious effects of the drugs.

Sex hormone replacement therapy for PMS, peri-menopause, and menopause symptoms is similar. Natural estrogen, derived from many plant foods,[276][294] and progesterone synthesized from wild yam and soy are now available for treatment.[102][276] These plant-derived hormones are identical to those in the human body. Because the hormones are identical to those synthesized in the body, they are rapidly-metabolized, exert gentler effects, and are free from adverse effects.[276,pp.39-40]

Progesterone Replacement Therapy

A cadre of clinicians today promotes the use of natural progesterone for preventing or treating PMS, peri-menopause, and menopause. This cadre and its followers face an uphill battle against the entrenched forces chanting "estrogen deficiency, estrogen deficiency!" Lee wrote, "Given the complexity and heterorgenicity (i.e., multiple factors) of cause and effect in the intricate arrangement of stress, diet, hypothalamic and pituitary function, and normal hormones, the prevailing attitude that female health concerns are merely a matter of 'estrogen deficiency' is flawed, oversimplified, and ultimately dangerous."[102,pp.112-113] So convinced are most conventional clinicians that an estrogen deficiency is practically the only potential problem with female health problems that few ever measure progesterone levels. As a result, as Lee also wrote, they are unaware that many of their menstruating patients are progesterone deficient.[102,pp.112-113] Studies I review above (see section titled "Luteinization") show that inadequate thyroid hormone regulation of the ovaries can result in failed ovulation and an array of conditions such as PMS and luteal phase defect. When ovulation does not occur, a corpus luteum does not form, and the woman is therefore progesterone deficient during the luteal phase of the menstrual cycle. Such research findings support those who argue that progesterone deficiency is a major contribution to female sex-related health problems.

Lee is probably the most vocal of the progesterone replacement advocates. He wrote that the fundamental problem underlying menopausal symptoms is estrogen dominance (estrogen unopposed or not balanced by progesterone) due to a progesterone deficiency.[102,p.128]

Laux and Conrad wrote that synthetic progestins are more potent than natural progesterone and are more likely to inhibit endogenous progesterone production. Natural progesterone is less likely to suppress endogenous progesterone production.[276,p.98] This is an important consideration because progestins do not

have exactly the same effect on the body as do natural progesterone. On principle, in replacement therapy, a duplication of the effects of natural progesterone seems most desirable. Also, exogenous progesterone would best *supplement* endogenous progesterone rather than *suppress* its production, as progestins are likely to do.

For details of treatment using natural progesterone, I recommend *What Your Doctor May Not Tell You About Menopause* (Warner Books, New York, 1996) by John R. Lee, and *Natural Woman, Natural Menopause* (Harper Perennial, New York, 1998) written by Marcus Laux and Christine Conrad.[276]

Estrogen Replacement Therapy

Estrogen replacement therapy may be necessary to maintain physiological balance in some women who have not reached menopause. Estrogen replacement may be necessary to relieve estrogen deficiency and to preserve secondary sex characteristics (such as breast size), the turgor and lubricating capacity of the vagina and vulva, to prevent coronary artery disease, and maintain a sense of well-being.[74,p.277]

Some women will comply with the conventional clinician's prompting to begin estrogen replacement therapy with synthetic pharmaceutical preparations. These women would be wise to assess the risks, such as endometrial and breast cancer, against the likely advantages, such as slowing of bone loss and prevention of osteoporosis.[328] The clinician should forthrightly discuss these matters with the woman so that she can make a choice regarding therapy that is consistent with her personal values.[74,p.285]

Sonkin wrote that menopause and thyroid deficiency are the endocrine disorders most commonly associated with myofascial pain and trigger points.[1,pp.55&58] During menopause, most women also have flushes, sweats, anxiety, weakness, fatigue, depression, impaired ability to cope, loss of creativity and libido. On the other hand, he wrote, the only symptoms of estrogen deficiency may be muscle or joint pains. Regardless, he continued, the symptoms rapidly improve with adequate estrogen replacement. Some pain, however, may result from associated postural changes due to microfractures or collapse of osteoporotic vertebrae.[1,p.55]

According to Lee, progesterone supplementation alone improves most menopausal symptoms. He qualified, however, that if progesterone does not improve the symptoms, the woman may require low-dose estrogen supplementation for several years. Afterward, she can gradually withdraw from the estrogen supplementation without the symptoms recurring.[102,p.82] As Laux and Conrad and Cabot explained, however, natural estrogens are more effective and safer.[276,p.68][294,pp.93-94]

For many women, adopting a diet that provides enough phytoestrogens can relieve or prevent estrogen deficiency symptoms. However, for many women, the situation is not that simple. Estrogen secretion by the ovaries decreases during peri-menopause, as the number of follicles decreases, and during menopause, after the ovaries no longer secrete estrogen. However, for a variety of reasons, many women may be estrogen dominant rather than deficient. For example, the women may consume a high concentration of fatty foods that contain lipophilic PCBs, dioxins, and furans. Many of these man-made contaminants are estrogenic—that is, they bind to estrogen receptors in tissues and either stimulate or inhibit estrogenic effects. Whether they stimulate or inhibit estrogenic effects, they block endogenous estrogen from exerting its ordinary effects. (See section above titled "Effects of Xenoestrogens.") In addition, inadequate thyroid hormone regulation of liver function may cause abnormally slow clearance of estrogen from the body, resulting in elevated circulating estrogen levels[78,p.905] (see subsection above titled "Estrogen Dominance").

For those considering the use of estrogen replacement therapy rather than progesterone replacement, I recommend *Smart Medicine for Menopause* (published by Avery Publishing Group, Garden City Park, 1995) written by Sandra Cabot. While she advocates estrogen replacement therapy, she prefers the use of natural estrogens such as those derived from plant foods.

Often, clinicians prescribe estrogen therapy without ordering laboratory tests, or the correct tests, to learn a woman's hormonal status. Hormonal status can best be determined by ordering an estrogen panel, progesterone, testosterone, FSH, LH, DHEA, and thyroid hormone function tests, possibly including a TRH stimulation test. Testing may show that a woman is already estrogen dominant, providing an explanation for her fluid retention, depression, headaches, and urinary tract infections. Adding additional estrogen can worsen such adverse effects from a dominance of the hormone. Laux and Conrad quote Hanley, a family physician, who sees women patients who have reacted badly to prescribed estrogen. The estrogen complicates the symptoms of the women who are estrogen dominant before beginning use of the prescribed estrogen. She improves the patients' status by switching them to natural progesterone. The progesterone can be converted to estrogen, if an estrogen deficiency exists. Laux

and Conrad, wrote that for the peri-menopausal woman, natural progesterone can therefore be the best first line of treatment.[276,p.116]

Thyroid Hormone Therapy

For fibromyalgia patients with symptoms related to female sex hormonal changes and the menstrual cycle, the use of progesterone and/or estrogen usually is not enough to provide relief. As Waxman and Zatakis wrote of female fibromyalgia patients, "Restoration of a premenopausal state with cyclic estrogen and progesterone therapy aids in patient management. Improvement regularly occurs in this setting, but cures are nonexistent: a state of chronic pain that is partially controlled is the usual outcome."[77,p.171] Usually, more comprehensive metabolic rehabilitation, including the use of thyroid hormone, is necessary (see Chapter 5.2). The strategic use of estrogen and progesterone, calculated on an individual basis, should be a part of most female patients' individualized metabolic rehabilitation regimen.

Sonkin reported that women may improve only slowly when they have fibromyalgia and/or myofascial pain syndrome and require both estrogen and thyroid hormone therapy. Raising their metabolic rate may relieve their muscle symptoms only after months or even a year has passed.[88,p.165] In my experience, such slow responsiveness occurs only when the thyroid hormone used during treatment has been T_4. When patients use a T_4/T_3 combination or T_3 alone, improvement or recovery occurs much more quickly.

● FACTORS POSSIBLY RESPONSIBLE FOR THE HIGHER INCIDENCE OF FIBROMYALGIA AMONG FEMALES

In general, men exposed to the same precipitators do not develop fibromyalgia. Why?

LOWER METABOLIC RATE OF WOMEN: A PREDISPOSING FACTOR FOR THE DEVELOPMENT OF FIBROMYALGIA

On average, the metabolic rates of women and their 24-hour energy expenditure are lower than those of men.[241] A woman's metabolic rate is even lower when she has inadequate thyroid hormone regulation of cell function due to hypothyroidism or resistance to thyroid hormone. When her metabolic rate declines below a critical threshold, she will develop symptoms and signs of hypometabolism. The particular symptoms and signs that develop will depend on the tissue most affected by the hypometabolism.

The lower metabolic rate of women is caused partly by lower androgen activity in their bodies. Administering male sex hormone increases the metabolic rate by 10%-to-15%. In contrast, administering female sex hormone raises the metabolic rate only a small and insignificant amount.[78,p.795]

Role of Gender Differences in Women's Lower Metabolic Rate

Whether or not gender differences account for the lower metabolic rates of women is controversial. Sanborn and Jankowski reported that the difference in resting metabolic rate of women and men is not due to gender. They note that women have a larger surface area to mass ratio, which may be advantageous in dry heat. Compared to men, they generally have more body fat and less lean muscle mass. They concluded that because fat is less metabolically active than muscle, the higher fat content of women accounts for their lower resting metabolic rate. In summary, they wrote, "The lower resting metabolic rate is not related to gender *per se*."[28]

However, Arciero et al. found evidence of a gender difference in resting metabolic rate. The difference in metabolic rate was independent of the difference in the muscle mass of men and women. The researchers controlled for differences due to body composition (muscle and fat mass) and aerobic fitness. They tested 328 men aged from 17-to-80 years, and 194 women aged 18-to-81 years. The mean resting metabolic rate of men was 23% higher than that of women. The investigators used multiple regression analysis to analyze their data. The outcome indicated that 84% of individual variation in the resting metabolic rate resulted from fat-free (muscle, bone, connective tissue) mass, fat mass, peak VO_2 max, and gender. When they controlled for fat-free mass, fat mass, and peak VO_2, women still had a 3% lower resting metabolic rate. The mean adjusted resting metabolic rate for women was 1,563 kcal/day, and for men it was 1,613 kcal/day. The adjusted resting metabolic rate of premenopausal and postmenopausal women was also lower than men of roughly the same age.[29]

Greater Predisposition of Women to Develop Syndromes of Hypometabolism

Whatever the mechanism(s) of women's lower metabolic rates, most women do have lower metabolic rates than men. It is highly probable that women's lower metabolic rates predispose them to develop syndromes of hypometabolism. Fibromyalgia is one of those syndromes.

The major hypothesis I present in this book is that fibromyalgia is a condition of hypometabolism. Inadequate thyroid hormone regulation of cell function is not essential to the hypothesis. Instead, the proposal that inadequate thyroid hormone regulation of cell function is a corollary hypothesis—it explains one underlying mechanism of fibromyalgia as a condition of hypometabolism. The hypometabolism hypothesis of fibromyalgia posits this: Anything that impedes metabolism enough in tissues peculiar to the fibromyalgia clinical phenotype can be the sole underlying factor or a contribution to fibromyalgia in some cases. The lower metabolic rate of women, due to the predominant influence of female over male sex hormones in them, appears to serve as a predisposing factor. It renders women more susceptible to fibromyalgia. They are thus more likely to develop fibromyalgia when one or more other metabolism-impeding factors, such as mild hypothyroidism or thyroid hormone resistance, impinges on them. Similarly, they are more likely to develop fibromyalgia symptoms and signs in response to other metabolism-impeding factors, such as physical deconditioning, the use of β-adrenergic blocking medications, or exposure to acetylcholinesterase inhibitors (see Glossary).

Hypothyroidism and the Female

Hypothyroidism affects the reproductive system in women more than in men,[212,p.1195] and women are far more susceptible to developing hypothyroidism than are men. Cooper wrote that about 5% of the population has the mildest form of hypothyroidism, subclinical hypothyroidism, manifested only by an elevated TSH.[20,p.246][21][22] With advancing age, the incidence of subclinical hypothyroidism increases. Rosenthal et al. reported that among seemingly healthy, elderly individuals, 13.2% had subclinical hypothyroidism. However, women are far more susceptible to hypothyroidism. They are almost twice as likely to have elevated TSH levels than men of the same age,[19][20,p.246][21][22] and hypothyroidism occurs 4-to-7 times as often in women as in men.[207,p.553] The prevalence of hypothyroidism in women over age 60 approaches 15%.[21][22]

The increased incidence of hypothyroidism (and probably thyroid hormone resistance) among women as they age, and the usual onset of fibromyalgia during the middle years, suggests a possible relationship. Felson wrote that the age of onset of fibromyalgia among patients varies from 12-to-45 years, but the mean age of onset for most patients is 40-to-55 years. He wrote that few patients develop the condition after age 60.[18,p.8] Similarly, Guler et al. reported that fibromyalgia is common between the ages of 30 and 60 years.[79] If a woman's HPG axis becomes inadequately regulated by thyroid hormone when peri-menopause is occurring, her reactions to peri-menopausal changes in hormone levels might be exaggerated. Moreover, if the metabolism of her fibromyalgia related tissues is only marginally sufficient, the hormonal changes associated with PMS, peri-menopause, and menopause may constitute stresses that result in even slower metabolism with the generation of symptoms of hypometabolism (see subsection above titled "Surgical Menopause and Traumatic Onset of Fibromyalgia," and Chapter 3.5, section titled "A Putative Etiological and Exacerbating Role for Increased Cortisol Levels").

Women may be more responsive to subtle decreases in thyroid hormone regulation of cell function. In turn, they may be more responsive than men to increased thyroid hormone exposure. Prange et al. found that T_3 treatment for depression was more effective for women.[223] They conjectured that women may be more responsive than men to thyroid hormone.[220]

Estrogen

Estrogen has some anti-thyroid effects. Because of this, if a woman is estrogen dominant, she may develop symptoms typical of hypothyroidism.

Increased Estrogen Levels May Lower Circulating Thyroid Hormone Levels and Inhibit T_4 to T_3 Conversion. Bennett suggested that estrogens account in some way for the higher incidence of fibromyalgia in women.[3,pp.145-146] There are a number of possibilities.

Normally, women have a stronger TSH reaction than men when injected with TRH[4] (see Chapter 4.2, section titled "TRH-Stimulation Test"). The TSH response to injected TRH is greater during the follicular phase of the menstrual cycle, just before ovulation, when estrogen secretion is highest (see Figure 3.6.2). The TSH response to TRH is lower during the luteal phase when the progesterone level is highest and the estrogen level is considerably lower. In women taking estrogen-containing oral contraceptives, the TSH response to injected TRH is greater than in women not taking the contraceptives.[5] These TRH stimulation test results suggest that elevated levels of estrogen suppress circulating thyroid hormone levels. This is suggested because the lower the circulating thyroid

hormone levels are, the more responsive is the anterior pituitary gland to TRH.

In addition, however, estrogen may inhibit the conversion of T_4 to T_3. This is indicated by increased levels of reverse-T_3 in the serum of oral contraceptive users.[5][6]

It appears from these two sets of findings that elevated estrogen levels decrease thyroid hormone levels. If so, elevated estrogen levels may also lower the metabolic rate of women. Thus, we might predict that women with chronically higher estrogen levels are more susceptible to fibromyalgia. Also, we might expect fibromyalgic women to have worse symptoms when estrogen levels are highest during the menstrual cycle.

I do not believe, however, that predicting the fibromyalgic woman's status during the menstrual cycle is this simple. If inadequate thyroid hormone regulation of cell function is the underlying cause of a woman's fibromyalgia, and if inadequate thyroid hormone regulation of the HPG axis underlies her sex-related abnormalities, estrogen may be only one sex hormone the levels of which adversely affect her fibromyalgia status. For example, if the inadequate thyroid hormone regulation of the axis results in failed luteinization, the corpus luteum may not develop, may degenerate, and as a result, fail to secrete normal amounts of progesterone during the luteal phase of the cycle. Normally, during the luteal phase, progesterone increases metabolism enough to elevate body temperature by 0.5° F, beginning abruptly at the time of ovulation.[78,p.913][228,p.607] The temperature increase in the luteal phase is consistent with luteal phase increases in basal metabolic rate,[261] oxygen consumption,[263] and protein catabolism.[264] At the end of the luteal phase, when estrogen and progesterone levels precipitously decrease, the basal metabolic rate decreases and remains low throughout menstruation. It is noteworthy that in the follicular phase, when estrogen levels rise considerably but progesterone levels remain low, the basal metabolic rate is low, and it reaches its lowest level just before ovulation. In women who suffer from subnormal metabolism (fibromyalgia) due to inadequate thyroid hormone regulation of cell function, one might expect their fibromyalgia status to improve in the early and mid-luteal phase when progesterone levels accelerate metabolism. But inadequate thyroid hormone regulation of the HPG axis is likely to deprive the women of the progesterone-induced increase in metabolism by causing failed luteinization. Besides depriving them of this normal time of increased metabolism, it might also cause excessive menstrual bleeding due to failure to ovulate, infertility, or habitual abortions. From inadequate thyroid hormone regulation, women are likely not only to have a normal follicular phase slowing of metabolism (due to suppression of thyroid hormone by estrogen), but they are also likely to fail to experience the normal luteal phase increase of metabolism due to a progesterone deficiency.

A potential outcome of the absence of the luteal phase increase in metabolism is a lack of psychological and physiological preparation for the precipitous drop of estrogen and progesterone levels just before the beginning of menstruation. An absence of the normal increase in metabolism during the luteal phase may leave the woman highly vulnerable to adverse effects from the low metabolic rate,[261] low oxygen consumption,[263] low protein catabolism, and the low carbohydrate use (decreased carbohydrate tolerance) during menstruation.[264]

The thyroid hormone-lowering effect of the estrogen may not be obvious to all clinicians from laboratory thyroid function testing. In fact, because the woman's total T_4 may be elevated, some clinicians may assume that she is on the high end of circulating thyroid hormone levels and is therefore somewhat hypermetabolic. But a patient may have a high-normal T_4 level because her elevated estrogen level is increasing the circulating level of the main protein that transports thyroid hormone, thyroxine binding globulin. In most women, the use of exogenous estrogen (as in oral contraceptives) elevates the circulating level of thyroxine-binding globulin (see Chapter 4.2, section titled "Estrogens," and Table 4.2.5). Elevated estrogen levels during pregnancy have the same effect.[71] The body adapts to the higher level of the transport protein. The T_3 and T_4 bound to the protein reach new, higher steady-state concentrations, but the free T_3 and free T_4—which are most readily available to stimulate metabolism—remain at normal levels, except for brief alterations in the free T_4 level.[72,p.830] Thus, while thyroid hormone levels may be depressed by elevated estrogen levels, an increased level of thyroxine binding globulin may result in a high-normal T_4 level that is not associated with an increase in metabolism.[73] Of interest, in contrast to exogenous estrogen, some synthetic progestins, such as norethindrone, reduce serum thyroxine-binding globulin levels and T_4 levels.[75]

Indications of Estrogen Inhibition of Thyroid Function During the Follicular Phase. In normal women, several measures indicate that metabolism accelerates during the luteal phase of the menstrual cycle. The metabolic acceleration is commonly ascribed to

elevated progesterone levels. That progesterone takes part in increasing metabolism during the luteal phase is suggested by studies such as that by Bisdee et al. They found that the increased metabolic rate of women during sleep in the luteal phase did not correlate with various hormone measures including thyroid hormone. However, the metabolic rate during sleep was inversely related to the falling ratio of urinary metabolites of estrogen to progesterone (estrone-3-glucuronide and pregnanediol-3α-glucuronide)—that is, as the ratio of estrogen to progesterone decreased, the metabolic rate increased.[265] However, some studies suggest that thyroid hormone contributes to the metabolic speed up.

For example, Lariviere et al. found that in 8 healthy women, oxidative metabolism of the amino acid leucine was higher during the luteal phase of the cycle than in the follicular phase. Resting energy expenditure was also higher in the luteal phase. They also found that during the luteal phase, the plasma free T_3 and ratio of T_3 to reverse-T_3 were significantly higher. The researchers noted that the concomitant increase in leucine metabolism and circulating free T_3 raises the possibility of a causal relation: reduced protein metabolism and thyroid hormone levels during the follicular phase, and increased protein metabolism and thyroid hormone levels during the luteal phase of the cycle.[262]

Conversely, in the section above titled "Inadequate Thyroid Hormone Regulation in PMS," I described several studies in which PMS was associated with laboratory evidence of low thyroid hormone function. The metabolic slow down during the follicular phase may be the result of thyroid system suppression due to elevated estrogen levels.

Solomon et al. measured the basal metabolic rates of 6 healthy young women during the menstrual cycle. Throughout the cycle, their metabolic rates varied significantly. The basal metabolic rate decreased at menstruation. The rate reached its lowest level about 1 week before ovulation, the time during which estrogen is at its highest during the cycle. After ovulation, the metabolic rate increased until menstruation began again.[261]

Das and Jana measured the basal total body oxygen consumption, another measure of metabolic rate, of 32 women between 17 and 28 years old. The measures were done during menstruation, during the rest of the follicular phase, and during the luteal phase. Oxygen consumption was almost identical during menstruation and the rest of the follicular phase, but it was significantly higher during the luteal phase. Das and

Jana wrote that the rise of oxygen consumption was a post-ovulatory phenomenon mediated by hormones, mainly progesterone[263] and thyroid hormone.

In 8 women who maintained a constant diet through a menstrual cycle, creatinine and nitrogen excretion in the urine was higher in the luteal phase. This suggests higher protein catabolism during the luteal phase. Also, carbohydrate use was less in the early follicular phase, suggesting that the low estrogen levels decreased carbohydrate tolerance.[264] However, reduced thyroid hormone regulation of cell function could also contribute to reduced carbohydrate use during the follicular phase. (See Chapter 3.1, section titled "Thyroid Status and the Sympathetic-Catecholamine-Adrenoceptor Axis," and Chapter 3.4, subsection titled "Impaired Aerobic and Anaerobic Metabolism in Fibromyalgia: Possible Effect of Increased α- and Decreased β-Adrenergic Receptors.")

Androgens

Females produce less androgenic steroids than males do.[7] As a result, women generate less myofibrillar and sarcoplasmic protein.[8][9] For instance, studies show that the cross-sectional areas of the paraspinal muscles of men are larger than those of women, indicating greater muscle bulk in relation to body weight in men.[26,p.393] A lower protein content and less bulk may make women's muscles more susceptible to microtrauma, leading to myofascial tenderness. (See subsection above titled "Actions of Androgens.")

The ovaries secrete testosterone, and normal amounts of this androgen are necessary for many body functions, both peripherally and in the central nervous system. (See section above titled "Reduced Sex Drive.") Normally lower production in women may make them more susceptible to pernicious effects from the testosterone-lowering impact of hypothyroidism and/or thyroid hormone resistance.

● INADEQUATE THYROID HORMONE REGULATION OF THE MALE HYPOTHALAMIC-PITUITARY-GONADAL AXIS

EFFECTS OF HYPOTHYROIDISM ON MALE SEX FUNCTION

The low libido, reduced sexual activity, and impotence reported by some men with chronic fatigue syndrome[349,pp.59,137,203] may be a result of inadequate thyroid hormone regulation of the HPG axis. Some medical writers such as Lateiwish et al. have listed subnormal libido as a feature of hypothyroidism.[161] Velazquez et al. reported that despite normal basal free testosterone levels, 70% of hyperthyroid men and 60% of hypothyroid men complained of decreased libido.[166] Johnson et al. noted that hypothyroidism has been cited as a cause of infertility, abnormal semen quality, and low libido in humans and other animals.[191] Wortsman et al. wrote that hypothyroid men may be infertile and impotent.[195]

Baskin evaluated 600 impotent men for androgen deficiency, high prolactin levels, and thyroid hormone deficiency. Of the 600, 192 (32%) had hormonal abnormalities. Of the 192 men with hormonal abnormalities, 12 (6%) had unsuspected hypothyroidism. Baskin considered hypothyroidism common among the impotent men, and he wrote that thyroid hormone therapy relieved the hypothyroid men's impotence.[194]

EFFECTS OF HYPOTHYROIDISM ON MALE SEX HORMONES

A deficiency or excess of thyroid hormone may adversely affect sex-related function of men. A lack of thyroid hormone in men may cause a complete lack of libido, while excessive amounts of thyroid hormone may cause impotence.[78,p.836] If a man's thyroid hormone deficiency causes a severe enough testosterone deficiency, he may also become impotent.

Wortsman et al. concluded from their studies that abnormalities of gonadal function are common in men with primary hypothyroidism.[195] Velazquez et al. studied the effects of thyroid dysfunction on the pituitary-gonadal axis in 10 men with Graves' disease and 5 with hypothyroidism. The findings in men who were hyperthyroid due to Graves' disease were the following: (1) normal serum free-testosterone levels, (2) reduced testosterone response to hCG stimulation, and (3) an exaggerated response of LH to GnRH. When treatment provided normal free T_4 levels, these abnormal values became normal. The findings in hypothyroid men were as follows: (1) normal testosterone response to hCG, (2) reduced LH response to GnRH, and (3) a positive correlation between the free T_4 level and the LH response to GnRH—the lower the free T_4 level, the lower the LH response to GnRH. These abnormalities in hypothyroid men improved with T_4 treatment. The researchers concluded that hypothyroid men have a defective LH response to GnRH.[166] The reader should recall that LH stimulates the Leydig cells to produce testosterone, and subnormal LH stimulation of the Leydig cells is likely to result in subnormal testosterone production. In one study, fibromyalgia patients had subnormal pituitary LH secretion in response to injected GnRH. The patients also had low T_3 levels.[331] This pattern of values is close to that of the hypothyroid men in the study by Wortsman et al.[195]

In another study, Wortsman et al. studied two groups of men. One group had "hypergonadotropic hypogonadism." In this condition, men have subnormal structure and/or function of the gonads (measured as low testosterone levels) due to a primary problem with the gonads. The blood and urine have increased levels of the pituitary gonadotropins, FSH and LH. I will refer to this condition as "primary hypogonadism." The other group of men had "hypogonadotropic hypogonadism." These patients have subnormal gonadal development and/or function (low testosterone levels) that results from deficient secretion of FSH and LH. I will refer to this condition as "secondary hypogonadism." Low testosterone levels suggest hypogonadism. High levels of FSH and LH accompanying low testosterone levels suggest primary subnormal gonadal function—the testicles have a primary dysfunction that does not permit them to respond with increased testosterone secretion even when exposed to high levels of FSH and LH. On the other hand, low levels of FSH and LH suggest secondary subnormal gonad function—the testicles are secreting too little testosterone because of deficient exposure to FSH and LH. Wortsman et al. found that of 19 men with primary hypogonadism, 9 (47%) had thyroid disease: benign and malignant thyroid gland tumors, hypothyroidism due to Hashimoto's thyroiditis, or hypothyroidism due to amiodarone therapy. Among patients with secondary hypogonadism, only 1 had thyroid disease: hypothyroidism due to Hashimoto's thyroiditis. Patients with primary hypogonadism were significantly older (mean age: 51±4 years) than those with secondary hypogonadism (mean age: 37±4 years). Also, patients with thyroid diseases were significantly older (mean age: 60±6 years) than those without (mean age: 43±6 years). The researchers advised clinicians to evaluate thyroid gland structure and function of older patients with hypogonadism, especially those who have had long-sustained elevations of FSH and LH.[192]

In another study, 9 of 15 boys (60%) who had severe long-standing primary hypothyroidism also had enlarged testicles. All 15 boys had elevated TSH levels. But only boys with enlarged testicles had high serum prolactin and gonadotropin levels. The boys had blunted responses to GnRH, differing in this respect from children with true precocious puberty. Despite their elevated LH levels, their serum testosterone levels were in the range typical of prepubertal boys. Their testosterone levels, which were lower than pubertal boys, accounted for the absence of secondary sex characteristics (such as facial and pubic hair) normally induced by testosterone. The boys' prolactin levels decreased and their testosterone levels increased when they used bromocriptine. (Bromocriptine is an ergot derivative that inhibits prolactin secretion and release of prolactin in response to TRH. Clinicians use bromocriptine to inhibit the growth of tumors that secrete prolactin, thus lowering the circulating prolactin level.) The positive response to bromocriptine suggests that the boys' elevated prolactin levels were inhibiting the action of LH on the Leydig cells of the testicles. The researchers concluded that the boys' testicular enlargement resulted from continuous FSH stimulation. Therefore, they contended that unless the boys' HPG axes are at the pubertal stage, the term "true precocious puberty" is not proper in boys with hypothyroidism and testicular enlargement.[193]

Mann et al. used mouse Leydig tumor cells to assess the effectiveness of T_3 in stimulating sex hormone synthesis. T_3 induced a 3.6-fold increase in the gene expression of the mRNA for steroidogenic acute regulatory protein. This protein helps regulate the production of steroid hormones. T_3 also induced an acute 4.0-fold increase in steroid hormone production, probably mediated by the increase in production of the acute regulatory protein. T_3 also significantly increased testosterone production. Mann et al. concluded that thyroid hormone induced a regulatory cascade that results in testosterone production in Leydig cells.[153]

Inducing hypothyroidism in male rats increased the time before they inserted their penises in female rats and reduced the rate of ejaculation. These behavioral changes occurred although the rats' testosterone levels were still normal. The behaviors became normal again when the researchers gave the rats thyroid hormone.[320] In another study, hypothyroid male rats had blunted pituitary LH secretion to GnRH stimulation.[321]

Not all studies have confirmed a relation between hypothyroidism and sex function. Johnson et al., for example, studied the effects of hypothyroidism on the reproductive function of dogs. Dogs that received ^{131}I became hypothyroid. Afterward, the dogs' serum levels of thyroid hormones were consistently below the lower limit of normal. However, the researchers found no difference between the reproductive function of hypothyroid and euthyroid dogs.[191]

ANDROPAUSE

The testicles continue to function fairly normally into old age, but in some older men, due to disease and lifestyle, testicular function declines.[2] In contrast to the female menopause, the male andropause has a slower onset. Gradually, however, production of testosterone by the Leydig cells of the testicles may decrease enough so that symptoms and signs of testosterone deficiency develop. Potential symptoms include fatigue; weakness; reduced libido, difficulty reaching orgasm, and impotence; depression; apathy; and a loss of drive, self-confidence, and competitiveness. The muscles, testicles, and penis may atrophy, and the testicles may soften. The rate of facial and body hair growth usually decreases, and the man may need to shave less often.[1,p.55][294,p.168]

In the adult male, manifestations of decreased testosterone secretion are difficult to distinguish during a clinical examination. Loss of libido and impotence are not specific to diminished testosterone secretion and occur most often in men whose Leydig cells function normally. The clinician may be able to determine that the symptoms are due to male hypogonadism based on two phenomena. One is signs of testosterone deficiency: softening of the testis, a decreased need to shave, and early soft wrinkling of the face. The other is a low serum testosterone level (normal = 0.3-to-1.0 μg/dL). However, impotence and loss of libido do not correlate with testosterone levels > 0.3 μg/dL.[104,p.2074]

During andropause, men have an increased ratio of estradiol to testosterone. The increased ratio of estradiol to testosterone increases insulin resistance.[115] The resistance may render some men more susceptible to energy deficient muscle contractures and resulting treatment resistant myofascial pain.[1,p.55]

A testosterone deficiency favors the development of coronary atherosclerosis. Testosterone is a functional regulator of the vascular tonus. Infusing testosterone into canine coronary arteries dilates the main and the small vessels. The vasodilation appears to result in part through induction of nitric oxide synthetase and activation of ATP-dependent potassium channels. Considerable data suggest that normalizing testosterone levels corrects the abnormalities associated with low androgen levels.[115]

TREATMENT

If the male patient has undergone andropause, perhaps much earlier than for other men, his androgen deficiency must be corrected. Laboratory tests may reveal low testosterone and/or DHEA levels. It is possible that the man's testosterone levels will be normal. If the patient does not have a deficiency of testosterone, the clinician should consider whether his tissues are partially resistant to the hormone. Also, a GnRH stimulation test may show that his pituitary gland has a blunted LH response to the GnRH.

Cabot recommends that males experiencing symptoms of andropause use nutritional medicine, lifestyle changes, and possibly hormone replacement therapy.[294,p.168]

If it is effective, the patients should use dehydroepiandrosterone (DHEA) rather than synthetic androgens. Synthetic androgens have serious potential adverse effects, such as prostatic hypertrophy and liver cancer.[23][350][351][352] DHEA is a natural alternative to synthetic testosterone medications. It may effectively increase testosterone levels. DHEA use is likely to be safe when the patient uses the lowest effective daily dosage. Several books are available that describe recommended dosage amounts and schedules. In the body, DHEA is enzymatically converted to androstenedione and androstenediol, and each of these androgens is then converted to testosterone.[228,p.580]

The clinician should advise the man that until androgen replacement therapy takes effect, it may be best to avoid or minimize the use of alcohol because of its testosterone lowering effect. This caution is important with many males because of their tendency to increase their alcohol consumption as a method of assuaging their troubling preoccupations, anxieties, and apprehensions.

If androgen replacement therapy does not improve the patient's status, despite his also exercising to tolerance, eating a wholesome diet, and taking nutritional supplements, the clinician should consider whether the patient has hypothyroidism and/or thyroid hormone resistance. Hypothyroidism or thyroid hormone resistance is a likely underlying condition if the patient meets the criteria for fibromyalgia. In this case, the patient should undergo metabolic rehabilitation involving the use of thyroid hormone, and androgen replacement therapy may need to be included for a successful outcome.

REFERENCES

1. Sonkin, L.S.: Myofascial pain due to metabolic disorders: diagnosis and treatment. In *Myofascial Pain and Fibromyalgia: Trigger Point Management*. Edited by E.S. Rachlin, St. Louis, Mosby, 1994, pp.45-60.
2. Longcope, C.: The effects of age on secretion and concentration of gonadal hormones. In *Atherogenesis and Aging*. Edited by S.R. Bates and Gangloff, E.C., New York, Springer-Vrelag, 1987, p.198.
3. Bennett, R.M.: Muscle physiology and cold reactivity in the fibromyalgia syndrome. *Rheu. Dis. Clin. N. Amer.*, 15: 135-147, 1989.
4. Noel, G.L., Dimond, R.C., Wartofsky, L., Earl, J.M., and Frantz, A.G.: Studies of prolactin and TSH secretion by continuous infusion of small amounts of thyrotropin-releasing hormone. *J. Clin. Endocrinol. Metab.*, 39:6, 1974.
5. Ramey, J.N., Burrow, G.N., Polackwich, R.J., and Donabedian, R.K.: The effect of oral contraceptive steroids on the response of thyroid-stimulating hormone to thyrotropin-releasing hormone. *J. Clin. Endocrinol. Metab.*, 40: 712, 1975.
6. Pansini, F., Bassi, P., and Cavallini, A.R.: Effect of the hormonal contraception on serum reverse triiodothyronine levels. *Gynecol. Obstet. Invest.*, 23:133, 1987.
7. Nicoloff, J.T., Fisher, D.A., and Appleman, M.D.: The role of glucocorticoids in the regulation of thyroid function in man. *J. Clin. Invest.*, 49:1922, 1970.
8. Iranmanish, A., Lizarralde, G., Johnson, M.L., and Veldhuis, J.D.: Dynamics of 24-hour endogenous cortisol secretion and clearance in primary hypothyroidism assessed before and after partial thyroid hormone replacement. *J. Clin. Endocrinol. Metab.*, 70:155, 1990.
9. Peterson, R.E.: The influence of the thyroid on adrenal cortical function. *J. Clin. Invest.*, 37:736, 1958.
10. Lowe, J.C.: A case of debilitating headache complicated by hypothyroidism: its relief through myofascial therapy. *Dig. Chir. Econ.*, 31:73-75, 1988.
11. Lowe, J. C.: How—and how not—to use combination therapy. *Dyn. Chir.*, April 11, 1990, pp.10-11.
12. Raspe, H. and Baumgartner, C.: The epidemiology of fibromyalgia syndrome (fibromyalgia) in a German town. (Myopain '92, Copenhagen, Denmark, August 17-20, 1992), *Scand. J. Rheumat.*, 94(Suppl.):8, 1992.
13. Prescott, E., Jacobsen, S., Kjoller, M., Bulow, P., Danneskiold-Samsöe, B., and Kamper-Jorgensen, F.: Prevalence of fibromyalgia in the adult Danish population. (Myopain '92, Copenhagen, Denmark, August 17-20, 1992), *Scand. J. Rheumat.*, 94(Suppl.):8, 1992.
14. Croft P.R., Schollum, J., Rigby, A.S., Boswell, R.F., and Silman, A.J.: Chronic widespread pain in the general population. (Myopain '92, Copenhagen, Denmark, August 17-20, 1992), *Scand. J. Rheumat.*, 94(Suppl.):8, 1992.
15. Romano, T.J.: Presence of fibromyalgia (FS) in osteoar-
thritis (OA) patients. (Myopain '92, Copenhagen, Denmark, August 17-20, 1992), *Scand. J. Rheumat.*, 94 (Suppl.):11, 1992.
16. Romano, T.J.: Incidence of fibromyalgia syndrome (FS) in rheumatoid arthritis (RA) patients in a general rheumatology practice. (Myopain '92, Copenhagen, Denmark, August 17-20, 1992), *Scand. J. Rheumat.* 94(Suppl.):11, 1992.
17. Campbell, S.M., Clark, S., Tindall, E.A., and Bennett, R.M.: Clinical characteristics of fibrositis: I. A "blinded" controlled study of symptoms and tender points. *Arthritis Rheum.*, 26:817-824, 1983.
18. Felson, D.T.: Epidemiologic research in fibromyalgia. *J. Rheum.*, 16(Suppl.19):7-11, 1989.
19. Poehlman, E.T., McAuliffe, T.L., Van Houten, D.R., and Danforth, E., Jr.: Influence of age and endurance training on metabolic rate and hormones in healthy men. *Amer. J. Physiol.*, 259 (1 Pt.1):E66-E72, 1990.
20. Rosenthal, M.J., Hunt, W.C., and Garry, P.J.: Thyroid failure in the elderly:microsomal antibodies as discriminant for therapy. *J.A.M.A.*, 258:209-213, 1987.
21. Tunbridge, W.M.G., Evered, D.C., and Hall, R.: The spectrum of thyroid disease in a community survey. *Clin. Endocrinol.*, 7:481-493, 1977.
22. Sawin, C.T, Chopra, D., and Azizi, F.: the aging thyroid: increased prevalence of elevated serum thyrotropin levels in the elderly. *J.A.M.A.*, 242:247-250, 1979.
23. Moldawer, M.: Anabolic agents: clinical efficacy versus side effects. *J. Amer. Med. Womens Assoc.*, 23(4):352-369, 1968.
24. Lowe, J. C.: Oral contraceptives and myofascial pain. *Dig. Chir. Econ.*, 34:100-101, 1991.
25. Lowe, J. C.: Myofascial pain and "The Pill." *J. Nat. Assoc. Trigger Point Myother.*, 5.1:5, 1992.
26. Cooper, R.G., Forbes, W. St. Clair, and Jayson, M.I.V.: Radiographic demonstration of paraspinal muscle wasting in patients with chronic low back pain. *Brit. J. Rheumatol.*, 31:389-394, 1992.
27. Tkachenko, N.N., Potin, V.V., Beskrovnyi, S.V., and Nosova, L.G.: Hypothyroidism and hyperprolactinemia: *Akush. Ginekol.*, 10:40-43, 1989.
28. Sanborn, C.F. and Jankowski, C.M.: Physiologic considerations for women in sports. *Clin. North Amer.*, 13(2):315-327, 1994.
29. Arciero, P.J., Goran, M.I., and Poehlman, E.T.: Resting metabolic rate is lower in women than in men. *J. Appl. Physiol.*, 75(6):2514-2520, 1993.
30. Tepperman, J. and Tepperman, H.M.: *Metabolic and Endocrine Physiology*, 5th edition. Chicago, Year Book Medical Publishers, Inc., 1987.
31. Welshons, W.V. and Gorski, J.: Nuclear location of estrogen receptors. In *The Receptors*. Edited by P.M. Conn, New York, Academic Press, 1986.
32. Migeon, C.: Adrenal androgens in man. *Amer. J. Med.*, 53: 606, 1972.
33. Baxter, J.D. and Tyrrell, J.B.: The adrenal cortex. In *Endocrinology and Metabolism*, 2nd edition. Edited by P. Felig, J.D. Baxter, A. Broadus, and L.A. Frohman, New York, McGraw-Hill Book Co., 1987, pp.511-650.
34. MacDonald, P., Grodin, J., and Siiteri, P.: Dynamics of androgen and estrogen secretion. In *Control of Gonadal*

Steroid Secretion. Edited by D. Baird and J. Strong, Baltimore, Williams and Wilkins, 1971.

35. Ito, T. and Horton, R.: The source of plasma dihydrotestosterone in man. *J. Clin. Invest.*, 50:1621, 1971.

36. Horton, R.J.: Testicular steroid transport, metabolism and effects. In *Endocrinology and Metabolism*, 2nd edition. Edited by P. Felig, J.D. Baxter, A. Broadus, and L.A. Frohman, New York, McGraw-Hill Book Co., 1987, pp.937-942.

37. Johnson, M.P., Young, C.Y., Rowley, D.R., and Tindall, D.J.: A common molecular weight of the androgen monomer in different target tissues. *Biochemistry*, 26:3174, 1987.

38. Trapman, J., Klaassen, P., Kuiper, G., van der Korput, J., and Brinkman, A.: Cloning, structure, and expression of a cDNA encoding the human androgen receptor. *Biochem. Biophys. Res. Commun.*, 153:241, 1988.

39. Philips, N. and Duffy, T.: One-hour glucose tolerance in relation to the use of contraceptive drugs. *Amer. J. Obstet. Gynecol.*, 116:91-100, 1973.

40. Kalkhoff, R.K.: Effects of oral contraceptive agents on carbohydrate metabolism. *J. Steroid Biochem.*, 6:949-956, 1975.

41. Perlman, J.A., Russell-Briefel, R., and Lieberknecht, G.: Oral glucose tolerance and the potency of contraceptive progestins. *J. Chronic Dis.*, 38:857-864, 1985.

42. Wingrave, S.J., Kay, C.R., and Vessey, M.P.: Oral contraceptives and diabetes. *Br. Med. J.*, 1:23, 1979.

43. Duffy, T.J. and Ray, R.: Oral contraceptive use: prospective follow-up of women with suspected glucose intolerance. *Contraceptive*, 30:197-208, 1984.

44. Kalkhoff, R.K., Kim, H.F., and Stoddard, F.J.: Acquired subclinical diabetes mellitus in women receiving oral contraceptive agents. In *Metabolic Effects of Gonadal Hormone and Contraceptive Steroids*. Edited by H.A. Salhanick, D.M. Kipnis, and R.L. Vande Wiele, New York, Plenum Press, 1969, pp.193-203.

45. Gaspard, U.J. and Lefebvre, P.J.: Clinical aspects of the relationship between oral contraceptives, abnormalities in carbohydrate metabolism, and the development of cardiovascular disease. *Amer. J. Obstet. Gynecol.*, 163(1 Pt.2): 334-343, 1990.

46. Skouby, S.O., Andersen, O., Saurbrey, N., and Kuhl, C.: Oral contraception and insulin sensitivity: *in vivo* assessment in normal women and in women with previous gestational diabetes. *J. Clin. Endocrinol. Metab.*, 64:519-526, 1987.

47. Fontbonne, A. and Eschwege, E.: Diabetes, hyperglycaemia, hyperinsulinaemeia and atherosclerosis: epidemiological data. *Diabete et Metabollisme* (Paris), 13:350-353, 1987.

48. Beck-Nielsen, H., Nielsen, O.H., Damsbo, P., Vaag, A., Handberg, A., and Henriksen, J.E.: Impairment of glucose tolerance: mechanisms of action and impact on the cardiovascular system. *Amer. J. Obstet. Gynecol.*, 163(1): 292-295, 1990.

49. Spellacy, W.N., Facog, W.C., Buhi, M.S., and Birk, S.A.: Effects of norethindrone on carbohydrate and lipid metabolism. *Obstretics and Gynecology*, 46:560-563, 1975.

50. Fuller, J.J., Shippley, M.J., Rose, G., Jarrett, R.J., and Keen, H.: Mortality from coronary heart disease and stroke in relation to degree of glycaemia: the Whitehall study. *Br. Med. J.*, 287:867-870, 1983.

51. Eschwege, E., Ducimetiere, P., Claude, J.R., and Richard, J.L.: Blood glucose and coronary heart disease. *Lancet*, II: 472-473, 1980.

52. Ducimetiere, P., Eschwege, E., Papoz, L., Claude, J.R., and Rosselin, G.E.: Relationship of plasma insulin levels to the incidence of myocardial infarction and coronary heart disease mortality in a middle-aged population. *Diabetology*, 19:205-210, 1980.

53. Welborn, T.A. and Wearne, K.: Coronary heart disease incidence and cardiovascular mortality in Busselton with reference to glucose and insulin concentrations. *Diabetes Care*, 2:154-160, 1979.

54. Pyorala, K., Savolainen, E., Kaudola, S., and Haapakoski, J.: High plasma insulin as coronary heart disease risk factor. In *Advances in Diabetes Epidemiology*. Edited by E. Eschwege, (Inserm Symposium No.22.), Amsterdam, Elsevier Biomedical Press, 1982.

55. Stout, R.W.: Insulin and atheroma: an update. *Lancet*, 1: 1077-1079, 1987.

56. Reaven, G.M.: Non-insulin-dependent diabetes mellitus, abnormal lipoprotein metabolism and atherosclerosis. *Metabolism*, 36:1-8, 1987.

57. Laakso, M., Pyorala, K., Voutilainen, E., and Marniemi, J.: Plasma insulin and serum lipids and lipoproteins in middle-aged non-insulin-dependent diabetic and non-diabetic subjects. *Amer. J. Epidemiol.*, 125:611-621, 1987.

58. Spellacy, W.N., Buhi, W.C., and Birk, S.A.: The effects of two years of mestranol treatment on carbohydrate metabolism. *Metabolism*, 31:1006-1008, 1982.

59. Spellacy, W.N., Buhi, W.C., and Birk, S.A.: The effect of estrogens on carbohydrate metabolism: glucose, insulin, and growth hormone studies on one hundred seventy-one women ingesting Premarin, mestranol and ethinylestradiol for six months. *Amer. J. Obstet. Gynecol.*, 114:378-390, 1972.

60. Spellacy, W.N.: Carbohydrate metabolism during treatment with estrogen, progestogen, and low-dose oral contraceptives. *Amer. J. Obstet. Gynecol.*, 142:732-734, 1982.

61. Wynn, V.: Effects of progesterone and progestins on carbohydrate metabolism. In *Progesterone and Progestins*. Edited by C.W. Bardin, E., Milgrom, and P. Mauvais-Jarvis, New York, Raven Press, 1983.

62. Godsland, I.F., Crook, B.A., and Wynn, V.: Low-dose oral carbohydrates and carbohydrate metabolism. *Amer. J. Obstet. Gynecol.*, 163:348-353, 1990.

63. Wynn, V., Godsland, I., and Simpson, R.: Carbohydrate and lipid metabolism in low-dose oral contraceptives. In *Proceedings of the 12th World Congress of Obstetrics and Gynecology*. Edited by P. Belfort, J.A. Pinotii, and T.K.A.B. Eskes, Carnforth, Parthenon Publishing, 1989.

64. Reaven, G.M.: Role of insulin resistance in human disease. *Diabetes*, 37:1595-1608, 1988.

65. Skouby, S.O., Andersen, O., Petersen, K.R., and Molsted-Pedersen, L.: Mechanism of action of oral contraceptives on carbohydrate metabolism at the cellular level. *Amer. J. Obstet. Gynecol.*, 163:343-348, 1990.

66. Falht, K., Cutfield, R., Alejandro, R., Heding, L, and Mintz, D.: The effects of hyperinsulinemia on arterial wall and peripheral muscle cell metabolism in dogs. *Metabo-*

lism, 34:1146-1149, 1985.

67. Beck-Nielsen, H. and Hother-Nielsen, O.: Insulin resistance. In *The Diabetes Annual/4.* Edited by K.G.M.M. Aalberti and I.P. Krall, New York, Elsevier Science Publishers, 1988.

68. Caro, J.F., and Sinha, M.K.: Insulin receptor kinase in human skeletal muscle from obese subjects with and without noninsulin dependent diabetes. *J. Clin. Invest.*, 79:1330-1337, 1987.

69. Freidenberg, G.R., Henry, R.R., and Klein, H.H.: Decreased kinase activity of insulin receptors from adipocytes of non-insulin-dependent diabetic subjects. *J. Clin. Invest.*, 79:240-246, 1987.

70. Damsbo, P., Vaag, A., Hother Nielsen, O., Falholt, K., and Beck-Nielsen, H.: Lack of glycogen synthetase activation at physiological insulin concentrations in skeletal muscle from NIDDM patients. *Diabetes*, 38:88A, 1989.

71. Ain, K.B., Mori, Y., and Refetoff, S.: Reduced clearance rate of thyroxine-binding globulin (TBG) with increased sialylation: a mechanism for estrogen-induced elevation of serum TBG concentration. *J. Clin. Endocrinol. Metab.*, 65:689, 1987.

72. Longcope, C.: The male and female reproductive systems in thyrotoxicosis. In *Werner and Ingbar's The Thyroid: A Fundamental and Clinical Text*, 6th edition. Edited by L.E. Braverman and R.D. Utiger, Philadelphia, J.B. Lippincott Co., 1991, pp.828-835.

73. Beck, R.P., Fawcett, D.M., and Morcos, F.: Thyroid function studies in different phases of the menstrual cycle and in women receiving norethindrone with or without estrogen. *Amer. J. Obstet. Gynecol.*, 112:369, 1972.

74. Frohman, L.A.: Diseases of the anterior pituitary. In *Endocrinology and Metabolism*, 2nd edition. Edited by P. Felig, J.D. Baxter, A. Broadus, and L.A. Frohman, New York, McGraw-Hill Book Co., 1987, pp.247-337.

75. Bartalena, L.: Recent achievements in studies on thyroid hormone-binding proteins. *Endocr. Rev.*, 11:47, 1990.

76. Russell, I.J.: Neurohormonal aspects of fibromyalgia syndrome. *Rheum. Dis. Clin. N. Amer.*, 15:149-168, 1989.

77. Waxman, J. and Zatzkis, S.M.: Fibromyalgia and menopause: examination of the relationship. *Postgrad. Med.*, 80:165-171, 1986.

78. Guyton, A.C.: *Textbook of Medical Physiology*, 8th edition. Philadelphia, W.B. Saunders Co., 1991.

79. Guler, M., Kirnap, M., Bekaroglu, M., Uremek, G., and Onder, C.: Clinical characteristics of patients with fibromyalgia. *Isr. J. Med. Sci.*, 28(1):20-23, 1992.

80. Dellovade, T.L., Y.-S., Zhu., and Pfaff, D.W.: Potential interactions between estrogen receptor and thyroid hormone receptor relevant for neuroendocrine systems. *J. Steroid Biochem. Molec. Biol.*, 53(1-6):27-31, 1995.

81. Lurie, S. and Borenstein, R.: The premenstrual syndrome. *Obstet. Gyn. Surv.*, 45(4):220-228, 1990.

82. Michnovicz, J.J. and Galbraith, R.A.: Effects of exogenous thyroxine on C-2 and C-16α hydroxylations of estradiol in humans. *Steroids*, 55:22-26, 1990.

83. Maruo, T., Katayama, K., Barnea, E.R., and Mochizuki, M.: A role for thyroid hormone in the induction of ovulation and corpus luteum function. *Horm. Res.*, 37(Suppl.1): 12-18, 1992.

84. Mattheij, J.A.M., Swarts, J.J.M., Lokerse, P., van Kampen, J.T., and Van der Heide, D.: Effect of hypothyroidism on the pituitary-gonadal axis in the adult female rat. *J. Endocrinology*, 146:87-94, 1995.

85. Wakim, A.N., Polizotto, S.L., and Burholt, D.R.: Augmentation by thyroxine of human granulosa cell gonadotrophin-induced steroidogenesis. *Human Reproduct.*, 10(11): 2845-2848, 1995.

86. Maruo, T., Hayashi, M., Matsuo, H., Yamamoto, T., Okada, H., and Mochizuki, M.: The role of thyroid hormone as a biological amplifier of the actions of follicle-stimulating hormone in the functional differentiation of cultured porcine granulosa cells. *Endocrinology*, 121(4):1233-1241, 1987.

87. Colborn, T., Dumanoski, D., and Myers, J.P.: *Our Stolen Future.* New York, Penguin Books, Inc., 1996.

88. Sonkin, L.S.: Endocrine disorders and muscle dysfunction. In *Clinical Management of Head, Neck and TMJ Pain and Dysfunction.* Edited by B. Gelb, Philadelphia, W.B. Saunders Co., 1985, pp.137-170.

89. Lowe, J. C.: When nothing else stops trigger point pain. *Dyn. Chir.*, October 24, 1990, p.38.

90. Lowe, J.C.: *The Purpose and Practice of Myofascial Therapy*, (6-tape audio-cassette album). Houston, McDowell Publishing Co., 1989.

91. Lowe, J.C. and Honeyman-Lowe, G.: Facilitating the decrease in fibromyalgic pain during metabolic rehabilitation: an essential role for soft tissue therapies. *J. Bodywork Movem. Ther.*, 2(4):208-217, 1998.

92. Lowe, J.C. and Honeyman-Lowe, G.: Ultrasound treatment for trigger points: differences in technique for myofascial pain syndrome and fibromyalgia patients. *Lyon Méditerranée Médcal: Méd. Sud-Est.*, 2:12-15, 1999.

93. Lowe, J.C.: Treatment-resistant myofascial pain syndromes. In *Functional Soft Tissue Examination and Treatment by Manual Methods: The Extremities.* Edited by W.I. Hammer, Gaithersburg, Aspen Publications, 1991, pp.229-234.

94. Mendelsohn, R.S.: *MalePractice: How Doctors Manipulate Women.* Chicago, Contemporary Books, 1981.

95. Travell, J.G. and Simons, D.G.: *Myofascial Pain and Dysfunction: The Trigger Point Manual*, Baltimore, Williams & Wilkins, 1983.

96. Simons, D.G., Travell, J.G., and Simons, L.S.: *Travell & Simons' Myofascial Pain and Dysfunction: The Trigger Point Manual, Vol.1, Upper Half of Body.* Baltimore, Williams & Wilkins, 1999.

97. Lowe, J. C.: The neglected mechanism. *Dyn. Chir.*, August 29, 1990, p.35.

98. Lowe, J. C.: The most common source of pain. *Chir. J. N, Carolina*, 75(7):26-27, 1992.

99. Lowe, J.C.: Litigation-chronic pain syndrome: Weintraub's unproven entity. *Amer. J. Pain Manag.*, 3(3):131-136, 1993.

100. Lowe, J.C.: The most common source of musculoskeletal pain. *Amer. J. Clin. Chiro.*, Aug., 1993, pp.26-27.

101. Lowe, J.C.: Repetition of Bogduk's erroneous conclusion. *Amer. J. Clin. Chiro.*, Nov., 1994, p.14.

102. Lee, J.R.: *What Your Doctor May Not Tell You About Menopause.* New York, Warner Books, Inc., 1996.

103. Harvey, R.A. and Champe, P.C.: *Pharmacology.* Philadelphia, J.B. Lippincott Co., 1992.

104. Shoupe, D.: Contraception in the 1990s. *Curr. Opin. Obstet. Gynecol.,*. 8(3):211-215, 1996.

105. Tyrer, L.: Introduction of the pill and its impact. *Contraception,* 59(1 Suppl.):11S-16S, 1999.

106. Davis, A. and Wysocki, S.: Clinician/patient interaction: communicating the benefits and risks of oral contraceptives. *Contraception,* 59(1 Suppl.):39S-42S, 1999.

107. Fuchs, N., Prinz, H., and Koch, U.: Attitudes to current oral contraceptive use and future developments: the women's perspective. *Eur. J. Contracept. Reprod. Health Care,* 1(3):275-284, 1996.

108. Jones, K.P.: Oral contraception: current use and attitudes. *Contraception,* 59(1 Suppl.):17S-20S, 1999.

109. Sherif, K.: Benefits and risks of oral contraceptives. *Amer. J. Obstet. Gynecol.,* 180(6 Pt.2):S343-S348, 1999.

110. Womack, J. and Beal, M.W.: Use of Norplant in women with or at-risk for noninsulin-dependent diabetes. *J. Nurse Midwifery,* 41(4):285-296, 1996.

111. Panay, N. and Studd, J.: Progestogen intolerance and compliance with hormone replacement therapy in menopausal women. *Hum. Reprod. Update,* 3(2):159-171, 1997.

112. Brussaard, H.E., Gevers-Leuven, J.A., Frolich, M., Kluft, C., and Krans, H.M.: Short-term oestrogen replacement therapy improves insulin resistance, lipids and fibrinolysis in postmenopausal women with NIDDM. *Diabetologia,* 40 (7):843-849, 1997.

113. Spencer, C.P., Godsland, I.F., and Stevenson, J.C.: Is there a menopausal metabolic syndrome? *Gynecol. Endocrinol.,* 11(5):341-355, 1997.

114. Colacurci, N., Zarcone, R., Mollo, A., Russo, G., Passaro, M., de Seta, L., and de Franciscis, P.: Effects of hormone replacement therapy on glucose metabolism. *Panminerva Med.,* 40(1):18-21, 1998.

115. Medras, M. and Jankowska, E.: Testosterone and atherosclerosis in males during andropause. *Pol. Merkuriusz Lek.,* 6(34):205-207, 1999.

116. Raudaskoski, T., Tomas, C., and Laatikainen, T.: Insulin sensitivity during postmenopausal hormone replacement with transdermal estradiol and intrauterine levonorgestrel. *Acta. Obstet. Gynecol. Scand.,* 78(6):540-545, 1999.

117. Kimmerle, R., Heinemann, L., Heise, T., Bender, R., Weyer, C., Hirschberger, S., and Berger M.: Influence of continuous combined estradiol-norethisterone acetate preparations on insulin sensitivity in postmenopausal nondiabetic women. *Menopause,* 6(1):36-42, 1999.

118. Escalante-Pulido, J.M. and Alpizar-Salazar, M.: Changes in insulin sensitivity, secretion and glucose effectiveness during menstrual cycle. *Arch. Med. Res.,* 30(1):19-22, 1999.

119. Wu, J., Bi, Y., and Wang, H.: The effects of ethinyl estradiol on glucose metabolism in postmenopausal women. *Chung Hua. Fu. Chan. Ko. Tsa. Chih.,* 32(9):528-531, 1997.

120. Hulman, S., Brodsky, N., Miller, J., Donnelly, C., Helms, J., and Falkner, B.: Effect of estrogen withdrawal on blood pressure and insulin resistance in sucrose-fed juvenile rats. *Amer. J. Hypertens.,* 9(12 Pt.1):1200-1205, 1996.

121. Gossain, V.V., Sherma, N.K., Michelakis, A.M. and Rovner, D.R.: Effect of oral contraceptives on plasma glucose, insulin and glucagon levels. *American Journal of Obstetrics and Gynecology,* 147:618-623, 1983.

122. Ramamoorthy, R., Saraswathi, T.P. and Kanaka, T.S.: Carbohydrate metabolic studies during twelve months of treatment with a low-dose combination oral contraceptive. *Contraception,* 40(5):563-569, 1989.

123. De Pirro, R., Forte, F., Dertoli, A., Greco, A.V. and Lauro, R.: Changes in insulin receptors during oral contraception. *J. Clin. Endocrin. Metab.,* 52:29-33, 1981.

124. Botella-Llusia, J.: Influence of other endocrine glands on sex. In *Endocrinology of Women.* Edited by J. Botella-Llusia, Philadelphia, W.B. Saunders, 1973, p.187.

125. Greenspan, F.S.: Thyroid-gonadal interrelationship. In *Gynecologic Endocrinology,* 3rd edition. Edited by J.J. Gold and J.B. Josimovich, Cambridge, Harper & Row, 1980, p.175.

126. Bixton, C.L. and Herrmann, W.L.: Effect of thyroid therapy on menstrual disorders and sterility. *J.A.M.A.,* 155: 1035, 1954.

127. Mochizuki, M.: Thyroid gland and menstrual disorders. *Obstet. Gynecol. Ther.,* 33:641, 1977.

128. Ueda, Y., Hayashi, K., Kishimoto, Y., and Mizusawa, S.: Sexual function in women with diseases of the thyroid gland. *Acta Obstet. Gynecol. Jpn.,* 11:48, 1965.

129. Fredrikson, H. and Ryden, H.: The thyroid-ovarian correlation in the rabbit. *Acta Physiol. Scand.,* 14:136, 1947.

130. Folley, S.J.: Experiments on the relation between the thyroid gland and lactation in the rat. *J. Physiol.,* 93:401, 1938.

131. Krohn, P.L.: The effect of thyroidectomy on reproduction in the female rabbit. *J. Endocrinol.,* 7:307, 1951.

132. Williams, R.H., Weinglass, A.R., Russell, G.W., and Peters, J.: Anatomical effects of thiouracil. *Endocrinology,* 34:317, 1944.

133. Channing, C.P., Tsai, V., and Sachs, D.: Role of insulin, thyroxine, and cortisol in luteinization of porcine granulosa cells grown in chemically defined media. *Biol. Reprod.,* 15:235, 1976.

134. Hayles, A.B. and Cloutire, M.D.: Clinical hypothyroidism in the young: a second look. *Symp. Endocr. Disorders,* 56: 871, 1972.

135. Van Wyk, J. and Grumbach, M.M.: Syndrome of precocious menstruation and galactorrhea in juvenile hypothyroidism: an example of hormonal overlap pituitary feedback. *J. Pediatr.,* 57:416, 1960.

136. Kendle, F.: Case of precocious puberty in a female cretin. *Br. Med. J.,* 1:246, 1905.

137. Thomas, R. and Reid, R.L.: Thyroid disease and reproductive dyfunction: a review. *Obstet. Gynecol.,* 70(5):789-798, 1987.

138. Erickson, G.F., Wang, C., and Hsueh, A.J.W.: FSH induction of functional LH receptors on granulosa cells cultured in a chemically defined medium. *Nature,* 279:336, 1979.

139. Rani, C.S.S., Salhanick, A.R., and Armstrong, D.T.: Follicle stimulating hormone induction of luteinizing hormone receptor in cultured rat granulosa cells: an examination of the need for steroids in the induction process. *Endocrinology,* 108:1379, 1981.

140. Channing, C.P.: Follicle stimulating hormone stimulation of [^{125}I]-human chorionic gonadotropin binding in porcine granulosa cell culture. *Proc. Soc. Exp. Biol. Med.,* 149: 238, 1975.

141. Nimrod, A., Tsafriri, A., and Lindler, H.R.: *In vitro* induc-

tion of binding sites for human chorionic gonadotropin in rat granulosa cells by follicle-stimulation hormone. *Nature*, 267:232, 1977.

142. Jones, P.B.C. and Hsueh, A.J.W.: Regulation of 3β-hydroxysteroid dehydrogenase by gonadotropin-releasing hormone and follicle-stimulating hormone in cultured rat granulosa cells. *Endocrinology*, 110:1663, 1982.

143. Biswas, R., Bandyopadhyay, A., Guin, S., and Bhattacharya, S.: Binding of thyroid hormone to mouse granulosa cell nuclei and its biological relevance. *J. Biosci.*, 18:327-335, 1993.

144. Wakim, A.N., Polizotto, S.L., Buffo, M.J., Marrero, M.A., Burholt, D.R.: Thyroid hormones in human follicular fluid and thyroid hormone receptors in human granulosa cells. *Fertil. Steril.*, 59(6):1187-1190, 1993.

145. Wakim, N.G., Ramani, N., and Rao, C.V.: Triiodothyronine receptors in porcine granulosa cells. *Amer. J. Obstet. Gynecol.*, 156(1):237-240, 1987.

146. Wakim, A.N., Jasnosz, K.M., Alhakim, N., Brown, A.B., and Burholt, D.R.: Thyroid hormone receptor messenger ribonucleic acid in human granulosa and ovarian stromal cells. *Fertil. Steril.*, 62(3):531-534, 1994.

147. Wakim, A.N., Polizotto, S.L., and Burholt, D.R.: α_1 and β_1-Thyroid hormone receptors on human granulosa cells. *Recent Prog. Horm. Res.*, 49:377-381, 1994.

148. Maruo, T., Hiramatsu, S., Otani, T., Hayaski, M., and Mochizuki, M.: Increase in the expression of thyroid hormone receptors in porcine granulosa cells early in follicular maturation. *Acta Endocrinol.*, 127:152-160, 1992.

149. DiZerega, G.S. and Hodgen, G.D.: Luteal phase dysfunction infertility: a sequel to aberrant folliculogenesis. *Fertil. Steril.*, 35:489, 1981.

150. Goldman, S., Dirnfeld, M., Abramovici, H., and Kraiem, Z.: Triiodothyronine and follicle-stimulating hormone, alone and additively together, stimulate production of the tissue inhibitor of metalloproteinases-1 in cultured human luteinized granulosa cells. *J. Clin. Endocrinol. Metab.*, 82 (6):1869-1873, 1997.

151. Goldman, S., Dirnfeld, M., Abramovici, H., and Kraiem, Z.: Triiodothyronine (T_3) modulates hCG-regulated progesterone secretion, cAMP accumulation and DNA content in cultured human luteinized granulosa cells. *Mol. Cell. Endocrinol.*, 96(1-2):125-131, 1993.

152. Wolfe, F.: Diagnosis of fibromyalgia. *J. Musculoskeletal Med.*, 7:54, 1990.

153. Manna, P.R., Tena-Sempere, M., and Huhtaniemi, I.T.: Molecular mechanisms of thyroid hormone-stimulated steroidogenesis in mouse leydig tumor cells. Involvement of the steroidogenic acute regulatory (StAR) protein. *J. Biol. Chem.*, 274(9):5909-5918, 1999.

154. Mochizuki, M., Maruo, T., Matsuo, H., Samoto, T., and Ishihara, N.: Biology of human trophoblast. *Int. J. Gynaecol. Obstet.*, 60(Suppl.1):S21-S28, 1998.

155. la Marca, A., Morgante, G., and De Leo, V.: Human chorionic gonadotropin, thyroid function, and immunological indices in threatened abortion. *Obstet. Gynecol.*, 92(2): 206-211, 1998.

156. Matsuo, H., Maruo, T., Hayashi, M., and Mochizuki, M.: Modification of endocrine function of trophoblasts by thyroid hormone. *Nippon Sanka Fujinka Gakkai Zasshi,* 43 (11):1533-1538, 1991.

157. Mochizuki, M. and Maruo, T.: Biology of trophoblast and its endocrinological profiles. *Nippon Naibunpi Gakkai Zasshi*, 68(8):724-735, 1992.

158. Kol, S., Karnieli, E., Kraiem, Z., Itskovitz-Eldor, J., Lightman, A., and Ish-Shalom, S.: Thyroid function in early normal pregnancy: transient suppression of thyroid-stimulating hormone and stimulation of triiodothyronine. *Gynecol. Obstet. Invest.*, 42(4):227-229, 1996.

159. Maruo, T., Matsuo, H., and Mochizuki, M.: Thyroid hormone as a biological amplifier of differentiated trophoblast function in early pregnancy. *Acta Endocrinol.* (Copenh.), 125(1):58-66, 1991.

160. Skjoldebrand, L., Brundin, J., Carlstrom, A., and Pettersson, T.: Thyroxine-binding globulin in spontaneous abortion. *Gynecol. Obstet. Invest.*, 21(4):187-192, 1986.

161. Lateiwish, A.M., Feher, J., Baraczka, K., Racz, K., Kiss, R., and Glaz, E.: Remission of Raynaud's phenomenon after L-thyroxine therapy in a patient with hypothyroidism. *J. Endocrinol. Invest.*, 15(1):49-51, 1992.

162. Ross, H.A., Exalto, N., Kloppenborg, P.W., and Benraad, T.J.: Thyroid hormone binding in early pregnancy and the risk of spontaneous abortion. *Eur. J. Obstet. Gynecol. Reprod. Biol.*, 32(2):129-136, 1989.

163. Maruo, T., Katayama, K., Matuso, H., Anwar, M., and Mochizuki, M.: The role of maternal thyroid hormones in maintaining early pregnancy in threatened abortion. *Acta Endocrinol.* (Copenh.), 127(2):118-122, 1992.

164. Winikoff, D. and Malinek, M.: The predictive value of thyroid "test profile" in habitual abortion. *Br. J. Obstet. Gynaecol.*, 82(9):760-766, 1975.

165. Skjoldebrand, L. and Sparre, L.S.: Maternal free thyroxine and thyroxine-binding globulin during pregnancy ending in congenital malformations in the offspring. *Gynecol. Obstet. Invest.*, 27(1):19-21, 1989.

166. Velazquez, E.M. and Bellabarba-Arata, G.: Effects of thyroid status on pituitary gonadotropin and testicular reserve in men. *Arch. Androl.*, 38(1):85-92, 1997.

167. Smith, S.C. and Bold, A.M.: Interpretation of *in vitro* thyroid function tests during pregnancy. *Br. J. Obstet. Gynaecol.*, 90(6):532-534, 1983.

168. Davis, L.E., Leveno, K.J., and Cunningham, F.G.: Hypothyroidism complicating pregnancy. *Obstet. Gynecol.*, 72: 108, 1988.

169. Burrow, G.N.: The thyroid gland and reproduction. In *Reproductive Endocrinology.* Edited by S.S.C. Yen and R.B. Jaffe, Philadelphia, W.B. Saunders, 1986, p.424.

170. Nikolai, T.F., Mulligan, G.M., Gribble, R.K., Harkins, P.G., Meier, P.R., and Roberts, R.C.: Thyroid function and treatment in premenstrual syndrome. *J. Clin. Endocrinol. Metab.*, 70:1108, 1990.

171. Vulsma, T., Gons, M.H., and De Vijder, J.: Maternal-fetal tranfer of thyroxine in congenital hypothyroidism due to a total organification defect or thyroid agenesis. *N. Engl. J. Med.*, 321(1):13-16, 1989.

172. Sack, J., Kaiserman, I., and Siebner, R.: Maternal-fetal T_4 transfer does not suffice to prevent the effects of in utero hypothyroidism. *Horm. Res.*, 39(1-2):1-7, 1993.

173. Utiger, R.D.: Therapy of hypothyroidism: when are changes needed. *N. Engl. J. Med.*, 323:126, 1990.

174. Mandel, S.J., Larsen, P.R., Seely, E.W., and Brent, G.A.: Increased need for thyroxine during pregnancy in women

with primary hypothyroidism. *N. Engl. J. Med.*, 323(2):91-96, 1990.

175. Emerson, C.H.: Thyroid disease during and after pregnancy. In *Werner and Ingbar's The Thyroid: A Fundamental and Clinical Text*, 6th edition. Edited by L.E. Braverman and R.D. Utiger, Philadelphia, J.B. Lippincott Co., 1991, pp.1263-1279.

176. Gardiner-Hill, H.: Pregnancy complicating simple goitre and Graves' disease. *Lancet*, 1:120, 1929.

177. Momotani, N., Ito, K., Hamada, N., Ban, Y., Nishikawa, Y., and Mimura, T.: Maternal hyperthyroidism and congenital malformations in the offspring. *Clin. Endocrinol.* (Oxf.), 20:695, 1984.

178. Cove, D.H. and Johnston, P.: Fetal hyperthyroidism: experience of treatment in four siblings. *Lancet*, 1:430, 1985.

179. LaFranchi, S. and Mandel, S.H.: Graves' disease in the neonatal period and childhood. In *Werner and Ingbar's The Thyroid: A Fundamental and Clinical Text*, 6th edition. Edited by L.E. Braverman and R.D. Utiger, Philadelphia, J.B. Lippincott Co., 1991, pp.1237-1246.

180. Fisher, D.A.: Thyroid physiology in the perinatal period and during childhood. In *Werner and Ingbar's The Thyroid: A Fundamental and Clinical Text*, 6th edition. Edited by L.E. Braverman and R.D. Utiger, Philadelphia, J.B. Lippincott Co., 1991, pp.1207-1218.

181. Niswander, K.R.: Metabolic and endocrine conditions. In *Women and Their Pregnancies*. Edited by K.R. Niswander and M. Gordon, Philadelphia, W.B. Saunders, 1972, p.246.

182. Davis, L.E., Leveno, K.J., and Cunningham, F.G.: Hypothyroidism complicating pregnancy. *Obstet. Gynecol.*, 72:108, 1988.

183. Montoro, M., Collea, J.V., Frasier, S.D., and Mestman, J.H.: Sucessful outcome of pregnancy in women with hypothyroidism. *Ann. Intern. Med.*, 94:31, 1981.

184. Greenman, G.W., Gabrielson, M.O., Howard-Flanders, J., and Wessel, M.A.: Thyroid dysfunction in pregnancy. *N. Engl. J. Med.*, 267:426, 1962.

185. Carr, E.A., Jr., Beierwaltes, W.H., Raman, G., et al.: The effect of maternal thyroid function on fetal thyroid function and development. *J. Clin. Endocrinol. Metab.*, 19:1, 1959.

186. McDougall, I.R. and Maclin, N.: Hypothyroid women need more thyroxine when pregnant. *J. Fam. Pract.*, 41 (3):238-240, 1995.

187. Vojvodic, L., Sulovic, V., Milacic, D., and Terzic, M.: The course and outcome of pregnancy in pregnant women with hypothyroidism. *Srp. Arh. Celok. Lek.*, 121(3-7):62-64, 1993.

188. Gerber, P.: Thyroid and pregnancy. *Schweiz. Rundsch. Med. Prax.*, 82(32):854-857, 1993.

189. Leung, A.S., Millar, L.K., Koonings, P.P., Montoro, M., and Mestman, J.H.: Perinatal outcome in hypothyroid pregnancies. *Obstet. Gynecol.*, 81(3):349-353, 1993.

190. Wilansky, D.L. and Greisman, B.: Early hypothyroidism in patients with menorrhagia. *Amer. J. Obstet. Gynecol.*, 160(3):673-677, 1989.

191. Johnson, C., Olivier, N.B., Nachreiner, R., and Mullaney, T.: Effect of 131I-induced hypothyroidism on indices of reproductive function in adult male dogs. *J. Vet. Intern. Med.*, 13(2):104-110, 1999.

192. Wortsman, J., Moses, H.W., and Dufau, M.L.: Increased incidence of thyroid disease among men with hypergonadotropic hypogonadism. *Amer. J. Med.*, 80(6):1055-1059, 1986.

193. Castro-Magana, M., Angulo, M., Canas, A., Sharp, A., and Fuentes, B.: Hypothalamic-pituitary gonadal axis in boys with primary hypothyroidism and macroorchidism. *J. Pediatr.*, 112(3):397-402, 1988.

194. Baskin, H.J.: Endocrinologic evaluation of impotence. *South. Med. J.*, 82(4):446-449, 1989.

195. Wortsman, J., Rosner, W., and Dufau, M.L.: Abnormal testicular function in men with primary hypothyroidism. *Amer. J. Med.*, 82(2):207-212, 1987.

196. Man, E.B. and Jones, W.S.: Thyroid function in human pregnancy. V. Incidence of maternal serum low butanol-extractable iodines and of normal gestational TBG and TBPA capacities; retardation of 8-month-old-infants. *Amer. J. Obstet. Gynecol.*, 104:898, 1969.

197. Man, E.B. and Serunian, S.A.: Thyroid function in human pregnancy. IX. Development of retardation of 7-year-old progeny of hypothyroxinemic women. *Amer. J. Obstet. Gynecol.*, 125:949, 1976.

198. Varma, S.K., Murray, R., and Stanbury, J.B.: Effects of maternal hypothyroidism and triidothyronine on the fetus and newborn in rats. *Endocrinology*, 102:24, 1978.

199. Goldsmith, R.E., Sturgis, S.H., Lerman, J., and Stanbury, J.B.: The menstrual pattern in thyroid disease. *J. Clin. Endocrinol. Metab.*, 12:846, 1952.

200. Bonet, B. and Herrera, E.: Different responses to maternal hypothyroidism during the first and second half of gestation in the rat. *Endocrinology*, 122:450, 1988.

201. Potter, B.J., McIntosh, G.H., Mano, M.T., et al.: The effect of maternal thyroidectomy prior to conception on foetal brain development in sheep. *Acta Endocrinol.* (Copenh.), 112:93, 1986.

202. Peterson, R.R., Webster, R.C., Rayner, B., and Young, W.C.: The thyroid and reproductive performance in the adult female guinea pig. *Endocrinology*, 51:504, 1952.

203. Thomas, D.K., Storlien, L.H., Bellingham, W.P., and Gillette, K.: Ovarian hormone effects on activity, glucoregulation, and thyroid hormone in rats. *Physiol. Behav.*, 36 (3):567-573, 1986.

204. Kamei, Y., Tsutsumi, O., Yamakawa, A., Oka, Y., Taketani, Y., and Imaki, J.: Maternal epidermal growth factor deficiency causes fetal hypoglycemia and intrauterine growth retardation in mice: possible involvement of placental glucose transporter GLUT3 expression. *Endocrinology*, 140(9):4236-4243, 1999.

205. Morrish, D.W., Dakour, J., and Li, H.: Functional regulation of human trophoblast differentiation. *J. Reprod. Immunol.*, 39(1-2):179-195, 1998.

206. Kimball, O.P.: Clinical hypothyroidism. *Kentucky Med. J.*, 31:488-495, 1933.

207. DeGroot, L.J., Larsen, P.R., Refetoff, S., and Stanbury, J.B.: *The Thyroid and Its Diseases*, 5th edition. New York, John Wiley & Sons, 1984.

208. Kirk, E. and Kvorning, S.A.: *Hypometabolism: A Clinical Study of 308 Consecutive Cases*. Copenhagen, Einar Munksgaard, Publisher, 1946.

209. Thurmon, F.M. and Thompson, W.O.: Low basal metabolism with myxedema. *Arch. Intern. Med.*, 46:879-897,

1930.

210. Kurland, G.S., Hamolsky, M.W., and Freedberg, A.S.: Studies in non-myxedematous hypometabolism. I. The clinical syndrome and the effects of triiodothyronine, alone or combined with thyroxine. *J. Clin. Endocrinol.*, 15: 1354, 1955.

211. Morton, J.H.: Sodium lithyronine in metabolic insufficiency syndrome and associated disorders. *J.A.M.A.*, 165:124-129, 1957.

212. Longcope, C.: The male and female reproductive systems. In *The Thyroid*, 4th edition. Edited by S.C. Werner and S.H. Ingbar, New York, Harper and Row Publishers, 1987, pp.1194-1198.

213. Rogers, J.: Medical progress: menstruation and systemic disease, thyroid disorders. *N. Engl. J. Med.*, 259:721, 1958.

214. Scott, J.C. and Mussey, E.: Menstrual patterns in myxedema. *Am. J. Obstet. Gynecol.*, 90:161, 1964.

215. Boroditsky, R.S. and Faiman, C.: Galactorrhea-amenorrhea due to primary hypothyroidism. *Amer. J. Obstet. Gynecol.*, 16:661, 1973.

216. Edwards, C.R.W., Forsyth, I.A., and Besser, G.M.: Amenorrhea, galactorrhea and primary hypothyroidism with high circulating levels of prolactin. *Br. Med. J.*, 3:462, 1971.

217. Guinet, P., Tourniaire, J., Orgiazzi, J., and Robert, M.: Peripheral myxedema: amenorrhea-galactorrhea; radiologic picture of hypophysial adenoma; inhibition of excessive TSH secretion. *Ann. Endocrinol.* (Paris), 33:376, 1972.

218. Kinch, R.A.H., Plunkett, E.R., and Devlin, M.C.: Postpartum amenorrhea-galactorrhea of hypothyroidism. *Amer. J. Obstet. Gynecol.*, 105:766, 1969.

219. Ross, G.T., Scholz, D.A., Lambert, E.H., and Geraci, J.E.: Severe uterine bleeding and degenerative skeletal-muscle changes in unrecoginized myxedema. *J. Clin. Endocrinol. Metab.*, 18:496-497, 1958.

220. Buchanan, G.C., Tredway, D.R., Pittard, J.C., and Daane, T.A.: Gonadotrophin secretion and hypothyroidism. *Obstet. Gynecol.*, 50:392-396, 1977.

221. Nichols, A.J. and Ruffolo, R.R., Jr.: Functions mediated by α-adrenoceptors. In α-*Adrenoceptors: Molecular Biology, Biochemistry and Pharmacology*. Basel, Karger, 1991, pp.113-179.

222. Hodges, R.E., Hamilton, H.E. and Keetel, W.C.: Pregnancy in myxedema. *Arch. Intern. Med.*, 90:863, 1952.

223. Prange, A.J., Wilson, I.C., Rabon, A.M., and Lipton, M.A.: Enhancement of imipramine antidepressant activity by thyroid hormone. *Amer. J. Psychiat.*, 126:39-51, 1969.

224. Bruni, J.F., Marshall, S., Dibbet, J.A., and Meites, J.: Effects of hyperthyroidism and hypothyroidism on serum LH and FSH levels in intact and gonadectomized male and female rats. *Endocrinology*, 97:558-563, 1975.

225. Dunn, J., Peppler, R., Hess, M., and Johnson, D.C.: Proestrous gonadotropin levels in thyroparathyroidectomized female rats. *Experimentia*, 32:1342-1344, 1976.

226. Peppler, R.D., Hess, M., and Dunn, J.D.: Compensatory ovulation after unilateral ovariectomy in thyoidectomized rats. *J. Endocrinol.*, 66:137-138, 1975.

227. Hagino, N.: Influence of hypothyroid state on ovulation in rats. *Endocrinology*, 88:1332-1336, 1971.

228. Berne, R.M. and Levy, M.N.: *Principles of Physiology*. St. Louis, C.V. Mosby Company, 1990.

229. Phifer, R.F., Midgley, A.R., and Spicer, S.S.: Immunohistologic and histologic evidence that FSH and LH are present in the same cell type in the human pars distalis. *J. Clin. Endocrinol. Metab.*, 36:125, 1973.

230. Colon, J.M., Lessing, J.B., Yavetz, C., Peyser, M.R., Ganguly, M., and Weiss, G.: The effect of thyrotropin-releasing hormone stimulation on serum levels of gonadotropins in women during the follicular and luteal phases of the menstrual cycle. *Fertil. Steril.*, 49(5):809-812, 1988.

231. Benelli, C., Michel, O., and Michel, R.: Effect of thyroidectomy on pregnenolone and progesterone biosynthesis in rat adrenal cortex. *J. Steroid Biochem.*, 16:749-754, 1982.

232. Bandyopadhyay, A., Roy, P., and Bhattacharya, S.: Thyroid hormone induces the synthesis of a putative protein in the rat granulosa cell which stimulates progesterone release. *J. Endocrinol.*, 150(2):309-318, 1996.

233. Soules, M.R., Clifton, D.K., Cohen, N.L., Bremner, W.J., and Steiner, R.A.: Luteal phase deficiency: abnormal gonadotropin and progesterone secretion patterns. *J. Clin. Endocrinol. Metab.*, 69:813, 1989.

234. McNeely, M.J. and Soules, M.R.: The diagnosis of luteal phase deficiency: a critical review. *Fertil. Steril.*, 50:1, 1988.

235. Reuters Health, 1999, <http://www.intelihealth.com/enews?207582>

236. Daly, D.C., Walters, C.a., Soto-Albors, C.E., and Riddick, D.H.: Endometrial biopsy during treatment of luteal phase defects is predictive of therapeutic outcome. *Fertil. Steril.*, 40(3):305-310, 1983.

237. Hayashi, M., Maruo, T., Matsuo, H., and Mochizuki, M.: The biocellular effect of thyroid hormone on functional differentiation of porcine granulosa cells in culture. *Nippon Naibunpi Gakkai Zasshi*, 61(10):1189-1196, 1985.

238. Ballinger, C.B., Browning, M.C., and Smith, A.H.: Hormone profiles and psychological symptoms in peri-menopausal women. *Maturitas*, 9(3):235-251, 1987.

239. Hayashi, M., Maruo, T., Matsuo, H., and Mochizuki, M.: Effect of thyroid hormone on steroidogenic enzyme induction in porcine granulosa cells cultured *in vitro*. *Nippon Naibunpi Gakkai Zasshi*, 63(10):1231-1240, 1987.

240. Griggs, R.C., Kingston, W., Jozefowicz, R.F., Forbes, G., and Halliday, D.: Effect of testosterone on muscle mass and muscle protein synthesis. *J. Appl. Physiol.*, 66:498-503, 1989.

241. Ferraro, R., Lillioja, S., Fontvielle, A., Rising, R., Bogardus, C., and Ravussin, E.: Lower sedentary metabolic rate in women compared with men. *J. Clin. Invest.*, 90:780-784, 1992.

242. Forbes, G.B.: The effect of anabolic steroids on lean body mass: the dose response curve. *Metabolism*, 34:571-573, 1985.

243. Herver, G.R., Knibbs, A.V., Burkinshaw, L., et al.: Effects of methandienone on the performance and body composition of men undergoing athletic training. *Clin. Sci.* (Lond.), 60:457-461, 1981.

244. Seligmann, J., Friday, C., and Wingert, P.: Menopause. *Newsweek*, May 25, 1992.

245. Hargrove, J.T. and Abraham, G.E.: The ubiquitousness of premenstrual tension in gynecologic practice. *J. Reproduct. Med.*, 28(7):435-437, 1983.

246. Moos, R.H.: The development of a premenstrual distress questionnaire. *Psychosom. Med.*, 30:853, 1969.

247. Woods, N.F., Most, A., Hahn, L., et al.: Prevalence of premenstrual symptoms. *Amer. J. Public Health*, 72:1257, 1982.

248. Sampson, G.A. and Prescott, P.: The assessment of the symptoms of premenstrual syndrome and their response to therapy. *Br. J. Psychiat.*, 138:399, 1981.

249. Bickers, W. and Woods, M.: Premenstrual tension: rational therapy. *Tex. Rep. Biol. Med.*, 9:406, 1951.

250. Sutherland, H. and Stewart, I.: A critical analysis of the premenstrual syndrome. *Lancet*, 1:1180, 1965.

251. O'Brian, P.M.S.: The premenstrual syndrome: a review. *J. Reproduct. Med.*, 30:113, 1985.

252. Frank, R.T.: Hormonal causes of premenstrual tension. *Arch. Neurol. Psychiat.*, 26:1053, 1931.

253. Merriam, G.R., Brody, S.A., and Almeida, O.: Endocrinology of the menstrual cycle: implications for premenstrual syndrome. In *Proceedings of the National Institute of Mental Health Premenstrual Syndrome Workshop*, National Institute of Mental Health. Bethesda, MD, 1983.

254. Herman, W.M. and Beach, R.C.: Experimental and clinical data indicating the psychotropic properties of progestagens. *Postgrad. Med.*, 54(Suppl.2):82, 1978.

255. Landau, R.L. and Lugibihi, K.: The catabolic and natriuretic effects of progesterone in man. *Rec. Prog. Horm. Res.*, 17:249, 1961.

256. Green, R. and Dalton, K.: Premenstrual syndrome. *Br. Med. J.*, 1:1007, 1953.

257. Dalton, K.: *Once a Month*. Claremont, Hunter House, 1990.

258. Schmidt, P.J., Rosenfeld, D., Muller, K.L., Grover, G.N., and Rubinow, D.R.: A case of autoimmune thyroiditis presenting as menstrual related mood disorder. *J. Clin. Psychiat.*, 51(10):434-436, 1990.

259. Roy-Byrne, P.P., Rubinow, D.R., Hoban, M.C., Grover, G.N., and Blank, D.: TSH and prolactin responses to TRH in patients with premenstrual syndrome. *Amer. J. Psychiat.*, 144(4):480-484, 1987.

260. Ostensen, M., Rugelsjoen, A., and Wigers, S.H.: The effect of reproductive events and alterations of sex hormone levels on the symptoms of fibromyalgia. *Scand. J. Rheumatol.*, 26(5):355-360, 1997.

261. Solomon, S.J., Kurzer, M.S., and Calloway, D.H.: Menstrual cycle and basal metabolic rate in women. *Amer. J. Clin. Nutr.*, 36(4):611-616, 1982.

262. Lariviere, F., Moussalli, R., and Garrel, D.R.: Increased leucine flux and leucine oxidation during the luteal phase of the menstrual cycle in women. *Amer. J. Physiol.*, 267(3 Pt.1):E422-E428, 1994.

263. Das, T.K. and Jana, H.: Basal oxygen consumption during different phases of menstrual cycle. *Indian J. Med. Res.*, 94:16-19, 1991.

264. Bisdee, J.T., Garlick, P.J., and James, W.P.: Metabolic changes during the menstrual cycle. *Br. J. Nutr.*, 61(3):641-650, 1989.

265. Bisdee, J.T., James, W.P., and Shaw, M.A.: Changes in energy expenditure during the menstrual cycle. *Br. J. Nutr.*, 61(2):187-199, 1989.

266. Girdler, S.S., Pedersen, C.A., and Light, K.C.: Thyroid axis function during the menstrual cycle in women with pre-menstrual syndrome. *Psychoneuroendocrinology*, 20(4):395-403, 1995.

267. Schmidt, P.J., Grover, G.N., Roy-Byrne, P.P., and Rubinow, D.R.: Thyroid function in women with premenstrual syndrome. *J. Clin. Endocrinol. Metab.*, 76(3):671-674, 1993.

268. Girdler, S.S., Pedersen, C.A., Stern, R.A., and Light, K.C.: Menstrual cycle and premenstrual syndrome: modifiers of cardiovascular reactivity in women. *Health Psychol.*, 12(3):180-192, 1993.

269. Nikolai, T.F., Mulligan, G.M., Gribble, R.K., Harkins, P.G., Meier, P.R., and Roberts, R.C.: Thyroid function and treatment in premenstrual syndrome. *J. Clin. Endocrinol. Metab.*, 70(4):1108-1113, 1990.

270. Korzekwa, M.I., Lamont, J.A., and Steiner, M.: Late luteal phase dysphoric disorder and the thyroid axis revisited. *J. Clin. Endocrinol. Metab.*, 81(6):2280-2284, 1996.

271. Faughnan, M., Lepage, R., Fugere, P., Bissonnette, F., Brossard, J.H., and D'Amour, P.: Screening for thyroid disease at the menopausal clinic. *Clin. Invest. Med.*, 18(1):11-18, 1995.

272. Casper, R.F., Patel-Christopher, A., and Powell, A.M.: Thyrotropin and prolactin responses to thyrotropin-releasing hormone in premenstrual syndrome. *J. Clin. Endocrinol. Metab.*, 68(3):608-612, 1989.

273. Gerhard, I., Becker, T., Eggert-Kruse, W., Klinga, K., and Runnebaum, B.: Thyroid and ovarian function in infertile women. *Hum. Reprod.*, 6(3):338-345, 1991.

274. London, R.S., Bradley, L., and Chiamori, N.Y.: Effect of a nutritional supplement on premenstrual symptomatology in women with premenstrual syndrome: a double-blind longitudinal study. *J. Amer. Coll. Nutr.*, 10(5):494-499, 1991.

275. Tiemstra, J.D. and Patel, K.: Hormonal therapy in the management of premenstrual syndrome. *J. Amer. Board Fam. Pract.*, 11(5):378-381, 1998.

276. Laux, M. and Conrad, C.: *Natural Woman, Natural Menopause*. New York, Harper Perenial, 1997.

277. Young, E. and Korszun, A.: Psychoneuroendocrinology of depression: hypothalamic-pituitary-gonadal axis. *Psychiatr. Clin. N. Amer.*, 21(2):309-323, 1998.

278. Arpels, J.C.: The female brain hypoestrogenic continuum from the premenstrual syndrome to menopause. A hypothesis and review of supporting data. *J. Reprod. Med.*, 41(9):633-639, 1996.

279. Arafat, E.S., Hargrove, J.T., Maxson, W.S., Desiderio, D.M., Wentz, A.C., and Andersen, R.N.: Sedative and hypnotic effects of oral administration of micronized progesterone may be mediated through its metabolites. *Amer. J. Obstet. Gynecol.*, 159(5):1203-1209, 1988.

280. Redmond, G.: Mood disorders in the female patient. *Int. J. Fertil. Womens Med.*, 42(2):67-72, 1997.

281. Rosie, R., Grace, O., Quinn, J.P., Fink, G., and Sumner, B.E.: Estrogen control of central neurotransmission: effect on mood, mental state, and memory. *Cell. Mol. Neurobiol.*, 16(3):325-344, 1996.

282. Pearlstein, T.B.: Hormones and depression: what are the facts about premenstrual syndrome, menopause, and hormone replacement therapy? *Amer. J. Obstet. Gynecol.*, 173(2):646-653, 1995.

283. Severino, S.K. and Moline, M.L.: Premenstrual syndrome.

Identification and management. *Drugs,* 49(1):71-82, 1995.

284. Karakanias, G.B., Li, C.S., and Etgen, A.M.: Estradiol reduction of α_2-adrenoceptor binding in female rat cortex is correlated with decreases in $\alpha_{2A/D}$-adrenoceptor messenger RNA. *Neuroscience,* 81(3):593-597, 1997.

285. Pert, C.: *Molecules of Emotion.* New York, Scribner, 1997.

286. Lee, K.A., Shaver, J.F., Giblin, E.C., and Woods, N.F.: Sleep patterns related to menstrual cycle phase and premenstrual affective symptoms. *Sleep,* 13(5):403-409, 1990.

287. Goldberg, M.: Diagnosis of euthyroid hypometabolism. *Amer. J. Obst. & Gynec.,* 81(5):1053-1058, May, 1961.

288. DeGowin, R.L. and DeGowin, E.L.: *Bedside Diagnostic Examination,* 3rd edition. New York, Macmillan Publishing Co., 1976.

289. ter Borg, E.J., Gerards-Rociu, E., Haanen, H.C., and Westers, P.: High frequency of hysterectomies and appendectomies in fibromyalgia compared with rheumatoid arthritis: a pilot study. *Clin. Rheumatol.,* 18(1):1-3, 1999.

290. Graeff, F.G., Brandao, M.L., Audi, E.A., and Schutz, M.T.: Modulation of the brain aversive system by GABAergic and serotonergic mechanisms. *Behav. Brain Res.,* 22(2):173-180, 1986.

291. Mortola, J.F.: Assessment and management of premenstrual syndrome. *Curr. Opin. Obstet. Gynecol.,* 4(6):877-885, 1992.

292. Mortola, J.F.: Applications of gonadotropin-releasing hormone analogues in the treatment of premenstrual syndrome. *Clin. Obstet. Gynecol.,* 36(3):753-763, 1993.

293. Dhar, V. and Murphy, B.E.: The premenstrual syndrome and its treatment. *J. Steroid Biochem. Mol. Biol.,* 39(2):275-281, 1991.

294. Cabot, S.: *Smart Medicine for Menopause.* Garden City Park, Avery Publishing Group, 1995.

295. Gerhard, I., Eggert-Kruse, W., Merzoug, K., Klinga, K., and Runnebaum, B.: Thyrotropin-releasing hormone (TRH) and metoclopramide testing in infertile women. *Gynecol. Endocrinol.,* 5(1):15-32, 1991.

296. Giangrande, P.H. and McDonnell, D.P.: The A and B isoforms of the human progesterone receptor: two functionally different transcription factors encoded by a single gene. *Recent Prog. Horm. Res.,* 54:291-313, 1999.

297. Pau, K.Y. and Spies, H.G.: Neuroendocrine signals in the regulation of gonadotropin-releasing hormone secretion. *Chin. J. Physiol.,* 40(4):181-196, 1997.

298. Moutsatsou, P. and Sekeris, C.E.: Estrogen and progesterone receptors in the endometrium. *Ann. N.Y. Acad. Sci.,* 816:99-115, 1997.

299. Wiebe, J.P.: Nongenomic actions of steroids on gonadotropin release. *Recent Prog. Horm. Res.,* 71-99, 1997.

300. Joels, M.: Steroid hormones and excitability in the mammalian brain. *Front. Neuroendocrinol.,* 18(1):2-48, 1997.

301. Leung, P.C. and Peng, C.: Gonadotropin-releasing hormone receptor: gene structure, expression and regulation. *Biol. Signals,* 5(2):63-69, 1996.

302. Katzenellenbogen, B.S.: Estrogen receptors: bioactivities and interactions with cell signaling pathways. *Biol. Reprod.,* 54(2):287-293, 1996.

303. Camacho-Arroyo, I., Pasapera, A.M., Perez-Palacios, G., and Cerbon, M.A.: Progesterone and its metabolites in central nervous system function. *Rev. Invest. Clin.,* 47(4):329-340, 1995.

304. Keys, J.L. and King, G.J.: Effects of topical and systemic estrogen on morphology of porcine uterine luminal epithelia. *Biol. Reprod.,* 46(6):1165-1175, 1992.

305. Shimoya, K., Tomiyama, T., Hashimoto, K., et al.: Endometrial development was improved by transdermal estradiol in patients treated with clomiphene citrate. *Gynecol. Obstet. Invest.,* 47(4):251-254, 1999.

306. Perez, J.F., Conley, A.J., Dieter, J.A., Sanz-Ortega, J., and Lasley, B.L.: Studies on the origin of ovarian interstitial tissue and the incidence of endometrial hyperplasia in domestic and feral cats. *Gen. Comp. Endocrinol.,* 116(1):10-20, 1999.

307. Magarelli, P.C., Zachow, R.J., and Magoffin, D.A.: Developmental and hormonal regulation of rat theca-cell differentiation factor secretion in ovarian follicles. *Biol. Reprod.,* 55(2):416-420, 1996.

308. Conley, A.J., Howard, H.J., Slanger, W.D., and Ford, J.J.: Steroidogenesis in the preovulatory porcine follicle. *Biol. Reprod.,* 51(4):655-661, 1994.

309. Bergh, C., Olsson, J.H., Selleskog, U., and Hillensjo, T.: Steroid production in cultured thecal cells obtained from human ovarian follicles. *Biol. Reprod.,* 8(4):519-524, 1993.

310. Reilly, C.M., Cannady, W.E., Mahesh, V.B., Stopper, V.S., De Sevilla, L.M., and Mills, T.M.: Duration of estrogen exposure prior to follicle-stimulating hormone stimulation is critical to granulosa cell growth and differentiation in rats. *Biol. Reprod.,* 54(6):1336-1342, 1996.

311. Klein, N.A., Battaglia, D.E., Miller, P.B., Branigan, E.F., Giudice, L.C., and Soules, M.R.: Ovarian follicular development and the follicular fluid hormones and growth factors in normal women of advanced reproductive age. *J. Clin. Endocrinol. Metab.,* 81(5):1946-1951, 1996.

312. Illingworth, P.J., Reddi, K., Smith, K.B., and Baird, D.T.: The source of inhibin secretion during the human menstrual cycle. *J. Clin. Endocrinol. Metab.,* 73(3):667-673, 1991.

313. Mango, D., Ricci, S., Manna, P., Olleja, L., Tripodi, R., Tropeano, G., and Lucisano, A.: Ultrasonic and endocrinologic aspects in gonadotropin releasing hormone induction of ovulation. *J. Endocrinol. Invest.,* 14(5):361-366, 1991.

314. Check, J.H., Dietterich, C., and Houck, M.A.: Ipsilateral versus contralateral ovary selection of dominant follicle in succeeding cycle. *Obstet. Gynecol.,* 77(2):247-249, 1991.

315. Conard, J.: Modifications of the hemostatic balance during estrogen treatments: menopause and its treatment. *Therapie,* 54(3):363-367, 1999.

316. Wong, S. and Wong, J.: Is physical activity as effective in reducing risk of cardiovascular disease as estrogen replacement therapy in postmenopausal women? *Int. J. Nurs. Stud.,* 36(5):405-414, 1999.

317. Cook, M.J.: Perimenopause: an opportunity for health promotion. *J. Obstet. Gynecol. Neonatal Nurs.,* 22(3):223-228, 1993.

318. Gambacciani, M., Spinetti, A., Cappagli, B., et al.: Hormone replacement therapy in perimenopausal women with a low dose oral contraceptive preparation: effects on bone mineral density and metabolism. *Maturitas,* 19(2):125-

131, 1994.

319. Burger, H.G.: The endocrinology of the menopause. *J. Steroid Biochem. Mol. Biol.*, 69(1-6):31-35, 1999.

320. Tohei, A., Watanabe, G., and Taya, K.: Effects of thyroidectomy or thiouracil treatment on copulatory behavior in adult male rats. *J. Vet. Med. Sci.*, 60(3):281-285, 1998.

321. Tohei, A., Akai, M., Tomabechi, T., Mamada, M., and Taya, K.: Adrenal and gonadal function in hypothyroid adult male rats. *J. Endocrinol.*, 152(1):147-154, 1997.

322. Burt, V.K., Altshuler, L.L., and Rasgon, N.: Depressive symptoms in the perimenopause: prevalence, assessment, and guidelines for treatment. *Harv. Rev. Psychiatry*, 6(3): 121-132, 1998.

323. LeBoeuf, F.J. and Carter, S.G.: Discomforts of the perimenopause. *J. Obstet. Gynecol. Neonatal Nurs.*, 25(2): 173-180, 1996.

324. Sulak, P.J.: The perimenopause: a critical time in a woman's life. *Int. J. Fertil. Menopausal. Stud.*, 41(2):85-89, 1996.

325. Li, S., Lanuza, D., Gulanick, M., Penckofer, S., and Holm, K.: Perimenopause: the transition into menopause. *Health Care Women Int.*, 17(4):293-306, 1996.

326. American College of Obstetricians and Gynecologists: ACOG technical bulletin: health maintenance for perimenopausal women. *Int. J. Gynaecol. Obstet.*, 51(2):171-181, 1995.

327. Mishell, D.R., Jr.: Estrogen replacement therapy: an overview. *Amer. J. Obstet. Gynecol.*, 161(6 Pt.2):1825-1827, 1989.

328. Samsioe, G.: The menopause revisited. *Int. J. Gynaecol. Obstet.*, 51(1):1-13, 1995.

329. Matthews, K.A., Wing, R.R., Kuller, L.H., Meilahn, E.N., and Plantinga, P.: Influence of the perimenopause on cardiovascular risk factors and symptoms of middle-aged healthy women. *Arch. Intern. Med.*, 154(20):2349-2355, 1994.

330. Dessein, P.H., Shipton, E.A., Joffe, B.I., Hadebe, D.P., Stanwix, A.E., and Van der Merwe, B.A.: Hyposecretion of adrenal androgens and the relation of serum adrenal steroids, serotonin and insulin-like growth factor-1 to clinical features in women with fibromyalgia. *Pain*, 83(2): 313-319, 1999.

331. Riedel, W., Layka, H., and Neeck, G.: Secretory pattern of GH, TSH, thyroid hormones, ACTH, cortisol, FSH, and LH in patients with fibromyalgia syndrome following systemic injection of the relevant hypothalamic-releasing hormones. *Z. Rheumatol.*, 57(Suppl.2):81-87, 1998.

332. Fransen, J. and Russell, I.J.: *The Fibromyalgia Help Book: Practical Guide to Living Better with Fibromyalgia.* Saint Paul, Smith House Press, 1996.

333. Anderberg, U.M., Marteinsdottir, I., Hallman, J., and Bäckström, T.: Variability in cyclicity affects pain and other symptoms in female fibromyalgia syndrome patients. *J. Musculoskel. Pain*, 6(4):5-22, 1998.

334. Anderberg, U.M., Marteinsdottir, I., Hallman, J., Ekselius, L, and Bäckström, T.: Symptom perception in relation to hormonal status in in female fibromyalgia syndrome patients. *J. Musculoskel. Pain*, 7(3):21-38, 1999.

335. Kuczmierczyk, A.R., Adams, H.E., Calhoun, K.S., et al.: Pain responsivity in women with premenstrual syndrome across the menstrual cycle. *Percept. Mot. Skills*, 63(2

Pt.1):387-393, 1986.

336. Hallman, J.: The premenstrual syndrome: an equivalent of depression? *Acta Psychiatr. Scand.*, 73:403-411, 1986.

337. Andersch, B.: Epidemiological, hormonal, and water balance in studies in premenstrual tension. Thesis: Department of Gynecology and Psychiatry, Unversity of Gothenburg, Sweden, 1980.

338. Bäckström, T.: Neuroendocrinology of premenstrual syndrome. *Clin. Obstet. Gynaecol.*, 35(3):612-628, 1992.

339. Sherwin, B.B. and Gelfand, M.M.: Sex steroids and affect in the surgical menopause: a double-blind and cross-over study. *Psychoneuroendocrinology*, 10:325-335, 1985.

340. Montgomery, J.C., Appleby, L., Brincat, M., et al.: Effect of estrogen and testosterone implants on psychological disorders in the climacteric. *Lancet*, 7:297-299, 1987.

341. Dennerstein, L., Burrows, G.D., Hyman, G.J., and Sharpe, K.: Hormone therapy and affect. *Maturitas*, 1:247-259, 1979.

342. Ditcoff, E.J., Crary, W.G., Cristo, M., and Lobo, R.A.: Estrogen improves psychological function in asymptomatic postmenopausal women. *Obstet. Gynecol.*, 78:991-995, 1991.

343. Basson R.: Androgen replacement for women. *Can. Fam. Physician*, 45:2100-2107, 1999.

344. Sarrel, P.M.: Psychosexual effects of menopause: role of androgens. *Amer. J. Obstet. Gynecol.*, 180(3 Pt.2):319-324, 1999.

345. Sarrel, P., Dobay, B., and Wiita, B.: Estrogen and estrogen-androgen replacement in postmenopausal women dissatisfied with estrogen-only therapy. Sexual behavior and neuroendocrine responses. *J. Reprod. Med.*, 43(10):847-856, 1998.

346. Riley, A.J.: Life-long absence of sexual drive in a woman associated with 5-dihydrotestosterone deficiency. *J. Sex Marital Ther.*, 25(1):73-78, 1999.

347. Longcope, C.: The male and female reproductive systems in hypothyroidism. In *Werner and Ingbar's The Thyroid: A Fundamental and Clinical Text*, 6th edition. Edited by L.E. Braverman and R.D. Utiger, Philadelphia, J.B. Lippincott Co., 1991, pp.1052-1055.

348. *Merck Manual of Diagnosis and Therapy*, 15th edition. Edited by R. Berkow and A.J. Fletcher, Rahway, Merck, Sharp & Dohme Research Laboratories, 1987.

349. Berne, K.: *Running on Empty: The Complete Guide to Chronic Fatigue Syndrome.* Alameda, Huter House, Inc., Publishers, 1995.

350. Boyd, .P.R and Mark, G.J.: Multiple hepatic adenomas and a hepatocellular carcinoma in a man on oral methyl testosterone for eleven years. *Cancer*, 40(4):1765-1770, 1977.

351. Pope, H.G. and Katz, D.L.: Affective and psychotic symptoms associated with anabolic steroid use. *Amer. J. Psychiat.*, 145(4):487-490, 1988.

352. Longson, D.: Androgen therapy. *Practitioner*, 208(245): 338-348, 1972.

353. Skene, S.A., Dewhurst, I.C., and Greenberg, M.: Polychlorinated dibenzo-*p*-dioxins and polychlorinated dibenzofurans—the risks to human health: a review. *Human Toxicol.*, 8:173-203, 1989.

354. Safe, S.: Polychlorinated biphenyls and polybrominated biphenyls (PBBs): biochemistry, toxicology, and mecha-

nism of action. *Crit. Rev. Toxicol.*, 13:319-395, 1984.

355. Ruh, M.F., Ruh, T.S., and Klitgaard, H.M.: Uptake and retention of estrogens by uteri from rats in various thyroid states. *Proc. Soc. Exp. Biol. Med.*, 134:558-561, 1970.

356. Gardner, R.M., Kirkland, J.L., Ireland, J.S., and Stancel, G.M.: Regulation of the uterine response to estrogen by thyroid hormone. *Endocrinology,* 103:1164-1172, 1978.

357. Bronson, F.H.: Mammalian reproduction: an ecological perspective. *Biol. Reprod.*, 32:1-26, 1985.

358. Schneider, J.E. and Wade, G.N.: Decreased availability of metabolic fuels induces anestrus in golden hamsters. *Amer. J. Physiol.*, 258:R750-R755, 1990.

359. Gurguis, G.N., Yonkers, K.A., Phan, S.P., Blakeley, J.E., Williams, A., and Rush, A.J.: Adrenergic receptors in premenstrual dysphoric disorder: I. Platelet α_2-receptors: G_i protein coupling, phase of menstrual cycle, and prediction of luteal phase symptom severity. *Biol. Psychiat.*, 44(7): 600-609, 1998.

360. Jones, S.B., Bylund, D.B., Rieser, C.A., Shekim, W.O., Byer, J.A., and Carr. G.W.: α_2-Adrenergic receptor binding in human platelets: alterations during the menstrual cycle. *Clin. Pharmacol. Ther.*, 34(1):90-96, 1983.

361. Bennett, R.M., Clark, S.R., Campbell, S.M., et al.: Symptoms of Raynaud's syndrome in patients with fibromyalgia: a study utilizing the Nielsen test, digital photoplethysmography and measurements of platelet α_2-adrenergic receptors. *Arthritis and Rheumatism*, 34:264-269, 1991.

362. Seippel, L. and Backstrom, T.: Luteal-phase estradiol relates to symptom severity in patients with premenstrual syndrome. *J. Clin. Endocrinol. Metab.*, 83(6):1988-1992, 1998.

363. Redei, E. and Freeman, E.W.: Daily plasma estradiol and progesterone levels over the menstrual cycle and their relation to premenstrual symptoms. *Psychoneuroendocrinology*, 20(3):259-267, 1995.

364. Hammarback, S., Damber, J.E., and Backstrom, T.: Relationship between symptom severity and hormone changes in women with premenstrual syndrome. *J. Clin. Endocrinol. Metab.*, 68(1):125-130, 1989.

365. Wang, M., Seippel, L., Purdy, R.H., and Backstrom, T.: Relationship between symptom severity and steroid variation in women with premenstrual syndrome: study on serum pregnenolone, pregnenolone sulfate, 5 α-pregnane-3,20-dione and 3 α-hydroxy-5 α-pregnan-20-one. *J. Clin. Endocrinol. Metab.*, 81(3):1076-1082, 1996.

366. Nakayama, K., Nakagawa, T., Hiyama, T., Katsu, H., Wakutsu, N., Koga, M., and Usijima, S.: Circadian changes in body temperature during the menstrual cycle of healthy adult females and patients suffering from premenstrual syndrome. *Int. J. Clin. Pharmacol. Res.*, 17(4):155-164, 1997.

Section III

Interpretation of Fibromyalgia Symptoms and Objective Findings as Manifestations of Inadequate Thyroid Hormone Regulation

B. Mechanisms Underlying Particular Symptoms, Signs, and Findings

3.9

Cold and Heat Intolerance

Cold intolerance is common among fibromyalgia patients. Many patients report that they feel cold throughout most of their body, but more often, they complain of cold fingers and toes. Cold fingers and toes are called Raynaud's phenomenon or disease.

Normally, the sympathetic nervous system and the thyroid system interact to regulate body heat. In response to reduced environmental or core body temperature, the sympathetic nervous system becomes more active, and sympathetic nerve endings secrete more norepinephrine. The norepinephrine binds to α_2-adrenergic receptors on arterioles and arteries in the skin, inducing vasoconstriction. The vasoconstriction reduces blood flow. The reduced flow cools the skin by reducing heat loss from the blood. As a result, the heat of the general circulation is maintained.

Cold exposure also normally increases thyroid hormone secretion by the thyroid gland and conversion of T_4 to T_3. The increased availability of T_3 accelerates the metabolic rate of cells with heat production as a byproduct. The T_3 also induces a dramatic increase in heat generation by brown fat tissue. Because thyroid hormone potently stimulates the generation of heat, it is said to be "calorigenic" and "thermogenic" (heat producing).

Individuals with inadequate thyroid hormone regulation of cell function, due either to hypothyroidism or cellular resistance to thyroid hormone, typically feel too cold. Also, they are highly sensitive to relatively small reductions in environmental temperature. Their coldness and cold reactivity result from several mechanisms. First, their cells generate a subnormal amount of heat because of a reduced rate of meta-

bolism. The increase in α-adrenergic receptors contributes at several body loci. An increase in the density of the receptors in certain central nervous system centers and the sympathetic ganglia causes subnormal sympathetic nervous system responsiveness to stress such as cold. An increase in the density of receptors on the arterioles and arteries in the skin constricts the vessels and results in cold skin. Also, reduced regulation of many genes by thyroid hormone reduces the synthesis and breakdown of proteins. The reduction decreases the generation of body heat. Among the proteins that are synthesized in lower quantity are several enzymes that normally contribute substantially to body heat. The most important of these enzymes are α-glycerophosphate dehydrogenase, Na^+/K^+-ATPase, malic enzyme, and glucose-6-phosphate dehydrogenase.

During sleep, the temperature of patients with inadequate thyroid hormone regulation becomes even lower than when they are awake. This results from the patients' subnormal metabolism due to inadequate regulation by thyroid hormone being compounded by the normal 10%-to-15% reduction, on average, in metabolic rate during sleep. The sleep-related reduction in metabolism results from reduced activity of skeletal muscle and the sympathetic nervous system. This compounded cooling of patients is likely to result in some degree of heat generating (thermogenic) muscle contractions during sleep. The contractions may shorten tendons that cross joints, resulting in the perception of joint stiffness when the patient awakes. The perception would subside after the body warms when the person becomes active after rising from bed.

Thermogenic contractions in patients with a low

core temperature may compress trigger points in skeletal muscles. Nociceptive nerve signals from the trigger points may contribute to the patient's perception of fibromyalgic pain. These signals are also likely to contribute to sleep disturbance by activating the brain stem reticular activating system.

Excessive sensitivity to cold, termed cold intolerance, is common among fibromyalgia patients. Bennett wrote of a growing consensus that fibromyalgia patients, compared to the normal population, have an exaggerated response to cold. He suggested that the patients' exaggerated response to cold may account for their reporting that cold, damp weather intensifies their symptoms.[11,p.145]

A minority of fibromyalgia patients report heat intolerance.

● COLD INTOLERANCE IN FIBROMYALGIA

Fibromyalgia patients commonly report discomfort in response to temperatures that for most people are comfortable. An environment others consider cold, fibromyalgia patients may consider painfully cold. Many patients report feeling cold over most or all of the body. The thermal clothing used by some patients is testimony to their extraordinary cold sensitivity. Some patients are cold nearly all the time, even when wearing thermal clothing in a warm atmosphere. In the oppressive weather conditions of Texas, for example, many cold intolerant fibromyalgia patients experience as genial warmth the fierce summer heat that virtually melts the rest of humanity.

Fibromyalgia researchers have given particular attention to patients' cold fingers and toes, a symptom typical of Raynaud's phenomenon or disease (see next section). The patient's fingers and toes are usually the coldest body parts.

RAYNAUD'S PHENOMENON AND DISEASE

Raynaud's phenomenon is a distinct pathophysiological process characterized by constriction or spasm of arterioles and arteries.[6,p.333] The term Raynaud's phenomenon is used when the symptoms and objective findings of the condition are known to be secondary to another condition, such as trauma, thoracic outlet syn-

drome, or ergot toxicity.[19,p.563] When the cause is unknown (idiopathic), the term "Raynaud's disease" is used. Patients with either Raynaud's disease or phenomenon respond to cold exposure or emotional arousal with pallor and numbness, and possibly tingling and burning, of the digits of the hands and feet. These symptoms are usually followed by bluish or purplish coloration of the skin (cyanosis) which suggests inadequately oxygenated blood. The digits then turn red before resuming their normal color.

REPORTS OF RAYNAUD'S SYMPTOMS IN FIBROMYALGIA

Bengtsson and associates reported that 38% of their 55 fibromyalgia patients had the symptoms of Raynaud's phenomenon.[7] Vaerøy et al. reported that 53.3% of their fibromyalgia patients had a Raynaud's-like phenomenon in the toes, fingers, or both.[10] Dinerman et al. reported the symptoms in 30% of their fibromyalgia patients.[8] Ingram et al. reported an incidence of 20%-to-30% among their patients.[9] Bennett wrote that this 20%-to-30% compares with a 10% prevalence in the normal population.[11] Ingram and his group also reported that of 28 fibromyalgia patients in their study, 39% showed objective evidence of cold sensitivity.[9]

COLD SKIN IN FIBROMYALGIA PATIENTS

In a study of 42 fibromyalgia patients, Scudds et al. used infrared thermography to measure the resting temperatures of the patients' exposed backs. The researchers measured the temperature after a 20-minute stabilization period. They compared the result with the mean back temperature of myofascial pain patients. The mean resting back temperature of fibromyalgia patients' was significantly lower than that of myofascial pain patients. The mean temperature of fibromyalgia patients was 0.65° lower.[31]

Hau et al. found that compared to a healthy control group, fibromyalgia patients had a significantly lower baseline mean back temperature. The researchers wrote, "The significantly lower skin temperature in the FM [fibromyalgia] group implies that adrenergic sympathetic nerve activity in FM patients may be increased at rest."[32] The conjecture of increased sympathetic activity is based on the presumption that the patients' sympathetic nerves secrete an increased amount of norepinephrine. Normally, this occurs in response to reduced core body and environmental temperature.[69,p.799] The norepinephrine would bind to α_2-adrenergic receptors on skin blood vessels and induce vasoconstriction. The resulting reduced blood flow would cool the skin.

● COLD INTOLERANCE IN HYPOTHYROID AND EUTHYROID HYPOMETABOLIC PATIENTS

Hypothyroid patients commonly complain of cold sensitivity,[12][13,p.577][14] and many have Raynaud's symptoms.[19,p.563] Table 3.9.1 shows the percentage of hypothyroid patients and normal control subjects with symptoms and signs related to abnormal cold sensitivity in two studies. Several authors have reported cold sensitivity or coldness of the extremities in euthyroid hypometabolic patients.[15][16][17][18] In my clinical experience, roughly an equal percentage of hypothyroid and euthyroid hypometabolic fibromyalgia patients complain of cold intolerance.

INADEQUATE THYROID HORMONE REGULATION OF THERMOGENIC SYSTEMS OF THE BODY: MECHANISMS OF LOW BODY TEMPERATURE

Normal Interaction of the Sympathetic-Catecholamine-Adrenoceptor System and Thyroid Hormone

Normally, the sympathetic-catecholamine-adrenoceptor axis and thyroid hormone interact to maintain normal body temperature as a part of homeostasis.[20,p.176][33] When metabolic demand increases, as during exposure to cold, the sympathetic nervous system produces a rapid increase in metabolism. Sympathetic nerves release norepinephrine which binds to β-adrenergic receptors on cell membranes. As a result, cell metabolism accelerates and body heat simultaneously increases.

More gradual increases in metabolism occur through increases in thyroid hormone production and release, and by increased conversion of T_4 to T_3. Increased exposure of the adrenergic genes to T_3 increases transcription for β-adrenergic receptors and decreases transcription for α-adrenergic receptors. When the density of β-adrenergic receptors on cell

membranes increases, exposure of the cells to norepinephrine and epinephrine increases metabolism. Binding of β-adrenergic receptors to catecholamines increases glucose metabolism.[33] All the steps necessary for the release of energy from glucose increase. The steps include gluconeogenesis, glycogenolysis, glycolysis, an increase in blood glucose levels, and the peripheral tissue metabolism of glucose.[20,pp.168-169] Body heat increases from the acceleration of heat-liberating energy metabolism.

Table 3.9.1. Incidence of symptoms and signs related to abnormal cold sensitivity in hypothyroidism.*

SYMPTOMS & SIGNS	STUDY A % OF 77 CASES	STUDY B % OF 100 CASES	CONTROL SUBJECTS % OF 100
Sensation of cold	89	95	39
Decreased sweating	89	68	17
Cold skin	83	80	33
Pallor of skin	67	50	14
Pallor of lips	57	50	—†
Cyanosis‡	7	—	—

*The Thyroid and Its Diseases, by L.J. DeGroot, P.R. Larsen, S. Refetoff, and J.B. Stanbury, New York, John Wiley & Sons, 1984, pp.577-578.
†Dash indicates that the symptom or sign was not reported in the study.
‡Bluish or purplish coloration of the skin and mucous membranes.

When metabolic demand decreases, both the sympathetic-catecholamine-adrenoceptor axis and the thyroid system act independently to slow metabolism. Metabolic demand is low, for example, during fasting, starvation, or severe illness. During these times, sympathetic nerves decrease secretion of catecholamines; and thyroid hormone production, secretion, and conversion of T_4 to T_3 decrease. Decreased exposure of the adrenergic genes to T_3 decreases transcription for β-adrenergic receptors and increases transcription for α-adrenergic receptors. As a result, the density of β-adrenergic receptors on cell membranes decreases, and the density of α-adrenergic receptors increases. In this case, exposure of the cells to catecholamines decreases metabolism. Binding of α-adrenergic receptors to catecholamines decreases glucose metabolism. All the steps necessary for the release of energy from glucose decrease. Body heat decreases from the slowing of heat-liberating energy metabolism.

Impaired Metabolic Adaptation to Cold Exposure in Hypothyroidism: Contributing Mechanisms

In normal humans, exposure to cold induces nonshivering (facultative) thermogenesis. During this thermogenic process, an increased amount of energy is expended specifically to generate heat.[68,p.492] The mechanism of nonshivering thermogenesis is sympathetic nerve stimulation of brown adipose tissue[69,p.794] (see subsection below titled "Brown Adipose Tissue (BAT)"). In response to the increased sympathetic innervation, an increased amount of T_3 also becomes available to cells. During cold exposure in hypothyroid humans, however, the sympathetic-catecholamine-adrenoceptor axis and the thyroid system fail to induce adequate metabolic adjustments. As a result, body heat may not increase sufficiently to maintain comfort and homeostasis, and adaptation to cold is inadequate.[61][62]

Also in hypothyroidism, heat-generating enzymes that normally increase during cold exposure may not increase appropriately. For example, in hypothyroid individuals, malic enzyme and glucose-6-phosphate dehydrogenase (two NADPH-generating lipogenic enzymes) may not adequately increase during exposure to cold. In normal rats, cold exposure caused a time-dependent increase in the activity of the two enzymes in brown fat. The fat generating function of the enzymes is presumably to provide fat for heat production during whole-body cold exposure. After 96 hours of cold exposure, malic enzyme activity had increased 5.2-fold and glucose-6-phosphate dehydrogenase activity 3-fold. In hypothyroid rats, cold exposure did not increase the activity of the enzymes. Physiologic doses of T_4 restored the cold-induced increase in enzyme activity, but interestingly, T_3 did not.[35] (For low activity of other important heat-generating enzymes in hypothyroidism, see section immediately below.)

The increase in α-adrenergic receptors on cell membranes in hypothyroidism is perhaps the main underlying molecular mechanism responsible for the individual's inadequate adaptation to cold. An increased density of α-adrenergic receptors on the membranes of neural cells that regulate sympathetic nervous system activity causes subnormal sympathetic responsiveness to stress (see Chapter 3.1, subsection titled "Subnormal Sympathetic Response to Stresses in Hypothyroid and Fibromyalgia Patients"). In addition, the increased density of α-adrenergic receptors on the cell membranes of most peripheral tissue cells inhibits energy metabolism in the cells. The decreased sympathetic drive and decreased energy metabolism resulting from the increased density of α-adrenergic receptors result

in subnormal body temperature. Reduced core body temperature and vasoconstriction of blood vessels in the skin (mediated by α_2-adrenergic receptors presumably to conserve body heat) cause the patient to perceive being cold.

Regulation of Protein Synthesis and Degradation. Increased oxygen consumption and heat production accompany thyroid hormone stimulation of protein synthesis.[20,p.175] Chemical agents that block protein-producing transcription or translation decrease thermogenesis.[62] Danforth and Burger estimated that increased whole body protein turnover may account for as much as 70% of the calorigenic effects of thyroid hormone.[58] Thus, reduced protein turnover during inadequate thyroid hormone regulation of gene transcription may markedly reduce body heat production.

Among the proteins that cells produce in lower quantities during inadequate thyroid hormone regulation of transcription are four enzymes that contribute substantially to the production of body heat (see next section).

Regulation of Enzymes with Thermogenic Function. Thyroid hormone regulates the levels and activity of many enzymes. Two of the enzymes that have a strong thermogenic function are Na^+/K^+-ATPase and α-glycerophosphate dehydrogenase (see Chapter 2.2, subsection titled "Thyroid Hormone and Membrane Na^+/K^+-ATPase Activity," and subsection titled "Production of ATP").

Sodium/Potassium-ATPase *(Na^+/K^+-ATPase).* The enzyme probably most responsible for increasing body heat is Na^+/K^+-ATPase.[33] This enzyme uses cytoplasmic ATP to catalyze activity of the Na^+/K^+ pump. The pump is one of the main energy-using mechanisms of the cell. It accounts for 5%-to-40% of steady-state energy expenditure.[70] Heat is released as a by-product of the enzymatic activity. Thyroid hormone regulates genetic expression of Na^+/K^+-ATPase[71] (see Chapters 2.2 and 2.3). As exogenous thyroid hormone increases production of the enzyme, enzymatic activity increases. Body temperature rises as a result of the enzymatic activity.

α-Glycerophosphate Dehydrogenase. Thyroid hormone regulates levels of the mitochondrial enzyme, α-glycerophosphate dehydrogenase. This enzyme plays a key role in thermogenesis during cold exposure.[20,p.177][55] (See Chapter 2.2, subsection titled "Mitochondrial Energy Processes: Production of ATP.") Some researchers attribute most of the calorigenic (heat-producing) effects of thyroid hormone to the combined increase in α-glycerophosphate dehydrogenase and Na$^+$/K$^+$-ATPase.[59,p.207][60] Administration of thyroid hormone increases both these enzymes; thyroid hormone deficiency decreases them. Body heat rises secondarily to the thyroid hormone-induced production of the enzymes.

Inhibitory Molecules. Inadequate thyroid hormone regulation of gene transcription increases cellular production of three inhibitory molecules: α-adrenergic receptors, phosphodiesterase, and inhibitory G$_i$ proteins. (See Chapter 2.2, section titled "Molecular Byproducts that Mediate Hypometabolism: α-Adrenergic Receptors, Phosphodiesterase, and G$_i$ Proteins," and subsections titled "Interpretation of Fibromyalgia Features as Manifestations of Low β-Adrenergic Receptor and High α-Adrenergic Receptor Density," "Phosphodiesterase," and "G$_i$ Proteins.") Increases in these molecules account for most of the metabolic slow-down and hypothyroid-like symptoms and signs associated with inadequate thyroid hormone regulation of cell function. By slowing metabolism, these molecules secondarily contribute to reduced body temperature. When a hypothyroid patient takes enough exogenous thyroid hormone, the production of the inhibitory molecules decreases. As a result, cell metabolism increases and body temperature rises.

Increased α$_2$-Adrenergic Receptors. The cold skin of fibromyalgia patients is best accounted for by an increase in the density of α$_2$-adrenergic receptors on cutaneous blood vessels. I base this conjecture on the finding of an increased density of α$_2$-adrenergic receptors on the platelets of fibromyalgia patients.[29]

Brown Adipose Tissue (BAT). BAT, or brown fat, is a key thermogenic tissue in many mammals. The quantity of the tissue increases in cold adaptation or as a prelude to hibernation in some small mammals.[20,p.176]

The high thermogenic capacity of BAT results from its high heat production compared to ATP synthesis. Brown fat consists of many small fat globules rather than fewer large fat globules as in other adipose tissue. Brown fat cells contain a large number of mitochondria. Oxidative phosphorylation in the mitochondria is mainly "uncoupled." (For an explanation of the concept of coupling in relation to heat release, see Chapter 2.2, subsection titled "Mitochndrial Energy Processes: Production of ATP.") When sympathetic nerves secrete norepinephrine in BAT, the mitochondria produce virtually no ATP but produce large amounts of heat; practically all the oxidative energy promptly becomes heat.[69,p.794] The high heat production in relation to ATP synthesis occurs because of the activity of uncoupling protein (thermogenin) in the in-

ner mitochondrial membrane of BAT cells. The protein triggers uncoupled mitochondrial respiration. Ludvik wrote that uncoupling protein stimulates the release of stored energy as heat by dissipating the proton gradient.[43] The uncoupled respiration is a unique feature of BAT and permits an extraordinarily high capacity for heat production.[63][64]

Sympathetic Nervous System Innervation of BAT. The sympathetic nervous system strongly regulates BAT. Sympathetic nerves release norepinephrine in BAT. Binding of the norepinephrine to adrenergic receptors, mainly the β$_3$ subtype, dramatically increases BAT cell metabolism.[58]

β$_3$-Adrenergic Receptors. Of the β-adrenergic receptors in BAT, about 80% are the β$_3$-adrenergic receptor subtype.[44] In studies with laboratory animals, activation of β$_3$-adrenergic receptors causes significant weight loss. In humans, β$_3$-adrenergic receptor agonists have failed to stimulate significant energy expenditure and weight loss. Ludvik conjectured that the failure is due to the relatively small amount of brown fat in humans.[43] The amount of brown fat in humans varies considerably. When I took human dissection during my freshman year of chiropractic college, I had the opportunity to observe the cadaver of a 5-year-old girl (killed in an automobile accident) who had an extraordinary density of brown fat spread through her back torso. Most humans, however, have much less brown fat. The smaller quantity of brown fat in humans may contribute to less energy expenditure and heat production upon activation of β$_3$-adrenergic receptors. Nonetheless, the smaller quantity of BAT is probably not the only cause. Instead, a fairly rapid down regulation of β$_3$-adrenergic receptors may also contribute. Jockers et al. found that "prolonged treatment" (30-to-40 hours) with β$_3$-adrenergic receptor agonists completely "desensitized" the receptor response; that is, treatment with the agonist resulted in a rapid cessation of activation of adenyl cyclase in brown fat cell membranes by β$_3$-adrenergic receptors.[44] This finding suggests that rapid down regulation of β$_3$-adrenergic receptors, combined with a sparsity of BAT in humans, contributes to the limited usefulness of β$_3$-adrenergic receptor agonists in heat production and weight loss.

Increases of T$_3$ in BAT Induced by Sympathetic Innervation During Cold Exposure. The enzyme BAT T$_4$-5'-type II-deiodinase, which converts T$_4$ to T$_3$, plays a central role in controlling heat production in BAT. Cold exposure increases secretion of norepinephrine in BAT by sympathetic nerves. The norepinephrine increases heat production.[20,pp.176-177][33] An intermediate step in the increased heat production is an increase in the activity of T_4-5'-deiodinase in response to the increased exposure to norepinephrine.[53][65] Increased activity of the enzyme markedly increases the amount of T_3 in the fat cells of the tissue. Some of the T_3 escapes into the circulation and stimulates the metabolism of other peripheral tissues, increasing their contribution to thermogenesis during cold exposure.[66][67] The increased quantity of T_3 in BAT saturates the T_3-receptors in the nuclei of the fat cells, resulting in acceleration of mitochondrial respiration and heat production.

Inhibition of the enzyme by T_4 in hyperthyroidism appears to diminish thermogenesis by BAT. Brown fat heat production may also be diminished by a reduction in β_3-adrenergic receptors in BAT during thyrotoxicosis. Thyrotoxicosis uniquely reduces the expression of β_3-adrenergic receptors in brown adipose tissue. Silva wrote that the increased obligatory thermogenesis (necessary to maintain a constant high body temperature) in thyrotoxicosis, via afferent neural pathways, may reduce the hypothalamic stimulation of brown fat. The reduced hypothalamic stimulation would provide a second mechanism that limits BAT thermogenesis in hyperthyroidism.[33]

Decreased Transcription for Uncoupling Protein in Hypothyroidism. Ludvik reported that β_3-adrenergic receptor agonists have not been effective in increasing energy expenditure and weight loss in obese humans (see section immediately above). He suggested that uncoupling protein subtypes $_2$ and $_3$ might be more effective because they "dissipate the proton gradient, thereby releasing stored energy as heat."[43]

In BAT, norepinephrine release by the sympathetic nerve endings and increased T_4 to T_3 conversion induce expression of uncoupling protein.[53][54][55][56] Mitochondrial uncoupling protein is exclusively expressed in fat cells of brown adipose tissue.[46] Increases in uncoupling protein maximize heat production during metabolic stimulation by the sympathetic nervous system.[53][54][55][56] Norepinephrine and T_3 regulate transcription of the uncoupling gene. Norepinephrine provides the gene with the primary signal, and T_3, upon binding to T_3-receptors on the gene, stimulates transcription of uncoupling protein mRNA within a couple of hours. However, in hypothyroidism, increased transcription of uncoupling protein does not occur. This finding suggests that in hypothyroidism, the main mechanism of inadequate heat production by BAT during cold exposure is too little T_3 to activate transcription of uncoupling protein.[20,p.177][57]

Hermann et al. wrote that the unique presence of uncoupling protein permits BAT to expend calories unrelated to the performance of work. The expenditure causes higher heat generation than other tissues are capable of. Hermann et al. created mice with BAT deficiency. As a result, the mice had reduced energy expenditure and marked obesity, especially when fed the equivalent of a "Western diet" consisting of 41% fat. The researchers concluded that the thermogenic function of BAT is necessary for protection from diet induced obesity.[45]

Low Thyroid Hormone Receptor Density

Guernsy and Moroshige have shown that ob/ob mice have a low density of nuclear T_3 receptors in liver and lung tissues. The mice have normal circulating levels of thyroid hormones. Probably as an adaptation, they have superefficient metabolism. Yet they have blunted end organ responses to thyroid hormone. They have low resting oxygen consumption, and they cannot increase thermogenesis on exposure to cold. They thus have an inadequate ability to adapt to cold.[30,p.324]

Increased Cellular Sensitivity to Adenosine in Hypothyroidism

Cells have an increased sensitivity to adenosine in hypothyroidism. The increased sensitivity appears to result from the increase in G_i (inhibitory G protein) that occurs in hypothyroidism. (For descriptions of G_i, see Chapter 3.1, sections titled "Biochemical Factors Other than T_3 that Augment α-Adrenergic Responsiveness and Decrease β-Adrenergic Responsiveness of Cells in Hypothyroidism," and "Post-Adrenergic Receptor Mechanisms in the Cell Membrane that Mediate Catecholamine-Adrenoceptor Signals.") Apparently, the adenosine receptor, upon binding to adenosine, interacts with G_i to inhibit activation of adenylate cyclase.[40][41] In euthyroid rats, G_i is not increased, and when adenosine binds to adenosine receptors, the combination affects cells in a different way, interacting probably with G_s rather than increased G_i.

The increased sensitivity to adenosine in hypothyroidism has physiological consequences. For example, adenosine infusions into the kidneys of normal rats caused vasoconstriction and decreased glomerular flow. In hypothyroid rats, adenosine caused vasodilation and increased glomerular flow.[38] In hypothyroidism, white adipose tissue is more sensitive than normal to the inhibitory effects of adenosine.[39,p.1050]

Increased sensitivity of cells to adenosine may contribute to low body temperature of patients with inadequate thyroid hormone regulation of cell function. To appreciate the temperature lowering effect of increased cellular sensitivity to adenosine, it is interesting to consider an opposite effect—increased body temperature through the adenosine blocking effects of caffeine.

Effects of Caffeine on Body Temperature. In mice, intraperitoneal injections of caffeine (60 mg/kg) significantly elevated the temperature of brown adipose tissue, with a lower rise in core temperature. Oxygen consumption increased in the mitochondria of brown adipose tissue, and the resting metabolic rate increased. The investigators concluded that caffeine increases brown adipose tissue thermogenesis, and that this may contribute to increases in the metabolic rate.[3]

Koot and Deurenberg had young men consume 150 mL of decaffeinated coffee. Caffeine (200 mg) was added to some of the coffee. Measures were taken before coffee consumption (the fasting state) and up to 3 hours afterward. After caffeine-containing coffee was consumed, resting metabolic rate increased immediately (a mean of 0.2 kj/min) and remained increased for the 3 hours that measurements were taken. Mean caffeine-induced thermogenesis was 0.3 kj/min. This converts to a mean increase in metabolic rate of 7% during the 3 hours of measurements. Internal temperature began increasing after the coffee with or without caffeine was consumed, and at 2 hours, the temperature of subjects drinking caffeine-laced coffee was significantly different. Mean skin temperature increased after coffee consumption, and at 90 minutes post-consumption, those with caffeine in their coffee had a significantly elevated temperature compared to those without. The authors wrote that after caffeine consumption, energy expenditure increases first, and after some delay, internal and skin temperature also increase. Correlation between changed metabolic rate and increased skin temperature after caffeine consumption was low (r=0.38; P=0.06). They argued that based on their findings, using skin temperature to measure changes in energy expenditure is not justified.[2]

A single-dose oral intake of 100 mg of caffeine was shown to increase the resting metabolic rate of both lean individuals and those who had previously been obese (postobese subjects). There was a 3%-to-4% rise over 150 minutes. The postobese subjects had defective diet-induced thermogenesis that was improved by the caffeine-induced increase in metabolic rate. Repeated intake of 100 mg. of caffeine at 2-hour intervals over a 12-hour period during the day increased energy expenditure of both lean and postobese

subjects by 8% to 11% during that time. The subsequent night-time 12-hour resting metabolic rate was not influenced by the prior caffeine consumption. Lean subjects had a 150 kcal increase in daily energy expenditure, and postobese subjects had a 79 kcal increase. The investigators wrote, "Caffeine at commonly consumed doses can have a significant influence on energy balance and may promote thermogenesis in the treatment of obesity."[4]

Improvement of Raynaud's Symptoms with T_3

In some patients, Raynaud's symptoms are underlain by inadequate thyroid hormone regulation of the adrenergic genes and body temperature. This proposition is supported by recent studies showing that T_3 effectively improves Raynaud's symptoms. Dessein and Gledhill conducted a pilot study in which they found evidence that T_3 was an effective treatment for some patients with Raynaud's.[36] They subsequently conducted three other studies that showed the treatment to be effective.[34][37][42] They found that T_3 significantly reduced the frequency, duration, and severity of attacks of Raynaud's symptoms, and skin temperature in the hands significantly increased. Also, the time needed for skin temperature to rise to normal after exposure to cold significantly shortened.[34] The skin ulcers of 6 patients healed. The researchers used 60 μg-to-80 μg of T_3 to control "vasospastic attacks" in Raynaud's patients.[42] The improvement of patients' Raynaud's symptoms with the use of T_3 most likely resulted from a decrease in α_2-adrenergic receptors on the blood vessels of the skin (see Chapter 3.1, subsection titled "Pain").

OTHER THERMOGENIC REGULATORS THAT MAY BE INVOLVED IN LOW BODY TEMPERATURE

Lower Metabolic Rate in Females

Fibromyalgia appears to result from hypometabolism of specific tissues. Every fibromyalgia patient I have seen was hypometabolic, and I have never seen credible evidence of fibromyalgia in a hypermetabolic person. If a lowering of metabolism in certain tissues gives rise to fibromyalgia, then it becomes clear why women are more susceptible than men to develop fibromyalgia: The metabolism of women is normally lower than that of men, and less additional lowering of their metabolism is necessary to reach the threshold for generation of hypometabolism symptoms.

The difference in the metabolic rates of women and men is a result of differences in their sex hormones. Administration of male sex hormone increases the metabolic rate by 10%-to-15%; female sex hormone raises the metabolic rate a small but usually insignificant amount.[69,p.795] (See Chapter 3.6.) Although the metabolic rate of women is lower than that of men, body temperature of women may not be lower, probably because of their higher fat to lean tissue ratio.

According to Glickman-Weiss et al., males with higher percentages of body fat maintain higher core temperatures. Their aerobic metabolic rates are lower than males with lower percentages of body fat. The researchers wrote that this finding verifies that body fat has an "insulatory benefit." For example, because females have more body fat and less muscle than males, they are able to maintain rectal temperature at a lower energy cost. Glickman-Weiss et al. tested women with high and low body fat for thermal responses to acute exposure (120 minutes) to temperatures of 41° F (5° C) and 80.6° F (27° C). Rectal temperature was lower in women with low body fat. The investigators concluded that higher body fat provided significantly more insulation, enabling the subjects with high body fat to maintain higher rectal temperatures.[5]

McLellan subjected males and females to heat stress. He had them wear nuclear, biological, and chemical protective clothing while they engaged in intermittent walking and seated rest. The environmental temperature was maintained at 104° F (40° C) at 30% relative humidity. The mean heart rate of females was higher throughout the study. Their mean skin temperature was higher and their sweat and evaporation rates from the clothing were lower than those of males. The rectal temperature of the females increased faster, and they tolerated the heat for a shorter time. McLellan concluded that the females were at a thermoregulator disadvantage compared to the males under the test conditions. He attributed the disadvantage to two factors: (1) the lower specific heat of fat tissue versus lean tissue (specific heat is the amount of heat required to raise the temperature of any substance by 1° compared with that required to raise the temperature of the same volume of water 1°), and (2) the higher percentage of body fat in females.[73]

Despite the differences in how females and males respond to cold based on dissimilarity in the percentage of body fat, the differences are also significantly influenced by other factors. Pettit et al., based on their findings, concluded that males and females exhibit striking differences in cardiovascular and metabolic responses to cold air exposure. The researchers also concluded that the percentage of body fat did not account for the differences. When exposed to 41° F (5° C), males had a greater increase in heart stroke volume than did females. Also, males had greater decreases in heart rate and skin temperature. Moreover, the contribution of carbohydrates and fats to total energy expenditure differed. The carbohydrate to fat ratio of men was 47:53; that of women was 36:64.[28]

Sleep

The metabolic rate decreases by 10%-to-15% during sleep. According to Guyton, the decrease occurs because of reduced skeletal muscle tone and lowered sympathetic nervous system activity during sleep.[69,p.795] The decrease in the metabolic rate during sleep worsens the status of the patient who is symptomatic while awake due to hypometabolism caused by inadequate thyroid hormone regulation. The reduced body heat during sleep probably contributes to the shortening of muscles during sleep so that the patient perceives stiffness upon awakening (see Chapter 3.20, section titled "Possible Mechanisms of Stiffness in Fibromyalgia Patients: Thermogenic Contractions").

Landis et al. found that after one night of sleep deprivation, the esophageal and rectal temperatures of 6 young healthy women were decreased. Warming the women's skin to 104° F (38° C) resulted in an attenuated dilation of cutaneous blood vessels. Following a mild increase in skin temperature with the heat, the skin was cooled and held at 89.6° F (32° C). The cooling caused a rapid decrease in esophageal and rectal temperature. The researchers wrote that sleep deprivation caused the women to lose heat rapidly in response to mild cooling stimulus. They speculated that sleep-deprived humans (1) are more vulnerable to heat loss, and (2) they have a diminished ability to warm at temperatures that are normally comfortable to humans.[72] The outcome of this study raises the possibility that fibromyalgia patients' sleep disturbance and deprivation may contribute to their cold sensitivity.

Feasting and Thermogenesis

Feasting on a balanced meal of carbohydrate, fat, and protein increases resting metabolic rate, respiratory quotient, and body temperature.[1] Consumption of the average meal also transiently increases body temperature (postprandial thermogenesis). Some patients with inadequate thyroid hormone regulation of cell function may consume large amounts of food at a sitting. The resulting postprandial thermogenesis may provide them brief relief from the discomfort of a low body temperature. However, hypothyroid patients typically have a reduced appetite and lower than normal food intake.

THERMOGENIC MUSCLE CONTRACTIONS: POSSIBLE ACTIVATOR OF MYOFASCIAL TRIGGER POINT PAIN

The patient who is sensitive to cold may consciously tighten various muscles as an instinctive method of increasing body heat. Muscles also contract involuntarily as part of "shivering thermogenesis." (Shivering thermogenesis is invoked when cold signals from the skin and spinal cord activate the primary motor center for shivering in the posterior hypothalamus. Signals from the center descend through bilateral tracts in the brain stem and the lateral columns of the spinal cord and synapse with ventral horn cells. Signals from the ventral horns are then transmitted to skeletal muscles throughout the body. Shivering of the muscles occurs when their tone increases sufficiently. The shivering can increase body heat 4-to-5 times normal.[69,p.803]) The muscle contractions increase the metabolism of the muscle cells and increase their heat production. (See Chapter 3.20, section titled "Possible Mechanisms of Stiffness in Fibromyalgia Patients: Thermogenic Contractions.")

When an irritable trigger point is housed in a muscle that contracts to generate heat, the pressure in the muscle may increase sufficiently to further irritate the trigger point. If the trigger point was latent (was not actively referring pain) before the contractions, it may become active. If the point was mildly active before the contractions, the referral of pain may intensify. (See Chapter 3.16, subsection titled "Trigger Points as a Source of Paresthesia: Hypometabolism as a Perpetuating Factor.")

POSSIBLE MECHANISM OF COLD INTOLERANCE IN FIBROMYALGIA

Bennett pointed out that catecholamines produce relative dilation of myofascial arterioles but, in contrast, the hormones induce constriction of skin arterioles.[11,pp.145-146] He also noted that catecholamines stimulate cutaneous vasoconstriction upon binding to α_2-adrenergic receptors on skin arterioles.[11,p.146] Bennett also wrote that the possible relation of cold sensitivity to the pathogenesis of fibromyalgia is obscure.[11,p.145] I contend that the possible relation is clear—inadequate thyroid hormone regulation of the

α_2-adrenergic gene plausibly accounts for the increase in α_2-adrenergic receptors on the platelets of fibromyalgia patients,[29] their Raynaud's symptoms, and in part, for their general cold sensitivity and cold intolerance.

The metabolic rate decreases during inadequate thyroid hormone regulation of cell function, and the decreased metabolism reduces heat generation. Some physiological adjustments occur that conserve body heat. For example, skin blood vessels constrict, reducing heat loss from the blood through the skin. The sympathetic nervous system of some patients compensates for low body temperature[23,p.904] by increasing circulating norepinephrine.[24][25][26] The elevated norepinephrine binds to the increased numbers of α_2-adrenergic receptors, increasing constriction of skin blood vessels.[27,p.198] The vasoconstriction lowers the temperature of the skin and the patient feels cold.[21][22] Despite the reduced heat loss through vasoconstriction, in most patients body temperature is usually reduced due to subnormal function of other physiological mechanisms. Specifically, cold adaptation is subnormal because of impairment of the sympathetic nervous system and the thyroid system.[20,p.202] As a result, the patient is excessively sensitive to relatively mild environmental cold.

● HEAT INTOLERANCE

Some fibromyalgia patients are heat rather than cold intolerant. Their heat intolerance is consistent with heat intolerance in a minority of hypothyroid patients. In a study of 100 hypothyroid patients, 2% were heat intolerant. Among euthyroid subjects, 12% were heat intolerant.[13,p.578] Corman described heat intolerance and agitation in hypothyroidism,[48] and Bodnar et al. described the heat intolerance as an "atypical manifestation" of hypothyroidism.[50] Garcia et al. wrote that the symptom is a rare feature of hypothyroidism that may suggest the opposite condition, hyperthyroidism.[51]

We can only speculate about why some hypothyroid patients are heat sensitive. I can find no studies that specifically address the issue. It is possible that in these individuals, the mechanisms of heat production and heat loss are not synchronous. Thus, in general terms, heat loss may be subnormal enough so that heat production, although subnormal, keeps the core temperature high enough for the patient to find environmental heat uncomfortable. McNabb speculated in a similar respect regarding hyperthyroid patients who do not have heat intolerance. She wrote that alterations in heat loss may compensate for increased heat production, resulting in a constant, normal body temperature.[20,p.166]

HEAT INTOLERANCE FROM EXCESS THYROID HORMONE INTAKE AND MENOPAUSE

Heat intolerance occurs in many patients who take dosages of thyroid hormone that are excessive for them. The perception of excessive body heat is for the most part persistent, although the perception may be more intense during physical exertion and exposure to environmental heat. The clinician must be able to distinguish the fairly persistent perception of excess body heat from excess thyroid hormone from the hot flashes of menopause. Hot flashes are common among menopausal women. For example, among 614 menopausal Thai women, 347 (57%) reported hot flushes. Heat intolerance was also common among the 614 women.[52]

OTHER FACTORS THAT MAY CAUSE OR CONTRIBUTE TO HEAT INTOLERANCE

Kenny listed among correlates of heat intolerance (1) a history of heat illness, (2) previous difficulty in acclimating or reacclimating to heat, (3) low aerobic fitness level, (4) age, (5) hypertension, (6) high body fat content, (7) small body size, (8) alcohol consumption, and (9) use of narcotics and other prescription drugs.[47] The clinician should consider such correlates with an aim to controlling them to relieve heat intolerance in the fibromyalgia patient whose intolerance is not improving during metabolic rehabilitation.

Of special interest is the possibility that antidepressant medications, which clinicians commonly prescribe for fibromyalgia patients, may cause heat intolerance. Epstein et al. described a case in which fluoxetin (Prozac) and lithium carbonate induced heat intolerance that resulted in heat stroke when the patient worked for 4 hours in a hot and dry climate. A year later, the patient had atrophy of the cerebellum and residual cerebellar symptoms. The authors stated that to their knowledge, theirs was the first description of a patient developing heat intolerance from the use of combined fluoxetin and lithium.[49]

REFERENCES

1. Owen, O.E., Reichard, G.A., Jr., Patel, M.S., and Boden, G.: Energy metabolism in feasting and fasting. *Adv. Exper. Med. Biol.*, 111:169-188, 1979.

2. Koot, P. and Deurenberg, P.: Comparison of changes in energy expenditure and body temperatures after caffeine consumption. *Ann. Nutri. Metab.*, 39(3):135-142, 1995.

3. Yoshioka, K., Yoshida, T., Kamanaru, K., Hiraoka, N., and Kondo, M.: Caffeine activates brown adipose tissue thermogenesis and metabolic rate in mice. *J. Nutri. Sci. Vitaminology*, 36(2):173-178, 1990.

4. Dulloo, A.G., Geissler, C.A., Horton, T., Collins, A., and Miller, D.S.: Normal caffeine consumption: influences on thermogenesis and daily energy expenditure in lean and postobese human volunteers. *Amer. J. Clin. Nutri.*, 49(1): 44-50, 1989.

5. Glickman-Weiss, E.L., Nelson, A.G., Hearon, C.M., Prisby, R., and Caine, N.: Thermal and metabolic responses of women with high fat versus low fat body composition during exposure to 5° and 27° C for 120 min. *Aviat. Space Environ. Med.*, 70(3 Pt.1):284-288, 1999.

6. Chandrasoma, P. and Taylor, C.R.: *Concise Pathology.* Appleton & Lange, Norwalk, 1991.

7. Bengtsson, A., Henriksson, K.G., Jorfeldt, L., Kagedal, B., Lennmarken, C., and Lindstrom, F.: Primary fibromyalgia: a clinical and laboratory study of 55 patients. *Scan. J. Rheumatol.*, 15:340-347, 1986.

8. Dinerman, H., Goldenberg, D.L., and Felson, D.T.: A prospective evaluation of 118 patients with the fibromyalgia syndrome: prevalence of Raynaud's phenomenon, sicca symptoms, ANA, low complement and Ig disposition at the dermal-epidermal junction. *J. Rheumatol.*, 13:368-373, 1986.

9. Ingram, S., Nelson, D., Porter, J., et al: An association of cold induced vasospasm and fibrositis. *Arthritis Rheumat.*, 30:513, 1987.

10. Vaerøy, H., Helle, R., Øystein, F., Kåss, E., and Terenius, L.: Elevated CSF levels of substance P and high incidence of Raynaud's phenomenon in patients with fibromyalgia: new features for diagnosis. *Pain*, 32:21-26, 1988.

11. Bennett, R.M.: Muscle physiology and cold reactivity in the fibromyalgia syndrome. *Rheumat. Dis. Clin. N. Amer.*, 15:135-147, 1989.

12. Kirk, E. and Kvorning, S.A.: *Hypometabolism: A Clinical Study of 308 Consecutive Cases.* Copenhagen, Einar Munksgaard, Publisher, 1946.

13. DeGroot, L.J., Larsen, P.R., Refetoff, S., and Stanbury, J.B.: *The Thyroid and Its Diseases,* 5th edition. New York, John Wiley & Sons, Inc., 1984.

14. Watanakunakorn, C., Hodges, R.E., and Evans, T.C.: Myxedema: a study of 400 cases. *Arch. Intern. Med.*, 116:183-190, 1965.

15. Thurmon, F.M. and Thompson, W.O.: Low basal metabolism with myxedema. *Arch. Intern. Med.*, 46:879-897, 1930.

16. Kurland, G.S., Hamolsky, M.W., and Freedberg, A.S.: Studies in non-myxedematous hypometabolism: I. The clinical syndrome and the effects of triiodothyronine, alone or combined with thyroxine. *J. Clin. Endocrinol.*, 15:1354, 1955.

17. Fields, E.M.: Treatment of metabolic insufficiency and hypothyroidism with sodium liothyronine. *J.A.M.A.*, 163:817, 1957.

18. Tittle, C.R.: Effects of 3,5,3' l-triiodothyronine in patients with metabolic insufficiency. *J.A.M.A.*, 162:271, 1956.

19. *The Merck Manual of Diagnosis and Therapy*, 15th edition. Edited by R. Berkow and A.J. Fletcher, Rahway, Merck, Sharp & Dohme Research Laboratories, 1987.

20. McNabb, F.M.A.: *Thyroid Hormones.* Englewood Cliffs, Prentice Hall, 1992.

21. Fregly, M.F., Nelson, E.L., and Resch, G.E.: Reduced beta-adrenergic responsiveness in hypothyroid rats. *Amer. J. Physiol.* 229:916, 1975.

22. Grill, V. and Rosenquist, U.: Inhibition of the noradrenaline induced adenyl cyclase stimulation by augmented and adrenergic response in subcutaneous adipose tissue from hypothyroid subjects. *Acta Med. Scand.*,194:129, 1973.

23. Guyton, A.C.: *Textbook of Medical Physiology*, 7th edition. W.B. Saunders Co., Philadelphia, 1986.

24. Wahi, R.S., Chansouria, J.P.N., and Udupa, K.N.: Normal levels of norepinephrine in short term hypothyroidism. *J. Clin. Endocrinol. Metab.*, 51:934-935, 1980.

25. Lipton, M.A., Prange, A.J., Dairman, W., and Udenfriend, S.: Increased rate of norepinephrine biosynthesis in hypothyroid rats. *Fed. Proc.*, 27:399, 1968.

26. Prange, A.J., Jr., Meed, J.L., and Lipton, M.A.: Catecholamines: diminished rate of norepinephrine biosynthesis in rat brain and heart after thyroxine pretreatment. *Life Sci.*, 9:901, 1970.

27. deVries, H.A.: *Physiology of Exercise*, 4th edition. Dubuque, Wm. C. Brown Publishers, 1986.

28. Pettit, S.E., Marchand, I., and Graham, T.: Gender differences in cardiovascular and catecholamine responses to cold-air exposure at rest. *Can. J. Appl. Physiol.*, 24(2):131-147, 1999.

29. Bennett, R.M., Clark, S.R., Campbell, S.M., et al.: Symptoms of Raynaud's syndrome in patients with fibromyalgia. A study utilizing the Nielsen test, digital photoplethysmography and measurements of platelet α_2-adrenergic receptors. *Arthritis Rheum.*, 34(3):264-269, 1991.

30. Tepperman, J. and Tepperman, H.M.: *Metabolic and Endocrine Physiology*, 5th edition. Chicago, Year Book Medical Publishers, Inc., 1987.

31. Scudds, R.A., Heck, C., Delaney, G., and Teassell, R.W.: A comparison of referred pain, resting skin temperature, and other signs in fibromyalgia (FM) and myofascial pain syndrome (MPS). *J. Musculoskel. Pain*, 3(1):121, 1995.

32. Hau, P.P., Scudds, R.A., and Harth, M.: The measurement of mechanically induced erythema by thermography in patients with fibromyalgia. *J. Musculoskel. Pain*, 3(Suppl.1): 98, 1995.

33. Silva, J.E.: Thyroid hormone control of thermogenesis and energy balance. *Thyroid,* 5(6):481-492, 1995.

34. Dessein, P.H., Morrison, R.C., Lamparelli, R.D., and van der Merwe, C.A.: Triiodothyronine treatment for Raynaud's phenomenon: a controlled trial. *J. Rheumatol.*, 17: 1025-1028, 1990.

35. Carvalho, S.D., Negrao, N., and Bianco, A.C.: Hormonal regulation of malic enzyme and glucose-6-phosphate dehydrogenase in brown adipose tissue. *Amer. J. Physiol.*, 264 (6 Pt.1):E874-E881, 1993.

36. Dessein, P.H. and Gledhill, R.F.: Treatment of Raynaud's phenomenon with large doses of triiodothyronine: a pilot study. *Ann. Rheum. Dis.*, 46(12):944-945, 1987.

37. Dessein, P.H. and Gledhill, R.F.: Triiodothyronine in Raynaud's phenomenon: further objective evidence of its beneficial effect. *Br. J. Rheumatol.*, 27(3):244-246, 1988.

38. Franco, M., Bobadilla, N.A., Suarez, J., Tapia, E., Sanchez, L., and Herrera-Acosta, J.: Participation of adenosine in the renal hemodynamic abnormalities of hypothyroidism. *Amer. J. Physiol.*, 270(2 Pt.2):F254-F262, 1996.

39. Silva, J.E. and Landsberg, L.: Catecholamines and the sympathoadrenal system in hypothyroidism. In *Werner's The Thyroid: A Fundamental and Clinical Text*, 6th edition. Edited by L.E. Braverman and R.D. Utiger, Philadelphia, J.B. Lippincott Co., 1991, pp.1050-1051.

40. Mazurkiewicz, D. and Saggerson, E.D.: Inhibition of adenylate cyclase in rat brain synaptosomal membranes by GTP and phenylisopropyladenosine is enhanced in hypothyroidism. *Biochem. J.*, 263(3):829-835, 1989.

41. Malbon, C.C., Rapiejko, P.J., and Mangano, T.J.: Fat cell adenylate cyclase system. Enhanced inhibition by adenosine and GTP in the hypothyroid rat. *J. Biol. Chem.*, 260 (4):2558-2564, 1985.

42. Gledhill, R.F., Dessein, P.H., and van der Merwe, C.A.: Treatment of Raynaud's phenomenon with triiodothyronine corrects co-existent autonomic dysfunction: preliminary findings. *Postgrad. Med. J.*, 68(798):263-267, 1992.

43. Ludvik, B.: Weight loss by increasing energy consumption and thermogenesis. *Acta Med. Austriaca.*, 25(4-5):136-137, 1998.

44. Jockers, R., Issad, T., Zilberfarb, V., de Coppet, P., Marullo, S., and Strosberg, A.D.: Desensitization of the β-adrenergic response in human brown adipocytes. *Endocrinology*, 139(6):2676-2684, 1998.

45. Hamann, A., Flier, J.S., and Lowell, B.B.: Obesity after genetic ablation of brown adipose tissue. *Z. Ernährungswiss*, 37(Suppl.1):1-7, 1998.

46. Oberkofler, H., Dallinger, G., Liu, Y.M., Hell, E., Krempler, F., and Patsch, W.: Uncoupling protein gene: quantification of expression levels in adipose tissues of obese and non-obese humans. *J. Lipid Res.*, 38(10):2125-2133, 1997.

47. Kenney, WL. Physiological correlates of heat intolerance. *Sports Med.*, 2(4):279-286, 1985.

48. Corman, L.C.: Agitation and heat intolerance in hypothyroidism. *Arch. Intern. Med.*, 141(7):959-960, 1981.

49. Epstein, Y., Albukrek, D., Kalmovitc, B., Moran, D.S., and Shapiro, Y.: Heat intolerance induced by antidepressants. *Ann. N.Y. Acad. Sci.*, 813:553-558, 1997.

50. Bodnar, P.N., Donish, R.M., and Romashkan, S.V.: Atypical manifestations of hypothyroidism. *Klin. Med.* (Mosk.), 64(5):86-92, 1986.

51. Garcia Zamalloa, A., Ojeda Perez, E., Vargas Cerdan, M., Suarez Munoz, F., and Isaba Senosiain, L.: Hypothyroidism state with psychomotor agitation and fast atrial fibrillation: a rare form of presentation. *An. Med. Interna.*, 9(8): 391-392, 1992.

52. Sukwatana, P., Meekhangvan, J., Tamrongterakul, T., Tanapat, Y., Asavarait, S., and Boonjitrpimon, P.: Menopausal symptoms among Thai women in Bangkok. *Maturitas*, 13 (3):217-228, 1991.

53. Bianco, A.C. and Silva, J.E.: Optimal response of key en-

zymes and uncoupling protein to cold in BAT depends on local T_3 generation. *Amer. J. Physiol.*, 253:E255-E263, 1987.

54. Bianco, A.C. and Silva, J.E.: Intracellular conversion of thyroxine to triiodothyronine is required for the optimal thermogenic function of brown adipose tissue. *J. Clin. Invest.*, 79:295-300, 1987.

55. Bianco, A.C. and Silva, J.E.: Nuclear 3,5,3'-triiodothyronine (T_3) in brown adipose tissue: receptor occupancy and sources of T_3 as determined by *in vivo* techniques. *Endocrinology*, 120:55-62, 1987.

56. Bianco, A.C. and Silva, J.E.: Cold exposure rapidly induces virtual saturation of brown adipose tissue nuclear T_3 receptors. *Amer. J. Physiol.*, 255:E496-E503, 1988.

57. Bianco, A.C., Sheng, X., and Silva, J.E.: Triiodothyronine amplifies norepinephrine stimulation of uncoupling protein gene transcription by a mechanism not requiring protein synthesis. *J. Biol. Chem.*, 263:18168-18175, 1988.

58. Danforth, E., Jr. and Burger, A.: The role of thyroid hormones in the control of energy expenditure. *Clin. Endocrinol. Metab.*, 13:581-595, 1984.

59. Shambaugh, III, G.E.: Biologic and cellular effects. In *The Thyroid: A Fundamental and Clinical Text*, 5th edition. Edited by S.C. Werner and S.H. Ingbar, New York, Harper and Row, Publishers, 1986.

60. Bronk, J.R. and Bronk, M.S.: The influence of thyroxine on oxidative phosphorylation in mitochondria from thyroidectomized rats. *J. Biol. Chem.*, 237:897, 1962.

61. Van Hardeveld, C.: Effects of thyroid hormone on oxygen consumption, heat production, and energy economy. In *Thyroid Hormone Metabolism.* Edited by G. Hennemann, New York, Marcel Dekker, 1986, pp.579-808.

62. Hock, F.L.: Metabolic effects of thyroid hormones. In *Handbook of Physiology*, Vol. III: Section 7, Endocrinology: Thyroid. Edited by M.A. Greer and D.H. Solomon, Washington, D.C., Amer. Physiol. Society, 1974, pp.391-411.

63. Cannon, B. and Bedergaard, J.: The biochemistry of an inefficient tissue: brown adipose tissue. *Essays Biochem.*, 20:110-163, 1985.

64. Nicholls, D.G. and Locke, R.M.: Thermogenic mechanisms in brown fat. *Physiol. Rev.*, 64:1-64, 1984.

65. Silva, J.E. and Larsen, P.R.: Adrenergic activation of triiodothyronine production in brown adipose tissue. *Nature*, 305:712-713, 1983.

66. Silva, J.E. and Larsen, P.R.: Potential of brown adipose tissue type II thyroxine (T_4) 5'-deiodinase as a local and systemic source of triiodothyronine (T_3) in rats. *J. Clin. Invest.*, 76(6):2296-2305, 1985.

67. Fernandez, J.A., Mampel, T., Villarroya, F., and Iglesias, R.: Direct assessment of brown adipose tissue as a site of systemic triiodothyronine production in the rat. *Biochem. J.*, 243:281-284, 1987.

68. Berne, R.M. and Levy, M.N.: *Principles of Physiology*. St. Louis, C.V. Mosby Company, 1990.

69. Guyton, A.C.: *Textbook of Medical Physiology*, 8th edition. Philadelphia, W.B. Saunders, 1991.

70. Ismail-Beigi, F. and Edelman, I.S.: The mechanism of the calorigenic action of thyroid hormone. Stimulation of Na^+-K^+-activated adenosinetriphosphatase activity. *J. Gen. Physiol.*, 57(6):710-722, 1971.

71. Ismail-Beigi, F.: Thyroid hormone regulation of Na^+-K^+-ATPase expression. *Trends Endocrinol. Metab.*, 4:152-155, 1993.

72. Landis, C.A., Savage, M.V., Lentz, M.J., and Brengelmann, G.L.: Sleep deprivation alters body temperature dynamics to mild cooling and heating but not sweating threshold in women. *Sleep*, 21(1):101-108, 1998.

73. McLellan, T.M.: Sex-related differences in thermoregulatory responses while wearing protective clothing. *Eur. J. Appl. Physiol.*, 78(1):28-37, 1998.

3.10

Depression, Anxiety, and Cognitive Dysfunction

Psychological Status of Fibromyalgia Patients

Studies of the psychological status of fibromyalgia patients show that the prevalence of psychological disorders is about the same as in rheumatoid arthritis patients. One study showed that the incidence of psychological disorders of fibromyalgia patients in a primary health care facility was no different from other clinic patients used as controls. The incidence of psychological disorders apparently increases in patients referred to speciality clinics. This indicates that the protracted and intense suffering of fibromyalgia patients referred to such clinics is responsible for the increase in occurrence of psychological disturbances. It also indicates that psychological disturbances are not the cause of fibromyalgia. Researchers have determined that psychological abnormalities are not essential to the diagnosis of fibromyalgia.

Adverse Psychosocial Consequences of Having Fibromyalgia

Many fibromyalgia patients have adverse psychosocial consequences from having fibromyagia. These range from a lack of understanding and sympathy of loved ones, coworkers, and clinicians. Some people may show annoyance and harshly judge the patient for claiming to have symptoms of a disorder for which there is no visible evidence. Other patients suffer distress resulting from dwindling or exhausted financial reserves from paying for diagnostic services and failed treatments and from an inability to work.

Depression in Fibromyalgia

In a primary care clinic, fibromyalgia patients were no more depressed than control patients. In specialty clinics, a higher than normal percentage of fibromyalgia patients had depression in the past and present depression, but the prevalence of depression is no higher than that of rheumatoid arthritis patients. Several possible mechanisms may underlie the depression of fibromyalgia patients who are hypothyroid and/or thyroid hormone resistant: (1) an increase of α_2-adrenergic receptors, (2) a decrease of β-adrenergic receptors, (3) decreased serotonin secretion, (4) increased monoamine oxidase activity, and (5) too little vigorous physical activity. Each of these mechanisms can result from inadequate thyroid hormone regulation of cell function.

Anxiety in Fibromyalgia

It appears that fibromyalgia patients in primary care clinics do not have a higher incidence or intensity of anxiety than other patients used as controls. However, in speciality clinics, fibromyalgia patients have an increased prevalence and intensity of anxiety. The greater prevalence and intensity of anxiety are probably features of the increase in psychological disturbance associated with more severe or protracted suffering from fibromyalgia.

In patients whose fibromyalgia is a result of severe hypothyroidism or thyroid hormone resistance, anxiety may result from excessive sympathetic nervous system activity as a compensation for severe hypometabolism. The increased density of α_2-adrenergic receptors in sympathetic nerve cell bodies would increase the resistance of the sympathetic nervous system from activating except by strong stimuli. Strong stimuli, however, would cause sudden surges of sympathetic activity. Against the background of a precarious prognosis and other occupational and social concerns, the patient may perceive the generalized sympathetic arousal to be anxiety.

Cognitive Dysfunction in Fibromyalgia

The patient whose fibromyalgia is underlain by inadequate thyroid hormone regulation of cell function is likely to have cognitive dysfunction. The inadequate regulation may cause the dysfunction by increasing the density of α-adrenergic receptors and decreasing the density of β-adrenergic receptors on brain cells and cerebral blood vessels. The results of these changes are subnormal brain cell metabolism and reduced brain blood flow. The brain has a higher metabolic rate than other tissues, and insufficient delivery of oxygen, glucose, and other metabolic substrates to brain cells is likely to result in their dysfunction. The dysfunction is likely to occur because the use of brain cells, as during thinking, increases their metabolic rate and the flow of blood to them through local vessels. The changes induced by inadequate thyroid hormone regulation impede both of these physiological accompaniments of thinking. Cognitive dysfunction is likely to result despite reduced metabolic demand of the cells due to the change in the density of adrenergic receptor types on their membranes.

Adverse Psychological
Effects of Hypothyroidism

Medical writers described the adverse psychological effects of hypothyroidism as far back as the late 19th century. The two main effects include depression and cognitive dysfunction. However, adult patients may have emotional lability, mental sluggishness, diminished spontaniety and indifference, and self-accusatory ruminations. In more severe cases, patient may have suspiciousness, delusions with ideas of persecution, and delirium ("myxedema madness"). Children may also have learning problems and generally delayed development. The range and severity of symptoms usually progressively increase with untreated hypothyroidism of more severe degrees. However, severe psychological symptoms often accompany the

mildest degree of thyroid hormone deficiency. In addition, clinical experience shows some patients with mild thyroid hormone resistance also have severe psychological symptoms.

The psychological abnormalities of fibromyalgia patients appear to be caused by two main factors. One is inadequate thyroid hormone regulation of cell function, and the other is the adverse psychosocial consequences of living with ineffectively treated fibromyalgia.

● PSYCHOLOGICAL STATUS OF FIBROMYALGIA PATIENTS

Hugh Smythe is a rheumatologist who has been highly active in fibromyalgia research. In 1972, a chapter he wrote on fibromyalgia (then called "fibrositis") was published in a rheumatology textbook. In the chapter, Smythe cautiously discussed the putative role of psychogenesis in fibromyalgia. He wrote: "The use of the term 'psychogenic rheumatism' as a synonym for fibrositis has drawn attention to an important contributing factor . . . but has not served the patients well. Most patients and many doctors have understood this term to imply that the pain is imaginary or hysterical in origin, which is very rarely the case."[1,pp.874-875]

Smythe made some distinctions between fibromyalgia and what might be considered "psychogenic pain." He wrote: "The fibrositis syndrome lacks the bizarre features of symbolic psychogenic regional pain. The symptoms are similar from patient to patient, and the tender points predictable and relatively constant in location. The term 'tension rheumatism' more accurately describes the psychogenic mechanism involved, but fails to account for the pain and tenderness found over bony promenences and other non-muscular areas."[1,p.875]

In 1977, in collaboration with Moldofsky, Smythe dropped the word "psychogenic," even as a conservatively applied qualifier and redefined fibromyalgia as a nonrestorative sleep syndrome.[28] His decision to drop the term as a qualifier has since been supported by studies of the psychological status of fibromyalgia patients. Researchers have found that fibromyalgia patients have about the same prevalence of psychological disorders as other chronic pain patients. The prevalence increases for the most part only in patients reaching tertiary facilities. This indicates that their prolonged and intense suffering are the cause of their higher incidence of psychological disturbances, and the psychological disturbances are not the cause of fibromyalgia.

Three studies in the 1980s, in which researchers used the Minnesota Multiphasic Personality Inventory, showed that about one-third of the fibromyalgia patients had significant psychological disturbance.[6][7][8] In one study, investigators claimed that the patients' fibromyalgia symptoms (pain, fatigue, and sleep disturbance) did not explain the abnormal MMPI test results.[8] This is a dubious interpretation of the study results.

In 1994, Yunus studied the psychological factors in fibromyalgia. He reported that two factors distinguish fibromyalgia from psychogenic rheumatism: the consistent finding of tender points and a demonstrable aberrant central pain mechanism.[2][3] He pointed out that some 25%-to-35% of patients in specialty rheumatology clinics have significant psychological distress. In contrast, a study in a primary care internal medicine clinic assessing the psychological status of fibromyalgia patients showed no differences between fibromyalgia patients and clinic controls. Yunus concluded, "Presently available data indicate that [fibromyalgia] is not a psychiatric condition."[4]

Researchers have compared the psychological status of fibromyalgia patients to that of other chronic pain patients. They used several methods of assessment, including a standardized interview, the Illness Behavior Questionnaire, Chronic Illness Problem Inventory, and the Symptom Check List. The status of fibromyalgia patients was similar to that of other chronic pain patients.[18] Psychological profiles of fibromyalgia patients did not correlate with several fibromyalgia features: number of painful body sites, number of tender points, sleep disturbance, fatigue, subjective swelling, paresthesia, or the description "I hurt all over." The severity of pain, however, was associated with psychological disturbance.[5] The intensity of rheumatoid arthritis patients' pain is also associated with their degree of psychological disturbance.[29] In another study, researchers found no significant difference between fibromyalgia and rheumatoid arthritis patients in any lifetime psychological abnormality, including anxiety, depression, or somatization.[11] These findings justify the conclusion from 1987[4] and 1991[5] studies that psychological abnormalities are not essential to the diagnosis of fibromyalgia.

ADVERSE PSYCHOSOCIAL CIRCUMSTANCES ASSOCIATED WITH HAVING FIBROMYALGIA

Yunus wrote that the higher incidence of psychological distress among fibromyalgia patients at specialty clinics (rheumatology clinics, for example, as opposed to primary clinics such as family medicine practices) may represent referral bias; that is, perhaps clinicians more readily refer psychologically troubled fibromyalgia patients to specialty facilities.[4] In addition to referral bias, it is likely that patients referred to specialty clinics have more severe and prolonged fibromyalgia. Their more intense and protracted suffering might lead to psychological symptoms for several reasons. One is the frustration of more failed treatments. Another is impatience of or harsh accusations from loved ones, coworkers, and clinicians over the patients' complaints and dysfunction despite the absence of visible evidence of disease.

Goldstein described well the adverse psychosocial consequences of patients having chronic fatigue syndrome, which he,[119] as I, believes are probably the same as fibromyalgia patients: "Husbands have beaten their wives because they thought they were lazy, and divorces have occurred because the spouse did not understand the illness and/or could not handle the pressures of living with a person who had a chronic, disabling illness which could not be authentically demonstrated to much of the medical profession. The general public, relatives, friends, and neighbors may be afraid of 'catching it.' Patients may withdraw from social interactions not just because of fatigue, but because friends do not understand chronic fatigue syndrome, and the patient gets tired of making up excuses for unavailability."[19,p.54]

One study recently showed that in several countries, chronic pain patients had a significantly higher percentage of psychological disturbance. Oye et al., in a World Health Organization study, sought to determine the impact of persistent pain on primary care patients. Fifteen primary care centers were included. The centers were located in Asia, Africa, Europe, and the Americas. Of 25,916 patients, ranging in age from 18-to-65 years, 5,438 were interviewed. Across the 15 centers, 22% of patients reported persistent pain, defined as the experience of pain most of the time for 6 months or more during the previous year. The incidence of pain across the centers varied from 5.5%-to-33.0%. Researchers conducted standard tests to assess the incidence of psychological disturbance, lability, and limitation of activity among the patients. Compared to patients without persistent pain, those with persistent pain had a significantly higher incidence of anxiety and depressive disorders, limited activity, and perceptions of poor health. The researchers wrote that the relationship between anxiety and depressive disorders and persistent pain occurred among patients in all 15 centers.[49,p.1222] In that fibromyalgia patients have chronic widespread pain, it is reasonable to expect adverse psychological effects in some, as with the chronic pain patients described in this study.

Table 3.10.1. Ten common psychological symptoms in hypothyroidism.

1. Depression
2. Emotional lability
3. Mental sluggishness
4. Diminished spontaniety and indifference
5. Self-accusatory ruminations
6. Suspiciousness
7. Delusions with ideas of persecution
8. Delirium ("Myxedema Madness")
9. Coma
10. In children, learning problems and overall delayed development

*From Walker, S., III.: *Psychiatric Signs and Symptoms Due to Medical Problems.* Springfield, Charles C. Thomas, Publisher, 1967.[58,pp.112-113]

Among the population of patients with chronic pain, fibromyalgia patients are especially likely to be subjected to a condition that appears especially to engender psychological disturbance—financial strain. In my experience, many fibromyalgia patients find themselves impecunious because they have spent tens of thousands of dollars pursuing relief through clinical care. Not only do some patients no longer have expendable money, but they still have fibromyalgia symptoms that impede their ability to work and generate more money.

Weich and Lewis, in a study of 7,726 adults in England, Wales, and Scotland, recently found that financial strain was strongly associated with both the onset and maintenance of common mental disorders. They wrote that unemployment and poverty increased the prevalence of mental disorders by sustaining them.[167] This result supports the common observation that fibromyalgia patients who are unemployed and in poverty have anxiety and depression. In some patients, dwindling financial resources and the inability to work

exacerbate and/or prolong psychological disorders associated with the fibromyalgia patient's prolonged illness, failed treatment, and lack of social support.

● PSYCHOLOGICAL EFFECTS OF HYPOTHYROIDISM

As I have shown in various chapters of this book, hypothyroidism may profoundly affect both the nervous system and endocrine system, the two main regulatory systems of the body. Hypothyroidism can also profoundly affect the brain, where the regulatory centers of the nervous and endocrine systems reside. The brain effects include depression, anxiety, and cognitive dysfunction. Table 3.10.1 lists the most common psychological symptoms associated with hypothyroidism.

PSYCHOLOGICAL SYMPTOMS AND HYPOTHYROIDISM

In the 1960s, American psychology was dominated by a behaviorist model that largely ignored biological influences on thought, emotion, and behavior. In the 1970s, cognitive psychology, which also largely neglected biological factors, became more prominent. Over the past 30 years, however, most scientists and clinicians from diverse disciplines have come to accept that biological and psychological functions intricately interact.[40,pp.vii-viii][41][42]

It is surprising that this understanding of biological/psychological interaction came so slowly, for, as Walker showed in 1967, many psychological symptoms are common features of medical diseases. He also described the common psychological symptoms of hypothyroid patients.[58] Other medical writers began describing adverse mental, emotional, and overt behavioral effects typical of untreated hypothyroidism in the late 19th century.[41][43][44][45][46][48][148] For the clinician familiar with the psychological effects of hypothyroidism, the diagnosis is easy to make when psychological changes are extreme and clear-cut. When the patient also has classic physical features of hypothyroidism, the diagnosis is especially easy. The clinician should note, however: (1) in either mild or severe hypothyroidism, the psychological changes may be subtle, and (2) psychological changes may be the earliest or most prominent feature of hypothyroidism of any severity.[47,p.911]

Psychological Changes in Hypothyroidism

Weiner has described the progression of psychological symptoms as hypothyroidism becomes more severe. Initially, the patient may complain of vague symptoms such as "weakness" and "lack of interest in things." As the changes progress, she may complain of many symptoms. She may have trouble concentrating; sluggish thinking; and diminished ability to calculate mentally, answer questions, or recall the proper word to express herself. Her memory for recent events may be poor, and after awhile she may lose her memory for remote events. As the severity of the thyroid hormone deficiency progresses, her ability to perform daily, routine tasks may diminish. She may become less attentive and responsive to others, lack interest in her surroundings, and she may lose her capacity for learning and performing new tasks. She may speak less and, when she does talk, she tends to repeat herself. Her actions are likely to be slow and the accuracy of her perceptions diminished. She may also form illusions, and as her condition worsens, she may have visual and other hallucinations.[47,p.911] These mental/perceptual tendencies may progress to paranoid ideas and behavior. If her hypothyroidism becomes more severe, she is likely to be drowsy and lethargic. In extremely severe hypothyroidism, the patient may lapse into a stupor and coma.[49,p.1222] A similar sequence of symptoms is likely to occur in patients with progressively worsening cellular resistance to thyroid hormone.

Some features of this clinical progression of symptoms may easily lead to a diagnosis of endogenous depression or depressive mood state.[47,p.911] At this time, a psychiatrist or other clinician are likely to neglect to make a proper differential diagnosis and select a *DSM* label that describes patients' sets of symptoms. Then he will prescribe one or more psychotropic medications "appropriate" to the label,[150] leaving the hypothyroidism uncorrected , enabling it to exert a variety of adverse effects, while relieving the patient to some degree of annoyance by its psychological effects.

Hypothyroidism may indeed cause a melancholic disorder.[50] The patient may cry easily, have little desire for food, suffer from constipation, sleep poorly, obsessively reproach herself, and ponder suicide. Paradoxically, some patients develop a disorganized agitated state rather than depression.[51][52][53][54] They may be unable to sleep, hyperactive, irritable, and angry. Some patients have auditory and visual hallucinations. Other patients are fearful, suspicious, and delusional. Depression predominates, but the specific mental state and thought content varies with the individual patient.[49,p.1222] "The changes in mood and content of thought," Weiner wrote, "are characteristic of the individual patient, whereas the alterations in attention, concentration, perception, and form and speed of thought and action are common to all."[47,p.911]

Cerebellar Involvement

Severe hypothyroidism may cause impairing and even devastating central nervous system signs and symptoms. These include coma, convulsions[30][31][32] and psychosis. The patient may have impaired cranial nerve function, and his cerebrospinal fluid may contain elevated levels of protein and gamma globulin.

Some of the earliest literature on adult hypothyroidism mentions unsteady gait. In 1910, Soederbergh identified the condition as true cerebellar ataxia.[34] Recently, investigators have again focused attention on the condition.[35] In most reports, patients have been middle-aged or elderly, and their gait became ataxic over a period of months or years. In some cases, the patient could not stand or walk without help.

The patient walks in shuffling steps. She has an intention tremor of her upper extremities and her alternating movements are slow. She is uncoordinated, and she makes rapid and brusque movements with more force than necessary (dysmetria). She may have difficulty speaking and her speech may be defective because of impaired speech muscles (dysarthria).

Some ataxic patients are mentally alert. This suggests that they have a cerebellar deficit rather than psychomotor retardation or lethargy. Researchers have not definitely determined the lesion responsible for the ataxia. The lesion is probably molecular. The reversibility of the condition with treatment indicates this. The use of T$_4$ has restored normal or near normal motor function in most patients.[37,p.904] If the lesion involved large portions of the cerebellar tissue, the ataxia would not respond so well to treatment.

Dementia

In extremely severe hypothyroidism, the patient's cerebral function may seriously deteriorate. She may gradually lose effectiveness at sensing, thinking, and moving. She talks less and ceases to respond much to her environment, and her mental activity diminishes. She may express abnormal ideas and behave in bizarre ways. Of particular interest is her extreme tendency to sleep called somnolence. She lies inert, either drowsy or asleep, most of the day. One of Adams and Rosman's patients slept 21 or 22 hours each day. Others had to prod him to eat. His state approached myxedematous coma, yet a detailed neurologic exam revealed no abnormalities. Adams and Rosman pointed out that this type of patient usually has well-coordinated movements. Typically, her body temperature is low and she has slowed tendon reflexes.[37,pp.904-905] The patient's EEGs usually substantiate that she had impaired cerebral function.[38]

No one has confirmed an association between a specific lesion and hypothyroid dementia, but researchers implicate slowed cerebral blood flow and metabolism.[39] The lesions may be functional and not structural. There are two reasons for concluding this: (1) the use of exogenous thyroid hormone reverses the patient's dementia, and (2) no one has identified visible ischemic cortical lesions,[37,p.905] suggesting that structural damage of brain tissue has not occurred.

IMPLICATIONS OF THE BRAIN EFFECTS OF HYPOTHYROIDISM

The extreme cerebellar and cerebral effects of severe hypothyroidism make one point clear— neurological abnormalities are an important part of the thyroid hormone deficiency, and they are probably also a part of cellular resistance to thyroid hormone. Milder degrees of hypothyroidism usually cause less clear-cut and less severe central nervous system abnormalities. These may not debilitate a patient, as severe hypothyroidism may. Still, though, they may diminish her performance and quality of life. A sluggish mind and faulty memory, for example, impose costly social, academic, and occupational limitations on an individual. And the depression that may afflict a patient with only mild hypothyroidism can sabotage the patient's potential to live a normal life, and it can lead to her suicide. When hypothyroidism or thyroid hormone resistance underlies a patient's fibromyalgia, she is as likely as other hypothyroid patients to suffer from these psychological abnormalities.

● DEPRESSION

DEPRESSION IN FIBROMYALGIA

Wolfe reported that 31.5% of U.S. fibromyalgia patients have had prior depression.[25] By contrast, researchers reported that of 47 Brazilian women with fibromyalgia, 80% had depression.[26] This high percentage may have resulted from sampling error and is not representative of the wider population of fibromy-

algia patients in Brazil. Only 12% of control subjects had depression. Of three other studies,[9][10][11] only one showed significant past or present depression in fibromyalgia patients compared to rheumatoid arthritis patients.

Other writers have reported different percentages of depression, depending on the methods of evaluation used. Hudson, for example, reported that 29% of fibromyalgia patients were experiencing significant depression.[9] Goldenberg found that of 31 fibromyalgia patients, 71% had prior depression. At the time of Goldenberg's study, only 26% of the patients were depressed. In another sample of 82 fibromyalgia patients, he found that 46% had depression in the past, and 13% were presently depressed.[103,p.69] When evaluated with the Zung Self-Rating Depression Scale, fibromyalgia patients were not more depressed than rheumatoid arthritis patients.[12] Similarly, when assessed with the Beck Depression Inventory, fibromyalgia patients in a primary care clinic were not more depressed than control patients.[4]

Yunus argued that it is not appropriate to apply the diagnostic term "affective spectrum disorder" to fibromyalgia patients,[2,p.89] as others suggested.[15] In support of his argument, he cited a study showing nonsuppression of cortisol by dexamethasone in only 25% of fibromyalgia patients[16] and another study showing that 3H-imipramine binding in fibromyalgia patients is different from binding in depressed patients.[17] He concluded, "Taken together, it appears fairly clear that fibromyalgia is not primarily due to depression, and these two conditions are biochemically different."[2,p.89] Mountz and coworkers found that fibromyalgia patients had higher depression scores than controls. He attributed the depression to the significantly reduced blood flow through thalamus and caudate nuclei of patients.[27]

Many fibromyalgia patients have a history of depression before the onset of their fibromyalgia.[36,pp.45-46][104,p.62][168] In Goldenberg's sample of 31 fibromyalgia patients, 64% had depression before the onset of fibromyalgia. The average number of years between the onset of depression and the onset of fibromyalgia was 11 years. The range was 1-to-30 years. Of another sample of 14 fibromyalgia patients with a history of major depression, depression preceded the onset of fibromyalgia by an average of 6.7 years.[103,p.69] The range was 1-to-14 years.[9,p.443] Many fibromyalgia patients, upon careful questioning, recall experiencing several symptoms characteristic of inadequate thyroid hormone regulation, only one of which was depression, long before the onset of fibromyalgia.

I believe this is evidence that many patients have a history of borderline sufficient or insufficient metabolism, manifested as depression and other symptoms, intermittently or chronically, before developing fibromyalgia. They appear to be predisposed to develop the full array of fibromyalgia symptoms and signs upon the occurrence of some precipitating event. I have explained this putative mechanism in detail in Chapter 3.5 (see the section titled "A Putative Etiological and Exacerbating Role for Increased Cortisol Levels").

In two studies, investigators found that family members of fibromyalgia patients had a higher incidence of major depression than those of patients with rheumatoid arthritis.[9,p.443][103,p.69] This finding may represent common learned behaviors, but it may also represent the mood effect of genetically-determined hypothyroidism and/or resistance to thyroid hormone. One or both inherited mechanisms may affect multiple members of families, causing depression. However, only some family members may have the full spectrum of fibromyalgia symptoms and signs.

A Linking Physiological Mechanism

Goldenberg wrote that his test results suggest a relationship between fibromyalgia and depression.[103,p.69] He notes that 26% of his study patients were depressed at the onset of their fibromyalgia symptoms. To him, this indicated a common psychobiological association between depression and fibromyalgia, but not necessarily a causal connection. He also noted that fibromyalgia patients and depressed patients have other features in common: sleep disturbance, anxiety, "tension" headaches, fatigue, irritable bowel syndrome, and dry eyes. "Such symptoms," he wrote, "may be linked in some physiological fashion." It is likely that the link is the mechanism proposed in this book—inadequate thyroid hormone regulation of cell function—as ample evidence shows that this mechanism can generate the entire array of symptoms and signs shared by fibromyalgia and depressed patients.

DEPRESSION IN HYPOTHYROIDISM

For many patients, the first symptoms of hypothyroidism are depression and cognitive dysfunction.[47,p.911] Deep depression may result from even occult hypothyroidism.[56][57] Not all hypothyroid patients have depression, but the symptom is common among thyroid hormone deficient patients.[132] Some researchers have reported that hypothyroidism pre-

disposes patients to depression, and correction of the hypothyroidism improves or relieve the depression.[76] In a study of 100 hypothyroid patients, 60% were depressed.[133,p.578] One writer reported depression as a symptom in 23% of euthyroid hypometabolic patients.[134] The authors of these reports did not specify whether patients' depression was mild, moderate, or severe; nor did they state whether their patients' depression was prior or present. Loosen and Prange reported that 25% of depressed patients may have occult thyroid dysfunction.[56]

Deep Depression in Borderline Hypothyroidism and Thyroid Hormone Resistance

The hypothyroidism of a depressed patient may be so mild that even an astute clinician may overlook it. Some authors have proposed that some 25% of depressed patients have occult hypofunction of the thyroid gland.[56]

Gewirtz et al. suggested that some depressed patients' tissues have a blunted response to T_3 and T_4. They conjectured that the blunted responsiveness is due to faulty binding of thyroid hormone to thyroid hormone receptors. This, of course, is one mechanism of thyroid hormone resistance (see Chapter 2.5). Because tests for nuclear binding of thyroid hormone were not readily available at the time, they used other laboratory methods to evaluate 15 patients with refractory depression. All patients had clinical indications of hypothyroidism: they were overweight, sluggish, bothered by obsessional ruminations, and had slow thought processes. The researchers found that 6 of the patients had laboratory evidence of hypothyroidism. Their T_3 and T_4 blood levels were within the normal range, but their metabolic rates were low and their TSH levels elevated. Exogenous thyroid hormone relieved the patients' depression. The researchers concluded that checking the circulating levels of T_3 and T_4 is of little value in detecting the hypothyroidism of such patients. The diagnostic methods they recommended, in addition to clinical judgement of the patient's condition, were the TSH level, antithyroid antibody titer, and the basal metabolic rate.[57]

Possible Mechanisms

Possible mechanisms underlying depression in hypothyroid and/or thyroid hormone resistant fibromyalgia patients include an increase of α_2-adrenergic receptors, a decrease of β-adrenergic receptors, decreased serotonin secretion, increased monoamine oxidase activity, and insufficient vigorous physical activity. Each of these mechanisms can result from inadequate thyroid hormone regulation of cell function.

Increased α_2-Adrenergic Receptors. Nichols and Ruffolo defined depression as a disturbance of mood "severe enough to alter cognition, judgment, and interpersonal relationships."[135,p.123] One important regulator of mood is norepinephrine-secreting neurons from locus ceruleus in the brain stem that pass to and innervate the hippocampus, which is a part of the limbic system.[136] Stimulating the hippocampus causes hyperexcitability.[137] Injecting norepinephrine locally into the structure increases the activity of rats in the open field and in laboratory tests.[136] Neurons of the locus ceruleus have a low resting rate of secretion of norepinephrine. The low secretory rate may result from ongoing tonic α_2-adrenergic receptor inhibition of neuronal firing. Blocking of α_2-adrenergic receptor activity stimulates norepinephrine secretion by noradrenergic neurons.[138] Activation of α_2-adrenergic receptors in locus ceruleus noradrenergic neurons that terminate in the hippocampus inhibits their secretion of norepinephrine. The inhibition of norepinephrine secretion causes behavioral depression. In addition, as Nichols and Ruffolo noted, release of norepinephrine from the terminals of locus ceruleus neurons in the hippocampus is controlled by α_2-adrenergic receptors on the terminals. Activating the receptors reduces release of norepinephrine, and inhibiting them increases norepinephrine release.[135,pp.123-124]

It is likely that depression in fibromyalgia patients who have hypothyroidism and/or thyroid hormone resistance is mediated in part by inhibited norepinephrine secretion in the hippocampus. This is highly probable because inadequate thyroid hormone regulation of transcription of the adrenergic genes increases the density of α_2-adrenergic receptors on cell membranes.

Decreased β-Adrenergic Receptors. Thyroid hormone regulates adrenergic receptor isoforms. In thyroid hormone deficiency, β-adrenergic receptor density on cell membranes decreases. The decrease of β-adrenergic receptors results in a dominance of α-adrenergic receptor-mediated effects on cells. The main effects are a slowing of intracellular metabolic processes. (See Chapter 3.1.)

Most physiological and biochemical responses to catecholamines are reduced in hypothyroid tissues.[115,p.385] Most hypothyroid patients are distinctly hypoadrenergic (cool, sluggish, anergic, hypotensive, and depressed), as though they have undergone a biochemical sympathectomy at the receptor level. This effect results in part from the finding that hypothyroid rats have a decreased density of β-adrenergic receptors in brain tissues such as the cerebral cortex[110][112] and the cerebellum.[113]

The increased synthesis of norepinephrine in severe hypothyroidism is probably a less than complete compensation for the decreased number of β-adrenergic receptors.[117] Upon finding that T_3 increased the effectiveness of imipramine (a drug that increases norepinephrine at synapses by blocking its inactivation),[107,p.408] Prange et al. wrote that their patients were probably hypometabolic because of borderline hypothyroidism or from some non-thyroidal mechanism. In either case, T_3 enhanced adrenergic receptor responses to whatever amount of neural transmitter (norepinephrine) was present at the synaptic cleft. This corresponds to other studies showing that T_3 heightens nerve tissue responses to tricyclic antidepressants (shown by increased postsynaptic cyclic AMP).[111,p.243] Prange et al. wrote, "We propose that slight shifts in thyroid state toward hypothyroidism, although still within the statistical range of normality, affect nervous tissue—and perhaps only nervous tissue—in such a fashion as to produce a predisposition to retarded depression."[116]

One clinical effect of a subnormal density of β-adrenergic receptors on brain cell membranes is depression. Depression is an adverse effect of some patients taking β-adrenergic receptor blocking drugs that pass the brain blood barrier. By inhibiting β-adrenergic receptors in various brain regions, the drugs produce fatigue, sleep disturbance, and mental depression.[107,p.239] This set of symptoms, of course, is typical of fibromyalgia patients. This observation supports the hypothesis that inadequate thyroid hormone regulation of the adrenergic genes, by decreasing the density of β-adrenergic receptors on brain cell membranes, produces some features of fibromyalgia—fatigue, disturbed sleep, and depression. Another finding supports the hypothesis: that depression associated with low norepinephrine or serotonin levels can be reduced or relieved by β_2-adrenergic agonist drugs such as salbutamol, which increase both noradrenergic and serotonergic activity.[97]

A word about norepinephrine levels in fibromyalgia patients is in order here. According to the catecholamine hypothesis of mood or emotional disorders, an inadequacy of norepinephrine in the central nervous system may cause depression.[76][77,p.509] This hypothesis is relevant to depression in fibromyalgia patients because of the finding of low cerebrospinal fluid levels of the metabolite of norepinephrine in fibromyalgia patients.[114] Even when the norepinephrine level is not low, however, the same effect, depression, is expected from a subnormal density of β-adrenergic receptors on brain cell membranes. The overall body of information contained in this book, information which includes the finding of an increased density of α_2-adrenergic receptors on the platelets of fibromyalgia patients,[80] argues strongly that inadequate thyroid hormone regulation of cell function is the main underlying mechanism of fibromyalgia. One effect of the inadequate regulation is a decreased density of β-adrenergic receptors on brain cell membranes. A decreased density of these receptors, combined with a decreased brain level of norepinephrine, almost guarantees that the result for fibromyalgia patients will be depression.

Low Serotonin Levels. Serotonin is a neurotransmitter that is important in emotional states,[79] and impaired serotonergic mechanisms may play a role in the depression of hypothyroid patients. Abnormalities of the serotonin system may be involved in the pathophysiology of depression of many patients.[120][121][122][123] Several of the anatomical projections of serotonergic fibers from the brain stem innervate brain regions that control a variety of "mood-related" behaviors, such as appetite, sleep, and attention.[120][122] The simultaneous alteration of these behaviors in depressed patients suggests a close link between the serotonin system and depression.[124] Through models constructed to explain the effects of antidepressant treatments, researchers have concluded that intensification of serotonergic function is the common underlying factor in most treatments.[125]

Serotonin, Thyroid Hormone, and α_2-Adrenergic Receptors. Thyroid hormone plays an important role in the regulation of serotonin levels.[78] Central serotonin function may be decreased in hypothyroidism.[126][127][128] Among the types of serotonin receptors in the brain, the 5-HT$_{1A}$ receptor is principally involved in mediating anxiety and depression.[121] This receptor is abundant in the nucleus raphe dorsalis and limbic areas such as the cortex and hippocampus.[122] These brain areas also have high level gene expression for the three types of c-*erb*Aα thyroid hormone receptors and the c-*erb*Aβ$_1$ thyroid hormone receptor.[129][130] Tejani-Butt et al. found that at 7 and 35 days after thyroidectomy in rats, binding of a highly specific radioactive ligand to 5-HT$_{1A}$ receptors significantly increased in the cortex and hippocampus. Thyroidectomy did not increase 5-HT$_{1A}$ receptor binding in the hypothalamus where the density of the receptors is normally low. It also did not increase binding in the nucleus raphe dorsalis. High doses of T$_4$ for 28 days

returned binding to normal levels in the cortex. Binding increased in the hippocampus and hypothalamus, and did not change in the dorsal raphe nucleus. The investigators wrote: "These results suggest that a neuromodulatory link may exist between the hypothalamic-pituitary-thyroid axis and 5-HT$_{1A}$ receptors in the limbic regions of the rat brain. Depending on the brain region examined, a differential response to circulating levels of thyroid hormone was observed."[124,p.1011]

Whatever the direct effects of thyroid hormone on serotonin levels, the hormone exerts indirect control over serotonin secretion through adrenergic receptors on serotonin-secreting neurons. Activation of β$_2$-adrenergic receptors increases the activity of serotonin-secreting neurons.[97] Activation of α$_2$-adrenergic receptors inhibits serotonin secretion (see Chapter 2.3, section titled "Serotonin"). Such findings indicate that the decreased density of β-adrenergic receptors and the increase in the density of α$_2$-adrenergic receptors occur when transcription of the adrenergic genes by thyroid hormone potentially decreases serotonin secretion.[55][81][82][118] The decreased secretion may contribute to the depression of hypothyroid and/or thyroid hormone resistant fibromyalgia patients.

Antidepressant Medications as a Fibromyalgia Treatment. Some antidepressant medications lengthen the sojourn of serotonin in serotonergic neural synapses. In doing so, the medications may relieve the depression caused by hypothyroidism. In some cases, the depression relief is lifesaving. In many other cases, however, in which thyroid hormone deficiency or resistance underlies the depression, relief through the medication is a potentially costly expediency. As a rule, clinicians today are trained and pressured to quickly pick a *DSM* label that is descriptive of the patient's set of symptoms or main symptom, such as depression. They are also trained to prescribe for the patient, in cookbook fashion, a medication recommended by drug manufacturers and researchers whose work the manufacturers fund. This convenient way to "diagnose" and treat has led to diagnostic laziness and a failure to perform proper differential diagnoses.[150] When a clinician fails to differentially diagnose a patient's hypothyroidism or thyroid hormone resistance and merely diminishes or relieves a patient's depression by antidepressant medication, other pathologic effects of the undiagnosed and untreated thyroid hormone deficiency or resistance will continue apace. One pathological effect that may end a patient's life prematurely is atherosclerotic cardiovascular disease (see Chapter 4.4, section titled "Harm from Untreated and Undertreated Hypothyroidism"). Such long-range risks would best be a serious concern of patients and clinicians who wish to practice according to the Hippocratic admonition, "First, do no harm." Tragically, in that most patients' fibromyalgia is underlain mainly by inadequate thyroid hormone regulation of cell function, the widespread use of antidepressant medications as the main fibromyalgia treatment raises serious ethical and humanitarian concerns. This is all the more so in that antidepressant treatment is ineffective as a fibromyalgia treatment.

Monoamine Oxidase (MAO) Activity. When norepinephrine (or epinephrine) is released at synapses, much of it is removed by deamination (removal of its single amino radical, or NH_2). The mitochondrial enzyme MAO catalyzed the deamination.[107,pp.103&415] (See Chapter 3.1, section titled "Metabolic Degradation of Catecholamines," and the subsection titled "Inhibition of Monoamine Oxidase.")

In hypothyroidism, MAO activity increases. Conversely, activity of the enzyme decreases in hyperthyroidism.[108][109] Increased activity of MAO reduces the quantity of norepinephrine available at synapses, reducing noradrenergic drive. MAO inhibitors reduce the breakdown of norepinephrine, increasing the amount of the neurotransmitter in synapses. MAO inhibitors are as effective as more modern tricyclic antidepressants. They are seldom used, however, because of unpredictable adverse effects when they interact with many drugs and amines in foods.[107,p.414] The potentiation of the antidepressant effects of MAO inhibitors, such as phenelzine (Nardil),[105][106] by T_3 may result from induction of the MAO inhibitor by T_3. (See Chapter 2.3, subsection titled "Thyroid Hormone-Inducible Monoamine Oxidase (MAO) Inhibitor.")

Thyroid hormone administration decreases MAO activity. This increases the amount of norepinephrine available at synapses of neural pathways that mediate normal mood. In patients whose fibromyalgia is caused by hypothyroidism or thyroid hormone resistance, MAO activity may be high. The high MAO activity would be expected to reduce the patients' norepinephrine levels. High MAO activity may be the mechanism responsible for low norepinephrine levels in the cerebrospinal fluid of some fibromyalgia patients.[114] The expected result of the low norepinephrine levels is depression and cognitive dysfunction.

Deficient Vigorous Physical Activity. For reasons I explain in Chapter 3.4, inadequate thyroid hormone regulation of cell function leaves patients lacking the motor drive and inclination to engage in vigorous physical activity. Their low level of physical activity can contribute to their depression. Researchers have massively documented that exercise potently improves psychological status, as I described in two previous publications.[88][89] (See Chapter 5.5, section titled "Indications of the Role of Suboptimal Metabolism in Fibromyalgia.") Investigators have shown that brief exercise can significantly reduce depression.[98] Ten weeks of jogging significantly improved various depressive disorders.[99] Research has shown a relationship between fitness level and emotional stability in middle-aged men,[100] and daily exercise improved both the physical and psychiatric status of institutionalized elderly mental patients.[101] As deVries put it, "The wisdom of the ages that suggested that vigorous exercise makes you feel good is now supported by laboratory evidence."[102,p.249] We have found that in fibromyalgia patients who undergo metabolic rehabilitation including thyroid hormone, results are virtually always less than satisfying if the patients fail to engage in exercise to tolerance. Although many patients are not able to exercise before beginning the use of thyroid hormone, when they reach an effective dosage, their tolerance for exercise increases progressively. Eventually, they are able to exercise as vigorously as other healthy individuals.

Thyroid Hormone
Treatment for Depression

Depressed hypothyroid patients respond well to thyroid hormone therapy, usually with partial or complete relief of their depression.[83][84][85] Prange et al. studied the effects of combining thyroid hormones with a tricyclic antidepressant drug, imipramine. They found that depressed patients improved most when they took a small dose of T_3 combined with the usual dose of imipramine.[89] Imipramine alone did not produce the improvements that the combined treatment did. Combining the two treatments did not increase drug toxicity. The investigators proposed that: (1) T_3 increases the sensitivity of adrenergic receptors to neurotransmitters such as norepinephrine, and (2) imipramine sustains a higher concentration of norepinephrine in the synapses. They suggested that women are more responsive to the combination therapy. The greater responsiveness of women is in line with the finding that brains of female rats take up T_3 more efficiently than do brains of male rats.[90]

Whybrow found that all patients with hypothyroidism and hyperthyroidism showed mental deficits. The deficits always gradually improved as the thyroid state improved.[49] Whybrow's finding confirmed those of Asher. Their patients with long-standing hypothyroidism often showed residual signs of organic brain disease after the function of other tissues returned to normal.[51]

Whybrow wrote that mild hypothyroidism may complicate depression due to some other cause. In such cases, he recommended that the therapeutic goal should be to provide a thyroid dosage sufficient to reduce the serum TSH level to normal. This dosage, however, may not be enough to relieve the patient's depression. In this case, he recommended that the patient should undergo other therapeutic measures, such as psychotherapy.[49] In other cases, Whybrow pointed out, T_3 may mitigate or relieve severe depression—even when there is no clear evidence of hypothyroidism. He recommended 25-to-50 µg daily. This is especially helpful in drug-resistant depression and in women.[93][94][95]

I have found that the depression of fibromyalgia patients with hypothyroidism and/or thyroid hormone resistance markedly improves or is completely relieved by the use of thyroid hormone as a part of their metabolic rehabilitation. Fortunately, some progressive endocrinologists, such as Ridha Arem, now recognize that depression is a common symptom of hypothyroid patients and that the proper treatment is thyroid hormone therapy.[61]

● ANXIETY

OCCURRENCE IN FIBROMYALGIA

Researchers have reported that 47.8% of FMS patients report having anxiety.[25] Use of the Hassles scale[12][13] and the Life Events Inventory[6] in studies of fibromyalgia patients at speciality clinics suggest that they have more intense mental stress than do rheumatoid arthritis patients or normal controls. Another study of specialty clinic fibromyalgia patients using the Spielberger State and Trait Anxiety Inventory showed higher anxiety than that of controls.[14] Similar, three MMPI studies suggested that a subgroup of fibromyalgia patients at specialty clinics have high levels of anxiety.[6][7][8] Mountz reported higher anxiety scores in fibromyalgia patients than controls. He proposed that the patients' anxiety is a function of their significantly reduced blood flow through thalamus and caudate nuclei of the patients.[27] Wolfe reported that 31.5% of U.S. fibromyalgia patients have anxiety,[25] and Martenz reported that 63.8% of 47 Brazilian women with fibromyalgia had anxiety.[26] In the latter

study, only 16% of control subjects had anxiety.

It is noteworthy that a study of fibromyalgia patients of a primary care clinic showed that they did not have significantly higher anxiety levels than other patients used as controls.[4] This finding, in view of those in the previous paragraph, suggests that patients whose fibromyalgia is so severe or prolonged as to require referral by primary care physicians to specialists have a higher incidence or intensity of anxiety.

OCCURRENCE IN HYPOTHYROIDISM

A significant percentage of hypothyroid patients are nervous and apprehensive.[133,p.574] In a study of 77 hypothyroid patients, 35% were nervous. In another study of 100 hypothyroid patients, 51% were nervous.[133,p.577] Several writers report anxiety or nervousness as a symptom of euthyroid hypometabolism.[134][140][141][142][143]

Kimball wrote in 1933,[139,p.489] after a 10-year study of hypothyroid patients, "I have found that a rather sudden drop in metabolism may have about the same devastating effect on the sympathetic nervous system, *producing very similar nervous manifestations* [italics mine], as a sudden rise, such as is seen in acute exophthalmic goiter. I have seen quite a few such cases diagnosed as acute hyperthyroidism."

POSSIBLE MECHANISM OF HYPOMETABOLISM

Surges of sympathetic nervous system activity as an overcompensation for subnormal metabolism may account for the hypothyroid patients' nervousness and anxiety, and the same mechanism would apply to hypothyroid fibromyalgia patients.

Compensatory Sympathetic Arousal
Early thyroidology researchers considered that in hypothyroidism, noradrenergic receptors are "dulled." This concept of "dulled" receptors was used to explain what we now know to be a decreased density of β-adrenergic receptors on cell membranes, resulting in a subnormal response of the cells to catecholamines. (See Chapter 3.1, section titled "Inadequate Thyroid Hormone Regulation of Adrenergic Gene Transcription.") When hypothyroidism is severe, but probably not when mild or moderate, the sympathetic nervous system compensates for the subnormal metabolism of

cells by secreting increased amounts of norepine-phrine. In fact, in severe hypothyroidism, the sympathetic system tends to be overly active.[144,p.934] Both animal and human studies have shown this relationship.[117][145][146][147] For example, the adrenal medullae of the hypothyroid rat respond with exaggerated vigor to an intense hypoglycemic stimulus (such as the administration of the sugar 2-deoxyglucose).[107] This heightened sympathetic activity is mediated at least in part through the central nervous system.[161] This is indicated by the increased turnover of norepinephrine in the brain stem of severely hypothyroid rats.[144,p.934] It may also be mediated by exaggerated stress-induced ACTH secretion or secondary high peaks in cortisol secretion by the adrenal cortex. ACTH has been shown to stimulate epinephrine and norepinephrine secretion in humans,[155] and corticosteroids (in amounts secreted in response to ACTH) stimulate catecholamine release.[156] Both hypothyroid[157] and fibromyalgia[158] patients have exaggerated ACTH responses to stress. Some studies have shown elevations in cortisol levels in hypothyroidism[159] and fibromyalgia,[160] although other evidence suggests subnormal adrenocorticol function in both conditions (see Chapter 3.5).

Aversive psychological stimuli and chemicals such as caffeine may produce surges of catecholamines that activate β-adrenergic receptors in some tissues, causing psychophysiological arousal that the patient perceives as anxiety. The effect might resemble that of an excessive dosage of desipramine causing excess secretion of norepinephrine at synapses.[107,p.405] The anxiety or nervousness listed as symptoms of hypometabolic patients in early studies may be due to such catecholamine surges. For example, Thompson and Thompson wrote of patients with low metabolic rates who had headaches, weakness, chronic fatigue, and nervousness. They wrote, "In fact, the nervousness is often so marked that it suggests mild hyperthyroidism rather than hypothyroidism."[141,p.495] Thurman and Thompson cited marked nervousness among other hypometabolic patients. The patients had palpitations and emotional upsets *at the slightest provocation*. The investigators pointed out that such symptoms resemble hyperthyroidism, although the patients' BMRs are not high and in fact may be low.[140,pp.883-884]

Hyperpolarization of Sympathetic Ganglia Due to Increased α-Adrenergic Receptor Density on Ganglion Cells

Both central and peripheral administration of α_2-adrenergic receptor agonists, such as norepinephrine

and the drug clonidine, induce hypotension and brady-cardia.[162] These effects are mediated in part by an increase of presynaptic α_2-adrenoceptor activity in the sympathetic ganglia. The use of clonidine as an α_2-adrenergic receptor agonist has shown that increased α_2-adrenoceptor activity hyperpolarizes sympathetic ganglionic cells.[163] The hyperpolarization is similar to the "relative" refractory period of nerve fibers rather than an "absolute" refractory period.

Following an action potential and a subsequent absolute refractory period, during which even strong stimuli cannot set off another action potential, some voltage-activated sodium channels are in an inactive state, blocking further entry of sodium ions (Na^+) into the cells. The potassium channels are wide open, permitting and excess of potassium ions (K^+) to flow out of the cells, temporarily leaving the insides of the cells in extreme negativity (hyperpolarized). The hyperpolarization renders the cells more resistant than normal to the initiation of action potentials. But whereas even strong stimuli cannot initiate an action potential during an absolute refractory period, they can do so during a relative refractory period.[20,p.64] The inability of the sympathetic ganglia to be activated by mildly or moderately intense stimuli may account for the failure of the fibromyalgia patient's cardiorespiratory system to activate and meet the demands for increased oxygen delivery to muscle exercising at mild or moderate levels of intensity. The lower heart rates and cardiac output during exercise in some fibromyalgia patients[5,p.37] may be mediated in part by this mechanism. However, strong stimuli may overcome the resistance of sympathetic ganglia to the initiation of action potentials during α-adrenergic receptor-induced hyperpolarization. The result would be a sudden sympathetic nervous system discharge that the patient perceives as anxiety or panic. (For a more complete description of this mechanism, see Chapter 3.4, subsection titled "Hyperpolarization of Sympathetic Neurons and Facilitation of Parasympathetic Neurons by an Increased Density of α-Adrenergic Receptors.")

Perceptual or Cognitive Set as a Cause of Anxiety in Fibromyalgia Patients

Anxiety in fibromyalgia patients may be interpreted as surges of sympathetic arousal in response to strong stimuli against a perceptual backdrop of a threatening plight. Patients may interpret their sympathetic surges as "anxiety" because they perceive their plight as precarious and threatening. Behavioral researchers have shown that when a subject's sympathetic nervous system is aroused due to the intake of a strong sympathetic stimulant, the emotion experienced is not determined by the sympathetic arousal, *per se*. Instead, social/psychological cues determine the emotion.[151][152][153] In the typical study, a group of subjects was given electric shock or chemical sympathetic stimulants to generally arouse them. After the stimulation, in different phases of the study, they exhibited emotions as diverse as anger and euphoria. What determined their particular emotional reaction was not the original arousing stimulus. Instead, it was the suggestive influence of a particular emotional behavior exhibited by a "plant," a member of the groups who was, unbeknown to the subjects, actually an experimenter. Bandura reviewed the relevant studies and wrote, "Results of both physiological and psychological studies support the conclusion that a common diffuse state of physiological arousal mediates diverse forms of emotional behavior and that *different emotional states are identified and discriminated primarily in terms of external stimuli rather than internal somatic cues* [italics mine]."[154,p.488]

Many fibromyalgia patients contemplate their uncertain prognosis and the adverse occupational and social ramifications of their illness. Hence, while in the throes of fibromyalgia, their "environment" is replete with threatening stimuli. With these stimuli dominating their perception, they may interpret surges of sympathetic arousal as anxiety or even panic.

● **COGNITIVE DYSFUNCTION**

Several studies have now shown cognitive dysfunction in fibromyalgia patients.[20][21][22][23][24] Some well-known clinicians who treat chronic fatigue syndrome patients will not make the diagnosis unless the patient has confirmed intellectual impairment.[19,p.46] These cognitive dysfunctions mainly include deficits of memory and sustained concentration. Even before the first study appeared, I was convinced that the vast majority of my fibromyalgia patients had poor memory and concentration. For some patients, such as CPAs and attorneys, the dysfunction was so severe that they lost their professional positions with companies. For other patients, the dysfunction was frustrating, annoying, or diminished their self-confidence and self-esteem. Based on my clinical experience, I agree with Goldstein's statement, "I now believe that if patients are told that their neuropsychological testing does not reveal any cognitive deficit, then there is a problem

with the instruments being used or with the sophistication of the psychologist's interpretation of the results."[19,p.52]

In many cases, cognitive dysfunction is the first symptom of hypothyroidism. The patients usually also have depression.[47,p.911] Other psychological symptoms may also occur (see Table 3.10.1).

POSSIBLE MECHANISMS OF COGNITIVE DYSFUNCTION

Inadequate thyroid hormone regulation of cell function can cause cognitive dysfunction by at least three mechanisms: (1) reduction of brain blood flow, (2) an increase in the density of α-adrenergic receptors on brain cells, and (3) a decreased density of β-adrenergic receptors on brain cells.

Reduced Brain Blood Flow

Studies I include in Chapter 3.2 (section titled "Decreased Brain Blood Flow in Fibromyalgia") document decreased brain blood flow in fibromyalgia patients. In many cases, the reduced blood flow is so severe as to constitute ischemia. It is highly likely that the decreased blood flow contributes to patients' cognitive dysfunction. By three main mechanisms, inadequate regulation by thyroid hormone plausibly explains the reduced brain blood flow of fibromyalgia patients (see Chapter 3.2, section titled "Reduced Cerebral Blood Flow").

Increased Density of α-Adrenergic Receptors on Brain Cells

As I explain in Chapter 3.2, one means by which inadequate thyroid hormone regulation of cell function reduces the flow of blood to the brain is by increasing the density of α-adrenergic receptors on cerebral blood vessels. (See section titled "Role of Adrenergic Receptors in Vascular Resistance and Blood Flow in Hypothyroidism," and the section titled "Reduced Cerebral Blood Flow.") In addition, however, an increased density of α-adrenergic receptors on most brain cells inhibits their metabolism.

Stimulating nerve signals reaching the neurons of the locus ceruleus in the brain stem induce secretion of norepinephrine. The norepinephrine is secreted in brain structures distant from the brain stem (see Chapter 3.1, section titled "Locations of Catecholaminergic Neurons"). When thyroid hormone regulation of transcription of the adrenergic receptor genes is inadequate, transcription for the receptors increases. As a result, the density of α_2-adrenergic receptors on cell membranes increases. When norepinephrine is secreted and binds with the increased density of these receptors on brain cells, metabolism of the cells is impeded. In addition, brain neurons become hyperpolarized and less excitable, resulting in decreased neural signals to various brain structures.[131] These underlying molecular events are likely to manifest clinically as cognitive dysfunction and depression.

Researchers recently found that low estrogen levels increase the density of α_2-adrenergic receptors in the frontal region of the cortex of female rats. Administering estradiol to the rats decreased the density of the receptors.[86] This finding may explain the cognitive dysfunction of some women during the late luteal phase (the premenstrual period) of the menstrual cycle when estrogen levels are low. An increase of estrogen levels a week or so after menstruation during the follicular phase of the cycle probably reduces the density of the receptors in the frontal region, relieves cognitive dysfunction, and provides a transient euphoria for some women. (See Chapter 3.6, section titled "Amplifying of Estradiol-Induced Cerebral Cortex Inhibition by Inadequate Thyroid Hormone Regulation of Adrenergic Gene Transcription.") Inadequate thyroid hormone regulation of the adrenergic genes increases the density of α_2-adrenergic receptors on cell membranes. In women whose fibromyalgia is mainly due to inadequate thyroid hormone regulation, the resulting increase in α_2-adrenergic receptors would compound increased density due to low estrogen levels during the luteal phase of the menstrual cycle. Thus, these fibromyalgic women may have especially severe cognitive dysfunction as a PMS symptom.

Decreased Density of β-Adrenergic Receptors

In addition, inadequate thyroid hormone transcription regulation of the β-adrenergic receptor genes results in decreased synthesis of this type of adrenergic receptor. Decreased binding of catecholamines to β-adrenergic receptors on cell membranes slows cell metabolism, as does binding of catecholamines to α-adrenergic receptors on the cell membranes. Decreased binding of catecholamines to β-adrenergic receptors and increased binding of catecholamines to α-adrenergic receptors in the hippocampus, a part of the limbic system, interferes with memory. The hippocampus is a target of noradrenergic neurons from the locus ceruleus. Normally, norepinephrine, secreted by the noradrenergic neurons, increases the excitability of

hippocampal cells upon binding to β-adrenergic receptors. The binding is followed by activation of cAMP-dependent protein kinase, resulting in inhibition of Ca^{2+}-activated K^+ conductance.[165] Berne and Levy wrote that the hippocampus is important in recent memory. While lesions of the hippocampus may not interfere with either short- or long-term memory, lesions may disrupt the process by which short-term memories are permanently stored. Also, lesions may disrupt the process of recollection of memories.[166,pp.143-144] Decreased binding of catecholamines to β-adrenergic receptors and increased binding of catecholamines to α-adrenergic receptors constitutes a molecular lesion.

COGNITIVE EFFECTS OF THE EFFECTS OF HYPOTHYROID-RELATED MECHANISMS

Thyroid hormone is critical to normal brain function. Compared to other tissues, the brain has a higher concentration of thyroid hormone receptors. When investigators measured the amount of messenger RNA in various tissues that code for thyroid hormone receptors, the brain has the highest concentration. Among tissues examined, the highest concentration of messenger RNA coded for c-*erb*Aβ_1 thyroid hormone receptors was in the brain.[59,p.212]

Attempts to define a clear, generalized thyroid defect in emotional disorders have failed.[60] As a result, there has been much debate over the metabolic basis of depression in hypothyroidism Prange et al. wrote, "We propose that slight shifts in thyroid state toward hypothyroidism, although still within the statistical range of normality, affect nervous tissue—and perhaps only nervous tissue—in such a fashion as to produce a predisposition to retarded depression." Whybrow wrote in detail of the various likely mechanisms.[49,pp.1223-1224]

The brain normally has a higher metabolic rate than other tissues (see Chapter 3.2, subsection titled "High Brain Requirement for Blood Flow and Oxygen"). Psychological abnormalities in hypothyroidism probably result from subnormal metabolism mediated by the three mechanisms I described in the above section. The metabolic rate is higher in the gray matter than in the white matter, and higher in the brain than in the spinal cord. The metabolic rate of the brain, based on oxygen consumption, is about 20% of the body's 250 ml oxygen/min at rest. This is a disproportionately high rate of oxygen consumption for its size in relation to the rest of the body. This means that the metabolism of the brain's neurons and glia consumes about 50 ml of oxygen per minute. The cerebral cortex is the most voracious consumer (8 ml oxygen/100 g tissue per minute). This rate is 8 times the oxygen consumption of the white matter below the cortex.[62,pp.282-284]

The hypothyroid patient's impaired cognitive function may be related to a significant neurophysiological phenomenon. During thinking, reading, counting, or speaking, particular regions of the cerebral cortex become active. Within seconds, the oxygen consumption of local brain cells in these regions increases. The local blood flow simultaneously increases. The regionally increased neuronal activity elevates the metabolic activity of the neurons. The acid metabolic by-products induce local vasodilation and increased blood flow. If the circulation is impaired due to a high density of α-adrenergic receptors on cerebral blood vessels (in turn, due to inadequate thyroid hormone regulation of the adrenergic genes), the increased requirement of the brain cells for oxygen, glucose, and other metabolic substrates may not be met. The deficient supply of metabolic substrates may contribute to the hypothyroid patient's cognitive impairment. As Schmidt noted, we do not have a decisive experimental method for showing how the "mind" and neuronal activity are linked. Yet the actions and statements of human experimental subjects make one thing clear: "*Mental performance* is always accompanied by certain highly specific forms of *neuronal activity* and *does not occur in their absence* [italics by Schmidt]."[62,p.284] In hypothyroidism, gradations of impaired brain cell activity must occur, with commensurate degrees of impaired mental function.

Thyroid hormone is vital to the normal development of the central nervous system. Thyroid hormone deficiency in neonates causes marked changes in protein[63] and nucleic acid[65] metabolism. Deficiency also causes changes in the activity of enzymes in the central nervous system.[64] Replacement therapy reverses these changes when it is begun early enough. Delaying treatment permanently impairs the child's brain function.

By contrast, physiological changes in adults due to hypothyroidism are usually reversible. Studies using a nitrous oxide technique showed that cerebral blood flow in hypothyroid patients was 38% below normal.

Their oxygen and glucose consumption was also reduced to 27% below normal. Their cerebral blood vessels had double the normal resistance to blood flow.[297] The patients also had reduced brain oxygen consumption. This is an interesting finding in that laboratory animals' brain oxygen consumption did not vary with thyroid hormone excess or deficiency.[166,p.170] All hypothyroid patients had impaired cognition. Three patients studied again after their recovery of normal thyroid status showed a return toward normal physiological values. These changes, along with abnormal EEGs,[33] suggest that impaired cognition in hypothyroidism is a nonspecific final common pathway of mental dysfunction.

The findings I described in the previous paragraphs contradict Oppenheimer's statement that administering thyroid hormone does not increase the brain's consumption of oxygen.[59,p.212] It is common to read such statements in the thyroidology literature. Dembi et al. provided an explanation.[66,p.212] They wrote that the belief that administering thyroid hormone does not increase brain oxygen consumption arose when researchers in the 1950s[67][68] injected rats with pharmacologic dosages of T_4, sacrificed the animals, and found that brain slices from them did not show evidence of increased oxygen consumption. Referring to one of these studies,[67] Loeb stated, "In experimental thyrotoxicosis [post-injection of T_4] an enhanced rate of oxygen consumption is demonstrated in nearly all tissues with the exception of spleen, testis, and adult brain."[69,p.845] Dembi et al. wrote that because of these studies, researchers thought that thyroid hormone penetrated the brain poorly and had no metabolic effects on it.[66,p.221]

However, in the late 1970s, transthyretin (previously called prealbumen) was found to transport T_3 and T_4 across the blood-brain barrier into the brain.[70][71][72] In addition, researchers found that the adult brain contains considerable amounts of T_3[73] and specific T_3-receptors in brain cell nuclei.[74][75] These findings made it unlikely that thyroid hormone played no role, or even a little role, in the metabolism and metabolism-related functions of the brain. Indeed, thyroid hormone has substantial effects on the brain. For example, Dembi et al. found that compared to euthyroid rats, the basal metabolic rate of the brain of hypothyroid rats (at 5 days after thyroidectomy) decreased by 17%. At 10 days, the basal metabolic rate had decreased by 38%, and at 60 days by 47%.[66]

● OTHER THYROID HORMONE-RELATED PSYCHOLOGICAL ABNORMALITIES

ASSERTIVENESS AND AGGRESSIVENESS

A small percentage of fibromyalgia patients who have been under my care and that of Honeyman-Lowe, before undergoing metabolic rehabilitation, have had an extraordinarily low threshold for anger, hostility, and aggressive behavior. Some patients were hypothyroid and others were thyroid hormone resistant. Ahles et al. reported that in assertiveness and aggressiveness scores, fibromyalgia patients resemble patients with rheumatoid arthritis and normal controls.[6] While the prevalence of hostility and aggressiveness may not differ from that of normal controls, some fibromyalgia patients, before undergoing metabolic rehabilitation, are barely capable of controlling frequent surges of anger and aggressiveness; some are incapable of doing so. The intensity of the anger and aggressive behavior of a very small minority of patients has been so extremely severe that these patients were incapable of working with my staff and me long enough to benefit from metabolic rehabilitation. Fortunately, most such patients eventually complete treatment, and during the course of their recovery, their threshold for hostility and aggressive behavior increases sufficiently so that these tendencies cease to be a problem. What before was excessive aggressiveness has usually turned out within a few months to be a playful social tendency that has made the patients delightful to interact with.

ADVERSE REACTIONS IN PSYCHOTIC PATIENTS

Clinicians should be cautious while treating the psychotic patient with exogenous thyroid hormone because the treatment may worsen the psychosis.[96] In some patients who are not actively psychotic, thyroid replacement therapy may cause psychotic delirium. An initial dosage of thyroid hormone that is too large may instigate this reaction. Chlorpromazine may be helpful in reducing dangerously excitatory behavior or assaults by a patient until the clinician can take other appropriate therapeutic measures.

REFERENCES

1. Smythe, H.A.: Non-articular rheumatism and the fibrositis syndrome. In *Arthritis and Allied Conditions*, 8th edition. Edited by J.L. Hollander and D.J. McCarty, Philadelphia, Lea & Febiger, 1972, pp.874-884.
2. Yunus, M.B.: Psychological factors in fibromyalgia syndrome: an overview. *J. Musculoskeletal Pain*, 2(1):87-91, 1994.
3. Yunus, M.B.: Towards a model of pathophysiology of fibromyalgia: aberrant central pain mechanisms with peripheral modulation. *J. Rheumatol.*, 19:846-850, 1992.
4. Clark, S., Campbell, S.M., Forehand, M.E., Tindall, E.A., and Bennett, R.M.: Clinical characteristics of fibrositis. II. A "blinded" controlled study using standard psychological tests. *Arthritis Rheum.*, 28:132-137, 1985.
5. Yunus, M.B., Ahles, T.A., Aldag, J.C., and Masi, A.T.: Relationship of clinical features with psychological status in primary fibromyalgia. *Arthritis Rheum.*, 34:15-21, 1991.
6. Ahles, T.A., Yunus, M.B., Railey, S.D., et al.: Psychological factors associated with primary fibromyalgia syndrome. *Arthritis Rheum.*, 27:1101-1106, 1984.
7. Wolfe, F., Cathey, M.A., Kleinheksel, S.M., et al.: Psychological status in primary fibrositis and fibrositis associated with rheumatoid arthritis. *J. Rheumatol.*, 11: 500-506, 1984.
8. Leavitt, F. and Katz, R.S.: Is the MMPI invalid for assessing psychological disturbance in pain related organic conditions? *J. Rheumatol.*, 16:521-526, 1989.
9. Hudson, J.I., Hudson, M.S., Pliner, L.F., et al.: Fibromyalgia and major affective disorders: a controlled phenomenology and family history study. *Amer. J. Psychiat.*, 142:441-446, 1985.
10. Kirmayer, L.J., Robbins, J.M., and Kapusta, M.A.: Somatization and depression in fibromyalgia syndrome. *Amer. J. Psychiat.*, 145:950-954, 1988.
11. Ahles, T.A., Khan, S.A., Yunus, M.B., et al.: Psychiatric status of primary fibromyalgia and rheumatoid arthritis patients and nonpain controls: a blinded comparison of *DSM-III* diagnoses. *Amer. J. Psychiat.*, 148:1721-1726, 1991.
12. Dailey, P.A., Bishop, G.D., Russell, I.J., and Fletcher, E.M.: Psychological stress and the fibrositis/fibromyalgia syndrome. *J. Rheumatol.*, 17:1380-1385, 1990.
13. Uveges, J.M., Parker, J.C., Smarr, K.L., et al.: Psychological symptoms in primary fibromyalgia syndrome: relationship to pain, life stress, and sleep disturbance. *Arthritis Rheum.*, 33:1279-1283, 1990.
14. Yunus, M.B., Dailey, J.W., Aldag, J.C., et al.: Plasma and urinary catecholamines in primary fibromyalgia: a controlled study. *J. Rheumatol.*, 19:95-97, 1992.
15. Hudson, J.I. and Pope, H.G.: Fibromyalgia and psychopathology: is fibromyalgia a form of "affective spectrum disorder"? *J. Rheumatol.*, 25:1551-1556, 1988.
16. Ferraccioli, G., Cavalieri, F., Salaffi, F., et al.: Neuroendocrine findings in primary fibromyalgia and in other chronic rheumatic conditions (rheumatoid arthritis, low back pain). *J. Rheumatol.*, 17:869-873, 1990.
17. Kravitz, H.M., Katz, R., Kot, E., et al.: Biochemical clues to a fibromyalgia-depression link: imipramine binding in

patients with fibromyalgia or depression and in healthy controls. *J. Rheumatol.*, 19:1428-1432, 1992.

18. Birnie, K.J., Knipping, A.A., Van Rijswijk, M.H., et al.: Psychological aspects of fibromyalgia compared with chronic and nonchronic pain. *J. Rheumatol.*, 18:1845-1848, 1991.

19. Goldstein, J.A.: *Chronic Fatigue Syndrome: The Limbic Hypothesis.* New York, Haworth Medical Press, 1993.

20. Nielson, W.R., Grace, G.M., Hopkins, M., and Berg, M.: Concentration and memory deficits in patients with fibromyalgia syndrome. *J. Musculoskeletal Pain*, 3(Suppl.1): 123, 1995.

21. Bujak, D.I., Dornbush, R.L., and Weinstein, A.: Fibromyalgia and cognitive abnormalities induced by Lyme disease. *J. Musculoskeletal Pain*, 3(Suppl.1):63, 1995.

22. Goldstein, J.A.: Decreased event-related potential N-100: a possible neurologic marker for CFS impairment. *J. Musculoskeletal Pain*, 3(Suppl.1):115, 1995.

23. Romano, T.J., Stiller, J.W., Vasey, F.B., and Bradley, P.J.: The development of fibromyalgia after silicone breast implants: the Korean experience. *J. Musculoskeletal Pain*, 3(Suppl.1):108, 1995.

24. Sandman, C.A., Barron, J.L., Nackoul, K., Goldstein, J., and Fidler, F.: Memory deficits associated with chronic fatigue immune dysfunction syndrome. *Biol. Psychiat.*, 33(8-9):618-623, 1993.

25. Wolfe, F.: Diagnosis of fibromyalgia. *J. Musculoskeletal Med.*, 7:54, 1990.

26. Martenz, J.E., Ferraz, M.B., Fontana, A.M., and Atra, E.: Psychological aspects of Brazilian women with fibromyalgia. *J. Psychosomatic Res.*, 39:167-174, 1995.

27. Mountz, J.N., Bradley, L.A., Modell, J.G., Alexander, R.W., et al.: Fibromyalgia in women: abnormalities of regional cerebral blood flow in the thalamus and the caudate nucleus are associated with low pain thresholds. *Arthritis Rheumatol.*, 38:926-938, 1995.

28. Smythe, H.A. and Moldofsky, H.: Two contributions to understanding of the "fibrositis" syndrome. *Bull. Rheum. Dis.*, 28:928-931, 1977.

29. Parker, J., Frank, R., Beck, N., et al.: Pain in rheumatoid arthritis: relationship to demographic, medical, and psychological factors. *J. Rheumatol.*, 15:433-437, 1988.

30. Nickel, S.N. and Frame, B.: Neurologic manifestations of myxedema. *Neurology*, 8:511, 1958.

31. MacDonald, D.W.: Hypothermic myxedema coma: three case reports. *Brit. M. J.*, 2:1144, 1958.

32. Levin, M.E. and Daughaday, W.H.: Fatal coma due to myxoedema. *Amer. J. Med.*, 18:1017, 1955.

33. Browning, T.B., Atkins, R.W., and Weiner, H.: Cerebral metabolic disturbances in hypothyroidism: clinical and electroencephalographic studies in the psychosis of myxoedema and hypothyroidism. *A.M.A. Arch. Intern. Med.*, 93:938, 1954.

34. Soederbergh, G.: Faut-il attribuer a une perturbation des fonctions cerebelleuses certain troubles moteur du myxoedeme? *Rev. Neuro.* (Paris), 2:487, 1910.

35. Jellinek, E.H. and Kelly, R.E.: Cerebellar syndrome in myxedema. *Lancet*, 2:225, 1960.

36. Goldenberg, D.L.: Psychiatric illness and fibromyalgia. *J. Musculoskeletal Pain*, 2(3):41-49, 1994.

37. Adams, R.D. and Rosman, N.P.: Neuromuscular system. In *The Thyroid*, 4th edition. Edited by S.C. Werner and S.H. Ingbar, New York, Harper and Row Publishers, 1987.

38. Spiro, A.J., Kirano, A., Beilin, R.L., and Finkelstein, J.W.: Cretinism with muscular hypertrophy (Kocher-Debre-Semelaigne syndrome). *Arch. Neurol.*, 23:340-349, 1970.

39. Scheinberg, P.: Correlative observations of cerebral metabolism and cardiac output in myxedema. *J. Clin. Invest.*, 29:1139, 1950.

40. Thayer, R.E.: *The Biopsychology of Mood and Arousal.* New York, Oxford University Press, 1989.

41. Franklin, J.: *Molecules of the Mind.* Dell Publishing Co., 1987.

42. Barondes, S.H.: *Molecules and Mental Illness.* New York, Scientific American Library, 1993.

43. Gull, W.W.: On a cretinoid state supervening in adult life in women. *Trans. Clin. Soc.* (Lond.), 7:180, 1874.

44. Inglis, T.: Two cases of myxeodema. *Lancet*, 2:496, 1880.

45. Committee of the Clinical Society of London. Report on myxedema. *Trans. Clin. Soc.* [Suppl] (Lond.), 21:18, 1888.

46. Savage, G.H.: Myxoedema and its nervous symptoms. In *J. Ment. Sci.*, 25:417, 1880.

47. Weiner, H.: Emotions and mentation. In *The Thyroid*, 4th edition. Edited by S.C. Werner and S.H. Ingbar, New York, Harper and Row Publishers, 1987.

48. Murray, G.R.: Note on the treatment of myxoedema by hypodermic injections of an extract of the thyroid gland of a sheep. *Br. Med. J.*, 2:796, 1891.

49. Whybrow, P.C.: Behavioral and psychiatric aspects. In *Werner's The Thyroid: A Fundamental and Clinical Text*, 5th edition. Edited by S.H. Ingbar and L.E. Braverman, Philadelphia, J.B. Lippincott Co., 1986, pp.1222-1224.

50. Shaw, C.: Case of myxedema with restless melancholia treated by injection of thyroid juice: recovery. *Brit. Med. J.*, 2:451, 1892.

51. Asher, R.: Myxoedematous madness. *Brit. Med. J.*, 2:555, 1949.

52. Easson, W.M.: Myxedema with psychosis. *Arch. Gen. Psychiat.*, 14:277, 1966.

53. Karnosh, I.J. and Stout, R.E.: Psychoses of myxoedema. *Amer. J. Psychiat.*, 91:1263, 1934.

54. Treadway, C.R., Prange, A.J., Doehne, E.F., Edens, C.J., and Whybrow, P.C.: Myxedema psychosis: clinical and biochemical changes during recovery. *J. Psychiat. Res.*, 5:289, 1967.

55. Maura, G., Gemignani, A., and Raiteri, M.: Noradrenaline inhibits central serotonin release through α_2-adrenoceptors located on serotonergic nerve terminals. *Naunyn-Schmiedeberg's Arch. Pharmacol.*, 320:272-274, 1982.

56. Loosen, P.T. and Prange, A.J., Jr.: Serum thyrotropin response to thyrotropin-releasing hormone in psychiatric patients: a review. *Amer. J. Psychiat.*, 139:405-416, 1982.

57. Gewirtz, G.R., Malaspina, D., Hatterer, J.A., Feureisen, S., Klein, D., and Gorman, J.M.: Occult thyroid dysfunction in patients with refractory depression. *Amer. J. Psychiat.*, 145(8):1012-1014, 1988.

58. Walker, S., III: *Psychiatric Signs and Symptoms Due to Medical Problems.* Springfield, Charles C. Thomas, Publisher, 1967, pp.112-113.

59. Oppenheimer, J.H.: Thyroid hormone action at the molecular level. In *Werner's The Thyroid: A Fundamental and Clinical Text*, 6th edition. Edited by L.E. Braverman and R.D. Utiger, Philadelphia, J.B. Lippincott Co., 1991, pp.204-224.

60. Gibson, J.G.: Emotions and the thyroid gland: a critical appraisal. *J. Psychosom. Res.*, 6:93-116, 1962.

61. Arem, R.: *The Thyroid Solution*. New York, Ballantine Books, 1999.

62. Schmidt, R.F.: Integrative functions of the central nervous system. *Fundamentals of Neurophysiology*, 3rd edition. New York, Springer-Verlag, 1985, pp.270-316.

63. Geel, S.E., Valcana, T., and Timiras, P.S.: Effect of neonatal hypothyroidism and of thyroxine on L[14C] leucine incorporation in protein *in vivo* and the relationship to ionic levels in the developing brain of the rat. *Brain Res.*, 4:143, 1967.

64. Singhall, R.L. and Rastogi, R.B.: Neurotransmitter mechanisms during mental illness induced by alterations in thyroid function. In *Advances in Pharmacology and Chemotherapy*, Vol. 15. Edited by S. Garratini, A. Golding, F. Hawking, and I.J. Kopin, New York, Academic Press, 1978.

65. Geel, S.E. and Timiras, P.S.: The influence of neonatal hypothyroidism and of thyroxine on the ribonucleic acid and deoxyribonucleic acid concentrations of rat cerebral cortex. *Brain Res.*, 4:135, 1967.

66. Dembri, A., Belkhiria, M., Michel, O., and Michel, R.: Effects of short- and long-term thyroidectomy on mitochondrial and nuclear activity in adult rat brain. *Molec. Cell. Endocrinol.*, 33:211-223, 1983.

67. Barker, S.B. and Klitgaard, H.M.: Metabolism of tissues excised from thyroid-injected rats. *Amer. J. Physiol.*, 179:81-88, 1952.

68. Barker, S.B.: *Proc. Soc. Exp. Biol.*, 90:1372-1378, 1955.

69. Loeb, J.N.: Metabolic changes in thyrotoxicosis. In *Werner and Ingbar's The Thyroid: A Fundamental and Clinical Text*, 6th edition. Edited by L.E. Braverman and R.D. Utiger, New York, J.B. Lippincott Co., 1991, pp.845-853.

70. Blake, C.C.F., Geisow, M.J., and Swan, I.D.A.: Structure of human plasma prealbumin at 2.5A resolution: a preliminary report on the polypeptide chain conformation quaternary structure and thyroxine binding. *J. Mol. Biol.*, 88:1, 1974.

71. Blake, C.C.F. and Oatley, S.J.: Protein-DNA and protein-hormone interactions in prealbumin: a model of the thyroid hormone nuclear receptor? *Nature*, 268:115, 1977.

72. Blake, C.C.F., Burridge, J.M., and Oatley, S.J.: Binding interactions with TBPA. In *Endocrinology*. Edited by T.A. Cumming, J.W. Funder, and F.A.O. Mendelsohn, Canberra, Australian Academy of Science, 1980, p.417.

73. Obregon, M.J., Morreale de Escobar, G., and Escobar del Rey, F.: *Endocrinology*, 103:2145-2153, 1978.

74. Oppenheimer, J.H., Schwartz, H.L., and Surks, M.I.: *Endocrinology*, 95:897-903, 1974.

75. Schwartz, H.L. and Oppenheimer, J.H.: *Endocrinology*, 103:267-273, 1978.

76. Whybrow, P.C. and Prange, A.J.: A hypothesis of thyroid-catecholamine-receptor interaction: its relevance to affective illness. *Arch. Gen. Psychiat,*, 38:108, 1981.

77. Shildkraut, J.J.: The catecholamine hypothesis of affective disorders: a review of supporting evidence. *Amer. J. Psychiat.*, 122:509-522, 1965.

78. Schwark, W.S. and Keesey, R.R.: Thyroid hormone control of serotonin in developing rat brain. *Res. Commun. Chem. Pathol. Pharmacol.*, 10:37, 1975.

79. Prange, A.J. Jr., Wilson, I.C., Lynn, C.W., Alltop, L.B., and Stikeleather, R.A.: L-tryptophan in mania: contribution to a permissive hypothesis of affective disorders. *Arch. Gen. Psychiat.*, 30:56, 1974.

80. Bennett, R.M., Clark, S.R., Campbell, S.M., et al.: Symptoms of Raynaud's syndrome in patients with fibromyalgia: a study utilizing the Nielsen test, digital photoplethysmography and measurements of platelet α_2-adrenergic receptors. *Arthritis and Rheumatism*, 34:264-269, 1991.

81. Svensson, T.H., Bunney, B.S., and Aghajanian, G.K.: Inhibition of both noradrenergic and serotonergic neurons in brain by the α-adrenergic agonist clonidine. *Brain Res.*, 92:291, 1975.

82. Trendelenburg, A.U., Trendelenburg, M., Starke, K., and Limberger, N.: Release-inhibiting α_2-adrenoceptors at serotonergic axons in rat and rabbit brain cortex: evidence for pharmacological identity with α_2-autoreceptors. *Naunyn-Schmiedeberg's Arch. Pharmacol.*, 349:25-33, 1994.

83. Coppen, A., Whybrow, P.C., Noguera, R., Maggs, R., and Prange, A.J.: The comparative antidepressant value of L-tryptophan and imipramine with and without attempted potentiation by liothyronine. *Arch. Gen. Psychiat.*, 26:234, 1972.

84. Goodwin, F.K., Prange, A.J., Post, R.M., Muscettola, G., and Lipton, M.A.: Potentiation of antidepressant effects by thyronine in tricyclic nonresponders. *Amer. J. Psychiat.*, 139:34, 1982.

85. Prange, A.J., Jr., Wilson, I.C., Rabon, A.M., and Lipton, M.A.: Enhancement of imipramine antidepressant activity by thyroid hormone. *Amer. J. Psychiat.*, 126(4):457-469, 1969.

86. Karakanias, G.B., Li, C.S., and Etgen, A.M.: Estradiol reduction of α_2-adrenoceptor binding in female rat cortex is correlated with decreases in $\alpha_{2A/D}$-adrenoceptor messenger RNA. *Neuroscience,* 81(3):593-597, 1997.

87. Lowe, J.C.: Physical activity: a form of physiopsychotherapy. *Digest Chiro. Economics*, 21(2):33-37, Sept-Oct, 1978.

88. Lowe, J.C.: Psychological benefits of physical activity. *ACA J. Chiro.*, 13(1):S1-S6, 1979.

89. Prange, A.J., Wilson, I.C., Rabon, A.M., and Lipton, M.A.: Enhancement of imipramine antidepressant activity by thyroid hormone. *Amer. J. Psychiat.*, 126:464, 1969.

90. Magnus-Levy, A.: Energy metabolism in health and disease. *J. Hist. Med.*, 2:307, 1947.

91. Mangieri, C.N. and Lund, M.H.: Potency of United States Pharmacopeia desiccated thyroid tablets as determined by the antigoitrogenic assay in rats. *J. Clin. Endocrinol. Metab.*, 30:102, 1970.

92. Wiberg, G.S., Devlin, W.F., and Stephenson, N.R.: A comparison of the thyroxine: tri-iodothyronine content and biological activity of thyroid from various species. *J. Pharm. Pharmacol.*, 14:777, 1962.

93. Sawin, C.T., Surks, M.I., and London, M.: Oral thyroxine: variation in biologic action and tablet content. *Ann.*

Intern. Med., 100:641, 1984.

94. Surks, M.I., Schadlow, A.R., and Oppenheimer, J.H.: A new radioimmunoassay for plasma L-thyronine: measurement in thyroid disease and in patients maintained on hormonal replacement. *J. Clin. Invest.*, 51:3104, 1972.

95. Jackson, I.M.D. and Cobb, W.E.: Why does anyone still use desiccated thyroid USP? *Amer. J. Med.*, 64:284, 1978.

96. Bernstein, R.S. and Robbins, J.: Intermittent therapy with L-thyroxine. *N. Engl. J. Med.*, 281:1444, 1969.

97. Hallberg, H., Almgren, O., and Svensson, T.H.: Increased brain serotonergic and noradrenergic activity by the β_2-agonist salbutamol: a putative antidepressant drug. *Psychopharmacology*, 73:201, 1981.

98. Morgan, W.P. and Horstman, D.H.: Anxiety reduction following acute physical activity. Abstracted in *Med. Sci. Sports*, 8:62, 1976.

99. Brown, R.S., Ramirez, D.E., and Taub, J.M.: The prescription of exercise for depression. Paper read at ACSM meeting, May 24, 1978, Washington, D.C.

100. Young, R.J. and Ismael, A.H.: Relationship between anthropometric, physiological, biochemical and personality variables before and after a four-month conditioning program for middle-aged men. *J. Sports Med. Phys. Fitness*, 16:267-276, 1976.

101. Stamford, B.A., Hambacher, W., and Fallica, A.: Effects of daily physical exercise on the psychiatric state of institutionalized geriatric mental patients. *Res. Quart.*, 45:34-41, 1974.

102. deVries, H. A.: *Physiology of Exercise*, 4th edition. Dubuque, Wm. C. Brown Publishers, 1986.

103. Goldenberg, D.L.: Psychologic studies in fibrositis. *Amer. J. Med.*, 81(Suppl.3A):67-70, 1986.

104. Straus, S.E.: Chronic fatigue syndrome. *J. Musculoskel. Pain*, 2(3):57-63, 1994.

105. Hullett, F.J. and Bidder, T.G.: Phenelzine plus triiodothyronine combination in a case of refractory depression. *J. Nerv. Ment. Dis.*, 171:318-321, 1983.

106. Joffe, R.T.: Triiodothyronine potentiation of the antidepressant effect of phenelzine. *J. Clin. Psychiatry*, 49:409-410, 1988.

107. Gilman, A.G., Rall, T.W., Nies, A.S., and Taylor, P.: *The Pharmacological Basis of Therapeutics*, 8th edition. New York, Pergamon Press, 1990.

108. Levine, R.J., Oates, J.A., Vendsalu, A., and Sjoerdsma, A.: Studies on the metabolism of aromatic amines in relation to altered thyroid function in man. *J. Clin. Endocrinol.*, 22:1242-50, 1962.

109. Spinks, A. and Burn, J.H.: Thyroid activity and amine oxidase in the liver. *Brit. J. Pharmacol.*, 7:93-8, 1952.

110. Gross, G., Brodde, O.E., and Schumann, J.H.: Decreased number of β-adrenoreceptors in cerbral cortex of hypothyroid rats. *Euro. Pharmacol.*, 61:191-194, 1980.

111. Emerson, C.H., Liberman, C., and Braverman, L.E.: Hypothyroidism. In *The Thyroid*. Edited by W.L. Green, New York, Elsevier, 1987.

112. Gross, G. and Schumann, H.J.: Reduced number of α_2-adrenoceptors in cortical brain membranes of hypothyroid rats. *J. Pharmacy Pharmacol.*, 33:552, 1981.

113. Smith, R.M., Patel, A.J., Kingsbury, A.E., Hunt, A., and Balazs, R.: Effects of thyroid state on brain development: β-adrenergic receptors and 5'-nucleotidase activity. *Brain Res.*, 198:375, 1980.

114. Russell, I.J., Vaerøy, H., Jabors, M., and Nyberg, F.: Cerebrospinal fluid biogenic amine metabolites in fibromyalgia/fibrositis syndrome in rheumatoid arthritis. *Arthritis Rheumat.*,35:550-556, 1992.

115. Bilezikian, J.P. and Loeb, J.N.: The influence of hyperthyroidism and hypothyroidism on α- and β-adrenergic receptor systems and adrenergic responsiveness. *Endocrine Rev.*, 4:378-388, 1983.

116. Prange, A.J., Wilson, I.C., Rabon, A.M., and Lipton, M.A.: Enhancement of imipramine antidepressant activity by thyroid hormone. *Amer. J. Psychiatry*, 126:39-51, 1969.

117. Lipton, M.A., Prange, A.J., Dairman, W., and Udenfriend, S.: Increased rate of norepinephrine biosynthesis in hypothyroid rats. *Fed. Proc.*, 27:399, 1968.

118. Limberger, N., Bonanno, G., Späth, L., and Starke, K.: Autoreceptors and α_2-adrenceptors at the serotonergic axons of rabbit brain cortex. *Naunyn-Schmiedeberg's Arch. Pharmacol.*, 332:324-331, 1986.

119. Goldstein, J.A.: *Betrayal by the Brain.* New York, Haworth Medical Press, 1996.

120. Willner, P.: Antidepressants and serotonergic neurotransmission: an integrative review. *Psychopharmocology*, 85:387-404, 1985.

121. Hamon, M., Gozlan, H., Mestikawy, S.E., Emerit, M.B., Gozlan, H., and Schechter, L.: The central 5-HT$_{1A}$ receptors: pharmacological, biochemical, functional, and regulatory properties. *Ann. N.Y. Acad. Sci.*, 600:114-131, 1990.

122. Gothert, M.: 5-Hydroxytryptamine receptors: an example for the complexity of chemical transmission of information in the brain. *Arzneimittelforschung*, 2:238-249, 1992.

123. Van de Kaar, L.D.: Neuroendocrine aspects of the serotonergic hypothesis of depression. *Neurosci. Biobehav. Rev.*, 13:237-246, 1989.

124. Tejani-Butt, S.M., Yang, J., and Kaviani, A.: Time course of altered thyroid states on 5-HT$_{1A}$ receptors and 5-HT uptake sites in rat brain: an autoradiographic analysis. *Neuroendocrinology*, 57:1011-1018, 1993.

125. Blier, P., de Montigny, C.D., and Chaput, Y.: Modifications of the serotonin system by antidepressant treatments: implications for the therapuetic response in major depression. *J. Clin. Psychopharmacology*, 7(6 Suppl.): 24S-35S, 1987.

126. Savard, P., Merand, Y., Paolo, T.D., and Dupont, A.: Effect of neonatal hypothyroidism on the serotonin system of the rat brain. *Brain Res.*, 292:99-108, 1984.

127. Vaccari, A.: Decreased central serotonin function in hypothyroidism. *Eur. J. Pharmacol.*, 82:93-95, 1982.

128. Singhal, R.L., Hrdina, P.D., and Rastogi, R.B.: Brain biogenic amines and altered thyroid function. *Life Sci.*, 17: 1617-1626, 1975.

129. Bradley, D.J., Young, W.S., III, and Weinberger, C.: Differential expression of α and β thyroid hormone receptor genes in rat brain and pituitary. *Proc. Natl. Acad. Sci.* (USA), 86:7250-7254, 1989.

130. Cook, C.B. and Koenig, R.J.: Expression of erbAα and β mRNAs in regions of adult rat brain. *Mol. Cell. Endocrinol.*, 70:13-20, 1990.

131. Williams, J.T., Surprenant, A.M., and North, R.A.: Inhibitory synaptic transmission mediated by catecholamines. VI. Adrenergic neuron electrophysiology and behavior. In *Epinephrine in the Central Nervous System*. Edited by P. Stolk, E. U'Prichard, and J. Fuxe, New York, Oxford University Press, 1988, pp.252-258.

132. Joffe, T.R.: A perspective on the thyroid and depression. *Can. J. Psychiatry*, 35:754-759, 1990.

133. DeGroot, L.J., Larsen, P.R., Refetoff, S., and Stanbury, J.B.: *The Thyroid and Its Disease*, 5th edition. New York, John Wiley & Sons, 1984.

134. Morton, J.H.: Sodium lithyronine in metabolic insufficiency syndrome and associated disorders. *J.A.M.A.*, 165: 124-129, 1957.

135. Nichols, A.J. and Ruffolo, R.R., Jr.: Functions mediated by α-adrenoceptors. In *α-Adrenoceptors: Molecular Biology, Biochemistry and Pharmacology*. Basel, Karger, 1991, pp.113-179.

136. Kostowski, W., Plaznik, A., and Danysz, M.A.: The role of the locus coeruleus-limbic noradrenergic transmission in the action of antidepressant drugs. *Psychopharmacol. Bull.*, 22:512-522, 1986.

137. Koizumi, K. and Brooks, C.M.: The autonomic nervous system and its role in controlling body functions. In *Medical Physiology*. Edited by Mountcastle, St. Louis, Mosby, 1980, pp.893-922.

138. Simson, P.E., Cierpial, M.A., Heyneman, L.E., and Weiss, J.M.: Pertussis toxin blocks the effects of α₂-agonists and antagonists on locus coeruleus activity *in vivo*. *Neurosci. Lett.*, 89:361-366, 1988.

139. Kimball, O.P.: Clinical hypothyroidism. *Kentucky Med. J.*, 31:488495, 1933.

140. Thurmon, F.M. and Thompson, W.O.: Low basal metabolism with myxedema. *Arch. Intern. Med.*, 46:879-897, 1930.

141. Thompson, W.O. and Thompson, P.K.: Low basal metabolism following thyrotoxicosis. *J. Clin. Invest.*, 5:471-501, 1928.

142. Kurland, G.S., Hamolsky, M.W., and Freedberg, A.S.: Studies in non-myxedematous hypometabolism: I. The clinical syndrome and the effects of triiodothyronine, alone or combined with thyroxine. *J. Clin. Endocrinol.*, 15:1354, 1955.

143. Goldberg, M.: Diagnosis of euthyroid hypometabolism. *Amer. J. Obst. & Gynec.*, 81(5):1057-1058, 1961.

144. Landsberg, L.: Catecholamines and the sympathoadrenal system. In *The Thyroid*, 4th edition. Edited by S.C. Werner and S.H. Ingbar, New York, Harper and Row Publishers, 1987.

145. Harrison, T.S.: Adrenal medullary and thyroid relationships. *Physiol. Rev.*, 44:161, 1964.

146. Prange, A.J.Jr., Meed, J.L., and Lipton, M.A.: Catecholamines: diminished rate of norepinephrine biosynthesis in rat brain and heart after thyroxine pretreatment. *Life Sci.*,9:901, 1970.

147. Wahi, R.S., Chansouria, J.P.N. and Udupa, K.N.: Normal levels of norepinephrine in short term hypothyroidism. *J. Clin. Endocrinol. Metab.*, 51:934-935, 1980.

148. MacKenzie, H.W.G.: A case of myxoedema treated with great benefit by feeding with fresh thyroid glands. *Br. Med. J.*, 2:940, 1892.

149. Johnson, D.G.: Adrenomedullary response to 2-deoxyglucose in the hypothyroid, euthyroid and hyperthyroid rat. *Acta Physiol. Scand.*, 65:337, 1965.

150. Walker, S., III: *A Dose of Sanity*. New York, John Wiley & Sons, Inc., 1996.

151. Renold, A.E., Quigley, T.B., Kenard, H.E., and Thorn, G.W.: Reaction of the adrenal cortex to physical and emotional stress in college oarsmen. *New Eng. J. Med.*, 244: 754-757, 1951.

152. Schachter, J.: Pain, fear and anger in hypertensives and normotensives: a psychophysiological study. *Psychosom. Med.*, 19:17-29, 1957.

153. Schachter, S. and Singer, J.E.: *Psychol. Rev.*, 69:379-399, 1962.

154. Bandura, A.: *Principles of Behavior Modification*. New York, Holt, Rinehart and Winston, Inc., 1969.

155. Valenta, L.J., Elias, A.N., and Eisenberg, H.: ACTH stimulation of adrenal epinephrine and norepinephrine releases. *Horm. Res.*, 23:16-20, 1986.

156. Ungar, A. and Phillips, J.H.: Regulation of the adrenal medulla. *Physiol. Rev.*, 63:787-843, 1983.

157. Kamilaris, T.C., DeBold, C.R., Pavlou, S.N., et al.: Effect of altered thyroid hormone levels on hypothalamic-pituitary adrenal function. *J. Clin. Endocrinol. Metab.*, 65: 994-999, 1987.

158. Griep, E.N., Boersma, J.W., and deKloet, E.R.: Altered reactivity of the hypothalamic-pituitary-adrenal axis in the primary fibromyalgia syndrome. *J. Rheumatol.*, 20:469-474, 1993.

159. Iranmanish, A., Lizarralde, G., Johnson, M.L., and Veldhuis, J.D.: Dynamics of 24-hour endogenous cortisol secretion and clearance in primary hypothyroidism assessed before and after partial thyroid hormone replacement. *J. Clin. Endocrinol. Metab.*, 70:155, 1990.

160. Crofford, L.J.: The hypothalamic-pituitary-adrenal axis in the fibromyalgia syndrome. *J. Musculoskel. Pain*, 4(1/2): 181-200, 1996.

161. Landsberg, L and Axelrod, J.: Influence of pituitary, thyroid, and adrenal hormones on norepinephrine turnover and metabolism in the rat heart. *Circ. Res.*, 22(5):559-571, 1968.

162. Head, G.A. and Burke, S.: Importance of central noradrenergic and serotonergic pathways in the cardiovascular actions of rilmenidine and clonidine. *J. Cardiovacular Pharmacol.*, 18(6):819-826, 1991.

163. Brown, D.A. and Caulfield, M.P.: Hyperpolarizing α₂-adrenoceptors in rat sympathetic ganglia. *Br. J. Pharmacol.*, 65:435-445, 1979.

164. Guyton, A.C.: *Textbook of Medical Physiology*, 8th edition. Philadelphia, W.B. Saunders Co., 1991.

165. Nicoll, R.A.: The coupling of neurotransmitter receptors to ion channels in the brain. *Science*, 241:545-551, 1988.

166. Berne, R.M. and Levy, M.N.: *Principles of Physiology*, St. Louis, C.V. Mosby Co., 1990.

167. Weich, S. and Lewis, G.: Poverty, unemployment, and common mental disorders: population based cohort study. *Brit. Med. J.*, 317(7151):115-119, 1998.

168. Bradley, L.A., Alcarcón, G.S., Triana, M., et al.: Health care seeking behavior in fibromyalgia: associations with pain thresholds, symptoms severity, and psychiatric morbidity. *J. Musculoskel. Pain*, 2(3):79-87, 1994.

3.11

Fatigue and
Flexed Posture

Fatigue is a major symptom of fibromyalgia patients. It is also a major symptom of hypothyroid and euthyroid hypometabolic patients. The concept of anergy, the perception of a lack of energy, is useful for exploring possible mechanisms of fatigue. In this chapter, fatigue and anergy are considered synonymous.

In hypothyroidism, anergy may result from several mechanisms. One is decreased dopamine production which can decrease locomotor drive and activity. In one study, fibromyalgia patients had low cerebrospinal fluid levels of the dopamine metabolite, 3-methoxy-4-hydroxyphenethylene. This finding suggests that dopamine secretion is reduced in fibromyalgia, as would be predicted from inadequate thyroid hormone regulation of dopaminergic cells.

Another mechanism of anergy in hypothyroidism is decreased energy metabolism. Researchers have found low ATP concentrations in red blood cells from fibromyalgia patients. This finding indicates that the patients had impaired energy metabolism.

The third mechanism of anergy in hypothyroidism is increased production of three inhibitory molecules: α-adrenergic receptors, phosphodiesterase, and G_i proteins. The increase in G_i proteins increases the sensitivity of cells to the inhibitory effects of adenosine/adenosine receptor binding. The three inhibitory molecules and the increased sensitivity to adenosine, in concert, substantially contribute to the perception of fatigue. Fibromyalgia patients in one study had an increased density of α-adrenergic receptors on their platelets. This finding raises the possibility that the patients have α-adrenergic dominance. A fourth mech-

anism of anergy in hypothyroidism is non-restorative sleep. This, of course, is a major problem for fibromyalgia patients.

Fatigue resulting from inadequate thyroid hormone regulation of cell function may lead to slumping or flexed posture. The patient may not have the energy and motor drive to resist the ceaseless downward pull of gravity and maintain an erect posture when sitting or standing. The musculoskeletal dynamics of flexed posture may produce fibromyalgia tender points or worsen their sensitivity to pressure. Biomechanical stresses associated with flexed posture may cause increased sensory input to the central nervous system. Because of an impaired central nervous system pain modulating system, the patient may perceive the input as tenderness or pain (see Chapter 3.15).

Snorrason and coauthors defined fatigue in chronic fatigue syndrome patients. It is, they wrote, the experience of fatigue for more than 50% of the patient's waking hours and lasting more than 6 months.[12,p.37] To my knowledge, no one has officially defined fatigue in fibromyalgia. Fatigue, however, is a major symptom of fibromyalgia, though not all patients have fatigue. Wolfe reported the incidence of fatigue in fibromyalgia patients as 81.4%.[1]

Four studies list the incidence of fatigue in hypothyroid patients: 91.0% of 77 patients, 85.0% of 100 patients,[13,p.577] 100% of 86 patients,[2,p.11] and 69.75% of 400 patients.[3,p.185] Several authors have reported fatigue as a symptom of euthyroid hypometabolism.[4][5][6][7][8][9][10][11]

● FATIGUE DUE TO INADEQUATE THYROID HORMONE REGULATION OF CELL FUNCTION: MECHANISMS

Fatigue is a feature of numerous conditions. These include some rheumatic and hematological diseases, multiple sclerosis, myasthenia gravis, substance abuse, and eating disorders.[12,p.37] Probably the most common cause of fatigue is inadequate thyroid hormone regulation of cell function. Inadequate thyroid hormone regulation can cause fatigue by several mechanisms. As with the other symptoms and objective findings in Section III of this book, I draw on the hypothyroidism literature in proposing mechanisms. The vast majority of studies of the effects of inadequate thyroid hormone regulation of cell function have involved hypothyroidism. Hypothyroidism is therefore our prototype for cellular hypometabolism.

DECREASED DOPAMINE, LOW LOCOMOTOR DRIVE, AND LOW MOTOR ACTIVITY IN HYPOTHYROIDISM

Some fibromyalgia patients have low cerebrospinal fluid concentrations of the dopamine metabolite, 3-methoxy-4-hydroxyphenethylene. Concentrations of the metabolite were significantly lower in fibromyalgia patients than in rheumatoid arthritis patients and control subjects.[94] (See Chapter 3.4, subsection titled "Lower Central Nervous System Dopamine Levels" and the section titled "Features of Hypothyroidism that May Mediate Low Fitness Levels and Post-Exercise Symptom Exacerbation in Fibromyalgia.")

Thyroid hormone regulates dopamine synthesis by controlling the concentration of its precursor, DOPA, available for conversion to dopamine.[24,p.227][25][26][27] Hypothyroid patients and laboratory animals have decreased levels of dopamine.[28][29][30][31]

Hypothyroidism decreased the locomotor activity of young rats.[14] It is well established that dopaminergic neurons in the mesolimbic and nigrostriatal dopamine-containing pathways control locomotor activity.[15][16][18][19][20][21][22][23] Diarra et al. found that reduced synthesis of dopamine in the striatum accounted for impaired locomotor activity of developing rats that are hypothyroid.[17]

Modulation of the Effect of Lowered Dopamine on Locomotor Activity by α-Adrenergic Receptors

Decreased dopamine secretion by dopaminergic

neurons due to inadequate T_3 regulation of transcription lowers locomotor drive and activity. Another factor may compound the low locomotor drive due to inadequate T_3 regulation—a simultaneously increased density of α_2-adrenergic receptors on cell membranes. In most cells, T_3 binding to T_3-receptors represses transcription of the α_2-adrenergic receptor gene. When T_3 is not present or does not effectively bind to T_3-receptors on the gene, transcription activates and cells increase their synthesis of α_2-adrenoceptors. These receptors become positioned in high density on cell membranes. In one study, the platelets of fibromyalgia patients had an increased density of α_2-adrenergic receptors.[32] (See Chapter 3.1, section titled "Increased Density of α_2-Adrenergic Receptors on Platelets of Fibromyalgia Patients.") The α_2-adrenoceptor agonist clonidine inhibited both normal[33][34][35] and amphetamine-driven[36] locomotor activity.

Whether locomotor activity increases or decreases, however, depends on the type of α-adrenergic receptor increased or decreased by inadequate T_3 transcription regulation. In contrast to the inhibiting effect of α_2-adrenoceptor activation, α_1-adrenergic receptor agonists (phenylephrine and methoxamine) increased locomotor activity.[33][37]

Stereotyped Behaviors and Accompanying Low Motor Drive and Locomotion

Stereotyped behavior (stereotypy) is invariant, repetitive behavior with no apparent practical utility. If fibromyalgia patients with low motor drive exhibit behaviors that clinicans diagnose as "obsessive-compulsive," the behaviors may be sterotypy associated with subnormal dopamine levels due to inadequate thyroid hormone regulation of dopaminergic neurons.

Stereotyped rat behavior most often involves head movements, licking, biting, gnawing, and sniffing.[38,p.521] After lesioning of rat brain norepinephrine neurons, locomotor activity decreased but stereotyped behavior increased.[38] Kowstowski et al. found that electrically lesioning the locus ceruleus norepinephrine neurons in the brain stem decreased locomotor and exploratory behavior of rats. But the lesioning potentiated stereotypy induced by a dopamine agonist (apomorphine).[39] Dickinson et al., based on their studies, proposed that norepinephrine facilitates locomotor behaviors and inhibits stereotypic behaviors, and conversely, low norepinephrine levels inhibit locomotor behaviors and increase stereotypic behaviors.[38,p.526]

The α_2-adrenoceptor agonist clonidine potentiated stereotyped behaviors induced by dopamine or norepinephrine agonists.[36][41] α_2-Adrenoceptor antagonists inhibited sterotyped behaviors.[41][42] Dickinson et al. found that while α_1-adrenergic receptor activation inhibits stereotypic behaviors, α_2-adrenoceptor activation faciliates them.[38]

The finding of increased α_2-adrenergic receptors on the platelets of fibromyalgia patients[32] may make these researchers' findings relevant to fibromyalgia. Increased α_2-adrenergic receptors and subnormal dopamine levels due to inadequate thyroid hormone regulation may be the mechanisms behind stereotyped behaviors and accompanying low motor drive and locomotion in fibromyalgia.

FATIGUE DUE TO IMPAIRED ENERGY METABOLISM IN HYPOTHYROIDISM

Impaired Energy Production

Decreased energy production in hypothyroidism leads to anergy (fatigue, or the perception of a lack of energy). The degree of anergy varies with the severity of the thyroid hormone deficiency. Eisinger et al. found decreased ATP concentrations in the erythrocytes of fibromyalgia patients.[88,p.4] ATP is the energy "currency" of the cell, and we expect the patient with low ATP levels to have anergy (see Chapter 2.2, section titled "Energy-Yielding Processes in the Cytoplasm and Mitochondria").

Decreased Protein Synthesis

In hypothyroidism, the protein content of some tissues increases. Protein in the cerebrospinal fluid, for example, may double. Increased protein synthesis, however, does not cause the increase in the protein content of cerebrospinal fluid—increased capillary permeability does. Highly permeable capillaries allow blood proteins to "leak" into the cerebrospinal fluid.[69] Another example of increased tissue content of protein is collagen in connective tissues of the hypothyroid patient. The net content of the protein collagen in connective tissues increases. The net collagen increase results from slowed catabolism of collagen; its synthesis remains about normal.[70]

Despite increases in the protein content of some tissues, protein synthesis decreases throughout the body overall in hypothyroidism. A particularly important protein decrease is that of apoenzyme. Apoenzyme is the protein constituent of enzymes. Most enzymes also contain non-protein components called coenzymes. Vitamins B_1, B_2, B_3, and B_6 are coenzymes.

Coenzymes, which are smaller than apoenzymes, are either indispensable to the activity of enzymes or enhance their activity. A coenzyme binds to an apoenzyme; the combination is an enzyme. In hypothyroidism, amounts of a variety of enzymes in the cytoplasm and mitochondria decrease[71] (see Chapter 2.2, sections titled "Thyroid Hormone and Membrane Na^+/K^+-ATPase Activity," and "Energy-Yielding Processes in the Cytoplasm and Mitochondria"). Some enzymes whose amounts decrease are necessary for normal energy metabolism; a short supply of them may contribute to a patient's fatigue and listlessness. Reduced energy production in hypothyroidism directly relates to decreased synthesis of some enzymes.

FATIGUE DUE TO INCREASED PRODUCTION OF THREE INHIBITORY MOLECULES IN HYPOTHYROIDISM

In hypothyroidism, cells increase their synthesis of three inhibitory molecules: α-adrenergic receptors (see section below), phosphodiesterase, and G_i (inhibitory G) proteins. The increase in these molecules is the byproduct of inadequate thyroid hormone regulation of transcription of the genes that code for the molecules. These three molecules contribute to cellular hypometabolism through different mechanisms (see Chapter 2.3, section titled "Molecular Byproducts of Thyroid Hormone-Regulated Transcription: Relevance to Fibromyalgia"). The increase in G_i proteins increases the sensitivity of cells to the inhibitory effects of adenosine/adenosine receptor binding. The three inhibitory molecules, and the increased sensitivity to adenosine, in concert substantively contribute to the perception of fatigue.

Decreased Adrenergic Drive Due to α-Adrenergic Dominance

Decreased adrenergic drive may result in symptoms such as drooping eyelids, bradycardia, and the perception of weakness or a low energy level.[49,p.1043] Weakness and anergy, however, are the only symptoms some patients have.[50,p.1919] Writers have described two putative mechanisms of decreased adrenergic drive: (1) decreased sensitivity of adrenergic receptors, and (2) a shift in the balance of β- and α-adrenergic receptors to a predominance of α-adrenoceptors.

The belief that hypothyroidism reduces the sensitivity of adrenergic receptors was controversial for a time.[51][52] Studies and observations of clinicians had indicated that administering thyroid hormone enhanced β-adrenergic responses.[53,p.912] To some researchers, this suggested that thyroid hormone increased the sensitivity of β-adrenoceptors. Kunos et al. believed that the increased sensitivity resulted from an allosteric change in the structure of the receptors. They proposed that α- and β-adrenergic receptors were the same macromolecule that different conditions converted from one form to the other. They also proposed that thyroid hormone was the main control of the form the receptors assumed.[54][55][56] Studies later determined, however, that in most tissues, thyroid hormone increases transcription for β-adrenergic receptors and represses transcription of α-adrenergic receptors. Absence of thyroid hormone from the β- and α-adrenergic genes has the opposite effects—repression of transcription for β-adrenergic receptors and activation of transcription of α-adrenergic receptors. In a few cell types, such as hepatocytes and lymphocytes, the transcriptional effects of thyroid hormone at the different adrenergic genes are opposite to that in most tissues.[57][58][59,p.345] Thyroid hormone, then, regulates transcription for and synthesis of the different forms of adrenergic receptors, altering their relative count on cell membranes.

In most tissues, binding of catecholamines to β-adrenergic receptors accelerates metabolic processes; binding of catecholamines to α-adrenergic receptors slows metabolism. By increasing the β-adrenergic receptor density on cell membranes, thyroid hormone increases glygenolysis and glycolysis (see Chapter 2.2, subsection titled "Thyroid Hormone Regulation of Glycogenolysis"). Partly through increasing the rate of these pathways in the cytoplasm, and partly through increasing the rates of other pathways in the mitochondria, thyroid hormone increases ATP production and has a positive general effect on energy metabolism (see Chapter 2.2, section titled "Energy-Yielding Processes in the Cytoplasm and Mitochondria").

When an individual is physically or emotionally aroused and secretes large amounts of catecholamines, β-adrenergic receptors mediate responses such as tachycardia. (See Chapter 2.2, subsection titled "Thyroid Hormone Regulation of Glycogenolysis" and Chapter 3.1, sections titled "Different Adrenergic Receptor Types are Distinctly Different Molecules that are Products of Separate Genes" and "Inadequate Thyroid Hormone Regulation of Adrenergic Gene Transcription.") Taking a dosage of thyroid hormone that is excessive for an individual produces similar effects even without her being aroused. β-Adrenergic blocking drugs such as propranolol inhibit such β-adreno-

ceptor-mediated responses as nervousness, tremors, and rapid heart rate. The drugs do this by competing with catecholamines for binding sites on β-adrenergic receptors. Some clinicians prescribe β-adrenergic receptor blocking drugs to control situational anxiety or to stop tissue overstimulation from excessive exposure of cells to thyroid hormone.[60]

In hypothyroidism, the count of β-adrenergic receptors on cell membranes of most tissues decreases. For instance, thyroidectomy decreased the density of β-adrenergic receptors on rat heart membranes by 30%-to-40%.[52] One result of the reduced receptor count is that norepinephrine loses some of its ability to break down fat. To mediate lipolysis, norepinephrine must attach to fat cell β-adrenergic receptors. The reduced numbers of these receptors in hypothyroidism reduce the ability of norepinephrine to break down fat.[62] After researchers removed rats' thyroid glands and the β-adrenoceptor count decreased, doses of T_3 increased by fourfold the number of β-adrenergic receptors in the rats' salivary glands.[63]

Animal and human studies point to the same conclusions: In hypothyroidism α-adrenergic function predominates; in hyperthyroidism β-adrenergic function predominates.[64][65] In hyperthyroid rats, the number of β-adrenergic receptors in heart tissue approximately doubles.[66] Some investigators report that the brains of hypothyroid rats contain fewer than normal β-adrenergic receptors, but they found no obvious changes in the structure or function of the remaining β-adrenergic receptors present.[67] In one study of hypothyroid rats, however, the inhibitor Purkinje neurons of the cerebellum were somewhat insensitive to norepinephrine electrically driven in by iontophoresis. (These large neurons send dendrites to the molecular layer of the cerebral cortex and to the cerebellar white matter.) The investigators proposed that the reduced sensitivity of the neurons was due to hypothyroid-induced allosteric changes in β-adrenergic receptors, reducing their affinity for norepinephrine. Based on more recent data, however, we know that the reduced sensitivity of the neurons resulted from a decreased count of β-adrenergic receptors on the neuronal membranes. Administering T_3 returned to normal the sensitivity of the neurons to norepinephrine.[68]

Fatigue Mediated by α$_2$-Adrenergic Receptors. In hypothyroidism and cellular resistance to thyroid hormone, the increased density of α$_2$-adrenergic receptors may contribute to fatigue. α$_2$-Adrenergic receptor activation may contribute to the chronic fatigue of fibromyalgia patients, although in this sense, we must use "fatigue" as synonymous with "sedation." In the initial trials of clonidine (an α_2-adrenergic receptor agonist), patients were commonly sedated, so researchers noted sedation as a side effect of the drug.[44][45][46] Not only do α_2-adrenergic receptor agonists such as clonidine decrease motor activity; they also potentiate anesthesia and can induce sleep.[47]

α_2-Adrenergic receptor activation may mediate sedation and decreased motor activity by affecting two central nervous system sites. One site is the locus ceruleus. There, α_2-adrenergic receptor activation decreases neuronal firing and thereby decreases the amount of norepinephrine released in the thalamus and cerebral cortex. This phenomenon reduces the activity level of cortex cells, rendering them less receptive to sensory input. The second site is the axon terminals of locus ceruleus neurons in the thalamus and cerebral cortex. At these terminals, presynaptic α_2-adrenergic receptors inhibit release of norepinephrine. Nichols and Ruffolo contend that it is the second site that predominantly mediates sedation.[43,p.124]

Anergy Due to Increases in Phosphodiesterase and Inhibitory G Proteins (G_i)

Thyroid hormone regulates cellular concentrations of the inhibitory compounds phosphodiesterase and inhibitor G proteins (G_i). When properly regulated by thyroid hormone, phosphodiesterase and G_i—like a proper balance of α- and β-adrenergic receptors—help maintain normal metabolism. In hypothyroidism, however, phosphodiesterase and G_i increase and excessively inhibit cell processes. (See Chapter 2.3, section titled "Molecular Byproducts of Thyroid Hormone-Regulated Transcription: Relevance to Fibromyalgia: Molecular Byproducts that Mediate Hypometabolism: α-Adrenergic Receptors, Phosphodiesterase, and G_i Proteins.")

Anergy Due to an Augmented Inhibitory Effect of Adenosine in Hypothyroidism

Hypothyroidism increases the inhibitory effects of adenosine on cells. Studies suggest that hypothyroidism does not increase the sensitivity of cells to adenosine by increasing the density of adenosine receptors on cell membranes; rather, it does so by increasing the concentration of inhibitory G proteins (G_i) within cell membranes. G_i augments the inhibitory effect on the cell of adenosine/adenosine receptor binding. (For a detailed description of the roles of G proteins in cell membranes, see Chapter 3.1, section titled "Post-Adrenergic Receptor Mechanisms in the Cell Membrane

that Mediate Catecholamine-Adrenoceptor Signals.")

In 1991, Silva and Landsberg wrote that hypothyroidism increased the sensitivity of white adipose tissue to the inhibitory effects of adenosine.[61,p.1050] They referenced a study by Malbon et al. These researchers found that in fat cells of hypothyroid rats, an adenosine agonist (N6-phenylisopropyladenosine) inhibited experimentally-stimulated adenylate cyclase activity. The agonist was specific for A_1 adenosine receptors. The researchers also found that hypothyroidism did not increase the number of adenosine receptors in the membranes of rat fat cells. Hypothyroidism also did not increase the affinity of adenosine receptors for adenosine. Hypothyroidism did, however, increase the inhibition of adenylate cyclase by guanosine 5'-triphosphate (GTP) in the cell membrane. The researchers wrote that this suggests that hypothyroidism increased the inhibitory guanine nucleotide regulatory unit—inhibitory G protein signified by "G_i."[40] They concluded that the amplified inhibition of fat cells by adenosine is due to a specific increase in the activity and abundance of G_i with which adenosine interacts upon binding to an adenosine receptor.[100]

Kaasik et al. isolated left atria from rats. They administered isoproterenol, a β-adrenoceptor agonist, to the atria of hypothyroid rats, euthyroid rats, and rat atria saturated with thyroid hormone. Isoproterenol increased the developed tension, maximal rate of tension developed, and tension fall of atria. These effects of isoproterenol were greatest in the atria from hypothyroid rats and lowest in atria saturated with thyroid hormone. In atria stimulated with isoproterenol, an adenosine A_1-receptor agonist, N6-(phenylisopropyl)-adenosine, had a powerful negative inotropic effect—the agonist weakened atrial contractions. The contraction-weakening effects of the agonist were greatest in atria from hypothyroid rats. The number of adenosine receptors in hypothyroid atria were not increased. The investigators measured the amount of total G_i-like protein in the atria: they estimated the amounts of G_{i2} and G_{i3} and the amounts of low and high molecular weight forms of G_s (stimulatory G protein). Hypothyroid atria had slightly lower G_{i2} and G_{i3} concentrations, but the amounts of both forms of G_s (per mg of protein) were 50% lower than in euthyroid rat atria. Thus, the ratio of G_i to G_s was high. They wrote, "The levels of G_{i2} and G_{i3} were greatly elevated as compared to G_s as membrane marker. These changes were reversed by treatment of the hypothyroid rats with thyroid hormones." They concluded that their results showed an enhanced negative inotropic effect of adenosine. G_i mediated the effect.[81]

Stein, Clark, and Delaney studied the effects of chronic (14-day) changes in thyroid function on the adrenergic system in the brain. Other researchers had previously studied the effects of altering thyroid function on adenosine receptors in adipocytes (a type of peripheral tissue). Stein's study was the first of the effects in brain tissue. The researchers made some rats hypothyroid, kept some euthyroid, and rendered others "hyperthyroid" with T_3 injections. None of the treatments affected binding of an adenosine A_1-receptor antagonist to homogenate from cerebral cortex, cerebellum, or hippocampus. Moreover, the treatments had no effect on binding of an adenosine A_2-receptor agonist to homogenate from the striatum. The researchers found no consistent regional alterations unique to either hypothyroid or T_3-treated rats. They concluded, "These preliminary findings suggest that alterations in brain adenosine receptors or G-protein-receptor coupling are unlikely to be requisite correlates of abnormal thyroid hormone levels."[93]

Mazurkiewicz and Saggerson, however, did find changes in rat brain synaptosomes. They found that GTP (guanosine 5'-triphosphate) was involved in the increased inhibition of adenylate cyclase by adenosine in hypothyroidism. They tested synaptosomes (see Glossary) isolated from hypothyroid rats. They found that hypothyroidism increased the inhibition of adenylate cyclase by the A_1 adenosine receptor agonist phenylisopropyladenosine. They determined that hypothyroidism did not increase binding of the agonist to synaptosomal membranes; in fact, maximum binding was decreased somewhat. They concluded that in hypothyroidism, the adenosine-induced decrease in adenylate cyclase occurs because of an increase in G_i.[87]

Gur et al. exposed isolated left atria from hypothyroid rats to adenosine. They found that adenosine weakened atrial muscle contractions. This weakened strength of contraction is termed a negative inotropic effect. Inducing hypothyroidism also had an anti-adrenergic effect, reducing the responsiveness of the muscle to stimulation by catecholamine/adrenergic receptor binding. Treatment with T_3 relieved the inotropic and anti-adrenergic effects.[101]

Franco et al. found that adenosine infusions into the kidneys of normal rats caused vasoconstriction measures that indicated decreased glomerular flow. In hypothyroid rats, adenosine caused vasodilation; measures indicated increased glomerular flow. Specifically, the investigators found increased glomerular filtration rate through single nephrons, glomerular blood flow, and ultrafiltration coefficient.[74] This suggests that increased urinary frequency in fibromyalgia patients may

result in part from increased sensitivity to adenosine due to increases in G_i as a product of inadequate thyroid hormone regulation of cell function (see Chapter 3.21: Model for Urinary Urgency and Frequency).

SLEEP DISTURBANCE AND ANERGY

Too little restorative sleep contributes to the hypothyroid patient's anergy. Impaired muscle energy metabolism may cause energy deficiency muscle contractures (see Chapter 3.18). Noxious afferent signals generated at the site of these contractures ascend the spinal cord and stimulate the reticular activating system. Increased activity of the reticular activating system interferes with stage 4 restorative sleep[48] (see Chapter 3.15). The resulting lack of rest causes anergy or adds to it.

● POSTURE

TOTAL T_4 CONCENTRATION, POSTURE, AND PHYSICAL ACTIVITY

The total concentration of circulating T_4 undergoes two types of rhythmic variation. First, small random and brief changes occur. We can observe these by taking serum samples every 20 minutes.[84][85] Next, there are circadian variations of 7%-to-34%, with peak levels around 12 noon and the lowest point at about 2 am.[86] Alterations in the protein concentration of blood appear to cause these rhythmic changes. The protein alterations result from a hemodynamic response to changes in posture and possibly physical activity.[13,p.254] They are probably of no consequence to the metabolic rate. The basis for this conjecture is that due to its long circulation time, daily variations in the circulating T_4 level do not have an immediate effect on cellular metabolism (see Chapters 2.1 and 5.3).

FLEXED POSTURE

Some individuals have flexed posture because of inherited structural abnormalities such as a severely swayed low back. Other individuals simply do not practice "good" posture. Still others have flexed posture because they are too fatigued to resist the relentless pull of gravity when they are sitting or standing. The fatigue that encourages flexed posture may result from inadequate thyroid hormone regulation of cell function. (See section above: "Fatigue Due to Inadequate Thyroid Hormone Regulation of Cell Function: Mechanisms.")

Tender Points

Russian cosmonauts have described the effects of gravity upon reentering our atmosphere from outer space. "We have entered the atmosphere," said Anatoli Berezovoy. "The pressure is growing and pushes you into your seat."[79,p.122] "As we descended further," Valeri Ryumin said, "the pressure on our bodies mounted. The engine of the soft landing started up, and we hit the ground and turned to one side. The hatch opened and we saw the sky and human faces peeking in. I had lost coordination. My body, arms, and legs were terribly heavy. Dear Earth, how heavy you are, sitting on my shoulders."[79,p.124] The pull of gravity ceaselessly coaxes the human being toward a slouching posture. The weaker an individual's muscles (the lower his work capacity), the less he resists the pull.

Imagine observing a standing man throughout his life, with the observation compressed into a 5-minute time-lapse movie of him. This would dramatically show how gravity pulls his body down. He would quickly re-mold into a slumped caricature of himself as the least resisting body parts descend toward the ground. Eventually, submission to gravity leads to a slouching "old man" posture. He uses his back muscles less. To balance himself, he locks his knees in extension, creating the "sabre-leg" distortion. This backward bowing of the lower extremities forces the top of the pelvis to nod forward. The spinal column compensates by repositioning itself. The lumbar anterior curve, the thoracic posterior curve, and the cervical anterior curve accentuate. As a result, the person has a short and deep lumbar lordosis, a long extreme thoracic kyphosis, and a short deep cervical lordosis. This person also leans backward from the lumbosacral junction.[73,p.56]

In contrast to the hypothyroid patient, the hyperthyroid individual's muscles are constantly exercising. This may not be visible, but shows up on an EMG. When he does consciously work his muscles, the activity is superimposed on a constantly existing muscular load.[83,p.170] The reverse is true of the individual whose muscle fibers are hypometabolic. He is weak to begin with. Any additional muscle load, as when standing, may nullify any resolve he has to stand up straight. The weight of his own body may pull him into a flexed, slumping posture.

Slumping posture militates against muscle bal-

ance, and it positions some joints at their physiologic limit of articulation. Ligaments that support the joints may stretch to the extreme. The ligaments may become edematous, deformed and painful. The patient may feel pain at the strained joint or in the overlying skin.[78] Muscles chronically tightened to support malaligned joints may drain energy.

Regional dysfunctions also develop. Littlejohn reported that he examined 50 process workers who had no symptoms of noteworthy neck or arm pain or disability. In 30 of them, he found a restricted cervical range of motion and regional tender points, usually on the dominant side. He conjectured that these individuals are predisposed to develop what he termed "regional FS" (fibromyalgia) when other stresses, such as psychological factors, compound the cervical abnormalities he found.[80,p.56] Littlejohn's observation corresponds to a finding of Denslow and Korr. They found that the spinal cord at spinal transition areas (occipito-atlantal, cervico-thoracic, thoraco-lumbar, and lumbosacral junctions) were irritated. Also, the neuromuscular tissues innervated by the cord at those areas were irritated.[95][96][97][98][99] Slumping posture heightens this irritability and predisposes to segmentally-related tissue abnormalities when other stresses add to the aberrant physiology at these regions.

In addition, movement of the shoulder (glenohumeral) joint is suboptimal with a round-shouldered posture. The overhanging acromion shifts anteriorly and the arm internally rotates. This favors rotator cuff entrapment and attrition. In addition, the elongated infraspinatus muscles may form trigger points.[75,pp.133-134]

Hiemeyer and his associates called this posture "flexed." They hypothesized that the posture produces tender points in fibromyalgia.[72] They conducted a study of fibromyalgia patients with flexed posture. They divided patients into two groups. Those in "stage I flexed posture" could reverse their posture to erect. Those in "stage II flexed posture" were not able to resume an erect posture. When the investigators reversed the posture of stage I patients, 94% of the patients' tender points became less painful. When they partially reversed the posture of stage II patients to erect, 69% of their tender points became less painful.[72,p.172] Table 3.11.1 shows the values from the study.

The flexed posture reported by Hiemeyer et al. may create tender points or worsen their sensitivity by the effects of the posture on musculoskeletal tissues. The posture makes some tissues that have myofascial tender points lax. The tendinous attachment of the piriformis muscle to the greater trochanter is an example. The intratendinous substance may become "bunched up" with chronic shortening and compress the paltry number of blood vessels that traverse the tendon. In addition, as I have described elsewhere,[89] chronic minimal mobility of the connective tissues of the tendon leads to excessive cross-linking of the collagen fibers of the tissues. The tendinous tissue polymerizes and loses its flexibility after only 3 weeks of minimal motion.[90][91] The helical collagen fibers and the cross-bindings connecting them shorten or coil in on themselves when not regularly lengthened through movement.[92] The shortening, called "physiological creep," increases the pressure within the tissues and further compresses blood vessels that travel through them. When veins and lymphatic channels are compressed, metabolic wastes are not eliminated at a normal rate. The higher concentration of wastes lowers the threshold of receptors within the tendon.[48] The patient may more easily perceive the signals from these receptors as tender or painful because of an impaired central nervous system pain modulating system. This process may be the basis of tender points associated with flexed posture.

Table 3.11.1. Pain at tender points before and after correcting posture.*

	STAGE OF FLEXED POSTURE	
	I	II
Number of patients	6	34
Number of tender points tested	48	272
Painful tender points in flexed posture	38	182
Decreased pain at tender points in erect posture	36 (94%)	125 (69%)

*From Hiemeyer, K., Lutz, R., and Menninger, H.: Dependence of tender points upon posture: a key to the understanding of fibromyalgia syndrome. *J. Manual Med.*, 5:169-174, 1990.[72,p.172]

Visceral Prolapse. Goldthwait wrote that the diaphragm and abdominal muscles are the main supports that hold the abdominal viscera in place. In faulty posture, however, these two structures relax and become lax as supports. A low diaphragm and sagging organs impede circulation through abdominal tissues, and may cause passive congestion in one or all abdominal and pelvic organs. The drooping tissues may also impede general circulation. This happens because the diaphragmatic pump loses its efficiency. Congested, sagging organs apply pressure to both their nerves and

the sympathetic ganglia and plexuses. This may cause irregularities in the organs' functions, ranging from partial paralysis to activation of pressure receptors.[76,p.87]

Shafer wrote that poor body mechanics predispose to visceral disorders. He cautioned, however, that it is difficult to determine how much postural distortion is critical for impairing visceral function. In erect body posture, the abdominal viscera are held in optimal position. Connective tissue ledges and shelves partially support the abdominal organs. The adequacy of these supports decreases during a slumping posture as the lumbar lordosis and thoracic kyphosis increase and the abdominal muscles loosen.[75,p.134]

When the abdominal cavity shortens longitudinally, it compresses the viscera, secreting glands, and nerve ganglia.[77,pp.235-236] Increased tension on the superior mesenteric vessels may cause duodenal stasis. Correcting posture and relieving visceroptosis relieved symptoms of duodenal obstruction in 65% of patients. The corrected posture also relieved the gastric distress, nausea, and abdominal pain of 75% of patients.[75,p.135]

Some 26.3% of fibromyalgia patients report urinary urgency.[1,p.54] Visceroptosis associated with a slumping posture may contribute to this symptom in some patients (see Chapter 3.21, section titled Biomechanical Influence on Urinary Urgency). As the upper abdominal viscera press downward, the movement eventually compresses the urinary bladder. (This is similar to the effect of the growing baby *in utero* during late pregnancy.) The compression decreases ability of the bladder to expand normally. As relatively small amounts of urine collect in the bladder, the patient senses the need to urinate. Urinary frequency in fibromyalgia, however, is more likely due primarily to inadequate thyroid hormone regulation of the adrenergic genes (see Chapter 3.21: Model for Urinary Urgency and Frequency).

Segmentally-Related Physiological Aberrance. I mentioned above that Littlejohn found restricted cervical range of motion and regional tender points in 60% of essentially asymptomatic workers. He speculated that these individuals are predisposed to develop localized fibromyalgia (of the shoulder and arm) when other stresses impinge on their cervical spines. According to him, the critical link in initiating the fibromyalgia is a tissue injury neurologically related to the compromised part of the spine. He also wrote that the patient's psychological response to the injury complicates the injury. The tissue injury causes noxious signals to reach the dorsal horns of the spinal cord through small type C nerve fibers. He considered that these fibers "are intrinsic to the development of the predictable clinical features which characterize the syndrome." He proposed that segmental activation by pain signals causes reflex changes in organs that produce the characteristic features of fibromyalgia.[80,pp.56-57]

Littlejohn's description of this mechanism duplicates my more detailed description in *The Purpose and Practice of Myofascial Therapy*.[48] Of special importance to this model is the chronic central excitatory state of various spinal levels. This tends to occur particularly at spinal levels with dormant physiological abnormalities. These abnormalities include restricted ranges of joint motion and latent trigger points in paraspinal muscles. Noxious neural signals at these facilitated segments appear to augment any segmentally-related abnormalities that already exist. Experimentally intensifying the noxious input (creating an artificial trigger point by injecting an irritating chemical) increases segmentally-related abnormalities such as increased muscle tension, vasoconstriction, or changes in internal organs.[82] Korr found this when he injected an irritating chemical (6% NaCl) into the erector spinae or intercostal myofascia. This stoked up activity at subluxated (lesioned or irritable) spinal segments, although he injected the irritant far away from the spine. He had artificially created a myofascial trigger point, and he showed that the trigger point agitated the subluxated segments.[98][99]

REFERENCES

1. Wolfe, F.: Diagnosis of fibromyalgia. *J. Musculoskel. Med.*, 7:54, 1990.
2. Kirk, E. and Kvorning, S.A.: *Hypometabolism: A Clinical Study of 308 Consecutive Cases.* Copenhagen, Einar Munksgaard, Publisher, 1946.
3. Watanakunakorn, C., Hodges, R.E., and Evans, T.C.: Myxedema: a study of 400 cases. *Arch. Intern. Med.*, 116: 183-190, 1965.
4. Thurmon, F.M. and Thompson, W.O.: Low basal metabolism with myxedema. *Arch. Intern. Med.*, 46:879-897, 1930.
5. Thompson, W.O. and Thompson, P.K.: Low basal metabolism following thyrotoxicosis. *J. Clin. Invest.*, 5:471-501, 1928.
6. Kurland, G.S., Hamolsky, M.W., and Freedberg, A.S.: Studies in non-myxedematous hypometabolism: I. the clinical syndrome and the effects of triiodothyronine, alone or combined with thyroxine. *J. Clin. Endocrinol.*, 15:1354, 1955.
7. Goldberg, M.: Diagnosis of euthyroid hypometabolism. *Am. J. Obst. & Gynec.*, 81(5):1057-1058, May, 1961.
8. Morton, J.H.: Sodium liothyronine in metabolic insuffi-

ciency syndrome and associated disorders. *J.A.M.A.*, 165: 124-129, 1957.
9. Freedberg, A.S., Kurland, G.S., and Hamolsky, M.W.: Effect of l-tri-iodothyronine alone and combined with l-thyroxine in nonmyxedematous hypometabolism. *N. Engl. J. Med.*, 253:57-60, 1955.
10. Fields, E.M.: Treatment of metabolic insufficiency and hypothyroidism with sodium liothyronine. *J.A.M.A.*, 163: 817, 1957.
11. Tittle, C.R.: Effects of 3,5,3' l-triiodothyronine in patients with metabolic insufficiency. *J.A.M.A.*, 162:271, 1956.
12. Snorrason, E., Geirsson, A., and Stefansson, K.: Trial of a selective acetylcholinesterase inhibitor, galanthamine hydrobromide, in the treatment of chronic fatigue syndrome. *J. Chronic Fatigue*, 2(2/3):35-54, 1996.
13. DeGroot, L.J., Larsen, P.R., Refetoff, S., and Stanbury, J.B.: *The Thyroid and Its Diseases*, 5th edition. New York, John Wiley & Sons, Inc., 1984.
14. Rastogi, R.B., Lapierre, Y., and Singhal, R.L.: Evidence for the role of brain biogenic amines in depressed motor activity seen in chemically thyroidectomized rats. *J. Neurochem.*, 26:443-449, 1976.
15. Heffner, T.G. and Seiden, L.S.: Synthesis of catecholamines from [3H]tyrosine in brain during the performance of operant behavior. *Brain Res.*, 183:403-419, 1980.
16. Plaznik, A. and Kostowski, W.: The interrelationship between brain noradrenergic and dopaminergic neuronal systems in regulating animal behavior: possible clinical implications. *Psychopharmacol. Bull.*, 19:5-11, 1983.
17. Diarra, A., Lefauconnier, J.M., Valens, M., Georges, P., and Gripois, D.: Tyrosine content, influx, and accumulation rate, and catecholamine biosynthesis measured *in vivo*, in the central nervous system and in peripheral organs of young rats: influence of neonatal hypo- and hyperthyroidism. *Arch. Intern. Physiol. Biochem.*, 97:317-332, 1989.
18. Creese, I. and Iversen, S.D.: The pharmacological and anatomical substrates of the amphetamine response in the rat. *Brain Res.*, 83:419-436, 1975.
19. Jackson, D.M., Anden, N.-E., and Dahlstrom, A.: A functional effect of dopamine in the nucleus accumbens and in some other dopamine-rich parts of the rat brain. *Psychopharmacology*, 45:139-149, 1975.
20. Kelly, P.H., Seviour, P.W., and Iversen, S.D.: Amphetamine and apomorphine responses in the rat following 6-OHDA lesions of the nucleus acccumbens septi and corpus striatum. *Brain Res.*, 94:507-522, 1975.
21. Pijnenburg, A.J.J., Honig, W.M.M., and Van Rossum, J.M.: Effects of antagonists upon locomotor stimulation induced by injection of dopamine and noradrenaline into the nucleus accumbens of nialamide-pretreated rats. *Psychopharmacology*, 41:175-180, 1975.
22. Costall, B., Marsden, C.D., Maylor, R.J., and Pycock, C.J.: Sterotyped behavior patterns and hyperactivity induced by amphetamine and apomorphine after discrete 6-hydroxydopamine lesions of extrapyramidal and mesolimbic nuclei. *Brain Res.*, 123:89-111, 1977.
23. Makanjuola, R.O.A., Dow, R.C., and Ashcroft, G.W.: Behavioural responses to stereotactically controlled injections of monoamine neurotransmitters into the accumbens and caudate-putamen nuclei. *Psychopharmacol.*, 71:227-

235, 1980.

24. Cooper, J.R., Bloom, F.E., and Roth, R.H.: *The Biochemical Basis of Neuropharmacology*, 6ᵗʰ edtion. New York, Oxford University Press, 1991.

25. Mason, G.A., Bondy, S.C., Nemeroff, C.B., Walker, C.H., and Prange, A.J., Jr.: The effects of thyroid state on β-adrenergic and serotonergic receptors in rat brain. *Psychoneuroendocrinol.*, 12:261-270, 1987.

26. Engstrom, G., Svensson, T.H., and Waldeck, B.: Thyroxine and brain catecholamines: increased transmitter synthesis and increased receptor sensitivity. *Brain Res.*, 77:471-483, 1974.

27. Strombom, U., Svensson, T.H., Jackson, R.M., and Engstrom, G.J.: Hyperthyroidism: specifically increased response to central NA-(alpha)-receptor stimulation and generally increased monoamine turnover in brain. *J. Neural Transm.*, 41:73-92, 1977.

28. Puymirat, J., Luo, M., and Dussault, J.H.: Immunocytochemical localization of thyroid hormone nuclear receptors in cultured hypothalamic dopaminergic neurons. *Neuroscience*, 30(2):443-449, 1989.

29. Puymirat, J.: Effects of dysthyroidism on central catecholaminergic neurons. *Neurochem. Int.*, 7:969-978, 1985.

30. Puymirat, J., Barret, A., Picart, R., et al: Triiodothyronine enhances the morphological maturation of dopaminergic neurons from fetal mouse hypothalamus cultured in serum-free medium. *Neuroscience*, 10:801-810, 1983.

31. Puymirat, J., Barret, A., Faivre-Bauman, A., and Tixier-Vidal, A.: Biochemical characterization of the uptake and release of ³H-dopamine by dopaminergic neurons: a developmental study using serum-free cultures. *Devel. Biol.*, 119:75-84, 1987.

32. Bennett, R.M., Clark, S.R., Campbell, S.M., et al.: Symptoms of Raynaud's syndrome in patients with fibromyalgia: a study utilizing the Nielsen test, digital photoplethysmography and measurements of platelet α₂-adrenergic receptors. *Arthritis Rheum.*, 34:264-269, 1991.

33. Clineschmidt, B.V., Flataker, L.M., Faison, E., and Holmes, R.: An *in vivo* model for investigating α₁- and α₂-receptors in the CNS: studies with mianserin. *Arch. Int. Pharmacodyn. Ther.*, 242(1):59-76, 1979.

34. Delini-Stula, A., Baumann, P., and Buch, O.: Depression of exploratory activity by clonidine in rats as a model for the detection of relative pre- and postsynaptic central noradrenergic receptor selectivity of α-adrenolytic drugs. *Naunyn Schmiedeberg's Arch. Pharmacol.*, 307:115-122, 1979.

35. Drew, G.M., Gower, A.J., and Marriott, A.S.: α₂-Adrenoceptors mediate clonidine-induced sedation in the rat. *Br. J. Pharmacol.*, 67:133-141, 1979.

36. Mueller, K. and Nyhan, W.I.: Modulation of the behavioral effects of amphetamine in rats by clonidine. *Eur. J. Pharmacol.*, 83:339-342, 1982.

37. Pifl, Ch.F. and Hornykiewicz, O.: α-Noradrenergic involvement in locomotor activity. *Naunyn Schmiedeberg's Arch. Pharmacol.*, 330(Suppl.):R71, 1985.

38. Dickinson, S.L., Gadie, B., and Tulloch, I.F.: α₁- and α₂-Adrenoreceptor antagonists differentially influence locomotor and stereotyped behaviour induced by *d*-amphetamine and apomorphine in the rat. *Psychopharmacol.*, 96:521-527, 1988.

39. Kostowski, W., Jerlicz, M., Bidzinski, A., and Hauptmann, M.: Evidence for the existence of two opposite noradrenergic brain systems controlling behaviour. *Psychopharmacol.*, 59:311-312, 1978.

40. Segal, J.: Calmodulin modulates thymocyte adenylate cyclase activity through the guanine nucleotide regulatory unit. *Mol. Cell. Endocrinol.*, 64:95, 1989.

41. Thomas, K.V. and Handley, S.L.: Modulation of dexamphetamine-induced compulsive gnawing including the possible involvement of presynaptic α-adrenoreceptors. *Psychopharmacol.*, 56:61-67, 1978.

42. Zetler, G.: Clonidine sensitizes mice for apomorphine-induced stereotypic gnawing: antagonism by neuroleptics and cholecytokinin-like peptides. *Eur. J. Pharmacol.*, 111: 309-318, 1985.

43. Nichols, A.J. and Ruffolo, R.R., Jr.: Functions mediated by α-adrenoceptors. In α-*Adrenoceptors: Molecular Biology, Biochemistry and Pharmacology*. Basel, Karger, 1991, pp.113-179.

44. Bock, K.D., Heimsoth, V., Merguet, P. and Schoenermark, J.: Klinische und klinische-experimentelle Untersuchungen mit einer neuen blutdrucksenkenden Substanz: Dichlorophenylaminoimidazolin. *Dt. Med. Wschr.*, 91: 1761-1770, 1966.

45. Michel, D., Zimmerman, W., Nassehi, A., and Seraphim, P.: Erste Beobachtungen über einen antihypertensiven effekt von 2-(2-6-Dichlorphenyl-amino)-2-imidazolin hydrochlorid am menschen. *Dt. Med. Wschr.*, 91:1540-1547, 1966.

46. Davidov, M., Kakaviatos, N., and Finnerty, F.A.: The antihypertensive effects of an imidazoline compound. *Clin. Pharmacol. Ther.*, 8:810-816, 1967.

47. Miso, Y. and Kubo, T.: Central and peripheral cardiovascular responses of rats to guanabenz and clonidine. *Jap. J. Pharmacol.*, 40:87-119, 1982.

48. Lowe, J.C.: *The Purpose and Practice of Myofascial Therapy* (audio cassette training album). Houston, McDowell Publishing Co., 1989, tapes 1 and 2.

49. *The Merck Manual of Diagnosis and Therapy*, 15ᵗʰ edition. Edited by R. Berkow and A.J. Fletcher, Rahway, Merck, Sharp & Dohme Research Laboratories, 1987.

50. Gold, M.S., Pottash, A.L.C., and Extein, I.: Hypothyroidism and depression: evidence from complete thyroid function evaluation. *J.A.M.A.*, 245:1919, 1981.

51. Levey, G.S.: Catecholamine sensitivity, thyroid hormone and the heart. *Amer. J. Med.*, 50:413-420, 1971.

52. McConnaughey, M.M., Jones, L.R., Watanabe, A.M., Besch, H.R., Jr., Williams, L.T., and Lefkowitz, R.J.: Thyroxine and propylthiouracil effects on α- and β-adrenergic receptor number, ATPase activities, and sialic acid content of rat cardiac membrane vesicles. *J. Cardiovasc. Pharmacol.*, 1:609-623, 1979.

53. Landsberg, L. and Young, J.B.: Catecholamines and the sympathoadrenal system. In *Werner's The Thyroid: A Fundamental and Clinical Text*, 5ᵗʰ edition. Edited by S.H. Ingbar and L.E. Braverman, Philadelphia, J.B. Lippincott Co., 1986, pp.1223-1224.

54. Kunos, G., and Nickerson, M.: Effects of sympathetic innervation and temperature on the properties of rat heart adrenoceptors. *Br. J. Pharmacol.*, 59:603-614, 1977.

55. Kunos, G., Vermes-Kunos, I., and Nickerson, M.: Effects

of thyroid state on adrenoceptor properties. *Nature* (London), 250:779-781, 1974.

56. Kunos, G.: Thyroid hormone-dependent interconversion of myocardial α- and β-adrenoceptors in the rat. *Br. J. Pharmacol.*, 59(1):177-189, 1977.

57. Williams, R.S., Guthrow, C.E., and Lefkowitz, R.J.: β-Adrenergic receptors of human lymphocytes are unaltered by hyperthyroidism. *J. Clin. Endocrinol.*, 48:503-505, 1979.

58. Malbon, C.C., Li, S., and Fain, J.N.: Hormonal activation of glycogen phosphorylase in hepatocytes from hypothyroid rats. *J. Biol. Chem.*, 253:8820-8825, 1978.

59. Williams, R. S. and Lefkowitz, R.J.: The effects of thyroid hormone on adrenergic receptors. In *Molecular Basis of Thyroid Hormone Action*. Edited by J.H. Oppenheimer and H.H. Samuels, New York, Academic Press, Inc., 1983, pp.325-349.

60. Sterling, K. and Hoffenberg, R.: β-Blocking agents and antithyroid drugs as adjuncts to radioiodine therapy. *Semin. Nucl. Med.*, 1:422, 1971.

61. Silva, J.E. and Landsberg, L.: Catecholamines and the sympathoadrenal system in hypothyroidism. In *Werner's The Thyroid: A Fundamental and Clinical Text*, 6th edition. Edited by L.E. Braverman and R.D. Utiger, Philadelphia, J.B. Lippincott Co., 1991, pp.1050-1051.

62. Rosenquist, U.: Noradrenaline-induced lipolysis in subcutaneous adipose tissue from hypothyroid subjects. *Acta Med. Scand.*, 192:361-369, 1972.

63. Pointon, S.E. and Banergee, S.P.: Adrenergic and muscarinic cholinergic receptor in rat submaxillary glands: effects of thyroidectomy. *Biochim. Biophys. Acta*, 583:129, 1979.

64. Fregly, M.F., Nelson, E.L., and Resch, G.E.: Reduced β-adrenergic responsiveness in hypothyroid rats. *Amer. J. Physiol.*, 229:916, 1975.

65. Grill, V. and Rosenquist, U.: Inhibition of the noradrenaline induced adenyl cyclase stimulation by augmented and adrenergic response in subcutaneous adipose tissue from hypothyroid subjects. *Acta Med. Scand.*,194:129, 1973.

66. Bilezikian, J.P. and Loeb, J.N.: The influence of hyperthyroidism and hypothyroidism on α- and β-adrenergic receptor systems and adrenergic responsiveness. *Endocrine Rev.*, 4:378, 1983.

67. Gross, G., Brodde, O.E., and Schumann, H.J.: Decreased number of β-adrenoceptors in cerebral cortex of hypothyroid rats. *Eur. J. Pharmacol.*, 61:191, 1980.

68. Marwaha, J. and Prasad, K.N.: Hypothyroidism elicits electrophysiological noradrenergic subsensitivity in rat cerebellum. *Science*, 214:675, 1981.

69. Bronsky, D., Shrifter, H., and De La Heurga, J.: Cerebrospinal fluid proteins in myxedema, with special reference to electrophoretic partition. *J. Clin. Endocrinol. Metab.*, 18:470, 1958.

70. Fink, C.W., Ferguson, J.L., and Smiley, J.D.: Effect of hyperthyroidism and hypothyroidism on collagen metabolism. *J. Lab. Clin. Med.*, 69:950, 1967.

71. Pitot, H.C. and Yatvin, M.B.: Interrelationships of mammalian hormones and enzyme levels *in vivo*. *Physiol. Rev.*, 53:228, 1973.

72. Hiemeyer, K., Lutz, R., and Menninger, H.: Dependence of tender points upon posture: a key to the understanding of fibromyalgia syndrome. *J. Manual Med.*, 5:169-174, 1990.

73. Homewood, A.E.: *The Neurodynamics of the Vertebral Subluxation,* 2nd edition. St. Petersburg, Valkyrie Press, 1977.

74. Franco, M., Bobadilla, N.A., Suarez, J., Tapia, E., Sanchez, L., and Herrera-Acosta, J.: Participation of adenosine in the renal hemodynamic abnormalities of hypothyroidism. *Am. J. Physiol.*, 270(2 Pt.2):F254-F262, 1996.

75. Schafer, R.C.: *Clinical Biomechanics: Musculoskeletal Actions and Reactions*, 2nd edition. Baltimore, Williams & Wilkins, 1987.

76. Goldthwait, J.E.: *Essentials of Body Mechanics in Health and Disease,* 5th edition. Philadelphia, J.B. Lippincott, 1952.

77. Verner, J.R.: *The Science and Logic of Chiropractic.* Englewood, published by author, 1941.

78. Kendall, H.O. and Kendall, F.P.: Developing and maintaining good posture. *J. Am. Phys. Ther. Ass.*, 48:319-336,1968.

79. Kelley, K.W. (Editor): *The Home Planet.* Moscow, Mir Publishers, 1988.

80. Littlejohn, G.O.: Fibrositis/fibromyalgia syndrome in the workplace. *Rheum. Dis. Clin. North Am.*, 15:45-60, 1989.

81. Kaasik, A., Seppet, E.K., and Ohisalo, J.J.: Enhanced negative inotropic effect of an adenosine A_1-receptor agonist in rat left atria in hypothyroidism. *J. Mol. Cell. Cardiol.*, 26(4):509-517, 1994.

82. Lowe, J.C.: The subluxation and the trigger point: measuring how they interact. *Chiro. J.*, Oct., 1992.

83. Tepperman, J. and Tepperman, H.M.: *Metabolic and Endocrine Physiology*, 5th edition. Chicago, Year Book Medical Publishers, Inc., 1987.

84. O'Connor, J.F., Wu, G.Y., Gallagher, T.F., and Hellman, L.: The 24-hour plasma thyroxin profile in normal man. *J. Clin. Endocrinol. Metab.*, 39:765, 1974.

85. Azukizawa, M., Pekary, A.E., Hershman, J.M., and Parker, D.C.: Plasma thyrotropin, thyroxine, and triiodothyronine relationships in man. *J. Clin. Endocrinol. Metab.*, 43:533, 1976.

86. DeCostre, P., Buhler, U., DeGroot, L.J., and Refetoff, S.: Diurnal rhythm in total serum thyroxine levels. *Metabol.*, 20:782, 1971.

87. Mazurkiewicz, D. and Saggerson, E.D.: Inhibition of adenylate cyclase in rat brain synaptosomal membranes by GTP and phenylisopropyladenosine is enhanced in hypothyroidism. *Biochem. J.*, 263(3):829-835, 1989.

88. Eisinger, J.: Metabolic abnormalities in fibromyalgia. *Clin. Bull. Myofascial Ther.*, 3(1):3-21, 1998.

89. Lowe, J.C.: Hypertonic fascia. *Dyn. Chiro.*, 8:28, 1990.

90. Akeson, W.H., Amiel, D., LaViolette, D., et.al.: The connective tissue response to immobility: an accelerated aging response? *Experi. Geront.*, 3:289-301, 1968.

91. Amiel, D., Akeson, W.H., Harwood, F.L., and Mechanic, G.L.: The effect of immobilization on the types of collagen synthesized in periarticular connective tissue. *Connect. Tiss. Res.*, 8:27, 1980.

92. Guyton, A.C.: Personal communication., November 30, 1989.

93. Stein, M.B., Clark, M., and Delaney, S.M.: Chronic changes in thyroid hormones do not affect brain adenosine receptors. *Prog. Neuropsychopharmacol. Biol. Psychiat.*,

17(6):1037-1047, 1993.

94. Russell, I.J., Vaeroy, M., Jabors, M., and Nyberg, F.: Cerebrospinal fluid biogenic metabolites in fibromyalgia/fibrositis syndrome in rheumatoid arthritis. *Arthritis Rheum.*, 35:550-556, 1992.

95. Denslow, J.S., Korr, I.M, and Drems, A.D.: Quantitative studies of chronic facilitation in human motoneuron pools. *Amer. J. Physiol.*, 150(2):229-238, 1947.

96. Denslow, J.S. and Hassett, C.C.: Spontaneous and induced spasm in structural abnormalities. *J. Am. Osteopathic. Assoc.*, 42:207-212, 1943.

97. Denslow, J.S.: An analysis of the irritability of spinal reflex arcs. *J. Am. Osteopathic Assoc.*, 44:357-362, 1945.

98. Korr, I.M.: Personal communication. March, 1989.

99. Korr, I.M.: Experimental alterations in segmental sympathetic (sweat gland) activity through myofascial and postural disturbances. *Fed. Proc.*, 8:88, 1949.

100. Malbon, C.C., Rapiejko, P.J.,and Mangano, T.J.: Fat cell adenylate cyclase system. Enhanced inhibition by adenosine and GTP in the hypothyroid rat. *J. Biol. Chem.*, 260 (4):2558-2564, 1985.

101. Gur, S., Ari, N., and Ozturk, Y.: Increased responses to adenosine in isolated left atria from streptozotocin-diabetic rats: evidence for the involvement of hypothyroidism. *J. Cardiovasc. Pharmacol.*, 29(2):174-179, 1997.

3.12

Growth Hormone and Somatomedin C

Anterior pituitary cells termed somatotrophs synthesize and secrete growth hormone. Secretion of growth hormone by the pituitary is stimulated by growth hormone-releasing hormone from the hypothalamus. Many stimuli increase growth hormone secretion by increasing the secretion of growth hormone-releasing factor (hormone) by hypothalamic cells. About 70% of growth hormone secretion occurs during slow wave sleep in the early hours of sleep. Circulating levels of growth hormone are minuscule and have a short half-life.

Growth hormone is an anabolic hormone; it stimulates synthesis of proteins and proteoglycans in tissues. Another class of hormones, somatomedins, mediate the protein-enhancing effects of growth hormone in target tissues. In some tissues, growth hormone and somatomedins may act in unison to exert anabolic effects.

Growth hormone also exerts glucose sparing and storing effects. It increases insulin secretion, diminishes the use of glucose for energy, and increases glucose storage as glycogen.

Somatomedins inhibit growth hormone secretion by the pituitary somatotrophs. Somatomedin C also indirectly inhibits the somatotrophs by decreasing hypothalamic secretion of growth hormone-releasing factor. Growth hormone also inhibits its own secretion in a fine tuning negative feedback loop: It inhibits hypothalamic secretion of growth hormone-releasing factor and increases the hypothalamic release of somatostatin. Somatostatin directly inhibits growth hormone secretion by the pituitary.

Thyroid hormone potently regulates the synthesis and secretion of all components of the growth hormone-related axis—growth hormone-releasing factor, growth hormone, somatomedins (including somatomedin C), somatomedin receptors, and the somatomedin-binding proteins that transport somatomedins through the circulation.

Growth hormone levels are low in some fibromyalgia patients. Researchers have inferred that growth hormone levels are low from the patients' measurable low somatomedin C levels. Growth hormone injections increased the low somatomedin C levels in one group of fibromyalgia patients; the patients' scores on the Fibromyalgia Impact Questionnaire improved, and their myalgic scores and numbers of tender points decreased.

It is highly unlikely that low growth hormone and/or somatomedin C levels are a primary pathophysiologic mechanism of fibromyalgia. Improvement in some features of fibromyalgia—those typical of growth hormone or somatomedin C deficiency—is predictable for patients with low somatomedin C levels using replacement dosages of growth hormone. Growth hormone and somatomedin C levels, however, do not account for most symptoms and objective findings in fibromyalgia. In addition, some objective findings in fibromyalgia are inconsistent with low growth hormone levels. To wit: (1) In growth hormone deficiency, the use of glucose for energy increases, but in fibromyalgia, glycolysis is impaired, indicating a decreased use of glucose for energy; (2) in growth hormone deficiency, cellular glycogen deposition decreases, yet biopsies of tissues from fibromyalgia patients show increased glycogen deposition.

Low growth hormone and somatomedin C levels in some fibromyalgia patients are best accounted for by a hypothesis of inadequate thyroid hormone regulation of the genes that code for growth hormone-releasing factor, growth hormone, and somatomedin C. In the study in which growth hormone injections increased somatomedin C levels in fibromyalgia patients, 28% of the patients developed carpal tunnel syndrome as an adverse effect. Only 4% of placebo patients developed the syndrome. Carpal tunnel syndrome is a common feature of hypothyroidism and resistance to thyroid hormone due to T_3-receptor mutations. The cause of the syndrome is inadequate thyroid hormone regulation of fibroblasts. During inadequate regulation, fibroblasts increase their release of glycosaminoglycans into the ground substance of the connective tissues, including the flexor retinacula of the wrists. (The retinacula are the retaining band-like ligaments of the wrists.) As a result of the increase in glycosaminoglycans, the retinacula accumulate more water and swell. The swelling compresses the median nerve in the wrist. The symptoms result from the compression. Growth hormone increases production of glycosaminoglycans. It is possible that the injections, by increasing glycosaminoglycan accumulation, compounded a previously existing excess of glycosaminoglycans in the flexor retinacula of the wrists of 28% of the patients—an existing excess caused by inadequate thyroid hormone regulation of fibroblasts in the retinacula.

A corollary hypothesis is that inadequate thyroid hormone regulation of the adrenergic genes in the hypothalamic cells that produce growth hormone-releasing factor results in a decreased density of α_2-adrenergic receptors and an increased density of β-adrenergic receptors on the cell membranes (the opposite effects from those in most other tissues). The effect of this would be inhibition of growth hormone-releasing factor and growth hormone secretion. The decrease in α_2-adrenergic receptors in the hypothalamus may account for the decreased release of growth hormone in fibromyalgia patients in response to administration of clonidine (an α_2-adrenergic receptor agonist that normally increases growth hormone secretion).

The inadequate thyroid hormone regulation hypothesis provides a plausible starting point for low growth hormone and somatomedin C levels in fibromyalgia. The hypothesis thus accounts for the objective findings of low growth hormone and somatomedin C, as it does for the other objective findings and symptoms of fibromyalgia.

rowth hormone levels are low in a minority of fibromyalgia patients. Bennett reported low levels in 30% of patients.[74] That only a minority of patients have low levels makes it unlikely that the low levels underlie the features of fibromyalgia in most patients with the diagnosis. Nevertheless, some features of fibromyalgia may be mediated by low growth hormone and/or low somatomedin C levels. The low levels of growth hormone and somatomedin C are accounted for by inadequate thyroid hormone regulation of cells in the hypothalamus, pituitary, and peripheral tissues that produce somatomedin C. Finding low levels of these two hormones in fibromyalgia is powerfully favorable to the hypothesis that inadequate thyroid hormone regulation of cell function underlies many patients' fibromyalgia.

● GROWTH HORMONE AND SOMATOMEDIN C

Anterior pituitary cells termed somatotrophs synthesize and secrete the peptide molecule called growth hormone. The hormone is held in the granules of these cells until secreted. Some 15%-to-20% of growth hormone in the circulation is bound to transport proteins.[50] For the most part, growth hormone exerts its metabolic effects through mediation of somatomedins (see section below titled "Somatomedins").

SECRETION OF GROWTH HORMONE

Basal blood levels of growth hormone are minuscule and the hormone has a short half-life. For these reasons, the circulating hormone may not be detectable without a test that provokes the pituitary somatotrophs to secrete more. Provoking somatotroph secretion may be the most direct way to learn whether a patient has a growth hormone deficiency.[41,p.125] Growth hormone levels vary widely among individuals. The variation in blood levels is due to the fact that minimal exercise or physical or psychological stress increases growth hormone levels. Women typically have slightly higher levels.[64] Their levels are higher because their hormonal dynamics (particularly in relation to estrogen) heighten their sensitivity to stimuli that cause growth hormone release.[51][52]

Most stimuli provoke growth hormone release

through a three-step neural circuit. First, stimuli affect one or more of three brain centers (the ventromedial nucleus, arcuate nucleus, and limbic system). Stimulation of these centers causes release of neurotransmitters that act at a common site, the median eminence of the hypothalamus. Action of the neurotransmitters at this site causes release of growth hormone-releasing factor into the portal vessels. (Growth hormone-releasing factor is a peptide hormone. Researchers generally refer to it as growth hormone-releasing hormone and "somatoliberin." I use the older term growth hormone-releasing "factor" as an aid—albeit a modest one—to reader comprehension.) These vessels deliver growth hormone-releasing factor to the anterior pituitary. The somatotrophs of the pituitary gland respond to growth hormone-releasing factor by secreting growth hormone.[41,p.125][79]

Somatostatin

Growth hormone-releasing factor causes release of growth hormone from the pituitary gland; the peptide hormone somatostatin inhibits growth hormone release. Somatostatin is an inhibitory compound secreted by the hypothalamus but also by some peripheral tissues.[53] The effects of growth hormone-releasing factor and somatostatin are complicated because the pituitary has two functional storage sites of growth hormone. One releases the hormone immediately upon stimulation, and the other responds only to prolonged chemical prodding.[54][55]

A host of stimuli increase growth hormone secretion through growth hormone-releasing factor or decrease it through somatostatin. Some stimuli that increase secretion of growth hormone are hypoglycemia, vasopressin, the amino acid arginine, α-adrenergic stimulants, and protein depletion from the body. Chlorpromazine (Thorazine) decreases secretion through postsynaptic inhibition of a dopamine receptor.[41,p.126] Glucocorticoids also inhibit growth hormone secretion.[66,p.589] Chronic use of exogenous glucocorticoids inhibits growth hormone release.[41,p.126]

It is interesting that somatostatin may also suppress TSH secretion. Somatostatin lowers TSH in hypothyroid patients although their TSH is ordinarily high.[62] This means its influence over the thyrotrophs is strong because in hypothyroidism the thyrotrophs are disinhibited by the low levels of thyroid hormone and hyper-responsive to stimuli that provoke TSH release. Although somatostatin suppresses growth hormone and TSH secretion, it does not inhibit release of prolactin.[35,p.1585]

GROWTH HORMONE RELEASE DURING SLEEP

Careful studies of the relationship of slow wave sleep and growth hormone secretion indicate that the two phenomena are not closely linked through the neural mechanisms necessary for slow wave sleep. Slow wave sleep and growth hormone secretion ordinarily occur concomitantly. About 70% of growth hormone secretion occurs during deep or slow wave sleep (synonymous with stages 3 and 4 sleep). The hormone is released in bursts or "spikes." The bursts occur during the early hours of sleep; there is virtually no growth hormone secretion during later hours of sleep.[41,p.126][56] If early slow wave sleep is prevented by awakening the subject, no growth hormone is secreted.[29,p.267]

Researchers reported that preventing growth hormone secretion did not block slow wave sleep. Slow wave sleep occurred normally in patients taking drugs that inhibit growth hormone secretion (imipramine, flurazepam, methylscopolamine, and medroxyprogesterone).[29,p.267]

SOMATOMEDINS

Growth hormone stimulates the mesenchymal cells of liver, kidney, and other tissues to synthesize and secrete somatomedins. Somatomedins are polypeptide hormones. Researchers call somatomedins "insulin-like growth factors" because the hormones have structural and biologic properties similar to insulin.[35,p.1586] The hormones have insulin-like metabolic effects, particularly in fat tissues.[75] Somatomedin C and insulin growth factor-I are synonymous terms for the same peptide. Growth hormone largely regulates secretion of somatomedin C, but growth hormone has only minimal control over secretion of insulin-like growth factor-II.[75]

Somatomedins mediate the effects of growth hormone on target tissues. To illustrate, growth hormone induces the uptake of sulfate by cartilage proteoglycans[58] and the incorporation of amino acids into muscle proteins.[59] Growth hormone exerts these effects indirectly through somatomedins rather than through direct action on the proteoglycan and protein molecules. In some tissues, though, growth hormone and somatomedins may act in unison to exert anabolic effects.[41,p.127]

The term somatomedin implies "mediator of growth hormone."[35,p.1586] ("Somatotropin" is a synonym for growth hormone.) Somatomedins stimulate cartilage growth and mitosis and growth of many types of extraskeletal cells. Somatomedins are important in the diagnosis of growth disturbances secondary to pituitary disease. Plasma levels are low in pituitary dwarfism and high in acromegaly.[75]

Somatomedin C and
Growth Hormone Secretion

Circulating somatomedins largely govern growth hormone secretion[75] by inhibiting somatotroph secretion. Somatomedin C appears to indirectly inhibit the somatotrophs by inhibiting hypothalamic secretion of growth hormone-releasing factor. Inhibition of pituitary growth hormone secretion by affecting the hypothalamus is a long-loop feedback mechanism for control of growth hormone secretion. The increase in growth hormone secretion with protein depletion from the body may be due to decreased secretion of somatomedin C.[41,p.126]

Growth hormone also inhibits its own release as its levels become elevated. Through a negative feedback loop, it suppresses its own secretion by two effects on the hypothalamus: (1) inhibition of secretion of growth hormone-releasing factor[41,p.126] and (2) stimulation of secretion of somatostatin.[60] The decrease in growth hormone-releasing factor and increase in somatostatin inhibit pituitary secretion of growth hormone. This is a short-loop pituitary-hypothalamus-pituitary feedback mechanism. The loop probably functions to fine tune more potent regulation through long-loop somatomedin C regulation.[61,p.41]

METABOLIC EFFECTS
OF GROWTH HORMONE

Protein Deposition

Growth hormone is an anabolic hormone; it enhances protein synthesis.[35,p.1585] Administering growth hormone increased incorporation of radioactively labeled leucine (an amino acid) into muscle protein; absence of growth hormone decreased incorporation of the amino acid.[57] Merimee and Grant wrote, "It is now evident that [growth hormone] can promote amino acid uptake by muscle, cartilage, and isolated hepatic cells, and that an increased synthesis of protein usually follows this uptake."[41,p.126] Guyton listed the four effects of growth hormone on protein metabolism (see Table 3.12.1). The hormone increases nearly all aspects of amino acid uptake and protein synthe-

sis by cells. It also reduces the breakdown of proteins.[68,pp.822-823]

Carbohydrate Metabolism

As Tables 3.12.2 and 3.12.3 show, growth hormone has glucose-sparing and -storing effects in cells. Growth hormone deficiency has the opposite effects—increased glucose mobilization and use.

● LOW GROWTH HORMONE AND SOMATOMEDIN C IN FIBROMYALGIA PATIENTS

In 1988, Tilbe et al. reported finding a loss of the normal diurnal variation in growth hormone levels in fibromyalgia patients.[38] A year later, however, Tilbe reported not finding the abnormal diurnal variation in another group of fibromyalgia patients.[23] Several years later, other researchers reported low levels of somatomedin C in some fibromyalgia patients. The researchers inferred from this finding that growth hormone levels are also low in some patients.[3][4][5][6][7]

Buchwald et al., however, did not find the disruption of the growth hormone-somatomedin C axis previously reported in fibromyalgia patients. The researchers measured the levels of both somatomedin C and its binding protein in four groups of people: (1) 15 presumably healthy controls, (2) 15 patients with chronic fatigue syndrome, (3) 27 patients with fibromyalgia, and (4) 15 patients who met the criteria for both fibromyalgia and chronic fatigue syndrome. Investigators found no difference between the groups in the mean concentration of somatomedin C or its binding protein. In addition, they found no difference between the groups in the proportion of subjects with values for somatomedin C or its binding protein above or below the laboratory reference range.[1] Selection bias may have influenced the outcome of this study. This is suggested by the finding of other investigators that a minority of fibromyalgia patients have low growth hormone or somatomedin C levels.

Bennett reported that 30% of fibromyalgia patients have low growth hormone levels.[74] Beaufort and colleagues concluded from their study of somatomedin C levels in fibromyalgia patients: "Even if not significantly, growth hormone is decreased in fibromyalgia, peculiarly in a subgroup (36% of fibromyalgia patients). This could require appropriate therapy such as growth hormone or arginine." The researchers found that the mean growth hormone level for control subjects was 5.8±4.8 mU/L. The level for hypothyroid patients was 4.0±3.4 mU/L (not significantly different from control subjects), and 3.7±4.0 mU/L for fibromyalgia patients (P=0.05). Somatomedin C was normal in fibromyalgia patients (193±54 ng/mL) and was significantly decreased in hypothyroid patients (126±74 ng/mL, p<0.01).[8]

● THE GROWTH HORMONE HYPOTHESIS OF FIBROMYALGIA

The growth hormone deficiency hypothesis of fibromyalgia can account for only a few of the features of fibromyalgia. Growth hormone deficiency in children may result in delayed skeletal maturation.[44,p.974] This is evident in the dramatic growth retardation in hypothyroid children.[45,p.1040] In adults, however, growth hormone deficiency has few manifestations.[44,p.974] However, adult patients may have subnormal tissue repair. Fibromyalgia patients have "detrained" musculoskeletal tissues.[24] The detraining results largely from the inability to engage in sufficient physical activity (see Chapter 3.4), but growth hormone and somatomedin C deficiencies may contribute to the low work capacity of some patients. Deficiencies of the hormones may also contribute to the adverse reactions of some patients to physical exercise. For example, repair of microdamage to muscles and connective tissues may be impaired. As a result, the patients may recover only at an abnormally slow rate from the associated symptoms of the microdamage.

The hypothesis that growth hormone deficiency is a major underlying mechanism of fibromyalgia breaks down at several points. The hypothesis is inconsistent with the decreased glycolysis documented in fibromyalgia patients by Eisinger et al.[9][73][76] (growth hormone deficiency increases glycolysis). The hypothesis is also inconsistent with the increased cellular glycogen deposition reported by others.[70][71] Growth hormone deficiency is associated with the opposite phenomenon—increased glucose use.

Growth hormone has four effects on carbohydrate metabolism (see Table 3.12.2). An understanding of these effects, and their opposite effects in growth hormone deficiency (see Table 3.12.3), does not favor the growth hormone hypothesis of the etiology of fibromyalgia. The increased use of glucose for energy in growth hormone deficiency may result from the de-

creased availability of fatty acids for production of acetyl-CoA. The decreased availability of fatty acids may result in feedback effects to increase the breakdown of glycogen and glucose.[68,p.823] This effect contradicts the abnormalities in carbohydrate metabolism reported by Eisinger.[73] For example, he reported that the "energy crisis" in fibromyalgia is linked more to impaired glycolysis than to mitochondrial function. The impairment results in increased blood pyruvate levels and low muscle and erythrocyte ATP concentrations.

Also, in growth hormone deficiency, glucose and glycogen are used for energy at a faster rate. As a result, more glucose enters cells and is metabolized for energy release; less is deposited as glycogen.[68,p.823]

Table 3.12.1. Metabolic effects of growth hormone on protein deposition.*

1. Increased amino acid transport through cell membranes.
2. Increased transcription of DNA to synthesize RNA.
3. Increased RNA translation to promote protein synthesis by ribosomes.
4. Reduced catabolism of proteins and amino acids.

*After Guyton, A.C.: *Textbook of Medical Physiology*, 8th edition. Philadelphia, W.B. Saunders Co., 1991, pp.822-823.[68]

Table 3.12.2. Metabolic effects of growth hormone on carbohydrate metabolism.*

1. Decreased use of glucose for energy.
2. Increased cellular glycogen deposition.
3. Initial increased cellular uptake of glucose followed by decreased uptake of glucose and increased blood glucose concentrations (when excessive, termed "pituitary diabetes").
4. Increased insulin secretion ("diabetogenic effect").

*After Guyton, A.C.: *Textbook of Medical Physiology*, 8th edition. Philadelphia, W.B. Saunders Co., 1991, p.823.[68]

Table 3.12.3. Metabolic effects of growth hormone deficiency on carbohydrate metabolism.*

1. Increased use of glucose for energy.
2. Decreased cellular glycogen deposition.
3. Increased uptake of glucose and decreased blood glucose concentrations.
4. Decreased insulin secretion.

*After Guyton, A.C.: *Textbook of Medical Physiology*, 8th edition. Philadelphia, W.B. Saunders Co., 1991, p.823.[68]

This effect, decreased glycogen deposition, is contrary to the reports by Kalyan-Raman et al.[69] and Awad.[70][71] They found increased glycogen deposition in fibromyalgia, as is typically found in hypothyroidism.

Based on the findings in the above paragraphs, the growth hormone hypothesis must logically yield to the most useful alternate hypothesis, that of inadequate thyroid hormone regulation of cell function. This alternate hypothesis elegantly explains the glycolysis impairment and the increased glycogen deposition in fibromyalgia. Moreover, it can also explain the growth hormone and somatomedin C deficiencies (see sections below titled "Thyroid Hormone Regulation of Levels of Growth Hormone-Releasing Factor and Growth Hormone" and "Thyroid Hormone Regulation of Levels of Somatomedins").

Bennett et al. compared the effects of 6 months of daily growth hormone injections with the effects of placebo injections in female fibromyalgia patients. Before treatment, all patients had low somatomedin C levels. Compared to placebo patients, patients who received daily growth hormone injections began significantly improving after 4-to-6 months. Their improvement was shown by changes in the Fibromyalgia Impact Questionnaire, tender points, and myalgic score. The investigators wrote that 25% of the patients who received growth hormone dramatically improved. They also wrote that impaired growth hormone secretion is a feature of fibromyalgia that is currently treatable with growth hormone replacement therapy. This is true, and we can expect growth hormone injections to correct the features of fibromyalgia caused by growth hormone and somatomedin C deficiencies. However, if the inadequate thyroid hormone regulation of the growth hormone-somatomedin C axis is the cause of the deficiencies of the two hormones, correcting the deficiencies with the proper form and dosage of thyroid hormone is more appropriate.

Patients do not have adverse effects to proper thyroid hormone therapy. By comparison, three adverse effects occurred in patients in the Bennett et al. study: Fluid retention (growth hormone group, 24%; placebo group, 24%), arthralgias (growth hormone group, 60%; placebo group, 43%), and carpal tunnel syndrome (growth hormone group, 28%; placebo group, 4%). Carpal tunnel syndrome may have resulted from an increase in glycosaminoglycan production in the flexor retinaculum (the ligament around the wrist) induced by growth hormone and somatomedin C. An increase in glycocosaminoglycans may have compounded a preexisting excess of glycosaminoglycans in the ligaments of patients whose fibroblasts were already inadequately regulated by thyroid hormone. The consequence would be enough glycosaminoglycans to cause the adverse effects in Bennett's patients (see Chapters 3.3 and 3.16).

LOW GROWTH HORMONE LEVELS DUE TO INADEQUATE PHYSICAL ACTIVITY OR STAGES 3 AND 4 SLEEP

Bennett suggested that the loss of slow wave sleep and the absence of the stress of exercise cause growth hormone levels to decrease in fibromyalgia patients.[10,p.188] In general, disturbed sleep and lack of exercise do contribute to low growth hormone levels.[12][30] Growth hormone blood levels increase with exercise of moderate intensity and sufficient stages 3 and 4 (slow wave) sleep.[30][31] Conversely, growth hormone levels decrease with insufficient physical activity or loss of stages 3 or 4 sleep.[29,p.267] When lack of exercise or loss of slow wave sleep lower growth hormone levels, less protein is likely to be deposited in tissues. The decreased protein deposition may impair tissue repair and reduce connective tissue tone in fibromyalgia patients.[10,p.188]

Older et al. studied the effects of interrupted slow wave sleep on somatomedin C levels in 13 healthy volunteers. The investigators measured somatomedin C levels before and after three nights of interrupted slow wave sleep. No difference was found in somatomedin C levels before and after the three nights of interrupted sleep. Older et al. conjectured that fibromyalgia patients' low levels of somatomedin C may result from chronic rather than acute interruption of slow wave sleep. Alternatively, they speculated that factors other than disturbances of slow wave sleep cause the low levels.[28]

The best candidate for this other "factor" is inadequate thyroid hormone regulation of the cells that synthesize and secrete growth hormone-releasing factor, growth hormone, and somatomedins (see section below: "Possible Role of Thyroid Hormone in the Low Growth Hormone and Somatomedin C Levels in Fibromyalgia"). Inadequate thyroid hormone regulation of cell function can directly lower the synthesis and secretion of growth hormone and somatomedin. In addition to this direct effect, inadequate thyroid hormone regulation can account—through other mechanisms—for both low physical activity and inadequate slow wave sleep in fibromyalgia patients (see Chapters 3.4 and 3.18). Low physical activity and deficient slow wave sleep are themselves growth hormone- and somatomedin-lowering factors. Thus, inadequate thyroid hormone regulation has both direct and indirect effects on the synthesis and secretion of growth hormone and somatomedin.

DECONDITIONING AND IMPAIRED TISSUE REPAIR IN FIBROMYALGIA: DECREASED PROTEIN SYNTHESIS IN HYPOTHYROIDISM

The "deconditioned" state and impaired capacity for tissue repair of many fibromyalgia patients may be in part related to a well-established finding—the decreased rate of protein synthesis in hypothyroidism.[33] In one study in which rats were made hypothyroid by chemical ablation, protein synthesis decreased 20% compared to control rats.[34,p.329] One mechanism of decreased protein synthesis may be low growth hormone and somatomedin levels in hypothyroid patients. Another mechanism may be inadequate transcription regulation for many proteins by thyroid hormone. Thyroid hormone positively regulates transcription of many genes. Inadequate thyroid hormone regulation of the genes reduces the levels of mRNAs and production of the proteins the genes code for (see Chapters 2.2 and 2.3).

● POSSIBLE ROLE OF THYROID HORMONE IN THE LOW GROWTH HORMONE AND SOMATOMEDIN C LEVELS IN FIBROMYALGIA

Thyroid hormone is a potent regulator of the production of growth hormone-releasing factor, growth hormone, and somatomedins. Inadequate thyroid hormone regulation of genes in hypothalamic, pituitary, and several peripheral tissue cells may account for the low growth hormone and somatomedin C levels in fibromyalgia.

GENETIC CONTROL BY THYROID HORMONE

Growth Hormone-Releasing Factor and Growth Hormone

The genomic hypothesis of thyroid hormone action posits that the interaction between T_3 and its receptors regulates the transcription rate of "target genes."[42,p.215] The growth hormone gene is the most studied gene whose transcription is a target of thyroid hormone.

In fibromyalgia, inadequate slow wave sleep and reduced physical exercise may contribute to low growth hormone levels.[12][30] These two factors, however, may only compound low growth hormone levels caused by inadequate thyroid hormone regulation of transcription of the growth hormone gene.[13][14][43]

Seo et al. reported that T_3 increased growth hormone mRNA in pituitary tumor cells (GH_3 cells). They wrote that their data suggest that thyroid hormone stimulates growth hormone synthesis by inducing transcription of the growth hormone gene.[13] Yaffe and Samuels found that the rate of transcription of the growth hormone gene was proportional to the levels of chromosomal T_3-receptors occupied by thyroid hormone.[43]

Miki et al. reported that thyroid deficiency following thyroidectomy reduced growth hormone-releasing factor mRNA levels in the hypothalamus by up to 65%. Administering T_4 increased levels of the mRNA. The levels of pituitary growth hormone varied parallel to levels of growth hormone-releasing factor; growth hormone levels decreased after thyroidectomy and increased upon T_4 administration.[16] T_3 and T_4 increased expression of growth hormone receptor mRNA and potentiated the expression of somatomedin C mRNA in the presence of growth hormone.[17] In the absence of thyroid hormone, growth hormone mRNA levels decreased more than 98%.[13][14][18][19]

Tam et al. noted that adequate thyroid hormone levels are necessary for normal growth in mammals, and the hormone promptly stimulates the rate of growth hormone gene transcription in pituitary somatotroph cells. They conducted a study to learn the stage at which thyroid hormone exerts its genetic effect of increasing growth hormone secretion—gene expression of growth hormone-releasing factor, somatostatin, growth hormone-releasing factor receptors, or somatostatin receptor subtype 2. Growth hormone mRNA in the anterior pituitary was significantly decreased after rats were rendered hypothyroid with antithyroid treatment. After 1 week of antithyroid treatment, the amount of growth hormone-releasing factor mRNA in the pituitary was decreased. After 3 weeks of antithyroid treatment, growth hormone-releasing factor mRNA in the hypothalamus increased 2-fold. At 12 weeks, the mRNA had increased 4-fold. However, after 12 weeks, the content of growth hormone-releasing factor had decreased compared to that of control rats. After 12 weeks, the total amounts of somatostatin mRNA and somatostatin in the hypothalamus were significantly decreased, showing a reduction in somatostatin gene expression. The amount of somatostatin receptor subtype 2 was not reduced. The investigators concluded that hypothyroidism reduced gene expression of growth hormone-releasing factor receptors and somatostatin. They wrote: "Our results suggest that the changes in hypothalamic growth hormone-releasing factor and somatostatin gene expression in hypothyroid rats may be compensatory in nature and may be secondary to the reduction in growth hormone synthesis and secretion in these animals. The reduction in basal and growth hormone-releasing factor-stimulated growth hormone secretion in hypothyroidism can be explained by the observed reduction in growth hormone and growth hormone-releasing factor receptor gene expression."[77]

Copp and Samuels identified a cAMP-responsive region in the rat growth hormone gene. cAMP and thyroid hormone appear to exert independent and synergistic effects at the region and thereby regulate expression of the gene. The researchers wrote that sequences in the growth hormone gene that mediate thyroid hormone activation are located between -208 and -160.[27]

Other investigators have mapped the elements of the growth hormone gene where thyroid hormone exerts both basal and regulated effects on gene expression. Studies show that T_3 regulates transcription of the gene through mediation of sequences in the 5'-flanking DNA region.[81][82][84][88][90][91]

Somatomedin C

In general, thyroid hormone increases the production of somatomedin C and somatomedin C receptors. Most of the effects on the peptide hormone and its binding proteins are mediated by direct control by thyroid hormone of the growth hormone gene in the pituitary. However, Vetter and Teller wrote that in hypothyroidism and several other conditions (low-calorie malnutrition, malabsorption, various storage diseases, and chronic liver and kidney diseases), even if the growth hormone level is high (in most cases it is low), plasma somatomedin C levels are nonetheless low.[75]

Moreno et al. studied the effect of thyroid hormone deficiency on expression of the somatomedin C receptor gene in heart and lung. They found that in heart and lung cells of adult animals, thyroid hormone exerted a negative effect on expression of the receptor gene. In the presence of thyroid hormone, expression of the receptor gene decreased, and in the absence of thyroid hormone, expression increased. The investi-

gators noted that in general, the somatomedin C/somatomedin C receptor system is depressed in hypothyroid animals, so the specific increase in the number of somatomedin C receptors in the lung and heart of their hypothyroid animals probably "represents a mechanism to ameliorate the negative effects of hypothyroidism on these important organs." In heart cells, regulation of gene expression occurred at a stage preceding translation of receptor mRNA into the receptor protein. Parallel changes occurred in somatomedin C transcripts and the number of cell membrane somatomedin C receptors. In lung cells, however, thyroid hormone did not change the amount of somatomedin C transcripts. Instead, the hormone exerted effects on the receptors at or following translation. Growth hormone did not appear to mediate the effects of T_3 on the receptor gene.[85]

THYROID HORMONE REGULATION OF LEVELS OF GROWTH HORMONE-RELEASING FACTOR AND GROWTH HORMONE

Hypothyroidism impairs growth hormone secretion directly by inhibiting the somatotroph cells of the pituitary gland.[46][47] In the absence of thyroid hormone, growth hormone mRNA decreases more than 98%.[18][19][29][36] Both spontaneous and stimulated growth hormone secretion are reduced in thyroid hormone deficiency.[15][67] Hypothyroid patients also have a blunted growth hormone response to insulin-induced hypoglycemia,[35] indicating inhibited somatotroph function. The impairment of somatotroph function results in reduced somatomedin levels (see section below titled "Thyroid Hormone Regulation of Levels of Somatomedins").

Thyroid hormone deficiency directly reduces growth hormone secretion by the pituitary gland.[37] Pimentel-Filho et al. found that in patients with primary hypothyroidism, pituitary secretion of growth hormone stimulated by growth hormone-releasing hormone was blunted. The blunted response suggests that thyroid hormone deficiency impairs synthesis and release of growth hormone by the pituitary somatotrophs.[67] Davies et al. reported that thyroid hormone treatment of hypothyroid patients increased pituitary growth hormone secretion in response to growth hormone-releasing factor.[11] Moreno et al. found that the growth hormone level was much lower in hypothyroid rats than in euthyroid rats. T_3 treatment increased the growth hormone level 5-fold—restoring the level to that of euthyroid rats.[49]

Thyroid hormone deficiency reduces pituitary growth hormone secretion indirectly by reducing hypothalamic production of growth hormone-releasing factor.[37][40][48] Mitsuhashi et al. found that in patients with primary hypothyroidism, peak levels of plasma growth hormone-releasing factor and growth hormone were significantly lower than those in normal subjects.[40]

THYROID HORMONE REGULATION OF LEVELS OF SOMATOMEDINS

Somatomedin C levels are reduced in growth hormone deficiency and in hypothyroidism.[20] Westermark et al. investigated the influence of thyroid hormone levels on two growth factors: serum levels of somatomedin C and urine levels of epidermal growth factor. The researchers concluded: "Data from the present study thus demonstrate that the hyper- and hypothyroid states are accompanied by changes in serum and urine levels of growth factors and that these are affected by the treatment for these conditions. This conforms with the view that the growth promoting effect of thyroid hormones involves a stimulated synthesis or release of the classic growth factors."[26,p.420]

Impaired pituitary somatotroph cell function during hypothyroidism results in decreased liver production of somatomedin C. Reduced somatomedin C levels impede the response of cartilage to somatomedin C.[45,p.1041] Mosier et al. found that during chemically-induced hypothyroidism in rats, pituitary concentration of growth hormone decreased. Somatomedin levels were also reduced, and the incorporation of sulfate into cartilage decreased. Moreover, growth rates of body weight and tail length decreased.[15]

After Lewinson et al. chemically induced hypothyroidism in young rats, the width of the rats' epiphyseal growth plate cartilage decreased by 27% and the width of the articular cartilage decreased by 35%. The volume of epiphyseal trabecular bone decreased by 30%, and the volume of metaphyseal trabecular bone decreased by 66%. T_4 treatment resulted in "full recovery of the epiphyseal growth plate cartilage morphology." T_4 treatment also fully restored the epiphyseal trabecular bone; in fact, the volume of epiphyseal trabecular bone surpassed that of normal rats by 40%. The width of articular cartilage returned to normal values. However, the volume of metaphyseal trabecular bone only reached 68% of normal (a 2% increase from the volume in hypothyroidism). In contrast, although growth hormone treatment restored epiphyseal trabecular bone

to almost normal, the treatment did not improve the epiphyseal growth plate cartilage or articular cartilage. Metaphyseal trabecular bone improved with growth hormone treatment to a small though significant level.[98]

Decreased growth potential during low growth hormone and somatomedin levels is shown by the dramatic growth retardation in hypothyroid children.[45,p.1040] In hypothyroid adults, the low levels of the hormones have few manifestations.[44,p.974] Adults may, however, have impaired ability to repair damage to musculoskeletal tissues. The impaired ability may contribute to the adverse effects of exercise on fibromyalgia patients (see Chapter 3.4).

Chernausek et al. found that plasma levels of somatomedin C were low in 11 of 12 hypothyroid patients. With thyroid hormone treatment, the mean level increased 4-fold. In untreated hypothyroid patients, a single injection of growth hormone increased plasma somatomedin C levels 4-fold within 28 hours. The investigators wrote that the low somatomedin C levels appeared to result from low growth hormone secretion or a direct effect of hypothyroidism on somatomedin production.[63]

Takano et al. reported that the levels of somatomedin A were low in patients with primary hypothyroidism. The levels become normal with thyroid hormone treatment. In hypothyroid rats, thyroid hormone treatment increased the somatomedin A response to growth hormone by 42.2%. The researchers concluded that thyroid hormone increases both the synthesis and secretion of somatomedin A.[65]

Thyroid hormone appears to both directly and indirectly regulate the levels of somatomedin-binding proteins (the proteins that transport somatomedins in the circulation). Nanto-Salonen et al. found that in adult hypothyroid rats, the mean serum somatomedin C level was only 51% of that of euthyroid rats. Administering growth hormone increased the level up to 79% of that of euthyroid rats. Thus, growth hormone did not completely correct the reduced mean somatomedin C level. In the hypothyroid rats, the mean serum level of somatomedin-binding protein-3 was reduced to 80% of euthyroid rats. The levels of liver mRNA for the binding protein were only 50% of those of euthyroid rats. Administering growth hormone normalized levels of both the protein in the serum and mRNA in the liver. The mean level of somatomedin-binding protein4 in hypothyroid rats was only 50% of that in euthyroid rats. Growth hormone treatment did not increase the levels of this binding protein. Thyroid hormone therapy, however, normalized all the mean levels of all the measured factors—mean somatomedin C and somatomedin-binding protein-$_2$, -$_3$, and -$_4$. The investigators concluded that the effects of thyroid hormone on serum somatomedin levels and somatomedin-binding protein-$_3$ expression seem to be mediated indirectly via growth hormone. But increases in expression of binding protein-$_2$ and -$_4$ in adult rats may be direct thyroid hormone effects.[22]

Interestingly, Nanto-Salonen et al. found that hypothyroidism did not alter liver mRNA levels for types 1 and 2 somatomedin receptors. Administering thyroid hormone or growth hormone did not affect the two types of receptors. The researchers also reported that administering growth hormone alone only partially corrected the diminished somatic growth of hypothyroid adult and pup rats.[22]

THYROID HORMONE, ADRENERGIC RECEPTOR TYPE, AND REGULATION OF GROWTH HORMONE-RELEASING FACTOR AND GROWTH HORMONE SECRETION

In most tissues, normal thyroid hormone regulation of transcription of the adrenergic genes has two reliable effects on the adrenergic receptor density of cell membranes: an increase in β-adrenergic receptor density and a decrease in α-adrenergic receptor density. During subnormal thyroid hormone regulation of the adrenergic genes, as in hypothyroidism, the density of β-adrenergic receptors on membranes decreases; the density of α-adrenergic receptors increases.

In the liver and some neurons of the hypothalamus, normal thyroid hormone regulation of the adrenergic genes increases α-adrenergic receptors and decreases β-adrenergic receptors—the opposite effects from those in most other tissues. (See Chapter 2.3, section titled "Interpretation of Fibromyalgia Features as Manifestations of Low β-Adrenergic Receptor and High α-Adrenergic Receptor Density," subsection: "Effects of Thyroid Hormone on α- and β-Adrenergic Receptor Isoforms are Tissue Specific.")

When the adrenergic genes of some hypothalamic neurons are exposed to normal amounts of thyroid hormone, the density of α_1- and α_2- adrenergic receptors on the neuronal membranes increases. Stimulation of α_2-adrenergic receptors by agonists such as clonidine and norepinephrine increases secretion of growth hormone-releasing factor by hypothalamic cells.[2][35,p.1585][92] Stimulation of the α_2-adrenergic receptors also seems to inhibit somatostatin secretion.[2]

Growth hormone-releasing factor stimulates pituitary growth hormone secretion; somatostatin inhibits the secretion. Thus, by increasing the release of growth hormone-releasing factor and decreasing release of somatostatin, activation of α_2-adrenergic receptors stimulates pituitary secretion of growth hormone.[2][25] α-Adrenergic receptor antagonists, such as phentolamine, decrease secretion of growth hormone-releasing factor.[35,p.1585]

In several *in vivo* studies, stimulation of β-adrenergic receptors inhibited growth hormone release.[80][86][94] The inhibition probably resulted from stimulation of somatostatin-secreting neurons through activation of β-adrenergic receptors.[2][93,p.1258][95]

Excessive amounts of glucocorticoids (as in hypercortisolism) inhibit growth hormone release. The excess glucocorticoids inhibit growth hormone release through increasing secretion of somatostatin by hypothalamic neurons. Increased somatostatin secretion seems to result from the excess glucocorticoids causing a shift from α_2- to β-adrenergic receptor responsiveness of hypothalamic neurons. The shift to β-adrenergic receptor responsiveness decreases secretion of growth hormone-releasing factor and increases secretion of somatostatin. (By contrast, normal amounts of glucocorticoids increase the synthesis of growth hormone-releasing factor and growth hormone gene transcription. Excessive amounts of glucocorticoids, however, inhibit growth in all species studied.[97]) In one study, the β-adrenergic receptor antagonist propranolol increased growth hormone secretion.[2] The increase in growth hormone secretion may have occurred because the blocking of β-adrenergic receptors decreased somatostatin secretion; the decreased somatostatin would disinhibit the pituitary somatotrophs, resulting in an increase in growth hormone secretion.

Tritos et al. subjected rats to the stress of combined forced swimming and confinement. The stress presumably induced catecholamine release. The researchers found that β_2-adrenergic receptors in the rats inhibited somatomedin C secretion in the cerebellum. Somatomedin C release was not affected in the cerebral cortex or hippocampus.[96] This finding shows that β_2-adrenergic receptors mediate inhibition in some intracranial structures other than the hypothalamus.

Administering thyroid hormone increases growth hormone secretion.[17][78][89] In hypothyroidism, growth hormone secretion decreases.[13][14][18][19][46][83][85][87][89] In hypothyroidism, secretion of growth hormone-releasing factor decreases. Secretion becomes normal again with thyroid hormone treatment.[89] (See next section.) These findings, in view of the study results in the paragraphs above, suggest that thyroid hormone decreases β-adrenergic receptors in the hypothalamic cells that secrete growth hormone-releasing factor.

Bennett recently wrote that decreased growth hormone secretion in fibromyalgia patients appears to be due to increased somatostatin secretion by the hypothalamus. He suggested that intermittent hypercortisolemia may be the cause of the dysfunctional growth hormone secretion. Increased cortisol levels would increase the density of β-adrenergic receptors in hypothalamic cells. The increase in β-adrenergic receptors would increase somatostatin secretion by the hypothalamic cells. In turn, the increased somatostatin would inhibit growth hormone secretion by the pituitary.[74]

Evidence I present in this section supports Bennett's view: an increase in β-adrenergic receptors in the hypothalamus increases somatostatin release, and the increased somatostatin levels inhibit growth hormone secretion. Evidence also shows that high levels of cortisol can induce a shift toward β-adrenergic receptor dominance in hypothalamic cells. The shift results in an increase in somatostatin release and a decrease in growth hormone release. However, the proposal is dubious that fibromyalgia patients have intermittent high cortisol levels that cause a shift toward β-adrenergic receptor dominance in the hypothalamus (see Chapter 3.5). Far more likely is a shift toward β-adrenergic receptor dominance due to inadequate thyroid hormone regulation of the adrenergic genes in somatostatin-secreting cells of the hypothalamus.

Another finding of Bennett et al. supports the possibility of the role of inadequate thyroid hormone regulation. They reported that in fibromyalgia patients, growth hormone secretion was blunted after they administered clonidine, an α_2-adrenoceptor agonist.[3] In that activation of α_2-adrenergic receptors normally increases growth hormone secretion, growth hormone secretion in response to clonidine may have been impeded by another factor. In the hypothalamic cells that secrete growth hormone-releasing factor and somatostatin, we expect inadequate thyroid hormone regulation of transcription of the adrenergic genes to decrease the density of α-adrenergic receptors. A decrease in the density of these receptors can account for a decrease in the secretion of growth hormone-releasing factor and an increase in secretion of somatostatin. The expected result would be subnormal secretion of growth hormone by the pituitary in response to α_2-adrenergic receptor activation by clonidine.

GROWTH HORMONE AND SOMATOMEDIN LEVELS INCREASE DURING ADEQUATE THYROID HORMONE TREATMENT

In patients with primary or central hypothyroidism, pituitary hormones other than TSH may be deficient. Specific basal and stimulation tests can determine this. Martino et al. recommended basal and stimulation tests to evaluate growth hormone. They noted that abnormal results in the growth hormone tests are common for patients with central hypothyroidism, and the thyroid hormone deficiency may be the cause of the abnormal growth hormone test results.[32,p.787]

Thyroid hormone treatment usually restores growth hormone levels to normal.[32,p.787] Santini et al. found that thyroidectomized rats had markedly reduced serum levels of growth hormone; the levels became normal after treatment with low dose T_3.[21] Moreno et al. reported that growth hormone levels were much lower in hypothyroid rats than in euthyroid rats; administering T_3 increased the growth hormone levels to those of euthyroid rats. Treating the hypothyroid rats with 3,5-T_2 raised growth hormone levels to normal as T_3 did.[49] In rats with chemically-induced hypothyroidism, growth hormone and somatomedin levels decreased. (Growth rate also decreased.) Levels increased with thyroid hormone treatment.[15]

T_3 induces new growth hormone mRNA and synthesis of growth hormone.[13] The presence of glucocorticoids simultaneously with thyroid hormone induces growth hormone mRNA and growth hormone.[39,p.174] Although glucocorticoids facilitate production of growth hormone mRNA, chronic use of exogenous glucocorticoids inhibits growth hormone release.[41,p.126] High levels of endogenous glucocorticoids during intense stress may also inhibit growth hormone release.

Takano et al. reported that the low levels of somatomedin A in patients with primary hypothyroidism increased to normal with thyroid hormone therapy.[65] Thyroid hormone treatment of hypothyroid rats normalized the levels of all somatomedin-binding (transport) proteins that were low during hypothyroidism.[22]

REFERENCES

1. Buchwald, D., Umali, J., and Stene, M.: Insulin-like growth factor-I (somatomedin C) levels in chronic fatigue syndrome and fibromyalgia. *J. Rheumatol.*, 23:739-742,1996.
2. Muller, E.E., Locatelli, V., Ghigo, E., Cella, S.G., Loche, S., Pintor, C., and Camanni, F.: Involvement of brain

catecholamines and acetylcholine in growth hormone deficiency states. Pathophysiological, diagnostic and therapeutic implications. *Drugs,* 41(2):161-177, 1991.

3. Bennett, R.M., Clark, S.R., Burckhardt, C.S., and Cook, D.: IGF-1 assays and other GH tests in 500 fibromyalgia patients. *J. Musculoskel. Pain* (Abstract), 3(Suppl.1):109, 1995.

4. Bennett, R.M., Clark, S.R., Burckhardt, C.S., and Walczyk, J.: A double-blind placebo-controlled study of growth hormone therapy in fibromyalgia. *J. Musculoskel. Pain* (Abstract), 3(Suppl.1):110, 1995.

5. Stratz, T., Schochat, T., Faber, L., Schweiger, C., and Müller, W.: Are there subgroups in fibromyalgia? *J. Musculoskel. Pain* (Abstract), 3(Suppl.1):110, 1995.

6. Bennett, R.M., Clark, S.R., Campbell, S.M., and Burckhardt, C.S.: Low levels of somatomedin C in patients with the fibromyalgia syndrome: a possible link between sleep and muscle pain. *Arthritis Rheum.*, 35:1113-1116, 1992.

7. Nørregaard, J., Bülow, P.M., Volkman, H., Mehlsen, J., and Samsøe, B.D.: Somatomedin-C and procollagen aminoterminal peptide in fibromyalgia. *J. Musculoskel. Pain,* 3(4):33-40, 1995.

8. Beaufort, M.C., Rinaldi, J.P., Gandolfo, C., Plantamura, A., and Eisinger, J.: Growth hormone and fibromyalgia. Unpublished summary of study results, April 17, 1996.

9. Eisinger, J., Dupond, J.L., and Cozzone, P.J.: Anomalies de la glycolyse au cours des fibromyalgies: etude biologiques et thérapeutique. *Lyon Méditerranée Méd.*, 32: 2180-2181, 1996.

10. Bennett, R.M.: Beyond fibromyalgia: ideas on etiology and treatment. *J. Rheumatology,* 16(Suppl 19):185-191, 1989.

11. Davies, R.R., Dagogo-Jack, S., Turner, S.J., et al.: The effect of thyroid status on the growth hormone response to growth hormone releasing hormone 1-44. *J. Endocrinol. Invest.*, 12(8):517-521, 1989.

12. Karagiorgos, A., Garcia, J.F., and Brooks, G.A.: Growth hormone response to continuous and intermittent exercise. *J. Appl. Physiol.*, 11:302-307, 1979.

13. Seo, H., Vassart, G., Brocas, H., and Refetoff, S.: Triiodothyronine stimulates specifically growth hormone mRNA in rat pituitary tumor cells. *Proc. Natl. Acad. Sci.* (USA), 74:2054-2058, 1977.

14. Seo, H., Refetoff, S., Martino, E., Vassart, G., and Brocas, H.: The differential stimulatory effect of thyroid hormone on growth hormone synthesis and estrogen on prolactin synthesis due to accumulation of specific messenger ribonucleic acid. *Endocrinology*, 104:1083, 1979.

15. Mosier, H.D., Jr, Dearden, L.C., Jansons, R.A., and Hill, R.R.: Growth hormone, somatomedin and cartilage sulfation in failure of catch-up growth after propylthiouracil-induced hypothyroidism in the rat. *Endocrinology*, 100 (6):1644-1651, 1977.

16. Miki, N., Ono, M., Murata, Y., et al.: Thyroid hormone regulation of gene expression of the pituitary growth hormone-releasing factor receptor. *Biochem. Biophys. Res. Comm.* 217(3):1087-1093, 1995.

17. Brameld, J.M., Weller, P.A., Saunders, J.C., Buttery, P.J., and Gilmour, R.S.: Hormonal control of insulin-like growth factor-1 and growth hormone receptor mRNA expression by porcine hepatocytes in culture. *J. Endocrinol.*

146(2):239-245, 1995.

18. Martial, J.A., Baxter, J.D., and Goodman, H.M.: Regulation of growth hormone messenger RNA by thyroid and glucocorticoid hormones. *Proc. Natl. Acad. Sci.*, 74:1816, 1977.

19. Shapiro, L.E., Samuels, H.H., and Yaffe, B.M.: Thyroid and glucocorticoid hormones synergistically control growth hormone mRNA in cultured GH-1 cells. *Proc. Natl. Acad. Sci.*, 75:45, 1978.

20. Sugisaki, T., Yamadam, T., Takamatsu, K., and Noguchi, T.: The influence of endocrine factors on the serum concentrations of insulin-like growth factor-I (IGF-I) and IGF-binding proteins. *J. Endocrinol.*, 138(3):467-477, 1993.

21. Santini, F., Hurd, R.E., Lee, B., and Chopra, I.J.: Thyromimetic effects of 3,5,3'-triiodothyronine sulfate in hypothyroid rats. *Endocrinology*, 133(1):105-110, 1993.

22. Nanto-Salonen, K., Muller, H.L., Hoffman, A.R., Vu, T.H., and Rosenfeld, R.G.: Mechanisms of thyroid hormone action on the insulin-like growth factor system: all thyroid hormone effects are not growth hormone mediated. *Endocrinology,* 132(2):781-788, 1993.

23. McCain, G.A. and Tilbe, K.S.: Diurnal hormone variation in fibromyalgia syndrome: a comparison with rheumatoid arthritis. *J. Rheumatol.*, 19(Suppl.):154-157, 1989.

24. Becker, K.I., Ferguson, R.H., and McConahey, W.M.: The connective-tissue diseases and symptoms associated with Hashimoto's thyroiditis. *New Eng. J. Med.*, 268(6): 177-280, 1963.

25. Thomas, G.B., Scott, C.J., Cummins, J.T., and Clarke, I.J.: Adrenergic regulation of growth hormone secretion in the ewe. *Domest. Anim. Endocrinol.*, 11(2):187-195, 1994.

26. Westermark, K., Alm, J., Skottner, A., and Karlsson, A.: Growth factors and the thyroid: effects of treatment for hyper- and hypothyroidism on serum IGF-I and urinary epidermal growth factor concentrations. *Acta Endocrinol.* (Copenh), 118:415-421, 1988.

27. Copp, R.P. and Samuels, H.H.: Identification of an adenosine 3',5'-monophosphate (cAMP)-responsive region in the rat growth hormone gene: evidence for independent and synergistic effects of cAMP and thyroid hormone on gene expression. *Molecular Endocrinol.*, 3(5):790-796, 1989.

28. Older, S.A., Battafarano, D.F., Danning, C.L., Ward, J.A., Grady, E.P., Derman, S., and Russell, I.J.: The effects of delta wave sleep interruption on pain thresholds and fibromyalgia-like symptoms in healthy subjects; correlations with insulin-like growth factor I. *J. Rheumatol.*, 25 (6):1180-1186, 1998.

29. Frohman, L.A.: Diseases of the anterior pituitary. In *Endocrinology and Metabolism*, 2nd edition. Edited by P. Felig, J.D. Baxter, A. Broadus, and L.A. Frohman, New York, McGraw-Hill Book Co., 1987, pp.247-337.

30. Hartley, L.H.: Growth hormone and catecholamine response to exercise in relation to physical training. *Med. Sci. Sports*, 7:34-36, 1975.

31. Karagiorgos, A., Garcia, J.F., and Brooks, G.A.: Growth hormone response to continuous and intermittent exercise. *J. Appl. Physiol.*, 11:302-307, 1979.

32. Martino, E., Bartalena, L., Faglia, G., and Pinchera, A.:

Central hypothyroidism. In *Werner and Ingbar's The Thyroid: A Fundamental and Clinical Text*, 7th edition. Edited by L.P. Braverman and R.D. Utiger, Philadelphia, Lippincott-Raven Publishers, 1996, pp.779-791.

33. Rall, J.E., Robbins, J., and Lewallen, C.G.: In *The Hormones*, Vol. 5. Edited by G. Pincus, K.V. Thimann, and E.B. Astwood, New York, Academic Press, 1964, pp.159-439.

34. Diarra, A., Lefauconnier, J.M., Valens, M., Georges, P., and Gripois, D.: Tyrosine content, influx, and accumulation rate, and catecholamine biosynthesis measured *in vivo*, in the central nervous system and in peripheral organs of young rats: influence of neonatal hypo- and hyperthyroidism. *Arch. Intern. de Physiologie et de Biochem.*, 97:317-332, 1989.

35. MacGillivary, M.H.: Disorders of growth and development. In *Endocrinology and Metabolism*, 2nd edition. Edited by P. Felig, J.D. Baxter, A. Broadus, and L.A. Frohman, New York, McGraw-Hill Book Co., 1987, pp.1581-1628.

36. Noel, G.L., Dimond, R.C., Wartofsky, L., Earl, J.M., and Frantz, A.G.: Studies of prolactin and TSH secretion by continuous infusion of small amounts of thyrotropin-releasing hormone. *J. Clin. Endocrinol. Metab.*, 39:6, 1974.

37. Martinoli, M.G. and Pelletier, G.: Thyroid and glucocorticoid hormone regulation of rat pituitary growth hormone messenger ribonucleic acid as revealed by in situ hybridization. *Endocrinology*, 125(3):1246-1252, 1989.

38. Tilbe, K., Bell, D.A., and McCain, G.A.: Loss of diurnal variation in serum cortisol, growth hormone, and prolactin in patients with primary fibromyalgia. *Arthritis Rheum.*, 31:4, 1988.

39. Tepperman, J. and Tepperman, H.M.: *Metabolic and Endocrine Physiology*, 5th edition. Chicago, Year Book Medical Publishers, Inc., 1987.

40. Mitsuhashi, S., Yamasaki, R., Miyazaki, S., Saito, H., and Saito, S.: Effect of oral administration of L-dopa on the plasma levels of growth hormone-releasing hormone (GHRH) in normal subjects and patients with various endocrine and metabolic diseases. *Nippon Naibunpi Gakkai Zasshi*, 63(8):934-946, 1987.

41. Merimee, T.J. and Grant, M.B.: Growth hormone and its disorders. In *Principles and Practice of Endocrinology and Metabolism*. Edited by K.L. Becker, J.P. Bilezinkian, W.J. Bremner, W. Hung, C.R. Kahn, D.L. Loriaux, R.W. Rebar, G.L. Robertson, and L. Wartofsky, Philadelphia, J.B. Lippincott Co., 1990, pp.125-134.

42. Oppenheimer, J.H.: Thyroid hormone action at the molecular level. In *Werner and Ingbar's The Thyroid: A Fundamental and Clinical Text*, 6th edition. Edited by L.E. Braverman and R.D. Utiger, Philadelphia, J.B. Lippincott Co., 1991, pp.204-223.

43. Yaffe, B. and Samuels, H.H.: Hormonal regulation of the growth hormone gene: relationship of the rate of transcription to the level of nuclear thyroid hormone-receptor complexes. *J. Biol. Chem.*, 259:6284, 1984.

44. Pinchera, A., Martino, E., and Faglia, G.: Central hypothyroidism. In *Werner and Ingbar's The Thyroid: A Fundamental and Clinical Text*, 6th edition. Edited by L.E. Braverman and R.D. Utiger, Philadelphia, J.B. Lippincott Co., 1991, pp.968-984.

45. Snyder, P.J.: The pituitary in hypothyroidism. In *Werner and Ingbar's The Thyroid: A Fundamental and Clinical Text*, 6th edition. Edited by L.E. Braverman and R.D. Utiger, Philadelphia, J.B. Lippincott Co., 1991, pp.1040-1044.

46. Valcavi, R., Dieguez, C., Preece, M., Taylor, A., Portioli, I., and Scanlon, M.F.: Effect of thyroxine replacement therapy on plasma insulin-like growth hormone releasing factor in hypothyroid patients. *Clin. Endocrinol.*, 27:85, 1987.

47. Williams, T., Maxon, H., Thorner, M.O., and Frohman, L.A.: Blunted growth hormone (GH) response to GH-releasing hormone in hypothyroidism resolves in the euthyroid state. *J. Clin. Endocrinol. Metab.*, 61:454, 1985.

48. Jahreis, G., Hesse, V., Rohde, W., Prange, H., and Zwacka, G.: Nitrate-induced hypothyroidism is associated with a reduced concentration of growth hormone-releasing factor in hypothalamic tissue of rats. *Exp. Clin. Endocrinol.*, 97(1):109-112, 1991.

49. Moreno, M., Lombardi, A., Lombardi, P., Goglia, F., and Lanni, A.: Effect of 3,5-diiodo-L-thyronine on thyroid stimulating hormone and growth hormone serum levels in hypothyroid rats. *Life Sci.*, 214(26):2369-2377, 1998.

50. Baumann, G., Amburn, K., and Shaw, M.A.: A circulating growth hormone (GH)-binding protein complex: a major constituent of plasma GH in man. *Endocrinology*, 122:976, 1988.

51. Merimee, T.J., Rabinowitz, D., and Fineberg, S.E.: Arginine initiated release of human growth hormone: factors modifying the response in normal man. *N. Engl. J. Med.*, 280:1434, 1969.

52. Frantz, A.C. and Rabkin, M.T.: Effects of estrogen and sex difference on secretion of human growth hormone. *J. Clin. Endocrinol. Metab.*, 25:1470, 1965.

53. Koerker, D.J., Ruch, W., and Chideckel, E.: Somatostatin: hypothalamic inhibitor of the endocrine pancreas. *Science*, 184:482, 1974.

54. Stachura, M.E.: Basal and dibutyryl cyclic AMP stimulated release of newly synthesized and stored GH from perfused rat pituitaries. *Endocrinology*, 98:580, 1976.

55. Stachura, M.E.: Potassium modification of the somatostatin effect on stimulated rat growth hormone release. *Endocrinology*, 108:1027, 1981.

56. Merimee, T.J. and Rabinowitz, D.: Isolated human growth hormone deficiency and related disorders. *Isr. J. Med. Sci.*, 9:1599, 1973.

57. Knobil, E.: The pituitary growth hormone: an adventure in physiology. *Physiologist*, 9:25, 1966.

58. Salmon, W.D., Jr. and Daughaday, W.H.: A hormonally controlled serum factor which stimulates sulfate incorporation by cartilage in vitro. *J. Lab. Clin. Med.*, 49:825, 1957.

59. Salmon, W.D., Jr. and Duvall, M.R.: In vitro stimulation of leucine incorporation into muscle and cartilage protein by a serum fraction with SF activity: differentiation of effects from those of growth hormone and insulin. *Endocrinology*, 87:1168, 1970.

60. Frohman, L.A. and Jansson, J.: Growth hormone-releasing hormone. *Endocr. Rev.*, 7(3):223-253, 1986.

61. Darlington, D.N. and Dallman, M.F,: Feedback control in endocrine systems. In *Principles and Practice of Endocrinology and Metabolism*. Edited by K.L. Becker, J.P.

Bilezinkian, W.J. Bremner, W. Hung, C.R. Kahn, D.L. Loriaux, R.W. Rebar, G.L. Robertson, and L. Wartofsky, Philadelphia, J.B. Lippincott Co., 1990, pp.38-44.

62. Morley, J.E.: Neuroendocrine control of thyrotropin secretion. *Endocr. Rev.*, 2:396, 1981.

63. Chernausek, S.D., Underwood, L.E., Utiger, R.D., and Van Wyk, J.J.: Growth hormone secretion and plasma somatomedin-C in primary hypothyroidism. *Clin. Endocrinol.* (Oxf.), 19(3):337-344, 1983.

64. Frohman, L.A. and Berelowitz, M.: Physiological and pharmacological control of anterior pituitary hormone secretion. In *Peptides, Hormones, and Behavior*. Edited by A. Dunn and C.B. Nemeroff, New York, Spectrum, 1984, pp.119-125.

65. Takano, K., Hasumi, Y., Hizuka, N., Kogawa, M., Tsushima, T., and Shizume, K.: Effect of thyroid hormone on the serum level of somatomedin A. *Endocrinol. Japn.*, 27 (5):643-652, 1980.

66. Pescovitz, O.H., Cutler, G.B., and Loriaux, D.L.: Synthesis and secretion of corticosteroids. In *Principles and Practice of Endocrinology and Metabolism*. Edited by K.L. Becker, J.P. Bilezinkian, W.J. Bremner, W. Hung, C.R. Kahn, D.L. Loriaux, R.W. Rebar, G.L. Robertson, and L. Wartofsky, Philadelphia, J.B. Lippincott Co., 1990, pp.579-591.

67. Pimentel-Filho, F.R., Ramos-Dias, J.C., Ninno, F.B., Facanha, C.F., Liberman, B., and Lengyel, A.M.: Growth hormone responses to GH-releasing peptide (GHRP-6) in hypothyroidism. *Clin. Endocrinol.*(Oxf.), 46(3):295-300, 1997.

68. Guyton, A.C.: *Textbook of Medical Physiology*, 8th edition. Philadelphia, W.B. Saunders Co., 1991.

69. Kalyan-Raman, U.P., Kalyan-Raman, K., Yunus, M.B., and Masi, A.T.: Muscle pathology in primary fibromyalgia syndrome: a light microscopic, histological and ultrastructural study. *J. Rheumatology*, 11:808-813, 1984.

70. Awad, E.A.: Pathological changes in fibromyalgia. *First International Symposium on Myofascial Pain and Fibromyalgia*. Minneapolis, Minnesota, May 9, 1989.

71. Awad, E.A.: Histopathological changes in fibrositis. In *Advances in Pain Research and Therapy*, Vol.17. Edited by J.R. Fricton and E.A. Awad, New York, Raven Press, Ltd., 1990, pp.249-258.

72. Ramsay, I.: *Thyroid Disease and Muscle Dysfunction*. Chicago, Year Book Medical Publishers, Inc., 1974, pp.147-151.

73. Eisinger, J.: Metabolic abnormalities in fibromyalgia. *Clin. Bull. Myofascial Ther.*, 3(1):3-21, 1998.

74. Bennett, R.M.: Disordered growth hormone secretion in fibromyalgia: a review of recent findings and a hypothesized etiology. *J. Rheumatol.*, (Suppl.) 2:72-76, 1998.

75. Vetter, U. and Teller, W.M.: Somatomedins and their significance in pediatrics. *Klin. Padiatr.*, 197(5):378-385, 1985.

76. Eisinger, J., Plantamura, A., and Ayavou, T.: Glycolysis abnormalities in fibromyalgia. *J. Amer. Coll. Nutri.*, 13: 144-148, 1994.

77. Tam, S.P., Lam, K.S., and Srivastava, G.: Gene expression of hypothalamic somatostatin, growth hormone-releasing factor, and their pituitary receptors in hypothyroidism. *Endocrinology*, 137(2):418-424, 1996.

78. Brent, G.A., Larsen, P.R., Harney, J.W., Koenig, R.J., and Moore, D.D.: Functional characterization of the rat growth hormone promoter elements required for induction by thyroid hormone with and without co-transfectant β type thyroid hormone receptor. *J. Biol Chem.*, 264:178-182, 1989.

79. Krulich, L., Mayfield, M.A., Steele, M.K., McMillen, B.A., McCann, S.M., and Koenig, J.I.: Differential effects of pharmacological manipulations of central α_1-adrenergic and α_2-adrenergic receptors on the secretion of thyrotropin and growth hormone in male rats. *Endocrinology*, 110:796-804, 1982.

80. Krieg, R.J., Perkins, S.N., Johnson, J.K., Rogers, J.P., Aarimura, A., and Cronin, M.J.: β-Adrenergic stimulation of growth hormone (GH) release *in vivo*, and subsequent inhibition of GH-releasing factor-induced GH secretion. *Endocrinology*, 122: 531-537, 1988.

81. Casanova, J., Copp, R.P., Janocko, L., and Samuels, H.H.: 5'-Flanking DNA of the rat growth hormone gene mediates regulated expression by thyroid hormone. *J. Biol. Chem.*, 260(21):11744-11748, 1985.

82. Flug, F., Copp, R.P., Casanova, J., Horowitz, Z.D., Janocko, L., Plotnick, M., and Samuels, H.H.: cis-Acting elements of the rat growth hormone gene which mediate basal and regulated expression by thyroid hormone. *J. Biol. Chem.*, 262(13):6373-6382, 1987.

83. Williams, T., Maxon, H., Thorner, M.O., and Frohman, L.A.: Blunted growth hormone (GH) response to GH-releasing hormone in hypothyroidism resolves in the euthyroid state. *J. Clin. Endocrinol. Metab.*, 61:454, 1985.

84. Samuels, H.H., Casanova, J., Copp, R.P., and Janocko, L.: 5'-Flanking DNA sequences of the growth hormone gene mediates thyroid hormone stimulation of growth hormone gene transcription. *Trans. Assoc. Amer. Physicians*, 98:55-65, 1985.

85. Moreno, B., Rodriguez-Manzaneque, J.C., Perez-Castillo, A., and Santos, A.: Thyroid hormone controls the expression of insulin-like growth factor I receptor gene at different levels in lung and heart of developing and adult rats. *Endocrinology*, 138(3):1194-1203, 1997.

86. Bluet-Pajot, M.T., Durand, D., Mounier, F., Schaub, C., and Kordon, C.: Interaction of β-adrenergic agonists and antagonists with the stimulation of growth hormone release induced by clonidine or by morphine in the rat. *J. Endocrinol.*, 94:327-331, 1982.

87. Noel, G.L., Dimond, R.C., Wartofsky, L., Earl, J.M., and Frantz, A.G.: Studies of prolactin and TSH secretion by continuous infusion of small amounts of thyrotropin-releasing hormone. *J. Clin. Endocrinol. Metab.*, 39:6, 1974.

88. Samuels, H.H., Aranda, A., Casanova, J., et al.: Identification of the cis-acting elements and trans-acting factors that mediate cell-specific and thyroid hormone stimulation of growth hormone gene expression. *Recent Prog. Horm. Res.*, 44:53-114, 1988.

89. Miki, N., Ono, M., Murata, Y., et al.: Thyroid hormone regulation of gene expression of the pituitary growth hormone-releasing factor receptor. *Biochem. Biophys. Res. Comm.*, 217(3):1087-1093, 1995.

90. Samuels, H.H., Casanova, J., Copp, R.P., Janocko, L., Raaka, B.M., Sahnoun, H., and Yaffe, B.M.: Thyroid hormone receptors and action: the 5'-flanking region of the

rat growth hormone gene can mediate regulated gene expression. *Endocr. Res.*, 15(4):495-545, 1989.

91. Aranda, A., Copp, R.P., Pascual, A., and Samuels, H.H.: Influence of thyroid hormone on ADP-ribosylation of nuclear proteins in cultured GH1 cells. *FEBS Lett.*, 279(2): 179-183, 1991.

92. West, C.R., Gaynor, P.J., Lookingland, K.J., and Tucker, H.A.: Regulation of growth hormone-releasing hormone and somatostatin from perfused, bovine hypothalamic slices. I. α_2-Adrenergic receptor regulation. *Domest. Anim. Endocrinol.*, 14(5):334-348, 1997.

93. Jaffer, A., Daniels, W.M.U., Russell, V.A., and Taljaard, J.J.F.: Effects of α_2- and β-adrenoceptor agonists on growth hormone secretion following lesion of the noradrenergic system of the rat. *Neurochem. Res.*, 17(12):1255-1260, 1992.

94. Bluet-Pajot, M.T., Schaub, C., and Nasiet, J.: Growth hormone response to hypoglycemia under gamma-hydroxybutyrate narcoanalgesia in the rat. *Neuroendocrinol.*, 26:141-149, 1978.

95. Lima, L., Arce, V., Diaz, M.J., Tresguerres, J.A., and Devesa, J.: Glucocorticoids may inhibit growth hormone release by enhancing beta-adrenergic responsiveness in hypothalamic somatostatin neurons. *J. Clin. Endocrinol. Metab.*, 76(2):439-444, 1993.

96. Tritos, N., Kitraki, E., Phillipidis, H., and Stylianopoulou, F.: β-Adrenergic receptors mediate a stress-induced decrease in IGF-II mRNA in the rat cerebellum. *Cell. Mol. Neurobiol.*, 18(5):525-534, 1998.

97. Devesa, J., Barros, M.G., Gondar, M., Tresguerres, J.A., and Arce, V.: Regulation of hypothalamic somatostatin by glucocorticoids. *J. Steroid Biochem. Mol. Biol.*, 53(1-6): 277-282, 1995.

98. Lewinson, D., Harel, Z., Shenzer, P., Silbermann, M., and Hochberg, Z.: Effect of thyroid hormone and growth hormone on recovery from hypothyroidism of epiphyseal growth plate cartilage and its adjacent bone. *Endocrinology*, 124(2):937-945, 1989.

3.13

Immune Dysregulation

Inadequate Thyroid Hormone Regulation of the Immune System

The immune system defends the body against microorganisms and chemical toxins that can cause pathology. The initial defense of the body is by "innate immunity." This is resistance to microorganisms and toxins by general structures and processes of the body: skin, mucous membranes, gastric acids and digestive enzymes in the stomach and small intestine, and natural killer cells and other substances in the circulating blood. The second defense, termed "acquired immunity," is the formation of activated lymphocytes and antibodies against foreign organisms and toxins. Defenses can also be divided into cell-mediated immunity or T-lymphocyte immunity and antibody-mediated or B-lymphocyte immunity. In cell-mediated immunity, large numbers of activated lymphocytes are formed that are customized to destroy a specific foreign substance. In antibody-mediated immunity, antibodies are formed against specific antigens.

Immune System Abnormalities in Fibromyalgia and Hypothyroidism

Striving for a meaningful interpretation of the immune abnormalities of fibromyalgia in terms of inadequate thyroid hormone regulation of the immune system is difficult. The first problem is that the status of immune system abnormalities in fibromyalgia patients is not conclusively settled for several reasons: (1) differences in groups of patients studied, (2) uncertain diagnoses of patients and the health status of control subjects, (3) inadequate immunologic controls,

(4) testing of single blood samples rather than repeated samples that might show circadian changes, (5) reporting of statistically non-significant differences as different anyway, and (6) other methodological faults. The second problem in making a meaningful interpretation is the inconsistent and in some cases contradictory results of studies of some immune measures in hypothyroid laboratory animals and humans.

Despite these two classes of problems, however, reported results of some tests are comparable. While researchers reported that fibromyalgia patients had an increased CD4/CD8 ratio, hypothyroid patients had a decreased ratio. Researchers reported that both fibromyalgia and hypothyroid patients had reduced interleukin-2 secretion and low interleukin-2 receptor levels. Also, researchers reported that thyroid hormone increased natural killer cell activity. This suggests that inadequate thyroid hormone regulation of the immune system may result in a decrease of natural killer cells as reported in fibromyalgia patients.

Besides some overlap between the immune system abnormalities in fibromyalgia and hypothyroid patients, other evidence points to inadequate thyroid hormone regulation of the immune system as the underlying immune system disrupter in fibromyalgia. For example, some patients developed fibromyalgia after undergoing interleukin-2 therapy for cancer. It is possible that these patients' fibromyalgia is merely the signs and symptoms of undertreated or untreated hypothyroidism. This is possible in that interleukin-2 treatment induces hypothyroidism in 5%-to-10% of patients. Also, patients who have antithyroid antibodies but normal TSH and thyroid hormone levels, *especially women, have a significantly higher incidence of widespread musculoskeletal pain. This suggests that even undetectable subnormal thyroid hormone secretion may result in fibromyalgia symptoms. The finding is consistent with some patients developing symptoms of thyroid hormone deficiency before their thyroid function test results confirm subclinical hypothyroidism.*

Fibromyalgia and Chronic Fatigue Syndrome

The abnormalities reported in some fibromyalgia patients may be associated with impaired immunity. If so, these patients are likely to have an increased frequency and severity of infections and/or reactions to toxic chemicals. It is likely that the same underlying pathophysiologic mechanism, such as inadequate thyroid hormone regulation of cell function, is responsible for immune abnormalities in most fibromyalgia patients. Even so, within this homogeneous population of patients, the clinical effects of immune impairment are likely to be protean. This is likely because the immune system is extremely complex, and the complexity increases the possibilities for variable responsiveness to immune system disregulators such as too little thyroid hormone.

Study results show that chronic fatigue syndrome patients have more immune system abnormalities than do fibromyalgia patients. The two diagnostic groups of patients may represent separate diseases, one with more immune system involvement. Conversely, the similarities of the two groups of patients are so substantial that they are more homogeneous than heterogeneous. The predominant symptom of fatigue and more distinguishable immune involvement leads to a diagnosis of chronic fatigue syndrome. On the other hand, the predominant symptom of pain without distinguishable immune involvement leads to a diagnosis of fibromyalgia. The substantial immune system abnormalities with immune impairment in chronic fatigue syndrome patients are likely to result in a greater incidence of infections and toxic reactions. The greater incidence in this group would account for the diligent search of some investigators for responsible microbes and antimicrobial treatments. However, as Barnes and Galton so clearly argued, a subset of hypothyroid patients, due to inadequate thyroid hormone regulation of the immune system, is highly susceptible to infections. This is also true of a subset of patients with cellular resistance to thyroid hormone. If the predominant symptom of a subset of these patients is pain, they are likely to receive a diagnosis of fibromyalgia, although they are as prone to infections as are chronic fatigue syndrome patients.

One must bear in mind that the finding of immune system abnormalities or infection among some fibromyalgia patients does not necessarily mean that these are the cause of fibromyalgia. If inadequate thyroid hormone regulation of the cell function is the underlying mechanism of fibromyalgia, it is tenable that the inadequate regulation also underlies patients' immune system abnormalities and infections. Hypotheses that infections by particular microorganisms are the cause of fibromyalgia have two major weaknesses: all fibromyalgia patients do not have the infections and the treatments based on the hypotheses are typically ineffective. Other hypotheses that various infectious agents complicate fibromyalgia are reasonable in that the infections are most likely secondary to the underlying mechanism of fibromyalgia. Even when a treatment relieves an infection and appears to have relieved the patients' symptoms and signs, the conclusion that the infection caused the patients' fibromyalgia must be cautiously considered: long-term follow-up should show that the patients do not have recurrences of the infections and that, according to objective measures of fibromyalgia status, patients remain free from fibromyalgia.

Model of Immune System Dysregulation in Fibromyalgia

The hypothesis posited in this chapter is that the immune system abnormalities of some fibromyalgia patients are epiphenomena that occur secondary to inadequate thyroid hormone regulation of the immune system. Infections that occur secondary to the immune system abnormalities are tertiary consequences of inadequate thyroid hormone regulation.

Studies published since Barnes' views appeared in print vindicate his position on the relation of thyroid hormone and infection. The available studies show that susceptible individuals with inadequate thyroid hormone regulation of the immune system have abnormal results of various immune system tests. The results suggest immune system abnormalities, reduced resistance to infection, and adverse effects from toxic agents. The studies also suggest that in these susceptible individuals, adequate thyroid hormone regulation of the immune system can increase the effectiveness of the system in defending the body against microorganisms and toxins.

Subnormal Glucocorticoids

Glucocorticoids, such as cortisol, are the most

potent endogenous immunosuppressive substances. Cortisol levels are subnormal in some patients with fibromyalgia, chronic fatigue syndrome, hypothyroidism, and thyroid hormone resistance. When cortisol levels are subnormal, increased immune system activation occurs, as shown by various immune measures. Patients are likely to have an increased tendency toward inflammation, increased levels of interleukin-1 and interleukin-2, destabilization of lysosomes with the release of lysosomal enzymes that degrade organic compounds, increased recruitment of white blood cells, increased mobilization of T-lymphocytes, and increased production of antibodies by B-lymphocytes.

These measurable indicators of generalized immune system mobilization are found in laboratory animals that have adrenal insufficiency due to hypothyroidism. The indicators are more likely to be found in fibromyalgia and chronic fatigue syndrome patients who have subnormal cortisol secretion. Subnormal cortisol secretion in fibromyalgia may lower the resistance of some patients to infection, increasing their likelihood of infection with microorganisms such as mycoplasmas and Borrelia burgdorferi *(the spirochete responsible for Lyme diseases.) Long-term or repetitive antibiotic treatment may leave some patients with complicating symptoms due to overgrowth of* Candida albicans. *Subnormal cortisol may account for increased titers of various antibodies, such as anti-polymer antibodies. It is possible that subnormal cortisol levels may result in exaggerated responses of the immune system to antigens, leading to a diagnosis of multiple chemical sensitivity syndrome.*

Mast Cells

While subnormal cortisol may contribute to multiple chemical sensitivity syndrome, inadequate thyroid hormone regulation of the adrenergic genes may also contribute to the syndrome. Inadequate thyroid hormone regulation of the genes results in a decreased density of β-adrenergic receptors and an increased density of α-adrenergic receptors on cell membranes. Decreased β-adrenergic receptors and increased α-adrenergic receptors on mast cells increases the cells' secretion of inflammatory substances. Moreover, in hypothyroidism, the number of mast cells in tissues increases. The increased number of mast cells and an increase in their secretions, against a background of a hyper-responsive immune system due to subnormal cortisol, is a plausible mechanism for multiple chemical sensitivity syndrome. This mechanism may also explain the increase in rhinitis symptoms in fibromyalgia and chronic fatigue syndrome.

Silicone Breast Implants

Many patients with silicone breast implants have symptoms characteristic of fibromyalgia due to inadequate thyroid hormone regulation of cell function. Some of the patients also have positive immune function test results, especially elevated titers of anti-nuclear antibodies. The positive immune test results are not specific for any organ system. Patients with fibromyalia symptoms and positive immune test results are said to have "silicone implant-associated syndrome" (SIAS). Results of epidemiological studies have not shown a statistically significant increase in well-recognized diagnosable rheumatologic diseases in SIAS patients. However, published reports make it clear that ruptures, leaks, and bacterial colonization of silicone implants are common. That fibromyalgia is a previously established disease does not rule out silicone breast implants or something associated with them as a factor contributing to patients' fibromyalgia symptoms. The implants or something associated with them may contribute as a precipitator in women who were predisposed to fibromyalgia by inadequate thyroid hormone regulation of cell function. Also, silicone implants or something associated with them may contribute as an exacerbator in women who had fibromyalgia before receiving breast implants.

The immune system protects the body from microorganisms and toxins that can cause disease. In the spring of 1881, Pasteur used a logical procedure to prove the truth of his hypothesis that anthrax vaccination produces immunity to anthrax.[104,p.403] Since then, the pursuit of microbial infections as the cause of disease has been a bustling enterprise among medical researchers. Sometimes, the enterprise has benefitted society. As Illich wrote, chemotherapy played a significant role in controlling pneumonia, gonorrhea, and syphilis. Drug therapies can easily and quickly cure malaria, syphilis, yaws, and typhoid. Immunization contributed to the decrease in whooping cough and measles, and it has virtually eliminated paralytic poliomyelitis. Illich continued, however: "For most infections, however, medicine has not been equally effective. Drug treatment has helped to reduce mortality from tuberculosis, tetanus, diphtheria, and scarlet fever, but in the total decline of mortality and morbidity from these diseases, chemotherapy played a minor and possibly insignificant role."[99,pp.22-23] New infections replace old ones, but the overall rate of infections does not change.[100][101]

Moreover, treatments that militate against one infection abet others.[102]

Government officials and the public seem ever eager to fund research that is likely to lead to the identification and elimination of pathogenic microbes. Often, however, the willingness of some people to fund such research and the eagerness of others to profit from the funding result in tragedy and waste. We have no better example than the invention of the AIDS virus by medical researchers. This invention has cost the public billions of dollars with nothing to show for it except immense amounts of information on a benign and dormant virus.[70]

History shows that the nucleus of the problem I describe here was present shortly after Pasteur's work became known. He advanced the concept that single infective agents cause specific diseases, and for most of the 20th century, allopathic physicians based their practices on this oversimplified view. Bechamps refuted the view of Pasteur, promoting the concept that lowered resistance to infection was the cause of disease. This latter concept is succinctly expressed as "the soil, not the seed."[103,p.7] The mode of practice of modern naturopathic physicians and holistic allopathic physicians represent a more balanced view. They work to increase the resistance of patients while using medications to eliminate particularly virulent microbes when the need arises.

"With the recent resurgence of preventative medicine," wrote Rosenbaum and Susser, "there is a renewed appreciation of the vital role played by host resistance. The immune system is highly complex and dynamic. Malnutrition, stress, and environmental pollution can damage the immune sensitive components and make us susceptible to infection." They also described the essence of their approach to aiding host resistance: "As a result of this new way of thinking, considerable efforts are being directed toward biological ways of modulating the immune response. Immunomodulation with drugs and nutrients which are called biological response modifiers has become the mainstay of our treatment approach."[103,p.7] One of the most effective biological modifiers of immune function is adequate thyroid hormone regulation of the immune system. Broda O. Barnes and Lawrence Galton most clearly expressed this finding. They convincingly showed that for many people, adequate thyroid hormone makes the critical difference in resistance to infective disease (see section below titled "Barnes' Views").

● OVERVIEW OF IMMUNITY

In this overview of immunity,[2,pp.105-129][48,pp.365-384][62,pp.4-11,291-303] I mainly include components of the immune system that studies have shown to be abnormal in fibromyalgia and thyroid hormone deficiency. Microorganisms perpetually occupy the surface of the human body. Bacteria, fungi, viruses, and parasites are teaming on the skin and on the mucous membranes of the mouth and eyes, and the respiratory, gastrointestinal, and urinary tracts. Microorganisms such as bacteria and viruses that do not normally reside on the skin and mucous membranes occasionally attempt to enter the body. Many microorganisms—both those that do and do not normally occupy the surface of the body—and various toxins may cause disease if they pass through the skin or mucous membranes and survive in the inner tissues of the body. However, the body resists damage by microorganisms and toxins through processes that we collectively call immunity.

"Innate immunity" is the resistance that general body structures and processes provide. On the surface of the body, the skin and mucous membranes provide innate immunity. These structures bar microbes and toxins from entering the deeper tissues. The acid and digestive secretions of the gastrointestinal tract are also a part of innate immunity. These secretions destroy microbes before they can enter the tissues. Within the body, white blood cells and tissue macrophages take part in innate immunity. These cells ingest and digest microorganisms, a process called "phagocytosis." In addition, several substances in the blood, such as natural killer cells, contribute to innate immunity.

In addition to innate immunity, "acquired immunity" helps protect the body from microorganisms and toxins. Acquired immunity involves antibodies and activated lymphocytes. These attack and destroy microorganisms and toxins. Overlapping both innate and acquired immunity are cell-mediated and antibody-mediated immunity. As the name implies, cell-mediated immunity involves cellular elements. Humoral immunity involves circulating antibodies. This latter classification is convenient for understanding how the immune system works.

LYMPHOCYTES

The lymphocyte system is the beginning point of both cell-mediated and antibody-mediated immunity. Lymphocytes mainly occupy the lymph nodes. They also occupy other lymph tissues, including the spleen, bone marrow, and tissues beneath the mucosa of the gastrointestinal tract. Two types of lymphocytes occupy lymph tissues: T- and B-cells or T- or B-lymphocytes. In addition, there are types of lymphocytes that are not T- or B-lymphocytes (see subsection below titled "Natural Killer Cells").

T-Lymphocytes

T-Lymphocytes produce the activated lymphocytes that provide cell-mediated immunity. Processing by the thymus gland is necessary before T-lymphocytes can produce activated lymphocytes, and it is for this reason that they are called T-lymphocytes.[86]

Researchers classify T-lymphocytes into several subsets. The subsets are based on different surface receptors on the lymphocytes that react with specific antibodies. Researchers use flow cytometry to measure lymphocyte subsets. Hernanz et al. listed the following subsets: CD3 (T-cells), CD19 (B-cells), CD16 (natural killer cells), CD4 (T helper/inducer cells), CD8 (T cytotoxic/suppressor cells), CD25 (interleukin-2 receptors), CD69 (activation inducer molecule markers), CD71 (transferrin receptors) and CD54 (ICAM-1). The ratio of CD4 to CD8 is also estimated.[131]

Different subsets of CD4 lymphocytes help B-lymphocytes develop into antibody-producing plasma cells. CD8 lymphocytes exert cytotoxic effects. Some subsets of CD8 lymphocytes destroy tumors and cells infected with viruses. Other CD8 lymphocytes inhibit B-lymphocyte production of antibodies. An imbalance in the number of active CD4 and CD8 lymphocytes severely impairs cellular immune function. When the ratio of CD4/CD8 cells is less than 1, the individual is highly susceptible to opportunistic infections and tumors.

B-Lymphocytes

B-Lymphocytes produce the antibodies that provide humoral immunity. In fetal life, before B-lymphocytes produce antibodies, they undergo processing first in the liver and then in the bone marrow. They are called B-lymphocytes because researchers first discovered them in birds in which the preprocessing occurs in the *bursa of Fabricius*. The processing of B-lymphocytes in the liver and bone marrow prepares them for later production of antibodies.

After a series of developmental steps, B-lymphocytes develop into plasma cells that form antibodies. Antibodies are also called immunoglobulins. Antibodies have unique amino acid sequences and tertiary structures that bind to complementary structures on antigen molecules.

CELL-MEDIATED IMMUNITY

Cell-mediated immunity (also called T-cell immunity) involves the formation of large numbers of activated lymphocytes customized to destroy a specific foreign substance. The activated lymphocytes are formed in lymphoid tissues.

In microbial infections, antibodies play a role in the immune response, but cell-mediated immunity is most important in providing resistance and facilitating recovery. The effect of suppressed cell-mediated immunity is well known today through experience with AIDS.[2,p.115] Chronic, heavy recreational drug use is the most probable cause of AIDS. Patients with severely advanced AIDS usually die. In many individuals, AIDS is iatrogenic, caused by the use of prescribed AZT—a poison that virtually ensures death through AIDS-related disease. AZT kills dividing cells in all tissues of the body. It causes ulcerations and hemorrhaging, damage to hair follicles and skin, the death of mitochondria, wasting of muscles, and destruction of the immune system and other blood cells.[13][37][70,p.301] The iatrogenic deaths due to AZT poisoning are then falsely ascribed to the innocuous and dormant virus HIV.[70,pp.300-359] The drug-induced deaths result from impaired immunity and overwhelming and devastating infections and tumors.

Natural Killer Cells

Natural killer cells are lymphocytes, but they are not T- or B-lymphocytes. They circulate in the blood and recognize and destroy foreign cells, tumor cells, and some infected cells.

Some Cytokines

Cytokines are soluble proteins produced mainly by macrophages and activated lymphocytes. The cytokines affect other immune-related cells, modulating the intensity of the inflammatory or immune response.

Lymphokines. Lymphokines are cytokines that affect lymphocytes. When secreted by a T-lymphocyte specific for a particular antigen, lymphokines activate many additional lymphocytes. The two lymphokines touched on in this chapter are interleukin-1 and interleukin-2.

Interleukin-1. Interleukin-1 is a polypeptide synthesized primarily by macrophages. Along with interferon-γ and tumor necrosis factor, interleukin-1 is an inflammatory cytokine. It induces fever by affecting the hypothalamus. It also induces sleep, anorexia, and inflammation. It activates T- and B-lymphocytes, neutrophils, eosinophils, and basophils, and fibroblasts. It also stimulates T-lymphocytes to release interleukin-2.

Interleukin-2. Interleukin-2 is a polypeptide secreted mainly by CD4 cells (the subpopulations of T-lymphocytes with CD4 surface glycoprotein receptors that react with specific antibodies). Interleukin-2 stimulates T-lymphocyte growth, co-stimulates B-lymphocyte growth and differentiation, and increases natural killer cell activity.

Interferons: Macrophage-Affecting Cytokines. Interferons are cytokines that increase the activity of macrophages.

Interferon-α. White blood cells produce interferon-α in response to viruses and double-stranded RNA. Interferon-α inhibits replication of viruses and tumor growth, and it increases the activity of natural killer cells and macrophages. It also increases the expression of major histocompatibility complex (see section below titled "Human Leukocyte Antigens (HLA)").

Interferon-γ. T-lymphocytes produce interferon-γ in response to antigen exposure. Like interkeulin-1 and tumor necrosis factor, interferon-γ is an inflammatory cytokine. Interferon-γ potentiates the activation of macrophages, and it increases the activity of natural killer cells and class I and class II major histocompatibility complex (see section below titled "Human Leukocyte Antigens (HLA)"). It also co-stimulates the growth and differentiation of B-lymphocytes. Moreover, it decreases interleukin-4-induced CD23 and IgE secretion (see subsection below titled "Classes of Immunoglobulins: IgE" and section titled "Allergy").

Tumor Necrosis Factor. Macrophages release tumor necrosis factor. The cytokine then activates neutrophils and takes part in endotoxin-stimulated septic shock.

ANTIBODY-MEDIATED (B-CELL, HUMORAL) IMMUNITY

Antibody-mediated immunity is also called B-cell and humoral immunity. It is immunity acquired by the formation of antibodies in response to antigens. Lymphoid tissues are the sites of antibody formation.

Antigens are substances that combine with antibodies and elicit specific immune responses. The term "antigen" comes from the fact that the substance *gen*erates *anti*bodies. An alternate term for antigenic (stimulating antibody formation) is "immunogenic." A substance is antigenic or immunogenic if it is sufficiently large and the immune system is capable of

recognizing it as foreign to the body. A "hapten" is a substance that reacts with antibodies but is too small to function as an antigen in stimulating antibody formation. Haptens can induce antibody formation by binding to a carrier protein. For example, penicillin is a hapten that can induce antibody formation by combining with albumin.

Upon exposure of the body to an antigen for the first time, antibodies to the antigen appear in the serum within days or weeks. Upon first exposure to the antigen, the level of the antibodies rises for several weeks and then decreases. IgM antibodies form first, then IgG and/or IgA antibodies. Usually, IgM antibody levels decrease sooner than IgG levels. For example, early during hepatitis A infection, IgM antibodies appear. Levels decrease within several weeks. About the same time, IgG levels rise and may persist for life. Thus, IgM is a marker for acute hepatitis A infection, and IgG suggests previous exposure.

Classes of Immunoglobulins

Antibodies are complex glycoproteins called immunoglobulins. There are several types.

IgM. IgM is a large molecule that is the main immunoglobulin during exposure to a new antigen. Its ten antigen binding sites make it the most rapacious immunoglobulin in antigen-antibody reactions. It provides potent defense against bacteria and viruses. IgM is much more effective at activating complement than is IgG. IgM molecules facilitate processes called opsonization and agglutination that aid phagocytes in engulfing microorganisms. In opsonization, microbes are altered so that phagocytes more easily ingest them (see section below titled "The Complement System"), and in agglutination, microbes adhere in clumps.

IgG. IgG is the most prevalent of the immunoglobulins. IgG is produced when IgM titers begin decreasing after initial contact with an antigen. IgG is the most important antibody in the secondary immune response. In the plasma and extra-vascular spaces, it provides an effective defense against viruses and bacteria, particularly encapsulated bacteria.

IgE. IgE is known as the skin-sensitizing or anaphylactic antibody. It is found mainly in mucous secretions of the respiratory and gastrointestinal tracts. Its serum levels are much lower than those of other immunoglobulins, and especially sensitive techniques are needed to measure its levels. IgE has a locus termed the "Fc region" that binds to the surface of mast cells and basophils. The IgE level is elevated in allergic asthma, hay fever, atopic dermatitis, and parasitic diseases.

Autoimmune Disorders

In autoimmune disorders, autoantibodies form to endogenous antigens. Tissue damage results.

Several possible mechanisms may be instrumental in autoimmunity. (1) An endogenous substance normally sequestered in the cells of a tissue may escape upon trauma to the tissue. When sequestered within the tissue, autoantibodies may not have access to the antigen. Activated T-lymphocytes, however, may have better access to the antigen within the tissue and react with it. (2) A chemical, physical, or biologic alteration of a substance may be immunogenic. For example, when some substances that are not normally antigenic combine with proteins, the combination may be antigenic. Ultraviolet light may alter a skin protein and autoantibodies may then form and react with it. (3) Cross reactions can occur between a foreign antigen and an endogenous substance. For example, following rabies vaccination, encephalitis may result from a cross-reaction between constituents of the individual's brain cells and constituents of animal brain cells in the vaccine. (4) Autoimmunity may result from autoantibodies reacting to mutant cells. (5) Reduced function of suppressor T-lymphocytes may result in autoimmune disease. Normally, T-lymphocytes limit immune responses to endogenous antigens. When T-lymphocyte function diminishes, antibodies to endogenous substances may form, resulting in autoimmunity.

Hashimoto's thyroiditis is associated with autoantibodies against various thyroid gland components such as thyroglobulin and thyroid peroxidase. The usual results are thyroid tissue damage and hypothyroidism. Autoimmune thyroiditis is the most common cause of primary hypothyroidism. Both cell-mediated and antibody-mediated autoimmunity are involved (see Chapter 2.4).

In Graves' disease, thyroid-stimulating antibodies react with TSH receptors on the thyroid gland. The reaction causes excess secretion of thyroid hormones and results in thyrotoxicosis. Roughly 10% of Graves' patients spontaneously become hypothyroid, and others become hypothyroid after chemical or surgical ablation of the thyroid gland. (See Chapter 2.4)

Environmental factors appear to induce autoimmune disease in predisposed individuals. Predisposition appears to be genetically based. Commonly, relatives of patients with autoimmune disease have the same types of autoantibodies. Identical twins have a higher incidence of autoimmune disease than fraternal twins. A high familial incidence of autoimmune disease may be associated with human leukocyte antigens (see HLA).

Human Leukocyte Antigens (HLA). Normally, the immune system can distinguish substances that are "of the body" from those that are not. This ability is determined mainly by products of the major histocompatibility complex (MHC), the genes of which are located on chromosome 6. The genes belong to the Ig superfamily. Susceptibility to some diseases appears to be linked to genes closely related to the MHC.

MHC is a cluster of closely situated genes that code for antigens involved in immune reactions to transplanted organs. Whether a transplanted organ is histocompatible is largely determined by whether the donor and recipient have in common antigens coded by genes within the MHC. Most of the antigens are glycoproteins located on cell surfaces. Identical twins share antigens, so organ grafts between them are usually not rejected by the immune system.

Some researchers refer to the genes within the MHC as MHC genes. Others call them HLA genes, and they refer to the antigens they code for as HLA antigens. HLA genes within the MHC code for "human leukocyte antigens." These antigens on the leukocytes of one person cause antibodies to form in another person. Each person inherits a set of HLA genes from each parent, and each HLA gene is termed a histocompatibility locus.

Class-I HLA antigens are coded by the HLA-A, HLA-B, and HLA-C genes with the MHC. About 150 different class-I antigens reside on cell membranes. Cytotoxic T-lymphocytes recognize and react with these antigens. Class-I HLA antigens are largely responsible for graft rejections because they are present on virtually all body cells.

Class-II HLA antigenic molecules (HLA-DR, HLA-DQ, and HLA-DP) are coded by several genes in the HLA-D region. Helper T-lymphocytes recognize and react with them. If cytotoxic or helper T-lymphocytes react with HLA antigens on cell membranes of a transplanted organ, graft rejection usually occurs. The class II HLA antigenic molecules are expressed on various antigen presenting cells. Peptide fragments that match peptide-binding grooves on class II HLA antigenic molecules are expressed on the surfaces of antigen presenting cells. The peptides bind to HLA molecules and are therefore called "anchors." T-lymphocyte receptors "recognize" and react to these peptides on HLA molecules.[87]

Susceptibility to some diseases appears to be related to genes within the HLA regions on chromosome 6. However, investigators have not determined how susceptibility to specific diseases is related to the specific HLA genes. It is possible that HLA antigens cross-react with the antigenic components of microorganisms and trigger autoimmune responses. It is also possible that HLA antigens function as receptors on the surfaces of microorganisms. For example, HLA antigens may become incorporated into the protein coat of a virus.

THE COMPLEMENT SYSTEM

The complement system overlaps innate and acquired immunity. It consists of about 20 proteins that circulate in the serum, several of which are precursors of enzymes. Researchers designate the main proteins as B, C1 through C9, and D. All circulate and escape from capillaries into the tissue spaces. About 10% of serum proteins are complement proteins.

The complement system has two main effects: the breakdown of microbes and tumor cells, and the induction of substances that take part in inflammation and attract phagocytes. The protein precursors are usually inactive. They are activated by antigen-antibody reactions and molecules such as endotoxins, both of which set off a sequence of reactions. In one reaction of the complement system, microbes or toxins activate the enzyme C3 convertase. This enzyme acts on C3, which is the highest-concentration complement system protein in the circulation. Activity of the enzyme produces C3b. Neutrophils and macrophages have C3b receptors on their surfaces. Binding of C3b to the receptors of these phagocytes enables them to attach to and engulf cells and antigen-antibody complexes. This process, which facilitates phagocytosis, is called "opsonization," and it can increase by a hundred-fold the number of engulfed bacteria. In another reaction, complement products attack constituents of virulent viruses and render them harmless.

In still another reaction of the complement system, fragments of C3a, C4a, and C5 activate mast cells and basophils. Upon activation these cells release histamine and other substances into the circulating blood. These substances increase blood flow, passage of fluid and plasma into tissue spaces, and other tissue reactions that neutralize antigens. These processes are part of inflammatory and allergic reactions. (See section below titled "Allergy.")

ALLERGY

An allergy is the collection of secondary effects of an immune system reaction to an antigen. An antigen is called an "allergen" when it sets off an allergic reaction.

Atopic Allergy

Atopic allergy refers to allergic tendencies resulting from an unusual response of the immune system. An allergic tendency is transmitted genetically. The patient who develops an atopic allergy has an inherited predisposition to develop hypersensitivity to a particular antigen. IgE antibodies mediate the hypersensitivity. The patient has large amounts of circulating IgE immunoglobulins called sensitizing antibodies. IgE reacts with an allergen and results in the allergic reaction.

In inducing the allergic reaction, IgE binds to mast cells and basophils. The membranes of the mast cells and basophils undergo changes and rupture, and the granules and various substances of the cells escape. Among the substances released are histamine and slow-reacting anaphylaxis substance. The mixture of these substances, which are called leukotrienes, is toxic. The substances released from the cells cause local blood vessels to dilate and capillaries to become more permeable. As a result, fluid passes from the vessels to the tissue that sustains the damage. The substances also attract neutrophils and eosinophils.

The symptoms and signs of the patient depend on the tissues affected. An allergic reaction of the skin results in urticaria; of the nose, mouth, and pharynx, hay fever; of the eyes, allergic conjunctivitis; and of the bronchioles, asthma.

Delayed-Reaction Allergy

A delayed-reaction allergy is mediated by activated T-lymphocytes. Repeated exposure to a toxin causes production of activated helper and cytotoxic T-lymphocytes. After another exposure to the toxin, the T-lymphocytes migrate into the involved tissue and stimulate a cell-mediated immune reaction. During this process, T-lymphocytes release toxic substances into the tissue, and macrophages invade the tissue. The process can severely damage the involved tissue.

● IMMUNE ABNORMALITIES IN FIBROMYALGIA

Reports of the results of immune system studies of fibromyalgia patients have been inconsistent. The inconsistencies could be a product of the variable effects of inadequate thyroid hormone regulation of the immune system in different individuals.

ALLERGY AND FIBROMYALGIA

Enestrom et al. examined skin biopsies from 25 fibromyalgia patients, 8 rheumatoid arthritis patients, 9 whiplash pain patients, and 5 normal control subjects. They examined for IgG deposits, collagen types, and skin connective tissue mast cells. The dermis and blood vessel walls of fibromyalgia patients had significantly more IgG deposits and a higher mean number of mast cells. The dermis and vessels also had higher reactivity for collagen III. The researchers reported a correlation between the patients' IgG scores and the percentage of degranulated mast cells. They wrote that their findings support a hypothesis of neurogenic inflammation in fibromyalgia.[45]

Baraniuk et al. reported positive allergy skin test results in 35% of chronic fatigue syndrome patients and 44% of normal subjects. The difference, however, was not statistically significant. The investigators wrote that 30% of chronic fatigue syndrome patients had positive allergy skin tests suggesting a potential for allergic rhinitis. The percentage of patients with positive skin test results did not statistically differ from the percentage of normal controls with positive results. Of those with a positive skin test, 83% complained of rhinitis. Also, 46% had non-allergic rhinitis. They suggested that the mechanism of the non-allergic rhinitis may offer insights into the pathogenesis of chronic fatigue syndrome.[42]

Baraniuk et al. also reported that about 70% of fibromyalgia and chronic fatigue syndrome patients have symptoms of rhinitis. Yet only 35%-to-50% have positive skin allergy test results. The researchers speculated that this finding suggests that non-allergic mechanisms are involved in the patients' rhinitis. They performed lavages to obtain nasal mucous samples from 27 patients with fibromyalgia/chronic fatigue syndrome, 7 allergic rhinitis patients, 7 cystic fibrosis patients, and 9 healthy subjects. Nasal mucous constituents provide evidence of ongoing secretory processes. Allergic rhinitis patients had higher IgG counts and vascular permeability. The fibromyalgia/chronic fatigue syndrome patients had no markers indicative of allergy rhinitis. In addition, the researchers found no difference between the lavage mucous of fibromyalgia/chronic fatigue syndrome patients and normal subjects.[38] The results did not determine what may underlie the rhinitis symptoms of fibromyalgia/chronic fatigue syndrome.

AUTOIMMUNE DISEASE AND FIBROMYALGIA

Researchers have studied the levels of several types of antibodies in fibromyalgia patients.

Antibodies to Epstein-Barr Virus and Parvovirus

Wallace et al. reported that the subclasses of IgG were normal in 16 fibromyalgia patients. Titers of antibodies to Epstein-Barr virus capsid antigen (IgG and IgM) were no different from apparently normal control subjects.[113,p.284]

Branco et al. compared the titers of specific IgG antibodies against parvovirus B19 in 52 fibromyalgia patients and 39 controls. The mean of positive titers among the patients was not signficiantly different from that of controls. Branco et al. concluded that their results did not support a causative role for parvovirus B19 infection in fibromyalgia.[132]

Anti-Serotonin Antibodies

Klein et al. tested the sera of 50 fibromyalgia patients for both organ-specific and non-organ-specific antibodies. They reported finding no common antibodies against nuclei, mitochondria, or microsomes. However, 74% of the patients had antibodies against serotonin and gangliosides (glycosphingolipids are found mainly in nerve and spleen tissue, and they are an important constituent of serotonin receptors[19]). The patients had elevated titers of both IgG and IgM anti-serotonin antibodies. The antibodies cross-reacted with tryptophan. The researchers noted that anti-serotonin antibodies are not found in rheumatic disorders such as rheumatoid arthritis, polymyalgia rheumatica, and collagen diseases. They conjectured that the antibodies they found in fibromyalgia patients may be anti-receptor antibodies, in that the gangliosides are structural components of serotonin receptors. They proposed that the low serum levels of serotonin in fibromyalgia patients result from an autoimmune process.[18]

An attempt to replicate the finding was not successful. The sera of 30 fibromyalgia patients did not contain IgG or IgM antibodies to serotonin or the gangliosides that are components of serotonin receptors. In fact, the mean level of IgM antibodies against serotonin was actually significantly lower (P=0.03) than in normal controls.[20] Similarly, Vedder and Bennett did not find laboratory evidence of serotonin receptor antibodies in fibromyalgia patients.[21]

Antinuclear Antibodies

Dinerman et al. reported that fibromyalgia patients who had Raynaud's phenomenon were positive for antinuclear antibodies.[129] However, Bengtsson et al. evaluated 48 fifty-year-old fibromyalgia patients 8 years after their initial diagnosis of fibromyalgia. The researchers wrote that at follow-up, antinuclear antibody titers were slightly higher than 8 years earlier, but the levels were still within the normal range.[33] The higher incidence of elevated antinuclear antibody titers may have resulted from the older age of the patients.[34] In a study of many fibromyalgia patients, Yunus et al. found that the prevalence of antinuclear antibodies in the patients was similar to that of normal control subjects.[130]

Antipolymer Antibodies

Wilson et al. reported that the prevalence of sero-activity for antipolymer antibodies was higher in fibromyalgia patients than other patients. They reported seroactivity in 22 of 47 fibromyalgia patients (47%), 3 of 16 osteoarthritis patients (19%), 1 of 13 rheumatoid arthritis patients (8%), and 4 of 21 control subjects (19%). The prevalence of seroactivity was significantly higher in patients with severe fibromyalgia than in those with mild fibromyalgia. Of 28 patients with severe fibromyalgia, 17 (61%) were seroactive. Of 37 patients with mild fibromyalgia, 11 (30%) were seroactive. Wilson et al. also reported that the mean threshold and mean tolerance algometer scores of fibromyalgia patients were lower in those who were seropositive than in those who were seronegative. (Lower algometer scores show higher pressure/pain sensitivity of tender points.) The researchers concluded that a subset of fibromyalgia patients have an immunological response involving formation of antipolymer antibodies. They also wrote that their results suggest that the antipolymer antibody assay may serve as an objective marker in the diagnosis and assessment of fibromyalgia.[39] (See my comments on the findings in the study in the section below titled "Autoimmune Disease and Thyroid Function.") Antipolymer antibodies were elevated in symptomatic silicone breast implant patients, many of whom have fibromyalgia symptoms (see section below titled "Silicone Breast Implants and Fibromyalgia").

HLA

Yunus noted that fibromyalgia commonly occurs in more than one member of a family, but evidence for a genetic basis for the condition is limited. He also pointed out that a few researchers have reported familial aggregation and an association with HLA (see subsection above title "Human Leukocyte Antigens (HLA)"). He reported studying a possible genetic linkage of fibromyalgia in "multicase" families and found a weak linkage (p<0.029) of fibromyalgia with HLA.[43]

The following year, Yunus et al. published the results of further testing for a linkage. They studied 40 Caucasian multicase families in which 2 or more first degree relatives had diagnoses of fibromyalgia. Of 41 sibships (brothers and sisters of a single family), 85 members were affected and 21 were unaffected. HLA typing was run for A, B, and DRB 1 alleles and haplotypes were determined. The researchers evaluated sibships in the multicase families by looking for a genetic linkage to the HLA region. They reported that sibship analysis revealed a significant linkage of fibromyalgia to the HLA region (p=0.028). They concluded that their results showed that within their 40 multicase families, a possible gene for fibromyalgia was linked to the HLA region.[44]

Researchers have not determined how a link to HLA genes may be associated with diseases (see subsection above titled "Human Leukocyte Antigens (HLA)").

CYTOKINES

Wallace et al. found that cytokines were normal in fibromyalgia patients compared to apparently normal control subjects. The percentage of patients with cytokines within the detectable range and the mean cytokine levels were not significantly different from those of controls.[113,p.285]

Wallace reported that patients who had undergone treatment for cancer with intravenous interleukin-2 had features of fibromyalgia.[114] (See subsection below titled "Cytokines: Interleukin-2 Therapy and Hypothyroidism.")

King et al. conducted a study of 10 fibromyalgia patients, 10 myofascial pain syndrome patients, and 10 healthy controls to determine their serum levels of two cytokines: interleukin-1β and tumor necrosis factor-α. The researchers found that the mean levels of tumor necrosis factor-α of fibromyalgia and myofascial pain syndrome patients did not significantly differ from the mean level of the healthy controls. They found that serum interleukin-1β levels were undetectable in all groups—patients and healthy controls. They wrote that the study results did not suggest that fibromyalgia and myofascial pain syndrome were related to "cytokine-induced soft tissue sensitization."[36]

LYMPHOCYTES

Wallace reported that in fibromyalgia patients compared to controls, analysis of lymphocyte subsets showed an increased mean CD4/CD8 ratio. Of 15 patients whose CD4/CD8 ratios were measured 3-to-5 times during a 6-month period, 9 had at least one measure above the upper limit of the range of normal. During the 6-months, 4 of the 9 patients had elevated CD4/CD8 ratios at each evaluation.[113,pp.279-280] An imbalance in the numbers of active CD4 to CD8 cells severely impairs cellular immune function (see subsection above titled "Lymphocytes: T-Lymphocytes").

MYCOPLASMAL INFECTIONS

Mycoplasmas are the smallest and simplest free-living and self-replicating organisms.[2,p.268][49][50] Their diameter, 125-to-300 nm (a nanometer is one billionth of a meter), is similar to that of other small bacteria such as *Chlamydiae* and large viruses.[2,p.268][50] They can pass through filters with a pore size of 45–nm and smaller and thus can escape filtration procedures used to prevent contamination. Although researchers classify mycoplasmas as bacteria,[2,p.268] they do not possess a rigid cell wall found in most types of bacteria. They probably evolved by reductive evolution from Gram-positive bacteria with low guanine-to-cytosine genomes.[49][51] Because of genetic analyses of some bacteria that lack cell walls, such as *Haembartonella*, researchers are reclassifying mycoplasmas. These hemotropic organisms apparently represent a new group of pathogens.[1]

Mycoplasmas can occur in multiple structural forms. This "polymorphism" is possible because of their triple-layered plasma membrane that lacks the rigidity of bacterial cell walls.[50] The mycoplasma cell membrane contains a sterol (a steroid of 27 or more carbon atoms with 1 alcohol or OH group). Since they do not have a polysaccharide cell wall, they are resistant to penicillin. However, certain antibiotics, such as tetracycline and erythromycin generally inhibit the metabolism and growth of mycoplasmas.[2,p.268]

Molecular Biology

Mycoplasmas contain ribosomes and a circular, double-stranded DNA molecule. Investigators have now completely sequenced the genomes of *Mycoplasma genitalium* and *Mycoplasma pneumoniae*,[51] and the genomes contain far fewer genes than most bacteria. For example, the genome of *Mycoplasma genitalium* is only 580 kb long and contains only 470 genes. By comparison, the genome of *E. coli* contains about 4000 genes. *Mycoplasma genitalium* are considered one of the smallest organisms with a minimal set of genes capable of independent life. *Mycoplasma genitalium* evolved without their cell wall and ability to synthesize certain metabolites and macromolecule precursors. To survive, they must associate with host cells that synthesize these molecules. They are completely dependent on their hosts for fatty acids and cholesterol because they lack genes needed for the synthesis of fatty acids and sterol. They have only one gene that codes for amino acid synthesis, and they are thus almost completely dependent on host amino acids for protein synthesis. In addition, they have few genes encoding vitamin and nucleic acid precursors as well as those that code for products related to energy metabolism. They thus are dependent on a limited supply of ATP for their parasitic lifestyle. The lack of a rigid cell wall also relieves them of the requirement to synthesize molecules for transport across the cell wall. Razin suggested that a genomic price must have been paid to maintain parasitism, which might explain why a significant number of mycoplasmal genes is devoted to adhesion molecules (adhesins), attachment organelles and variable membrane surface antigens directed toward evasion of the host immune system.[49] Highly pathogenic mycoplasmas are found at intracellular sites sequestered away from the immune system, and their surface molecules are needed for host cell entry. In addition, such mycoplasmas are usually very slow-growing, and this may account for the chronic nature of the illness associated with the infection in individuals with impaired immune systems, as argued by Nicolson.[4]

Mycoplasmas have evolved with remarkable mechanisms to increase their chances of survival as parasites. For example, they can expand their repertoire of antigens by producing antigens of different structures. This process can quickly generate host antigen mimics or antigens that the host's immune system cannot recognize as foreign. The genes in mycoplasmas' encoding surface antigens are compressed into minimal genomic coding sequences. Because they do not have a cell wall, most mycoplasmas' antigens are lipoproteins. These lipoproteins can provide specific defenses against the host immune system by modifying host responses. Moreover, the host immune system can become involved in the development of pathogenic effects caused by mycoplasmas and in worsening mycoplasma-induced diseases. Thus mycoplasmas can be involved as causal agents in illnesses, or as cofactors that stimulate progression of illness or as opportunistic infections when host immune responses are compromised.[203]

Mycoplasmas can affect immune responses. For example, they can stimulate or suppress various subsets of lymphocytes, and they can also alter the activities of monocytes/macrophages and natural killer cells. They can also stimulate production of cytokines and chemokines that can regulate immune responses, including inflammation-promoting cytokines, such as tumor necrosis factor alpha, interleukin-1, and interleukin-6 by macrophages. In addition, mycoplasmas can stimulate up-regulation of cytokines released by mitogenically-stimulated lymphocytes. So, mycoplasmas may markedly modulate a host's immune system and alter inflammatory responses.[51]

Mycoplasmal Infections

Mycoplasmas are members of the normal flora of the mouth. They can be grown from normal saliva, oral mucous membrane cells, sputum, and tonsillar tissues.[2,p.289] At these superficial sites, however, they are not usually considered pathogenic.[203] When mycoplasmas invade into the blood or tissues, they can enter sites where they can be potential pathogens. Certain mycoplasmas have a predilection for attachment to the host cell membranes of mammals,[2,p.268] and when this occurs, mycoplasmas can eventually enter host cells. According to Nicolson, individuals whose immune systems have been impaired by a virus, radiation, or chemical pollutants may have the highest likelihood of developing a mycoplasmal infection.[4]

That an impaired immune system may result in a mycoplasmal infection suggests that mycoplasmas are opportunistic organisms. Consequently, some writers have called them "parasitic"[2,p.269] and referred to their "parasitic mode of life."[49] Mycoplasmas have been isolated from the oral cavity and various mucous membranes and tissues, especially from the genital, urinary, and respiratory tracts. They have also been isolated from brain abscesses and pleural joint effusions.[2,p.269] Haier et al. reported that a high percentage of rheumatoid arthritis patients had multiple systemic mycoplasmal infections. These investigators concluded that mycoplasmal infections may be an important cofactor in the pathogenesis of rheumatoid arthritis.[197]

Chronic Fatigue Syndrome/Fibromyalgia Patients. Although Komaroff et al. reported an absence

of antibodies to *Mycoplasma fermentans* in chronic fatigue syndrome patients,[52] genetic studies by Nicolson et al. with Forensic Polymerase Chain Reaction, a much more sensitive technique, found strong evidence for mycoplasmal infections in more than 144 of 203 patients, and of these, most were *Mycoplasma fermentans* infections. Fewer than 9% of healthy individuals showed evidence of mycoplasmal infections.[204] Similarly, Choppa et al. detected the presence of *Mycoplasma genus* DNA sequences in cell cultures as well as in the blood of patients with chronic fatigue syndrome. They could distinguish between three pathogenic species of mycoplasma (*M. fermentans, M. hominis, and M. penetrans*). Among 100 chronic fatigue syndrome patients, 52% had *Mycoplasma genus* infection. *Mycoplasma fermentans* was involved in 32% of patient infections, *Mycoplasma hominis* in 9%, and *Mycoplasma penetrans* in 6%. Only 15% of 100 healthy individuals had any mycoplasmal infection. Of these, *Mycoplasma fermentans* was found in 8% of healthy individuals' blood infections, *Mycoplasma hominis* in 3%, and *Mycoplasma penetrans* in 2%.[54]

In another study, Vojdani et al. reported finding that of 100 chronic fatigue syndrome patients, 52% had genetic evidence of *Mycoplasma genus*, and 34% had evidence of *Mycoplasma fermentans*. In contrast, 14% of 50 healthy subjects had genetic evidence of *Mycoplasma genus*, and 8% had evidence of *Mycoplasma fermentans*. Individuals with high genome copy numbers of *Mycoplasma fermentans* had higher IgG and IgM antibodies against the organism.[55]

Ginsburg et al. compared the incidence of genitourinary mycoplasmal infections in 49 women with system lupus erythematosus and 22 patients with chronic fatigue syndrome. The incidence in lupus was 63% and in chronic fatigue syndrome, 4.5%.[53]

More recent studies have reported a high incidence of multiple mycoplasmal infections, and probably other infections as well, in chronic fatigue syndrome and fibromyalgia patients. When Nicolson et al. examined chronic fatigue syndrome/fibromyalgia patients for *M. fermentans, M. pneumoniae, M. penetrans* and, *M. hominis* infections, they found multiple infections in more than 50% of 93 patients. More than 30% of chronic fatigue syndrome/fibromyalgia patients had double mycoplasmal infections and more than 20% had triple mycoplasmal infections, but only when one of the species was *M. fermentans* or *M. pneumoniae*. Higher scores for increases in the severity of signs and symptoms were also found in patients with multiple infections. Chronic fatigue syndrome/fibromyalgia patients infected with different mycoplasma species generally had a longer history of illness. The longer history suggests that patients may have contracted additional infections over time.[203] Nicolson et al. also reported that the mycoplasmal infections were similar to those found in patients with Gulf War illness and account for considerable morbidity in these patients.[56]

Treatment for Mycoplasmal Infection

Specific antibodies inhibit the growth of mycoplasmas, and the levels of specific antibodies (at least against *Mycoplasma pneumoniae*) rise during infection. In a *Mycoplasma pneumoniae* infection, the white cell and differential counts are within normal limits.[2,pp.268&270] The effects of mycoplasmas on the host immune system may militate against an effective host immune response to mycoplasmal infection (see above subsection titled "Molecular Biology").

One treatment protocol for mycoplasmal infections includes multiple cycles of antibiotics and nutritional support.[205] Nicolson explained that patients' symptoms may include the fatigue, headaches, soreness, and joint pain that overlap many chronic illnesses.[4] But what distinguishes mycoplasmal infections are the severity of some signs and symptoms and the response to certain antibiotics.[199]

Since mycoplasmas do not have a cell wall, they are resistant to antibiotics that act on cell wall synthesis machinery. For example, mycoplasmas are resistant to penicillins and other antibiotics that act on constituents of bacterial cell walls.[50] They are also resistant to rifampicins.[50] Nonetheless, mycoplasmas are susceptible to several broad-spectrum antibiotics. Most of these antibiotics inhibit the replication of mycoplasmas rather than exerting a cytotoxic effect. Tetracyclines are particularly effective, especially for genital tract mycoplasmal infections. Macrolides are particularly effective for respiratory tract mycoplasmal infections, but tetracycline, erythromycin, and ketolides and quinolones are equally effective, and the latter tend to kill the microorganisms. In time, mycoplasmas may develop resistance to antibiotics such as tetracyclines.[50] Taylor-Robinson and Bebear noted that their relative resistance to antibiotics may make mycoplasmas difficult to eliminate from human hosts.[50]

Nicolson and Rosenberg-Nicolson recommended antibiotic therapy for patients with mycoplasmal infections,[199][205] including Gulf War illness patients who have fibromyalgia and chronic fatigue syndrome.[198] According to Nicolson, however, eliminating mycoplasmas may be especially difficult in immunosuppressed or immunodeficient individuals.[4] This is especially true of those with decreased levels of the gamma fraction of serum globulin or a general decrease in the quantity of immunoglobulins (hypogammaglobulinemia), with an increased susceptibility to puss-forming infections.[50] In addition to antibiotics, vitamins, minerals, immune enhancers, and other supplements are necessary for recovery.[205]

Appropriate treatment of mycoplasmal infections found in chronic illnesses has been useful in facilitating recovery from the illnesses. For example, of 87 Gulf War illness patients who tested positive for mycoplasmal infections, all patients relapsed after the first 6-week cycle of antibiotic therapy. But after up to 6 cycles of therapy, 69 of the 87 patients recovered and returned to active duty.[56] The clinical responses were not due to placebo effects, and they were not due to immunosuppressive effects that can occur with some recommended antibiotics. Interestingly, chronic fatigue syndrome, fibromyalgia, and Gulf War illness patients who slowly recovered after several cycles of antibiotics were generally less environmentally sensitive. The lower sensitivity of these patients suggests that their immune systems might have been returning to pre-illness states.[30] If such patients had illnesses caused by psychological problems or solely by chemical exposures, they should not respond to the recommended antibiotics and slowly recover. In addition, if such treatments were just reducing autoimmune responses, then patients would relapse after stopping treatment.[203] Similarly, most chronic fatigue syndrome/fibromyalgia patients who tested positive for mycoplasmal infections also responded to the antibiotic therapy.[206] Most of these clinical studies were not controlled. However, the results of two double-blind placebo-controlled studies comparing placebos with the use of minocycline suggest that this antibiotic is clinically effective for rheumatoid arthritis patients.[9][10] These results strongly suggest the involvement of mycoplasmal infections in some chronic illnesses, including many cases of fibromyalgia. According to Nicolson, the results also suggest that treatment for mycoplasmal infections enable patients to effectively overcome these illnesses.[30]

Virtually no information is available on the possible interaction of inadequate thyroid hormone regulation of immune function and susceptibility to mycoplasmal infections and resistance to treatment for the infections. Of Nicolson's patients in the study I cited above, 79% returned to active duty following 6 cycles of therapy for mycoplasmal infections.[56] Some study subjects were fibromyalgia patients. If fibromyalgia patients have severely inadequate thyroid hormone regulation of the immune system, infections relieved by antibiotic therapy would most likely re-occur.

Some infected fibromyalgia patients improve and become functional following cycles of antibiotics as part of the treatment protocol of Nicolson et al.[30] It is possible that these patients, before acquiring mycoplasmal infections, had marginally sufficient metabolism due to inadequate thyroid hormone regulation of cell function, and their metabolic insufficiency predisposed them to the infections. It is also possible that their metabolic status improved due to various features of Nicolson's exemplary broad scope treatment protocol. In addition to antibiotic therapy, the patients also undergo various other interventions that may improve their metabolic status despite continuing inadequate thyroid hormone regulation of cell function. For example, patients may undergo treatment with hyperbaric oxygen, peroxide baths, cessation of the intake of high sugar and high fat foods, adoption of a wholesome, health-inducing diet, use of a wide array of nutritional supplements, replacement of the normal gut flora, herbal therapies, and exercise to tolerance. Nicolson noted that patients must continue various supplements to maintain immune system efficiency.[205] Do these features of the protocol improve metabolic status and secondarily improve immune system efficiency so the infections relieved through antibiotic therapy do not recur? This is a question for which no definite answer is available at this time.

Information on treatment for mycoplasmal infections is available through the Institute for Molecular Medicine with which Professor Garth L. Nicolson is affiliated.[22] For more information on antifungal treatment, see the section below titled "Fungal Infection."

SILICONE BREAST IMPLANTS AND FIBROMYALGIA

Many patients who have silicone breast implants suffer from symptoms and positive immune test results. The symptoms and positive test results are called "silicone implant-associated syndrome" or "SIAS." The term SIAS, proposed by Bridges,[191] is a synonym for "human adjuvant disease," "silicone associated disorder," and "siliconosis."

Silicone Breast Implants and SIAS

Breast implants containing silicone have been used since 1962 for cosmetic breast augmentation or breast reconstruction after mastectomy.[163][164][165][166][169][184][201] Eventually, well-publicized case reports

stimulated concern over the safety of silicone in breast implants, and accumulating evidence suggested that silicone from the implants induces systemic disease. Some medical writers had reported serious local complications associated with the implants. These included contracture of the scar capsule that formed around the implants, foreign body granulomas in the capsular tissue and in lymph nodes, rupture of the implants, gel "bleed" from them, and spread of the silicone to regional lymph nodes. Also, magnetic resonance spectroscopy and atomic emission spectroscopy revealed silicon compounds in the blood of some women with silicone breast implants. Silicone was also found in the livers of some women.[166]

Other researchers expressed concern over an increased risk for autoimmune disease, especially the rare but occasionally fatal disease scleroderma. Growing concern and a lack of evidence for the safety of silicone implants resulted in a response in 1992 of the Food and Drug Administration. The FDA requested a voluntary moratorium on the implantation of silicone gel in breasts. The request stipulated that silicone implants should be used only in reconstructive surgery and as part of clinical trials.[165][169] The action of the FDA stimulated a surge of studies on the reactions of the body to silicone and clinical observations of patients with silicone implants.

The question of the safety of silicone breast implants appears to have polarized the opinions of medical writers. Vayssairat et al. wrote in 1997, for example, "The silicone implant controversy wavers between reassuring epidemiological studies and about 300 case reports of patients developing a definite or incomplete/atypical connective tissue disease after receiving silicone gel-filled breast implants."[167]

Reports that Silicone Implants are Not Harmful. Among those who have published reassuring statements is Blackburn. In 1993, Blackburn et al. wrote, "In general, the implants have been well tolerated and reports have indicated a high degree of patient satisfaction." In 1997, Blackburn et al. wrote, "In general, the implants have been well tolerated and reports have indicated a high degree of patient satisfaction. Nonetheless, there have been anecdotal reports of patients with musculoskeletal complaints that have been attributed to silicone breast implants."[163] In 1997, Blackburn and Everson wrote again of anecdotal reports that suggested a relation between silicone breast implants and rheumatic diseases. "Fortunately," they wrote, "this issue has now been extensively addressed by controlled studies, which demonstrate no association between breast implants and rheumatoid arthritis, systemic lupus erythematosus, and scleroderma. More-over, several studies that now have addressed the issue of 'atypical connective tissue disease' indicate no association between a number of rheumatic complaints and silicone breast implants. Additionally, several controlled studies show no evidence of chronic inflammation in patients with silicone breast implants." As if to allay patients' and clinicians' concerns, they concluded, "These observations should be reassuring to women with breast implants and the individuals who care for them."[168] Similarly, Noone wrote in 1997 that the medical literature failed to support a relation of silicone gel breast implants to systemic diseases. He also wrote, "Silicone gel breast implants may rupture and cause local symptoms, but they have not been demonstrated to be a systemic health hazard for patients who have undergone augmentation mammaplasty or post-mastectomy reconstruction."[169]

Studies Indicating Adverse Effects. Researchers such as Naim et al. do not agree that silicone is an inert and nontoxic substance in the human body. They wrote that most studies suggest that silicones are stable compounds, but they nonetheless can elicit benign inflammatory responses. Their animal experiments showed that silicone gel from commercial breast implants has the potential as an immunological "adjuvant." (In immunology, an adjuvant is a substance that increases antigenicity or immune reactions.) Their studies showed that silicone-gel is a potent antibody adjuvant and elicited auto-antibodies against rat thyroglobulin and bovine collagen II. They discussed the advisability of replacing silicone-gel in implants with a more hydrophilic material.[164]

Brautbar and coauthors wrote that according to established medical criteria for causation, silicone breast implants cause immunological disease. They itemized several findings from *in vivo* and *in vitro* studies, case reports, and population studies: (1) silicone is immunogenic in humans; (2) silicone is biodegradable and transported via the reticuloendothelial system to distant body sites; (3) silicone breast implants leak, allowing silicone to migrate from the breast implants; (4) studies document an autoimmune reaction and immunological dysfunction in patients with silicone breast implants; and (5) for 50%-to-70% of patients, the immunological abnormalities and symptoms are reversible upon removal of the breast implants.[182]

A report by Peters et al., to my mind, settles the question of the potential for silicone implants to adversely affect women. They studied 100 consecutive women seen between 1992 and 1995 who requested

removal of their silicone implants. Rheumatologists had referred 18 of the patients with diagnoses of autoimmune or rheumatic diseases. Of these 18 patients, 6 had autoimmune diseases: 2 patients had systemic lupus, 2 had rheumatoid arthritis, 1 had multiple sclerosis, and 1 had Raynaud's disease. Twelve patients had rheumatic diseases: 2 had inflammatory arthritis and 10 had fibromyalgia. (These authors incorrectly classified fibromyalgia as rheumatic disease.) All 18 patients had developed symptoms of the diseases after receiving implants.[171]

Of the 186 implants Peters et al. removed, 106 (57%) had ruptured or were leaking. However, only 3.2% of the implants were exuding silicone outside the capsules that encased the implants. The capsules of 25% of the implants were calcified and had visible calcium plaques on their inner surfaces. Bacteria were colonizing 42% of the implants. The prevalence of significant contractures of the capsules around implants was 61%. Significant contractures were related to implant location, duration of implantation, and calcification of the capsule.[171]

Peters et al. evaluated questionnaires completed by 75 of the 100 women. The researchers sent a questionnaire to a patient an average of 2.7 years (a range of 1-to-5 years) after removing her implants. The mean duration of implantation was 12 years, with a range of 1-to-27 years. According to responses to the questionnaires, 36 patients had undergone at least one "closed capsulotomy" (disruption of the scar formed around an implant without an incision through the skin), and 54% had undergone at least one "open capsulotomy" (disruption of a scar formed around an implant by surgical entry of the breast). The women gave the reasons they had requested removal of the implants: 76% suspected silicone-related health problems, 59% suspected implant rupture, 36% had breast firmness, 36% had breast pain, and 23% had musculoskeletal pain. Lost nipple sensitivity was a complaint of 75%, and 36% complained of complete loss of nipple sensation. Nipple sensitivity improved in 38% of patients after explantation. Of the 75 women who responded to the questionnaire, 45% believed that their implants had caused permanent health problems. After removal of the implants, 3 women reported breast sensitivity decreased, and 3 reported breast pain. Of women who did not have the silicone implants replaced by saline implants, 15% believed the appearance of their breasts was improved, 36% were "pleased," 33% were disappointed, and 13% felt "mutilated." Fifty-six percent believed that the surgeons who did the implantations had failed to give them adequate informed consent, especially concerning potential implant rupture and a possible relationship to disease.[171]

Vasey et al. studied the clinical findings in 50 consecutive symptomatic women with silicone breast implants and rheumatic diseases. The most common findings were chronic fatigue, muscle pain, joint pain, joint swelling, and lymphadenopathy. Of the 50 women, 17 did not have the implants removed. A mean of 14 months later, their symptoms had not changed. The remainder of the women, 33, had their implants removed. The implants of 12 of the 33 women (36%) had ruptured. During a mean follow-up of 22 months, 24 of the women reported that they had improved clinically, 8 reported no change, and 1 reported being worse off clinically. Vasey et al. wrote, "We believe this series supports a relationship between silicone breast implants and rheumatic disease signs and symptoms." Based on their findings, the researchers advised physicians to inform women about the possible benefits of having their implants removed.[183]

Thomas et al. wrote that in the recent medical literature and popular media, writers had reported that silicone gel-filled breast implants induced clinical problems. The problems included capsular formation, granulomatous disease, arthritis, arthralgia, fibromyalgia, autoimmune collagen vascular disease, human adjuvant disease, siliconosis, silicone-related disease, and SIAS. They conducted a study of 25 patients referred to them to have their silicone implants removed. The patients' symptoms and signs included breast pain, joint pain, fibromyalgia, dry eyes, dry mouth, abnormal sensitivity to sensory stimuli such as touch, and unilateral decreased visual acuity (amblyopia). They used clinical examination and mammography to reveal implant rupture. Most of the patients had their silicone implants replaced with saline-filled implants. The investigators wrote, "Histopathologic analyses of all tissue samples revealed chronic inflammation." Patients reported that their symptoms improved over months. Thomas et al. wrote that based on their 25 patients and a review of the relevant literature, they needed to express five points: (1) a small percentage of patients who have implants removed will have chronic sickness, and predicting which patients will be ill is problematic; (2) that silicone gel induces illness is not proven but is implied; (3) patients with silicone implants should consider having them removed, with full knowledge of possible illness associated with the surgical procedure; (4) women considering undergoing implantation should consider opting for saline-filled implants; and (5) patients and their physicians should discuss the potential risks and benefits before implan-

tation.[184]

Symptoms of patients with SIAS

Several researchers have reported that the prevalence of SIAS symptoms is high among silicone breast implant patients.[174][177][183][188][189][190] Symptoms that are common among silicone breast implant patients are remarkably similar to those of fibromyalgia/chronic fatigue syndrome.

Freunlich et al. reported the most prominent complaints of 50 consecutive women with silicone breast implants: 89% had fatigue, 75% had generalized stiffness, 71% had poor sleep, 78% arthralgias, and 50% had dry eyes and mouths. Other complaints were hair loss, adenopathy, night sweats, and frequent sore throats.[177] Vasey et al. reported that the most common clinical findings among women with silicone breast implants are chronic fatigue, muscle pain, joint pain, joint swelling, and lymphadenopathy.[183] A year later, Vasey wrote that several findings are consistent in the clinical observation of patients with silicone implants: chronic fatigue, muscle pain, joint pain, lymphadenopathy, peripheral neuritis and bladder dysfunction syndrome.[178] (See subsection below titled "Fibromyalgia-Like Symptoms Among SIAS Patients.") Wolfe described the major symptoms of SIAS (joint and muscle pain, fatigue, paresthesia, cognitive dysfunction, eye and mouth dryness, and hair loss) as features of fibromyalgia.[187]

Immune Abnormalities in SIAS

The evidence is clear that silicone is immunogenic in the human body.[164][182] Freundlich et al. studied implant patients who had symptoms resembling those of fibromyalgia/chronic fatigue syndrome. Among the symptoms were dry eyes and mouth. Biopsies of salivary glands from some patients revealed mononuclear cell infiltrates consistent with Sjögren's syndrome. However, the infiltrating cells were not typical of those found in Sjögren's patients. Of the women included in the study, 38% tested positive for antinuclear antibodies. The researchers suggested that the immune system findings and musculoskeletal symptoms suggest a unique syndrome.[177]

Lewy and Ezrailson wrote that the most commonly cited abnormal test result in women with silicone breast implants is antinuclear antibodies. They compared the rate of positive antinuclear antibody test results in 3380 breast implant recipients with normal controls. Compared to the controls, implant patients had a 6-fold increase in positive test results. The increased risk was not related to age, but it was related at least partly to the length of time the patient had implants.[175]

Bridges et al. assessed the prevalence of antinuclear antibodies in women with silicone implants and controls. Antibody tests were positive in 30% of patients with silicone implants and rheumatic symptoms, 28% of women with silicone implants but no rheumatic symptoms, 25% of women with fibromyalgia, and 8% of age-matched normal women. The researchers concluded that comparatively, a larger percentage of women with silicone implants have autoantibodies. This result indicates immune activation in women with silicone implants.[181]

Zazgornik et al. conducted a retrospective study in which they compared 36 women with silicone implants with sex- and age-matched controls. Among controls, 3 women (8%) had a raised antinuclear antibody titer, and 1 (3%) had antithyroid (microsomal) antibodies. Among implant patients, 12 (33%) had raised antinuclear antibody titers. The difference between the mean titers of control subjects and patients was statistically significant. Of the 12 patients with raised titers, 1 had anti-smooth muscle antibodies, 2 had anti-neutrophilic cytoplasm antibodies, 1 was positive for rheumatoid factor, and 2 had antithyroid (microsomal) antibodies. Among the patients, then, a total of 14 women (39%) had detectable autoantibodies. Zazgornik et al. wrote that most of the detected autoantibodies were not specific to any organ, and most of the raised antinuclear antibodies were of the heterogenous type and not related to distinct diseases. Only 1 patient had musculoskeletal symptoms.[192]

Naim et al. found that silicone gel from commercial breast implants elicited auto-antibodies against rat thyroglobulin and bovine collagen II. They wrote that despite the antibodies, they found no tissue evidence of thyroiditis or arthritis.[164] Kaiser and colleagues reported the case of a 42-year-old woman who developed arthritis 11 years after receiving silicone implants. She had antinuclear antibodies and cytoplasmic thyroid antibodies. Her erythrocyte sedimentation rate was constantly increased. She had signs of silicone mastitis and a CT scan showed infiltration of the right breast implant.[176]

Vayssairat et al. wrote that few researchers have reported Hashimoto's thyroiditis as a result of silicone breast implants. They described 2 patients who developed Hashimoto's after receiving bilateral silicone breast implants for cosmetic purposes. One 45-year-old patient underwent implantation in 1976. In 1991, she developed Hashimoto's that evolved into thyroid hormone deficiency. Although she was using T_4, she

complained of fatigue, joint pain, morning stiffness, and sicca syndrome for which she used artificial tears. In 1995, she had a raised titer of antinuclear antibodies and a high level of antithyroid microsomal antibodies. Her gamma globulin level was elevated by 22.6%. Her thyroid gland was diffusely enlarged. Because her implants were painful, she had them removed in 1996. Microscopic examination revealed a fibrous capsule with extremely dense connective tissue and fibrosis. The second patient was 55 years old. She received silicone breast implants in 1984. In 1995, she developed Hashimoto's. Her thyroid gland was painful and tender to palpation. She had mild hyperthyroidism and positive antithyroglobulin antibodies. She underwent corticosteroid treatment for 5 months. In 1996, she had positive antinuclear antibodies. Because her implants were painful, she had them removed. Vayssairat et al. wrote that Hashimoto's thyroiditis is only rarely associated with silicone breast implants, and they conceded that it is possible that there may have been no relation between the thyroiditis and the implants.[167]

No Well-Defined Rheumatologic Diseases Associated with SIAS

Substantial evidence shows that many women have adverse effects from silicone implants or something associated with them. Despite this, studies have not shown that a significant percentage of women with the implants meet the criteria for generally recognized and diagnosable diseases such as rheumatoid arthritis, systemic lupus erythematosus, and scleroderma.

Epidemiologic studies of the potential adverse effects of silicone breast implants have concentrated mainly on cancer and connective tissue disorders.[179] After reviewing 88 published studies, Noone wrote in 1997 that the conclusions of comprehensive epidemiologic studies were that there is no connection between breast implants and the known connective tissue diseases.[169] Blackburn et al. studied silicone breast implant patients who complained of musculoskeletal symptoms such as muscle pain. They tested for substances related to systemic inflammatory rheumatic disorders. These included interleukin-6, interleukin-8, tumor necrosis factor-alpha, soluble intercellular adhesion molecule-1, and soluble interleukin-2 receptor. They reported that the patients' levels of the substances did not differ from those of normal subjects. They also reported that the patients' levels were significantly lower than levels of patients with chronic inflammatory disorders such as rheumatoid arthritis and systemic lupus erythematosus. They concluded, "Our clinical and laboratory evaluation of symptomatic breast implant patients argues against an association of silicone breast implants with a distinctive rheumatic disease or a systemic inflammatory disorder."[163] In Sweden, Nyren et al. conducted a nationwide retrospective study of the risk of connective tissue diseases and related disorders in breast implant patients. They concluded that their data did not show an association between implants and connective tissue diseases.[170] Gabriel et al. studied all women in Olmsted County, Minnesota, who had received breast implants between 1964 and 1991. Each breast implant subject was matched with a control subject who did not have implants. The researchers followed 749 breast implant subjects for 7.8 years and their matched non-implant subjects for 8.3 years. During these times, 5 implant subjects and 10 non-implant subjects received diagnoses of a specific connective tissue disease. Symptoms of arthritis developed in 25 implant subjects and 39 non-implant subjects. The researchers reported that the only symptom that was more common in implant subjects was morning stiffness. They concluded that they found no association between breast implants and connective tissue diseases.[193]

Freundlich et al. reported that Japanese women injected with raw silicone developed features of a collagen vascular disease, but they did not meet the criteria for a specific diagnosable disease.[177] However, such studies have raised the possibility that silicone implants cause or contribute to an "atypical" disease, one for which there are no generally accepted diagnostic criteria. Brown et al. wrote in 1998 that epidemiologic studies had ruled out a large increase in the risk of connective tissue disease overall in women with breast implants. They qualified, however, that studies were too small and methodologically weak to rule out an increase in rare connective tissue diseases or atypical syndromes.[165] Lewy et al. reported that silicone breast implants have been associated with abnormal laboratory test results that suggest an atypical autoimmune disease.[175] Bridges et al. studied 156 women with silicone breast implants whom clinicians referred for complaints of rheumatic symptoms. They compared their serologic test results with those of women with silicone implants but no complaints of rheumatic symptoms. The researchers reported that because most women with implants and rheumatic complaints had nonspecific symptoms and normal serologic test results, it did not appear that they had serious connective tissue diseases. But a subset of women had serologic test results and clinical signs that were unusual for referred patients. They concluded, "These observations suggest, but cannot establish, that some women with

silicone breast implants may develop atypical immunologic reactions."[174]

Although large epidemiologic studies have not found a statistically significant relation between silicone breast implants and diagnosable diseases, isolated reports of diagnosable diseases have been published. Sahn et al., for example, wrote of a 46-year-old woman who developed localized scleroderma after her silicone gel-filled breast prostheses were surgically manipulated. Firm, shiny plaques appeared first on her legs and then on her thighs. Scleroderma was confirmed through histopathologic examination of a deep-skin biopsy specimen. She had her silicone implants removed and replaced with saline-filled implants. Gradually, the scleroderma resolved. Examination of the removed implant capsules revealed silicone leakage.[173] Such reports make it likely that diagnosable diseases do develop in a minority of susceptible silicone breast implant patients.

As Teuber et al. wrote, "Development of disease due to implants would depend on the interaction of genetic host factors so that only a few patients would potentially be at risk. Based on the example of other chemically mediated disorders, such as scleroderma in association with silica exposure, latency periods of more than 30 years before disease develops may be possible."[180] If this long a latency period is required, it may be some time yet until we know the full impact of the adverse effects of silicone implants. It was only in the 1980s that silicone breast implantation markedly increased.

Fibromyalgia-Like Symptoms Among SIAS Patients

Nyren et al. conducted a nationwide retrospective study in Sweden of the risk of connective tissue diseases and related disorders in breast implant patients. They included 7442 women with silicone breast implants. They reported finding no significant increase in the risk for patients developing polymyalgia rheumatica, several related disorders, or fibromyalgia.[170] The conclusions of several other studies, however, conflict with that of Nyren et al.

Peters et al. wrote that of 100 consecutive women requesting removal of their silicone breast implants, 10 of the patients had fibromyalgia that had developed after they had received implants.[172] Blackburn et al. wrote of anecdotal reports of musculoskeletal symptoms related to patients' silicone breast implants. They studied 70 women with implants who gave musculoskeletal complaints. Many had muscle pain. Blackburn et al. wrote that clinical examination showed that most of the patients had fibromyalgia, osteoarthritis, or soft-tissue rheumatism. One patient had rheumatoid arthritis that she had before getting implants and one had Sjögren's. They did not find laboratory evidence of inflammatory disorders in the women and concluded that their symptoms were related to "well-delineated noninflammatory musculoskeletal syndrome."[163] Bennett wrote that an increased prevalence of anti-polymer antibodies was found in symptomatic silicone breast implant recipients who often have fibromyalgia.[171]

Cuellar et al. studied 300 women with silicone implants whom clinicians had referred to an arthritis clinic for various musculoskeletal complaints. The women ranged in age from 25-to-69, and their mean age was 44.4. Symptoms developed on the average 6.8 years after the women received their implants. The range of onset time was from 6 months to 19 years. Cuellar et al. wrote that the clinical features of 250 of the women (83.3%) strongly suggested an underlying connective tissue disease. Of the 300, 33 (11%) had distinctive connective tissue diseases, 32 (10.6%) had undifferentiated connective tissue disease or human adjuvant disease, and 162 (54%) met the criteria for fibromyalgia and/or chronic fatigue syndrome. Patients also had other symptoms: recurrent unexplained low grade fever, hair loss, skin rash, sicca symptoms, Raynaud's phenomenon, carpal tunnel syndrome, memory loss, headaches, chest pain, and shortness of breath. Of the women who had their implants removed, 70% reported that their symptoms improved. The researchers concluded, "A significant proportion of [silicone breast implant] patients referred for rheumatic evaluation have clinical manifestations highly suggestive of an underlying connective tissue disease."[194]

Two Fibromyalgia Studies Related to SIAS. Wolfe conducted a study to learn if the various symptoms and the frequency of symptoms of fibromyalgia patients are similar to those of patients with SIAS. His aim was to decide whether the silicone syndrome is a new disease or may actually be fibromyalgia. Based on responses to a survey mailed to 901 fibromyalgia patients, he reported that the symptoms typical of SIAS were as frequent or more frequent than in fibromyalgia. Among fibromyalgia patients, 37% had joint pains, muscle pain, sicca complex, atypical rash, and peripheral neuropathy symptoms. Of the patients who responded, 55.2% had 4 of the 5 features reported of typical silicone syndrome. Wolfe wrote in conclusion, "These data do not suggest that SIAS is an unrecognized new disease, but suggest the opposite, that such symptoms are well-known and previously recognized, and are common among those with muscu-

loskeletal complaints and those seen in rheumatology clinics."[187]

In the above study, Wolfe found that the symptoms reported to be typical of SIAS are common among fibromyalgia patients. He concluded from this finding that the symptoms of implant patients do not signify a previously unrecognized disease related to the implants.[187] I do not believe this conclusion is justified.

His conclusion implies that because patients with established rheumatologic disorders have symptoms typical of implant patients, the implants could not be generating a new set of patients who share the same symptoms. The fact that the symptoms are similar does not rule out a new mechanism generating the symptoms. Wolfe's conclusion presupposes that a particular set of symptoms (such as those of SIAS) can be the exclusive product of one and only one underlying mechanism. However, different causative agents can produce symptoms that are similar to or the same as those produced by another causative agent. For example, multiple B complex vitamin deficiencies can produce symptoms in patients that overlap with the symptoms of some patients who are hypothyroid, some who use large daily doses of β-blockers, some who have cellular resistance to thyroid hormone, and some with severe physical deconditioning. The symptoms of these different groups of patients may overlap extensively—so much in fact that even a skilled diagnostician has trouble distinguishing the underlying cause based on the symptoms. It is possible, then, that silicone from breast implants has produced a new set of patients (those with SIAS) who have symptoms overlapping or duplicating symptoms of older, more generally accepted diseases. Thus, some rheumatology patients without silicone implants have symptoms typical of patients with SIAS, but this does not exclude the possibility that silicone is instrumental in producing the symptoms of SIAS patients.

Wolfe and Anderson conducted another study related to SIAS and fibromyalgia. Their purpose was to test the hypothesis that silicone implants are a cause of fibromyalgia. They compared 508 fibromyalgia patients with 1228 control subjects, assessing a possible relationship between silicone implants and fibromyalgia. Wolfe and Anderson acquired information on the type of implant and the relation of the time of implantation to the onset of fibromyalgia. After analyzing their data, they reported finding no statistically significant relationship between silicone implants and subsequently developed fibromyalgia. They noted that one-third of the fibromyalgia patients underwent breast implantation after developing fibromyalgia. They also wrote, "When all implants regardless of temporal relationship were considered, the overall relationship between any implant and the diagnosis of FM was significant," and "implants appear to be more common in patients with than in those without fibromyalgia."[186]

Wolfe and Anderson looked at the temporal relationship between patients undergoing implantation and the onset of their fibromyalgia. One-third of the patients with implants had fibromyalgia before receiving implants.[186] This shows with certainty that the implants were not the single cause of the fibromyalgia of this one-third. This result, however, does not rule out the possibility that implants or something associated with them contributed to some patients' fibromyalgia. We do not know whether the patients' fibromyalgia worsened after they received the implants. (This is a relevant question in view of the reported incidence of ruptures or leaks of silicone implants. In one study, of 186 implants removed from symptomatic patients, 106 (57%) had ruptured or were leaking.[171] In another study, the implants of 12 of 33 patients (36%) had ruptured.[183]) If the patients' fibromyalgia did worsen, this would suggest that the implants or something associated with them contributed to the fibromyalgia.

Based on my intense questioning of fibromyalgia patients over the years, I believe that many have mild, intermittent symptoms of hypometabolism (fibromyalgia symptoms) for many years before developing full-blown fibormyalgia. The mild, intermittent symptoms suggest to me that these patients have marginally sufficient tissue metabolism, and that on occasion, their metabolism slows more, causing symptoms of hypometabolism for a while. Eventually, these individuals have physical, emotional, biochemical, or microbial traumas and soon after develop chronic, severe fibromyalgia. Trauma causes the adrenal gland to secrete increased amounts of cortisol, and the cortisol inhibits the thyroid system at two critical points. Inhibition of the thyroid system slows their metabolism enough so that they develop constant, severe symptoms of hypometabolism for which they receive a diagnosis of fibromyalgia. The inhibition of the thyroid system by cortisol is a transient phenomenon, but while patients are physically inactive due to their symptoms, they are likely to lose muscle mass. The lost muscle mass causes metabolism to remain slow—slow enough in many patients to sustain the fibromyalgia symptoms. (See Chapter 3.5, section titled "A Putative Etiological and Exacerbating Role for Increased Cortisol Levels.") It is plausible that silicone breast implants or something associated with them serves a role similar to that of

elevated cortisol during stress, functioning as a precipitating factor that induces symptoms of fibromyalgia in patients predisposed by marginally sufficient tissue metabolism. It is possible, then, that for some patients, silicone breast implants or something associated with them contributes to the onset of chronic fibromyalgia after these women receive implants. It is also possible that for other women, the implants or something associated with them exacerbates fibromyalgia that existed before the patients received the implants.

Speculations that Psychosocial Factors Underlie Fibromyalgia-Like Symptoms in SIAS. Wolfe and Anderson reported that they found an overall significant relationship between silicone breast implants and fibromyalgia. Possibly to account for the overall significant relationship, they wrote, "A common, predisposing set of psychosocial characteristics may be shared between those who have fibromyalgia and those who undergo silicone breast implants."[186] Peters et al. reported the reasons 100 women gave for their opting for breast implantations: 75% for augmentation, 11% for lifting, 12% for reconstruction, and 2% for congenital aplasia.[171] Although most implantations were for cosmetic purposes, the suggestion of some predisposing set of psychosocial characteristics among these women is mere speculation with no basis in credible scientific evidence. Unfortunately, speculations that health problems have psychosocial causes are a common unscientific cognitive refuge for medical researchers who have failed to find biological causes of the problems. This refuge is a *non sequitur*. It simply does not follow logically that because no one has established the biological basis of a health problem that the cause must therefore be a psychosocial one. (See Chapter 1.2, section titled "Logical Analysis of the Putative Somatoform Disorders and Their Hypothesized Underlying Psychogenic Mechanisms.")

While authors such as Wolfe and Anderson waft across the possibility of a psychosocial cause, others embroider elaborate psychosocial explanations for conditions such as SIAS. Barsky and Borus are an example. They included "the side effects of silicone breast implants" among "functional somatic syndromes." (The term "functional" means not of organic origin. Some writers use the term as a synonym for "neurosis." They believe the patient uses functional behavior to cope with underlying anxiety. The notion of functional syndromes is highly speculative and subject to great abuse by clinicians. Because of its potential for abuse and its highly dubious value, clinicians should abandon the notion. See Chapter 1.2.) They also included Gulf War syndrome, chronic whiplash, chronic fatigue syndrome, irritable bowel syndrome, and fibromyalgia. What these conditions have in common, they wrote, is that they are "characterized more by symptoms, suffering, and disability than by consistently demonstrable tissue abnormality." The writers conceded that biological causes may eventually be found for some patients' symptoms. Nevertheless, they wrote, "the suffering of these patients is exacerbated by a self-perpetuating, self-validating cycle in which common, endemic, somatic symptoms are incorrectly attributed to serious abnormality, reinforcing the patient's belief that he or she has a serious disease." They speculate that four psychosocial factors "propel this cycle of symptom amplification: (1) the belief that one has a serious disease; (2) the expectation that one's condition is likely to worsen; (3) the 'sick role,' including the effects of litigation and compensation; and (4) the alarming portrayal of the condition as catastrophic and disabling." They also listed several influences that worsen and perpetuate the "somatic distress" of the patient with a functional somatic syndrome: "sensationalized media coverage, profound suspicion of medical expertise and physicians, the mobilization of parties with a vested self-interest in the status of functional somatic syndromes, litigation, and a clinical approach that overemphasizes the biomedical and ignores psychosocial factors." According to them, these influences intensify the patient's fears and pessimistic expectations. They also prolong his or her disability and reinforce the patient's sick role.[185]

Despite diligent searching, I have found no credible scientific evidence to justify such an explanation. Conjecturing is an essential step in scientific inquiry. However, conjecturing psychosocial mechanisms to explain syndromes with no established biological basis has become a threadbare mental exercise during the 20th century. As long as humans suffer from symptoms that have no established biological basis, some medical writers will relentlessly embroider fanciful psychosocial explanations to account for the symptoms. But patients and clinicians should bear in mind the failure of such writers to offer credible scientific evidence to support their explanations.

Conclusions About SIAS

Results of epidemiological studies suggest that silicone breast implants do not significantly increase the incidence of generally accepted diagnosable rheumatologic diseases. Despite this, it is clear that many women with silicone implants develop immunological abnormalities and symptoms and signs typical of fibromyalgia. The silicone breast implant patients with

these abnormalities, signs, and symptoms are said to have SIAS. A review of the available evidence compels me to conclude that many women are likely to incur substantial adverse health effects from silicone breast implants or something associated with them.

Most women's SIAS symptoms improve after removal of the implants. In these women, it is highly likely that silicone implants or something associated with them caused their SIAS symptoms. More than half the women with SIAS who have their silicone implants removed experience improvement or relief of their musculoskeletal symptoms. Brautbar et al. wrote that for 50%-to-70% of patients, removal of breast implants reverses the symptoms and immunological abnormalities.[182] Improvement usually occurs months after removal.[184] Vasey et. al. reported that for 33 patients, improvement occurred an average of 22 months after the patients had their implants removed. Of the 33 women, 24 women were clinically improved, 8 reported no improvement, and 1 reported that she was worse.[183] The improvement of many women after removal of their implants suggests that the implants played a substantial role in generating and sustaining the women's symptoms. That some women do not completely improve after removal of the implants, and that some women do not improve at all after removal, suggests three possibilities: (1) silicone that migrated from the implants into other body tissues contributes to continuation of the symptoms, (2) the implants or something associated with them set into motion immune or other body processes that sustain the symptoms even after implant removal, and (3) the implants contributed to symptoms that are mainly a product of a more influential underlying mechanism such as inadequate thyroid hormone regulation of cell function.

My opinion is that women with silicone implants and their clinicians should be wary of assurances by some researchers that the implants are harmless. That epidemiological studies have not found a significant increase in the incidence of well-recognized diseases in breast implant patients is not proof that the implants are not associated with development of disease in susceptible individuals. Patients and their clinicians should also consider as completely lacking in scientific credibility suggestions of some medical writers that the fibromyalgia-like symptoms of many recipients of silicone breast implants are a product of psychosocial mechanisms. While the scientific evidence that silicone implants cause adverse health effects is controversial, scientific evidence that psychosocial mechanisms generate the symptoms of SIAS or fibromyalgia is completely lacking.

VIRAL INFECTION

Some researchers have proposed that the cause of fibormyalgia is a viral infection. Researchers have studied the prevalence of positive tests for Epstein-Barr virus, parvovirus, and hepatitis C virus in fibromyalgia patients.

Viral Infection: Proposed Cause of Fibromyalgia

As with other chronic conditions without a generally accepted etiology, some researchers have proposed that fibromyalgia is caused by a virus. Lund-Olesen and Lund-Olesen made this proposal.[26] On the questionable assumption that fibromyalgia is primarily a muscle disease, they cited evidence that viruses can injure muscle cells. Specifically, they cited epidemic pleuradynia (Bornholm disease),[27] also termed epidemic myalgia.[28] Lund-Olesen and Lund-Olesen hypothesized that a putative fibromyalgia-causing virus damages the calcium channels in striatal muscle cells. According to them, the damage results in abnormally large amounts of calcium ions in the sarcoplasmic fluids. They proposed that the excess calcium heightens muscle tone ". . . so much so," they continued, "that the individual cells, as well as the muscle as a whole, develop a state comparable to that following static muscular work." They proposed that if this viral-induced mechanism does underlie fibromyalgia, then treatment with a calcium channel blocker would be therapeutically effective. They reported striking improvement in one patient with the use of 7.5 mg daily of the calcium antagonist isradipine.[26] My observation of patients using calcium channel blockers who simultaneously had severe fibromyalgia argues against this therapeutic proposal.

Lund-Olesen and Lund-Olesen listed fibromyalgia/chronic fatigue syndrome symptoms that could be associated with post-viral syndrome. These include extreme lethargy, generalized muscle pain and stiffness, soreness of muscles lasting more than 3 months, recurrent fever, pharyngitis, conjunctivitis, irritable bowel syndrome, sleep disturbances, and poor concentration and memory. Then the authors imply that these may result from a viral infection.[26,p.55] They wrote that virological studies[27][31][32] suggest that the patients have abnormal serological profiles, suggesting that viral infections play a pathogenic role. For example, 22% of 76 patients with chronic fatigue syndrome in one study had positive cultures for enteroviruses.[31] However, the researchers conceded, in concert with others,[29]

that a relationship of the syndrome to viral involvement is not certain.

The symptoms Lund-Olesen and Lund-Olesen list above may indeed accompany some acute viral infections. However, patients who have these symptoms during viral infections typically recover after a short time. I am aware of no evidence that chronic viral infections perpetuate the symptoms. It appears more likely that continuation of some patients' symptoms after the acute phase of the infection is a product of chronic hypometabolism of various tissues. The chronic hypometabolism may occur in individuals who, before the infections, had borderline sufficient metabolism. It is possible that elevated cortisol levels and physical inactivity during the infection and recovery period lowers the patients' metabolism further—below the threshold for generation of symptoms characteristic of hypothyroidism. If the patients do not accelerate their metabolism, perhaps by increasing their lean muscle mass through exercise, the symptoms may continue and they may receive a diagnosis of fibromyalgia.

Antibodies to Epstein-Barr Virus and Parvovirus

Fibromyalgia patients' titers of antibodies to Epstein-Barr virus were no different from apparently healthy control subjects.[113,p.284] Also, fibromyalgia patients' mean titer of antibodies against parvovirus B19 was no different from that of normal controls.[132] See section above titled "Autoimmune Disease and Fibromyalgia: Antibodies to Epstein-Barr Virus and Parvovirus."

Prevalence of Hepatitis C Virus Infection in Fibromyalgia

Hepatitis C is a single-stranded flavivirus-like RNA virus. The virus is involved in about 80% of post-transfusion hepatitis and a high percentage of spontaneous hepatitis. A high percentage of patients with hepatitis C virus infections are intravenous drug users. Accordingly, the most common route of infection appears to be parenteral.

Onset of hepatitis C virus infection is insidious. Serum antibodies to the virus may take several months to appear after the acute infection. Afterward, antibody titers slowly decline unless the infection becomes chronic. The liver enzyme alanine aminotransferase (ALT, formerly known as SGPT) remains elevated from 1-to-6 months or more. About 50% of patients develop chronic hepatitis. Clinically, the infection is usually mild. Patients are seldom hospitalized and some 75% of patients do not have jaundice. Most patients do not have symptoms.[48,p.900][62,pp.454-458]

Rivera et al. conducted tests to learn the prevalence of hepatitis C virus infection in 112 fibromyalgia patients compared to rheumatoid arthritis patients. Hepatitis C virus antibodies were present in 17 fibromyalgia patients (15.2%) and 6 rheumatoid arthritis patients (5.3%). The difference was statistically significant. The liver enzyme ALT was normal in the serum of 8 fibromyalgia patients (47%), although 4 of them (50%) had detectable hepatitis C virus-RNA.[35]

Rivera et al. also examined 58 patients who had chronic hepatitis C virus infection to learn what percentage of them met the criteria for fibromyalgia. All the patients had detectable serum hepatitis C virus-RNA and antibodies. Thirty-one (53%) had diffuse musculoskeletal pain, but only 6 (10%) meet the diagnostic criteria for fibromyalgia. In the control group of 58 subjects, 13 (22%) had diffuse musculoskeletal pain and only 1 (1.7%) fulfilled the criteria for fibromyalgia Patients with chronic hepatitis C virus infection who did not meet the criteria for fibromyalgia had a mean serum ALT level of 122±76.3. By comparison, infected patients who did meet the fibromyalgia criteria had a mean serum ALT of 51.7±38.4. Autoimmune markers did not differ between patients who had and who did not have fibromyalgia. From their study results, Rivera et al. concluded that a relation between active hepatitis C virus and fibromyalgia existed in some of their patients. However, they wrote that the infected patients did not have liver damage or autoimmune markers.[35] They advised clinicians to consider hepatitis C virus infection in fibromyalgia patients even though their ALT levels are not elevated.[35] Buskila reported that of 90 patients with hepatitis C virus infection, 14 (16%) met the criteria for fibromyalgia.[133][134]

Neopterin and Biopterin: Other Indicators of Viral Infection

Bonaccorso et al. measured the neopterin and biopterin excretion in 24-hour urine samples of fibromyalgia patients. They compared the results with samples from normal volunteers and patients with major depression. (See immediately below for descriptions of neopterin and biopterin.) The mean concentrations of neopterin and biopterin in urine samples of fibromyalgia patients were no different from those of normal volunteers. Patients with major depression had higher neopterin concentrations. Based on the results, the investigators wrote that activation of cell-mediated immunity may not be a feature of fibromyalgia. They

cautioned, however, that researchers should test for other immune markers before reaching a final conclusion about immune involvement.[40]

Note on Neopterin and Biopterin: Human monocytes/macrophages produce neopterin during viral infections in response to interferon-γ. During viral infections, levels of neopterin increase in serum and urine. Clinicians can use elevated levels to differentiate between viral and bacterial infections. Neopterin enhances cytotoxicity and elimination of single cells by fragmenting them into membrane-bound particles that phagocytes can ingest and digest (a process called apoptosis).[89]

Biopterin serves immune system-related functions as (6R)-5,6,7,8-tetrahydrobiopterin or H4-biopterin. It is an antioxidant in cells and is an important regulator of the function of nitric oxide synthase. Nitric oxide synthase generates nitric oxide, and nitric oxide regulates vascular tone and is involved in immune surveillance.[97] The nitric oxide molecule has several amino acids critical for binding of biopterin. Biopterin exerts an allosteric action (see Glossary) on the nitric oxide molecule, stabilizing the molecule for several biochemical functions such as binding of its substrate L-arginine.[91][95] When biopterin is deficient, however, nitric oxide synthase generates the cytotoxic reactive species superoxide anion and hydrogen peroxide. When biopterin is deficient, secreted nitric oxide reacts with superoxide anion and hydrogen peroxide. The reaction forms peroxynitrite, singlet oxygen, and a hydroxyl radical which are highly toxic. Nitric oxide and the reactive species may be involved in pathological conditions such as inflammation, diabetes mellitus, and ischemia-reperfusion injury. When biopterin levels in cells are sufficient, nitric oxide synthase produces more nitric oxide and less of the reactive species. Thus, sufficient levels of biopterin protect cells against injury from the results of the neopterin-deficient function of nitric oxide synthase. Biopterin also protects against cytotoxity by serving as a scavenger for reactive oxygen species.[96] Biopterin is also linked to immune system function in mood disorders and stress as a cofactor in the synthesis of neurotransmitters and as a modulator of the hypothalamic-pituitary-adrenal axis.[97]

LYME DISEASE: *BORRELIA BURGDORFERI* SPIROCHETE INFECTION

Infection with the spirochete *Borrelia burgdorferi* causes the illness called Lyme disease. It is the most common arthropod-borne infection. Most cases occur in the Northeast, the Midwest, and California.[136] The word "Lyme" is taken from the town of Lyme, Connecticut. This is the location where clusters of cases of the infection were first identified. The bite of a small tick of the genus *Ixodes* transmits the spirochetes to humans.[2,p.284]

In the early phase of the illness, patients have a distinctive skin lesion termed "erythema chronicum migrans." The lesion begins in 50%-to-70% of patients with a reddened area near the bite.[152] It slowly expands with central clearing.[2,p.285] Most patients have flu-like symptoms with fever, chills, headaches, and muscle pain. The symptoms often resemble those of a "summer cold" or viral infection.[152] In the late phase, which may be confused with fibromyalgia, the patient usually has arthritis and joint pain and neurological effects such as painful radiculopathy.[2,p.285][152] Researchers have now expanded the clinical features of Lyme disease to include a flu-like illness without the skin lesion and persistence of antibodies to the spirochete after antibiotic treatment.[136]

Lyme disease involves multiple systems of the body, and the clinical effects overlap those of several other diseases. The clinician often has difficulty distinguishing the late-phase neurologic abnormalities of Lyme disease from fibromyalgia and chronic fatigue syndrome.[139][150] As a result, clinicians often misdiagnose some fibromyalgia and chronic fatigue syndrome patients as having "chronic Lyme disease"[139] (see subsection below titled "Putative Chronic Lyme Disease"). Steere wrote that the misdiagnosis of other conditions such as fibromyalgia as Lyme disease may be giving a false impression that Lyme disease is spreading.[146]

Rahn and Felz wrote that the clinician must learn to distinguish fibromyalgia from late-phase Lyme disease. The importance in this is that fibromyalgia is the condition most commonly misdiagnosed as Lyme disease.[137] According to Steere, diagnostic confusion results from the lack of standardized serologic tests and the varying clinical features of Lyme disease. He stipulated, however, that clinicians can distinguish Lyme disease from "look-alike disorders," such as fibromyalgia and chronic fatigue syndrome.[146] Evans and Schoen wrote that recognition of fibromyalgia occurring after infection with *Borrelia burgdorferi* allows more appropriate treatment in late-phase Lyme disease.[145]

Several authors have written that fibromyalgia/chronic fatigue syndrome may occur following effectively treated Lyme disease, may mimic Lyme disease,

or may be a complication of Lyme disease.[141][142][156] Frey et al. reported detecting DNA of *Borrelia burgdorferi* in the muscle of a fibromyalgia patient.[138]

Dinerman and Steere described patients with fibromyalgia associated with Lyme disease. They reported that of 287 patients with Lyme disease examined over a 3.5-year period, 22 (8%) also had fibromyalgia. Fifteen of these patients (5% of the 287) participated in the study. During 1.7 months after early-phase Lyme disease, 9 of the 15 patients developed widespread pain, tender points, dysesthesia, impaired memory, and debilitating fatigue. The other 6 patients developed these symptoms while they had arthritis due to Lyme disease. During late-phase Lyme disease, all 15 patients had some positive immune test results related to *Borrelia burgdorferi*. Antibiotic therapy relieved the signs of Lyme disease except for one patient whose knee swelling continued. At the end of the study, only one patient was completely free from symptoms. Dinerman and Steere concluded that Lyme disease may trigger fibromyalgia and that the fibromyalgia does not seem to respond to antibiotic treatment.[149] Burdge and O'Hanlon studied 65 patients referred for suspected Lyme disease. The researchers judged that only 2 of the 65 patients had probable Lyme disease. The other 63 patients received other diagnoses. Of the 65 referred patients, 11 (17%) received probable diagnoses of fibromyalgia or chronic fatigue syndrome.[147] It appears, then, that infection with the spirochete *Borrelia burgdorferi* occasionally triggers fibromyalgia, and the fibromyalgia does not improve with antibiotic therapy.[135]

On the other hand, Brier described a patient whose initial diagnosis was cervical facet joint syndrome. After a course of chiropractic manipulative therapy, the patient had a recurrence of cervical pain and developed spinal myofascitis, dermatitis, and migratory arthropathy. Other specialists subsequently diagnosed psoriatic arthritis and fibromyalgia. A follow-up blood test resulted in a diagnosis of Lyme disease.[153] Paparone described an unusual case of Lyme disease superimposed on severe primary hypothyroidism. The hypothyroidism was so severe and prominent that a clinician could easily have missed the diagnosis of Lyme disease.[157]

Several authors have written of the difficulties in differentiating Lyme disease from other diseases.[158][159][160][161] Emphasizing the difficulties in distinguishing Lyme disease from other disease, such as hypothyroidism, Bianconcini et al. wrote, "Lyme disease, involving skin, heart, nervous system and joints, is frequently protean and misdiagnosed, so that it was called 'the new great imitator.'"[162] Clinicians may misinterpret the symptoms of some patients with hypothyroidism or thyroid hormone resistance as those of Lyme disease.

Putative Chronic Lyme Disease

After antibiotic treatment, some patients have a post-Lyme disease syndrome that resembles fibromyalgia. Bujak et al. described a "post-Lyme syndrome" involving persistent joint pain, fatigue, and subjective memory loss. They studied 23 patients with the syndrome and 23 matched patients who appeared to have completely recovered from Lyme disease. Of the 23 patients with the syndrome, 7 (30%) had fibromyalgia, 3 (13%) had chronic fatigue syndrome, and 10 (43%) had mild symptoms of either condition but did not meet the criteria for each. (The diagnostic criteria for fibromyalgia and chronic fatigue syndrome are not likely to identify patients with very mild features of the conditions. Because of this, virtually all the patients in this study considered to have post-Lyme disease syndrome could actually have had fibromyalgia/chronic fatigue syndrome.) According to objective tests, patients with the post-Lyme disease syndrome had significantly lower attention and concentration than recovered patients. Fifty-two percent of patients with the syndrome and 35% of recovered patients had significantly lower verbal memory scores than visual memory scores. The researchers wrote that despite antibiotic therapy, a sequella of Lyme disease may be post-Lyme syndrome, including joint pain, fatigue, and impaired neurocognitive function.[140]

Hsu et al. reviewed the charts of patients referred for a persistent nonspecific musculoskeletal and/or neurological syndrome considered features of "chronic Lyme disease." Of nearly 800 patients, 77 met the criteria for fibromyalgia. Hus et al. wrote that the fibromyalgia accounted for the symptoms clinicians had attributed to ongoing Lyme disease. They also wrote, "Many had received multiple courses of antibiotic therapy for symptoms of fibromyalgia mistakenly attributed to chronic Lyme disease. No patient reported permanent and/or total resolution of fibromyalgia symptoms following antibiotic therapy." The conclusion of these authors is perplexing. They wrote, "Appropriate therapy for fibromyalgia in those who remained compliant, however, was often effective in improving some if not all of the chronic symptoms." They also wrote, "Fibromyalgia is a treatable and potentially curable disorder, and should be considered in the evaluation of patients with 'refractory Lyme disease.'"[143] This conclusion conflicts with the evidence

that short-term, conventional medical treatment for fibromyalgia provides some faint benefit, but long-term, the treatment is no more effective than placebos (See Chapter 5.1). While antibiotic therapy may be ineffective with fibromyalgia patients unless they have ongoing infections sensitive to the antibiotics used, conventional medical treatment for fibromyalgia is no more effective than inappropriate antibiotic therapy. Similarly perplexing, Sigal and Patella wrote that repeated and/or long-term antibiotic therapy prescribed for "chronic Lyme disease" has not cured the symptoms of fibromyalgia, but "Fibromyalgia is a potentially treatable and curable cause of chronic complaints and should be considered in the differential diagnosis of 'refractory Lyme arthritis.'"[148]

Improper Treatment

Huppertz and Karch wrote that without better diagnostic criteria, arthritis of a single joint (monarthritis) not otherwise explained and a positive Lyme serology is sufficient for a diagnosis of Lyme arthritis. They wrote that after the diagnosis is confirmed, clinicians should treat children without delay. Many clinicians share the point of view that patients with a positive serology and one or more symptoms of Lyme disease should with dispatch undergo antibiotic therapy.[154]

Others, however, believe that antibiotic therapy may be unjustified unless the clinician has made a more conservative diagnosis of Lyme disease. Schned and Williams wrote that many patients fear having Lyme disease. A positive test result in patients with vague symptoms may become problematic. They advised clinicians to explain to patients the phenomenon of "background" seropositivity in different locations. They also advised clinicians to explain drawbacks in using unnecessary antibiotic therapy when the patients' presumed chronic Lyme disease is actually fibromyalgia that developed over time after the Lyme disease.[151] Sigal wrote, "Of major consequence to the practitioner and patient is the possibility that persistent symptoms (e.g., fibromyalgia) may be caused by a process which is no longer antibiotic-sensitive. Special care in the management of so-called 'chronic Lyme disease' is crucial lest the clinician prescribes prolonged or unending courses of antibiotics for such noninfectious problems."[152]

Sigal summarized the cases of 100 patients referred to a Lyme disease referral clinic. He wrote that patients with an incorrect diagnosis of Lyme disease often undergo unnecessary prolonged or repeated intravenous antibiotic therapy. Current or preceding

Lyme disease explained the complaints of only 37 of the patients. Many of the patients had joint diseases unrelated to Lyme disease, and 25 of the patients met the criteria for fibromyalgia. Sigal wrote, "Approximately half of the 91 courses of antibiotic therapy given to these 100 patients before referral were probably unwarranted." He concluded, "Persistence of mild to moderate symptoms after adequate therapy and misdiagnosis of fibromyalgia and fatigue may incorrectly suggest persistence of infection, leading to further antibiotic therapy. Attention to patient anxiety and increased awareness of these musculoskeletal problems after therapy should decrease unnecessary therapy of previously treated Lyme disease."[155]

Lightfoot et al. studied the cost-effectiveness of empirical parenteral antibiotic therapy for patients who had chronic muscle pain and fatigue and a positive serologic test result for Lyme disease but who did not have the classic features of the disease. He reported that in endemic Lyme disease regions, the incidence of false-positive test results in the described patients was four times the incidence of true-positive test results. For each true-positive patient treated, the cost of treatment of patients with false-positive results was $86,221. Moreover, the empirical approach to treatment resulted in 29 cases of drug toxicity for each case treated by a more conservative strategy. The author concluded that the risks and costs of empirical parenteral antibiotic treatment exceeded the benefits in treating patients with nonspecific fatigue and muscle pain.[144]

● POSSIBLE MECHANISMS OF IMMUNE ABNORMALITIES RELATED TO INADEQUATE THYROID HORMONE REGULATION OF CELL FUNCTION

As an extension of the views of Barnes described below, I agree with Clauw and Chrousos: The immune abnormalities of fibromyalgia are epiphenomena rather than the cause of the illness.[17] They proposed that the mechanism of fibromyalgia, and of the immune system epiphenomena, is dysfunction of the central nervous system due to interacting genetic and environmental factors. This putative mechanism can plausibly explain some of the immune abnormalities of fibromyalgia. However, their proposed mechanism lacks specificity and fails to cogently account for too many other features of fibromyalgia. Conversely, the hypothesis I

posit in this book, inadequate thyroid hormone regulation of cell function, is more useful. It plausibly and specifically accounts for virtually every feature of fibromyalgia, including the reported immune system abnormalities.

That inadequate thyroid hormone regulation of the immune system results in a high frequency of severe and tenacious infections in some patients was best expounded by Barnes and his coauthor, Lawrence Galton.[75,pp.86-100] Among other medical writers whose views concur with those of Barnes are Greco and Harpold. They recently wrote that hypothyroidism is among the endocrine deficiency conditions that may cause abnormal cell-mediated or antibody-mediated immunity. The immune abnormalities can lead to various viral, bacterial, and fungal infections.[98] So sensible were Barnes' views of this phenomenon that I will summarize them immediately below, after which I will review some relevant studies published subsequent to his views.

BARNES' VIEWS

Barnes and Galton expressed with great clarity Barnes' highly credible views of thyroid hormone deficiency and infection. His views were based on his early experiments with thyroid hormone deficient laboratory animals, his personal health history, and his extensive clinical experience and highly clinical systematic observations.[75,pp.86-100] The results of many recent studies substantiate Barnes' views.

While working on his PhD degree, Barnes studied the adverse effects of thyroidectomy on baby rabbits. He reported that among other signs, they had chronic sniffles, recurrent acute infections, and early death from pneumonia. After medical school, when Barnes recognized his cold intolerance, he also realized that hypothyroidism underlaid his lifelong history of a high susceptibility to infection, which his family members shared. His infections included coryza, sore throats, boils, carbuncles, respiratory infections, and tonsillitis. When he began using exogenous thyroid hormone, he ceased to be troubled with infections. He also found that the use of exogenous thyroid hormone also relieved his immediate family of a strong tendency toward infections. Moreover, he found that infection-prone patients who had clinical indications of too little thyroid hormone stimulation were relieved of the tendency by their use of exogenous thyroid hormone.[75,pp.87-88]

Of this therapeutic outcome, he wrote, "As long as

our resistance is high, we don't provide the conditions under which infectious agents can multiply to the point of producing illness." He acknowledged that many factors can lower resistance, including too little sleep, poor nutrition, excessive stress, and low thyroid function. "If thyroid function is low enough," he wrote, "this in itself can be enough to open the door to repeated bacterial and viral invasions. And mild degrees of hypothyroidism can set the stage so that a brief loss of adequate sleep or a brief period of undue stress may do what it would not otherwise be capable of doing in anyone with normal thyroid function: add just enough to the lowering of resistance to permit infection." He wrote further, "Mild hypothyroidism may also set the stage so that exposure to another person with an infectious disease may lead to infection that would not 'take' in a person with normal thyroid function who is similarly exposed."[75,pp.90-91]

Barnes observed that in laboratory animals (rats, rabbits, and pigs) and human patients of all ages, exogenous thyroid hormone conferred an increase in resistance to infection. In 1953, he published a report of the association of low thyroid function with a high susceptibility to respiratory infections in 150 patients.[76] He wrote that at follow-up, after the patients had been using exogenous thyroid hormone, they felt more vigorous and in better health, and had fewer infections.[75,p.92]

In 1965, he presented a scientific exhibit at a meeting of the American Medical Association in New York. He presented data on the results of the use of exogenous thyroid hormone by a large group of patients. He reported that although Colorado (where he practiced) was one of the geographic regions with the highest incidence of rheumatic fever (caused by group A streptococcal infection), not one child taking thyroid hormone had acquired the infection. Children who had often been absent from school because of upper respiratory infections had improved and had only one or two colds per year. Few children taking thyroid hormone had ear infections. The low incidence of otitis media in children taking the hormone is particularly noteworthy. In 1960, 15 years after the advent of antibiotics, the use of the medications had not reduced the incidence of otitis media in children, and today, otitis media is rampant among pediatric patients despite over-prescribing of antibiotics by pediatricians. Rarely did children taking thyroid hormone develop pneumonia. Both children and adults taking thyroid hormone were more resistant to pneumonias and influenza, and vaccinations against influenza became unnecessary for elderly individuals.[75,pp.95-96]

Barnes also wrote that in susceptible patients with low thyroid function, bladder infections are common, sometimes resulting in kidney failure. He reported that in the last 25 years of his practice, after beginning the use of thyroid hormone, no patient with low thyroid function who had previously been prone to urinary tract infections had experienced repeated infections or had deteriorated kidney function.[75,p.97]

I strongly urge clinicians, researchers, and patients with hypothyroidism and cellular resistance to thyroid hormone to read Barnes' views of the relation of low resistance to infection to low thyroid function.[75]

STUDIES OF THE EFFECTS OF THYROID HORMONE DEFICIENCY ON IMMUNE SYSTEM MEASURES

In this section, I cite studies in which researchers tested the role of thyroid hormone on various functions of the immune system. The studies are only representative of those available. Those I include here, however, are sufficient to show that in susceptible individuals, inadequate thyroid hormone regulation of the immune system can result in abnormalities of the system, a reduced resistance to infection, and adverse effects from toxic agents. The studies also indicate that adequate thyroid hormone regulation of the immune system can enhance the effectiveness of immunity.

Interpreting the results of studies of the immune system of fibromyalgia patients in terms of inadequate thyroid hormone regulation of the system is difficult. In fact, interpreting the findings in terms of any causative model is troublesome. As Moldofsky wrote, "There are difficulties in interpreting these immunologic results [from fibromyalgia studies] because of differences in the clinical populations, diagnostic uncertainties, lack of adequate immunologic controls, and the use of single blood samples with failure to recognize circadian or sleep-related influences on certain immune functions."[111] Many studies of the immune systems of euthyroid, hypothyroid, and hyperthyroid groups share such methodological problems. Because of this, matching findings between fibromyalgia and hypothyroid patients is an exceedingly difficult task. Further complicating the difficulties is the tendency of some fibromyalgia researchers to reach conclusions along the lines of, "The values of this immune factor were elevated in half the fibromyalgia patients, *although the mean value did not significantly differ from that of health control subjects.*" The point to a significance level is to tell us how likely it is that, as in the particular case, the increased or decreased mean value was due to chance variation. If the difference in values between patients and control subjects did not reach significance, it is highly likely that the difference was due to chance variation and not a real difference between the two groups. Such published conclusions complicate the difficulty of deciding what study results to compare with those from hypothyroid studies.

Cellular Immunity

Mayer and colleagues described a case of fulminating meningococcal meningitis and sepsis associated with severe hypothyroidism caused by Hashimoto's autoimmune thyroiditis.[60] Pillay reported the case of a pediatric patient with congenital hypothyroidism and immune deficiency. The child had severe and persistent lymphopenia with diarrhea and recurrent episodes of respiratory symptoms related to bronchiectasis (chronic dilation of the bronchi or bronchioles due to inflammatory disease). The child died from overwhelming infection. Pillay wrote, "It is proposed that the prolonged deficiency of thyroid hormone may be directly related to the impairment of the cellular immune system."[59]

Kinoshita et al. studied the effects of thyroid hormone deficiency and excess on the growth and development of spontaneous pulmonary metastasis of Lewis lung carcinoma (3LL) cells in mice. They noted that as the 3LL tumors growing in mice progressed, the serum levels of T_3 and T_4 significantly decreased. The decreased levels were possibly similar to euthyroid sick syndrome in humans (see Chapter 2.5, subsection titled "Euthyroid Sick Syndrome"). The researchers reduced the circulating thyroid hormone levels of the mice below normal by administering methimazole. Low circulating thyroid hormone levels resulted in a suppression of primary and metastatic growth of tumors and prolonged survival. They increased the circulating levels above normal by injecting T_3 and/or T_4. Interestingly, injections of T_4 accelerated primary tumor growth and promoted pulmonary metastasis of the 3LL cells. On the other hand, T_3 injections significantly inhibited spontaneous pulmonary metastasis and prolonged survival rates of the mice. After 4 weeks of T_3 and T_4 injections, cytotoxicity of alveolar macrophages against 3LL cells significantly increased. T_3 injections did not affect the natural killer cell activity of spleen cells, but T_4 injections caused much lower natural killer cell activity. The investigators concluded that their data suggested that changes in thyroid function may have important effects on natural host defenses against human primary and metastatic lung cancers.[69] It is possible that decreasing thyroid hormone levels with progression of tumor growth may have caused some immune impairment, and the impairment enabled the tumors to progress unfettered.

Fowles et al. induced thyroid hormone deficiency in adult male mallard ducks. Three measures of immunity were not altered: antibody formation to sheep red blood cells, natural killer cell action against tumor cells, and macrophage phagocytosis of the killed fungus *Saccaromyces cereviseae*. However, after 21 days of thyroid hormone deficiency, cellular cytotoxic activity against tumor cells (RP-9) was significantly decreased. (The cytotoxic activity was lectin-dependent. Lectin is a protein that binds to glycoproteins on cell surfaces and exerts effects similar to those of specific antibodies.) From these results, the researchers concluded that hypothyroidism may impair cell-mediated immunity.[65]

Allergies

Allergy involves the release of chemicals such as histamine from mast cells. Some studies indicate that inadequate thyroid hormone regulation of the adrenergic genes may increase the numbers of mast cells and increase their secretion of histamine. We would expect the affected individual to have an increased susceptibility to allergic reactions and possibly multiple chemical sensitivities.

Mast Cells, Thyroid Hormone, and Allergy. The mast cells of loose connective tissues are important components of the immune system. The cells are derived from bone marrow precursors and amass along small blood vessels. They have many small plasma membrane folds and contain an abundance of basophilic granules in their cytoplasm. They also have an extensive Golgi complex, which suggests a high potential for secreting substances.[23,p.62] They contain membrane-bound granules that are so abundant that they almost hide the nuclei of the cells. The granules contain several bioactive substances. Two particularly important substances are heparin, a strong anticoagulant, and histamine, a substance that induces vasodilation and increased permeability of capillaries and venules.[88,pp.55-56] In reacting to allergens, mast cells release the substance from its granules, and the substances induce the tissue phenomena associated with allergy.[88,pp.55-56]

During inadequate thyroid hormone regulation of the adrenergic genes, the density of β-adrenergic receptors on mast cells decreases, and the density of α-adrenergic receptors increases. This shift in the density of adrenergic receptor types on mast cells, particularly the decrease in β-adrenergic receptors, causes the cells to secrete excess amounts of substances such as histamine released during allergic reactions. As a result, the patient may suffer from increased allergy tendencies. This may be the basis of some patients' multiple chemical sensitivities.

Fibromyalgia patients were found to have a higher number of mast cells in skin biopsies compared to healthy controls and rheumatoid arthritis patients.[45] This finding corresponds to the increased numbers of mast cells in hypothyroid rats.[92] Sabria et al. found that treating rats up to 5 days old with thyroid hormone or TSH decreased the number of mast cells and the levels of histamine in the rats' brains. Treating them with an antithyroid chemical, rendering them hypothyroid, increased both the number of mast cells and histamine levels.[92] Therefore, inadequate thyroid hormone regulation of the adrenergic genes, with a decrease in β-adrenergic receptors and an increase in α-adrenergic receptors, may result in a reduced threshold for mast cell secretion of histamine.

β-Adrenergic Receptors. The mainstay of the treatment for asthma is β-adrenergic agonists. β2-Adrenergic agonists are preferentially used because they have a lower incidence of adverse cardiovascular effects. Epinephrine injections are the treatment of choice for relieving the effects of acute, severe allergic reactions. Relief occurs because the injected epinephrine activates β-adrenergic receptors on mast cells, decreasing the release of histamine and leukotrienes.[14,pp.216-217] Studies have shown that the activation of β-adrenergic receptors inhibits the mast cells' release of substances that mediate inflammation.[93,p.632] Testimony to the potent suppression of allergy-induced secretions of mast cells by β-adrenergic agonists is the emergency room treatment of *status asthmaticus* (life-threatening severe and prolonged asthma). For many years, the main medications used for such emergencies were the nonselective β-adrenergic agonist epinephrine and the xanthine aminophylline. More recently, emergency room physicians and respiratory therapists came to prefer the use of selective β2-adrenergic receptor agonists.[93,p.634] Many asthma patients use the bronchodilator albuterol (a selective β2-adrenergic receptor stimulant) for maintenance, and emergency room personnel use it in heavier dosages for treatment of *status asthmaticus*.[94]

Phillips et al. noted that there is conflicting evidence on which adrenergic receptor subtypes occupy mast cells and how the receptors modulate the release of substances from the cell. They studied the types of receptors present and their effects on mast cells using dog mastocytoma cells. The cells had a high density of β-adrenergic receptors, predominantly of the β2-receptor subtype. The researchers found no evidence of α-adrenergic receptors or cholinergic receptors.[90] This finding by Phillips et al. supports the hypothesis that inadequate thyroid hormone regulation of the adrenergic genes, with a resulting reduction in the density of β2-adrenergic receptors on mast cells, underlies the increased tendency toward allergies in some fibromyalgia patients. This mechanism is particular likely in patients with multiple chemical sensitivity syndrome.

α-Adrenergic Receptors. The results of early studies of α-adrenergic receptors on mast cells and histamine secretion were inconsistent.[90] Later studies, however, indicate that overall, α-adrenergic receptors favor increased secretion of inflammation-promoting substances by mast cells.

Anderson et al. reported that administering the α2-adrenergic receptor agonist clonidine reduced the wheal and flare reactions in guinea pigs sensitized to ovalbumin. Clonidine also reduced the degranulation of mast cells during hypersensitivity reactions. The reduced degranulation reduced the release of inflammation-promoting substances from the mast cells. During the reactions, fewer neutrophils and eosinophils were attracted to the involved tissue sites. Clonidine did not alter the arrival of basophil and mononuclear cells (mainly lymphocytes) at the sites in the late phase of the wheal and flare reaction. Clonidine had only a minimal effect on allergic contact delayed hypersensitivity reactions, and it had no effect on nonspecific inflammation induced by applying croton oil.[15]

Moroni et al. found that murine neoplastic mast cells released histamine when exposed to increasing amounts of phenylephrine (an α1-adrenergic receptor stimulant) and norepinephrine (a high-affinity α2-adrenergic receptor agonist). In contrast, isoprenaline (a β-adrenergic receptor agonist also called isoproterenol) did not increase histamine secretion. The release of histamine evoked by α-adrenergic receptor stimulants was inhibited by administering phentolamine (a α1- and α2-adrenergic receptor blocker). Moroni et al. concluded, "α-Adrenergic receptors may be valuable in evoking histamine release by murine neoplastic mast cells."[46]

When inhaled, prazosin (an α1-adrenergic receptor blocker) reduced the severity of post-exercise bronchoconstriction in asthmatic children. This finding suggests that activation of α1-adrenergic receptors facilitates the release of histamine from mast cells.[16]

IgE in Hypothyroidism. Receptors for IgE antibodies occupy the surfaces of mast cells and are involved in inflammatory responses.[23,p.62] Manzolli et al. gave subcutaneous injections of ovalbumin to thyroidectomized rats. Fourteen days later, they took bronchoalveolar lavages 24-hours after subjecting the rats to an ovalbumin antigen challenge. Compared to control rats, thyroidectomized rats had markedly decreased cell yields in the lavages. The researchers wrote that the impaired response was due to a decrease in the number of circulating leukocytes. The rats did have a substantial reduction in the level of anti-ovalbumin IgE compared with controls. IgG levels did not differ between thyroidectomized and control rats. The impaired response was corrected by 16 days of T_4 treatment. The researchers concluded that hypothyroidism caused the development of the inflammatory component of asthma. A decrease in the production of IgE was the apparent mechanism.[202] An increased level of IgE may be the mechanism of the improved status of asthma patients who use exogenous T_3.

Autoimmune Disease and Thyroid Function

Penhale and Young reported that rats subjected to thyroidectomy (presumably partial) and thyroid gland irradiation became susceptible to developing "experimental" autoimmune thyroiditis. The rats were less likely to develop autoimmune thyroiditis, however, when protected by antibiotics from exposure to pathogenic microbes. When the researchers gave the rats the normal gastrointestinal flora (as fresh, homogenized intestinal contents) from conventionally reared rats, they developed a profound susceptibility to autoimmune thyroiditis. Penhale and Young conjectured that the rats in this study developed autoimmune thyroiditis by antigenic cross-reactivity with thyroid tissue.[3] It is also possible, however, that infection from intestinal microbes contributed to the thyroiditis. This certainly is possible in that some of their rats were protected from developing thyroiditis by administered antibiotics. Perhaps, though, both infection and antigenic cross-reactivity were instrumental, although subnormal cortisol secretion may also have been involved (see subsection below titled "Autoimmunity Possibly Secondary to Low Cortisol Levels in Fibromyalgia"). Whatever the mechanism(s), the study showed that rats became more susceptible to developing autoimmune thyroiditis when made hypothyroid by thyroidectomy or irradiation.

Kotani et al. also conducted a study in which rats became more susceptible to developing autoimmune thyroiditis after they underwent thyroidectomy and sublethal irradiation. They wrote that their results suggested that a genetically determined reduction in the ability of T-lymphocytes to suppress autoimmune responsiveness was the mechanism of the thyroiditis. They also speculated that a gene of the major histocompatibility complex (see subsection above titled "Human Leukocyte Antigens (HLA)") and genetically determined sensitivity of the thyroid gland to irradiation were also involved. However, as in the study by Penhale and Young,[3] thyroid hormone deficiency increased susceptibility to autoimmune thyroiditis.[57]

Reports of natural killer cell activity in autoimmune thyroid disorders are mixed. Some researchers have reported that natural killer cell activity was significantly decreased in Graves' and Hashimoto's thyroiditis patients[72] and others reported that the activity was not decreased.[73] (See section below titled "Natural Killer Cell Activity and Thyroid Status.")

Antithyroid Antibodies and Musculoskeletal Pain. Aarflot and Bruusgaard, for example, tested a hypothesis based on their observations from general practice—that patients with antithyroid antibodies tend to have complaints of chronic widespread musculoskeletal pain. They included in their study 737 men and 771 women who ranged in age from 40-to-42 years. The researchers determined the prevalence of detected thyroid microsomal antibodies in subjects with and without chronic widespread musculoskeletal complaints. Those with chronic widespread musculoskeletal complaints had a significantly higher incidence of antibodies than did subjects without such complaints (16.0% versus 7.3%, p < 0.01). The prevalence of antibodies was significantly higher in women than men (20.4% versus 11.6%, p = 0.02). It is noteworthy that laboratory thyroid function test results did not differ significantly between the two groups. The investigators wrote, "The association between chronic widespread musculoskeletal pain complaints and thyroid antibodies in women may reflect a subgroup of patients in which thyroid autoimmunity, rather than thyroid function, is important." They discussed the possible relationship of thyroid antibodies to fibromyalgia. The results of this study suggest that patients with microsomal thyroid antibodies may have symptoms due to suboptimal thyroid hormone regulation of cell function before thyroid gland dysfunction is detectable by tests of thyroid hormone and TSH levels.[47]

Autoimmunity Possibly Secondary to Low Cortisol Levels in Fibromyalgia. In response to injury, ACTH from the pituitary gland stimulates the adrenal cortices to secrete cortisol. The increased amount of cortisol inhibits every step in the tissue response to injury, including inflammation. The elevation in cortisol is most valuable when an injury is so severe that the individual is at risk of disability or death.[11,pp.566-567]

Endogenous and exogenous glucocorticoids suppress the growth of all lymphoid tissues; by doing so, they decrease the production of T-lymphocytes and antibodies.[48,p.389] A glucocorticoid deficiency is thus likely to result in an exaggerated tissue response to injury or infection, with potentially devastating consequences. Even a mild deficiency of cortisol may have adverse immune consequences. Glucocorticoids such as cortisol are the strongest endogenous immune system suppressing agents,[5] and a mild-to-moderate deficiency may permit excessive and potentially damaging immune responses. This is of concern in the study of fibromyalgia because of evidence that some patients have a subnormal response of the adrenal cortices to stress (see Chapter 3.5).

Overall, cortisol excess results in immune suppression, and cortisol deficiency results in immune activation. A deficiency of cortisol can increase immune system activity in several ways. First, the deficiency may result in too little lipocortin production. Lipocortin inhibits phospholipase A_2. Too little lipocortin results in an increase in phospholipase A_2. The increased amount of this enzyme stimulates production of arachidonic acid. Arachidonic acid is a precursor for prostaglandins which are mediators of inflammation. Hence, patients may have an increased tendency toward inflammation. Second, cortisol deficiency is likely to result in increased production of interleukin-1 by macrophages due to insufficient repression of the lymphokine gene. Release of interkeukin-2 by lymphocytes is also likely to increase. The deficiency of cortisol would liberate the complete cascade of cell-mediated immunity and favor a tendency for fever. Third, cortisol deficiency is likely to result in destabilization of lysosomes. Consequently, lysosomal enzymes are more readily released to degrade foreign substances. Fourth, cortisol deficiency may allow recruitment of leukocytes by increasing their ability to bind to chemotactic peptides. Fifth, the deficiency may allow increased mobilization of T-lymphocytes and increased antibody production by B-lymphocytes.[11,p.567] Thus, a cortisol deficiency results in an overall increase in activity of the immune system.

Because some fibromyalgia patients have a glucocorticoid deficiency, Demitrack and Crofford suggested that some immunologic disturbances in fibromyalgia patients result from the deficiency.[5,p.69] They pointed out that the cessation of elevated circulating cortisol levels results in an exacerbation of

autoimmune thyroiditis,[6] with myalgias, arthralgias, and muscle weakness.[7]

Rittenhouse and Redei assessed the inflammatory response in hypothyroid rats to a streptococcal cell wall preparation serving as an antigen. They noted that when the glucocorticoid level is low, the inflammatory response to the preparation is greatly enhanced. This shows that glucocorticoids are immune suppressants. Because glucocorticoid production is reduced in hypothyroidism, they hypothesized that the inflammatory response in hypothyroid rats would be enhanced. Three days after they administered the cell wall preparation to normal rats, a dramatic increase occurred in the mRNAs for macrophage inflammatory protein1α and interleukin-1β. The increase was even greater in hypothyroid rats. Rats with above normal T_4 levels after T_4 administration, and with a consequent increase in glucocorticoid levels, had a significant inhibition of the inflammatory response to the preparation. The outcome thus showed that hypothyroidism is associated with an exaggerated inflammatory response to antigens.[71]

Deficient Cortisol and Multiple Chemical Sensitivity Syndrome. Ziem and McTamney wrote of considerable overlap between the clinical features of fibromyalgia, chronic fatigue syndrome, and chemical sensitivity syndrome. Chemical sensitivity is an excessive responsiveness to multiple chemicals at concentrations well tolerated by the healthy population. Common features of chemical sensitivity syndrome are headaches (migraine in many), chronic fatigue, musculoskeletal pain, chronic respiratory inflammation (rhinitis, sinusitis, laryngitis, asthma), attention deficit, and hyperactivity in younger children. Patients may also have tremors, seizures, and mitral valve prolapse. Chronic immune system activation is a possible mechanism underlying chemical sensitivity syndrome.[200]

Excess immune system activity in some chemical sensitivity patients may result from subnormal cortisol secretion due to inadequate thyroid hormone regulation of the hypothalamic-pituitary-adrenal axis (see Chapter 3.5). In addition, an increased allergic tendency might result from an increased number of mast cells and an increase in mast cells secretions. Inadequate thyroid hormone regulation of the adrenergic genes may underlie both the increased number and secretions of mast cells (see section above titled "Allergies: Mast Cells, Thyroid Hormone, and Allergy"). The combined effect of subnormal cortisol, increased numbers of mast cells, and increased mast cell secretions plausibly accounts for multiple chemical sensitivity syndrome in some patients. If so, chemical sensitivity syndrome in some patients is a distinct clinical phenotype of hypothyroidism and/or cellular resistance to thyroid hormone.

Galland wrote that among the abnormalities associated with multiple chemical sensitivity syndrome are autoimmune thyroiditis and hypothyroidism. Another abnormality common to chemical sensitivity patients that can be associated with hypothyroidism is mitral valve prolapse (see Chapter 3.3). Also, chemical sensitivity patients have impaired excretion of essential amino acids despite a high protein diet. Inadequate thyroid hormone regulation of gene transcription profoundly diminishes protein production in the body, an effect that may account for the low amino acid excretion in some chemical sensitivity patients.

Galland wrote that 25% of multiple chemical sensitivity patients markedly improved, and another 18% less markedly improved, when they underwent treatment for their low levels of antioxidants (selenium, vitamin C, zinc, and sulfur-containing amino acids). He wrote that the various abnormalities in chemical sensitivity syndrome may be the result of some unidentified fundamental metabolic or neuroendocrine disturbance.[24] The most likely candidate is inadequate thyroid hormone regulation of the adrenal cortices, the adrenergic genes (and through these genes, regulation of mast cells), and other components of the immune system. Failure to correct the inadequate thyroid hormone regulation could account for improvement in only 43% of patients after correction of antioxidant deficiencies. A high enough dosage of the proper form of thyroid hormone may be necessary to correct subnormal cortisol levels and to properly suppress mast cells secretions.

Adrenal Insufficiency: Not a Cause of Fibromyalgia. In one report, the authors wrote that severe fibromyalgia resulted when a patient's pituitary gland was removed. Before surgery, the patient had an elevated cortisol level due to excess ACTH secretion. Removal of the pituitary eliminated ACTH secretion and lowered the cortisol level. This report suggests that a cortisol deficiency instigated the fibromyalgia.[8] Such reports must be considered carefully. In this one, fibromyalgia probably resulted from inadequate thyroid regulation of cell function. It is highly likely that the patient's woefully inadequate thyroid hormone dosage induced and maintained her fibromyalgia. (For a description of this informative case of a 54-year-old woman, see the introductory section of Chapter 4.4.)

T-Lymphocytes, B-Lymphocytes, and Interferon

Setoguchi et al. measured interferon-α and interferon-γ activity levels, natural killer cell activity, and subsets of lymphocytes in the peripheral blood of three different groups of thyroid disease patients. They included 217 control subjects, 27 patients with Basedow's (Graves') disease, 8 with Hashimoto's thyroiditis, and 5 with idiopathic hypothyroidism. The patient groups were similar to the control group in interferon-α levels and natural killer cell activity. Compared to control subjects, however, patients with Hashimoto's disease had significantly higher levels of interferon-γ, and patients with Basedow's disease had significantly lower levels. Also compared to controls, patients with Basedow's had significantly lower levels of T-lymphocytes, and patients with idiopathic hypothyroidism had significantly higher levels.[74] Patients with Basedow's disease had a higher level of B-lymphocytes, and patients with hypothyroidism had the lowest level of all the groups.

Lymphocyte Subsets. Patients with mononucleosis from Epstein-Barr virus infection were found to have a decrease of CD4 lymphocytes and an increase of CD8 lymphocytes. Their CD4/CD8 ratio was therefore decreased.[115] If the increased CD4/CD8 lymphocyte ratio in fibromyalgia patients reported by Wallace et al.[113,pp.279-280] is typical of fibromyalgia patients at large, Epstein-Barr virus infection may be an unlikely etiologic agent among fibromyalgia patients.

Luo reported that the salivary glands of Sjögren's syndrome patients contained predominantly T-lymphocytes of the CD4 subset. CD8 lymphocytes were decreased. Thus, the CD4/CD8 ratio was increased.[116] This ratio is similar to the increased CD4/CD8 ratio in fibromyalgia patients reported by Wallace et al.[113,pp.279-280] Unfortunately, Wallace et al. did not report whether their patients had sicca symptoms possibly related to Sjögren's syndrome. (See Chapter 3.17.)

Lymphocyte Subsets in Hypothyroid Patients. Most studies indicate that thyroid hormone deficiency is associated with decreased CD4 lymphocyte activity and increased CD8 lymphocyte activity. This is contrary to the report by Wallace et al. of an increased CD4/CD8 ratio in fibromyalgia patients.[113] We cannot be certain, however, that the patients in the Wallace et al. study are typical of the fibromyalgia population. They reported that the increased CD4/CD8 ratio of 15 fibromyalgia patients was elevated compared to that of "55 apparently healthy individuals who attended a community health fair."[113,p.279] Uncertainty about the health status of these control subjects leaves doubt about the value of the CD4/CD8 ratio of the fibromyalgia patients.

Erf reported that mice with congenital hypothyroidism had a significantly subnormal weight of the thymus gland and spleen. Thymus CD8 lymphocytes were lower than normal and the ratio of CD4 to CD8 lymphocytes was increased. Spleen CD4 lymphocytes were increased. Erf concluded: "These data provide further evidence for the importance of normal thyroid function in the development, maintenance, and function of the immune system. It was concluded that not only congenital hypothyroidism results in altered immune development in young-adult mice, but also long-term effects on immune development occur in progeny of hypothyroid mothers."[122]

Johnson et al. found that in hypothyroid chickens, proliferation of peripheral blood lymphocytes stimulated by mitogen was subnormal. However, administering T_3 to the chickens increased lymphocyte proliferation and increased the ratio of CD4 to CD8 lymphocytes. Johnson et al. wrote, "These results suggest that thyroid factors and alterations of thymic status significantly affect the generation of specific thymus-derived lymphocyte populations and their functional capabilities, perhaps due to changes in the thymic microenvironment. These alterations may have important consequences for the development of immunocompetence and disease resistance in chickens."[124]

Oren et al. wrote that decreased thyroid hormone production is associated with a variety of immunological manifestations. Among the manifestations, they included reduced activation of CD4 lymphocytes and increased CD8 lymphocytes activity.[126]

Covas et al. reported that the levels of subsets of peripheral blood T-lymphocytes were related to thyroid status. Patients who were hyperthyroid due to Graves' disease had low levels of all subsets but an increased ratio of CD4 to CD8 lymphocytes. Patients who were hypothyroid due to Hashimoto's thyroiditis had a reduced ratio of CD4 to CD8 lymphocytes. The researchers wrote that the CD4/CD8 ratio may be a measure for differentiating hypothyroid from hyperthyroid patients with autoimmune thyroiditis.[125]

Ohashi et al. studied the subsets of peripheral blood lymphocytes in patients with Graves' disease, Hashimoto's thyroiditis, and subacute thyroiditis. Patients with Graves' disease and Hashimoto's thyroiditis had increased percentages of CD4 lymphocytes. Patients who were euthyroid or hypothyroid after treatment for Graves' disease had increased CD8 lymphocytes.[123]

Natural Killer Cell Activity and Thyroid Status

Some researchers have reported that natural killer cell activity is not decreased in autoimmune thyroid disorders.[73] However, others have reported that natural killer cell activity is significantly decreased in Graves' and Hashimoto's thyroiditis patients.[72] Stein-Streilein et al. reported that excess T_4 decreased natural killer cell activity in rats. It did so by interfering with the triggering mechanism of the targets of natural killer cells. Normally, the targets, when triggered, release cell destroying molecules from natural killer cells.[66]

Although *excessive* T_4 decreased natural killer cell activity, other researchers have reported that administering T_4 to mice increased natural killer cell activity in them.[67][68] Provinciali et al., for example, measured the *in vitro* effects of T_4 on basal and lymphokine-induced natural killer cell cytotoxicity in mice. They administered two lymphokines, interleukin-2 and interferon, to the mice. The lymphokines caused a substantial increase in natural killer cytotoxic activity of spleen cells. Administering both lymphokines together produced an additive effect. Incubating spleen cells with T_4 did not alter the basal activity or activity induced by interleukin-2. But the incubation with T_4 increased the natural killer cell cytotoxic activity induced by interferon. In addition, the incubation significantly increased the "maximal boosting effect" on natural killer cell activity of administering interferon and interleukin-2 simultaneously. The researchers concluded that thyroid hormone increases natural killer cell-mediated cytotoxicity, especially by increasing the sensitivity of natural killer cells to interferon.[68]

Fever

Ladenson et al. reported that hypothyroid patients are susceptible to an increased risk of several minor complications from surgery. Their group of 40 hypothyroid patients did not differ from control surgery patients in perioperative infection. However, fever was less frequent in hypothyroid patients: Only 35% of hypothyroid patients had fever compared to 79% of control patients.[64] Fever develops for several reasons in patients with infection. Bacterial toxins and many protein degradation products (as from degenerating tissue) stimulate fever and are called "pyrogens." Pyrogens stimulate the hypothalamus to raise its temperature set-point, thereby increasing body temperature. When white blood cells, tissue macrophages, and natural killer lymphocytes phagocytize bacteria and their breakdown products, the cells release interleukin-1. Interleukin-1 also stimulates the hypothalamus to increase its temperature set-point, contributing to the increase in body temperature. The effect of interleukin-1 on the hypothalamus, however, may be indirect. It increases the production of prostaglandins from arachidonic acid, and the prostaglandins may be responsible for increasing the set-point of the hypothalamus.[48,p.806]

Whether fever is beneficial during infection has been a subject of debate for a long time. Research data suggest that elevated temperature is beneficial during infection because it augments host defenses. Because of this, some writers recommend that we not routinely suppress fever. Possibly the only clinical studies that provide support for the benefits of fever are the early ones of fever therapy for syphilis.[62,p.9] However, Langer and Scheer presented an interesting line of argument for the benefits of fever. First, they noted that Sir William Osler argued that of the three great scourges of mankind—fever, famine, and war—fever was by far the worst. Some authors agreed with Osler, concluding that the research literature provided no convincing evidence that fever protects humans against microbes and infection.[78] But Langer and Scheer cited Kluger who refuted the opinion that fever is of no benefit. Kluger pointed out that lizards ("cold-blooded" animals that depend on external environmental heat to maintain body temperature), when infected, seek out hot environmental conditions that raise their body temperature to fever levels. Similarly, infected fish swim to warmer water to raise their body temperature. In addition, a 2° C increase in temperature is followed by a 2000% increase in T-lymphocytes and antibodies, and fever markedly increases antibody production in spleen cells.[78] Langer and Scheer also noted that interleukin-1 increases body temperature and that the increased temperature provides an ideal climate for the multiplication of defense cells. They wrote in conclusion, "If fever increases our ability to fight diseases, do subnormal temperatures make us more susceptible to them? Very likely. Hypothyroidism and its accompanying subnormal temperatures are stresses which lower the body's innate ability to fight off infection."[77,pp.37-38] Indeed, the hypothyroid patient may be unable to generate a sufficient increase in body temperature during infection due to an inflexibly low metabolic rate. If fever is beneficial during infection, an impaired ability to generate fever may increase the likelihood of the patient developing complications from infection.

Fungal Infection

The word "fungus" comes from the Latin term for mushroom. Included among fungi are many forms of yeasts and molds. Fungi, like bacteria, can decompose all organic substances. They contribute to the well-being of our ecosystem by taking part in the recycling of carbon. We humans use fungi as food and to catalyze fermentation during the production of alcohol and medicines such as antibiotics.

Fungi are far more pathogenic to plants than humans and induce far more infections in plants. Nevertheless, infection by fungi such as *Candida albicans* is severely problematic for some humans.

Ali tested chronic fatigue syndrome patients for the incidence of IgE antibodies with specificity for four yeasts. Of 200 patients, 97% had antibodies to cephalosporium, 96% to alternaria, 95% to aspergillus, and 83% to *Candida albicans*.[112,p.150]

A study by Yu and coworkers suggested that hypothyroid patients may have an increased susceptibility to fungal infections of the thyroid gland. The researchers reviewed 191 cases of suppurative (pus-forming) thyroiditis reported in the English-language literature between 1980 and 1997. They compared the results with another review of 224 cases between 1900 and 1980. Their aim was to learn the percentage of involvement of different microbes in the infections in relation to the thyroid status of patients. Based on the combined data, they wrote that 83.1% of patients who were euthyroid had bacterial infections. Of patients who were hyperthyroid, 50% had mycobacterial infections. (Mycobacterium is a genus of aerobic bacteria.) Of hypothyroid patients, 62.5% had fungal infections.[58]

Crook hypothesized that yeast overgrowth in humans results in a generalized suppression of the immune system.[196] Yeast overgrowth can certainly cause a wide variety of symptoms and signs, including those characteristic of fibromyalgia and chronic fatigue syndrome.[196,pp.177-193] As Teitelbaum explained, yeast overgrowth is favored by several factors: "One of the most prevalent is frequent antibiotic use. When the good bacteria in the bowel are killed off by antibiotics along with the bad bacteria, the yeasts no longer have competition and begin to overgrow. The body often is able to rebalance itself after one or several courses of antibiotics, but *after repeated or long-term course— and especially if the body has an underlying immune dysfunction—the yeast can get the upper hand* [italics mine]."[195,p.43] The individual whose immunity is impaired due to inadequate thyroid hormone regulation of the immune system may be especially susceptible to yeast overgrowth with the repetitive or prolonged use of antibiotics. Even if the antibiotics relieve symptoms and signs due to *Borrelia burgdorferi*, mycoplasmal, or other infections, nothing much may have been gained if the patient is left with yeast overgrowth.

In my clinical career, I have seen only one patient who met the criteria for fibromyalgia who, after undergoing a comprehensive anti-*Candida* regimen, no longer met the criteria. It is possible that in the past, however, chronic fungal infections were instrumental in the resistance of some fibromyalgia patients who failed to improve or recover with metabolic rehabilitation. I know of many cases in which prolonged or repeated antibiotic use has resulted in severe *Candida albicans* infections. These infections are likely to result in patients, for example, who undergo prolonged antibiotic therapy for Lyme disease. Some authors recommend as a rational approach to Lyme disease that the clinician tailor antibiotic therapy to the severity of the disease and limit it in most cases to 4 weeks.[137] I agree with this contention in that the patient undergoing prolonged antibiotic therapy may develop severe *Candida albicans* overgrowth even if simultaneously engaging in a sustained anti-candida regimen.

The essence of Crook's treatment for superficial *Candida albicans* is this: (1) azole drugs, such as Diflucan, Nizoral, or Sporanox until the patient begins to improve, (2) simultaneous or follow-up use of an antifungal medication that is not absorbed from the gastrointestinal tract, such as nystatin, caprylic acid and/or citrus seed extracts, (3) an appropriate diet, including limited consumption of simple carbohydrates, and (4) avoidance of chemical pollutants, provision of psychological support, and the use of nutritional supplements.[196,pp.478-480]

I strongly recommend Crook's book *The Yeast Connection and the Woman*[196] to men and women whose symptoms may be caused or complicated by fungal infections, and to their physicians.

For additional information on prevention of and treatment for fungal infections following antibiotic therapy, see the section above titled "Treatment for Mycoplasmal Infection."

Septic Shock: Role of Thyroid Hormone in Recovery

The adequacy of thyroid function may be critical for some patients' survival after septic shock. Septic shock occurs when an individual has inadequate tissue perfusion associated with live bacteria in the circulating blood (bacteremia), especially gram-negative bacteria such as meningococci. In about ⅓ of cases, gram-positive cocci or *Candida* organisms are involved. Patients often acquire the bacteria involved in septic shock in the hospital. Other patients acquire the

bacteria during trauma or a medical or dental procedure. Septic shock often occurs in patients with compromised immune function. Babies may be born with septicemia and go into septic shock, but babies and adults with septic shock often show up at emergency rooms. Acute circulatory failure occurs, usually with hypotension, and multiple organs fail.[62,p.71] Usually, patients have respiratory distress syndrome (difficulty exchanging oxygen and carbon dioxide, resulting in acidosis). Patients may require intubation and ventilation to improve oxygen and carbon dioxide exchange and to relieve acidosis.[61] Acute kidney failure may also occur. Most patients die when treatment is not begun soon enough.[62,pp.71&73]

Leon-Sanz et al. studied the time course of functional thyroid abnormalities and their relation to case outcome for 27 consecutive patients with septic shock. They compared thyroid function of patients who survived the illness and those who died of septic shock after the thyroid testing. The patients, who had a mean age of 50 years, were in an intensive care unit of a university hospital. Reseachers measured the total T_4 and total T_3 on the 1st and 5th days after admission. Also, on these days, TSH levels were measured at 8 am, 8 pm, and 1 am, and the TSH response to TRH was measured on the 2nd and 6th days. All patients had low T_4 and T_3 levels on the 1st day. Only patients who survived the illness had significant increases in their T_4 and T_3 levels on the 5th day. On the 2nd day, patients who survived had a higher mean basal TSH (survivors, 0.89 ± 0.63 µIU/mL; nonsurvivors, 0.34 ± 0.42 µIU/mL). Survivors also had a higher mean TSH response to TRH injections (survivors, 229 ± 157 µIU/mL; nonsurvivors, 101 ± 101 µIU/mL). On the 1st day, the normal nocturnal TSH surge at 1 am (defined as the difference between the TSH level at 1 am and 8 am) was absent in both survivors and nonsurviors. On the 5th day, only survivors had recovered the normal nocturnal surge. The researchers concluded that patients with septic shock have an altered hypothalamic-pituitary-thyroid axis. (This is expected due to a rise in cortisol levels. The elevated cortisol inhibits TSH secretion. The resulting reduced TSH level in turn decreases thyroid gland secretion of T_4 and T_3. Also, the elevated cortisol inhibits T_4 to T_3 conversion. See Chapter 2.1, section titled "The Hypothalamus and TRH as a Fine Control for TSH Secretion." Also see Chapter 2.5, section titled "Disorders Involving Inhibition of T_4 to T_3 Conversion," and section titled "Proposal of a Sustained Euthyroid Sick Syndrome Under the Expropriated Name 'Wilson's Syndrome.'") The researchers wrote that their data suggest a less deranged hypothalamic-pituitary-thyroid axis in patients who survived septic shock. Hence, because the axis was less deranged in those who survived, their thyroid function improved. Because the axis was more deranged in those who later died, their thyroid function did not improve.[63]

Two different interpretations of the results of this study by Leon-Sanz et al. are evident. First, the patients whose thyroid function remained suppressed had such severe organ damage that their cortisol levels remained high, and the sustained high cortisol levels continued to suppress their thyroid function. The patients may have died from the more severe organ damage, and their suppressed thyroid function may have been an inconsequential secondary effect.

Second, in the patients whose thyroid function remained low after the first few days of illness, the thyroid systems lacked capacity to markedly increase their function. Consequently, the insufficient thyroid function was critically instrumental in the patients' deaths. Unfortunately, we do not know the thyroid status of the patients before they developed septic shock, and so we cannot determine whether this second interpretation is probable. We have reason to suspect, however, that lower thyroid hormone levels may compromise patients' recovery from severe illness. Hypothyroid patients were reported to be more susceptible to several minor complications from surgery. Although they did not have a higher infection rate, some patients were not able to develop fever when appropriate, and this inability may have made some patients more susceptible to infection. Hypothyroid patients undergoing noncardiac surgery had a higher incidence of low blood pressure, and they had a higher incidence of heart failure during cardiac surgery. After surgery, hypothyroid patients had a higher incidence of gastrointestinal complaints, and they had more neuropsychiatric complaints. (See Chapter 4.4, section titled "Complications of Surgery.") Moreover, ill patients who have thyroid hormone deficiency (and undoubtedly those with cellular resistance to thyroid hormone) are at risk for a poorer outcome due to impaired hemodynamics and cardiac function (See Chapter 4.4, "Improved Cardiovascular Status with Thyroid Hormone Therapy"). Schultz et al. reported that continuation of euthyroid sick syndrome (with low circulating T_3 levels) in bone marrow transplantation patients increased the chances of a fatal outcome. Of 100 transplantation patients, 22 died before 140 days after the transplant, 21 patients died between 140 and 365 days, and 57 patients survived longer than 365 days. By the 14th day after surgery, T_3 levels decreased and reverse-T_3 levels

and reverse-T_3/T_3 ratios increased in all patients. At the 28th day after surgery, the 57 patients who survived longer than 365 days had an increase in T_3 levels and decreases in reverse-T_3 and the reverse-T_3/T_3 ratio. This recovery of presurgery thyroid hormone measures did not occur in the patients who died within 140 days and between 140 and 365 days. The investigators reported that a failure to recover from euthyroid (low T_3) sick syndrome is associated with a higher probability of a fatal outcome from bone marrow transplantation.[82]

Cytokines

At least two cytokines, interleukin-1β and interferon-γ, are regulated in part by thyroid hormone. Regulation of interleukin-1β may be mediated mainly through β-adrenergic receptors. Thyroid hormone regulation of the β-adrenergic genes potently regulates the density of β-adrenergic receptors on cell membranes. Thyroid hormone regulation of interferon-γ activity is probably more direct, resulting from thyroid hormone binding to cell membranes and not to T_3-receptors in cell nuclei.

Levels of Interleukin-2 in Hypothyroidism. Cheney et al. reported that chronic fatigue syndrome patients had increased serum interleukin-2 levels.[127] Hader et al., however, reported that in response to mitogen stimulation, T-lymphocytes and CD4 cells from 12 fibromyalgia patients secreted a subnormal amount of interleukin-2. A higher amount of mitogen was needed to induce optimal secretion in the fibromyalgia patients, and optimal secretion was delayed.[128] The reduced secretion in fibromyalgia patients is similar to reduced interleukin-2 in hypothyroidism.

Inducing hypothyroidism in mice with methimazole suppressed production of interleukin-2 in the spleen. The suppression of interleukin-2 levels interfered with the normal proliferation of T-lymphocytes.[106] Komorowski studied cytokine blood levels in hypothyroid patients. He compared the levels in 7 primary hypothyroid patients and 8 euthyroid healthy controls. Compared to the controls, patients had normal levels of interleukin-1β but significantly lower levels of interleukin-2.[109]

Interleukin-2 Receptors in Hypothyroidism. Hernanz et al. found that fibromyalgia patients had low levels of interleukin-2 receptors (also termed CD25). They wrote that this suggests that the patients have impaired T-lymphocyte activation.[131] (The serum level of soluble interleukin-2 receptors is a marker of T-lymphocyte activation.[110]) As the studies below show, this corresponds to low interleukin-2 receptor levels and subnormal T-lymphocytes activation in hypothyroidism.

Lovicelli et al. reported that in patients who were hypothyroid due to autoimmune thyroiditis, levels of soluble interleukin-2 receptors were lower than in control subjects. When hypothyroid patients became "euthyroid" (presumably when they had TSH levels within the normal range) during T$_4$ treatment, their soluble interleukin-2 receptor levels increased to mean values similar to those of control subjects. The researchers concluded, "These results agree with those supporting a role for thyroid hormones in the regulation of the immune system." They noted that low interleukin-2 receptor levels are peculiar to hypothyroidism as an autoimmune disease. They also wrote that researchers and clinicians may use measures of soluble interleukin-2 receptors as a marker of the peripheral action of thyroid hormones.[107]

Koukkou et al. reported that soluble interleukin-2 receptor levels were significantly lower in hypothyroid patients. Levels were significantly higher in hyperthyroid patients. When patients became euthyroid, levels were normal. The investigators wrote that their findings suggest that high T$_4$ levels are associated with activation of human lymphocytes. They did not find a correlation between T$_3$ and T$_4$ levels and soluble CD8 levels and soluble interleukin-2 receptor levels.[108]

Mariotti et al. found that levels of soluble interleukin-2 receptors were highly correlated with thyroid hormone levels. They also found that in neither Graves' nor Hashimoto's patients did receptor levels correlate with anti-thyroglobulin, anti-thyroid peroxidase, or anti-TSH-receptor autoantibodies. Based on these findings, they concluded that thyroid hormone rather than autoimmunity is the main regulator of interleukin-2 receptors.[110]

Regulation of Interleukin-1β by β-Adrenergic Receptor Activation. In some tissues, thyroid hormone may regulate levels of interleukin-1β by controlling the density of β-adrenergic receptors on cell membranes. Maruta et al. reported that injecting the β-adrenoceptor agonist isoproterenol into the ventricles increased interleukin-1β mRNA in glial cells. (The term "glial" is from the Greek word for glue. Glia are cells in the central and peripheral nervous systems. They are distinct from nerve cells. They appear to serve both structural support and metabolic function in their occupancy between nerves and blood vessels. Projections from glial cells called "glial feet" press against capillary walls in the brain tissue, preventing overstretching of the capillaries during times of high arterial pressure.[48,p.681]) Lower doses of the β$_2$-adreno-

ceptor agonist procaterol caused a greater increase in the mRNA. The β$_1$-adrenoceptor agonist dobutamine increased the mRNA only in the meninges. These results indicate that increased activity of β-adrenergic receptors increases interleukin-1β gene expression in some brain tissues.[25]

Tomozawa et al. also found that β-adrenergic receptor activation by isoproterenol induced interleukin-1β mRNA in the hypothalamus and microglia, but not in astrocytes.[105] (Astrocytes and microglia are types of glial cells in the central nervous system.) In that thyroid hormone regulation of the β-adrenergic genes increases β-adrenergic density on cell membranes (see Chapter 3.1), inadequate thyroid hormone regulation of the adrenergic genes may result in decreased interleukin-1β levels in some brain regions.

Cytokines and the Sleep-Wake Cycle. According to Moldofsky, a reciprocal relationship exists between the immune system and the sleep-wake system. He wrote, "Interference either with the immune system (e.g. by a viral agent or by cytokines such as alpha-interferon or interleukin-2) or with the sleep-waking brain system (e.g. by sleep deprivation) has effects on the other system and will be accompanied by the symptoms of the chronic fatigue syndrome."[12] He wrote of evidence suggesting that fibromyalgia and chronic fatigue syndrome patients have disordered chronobiology (timing of repetitive or cyclic biological events). The evidence includes a relationship between interleukin-1 and the sleep-wake cycle. Whether and how such factors interact in fibromyalgia patients cannot be determined at this time; data is too scant and the methodology of the available studies varies too much.[11,pp.39&48] As a part of the disordered chronobiology of fibromyalgia patients, disturbed sleep (due to hypothyroidism or cellular resistance to thyroid hormone) could contribute to the immune abnormalities reported to occur in fibromyalgia (see Chapter 3.18).

Interleukin-2 Therapy and Hypothyroidism. Wallace described patients who had undergone treatment for cancer with intravenous interleukin-2 and subsequently developed features of fibromyalgia.[114] Interleukin-2 therapy induces hypothyroidism in some 5%-to-10% of patients.[117][118][119][120][121] It is possible that the fibromyalgia features in the patients Wallace et al. described were the symptoms and signs of thyroid hormone deficiency in the patients.

Viral Infection, Interferon-γ, and Thyroid Hormone

Studies by Lin and his colleagues have shown that thyroid hormone increases the antiviral activity of interferon-γ. For a description of interferon-γ, its source, and its major effects on the immune system, see the section above titled "Macrophage Affecting Cytokines: Interferon-γ."

Lin et al. found that T_4 and T_3 potentiated the antiviral activity of human interferon-γ in HeLa cells. (HeLa cells are a strain of cells continuously cultured from a patient's carcinoma of the cervix. Investigators named the cells according to the first two letters of the patient's first and last names, which are "Henrietta" and "Lacks." Researchers use the cultured cells to study the growth of other cells, the activity of viruses, and the effects of different agents on viral function.) T_3 was as effective as T_4 in increasing the activity of interferon-γ when incubated with cells long enough. Interestingly, reverse-T_3 also potentiated the antiviral action of interferon-γ. It did so, however, only in a preincubation model. When T_3 and reverse-T_3 were preincubated together, the effects of the two hormones were additive. The additive effect caused a 100-fold potentiation of the antiviral effects of interferon-γ. Lin et al. wrote that thyroid hormone potentiated the antiviral effects of interferon-γ by two mechanisms. One is a mechanism dependent on protein synthesis, indicating an effect of thyroid hormone on gene transcription. A fascinating finding is that this mechanism was responsive to reverse-T_3 which researchers previously thought had no effect on protein synthesis or metabolism. A second mechanism is a post-translational process that is independent of protein synthesis. The researchers do not know the details of the post-translational mechanism.[83]

Lin et al. reported that T_4 potentiated expression of the HLA-DR gene (see section above titled "Human Leukocyte Antigens (HLA)") induced by human interferon-γ. T_4 increased interferon-γ-induced HLA-DR mRNA 4-fold and HLA-DR protein 2.2-fold. Interferon-γ induction of HLA-DR expression requires activation of STAT1α and induction of the class II transactivator CIITA. In the presence of interferon-γ, T_4 enhanced cytokine activation of STAT1α. HeLa and CV-1 cells treated with T_4 resulted in activation of STAT1α cells. HeLa and CV-1 cells do not have thyroid hormone receptors. Because of this, the researchers proposed that the increased interferon-γ induction of HLA-DR in response to T_4 suggests early hormone recognition at the surfaces of HeLa and CV-1 cells. They wrote that this early recognition is distinct from thyroid hormone receptors in the nuclei of the cells. This means that the thyroid hormone potentiation of transcription of HLA-DR by interferon-γ is mediated by a cell membrane thyroid hormone binding site, with

activation of STAT1α and increased induction of CIITA.[81] It is noteworthy that Lin et al. found that blocking 5'-deiodinase (which converts T_4 to T_3) with 6-n-propel-2-thiouracil did not interfere with the potentiation of transcription. This means that T_4 itself rather than T_3 was responsible for the measured effects. Lin et al. found that milrinone, a compound structurally similar to thyroid hormone, had the same effects as T_4, yet milrinone does not interact with c-*erb*Aβ receptors in cell nuclei.[85] (c-ErbAβ receptors are the thyroid hormone receptors that mediate most cellular effects of thyroid hormone. See Chapter 2.6.)

Lin and his colleagues have continued to elucidate the exceedingly complex genetic mechanisms underlying the molecular step by which thyroid hormone increases the antiviral activity of interferon-γ.[41][84] For example, they have reported that T_4 potentiated interferon-γ action in wild-type (non-mutated) STAT1α cells but not in STAT1αA727 cells. STAT1αA727 are cells that contain STAT1α but with an alanine-for-serine substitution at residue 727. This mutation resulted in T_4 only minimally stimulating STAT1α activation.[84]

Cytomegalovirus Infection and Thyroid Hormone Resistance. Hirano and colleagues studied an infant with congenital cytomegalovirus infection who had a clinical picture consistent with general resistance to thyroid hormone. At 3 weeks of age, the infant's serum total and free T_3 and T_4 were above normal despite a high TSH level of 154 μU/mL. She did not have clinical features of thyrotoxicosis despite the high thyroid hormone levels. This suggests that she had general cellular resistance to the hormone. Only supraphysiologic doses of T_3 (16 μg/kg body weight) suppressed the high TSH to a normal level. While inherited general resistance is permanent, all thyroid function test results returned to normal in this patient. The child had normal bone development, but she had mild psychomotor retardation, sensory hearing loss, and microcephaly.[79] Refetoff and coauthors surmised that the transient viremia caused a reduction in the concentration of T_3-receptors or a reduction of cofactors that resulted in transient general resistance to thyroid hormone.[80,p.387] The transient resistance, however, apparently resulted in permanent abnormalities.

● **A MODEL TO EXPLAIN IMMUNE ABNORMALITIES IN FIBROMYALGIA**

A thesis of this chapter is in the same vein as Bechamps' late 19th century retort to Pasteur: "the soil, not the seed."[103,p.7] The thesis is that for many people, inadequate thyroid hormone regulation of the immune system results in reduced resistance to infection and toxin-induced disease. For them, adequate thyroid hormone is a critically important immune system modulator. One or more components of the immune system will be dysregulated, and the individual will react to microbes and toxins in an idiosyncratic way. How individuals react to infectious agents and toxins varies tremendously. As Teibelbaum put it: "Everyone's immune system has strong spots as well as weak spots. Some people never get colds but have frequent bouts with athlete's foot or another skin fungal infection. Other people never get fungal infections but tend to get bowel infections."[195,p.42]

Of course, some microbes are so virulent and some substances so toxic that they can overcome the innate and acquired resistance of most any individual and induce disease. Unfortunately, though, many clinicians and researchers still maintain an overzealous and purist Pasteurian posture—to them, the presence of an infection in fibromyalgia patients is proof positive that the responsible microbe is the cause of fibromyalgia. Their intention is good in that identifying a microbe that is the cause of a disease usually points to an effective treatment. But the caution expressed by Ali should be observed: The infection may be secondary to another condition that has lowered resistance and enabled the microbe to infect the patient.[112,pp.154&569] One condition that lowers the resistance of many individuals is inadequate thyroid hormone regulation of the immune system. Various immune system impairments in these individuals render them more susceptible to infections and toxicity than others who have adequate thyroid hormone regulation of the immune system. For those with inadequately regulated systems, proper diet and nutrition, rest and recreation, and ordinary steps to avoid toxins and infective agents may not be enough for them. Inadequate thyroid hormone regulation of the immune system is the critical missing link in immunocompetence that keeps their resistance low.

Clearly, some individuals with borderline sufficient metabolism (due to hypothyroidism and/or cellular resistance to thyroid hormone) have impaired immune systems. Depending on which parts of the immune system are impaired, an individual will be more susceptible to infection by some microorganisms or vulnerable to adverse effects from some classes of toxins. When she acquires an infection, or she is adversely affected by toxins, her illness may be severe enough to reduce her level of physical activity. The reduced activity, if sustained for even a short time, is likely to reduce her skeletal muscle mass. The reduced mass will further lower her metabolic rate, perhaps below the threshold for the onset of symptoms of hypometabolism. These symptoms, if they occur during the infection or toxic reaction, will complicate those of the infection or toxic reaction. After resolution of the infection or relief from the toxic reaction, the symptoms of hypometabolism are likely to persist because of her reduced muscle mass. Her symptoms of hypometabolism are likely to be more persistent and more severe than in times past, leading to the diagnosis of fibromyalgia.

I suspect that those who most easily fall prey to *Borrelia burgdorferi* and mycoplasmal infections have health histories and medical records showing recurrent complaints of symptoms characteristic of hypometabolism. These individuals are also likely to have histories of frequent and/or severe infections. The symptoms of hypometabolism are likely to be a product of inadequate thyroid hormone regulation of fibromyalgia-related tissues, and the infection a product of inadequate thyroid hormone regulation of the immune system. In some of these patients, toxic reactions to repetitious or prolonged antibiotic therapy and/or secondary fungal infections may contribute to symptoms that lead to a diagnosis of fibromyalgia.[144] Secondary *Candida albicans* infections due to antibiotic therapy may also contribute. The typical patient will never have had a diagnosis of hypothyroidism or resistance to thyroid hormone. If the patient received a diagnosis of hypothyroidism and underwent thyroid hormone treatment, the clinician will have prescribed T_4 alone and titrated the dosage according to the TSH level. Upon the failure of this regimen of thyroid hormone therapy, the prescribing clinician is likely to have concluded that the patient's continuing illness has nothing to do with hypothyroidism. Almost universally for such patients, the repeated or prolonged use of various medications intended to control their symptoms complicate the symptoms and speed their descent into progressively poorer health.

REFERENCES

1. Neimark, H. and Kocan, K.M.: The cell wall-less rickettsia Eperythrozoon wenyonii is a Mycoplasma. *FEMS Microbiol. Lett.*, 156(2):287-291, 1997.
2. Brooks, G.F., Butel, J.S., and Ornston, L.N.: Jawetz, Melnick & Adelberg's *Medical Microbiology*, 9th edition. Norwalk, Appleton & Lange, 1991.

3. Penhale, W.J. and Young, P.R.: The influence of the normal microbial flora on the susceptibility of rats to experimental autoimmune thyroiditis. *Clin. Exp. Immunol.*, 72: 288-292, 1988.

4. Vergano, D.: Bacteria tied to chronic illnesses. *Med. Sentinel*, 4:172-176, 1999.

5. Demitrack, M.A. and Crofford, L.J.: Hypothalamic-pituitary-adrenal axis dysregulation in fibromyalgia and chronic fatigue syndrome: an overview and hypothesis. *J. Musculoskeletal Pain*, 3(2):67-79, 1995.

6. Takasu, N., Komiya, I., Nagasawa, Y., Asawa, T., and Yamada, T.: Exacerbation of autoimmune thyroid dysfunction after unilateral adrenalectomy in patients with Cushing's syndrome due to an adrenocortical adrenoma. *N. Engl. J. Med.*, 322(24):1708-1712, 1990.

7. Dixon, R.B. and Christy, N.P.: On various forms of corticosteroid withdrawal syndrome. *Am. J. Med.*, 68(2):224-230, 1980.

8. Disdier, P., Harle, J.-R., Brue, T., Jaquet, P., Chambourlier, P., Grisoll, F., and Weiller, P.-J.: Severe fibromyalgia after hypophysectomy for Cushing's disease. *Arthritis Rheum.*, 34(4):493-495, 1991.

9. O'Dell, J.R., Paulsen, G., Haire, C.E., et al.: Treatment of early seropositive rheumatoid arthritis with minocycline: four-year follow-up of a double-blind, placebo-controlled trial. *Arthritis Rheumat.*, 42:1691-1695, 1999.

10. Tilley, B.C., Alarcon, G.S., Heyse, S.P., et al.: Minocycline in rheumatoid arthritis: a 48-week, double-blind, placebo-controlled trial. *Ann. Intern. Med.*, 122:81-89, 1995.

11. Berne, R.M. and Levy, M.N.: *Principles of Physiology.* St. Louis, C.V. Mosby Company, 1990.

12. Moldofsky, H.: Fibromyalgia, sleep disorder, and chronic fatigue syndrome. *Ciba Found. Sympos.*, 173:262-271, 1993.

13. Chiu, D. and Duesberg, P.H.: The toxicity of azidothymidine (AZT) on human and animal cells in culture at concentrations used for antiviral therapy. *Genetica*, 95: 103-109, 1995.

14. Hoffman, B.B. and Lefkowitz, R.J.: Catecholamines and sympathomimetic drugs. In *Goodman and Gilman's The Pharmacological Basis of Therapeutics*, 8th edition. New York, Pergamon Press, 1990, pp.187-220.

15. Anderson, C.D., Lindgren, B.R., and Andersson, R.G.: Effects of clonidine on the dermal inflammatory cell response of experimental toxic and allergic contact reactions and intradermal hypersensitivity. *Int. Arch. Allergy Appl. Immunol.*, 83(4):371-376, 1987.

16. Barnes, P.J., Wilson, N.M., and Vickers, H.: Prazosin, an α_1-adrenoceptor antagonist, partially inhibits exercise-induced asthma. *J. Allergy Clin. Immunol.*, 68(6):411-415, 1981.

17. Clauw, D.J. and Chrousos, G.P.: Chronic pain and fatigue syndromes: overlapping clinical and neuroendocrine features and potential pathogenic mechanisms. *Neuroimmunomodulation*, 4(3):134-153, 1997.

18. Klein, R., Bansch, M., and Berg, P.A.: Clinical relevance of antibodies against serotonin and gangliosides in patients with primary fibromyalgia syndrome. *Psychoneuroendocrinology*, 17(6):593-598, 1992.

19. Baba, H., Kaune, G.C., Ilyas, A.A., et al.: AntiGm1 gang-

lioside antibodies with differing fine specificities in patients with multifocal motor neuropathy. *J. Neuroimmunology*, 25:143-150, 1989.

20. Russell, I.J., Vodjani, A., Michalek, J.E., Vipraio, G.A., Lopez, Y., and MacKillip, F.: Circulating antibodies to serotonin in fibromyalgia syndrome, rheumatoid arthritis, osteoarthrosis, and healthy normal controls. (Abstract) *J. Musculoskel. Pain*, 3(Suppl.1):143, 1995.

21. Vedder, C.I. and Bennett, R.M.: An analysis of antibodies to serotonin receptors in fibromyalgia. *J. Musculoskel. Pain*, 3(Suppl.1):73, 1995.

22. Institute for Molecular Medicine. <www.immed.org> Immediate Fax-Back information: (714) 903-2900.

23. Pausen, D.F.: *Basic Histology.* Norwalk, Appleton & Lange, 1990.

24. Galland, L.: Biochemical abnormalities in patients with multiple chemical sensitivities. *Occup. Med.*, 2(4):713-720, 1987.

25. Maruta, E., Yabuuchi, K., Nishiyori, A., Takami, S., Minami, M., and Satoh, M.: β_2-adrenoceptors on the glial cells mediate the induction of interleukin-1β mRNA in the rat brain. *Brain Res. Mol. Brain Res.*, 49(1-2):291-294, 1997.

26. Lund-Olesen, L.H. and Lund-Olesen, K.: The etiology and possible treatment of chronic fatigue syndrome/fibromyalgia. *Med. Hypotheses*, 43:55-58, 1994.

27. Behan, P.O., Behan, W.M.H., and Bell, E.J.: The postviral fatigue syndrome:an analysis of the findings in 50 cases. *J. Infect.*, 10:211-222, 1985.

28. Young, N.A.: Enteroviral diseases: epidemic pleuradynia (Bornholm disease, epidemic myalgia, Devil's grip, Sylvests disease). In *Textbook of Medicine*, 15th edition. Edited by P.B. Beeson, W. McDermott, and J. B. Wyngaarden, Philadelpha, W.B. Saunders, 1979, pp.227-271.

29. Straus, S.E., Tosato, G., Armstrong, G. et. al.: Persisting illness and fatigue in adults with evidence of Epstein-Barr virus infection. *Ann. Intern. Med.*, 102:7-16, 1985.

30. Nicolson, G.L.: Personal written communication. October 26, 1999.

31. Landay, A.L., Jessop, C., Lennette, E.T., and Levy, J.A.: Chronic fatigue syndrome: clinical condition associated with immune activation. *Lancet*, ii:708-712, 1991.

32. Yosef, G.E., Bell, E.J., Mann, G.F., et al.: Chronic enterovirus infection in patients with postviral fatigue syndrome. *Lancet*, i:146-150, 1988.

33. Bengtsson, A., Bäckman, E., Lindblom, B., and Skogh, T.: Long term follow-up of fibromyalgia patients: clinical symptoms, muscular function, laboratory tests: an eight year comparison study. *J. Musculoskel. Pain*, 2(2):67-80, 1994.

34. Vrethem, M., Skogh, T., Berlin, G., and Ernerud, J.: Autoantibodies versus clinical symptoms in blood donors. *J. Rheumatol.*, 19:1919-1921, 1992.

35. Rivera, J., Dediego, A., Trinchet, M., and Monforte, G.: Fibromyalgia-associated hepatitis C virus infection. *Brit. J. Rheumatol.*, 36(9):981-985, 1997.

36. King, S., Fisher, B., Burnham, R., Maclean, I., Bell, G., and Warren, S.: Tumor necrosis factor, interleukin-1-β, and tissue oxygen levels in myofascial pain and fibromyalgia syndromes. *J. Musculoskel. Pain*, 5(3):53-66, 1997.

37. Duesberg, P.H.: AIDS acquired by drug consumption and

other noncontagious risk factors. *Pharmacol. Ther.*, 55(3): 201-277, 1992.

38. Baraniuk, J.N., Clauw, D., Yuta, A., et al.: Nasal secretion analysis in allergic rhinitis, cystic fibrosis, and nonallergic fibromyalgia/chronic fatigue syndrome subjects. *Amer. J. Rhinol.*, 12(6):435-440, 1998.

39. Wilson, R.B., Gluck, O.S., Tesser, J.R., Rice, J.C., Meyer, A., and Bridges, A.J.: Antipolymer antibody reactivity in a subset of patients with fibromyalgia correlates with severity. *J. Rheumatol.*, 26(2):402-407, 1999.

40. Bonaccorso, S., Lin, A.H., Verkerk, R., et al.: Immune markers in fibromyalgia: comparison with major depressed patients and normal volunteers. *J. Affect Disord.*, 48(1): 75-82, 1998.

41. Lin, H.Y., Thacorf, H.R., Davis, F.B., and Davis, P.J.: Potentiation by thyroxine of interferon-gamma-induced antiviral state requires PKA and PKC activities. *Amer. J. Physiol.*, 271(4 Pt.1):C1256-C1261, 1996.

42. Baraniuk, J.N., Clauw, D.J., and Gaumond, E.: Rhinitis symptoms in chronic fatigue syndrome. *Ann. Allergy Asthma Immunol.*, 81(4):359-365, 1998.

43. Yunus, M.B.: Genetic factors in fibromyalgia syndrome. *Z. Rheumatol.*, 57(Suppl.2):61-62, 1998.

44. Yunus, M.B., Khan, M.A., Rawlings, K.K., Green, J.R., Olson, J.M., and Shah, S.: Genetic linkage analysis of multicase families with fibromyalgia syndrome. *J. Rheumatol.*, 26(2):408-412, 1999.

45. Enestrom, S., Bengtsson, A., and Frodin, T.: Dermal IgG deposits and increase of mast cells in patients with fibromyalgia: relevant findings or epiphenomena? *Scand. J. Rheumatol.*, 26(4):308-313, 1997.

46. Moroni, F., Fantozzi, R., Masini, E., and Mannaioni, P.F.: The modulation of histamine release by α-adrenoceptors: evidences in murine neoplastic mast cells. *Agents Actions*, 7(1):57-61, 1977.

47. Aarflot, T. and Bruusgaard D.: Association between chronic widespread musculoskeletal complaints and thyroid autoimmunity. Results from a community survey. *Scand. J. Prim. Health Care*, 14(2):1111-1115, 1996.

48. Guyton, A.C.: *Textbook of Medical Physiology*, 8th edition. Philadelpha, W.B. Saunders Company, 1991.

49. Razin, S.: The minimal cellular genome of mycoplasma. *Indian J. Biochem. Biophys.*, 34(1-2):124-130, 1997.

50. Taylor-Robinson, D. and Bebear, C.: Antibiotic susceptibilities of mycoplasmas and treatment of mycoplasmal infections. *J. Antimicrob. Chemother.*, 40(5):622-630, 1997.

51. Razin, S., Yogev, D., and Naot, Y.: Molecular biology and pathogenicity of mycoplasmas. *Microbiol. Mol. Biol. Rev.*, 62(4):1094-1156, 1998.

52. Komaroff, A.L., Bell, D.S., Cheney, P.R., and Lo, S.C.: Absence of antibody to Mycoplasma fermentans in patients with chronic fatigue syndrome. *Clin. Infect. Dis.*, 17 (6):1074-1075, 1993.

53. Ginsburg, K.S., Kundsin, R.B., Walter, C.W., and Schur, P.H.: Ureaplasma urealyticum and Mycoplasma hominis in women with systemic lupus erythematosus. *Arthritis Rheum.*, 35(4):429-433, 1992.

54. Choppa, P.C., Vojdani, A., Tagle, C., Andrin, R., and Magtoto, L.: Multiplex PCR for the detection of Mycoplasma fermentans, M. hominis and M. penetrans in cell cultures and blood samples of patients with chronic fatigue

syndrome. *Mol. Cell. Probes*, 12(5):301-308, 1998.

55. Vojdani, A., Choppa, P.C., Tagle, C., Andrin, R., Samimi, B., and Lapp, C.W.: Detection of Mycoplasma genus and Mycoplasma fermentans by PCR in patients with Chronic Fatigue Syndrome. *FEMS Immunol. Med. Microbiol.*, 22 (4):355-365, 1998.

56. Nicolson, G.L., Nicolson, N.L., and Nasralla, M.: Mycoplasmal infections and chronic fatigue illness (Gulf War illness) associated with deployment to Operation Desert Storm. *Intern. J. Med.*, 1:80-92, 1998.

57. Kotani, T., Komuro, K., Yoshiki, T., Itoh, T., and Aizawa, M.: Spontaneous autoimmune thyroiditis in the rat accelerated by thymectomy and low doses of irradiation: mechanisms implicated in the pathogenesis. *Clin. Exp. Immunol.*, 45(2):329-337, 1981.

58. Yu, E.H., Ko, W.C., Chuang, Y.C., and Wu, T.J.: Suppurative Acinetobacter baumanii thyroiditis with bacteremic pneumonia: case report and review. *Clin. Infect. Dis.*, 27 (5):1286-1290, 1998.

59. Pillay, K.: Congenital hypothyroidism and immunodeficiency: evidence for an endocrine-immune interaction. *J. Pediatr. Endocrinol. Metab.*, 11(6):757-761, 1998.

60. Mayer, D., Miller-Hanisch, B., Bockh, A., and Hehrmann, R.: Fulminant meningococcal meningitis and sepsis associated with severe hypothyroidism caused by autoimmune (Hashimoto's) thyroiditis. *Exp. Clin. Endocrinol. Diabetes*, 105(Suppl.4):80, 1997.

61. Honeyman-Lowe, G.: Personal communication, September 11, 1999.

62. *Merck Manual of Diagnosis and Therapy*, 16th edition. Edited by R. Berkow, A.J. Fletcher, and M.H. Beers, Rahway, Merck Research Laboratories, 1992.

63. Leon-Sanz, M., Lorente, J.A., Larrodera, L., Ros, P., Alvarez, J., Esteban, A.E., and Landin, L.: Pituitary-thyroid function in patients with septic shock and its relation with outcome. *Eur. J. Med. Res.*, 2(11):477-482, 1997.

64. Ladenson, P.W., Levin, A.A., Ridgway, E.C., and Daniels, G.H.: Complications of surgery in hypothyroid patients. *Amer. J. Med.*, 77(2):261-266, 1984.

65. Fowles, J.R., Fairbrother, A., and Kerkvliet, N.I.: Effects of induced hypo- and hyperthyroidism on immune function and plasma biochemistry in mallards (Anas platyrhynchos). *Comp. Biochem. Physiol. C. Pharmacol. Toxicol. Endocrinol.*, 118(2):213-220, 1997.

66. Stein-Streilein, J., Zakarija, M., Papic, M., and McKenzie, J.M.: Hyperthyroxinemic mice have reduced natural killer cell activity: evidence for a defective trigger mechanism. *J. Immunol.*, 139(7):2502-2507, 1987.

67. Sharma, S.D., Tsai, V., and Proffitt, M.R.: Enhancement of mouse natural killer cell activity by thyroxine. *Cell Immunol.*, 73(1):83-97, 1982.

68. Provinciali, M., Muzzioli, M., and Fabris, N.: Thyroxine-dependent modulation of natural killer activity. *J. Exp. Pathol.*, 3(4):617-622, 1987.

69. Kinoshita, S., Sone, S., Yamashita, T., Tsubura, E., and Ogura, T.: Effects of experimental hyper- and hypothyroidism on natural defense activities against Lewis lung carcinoma and its spontaneous pulmonary metastases in C57BL/6 mice. *Tokushima J. Exp. Med.*, 38(1-2):25-35, 1991.

70. Duesberg, P.H.: *Inventing the AIDS Virus*. Washington,

DC, Regnery Publishing, Inc., 1996.

71. Rittenhouse, P.A. and Redei, E.: Thyroxine administration prevents streptococcal cell wall-induced inflammatory responses. *Endocrinology,* 138(4):1434-1439, 1997.

72. Wenzel, B.E., Chow, A., Baur, R., Schleusener, H., and Wall, J.R.: Natural killer cell activity in patients with Graves' disease and Hashimoto's thyroiditis. *Thyroid,* 8 (11):1019-1022, 1998.

73. Pedersen, B.K., Feldt-Rasmussen, U., Bech, K., Perrild, H., Klarlund, K., and Hoier-Madsen, M.: Characterization of the natural killer cell activity in Hashimoto's and Graves' diseases. *Allergy,* 44(7):477-481, 1989.

74. Setoguchi, J., Nakano, K., Tsutsumi, Y. et al.: Interferon-α and -γ product in peripheral blood of patients with thyroid diseases. *Nippon Naibunpi Gakkai Zasshi,* 67(5):630-635, 1991.

75. Barnes, B.O. and Galton, L.: *Hypothyroidism: The Unsuspected Illness.* New York, Harper & Row, Publishers, 1976.

76. Barnes, B.O.: Etiology and treatment of lowered resistance to upper respiratory infection. *Fed. Proc.,* 12:10, 1953.

77. Langer, S.E. and Scheer, J.F.: *Solved: The Riddle of Illness.* New Canaan, Keats Publishing, Inc., 1984.

78. Atkins, A.: Fever—new perspectives on an old phenomenon. *N. Engl. J. Med.,* 308(16):958-969, 1983.

79. Hirano, T., Jogamoto, M., and Chin, I.: Syndrome of resistance to thyroid hormone in an infant with congenital cytomegalovirus infection. *Acta Paediatr. Japan,* 31:504-508, 1989.

80. Refetoff, S., Weiss, R.E., and Usala, S.J.: The syndromes of resistance to thyroid hormone. *Endocrine Rev.,* 14:348-399, 1993.

81. Lin, H.Y., Martino, L.J., Wilcox, B.D., Davis, F.B., Gordinier, J.K., and Davis, P.J.: Potentiation by thyroid hormone of human IFN-gamma-induced HLA-DR expression. *J. Immunol.,* 161(2):843-849, 1998.

82. Schulte, C., Reinhardt, W., Beelen, D., Mann, K., and Schaefer, U.: Low T$_3$-syndrome and nutritional status as prognostic factors in patients undergoing bone marrow transplantation. *Bone Marrow Transplant.,* 22(12):1171-1178, 1998.

83. Lin, H.Y., Thacore, H.R., Davis, F.B., and Davis, P.J.: Thyroid hormone analogues potentiate the antiviral action of interferon-gamma by two mechanisms. *J. Cell. Physiol.,* 167(2):269-276, 1996.

84. Lin, H.Y., Davis, F.B., Gordinier, J.K., Martino, L.J., and Davis, P.J.: Thyroid hormone induces activation of mitogen-activated protein kinase in cultured cells. *Amer. J. Physiol.,* 276(5 Pt.1):C1014-C1024, 1999.

85. Lin, H.Y., Yen, P.M., Davis, F.B., and Davis, P.J.: Protein synthesis-dependent potentiation by thyroxine of antiviral activity of interferon-gamma. *Amer. J. Physiol.,* 273(4 Pt.1):C1225-C1232, 1997.

86. Bodey, B., Bodey, B., Jr., Siegel, S.E., and Kaiser, H.E.: Molecular biological ontogenesis of the thymic reticulo-epithelial cell network during the organization of the cellular microenvironment. *In Vivo,* 13(3):267-294, 1999.

87. Matsushita, S.: HLA-peptide complex and immunity-related diseases. *Rinsho Byori,* 47(6):511-518, 1999.

88. Krause, W.J. and Cutts, J.H.: *Concise Textbook of Histology,* 2nd edition. Baltimore, Williams and Wilkins, 1986.

89. Hamerlinck, F.F.: Neopterin: a review. *Exp. Dermatol.,* 8 (3):167-176, 1999.

90. Phillips, M.J., Barnes, P.J., and Gold, W.M.: Characterization of purified dog mastocytoma cells: autonomic membrane receptors and pharmacologic modulation of histamine release. *Am. Rev. Respir. Dis.,* 132(5):1019-1026, 1985.

91. Boucher, J.L., Moali, C., and Tenu, J.P.: Nitric oxide biosynthesis, nitric oxide synthase inhibitors and arginase competition for L-arginine utilization. *Cell. Mol. Life Sci.,* 55(8-9):1015-1028, 1999.

92. Sabria, J., Ferrer, I., Toledo, A., Sentis, M., and Blanco, I.: Effects of altered thyroid function on histamine levels and mast cell number in neonatal rat brain. *J. Pharmacol. Exp. Ther.,* 240(2):612-616, 1987.

93. Rall, T.W.: Drugs used in the treatment of asthma: the methylxanthines, cromolyn sodium, and other agents. In *Goodman and Gilman's The Pharmacological Basis of Therapeutics,* 8th edition. New York, Pergamon Press, 1990, pp.618-637.

94. Honeyman-Lowe, G.: Personal communication. September 18, 1999.

95. Werner, E.R., Werner-Felmayer, G., and Mayer, B.: Tetrahydrobiopterin, cytokines, and nitric oxide synthesis. *Proc. Soc. Exp. Biol. Med.,* 219(3):171-182, 1998.

96. Shimizu, S., Ishii, M., Momose, K., and Yamamoto, T.: Role of tetrahydrobiopterin in the function of nitric oxide synthase, and its cytoprotective effect. *Int. J. Mol. Med.,* 2 (5):533-540, 1998.

97. van Amsterdam, J.G. and Opperhuizen, A.: Nitric oxide and biopterin in depression and stress. *Psychiat. Res.,* 85 (1):33-38, 1999.

98. Greco, D.S. and Harpold, L.M.: Immunity and the endocrine system. *Vet. Clin. N. Amer. Small Anim. Pract.,* 24 (4):765-782, 1994.

99. Illich, I.: *Medical Nemesis: The Expropriation of Health.* New York, Pantheon Books, 1976.

100. Alston, J.H.: *A New Look at Infectious Disease.* London, Pitman, 1967.

101. Sofoluwe, G.O.: Promotive medicine: a boost to the economy of developing countries. *Trop. Geogr. Med.,* 22(2): 250-254, 1970.

102. Mellanby, K.: *Pesticides and Pollution.* New York, Collins, 1967.

103. Rosenbaum, M. and Susser, M.: *Solving the Puzzle of Chronic Fatigue Syndrome.* Tacoma, Life Sciences Press, 1992.

104. Copi, I.M.: *Introduction to Logic,* 2nd edition. New York, The MacMillan Company, 1961.

105. Tomozawa, Y., Yabuuchi, K., Inoue, T., and Satoh, M.: Participation of cAMP and cAMP-dependent protein kinase in beta-adrenoceptor-mediated interleukin-1 beta mRNA induction in cultured microglia. *Neurosci. Res.,* 22 (4):399-409, 1995.

106. Liu, W.K., Tsui, K.W., Lai, K.W., and Xie, Y.: Sister-chromatid exchanges in lymphocytes from methimazole-induced hypothyroid mice. *Mutat. Res.,* 326(2):193-197, 1995.

107. Loviselli, A., Calia, M.A., Murenu, S., Mossa, P., Cambosu, M.A., and Caradonna, A.: Circulating soluble IL-2 receptor levels are low in patients with hypothyroid auto-

immune thyroiditis. *Horm. Metab. Res.*, 26(11):548-551, 1994.

108. Koukkou, E., Panayiotidis, P., Alevizou-Terzaki, V., and Thalassinos, N.: High levels of serum soluble interleukin-2 receptors in hyperthyroid patients: correlation with serum thyroid hormones and independence from the etiology of the hyperthyroidism. *J. Clin. Endocrinol. Metab.*, 73(4): 771-776, 1991.

109. Komorowski, J.: Increased interleukin-2 level in patients with primary hypothyroidism. *Clin. Immunol. Immunopathol.*, 63(2):200-202, 1992.

110. Mariotti, S., Caturegli, P., Barbesino, G., et al.: Thyroid function and thyroid autoimmunity independently modulate serum concentration of soluble interleukin 2 (IL-2) receptor (sIL-2R) in thyroid diseases. *Clin. Endocrinol.* (Oxf.), 37(5):415-422, 1992.

111. Moldofsky, H.: Sleep, neuroimmune and neuroendocrine functions in fibromyalgia and chronic fatigue syndrome. *Adv. Neuroimmunol.*, 5:39-56, 1995.

112. Ali, M.: *The Canary and Chronic Fatigue.* Denville, Life Span Press, 1995.

113. Wallace, D.J., Peter, J.B., Bowman, R.L., Wormsley, S., and Silverman, S.: Fibromyalgia, cytokines, fatigue syndromes and immune regulation. In *Advances in Pain Research and Therapy*, Vol. 17. Edited by J.R. Fricton and E. Awad,, New York, Raven Press, 1990, pp.277-287.

114. Wallace, D.J., Margolin, K., and Waller, P.: Fibromyalgia and interleukin-2 therapy for malignancy. *Ann. Intern. Med.*, 108(6):909, 1988.

115. Zidovec, S., Culig, Z., Begovac, J., and Jeren, T.: Comparison of lymphocyte subpopulations in the peripheral blood of patients with infectious mononucleosis and human immunodeficiency virus infection: a preliminary report. *J. Clin. Lab. Immunol.*, 50(2):63-69, 1998.

116. Luo, F., Zhang, H., and Zhou, Z.: A study of immunopathology on salivary gland of Sjögren's syndrome. *Chung Hua Yen Ko Tsa Chih.*, 33(5):363-365, 1997.

117. van Liessum, P.A., de Mulder, P.H., Mattijssen, E.J., Corstens, F.H., and Wagener, D.J.: Hypothyroidism and goitre during interleukin-2 therapy without LAK cells. *Lancet*, 1(8631):224, 1989.

118. Beuzeboc, P., Escourolle, H., Dorval, T., Dieras, V., Mastorakos, G., Luton, J.P., and Pouillard, P.: Hypothyroidism after treatment with interleukin-2. *Presse Med.*, 18(14): 727, 1989.

119. Berthaud, P., Schlumberger, M., Comoy, E., Avril, M.F., Le Chevalier, T., Spielmann, M., and Tursz, T.: Hypothyroidism and goiter during interleukin-2 therapy. *J. Endocrinol. Invest.*, 13(8):689-690, 1990.

120. Hartmann, L.C., Urba, W.J., Steis, R.G., Smith, J.W., II, VanderMolen, L., Creekmore, S.P., and Longo, D.L.: Hypothyroidism after interleukin-2 therapy. *J. Clin. Oncol.*, 7(5):686-687, 1989.

121. Vialettes, B., Guillerand, M.A., Viens, P., et al.: Incidence rate and risk factors for thyroid dysfunction during recombinant interleukin-2 therapy in advanced malignancies. *Acta Endocrinol.* (Copenh.), 129(1):31-38, 1993.

122. Erf, G.F.: Immune development in young-adult C.RF-hyt mice is affected by congenital and maternal hypothyroidism. *Proc. Soc. Exp. Biol. Med.*, 204(1):40-48, 1993.

123. Ohashi, H., Okugawa, T., and Itoh, M.: Circulating ac-

tivated T-cell subsets in autoimmune thyroid diseases: differences between untreated and treated patients. *Acta Endocrinol.* (Copenh.), 125(5):502-509, 1991.

124. Johnson, B.E., Marsh, J.A., King, D.B., Lillehoj, H.S., and Scanes, C.G.: Effect of triiodothyronine on the expression of T-cell markers and immune function in thyroidectomized White Leghorn chickens. *Proc. Soc. Exp. Biol. Med.*, 199(1):104-113, 1992.

125. Covas, M.I., Esquerda, A., Garcia-Rico, A., and Mahy, N.: Peripheral blood T-lymphocyte subsets in autoimmune thyroid disease. *J. Investig. Allergol. Clin. Immunol.*, 2(3): 131-135, 1992.

126. Oren, R., Maaravi, Y., Karmeli, F., Kenet, G., Zeidel, L., Hubert, A., and Eliakim, R.: Anti-thyroid drugs decrease mucosal damage in a rat model of experimental colitis. *Aliment. Pharmacol. Ther.*, 11(2):341-345, 1997.

127. Cheney, P.R., Dorman, S.E., and Bell, D.S.: Interleukin-2 and the chronic fatigue syndrome. *Ann. Intern. Med.*, 110: 321, 1989.

128. Hader, N., Rimon, D., Kinarty, A., and Lahat, N.: Altered interleukin-2 secretion in patients with primary fibromyalgia. *Arthritis Rheum.*, 34:866-872, 1991.

129. Dinerman, H., Goldenberg, D.L., and Felson, D.T.: A prospective evaluation of 118 patients with the fibromyalgia syndrome: prevalence of Raynaud's phenomenon, sicca symptoms, ANA, low complement and Ig deposition at the dermal-epidermal junction. *J. Rheumatol.*, 13:368-373, 1986.

130. Yunus, M.B., Hussey, F.X., and Aldag, J.C.: Antinuclear antibodies and connective tissue disease features in fibromyalgia syndrome: a controlled study. *J. Rheumatol.*, 20: 1557-1560, 1993.

131. Hernanz, W., Valenzuela, A., Quijada, J., et al.: Lymphocyte subpopulations in patients with primary fibromyalgia. *J. Rheumatol.*, 21(11):2122-2124, 1994.

132. Branco, J.C., Tavares, V., Abreu, I., and Humbel, R.L.: Viral infection and fibromyalgia. *Acta Med. Port.*, 7(6): 337-341, 1994.

133. Buskila, D., Shnaider, A., Neumann, L., Zilberman, D., Hilzenrat, N., and Sikuler, E.: Fibromyalgia in hepatitis C virus infection. Another infectious disease relationship. *Arch. Intern. Med.*, 157(21):2497-2500, 1997.

134. Buskila, D., Shnaider, A., Neumann, L., et al.: Musculoskeletal manifestations and autoantibody profile in 90 hepatitis C virus infected Israeli patients. *Semin. Arthritis Rheum.*, 28(2):107-113, 1998.

135. Steere, A.C.: Musculoskeletal manifestations of Lyme disease. *Amer. J. Med.*, 98(4A):44S-48S, 1995.

136. Evans, J.: Lyme disease. *Curr. Opin. Rheumatol.*, 6(4): 415-422, 1994.

137. Rahn, D.W. and Felz, M.W.: Lyme disease update. Current approach to early, disseminated, and late disease. *Postgrad. Med.*, 103(5):51-54, 57-59, 63-64, 1998.

138. Frey, M., Jaulhac, B., Sibilia, J., Monteil, H., Kuntz, J.L., and Vautravers, P.: Detection of Borrelia burgdorferi DNA by gene amplification in the muscle of a patient with fibromyalgia. *Presse Med.*, 24(34):1623, 1995.

139. Steere, A.C.: Lyme disease: a growing threat to urban populations. *Proc. Natl. Acad. Sci. U.S.A.*, 91(7):2378-2383, 1994.

140. Bujak, D.I., Weinstein, A., and Dornbush, R.L.: Clinical

and neurocognitive features of the post-Lyme syndrome. *J. Rheumatol.*, 23(8):1392-1397, 1996.

141. Goldenberg, D.L.: Fibromyalgia, chronic fatigue syndrome, and myofascial pain syndrome. *Curr. Opin. Rheumatol.*, 7(2):127-135, 1995.

142. Lesniak, O.M. and Belikov, E.S.: The classification of Lyme borreliosis. *Ter. Arkh.*, 67(11):49-51, 1995.

143. Hsu, V.M., Patella, S.J., and Sigal, L.H.: "Chronic Lyme disease" as the incorrect diagnosis in patients with fibromyalgia. *Arthritis Rheum.*, 36(11):1493-1500, 1993.

144. Lightfoot, R.W., Jr., Luft, B.J., Rahn, D.W., et al.: Empiric parenteral antibiotic treatment of patients with fibromyalgia and fatigue and a positive serologic result for Lyme disease: a cost-effectiveness analysis. *Ann. Intern. Med.*, 119(6):503-509, 1993.

145. Evans, J. and Schoen, R.T.: Lyme disease. *Curr. Opin. Rheumatol.*, 5(4):454-460, 1993.

146. Steere, A.C.: Current understanding of Lyme disease. *Hosp. Pract.* (Off Ed), 28(4):37-44, 1993.

147. Burdge, D.R. and O'Hanlon, D.P.: Experience at a referral center for patients with suspected Lyme disease in an area of nonendemicity: first 65 patients. *Clin. Infect. Dis.*, 16(4):558-560, 1993.

148. Sigal, L.H. and Patella, S.J.: Lyme arthritis as the incorrect diagnosis in pediatric and adolescent fibromyalgia. *Pediatrics*, 90(4):523-528, 1992.

149. Dinerman, H. and Steere, A.C.: Lyme disease associated with fibromyalgia. *Ann. Intern. Med.*, 117(4):281-285, 1992.

150. Kaplan, R.F., Meadows, M.E., Vincent, L.C., Logigian, E.L., and Steere, A.C.: Memory impairment and depression in patients with Lyme encephalopathy: comparison with fibromyalgia and nonpsychotically depressed patients. *Neurology*, 42(7):1263-1267, 1992.

151. Schned, E.S. and Williams, D.N.: Special concerns in Lyme disease. Seropositivity with vague symptoms and development of fibrositis. *Postgrad. Med.*, 91(7):65-68, 1992.

152. Sigal, L.H.: Current recommendations for the treatment of Lyme disease. *Drugs*, 43(5):683-699, 1992.

153. Brier, S.R.: Lyme disease. *J. Manipulat. Physiol. Ther.*, 13(6):337-339, 1990.

154. Huppertz, H.I. and Karch, H.: Lyme arthritis in childhood: monarthritis of the knee joint, clinically indistinguishable from monarthritis of unknown origin. *Monatsschr. Kinderheilkd.*, 139(11):759-764, 1991.

155. Sigal, L.H.: Summary of the first 100 patients seen at a Lyme disease referral center. *Amer. J. Med.*, 88(6):577-581, 1990.

156. Kohler, J.: Lyme borreliosis in neurology and psychiatry. *Fortschr. Med.*, 108(10):191-193, 1990.

157. Paparone, P.W.: Hypothyroidism with concurrent Lyme disease. *J. Amer. Osteo. Assoc.*, 95(7):435-437, 1995.

158. Vladar, L., Markuljak, I., Kvetensky, J., et al.: Lyme disease in internal medicine. *Vnitr. Lek.*, 39(8):793-796, 1993.

159. Umicevic, P., Makevic, M., and Savanovic, V.: The most frequent neurologic manifestations of Lyme disease. *Glas. Srp. Akad. Nauka.* [Med], (43):219-223, 1993.

160. Coyle, P.K.: Neurologic complications of Lyme disease. *Rheum. Dis. Clin. N. Amer.*, 19(4):993-1009, 1993.

161. Sigal, L.H.: Persisting complaints attributed to chronic Lyme disease: possible mechanisms and implications for management. *Amer. J. Med.*, 96(4):365-374, 1994.

162. Bianconcini, G., Mazzali, F., Guidetti, D., Baratti, M., and Marcello, N.: Lyme disease. Case contribution and review of the literature. *Minerva Med.*, 85(1-2):43-50, 1994.

163. Blackburn, W.D., Jr. and Everson, M.P.: Lack of evidence of systemic inflammatory rheumatic disorders in symptomatic women with breast implants. *Plast. Reconstr. Surg.*, 99(4):1054-1060, 1997.

164. Naim, J.O., Lanzafame, R.J., and van Oss, C.J.: The effect of silicone-gel on the immune response. *J. Biomater. Sci. Polym. Ed.*, 7(2):123-132, 1995.

165. Brown, S.L., Langone, J.J., and Brinton, L.A.: Silicone breast implants and autoimmune disease. *J. Amer. Med. Womens' Assoc.*, 53(1):21-24, 1998.

166. Yoshida, S.H., Swan, S., Teuber, S.S., and Gershwin, M.E.: Silicone breast implants: immunotoxic and epidemiologic issues. *Life Sci.*, 56(16):1299-1310, 1995.

167. Vayssairat, M., Mimoun, M., Houot, B., Abuaf, N., Rouquette, A.M., and Chaouat, M.: Hashimoto's thyroiditis and silicone breast implants: 2 cases. *J. Mal. Vasc.*, 22(3):198-199, 1997.

168. Blackburn, W.D., Jr. and Everson, M.P.: Silicone-associated rheumatic disease: an unsupported myth. *Plast. Reconstr. Surg.*, 99(5):1362-1367, 1997.

169. Noone, R.B.: A review of the possible health implications of silicone breast implants. *Cancer*, 79(9):1747-1756, 1997.

170. Nyren, O., Yin, L., Josefsson, S., et al.: Risk of connective tissue disease and related disorders among women with breast implants: a nation-wide retrospective cohort study in Sweden. *B.M.J.*, 316(7129):417-422, 1998.

171. Bennett, R.: Fibromyalgia, chronic fatigue syndrome, and myofascial pain. *Curr. Opin. Rheumatol.*, 10(2):95-103, 1998.

172. Peters, W., Smith, D., Fornasier, V., Lugowski, S., and Ibanez, D.: An outcome analysis of 100 women after explantation of silicone gel breast implants. *Ann. Plast. Surg.*, 39(1):9-19, 1997.

173. Sahn, E.E., Garen, P.D., Silver, R.M., and Maize, J.C.: Scleroderma following augmentation mammoplasty: report of a case and review of the literature. *Arch. Dermatol.*, 126(9):1198-1202, 1990.

174. Bridges, A.J., Conley, C., Wang, G., Burns, D.E., and Vasey, F.B.: A clinical and immunologic evaluation of women with silicone breast implants and symptoms of rheumatic disease. *Ann. Intern. Med.*, 118(12):929-936, 1993.

175. Lewy, R.I. and Ezrailson, E.: Laboratory studies in breast implant patients: ANA positivity, gammaglobulin levels, and other autoantibodies. *Curr. Top. Microbiol. Immunol.*, 210:337-353, 1996.

176. Kaiser, W., Biesenbach, G., and Zazgornik, J.: Autoimmune phenomena after silicone implantation. *Dtsch. Med. Wochenschr.*, 112(36):1376-1379, 1987.

177. Freundlich, B., Altman, C., Snadorfi, N., Greenberg, M., and Tomaszewski, J.: A profile of symptomatic patients with silicone breast implants: a Sjögrens-like syndrome. *Semin. Arthritis Rheum.*, 24(1 Suppl.1):44-53, 1994.

178. Vasey, F.B.: Observation on women with breast implants.

J. Fla. Med. Assoc., 82(5):348-351, 1995.

179. Silverman, B.G., Brown, S.L., Bright, R.A., Kaczmarek, R.G., Arrowsmith-Lowe, J.B., and Kessler, D.A.: Reported complications of silicone gel breast implants: an epidemiologic review. *Ann. Intern. Med.*, 124(8):744-756, 1996.

180. Teuber, S.S., Yoshida, S.H., and Gershwin, M.E.: Immunopathologic effects of silicone breast implants. *West J. Med.*, 162(5):418-425, 1995.

181. Bridges, A.J., Anderson, J.D., Burns, D.E., Kemple, K., Kaplan, J.D., and Lorden, T.: Autoantibodies in patients with silicone implants. *Curr. Top. Microbiol. Immunol.*, 210:277-282, 1996.

182. Brautbar, N., Campbell, A., and Vojdani, A.: Silicone breast implants and autoimmunity: causation, association, or myth? *J. Biomater. Sci. Polym. Ed.*, 7(2):133-145, 1995.

183. Vasey, F.B., Havice, D.L., Bocanegra, T.S., Seleznick, M.J., Bridgeford, P.H., Martinez-Osuna, P., and Espinoza, L.R.: Clinical findings in symptomatic women with silicone breast implants. *Semin. Arthritis Rheum.*, 24(1 Suppl.1):22-28, 1994.

184. Thomas, W.O., III, Harper, L.L., Wong, S.W., Michalski, J.P., Harris, C.N., Moore, J.T., and Rodning, C.B.: Explantation of silicone breast implants. *Am. Surg.*, 63(5): 421-429, 1997.

185. Barsky, A.J. and Borus, J.F.: Functional somatic syndromes. *Ann. Intern. Med.*, 130(11):910-921, 1999.

186. Wolfe, F. and Anderson, J.: Silicone filled breast implants and the risk of fibromyalgia and rheumatoid arthritis. *J. Rheumatol.*, 26(9):2025-2028, 1999.

187. Wolfe, F.: "Silicone related symptoms" are common in patients with fibromyalgia: no evidence for a new disease. *J. Rheumatol.*, 26(5):1172-1175, 1999.

188. Kossovsky, N., Gornbein, J.A., Zeidler, M., et al.: Self-reported signs and symptoms in breast implant patients with novel antibodies to silicone surface associated antigens [anti-SSAA(x)]. *J. Appl. Biomater.*, 6:305, 1995.

189. Borenstein, D.: Siliconosis: a spectrum of illness. *Semin. Arthritis Rheum.*, 24(Suppl.1):1-7, 1994.

190. Solomon, G.: A clinical and laboratory profile of symptomatic women with silicone breast implants. *Semin. Arthritis Rheum.*, 24(Suppl.1):29-37, 1994.

191. Bridges, A.J.: Rheumatic disorders in patients with silicone implants: a critical review. *J. Biomater. Sci. Polym. Ed.*, 7:147-157, 1995.

192. Zazgornik, J., Piza, H., Kaiser, W., et al.: Autoimmune reactions in patients with silicone breast implants. *Wien. Klin. Wochenschr.*, 108(24):781-787, 1996.

193. Gabriel, S.E., O'Fallon, W.M., Kurland, L.T., Beard, C.M., Woods, J.E., and Melton, L.J.: Risk of connective tissue diseases and other disorders after breast implantation. *N. Engl. J. Med.*, 330(24):1697-1702, 1994.

194. Cuellar, M.L., Gluck, O., Molina, J.F., Gutierrez, S., Garcia, C., and Espinoza, R.: Silicone breast implant-associated musculoskeletal manifestations. *Clin. Rheumatol.*, 14 (6):667-672, 1995.

195. Teitelbaum, J.: *From Fatigued to Fantastic!* Garden City Park, Avery Publishing Group, 1996.

196. Crook, W.G.: *The Yeast Connection and the Woman.* Jackson, Professional Books, Inc., 1998.

197. Haier, J., Nasralla, M., Franco, A.R., and Nicolson, G.L.: Detection of mycoplasmal infections in blood of patients with rheumatoid arthritis. *Rheumatology* (Oxf.), 38(6): 504-509, 1999.

198. Nicolson, G.L. and Nicolson, N.L.: Gulf War illnesses: complex medical, scientific and political paradox. *Med. Confl. Surviv.*, 14(2):156-165, 1998.

199. Nicolson, G.L. and Rosenberg-Nicolson, N.L.: Doxycycline treatment and Desert Storm. *J.A.M.A.*, 273(8):618-619, 1995.

200. Ziem, G. and McTamney, J.: Profile of patients with chemical injury and sensitivity. *Environ. Health Perspect.*, 105(Suppl.2):417-436, 1997.

201. Sanchezguerrero, J.: Auto-antibody testing in patients with silicone implants. *Clin. Lab. Med.*, 17(3):341, 1997.

202. Manzolli, S., Macedo-Soares, M.F., Vianna, E.O., and Sannomiya, P.: Allergic airway inflammation in hypothyroid rats. *J. Allergy. Clin. Immunol.*, 104(3 Pt.1):595-600, 1999.

203. Nicolson, G.L., Nasralla, M, Haier, J., Erwin, R., Nicolson, N.L., and Ngwenya, R.: Mycoplasmal infections in chronic illnesses: fibromyalgia and chronic fatigue syndromes, Gulf War illness, HIV-AIDS, and rheumatoid arthritis. *Med. Sentinel*, 4:172-176, 1999.

204. Nicolson, G.L., Nasralla, M., Haier, J., and Nicolson, N.L.: Diagnosis and treatment of chronic mycoplasmal infections in fibromyalgia syndrome and chronic fatigue syndrome: relationship to Gulf War illness. *Biomed. Therapy*, 16:266-271, 1998.

205. Nicolson, G.L.: Considerations when undergoing treatment for chronic infections found in chronic fatigue syndrome, fibromyalgia syndrome and Gulf War illnesses. (Part 1). Antibiotics recommended when indicated for treatment of Gulf War illness/CFIDS/FMS (Part 2). *Intern. J. Med.*, 1:115-117, 123-128, 1998.

206. Nicolson, G.L.: The role of microorganism infections in chronic illnesses: support for antibiotic regimens. *CFIDS Chronicle*, 12(3):19-21, 1999.

3.14

Irritable Bowel Syndrome

The main features of irritable bowel syndrome (IBS) are abdominal pain and altered bowel function. Altered bowel function may be of the diarrhea-type, with loose, watery stools, or the constipation-type, with straining at stool.

Some researchers consider IBS a "functional" disorder, meaning that it does not involve a disease process. Instead, to some of them, IBS is altered physiology in response to stress, or it is a heightening of the patient's perception of normal bowel stimuli. IBS can be modulated by stress, but the view that the condition is purely a product of chronic stress is poorly formulated and lacks supporting evidence.

IBS is common among fibromyalgia patients. Estimates of the incidence range from 29.6%-to-70%. In one study, 72% of chronic fatigue syndrome patients had IBS.

Hypothyroid patients may have the abdominal pain and altered bowel function that lead to the diagnosis of IBS. Clinicians may give them a diagnosis of functional bowel disease, spastic colon, or irritable bowel syndrome, each of which is a synonym for the others. The patient's hypothyroidism goes untreated or undertreated, and she responds poorly to medications calculated to relieve the symptoms of the bowel condition. Many hypothyroid and euthyroid hypometabolic fibromyalgia patients receive a diagnosis of IBS (or one of its synonyms) and undergo ineffective treatments based on the misdiagnosis.

In 1993, Mayer and Gebhart argued that the mechanism of IBS is not abnormal motility of the gastrointestinal tract.[34] In 1999, however, Scar-pignato and Pelosini wrote that "many believe that IBS constitutes the clinical expression of an underlying motility disorder, affecting primarily the mid- and lower gut. Indeed, transit and contractile abnormalities have been demonstrated with sophisticated techniques in a subset of patients with IBS." As a result of the belief that disordered motility underlies IBS, clinicians often treat the pain and altered bowel function of IBS with drugs that affect gastrointestinal motility. Different medications are used, depending on whether the patient has constipation-type IBS or diarrhea-type IBS. Drug therapy has not been particularly effective, and patients often have adverse effects to the drugs.[29]

Scarpignato and Pelosini also wrote that researchers are not clear on what IBS represents: a normal perception of abnormal gastrointestinal function, or an abnormal perception of normal function.[29] Some clinicians use functional bowel disease, spastic colon, or irritable bowel syndrome as synonymous diagnostic terms.[38]

Some writers have contended that IBS results from chronic stress. No doubt, stress modulates IBS as it does most other health conditions. However, the stress hypothesis is poorly formulated and lacks evidential support.[3,p.119][42][46]

● **IRRITABLE BOWEL SYNDROME IN FIBROMYALGIA**

Wolfe gave the incidence of IBS in fibromyalgia patients as 29.6%.[1] Use of a valid bowel symptom questionnaire indicated that 72% of tested chronic fatigue syndrome patients had functional bowel disease.[52]

Chang wrote that functional gastrointestinal disorders are common among fibromyalgia patients. He also noted that the common association of gastrointestinal disorders and fibromyalgia suggests a common etiology. According to him, 60% of patients with functional bowel disorders have fibromyalgia. In addition, some 50% of fibromyalgia patients report symptoms typical of functional dyspepsia, and 70% complain of symptoms of IBS. He described four clinical characteristics common to the two conditions (although the last two are patently false in regard to fibromyalgia): (1) most patients associate stressful life events with the onset or worsening of symptoms, (2) most patients report disturbed sleep and fatigue, (3) psychotherapy and behavioral therapies are effective in treating patients' symptoms, and (4) low-dose tricyclic antidepressant medications improve symptoms. He wrote that in spite of similarities between patients with fibromyalgia and those with functional gastrointestinal disorders, the two types of patients have different perceptions in response to somatic and visceral stimuli. First, in response to mechanical stimuli, fibromyalgia patients have somatic hyperalgesia, but IBS patients without coexistent fibromyalgia have somatic hypoalgesia. Visceral distention (as in the study by Chun et al.,[12] see next paragraph) produces different perceptions in fibromyalgia and IBS patients.[51]

Chun et al. wrote that IBS patients typically have visceral hyperalgesia. To compare visceral pain perception of fibromyalgia patients with that of IBS patients, the researchers distended the rectum of patients to induce the perception of rectal pain. IBS patients had a lower rectal pain threshold than normal controls. The rectal pain threshold of fibromyalgia patients did not differ from that of controls. The visceral algesia of fibromyalgia patients, according to rectal distention, was normal.[12]

In publications, clinicians usually do not specify the criteria they used to diagnosis IBS in fibromyalgia patients. They also do not describe the features of IBS the patients complain of. Whether the IBS symptoms include constipation or diarrhea, however, inadequate thyroid hormone regulation may be the cause.

● GASTROINTESTINAL EFFECTS OF HYPOTHYROIDISM

Thyroid hormone affects the structure, motility, and secretions of the gastrointestinal tract. Watanaku-nakorn et al. reported that 30% of hypothyroid patients complain of constipation,[33] but Wall et al. reported that up to 60% of patients register the complaint.[35] Constipation may develop early during hypothyroidism as a mild disturbance of motility, especially in infants. However, constipation may become severe.[7][47] Gastrointestinal disturbance is so early and prominent a feature of hypothyroidism that Javitt wrote, "Hopefully the early symptomatology will lead the physician to recognition of the underlying problem."[30,p.854]

The tongue may enlarge so that swallowing is difficult.[49] Swallowing may become more troublesome as saliva becomes more viscous and its volume decreases.[48]

Motility of the esophagus or stomach may not usually slow enough to produce symptoms (see section below titled "Impaired Intestinal Motility"). On the other hand, the stomach emptying time decreases.[13] Javitt wrote that two factors may impair the motility of the stomach. One factor is atrophy of the gastric mucosa; the other is a decrease in both the size and number of gastric cells.[30,p.869] Acid secretion decreases,[9] possibly enough to impair digestion. As a result, the pH may stay too high for calcium to dissociate properly, reducing its absorption. The pH may also be too high to activate protein hydrolyzing enzymes in the stomach, impairing release of amino acids from protein during digestion. Reduced calcium and amino acid absorption may result in nutritional deficiencies, complicating the patient's condition.

Malabsorption may occur in hypothyroidism. Rat studies show the mechanism of malabsorption. When deprived of thyroid hormone, the rat's intestinal villi decrease in height. This decreases the weight of the intestinal tract and thins the mucosal lining, decreasing its absorptive surface area.[35] The amount of glucose absorbed varies with the total absorptive surface of the gastrointestinal tract, so fewer glucose molecules enter the circulation from the gastrointestinal tract. Slower motility of the gastrointestinal tract in hypothyroidism, however, compensates somewhat for the reduced amount of glucose absorbed by the smaller absorptive surface. Slowed motility allows glucose a longer total time in contact with the absorptive mucosal lining. The longer exposure time enables more glucose to traverse the mucosa and enter the blood. Changes in the glucose tolerance curves of hypothyroid patients[13] are therefore a function of three factors: (1) slowed gastric emptying, (2) slowed absorption rates, and (3) a reduced total amount of absorbed glucose.[30,p.869]

Some hypothyroid patients have carotenemia (an increase of blood carotene, possibly with yellowing of the skin). Carotene is a red hydrocarbon found in many plant foods. It is a precursor of vitamin A. In hypothyroidism, carotenemia may occur when the cells of the intestinal mucosa convert carotene to vitamin A too slowly (see Chapter 4.3, "Serum Carotene"). Too much unconverted carotene then enters the patient's blood.[40]

IMPAIRED INTESTINAL MOTILITY

Disturbed motility is the most frequent and severe gastrointestinal effect of hypothyroidism.[9][10][11] The most frequent symptoms patients report are distention, flatulence, and constipation.

Goto et al. noted that in hypothyroidism, the patient may have megacolon (extreme dilation and hypertrophy of the colon) or severe constipation as in Hirschsprung's disease. They conducted a study of the effects of hypothyroidism and T$_4$ treatment on motility of the colon of rats. Hypothyroid rats had (1) impaired weight gain, (2) reduced daily stool volume, (3) dilation of the colon, (4) reduced anal canal pressure, (5) decreased frequency of rhythmic colonic activity, and (6) slowed transit time through the colon.[50]

The reduced basal electrical rhythm of the gastrointestinal tract in hypothyroid patients probably slows their gastrointestinal motility. The rhythm of activity of the duodenum varies with the level of thyroid activity.[6] A decrease in the basal rhythm of intestinal activity in hypothyroidism correlates well with the patients' reduced frequency of bowel movements.[7] The more severe the hypothyroidism, the weaker the patient's intestinal contractions. In severe hypothyroidism, the patient may develop paralytic ileus.[36] In many fatal cases of hypothyroidism, the patients had atonic bowels.[39]

Hypothyroid patients require less food than euthyroid individuals, and in general, the patients eat less than their euthyroid counterparts. The reduced food intake decreases peristaltic activity of their intestines, leading to constipation. The slowed transit time through the gastrointestinal tract enables bacteria to produce gas from food residue, causing persistent and troubling flatulent distention.[24,p.565]

IMPROPER TREATMENT FOLLOWING MISDIAGNOSIS

Javitt pointed out that when clinicians fail to recognize hypothyroidism, "diagnostic misadventure" can lead to unnecessary abdominal surgery.[30,p.870][31]

He wrote, "Thus cathartics and cleansing enemas may fail to remove feces that can mimic neoplastic filling defects on repeated barium examinations. The edema fluid has also been reported to be absorbed in excessive amounts and aggravate the tendency to fluid retention and hyponatremia (low sodium blood level) in advanced disease."[30,p.870][32] When serous fluid collects in the peritoneal cavity (ascites) in hypothyroidism, the clinician may make the erroneous diagnosis of abdominal tumor.[31][39]

Misdiagnosis of Irritable Bowel Syndrome

Thompson and Heaton wrote that clinicians often give the mildly hypothyroid patient with gastrointestinal dysfunction one of the most common diagnoses in gastroenterology practice: functional bowel disease, spastic colon, or irritable bowel syndrome—all variations of the same term.[38] The diagnosis is especially likely when the constipated patient also has lower abdominal pain due to flatulence. The clinician may prescribe bulking agents and tranquilizing, sedating, anticholinergic drugs.[37,pp.809-810]

Lake-Bakaar et al. reported observing 2 patients with functional bowel disease and elevated TSH levels whose bowel symptoms resolved after the patients began thyroid therapy. Over the next two years, the investigators screened 46 consecutive patients with functional bowel disease. They identified 4 with previously undiagnosed hypothyroidism. They gave the patients a battery of tests to rule out gastrointestinal pathology. All the patients responded well to thyroid hormone therapy. Lake-Bakaar wrote, "Hypothyroidism might be an important and treatable cause of functional bowel disease. Measurement of serum TSH should, therefore, be included in the work-up of all patients with functional bowel disease."[25] The serum basal TSH alone, however, is not sufficient for diagnosing hypothyroidism (see Chapter 4.2).

USE OF FIBER SUPPLEMENTS

Misdiagnosis often leads to a self-regulating measure—the use of supplemental fiber. I have seen many patients who used large quantities of bran and other forms of fiber to control constipation caused by undiagnosed hypothyroidism or euthyroid hypometabolism. After undergoing metabolic rehabilitation involving thyroid hormone, the same amount of supplemental fiber usually caused loose stools. To avoid this, the patients had to reduce or stop the supplements.

Hypothyroidism may cause abnormalities of the liver and pancreas. In the liver, the central vein may abnormally dilate and there may be pericentral scarring.[43] It is common to find abnormal liver enzyme values in patients with moderate-to-severe hypothyroidism. Liver failure, however, is rare.[45] The high serum amylase found in hypothyroid patients suggests mild chronic pancreatitis. According to Maclean et al., lowered body temperature is the likely mechanism because hypothermia is a cause of pancreatitis.[44]

"IRRITABLE BOWEL SYNDROME" IN HYPOTHYROIDISM

IBS due to hypothyroidism is a clinical phenotype of inadequate regulation of local gastrointestinal tissues and central nervous system tissues. The condition may be predominantly the constipation- or diarrhea-type.

Diarrhea-Type and Constipation-Type IBS

Some clinicians falsely believe that the only bowel feature of hypothyroidism is reduced motility and constipation. They also falsely believe that the only bowel feature of IBS is loose, watery stools. For these clinicians, the fact that a fibromyalgia patient has diarrhea-type IBS rules out the possibility of her having hypothyroidism. Such a distinction is only definitional, however, and is not legitimate: IBS can be either the diarrhea- or constipation-type, and the hypothyroid patient may suffer from either or both.

Thompson and Heaton conducted a study to learn the incidence of IBS in 301 otherwise healthy subjects. The subjects fell into one of three age categories: young, middle-aged, or elderly. Each group contained about 100 people with roughly equal numbers of males and females. *The investigators emphasized the heterogeneity of functional bowel disorders in their subjects.* Many subjects with the diagnosis of IBS had a diarrhea-type condition. However, 10.3% of the IBS subjects had significant constipation, defined as frequent straining at stool. In 6% of the subjects, mainly the elderly, constipation was painless.[2,p.287]

Cann reported a study of 63 IBS patients who answered a symptom questionnaire. Of those with moderate or worse symptoms, 23 reported diarrhea and 20 reported constipation. There is a tendency for some symptoms to predominate in one sex: diarrhea was more common in men, and constipation was more common in women.[8,p.70]

Constipation-type IBS closely resembles the con-

stipation of hypothyroidism. In patients with constipation-type IBS, gastric emptying time is slowed,[4,p.8] as it is in hypothyroid patients.[5] The constipation-type IBS patient has a slowed transit time through the small bowel,[4,p.8] as does the hypothyroid patient.[6][7] *The similarity is so close that IBS researchers screen to eliminate hypothyroid patients from their studies.* Some of the researchers make a dubious distinction, suggesting that constipation-type IBS is functional and constipation in hypothyroidism is organic.[8,p.68]

Goldin and Wengrower described a hypothyroid patient whose predominant symptom was chronic diarrhea. The result of a fasting breath hydrogen test was positive. This result suggested that the diarrhea resulted from bacterial overgrowth in her gastrointestinal system. Antibiotics successfully relieved the diarrhea. The clinicians wrote, "We conclude that bacterial overgrowth due to hypomotility may be the etiology of the diarrhea in such patients."[17] Unless this patient's hypothyroidism was effectively treated, it is likely that the bacterial overgrowth and diarrhea would reoccur after she stopped the antibiotic therapy.

Patel and Hughes described a 75-year-old man with severe hypothyroidism. His main symptom was intermittent diarrhea, bloating, and abdominal pain. His symptoms resolved with thyroid hormone therapy. The colonoscopic biopsy specimens the investigators took from the patient were consistent with chronic ischemia. They hypothesized that gross dilatation of his colon, due to his hypothyroidism, led to ischemia of the intestinal tissues. The ischemia was favorable to recurrent episodes of pseudo-membranous colitis. They wrote that the clinician should consider this unusual feature of hypothyroidism when a patient has diarrhea, bloating, and abdominal pain.[41]

According to Lake-Bakaar, the severity of IBS symptoms may vary with the severity of thyroid hormone deficiency. He wrote that severe hypothyroidism can produce gross constipation, megacolon and ileus. In less severe hypothyroidism, however, IBS symptoms may be far less severe. He observed two patients with IBS who had elevated TSH levels, indicating primary hypothyroidism. When the patients' use of exogenous thyroid hormone lowered their TSH levels to normal, the bowel symptoms resolved. He then screened 46 consecutive patients with IBS and found that 4 of them had previously undiagnosed hypothyroidism. He reported that in a small subset of IBS patients, hypothyroidism may be responsible for the bowel symptoms. He wrote, "These patients all respond well to thyroid hormone replacement therapy. The chronicity of the symptoms and the failure to respond to multiple other medications in the past argue against a placebo response."[25]

Some writers have reported constipation or gastrointestinal disturbance in euthyroid hypometabolic patients.[14][15] Some clinicians might diagnose these symptoms as IBS in these patients, especially if thyroid function test results show that the patients do not have primary hypothyroidism. In my clinical experience, patients with hypothyroid and euthyroid hypometabolic fibromyalgia are likely to have either the diarrhea- or constipation-type IBS. In both groups of patients, metabolic rehabilitation involving the use of exogenous thyroid hormone typically relieves the symptoms.

MECHANISMS OF IBS
IN HYPOTHYROIDISM

Constipation-Type IBS

Regarding gastrointestinal function in hypothyroid patients, Sellin et al. wrote, "the sluggish and slow response is characteristic of the myxedematous patients."[19,p.1156] According to Baker and Harvey, "The symptoms from the digestive system are essentially the expression of the slow rate at which the living machinery is turning over."[7]

Researchers have proposed several mechanisms for the sluggish intestinal activity in the gastrointestinal tract. These mechanisms include autonomic neuropathy, altered impulse transmission at myoneural junctions, and intestinal ischemia. Sellin and coauthors noted, however, that in hypothyroidism, intestinal tissue displays two important characteristics: (1) decreased electrical activity, and (2) failure to respond to bethanecol. (Bethanecol is a cholinergic drug used to treat paralytic ileus. The drug stimulates the smooth muscle lining of the bowel when it is hypomobile, as following surgery.[16,p.127]) These two phenomena strongly suggest a functional defect at the level of the intestinal muscle.[19,p.1157]

Slowed gastrointestinal motility in hypothyroid patients may result from reduced basal electrical rhythm of the tract. The electrical rhythm of the duodenum varies with the level of thyroid activity.[6] Also, a decreased basal rhythm in hypothyroidism correlates well with the patients' reduced frequency of bowel movements.[7] This mechanism makes sense when we consider that thyroid hormone regulates the electrical potential and, in turn, electrical rhythm of the gastrointestinal tract.

Cell membranes have a powerful sodium-potassi-um pump. The pump moves three sodium ions to the outside of the membranes for every two potassium ions it moves to the inside. As a result, each revolution of the pump removes a net of one positive charge from the interior of the cell to the outside. As a result, a positive charge develops outside the cell and a negative charge inside the cell (-80 to -90 μ volts at resting level). The difference in charge on the two sides of the membrane is the electrical potential. The pump is therefore electrogenic.[22,p.47][23,pp.32-36] In other words, by changing the composition of electrically charged ions between the intracellular and extracellular fluids, the pump creates an electrical potential across the cell membrane. The electrical potential is essential to nerve signal transmission and muscle contraction. Hypothyroidism reduces Na^+/K^+-ATPase activity. This reduces activity of the pump. As a result, nerve and muscle membranes do not polarize enough, and they discharge only sluggishly. The decreased activity of the electrogenic pump may be the main mechanism of depressed gastrointestinal function in hypothyroidism. Incidentally, it is partly through this mechanism that thyroid hormone generates body heat. The hormone stimulates activity of Na^+/K^+-ATPase in the liver, intestines, and other tissues. As the enzyme cleaves phosphate radicals from ATP molecules, converting them to ADP, part of the energy from the phosphate bond escapes as heat.[20][21]

Diarrhea-Type IBS

Diarrhea-type IBS in hypothyroid patients may result from bacteria overgrowth or ischemia-induced chronic colitis. The reports of Goldin and Wengrower[17] suggest that diarrhea-type IBS in hypothyroidism results from bacterial overgrowth from reduced intestinal motility.

In the case reported by Patel and Hughes (see above), diarrhea, bloating, and abdominal pain may not have resulted from bacterial overgrowth. Results from tests for clostridium difficile enterotoxin were variably positive and negative. Colon biopsy specimen findings suggested ischemia of the intestinal tissues. Patel and Hughes proposed that the ischemia was favorable to recurrent episodes of pseudo-membranous colitis. The patient's diarrhea may have resulted from the chronic colitis. The use of exogenous thyroid hormone relieved the patient's symptoms.[41]

Lu and Chou reported a hypothyroid woman who had severe secretory-type diarrhea. Systemic lupus erythematosus complicated her condition. She also had other severe conditions, including cystitis and an obstructive urinary tract condition. The diarrhea, cystitis, and urinary obstruction regressed with large doses of corticosteroids.[18] If this patient had colitis due to ischemia, as did the patient described by Patel and Hughes[41] (see above), the corticosteroid treatment would have relieved the patient's symptoms, at least transiently.

Contribution of Autonomic Nervous System Pathways to Constipation-Type and Diarrhea-Type IBS

Gervais Tougas wrote that immune and endocrine mechanisms enable communication between the brain and intestinal tract. In addition, he wrote that neural pathways enable communication along the brain-gut axis. The sympathetic and parasympathetic branches of the autonomic nervous system, through neural pathways, strongly contribute to the homeostasis of gut function. Studies have shown that different disorders of autonomic nervous system function are associated with different symptoms of functional bowel disorder. Patients whose symptoms result from slowed gastrointestinal motility (constipation) generally have two autonomic abnormalities: (1) decreased parasympathetic (vagal/cholinergic activity) outflow and (2) increased sympathetic outflow. Patients whose symptoms result from increased motility (loose stools and/or diarrhea) usually have (1) increased parasympathetic outflow and (2) decreased sympathetic outflow. Gervais Tougas noted that autonomic dysfunction may account for some common gastrointestinal complaints of fibromyalgia and chronic fatigue syndrome patients.[26]

Increased parasympathetic outflow and decreased sympathetic outflow may underlie diarrhea-like irritable bowel syndrome in fibromyalgia. The molecular mechanism of this autonomic imbalance may be the same that underlies bradycardia and hypotension (see Chapter 3.1, section titled "Bradycardia and Low Blood Pressure"): an increase in central nervous system α_2-adrenergic receptors due to inadequate thyroid hormone regulation of the α-adrenergic genes. Central nervous system α_2-adrenergic receptors can both reduce sympathetic outflow and increase parasympathetic nervous system outflow.[27][28]

AMPLIFICATION OF PERCEPTIONS OF GASTROINTESTINAL SENSATIONS BY ELEVATED SUBSTANCE P

Mayer and Gebhart proposed that in irritable bowel syndrome, the central nervous system may become sensitized to sensory signals reaching it from the abdominal viscera. Hyperalgesia would occur after the signals are processed through the dorsal horns and thalamus.[34] Fibromyalgia patients have elevated substance P in the central nervous system (see Chapter 3.19). Elevated substance P in the incoming dorsal roots of the spinal cord, which contain sensory fibers from viscera, might amplify the signals. After projection of the signals to the brain, the patient may perceive visceral pain or other abnormal visceral sensations. Such chemical/neural interaction in fibromyalgia may contribute to the patient's perception of abnormal gastrointestinal function.

REFERENCES

1. Wolfe, F.: Diagnosis of fibromyalgia. *J. Musculoskel. Med.*, 7:54, 1990.
2. Thompson, W.G. and Heaton, K.W.: Functional bowel disorders in apparently healthy people. *Gastroenterology*, 79(2):283-288, 1980.
3. Goldstein, J.A.: *Betrayal by the Brain*. New York, Haworth Medical Press, 1996.
4. Read, N.W.: Irritable bowel syndrome (IBS): definition and pathophysiology. *Scand. J. Gastroenter.*, 22:7-13, 1987.
5. Holdsworth, C.D. and Besser, G.M.: Influence of gastric emptying-rate and of insulin response on oral glucose tolerance in thyroid disease. *Lancet*, 2(7570):700-702, 1968.
6. Christensen, J., Clifton, J.A., and Schedl, H.P.: Variations in the frequency of the human duodenal basic electrical rhythm in health and disease. *Gastroenterology*, 51(2):200-206, 1966.
7. Baker, J.T. and Harvey, R.F.: Bowel habit in thyrotoxicosis and hypothyroidism. *Br. Med. J.*, 1(744):322-323, 1971.
8. Cann, P.A.: An approach to the design of therapeutic trials in IBS. *Scand. J. Gastroenterology*, 22:67-76, 1987.
9. Bacharach, T. and Evans, J.R.: Enlargement of the colon secondary to hypothyroidism. *Ann. Intern. Med.*, 47:121, 1957.
10. Brown, T.R.: The effect of hypothyroidism on gastric and intestinal function. *J.A.M.A.*, 97:511, 1971.
11. Lester, C.W.: Endocrine disturbances simulating surgical conditions of the abdomen. *NY State J. Med.*, 37:406, 1957.
12. Chun, A., Desautels, S., Slivka, A., Mitrani, C., Starz, T., DiLorenzo, C., and Wald, A.: Visceral algesia in irritable bowel syndrome, fibromyalgia, and sphincter of Oddi dysfunction, type III. *Dig. Dis. Sci.*, 44(3):631-636, 1999.
13. Holdsworth, C.D. and Besser, G.M.: Influence of gastric emptying-rate and of insulin response on oral glucose tolerance in thyroid disease. *Lancet*, 2:700-702, 1968.
14. Thurmon, F.M. and Thompson, W.O.: Low basal metabolism with myxedema. *Arch. Intern. Med.*, 46:879-897, 1930.
15. Goldberg, M.: Diagnosis of euthyroid hypometabolism.

Am. J. Obst. & Gynec., 81(5):1057-1058, 1961.

16. Gilman, A.G., Rall, T.W., Nies, A.S., and Taylor, P.: *The Pharmacological Basis of Therapeutics*, 8th edition. New York, Pergamon Press, 1990.

17. Goldin, E. and Wengrower, D.: Diarrhea in hypothyroidism: bacterial overgrowth as a possible etiology. *J. Clin. Gastroenterol.*, 12:98-99, 1990.

18. Lu, K.C. and Chou, C.T.: Systemic lupus erythematosus complicated with cystitis, obstructive uropathy and intractable diarrhea: report of a case. *Taiwan I Hsueh Hui Tsa Chih*, 90(7):700-704, 1991.

19. Sellin, J.H., Vassilopoulou-Sellin, R., and Lester, R.: The gastrointestinal tract and liver. In *The Thyroid*, 4th edition. Edited by S.C. Werner and S.H. Ingbar, N.Y., Harper and Row Publishers, 1987.

20. Liberman, A., Asano, Y., Lo, C., and Edelman, I.S.: Relationship between Na⁺ dependent respiration and thyroid hormone on rat jejunal mucosa. *Biophys. J.*, 27:127-144, 1979.

21. Edelman, I.S. and Ismail-Beigi, F.: Thyroid thermogenesis and active sodium transport. *Rec. Prog. Horm. Res.*, 30:235-237, 1974.

22. Guyton, A.C.: *Textbook of Medical Physiology*, 8th edition. Philadelphia, W.B. Saunders Co., 1991.

23. Schmidt, R.F.: *Fundamentals of Neurophysiology*, 3rd edition. New York, Springer-Verlag, 1985.

24. DeGroot, L.J., Larsen, P.R., Refetoff, S., and Stanbury, J.B.: *The Thyroid and Its Diseases*, 5th edition. New York, John Wiley & Sons, 1984.

25. Lake-Bakaar, G.: Hypothyroidism and functional bowel disease. *Amer. J. Med.*, 88(3):312-313, 1990.

26. Gervais Tougas, G.: The autonomic nervous system in functional bowel disorders. *Can. J. Gastroenterol.*, 13 (Suppl.A):15A-17A, 1999.

27. Connor, H.E., Drew, G.M., and Finch, L.: Clonidine-induced potentiation of reflex vagal bradycardia in anesthetized cats. *J. Pharm. Pharmacol.*, 34:22-26, 1982.

28. Kobinger, W.: Central α-adrenergic systems as targets for antihypertensive drugs. *Rev. Physiol. Biochem. Pharmacol.*, 81:39-100, 1978.

29. Scarpignato, C. and Pelosini, I.: Management of irritable bowel syndrome: novel approaches to the pharmacology of gut motility. *Can. J. Gastroenterol.*, 13(Suppl.A):50A-65A, 1999.

30. Javitt, S.B.: Gastrointestinal tract. In *The Thyroid*, 4th edition. Edited by S.C. Werner and S.H. Ingbar, New York, Harper and Row Publishers, 1987.

31. Haley, H.B., Leigh, C., Bronsky, D., and Waldstein, S.S.: Ascites and intestinal obstruction in myxedema. *Arch. Surg.*, 85:328-333, 1962.

32. Liechty, R.D., Miller, R.F., and Cohen, A.N.: Myxedema causing adynamic ileus, serous effusions and inappropriate secretion of antidiuretic hormone. *Surg. Clin. North Amer.*, 50:1087, 1970.

33. Watanakunakorn, C., Hodges, R.E., and Evans, T.C.: Myxedema. *Arch. Intern. Med.*, 116:183-190, 1965.

34. Myer, E.A. and Gebhart, G.F.: Functional bowel disorders and the visceral hyperalgesia hypothesis. In *Basic and Clinical Aspects of Chronic Abdominal Pain*. Edited by E.A. Mayer and H.E. Raybould. New York, Elsevier, 1993.

35. Wall, A.J., Middleton, W.R.J., and Pearse, A.G.E.: Intestinal mucosal hyperplasia following induced hyperthyroidism in the rat. (Abstract) *Virchows Arch.*, [Zellpathol], 6:79, 1970.

36. Boruchow, I.B., Miller, T.D., and Fitts, W.T., Jr.: Paralytic ileus in myxedema. *Arch. Surg.*, 92:960-963, 1966.

37. *The Merck Manual of Diagnosis and Therapy*, 15th edition. Edited by R. Berkow and A.J. Fletcher, Rahway, Merck, Sharp & Dohme Research Laboratories, 1987.

38. Thompson, W.G. and Heaton, K.W.: Functional bowel disorders in apparently normal people. *Gastroenterology*, 70:283-288, 1980.

39. Nickerson, J.F., Hill, S.R., Jr., McNeil, J.H., and Barker, S.B.: Fatal myxedema with and without coma. *J. Clin. Endocrinol. Metab.*, 53:475-493, 1960.

40. Escamilla, R.F.: Carotinemia in myxedema: explanation of the typical slightly icteric tint. *J. Clin. Endocrinol. Metab.*, 2:33, 1942.

41. Patel, R. and Hughes, R.W., Jr.: An unusual case of myxedema megacolon with features of ischemic and pseudomembranous colitis. *Mayo Clin. Proc.*, 67(4):369-372, 1992.

42. Gorard, D.A. and Farthing, M.J.: Intestinal motor function in irritable bowel syndrome. *Dig. Dis. Sci.*, 12:72-84, 1994.

43. Baker, A., Kaplan, M., and Wolfe, H.: Central congestive fibrosis of the liver in myxedema ascites. *Ann. Intern. Med.*, 77:927-929, 1972.

44. Maclean, D., Murison, J., and Griffiths, P.D.: Acute pancreatitis and diabetic ketoacidosis in accidental hypothermia and hypothermic myxedema. *Br. Med. J.*, 4:757, 1973.

45. Emerson, C.H., Liberman, C., and Braverman, L.E.: Hypothyroidism. In *The Thyroid*. Edited by W.L. Green, New York, Elsevier, 1987, p.243.

46. McIntyre, M.B. and Pemberton, J.H.: Pathophysiology of colonic motor disorders. *Surg. Clin. North Amer.*, 73(6):1225-1243, 1994.

47. Bentley, R.J. and Browne, R.J.S.: Paralytic ileus and dementia in a case of myxedema. *Postgrad. Med.*, 45:779, 1969.

48. Friedenwald, J. and Morrison, J.: Gastrointestinal disturbances associated with endocrinopathies. *Endocrinology*, 17:393, 1933.

49. Cohen, S.J.: Difficulty in swallowing as an early sign. *Clin. Pediatr.* (Phila.), 10(11):682, 1971.

50. Goto, S., Billmire, D.F., and Grosfeld, J.L.: Hypothyroidism impairs colonic motility and function: an experimental study in the rat. *Eur. J. Pediatr. Surg.*, 2(1):16-21, 1992.

51. Chang, L.: The association of functional gastrointestinal disorders and fibromyalgia. *Eur. J. Surg. Suppl.*, (583):32-36, 1998.

52. Diehl, D.L., Fullerton, S., and Mayer, E.A.: Functional bowel disease symptoms in patients with chronic fatigue syndrome (CFS): prevalence and quality of life. Presented at the American Gastroenterologic Association Digestive Disease Week, San Diego, May 14-17, 1995.

3.15

Pain

Fibromyalgia patients, like subsets of hypothyroid and thyroid hormone resistance patients, have chronic widespread pain and tenderness at multiple body sites. Normally, norepinephrine and serotonin, secreted by inhibitory neurons that descend from the brain stem to the dorsal horns of the spinal cord, decrease the flow of nociceptive signals into the central nervous system (CNS). The serotonin concentration of the cerebrospinal fluid of fibromyalgia patients was not significantly low. In addition, antidepressant medications that sustain the presence of serotonin in neuronal synapses are ineffective as fibromyalgia treatments. Therefore, it is highly unlikely that a deficiency of serotonin, at least in the CNS, is involved in the widespread pain and tenderness of fibromyalgia patients.

Researchers found that the metabolite of norepinephrine was low in the cerebrospinal fluid of patients. This points to two factors (both resulting from inadequate regulation by thyroid hormone) that may be responsible for impaired CNS pain modulation in fibromyalgia: (1) a low cerebrospinal concentration of norepinephrine, probably due to inadequate thyroid hormone regulation of the adrenergic genes in the CNS (see Chapter 3.1), and (2) high substance P levels, due to inadequate thyroid hormone transcription regulation of the preprotachykinin gene that codes for preprotachykinin-A (the precursor of substance P) and the substance P receptor (see Chapter 3.19).

Several studies have shown that correcting inadequate thyroid hormone regulation of cell function through the use of exogenous thyroid hormone during metabolic rehabilitation relieves the widespread pain and the tenderness of fibromyalgia.

Chronic, widespread pain, along with tenderness at certain anatomic sites, distinguishes fibromyalgia from other syndrome classifications. The view I express in this book is that pain is the symptom that distinguishes fibromyalgia as one phenotypic expression of hypothyroidism or thyroid hormone resistance.

● PAIN IN FIBROMYALGIA

According to the 1990 ACR criteria, for a patient to receive the diagnosis of fibromyalgia, she must have chronic, widespread pain, and tenderness at 11 of 18 potential tender point sites.[1] The criteria, as formulated by the ACR committee, do not permit precise, quantitative evaluation of the patient's fibromyalgia status. Because metabolic rehabilitation, as I describe it in this book, is highly effective in enabling patients to markedly improve or completely recover from fibromyalgia, I found it necessary to modify the ACR criteria in such as way as to permit quantitative evaluations of changing patient status during the treatment. I explain the modifications in Chapter 4.1.

Wolfe reported that 97.6% of fibromyalgia patients have widespread pain. He also reported that 52.8% of fibromyalgia patients complain of headaches.[32]

● PAIN IN HYPOTHYROIDISM

In 1979, Beetham wrote, "Myxedema can also cause diffuse aching and stiffness and should be ruled out by appropriate blood tests."[2,p.438] His statement echos those of many other medical writers.[3][4][5][6][7][8][9][10][11][12][13][14] Most of these writers noted the similarity of "rheumatic"-like symptoms of many hypothyroid patients to those of "fibrositis" or fibromyalgia patients. Other writers have described muscle and joint pains in euthyroid hypometabolic patients.[10][16][17]

My colleagues and I have found, through laboratory evidence, that most fibromyalgia patients are either hypothyroid or thyroid hormone resistant.[18][19] Most of both the hypothyroid and thyroid hormone resistant patients have recovered with metabolic rehabilitation including the use of exogenous thyroid hormone. This form of therapy has dramatically relieved their pain and tenderness. The effectiveness of the protocol in relieving patients' pain and tenderness among other symptoms has been documented in several open but systematic trials[20][21][22][25] and in several controlled studies.[23][24][26] One follow-up study showed that the improved or eliminated pain and tenderness have persisted throughout a 1-to-5 year time frame after treatment began.[27]

HEADACHES

Some writers report headaches as a symptom of euthyroid hypometabolism.[16][29] Thurman and Thompson reported headaches among the symptoms of nervous, worrying, easily fatigued patients who had low BMRs but showed no evidence of hypothyroidism.[16,p.883] Thompson and Thompson mentioned patients with low BMRs who had headaches, as well as dizziness, weakness, chronic fatigue and nervousness.[29,p.495] Some patients included in these latter two reports may have been hypothyroid, since laboratory thyroid function tests were not available then to distinguish hypothyroid from euthyroid hypometabolic patients. None of the investigations of hypothyroid symptoms I have had access to have reported the incidence of headaches. The symptom has certainly been common, however, among the hypothyroid fibromyalgia patients Honeyman-Lowe[30] and I[31] have treated.

● POSSIBLE PAIN MECHANISMS IN HYPOTHYROIDISM

For most patients, fibromyalgia is a clinical phenotype of inadequate thyroid hormone regulation of cell function in which central pain modulation is impaired. Several mechanisms may be involved in mediating the pain.

IMPAIRED CNS PAIN MODULATION SYSTEM

Serotonin and norepinephrine strongly influence pain perception.[33] They do so by indirectly decreasing the flow of nociceptive nerve signals from the dorsal horns of the spinal cord to the brain. (See Figure 3.15.1.) Researchers found the concentration of norepinephrine in the cerebrospinal fluid of fibromyalgia patients to be significantly low. However, the concentration of the metabolite of serotonin was not significantly low.[34] The finding of normal cerebrospinal concentrations of the metabolite of serotonin is a serious blow to the serotonin deficiency hypothesis of fibromyalgia. Even with a normal concentration of serotonin, a low concentration of norepinephrine would be expected to enhance pain perception and to lower the fibromyalgia patient's pain threshold.

Mense assessed the hypothesis that a dysfunction of the descending antinociceptive system underlies fibromyalgic pain. He noted that animal studies show that interruption of the system by spinal cord cooling results in: (1) an increase in ongoing pain, (2) lowering of stimulation threshold, and (3) an increase in the magnitude of responses to stimulation of nociceptive dorsal horn neurons. The descending inhibitory system more strongly modulates responses to input from deep tissue nociceptors than to input from skin nociceptors. Mense wrote that if similar changes occur in fibromyalgia patients, we can expect that impairment of the tonically active descending system should result in several changes: (1) spontaneous or ongoing pain, (2) tenderness (lowering of the pain threshold to mechanical stimuli), and (3) hyperalgesia (increased responsiveness to noxious stimuli). These changes, he concluded, should affect mainly pain signals arising primarily from deep tissues.[42]

Norepinephrine and Serotonin

A system of neurons that secrete norepinephrine descends from the brain stem to the dorsal horns of the spinal cord. When these noradrenergic neurons secrete norepinephrine in the dorsal horns, the neurotransmitter sets off a sequence of chemical events that cause dorsal horn neurons to secrete opiates.[35][36] The opiates hyperpolarize the incoming terminals of sensory fibers, inducing analgesia. Impaired CNS pain modulation in fibromyalgia probably results from two factors: (1) a low cerebrospinal fluid concentration of norepinephrine,[34] probably due to inadequate thyroid hormone regulation of the adrenergic genes in the CNS (see Chapter 3.1), and (2) high cerebrospinal fluid concentration of substance P (which facilitates the flow of nociceptive signals into the dorsal horns), due to inadequate thyroid hormone transcription regulation of the preprotachykinin gene that codes for preprotachykinin-A (the precursor of substance P) and the substance P receptor (see Chapter 3.19).

Neurons that secrete serotonin also descend from the brain stem to the dorsal horns of the spinal cord.[37] When these neurons release serotonin and it reaches dorsal horn neurons, the serotonin sustains opiate secretion by interneurons. The opiates inhibit the ability of dorsal horn neurons to transmit nociceptive signals. Also, when researchers apply serotonin directly to the spinal cord, analgesia results. In addition, drugs that block the reuptake of serotonin (which sustains opiate secretion) are antinociceptive in most humans.[38] Serotonin levels were not significantly low in the cerebrospinal fluid of fibromyalgia patients.[34] Also, medications that sustain the presence of serotonin in neuronal synapses are ineffective as fibromyalgia treatments (see Chapter 5.1, section titled "Antidepressant Drugs"). Therefore, it is highly unlikely that a deficiency of serotonin, at least in the CNS, is involved in the widespread pain and tenderness of fibromyalgia patients.

There is much evidence, however, that any serotonin abnormalities found in fibromyalgia may be related to inadequate thyroid hormone regulation. Synthesis and turnover of serotonin is decreased in hypothyroid neonatal animals and increased in hyperthyroid animals,[43][44][45] and central serotonin function is decreased in hypothyroidism.[48][49][50] Thyroxine has been shown to increase serotonin levels in rat skin and ilium,[46] and urinary levels of 5-HIAA were found to increase in thyrotoxicosis and decrease in hypothyroidism.[47]

Tóth and Csaba measured the serotonin levels, minus the blood serotonin content, in brain stems of rabbits that had either been thyroidectomized or fed thyroxine. Brain stem serotonin increased in thyroxine treated rabbits 56.5% and decreased in thyroidectomized animals 21.7%. Blood content of serotonin increased by the same amount in thyroxine-treated rabbits, but decreased markedly more in the thyroidectomized group. *The researchers proposed that peripheral symptoms of hyperthyroidism and hypothyroidism are in part the effects of thyroid hormone on the central nervous system metabolism of tryptophan*

and serotonin.[51]

Thyroid hormone regulates serotonin synthesis in the brain partly through controlling the concentration of the serotonin precursor tryptophan. Jacoby and coworkers[40] administered to hypothyroid rats a chemical that inhibits 5-hydroxytryptophan decarboxylase, the enzyme that removes a carboxyl (COOH) group from 5-hydroxytryptophan, converting it to serotonin.[15,pp.343-344] This procedure caused the accumulation of 5-hydroxytryptophan. Rats in the hypothyroid state accumulated this serotonin precursor at a lower rate than controls. After treatment with enough T_4 to induce hyperthyroidism, 5-hydroxytryptophan accumulated at a rate greater than would be expected merely from administration of the decarboxylase inhibitor.[40] This implies that thyroid hormone exerts an influence on brain tryptophan levels. (See Chapter 3.1, sections titled "Serotonin" and "Pain," and Chapter 2.3 section titled "Serotonin" and subsection titled "Thyroid Hormone Status and Serotonin.")

Low norepinephrine levels in the cerebrospinal fluid due to inadequate thyroid hormone regulation of the adrenergic genes in the CNS also affect serotonin. A recent study by Archer et al. shows the importance of low CNS norepinephrine levels. They found that depleting spinal norepinephrine reversed and/or abolished the analgesic effects of serotonin agonists during three measures of pain. They concluded that spinal norepinephrine exerts an important tonic modulating effect on the function of the descending serotonergic pathway.[41]

Dorsal Horns of the Spinal Cord. The serotonin- and norepinephrine-secreting neurons that descend from the brain stem release these neurotransmitters at two sites in the dorsal horns (see Figure 3.15.1). First, they contact the dendrites of neurons in the spinothalamic tracts. Spinothalamic tract neurons conduct signs from the dorsal horns to the thalamus and cortex of the brain. When spinothalamic neurons transmit signals from the dorsal horns to these structures, the individual perceives pain. These signals can be inhibited, however, by the serotonin- and norepinephrine-secreting neurons that contact the spinothalamic neurons.

Second, the descending neurons contact interneurons in the dorsal horns. (Interneurons conduct signals between two or more neurons in the spinal cord.) The descending neurons also inhibit transmission between these interneurons. The serotonin and norepinephrine secreted by the descending neurons cause the interneurons to secrete enkephalin and dynorphin. Enkephalin and dynorphin are opioid substances that have potent analgesic effects.

The interneurons secrete these opioids near the terminals of two types of sensory fibers: (1) those that conduct nociceptive signals into the spinal cord from peripheral parts of the body, such as muscle, and (2) those that receive these nociceptive signals. Once secreted, enkephalin and dynorphin appear to inhibit sensory neurons from bringing noxious signals into the dorsal horns from the peripheral tissues; that is, the opioids block the transmission of noxious signals from incoming sensory neurons to interneurons and spinothalamic neurons.

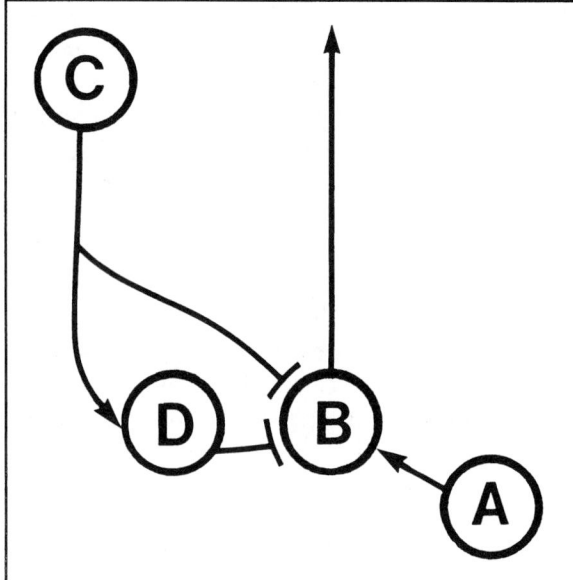

Figure 3.15.1. Primary sensory nerves (A) transmit nociceptive sensory signals (those that can give rise to the perception of pain) into the dorsal horns of the spinal cord. In the dorsal horns, the sensory nerves release chemicals such as glutamate and substance P. These chemicals induce spinothalamic nerves (B) to conduct the signals to the brain where they influence pain perception. Descending nerve fibers (C) release serotonin and norepinephrine in the dorsal horns. These neurotransmitter chemicals directly inhibit spinothalamic nerves (B). They also stimulate interneurons (D) to release opiates that in turn inhibit spinothalamic nerves. Serotonin and norepinephrine thus inhibit the transmission of nociceptive nerve signals to the brain.[28]

The opioids accomplish this "blocking" effect by inhibiting the release of several neurotransmitter substances from sensory neurons. Among these are glutamate and substance P. Enkephalin and dynorphin inhibit release of these transmitters from a sensory neuron when they bind to opiate receptors stationed on the sensory neurons. The binding of an opiate to its receptor triggers either or both of two phenomena: decreased calcium flow into the sensory nerve ending,

or increased potassium flow into the neuron. Increased potassium flow into the sensory neuron hyperpolarizes the neuron and makes it more difficult for the neuron to depolarize. The neuron's firing rate decreases, and this reduces the number of signals that reach the brain.[39,pp.396-397]

This blocking action—a result of serotonin and norepinephrine stimulating opiate release, with effects on calcium and potassium flow—when working well, provides an individual with normal pain perception. When the system is faulty, as during inadequate thyroid hormone regulation of the pain-modulating system, too many nociceptive signals reach the brain. As a result, the person has a heightened perception of pain. She may feel pain from sensory stimuli that ordinarily would not be considered "painful." The pressure on a body part from lying still for more than a few minutes may be painful to someone with a faulty pain-modulating system. This appears to be the plight of the fibromyalgia patient.

Familiarity with this pain control system and possible faults with it is important to understanding fibromyalgic pain. In years past, it was reasonable to hypothesize that the use of antidepressant medications would improve patients' fibromyalgia status by influencing this system. Once dorsal horn neurons secrete serotonin and norepinephrine into synapses between interneurons, various antidepressant medications slow the rate at which the neurons remove the transmitters from the synapses. The increased amounts of serotonin and norepinephrine left in the synapses are expected to increase the amounts of opioids that local interneurons release. The lack of pain relief from use of these medications by fibromyalgia patients is legend and has been confirmed (see Chapter 5.1, section titled "Antidepressants"). Because the use of the proper form and dosage of thyroid hormone, as a part of metabolic rehabilitation, relieves most fibromyalgia patients' pain and tenderness, it is highly likely that inadequate thyroid hormone regulation is the underlying mechanism.

REFERENCES

1. Wolfe, F., Smythe, H.A., Yunus, M.B., et al.: The American College of Rheumatology 1990 criteria for the classification of fibromyalgia: report of the multicenter criteria committee. *Arthritis Rheumatol.*, 33:160-172, 1990.
2. Beetham, W.P., Jr.: Diagnosis and management of fibrositis syndrome and psychogenic rheumatism. *Med. Clin. North Am.*, 63:433-439, 1979.
3. Alajouanine, T. and Nick, J.: De l'existence d'une myopathie d'origine hypothyroidienne. *Paris Med.*, 35:346, 1945.

4. Wilson, J. and Walton, J.N.: Some muscular manifestations of hypothyroidism. *J. Neurol. Neurosurg. Psychiat.*, 22:320-324, 1959.

5. Bergouignan, M., Vital, C., and Bataille, J.M.: Les myopathies hypothyroidiennes: aspects cliniques et histopathologiques. *Presse Med.*, 75:1551, 1967.

6. Fessel, W.J.: Myopathy of hypothyroidism. *Ann. Rheumatic Dis.*, 27:590-596, 1968.

7. Golding, D.N.: Hypothyroidism presenting with musculoskeletal symptoms. *Ann. Rheum. Dis.*, 29:10-14, 1970.

8. Wilke, W.S., Sheeler, L.R., and Makarowski, W.S.: Hypothyroidism with presenting symptoms of fibrositis. *J. Rheumat.*, 8:627-630, 1981.

9. Delamere, J.P., Scott, D.L., and Felix-Davies, D.D.: Thyroid dysfunction and rheumatic diseases. *J. Royal Soc. Med.*, 75:102,1982.

10. Sonkin, L.S.: Endocrine disorders and muscle dysfunction. In *Clinical Management of Head, Neck, and TMJ Pain and Dysfunction*. Edited by B. Gelb, Philadelphia, W.B. Saunders Co., 1985, pp.137-170.

11. Awad, E.A.: Pathological changes in fibromyalgia. *First International Symposium on Myofascial Pain and Fibromyalgia*. Minneapolis, Minnesota, May 9, 1989.

12. Awad, E.A.: Histopathological changes in fibrositis. In *Advances in Pain Research and Therapy*, Vol.17. Edited by J.R. Fricton and E.A. Awad, New York, Raven Press, Ltd., 1990, pp.249-258.

13. Aarflot, T. and Bruusgaard, D.: Association of chronic widespread musculoskeletal complaints and thyroid autoimmunity. Results from a community survey. *Scand. J. Prim. Health Care*, 14(2):111-115, 1996.

14. Rodolico, C., Toscano, A., Benvenga, S., et al.: Myopathy as the persistently isolated symptomatology of primary autoimmune hypothyroidism. *Thyroid*, 8(11):1033-1038, 1998.

15. Cooper, J.R., Bloom, F.E., and Roth, R.H.: *The Biochemical Basis of Neuropharmacology*, 6th edition. New York, Oxford University Press, 1991.

16. Thurmon, F.M. and Thompson, W.O.: Low basal metabolism with myxedema. *Arch. Intern. Med.*, 46:879-897, 1930.

17. Goldberg, M.: Diagnosis of euthyroid hypometabolism. *Amer. J. Obst. & Gynec.*, 81(5):1053-1058, 1961.

18. Lowe, J.C.: Thyroid status of 38 fibromyalgia patients: implications for the etiology of fibromyalgia. *Clin. Bull. Myofascial Ther.*, 2(1):47-64, 1997.

19. Lowe, J.C., Reichman, A., Honeyman, G.S., and Yellin, J.: Thyroid status of fibromyalgia patients. (Abstract) *Clin. Bull. Myofascial Ther.*, 3(1):69-70, 1998.

20. Lowe, J.C., Eichelberger, J., Manso, G., and Peterson, K.: Improvement in euthyroid fibromyalgia patients treated with T_3. *J. Myofascial Ther.*, 1(2):16-29, 1994.

21. Lowe, J.C.: T_3-induced recovery from fibromyalgia by a hypothyroid patient resistant to T_4 and desiccated thyroid. *J. Myofascial Ther.*, 1(4):26-31, 1995.

22. Lowe, J.C.: Results of an open trial of T_3 therapy with 77 euthyroid female fibromyalgia patients. *Clin. Bull. Myofascial Ther.*, 2(1):35-37, 1997.

23. Lowe, J.C., Garrison, R., Reichman, A., Yellin, J., Thompson, M., and Kaufman, D.: Effectiveness and safety of T_3 therapy for euthyroid fibromyalgia: a double-blind, place-bo-controlled response-driven crossover study, *Clin. Bull. Myofascial Ther.*, 2(2/3):31-57, 1997.

24. Lowe, J.C., Reichman, A., and Yellin, J.: The process of change during T_3 treatment for euthyroid fibromyalgia: a double-blind placebo-controlled crossover study. *Clin. Bull. Myofascial Ther.*, 2(2/3):91-124, 1997.

25. Honeyman, G.S.: Metabolic therapy for hypothyroid and euthyroid fibromyalgia: two case reports. *Clin. Bull. Myofascial Ther.*, 2(4):19-49, 1997.

26. Lowe, J.C., Garrison, R., Reichman, A., and Yellin, J.: Triiodothyronine (T_3) treatment of euthyroid fibromyalgia: a small-n replication of a double-blind placebo-controlled crossover study. *Clin. Bull. Myofascial Ther.*, 2(4):71-88, 1997.

27. Lowe, J.C., Reichman, A., and Yellin, J.: A case-control study of metabolic therapy for fibromyalgia: long-term follow-up comparison of treated and untreated patients. (Abstract) *Clin. Bull. Myofascial Ther.*, 3(1):23-24, 1998.

28. Lowe, J.C. and Honeyman-Lowe, G.: Facilitating the decrease in fibromyalgic pain during metabolic rehabilitation: an essential role for soft tissue therapies. *J. Bodywork Movem. Ther.*, 2(4):208-217, 1998.

29. Thompson, W.O. and Thompson, P.K.: Low basal metabolism following thyrotoxicosis. *J. Clin. Invest.*, 5:471-501, 1928.

30. Honeyman-Lowe, G.: Personal communication. January 11, 1998.

31. Lowe, J.C.: A case of debilitating headache complicated by hypothyroidism: its relief through myofascial therapy. *Dig. Chir. Econ.*, 31:73-75, Nov/Dec 1988.

32. Wolfe, F.: Diagnosis of fibromyalgia. *J. Musculoskel. Med.*, 7:54, 1990.

33. Lowe, J.C.: Loss of central pain control in fibromyalgia patients. *J. Myofascial Ther.*, 1(2):9-10, 1994.

34. Russell, I.J., Vaeroy, H., Javors, M., and Nyberg, F.: Cerebrospinal fluid biogenic amine metabolites in fibromyalgia/fibrositis syndrome and rheumatoid arthritis. *Arthritis Rheum.*, 35:550-556, 1992.

35. Dubner, R. and Bennett, G.J.: Spinal and trigeminal mechanisms of nociception. *Ann. Rev. Neurosci.*, 6:381, 1983.

36. Hammond, D.L.: Pharmacology of central pain-modulating networks (biogenic amines and nonopioid analgesics). In *Advances in Pain Research and Therapy*, Vol. 9. Edited by H.L. Fields, R. Dubner, and F. Cervero, New York, Raven Press, 1985, pp.499-511.

37. Hammond, D.L.: Control systems for nociceptive afferent processing: the descending inhibitory pathways. In *Spinal Afferent Processing*. Edited by T.L. Yaksh, New York, Plenum Press, 1986, pp.363-390.

38. Fields, H.L.: Neural mechanisms of opiate analgesia. In *Advances in Pain Research and Therapy*, Vol. 9. Edited by H.L. Fields, R. Dubner, and F. Cervero, New York, Raven Press, 1985, pp.479-486.

39. Jessell, T.M. and Kelly, D.D.: Pain and analgesia. In *Principles of Neural Science*, 3rd edition. Edited by E.R. Kandel, J.H. Schwartz, and T.M. Jessell, Norwalk, Appleton & Lange, 1991, pp.385-399.

40. Jacoby, J.K., Mueller, G., and Wurtman, R.J.: Thyroid state and brain monoamine metabolism. *Endocrinology*, 97:1332-1335, 1975.

41. Archer, T., Arwestrem, E., Jonsson, G., Minor, G., and

Post, C.: Noradrenergic-serotonergic interactions and nociception in the rat. *Eur. J. Pharmac.*, 120:295-307, 1986.

42. Mense, S.: Descending antinociception and fibromyalgia. *Z. Rheumatol.*, 57(Suppl.2):23-26, 1998.

43. Seo, H., Vassart, G., Bocas, H., and Refetoff, S.: Triiodothyronine stimulates specifically growth hormone in RNA in rat pituitary tumor cells. *Proc. Natl. Acad. Sci.* (USA), 74:2054-2058, 1977.

44. Tata, J.R., Ernster, L., and Lindberg, O.: The action of thyroid hormones at the cell level. *Biochem. J.*, 86:408-428, 1963.

45. Dillmann, W.H., Mendecki, J., and Koerner, D.: Triiodothyronine (T_3) stimulated formation of poly(A)-containing nuclear RNA and mRNA in rat liver. *Endocrinology*, 102:568-575, 1978.

46. Samuels, H.H., Tsai, J.S., and Casanova, J.: Thyroid hormone action: *in vitro* demonstration of putative receptors in isolated nuclei and soluble nuclear extracts. *Science*, 184:1188-1191, 1974.

47. Nakamura, M., Hamada, S., and Imura, M.: Sequential changes in rat liver nuclear triiodothyronine receptors and mitochondrial alpha-glycerophosphate dehydrogenase activity after administration of triiodothyronine. *Biochem. J.*, 182:377-382, 1979.

48. Savard, P., Merand, Y., Paolo, T.D., and Dupont, A.: Effect of neonatal hypothyroidism on the serotonin system of the rat brain. *Brain Res.*, 292:99-108, 1984.

49. Vaccari, A.: Decreased central serotonin function in hypothyroidism. *Eur. J. Pharmacol.*, 82:93-95, 1982.

50. Singhal, R.L., Rastogi, R.B., and Hedina, P.D.: Brain biogenic amines and altered thyroid function. *Life Sci.*, 17:1617-1626, 1975.

51. Tóth, S. and Csaba, B.: The effect of thyroid hormone on 5-hydroxytryptamine (5-HT) level of brain stem and blood in rabbits. *Experientia*, 22:755-756, 1966.

3.16

Paresthesia

Paresthesia, or abnormal sensation, is a common symptom of fibromyalgia patients, as it is of hypothyroid patients. Fibromyalgia patients experience a variety of abnormal sensations. The most common abnormal sensation is widespread pain, the subject of Chapter 3.15. Other common abnormal sensations of fibromyalgia patients are numbness, tingling, itching, burning, prickling, and lightening-like bolts of pain.

In one study, fibromyalgic women had a higher incidence of carpal tunnel syndrome than women in the population at-large. Carpal tunnel syndrome is an abnormality of a single nerve (mononeuropathy), the median nerve. Hypothyroid patients also have a high rate of carpal tunnel syndrome. The syndrome in most patients results from compression of the median nerve as it passes through the wrist. The compression in hypothyroid patients is caused by myxedematous swelling of the ligament around the wrist called the flexor retinaculum. The retinaculum is a strong fibrous band around the wrist and binds down the flexor tendons of the fingers and thumb. A minority of fibromyalgia patients have myxedema virtually identical to that of hypothyroid patients. This finding, shown on biopsies and in clinical experience, makes it likely that carpal tunnel syndrome in some fibromyalgia patients results from myxedema caused by inadequate thyroid hormone regulation of fibroblasts.

No studies of fibromyalgia patients are available to compare the incidence of nerve dysfunction and polyneuropathy with the incidence of these in hypothyroid patients.

Paresthesia in patients with inadequate thyroid hormone regulation of cell function may result from at least four mechanisms. First, paresthesia may be related in some way to the EMG-verified slow conduction rate of nerves and the slow relaxation of muscle

after contractions. Researchers have found that hypothyroid, euthyroid hypometabolic, and fibromyalgia patients have slow muscle relaxation after contractions. Second, axonal degeneration, found in muscle biopsies from hypothyroid patients, may account for some abnormal sensation. Third, myxedema, which a minority of hypothyroid and fibromyalgia patients have, may produce paresthesia by mechanically compressing nerves and thereby causing them to dysfunction. Fourth, myofascial trigger points due to muscle hypometabolism may refer abnormal sensation.

In my clinical experience, most patients describe their abnormal sensations as numbness and tingling. Others, however, have described a perception of burning. Although the subjective swelling some patients describe may be paresthesia, the perception may result from mild myxedematous connective tissue swelling (see Chapter 3.3). Paresthesia in hypothyroid and euthyroid fibromyalgia patients has improved or disappeared upon treatment with metabolic rehabilitation.[24][35][36][37][38]

● PARESTHESIA IN FIBROMYALGIA

PREVALENCE

In 1989, Wolfe wrote that paresthesia was among features of fibromyalgia that are present in more than 25% of cases.[38] In 1990, he specified that 62.8% of fibromyalgia patients reported paresthesias.[14] Other authors have stated of paresthesia that it "sometimes occurs" in fibromyalgia.[39] Simms and Goldenberg, in

1988, provided a detailed study of paresthesia in fibromyalgia. They included 161 fibromyalgia patients in their retrospective study. They found that 84% had complained of numbness or tingling at their initial evaluations. Most reported either bilateral upper extremity paresthesia or upper and lower extremity paresthesia. The investigators reported that none of the patients had concurrent diseases of which peripheral neuropathy is a feature. Of 36 patients with paresthesia who had undergone electromyography, 32 had normal results. At a mean of 25 months after the initial evaluations, 57 of the 161 patients underwent a second evaluation. Of these, 56 reported still having paresthesia. Simms and Goldenberg concluded, "Paresthesias are common in fibromyalgia and may mimic a neurologic disorder, although objective abnormalities are rare. Judicious use of neurodiagnostic tests is therefore indicated in the clinical setting of fibromyalgia."[40]

CARPAL TUNNEL SYNDROME: A MONONEUROPATHY IN FIBROMYALGIA

Perez-Ruiz et al. reported a high prevalence of undetected carpal tunnel syndrome among fibromyalgia patients. The investigators assessed the prevalence of carpal tunnel syndrome in 206 consecutive female fibromyalgia patients. The researchers used electromyography and nerve conduction velocity testing to assess 60 patients with dermatomal paresthesia. (A dermatome is an area of skin innervated by skin branches of a single spinal nerve. Not all dermatomal areas are anatomically clear cut; some overlap.) In 33 of the 60 patients (55%), findings were diagnostic for carpal tunnel syndrome. (These 33 patients are 16% of the 206 patients with dermatomal paresthesia.) Clinicians had previously diagnosed only 2 of the 33 patients as having carpal tunnel syndrome. The investigators noted that the incidence of carpal tunnel syndrome in the general population of women is 10.2%. Although the 16% in this study was higher, the difference was not statistically significant. They concluded that carpal tunnel syndrome in women fibromyalgia patients is as common as in the female population at-large. They also pointed out that the prevalence of undiagnosed carpal tunnel syndrome in the female fibromyalgia population is larger than in the general population. Because of this, they wrote that nerve conduction studies may be necessary to identify fibromyalgic women with dermatomal paresthesia due to carpal tunnel syndrome.[44]

ELECTROMYOGRAPHY (EMG) IN FIBROMYALGIA

The electrophysiological studies done on fibromyalgia patients have focused on muscle. I can find no published studies distinguishing the role of nerve dysfunction from that of muscle. In one study, 4 of 36 fibromyalgia patients with paresthesia had abnormal EMG results typical of neuropathy.[40] This one study is not sufficient for us to compare the prevalence of EMG abnormalities among fibromyalgia patients with that among hypothyroid patients.

Kraft et al. reported that EMG tests showed that the resting muscles of fibrositis patients were electrically silent.[67] Bengtsson reported the same result on EMG tests. She also reported another finding: When she electrically stimulated the adductor pollicis muscles of fibromyalgia patients, the force of muscle contraction was the same as in normal controls.[69] Stokes et al. reported the same finding of normal muscle strength when they tested fibromyalgia patients and controls. The investigators reported that the patients, who had fatigue and musculoskeletal pain, had "effort syndrome." Their muscle contractions were subnormal during voluntary efforts to contract the muscles, but their muscle contracted normally upon electrical stimulation.[68] Most of the patients in these studies were considered to have "fibrositis." We must temper interpretations of these results with the thought that some patients may not have met the criteria we use today to diagnose fibromyalgia. Bennett wrote of the study results: "These findings suggest a normal contractility of skeletal muscle and imply that the impaired performance during voluntary activity is due to a central mechanism, possibly lack of motivation, pain, or fear of pain—or in rare cases reflex inhibition due to afferent activity in relatively asymptomatic arthropathy."[66,p.56]

Contrasting with the results of the studies cited above are the results of a more recent study by Sprott et al. They used surface electrodes to test the EMG activity of the lumbar erector spinae muscles of fibromyalgia patients and controls. The researchers used mapping with a 16-channel EMG technique to distinguish any difference between muscle activity in fibromyalgia patients and the controls. Analysis showed that muscles of fibromyalgia patients (when the muscles were at rest) had higher EMG activity than muscles in control subjects. The differences in EMG activity of resting muscles in individual fibromyalgia patients were greater than the differences in controls.

During flexion of the upper body, the lumbar muscles of fibromyalgia patients had lower EMG activity than those of control subjects. The researchers concluded that fibromyalgia patients have increased EMG activity of the lumbar muscles at rest. They also concluded that the EMG activity of the lumbar muscles during flexion is lower than normal. This finding suggests that either (1) the alpha motor nerve supply to the muscles was lower than normal or (2) the muscles had a subnormal responsiveness to normal alpha motor innervation. The researchers noted a lower-than-normal mobility of the lumbar spinal region of fibromyalgia patients.[21]

In another study, Elert found that the muscle of fibromyalgia patients, after multiple contractions, did not return to resting EMG levels at a normal rate; that is, the muscle had a delayed relaxation time.[43] This finding corresponds to the delayed relaxation of muscle after stimulation in hypothyroid patients (see sections below titled "'Irritability' of Muscle in Hypothyroidism" and "Slowed Muscle Relaxation in Hypothyroidism").

RESTLESS LEG SYNDROME IN FIBROMYALGIA

Paresthesia is a feature of restless leg syndrome. I have found no published studies of the syndrome among fibromyalgia patients. However, a minority of my fibromyalgia patients have had restless leg syndrome. Uncomfortable paresthesia was one of their symptoms. Goldstein wrote that chronic fatigue syndrome patients and fibromyalgia patients commonly have restless leg syndrome and periodic limb movements during sleep. He also noted that the patients have dysesthesia in both legs and have uncontrollable urges to move them.[55,pp.61-62]

● PREVALENCE OF PARESTHESIA IN HYPOTHYROIDISM AND EUTHYROID HYPOMETABOLISM

PREVALENCE

Paresthesia often represents diffuse involvement of the peripheral nervous system in hypothyroidism.[1,p.1029] However, paresthesia may be largely isolated to anatomical regions. Some hypothyroid patients have only hand paresthesia as a symptom of carpal

tunnel syndrome. Hand paresthesia suggests involvement of the median nerve (see section below titled "Carpal Tunnel Syndrome in Hypothyroidism: A Mononeuropathy"). Other hypothyroid patients have paresthesia at the outer side of the lower thigh. This anatomical location suggests involvement of the lateral femoral cutaneous nerve. The area may be painful, and the patient may feel tingling, formication, or itch. The skin is typically hypersensitive to touch.[22]

According to Rao et al., of 20 unselected hypothyroid patients, 11 reported paresthesia.[47] In a study of 100 patients with hypothyroidism, 56% reported paresthesia. In another study with 15 cases, 13% had paresthesia.[7,p.578] In a fourth study, of 39 consecutive primary hypothyroid patients, 24 (64%) had subjective complaints, especially of paresthesia, that suggested polyneuropathy. The investigators in this last study examined the patients and found objective indications supporting a diagnosis of polyneuropathy in 13 patients (33%). Electrophysiological measures confirmed a diagnosis of polyneuropathy in 28 patients (72%).[2]

Some researchers have reported that the symptoms of peripheral neuropathy, including paresthesia, and neurophysiological parameters in hypothyroid patients uniformly improved upon treatment with thyroid hormone.[1,p.1029] Kraft and Vetter reported the case of a hypothyroid woman who had edema of the tissues around her eyes, and finger paresthesia. Another clinician had previously diagnosed the paresthesia as carpal tunnel syndrome. Her edema, paresthesia, and other indications of hypothyroidism improved with T_4 treatment.[9]

Thurmon and Thompson reported paresthesia as a symptom of euthyroid hypometabolism.[8] My records show that most euthyroid fibromyalgia patients, who are invariably hypometabolic, have paresthesia before treatment. Metabolic rehabilitation including the use of T_3 has relieved the paresthesia of nearly all of these euthyroid hypometabolic fibromyalgia patients.

CARPAL TUNNEL SYNDROME IN HYPOTHYROIDISM: A MONONEUROPATHY

Carpal tunnel syndrome often occurs secondarily to hypothyroidism.[4] In these patients, carpal tunnel syndrome is a mononeuropathy that results mainly from compression of the median nerve at the wrist.[4] Typically, patients report nocturnal paresthesia in a median nerve distribution. One or both hands may be symptomatic. Rarely, a patient has muscle weakness, atrophy, and sensory loss. If the carpal ligament of some patients is not incised, the symptoms become permanent.[1,p.1029]

Carpal tunnel syndrome is common in hypothyroid patients.[45] Rao et al. found that of 20 unselected hypothyroid patients, 6 (30%) had carpal tunnel syndrome. Five of the patients had increased sensory nerve latencies; one had an increased distal motor latency. ("Latency" refers to the time of inactivity between application of a stimulus and the response.) Increased nerve latency indicates slowed nerve conduction. An increased motor latency refers to a delayed muscle reaction to a stimulus.) In one study, 11 of 20 patients reported paresthesia. Nerve conduction was abnormal in 13 patients, and in 10 patients, conduction was abnormal predominantly in the median nerve.[47] In a study of 100 patients with hypothyroidism, 56% reported paresthesia. In a study of 15 cases, 13% had paresthesia.[7,p.578]

Kraft and Vetter reported the case of a hypothyroid woman with finger paresthesia previously diagnosed as carpal tunnel syndrome. Her muscles were generally weak, she was intolerant of cold, and her physical abilities were limited. Her skin was rough and cool, her serum TSH was high, and her thyroid hormone levels were low. She gradually improved with T_4 treatment.[9] The findings and results in this case are in line with other reported cases in which hand paresthesia was associated with carpal tunnel syndrome in hypothyroid patients.[4][6][10][11][12][13,p.904] Moosa and Dubowitz reported slow conduction velocity in the ulnar and posterior tibial nerves of children with untreated congenital hypothyroidism.[6]

POLYNEUROPATHY IN HYPOTHYROIDISM

Besides specific mononeuropathies in hypothyroidism, some medical writers have cited more diffuse involvement of the peripheral nervous system. Clinicians term a condition of multiple nerve abnormalities polyneuropathy.

Crevasse and Logue described a case of iatrogenic hypothyroidism and polyneuropathy. The patient became hypothyroid and developed an associated polyneuropathy after a surgeon removed her thyroid gland as a treatment for cardiac disease.[31] Beghi evaluated 39 consecutive primary hypothyroid patients. Of these, 25 (64%) had subjective complaints that suggested polyneuropathy, mainly paresthesia. Clinical examination indicated that 13 (33%) had polyneuropathy, and clinicians confirmed the diagnosis through electrophysiologic assessment in 28 cases (72%).[2] Adams

and Rosman reported polyneuropathy in 31 of 65 patients with spontaneous hypothyroidism. The most common complaints were paresthesia and "lancinating" and other types of pain in the legs. The researchers did not report whether the patients had weak muscles, absent reflexes, or sensory loss.[13,p.904] The symptoms ceased after the patients began using thyroid hormone.

Hypothyroidism and euthyroid hypometabolism may cause energy deficiency contractures and trigger points in muscle, and the trigger points can refer abnormal sensation. Trigger points in multiple muscles can mimic the clinical picture of polyneuropathy. In addition to abnormal sensation, the patient may have muscle weakness and weak or absent reflexes, completing the picture of polyneuropathy. The properly trained clinician can easily distinguish myofascial trigger points from polyneuropathy. He can also effectively stop referral from them. If the patient has either hypothyroidism or euthyroid hypometabolism, however, the metabolic condition will most likely have to be effectively treated before local physical trigger point therapy can provide enduring relief (see section below titled "Trigger Points as a Source of Paresthesia").

RESTLESS LEG SYNDROME IN HYPOTHYROIDISM

Some hypothyroid patients have restless leg syndrome. In fact, according to Bon et al., the presence of the syndrome is for some patients the initial indication of hypothyroidism.[41] The syndrome may occur in patients whose hypothyroidism is moderately severe.[42]

● POSSIBLE MECHANISMS OF PARESTHESIA AND RELATED SYMPTOMS IN FIBROMYALGIA

Inadequate thyroid hormone regulation of cell function underlies most patients' fibromyalgia. In these patients, paresthesia may be a manifestation of several mechanisms: nerve function abnormalities demonstrable by electrophysiological methods, axonal degeneration, myxedema, subnormal dopamine, and trigger points.

ELECTROMYOGRAPHY (EMG) STUDIES

Zampollo et al. reported diffuse anomalies of EMG parameters in hypothyroid patients with peripheral neuropathy. The anomalies included altered motor and sensitive nerve conduction velocity, F-wave, H-reflex, and H-index.[45] Rao et al. reported that 14 of 20 hypothyroid patients (70%) had reduced mean duration of motor unit potentials and reduced mean amplitude. These nerve conduction anomalies are consistent with myopathy. Five patients had increased sensory latencies, and 1 had increased motor latencies. The investigators wrote that these latter findings in median nerves indicated subclinical carpal tunnel syndrome.[47]

Several investigators noted that in hypothyroid animals and humans, peripheral nerves are less excitable. Horsten and Boeles recorded sciatic nerve conduction in hypothyroid patients. The optimal frequency of alternating current that provoked nerve activity was lower than in normal subjects. There was also a 50% rise in "chronaxie." The chronaxie is the minimum time necessary for a current (of a given strength) to pass through a nerve and cause a muscle contraction. Thus, it took longer for a current to stimulate a muscle contraction through its motor nerve.[23]

Moosa and Dubowitz tested the ulnar and posterior tibial nerves of children with untreated congenital hypothyroidism.[6] The nerves conducted signals at slowed velocities. Murray and Simpson used an EMG technique to determine the conduction velocity in the median and ulnar nerves of 11 hypothyroid patients. In 3 patients, the median nerve conducted signals at a slow rate from the elbow to the wrist. The investigators attributed the slow conduction rate to carpal tunnel syndrome.

"Irritability" of Muscle in Hypothyroidism

Studies have shown that hypothyroidism may be accompanied by "irritability" of skeletal muscle with delayed relaxation after stimulation. Investigators completely removed rabbits' thyroid glands and 4 weeks later performed needle EMGs on the animals' muscles. Inserting a needle electrode into the rabbits' muscles evoked trains of positive waves and spikes. These electrical patterns resembled those of myotonic muscle.[26,p.636] (Myotonic muscle remains contracted for a prolonged time after stimulation or after a strong contraction.)

Ross et al. performed a needle EMG on a hypothyroid patient whose only initial symptom was severe uterine bleeding. They examined her calf, anterior tibia, biceps brachii, first dorsal interosseous, and sacrospinal muscles. These muscles showed no involun-

tary twitching, quivering, or spontaneous contractions of individual fibers. When the patient consciously contracted the muscles, the motor-unit action potentials were normal. But when the investigators mechanically stimulated the muscle fibers by moving the needle electrode, fibers in some areas proved abnormally irritable. These irritable fibers, especially in the calf and sacrospinal muscles, occasionally reacted with trains of positive waves. In this respect, the fibers resembled the degenerating muscle fibers researchers found in thyroidectomized rabbits (see paragraph above).[26,p.636] The investigators biopsied the patient's left soleus muscle. The fibers were less irritable in an EMG exam 3 months after the patient began taking desiccated thyroid. The fibers were minimally (albeit abnormally) irritable. The researchers found both degenerating and regenerating muscle fibers. They found these fibers distributed inconsistently through the muscle and diffusely scattered throughout the muscle fascicles.[27]

The myotonic-like feature (delayed relaxation time) of hypothyroid muscle may have resulted from the same biochemical changes that cause hypothyroid patients to have a slowed relaxation of reflexes (see section below). The trains of positive waves of EMG activity of rabbit [26,p.636] and human[27] muscle upon irritation of the muscle with needle electrodes may be similar to the increased resting activity of lumbar muscles in fibromyalgia patients.[67] Fibromyalgia patients' muscles may be similarly "irritable." A possible explanation for such irritability may be a lowered threshold for firing of alpha motor neurons in the anterior horns of the spinal cord. The threshold could be low because increased substance P released by the dorsal root ganglia increases the afferent signals entering the dorsal horns, thus inducing segmental facilitation of the alpha motor neurons in the anterior horns. The result would be increased "irritability" or "excitability" of the muscle innervated by the alpha motor neurons. The increased excitability of the muscle would be detected as increased EMG activity.

Slowed Muscle Relaxation in Hypothyroidism

Studies show that hypothyroid patients and fibromyalgia patients have slowed muscle relaxation after multiple contractions. Ross et al. studied signal conduction in a patient's left ulnar nerve. When they stimulated the nerve, the electrical responses of the hypothenar and adductor pollicis muscles were normal. The nerve's motor fibers conducted signals at a normal rate. Before the patient began desiccated thyroid, however, a single stimulus applied to the ulnar nerve provoked a prolonged twitch of the adductor pollicis muscle. After treatment, the muscle twitched for a shorter time.[27] This prolonged activity of the muscle may have resulted from the low activity levels of calcium-ATPase and low ATP levels in hypothyroid muscle. These factors account for the slowed relaxation phase of hypothyroid muscle during reflex testing. Like hypothyroid patients, fibromyalgia patients were found to have slowed relaxation of muscle following voluntary contractions.[43] In my clinical experience and that of my colleagues such as Honeyman-Lowe, most fibromyalgia patients have a slow Achilles reflex relaxation phase before beginning metabolic rehabilitation. The speed of the relaxation phase increases to normal during treatment, serving as a valuable indicator of peripheral tissue metabolic status.

The same biochemical abnormality known to delay muscle relaxation in some hypothyroid patients—which is induced and sustained by inadequate thyroid hormone regulation of muscle cells—may account for slowed muscle relaxation in fibromyalgia patients. (See Chapter 4.3, section titled "Achilles Reflex Time.") Abnormally delayed relaxation of muscle may result in an increased conduction of sensory signals from the muscles to the central nervous system. The sensory signals would enter the dorsal horns of the spinal cord. Fibromyalgia patients appear to have an impaired ability to properly modulate sensory signals entering the central nervous system. As a result, the signals are likely to have an increased stimulatory and perceptual impact on the central nervous system. The impairment in fibromyalgia is due in part to increased central nervous system substance P levels (see Chapters 3.15 and 3.19).

The impaired modulation of incoming signals raises the possibility that any sensory signals—but especially those transmitted through type C and A delta fibers—may have undue access to the central nervous system. These signals may induce facilitation of spinal cord and brain stem neural pathways. Among those pathways are the spinothalamic tracts that conduct signals through secondary neurons to the brain stem and brain. We would expect these pathways, when facilitated, to conduct an excess of afferent signals (that originate in slightly myotonic muscles) to the brain stem and brain. During passage of the signals through the brain stem, collateral signals will be conducted to the reticular activating system. Activation of this system produces psychological and physical arousal. The arousal may interfere with sleep.[51] It may also provide

a state of alertness during waking that accentuates awareness of abnormal sensations resulting from excess sensory signals generated by the skeletal muscles. Thus, it is possible that the delayed relaxation of muscle may contribute to paresthesia.

AXONAL DEGENERATION: BIOPSY FINDINGS

Nerve biopsies have shown axonal degeneration of the sural nerve from hypothyroid patients with polyneuropathy.[3] Zampollo et al., for example, examined for pathology the sural nerve of two hypothyroid patients who had peripheral neuropathy. One patient had marked segmental demyelination and axonal degeneration.[45] Memni et al. found axonal degeneration during biopsies of sural nerve samples from four hypothyroid patients with polyneuropathy.[3]

Pollard et al. studied two hypothyroid patients with polyneuropathy. The patients had paresthesia, muscle pain, distal weakness, and sensory impairment. They also had lack of coordination of both upper and lower extremities, impaired gait, and depressed tendon reflexes. Upon electrophysiological testing, the researchers found a moderate slowing of motor conduction velocity and absent sensory potentials. They took samples of the sural nerve from both patients and studied them by light and electron microscopy. The nerves had a loss of myelinated fibers of all diameters, especially those of large diameter. By teasing out fibers for inspection, they found that the main abnormality was axonal degeneration. Upon electron microscopy, they found degenerating fibers, distinct cluster formations, mitochondrial abnormalities, and prominent glycogen deposits in the Schwann cells. There was a relative increase in the quantity of small diameter unmyelinated fibers. Pollard et al. concluded that the polyneuropathy of hypothyroidism results mainly from axonal degeneration.[46]

MYXEDEMA

Myxedematous Substance in Neural Tissue

Astrom, Kugelberg, and Muller reported that they detected no mucinous deposits in the endoneurium and perineurium of hypothyroid patients.[32] On the other hand, Nickel et al. found degenerated peripheral nerve fibers as a complication of hypothyroidism. They performed microscopic exams of the sural nerve. They found that an edematous substance had infiltrated the endoneurium and perineurium. The substance occupied the interstitial spaces (the spaces between the nerves and their connective tissues) and separated many of the nerve fibers. They also found multiple degenerated foci in the myelin sheaths and axis cylinders. These foci distorted the axons so their borders were nebulus and fragmented. They found fibrosis as well.[4]

Anderson and associates found subnormal myelination in sheep infected with a nonarbo togavirus,[18] a virus related to Rubella virus of man.[19] Anderson reported that it appeared that the hypomyelination was due to depressed levels of circulating thyroid hormones. They confirmed the results of Terpstra, which showed infection of the sheep pituitary and thyroid glands by the virus.[15] Anderson and colleagues innoculated pregnant sheep with the virus.[18] After the birth of affected lambs, researchers stained pituitary cells from the lambs. The staining revealed sparse antibodies for the virus in the cells. Staining also showed large numbers of the antibodies in thyroid gland follicular epithelial cells. The structure of the infected cells was normal. TSH levels were normal, but T_3 and T_4 levels were significantly low in infected lambs. This study confirmed virally-induced hypothyroidism in sheep.

Hypothyroidism[20] and retarded myelination[16][17] have been documented to result from congenital rubella syndrome, the nonarbo togavirus infection of human beings.[19] These data raise the possibility that infection with nonarbo togaviruses may, by inducing hypothyroidism, impair myelination. An accumulation of myxedematous substance (water-binding mucopolysaccharides) may impair myelination of the nerves.

Myxedematous Substance in Connective Tissues

Murray and Simpson believed that myxedematous substance in connective tissues causes the paresthesia (termed carpal tunnel syndrome) that is so common in hypothyroid patients' hands. The substance gathers under the flexor retinaculum, the ligamentous strap around the wrist that binds together the tendons of the hand muscles. The resulting swelling of the retinaculum compresses the median nerve, causing a compression neuropathy with hand paresthesia. The patient usually experiences abnormal sensations at night in a median nerve distribution in one or both hands. As the condition worsens, the syndrome may progress to sensory loss and muscle weakness and atrophy. These abnormalities may become permanent, but incising the carpal ligament early enough may relieve the symptoms.[25]

Murray and Simpson reached their conclusion after relieving their patients' symptoms by a surgical procedure. For example, they relieved the paresthesia of the thumb and second finger in one of their patients with carpal tunnel syndrome by cutting the flexor retinaculum.[25] Wayne provided support for this view of median nerve compression in 46 of 50 patients with hypothyroidism.[28]

Carpal tunnel syndrome due to median nerve compression is not the only mononeuropathy that is likely to occur during hypothyroidism. For instance, myxedematous substance may accumulate in the tight fallopian canal of the temporal bone. The accumulation causes swelling that compresses the facial nerve. As a result, the muscles of the face may weaken.[29] Earll and Kolb reported that in two cases of hypothyroidism, entrapment of the facial nerve in the tight fallopian canal of the temporal bone caused facial muscle weakness.[5]

Nickel and Frame pointed out, however, that this mechanism does not explain the general fading glove- and stocking-like sensory disturbance in both upper and lower extremities of many myxedematous patients. They offer an alternative explanation—that paresthesia and sensory loss result from swollen skin and subcutaneous tissues mechanically interfering with the sensory receptors imbedded in them.[12]

Suarez and Sabin reported a case of meralgia paresthetica in a hypothyroid 48-year-old woman. The meralgia paresthetica involved numbness, burning, and tingling in the anterolateral aspect of the patient's left thigh. The paresthesia had persisted for 2 months. The patient had no history of back pain. She was thin and had a patch of hypesthesia in the lateral aspect of the thigh. Her TSH was elevated and her T_4 was low. Her symptoms subsided and her blood tests were normal after 2 months of thyroid hormone replacement. The authors suggested a mechanism of the patient's symptoms: that water-binding mucopolysaccharides (myxedematous substance) had collected in the membranes (the perineurium and endoneurium) of the lateral femoral cutaneous nerve. The myxedematous substance presumably reduced the space available for the nerve as in the tunnel formed by the inguinal ligament and the iliac spine.[22]

Myxedema in Fibromyalgia

Awad performed biopsies of "fibrositic" muscle from patients[62][63][64] whom he considered in retrospect to be fibromyalgia patients.[62] He found myxedematous substance in the tissue samples. The substance was virtually identical to the accumulated mucopoly-saccharides found in myxedematous connective tissues from hypothyroid patients. Awad believed that the myxedematous substance he found pointed to inadequate thyroid hormone regulation of tissues in the etiology of fibromyalgia.[65]

The increased mucopolysaccharides in fibromyalgia patients reported by Awad are but one of the connective tissue abnormalities fibromyalgia patients share with hypothyroid patients. In fact, the two groups of patients share practically the same connective tissue abnormalities (see Chapter 3.3).

SUBNORMAL DOPAMINE PRODUCTION IN HYPOTHYROIDISM AND FIBROMYALGIA

Inadequate thyroid hormone regulation of dopaminergic cells decreases synthesis and secretion of dopamine. The mean cerebrospinal fluid level of the dopamine metabolite 3-methoxy-4-hydroxyphenethylene glycol (MHPG) was low in fibromyalgia patients.[34] (See Chapter 3.4, subsection titled "Thyroid Hormone Regulation of Dopamine Levels and Motor Drive.") Dopamine agonists are used to treat restless leg syndrome. For example, researchers have reported that pergolide, a long-acting agonist of D_1 and D_2 dopamine receptors, effectively reduces the symptoms of restless leg syndrome.[30][33] This therapeutic effect raises the possibility that the syndrome is due in part to subnormal dopamine levels.[55,p.153] Subnormal dopamine levels in fibromyalgia patients due to inadequate thyroid hormone regulation of dopaminergic neurons may account for their restless leg syndrome (see Chapter 3.1).

TRIGGER POINTS AS A SOURCE OF PARESTHESIA

Regional or widespread paresthesia may be referred sensation from one or more trigger points. A trigger point is a hypersensitive locus in a tissue. When a trigger point is sufficiently irritable, it spontaneously refers pain or other abnormal sensations.

Most fibromyalgia patients have trigger points. Gerwin reported that most of 25 fibromyalgia patients had myofascial trigger points.[70] Scudds et al. applied pressure to sensitive areas in the muscles of fibromyalgia patients. The pressure produced referred pain in half the patients (21 of 42).[71]

For some hypothyroid and euthyroid hypometabolic patients, myofascial trigger points are a source of paresthesia. The main abnormal sensations patients experience from trigger points are referred tenderness and pain. That patients experience such tenderness and pain is evidence of the strong clinical effects of trigger points on sensation.[49,p.23] However, some patients also experience itching, burning, pricking, or lightening-like bolts of pain.[49,p.43] Writers may refer to these sensations as "dysesthesia," by which they mean unpleasant abnormal sensations, whether spontaneous or induced.[49,p.3] Vecchiet et al. experimentally induced "algogenic" foci in the skeletal muscles of patients. These "artificial" trigger points caused altered cutaneous, subcutaneous, and muscular sensory thresholds.[50]

Trigger points in skin, mucous membranes, and scars are likely to refer burning, prickling, or lightening-like jabs of pain.[49,p.43] Trigger points in fibrotic myofascial tissues are likely to generate a dull, persistent aching and other sensations such as itching. (Fibrosis involves an accumulation of collagen fibers that cross-bind and coil roughly in a concentric direction, contracting the tissues in which they are embedded.[53][54]) Trigger points in fibrotic tissue are often housed in the large longissimus muscles parallel and adjacent to the thoracic spine. These trigger points are usually more resistant to treatment than trigger points in myofascial tissues that are not fibrotic. Usually, considerable skill is necessary to effectively relieve patients of pain or paresthesia generated by these trigger points.[53][54]

The inability of clinicians to accurately diagnose and effectively relieve myofascial trigger point pain has a particularly tragic consequence for some patients—over time, progressively more muscles may become involved so that the patient's symptoms become globalized and the patient debilitated.[59] Widespread pain due to trigger points in three or four quadrants of the body may mimic the pain of fibromyalgia.[70] In some cases, clinicians may misdiagnose patients' widespread myofascial pain as fibromyalgia.

Average Response to Treatment

Whatever the abnormal sensation referred from a trigger point, pressing a finger firmly into the point amplifies the abnormal sensation. In patients who do not have what Travell and Simons termed "perpetuating factors," the finger pressure, applied with expertise, may be sufficient to desensitize the trigger point. Desensitizing the point usually reduces local tenderness at the point and stops the referred sensation. In some cases, however, the clinician may have to use other procedures, such as continuous ultrasound, systematic stretching, and moist heat, to desensitize the point.[51][52] Optimal therapeutic effects usually necessitate that the patient take nutritional supplements.[60] In my clinical experience, the proper use of myofascial therapy techniques promptly relieves the pain and/or paresthesia of at least 80% of patients entering a chiropractic practice. Most clinicians, with a minimum of training and experience in the proper techniques, will have a high success rate conscientiously using trigger point therapy to treat patients.

On the Internet, patients commonly post a message that indicates a tragic circumstance: Their clinicians tell them that they have myofascial pain, but there is no treatment for it, and they must learn to live with it. This corresponds to my experience with clinicians in general, many of whom specialize in treating pain patients. Myofascial pain is the most common source of musculoskeletal pain.[56][57][58] Myofascial trigger points are the most common source of musculoskeletal pain in patients the clinicians will encounter in their careers. For clinicians in general not to know that *proper treatment readily relieves myofascial pain* is testimony to an inadequacy in their clinical training.

Hypometabolism as a Perpetuating Factor

Even expertly applied myofascial trigger point therapy may not stop referral of pain and/or paresthesia sustained by a perpetuating factor. Hypometabolism is a perpetuating factor for many patients. Hypometabolism of skeletal muscle may predispose a patient to respond with trigger point formation and activation to otherwise innocuous stimuli. In addition, hypometabolism may render skeletal muscle resistant to the most expertly administered myofascial therapy.

Simons et al. wrote, "Patients referred to us with MPS [myofascial pain syndrome] often arrive untreated for their slightly low thyroid function because they have only mild symptoms of hypothyroidism and borderline low, or low normal, thyroid tests." Regarding the role of hypometabolism in these patients' trigger points, they also wrote: "Experience has shown that these patients are more susceptible to myofascial TrPs [trigger points]; they obtain only temporary pain relief with specific myofascial therapy. This increased irritability of their muscles and their poor response to therapy are greatly improved by supplemental thyroid, if they have no other major perpetuating factor."[49,pp.213-214]

Simons et al. described an unpublished study by Gerwin in which he determined that 10% of myofascial pain patients were hypothyroid. (The study was later published as an abstract.[70]) Gerwin diagnosed

hypothyroidism based both on symptoms and T_3, T_4, free T_4, TSH or the TRH stimulation test. A prominent feature of the patients was the widespread myofascial trigger points.[70] As I noted above, widespread pain referred from trigger points in multiple muscles may lead to a misdiagnosis of fibromyalgia (see subsection above titled "Trigger Points as a Source of Paresthesia").

Simons et al. referred to an observation by Gerwin: that treating hypothyroidism renders trigger points more susceptible to therapy. They noted, however, that thyroid hormone treatment *alone* may not eliminate referral from myofascial trigger points, any more than trigger points would spontaneously "clear" in the euthyroid patient.[49,214] This corresponds to my clinical experience with hypothyroid and euthyroid hypometabolic patients, as I first reported in 1988.[61] More recently, Honeyman-Lowe and I similarly noted that to maximize the pain relief of fibromyalgia patients during metabolic rehabilitation, we must virtually always use physical treatment techniques. Myofascial trigger points are the most common lesions we must eliminate through the use of physical techniques.[48]

REFERENCES

1. DeLong, G.R. and Adams, R.D.: The neuromuscular system and brain in hypothyroidism. In *The Thyroid: A Fundamental and Clinical Text*, 6th edition. Edited by L.E. Braverman and R.D. Utiger, Philadelphia, J.B. Lippincott Co., 1991, pp.1027-1039.
2. Beghi, E., Delodovici, M.L., Boglium, G., et al.: Hypothyroidism and polyneuropathy. *J. Neurol. Neurosurg. Psychiatry*, 52:1420, 1989.
3. Memni, R., Bottacchi, E., Fazio, R., et al.: Polyneuropathy in hypothyroidism: clinical, electrophysiological, and morphological findings in four cases. *J. Neurol. Neurosurg. Psychiatry*, 50:1454, 1987.
4. Phalen, G.S.: The carpal-tunnel syndrome: 17 years experience in diagnosis and treatment of 654 hands. *J. Bone Joint Surg.*, 48:211, 1966.
5. Earll, J.M. and Kolb, F.O.: Facial paralysis occurring with hypothyroidism: a report of two cases. *Calif. Med.*, 106:56, 1967.
6. Moosa, A. and Dubowitz, V.: Slow nerve conduction velocity in cretins. *Arch. Dis. Child.*, 46:852, 1971.
7. DeGroot, L.J., Larsen, P.R., Refetoff, S., and Stanbury, J.B.: *The Thyroid and Its Diseases*, 5th edition. New York, John Wiley & Sons, 1984.
8. Thurmon, F.M. and Thompson, W.O.: Low basal metabolism with myxedema. *Arch. Intern. Med.*, 46:879-897, 1930.
9. Kraft, K. and Vetter, H.: Adynamia: finger paresthesias (clinical conference): *Schweiz. Rundsch. Med. Prax.*, 78:270-272, 1989.

10. Murray, I.P.C. and Simpson, J.A.: Acroparesthesia in myxedema. *Lancet*, 1:1360, 1958.

11. Wayne, E.J.: Hypothyroidism and the nervous system. *J.A.M.A.*, 172:1420, 1960.

12. Nickel, S.N. and Frame, B.: Nervous system in myxedema. In *Current Concepts in Hypothyroidism*. Edited by K.R. Crispell, New York, The Macmillan Co., 1963, p.167.

13. Adams, R.D. and Rosman, N.P.: Neuromuscular system. In *The Thyroid*, 4th edition. Edited by S.C. Werner and S.H. Ingbar, New York, Harper and Row Publishers, 1987.

14. Wolfe, F.: Diagnosis of fibromyalgia. *J. Musculoskel. Med.*, 7:54, 1990.

15. Terpstra, C.: Detection of Border disease antigen in tissues of affected sheep and in cell cultures by immunofluoresence. *Res. Vet. Sci.*, 25:350, 1978.

16. Naeye, R. and Blanc, W.: Pathogenesis of congenital rubella. *J. Am. Med. Assoc.*, 194:1277, 1965.

17. Rorke, L.B. and Spiro, A.J.: Cerebral lesions in congenital rubella syndrome. *J. Pediatr.*, 70:243, 1967.

18. Anderson, C.A., Higgins, R.J., Smith, M.E., and Osburn, B.I.: Border disease: virus-induced disease in thyroid hormone levels with associated hypomyelination. *Lab. Invest.*, 57(2):168-175, 1987.

19. Van Oirschot, J.T.: Congenital infections with nonarbo togaviruses. *Vet. Microbiol.*, 8:321, 1983.

20. Hanid, T.K.: Hypothyroidism in congenital rubella. *Lancet*, 2:854, 1978.

21. Sprott, H., Anders, C.H., Scholle, H.C.H., and Hein, G.: EMG-mapping in fibromyalgia. *J. Musculoskel. Pain*, 3(1):67, 1995.

22. Suarez, G. and Sabin, T.D.: Meralgia paresthetica and hypothyroidism. *Ann. Intern. Med.*, 112:149, 1990.

23. Horsten, G.P.M. and Boeles, J.T.F.: Influence of hypothyroidism on the excitability of peripheral nerves. *Arch. Internat. Pharnocodyn*, 78:93, 1949.

24. Lowe, J.C., Reichman, A.J., and Yellin, J.: A case-control study of metabolic therapy for fibromyalgia: long-term follow-up comparison of treated and untreated patients. *Clin. Bull. Myofascial Ther.*, 3(1):23-24, 1998.

25. Murray, I.P.C. and Simpson, J.A.: Acroparesthesia in myxedema. *Lancet*, 1:1360, 1958.

26. Lambert, E.H. and Sayre, G.P.: Myopathy in rabbits following thyroidectomy. *Amer. J. Physiol.*, 183:636-637, 1955.

27. Ross, G.T., Donald, M.D., Scholz, A., Lambert, E.H., and Geraci, J.E.: Severe uterine bleeding and degenerative skeletal-muscle changes in unrecognized myxedema. *J. Clin. Endocrinol.*, 18:496-497, 1958.

28. Wayne, E.J.: Hypothyroidism and the nervous system. *J.A.M.A.*, 172:1420, 1960.

29. Salick, A.I. and Pearson, C.M.: Electrical silence of myoedema. *Neurology* (Minneap.), 17(9):899-901, 1967.

30. Wetter, T.C., Stiasny, K., Winkelmann, J., et al.: A randomized controlled study of pergolide in patients with restless legs syndrome. *Neurology*, 52(5):944-950, 1999.

31. Crevasse, L.E. and Logue, R.B.: Peripheral neuropathy in myxedema. *Ann. Intern. Med.*, 50:1433, 1974.

32. Astrom, K-E., Kugelberg, E., and Muller, R.: Hypothyroid myopathy. *Arch. Neurol.*, 5:26-36, 1961.

33. Gunning, K. and Gay, C.: Treatment of restless leg syndrome with pergolide. *J. Fam. Pract.*, 48(4):250, 1999.

34. Russell, I.J., Vaeroy, M., Jabors, M., and Nyberg, F.: Cerebrospinal fluid biogenic metabolites in fibromyalgia/fibrositis syndrome in rheumatoid arthritis. *Arthritis Rheum.*, 35:550-556, 1992.

35. Lowe, J.C., Garrison, R.L., Reichman, A.J., Yellin, J., Thompson, M., and Kaufman, D.: Effectiveness and safety of T_3 (triiodothyronine) therapy for euthyroid fibromyalgia: a double-blind placebo-controlled response-driven crossover study. *Clin. Bull. Myofascial Ther.*, 2(2/3):31-58, 1997.

36. Lowe, J.C., Reichman, A.J., and Yellin, J.: The process of change during T_3 treatment for euthyroid fibromyalgia: a double-blind placebo-controlled crossover study. *Clin. Bull. Myofascial Ther.*, 2(2/3):91-124, 1997.

37. Lowe, J.C., Garrison, R.L., Reichman, A.J., and Yellin, J.: Triiodothyronine (T_3) treatment of euthyroid fibromyalgia: a small-N replication of a double-blind placebo-controlled crossover study. *Clin. Bull. Myofascial Ther.*, 2(4):71-88, 1997.

38. Wolfe F.: Fibromyalgia: the clinical syndrome. *Rheum. Dis. Clin. North Amer.*, 15(1):1-18, 1989.

39. Guler, M., Kirnap, M., Bekaroglu, M., Uremek, G., and Onder, C.: Clinical characteristics of patients with fibromyalgia. *Isr. J. Med. Sci.*, 28(1):20-23, 1992.

40. Simms, R.W. and Goldenberg, D.L.: Symptoms mimicking neurologic disorders in fibromyalgia syndrome. *J. Rheumatol.*, 15(8):1271-1273, 1988.

41. Bon, E., Rolland, Y., Laroche, M., Cantagrel, A., and Mazieres, B.: Hypothyroidism on Colchimax revealed by restless legs syndrome. *Rev. Rheum. Engl. Ed.*, 63(4):304, 1996.

42. Schlienger, J.L.: Restless leg syndrome due to moderate hypothyroidism. *Presse Med.*, 14(14):791, 1985.

43. Elert, I.E., Rantapää-Dahlqvist, S.B., Henriksson-Larsen, K., and Gerdle, B.: Increased EMG-activity during short pauses in patients with fibromyalgia. *Scand. J. Rheumatol.*, 18:321-323, 1989.

44. Perez-Ruiz, F., Calabozo, M., Alonso-Ruiz, A., Herrero, A., Ruiz-Lucea, E., and Otermin, I.: High prevalence of undetected carpal tunnel syndrome in patients with fibromyalgia syndrome. *J. Rheumatol.*, 22(3):501-504, 1995.

45. Zampollo, A., Cristofori, E., Zacchetti, O., and Spreafico, A.: Hypothyroid neuropathy: description of two cases. *Minerva Med.*, 74(5):165-172, 1983.

46. Pollard, J.D., McLeod, J.G., Honnibal, T.G., and Verheijden, M.A.: Hypothyroid polyneuropathy. Clinical, electrophysiological and nerve biopsy findings in two cases. *J. Neurol. Sci.*, 53(3):461-471, 1982.

47. Rao, S.N., Katiyar, B.C., Nair, K.R., and Misra, S.: Neuromuscular status in hypothyroidism. *Acta Neurol. Scand.*, 61(3):167-177, 1980.

48. Lowe, J.C. and Honeyman-Lowe, G.: Facilitating the decrease in fibromyalgic pain during metabolic rehabilitation: an essential role for soft tissue therapies. *J. Bodywork Movem. Ther.*, 2(4):208-217, 1998.

49. Simons, D.G., Travell, J.G., and Simons, L.S.: *Travell & Simons' Myofascial Pain and Dysfunction: The Trigger Point Manual, Vol. 1, Upper Half of Body*, 2nd edition. Baltimore, Williams & Wilkins, 1999.

50. Vecchiet, L., Galletti, R., Giamberardino, M.A., et al.: Modifications of cutaneous, subcutaneous, and muscular

sensory and pain thresholds after the induction of an experimental algogenic focus in the skeletal muscle. *Clin. J. Pain*, 4:55-59, 1988.

51. Lowe, J.C.: *The Purpose and Practice of Myofascial Therapy* (audio cassette album). Houston, McDowell Publishing Company, 1989.

52. Lowe, J. C.: How—and how not—to use combination therapy. *Dyn. Chiro.* April 11, 1990, pp.10-11.

53. Lowe, J. C.: When fibrosis complicates trigger points. *J. Nat. Assoc. Trigger Point Myotherap.*, 3.3:7-8, Fall, 1990.

54. Lowe, J. C.: Fascia and premenstrual headaches. *Mass. Ther. J.*, 30(2):21-24, Spring, 1991.

55. Goldstein, J.A.: *Chronic Fatigue Syndrome: The Limbic Hypothesis.* New York, Haworth Medical Press, 1992.

56. Travell, J.G. and Simons, D.G.: *Myofascial Pain and Dysfunction: The Trigger Point Manual, Vol. 1.* Baltimore, Williams and Wilkins, 1983.

57. Lowe, J. C.: The most common source of pain. *Chiro. J. North Carol.*, 75(7):26-27, 1992.

58. Lowe, J.C.: The most common source of musculoskeletal pain. *Amer. J. Clin. Chiro.*, August, 1993, pp.26-27.

59. Lowe, J. C.: Globalization of myofascial pain syndromes. *Dyn. Chiro.*, March 14, 1990, p.18.

60. Lowe, J.C.: The need for nutrition supplementation in myofascial pain syndromes. *Anabolism: J. Prevent. Med.*, 7 (2):5, 1988.

61. Lowe, J.C.: A case of debilitating headache complicated by hypothyroidism: its relief through myofascial therapy. *Dig. Chiro. Econ.*, 31:73-75, 1988.

62. Awad, E.A.: Pathological changes in fibromyalgia. *First International Symposium on Myofascial Pain and Fibromyalgia.* Minneapolis, Minnesota, May 9, 1989.

63. Awad, E.A.: Histopathological changes in fibrositis. In *Advances in Pain Research and Therapy*, Vol. 17. Edited by J.R. Fricton and E.A. Awad, New York, Raven Press, Ltd., 1990, pp.249-258.

64. Awad, E.A.: Interstitial myofibrositis: hypothesis of the mechanism. *Arch. Phy. Med. Rehabil.*, 54:449-453, 1973.

65. Awad, E.A.: Personal communication. April 6, 1992.

66. Bennett, R.M.: Myofascial pain syndromes and the fibromyalgia syndrome: a comparative analysis. In *Advances in Pain Research and Therapy*, Vol. 17. Edited by J.R. Fricton and E. Awad, New York, Ravel Press, 1990.

67. Kraft, G.H., Johnson, E.W., and LeBan, M.M.: The fibrositis syndrome. *Arch. Phys. Med. Rehabil.*, 49:155-162, 1968.

68. Stokes, M.J., Cooper, R.G., and Edwards, R.H.T.: Normal muscle strength and fatigability in patients with effort syndromes. *Brit. Med. J.*, 297(6655):1014-1017, 1988.

69. Bengtsson, A., Henriksson, K.G., Jorfeldt, L., Kagedal, B., Lennmarken, C., and Lindstrom, F.: Primary fibromyalgia. A clinical and laboratory study of 55 patients. *Scand. J. Rheumatol.*, 15(3):340-347, 1986.

70. Gerwin, R.D.: A study of 96 subjects examined both for fibromyalgia and myofascial pain. *J. Musculoskel. Pain*, 3 (1):121, 1995.

71. Scudds, R.A., Heck, C., Delaney, G., and Teassell, R.W.: A comparison of referred pain, resting skin temperature, and other signs in fibromyalgia (FM) and myofascial pain syndrome (MPS). *J. Musculoskel. Pain*, 3(1):121, 1995.

3.17

Sicca-Like Membranes and Dry Skin

Fibromyalgia patients commonly complain of dry mouth and eyes (termed sicca symptoms) and dry skin. Sicca symptoms may result from various medications (including antidepressant medications often prescribed for fibromyalgia), menopause, Sjögren's syndrome, and inadequate thyroid regulation. Some clinicians use the term Sjögren's syndrome for the symptoms of dry mouth and eyes despite the cause. Other clinicians restrict their use of the term to sicca symptoms resulting from an autoimmune process. Autoimmunity is a common underlying factor in some patients with both Sjögren's syndrome and primary hypothyroidism. However, even when autoimmunity is not involved, hypothyroid patients commonly have sicca symptoms and dry skin. The mechanism of the symptoms is reduced blood flow to mucous membranes and skin and reduced metabolism of mucous membrane and skin cells. Sicca symptoms and dry skin typically diminish or disappear during metabolic rehabilitation involving the use of thyroid hormone.

Many clinicians use the term "sicca" to refer to dry mouth and eyes. Clinicians can objectively verify these symptoms through the findings of a reduced "wetting" capacity of the salivary glands and reduced "tearing" capacity of the lacrimal glands of the eyes (a positive Schirmer's test[13][14]).

Sicca symptoms and dry skin are clinical features of hypothyroidism. Dry mouth may result from the use of various drugs such as the antidepressants many clinicians prescribe as a treatment for fibromyalgia. Dry mucous membranes may also accompany menopause. The clinician should distinguish the contribution of such factors to the patient's sicca symptoms. Treatment of fibromyalgia with metabolic rehabilitation involving the use of thyroid hormone usually diminishes or relieves sicca symptoms. When caused or amplified by drug use or a sex hormone deficiency, however, sicca symptoms are likely to persist until the clinician and patient take appropriate corrective action.

Sicca symptoms are the major feature of Sjögren's syndrome, alternately termed Gougerot-Sjögren disease and keratoconjunctivitis sicca. What is and what is not Sjögren's syndrome is not a settled issue. Who, Fox recently questioned, should clinicians diagnose as having Sjögren's syndrome—a small group of patients with abnormalities of secretory glands due to an autoimmune process, or a large group who have symptoms of dry eyes and mouth? He defined primary Sjögren's syndrome as a systemic autoimmune disease characterized by "keratoconjunctivitis sicca" and "xerostomia." (Xerostomia means dry mouth. Keratoconjunctivitis sicca means inflammation of the conjunctiva and of the cornea with reduced tearing. The conjunctiva is the mucous membrane that invests the anterior surface of the eyeball and the posterior surface of the eye lids.) Fox wrote that the xerostomia and keratoconjunctivitis sicca in primary Sjögren's syndrome result from lymphocytic infiltrates of the lacrimal and salivary glands. He noted that the diagnostic criteria for the condition remain controversial, "leading to confusion in the clinical and research literature."[15] The patient with primary Sjögren's has dry mouth and eyes due to atrophy of her salivary glands and the secretory epithelium of her eyes. The patient's lacrimal and salivary glands may be swollen because lymphoid tissue has infiltrated or replaced the normal glandular tissue. The patient most commonly is a menopausal woman, and has rheumatoid arthritis and Raynaud's phenomenon.[1,p.1249]

Fox also recently explained a suggested revision of the European diagnostic criteria for primary Sjögren's syndrome. It includes the use of the Sjögren's syndrome-A antibody or characteristic minor salivary gland biopsy findings. He wrote that investigators have not identified the antigens that initiate primary Sjögren's syndrome. However, studies have shown that patients with established primary Sjögren's syndrome have variously had immune reactivity against SS-A, SS-B, fodrin, α-amylase, and carbonic anhydrase. Sicca symptoms, including dryness and pain, may result from interference with any part of the functional anatomic unit involved in salivation and tearing: the mucosal surface (the site of inflammation), sensory nerve signals from the secretory glands to the midbrain (lacrimatory and salivatory nuclei), motor nerve signals from the brain to the secretory glands, or acinar/ductal structures in the gland.[16]

● SICCA-LIKE MEMBRANES AND DRY SKIN IN FIBROMYALGIA

Sicca symptoms are common in fibromyalgia.[5][11] Of patients who took part in the 1990 ACR consensus study of fibromyalgia, 35.8% reported sicca symptoms.[5] Dinerman et al. found that of 118 fibromyalgia patients, 21 (18%) had sicca symptoms.[13] Nishikai reported that 71% of Japanese fibromyalgia patients complained of sicca symptoms.[12] Of 72 fibromyalgia patients studied by Bonafede et al., 6.9% probably had Sjögren's syndrome and 11% possibly did.[14] Tishler et al. reported that of 65 patients with primary Sjögren's syndrome, 36 (55%) met the criteria for fibromyalgia. The researchers concluded that fibromyalgia is common in patients with primary Sjögren's syndrome.[17]

The rheumatologists who identified sicca symptoms in fibromyalgia patients taking part in the ACR consensus study used their usual methods for diagnosing conditions that patients had other than fibromyalgia. The clinicians may have assigned the diagnosis based on the patients' complaints of dryness, not based on laboratory test results indicating physical, histological, or autoimmune involvement. It is not certain, therefore, what the basis of the dryness was. The dryness may have been a feature of inadequate thyroid hormone regulation of the secretory glands and mucosal membranes.

● SICCA-LIKE MEMBRANES AND DRY SKIN IN HYPOTHYROIDISM

Dry skin and mucous membranes are common in hypothyroid patients. The hair of many hypothyroid patients is dry, brittle, sparse, and lacks shine. The hair follicles are hypoactive and hair growth is retarded. The scalp is cool, dry, and scaly. The skin is dry due to reduced secretion by sweat and sebaceous glands. The palms are cool and dry. The skin commonly scales, but not with the severity of scaling as in ichthyosis. (Ichthyosis is a congenital disease in which the patient's skin is dry and forms fish-like scales.) The nails are often thickened and brittle.[2,pp.558-559]

Dry skin and mucous membranes in hypothyroidism result partly because of vasoconstriction and reduced blood flow in skin and mucous membranes and subnormal metabolism of skin and mucous membrane cells.[2,pp.558-559] The cold intolerance and Raynaud's-like symptoms in fibromyalgia patients suggest cutaneous vasoconstriction.[3,p.145] In addition, the high count of α_2-adrenergic receptors found on the patients' platelets[4] indicates that the patients have vascular constriction typical of α_2-adrenergic receptor dominance in hypothyroidism. α_2-Adrenergic receptor dominance may result from inadequate thyroid hormone regulation of the α_2-adrenergic receptor gene. Inadequate regulation of the gene most likely results from hypothyroidism and/or cellular resistance to thyroid hormone. (See Chapter 3.1, section titled "Adrenergic Receptors.")

In addition to reduced blood flow and slowed metabolism, sicca-like symptoms may result from an underlying autoimmune process. Crown et al. found a highly significant association between thyroid autoantibodies and lacrimal gland dysfunction characteristic of sicca syndrome.[8] Rand et al. described a cat that developed spontaneous adult-onset hypothyroidism. Among the clinical features of the animal's thyroid hormone deficiency were poor hair growth and severe seborrhea sicca (dandruff, or an accumulation of dry scales on the skin, particularly the scalp). Histological studies showed hypertrophy of the horny layer of the epidermis.[10] Barnett and Sansom described keratoconjunctivitis sicca in dogs caused by hypothyroidism. They wrote that keratoconjunctivitis sicca appears to be an autoimmune disease which is similar to Sjögren's syndrome.[7]

Ayala et al. reported two cases of premature ovarian failure, hypothyroidism, and sicca syndrome. They noted that their report was the first of an association of sicca syndrome and ovarian and thyroid gland deficiency. They concluded that their findings of antibodies specific to the involved organs and antibodies to nonorgan antigens suggest that premature ovarian failure, hypothyroidism, and sicca syndrome share a common autoimmune pathogenesis.[9]

Wemeau et al. found that of 36 hypothyroid patients with thyroiditis, 9 had enlarged submaxillary and/or parotid glands and dryness of the mouth or eyes. The patients also had antisalivary duct antibodies. Histologic tests showed that 6 of the patients' minor salivary glands had foci of lymphocytes and plasmocytes. The investigators noted the similarities between autoimmune thyroiditis and Sjögren's syndrome and conjectured that patients may have a common genetic predisposition to the two conditions.[6]

Autoimmunity causes primary hypothyroidism through antibodies against the thyroid gland (see Chapter 4.2, "Thyroid Autoantibodies"). If a common autoimmune process in a patient causes both sicca syndrome and impaired thyroid gland function, we would expect to find the most severe sicca symptoms in patients with primary hypothyroidism. However, patients with central hypothyroidism or partial cellular resistance to thyroid hormone may also have sicca symptoms due to the reduced blood flow and slowed metabolism of skin and mucous membrane cells.

In my clinical experience, fibromyalgia patients' symptoms of dry mucous membranes and skin improve or disappear when the patients undergo metabolic rehabilitation involving the use of thyroid hormone. Improvement or recovery from the symptoms does not, however, indicate which of several possible therapeutic mechanisms are involved. The patients' use of thyroid hormone may improve circulation to skin, mucous membranes, and their secretory glands, increase the metabolism of the glands, or reverse underlying autoimmune processes.

● SKIN DISCOLORATION IN FIBROMYALGIA

Caro reported that the skin of 64% of fibromyalgia patients was discolored in a reticular fashion.[18] She wrote that the discoloration looks like a form of "livedo reticularis." (Livedo reticularis is a semipermanent purplish or bluish mottling or network-patterned discoloration of the skin. It is caused by dilation of the capillaries and venules of the skin and aggravated by exposure to cold.) In 40% of the fibromyalgia patients, discoloration was mild; in 24% it was moderate-to-marked. Caro wrote that the skin discoloration in fibromyalgia patients is so subtle that the clinician can easily overlook it. It is most visible along the inner parts of the arms and thighs. Exposing the patients to cold during the examination can intensify the discoloration.

Caro proposed that the phenomenon involves an abnormal collection of proteins. The proteins purportedly accumulate in the interstitial spaces of the dermal-epidermal junction in fibromyalgia patients. She concluded that enhanced vascular permeability best explains this cutaneous finding.[19,pp.46-47]

Recent findings related to capillary permeability may relate the skin phenomenon Caro wrote about to inadequate thyroid hormone regulation in fibromyalgia patients. Crone wrote that capillary endothelial cells contain arrays of actomyosin (contractile) filaments. These filaments make up about 35% of the cells' protein. The cytoplasm of the cells also contains cisterns (reservoirs) that are continuous with invaginations in the cell membranes. These cisterns resemble the transverse tubules (T-tubules) and cisterns of skeletal muscle cells. Also as in muscle cells, a sudden increase in free calcium in the cytoplasmic fluid is the central event in initiating contraction of the actomyosin in capillary epithelial cells. Contraction of the actomyosin increases the permeability of the capillary walls.[20,pp.17-18]

How may actomyosin contraction increase capillary permeability? The mechanism is suggested by the endothelial cells' structural role in the capillary wall. The endothelial cell has one, two, or three points of contact with adjacent endothelial cells in the capillary wall. Between these contacts are clefts through which macromolecules (such as the proteins Caro mentions) may escape from the inside (lumen) of the capillary to the interstitial spaces. This would occur only when the endothelial cells of the capillary contract, pulling back and expanding the clefts between themselves and their neighboring cells.[20,p.16]

Inadequate thyroid hormone regulation of energy metabolism of the capillary endothelial cells in the fibromyalgia patient may reduce the available ATP inside the cells. A sufficient amount of ATP within the cells is necessary for the contractile filaments to separate and lengthen. When ATP is deficient, the contractile filaments remain attached and shortened, with contraction of the cell. Contraction of multiple capillary endothelial cells would cause a sustained widening of the clefts between the cells. The widened clefts would permit proteins to escape from the capillary and enter the interstitial spaces. Thus, the capillary permeability that Caro proposed to underlie the reticular skin discoloration may result from inadequate thyroid hormone regulation of energy metabolism in the endothelial cells of capillary walls.

Energy deficiency contractures may also account for Fassbender's report of "swelling of endothelial cells" in muscle capillaries of fibrositis patients. He wrote that the changes in the cells were striking. He hypothesized that the increased content of organelles (such as secondary lysosomes) within the cells caused so much swelling that the cells protruded into the narrowed capillary lumen.[22,p.305] Other investigators have reported swollen capillary endothelial cells in biopsies of quadriceps muscle after they had induced ischemia in the muscle.[23] The ischemia, by reducing delivery of nutrients to the muscle cells, may have resulted in an energy deficit in the endothelial cells. This may have reduced the amount of ATP in the cells, allowing chronic contractions of the actomyosin with swelling of the cells.

It is possible that chronic contractions of the actomyosin, as they shorten the lateral dimensions of these normally flat cells, contribute to the increase in spherical shape. In a discussion I had with Guyton, he said that physiologists have not demonstrated that capillary endothelial cells contract strongly. The cells appear to contract faintly. This is in contrast to the smooth muscle fibers of the precapillary sphincter in humans and the small terminal lymphatics in the bat wing. He agreed, however, that theoretically, capillary endothelial cells may contract enough to make themselves so spherical that they protrude into the capillary lumen.[24]

It is also possible that increased substance P levels due to inadequate thyroid hormone regulation of central nervous system cells may contribute to livedo reti-

cularis in fibromyalgia patients. Substance P levels are increased in the central nervous system in thyroid hormone deficiency.[25] Substance P is transported from the spinal cord to peripheral tissues "antidromically."[26][27] (Antidromic transport refers to conduction of a substance in the direction opposite from normal. Sensory nerves, which transmit nerve impulses from peripheral tissues to the central nervous system, transport substance P from the central nervous system to peripheral tissues.) After nerves transport substance P to nerve endings in peripheral tissues, substance P is released into the tissue surrounding the nerve endings. There, substance P contacts blood vessels and causes them to dilate. The released substance P also stimulates mast cells to release histamine. The histamine then induces vasodilation and extravasation of plasma from the vessels. Fibromyalgia patients have been found to have a higher mean number of mast cells in skin biopsies than do healthy subjects and rheumatoid arthritis patients.[21] The increased density of mast cells may cause an exaggerated response to substance P.[4] An extraordinarily high substance P level would be necessary to cause extravasation: the amount of substance P needed to cause plasma extravasation is about 10 times the amount that causes vasodilation. This is consistent with the extraordinarily high substance P levels in fibromyalgia patients (see Chapter 3.19).

INCREASED CAPILLARY PERMEABILITY IN HYPOTHYROIDISM

Capillary permeability is increased in hypothyroidism. Loeb commented on the report of Bronsky et al.[28] that there is a near doubling in the mean protein content of the cerebrospinal fluid in hypothyroidism. He suggested that enhanced capillary permeability accounts for a portion of the increased protein content of the fluid. He also proposed that capillary permeability accounts in part for some of the increased protein content of intestinal fluids and serous effusions in the hypothyroid patient.[29,p.1066]

REFERENCES

1. *The Merck Manual of Diagnosis and Therapy*, 15th edition. Edited by R. Berkow and A.J. Fletcher, Rahway, Merck, Sharp & Dohme Research Laboratories, 1987.
2. DeGroot, L.J., Larsen, P.R., Refetoff, S., and Stanbury, J.B.: *The Thyroid and Its Diseases*, 5th edition. New York, John Wiley & Sons, 1984.
3. Bennett, R.M.: Muscle physiology and cold reactivity in

the fibromyalgia syndrome. *Rheum. Dis. Clinics North Amer.*, 15:135-147, 1989.

4. Bennett, R.M., Clark, S.M., and Campbell, S.M.: Symptoms of Raynaud's syndrome in patients with fibromyalgia: a study utilizing the Nielsen test, digital photoplethysmography and measurements of platelet α_2-adrenergic receptors. *Arthritis Rheum.*, 34:264-269, 1991.

5. Wolfe, F., Smythe, H.A., Yunus, M.B., et al.: The American College of Rheumatology 1990 criteria for the classification of fibromyalgia: report of the multicenter criteria committee. *Arthritis Rheumatol.*, 33:160-172, 1990.

6. Wemeau, J.L., Dessaint, J.P., Leonardelli, J., Rouget, J.P., Racadot, A., and Linquette, M.: Hypothyroidism and the Gougerot-Sjögren syndrome. *Ann. Med. Interne.* (Paris), 134(4):288-292, 1983.

7. Barnett, K.C. and Sansom, J.: Dry eye in the dog and its treatment. *Trans. Ophthalmol. Soc.*, 104(Pt.4):462-466, 1985.

8. Crowe, J.P., Christensen, E., Butler, J., Wheeler, P., Doniach, D., Keenan, J., and Williams, R.: Primary biliary cirrhosis: the prevalence of hypothyroidism and its relationship to thyroid autoantibodies and sicca syndrome. *Gastroenterol.*, 78(6):1437-1441, 1980.

9. Ayala, A., Canales, E.S., Karchmer, S., Alarcon, D., and Zarate, A.: Premature ovarian failure and hypothyroidism associated with sicca syndrome. *Obstet. Gynecol.*, 53(3 Suppl.):98S-101S, 1979.

10. Rand, J.S., Levine, J., Best, S.J., and Parker, W.: Spontaneous adult-onset hypothyroidism in a cat. *J. Vet. Intern. Med.*, 7(5):272-276, 1993.

11. Barton, A., Pal, B., Whorwell, P.J., and Marshall, D.: Increased prevalence of sicca complex and fibromyalgia in patients with irritable bowel syndrome. *Amer. J. Gastroenterol.*, 94(7):1898-1901, 1999.

12. Nishikai, M.: Fibromyalgia in Japanese. *J. Rheumatol.*, 19(1):110-114, 1992.

13. Dinerman, H., Goldenberg, D.L., and Felson, D.T.: A prospective evaluation of 118 patients with the fibromyalgia syndrome: prevalence of Raynaud's phenomenon, sicca symptoms, ANA, low complement, and Ig deposition at the dermal-epidermal junction. *J. Rheumatol.*, 13(2):368-373, 1986.

14. Bonafede, R.P., Downey, D.C., and Bennett, R.M.: An association of fibromyalgia with primary Sjögren's syndrome: a prospective study of 72 patients. *J. Rheumatol.*, 22(1):133-136, 1995.

15. Fox, R.I.: Sjögren's syndrome: controversies and progress. *Clin. Lab. Med.*, 17(3):431-444, 1997.

16. Fox, R.I., Tornwall, J., Maruyama, T., and Stern, M.: Evolving concepts of diagnosis, pathogenesis, and therapy of Sjögren's syndrome. *Curr. Opin. Rheumatol.*, 10(5):446-456, 1998.

17. Tishler, M., Barak, Y., Paran, D., and Yaron, M.: Sleep disturbances, fibromyalgia and primary Sjögren's syndrome. *Clin. Exp. Rheumatol.*, 15(1):71-74, 1997.

18. Caro, X.J.: Immunofluorescent detection of IgG at the dermal-epidermal junction in patients with apparent primary fibrositis syndrome. *Arthritis Rheum.*, 27(10):1174-1179, 1984.

19. Caro, X.J.: Immunofluorescent studies of skin in primary fibrositis syndrome. *Amer. J. Med.*, 81(Suppl.3A):43-49, 1986.

20. Crone, C.: When capillary permeability increases. *News Physiol. Sci.*, 2:16-18, 1987.

21. Enestrom, S., Bengtsson, A., and Frodin, T.: Dermal IgG deposits and increase of mast cells in patients with fibromyalgia: relevant findings or epiphenomena? *Scand. J. Rheumatol.*, 26(4):308-313, 1997.

22. Fassbender, H.G.: *Pathology of Rheumatic Diseases.* New York, Springer-Verlag, 1975.

23. Gidlöf, A., Hammersen, F., Larsson, J., Lewis, D.H., and Liljedahl, S.O.: Is capillary endothelium in human skeletal muscle an ischemic shock tissue? *Symposium on Induced Skeletal Muscle Ischemia in Man.* Linkoping, Sweden, November 6-7, 1980, pp.63-79.

24. Guyton, A.C.: Personal communication. July 14, 1992.

25. Vaeroy, H., Helle, R., Forre, O., Kåss, E., and Terenius, L.: Elevated CSF levels of substance P and high incidence of Raynaud phenomenon in patients with fibromyalgia: new features for diagnosis. *Pain*, 32(1):21-26, 1988.

26. Lembeck, F. and Donnerer, J.: Postocclusive cutaneous vasodilatation mediated by substance P. *Naunyn-Schmiedeberg's Arch. Exp. Path. Pharmak.*, 316:165-171, 1981.

27. Lembeck, F. and Holzer, P.: Substance P as neurogenic mediator of antidromic vasodilatation and neurogenic plasma extravasation. *Naunyn-Schmiedeberg's Arch. Exp. Path. Pharmacol.*, 310(2):175-183, 1979.

28. Bronsky, D., Shrifter, H., De la Huerga, J., et al.: Cerebrospinal fluid proteins in myxedema, with special reference to electrophoretic partition. *J. Clin. Endocrinol. Metab.*, 18:470, 1958.

29. Loeb, J.N.: Metabolic changes in hypothyroidism. In *Werner and Ingbar's The Thyroid: A Fundamental and Clinical Text*, 6th edition. Edited by L.E. Braverman and R.D. Utiger, Philadelphia, J.B. Lippincott Co., 1991, pp.1064-1071.

3.18

Sleep Disturbance

Sleep Physiology

Sleep is an altered state of consciousness that internal and external stimuli easily disrupt. Disruption of sleep, especially slow wave sleep, adversely affects humans. The electroencephalogram distinguishes the electrical brain waves of two waking stages, beta and alpha. Beta brain waves occur during intense mental activity, and alpha waves occur during quiet, resting wakefulness. Researchers divide the stages of sleep into two categories: rapid eye movement sleep (REM) and non-rapid eye movement sleep (NREM). When humans fall asleep, they enter NREM slow wave sleep and pass through four stages. Bursts of alpha waves normally intrude into stage 1 waves of slow wave sleep. Brain waves become progressively slower in stages 2, 3, and 4 sleep. Stage 4 is delta sleep. Alpha waves do not normally intrude into delta wave sleep. A minimal amount of delta wave sleep is necessary for the individual to feel rested and restored.

Sleep Disturbance in Fibromyalgia

Most fibromyalgia patients complain that their sleep is not restful and that they are fatigued. Several studies have shown that some fibromyalgia patients have intrusion of alpha waves into delta waves during sleep. Investigators term the intrusion "alpha-delta sleep" or "alpha anomaly." One study found that only 36% of patients had alpha intrusion into delta wave sleep. The presence of the sleep anomaly in this minority of patients did not correlate with the intensity of the patients' fibromyalgia. The patients' use of amitriptyline did not affect the anomaly.

The sleep disturbance that occurs in some fibromyalgia patients also occurs in some normal individuals and patients with rheumatoid arthritis, osteoarthritis, and hypothyroidism.

Sleep Disturbance Cycle

A variety of internal and external stimuli may disrupt sleep. Pain is probably the most common disrupter of sleep. The patient may experience pain as headaches; chronic, diffuse aching; or referral from myofascial trigger points.

Various medications may also disrupt sleep. Phenobarbital may disrupt sleep by increasing the rate of degradation of T_4, resulting in sleep disrupting effects of thyroid hormone deficiency. Xanthine chemicals used too close to bedtime commonly interfere with sleep. The theophylline used to control asthmatic symptoms, and the caffeine, theophylline, and theobromine in coffee and tea, are xanthines that commonly disrupt sleep. Whatever the source of the disrupted sleep, the usual consequence over time is symptoms and signs typical of fibromyalgia.

Thyroid Hormone

Some patients with hypothyroidism and cellular resistance to thyroid hormone have sleep disturbance that appears the same as or similar to that of fibromyalgia patients. Inadequate thyroid hormone regulation of cell function may cause disrupted, nonrestorative sleep through several mechanisms. First, inadequate thyroid hormone regulation of the adrenergic genes can increase the density of α_2-adrenergic receptors and decrease the density of β_1-adrenergic receptors on cell membranes. Increased α_2-adrenergic receptor activation may induce sedation and drowsy wakefulness, and it may inhibit deep slow wave NREM sleep and REM sleep. Decreased β_1-adrenergic receptor activation may increase drowsy wakefulness and decrease REM sleep.

Inadequate thyroid hormone regulation of energy metabolism in skeletal muscles results in sustained *contraction of the muscles. Compression of veins may decrease the evacuation of metabolic products that irritate nerve endings (reduce their activation thresholds) in the connective tissues of muscles. Activation of the nerves would result in the transmission of noxious signals to the central nervous system. Compression of arteries may reduce the supply of energy-yielding nutrients to muscle cells, inducing energy deficiency contractures. The result may be the formation and/or activation of trigger points, with transmission of highly nociceptive signals into the central nervous system. After entering the dorsal horns of the spinal cord, the signals are transmitted to the brain. While passing through the brain stem, the impulses stimulate collateral fibers to the reticular activating system. The resulting increase in neural activity of the system stimulates the brain in general, creating and sustaining arousal and wakefulness. Until relieved through effective myofascial therapy, the noxious impulses from myofascial tissues are likely to continue to disrupt sleep, leaving the patient with fibromyalgia symptoms.*

In patients with hypothyroidism or cellular resistance to thyroid hormone, symptoms and signs resulting from disturbed sleep compound, and may cyclically intensify, similar symptoms and signs resulting from inadequate thyroid hormone regulation of various body systems. For illustration, pain from inadequate thyroid hormone regulation of cell function may disturb sleep, and the disturbed sleep is likely to further lower the pain threshold, augmenting the patient's perception of pain.

Disturbed sleep is sometimes caused by occasional stimuli. For example, sleep in an unfamiliar bed on a short trip out of town can cause disturbed, nonrestful sleep. If no other sleep disrupting stimulus impinges on the individual, sleeping in her own bed should relieve the symptoms and signs associated with the disrupted sleep. However, if the individual has inadequate thyroid hormone regulation of cell function, the sleep disturbance is likely to persist despite otherwise optimal circumstances. Treatment with the proper form and dosage of thyroid hormone is a prerequisite to the individual getting consistently restful and restorative sleep.

Proposed Model of Disturbed Sleep

Moldofsky et al. conjectured that the external auditory stimulus they used to disrupt slow wave sleep and induce fibromyalgia symptoms parallels an internal arousal mechanism that disturbs sleep in fibromyalgia patients. They proposed that the internal

mechanism competes with the NREM sleep system and causes a deficiency of slow wave sleep. The adverse effect of the deficiency is the onset or worsening of fibromyalgia symptoms. Some researchers have speculated that a central nervous system serotonin deficiency is the ultimate source of deficient slow wave sleep. However, the available evidence suggests that fibromyalgia patients do not have a CNS serotonin deficiency. Also, some evidence suggests that a CNS serotonin deficiency causes only a transient reduction in slow wave and REM sleep, and that sleep soon returns to normal despite a sustained deficiency of serotonin.

In fibromyalgia patients with hypothyroidism or cellular resistance to thyroid hormone, the internal arousal mechanism Moldofsky et al. proposed is likely to have two components. One is a predictable increase in the density of α_2-adrenergic receptors and a decrease in the density of β_1-adrenergic receptors on cell membranes. These adrenergic receptor changes are sufficient to disturb patients' sleep, particularly slow wave sleep. The second component of the internal arousal mechanism is the increased pain perception that follows deficient slow wave sleep. Increased pain perception from disrupted sleep would compound aches and pains induced by other mechanisms resulting from inadequate thyroid hormone regulation of cell function. The compound source of pain perception (from disturbed sleep and inadequate thyroid hormone cell regulation) would further interfere with patients' slow wave sleep. Thus, disturbed sleep and increased pain perception—with inadequate thyroid hormone regulation of cell function as the starting point for both—are likely to cyclically exacerbate one another and progressively escalate the severity and complexity of the patient's fibromyalgia.

In one study of melatonin secretion in fibromyalgia, patients had lower than normal secretion compared to normal control subjects. Low melatonin levels in fibromyalgia could contribute to sleep disturbance, fatigue, and pain. However, inadequate thyroid hormone regulation of serotonin metabolism results in an increase in melatonin production. If future studies confirm the low levels, the finding would diverge from the hypothesis posited in this book: that inadequate thyroid hormone regulation of cell function is the underlying mechanism in most cases of fibromyalgia. At this time, a conclusion cannot be reached regarding the melatonin status of fibromyalgia patients. The number of patients and subjects in the study were too small to establish low melatonin levels as an objective finding in fibromyalgia. An un-

derstanding of melatonin secretion in fibromyalgia and its relation to the thyroid status of patients must await further studies involving more patients and subjects.

Sleep disturbance plays an important role in the induction of fibromyalgia in some patients. It can also result from inadequate thyroid hormone regulation of cell function and complicate and exacerbate the other resulting symptoms and signs.

Sleep is a state of altered consciousness rather than unconsciousness. This is evident from the ease with which environmental stimuli can disrupt sleep. Disruption of sleep, particularly deep slow wave (delta) sleep, adversely affects humans. Symptoms and signs typical of fibromyalgia may result.[46,pp.146-147]

A review of the brain waves during different stages of consciousness will make the information in this chapter more meaningful. Electrical recordings from the surface of the brain or the outer surface of the head show continuous electrical activity in the brain. The patterns and intensity of the waves depend mostly on the level of excitement of the brain. The level of excitement varies during the sleep-wake cycle. The frequency of the waves varies between 1 every several seconds to 50 or more per second. Sometimes, the waves are irregular. At other times, the waves are regular enough to be classified as alpha, beta, theta, or delta waves.[23,p.662]

Alpha waves occur when humans are awake and in a quiet, resting state. The frequency of alpha waves is 8-to-13 cycles per second. During deep sleep, alpha waves normally disappear completely. When the individual engages in mental activity, higher frequency asynchronous beta waves supplant the alpha waves. Beta waves occur during active cerebration. Their frequency is between 14 and 25 cycles or higher per second. The frequency of theta waves is between 4 and 7 cycles per second. In some individuals, theta waves occur during emotional upset, especially during disappointment or frustration. All waves below 3.5 cycles per second are considered delta waves. The frequency may slow to 1 cycle every 2 or 3 seconds. Delta waves occur during very deep slow wave sleep. Whereas separating the thalamus from the cerebral cortex eliminates alpha waves, it induces delta waves. This suggests that delta waves occur when the cortex is freed from the activating influence of the lower brain centers.[23,pp.662-663]

The two main stages of sleep are rapid eye movement (REM) sleep and non-rapid eye movement (NREM) sleep. REM sleep is deep sleep with a brain wave pattern more like that of waking states than of other states of sleep. Because of this waking-like brain wave pattern during deep sleep, REM sleep is also called paradoxical sleep.[46,p.147]

When we fall asleep, the initial sleep stage is NREM slow wave sleep. During NREM sleep, the electroencephalogram (EEG) is slower and more synchronized. As time passes, the depth of NREM increases, gradually descending through four stages. With lower stages, the EEG slows and the person becomes more difficult to arouse from sleep. Muscle tone and reflex activities diminish, blood pressure decreases, heart rate slows, and the pupils constrict. As humans age, they spend less time in the deepest stage of NREM sleep; by age 60, some humans spend no time in this deepest stage.[46,p.147] The first stage involves very light sleep in which bursts of alpha waves normally occur. During stages 2, 3, and 4 slow wave sleep, brain waves become progressively slower until they reach the delta wave frequency of 2-to-3 cycles per second.[23,p.663]

After roughly an hour and a half, the depth of sleep decreases and the person passes into REM sleep for 20 minutes or so. The EEG becomes desynchronized and the voltage decreases, much as it does during arousal.[46,p.147] The waves are irregular high frequency beta waves.[23,p.663] Muscle tone disappears and reflexes become inhibited. Brief contractions of muscle and rapid eye movements interfere with the inhibited muscle tone and reflexes. The EEG shows transient waves (pontine-geniculate-occipital) transmitted from the brain stem to the occipital cortex.[46,p.147]

● SLEEP DISTURBANCE IN FIBROMYALGIA

ALPHA-DELTA SLEEP ANOMALY

Most fibromyalgia patients with disturbed sleep complain of feeling unrested upon awakening and of chronic fatigue.[49][50] Moldofsky et al. first identified a brain wave EEG anomaly in fibromyalgia patients during sleep.[6][7] Other researchers have confirmed that fibromyalgia patients, albeit a minority, have the anomaly.[51][52][53]

The sleep brain wave anomaly in fibromyalgia patients is an intrusion of alpha waves into the slower waves of stages 2, 3, and 4 NREM sleep.[43,p.1211] Moldofsky et al. termed the anomaly "alpha-delta" sleep.[6]

In 1975, Moldofsky and his associates studied the effects of disturbed slow wave sleep on patients with fibromyalgia (then called "fibrositis") and healthy subjects. The researchers used brief bursts of an auditory stimulus (up to 20 seconds) to disturb the patients' and subjects' sleep. The stimulus initiated body movement. It also induced alpha intrusion into slow wave NREM sleep, contaminating it and causing a shift to stage 1 or stage 2 sleep or brief wakefulness.[6,p.349] The slow wave sleep deprivation caused healthy subjects to have temporary musculoskeletal and mood symptoms. These symptoms were similar to the chronic symptoms of the fibromyalgia patients in the study. The subjects also developed tender points. When the subjects were permitted undisturbed slow wave sleep, their symptoms remitted and their tender points disappeared.[6,p.349] These adverse effects of disturbed slow wave sleep are similar to those reported earlier by Agnew et al. After the experimenters disrupted slow wave sleep with electrical shocks, subjects "became physically uncomfortable, withdrawn, less aggressive, and manifested concern over vague physical complaints and changes in bodily feelings."[14]

Moldofsky et al. conjectured that the external auditory stimulus they used to disrupt slow wave sleep parallels an internal arousal mechanism that disturbs sleep. They proposed that the internal mechanism competes with the NREM sleep system. As a result, the mechanism impairs the presumably restorative function of NREM sleep and induces symptoms. They suggested that fibromyalgia is a "non-restorative sleep syndrome." They also speculated that disordered serotonin metabolism is the basis of the sleep disturbance and symptoms.[6]

In another study, Moldofsky and Scarisbrick deprived normal volunteers of slow wave sleep. The "subjects exhibited bursts of an alpha-like rhythm intermingled with delta-wave frequency only in response to the noise stimuli during the stage 4 deprivation condition."[7,p.42] From the slow wave disruption, the volunteers developed symptoms characteristic of fibromyalgia.[7]

The results of a study of healthy volunteers done by Older et at. were not as decisive as the results of the studies by Moldofsky et al. and Agnew et al. Older et al. assessed the production of low pain thresholds and fibromyalgia-like symptoms by disturbed slow wave sleep in healthy volunteers. The researchers used algometry to assess pain thresholds and a visual analog scale to assess symptoms. They disrupted the slow wave sleep of 13 volunteers on 3 consecutive nights. Six other volunteers whose sleep was not disrupted

served as controls. The mean pain threshold or symptoms did not significantly differ between the groups at baseline, during the 3 nights of disrupted sleep, or during recovery. In both groups, the pain threshold was lower in the mornings during all three conditions. The researchers wrote that symptoms were more apparent in those whose sleep was disrupted, and the symptoms were related to fatigue.[45]

The findings of Moldofsky et al. and Agnew et al. supported Hartmann's hypothesis that slow wave sleep (during NREM sleep), but not REM sleep, is instrumental in restoring physical functioning.[17] Justifiably, Moldofsky has continued to argue that the alpha-delta sleep anomaly plays an important role in fibromyalgia.[81][82] In a 1993 paper, Moldofsky wrote that disordered sleep physiology within NREM sleep, the alpha rhythm disturbance of slow wave sleep "that accompanies increased nocturnal vigilance and light, unrefreshing sleep" is common to both fibromyalgia and chronic fatigue syndrome. He noted that as a result, disturbed sleep is a feature of both conditions.[30]

Pain and psychologically distressing situations can induce the alpha-delta sleep anomaly.[47] Interestingly, however, individuals with chronic insomnia do not appear to have this sleep anomaly.[48] It is noteworthy that although a deficit of slow wave sleep during NREM sleep causes symptoms in healthy subjects, Vogel reported that deprivation of REM sleep had little adverse effect on healthy subjects.[13]

Carette et al. assessed the prevalence of the alpha-delta anomaly in 22 fibromyalgia patients. The researchers also studied whether the alpha anomaly in NREM sleep is a predictor of a therapeutic response to amitriptyline. They evaluated the patients during a 2-month double-blind, placebo-controlled crossover test of amitriptyline. At baseline and after 2 months, the patients underwent EEGs while they slept. At baseline, only 8 patients (36%) had the alpha-delta anomaly. These patients complained of trouble sleeping, but they differed in no other way from the patients who had trouble sleeping but did not have the anomaly. The researchers wrote that 6 patients (27%) treated with amitriptyline had some benefit. There was no difference in the degree of the anomaly between patients who benefitted from the use of amitriptyline and those who did not. (Scrutiny of the researchers' visual analog scale (VAS) data clearly shows that amitriptyline provided minimal improvement in pain, fatigue, sleep, and patient and physician global evaluations. There was no improvement in the myalgic score, that is, the sum of point tenderness at 10 points. At the end of the study, however, the VAS scores of patients who took amitriptyline significantly differed from those who took placebos, except for myalgia scores. Those who took amitriptyline were still symptomatic, and their mean sleep VAS score after treatment was only improved 25% from the baseline score. This is a case where we must distinguish between statistical significance and clinical significance. In other words, statistically significant "improvement" with treatment may not mean much in terms of improvement in the patients' clinical status. Although patients who took amitriptyline for 2 months in this study had a 25% improvement in sleep VAS scores, assessment for a longer time may have shown that amitriptyline provided no more improvement than did placebos. I base this conjecture on the outcome of another study by Carette et al.[77][78]) The researchers wrote that fibromyalgia patients have a higher incidence of the sleep anomaly than age- and sex-matched controls, but that 64% of the fibromyalgia patients (14 of 22) could not be distinguished from normal control subjects on the basis of the anomaly. Carette et al. concluded, "The alpha NREM sleep anomaly is present in only a small proportion of fibromyalgia patients. It does not correlate with severity nor is it affected by treatment with amitriptyline."[43]

This study by Carette is of interest regarding the common belief among rheumatology fibromyalgia researchers that antidepressants such as amitriptyline improve fibromyalgia patients' sleep. In a recent book for patients, Russell listed antidepressants in his Medication Guide, admitting that some have not been shown to be effective as treatments for fibromyalgia. (Actually, the available evidence indicates that none are effective.) He wrote, however, "The list of medications (see Medication Guide) includes some that will improve sleep quality."[44,p.36] In my years of study of fibromyalgia, I have never encountered a single case for which I found credible evidence of noteworthy improvement—even of improvement of sleep—or recovery through the use of these medications. (See Chapter 5.1, "Assessments of Antidepressant Treatment of Fibromyalgia.") I have communicated with many fibromyalgia patients who used antidepressants, especially amitriptyline and cyclobenzaprine, presumably to improve their sleep. Although their sleep appeared to be as disturbed as that of patients not taking antidepressants, many of the patients resisted stopping the antidepressants. The source of their resistance was a fear that their disturbed sleep would worsen if they stopped the medications. Based on such experiences, I remain doubtful that these medications improve the sleep of fibromyalgia patients.

SLEEP APNEA

Plantamura, Steinbauer, and Eisinger studied the incidence of fibromyalgia among 50 subjects with sleep abnormalities according to polysomnography and 31 control subjects. Of the 50 subjects with sleep abnormalities, 29 had sleep apnea and 21 had poor sleep without apnea. The researchers examined the patients to learn what percentage met the ACR criteria for fibromyalgia. Of the 29 sleep apnea subjects, 1 (3.4%) met the fibromyalgia criteria. Of the 21 subjects with poor sleep without apnea, 1 (4.8%) met the criteria. One control subject (3.2%) met the criteria. The results of this study suggest that there is only a low incidence of fibromyalgia among individuals with sleep abnormalities and particularly those with sleep apnea.[42]

● SLEEP DISTURBANCE IN HYPOTHYROIDISM

Most hypothyroid patients report that they tend to sleep too much. Watanakunakorn and his coworkers reported that of 400 hypothyroid patients, 25.25% reported that they were lethargic, and 25.25% reported sleepiness. On the other hand, 4.75% of their patients reported they had insomnia. This is to be expected in patients whose muscles are especially sensitive to inadequate thyroid hormone regulation of energy metabolism. As I wrote elsewhere, subnormal energy metabolism can lead to painful energy deficiency contractures, and nociceptive signals from the contractures can cause insomnia by stimulating the brain stem reticular activating system. Stimulation of this system produces alertness and can strongly interfere with sleep.[63] These investigators reported several types of pain that could disturb sleep in hypothyroid patients: headache (21.75%), abdominal pain (12.25%), arthritis (15.25%), cramps (10.25%), and backache (8.50%). In addition, 13.25% of their patients reported being nervous, which might interfere with sleep in the same fashion.[8,p.185]

RANGE OF SLEEP EFFECTS OF HYPOTHYROIDISM

The effects of hypothyroidism on alertness and sleep tendencies are well known. The literature contains descriptions of light nonrestorative sleep, psychomotor retardation, and lethargy. Lethargy may progress from a general psychophysiological sluggishness in mild hypothyroidism to coma in severe hypothyroidism.[62,p.901] Many patients have described to me that they sleep for prolonged times but not deeply enough, feel lethargic upon awakening, and lie in bed for a prolonged time half-awake or in a trance-like state, cogitating sluggishly about the need to get up, feeling guilty about not doing so, but being unable to muster the drive to get out of bed.

It may seem a paradox that in milder hypothyroidism, patients sleep lightly, yet in more severe hypothyroidism, patients may become comatose. A factor that may partly explain this range of sleep effects in hypothyroidism is alterations in serotonin secretion. The nucleus raphe dorsalis is the main site of serotonin synthesizing and secreting neurons in the central nervous system. In this nucleus, the effects of the α_2-adrenergic receptor activator clonidine on serotonin secretion varied, depending on the dosage used. A low dose of clonidine decreased the serotonin metabolite 5-hydroxyindole acetic acid (indicating reduced serotonin levels), and a high dose increased 5-hydroxyindole acetic acid (indicating increased serotonin secretion).[1][2][3] (See subsection below titled "Serotonin.") In mild hypothyroidism, inadequate thyroid hormone regulation of the adrenergic genes may be mild, with only a low increase in α_2-adrenergic receptors on serotonin-secreting neurons. The receptors would inhibit serotonin secretion, and the reduced secretion may contribute to sleep disturbance. In severe hypothyroidism, inadequate thyroid hormone regulation of the adrenergic genes may be extreme, with a high increase in α_2-adrenergic receptors on serotonin-secreting neurons. As with high dose clonidine activation of the receptors, serotonin secretion may be increased, contributing to the almost comatose status of the patient.

SIMILAR BRAIN WAVE PATTERNS OF FIBROMYALGIA AND HYPOTHYROID PATIENTS DURING SLEEP

In addition to some fibromyalgia patients, some healthy subjects[54] and some patients with rheumatoid arthritis,[55] osteoarthritis,[56] and hypothyroidism have disrupted stage 3 or stage 4 sleep. The abnormal brain wave patterns of fibromyalgia patients (see section above "Sleep Disturbance in Fibromyalgia") are virtually the same as those of hypothyroid patients.

Kales and others studied the pattern and quantity

of the stages of sleep in several hypothyroid patients. The patients had a deficiency of both stages 3 and 4 sleep. The researchers reevaluated the patients' sleep status after the patients had undergone thyroid hormone therapy. The reevaluations showed that the time the patients spent in the sleep stages had returned to normal.[9]

Wilke, Sheeler, and Makarowski reported that most of their fibromyalgia patients who were also hypothyroid complained of "poor, interrupted" or "restless" sleep before starting thyroid hormone therapy. With treatment, the patients' muscle pain and sleep disturbance disappeared at the same time. They wrote, "It is tempting for us to postulate that hypothyroidism in our patients impaired stage 4 sleep, which then resulted in myalgias typical of the fibrositis syndrome."[10,p.630]

Hayashi et al. noted sleep disturbance in children with acquired hypothyroidism.[18]

POSSIBLE MECHANISMS OF SLEEP DISTURBANCE FROM INADEQUATE THYROID HORMONE REGULATION OF CELL FUNCTION

Serotonin

According to Sternback, a central nervous system deficiency of serotonin results in disturbed sleep and lowered pain tolerance and depression.[40,p.243] Evidence does indicate that serotonin induces sleep,[11] and evidence suggests that a serotonin deficiency may at least *transiently* reduce slow wave sleep (see section immediately below). But whether a serotonin deficiency results in disturbed sleep may be a moot point regarding fibromyalgia patients. Only one study is available from which we can estimate the central nervous system level of serotonin in fibromyalgia. In this study, researchers measured fibromyalgia patients' cerebrospinal fluid concentration of the metabolite of serotonin, 5-hydroxyindole acetic acid (5-HIAA). The concentration did not significantly differ from that of normal control subjects.[80] The result of this study raises doubts that a CNS serotonin deficiency causes chronic sleep disturbance and nonrestorative sleep in fibromyalgia patients. The recent finding that amitriptyline did not improve the alpha-delta sleep anomaly in fibromyalgia (which some have proposed results from low CNS serotonin levels) reinforces the doubt of a CNS serotonin deficiency in fibromyalgia.[43]

Decreased Serotonin Levels May Only Temporarily Reduce REM and Slow Wave Sleep. Some researchers have argued that serotonin potently regulates slow wave sleep.[66][67] Because of this belief, the hypothesis that low CNS serotonin levels would cause fibromyalgia symptoms due to impaired slow wave sleep was for a time a plausible hypothesis. But it is questionable whether a CNS serotonin deficiency can account for *chronic* sleep disturbance of fibromyalgia patients.

Kelly wrote that a serotonin deficit may reduce REM or slow wave sleep only for a brief time.[29,p.800] He described a study in which Dement administered parachlorophenylalanine (PCPA) to a cat to inhibit its synthesis of serotonin. First, he measured the normal sleep of the cat for 4 days. Next, the cat received PCPA for 8 consecutive days. Dement then compared the effects of PCPA on the cat's REM and slow wave sleep with its normal sleep. Shortly after the cat began receiving PCPA, both REM and slow wave sleep sharply decreased. But on the 8th day, both types of sleep had resumed their normal levels. Despite this, serotonin levels remained at approximately zero throughout the time span of the PCPA treatment.[28] Kelly referred to findings such as this as "the crucial difficulty with the serotonin hypothesis of sleep." He noted that PCPA initially caused insomnia, but after only 1 week of injections of PCPA each day, both REM and slow wave sleep returned to 70% of normal. The return to normal sleep occurred despite *continued and complete suppression of serotonin synthesis*.[29,p.800]

Ware wrote that study results indicate that tricyclic antidepressants effectively relieve sleep disturbance related to depression, and in select cases, the drugs may prove effective in disturbed sleep related to fibromyalgia.[59] However, that the medications are effective even in select cases of fibromyalgia is dubious. For example, in one test of amitriptyline, fibromyalgia patients had minimal improvement after 2 months compared to patients taking placebos.[43] Longer term testing might have shown the antidepressant to be no more effective than the placebo. This was the outcome of the only long-term trial of amitriptyline and cyclobenzaprine. Short-term, patients had slight improvement, but long-term (3 and 6 months), the measured effects of the antidepressants did not statistically differ from those of placebos.[77][78] A safe assumption is that tricyclic antidepressants increase the concentration of serotonin in the CNS of fibromyalgia patients who use them. But if increased serotonin concentrations minimally improved sleep short-term and did not improve it long-term, it is not likely that a serotonin deficiency underlies chronic sleep disturbance in fibromyalgia. If we can extrapolate to humans the findings of the cat

study by Dement in the previous paragraph, reduced serotonin levels would cause only transient reduction in slow wave sleep. Some other factor, such as the sleep disrupting effects of inadequate thyroid hormone regulation of cell function, must account for patients' chronically reduced slow wave sleep.

Control of Serotonin Secretion by α_2-Adrenoreceptors. It is possible that future studies may contradict the one showing normal cerebrospinal levels of 5-HIAA (and presumably normal levels of serotonin) in fibromyalgia[80] and show that patients have low CNS serotonin levels. If so, the underlying mechanism of the low serotonin levels could be inadequate thyroid hormone regulation of the adrenergic genes, with an increase in α_2-adrenoreceptors on the membranes of serotonergic neurons (see section below titled "Increased α_2-Adrenergic and Decreased β_1-Adrenergic Receptors"). When catecholamines bind to α_2-adrenergic receptors on serotonergic neurons, the neurons synthesize and secrete reduced amounts of serotonin.[12,p.137] The resulting low serotonin level might result in disturbed and nonrestorative sleep. Inadequate thyroid hormone regulation of the adrenergic genes may thus mediate features of fibromyalgia caused by low CNS serotonin levels.

How much serotonin is secreted in the CNS, however, might depend in part on the degree of α_2-adrenergic receptor dominance on the membranes of serotonergic neuronal cells. The nucleus raphe dorsalis is the main site of serotonin synthesizing and secreting neurons in the CNS. In this nucleus, the effects of the α_2-adrenergic receptor agonist clonidine on the secretion of serotonin differed, depending on the dosage used. A low dose of clonidine decreased 5-HIAA, while a high dose increased it.[1][2][3] The decrease in 5-HIAA with low dose clonidine suggests reduced serotonin release by neurons of the nucleus raphe dorsalis. The decrease in 5-HIAA is consistent with the findings that low dose clonidine reduced slow wave sleep and REM sleep.[5] The increase in 5-HIAA with high dose clonidine suggests increased serotonin release by neurons of the nucleus. An increase in 5-HIAA is consistent with the finding that high dose clonidine induced sleep.[4] Possibly, decreased 5-HIAA (indicating decreased serotonin secretion) with low dose clonidine (suggesting low-level activation of α_2-adrenergic receptors), with reduced slow wave sleep, corresponds to disturbed and nonrestorative sleep in mild-to-moderate hypothyroidism. And, increased 5-HIAA (indicating increased serotonin secretion) with high dose clonidine (suggesting high-level activation of α_2-adrenergic receptors), with sedation and sleep induction, corresponds to the almost coma-like sleep of patients with severe hypothyroidism.

Increased α_2-Adrenergic and Decreased β_1-Adrenergic Receptors

The influences of different hormones, neurotransmitters, receptors, and receptor subtypes on sleep are complex, and researchers have not yet elucidated all the interactions involved. Overall, activation of β-adrenergic receptors increases physical and mental activities. The hyperactivity of untreated thyrotoxicosis illustrates in the extreme the excitatory effects of β-adrenergic receptor dominance. In general, α-adrenergic receptor activity slows mental and physical activity, as untreated hypothyroidism demonstrates. The specific influences of β- and α-adrenergic receptor subtypes on sleep and wakefulness, however, are not well understood at this time, although the interactions are clearly complex. Some data are available on the roles of different adrenergic receptor subtypes in some sleep and waking states, although some data are contradictory. In Table 3.18.1, I have included some effects on sleep and wakefulness of different adrenergic receptor subtypes found in the studies included in the rest of this section.

It appears that insufficient deep slow wave sleep and drowsy wakefulness, resulting in nonrestorative sleep, is promoted by increased α_2-adrenergic receptor activity and decreased β_1-adrenergic receptor activity. This dominant pattern of adrenergic receptor type activity is typical of inadequate thyroid hormone regulation of the adrenergic genes in hypothyroidism. The increased density of α_2-adrenergic receptors on the platelets of fibromyalgia patients[70] raises the possibility of the same pattern in fibromyalgia. (See Chapter 3.1, section titled "Altered Sleep Patterns.")

Makela and Hilakivi found that in rats, clonidine (an α_2-adrenergic receptor agonist) increased the proportion of time spent in the drowsy stage of wakefulness. The agonist also inhibited both REM sleep and deep slow wave sleep in NREM sleep. Clonidine did not affect light slow wave sleep or wakefulness. Yohimbine (an α_2-adrenergic receptor blocker) decreased the drowsy wakefulness induced by clonidine and increased aroused wakefulness. Phentolamine, another α_2-adrenergic receptor blocker, did not interfere with the α_2-adrenergic receptor-stimulating effects of clonidine. Prazosin, an α_1-adrenergic receptor blocker, prolonged the effects of clonidine (longer drowsy stage of wakefulness and inhibited deep slow wave NREM and REM sleep). Makela and Hilakivi concluded that the sedative effect of clonidine results from activation of α_2-adrenergic receptors, but a different subtype of α_2-adrenergic receptor may mediate the clonidine-induced inhibition of deep slow wave sleep and REM sleep.[60]

Hilakivi and Leppavuori studied the effects of α_1-adrenergic receptor blocking and activation on the stages of the sleep-waking cycle of the cat. The aim was to learn the levels of α_1-adrenergic transmission that are optimal for sleep and wakefulness. The α_1-adrenergic receptor agonist prazosin decreased the latency of REM sleep and increased the episodes of and time in REM sleep. Prazosin also potentiated the drowsiness induced by the α_2-adrenergic receptor agonist clonidine. Only the highest dosage of prazosin decreased REM and deep slow wave sleep. The α_1-adrenergic receptor blocker methoxamine decreased REM sleep and increased time in aroused wakefulness. The researchers wrote that moderate inhibition of cerebral α_1-adrenergic transmission facilitated REM sleep in the cat. They also noted that the level of cerebral α_1-adrenergic transmission is high during aroused waking and low during drowsy waking.[65]

Hilakivi found that in cats, the β_1-adrenergic receptor agonist prenalterol increased REM sleep. A β_1-adrenergic receptor blocker, metoprolol, increased drowsy waking, and at larger doses, decreased REM sleep. The β_2-adrenergic receptor agonist salbutamol decreased REM sleep. Propranolol, a β_1- and β_2-adrenergic receptor blocker, decreased the REM sleep that was increased by the α_1- and α_2-adrenergic receptor blocker phentolamine. Propranolol also potentiated the increased drowsy waking and decreased REM and deep slow wave sleep induced by the α_2-adrenergic receptor agonist clonidine. Hilakivi concluded that a high level of β-adrenergic receptor activity may facilitate REM sleep, and that a low level of activity (especially combined with a high level of α_2-adrenergic receptor activity) may facilitate drowsy waking.[5]

β-Adrenergic receptors in the medial preoptic area of the brain are involved in the regulation of sleep and wakefulness. In moving rats, microinjection of a β-adrenergic receptor agonist (isoproterenol) into the preoptic area induced arousal. In other rats, the researchers used 6-hydroxydopamine in the brain stem to destroy the norepinephrine-secreting neurons to the preoptic area. In these rats, without norepinephrine innervation of the area, the β-adrenergic receptor agonist did not induce arousal. The researchers wrote that their results suggest that microinjected isoproterenol acts at presynaptic β-adrenergic receptors of norepinephrine nerve endings that reach the preoptic area from the brain stem.[61]

Table 3.18.1. Effects of activation of inhibition of adrenergic receptor subtype on sleep and wakefulness.

Receptor subtype	Receptor activation	Receptor block	Effect on sleep or wakefulness
α_2-adrenoceptor	x		Induced sedation and drowsy wakefulness, and inhibited deep slow wave NREM and REM sleep.
α_2-adrenoceptor		x	Decreased the drowsy wakefulness induced by α_2-adrenergic receptor agonists.
α_1-adrenoceptor	x		Decreased latency of REM sleep, and increased episodes and time in REM sleep and aroused wakefulness.
α_1-adrenoceptor		x	Decreased REM sleep, and increased time in aroused wakefulness and drowsy wakefulness.
nonspecific β-adrenoceptor	x		Induced arousal (when injected into preoptic area of the brain).
β_1-adrenoceptor	x		Increased REM sleep.
β_1-adrenoceptor		x	Increased drowsy waking; and at larger doses, decreased REM sleep.
β_2-adrenoceptor	x		Decreased REM sleep.
β_1- and β_2-adrenoceptor		x	Decreased the REM sleep increased by α_1- and α_2-adrenergic receptor blocker, potentiated the increased drowsy waking induced by α_2-adrenergic receptor agonist, and decreased REM and deep slow wave sleep.

Possible Protective Effect of Increased Metabolism Associated with Physical Exercise

Moldofsky and Scarisbrick wrote that the musculoskeletal symptoms in study subjects deprived of slow wave sleep may not have resulted solely from the sleep deprivation. Physical fitness might also be an important variable.[7,p.43] None of the subjects in one study exercised regularly; they led sedentary lives as students. In a previous pilot study,[6,p.349] the researchers used 3 subjects who were "quite physically fit," 2 of whom ran 3-to-7 miles each day and continued their customary exercise schedule during the study. When deprived of slow wave sleep, these subjects did not develop fibromyalgia symptoms. In addition, their algometer tender point scores decreased (the algometer exam results showed a higher pressure/pain threshold or, in other words, lower tender point sensitivity). Moldofsky and Scarisbrick noted that in previous studies of sleep deprivation, researchers had not reported their subjects developing fibromyalgia symp-

toms.[6][7] He speculated that this result might have been due to the fitness levels of the subjects. The subjects were "young naval recruits who presumably would be quite physically fit and unlike our sedentary nonathletic university students."[7,p.43]

Moldofsky and Scarisbrick also pointed out that as far back as the 12th century, Maimonides had remarked on the tendency for sedentary people to develop musculoskeletal symptoms.[7,p.43] Maimonides wrote, "If one leads a sedentary life and does not take exercise, neglects the calls of nature, or is constipated—even if he eats wholesome food and takes care of himself in accordance with medical rules—he will, throughout his life, be subject to aches and pains and his strength will fail him."[16]

People today are no different: those with low levels of physical fitness have lower metabolic rates, and they are much more prone to develop fibromyalgia symptoms than are physically fit individuals. However, if an individual has inadequate thyroid hormone regulation of metabolism, her metabolism will still be subnormal, and even regular physical exercise is not likely to permanently protect the individual from the symptoms and signs of fibromyalgia (see Chapter 3.4).

Role of Internal and External Noxious Stimuli in Disturbed Sleep

Moldofsky wrote in 1975 that his observations on disturbed slow wave sleep suggest that a psychophysiological mechanism is involved in generating fibromyalgia symptoms. The intrusion of the alpha rhythm, a waking rhythm, into slow wave sleep, suggests "the operation of an internal arousal, alpha-induction mechanism in competition with the NREM (non-REM) sleep system." He speculated that alpha intrusion might impair the presumed restorative function of non-REM sleep and induce fibromyalgia. "This disturbance in sleep physiology could have been triggered in our patients by their traumatic or emotionally disturbing situations. The subsequent fatigue, irritability, depression, anxiety, and musculoskeletal aching and stiffness would become incorporated in a vicious, self-perpetuating, nonrestorative sleep cycle. Successful treatment of the clinical disorder might thus lie in the direction of improved sleep physiology."[6,pp.349-350]

Psychologically induced arousal is certainly an important cause of insomnia and nonrestful sleep. Berne and Levy wrote that emotional upset is the most common cause of insomnia.[46,p.148] Fibromyalgia patients typically suffer from emotional upset related to their condition. The uncertainty of their prognosis is emotionally disturbing to many. The inability to work and payment for useless medical treatments may lead to financial worries. In addition, many find it emotionally disturbing that relatives and clinicians imply or outright accuse them of not having a "real" illness and of being indolent. (See Chapter 1.2, sections titled "Iatrogenic Psychological Distress" and "Factors that May Account for Psychological Disturbance Among Fibromyalgia Patients.")

The results of recent studies strongly argue that pain serves as an internal stimulus that disrupts sleep in fibromyalgia patients. Tavares and Branco noted that sleep disturbance can be either the cause or the effect of fibromyalgia, or both. They conducted a study to clarify the relationship between tender points and pain with symptoms of disturbed sleep. Fifty-three women with a mean age of 45.7±8.0 years took part in the study. Patients answered questions about the time they went to sleep, how long it took to fall asleep, and the number of times they awoke from sleep. They also filled out a self-report questionnaire named the Post-sleep Inventory. The inventory is designed to assess symptoms that may occur before and during sleep and at the time of waking. The researchers assessed the patients' tender points according to the ACR method and pain intensity by a visual analog scale. Tavares and Branco found a positive correlation between pain intensity and the time it took to go to sleep (r=0.4; p<0.005), feelings of having had too little sleep (r=0.4; p<0.005), and physical discomfort upon awakening (r=0.325; p<0.05). They also found a positive correlation between the tender point count and subjective feelings of muscle tension when going to sleep (r=0.324; p<0.05). There was a negative correlation between the intensity of pain and how long patients slept (r=0.368; p<0.01). Tavares and Branco concluded that *increased pain intensity decreases the quality of sleep*.[68]

Hemmeter et al. reached a similar conclusion. They noted that chronic pain patients, including those with fibromyalgia, often suffer from disturbed sleep. The researchers recorded the sleep EEGs of 13 fibromyalgia patients to objectively characterize their sleep. Their aim was to learn the relationship between sleep abnormalities and pain intensity. Following this evaluation, they conducted a placebo-controlled study of the effects of ketanserine (a serotonin 5-HT$_2$-receptor blocker) on the patients because of its reported effectiveness in the regulation of sleep and pain. Hemmeter et al. concluded, "The results of our studies in patients with fibromyalgia show that *the alteration of sleep is mainly characterized by a disturbance of sleep continuity associated with the experience of pain intensity* [italics mine]." They also noted that the longer a patient has had fibromyalgia, the greater the intensity of her symptoms and the less successful the outcome of treatment.[69] This observation supports the notion of a continuing interaction of poor sleep and other symptoms resulting in a progressive deterioration of the patient's status.

The results of these studies support Moldofsky's argument that the successful treatment of fibromyalgia lies in the direction of improved sleep physiology.[6,pp.349-350] Improving sleep quality in patients with inadequate thyroid hormone regulation of cell function necessitates using the proper form and dosage of thyroid hormone. In addition, improving sleep physiology involves alleviating any psychological stimuli disturbing sleep, such as the interpretation of situations as aversive or threatening. Imaging a possible catastrophic nature of undiagnosed fibromyalgia symptoms is an example, as when a clinician tells the patient unjustifiably that she may have early, unverifiable systemic lupus erythematosus. Moreover, physical sources of sleep disturbance, such as trigger points, and chemical sources, such as various medications, must be controlled or eliminated. Below is a partial list of internal and external sources of sleep disturbance.

Internal Stimuli

A variety of internal stimuli can cause disturbed sleep, and secondarily, result in the various symptoms that accompany disturbed sleep.

Chronic Pain. Moldofsky suggested that pain and distressing psychological situations can induce the alpha EEG NREM sleep anomaly.[47] Disturbed sleep can increase an individual's susceptibility to acute pain.[41,p.288] Sleep disturbance, however, is the most common complaint of patients with continuous chronic pain. According to Sternbach, patients reported that before they developed pain, they slept well. After the pain developed, falling asleep became progressively more difficult because they could not get comfortable. Also, while trying to go to sleep, their minds were less preoccupied with other matters and their pain became their predominant perception. Finally, from exhaustion, they would slip into a restless sleep. During the sleep, when they changed position, pain would wake them. At some point, they might awaken and not be able to fall asleep again. Even if a patient slept until morning, her sleep was usually nonrestorative. Typically, the patient would feel fatigued and have cognitive dysfunction during the day, partly because of the disturbed sleep but also because the pain had eroded her sense of well-being. In addition to her sleep disturbance and fatigue, the patient usually had irritability, constipation, decreased libido and sexual activity, diminished activity level, and a low pain threshold.[37][38][39]

Headaches. Chronic headache sufferers often complain of fatigue, irritability, and disturbed sleep.[57][58] Drake et al. found that patients with intermittent migraine headaches had minimal sleep disturbance; those with chronic headaches were more likely to have disturbed sleep, and chronically poor sleep worsened the headaches. Also, patients with muscle contraction or tension headaches were more likely to have sleep alternations similar to those of fibromyalgia patients: they awoke frequently during sleep and had decreased slow wave sleep.[58]

Holroyd reported that of 245 subjects with chronic tension headaches, 70% had fatigue, headache-related anxiety and stress, and disturbed sleep. Sixty-six percent of the patients had headaches every day. On the physical and social functioning scales of the Medical Outcomes Study, 52% of the patients met criteria for

impairment. Holroyd concluded that the headaches disrupt the patients' lives. The sleep disturbance caused by the headaches most likely exacerbates the other symptoms, and the disturbed sleep may augment the tendency toward further headaches.[36]

Several studies suggest that sleep disturbance results in headaches in some individuals. For example, Paiva et al. found that nocturnal monitoring during sleep identified specific sleep disorders in 55% of subjects who had onset of headache during sleep. After treatment of the sleep disorder, all subjects with a sleep disorder reported improvement or absence of their headaches. The researchers concluded that headaches that occur during the night or early morning are often related to disturbed sleep.[35] In another study, Paiva et al. reported that morning or nocturnal headaches may indicate a sleep disturbance. They found that patients with substance abuse headaches mainly had insomnia, and the insomnia was relieved by stopping use of the substances.[34]

Such studies as those in this section suggest that headaches, like pain from trigger points, are likely to disturb sleep. In turn, sleep disturbance caused by headaches may result in more headaches.

Trigger Points. One of the most remarkable experiences I have had in clinical practice concerns the relation of myofascial trigger points to sleep. Uncountable times, when treating the trigger points of patients who had insomnia and other sleep disturbances, the patients have fallen into deep sleep on my treatment tables. Some awoke only after vigorous efforts to arouse them. Sometimes, my assistants and I have closed the treatment room doors and allowed the patients to get a long stretch of much needed sleep. These experiences have taught me that trigger points—whether actively referring pain or "latent"—often are a profound source of sleep disturbance, and desensitizing the points often results in profoundly restful sleep. I know of no studies of this phenomenon, but my common experience with it convinces me that each patient with sleep disturbance should be examined and treated for trigger points.

Patients with untreated hypothyroidism or cellular resistance to thyroid hormone are particularly prone to pain, excess physical and mental arousal, and disturbed sleep from myofascial trigger points. Neural impulses from a trigger point are transmitted to the spinal cord by type C and A delta nerve fibers. In their effect on the central nervous system, these impulses are especially noxious. Low level impulses from one trigger point are sufficient to cause severe sleep disturbance. After entering the cord, the impulses are transmitted to the brain. In passing through the brain stem, the impulses stimulate collateral fibers to the reticular activating system. Stimulation of the reticular system increases overall brain activity and creates an intense state of arousal and alertness. In this aroused and alert state, the individual cannot sleep until the impulses from the trigger point are halted, either spontaneously or by effective treatment.[63][64] The effects of sleep disturbance due to trigger points are no different than those caused by other sleep disrupting stimuli.

Medication. Among internal stimuli that can disturb sleep is medication. Although sleep-disturbing medication is an exogenous agent, it influences internal mechanisms that in turn disrupt sleep.

Goldman and Krings reported the case of a woman who developed fibromyalgia symptoms after changing her anticonvulsant medication for tonic/clonic seizures from hydantoin sodium to phenobarbital. The clinicians diagnosed the patient's condition as phenobarbital-induced fibromyalgia. The patient's fibromyalgic pain completely disappeared after she stopped taking phenobarbital. Goldman and Krings considered sleep disturbance as a mechanism by which the phenobarbital induced fibromyalgia symptoms.[31]

In rats, phenobarbital increases the rate of degradation of T_4 by both deiodination and excretion in the stool.[32] The drug increases the activity of glucuronyl transferase, resulting in an increase in T_4 glucuronide.[33] (T_4 glucuronide is a condensation product of glucuronic acid with T_4. The conjugation of T_4 and many catabolic products in the body with glucuronic acid occurs in the liver. Most glucuronides are excreted in the urine.) As a result of the conjugation of T_4 with glucuronic acid, the T_4 is eliminated from the body at an increased rate and the serum T_4 level decreases. McCain et al. suggested that an increase in TSH stimulated by the decreased T_4 level stimulates increased T_4 secretion by the thyroid gland, compensating for the phenobarbital-induced acceleration of T_4 clearance from the body.[33] It is possible that the pituitary-thyroid axis of Goldman and Krings' patient was not capable of increasing thyroid hormone secretion by the thyroid gland. Alternately, the phenobarbital may have had such an extraordinarily potent effect on glucuronyl transferase that the patient's pituitary-thyroid axis was not able to compensate.

Growth Hormone Deficiency. Some evidence suggests that growth hormone deficiency results in sleep disturbance. Hayashi et al. used polysomnography to test 3 female children with growth hormone deficiency. Rapid eye movement sleep was reduced before treatment with growth hormone and increased

afterward.[18][19] Young adults with growth hormone deficiencies had prolonged sleep time due to longer times in stage 1 and stage 2 sleep. They had a significant decrease in slow wave sleep time.[25] Intravenous administration of growth hormone in pulses during the first half of the night in normal young control subjects raised their plasma growth hormone levels and increased their slow wave sleep.[21] Pulsed growth hormone administration, resembling natural pulsatile secretion, promoted sleep more effectively than continuous administration.[21][22]

Growth hormone secretion is related to sleep. Jarrett et al. reported that in young adults and children, secretion of growth hormone at the onset of sleep is reliable and reproducible. They wrote that hormone secretion usually occurs during the first NREM period of sleep. They also wrote that they did not find a relationship between delta wave activity and growth hormone secretion. They suggested that sleep onset and growth hormone secretion are indirectly stimulated by complex mediating factors.[79]

Some researchers believe there is a close temporal relationship between growth hormone release and slow wave sleep.[19] Gronfier et al. found that growth hormone pulses coincided with peaks in slow wave sleep. The quantity of growth hormone secreted during pulses was correlated with the amount of concomitant slow wave activity. The researchers concluded that there is a close temporal and quantitative relationship between growth hormone secretion and slow wave activity, suggesting a common stimulatory mechanism.[20] Davidson et al. found that the normal nocturnal growth hormone surge disappeared in subjects deprived of sleep. When the subjects were permitted to sleep again, growth hormone secretion was prolonged, and some subjects had second secretory peaks that were not related to slow wave sleep. The researchers also found that growth hormone secretion was greater in slow wave sleep than in other sleep stages. They concluded that the nocturnal surge of growth hormone is sleep-dependent.[24]

Older et al. evaluated the effects of disrupted slow wave sleep on serum somatomedin C levels in healthy volunteers. The researchers disrupted the slow wave sleep of 13 volunteers on 3 consecutive nights. Six other volunteers whose sleep was not disrupted served as controls. At baseline, the somatomedin C levels of the two groups did not significantly differ. After the study, levels still did not differ between the two groups. The researchers wrote that the low somatomedin C levels in fibromyalgia patients may result from chronic rather than acute disruption of slow wave sleep. They allowed, however, that the low levels may depend on factors other than disrupted slow wave sleep.[45] Inadequate thyroid hormone regulation of growth hormone transcription and somatomedin C levels is the most plausible mechanism.

Thyroid hormone potently regulates growth hormone production. The hormone also regulates the levels of somatomedin C. It is likely that a growth hormone deficiency in fibromyalgia patients and deficient slow wave sleep related to the deficiency are secondary to inadequate thyroid hormone regulation of growth hormone gene transcription (see Chapter 3.12).

Histamine. Increased histamine secretion, by increasing alertness,[27] may interfere with sleep. Lin et al. found that administering an agent that inhibited the histamine-synthesizing enzyme decreased wakefulness and increased slow wave sleep. Histamine probably mediates arousal and pain perception that interferes with sleep.[26] Histamine secretion may be increased by binding of catecholamines to α_2-adrenergic receptors. Density of α_2-adrenergic receptors on cell membranes is increased during inadequate thyroid hormone regulation of transcription of the adrenergic receptor genes. (See Chapter 3.1, section titled "Altered Sleep Patterns.")

Sleep Apnea in Hypothyroidism. The term "apnea" means absence of breathing. Apnea during sleep is usually caused by an upper airway obstruction. The patient awakes frequently and as a result, usually has fatigue and sleepiness during waking hours.

Many hypothyroid patients have sleep apnea.[49] Teramoto et al. found that of 18 elderly hypothyroid patients (73.6±5.9 years old), 14 (78%) had sleep apnea.[71] Bai reported that of 21 hypothyroid patients, 11 (52%) had sleep apnea.[76] Abouganem et al. emphasized the importance of the clinician identifying hypothyroidism as a cause of sleep apnea. If a patient undergoes proper thyroid hormone therapy, the cardiovascular risks of prolonged apnea may be avoided.[15] Of course, hypothyroidism is itself a risk factor for cardiovascular disease independent of prolonged sleep apnea. Proper hormone treatment improves both the apnea and any cardiovascular disease underlain by thyroid hormone deficiency.

Reduced Hemoglobin Oxygenation During Sleep in the Arterial Blood of Fibromyalgia Patients with Sleep Apnea. Alvarez et al. studied 28 fibromyalgic females and 15 matched control subjects. All the patients and subjects had high scores on the Epworth Sleepiness Scale. The objective of the researchers was to measure $SaO_2\%$ in patients and subjects who had oxygen desaturation of hemoglobin

related to sleep apnea. These researchers measured the oxygen saturation of hemoglobin in the arterial blood ($SaO_2\%$) during sleep. Compared to control subjects, fibromyalgia patients had lower overnight minimum $SaO_2\%$ (90.7 ±0.9 versus 86.8 ±1.3). The conclusion was that the fibromyalgia patients had a fall in oxygen saturation of hemoglobin in arterial blood ($SaO_2\%$) during sleep.[73] This corresponds to the reduced SaO_2 of hypothyroid patients with sleep apnea.

Low SaO_2 in Hypothyroidism. Zaroulis et al. reported that the *in vitro* P50 values (the oxygen tension at half saturation of hemoglobin) were normal in hypothyroid and hyperthyroid patients. They wrote, "The known changes in oxygen consumption produced by alterations in thyroid hormone levels in patients with hypothyroidism or hyperthyroidism did not affect red blood cell oxygen transport function."[75] However, in more recent studies researchers found that low SaO_2 values in untreated hypothyroidism significantly increased following thyroid hormone therapy. Teramoto et al. found that after 3-to-6 months of treatment with thyroid hormone, elderly hypothyroid patients had a reduced incidence of sleep apnea. In addition, their lowest level of SaO_2 during sleep had significantly increased from the previous lowest level.[71]

Bai tested the respiratory function of 21 patients with primary hypothyroidism before and after thyroid hormone therapy. Nine of the patients were available for follow-up. Several measures of respiratory function were markedly improved after treatment: maximum apnea time, mean apnea time, respiratory disturbances index, and the lowest blood oxygen saturation ($SaO_2 \%$). Bai wrote, "We conclude that OSA [obstructive sleep apnea] in hypothyroidism showed the most satisfactory response to non-surgical treatment, and OSA syndrome could be cured as soon as hypothyroidism was controlled by desiccated thyroid."[76]

Possible Contribution of Weak Respiratory and Postural Muscles in Hypothyroidism. The respiratory and oxygen transport systems are complex. Many interactions and potential abnormalities at various levels within the systems may combine to make oxygen transport in the blood and the oxygen supply to tissues inadequate.[74] An effect of inadequate thyroid hormone regulation of cell function that may contribute to reduced oxygenation of the blood (low SaO_2) is weakness of the respiratory and postural muscles. Since the end of the 19th century, medical writers have described muscle weakness as a feature of hypothyroidism. The weak muscles of hypothyroid patients favor slumping or flexed posture. In this posture, which may continue during sleep, the diaphragm and abdominal organs sag. The sagging compresses tissues within the abdomen, impedes circulation, and causes passive congestion in one or all abdominal and pelvic organs. During this process, the diaphragmatic pump may lose its efficiency. The reduced efficiency is likely to restrict normal inspiration of air, possibly resulting in subnormal oxygenation of the blood.[72,p.87] (See Chapter 3.11, section titled "Visceral Prolapse.")

External Stimuli

Moldofsky and Scarisbrick used brief bursts of an auditory stimulus for up to 20 seconds to disturb the slow wave sleep of healthy volunteers. Those who were sedentary developed fibromyalgia-like symptoms.[6] This study showed that external stimuli are capable of disturbing normal sleep in such a way that fibromyalgia symptoms result.[7] Most people know of the effectiveness of other external stimuli, such as the crying of a baby, in disrupting sleep so that fatigue, stiffness, body discomfort and pain—cardinal symptoms of fibromyalgia—develop.

Some individuals have poor quality sleep due to inadequate thyroid hormone regulation of the adrenergic genes. The poor quality sleep may result from an increased density of α_2-adrenergic receptors on cell membranes and a decreased density of β_1-adrenergic receptors (see section above titled "Increased α_2-Adrenergic and Decreased β_1-Adrenergic Receptors"). The sleep of these individuals is likely to be more easily disrupted by external stimuli. Metabolically normal subjects deprived of sleep recover from the adverse effects after obtaining sufficient slow wave and REM sleep.[83] Those with increased α_2-adrenergic receptors and decreased β_1-adrenergic receptors due to inadequate thyroid hormone regulation of the adrenergic genes are not likely to recover until they undergo treatment with the proper form and dosage of thyroid hormone.

MELATONIN SECRETION POSSIBLY LOW IN FIBROMYALGIA PATIENTS

Melatonin is a metabolite of serotonin that is synthesized in the pineal gland.[89,p.74] Infusion of tryptophan (the amino acid precursor of serotonin) to healthy young men caused a dose-dependent rise in circulating melatonin.[90]

The one report of low melatonin secretion in fibromyalgia may be important. As Wikner et al. wrote, melatonin promotes sleep, and subnormal secretion may disturb patients' sleep. The disturbed sleep may

cause fatigue and pain. The researchers measured the serum and urinary levels of melatonin and calculated the total melatonin secretion of 8 fibromyalgia patients and 8 healthy sex- and age-matched controls. The patients had a 31% lower melatonin secretion during the hours of darkness (11 pm-to-7 am). The peak value of melatonin was also lower in the patients. The rate of secretion and peak secretion did not significantly differ between the groups. Wikner et al. noted that serum levels of the two precursors of melatonin, tryptophan and serotonin, were also low, and these low levels may also have contributed to sleep disturbance and increased pain perception.[84] (The levels of these precursors may be influenced by thyroid hormone.)

To establish an objective finding characteristic of fibromyalgia, the number of fibromyalgia patients and matched controls in this study—8 of each—were not sufficient, and we should consider the results those of a pilot study. Thus, we must await further studies with larger numbers of participants before accepting that fibromyalgia patients have significantly low melatonin secretion. I question that they do have low levels. I base my question on the results of studies of the influence of thyroid hormone on melatonin synthesis, secretion, and circulating levels. Overall, the studies suggest that thyroid hormone increases circulating melatonin levels.

Biochemical evidence suggests that increases or decreases in exposure of the pinealocytes to thyroid hormone affect melatonin synthesis and secretion. Rom-Bugoslavskaia and Bondarenko, for example, reported that thyroid hormone exerts a regulatory role over serotonin metabolism in pinealocytes. (Pinealocytes are the chief cells of the pineal gland. They synthesize melatonin from serotonin.) Rom-Bugoslavskaia and Bondarenko wrote that saturating the body with T_4 shifts serotonin processing toward a pathway that results in melatonin synthesis. First, acetylation of serotonin results in the formation of N-acetylserotonin. Second, ortho-methylation results in the formation of melatonin (also termed O-methyl serotonin). On the other hand, total thyroidectomy partially shifts serotonin processing away from this melatonin-synthesizing pathway. Consequently, while thyroid hormone is deficient, serotonin predominantly undergoes oxidative deamination with the formation of its major breakdown product, 5-hydroxyindole acetic acid. (If thyroid hormone regulation of pineal cells is inadequate, we would expect decreased 5-hydroxyindole acetic acid, as found in some fibromyalgia patients. Despite the shift away from melatonin production and toward production of 5-hydroxyindole acetic acid, we would nonetheless expect low production of 5-hydroxyindole acetic acid. The low levels would result from an increased density of α_2-adrenergic receptors on the membranes of serotonin-secreting neurons, and the increased density would result from inadequate thyroid hormone regulation of the adrenergic genes. The increased density of α_2-adrenergic receptors would inhibit serotonin secretion. Rom-Bugoslavskaia and Bondarenko concluded that thyroid hormone deficiency and excess have opposite effects on the pineal gland. They wrote that the formation of methoxyindoles (such as melatonin) is the process in the pineal gland most sensitive to thyroid hormone.[88]

Despite this description of serotonin pathways influenced by thyroid hormone, some researchers question the mechanism by which thyroid hormone influences melatonin secretion. Guerrero and Reiter published statements that question a role for T_3 in melatonin secretory rhythms. They wrote that no one has reported a role for α-adrenergic receptors (which increase during inadequate thyroid hormone regulation of adrenergic gene transcription) in the pineal gland of adults. Activity of 5'-deiodinase (which converts T_4 to T_3) in the pineal gland is well established, but few data are available concerning the physiological significance of the enzyme in the gland. In fact, according to Guerrero and Reiter, studies suggest that the secretory rhythms of melatonin by the pineal gland do not rely on the cyclic production of T_3.[87]

This conclusion is supported by the results of a study by Soszynski et al. They studied the circadian rhythm of melatonin in 16 women with altered thyroid status. Eight of the women had hypothyroidism and 8 had hyperthyroidism. Five healthy controls also took part. Women in all three groups had a significant melatonin circadian rhythm. None of the measures of melatonin (such as the secretory amplitude and time of greatest secretion) significantly differed between the groups. The researchers concluded that neither hypothyroidism nor hyperthyroidism altered the circadian rhythm of melatonin secretion. However, while the integrated 24-hour secretion of melatonin was similar between patients and controls, melatonin levels positively correlated with TSH levels in hypothyroidism and negatively correlated with T_3 levels in hyperthyroidism. Thus, while the rhythm of melatonin secretion was not affected, thyroid hormone deficiency increased melatonin levels and thyroid hormone excess decreased the levels.[92]

Other researchers have also reported increased melatonin secretion in hypothyroid patients. Rojdmark et al. reported that compared to normal subjects, hypo-

thyroid patients had higher serum peak melatonin values, total nighttime melatonin secretion, and excretion of melatonin in the urine.[85] Bals-Pratsch et al. measured the melatonin in pooled sera from 4 subclinical hypothyroid patients, 1 primary hypothyroid patient, and 4 normal control subjects every 30 minutes for 24 hours. The researchers wrote that the samples from patients had significantly higher melatonin values seven times during the night.[86]

Still other researchers have reported a conflicting finding—that melatonin secretion is not affected by thyroid hormone status. Bauer et al. rendered some rats hypothyroid through thyroidectomy and made others thyrotoxic by administering T_3 for 9 days. Despite clear-cut metabolic effects of the thyroid hormone deficiency or excess, thyroid hormone deficiency or excess did not alter the content of melatonin in the rats' pineal glands during the day or night.[91]

Future studies may determine that in fact most fibromyalgia patients do have low melatonin secretion. If so, the finding may constitute a proposition that diverges from the hypothesis I posit in this book: that fibromyalgia in most patients results from inadequate thyroid hormone regulation of cell function. First, however, further studies involving far greater numbers of fibromyalgia patients are necessary to substantiate or refute the results reported by Wikner et al.[84]

REFERENCES

1. Clement, H.-W., Gemsa, D., and Wesemann, W.: The effect of adrenergic drugs on serotonin metabolism in the nucleus raphe dorsalis of the rat, studied by *in vivo* voltammetry. *Euro. J. Pharmacol.*, 217:43-48, 1992.
2. Aslanian, V. and Renaud, B.: Changes in serotonin metabolism in the rat raphe magnus and cardiovascular modifications following systemic administration of clonidine and other central α_2-agonists: an *in vivo* voltammetry study. *Neuropharmacology*, 28:387, 1989.
3. Svensson, T.H., Bunney, B.S., and Aghajanian, G.K.: Inhibition of both noradrenergic and serotonergic neurons in brain by the α-adrenergic agonist clonidine. *Brain Res.*, 92:291, 1975.
4. Monti, J.M.: Catecholamines and the sleep-wake cycle. I. EEG and behavioral arousal. *Life Sci.*, 30:1145, 1982.
5. Hilakivi, I.: The role of β- and α-adrenoceptors in the regulation of the stages of the sleep-waking cycle in the cat. *Brain Res.*, 277:109-118, 1983.
6. Moldofsky, H., Scarisbrick, P., England, R., and Smythe, H.: Musculoskeletal symptoms and non-REM sleep disturbance in patients with "fibrositis syndrome" and healthy subjects. *Psychosomat. Med.* 37(4):341-351, 1975.
7. Moldofsky, H. and Scarisbrick, P.: Induction of neurasthenic musculoskeletal pain syndrome by selective sleep stage deprivation. *Psychosom. Med.*, 38:35-44, 1976.

8. Watanakunakorn, C., Hodges, R.E., and Evans, T.C.: Myxedema: a study of 400 cases. *Arch. Intern. Med.*, 116:183-190, 1965.

9. Kales, A., Heuser, G., and Jacobson, A.: All night sleep studies in hypothyroid patients, before and after treatment. *J. Clin. Endocrinol.*, 27:1593-1599, 1967.

10. Wilke, W.S., Sheeler, L.R., and Makarowski, W.S.: Hypothyroidism with presenting symptoms of fibrositis. *J. Rheum.*, 8:627-630, 1981.

11. Weinstock, W., Weiss, C., and Gitter, S.: Blockade of 5-hydroxytryptamine receptors in the central nervous system by β-adrenoceptor antagonists. *Neuropharmacology*, 16:273, 1977.

12. Frankhyzen, A. and Muller, A.: *In vitro* studies on the inhibition of serotonin release through α-adrenoreceptor activity in various regions of the rat CNS. *Abstract of 5th Catecholamine Symposium*, 1983, p.137.

13. Vogel, G.W.: REM deprivation. III. Dreaming and psychosis. *Arch. Gen. Psychiatry*, 18:312-329, 1968.

14. Agnew, H.W., Webb, W.B., and Williams, R.L.: Comparison of stage four and 1-REM sleep deprivation. *Percept. Mot. Skills*, 24:851-858, 1967.

15. Abouganem, D., Taylor, A.L., Donna, E., and Baum, G.L.: Extreme bradycardia during sleep apnea caused by myxedema. *Arch. Intern. Med.*, 147(8):1497-1499, 1987.

16. Maimonides, M.: Mishneh Torah. In *The Book of Knowledge*. Edited by M. Hyamson, Boys Town Jerusalem Publishers, 1962.

17. Hartmann, E.L.: *The Function of Sleep*. New Haven, Yale University Press, 1973.

18. Hayashi, M., Saisho, S., Suzuki, H., Shimozawa, K., and Iwakawa, Y.: Sleep disturbance in children with congenital and acquired hypothyroidism. *No To Hattatsu. Brain Dev.*, 20:294-300, 1988.

19. Hayashi, M., Saisho, S., Suzuki, H., Shimozawa, K., and Iwakawa, Y.: Sleep disturbance in children with growth hormone deficiency. *No To Hattatsu. Brain Dev.*, 14:170-174, 1992.

20. Gronfier, C., Luthringer, R., Follenius, M., et al.: A quantitative evaluation of the relationship between growth hormone secretion and delta wave electroencephalographic activity during normal sleep and after enrichment in delta waves. *Sleep*, 10(10):817-824, 1996.

21. Schier, T., Guldner, J., Colla, M., Holsboer, F., and Steiger, A.: Changes in sleep-endocrine activity after growth hormone-releasing hormone depend on time of administration. *J. Neuroendocrinol.*, 9(3):201-205, 1997.

22. Marshall, L., Molle, M., Boschen, G., Steiger, A., Fehm, H.L., and Born, J.: Greater efficacy of episodic than continuous growth hormone-releasing hormone administration in promoting slow wave sleep. *J. Clin. Endocrinol. Metab.*, 81(3):1009-1013, 1996.

23. Guyton, A.C.: *Textbook of Medical Physiology*, 8th edition. Philadelpha, W.B. Saunders Company, 1991.

24. Davidson, J.R., Moldofsky, H., and Lue, F.A.: Growth hormone and cortisol secretion in relation to sleep and wakefulness. *J. Psychiat. Neurosci.*, 16(2):96-102, 1991.

25. Asrom, C. and Lindholm, J.: Growth hormone-deficient young adults have decreased deep sleep. *Neuroendocrinology*, 51(1):82-84, 1990.

26. Lin, J.S., Sakai, K., and Jouvet, M.: Hypothalamo-preoptic histaminergic projections in sleep-wake control in the cat. *Eur. J. Neurosci.*, 6(4):618-625, 1994.

27. Nicholson, A.N., Pascoe, P.A., Turner, C., et al.: Sedation and histamine H_1-receptor antagonism: studies in man with the enantiomers of chlorpheniramine and dimethindene. *Brit. J. Pharmacol.*, 104(1):270-276, 1991.

28. Dement, W.C.: An essay on dreams: the role of physiology in understanding their nature. In *New Directions in Psychology, II*. New York, Holt, Rinehart, and Winston, 1965, pp.135-257.

29. Kelly, D.D.: Sleep and dreaming. In *Principles of Neural Science*, 3rd edition. Edited by E.R.Kandel, J.H. Schwartz, and T.M. Jessell, Norwalk, Appleton & Lange, 1991, pp.792-804.

30. Moldofsky, H.: Fibromyalgia, sleep disorder, and chronic fatigue syndrome. *Ciba Found. Sympos.*, 173:262-271, 1993.

31. Goldman, S.I. and Krings, M.S.: Phenobarbital-induced fibromyalgia as the cause of bilateral shoulder pain. *J. Amer. Osteop. Assoc.*, 95(8):487-490, 1995.

32. Oppenheimer, J.H., Bernstein, G., and Surks, M.I.: Increased thyroxine turnover and thyroidal function after stimulation of hepatocellular binding of thyroxine by phenobarbital. *J. Clin. Invest.*, 47:1399, 1968.

33. McClain, R.M., Leven, A.A., Posch, R., and Downing, J.C.: The effect of phenobarbital on the metabolism and excretion of thyroxine in rats. *Toxicol. Appl. Pharmacol.*, 99:216, 1989.

34. Paiva, T., Batista, A., Martins, P., and Martins, A.: The relationship between headaches and sleep disturbances. *Headache*, 35(10):590-596, 1995.

35. Paiva, T., Farinha, A., Martins, A., Batista, A., and Guilleminault, C.: Chronic headaches and sleep disorders. *Arch. Intern. Med.*, 157(15):1701-1705, 1997.

36. Holroyd, K.: Department of Psychology, Ohio University, 1998. < http://www.pslgroup.com/dg/8948a.htm >

37. Sternback, R.A.: *Pain Patients: Traits and Treatment*. New York, Academic Press, 1974.

38. Sternback, R.A.: Chronic pain as a disease entity. *Triangle*, 20:27, 1981.

39. Sternback, R.A.: Acute versus chronic pain. In *Textbook of Pain*. Edited by P.D. Wall and R. Melzack, London, Churchill Livingston, 1984, pp.173-177.

40. Sternback, R.A.: Acute versus chronic pain. In *Textbook of Pain*, 2nd edition. Edited by P.D. Wall and R. Melzack, London, Churchill Livingston, 1989, pp.242-246.

41. Cousins, M.: Acute versus chronic pain. In *Textbook of Pain*, 2nd edition. Edited by P.D. Wall and R. Melzack, London, Churchill Livingston, 1989, pp.284-305.

42. Plantamura, A., Steinbauer, J., and Eisinger, J.: Sleep apnea and fibromyalgia: the absence of correlation does not indicate an exclusive central hypothesis. *Rev. Med. Interne.*, 16(9):662-665, 1995.

43. Carette, S., Oakson, G., Guimont, C., and Steriade, M.: Sleep electroencephalography and the clinical response to amitriptyline in patients with fibromyalgia. *Arthritis Rheumatol.*, 38(9):1211-1217, 1995.

44. Fransen, J. and Russell, I.J.: *The Fibromyalgia Help Book: Practical Guide to Living Better with Fibromyalgia*. Saint Paul, Smith House Press, 1996.

45. Older, S.A., Battafarano, D.F., Danning, C.L., Ward, J.A.,

Grady, E.P., Derman, S., and Russell, I.J.: The effects of delta wave sleep interruption on pain thresholds and fibromyalgia-like symptoms in healthy subjects; correlations with insulin-like growth factor I. *J. Rheumatol.*, 25(6): 1180-1186, 1998.

46. Berne, R.M. and Levy, M.N.: *Principles of Physiology.* St. Louis, C.V. Mosby Company, 1990.

47. Moldofsky, H.: Sleep and fibrositis syndrome. *Rheum. Dis. Clin. North Amer.*, 15:91-103, 1989.

48. Saskin, P., Moldofsky, H., and Salem, L.: Sleep and symptoms in psychophysiologic insomnia and fibrositis. *Sleep Res.*, 16:421, 1987.

49. Campbell, S.M., Clark, S., Tindall, E.A., Forehand, M.E., and Bennett, R.M.: Clinical characteristics of fibrositis. I. A "blinded," controlled study of symptoms and tender points. *Arthritis Rheum.*, 26(7):817-824, 1983.

50. Wolfe, F., Hawley, D.J., Cathey, M.A., Caro, X., and Russell, I.J.: Fibrositis: symptom frequency and criteria for diagnosis: an evaluation of 291 rheumatic disease patients and 58 normal individuals. *J. Rheumatol.*, 12:1159-1163, 1985.

51. Ware, J.C., Russell, J., and Campos, E.: Alpha intrusions into the sleep of depressed and fibromyalgia syndrome (fibrositis) patients. *Sleep Res.*, 15:210, 1986.

52. Molony, R.R., MacPeek, D.M., Shiffman, P.L., Frank, M., Schwartzberg, M., and Seibold, J.R.: Sleep, sleep apnea, and fibromyalgia syndrome. *J. Rhematol.*, 13:797-800, 1986.

53. Schackell, B.S. and Horne, J.A.: The alpha-sleep anomaly and related phenomena. *Sleep Res.*, 16:432, 1987.

54. Scheuler, W., Kubicki, S., Marquardt, J., Scholz, G., Henkes, H., and Gaeth, L.: The alpha-sleep pattern: quantitative analysis and functional aspects. In *Sleep 1986.* Edited by W.P.Koella, F. Obal, H. Schultz, and P. Vissar, Stutgart, Fischer, 1988.

55. Hirsch, M., Carlander, B., Vergé, M., Tafti, M., Anaya, J.-M., Billiard, M., and Sany, J.: Objective and subjective sleep disturbances in patients with rheumatoid arthritis: a reappraisal. *Arthritis Rheum.*, 37:41-49, 1994.

56. Moldofsky, H., Lue, F.A., and Saskin, P.: Sleep and morning pain in primary osteoarthritis. *J. Rheumatol.*, 14:124-128, 1987.

57. Philips, H.C. and Jahanshahi, M.: The effects of persistent pain: the chronic headache sufferer. *Pain*, 21(2):163-176, 1985.

58. Drake, M.E., Jr., Pakalnis, A., Andrews, J.M., and Bogner, J.E.: Nocturnal sleep recording with cassette EEG in chronic headaches. *Headache*, 30(9):600-603, 1990.

59. Ware, J.C.: Tricyclic antidepressants in the treatment of insomnia. *J. Clin. Psychiat.*, 44(9 Pt.2):25-28, 1983.

60. Makela, J.P. and Hilakivi, I.T.: Evidence for the involvement of α_2-adrenoceptors in the sedation but not REM sleep inhibition by clonidine in the rat. *Med. Biol.*, 64(6): 355-360, 1986.

61. Sood, S., Dhawan, J.K., Ramesh, V., John, J., Gopinath, G., and Kumar, V.M.: Role of medial preoptic area β-adrenoceptors in the regulation of sleep-wakefulness. *Pharmacol. Biochem. Behav.*, 57(1-2):1-5, 1997.

62. Emerson, C.H., Liberman, C., and Braverman, L.E.: Hypothyroidism. In *The Thyroid*. Edited by W.L. Green, New York, Elsevier, 1987.

63. Lowe, J.C.: The myofascial genesis of unpleasant thoughts and emotions: its neural basis. *Dig. Chiro. Econ.*, 32(5): 78, 80-81, (Mar./Apr.) 1989.

64. Lowe, J.C.: The emotional effects of noxious myofascial stimulation. *Amer. Chiro. Mag.*, Jan. 22-24, 1989.

65. Hilakivi, I. and Leppavuori, A.: Effects of methoxamine, an α_1-adrenoceptor agonist, and prazosin, an α_1-antagonist, on the stages of the sleep-waking cycle in the cat. *Acta Physiol. Scand.*, 120(3):363-372, 1984.

66. Morgane, P.J.: Serotonin: twenty years later—monoamine theory of sleep: the role of serotonin: a review. *Psychopharmacol. Bull.*, 17:13-17, 1981.

67. Chase, T.N. and Murphy, D.L.: Serotonin and central nervous system function. *Ann. Rev. Pharmacol.*, 13:181-197, 1973.

68. Tavares, V. and Branco, J.: Relation of sleep related complaints with tender points and pain intensity in fibromyalgia syndrome. *J. Musculoskel. Pain*, 3(Suppl.1):138, 1995.

69. Hemmeter, U., Kocher, R., Ladewig, D., et al.: Sleep disorders in chronic pain and generalized tendomyopathy. *Schweiz. Med. Wochenschr.*, 125(49):2391-2397, 1995.

70. Bennett, R.M., Clark, S.R., Campbell, S.M., et al.: Symptoms of Raynaud's syndrome in patients with fibromyalgia. A study utilizing the Nielsen test, digital photoplethysmography and measurements of platelet α_2-adrenergic receptors. *Arthritis Rheum.*, 34(3):264-269, 1991.

71. Teramoto, S., Ohga, E., Katayama, H., et al.: Effects of thyroid hormone replacement therapy on nocturnal apnea in elderly patients with hypothyroidism. *Nihon Kokyuki Gakkai Zasshi*, 36(7):590-594, 1998.

72. Schafer, R.C.: *Clinical Biomechanics: Musculoskeletal Actions and Reactions*, 2nd edition. Baltimore, Williams & Wilkins, 1987.

73. Alvarez Lario, B., Alonso Valdivielso, J.L., Alegre Lopez, J., Martel Soteres, C., Viejo Banuelos, J.L., and Maranon Cabello, A.: Fibromyalgia syndrome: overnight falls in arterial oxygen saturation. *Amer. J. Med.*, 101(1):54-60, 1996.

74. Goldman, A.L.: Respiratory abnormalities in hypothyroidism. *Compr. Ther.*, 3(12):17-24, 1977.

75. Zaroulis, C.G., Kourides, I.A., and Valeri, C.R.: Red cell 2,3-diphosphoglycerate and oxygen affinity of hemoglobin in patients with thyroid disorders. *Blood*, 52(1):181-185, 1978.

76. Bai, Y.: Primary hypothyroidism with obstructive sleep apnea syndrome. *Chung Kuo I Hsueh Ko Hsueh Yuan Hsueh Pao*, 14(4):267-272, 1992.

77. Carette, S., Bell, M., Reynolds, W.J., et al.: A controlled trial of amitriptyline, cyclobenzaprine, and placebo in fibromyalgia. *Arthritis Rheum.*, 35(Suppl.9):112, 1992.

78. Carette, S., Bell, M., Reynolds, W.J., et al.: Comparison of amitriptyline, cyclobenzaprine, and placebo in the treatment of fibromyalgia. *Arthritis Rheum.*, 37(1):32-40, 1994.

79. Jarrett, D.B., Greenhouse, J.B., Miewald, J.M., Fedorka, I.B., and Kupfer, D.J.: A reexamination of the relationship between growth hormone secretion and slow wave sleep using delta wave analysis. *Biol. Psychiat.*, 27(5):497-509, 1990.

80. Russell, I.J., Vaeroy, H., Javors, M., and Nyberg, F.:

Cerebrospinal fluid biogenic amine metabolites in fibromyalgia/fibrositis syndrome and rheumatoid arthritis. *Arthritis Rheum.*, 35:550-556, 1992.

81. Moldofsky, H.: Sleep mechanisms and fibromyalgia. *First International Symposium on Myofascial Pain and Fibromyalgia.* Minneapolis, Minnesota, May 9, 1989.

82. Moldofsky, H.: The contribution of sleep-wake physiology to fibromyalgia. In *Advances in Pain Research and Therapy,* Vol.17. Edited by J.R. Fricton and E.A. Awad, New York, Raven Press, Ltd., 1990, pp.227-240.

83. Luden, A., Moses, J.M., Johnson, L.C., and Naitoh, P.: The recuperative effects of REM sleep and stage 4 sleep on human performance after complete sleep loss. *Psychophysiology*, 11:133-136, 1974.

84. Wikner, J., Hirsch, U., Wetterberg, L., and Rojdmark, S.: Fibromyalgia: a syndrome associated with decreased nocturnal melatonin secretion. *Clin. Endocrinol.* (Oxf), 49(2): 179-183, 1998.

85. Rojdmark, S., Berg, A., Rossner, S., and Wetterberg, L.: Nocturnal melatonin secretion in thyroid disease and in obesity. *Clin. Endocrinol.* (Oxf), 35(1):61-65, 1991.

86. Bals-Pratsch, M., De Geyter, C., Muller, T., et al.: Episodic variations of prolactin, thyroid-stimulating hormone, luteinizing hormone, melatonin and cortisol in infertile women with subclinical hypothyroidism. *Hum. Reprod.,*

12(5):896-904, 1997.

87. Guerrero, J.M. and Reiter, R.J.: Iodothyronine 5'-deiodinating activity in the pineal gland. *Int. J. Biochem.*, 24(10): 1513-1523, 1992.

88. Rom-Bugoslavskaia, E.S. and Bondarenko, L.A.: Effect of deficiency and excess of thyroid hormones in the body on indolamine metabolism in the rat epiphysis cerebri. *Probl. Endokrinol.* (Mosk), 30(5):82-85, 1984.

89. Theoharides, T.C.: Autocoids. In *Pharmacology.* Edited by T.C. Theoharides, Boston, Little, Brown and Company, 1992, pp.49-90.

90. Heuther, G., Hajak, G., Reimer, A., et al.: The metabolic fate of infused L-tryptophan in men: possible clinical implications of the accumulation of circulating tryptophan and tryptophan metabolites. *Psychopharmacology,* 109(4): 422-432, 1992.

91. Bauer, M.S., Poland, R.E., Whybrow, P.C., and Frazer, A.: Pituitary-adrenal and thyroid effects on melatonin content of the rat pineal gland. *Psychoneuroendocrinology,* 14 (3):165-175, 1989.

92. Soszynski, P., Zgliczynski, S., and Pucilowska, J.: The circadian rhythm of melatonin in hypothyroidism and hyperthyroidism. *Acta Endocrinol.* (Copenh), 119(2):240-244, 1988.

3.19

Substance P

Fibromyalgia patients have elevated cerebrospinal substance P levels. Inadequate regulation of gene transcription by thyroid hormone is the most plausible explanation for the elevated levels. Thyroid hormone regulates substance P in discrete nuclei of the brain, in the anterior pituitary, in the lumbar spinal cord, and in the dorsal root ganglia. Most significantly, however, thyroid hormone directly regulates transcription of the preprotachykinin gene. This gene codes for preprotachykinin-A (the precursor of substance P) and the substance P receptor. Studies confirm the negative regulation of substance P by thyroid hormone; that is, increased exposure of the gene to thyroid hormone decreases production of substance P; conversely, decreasing exposure of the gene to thyroid hormone increases production of substance P. Increased substance P levels within the central nervous system may mediate in large part the heightened perception of pain by fibromyalgia patients. (This chapter is based on a paper by Jackie Yellin.[40])

Until recently, low peripheral serotonin levels received most attention as a feature of fibromyalgia. Attention is now generally shared with high substance P levels, since researchers reported that the levels in fibromyalgia patients are extraordinarily high.[40]

A high substance P level is a distinctive laboratory finding. It substantially contributes to the cumulative evidence that inadequate thyroid hormone regulation of gene transcription is the underlying pathogenic factor in fibromyalgia.

Several studies have shown elevated levels of substance P in the cerebrospinal fluid of fibromyalgia patients.[1][2][3] By contrast, serum and urine substance P levels are usually normal.[4,p.74] The elevated cerebrospinal fluid levels appear to be a mediator of nociception in fibromyalgia patients.[8] One researcher recently stated that elevated cerebrospinal substance P in fibromyalgia ". . . is the most dramatically abnormal laboratory measure yet documented in these patients. It clearly distinguishes patients selected by the ACR criteria from healthy, normal individuals." He also stated that fibromyalgia is the only clinical disorder in which patients have profoundly elevated levels of cerebrospinal substance P.[4,p.76]

The same researcher, during a recent lecture in Houston, Texas,[6] stated that one study showed that substance P levels typically stay elevated in fibromyalgia patients over time. After learning of high substance P levels in the cerebrospinal fluid of fibromyalgia patients, he suspected that the enzyme that breaks down substance P might be catabolizing substance P too slowly. He measured the concentration of the enzyme and its activity level. The amount was normal. Its activity level, however, was slightly increased. The increased activity may be a positive feedback adaptation to lower the elevated levels of substance P. The researcher concluded that the enzyme is not involved, and "It's just that substance P is being produced at a greater rate than it should be."

Cullum, Graf, Yellin, and I previously proposed in *Medical Hypotheses* that inadequate thyroid hormone regulation of preprotachykinin gene transcription causes increased substance P levels. Substantial evidence supports this conjecture.[7]

● SUBSTANCE P

Substance P is a small neuropeptide that is excitatory to afferent pain-mediating neurons and motor neurons.[9][10][11][12][13][14] Evidence indicates that in the spinal cord, substance P acts in a background manner to aid transmission through powerful synaptic pathways that are involved in reflex activity.[14] Also, substance P facilitates sensory processing.[12][15][16] It particularly facilitates transmission of signals that give rise to pain perception.

● THYROID HORMONE REGULATION OF SUBSTANCE P IN WIDESPREAD, DISCRETE NUCLEI OF THE BRAIN

Dupont et al. measured changes in substance P content of discrete nuclei from various regions of the brain of neonatal rats after their thyroid glands were removed and after treatment with T_4. After removal of the gland, substance P levels markedly increased: substance P levels were 2.5 times higher in some brain areas than in control animals. The increases were statistically significant in 19 of the 32 brain nuclei dissected.[17,p.2042] By far, the greatest increase in substance P occurred in the substantia nigra zona reticulata (a midbrain structure). Administering T_4 to the rats decreased substance P levels.

THYROID HORMONE REGULATION OF SUBSTANCE P IN THE ANTERIOR PITUITARY GLAND

Substance P is also synthesized by cells in the anterior pituitary gland.[18][19] There, the neuropeptide may act as a local agent in controlling other pituitary secretions.[19][20,p.393] Thyrotrophs are cells in the anterior pituitary that secrete TSH, the hormone that stimulates the thyroid gland to release thyroid hormone. A subset of thyrotrophs contain substance P.[21] When the amount of thyroid hormone reaching the thyrotrophs decreases, gene transcription for both TSH and substance P is activated. Transcription for their respective mRNAs is increased, and the cells synthesize more TSH and substance P. This shows that substance P (at least in the rat pituitary) is negatively regulated by thyroid hormone—increased thyroid hormone exposure to the pituitary thyrotrophs decreases synthesis of substance P, and decreased exposure increases synthesis.[20,p.396] Studies have confirmed this negative regulation: Administering thyroid hormone decreases

substance P mRNA, and thyroidectomy increases substance P mRNA.[18][19][20][22][23]

THYROID HORMONE REGULATION OF SUBSTANCE P IN THE LUMBAR SPINAL CORD

In the spinal cord, substance P is present in the descending nerve pathways of the intermediolateral horn cells, and moderate amounts are present in the ventral horns.[24][25] It is more concentrated, however, in the dorsal horns,[26][27][28] principally in the superficial layers.[29] The dorsal root ganglia[26][27][28] and primary sensory neurons that connect to the dorsal horns[27][30][31][32] contain substance P. When Savard and colleagues made neonatal rats hypothyroid, substance P content in the rats' dorsal horns increased by 100%.[33] The "hypersensitivity" of hypothyroid animals is possibly related to the high concentrations of substance P in their dorsal horns.[33,p.266]

THYROID HORMONE REGULATION OF THE PREPROTACHYKININ GENE AND PREPROTACHYKININ-A mRNA

Thyroid hormone directly regulates transcription of the preprotachykinin gene.[18][19,p.339][34,p.2913] The preprotachykinin-A gene encodes both preprotachykinin-A (PPT-A), the precursor of substance P, and the substance P receptor.[35][36] Activation of the gene results in production of several preprotachykinins from which substance P derives through alternative mRNA splicing.[37][38] Removal of the thyroid gland increased PPT-A mRNA in the anterior pituitary.[18] During thyroid hormone deficiency, PPT-A mRNA increased 800%.[18] Giving T_4 to thyroid hormone-deficient animals decreased PPT-A mRNA relative to controls.[22] Excessive amounts of T_4 significantly reduced substance P levels.[20]

● ELEVATED SUBSTANCE P AND FIBROMYALGIA

Elevated substance P (combined with low serotonin levels) may account for fibromyalgia patients' pain and tenderness. The high level of substance P in the brain and dorsal horns of hypothyroid rats may correspond to the high cerebrospinal fluid levels in fibromyalgia patients who have inadequate thyroid hormone regulation of the preprotachykinin gene. The high cerebrospinal fluid levels of substance P may also contribute to sleep disturbance in fibromyalgia patients. This possibility is suggested by the finding of a positive correlation between high substance P levels and sleep disturbance.[8]

High substance P levels can account at least in part for pain and sleep disturbance in fibromyalgia. But the high levels do not account for other symptoms and objective findings. Among those the high levels do not explain are reduced brain blood flow and low levels of several regulatory substances: dopamine, norepinephrine, growth hormone, somatomedin C, corticotropin-releasing hormone, cortisol, and peripheral serotonin. Inadequate thyroid hormone regulation of cell function theoretically can account for all of these abnormalities, including high cerebrospinal fluid substance P.[7]

Thyroid hormone may fail to regulate the preprotachykinin gene for several reasons. Too little thyroid hormone may enter the central nervous system because the patient is hypothyroid due to hypothalamic, pituitary, or thyroid gland dysfunction.[5] Too little may enter because a subnormal amount binds to transthyretin, the protein that transports the hormone into the central nervous system. Subnormal binding of thyroid hormone may occur because dioxin and PCB molecules displace the hormone from transthyretin. The dioxin and PCB molecules bind to transthyretin and enter the brain in the place of thyroid hormone.[39] (See Chapter 2.4, subsection titled "Environmental Contaminants: Effects on Thyroid Hormone Transport Proteins.") Also, thyroid hormone receptors attached to the DNA of the preprotachykinin gene may be mutated and have too low an affinity for thyroid hormone.[7] (See Chapter 2.6) Whatever the mechanism, inadequate transcription regulation of the preprotachykinin gene may account for the elevated substance P levels in the cerebrospinal fluid of fibromyalgia patients.

REFERENCES

1. Vaerøy, H., Helle, R., Øystein, F., Kåss, E., and Terenius, L.: Elevated CSF levels of substance P and high incidence of Raynaud phenomenon in patients with fibromyalgia: new features for diagnosis. *Pain*, 32:21-26, 1988.
2. Russell, I.J., Orr, M.D., Littman, B., et al.: Elevated cerebrospinal levels of substance P in patients with the fibromyalgia syndrome. *Arthritis Rheum.*, 37:1593-1601, 1994.
3. Russell, I.J., Orr, M.D., Michalek, J.E., Nyberg, F., and Eriksson, U.: Substance P (SP), spendopeptidase activity (SP$_{1-7}$) in fibromyalgia syndrome (FS) cerebrospinal fluid (CSF). *J. Musculoskel. Pain* (Abstr.), 3(Suppl.1):5, 1995.
4. Russell, I.J.: Neurochemical pathogenesis of fibromyalgia syndrome. *J. Musculoskel. Pain*, 4(1/2):61-92, 1996.
5. Lowe, J.C.: Thyroid status of 38 fibromyalgia patients: implications for the etiology of fibromyalgia, *Clin. Bull. Myofascial Ther.*, 2(1):47-64, 1997.
6. Russell, I.J.: Current ideas about fibromyalgia (lecture on audio tape). Houston, Texas, Fibromyalgia Association of Houston, Inc., Sept. 24, 1996.
7. Lowe, J.C., Cullum, M.E., Graf, L.H., Jr., and Yellin, J.: Mutations in the c-*erb*Aβ$_1$ gene: do they underlie euthyroid fibromyalgia? *Med. Hypotheses*, 48(2):125-135, 1997.
8. Schwarz, M.J., Spath, M., Muller-Bardorff, H., Pongratz, D.E., and Bondy, B.: Relationship of substance P, 5-hydroxyindole acetic acid and tryptophan in serum of fibromyalgia patients. *Neurosci. Lett.*, 259(3):196-198, 1999.
9. Nicoll, R.A.: The action of thyrotropin-releasing hormone, substance P, and related peptides on frog spinal motoneurons. *J. Pharmacol. Exp. Ther.*, 207:817-824, 1978.
10. Henry, J.L., Krnjevic, K., and Morris, M.E.: Excitatory effects of substance P in the spinal cord. *Fed. Proc.*, 33:548, 1974.
11. Henry, J.L., Krnjevic, K., and Morris, M.E.: Substance P in spinal neurons. *Canad. J. Physiol. Pharmacol.*, 33:423-432, 1975.
12. Henry, J.L., Sessle, B.J., Lucier, G.E., and Hu, J.W.: Effects of substance P on nociceptive and non-nociceptive trigeminal brain stem neurons. *Pain*, 8:33-45, 1980.
13. Malmberg, A. and Yaksh, T.: Hyperalgesia mediated by spinal glutamate or substance P receptor blocked by spinal cyclooxygenase inhibition. *Science*, 257:1276-1279, 1992.
14. Nicoll, R.A.: Excitatory action of TRH on spinal motoneurons. *Nature* (Lond.), 265:242-243, 1977.
15. Henry, J.L.: Effects of substance P on functionally identified units in rat spinal cord. *Brain Res.*, 114:439-451, 1976.
16. Randic, M. and Miletric, V.: Effect of substance P in rat dorsal horn neurons activated by noxious stimuli. *Brain Res.*, 128:164-169, 1977.
17. Dupont, A., Dussault, J-H., Rouleau, D., et al.: Effect of neonatal thyroid deficiency of the catecholamine, substance P, and thyrotropin-releasing hormone contents of discrete rat brain nuclei. *Endocrinology*, 108(6):2039-2045, 1981.
18. Jonassen, J.A., Mullikin-Kirkpatrick, D., McAdam, A., and Leeman, S.E.: Thyroid hormone status regulates preprotachykinin-A gene expression in male rat anterior pituitary. *Endocrinology*, 121(4):1555-1561, 1987.
19. Jones, P.M., Ghatei, M.A., Steel, J., et al.: Evidence for neuropeptide Y synthesis in the rat anterior pituitary and the influence of thyroid hormone status: comparison with vasoactive intestinal peptide, substance P, and neurotensin. *Endocrinology*, 125(1):334-341, 1989.
20. Jones, P.M., Ghatei, M.A., Wallis, S.C., and Bloom, S.R.: Differential response of neuropeptide Y, substance P, and vasoactive intestinal polypeptide in the rat anterior pituitary gland to alterations in thyroid hormone status. *J. Endocrinol.*, 143(2):393-397, 1994.
21. DePalatis, L.R., Fiorindo, R.P., and Ho, R.H.: Substance

P immunoreactivity in the anterior pituitary gland of the guinea pig. *Endocrinology*, 110:282, 1982.

22. Lam, K.S., Lechan, R.M., Minamitani, N., Segerson, T.P., and Reichlin, S.: Vasoactive intestinal peptide in the anterior pituitary is increased in hypothyroidism. *Endocrinology*, 124:1077-1084, 1989.

23. Aronin, N., Morency, K., Leeman, S.E., Braverman, L.E., and Coslovsky, R.: Regulation by thyroid hormone of the concentration of substance P in the rat anterior pituitary. *Endocrinology*, 114(6):2138-2142, 1984.

24. Appel, N.M., Wessendorf, M.W., and Elde, R.P.: Thyrotropin-releasing hormone in spinal cord: coexistence with serotonin and with substance P in fibers and terminals apposing identified preganglionic sympathetic neurons. *Brain Res.*, 415:137-143, 1987.

25. Wessendorf, M.W., Appel, N.M., Molitor, T.W., and Elde, R.P.: A method for immunofluorescent demonstration of three coexisting neurotransmitters in rat brain and spinal cord, using the fluophores fluoescein, lissamine rhodamine, and 7-amino-4-methylcoumarin-3-acetic acid. *J. Histol. Cytol.*, 38:1859-1877, 1990.

26. Hökfelt, T., Kellerth, J.O., Nilsson, G., and Pernow, B.: Substance P: localization in the central nervous system and in some primary sensory neurons. *Science*, 190:889-890, 1975.

27. Hökfelt, T., Kellerth, J.O., Nilsson, G., and Pernow, B.: Experimental immunohistochemical studies on the localization and distribution of substance P in cat primary sensory neurons. *Brain Res.*, 100:135-252, 1975.

28. Hökfelt, T., Elde, R., Johansson, O., Luft, R., Nilsson, G., and Arimura, A.: Immunohistochemical evidence for separate populations of somatostatin-containing and substance P-containing primary afferent neurons in the rat. *Neurosci.*, 1:131-136, 1976.

29. Jancso, G., Hökfelt, T., Lundberg, J.M., et al.: Immunohistochemical studies of the effect of capsaicin on spinal and medullary peptide and monoamine neurons using antisera to substance P, gastrin/CCK, somatostatin, VIP, enkephaline, neurotensin, and 5-hydroxytryptamine. *J.*

Neurocytol., 10:963-980, 1981.

30. Theriault, E., Otsuka, M., and Jessell, T.: Capsaicin-evoked release of substance P from primary sensory neurons. *Brain Res.*, 170:209-213, 1979.

31. Harmar, A. and Keen, P.: Chemical characterization of substance P-like immunoreactivity in primary afferent neurons. *Brain Res.*, 220:203-207, 1981.

32. Hökfelt, T., Lundberg, J., Schultzberg, M., Johansson, O., Ljungdahl, A., and Rehfeld, J.: Co-existence of peptides and putative transmitters in neurons. In *Neural Peptides and Neuronal Communications*. Edited by E. Costa and M. Trabucci, New York, Raven Press, 1980, pp.1-23.

33. Savard, P., Mérand, Y., Bédard, P., Dussault, J-H., and Dupont, A.: Comparative effects of neonatal hypothyroidism and euthyroidism on TRH and substance P content of lumbar spinal cord in saline and PCPA-treated rats. *Brain Res.*, 277:263-268, 1983.

34. Aronin, N., Coslovsky, R., and Chase, K.: Hypothyroidism increases substance P concentrations in the heterotopic anterior pituitary. *Endocrinology*, 122(6):2911-2914, 1988.

35. Mendelson, S.C. and Quinn, J.P.: Characterization of potential regulatory elements within the rat preprotachykinin-A promoter. *Neuroscience Letters*, 184(2):125-128, 1995.

36. Too, H.P., Marriott, D.R., and Wilkin, G.P. Preprotachykinin-A and substance P receptor (NK1) gene expression in rat astrocytes in vitro. *Neuroscience Letters* 182(2):185-187, 1994.

37. Nawa, H., Kotani, H., and Nakanishi, S.: Tissue-specific generation of two preprotachykinin mRNAs from one gene by alternative splicing. *Nature*, 312:729, 1984.

38. Krause, J.E., Chirgwin, J.M., Carter, M.S., Xu, Z.S., and Hershey, A.D.: Three rat preprotachykinin mRNAs encode the neuropeptides substance P and neurokinin A. *Proc. Natl. Acad. Sci. (USA)*, 84:881, 1987.

39. Brouwer, A.: Inhibition of thyroid hormone transport in plasma of rats by polychlorinated biphenyls. *Arch. Toxicol.*, 13(Suppl.):440-445, 1989.

40. Yellin, J.: Why is substance P high in fibromyalgia? *Clin. Bull. Myofascial Ther.*, 2(2/3):23-30, 1997.

3.20

Swelling and Stiffness

Fibromyalgia patients commonly complain of swelling and stiffness. Some fibromyalgia researchers have reported the swelling as only "subjective swelling." The swelling in some patients, however, may result from fluid accumulation due to inadequate thyroid hormone regulation of fibroblast cells. The patient may be subjectively aware of slight swelling for at least two reasons: (1) her central nervous system is unable to normally modulate down incoming peripheral nerve signals, and (2) the patient may be highly vigilant of her body signals because of apprehension over the nature of the condition from which she suffers. Thus, the patient may perceive swelling that is too slight for clinicians to verify through inspection.

A minority of fibromyalgia patients have visible myxedematous swelling. Like classic myxedema, it is non-pitting and does not diminish with recumbency. It subsides and disappears when patients take high enough dosages of thyroid hormone.

Many fibromyalgia patients have extremely severe stiffness, most often upon rising from sleep. The stiffness may last from 15 minutes to hours. Some researchers consider stiffness prolonged when it lasts at least 15 minutes after the patient gets out of bed. Some patients report that their stiffness lasts for most of the day. Others complain that their stiffness intensifies after brief periods of inactivity.

Researchers have reported that hypothyroid and euthyroid hypometabolic patients complain of stiffness. Each of these classes of patients is likely to have inadequate thyroid hormone regulation of transcription and of cell function: hypothyroid patients because of a thyroid hormone deficiency; euthyroid hypometabolic patients because of partial cellular resistance to thyroid hormone.

Patients with inadequate thyroid hormone regulation may have stiffness because of one or more of four potential mechanisms. One mechanism is myxedematous swelling of the ground substance of the connective tissues of muscles and joints. This is a likely mechanism with regard to fibromyalgia in view of the extremely high serum hyaluronic acid levels of some fibromyalgia patients. Another mechanism is energy-deficiency contractures due to subnormal generation of ATP molecules in muscle cells.

Decreased Ca^{++}-ATPase activity is the third mechanism. Decreased Ca^{++}-ATPase activity in hypothyroid muscle results in insufficient removal of Ca^{++} from the sarcoplasmic fluid. The excess calcium ions in the fluid will become transient components of the troponin complex on actin filaments. Binding of the calcium ions to the complex keeps a high percentage of the active sites of actin available for the attachment of myosin cross-bridges. This attachment of the cross-bridges to actin results in sustained shortening of the actin and myosin filaments. Shortening of these filaments shortens muscle fibers, fascicles, and the muscle as a whole. As in ATP deficiency, this results in a mild, chronic rigor mortis-type shortening of muscle. From the shortened muscles, tension is transmitted through fascial sheets to tendons that cross joints. The increased tension of tendons across joints may reduce the flexibility and ease of movement of the joints. Patients are likely to perceive this as uncomfortable or painful stiffness.

A fourth possible mechanism of morning stiffness in fibromyalgia is sustained muscle contractions caused by subnormal generation of body heat during sleep. The muscle contractions generate heat (in response to the subnormal body heat) and are therefore termed "thermogenic." The contractions subside after the patient arises and becomes physically active. The activity generates body heat and stops the thermogenic contractions. Release of the contractions releases the *tension of tendons across joints. The release of tension permits easier joint mobility and stops the perception of stiffness.*

The relaxation phase of the Achilles reflex is slow in some 85% of hypothyroid patients. The reflex is slow in a roughly equal percentage of fibromyalgia patients. Two of the mechanisms mentioned above presumably mediate the slow relaxation phase: too few ATP molecules and subnormal Ca^{++}-ATPase activity in calf muscle cells. The Achilles reflex test illustrates well the sluggish or incomplete relaxation of skeletal muscle in both hypothyroid and euthyroid fibromyalgia patients.

A plausible model for the perception of stiffness by fibromyalgia patients involves two classes of phenomena: actual connective tissue swelling, and the three skeletal muscle mechanisms. Swelling is likely to occur because of increased accumulation of water-binding protein/carbohydrate molecules (proteoglycans) in the ground substance of patients' connective tissues. The three skeletal muscle mechanisms are (1) energy deficiency contractures due to decreases in high-energy phosphate production, especially ATP; (2) increased actin and myosin shortening due to decreased Ca^{++}-ATPase activity; and (3) thermogenic contractions due to low body temperature, especially throughout the metabolic slowing during sleep. Any or all of these mechanisms would induce sustained shortening of muscles with increased tension of their tendons across joints. This would reduce joint motion and cause the perception of stiffness. Actual swelling of the ground substance of muscle fascial sheets, tendons, and ligaments could compound the perception of stiffness. Increased muscle activity and metabolism upon rising from sleep would reverse the energy deficiency contractures and thermogenic contractions. Increased activity would also reduce or relieve the component of swelling due to any slowed fluid circulation associated with relative inactivity during sleep. Patients would then perceive a reduction or relief of stiffness, but only after a longer time than for normal individuals.

Myxedematous swelling would not subside with increased physical activity during waking hours. It would subside only when the patient's use of a high enough dosage of thyroid hormone suppresses secretory activity of fibroblasts in her connective tissues.

● SWELLING IN FIBROMYALGIA

Numerous researchers have reported "subjective swelling" as a symptom of fibromyalgia.[54][55][56][57]

[58][59][60] It is highly probable that the subjective swelling of fibromyalgia patients results from the accumulation of fluid in their connective tissues. I base this conjecture on two observations: (1) a small percentage of my hypothyroid and euthyroid fibromyalgia patients had myxedema that disappeared with thyroid hormone therapy, and (2) other fibromyalgia patients report to me that their subjective swelling was eliminated by metabolic rehabilitation involving the use of exogenous thyroid hormone.

MYXEDEMA AS A MECHANISM OF SWELLING AND STIFFNESS IN INADEQUATE THYROID HORMONE REGULATION

T_3 inhibits the amassing of water-binding proteoglycans, mainly hyaluronic acid, in the ground substance of connective tissues.[24] Some argue that the reduction in proteoglycans results from reduced synthesis rather than increased degradation.[25]

Myxedematous swelling involves the accumulation of water-binding molecules in the skin and other connective tissues.[20][21][22][23][24][25] Myxedema occurs in some patients with hypothyroidism[26][27][28][29] and thyroid hormone resistance syndromes.[30][31][32] Awad performed biopsies of "fibrositic" nodules of fibromyalgia patients and found what appeared to be localized myxedema.[33][34]

Some researchers have attributed transient pain, muscle cramps, and stiffness in hypothyroid patients to the separation of muscle fibers by "mucoedema."[22,p.571] This proposal is supported by the findings of Dorwart and Schumacher.[7] They reported that each of 12 hypothyroid patients complained of generalized stiffness. They found that the patients had thickened flexor tendon sheaths, and joint laxity and popliteal cysts. Needle biopsy showed only mild inflammation. Eight of the patients had synovial effusions. In 7 of these patients, the effusions were extremely viscous. Effusions in 6 patients contained calcium pyrophosphate crystals. We would expect the synovial effusions to contain a high concentration of hyaluronic acid. This is the main water-binding proteoglycan secreted by fibroblasts when insufficient thyroid hormone causes disinhibition of their activity (see Chapter 3.3). The increase in synovial water content, due to increases in hyaluronic acid, may account for the stiffness.

The swelling in connective tissues may result in impaired nerve function. Murray and Simpson used an EMG technique to determine the conduction velocity in the median and ulnar nerves of 11 hypothyroid patients. In 3 patients, the median nerve conducted signals too slowly from the elbow to the wrist. The investigators attributed the delay to carpal tunnel syndrome associated with myxedema.[19] In this syndrome, myxedematous swelling of the ligament surrounding the wrist compresses the median nerve. The patient usually experiences abnormal sensations at night in a median nerve distribution in one or both hands. As the condition worsens, the paresthesias may progress to sensory loss and muscle weakness and atrophy. These abnormalities may become permanent.

SODIUM AND FLUID RETENTION

The low blood pressure of fibromyalgia patients is likely to induce renin secretion by the juxtoglomerular cells adjacent to the glomeruli of the kidneys. The renin would be converted first to angiotensin I and then to angiotensin II, which is a powerful vasoconstrictor. Another effect of angiotensin II, however, is to stimulate aldosterone secretion by the adrenal cortices. Aldosterone is the most potent endogenous agent that stimulates the kidney tubules to reabsorb sodium. Aldosterone stimulates reabsorption of sodium and water from the kidney tubules into the blood. In some female patients, aldosterone secretion stimulated by angiotensin II may be disproportionately high compared to its vasoconstrictive effects. The result may be normal or subnormal blood pressure despite swelling due to the extracellular accumulation of sodium and water. (See Chapter 3.21, section titled "Kidney Vasoconstriction Induced by Increased Renin Secretion.")

● STIFFNESS IN FIBROMYALGIA

Wolfe reported that 77% of fibromyalgia patients complained of prolonged morning stiffness.[1] According to the ACR criteria, stiffness is prolonged if it lasts for 15 minutes or longer after the patient arises from sleep.[8] Researchers often include stiffness in their descriptions of fibromyalgia. Reiffenberger and Amundson [35] wrote, for example, "Fibromyalgia syndrome includes symptoms of widespread chronic musculoskeletal aching and stiffness and soft tissue tender points." Similarly, Cohen and Quintner wrote,[36] "Fibromyalgia syndrome is generally taken to denote a clinical state of widespread musculoskeletal pain, stiffness, and fatigue . . . ." And in discussing the possible

etiology of fibromyalgia, Neeck and Riedel wrote,[37] "Muscle pain, especially at the muscle-tendon junctions, fatigue, and stiffness are the first symptoms."

INADEQUATE THYROID HORMONE REGULATION OF CELL FUNCTION AS THE PUTATIVE CAUSE OF STIFFNESS IN FIBROMYALGIA

Fitzcharles and Esdaile[9] suggested that stiffness in fibromyalgia may actually be a manifestation of undiagnosed spondyloarthropathy. They wrote in 1997 that diffuse body pain in a woman is likely to lead to a diagnosis of fibromyalgia. Of 321 new rheumatology referrals, they found that clinicians had accurately diagnosed 35 (11%) as having fibromyalgia. The clinicians misdiagnosed another 11 patients (3%) as having fibromyalgia—the patients' symptoms were attributable to previously undiagnosed spondyloarthropathy. The authors noted that the symptoms of spondyloarthropathy considerably overlap those of fibromyalgia. Ten of the 35 fibromyalgia patients, for example, had spinal pain in at least two locations. Another 10 had pain at night that disturbed their sleep, and 9 had prolonged morning stiffness. The researchers concluded that clinicians are possibly making the diagnosis of primary fibromyalgia too freely and without consideration of other possible diagnoses. They are doing so especially when the patient has poorly-defined musculoskeletal pain.

We do not at this time have distinct criteria for distinguishing fibromyalgia from other conditions with overlapping features. Certainly, many clinicians often diagnose fibromyalgia without having adequately evaluated the patient for other diagnosable and treatable conditions that cause symptoms such as stiffness (see Chapter 1.1, section titled "Lack of Acceptance of Fibromyalgia by Many Physicians, and Its Use as a Waste-Basket Diagnosis"). The most frequently undiagnosed condition that can account for stiffness in fibromyalgia is inadequate thyroid hormone regulation of cell function.

STIFFNESS IN HYPOTHYROIDISM

Hypothyroid patients often complain that they have pain, and feel weak and stiff.[7][10][11][12][13][18] In 1874, Sir William Gull described 5 "cretinoid" women who complained of joint swelling and muscle stiffness.[13,p.180] Golding wrote of 9 hypothyroid patients with muscle symptoms. Rather than feeling weak, they complained of pain and stiffness.[11] Dorwart and Schumacher reported generalized stiffness as a symptom in 12 hypothyroid patients who had rheumatic signs and symptoms.[7] Other researchers have reported that hypothyroid patients complained of transient pain, muscle cramps, and stiffness. Dorwart and Schumacher speculated that these symptoms resulted from separation of muscle fibers by "mucoedema."[7]

Wilson and Walton wrote of the muscle symptoms in patients made hypothyroid by thyroidectomies performed to relieve hyperthyroidism.[10,p.320] One patient had carpopedal spasms, although her serum calcium and phosphate levels were normal. She felt cold, had dry skin, had hair loss, and her muscles were painful and stiff. Another patient reported that her face was slightly swollen and her fingers and facial muscles had been stiff. Her clinician thought that she was euthyroid. Because of her complaint of bizarre aches and pains affecting her limbs, he referred her to a psychiatrist. The psychiatrist found no psychological basis for her symptoms; however, he offered no satisfactory alternative explanation. The patient also saw a physician who mentioned that although she had gained "three stones" in weight post-operatively, she had no clinical signs of hypothyroidism. Another clinician referred her to one of the investigators because of the persistence of her muscular pain and aching. He observed that she had generalized muscle hypertrophy that was especially marked in the quadriceps and calves. All the patient's voluntary muscles were stiff and felt indurated. She performed movements slowly. On percussion of her deltoids and quadriceps, there was "dimpling" of the muscle. The "dimpling" lasted for more than 2 seconds and was similar to that seen in myotonia. Her pulse rate was 90 beats per minute, but she appeared myxedematous. She was lethargic and constipated, and to the clinician, her skin felt cold.

STIFFNESS IN EUTHYROID HYPOMETABOLISM

Other researchers have reported stiffness in patients who had euthyroid hypometabolism[2][3][4][5][17] (see Chapter 2.5). Occasionally, a clinician interprets the patient's swollen and stiff joints as rheumatoid arthritis, or he concludes that rheumatoid arthritis exists concurrently with hypothyroidism. The hypothyroid patient may, however, have swollen synovial tissues in joints in the absence of rheumatoid arthritis. Thyroid hormone therapy usually relieves the joint swelling

and associated stiffness.

STIFFNESS IN HYPOTHYROID AND EUTHYROID FIBROMYALGIA PATIENTS

Wilke, Sheeler and Makarowski described 8 hypothyroid patients who met Smythe's then-current criteria for fibromyalgia.[14] The criteria included (1) subjective aching and stiffness of more than 3 months' duration, (2) local point tenderness in at least 3 sites, and (3) normal laboratory values.[15] These clinicians' patients reported muscle and joint pain for at least 1 year. The clinicians diagnosed "subclinical" or "chemical" hypothyroidism based on at least a minimally elevated TSH level in each patient. Three of 4 patients tested had decreased T_4 levels, and 2 of 3 patients tested had a low free T_4 index.

My coauthors and I found that metabolic rehabilitation, including the use of supraphysiologic dosages of T_3, reduced or eliminated the stiffness of euthyroid fibromyalgia patients.[16][51][52][53]

● POSSIBLE MECHANISMS OF STIFFNESS IN FIBROMYALGIA PATIENTS

Inadequate thyroid hormone regulation of three skeletal muscle processes may contribute to stiffness in fibromyalgia. These processes are ATP production, Ca^{++}-ATPase activity, and thermogenic contractions due to low core body temperature, particularly during sleep. Myxedema, a connective tissue abnormality, may also contribute.

INADEQUATE ATP CONCENTRATIONS AS A CAUSE OF STIFFNESS IN INADEQUATE THYROID HORMONE REGULATION

Inadequate thyroid hormone regulation of muscle cell metabolism can impair production of the high energy phosphate compound ATP (see Chapter 2.2, section titled "Energy-Yielding Processes in the Cytoplasm and Mitochondria"). When energy metabolism in skeletal muscles is impaired, the contractile filaments of the muscles chronically shorten. When the contractile filaments shorten, they pull with them the fascial tissues that adhere to them. The force of pull on fascial planes transfers to the tendons that emerge from the planes. The force in turn, transmitted though the tendons, pulls the bones they attach to. The pull of tendons across joints can increase resistance to joint movement, generating the perception of stiffness.

INADEQUATE CA++-ATPASE ACTIVITY AS A CAUSE OF STIFFNESS IN INADEQUATE THYROID HORMONE REGULATION OF TRANSCRIPTION

Inadequate thyroid hormone regulation of cell function can reduce Ca^{++}-ATPase activity (see Chapter 2.2, section titled "Important Cell Membrane Effects of Thyroid Hormone: Thyroid Hormone, Membrane Ca^{2+}-ATPase Activity, and the Cell Content of Calcium").

When the action potential of an alpha motor neuron reaches a muscle cell and spreads over it, the sarcoplasmic reticulum releases calcium ions into the sarcoplasmic fluid. The calcium ions facilitate shortening of the actin and myosin filaments by making accessible the sites on actin filaments where myosin cross-bridges attach. Next, when sufficient Ca^{++}-ATPase is available in the sarcoplasm, the enzyme catalyzes reuptake of calcium ions by the reticulum. When the calcium ion concentration in the sarcoplasm decreases beyond some threshold, the actin and myosin filaments separate and the muscle lengthens or relaxes.[61]

When Ca^{++}-ATPase activity is decreased in muscle, as in hypothyroidism, removal of calcium ions from the sarcoplasmic fluid is not sufficient. The excess calcium ions in the fluid keep many active actin sites available for myosin filaments to attach to. The sustained attachment of actin and myosin results in chronic shortening of the actin and myosin complex. Shortening of the complex shortens muscle fibers, fascicles, and the muscle as a whole. From the shortened muscles, tension is transmitted through fascial sheets to tendons that cross joints. The increased tension of tendons across joints may reduce the flexibility and ease of movement of the joints. Patients are likely to perceive this as stiffness, and it may also be associated with pain.

ACHILLES REFLEX TIME AND INCOMPLETE MUSCLE RELAXATION: EFFECTS OF LOW CA++-ATPASE ACTIVITY AND DEFICIENT SKELETAL MUSCLE ATP

Researchers and clinicians have long considered a slow relaxation phase during the Achilles reflex a sign of hypothyroidism. Some have argued that the most characteristic physical sign of hypothyroidism is a sluggish relaxation phase of the tendon reflexes.[39] About 75% of hypothyroid patients have slowed reflexes.[38,p.487] In my clinical experience, most fibromyalgia patients have slowed Achilles reflexes that become normal with thyroid hormone therapy. With most patients, the clinician can use the Achilles reflex as one measure to assess the metabolic effect of thyroid hormone on skeletal muscle.[40][41]

I am aware of no studies other than mine in which investigators have measured the speed of the Achilles reflex of fibromyalgia patients. In one study, however, fibromyalgia patients had increased EMG activity in muscle during short pauses between contractions.[44] In another study, Elert et al.[42] looked for differences in surface electromyography recordings in fibromyalgia patients, myofascial pain syndrome patients, and healthy controls. The researchers made the recordings while the patients performed 100 repetitive shoulder flexions. The recordings did not detect differences in mechanical performance or muscle composition. However, no fibromyalgia patients were able to relax their muscles between contractions. Healthy subjects were able to do so. Only the myofascial pain syndrome patients with myalgic muscles were not able to relax between contractions. Bennett[43,p.149] commented that the inability of fibromyalgia patients to relax between contractions may indicate an important mechanism for the problem patients have in sustaining repetitive muscle contractions. This finding is relevant, however, to the slowed relaxation phase of the Achilles reflex found in most hypothyroid and fibromyalgia patients. The failure of fibromyalgic muscle to relax between repetitive contractions suggests that, as in hypothyroidism, the muscles have low levels of ATP and Ca^{++}-ATPase.

THERMOGENIC CONTRACTIONS

Another possible contribution to the perception of stiffness, especially upon arising from sleep, is shortening of muscles during thermogenic contractions. During the relative inactivity of sleep, ATPase cleaves fewer phosphate radicals from ATP to energize biochemical reactions. Of the energy liberated from the phosphate bond, roughly 50% escapes as heat. Hydrolysis of ATP in a variety of cellular processes contributes to heat production. These processes include ion transport (as with the Na^+/K^+ pump and the Ca^{++} pump in muscle cells), synthesis of various compounds (proteins, DNA, RNA, complex carbohydrates, and lipids), muscle contraction, secretion and absorption, and various metabolic pathways.[47,p.294] (See Chapter 2.2, section titled "Mitochondrial Energy Processes: Production of ATP" and Chapter 4.3, section titled "Basal Body Temperature.")

Thyroid hormone is a major regulator of thermogenesis.[46] When T_3 increases Na^+/K^+-ATPase concentration,[48] and the enzyme is active, it catalyzes conversion of ATP to ADP by breaking a phosphate bond. Breaking the bond liberates the energy of the bond. Part of the energy fuels the pump that moves sodium and potassium ions across cell membranes, as in nerve and muscle cells. Some energy also escapes as heat and warms the body. Some researchers contend that this pump accounts for much,[49] although not all,[50] of the energy expenditure and heat production from the action of thyroid hormones. When thyroid hormone fails to regulate these thermogenic processes, core body temperature decreases. This results in an even lower core body temperature during sleep, when relative inactivity further decreases thermogenic processes.

As the body cools during the relative inactivity of sleep, skeletal muscles and their fascia and tendons shorten. When the fibromyalgia patient awakes, she may perceive the shortening as stiffness. She is likely to perceive the stiffness as uncomfortable or painful because of her chronically heightened pain sensitivity. As she moves about after arising, her energy metabolism increases, warming her body. As she stretches her flesh intentionally or inadvertently as she goes about her daily routine, her body heat increases. As a result, her excess muscle tone and energy deficiency muscle contractures release somewhat. She then perceives relief of her stiffness.

Bennett et al. reported that fibromyalgia patients have an exaggerated reaction to cold, with cold-induced vasospasms. The researchers speculated that the increase in α_2-adrenergic receptor density on the patients' platelets was an upregulation due to the exaggerated reaction to cold.[45] It is more likely, however, considering the arguments I put forth in this book, that the increase in the density of α_2-adrenergic receptors results from inadequate thyroid hormone transcription regulation of the gene that codes for the α_2-adrenergic receptor. This would explain not only the increase in receptor density, but also lower body temperature. If the fibromyalgia patient's core body temperature is generally lower than normal, then during the relative inactivity of sleep, her body may cool sufficiently to induce thermogenic muscle contractions. The ther-

mogenic muscle contractions would cause increased tension of tendons across joints and produce the perception of stiffness.

MYXEDEMA AS A POSSIBLE MECHANISM OF THE PERCEPTION OF STIFFNESS

Myxedematous swelling may contribute to the perception of stiffness in patients whose fibromyalgia is a manifestion of inadequate thyroid hormone regulation. Myxedema is an actual swelling. The process may sufficiently affect the skin and underlying connective tissues to be visible to the patient and clinician as local or general puffiness. But it may be mild enough that its effects are not visible, although the patient reports a subjective feeling of swelling. Myxedematous swelling of connective tissues—especially of tissues with little capacity for expansion such as tendon sheaths, ligaments, and joint synovia—may be perceived as stiffness.

● A MODEL TO EXPLAIN SWELLING AND STIFFNESS IN FIBROMYALGIA

In those whose fibromyalgia is a manifestation of inadequate thyroid hormone regulation, the perception of stiffness may result from one or more of four possible mechanisms. One is actual swelling of the connective tissues due to increased proteoglycan accumulation. I expect this from the two objective findings in some fibromyalgia patients: (1) increased tissue levels of water-binding proteoglycans in biopsy samples, and (2) significantly increased serum levels of hyaluronic acid (the major proteoglycan)[6] (see Chapter 3.3). Sufficiently increased proteoglycans in the ground substance of fascial sheets of muscle, tendons, ligaments, and synovial joint linings cause a perception of swelling and resistance to musculoskeletal motion. In addition, swelling due to increased water-binding proteoglycans in ground substance can, above various thresholds, compress blood vessels and activate pain-mediating nerve endings that respond to pressure (such as type C and A delta mechanoreceptors). The swelling may be too slight for the patient or clinician to confirm by observation or palpation, or it may be visible as local or general myxedematous puffiness. The swelling may be most accentuated when the patient arises from sleep. At this time, connective tissues contain a high accumulation of fluid. The accumulation results from a decrease in fluid circulation through the tissues and blood vessels because of the reduced pumping action of skeletal muscles during the relative inactivity of sleep.

The other three possible mechanisms all entail abnormalities of skeletal muscle function due to inadequate thyroid hormone regulation. Each of these can cause skeletal muscles to shorten. The shortening transmits tension to the tendons that cross joints. The tension of the tendons can reduce mobility of the joints enough to contribute to the patient's perception of stiffness.

The first of these possible mechanisms is decreased production of high-energy phosphates (ATP and creatine phosphate) in skeletal muscle cells due to inadequate thyroid hormone regulation (see Chapter 2.2). A deficiency of ATP molecules can result in energy deficiency contractures of muscle fibers (see Chapter 3.4, section titled "Deficient Delivery of Oxygen to Muscle During Exercise"). During this process, muscles shorten, increasing tension at tendinous attachments.

The second possible skeletal muscle process is reduced activity of Ca^{++}-ATPase. This enzyme catalyzes reuptake of calcium ions by the endoplasmic reticulum after a muscle contraction. The resulting reduction in calcium ion concentration of the sarcoplasmic fluid is essential for complete separation of actin and myosin filaments. When Ca^{++}-ATPase activity is low—as it may be in inadequate thyroid hormone regulation—the sarcoplasmic fluid retains excess concentrations of calcium ions. This keeps the active sites on myosin filaments available for the attachment of actin filaments, increasing the ratchet-like interaction that shortens muscles.

A third skeletal muscle mechanism that may contribute to the perception of stiffness results from the combination of decreased ATP production and decreased cleavage of the third phosphate radical of the ATP molecule. Enzymatic cleavage of phosphate from ATP results in transfer of part of the energy of the cleaved phosphate bond to biochemical reactions. The cleavage also liberates part of the bond energy as heat. Decreased ATP production and decreased phosphate cleavage due to inadequate thyroid hormone regulation of gene transcription reduce body heat below normal in most affected patients. During sleep, their body heat declines even further because of decreased metabolic processes. The decreased body heat may increase thermogenic skeletal muscle contractions as a compensatory process to prevent critical lowering of the core body temperature during sleep. Sustained thermogenic

muscle contractions would exert tension on tendons that attach to the contracted muscles. The tendons that cross joints may reduce the mobility of the joints enough to impact the patient's perception. At the time of arising from sleep, the patient would perceive the reduced joint mobility as stiffness.

These three skeletal muscle processes could, singly or in combination, contribute to actual and perceived stiffness. Each could contribute to sustained shortening of muscles, with simultaneous tension exerted through tendons across joints. This would actually limit freedom of joint movement, causing the perception of stiffness. A good example is the often painful difficulty some patients report in walking upon first awakening from sleep. Calf muscles flex and extend the foot by means of tendons that attach to the periosteum of foot bones. In descending to their foot bone attachments, calf tendons cross the ankle. There, the retinacular ligaments bind them into a tight compartment, allowing longitudinal movement within their synovium-lubricated sheaths. (Retinacular ligaments are belt-like straps around the ankles and wrists. They compress and confine tendons passing over the joints into a small space. This confinement enables the pull exerted by the muscles the tendons extend from to move the foot or hand distal to the joint.) Shortening of the calf muscles during sleep (due to energy deficiency contractures, increased actin and myosin interaction from excessive exposure to calcium ions, and thermogenic contractions) would exert a simultaneous pull of the foot in the directions of extension and flexion. The counterforces would cancel actual extension and flexion at the ankle, and instead, actually restrict ankle movement. The patient would be likely to perceive this restriction as stiffness.

In addition, the ground substance of the patient's connective tissues may contain excessive amounts of water, due to the increased accumulation of proteoglycans. This actual swelling of the fascial sheaths of muscles, tendons, and retinacular ligaments could further accentuate the patient's perception of swelling and stiffness. Moreover, the increased intramuscular pressure from the contractions and contractures, and from the increased water-binding in the ground substance, might exceed the threshold for activation of type C and A delta mechano-receptors. Thus, type C and A delta nerve fibers would conduct nociceptive signals to the central nervous system, complicating the perception of stiffness with the perception of pain. Upon arising from sleep, increased energy metabolism associated with muscle contraction and movement, and the use of hot water by many patients, would reduce or completely relieve the muscle shortening temporarily. The movements and muscle contractions would also stimulate tissue fluid circulation and reduce actual tissue swelling. The patient would then experience some measure of relief from the swelling and stiffness. The time required to achieve relief, however, is in most cases longer than that for individuals without fibromyalgia.

REFERENCES

1. Wolfe, F.: Diagnosis of fibromyalgia. *J. Musculoskel. Med.*, 7:54, 1990.
2. Morton, J.H.: Sodium liothyronine in metabolic insufficiency syndrome and associated disorders. *J.A.M.A.*, 165: 124-129, 1957.
3. Freedberg, A.S., Kurland, G.S., and Hamolsky, M.W.: Effect of l-tri-iodothyronine alone and combined with l-thyroxine in nonmyxedematous hypometabolism. *N. Engl. J. Med.*, 253, 57-60, 1955.
4. Fields, E.M.: Treatment of metabolic insufficiency and hypothyroidism with sodium liothyronine. *J.A.M.A.*, 163: 817, 1957.
5. Tittle, C.R.: Effects of 3,5,3' l-triiodothyronine in patients with metabolic insufficiency. *J.A.M.A.*, 162:271, 1956.
6. Yaron, I., Buskila, D., Shirazi, I., Neumann, L., Elkayam, O., Paran, D., and Yaron, M.: Elevated levels of hyaluronic acid in the sera of women with fibromyalgia. *J. Rheumatol.*, 24(11):2221-2224, 1997.
7. Dorwart, B.B. and Schumacher, H.R.: Joint effusions, chondrocalcinosis and other rheumatic manifestations in hypothyroidism. A clinicopathologic study. *Amer. J. Med.*, 59(6):780-790, 1975.
8. Wolfe, F., Smythe, H.A., Yunus, M.B., et al.: The American College of Rheumatology 1990 criteria for the classification of fibromyalgia: report of the multicenter criteria committee. *Arthritis Rheumatol.*, 33:160-172, 1990.
9. Fitzcharles, M.A. and Esdaile, J.M.: The overdiagnosis of fibromyalgia syndrome. *Amer. J. Med.*, 103(1):44-50, 1997.
10. Wilson, J. and Walton, J.N.: Some muscular manifestations of hypothyroidism. *J. Neurol. Neurosurg. Psychiat.*, 22:320-324, 1959.
11. Golding, D.N.: Hypothyroidism presenting with musculoskeletal symptoms. *Ann. Rheum. Dis.*, 29:10-14, 1970.
12. Delamere, J.P., Scott, D.L., and Felix-Davies, D.D.: Thyroid dysfunction and rheumatic diseases. *J.Royal Soc. Med.*, 75:102, 1982.
13. Gull, W.W.: On a cretinoid state supervening in adult life in women. *Trans. Clin. Soc.* (Lond.), 7:180-185, 1874.
14. Wilke, W.S., Sheeler, L.R., and Makarowski, W.S.: Hypothyroidism with presenting symptoms of fibrositis. *J. Rheumat.*, 8:627-630, 1981.
15. Smythe, H.A.: Nonarticular rheumatism and the fibrositis syndrome. In *Arthritis and Allied Conditions*, 8th edition. Edited by J.L. Hollander and D.J. McCarty, Philadelphia, Lea and Febiger, 1972, pp.874-884.
16. Lowe, J.C., Eichelberger, J., Manso, G., and Peterson, K.: Improvement in euthyroid fibromyalgia patients treated

with T₃. *J. Myofascial Ther.*, 1(2):16-29, 1994.
17. Sonkin, L.S.: Myofascial pain due to metabolic disorders: diagnosis and treatment. In *Myofascial Pain and Fibromyalgia: Trigger Point Management.* Edited by E.S. Rachlin, St. Louis, Mosby, 1994, pp.45-60.
18. Watanakunakorn, C., Hodges, R.E., and Evans, T.C.: Myxedema: a study of 400 cases. *Arch. Intern. Med.*, 116: 185, 1965.
19. Murray, I.P.C. and Simpson, J.A.: Acroparesthesia in myxedema. *Lancet*, 1:1360, 1958.
20. Murata, Y., Ceccarelli, P., Refetoff, S., Horwitz, A.L., and Matsui, N.: Thyroid hormone inhibits fibronectin synthesis by cultured human skin fibroblasts. *J. Clin. Endocrinol. Metab.*, 64:334, 1987.
21. Asboe-Hansen, G.: The variability in the hyaluronic acid content of the dermal connective tissue under the influence of thyroid hormone. *Acta Dermato-Venereologica*, 30: 221-229, 1950.
22. Kohn, L.D.: Connective tissue. In *The Thyroid*, 4th edition. Edited by S.C. Werner and S.H. Ingbar, New York, Harper and Row Publishers, 1987.
23. Schiller, S.: Mucopolysaccharides in relation to growth and thyroid hormones. *J. Chronic Dis.*, 16:291, 1962.
24. Smith, T.J., Horwitz, A.L., and Refetoff, S.: The effect of thyroid hormone on glycosaminoglycan accumulation in human fibroblasts. *Endocrinol.*, 108:2397, 1981.
25. Smith, T.J., Murata, Y., Horwitz, A.L., Philipson, L., and Refetoff, S.: Regulation of glycosaminoglycan accumulation by thyroid hormone *in vitro. J. Clin. Invest.*, 70:1066, 1982.
26. Ramsay, I.: *Thyroid Disease and Muscle Dysfunction.* Chicago, Year Book Medical Publishers, Inc., 1974.
27. Gabrilove, J.L. and Ludwig, A.W.: The histogenesis of myxedema. *J. Clin. Endocrinol. Metab.*, 17:925, 1957.
28. Schiller, S., Slover, G.A., and Dorfman, A.: Effect of thyroid gland on metabolism of acid mucopolysaccharide in skin. *Biochem. Biophys. Acta.*, 58:27, 1962.
29. Von Knorring, J.: Changes in myocardial acid mucopolysaccharides in experimental hyper- and hypothyroidism in the rat. *Scand. J. Clin. Lab. Invest.*, [Suppl] 19(95):57, 1967.
30. Murata, Y., Refetoff, S., Horwitz, A.L., and Smith, T.J.: Hormonal regulation of glycosaminoglycan accumulation in fibroblasts from patients with resistance to thyroid hormone. *J. Clin. Endocrinol. Metab.*, 57:1233, 1983.
31. Ceccarelli, P., Refetoff, S., and Murata, Y.: Resistance to thyroid hormone diagnosed by the reduced response of fibroblasts to the triiodothyronine-induced supression of fibronectin synthesis. *J. Clin. Endocrinol. Metab.*, 65:242-246, 1987.
32. Refetoff, S., Degroot, L.J., Benard, B., and Dewind, L.T.: Studies of a sibship with apparent hereditary resistance to the intracellular action of thyroid hormones. *Metabol.*, 21: 723-756, 1972.
33. Awad, E.A.: Pathological changes in fibromyalgia. *First International Symposium on Myofascial Pain and Fibromyalgia*. Minneapolis, Minnesota, May 9, 1989.
34. Awad, E.A.: Histopathological changes in fibrositis. In *Advances in Pain Research and Therapy*, Vol.17. Edited by J.R. Fricton and E.A. Awad, New York, Raven Press, Ltd., 1990, pp.249-258.

35. Reiffenberger, D.H. and Amundson, L.H.: Fibromyalgia syndrome: a review. *Amer. Fam. Physician*, 53(5):1698-1712, 1996.

36. Cohen, M.L. and Quintner, J.L.: Fibromyalgia syndrome: a problem of tautology. *Lancet*, 342(8876):906-909, 1993.

37. Neeck, G. and Riedel, W.: Neuromediator and hormonal perturbations in fibromyalgia syndrome: results of chronic stress? *Baillieres Clin. Rheumatol.*, 8(4):763-775, 1994.

38. Klein, I.: Metabolic, physiologic, and clinical indexes of thyroid function. In *The Thyroid: A Fundamental and Clinical Text.* 6th edition. Edited by L.E. Braverman and R.D. Utiger, Philadelphia, J.B. Lippincott Co., 1991, pp.486-492.

39. Soloman, D.H.: Clinical examination of the thyroid. In *The Thyroid Gland: A Practical Clinical Treatise.* Edited by D.H. Soloman, Van Middlesworth, Chicago, Year Book Medical Publishers, Inc., 1986, pp.19-34.

40. Chaney, W.C.: Tendon reflexes in myxedema: a valuable aid in diagnosis. *J. Am. Med. Assoc.*, 82:2013-2016, 1924.

41. Lambert, E.H., Underdahl, L.O., Beckett, S., and Mederos, L.O.: A study of the ankle jerk in myxedema. *J. Clin. Endocrinol.*, 11:1186-1205, 1951.

42. Elert, J.E., Rantapää-Dahlqvist, S.B., Henriksson-Larsën, K., Lorentzon, R., and Gerdlë, B.: Muscle performance, electromyography and fibre type composition in fibromyalgia and work-related myalgia. *Scand. J. Rheumatol.*, 21:28-34, 1992.

43. Bennett, R.M.: Exercise and exercise testing in fibromyalgia patients: lessons learned and suggestions for future studies. *J. Musculoskel. Pain*, 2(3):143-152, 1994.

44. Elert, I.E., Rantapää-Dahlqvist, S.B., Henriksson-Larsën, K., and Gerdlë, B.: Increased EMG-activity during short pauses in patients with fibromyalgia. *Scand. J. Rheumatol.*, 18:321-323, 1989.

45. Bennett, R.M., Clark, S.R., Campbell, S.M., et al.: Symptoms of Raynaud's syndrome in patients with fibromyalgia: a study utilizing the Nielsen test, digital photoplethysmography and measurements of platelet α_2-adrenergic receptors. *Arthritis and Rheumat.*, 34:264-269, 1991.

46. Silva, J.E.: Thyroid hormone control of thermogenesis and energy balance. *Thyroid*, 5(6):481-492, 1995.

47. Guernsey, D.L. and Edelman, I.S.: Regulation of thermogenesis by thyroid hormones. In *Molecular Basis of Thyroid Hormone Action.* Edited by J.H. Oppenheimer and H.H. Samuels, New York, Academic Press, Inc., 1983, pp.293-324.

48. Lin, M.H. and Akera, T.: Increased Na,K-ATPase concentrations in various tissues of rats caused by thyroid hormone treatment. *J. Biol. Chem.*, 253:723-726, 1978.

49. Edelman, I.S.: Thyroid thermogenesis. *N. Engl. J. Med.*, 290:1303, 1974.

50. Fain, J.N. and Rosenthal, J.W.: Calorigenic action of triiodothyronine on white fat cells: effects of ouabain, oligomycin, and catecholamines. *Endocrinol.*, 89:1205, 1971.

51. Lowe, J.C., Garrison, R., Reichman, A., Yellin, J., Thompson, M., and Kaufman, D.: Effectiveness and safety of T_3 therapy for euthyroid fibromyalgia: a double-blind, placebo-controlled response-driven crossover study, *Clin. Bull. Myofascial Ther.*, 2(2/3):31-57, 1997.

52. Lowe, J.C., Reichman, A., and Yellin, J.: The process of change during T_3 treatment for euthyroid fibromyalgia: a double-blind placebo-controlled crossover study, *Clin. Bull. Myofascial Ther.*, 2(2/3):91-124, 1997.

53. Lowe, J.C., Garrison, R., Reichman, A., and Yellin, J.: Triiodothyronine (T_3) treatment of euthyroid fibromyalgia: a small-n replication of a double-blind placebo-controlled crossover study. *Clin. Bull. Myofascial Ther.*, 2(4):71-88, 1997.

54. Yunus, M., Masi, A.T., Calabro, J.J., Miller, K.A., and Feigenbaum, S.L.: Primary fibromyalgia (fibrositis): clinical study of 50 patients with matched normal controls. *Semin. Arthritis Rheumat.*, 11(1):151-171, 1981.

55. Wolfe, F.: The clinical syndrome of fibrositis. *Amer. J. Med.*, 81(3A):7-14, 1986.

56. Prescott, E., Jacobsen, S., Kjoller, M., et al.: Fibromyalgia in the adult Danish population: II. A study of clinical features. *Scand. J. Rheumatol.*, 22(5):238-242, 1993.

57. Jacobsen, S., Petersen, I.S., and Danneskiold-Samsøe, B.: Clinical features in patients with chronic muscle pain with special reference to fibromyalgia. *Scand. J. Rheumatol.*, 22(2):69-76, 1993.

58. Guler, M., Kirnap, M., Bekaroglu, M., Uremek, G., and Onder, C.: Clinical characteristics of patients with fibromyalgia. *Israel J. Med. Sci.*, 28(1):20-23, 1992.

59. Yunus, M.B., Masi, A.T., and Aldag, J.C.: Short term effects of ibuprofen in primary fibromyalgia syndrome: a double-blind, placebo-controlled trial. *J. Rheumat.*, 16(4):527-532, 1989.

60. Yunus, M.B., Holt, G.S., Masi, A.T., and Aldag, J.C.: Fibromyalgia syndrome among the elderly. Comparison with younger patients. *J. Amer. Geriat. Soc.*, 36(11):987-995, 1988.

61. Lowe, J.C.: *The Purpose and Practice of Myofascial Therapy* (audiocassette album). Houston, McDowell Publishing Company, 1989.

3.21

Urinary Frequency and Urgency

Some fibromyalgia patients report urinary urgency and urinate 10 or more times per day. (Urinary "urgency" is a compelling desire to urinate, and "frequency" is an increase in the number of times per day that the patient urinates.) In one study, the incidence of urgency was 26.3%, and in another it was 80%. In one study, fibromyalgia patients had elevated vasopressin (antidiuretic hormone) during changes in posture. Apparently, no other reports of the status of the hypothalamic-pituitary-kidney-bladder axis in fibromyalgia are available. The paucity of studies severely limits comparison of the axis in fibromyalgia with that in hypothyroidism. Thus, a high degree of conjecture is necessary in exploring the possible role of inadequate thyroid hormone regulation in urinary urgency and frequency in fibromyalgia.

Reports of the status of the hypothalamic-pituitary-kidney-bladder axis in hypothyroid patients vary. Most studies show decreased liquid consumption and decreased urine volume, although other studies report increased volume. Two factors may account for this discrepancy: (1) differences in research methods and (2) selective involvement in different patients of the various components of the hypothalamic-pituitary-kidney-bladder axis.

Osmolality is a measure of how concentrated dissolved substances are in a solution, such as blood. Normally, increased osmolality of the blood increases secretion of vasopressin by the pituitary gland. Vasopressin attaches to receptors on the collecting tubules of the kidneys and stimulates reabsorption of salt and water into the blood. The reabsorption of water increases the dilution of the blood (decreases its osmolality) and decreases the accumulation of water in the bladder.

Reports of vasopressin secretion in hypothyroidism vary. Some researchers report normal levels and others an increase. Other factors held constant, vasopressin decreases urine volume, urgency, and frequency. An increase should exaggerate these effects. However, the effects of vasopressin may be overridden in hypothyroidism by increases in the density of α-adrenergic receptors in the bladder and brain stem (see below). Researchers have reported low urine volume in some hypothyroid patients. The low volume in these patients might result from one or more phenomena: high vasopressin secretion; proper regulation of the adrenergic genes by thyroid hormone, resulting in a normal ratio of α- to β-adrenergic receptors in the bladder and brain stem; decreased liquid consumption, which is typical of hypothyroid patients; and vasoconstriction of the blood vessels in their kidneys with reduced water excretion, stimulated by low cardiac output and low blood volume.

One or more abnormalities in the function of the hypothalamic-pituitary-kidney-bladder axis may account for increased urgency and frequency among fibromyalgia patients who have inadequate thyroid hormone regulation of the axis. The most influential abnormality may be a shift from a balance of α- and β-adrenergic receptors toward a dominance of α_2-adrenergic receptors. This shift occurs when thyroid hormone regulation of transcription of the adrenergic receptor genes is inadequate.

745

Increased numbers of α_2-adrenergic receptors on the kidney tubules decrease the count of vasopressin receptors on the tubules. This decrease in vasopressin receptors renders the kidneys partially resistant to vasopressin. The resistance to vasopressin impedes the water-retaining effect of vasopressin, favoring increased excretion of water from the kidney into the urine.

Low blood pressure and blood volume may prevent excess loss of water in the urine of some fibromyalgia patients, as it does in some hypothyroid patients—but only if they have normal sympathetic nervous system drive. When sympathetic drive is normal in an individual, low blood pressure induces constriction of the afferent arterioles of the kidneys. Constriction of the arterioles reduces water loss in the urine. As a result, more water is retained in the blood and the blood pressure rises. Some fibromyalgia patients, however, have subnormal sympathetic drive. The subnormal drive reduces their cardiac output and blood pressure. In addition, the subnormal drive may also impede constriction of the kidney's afferent arterioles. As a result, constriction of the vessels may be insufficient to prevent excess loss of water in the urine. Consequently, the bladder may accumulate excess urine, increasing urgency and frequency of urination.

A patient may have normal vasopressin secretion, a normal vasopressin receptor count on kidney tubules, and sympathetic drive sufficient to induce normal kidney vasoconstriction. Even so, urinary urgency and frequency may result from α-adrenergic receptor dominance in the bladder and brain stem due to inadequate thyroid hormone regulation of the adrenergic genes. The external longitudinal muscle coat of the bladder walls is smooth muscle. α-Adrenergic receptors, upon binding to catecholamines, increase the tone or induce frank contraction of the muscle wall of the bladder (as with the smooth muscle lining of blood vessels). Conversely, β-adrenergic receptors, upon binding to catecholamines, relax the muscle wall of the bladder. In hypothyroidism, the decrease in β-adrenergic receptor density in the bladder wall, and a shift toward α-adrenergic dominance, increases the muscle tone of the bladder wall and can induce contractions. Increased tone, and especially frank contractions, reduces the internal volume of the bladder, reducing its capacity for storing urine. Also, increased α-adrenergic receptor density in the bladder trigone increases the tone of the trigone. (The trigone is a tri-

angular area on the lower posterior wall of the bladder. At its lowermost apex at the bottom of the bladder is the bladder neck. Urine passes through the neck into the urethra to be excreted from the body. At the uppermost angles of the trigone, the two ureters from the kidneys transport urine into the bladder). The increased tone contributes to the total increase in the tone of the bladder musculature. This further decreases the capacity of the bladder for filling. The reduced capacity for filling lowers the threshold for initiation of the urination reflex that induces urgency. This reflex, regulated at the brain stem level, is itself facilitated by α_1-adrenergic receptors. An increase in the count of these receptors in the brain stem center that regulates the reflex contributes to lowering of the threshold for the urination reflex. The lowered threshold favors urinary urgency and frequency.

Finally, fibromyalgia patients with reduced sympathetic drive due to inadequate thyroid hormone regulation may have subnormal sympathetic innervation of the ureters. They are also likely to have a concomitant increase in parasympathetic innervation of the ureters. The decrease in sympathetic innervation and the increase in parasympathetic innervation would increase peristaltic contractions of the ureters. The increased rate of contractions would accelerate the rate at which urine is transported to the bladder. The increased transport of urine would fill the bladder more rapidly. More rapid filling of a bladder with a reduced capacity for filling would readily activate the urination reflex, inducing urgency and frequency.

Most people urinate 4-to-6 times per day, mainly in the daytime.[1,p.1647] Normally, with increased liquid consumption, urine volume and frequency of urination also increase. When not due to increased urine volume, increased "frequency" (frequent urination) is a symptom of reduced filling capacity of the urinary bladder.[1,p.1647]

Frequency may be accompanied by "urgency," a compelling need to urinate. Chronic urgency can result from damage to the urinary bladder mucosa or its underlying structures. Infection, stones, tumors, or foreign bodies may damage the mucosa or submucosal structures. The damage usually involves inflammatory infiltration and edema of bladder tissues, with mild stretching and loss of bladder elasticity. Extensive damage can result in functional disease, pain, and urgency. In the patient with urgency, the amount of urine excreted at urination may be small. In severe cases, the patient may have a constant desire to urinate and may urinate involuntarily (incontinence).[1,p.1647]

● THE HYPOTHALAMIC-PITUITARY-KIDNEY-BLADDER AXIS

NORMAL HYPOTHALAMIC-PITUITARY-KIDNEY-BLADDER AXIS FUNCTION

Kidney Tubules

The kidneys are the major organ for both eliminating water from the body and conserving it when necessary. When liquid intake is low, or water is lost from the body by perspiration or diarrhea, the kidneys conserve water. They do so by reducing the volume of urine formed in the kidney tubules. (The kidney tubules are where water and other substances pass from the blood to the forming urine, or from the forming urine to the blood.) The tubules permit less water to escape to form urine, and this increases the osmolality of the urine relative to that of the plasma. (Osmolality is the concentration of a solution: the ratio of dissolved particles to the quantity of solution.)

When liquid consumption is high, the kidney tubules release more water in the urine. As a result, the bladder accumulates a larger volume of urine of low osmolality (urine with a higher ratio of water to dissolved particles). Urine volume normally varies from 0.5-to-20.0 L/day, and osmolality varies from 50-to-1200 mOsm/kg H_2O.[27,p.445]

Vasopressin and Vasopressin Receptors

Vasopressin is a hormone synthesized in hypothalamic cells. Nerve endings in the posterior pituitary store and release the hormone into the blood. Three main stimuli induce the pituitary to release vasopressin: an increase in osmolality of the blood, a decrease in blood volume, or a reduction in blood pressure.[27,p.446]

Blood osmolality increases when body fluids accumulate a high concentration of solutes, mainly sodium. Cells called "osmoreceptors" in the supraoptic and paraventricular nuclei of the hypothalamus—functioning as osmometers[27,p.445]—sense the increase in osmolality.[7,p.679] The osmoreceptor cells signal other hypothalamic neurons to synthesize vasopressin.[27,p.446] The axons of the vasopressin-synthesizing neurons descend from the hypothalamus through a funnel-shaped structure to the posterior pituitary gland. There,

the neuron terminals secrete vasopressin into the blood.[7,p.679]

After passing from the pituitary to the kidneys through the circulation, vasopressin attaches to vasopressin receptors on the membrane of collecting tubules of the kidneys. Vasopressin, bound to its receptors, activates adenylate cyclase and increases intracellular levels of cyclic adenosine monophosphate (cAMP). The increase in cAMP activates protein kinases that induce water channels to appear in the membrane. The channels increase permeability of the membrane to water. The increased permeability induces the tubules to reabsorb salt and water back into the blood from the urine forming in the tubules. The reabsorption of water decreases the osmolality of the blood, and it decreases dilution of the urine. Normally, when decreased amounts of vasopressin reach the kidneys, or there are too few vasopressin receptors on the tubules, the kidneys excrete a large volume of water in the urine. The greater excretion is termed "diuresis." When increased amounts of vasopressin bind to normal numbers of vasopressin receptors on the tubules, the kidneys reduce the volume of water they secrete in the urine. This water retaining process is termed "antidiuresis."

The main function of vasopressin and its receptors is to increase the permeability of the collecting tubules so that more water passes out of them and back into the blood. The hormone bound to its receptors also stimulates the ascending limb of Henle's loop and the collecting tubules to increase active reabsorption of NaCl.[27,p.447] Under the influence of vasopressin, the tubules reabsorb massive amounts of water back into the blood. The increased amount of water in the circulating blood dilutes the body fluids. The water of the body fluids accumulates waist substances. As the water and the substances circulate through the kidneys, the tubules accumulate and excrete them as urine by the bladder.

As the tubules reabsorb more water back into the blood and the blood becomes more dilute, osmoreceptors become less active. As a result, vasopressin-synthesizing neurons reduce their secretion of vasopressin. The reduced vasopressin level enables more water to accumulate in the tubules to be excreted in the urine.[7,p.679]

ABNORMAL HYPOTHALAMIC-PITUITARY-KIDNEY-BLADDER AXIS FUNCTION

For the kidneys to properly control the volume and

osmolality of blood and urine, two hypothalamic-pituitary processes must be normal. First, hypothalamic osmoreceptors must respond properly to highly concentrated blood. Second, the vasopressin-synthesizing neurons must secrete appropriate amounts of vasopressin from the posterior pituitary. Normally, vasopressin-synthesizing neurons secrete more of the hormone in response to decreases in blood pressure.[27,p.446]

Binding of catecholamines to increased numbers of α_2-adrenergic receptors in the posterior pituitary gland inhibits vasopressin secretion. This occurs in some hypothyroid patients (see below).[10] Induction of diuresis by clonidine suggests that activation of α_2-adrenergic receptors reduces vasopressin secretion. Clonidine is an α_2-adrenergic receptor agonist. According to Auriac et al., induction of diuresis by clonidine suggests that drug inhibits vasopressin secretion.[61]

Diuresis is essentially an increase in the volume of urine. It results from too little vasopressin reaching the kidney tubules to stimulate them to reabsorb a normal amount of water back into the circulation. Inordinate amounts of water accumulate in the tubules, and the water, as urine, leaves the kidneys through the ureters and collects in the bladder. As a result, the bladder fills more rapidly than normal. In extreme form, this phenomenon is called "diabetes insipidus."[7,p.427] This condition results from frank vasopressin deficiency. It is characterized by excessive thirst (polydipsia), weakness, dry skin, and excretion of excessive amounts of urine of normal chemical composition (polyuria).[27,p.450] In the milder form of vasopressin deficiency, the individual may merely complain of urinary urgency and frequent urination.

● URINARY ABNORMALITIES IN FIBROMYALGIA

URINARY URGENCY AND FREQUENCY

Some authors write of "irritable bladder syndrome" in some fibromyalgia patients.[58] Wolfe reported that 26.3% of fibromyalgia patients complain of urinary urgency.[3,p.54] Stormoken and Brosstad reported a much higher percentage: 80% of their fibromyalgia patients had urgency more than eight times per 24-hour period. The mean frequency of urination among their patients was 10 times per day.[4] These authors argued that urgency among fibromyalgia patients suggests a genetic predisposition to the condition and confirms that it is a "true" disease.

VASOPRESSIN LEVELS

Crofford et al. reported that vasopressin levels were not significantly different between fibromyalgia patients and control subjects. However, variability of levels was greater among fibromyalgia patients than controls. They found a trend toward increased AVP secretion following postural change in fibromyalgia patients. The increase in 5 of 12 patients (41%) was greater than two standard deviations above the highest value for a control patient.[41] Demitrack and Crofford reported that their preliminary data suggest increased vasopressin levels in fibromyalgia patients.[62,p.71]

INTERSTITIAL CYSTITIS

Interstitial cystitis is inflammation of the small spaces between the connective tissues (the "interstitium") of the bladder. Patients usually have pain in the bladder and pelvic region, and typically, they have urinary urgency and frequency.

Clauw et al. described the disorder as enigmatic. They pointed out that in interstitial cystitis, symptoms of the genital and urinary systems predominate. In comparison, in fibromyalgia, symptoms of musculoskeletal system predominate. Nonetheless, they noted that the two disorders are similar. They share demographics, natural history, exacerbating factors, and "allied conditions" such as irritable bowel syndrome and headaches. They hypothesized a substantial clinical overlap between interstitial cystitis and fibromyalgia. To test the hypothesis, they compared the range of current symptoms of patients with the two conditions. They questioned 60 fibromyalgia patients, 30 interstitial cystitis patients, and 30 age-matched healthy controls. The researchers assessed peripheral nociception in subjects by means of an algometer exam. Fibromyalgia and interstitial cystitis patients had a high frequency of similar current symptoms. Compared to controls, both groups of patients also had increased pain sensitivity at tender points and control points. The investigators concluded that the symptoms of interstitial cystitis and fibromyalgia significantly overlap. They also concluded that like fibromyalgia patients, interstitial cystitis patients have diffusely increased peripheral nociception. The researchers also speculated that the central mechanisms that mediate fibromyalgia symptoms also mediate interstitial cystitis symptoms.[40] The central mechanism they conjectured is at odds with the implication from conventional medical treatment that interstitial cystitis is a primary local bladder disorder.

POSSIBLE RELATION OF URINARY ABNORMALITIES IN FIBROMYALGIA TO INADEQUATE THYROID HORMONE REGULATION OF THE HYPOTHALAMIC-PITUITARY-KIDNEY-BLADDER AXIS

In fibromyalgia patients with inadequate thyroid hormone regulation of the hypothalamic-pituitary-kidney-bladder axis, several possible mechanisms that tend to occur in hypothyroidism may contribute to urinary urgency and frequency.

In one study, investigators found an increase in the density of α_2-adrenergic receptors on the platelets of fibromyalgia patients.[59] As I discuss in detail in Chapter 3.1, this finding provides the most important clue to the basis of symptoms and objective abnormalities in fibromyalgia. The finding alone provides a plausible basis for urinary urgency and frequency in some fibromyalgia patients. A possible increase in α-adrenergic receptors (due to inadequate thyroid hormone regulation of the α-adrenergic genes) is accordingly predominant in the proposed mechanisms in this section.

Table 3.21.1 is a comparison of axis abnormalities reported in fibromyalgia and hypothyroid patients.

VARIABILITY IN HYPOTHALAMIC-PITUITARY-KIDNEY-BLADDER AXIS FINDINGS IN HYPOTHYROIDISM

Considering the variability of hypothalamic-pituitary-kidney-bladder axis findings in hypothyroidism is important. Study results are inconsistent. No patterns of vasopressin secretion or urination are consistent across the entire population of hypothyroid patients. Many patients, for example, have decreased urine volume, others have normal volume, and others have increased volume. The pattern varies as do other features of hypothyroidism. For instance, most hypothyroid patients are intolerant of cold. But some are intolerant of heat, and others do not have temperature intolerances. (See Chapter 3.9.) Similarly, some patients are hypotensive, others are normotensive, and still others are hypertensive (see Chapter 3.2). We must bear in mind such variations when considering that features of fibromyalgia may result from inadequate thyroid hormone regulation of the hypothalamic-pituitary-kidney-bladder axis.

VASOPRESSIN SECRETION

Reports indicate that only some fibromyalgia patients have a trend toward increased vasopressin secretion.[41][62] Unfortunately, we have no reports at this time indicating whether fibromyalgia patients with increased vasopressin secretion have decreased, normal, or increased urgency and frequency.

We would expect increased vasopressin secretion to decrease urinary urgency and frequency. The decrease would occur, however, only if no other factor impinging on the hypothalamic-pituitary-kidney-bladder axis counterposed the increased vasopressin level and increased urgency and frequency. An increase in α-adrenergic receptors is possibly such a factor. An increase in α-adrenergic receptors and a decrease in β-adrenergic receptors can alone account for urgency and frequency in fibromyalgia. Because of this, the status of vasopressin secretion in patients (except in extreme cases) may be irrelevant to their urinary status.

If urgency and frequency are increased among fibromyalgia patients with normal vasopressin secretion, this would suggest that some factor other than vasopressin secretory status is responsible for the urinary symptoms. Again, however, no studies are available at this time showing the urinary status of fibromyalgia patients with normal vasopressin secretion.

Reports of Normal Vasopressin Levels in Hypothyroidism

Howard et al. found no changes in plasma or pituitary vasopressin levels in hypothyroid rats given an acute water load. Despite this, the rats had increased urine volume and lower than normal serum sodium and plasma osmolality. (The increased urine volume suggests that some factor other than vasopressin was affecting the hypothalamic-pituitary-kidney-bladder axis of the rats. An increase in α-adrenergic receptors and a decrease in β-adrenergic receptors were possibly responsible.) Steady-state vasopressin mRNA levels in the hypothalamus of the rats were not low. The researchers concluded that short-term chemically-induced hypothyroidism caused no detectable change in vasopressin synthesis. However, hypothyroidism exerted substantial effects on renal function and caused a modest central alteration in the plasma vasopressin-osmolality relationship.[26] Ali et al. also found no difference in vasopressin synthesis or blood levels between hypothyroid and euthyroid rats.[12]

Reports of Normal to Low Vasopressin Levels in Hypothyroidism

Failure in the past to detect abnormalities of vasopressin synthesis or secretion in hypothyroidism may have resulted from the use of laboratory tests that were less sensitive than later ones. Iwasaki et al. used a water-loading test to assess vasopressin secretion in 5 hypothyroid patients and 5 control subjects. The researchers used an RIA test, a more sensitive measure of vasopressin than tests used in the past. They found that basal levels of vasopressin were lower in hypothyroid patients than in normal subjects. The mean basal plasma vasopressin level in the patients (0.5±0.1 pmol/L) was significantly lower (P<0.01) than that in normal adults (2.5±0.5 pmol/L). The investigators infused saline intravenously to increase osmolality of the blood and provoke vasopressin release. The release was normal in some patients and low in others. Two patients' kidneys were not able to properly dilute urine and their blood sodium levels were low. (Their urine contained a high concentration of sodium.) In the basal state, 2 patients had mildly-to-moderately low blood sodium levels (hyponatremia). During water loading of their blood, they also had a mildly impaired ability to dilute urine. Both patients had suppressed plasma vasopressin levels. The investigators wrote that inappropriately high vasopressin levels are not common in hypothyroidism. They also wrote that impaired water excretion in some patients must be due to a mechanism other than high vasopressin levels.[13] Patients in this study who had low vasopressin levels may have had relative α-adrenergic inhibition of vasopressin release by the pituitary.

Ota et al. reported a tendency toward lower plasma vasopressin levels in hypothyroid patients. The levels did not properly fall following oral water loading of the blood. Their data suggested impaired release and increased metabolic breakdown of vasopressin.[30]

Vargus et al. studied urinary excretion of vasopressin in hyperthyroid and hypothyroid rats compared to normal rats. To stimulate vasopressin secretion, they used either of two stimuli that raised osmolality: water deprivation or a hypertonic saline load. Increased osmolality increased vasopressin excretion in hyperthyroid rats and decreased excretion in hypothyroid rats. Thus, hypothyroid rats had impaired secretion of vasopressin in response to osmotic stimuli.[29]

Carter et al. used propylthiouracil in drinking water to chemically induce hypothyroidism in rats. Hypothyroidism increased vasopressin mRNA levels in two structures: the supraoptic and paraventricular nuclei of the hypothalamus and in the neurointermediate lobe of the pituitary. However, when the researchers raised plasma osmolality, vasopressin mRNA levels did not increase. Interestingly, hypothyroidism induced by alternative procedures (surgical thyroidectomy or propylthiouracil injections) also did not increase the levels of vasopressin mRNA.[31]

In severe hypothyroidism, the thyroid hormone deficiency adversely affects most body tissues, including the kidney tubules.[14] The patient usually has impaired rather than excessive water excretion. The sodium content of his blood is low (hyponatremia), so much in fact that he may have water intoxication.[15,p.1013] Yet while vasopressin levels are high in some patients, levels in other patients are low.[13]

Reports of Elevated Vasopressin Levels in Hypothyroidism

As with fibromyalgia patients, researchers have reported that only a minority of patients with untreated hypothyroidism have increased vasopressin secretion. (See Chapter 3.5, subsection titled "Effects of Thyroid Hormone Deficiency on the Hypothalamic-Pituitary-Adrenal Axis: AVP.")

KIDNEY RESISTANCE TO VASOPRESSIN IN HYPOTHYROIDISM DUE TO A DEFICIT OF VASOPRESSIN RECEPTORS AND AN INCREASE IN α₂-ADRENERGIC RECEPTORS

Normally, when the blood pressure is low, vasopressin secretion increases. When the hormone reaches the kidneys, it binds to vasopressin receptors on the tubules. Binding of vasopressin to the receptors increases reabsorption of water back into the blood from the tubules. In hypothyroid patients, this kidney effect of vasopressin may be impaired due to a deficit of vasopressin receptors in the kidney tubules. The receptor deficit would result in a blunted response to vasopressin by the thick ascending Henle's loop in the medulla of the kidney. The blunted response would result in failure to absorb sufficient amounts of water back into the blood and loss of the water in the urine.

Vasopressin receptors in the loop may be defective or deficient, or the guanine protein that regulates the adenylate cyclase response to vasopressin may be faulty. Ali et al. found that in rats, hypothyroidism reduced the numbers of vasopressin receptors in the kidneys. Administering exogenous thyroid hormone corrected the receptor deficits.[12][23] "It can be concluded," they wrote, "that thyroid deficiency directly alters antidiuretic hormone [vasopressin] receptor biosynthesis in both liver and kidney, instead of acting via the depressed plasma antidiuretic hormone levels."[23]

An additional mechanism of the blunted response of the kidney tubules to vasopressin may be the increase in α_2-adrenergic receptor count that usually occurs in hypothyroidism. Activation of α_2-adrenergic receptors may decrease vasopressin secretion by the pituitary gland.[10] However, reduced vasopressin concentration in the plasma does not alone account for the diuretic action of α_2-adrenergic receptor agonists.[11] These receptors have a direct kidney effect. When they bind to catecholamines in the kidneys, they inhibit the action of vasopressin in the collecting tubules.[22,p.43] Catecholamine-α_2-adrenergic receptor binding in the kidneys of conscious rats increased sodium and water excretion. The mechanism of excretion was consistent with inhibition of vasopressin action on the kidney's cortical collecting tubules.[9] Binding of catecholamines to α_2-adrenergic receptors in the kidneys decreases vasopressin-stimulated adenylate cyclase activity.[16] The decrease in activity of the enzyme is compatible with diminished sodium transport back into the blood.[15,p.1014] The result is increased urine accumulation in the bladder, with urgency and frequency. In hypothyroid rats and in humans, the intake of sufficient exogenous thyroid hormone reverses the pituitary and kidney-bladder effects of increased α_2-adrenergic receptors.[15,p.1014]

URINE VOLUME IN HYPOTHYROIDISM

I know of no studies of urinary volume in fibromyalgia patients. Investigators have reported both decreased and increased urine volume in hypothyroid patients.

Reports of Decreased Urine Volume
Some authors have reported that hypothyroid patients usually drink small amounts of liquid, and possibly as a result, they have low urinary output.[5,p.566] Andersen et al. studied the urination patterns of 61 consecutive patients of different thyroid status: hyperthyroid, hypothyroid, and euthyroid. The researchers examined urination patterns after the patients' first visit to the hospital. They examined them again 6 months later, after treatment restored hyperthyroid and hypothyroid patients' thyroid hormone levels to normal. Hyperthyroid patients initially had increased nighttime urination (nocturia). On average, their initial urinary frequency was significantly higher than at follow-up. Hypothyroid patients initially had a low mean

frequency compared with follow-up. The investigators cautioned that the clinician should consider thyroid disease when patients have unexplained urinary frequency or retention.[28]

Ota et al. reported impaired water excretion in 5 hypothyroid patients after acute oral water loading. The impaired excretion was entirely relieved after 7 months of treatment with T_4.[30] Michael et al. measured the excretion of an oral water load in rats over a 3-hour period. They measured urinary excretion before and after administering T_3 in 12 hypothyroid and 7 age-matched control rats. At baseline, urinary excretion of hypothyroid rats' was low after water administration. In comparison to control rats, hypothyroid rats had a lower urine volume but higher urine osmolality. T_3 fully normalized all the observed abnormalities in the hypothyroid rats. The researchers concluded that thyroid hormone deficiency was directly responsible for the decreased urine excretion by the hypothyroid rats.[32]

Reports of Increased Urine Volume
Watanakunakorn et al. found that of 400 hypothyroid patients, 11.25% had excessive urination (polyuria), both during the day and night.[6,p.185] Howard et al. reported that hypothyroid rats had a delay in excretion of an acute water load and decreased urinary-concentrating ability. However, they had increased urine volume.[26]

INCREASED URINARY SODIUM EXCRETION IN HYPOTHYROIDISM

I am aware of no studies of urinary sodium excretion in fibromyalgia patients. As with urinary volume, however, studying the findings in hypothyroidism may provide a reference point for comparison with the results of future fibromyalgia studies.

Baseline urinary sodium excretion is usually normal in hypothyroid patients. But when subjected to stresses that normally induce sodium conservation by the kidneys, the patients' reabsorption of sodium from the tubules may be reduced. Vaamonde et al. quantified the increase in sodium excretion in hypothyroid humans. The researchers studied 14 patients and 13 normal subjects. They evaluated sodium balance when the patients and subjects had a 155 mEq sodium intake. The baseline excretion of sodium in the urine was comparable in patients and control subjects. They tested the response of the kidneys to acute salt loading. During the salt-loading tests, the excretion of sodium in the urine of hypothyroid patients was within the range of excreted sodium in control subjects. Patients had a significant 34% reduction in glomerular filtration (see Glossary), and the control subjects had a significant 37% reduction in filtration. This showed that both patients and controls excreted sodium in the urine in response to an acute sodium load that was within the same range.[17]

Vaamonde et al. also tested the response of the kidneys to two stimuli that induce rapid sodium conservation by the kidneys: (1) postural change, and (2) a larger than maximal dose of $_9\alpha$-fluorohydrocortisone.[17] ($_9\alpha$-Fluorohydrocortisone is fludrocortisone acetate, a highly potent synthetic glucocorticoid. Like the mineralocorticoid steroid hormones secreted by the adrenal cortices, $_9\alpha$-fluorohydrocortisone influences the metabolism of sodium and potassium. It also regulates circulating levels of these minerals by affecting the kidney tubules.)

The patients had less capacity to conserve sodium than did control subjects. Normally, engaging in the upright posture test markedly reduces the excretion of sodium in the urine. During the test, controls' sodium excretion decreased by 62%; hypothyroid patients' excretion decreased by only 28%. Normally, when researchers administer 2 mg of $_9\alpha$-fluorohydrocortisone to humans, sodium excretion markedly decreases. After the investigators administered $_9\alpha$-fluorohydrocortisone to normal subjects, their sodium excretion decreased by 72%. In comparison, the patients' excretion decreased by only 50%.

Hypothyroid patients had significantly increased sodium excretion before and during the saline loading test. They also had significantly increased excretion during their subnormal responses to both stimuli for acute sodium conservation. The patients' potassium excretion was lower than that of control subjects, even after $_9\alpha$-fluorohydrocortisone was administered. Thus, the hypothyroid patients' kidney tubules reabsorbed a subnormal amount of sodium. From this, the researchers concluded that thyroid hormone plays a role in normal sodium reabsorption.

THREE MECHANISMS THAT MAY AVERT INCREASED URINE VOLUME IN HYPOTHYROIDISM

One might expect that low or low-normal vasopressin secretion in some hypothyroid patients would permit excessive amounts of water and sodium to pass into the bladder, increase bladder volume, and increase urgency and frequency. Indeed, some hypothyroid patients do excrete excess sodium in their urine, as the studies in the previous section show. But the increased sodium excretion is not typically accompanied by increased water excretion. Patients may in fact have decreased water excretion. This seeming paradox may result in part from patients' lower liquid consumption. But three other mechanisms also avert excessive water excretion. One is constriction of kidney vessels induced by the activation of sympathetic nerves to the kidneys in response to lowered blood pressure. The other two mechanisms are the secretion of renin by the kidney and aldosterone by the adrenal cortices.

I can find no reports of the status of these three mechanisms in fibromyalgia patients. But examining the findings in hypothyroidism can provide a reference for comparing findings from future fibromyalgia studies.

Sympathetically-Mediated Kidney Vasoconstriction

Reduced glomerular filtration (see Glossary) usually averts excess water loss in hypothyroid humans and animals.[7,p.1012] Decreased cardiac output and low blood volume are the main stimuli that reduce glomerular filtration.[15,p.1012] These cardiovascular conditions activate the sympathetic nerves to the kidneys (see section below titled "Sympathetic and Parasympathetic Innervation of the Kidneys, Ureters, and Bladder"). Activation of the sympathetic nerves causes generalized constriction of kidney blood vessels.[18][19][20] This compensatory mechanism is potentially powerful. For example, excess transmission of sympathetic impulses to the kidney blood vessels may cause diastolic hypertension. Streeten et al. presumed that excess sympathetic transmission to the kidney vessels was the mechanism of diastolic hypertension in hypothyroid patients who made up 1.2% of referred hypertensive patients.[20] The increased resistance to blood flow in both afferent and efferent blood vessels of the kidneys has two effects: it reduces the rate of glomerular filtration and the flow of plasma through the kidneys.[21] The reduced filtration leaves more water in the blood, counteracting the potential hypotension from low cardiac output and/or low blood volume.

Several groups of researchers have reported impaired excretion of water in the urine in hypothyroidism.[5,p.566][28][30][32] The impaired excretion may be mediated by the increase in α-adrenergic receptors[27,p.453] caused by inadequate thyroid hormone regulation of the adrenergic receptor genes. During activation of sympathetic nerves to the kidneys, the nerve endings release norepinephrine. The norepinephrine binds to α-adrenergic receptors, and the binding induces constriction of kidney afferent arterioles. The constriction decreases glomerular filtrate and secretion of renin (see the section immediately below), and it increases NaCl reabsorption by the proximal tubules and Henle's loop.[27,p.453]

Kidney Vasoconstriction Induced by Increased Renin Secretion

When sodium excretion in the urine increases, water excretion also increases. The increased sodium and water excretion has two main effects on the general circulation: decreased levels of sodium and decreased fluid volume. As the extracellular fluid and plasma volume decrease, blood flow and blood pressure in the kidney arteries also decrease. Cells adjacent to the glomeruli (juxtaglomerular cells) respond to the decreased blood flow and pressure by secreting renin into the peripheral circulation.[27,p.569]

Renin is a small protein enzyme. When released into the blood, it catalyzes conversion of the plasma protein angiotensinogen to the peptide angiotensin I. Angiotensin I induces mild vasoconstriction. Within seconds, angiotensin I splits to release angiotensin II. This molecule is a powerful vasoconstrictor. It elevates arterial blood pressure, and to a lesser degree, venous pressure. The increased arterial pressure increases peripheral arterial resistance. The elevated venous pressure increases return of blood to the heart. The increased return of venous blood to the heart helps the heart to effectively pump against the increased arterial peripheral resistance. Angiotensin II also decreases the excretion of both salt and water. It does so partly by potently stimulating the synthesis and secretion of aldosterone (see Glossary) by the adrenal cortices (see subsection immediately below). The decreased salt and water excretion, which reduces urine volume, helps elevate arterial pressure by increasing extracellular fluid volume.[25,pp.211-212]

Normal Aldosterone-Kidney Physiology. The adrenal cortices secrete aldosterone mainly in response to reduced circulating fluid volume. The reduced volume normally results from lowered blood sodium levels and increased blood potassium levels.[27,p.569] Aldosterone binds to receptors on kidney tubular cells. The binding increases mRNAs and proteins that mediate the kidney actions of aldosterone. One of these actions is stimulation of sodium reabsorption from the urine in the distal tubules. The reabsorbed sodium passes through the tubular cells and back into the blood of the capillaries. The reabsorption decreases the net excretion of sodium in the urine, conserving the extracellular sodium of the body. Water is passively reabsorbed with the sodium so that the plasma sodium concentration (in relation to water content) increases only slightly. Thus, the extracellular fluid volume expands isotonically, averting excessive osmolality. While stimulating sodium excretion, aldosterone also stimulates active excretion of potassium from the tubular cells into the urine.[27,p.569]

Possible Reduced Aldosterone Secretion Due to Low-Normal Vasopressin Secretion. Secretion of aldosterone is not as direct a mechanism for immediately conserving body water as are the two other mechanisms I described above. Nevertheless, increased aldosterone secretion is involved in the conservation of body water. Hypothyroid patients who have reduced vasopressin secretion may also, as a result, have diminished aldosterone secretion. The reduced aldosterone secretion would result in increased excretion of water in the urine. The increased excretion would contribute to urgency and frequency.

Most neurons that secrete peptides secrete more than one type. The parvocellular neurons in the paraventricular nucleus that contain vasopressin also contain corticotropin-releasing hormone (CRH). The two hormones are released together from the median eminence. Vasopressin strongly potentiates the CRH-stimulated release of ACTH from the pituitary gland. This finding indicates a synergistic role for the two hormones.[16,p.418][24,p.743][33] Inhibition of secretion of the two hormones can result from two mechanisms during inadequate thyroid hormone regulation: (1) decreased transcription regulation of transcription for CRH, and (2) inhibition of hypothalamic synthesis of CRH and vasopressin due to decreased nerve impulse output from the superior cervical sympathetic ganglion. (See Chapter 3.5, subsection titled "Thyroid Hormone Status and the HPA Axis: CRH," and subsection titled "Indirect Effects of Inadequate Thyroid Hormone Regulation.") Inhibition of both CRH and vasopressin would cause subnormal ACTH secretion, or it might disrupt the secretory rhythm of ACTH. ACTH is a major activator of aldosterone secretion by the zona glomerulosa cells of the adrenal cortices.[39][48] Because of this, subnormal secretion of ACTH or disruption of its secretory rhythm might result in subnormal aldosterone secretion. ACTH normally regulates tonic secretion of aldosterone. Subnormal ACTH regulation diminishes the aldosterone response of the adrenal cortices to the primary stimulus of sodium depletion.

Inadequate Thyroid Hormone Regulation of the Sympathetic-Adrenergic System: A Source of Failure of the Three Mechanisms

Inadequate thyroid hormone regulation may cause failure of the three mechanisms that normally avert increased urine volume. Inadequate regulation does so through two mechanisms: decreased sympathetic nerve activity and α-adrenergic receptor dominance.

Decreased Sympathetic Activity. Subnormal sympathetic nervous system activity in hypothyroidism (see Chapter 3.1) may limit norepinephrine secretion at the kidney arterioles. The reduced secretion of norepinephrine would decrease the capacity of the kidney arterioles to constrict when blood pressure is low. As a result, glomerular filtration would increase with loss of more water in the urine (see subsection above titled "Sympathetically-Mediated Kidney Vasoconstriction").

α-Adrenergic Receptor Dominance. The shift from α- and β-adrenergic receptor balance to α-adrenergic receptor dominance that occurs in hypothyroidism would more potently impair the three mechanisms. Normally, when blood volume decreases sufficiently, β-adrenergic receptor stimulation of the kidneys increases the secretion of renin and aldosterone.[27,p.569] The secreted renin results in production of angiotensin II. This peptide raises blood pressure by causing arteries and veins to constrict, and it induces reabsorption of salt and water from the kidney tubules. (See subsection above titled "Kidney Vasoconstriction Induced by Increased Renin Secretion.") The secretion of aldosterone—stimulated by both β-adrenergic receptor activation and renin—induces reabsorption of sodium from the kidney tubules. (See subsection above titled "Normal Aldosterone-Kidney Physiology.")

α-Adrenergic receptor dominance in hypothyroidism may impede renin secretion and, in turn, aldosterone secretion. α₁-Adrenergic receptors, upon combining with catecholamines, inhibit renin release.[22,p.43] In that renin raises blood pressure partly by stimulating the release of aldosterone from the adrenal cortices, α-adrenergic receptor dominance may inhibit both renin and aldosterone secretion. Thus, during α-adrenergic receptor dominance, renin and aldosterone levels may not increase in response to low blood pressure. As a result, the kidney afferent arterioles would not constrict properly and glomerular filtrate would remain excessive. This could contribute to urinary urgency and frequency.

AUTONOMIC NERVOUS SYSTEM-ADRENERGIC RECEPTOR INNERVATION OF THE BLADDER

In patients with hypothyroidism or cellular resistance to thyroid hormone, thyroid hormone regulation of the adrenergic genes is usually inadequate. During inadequate regulation of the genes, the density of α-adrenergic receptors on cell membranes increases, and the density of β-adrenergic receptors decreases (see Chapter 3.1, section titled "Adrenergic Receptors"). This shift in the membrane density of the two types of receptors may potently alter kidney and bladder function. The alteration in function is alone sufficient to explain urinary urgency and frequency in fibromyalgia patients with inadequate thyroid hormone regulation of the adrenergic genes. In addition, inadequate thyroid hormone regulation of the autonomic nervous system may alter the autonomic innervation of the kidney, ureters, and bladder. Sympathetic innervation is likely to decrease and parasympathetic innervation is likely to increase. This shift in autonomic innervation would contribute to urgency and frequency.

Below, I describe the autonomic innervation of the bladder. Familiarity with the innervation is necessary for understanding how urgency and frequency are facilitated by a shift in adrenergic receptor type on membranes and a change in sympathetic/parasympathetic innervation. (For more details, I recommend the excellent review by Dodd and Role.[60,pp.773-774] I abstracted much of the overview below from their review, although some I wrote after Guyton's description.[25,p.352])

An Overview of the Autonomic Innervation of the Bladder

Bladder filling and urination are controlled by four types of nerves: sensory, sympathetic, parasympathetic, and skeletal muscle motor nerves. To help regulate bladder filling and urination, sympathetic nerves exert control by secreting norepinephrine which interacts with α- and β-adrenergic receptors. Parasympathetic nerves exert control by secreting acetylcholine which interacts with muscurenic and nicotinic receptors on cell membranes. Skeletal muscle (alpha) motor nerves exert control by secreting acetylcholine which binds to acetylcholine receptors on skeletal muscle membranes.

Sensory Nerves. The receptor endings of sensory nerves detect stretching of the bladder wall and posterior urethra. (The posterior urethra is the most proximal part of the urethra; it is also the neck of the lowermost part of the bladder.) The sensory nerves transmit impulses from the bladder to the dorsal horns of the spinal cord. In the cord, secondary impulses may synapse with and activate sympathetic or motor nerves. The secondary impulses also ascend to the brain stem and brain to act on other nerves involved in the control of urination. Stretch impulses from the posterior urethra are particularly strong, and these are primarily responsible for setting off the reflex that causes the bladder to empty.[25,p.352]

Parasympathetic, Sympathetic, and Skeletal Muscle Motor Nerves. The cell bodies of the parasympathetic nerves to the bladder are located in the intermediolateral (lateral) horns of the sacral spinal cord. These nerves secrete acetylcholine near or within the musculature that makes up the bladder wall. The cell bodies of the sympathetic nerves to the bladder reside in the intermediolateral (lateral) horns of the thoracic and upper lumbar spinal cord. The cell bodies of the skeletal muscle motor nerves to the bladder are situated in the ventral horns of the sacral spinal cord.

Spinal Cord and Supraspinal Controls Over Parasympathetic, Sympathetic, and Skeletal Muscle Motor Nerves that Regulate the Bladder. Activity of both spinal cord and supraspinal (brain stem and brain) cells partly controls the sympathetic, parasympathetic, and skeletal muscle motor nerves that help regulate bladder function. Researchers know little about the CNS innervation of the lower urinary tract. Studies have focused mostly on the spinal cord and the brain stem pontine urination center. To explore the neural connections of the bladder and the CNS, Zermann et al. injected pseudorabies virus into the bladder trigone of rats. (For a description of the trigone, see section below titled "Influence of Adrenergic Receptor Type on Bladder Function.") They described the virus as a self-amplifying and transneuronal tracer. Upon immunostaining for the virus, they learned the CNS centers are directly connected to the bladder. Spinal centers connected to the bladder included the intermediolateral cell column, the central autonomic nucleus, and the nucleus intercalatus at the spinal cord levels T12-L2 and L6-S2. Brain stem and brain centers connected to the bladder included the raphe pallidus et magnus, the A5 noradrenergic area, the pontine micturition center, the locus ceruleus, the periaquaductal gray, the nucleus para- et periventricularis of the hypothalamus, the red nucleus, the medial preoptic area, and the cortex. Zermann et al. concluded, "Lower urinary tract function is a complex multilevel and multineuronal interaction. It involves facilitation and inhibition at many levels of the CNS."[53]

Brain stem and brain neurons enable the individual to volitionally control urination, partly through voluntary control of the external bladder sphincter. Skeletal muscle motor nerves that reach the sphincter through the pudendal nerve control the voluntary skeletal muscle of the sphincter. The individual can prevent urination by contracting the sphincter even when the bladder, which is under involuntary control, is attempting to empty.[25,p.352]

Table 3.21.1. Urinary abnormalities in fibromyalgia and hypothyroid patients.

SYMPTOMS & URINARY FUNCTION	FIBROMYALGIA	HYPOTHYROIDISM
Vasopressin	Low-normal secretion in some (wider range than in controls)	Low-to-normal secretion & levels
Urgency	Some	Not known
Frequency	Some high	Some high
Nocturia	Not known (Some, if IC* patients included)	Some
Urine volume	Not known	Low, normal, or increased†
Urine dilution	Not known	Normal-to-impaired
Sodium excretion (during tests to provoke sodium conservation)	Not known	Increased

*IC: Intersititial cystitis
†Increases in volume are usually averted by renal vasoconstriction and reduced glomerular filtrate.

Parasympathetic Innervation. The preganglionic parasympathetic nerves that help regulate bladder function synapse on postganglionic parasympathetic nerves in the pelvic plexus of the lower abdomen. The postganglionic nerves release the neurotransmitter acetylcholine. Binding of the acetylcholine to muscarinic receptors (see Glossary) on the muscle cells of the bladder wall induces the cells to contract. During early filling of the bladder, parasympathetic nerves are inactive. Stretching of the bladder wall as urine accumulates initiates transmission of sensory signals from the bladder to the sacral spinal cord. After entering the spinal cord through the dorsal horns, these signals activate preganglionic parasympathetic neurons in the lateral horns. The neurons transmit signals to the pelvic ganglion where they synapse with and activate postganglionic parasympathetic nerves. The endings of the postganglionic nerves then release acetylcholine near the bladder wall. The acetylcholine binds to muscarinic receptors, inducing bladder wall contraction.

Sympathetic Innervation. During bladder filling, nerve impulses transmitted by sympathetic nerves from the spinal cord to the bladder induce the muscle lining of the bladder to relax. The sympathetic nerve impulses also inhibit transmission of parasympathetic impulses to the bladder. Low levels of bladder filling and distention initiate sensory signals that are transmitted to the spinal cord. After entering the dorsal horns of the cord, the signals activate preganglionic sympathetic nerves in the lateral horns. The sympathetic nerves transmit signals to the inferior mesenteric ganglion in the lower abdomen. In the ganglion, the impulses activate postganglionic sympathetic nerves. These nerves transmit impulses through postganglionic nerves to at least three sites: the bladder wall, the internal urethral sphincter, and the pelvic ganglion. The signals induce the endings of the sympathetic nerves to secrete norepinephrine at the sites. In the pelvic ganglion, the norepinephrine binds to α-adrenergic receptors. Binding to these receptors inhibits transmission of signals to the bladder through parasympathetic nerves. In the bladder wall, the norepinephrine binds to β-adrenergic receptors. The binding induces the muscle lining of the bladder to relax. Relaxation of the muscle lining increases the capacity of the bladder for filling. Binding of norepinephrine to β-adrenergic receptors also induces contraction of the internal urethral sphincter muscle, prohibiting the escape of urine from the bladder.

Skeletal Muscle Motor Innervation. During low level bladder filling and distention, sensory nerves transmit signals from the bladder to the spinal cord. The signals enter the dorsal horns of the cord and synapse with and activate somatic motor nerves in the ventral horns. The motor nerves transmit signals back to the bladder close to the external sphincter muscle. There, the nerve endings secrete acetylcholine. The acetylcholine binds to muscarinic receptors, thereby inducing contraction of the sphincter.

Inhibitory Brain Stem Innervation. With high levels of bladder filling and distention, brain stem neurons inhibit transmission of nerve signals to the bladder by both sympathetic and motor nerves. Inhi-

bition of the signals relieves the sympathetic nerve inhibition of parasympathetic nerves to the bladder. The resulting increased parasympathetic innervation of the bladder relaxes both the internal and external sphincters. The relaxation also allows the bladder to contract and expel the urine it holds.

Influence of Adrenergic Receptor Type on Bladder Function

Walden et al. studied the location of mRNAs and receptor binding sites for α_{1a}-, α_{1b}-, and α_{1d}-adrenergic receptor subtypes in the urinary bladder of rats, monkeys, and humans. They found only α_{1a}-adrenergic receptor subtype mRNA. All smooth muscle areas of the rat, monkey and human bladder contained α_{1a}-adrenergic receptor mRNA, and the bladder dome and base contained highest levels. In monkey bladder, more than 80% of the α_1-adrenergic receptors were the α_{1a}-adrenergic receptor subtype. The bladder dome, trigone, and base contained the receptor subtype. The epithelial lining of the bladder contained α_{1a}-adrenergic receptor mRNA, but α_{1a}-adrenergic receptors were not detectable. This finding suggests that genes of the epithelial cells transcribed the mRNA, but the mRNA was not translated into α_{1a}-adrenergic receptor proteins. Walden et al. concluded that α_{1a}-adrenergic receptors are the major subtype of adrenergic receptor in the smooth muscle of rat, monkey and human urinary bladder.[63]

Goepel et al. examined human and pig bladder neck and detrusor. (The bladder neck is the proximal portion of the urethra, the canal through which urine exits the body. The detrusor is the "body" or external longitudinal layer of the muscular coat of the bladder.) They found that these tissues are richly populated with α- and β-adrenergic receptors.[56] The order of abundance in human detrusor was β- > α_2- > α_1-. They found no major difference between the sexes or between the detrusor and bladder neck. α_2-Adrenergic receptors in all tissues were homogeneously of the α_{2A}-subtype. β-Adrenergic receptors represented a mixed population with a dominance of the β_2-subtype in all tissues.

Binding of norepinephrine to β-adrenergic receptors induces relaxation of the detrusor.[2,p.144] The selective β_2-adrenergic receptor agonist clenbuterol reduced spontaneous contractile force of rabbit bladder dome, bladder base, and proximal urethra.[52] Activation of β_2-adrenergic receptors with clenbuterol also inhibited induction of contractions by acetylcholine and electrical stimulation. Clenbuterol and the nonselective β-adrenergic receptor agonist isoproterenol potentiated contraction of the external urethral sphincter. The investigators concluded that clenbuterol may be useful in treating urinary incontinence by inhibiting detrusor contractions and facilitating contraction of the external urethral sphincter.

α-Adrenergic receptors increase the contraction of the bladder smooth muscle.[49] In normal rats, subcutaneous apomorphine induced bladder muscle contractions. (Apomorphine is derived from morphine by removal of one molecule of water. When injected, it induces vomiting by affecting the CNS to induce contractions of the smooth muscle lining of the stomach.) The contractions of the bladder were attenuated or abolished by chemically blocking α_1-adrenergic receptors. Researchers induced the receptor block by administering α_1-adrenergic receptor blockers (indoramin and doxazosin) to the spinal cord (intrathecally) or into bladder arteries.[54] This finding suggests that α_1-adrenergic receptors facilitate bladder contractions at both the spinal and local bladder tissue levels.

Activation of α-adrenergic receptors induces contractions of the trigone. The trigone is a triangular area on the lower posterior wall of the bladder. At its lowermost apex at the bottom of the bladder is the bladder neck. Urine passes through the neck into the urethra to be excreted from the body. At the uppermost angles of the trigone, the two ureters transport urine into the bladder from the kidneys.[25,p.351] The lower ends of the ureters enter the bladder at the trigone, travel obliquely through the trigone, and pass several centimeters beneath the bladder epithelium before opening into the bladder.

Some researchers believe that as the bladder fills, the pressure within the bladder vesicle compresses the ureters beneath the epithelial lining. The compression presumably prevents back flow when pressure mounts during urination.[25,p.352] Roshani et al., for example, wrote that the junction of the ureters with the bladder (ureterovesical-junction) serves a protective role—prevention of reflux of urine from the bladder into the upper urinary tract (the ureters and kidneys). They wrote that the protective mechanism is necessary because the pressure of the upper urinary tract is low. If the junction did not prevent reflux, urine would flow back through the ureters and possibly harm the kidneys. To study the anatomy of the junction, they examined ten bladders from fresh cadavers (24-hours postmortem). The anatomical structures they observed suggested the protective role of peristaltic contractions of the ureters. Urine travels through the lumen of each ureter to the junction. According to the researchers, the ureter shortens due to peristaltic contractions. The

shortening causes discharge of the urine into the cavity of the bladder. Peristaltic contraction of the ureter also constricts it, thickening the constricted portion. The thickening compresses the lumen, and the compression decreases the caliber of the lumen, preventing upstream leakage through the ureter. Also, distal spread of peristaltic contractions of the ureter in the superficial portion of the trigone increases the length of the ureter beneath the bladder mucosa. The lengthening contributes to the prevention of reflux.[64]

Two years after the Roshani et al. study, in 1998, Shafik wrote that the exact function of the trigone in the act of urination is unknown. He studied the electrical activity of the muscles of the detrusor and trigone. Using 9 volunteers, he measured the EMG activity of the muscles and bladder pressure before and during filling and voiding. At rest, the detrusor and trigone largely had slow electrical waves, but bursts of action potentials followed regular wave frequency. The frequency and amplitude of the waves in the trigone were significantly lower than in other parts of the bladder. As the bladder filled, neither bladder pressure nor electrical waves of the trigone and detrusor differed from resting measures. During voiding, however, electrical activity of the detrusor increased, exhibiting fast activity spikes and high-amplitude action potentials. Electrical activity of the trigone, however, did not differ from the activity before voiding began. This finding suggests that the trigone does not contract during voiding. Shafik wrote that the finding refutes reports that during voiding the trigone contracts to prevent reflux of urine into the ureters.[65]

Despite the finding of Shafik, α_{1a}-adrenergic receptors occupy cells of the trigone, and activation of the receptors induces contractions of the trigone. Rather than preventing reflux, trigone contractions may facilitate contractions of the detrusor in expelling urine from the bladder.

Effects of α-Adrenergic Receptor Dominance on Bladder Function. Inadequate thyroid hormone regulation of transcription of the adrenergic genes in bladder muscle cells presumably increases the ratio of α- to β-adrenergic receptors on the cell membranes. As in most other tissues, the increase establishes α-adrenergic receptor dominance on the cell membranes. α-Adrenergic dominance would increase tension of the detrusor and cause contractions of the trigone. Binding of norepinephrine to β_2-adrenergic receptors induces contraction of the internal urethral sphincter muscle,[52] prohibiting the escape of urine from the bladder. A decrease in β-adrenergic receptors (due to inadequate thyroid hormone regulation of the β-adrenergic genes) would relax the internal sphincter, permitting easier release of urine.

In fibromyalgia patients who have inadequate thyroid hormone transcription regulation of their adrenergic genes, increased tone of the detrusor, contractions of the trigone, and relaxation of the internal bladder sphincter could alone account for urinary urgency and frequency. High tone of the detrusor and contractions of the trigone would cause lower capacity for expansion during filling of the bladder. The lower expansion would lower the threshold for bladder-emptying. Relaxation of the internal sphincter would provide subnormal resistance to emptying. This mechanism of increased α-adrenergic receptors and increased β-adrenergic receptors fits the concept that urgency, without increased urine volume, represents decreased bladder capacity for expansion. This corresponds to a finding in interstitial cystitis patients, some of whom have fibromyalgia: uninhibited detrusor contractions were positively correlated with symptoms of urgency.[44] With lower bladder capacity, patients would have lower urine volumes at the first sensation to void.

Urination Reflex is Mediated by α₁-Adrenergic Receptors. During low levels of bladder filling and distention, sensory signals from the bladder synaptically activate skeletal muscle (alpha) motor nerves in the ventral horns of the spinal cord. The motor neurons transmit signals to the external bladder sphincter muscle. The signals cause the motor nerve endings to secrete acetylcholine. Upon binding to muscurenic receptors on sphincter muscle cell membranes, the acetylcholine induces contraction of the sphincter. The contraction blocks voiding of urine.

With high levels of bladder distention, sensory signals travel from the bladder to the CNS and initiate the urination reflex. The reflex involves activation of supraspinal efferent neurons. The descending efferent signals inhibit transmission of sympathetic impulses from the spinal cord to the bladder. The inhibition reverses the bladder relaxation induced by sympathetic nerve stimulation, permitting the bladder walls to contract.

The supraspinal efferent neurons also inhibit transmission of skeletal muscle motor nerve impulses from the spinal cord to the bladder. Inhibition of the motor impulses allows the external sphincter muscle to relax so that urine can descend through the urethra and escape from the body.

The supraspinal efferent signals also block sympathetic nerve inhibition of parasympathetic nerves to the bladder. The increase in parasympathetic nerve activity relaxes both the internal and external sphincters.

It also induces contraction of the bladder, inducing urination.[60,pp.773-774]

Spinal α₁-adrenergic receptors facilitate nerve transmission in the supraspinal efferent pathway. Ishizuka et al. conducted a study that showed the influence of α₁-adrenergic receptor activation in the spinal cord. They noted that bladder activity (contractions of the walls and relaxation of the sphincters) was stimulated by filling of the bladder with enough urine to distend the bladder walls. The bladder filling set off the urination reflex mediated by the supraspinal neurons. Two experimental procedures also stimulated bladder activity: (1) administering L-dopa to the spinal cord (intrathecally) and into bladder arteries, and (2) applying capsaicin (a cayenne pepper-like stimulant) to the inside of the bladder to irritate it. The investigators measured changes in bladder activity under each of the two stimulatory influences during spinal α₁-adrenergic receptor blockade. In short, their findings showed that blockade of α₁-adrenergic receptors decreased bladder activity (see Table 3.21.2). This shows that increased bladder activity is mediated by α₁-adrenergic receptors at the supraspinal level.[55]

When the researchers administered an α₁-adrenergic receptor blocker (indoramin) to the spinal cord and into bladder arteries, three changes were found: (1) an increase in bladder capacity, (2) and increase in the volume of urine in the bladder, and (3) a decrease in the pressure of urine in the bladder. One of 10 rats had dribbling incontinence due to urinary retention. These three changes suggest that blocking α₁-adrenergic receptors intrathecally and through bladder arteries decreases the bladder activity associated with urination.[55]

Ishizuka and colleagues also found that blocking α₁-adrenergic receptors by administering the blocker to the spinal cord attenuated bladder hyperactivity normally stimulated by administering L-dopa. These effects were similar to previous reports of the use of another α₁-adrenergic receptor blocker, doxazosin. In addition, when investigators applied the irritant capsaicin to the inside of the bladder, bladder activity increased. But when they administered the α₁-adrenergic receptor blocker to the spinal cord, the capsaisin-stimulated activity decreased. It is interesting that administering the α₁-adrenergic receptor blocker into bladder arteries *did not* reduce *capsaicin-stimulated* bladder activity. But administering the other α₁-adrenergic receptor blocker, doxazosin, into arteries moderately attenuated the capsaicin-stimulated activity.[55]

The researchers concluded that bladder filling triggers the supraspinal urination reflex, and the reflex is mediated in part by spinal α_1-adrenergic receptors. L-dopa stimulated bladder activity through a descending pathway. Transmission in the pathway, again, is partly mediated by spinal α_1-adrenergic receptors. Moreover, bladder hyperactivity evoked by applying capsaicin to the inside of the bladder elicits a vesicospinal-vesical reflex. α_1-Adrenergic receptors are less involved in this reflex than they are in the supraspinal voiding pathway and reflex. Nevertheless, blocking α_1-adrenergic receptors with one antagonist, doxazosin, decreased bladder activity stimulated by the local bladder irritant.[55]

The implication of this study is that if inadequate thyroid hormone regulation of the adrenergic receptor genes increases the density of α_1-adrenergic receptors in the spinal cord, brain stem, and in the tissues of the bladder, we can expect increased bladder activity associated with urination. The changes we would expect are (1) contraction of the bladder walls with decreased bladder capacity, (2) an increase in urine pressure in the bladder, and (3) decreases in the volume of urine in the bladder and of voided urine (see Table 3.21.2).

Incontinence in Women with Decreased α_1-Adrenergic Receptor Mediation of Bladder Function. "Outflow incontinence" or "overflow dribbling" is the opposite of urgency and frequency. The patient does not urinate at intervals but has urine dribbling. The dribbling is especially intense during stresses that compress the bladder by increasing abdominal pressure. Outflow incontinence occurs under several conditions. One is destruction of the sensory nerve fibers from the bladder to the spinal cord. Without intact sensory nerves, stretching of the bladder walls during filling does not trigger the urination reflex that is mediated by supraspinal neurons. Despite intact efferent fibers from the spinal cord to the bladder, the patient loses bladder control. The bladder does not empty at intervals but fills to capacity and overflows a few drops at a time into the urethra. This phenomenon was common among patients with syphilis. The infecting organism, Treponema pallidum, caused fibrosis of the dorsal nerve root fibers. The fibrosis causes constriction of the fibers, impeding their ability to transmit impulses into the dorsal horns of the spinal cord. Another cause of incontinence is injuries that crush the sacral spinal cord.[25,p.353]

Whereas an increase in α-adrenergic receptors may result in urgency and frequency, a decrease in α-adrenergic receptors or chemical blocking of them may cause incontinence. This phenomenon is illustrated by the results of a study by Dwyer and Teele. Clinicians use the α_1-adrenergic receptor blocker prazosin

as an antihypertensive drug. The drug is effective for this purpose because it relaxes smooth muscle and lowers peripheral vascular resistance. It also relaxes the smooth muscle of the urethra. Dwyer and Teele reported that of 1335 women with urinary incontinence and other urinary symptoms, 58 (4.3%) were taking prazosin. Of the 58 women taking prazosin, 45 (78%) had incontinence, and 50 women (86.2%) had "stress incontinence." (Stress incontinence is the inability to prevent escape of urine during stresses such as lifting, coughing, laughing, or sudden movement.) Only 65.7% of women not taking the drug had stress incontinence. Upon stopping use of the drug, 25 of the women had improvement or complete cessation of incontinence. More than 50% of the women had undergone surgeries intended to remedy their urinary symptoms. Withdrawal from prazosin increased functional urethral length, maximum urethral closure pressure, and abdominal pressure transmission.[51]

Bladder Capacity: Decreased by α_2-Adrenergic Receptor Agonists and Increased by α_2-Adrenergic Receptor Blockers. Ishizuka et al. studied the effects of α_2-adrenergic receptor agonists and antagonists on bladder activity in rats. They evaluated the effects with continuous cystometry. When the researchers administered a selective α_2-adrenergic receptor agonist (dexmedetomidine) to the spinal cord, all rats developed a complete inability to retain urine. The rats had extreme decreases in bladder capacity, urine pressure, volume of voided urine, and residual volume of urine in the bladder. When the researchers administered the α_2-adrenergic receptor agonist near the bladder, the effects were the same as when they administered it to the spinal cord: decreased bladder capacity, urine pressure, volume of voided urine, and residual urine in the bladder.[47] These results are consistent with the presumed effects of a predominance of α_2-adrenergic receptors in the spinal cord or the bladder due to inadequate thyroid hormone regulation of the α-adrenergic genes: increased bladder activity that favors urgency and frequency. The effects of the α_2-adrenergic receptor agonist were counteracted by administrating a selective α_2-adrenergic receptor blocker (atipamezole) to the spinal cord.

When the researchers administered the atipamezole to the spinal cord, changes included (1) increased bladder capacity, (2) urine pressure, (3) decreased volume of voided urine, and (4) increased residual urine in the bladder. They found similar changes when they administered the blocker into bladder arteries. Another selective α_2-adrenergic receptor blocker (rauwolscine) had effects similar to those of atipamezole.

From their overall results using agonists and blockers, Ishizuka et al. concluded that activated α_2-adrenergic receptors in the spine and bladder regulate urination in normal conscious rats (see Table 3.21.2). The activated receptors do this by increasing bladder activity associated with urination.[47]

Sympathetic and Parasympathetic Innervation of the Kidneys, Ureters, and Bladder

Normal Physiology. Sympathetic nerves innervate the afferent arterioles of the kidneys which transport blood to the glomeruli. The nerves also innervate the kidneys' efferent arterioles. The efferent arterioles transport blood that has already passed through the glomeruli to the capillary network that supplies the tubules. The capillaries allow exchange of substances between the blood and the tubules. Eventually, the efferent vessels loop back to and empty into the veins in the kidney cortices. The sympathetic nerves also innervate the cells of the kidney tubules.[25,p.287]

A decrease in blood pressure and a decrease in the fluid volume outside the cells of the body (extracellular fluid) activate the sympathetic nerves to the kidneys. Activation of the nerves causes the kidneys' afferent arterioles to constrict. The constriction decreases blood flow to the glomeruli and reduces the glomerular filtration rate. As a result, a reduced amount of water passes from the blood to the kidney tubules.

Decreased extracellular and plasma volume decreases blood flow and pressure in the kidneys' arteries. In response to the reduced blood flow and pressure, the juxtaglomerular cells of the afferent and efferent kidney arterioles release renin into the peripheral circulation. Release of renin leads to production of angiotensin II. Angiotensin II induces constriction of the kidney afferent arterioles. (See section above titled "Kidney Vasoconstriction Induced by Increased Renin Secretion.")

Vasoconstriction Mediated by α-Adrenergic Receptors, Mainly the α_1-Adrenergic Receptor Subtype. Sympathetic nerve activity and renin release cause the vessels of kidney and general circulation to constrict. As a result, plasma and extracellular fluid volume increase. The vasoconstriction is mediated mainly by α-adrenergic receptors.[27,p.453]

Kurooka et al. studied the quantity and distribution of α_1-adrenergic receptor subtype mRNA in human kidney cortex. They took specimens of kidney cortex tissue from 46 human patients during radical surgical excision of a kidney (nephrectomy) or total removal of a kidney and its ureter (nephroureterectomy). (The patients, who ranged in age from 59.0-to-14.7 years, had kidney cell carcinoma or a tumor in a kidney, the pelvis, or a ureter.) All arteries of the cortex expressed α_1-adrenergic receptor mRNAs for subtypes α_{1A}-, α_{1B}-, and α_{1D}-. The predominant mRNA was that of subtype α_{1A}. α_1-Adrenergic receptor subtype mRNAs were particularly predominant in the smooth muscle of artery walls. All three subtypes were weakly present in the endothelium of the glomeruli but could not be detected in the veins. The researchers concluded that most α_1-adrenergic receptors in the kidney cortex are in the arteries. They noted that no one knows what different cellular effects are mediated by activation of the different receptor subtypes.[66]

Numabe et al. studied the prolonged effects of α_1-adrenergic receptor blockade on the hemodynamics of the kidney. They administered a selective α_1-adrenergic receptor blocker (terazosin) to normal and spontaneously hypertensive rats. The blocker reduced resistance in arterioles, and it reduced the mean pressure of kidney arteries in spontaneously hypertensive rats. These results suggest that activation of α_1-adrenergic receptors increases resistance in arterioles and increases the mean pressure of kidney arteries.[57]

Edwards and Trizna studied postsynaptic α-adrenergic receptors in afferent and efferent arterioles in rabbit kidney cortex. They found that selective α_1-adrenergic receptor agonists induced vasoconstriction with a potency equal to that of norepinephrine. α_2-Adrenergic receptor agonists either did not induce vasoconstriction or induced constriction that was only 60% of that induced by norepinephrine or the α_1-adrenergic receptor agonists. They concluded that α-adrenergic receptors mediate vasoconstriction in the arterioles of the glomeruli, and the receptors are exclusively of the α_1-adrenergic receptor subtype.[67]

Effects of α-Adrenergic Receptor Predominance in Hypothyroidism: Differences Based on Putative Selective Tissue Involvement. In some patients with inadequate thyroid hormone regulation of the adrenergic genes, the blood vessels of the kidneys are most affected—the resulting predominance of α-adrenergic receptors on the vessels is more extreme than in other tissues. In these patients, secretion of minimal amounts of norepinephrine by sympathetic nerve endings will induce intense vasoconstriction.

In other patients, inadequate thyroid hormone regulation of the adrenergic genes most affects neural cells of the brain stem, brain, and sympathetic ganglia that regulate sympathetic nervous system drive—that is, the resulting predominance of α-adrenergic receptors on these cells is more extreme than on those of other tissues. As a result, exposure of the cells to minimal amounts of norepinephrine will inhibit neural output from the cells. The inhibition will result in sub-normal sympathetic drive.

The kidney blood vessels and the sympathetic nervous system regulating cells may both have an increased density of α-adrenergic receptors, but the increase is likely to be greater in one or the other. The effects on the kidney-bladder axis will be determined by whether the vessels or neural cells have the greater increased density of α-adrenergic receptors. The net effect on the axis, based on the intensity of involvement of the vessels and neural cells, will vary among patients. Below, I consider the effects of the exclusive involvement of each.

Predominance of α-Adrenergic Receptors on Kidney Arteries and Arterioles. In the patient with a selectively high expression of α-adrenergic receptors in the kidney arteries and arterioles, binding of the receptors to norepinephrine will cause exaggerated sympathetically-induced vasoconstriction. This phenomenon may account in part for decreased water excretion in some hypothyroid patients (see sections above

titled "Urine Volume in Hypothyroidism: Reports of Decreased Urine Volume" and "Effects of α-Adrenergic Receptor Dominance on Bladder Function").

Predominance of α-Adrenergic Receptors on Cells that Regulate Sympathetic Drive. Subnormal sympathetic innervation of the kidneys will result in too little vasoconstriction during times when extracellular fluid and plasma volume are low. The patients would have urgency and frequency and low blood pressure, all of which are common in fibromyalgia. In patients with subnormal sympathetic drive due to inadequate thyroid hormone regulation of the adrenergic genes, parasympathetic activity is likely to be relatively increased. For example, administering α_1- and α_2-adrenergic receptor agonists at the spinal level has a strong sympathetic blocking effect,[50] and the sympathetic blockade results in a relative increase in parasympathetic activity (see Chapter 3.1). Increased parasympathetic innervation of the ureters increases their peristaltic contraction, increasing their transport to the bladder. Thus, the combined effect of a decrease in sympathetic innervation of the kidney-bladder axis and an increase in parasympathetic innervation favors urgency and frequency.

Table 3.21.2. Effects of spinal and ganglia level α_1- and α_2-adrenergic receptor antagonists and agonists.

TYPE OF α-ADRENERGIC RECEPTOR LIGAND	EFFECT ON BLADDER CAPACITY	BLADDER URINE PRESSURE	VOLUME OF URINE IN THE BLADDER	VOLUME OF VOIDED URINE
ANTAGONIST	Increase	Decrease	Increase	Increase
AGONIST	Decrease	Increase	Decrease	Decrease

INTERSTITIAL CYSTITIS

Researchers state that they have not determined etiology and pathogenesis of interstitial cystitis. Interstitial cystitis is presently a diagnosis of exclusion—the clinician decides upon it by ruling out other disorders that cause similar symptoms. Recommended treatments for patients with severe, intractable symptoms include the use of transcutaneous electrical nerve stimulation units, medications such as opioids, and as a last resort, surgery to form a urinary diversion.[45]

Some researchers consider interstitial cystitis a syndrome rather than a specific disease of the bladder.[46] The similarities between the symptoms and signs of fibromyalgia and interstitial cystitis[40] raise

the possibility that the two conditions share the same pathophysiology. In some patients, inadequate thyroid hormone regulation of cell function may be the underlying cause of interstitial cystitis. Through a predominant selective involvement of the bladder tissues, interstitial cystitis may constitute a different clinical phenotype from fibromyalgia. The most chronic and intense features of this putative phenotype would involve pelvic pain, urinary urgency and frequency, and increased nighttime urination (nocturia).[42] Chronic hypertonicity of the detrusor and trigone of the bladder tissue, due to a shift toward α-adrenergic dominance, may induce pathophysiological changes that lead to symptoms of interstitial cystitis. Results of a study by Kirkemo et al. suggest this possibility. They found that

56 of 384 interstitial cystitis patients (14.6%) had un-inhibited detrusor contractions; the contractions were positively correlated with symptoms of urgency.[44] Inadequate thyroid hormone regulation of the kidney-bladder axis can account for the lowered bladder capacity and lower urine volumes at the first sensation to void in some interstitial cystitis patients. These symptoms would, of course, be more severe in patients with a Hunner's patch (a slow-to-heal ulcer of the bladder lining).[42] It is important to learn through cystoscopic examination whether the interstitial cystitis patient has a Hunner's patch so that proper treatment is begun.[43]

BRAIN INFLUENCES ON URGENCY

Goldstein suggested that lesions in the anterior cingulate gyrus may cause urinary urgency in chronic fatigue syndrome. He has frequently seen such lesions on PET scans, indicating metabolic impairment (PET is a measure of cell metabolism). He also wrote that SPECT scans often show decreased blood flow through the dorsolateral prefrontal region of the brain (SPECT is a measure of blood flow). He proposed that both these lesioned limbic areas may produce urinary urgency by affecting (through their descending fibers) the urination center in the ponto-mesencephalic tegmentum of the brain stem.[8,p.78]

Specific forebrain (and brain stem) areas are involved in the regulation of urination. When women withheld urine voiding, the blood flow decreased in the right anterior cingulate gyrus. Both the forebrain and brain stem urination sites were more active on the right than on the left side.[68] Another study involving PET, however, showed activation of the right anterior cingulate gyrus during sustained pelvic floor straining. Pelvic floor straining is an activity that might be involved in withholding urine voiding.[69]

Bladder emptying is subject to voluntary control involving brain activity. But the initiation of urination is an automatic supraspinal phenomenon called the urination (or micturition) reflex. Centers in the pons of the brain stem can both facilitate and inhibit the urination reflex. The cerebral cortex contains centers that mainly inhibit the reflex, but at times they facilitate it. Emptying of the bladder occurs primarily through the urination reflex, but the higher neural centers exercise final control.[7,p.462] Impaired metabolism of neurons in these centers (due to inadequate regulation by thyroid hormone) may reduce their normal inhibitory control of the urination reflex. The reduced inhibition might lower the threshold for the urination reflex and bladder emptying.

BIOMECHANICAL INFLUENCE ON URINARY URGENCY

The lower abdominal organs of a fibromyalgia patient with flexed posture may be drooping (visceroptosis) and compressed. The drooping and compression are especially likely if the patient's connective tissue tone is poor. Lax connective tissues may have underlain the excessively flexible joints of 65% of 210 fibromyalgia patients in one study, and the mitral value prolapse reported in some fibromyalgia patients (see Chapters 3.3 and 3.11).

Goldman speculated that both the hypermobility and mitral valve prolapse of some fibromyalgia patients are part of a more generalized connective tissue abnormality in these patients.[34] Klemp et al. did not find mitral valve prolapse in hypermobile ballet dancers,[35] but other researchers have found a high incidence of both mitral valve prolapse and joint hypermobility in the same patients.[36][37] Pelligrino et al. reported that 75% of fibromyalgia patients had mitral valve prolapse, and 33% had myxedematous degeneration (mucous connective tissue tumors).[38] These connective tissue abnormalities are impressively accounted for by two mechanisms: (1) inadequate thyroid hormone regulation of growth hormone and somatomedin C production, and (2) inadequate thyroid hormone regulation of the connective tissues (see Chapter 3.3).

The visceral peritoneum may not adequately support the abdominal organs of a patient who has generally lax connective tissues. (The peritoneum is a serous sac with a thin layer of connective tissue. It lines the abdominal cavity and covers most of the abdominal organs.) In addition, reduced muscle and fascial tone might allow the pelvic floor muscles to descend. The resulting descent of the abdominal viscera would compress and decrease the expansive capacity of the urinary bladder. Some parts of the walls of the compressed bladder, however, would expand and stretch. The stretching would activate stretch receptors, cause sensory signals to reach the spinal cord, and thereby initiate the urination reflex.[7,p.461]

Among my fibromyalgia patients with urgency and frequent urination, I recall only few who had extremely flexed postures or severely reduced connective tissue tone. These two factors may contribute to urgency and frequency in some patients, but my impression is that the percentage of patients is small.

Table 3.21.3. Factors related to inadequate thyroid hormone regulation that may increase or decrease the tendency toward urinary urgency and frequency in fibromyalgia.

EFFECTS ON THE TENDENCY TOWARD URGENCY AND FREQUENCY	
DECREASE	INCREASE
Vasopressin secretion	α_2-Adrenoceptor inhibition of kidney response to vasopressin Deficit of kidney vasopressin receptors
Hypotension-induced renin release	α_2-Adrenoceptor inhibition of renin release
Aldosterone secretion in response to low fluid volume and sodium levels	Suboptimal aldosterone release due to impaired HPA axis
Sympathetically-induced vasoconstriction in response to hypotension	Reduced vasoconstriction due to low sympathetic drive Hypertonicity of bladder detrusor due to low β-adrenoceptor density α_2-Adrenoceptor-induced hypertonicity and contractions of bladder detrusor Low threshold for urination reflex due to increased spinal α-adrenergic receptors
Normal rate of peristaltic waves of ureters	α_2-Adrenoceptor-induced parasympathetically-mediated increase in ureteral peristalsis

● MODEL FOR URINARY URGENCY AND FREQUENCY

A sense of urgency to urinate and frequent urination in some fibromyalgia patients may result from several possible mechanisms. Of minor importance as mechanisms are ptosis of the bladder and postural compression. Ptosis is a sinking of the bladder from its normal position in the lower abdominal cavity. The sinking results in compression of the bladder and a decrease in its capacity for filling. Bladder ptosis may result from lax connective tissue support. Postural compression may result from flexed posture, resulting in compression from abdominal contents above the bladder descending and applying pressure. The compression would result in a reduced capacity for filling.

Increased urinary frequency in fibromyalgia patients may also result in part from increased sensitivity to adenosine due to increases in G_i as a product of inadequate thyroid hormone regulation of cell function. (See Chapter 3.11, section titled "Anergy Due to an Augmented Inhibitory Effect of Adenosine in Hypothyroidism.")

Of more importance to urgency and frequency in fibromyalgia are two other potential mechanisms: (1) decreased sympathetic nervous system innervation of the kidney-ureter-bladder axis, and (2) an increase in α-adrenergic receptors and a decrease in β-adrenergic receptors involved in the regulation of urination.

DECREASED SYMPATHETIC DRIVE

When sympathetic innervation of the kidney arteries and arterioles is decreased, more water passes from the blood into the glomeruli and tubules. As a result, more water accumulates in the bladder as urine. Also, a concomitant relative increase in parasympathetic innervation would increase peristalsis of the ureters. The increased peristalsis would increase the amount of water transported from the kidneys to the bladder. This could cause more rapid filling of the bladder. A lower-level filling of the bladder would trigger sensory signals from the bladder to the spinal cord. Triggering of signals with lower level filling would result from a reduced capacity for filling caused by a shift toward α-adrenergic receptor dominance (see subsection immediately below). The sensory signals in response to stretching of the bladder would initiate the supraspinal urination reflex.

α-ADRENERGIC DOMINANCE

Several functional changes in the kidney-ureter-bladder axis due to a shift toward α-adrenergic receptor dominance would favor urinary urgency and frequency. The change in adrenergic receptor type is sufficient alone to account for urgency and frequency in some fibromyalgia patients.

First, at the level of the pituitary gland, the adrenergic shift could inhibit vasopression secretion, causing low-normal circulating levels. As a result, suboptimal amounts of vasopression may reach the kidneys. In the kidneys, the increase in α_2-adrenergic receptors could inhibit responsiveness of the collecting ducts to vasopressin. The receptors would do so by decreasing the density of vasopressin receptors on the kidney tubules. If the patient has deficient sympathetic drive, this would impede constriction of the kidney afferent arterioles. The impeded vasoconstriction would result in an increase in glomerular filtration and loss of water in the urine.

Even without the above effects, other effects of a shift toward α-adrenergic receptor dominance in the spine and bladder could effectively mediate urinary urgency and frequency in fibromyalgia. Sufficiently extreme α-adrenergic receptor dominance can cause urinary incontinence. We can view the incontinence as an extreme point on a continuum with urgency and frequency. Excessive α-adrenergic influence would cause hypertonicity of the bladder musculature. This would decrease the capacity of the bladder for filling, and it would lower the threshold for bladder emptying. The urination reflex mediated by the brain stem would also have a low threshold due to an increase in spinal and brain stem α-adrenergic receptors.

The increase in parasympathetic innervation of the ureters during α-adrenergic receptor dominance would increase peristalsis of the ureters. The increase in peristalsis would increase the transport of urine from the kidneys to the bladder. The increased transport would result in filling of the low-capacity bladder.

Urinary urgency and frequency would be the result of decreased sympathetic drive and a shift toward α-adrenergic receptor dominance due to inadequate thyroid hormone regulation of the kidney-bladder axis. Table 3.21.3 lists factors related to inadequate thyroid hormone regulation that may influence the tendency toward urinary urgency and frequency in fibromyalgia patients.

REFERENCES

1. *Merck Manual of Diagnosis and Therapy*, 16th edition. Edited by R. Berkow, A.J. Fletcher, and M.H. Beers, Rahway, Merck Research Laboratories, 1992.
2. Chusid, J.G.: *Correlative Neuroanatomy and Functional Neurology*, 6th edition. Los Altos, Lange Medical Publications, 1976.
3. Wolfe, F.: Diagnosis of fibromyalgia. *J. Musculoskel. Med.*, 7:53-69, 1990.
4. Stormorken, H. and Brosstad, F.: Fibromyalgia: family clustering and sensory urgency with early onset indicate genetic predisposition and thus a "true" disease. *Scand. J. Rheumatol.*, 21(4):207, 1992.
5. DeGroot, L.J., Larsen, P.R., Refetoff, S., and Stanbury, J.B.: *The Thyroid and Its Diseases,* 5th edition. New York, John Wiley & Sons, 1984.
6. Watanakunakorn, C., Hodges, R.E., and Evans, T.C.: Myxedema: a study of 400 cases. *Arch. Intern. Med.*, 116: 183-190, 1965.
7. Guyton, A.C.: *Textbook of Medical Physiology*, 7th edition. Philadelphia, W.B. Saunders Co., 1986.
8. Goldstein, J.A.: *Chronic Fatigue Syndrome: The Limbic Hypothesis*. New York, Haworth Medical Press, 1993.
9. Gellai, M. and Ruffolo, R.R., Jr.: Renal effects of selective α_1- and α_2-adrenoceptor agonists in conscious, normo-tensive rats. *J. Pharmacol. Exp. Ther.*, 240:723-728, 1987.
10. Roman, R.J., Cowley, A.W., Jr., and Lecherie, C.: Water diuretic and natriuretic effect of clonidine in the rat. *J. Pharmacol. Exp. Ther.*, 221:385-393, 1979.
11. Strandhoy, J.W., Morris, M., and Buckalew, V.M., Jr.: Renal effects of the antihypertensive, guanabenz, in the dog. *J. Pharmacol. Exp. Ther.*, 221:347-352, 1982.
12. Ali, M., Guillon, G., Cantau, B., Balestre, M.N., Chicot, D., and Clos, J.: A comparative study of plasma vasopressin levels and V1 and V2 vasopressin receptor properties in congenital hypothyroid rats under thyroxine or vasopressin therapy. *Horm. Metab. Res.*, 19:624-628, 1987.
13. Iwasaki, Y., Oisa, Y., Yamauchi, K., Takatsuki, K., Kondo, K., Hasegawa, H., and Tomita, A.: Osmoregulation of plasma vasopressin in myxedema. *J. Clin. Endocrinol. Metab.*, 70:534-539, 1990.
14. Skowsky, R.W. and Kikuchi, T.A.: The role of vasopressin in the impaired water excretion of myxedema. *Am. J. Med.*, 64:613, 1978.
15. Kleeman, C.R. and Mackovic-Basic, M.: The kidneys and electrolyte metabolism in hypothyroidism. In *Werner and*

Ingbar's The Thyroid: A Fundamental and Clinical Text, 6ᵗʰ edition. Edited by L.E. Braverman and R.D. Utiger, Philadelphia, J.B. Lippincott Co., 1991, pp.1009-1016.

16. Cooper, J.R., Bloom, F.E., and Roth, R.H.: *The Biochemical Basis of Neuropharmacology*, 6ᵗʰ edition. New York, Oxford University Press, 1991.

17. Vaamonde, C.A., Sebastienelli, M.J., Vaamonde, L.S., et al.: Impaired renal tubular reabsorption of sodium in hypothyroid man. *J. Lab. Clin. Med.*, 85(3):451, 1975.

18. Capasso, G., Giordano, D.R., Capodicasa, G., and De Santo, N.G.: The effect of atrial natriuretic factor on blood pressure and renal function of long-term hypothyroid rats. *Kidney Int.*, 24(Suppl.):S104, 1988.

19. Gay, R.G., Raya, T.E., Lancaster, L.D., Lee, R.W., Morkin, E., and Goldman, S.: Effects of thyroid state on venous compliance and left ventricular performance in rats. *Am. J. Physiol.*, 254:H81, 1988.

20. Streeten, D.H.P., Anderson, G.M., Howland, T., Chiang, R., and Smulyan, H.: Effect of thyroid function on blood pressure: recognition of hypothyroid hypertension. *Hypertension*, 11:78, 1988.

21. Bradley, S.E., Stephan, F., Coelho, J.B., and Reville, P.: The thyroid and the kidney. *Kidney*, 6:346, 1974.

22. Bilezikian, J.P.: Defining the role of adrenergic receptors in human physiology. In *Adrenergic Receptors in Man*. Edited by P.A. Insel, New York, Marcel Dekker, Inc., 1987, pp.37-67.

23. Ali, M., Guillon, G., Balestre, M.N., and Clos, J.: Effects of thyroid deficiency on the vasopressin receptors in the kidney of developing and adult rats. *Horm. Metab. Res.*, 19:115, 1987.

24. Kupfermann, I.: Hypothalamus and limbic system: peptidergic neurons, homeostasis, and emotional behavior. In *Principles of Neural Science*, 3ʳᵈ edition. Edited by E.R. Kandel, J.H. Schwartz, and T.M. Jessell, Norwalk, Appleton & Lange, pp.735-749.

25. Guyton, A.C.: *Textbook of Medical Physiology*, 8ᵗʰ edition. Philadelphia, W.B. Saunders Co., 1991.

26. Howard, R.L., Summer, S., Rossi, N., Kim, J.K., and Schrier, R.W.: Short-term hypothyroidism and vasopressin gene expression in the rat. *Amer. J. Kidney Dis.*, 19(6): 573-577, 1992.

27. Berne, R.M. and Levy, M.N.: *Principles of Physiology*. St. Louis, C.V. Mosby Co., 1990.

28. Andersen, L.F., Agner, T., Walter, S., and Hansen, J.M.: Micturition pattern in hyperthyroidism and hypothyroidism. *Urology*, 29(2):223-224, 1987.

29. Vargas, F., Baz, M.J., Luna, J.D., Andrade, J., Jodar, E., and Haro, J.M.: Urinary excretion of digoxin-like immunoreactive factor and arginine-vasopressin in hyper- and hypo-thyroid rats. *Clin. Sci.*, 81(4):471-476, 1991.

30. Ota, K., Kimura, T., Sakurada, T., et al.: Effects of an acute water load on plasma ANP and AVP, and renal water handling in hypothyroidism: comparison of before and after L-thyroxine treatment. *Endocrine J.*, 41(1):99-105, 1994.

31. Carter, D.A., Pardy, K., and Murphy, D.: Regulation of vasopressin gene expression: changes in the level, but not the size, of vasopressin mRNA following endocrine manipulations. *Cell. Mol. Neurobiol.*, 13(1):87-95, 1993.

32. Michael, U.F., Kelley, J., and Vaamonde, C.A.: Effects of aldosterone, methylprednisolone and triiodothyronine on the response to water loading in the conscious hypothyroid rat with diabetes insipidus. *Mineral Electrol. Metab.*, 10 (3):190-198, 1984.

33. Watabe, T., Tanaka, K., Kumagae, M., et al.: Role of endogenous arginine-vasopressin in potentiating corticotropin-releasing hormone-stimulated corticotropin secretion in man. *J. Clin. Endocrinol. Metab.*, 66(6):1132-1137, 1988.

34. Goldman, J.A.: Hypermobility and deconditioning: important links to fibromyalgia/fibrositis. *Southern Med. J.*, 84: 1192-1196, 1991.

35. Klemp, P., Stevens, J.E., and Isaacs, S.: A hypermobility study in ballet dancers. *J. Rheumatol.*, 11:692-696, 1984.

36. Pitcher, D. and Grahame, R.: Mitral valve prolapse and joint hypermobility: evidence for a systemic connective tissue abnormality? *Ann. Rheum. Dis.*, 41:352-354, 1982.

37. Grahame, R., Edwards, J.C., Pitcher, D., et al: A clinical and echocardiographic study of patients with the hypermobility syndrome. *Ann. Rheum. Dis.*, 40:541-546, 1981.

38. Pelligrino, M.J., Fossen, D.V., Gordon, C., et al: Prevalence of mitral valve prolapse in primary fibromyalgia: a pilot investigation. *Arch. Phys. Med. Rehabil.*, 70:541-543, 1989.

39. Gallo-Payet, N., Cote, M., Chorvatova, A., Guillon, G., and Payet, M.D.: Cyclic AMP-independent effects of ACTH on glomerulosa cells of the rat adrenal cortex. *J. Steroid Biochem. Mol. Biol.*, 69(1-6):335-342, 1999.

40. Clauw, D.J., Schmidt, M., Radulovic, D., Singer, A., Katz, P., and Bresette, J.: The relationship between fibromyalgia and interstitial cystitis. *J. Psychiat. Res.*, 31(1):125-131, 1997.

41. Crofford, L.J., Pillemer, S.R., Kalogeras, K.T., et al.: Hypothalamic-pituitary-adrenal axis perturbations in patients with fibromyalgia. *Arthritis Rheum.*, 37(11):1583-1592, 1994.

42. Nigro, D.A., Wein, A.J., Foy, M., et al.: Associations among cystoscopic and urodynamic findings for women enrolled in the Interstitial Cystitis Data Base (ICDB) Study. *Urology*, 49(5A Suppl):86-92, 1997.

43. Messing, E., Pauk, D., Schaeffer, A., et al.: Associations among cystoscopic findings and symptoms and physical examination findings in women enrolled in the Interstitial Cystitis Data Base (ICDB) Study. *Urology*, 49(5A Suppl): 81-85, 1997.

44. Kirkemo, A., Peabody, M., Diokno, A.C., et al.: Associations among urodynamic findings and symptoms in women enrolled in the Interstitial Cystitis Data Base (ICDB) Study. *Urology*, 49(5A Suppl):76-80, 1997.

45. Pontari, M.A., Hanno, P.M., and Wein, A.J.: Logical and systematic approach to the evaluation and management of patients suspected of having interstitial cystitis. *Urology*, 49(5A Suppl):114-120, 1997.

46. Haab, F. and Zimmern, P.: Interstitial cystitis: new concepts on etiology and diagnosis. *Progres. en Urologie*, 5 (5):653-660, 1995.

47. Ishizuka, O., Mattiasson, A., and Andersson, K.E.: Role of spinal and peripheral α_2 adrenoceptors in micturition in normal conscious rats. *J. Urology*, 156(5):1853-1857, 1996.

48. Chorvatova, A., Bilodeau, L., Chouinard, L., Gallo-Payet,

N., and Payet, M.D.: Characterization of an ACTH-induced chloride current in rat adrenal zona glomerulosa cells. *Endocr. Res.*, 25(2):173-178, 1999.

49. Maggi, C.A., Manzini, S., Grimaldi, G., Evangelista, S., and Meli, A.: High-cholesterol diet induces altered responsiveness of rabbit arterial smooth muscle to noradrenaline. *Pharmacol.*, 30(5):273-280, 1985.

50. Kooner, J.S., Birch, R., Frankel, H.L., Peart, W.S., and Mathias, C.J.: Hemodynamic and neurohormonal effects of clonidine in patients with preganglionic and postganglionic sympathetic lesions: evidence for a central sympatholytic action. *Circulation*, 84(1):75-83, 1991.

51. Dwyer, P.L. and Teele, J.S.: Prazosin: a neglected cause of genuine stress incontinence. *Obst. Gyn.*, 79(1):117-121, 1992.

52. Morita, T., Kihara, K., Nagamatsu, H., Oshima, H., and Kishimoto, T.: Effects of clenbuterol on rabbit vesico-urethral muscle contractility. *J. Smooth Muscle Res.*, 31 (4):119-127, 1995.

53. Zermann, D.H., Ishigooka, M., Doggweiler, R., and Schmidt, R.A.: Central autonomic innervation of the lower urinary tract: a neuroanatomy study. *World J. Urol.*, 16(6): 417-422, 1998.

54. Ishizuka, O., Mattiasson, A., Steers, W.D., and Andersson, K.E.: Effects of spinal α_1-adrenoceptor antagonism on bladder activity induced by apomorphine in conscious rats with and without bladder outlet obstruction. *Neurourol. Urodyn.*, 16(3):191-200, 1997.

55. Ishizuka, O., Pandita, R.K., Mattiasson, A., Steers, W.D., and Andersson, K.E.: Stimulation of bladder activity by volume, L-dopa and capsaicin in normal conscious rats—effects of spinal α_1-adrenoceptor blockade. *Naunyn-Schmiedebergs Arch. Pharmacol.*, 355(6):787-793, 1997.

56. Goepel, M., Wittmann, A., Rubben, H., and Michel, M.C.: Comparison of adrenoceptor subtype expression in porcine and human bladder and prostate. *Urological Res.*, 25(3): 199-206, 1997.

57. Numabe, A., Komatsu, K., and Frohlich, E.D.: Effects of ANG-converting enzyme and α_1-adrenoceptor inhibition on intrarenal hemodynamics in SHR. *Amer. J. Physiol.*, 266(5 Pt.2):R1437-R1442, 1994.

58. Ng, S.C.: The fibromyalgia syndrome. *Singapore Med. J.*, 33(3):294-295, 1992.

59. Bennett, R.M., Clark, S.R., Campbell, S.M., et al.: Symptoms of Raynaud's syndrome in patients with fibromyalgia. A study utilizing the Nielsen test, digital photoplethysmography and measurements of platelet α_2-adrenergic receptors. *Arthritis Rheum.*, 34(3):264-269, 1991.

60. Dodd, J. and Role, L.W.: The autonomic nervous system. In *Principles of Neural Science*, 3rd edition. Edited by E.R. Kandel, J.H. Schwartz, and T.M. Jessell, Norwalk, Appleton & Lange, 1991, pp.761-775.

61. Auriac, A., Azam, J., Dumas, J.C., Roux, G., and Montastruc, J.L.: Effects of clonidine on diuresis and water intake in normal and Brattleboro rats. *J. Pharmacol.*, 12(3): 277-288, 1981.

62. Demitrack, M.A. and Crofford, L.J.: Hypothalamic-pituitary-adrenal axis dysregulation in fibromyalgia and chronic fatigue syndrome: an overview and hypothesis. *J. Musculoskel. Pain*, 3(2):67-73, 1995.

63. Walden, P.D., Durkin, M.M., Lepor, H., Wetzel, J.M., Gluchowski, C., and Gustafson, E.L.: Localization of mRNA and receptor binding sites for the α_{1a}-adrenoceptor subtype in the rat, monkey and human urinary bladder and prostate. *J. Urol.*, 157(3):1032-1038, 1997.

64. Roshani, H., Dabhoiwala, N.F., Verbeek, F.J., and Lamers, W.H.: Functional anatomy of the human ureterovesical junction. *Anat. Rec.*, 245(4):645-651, 1996.

65. Shafik, A.: Role of the trigone in micturition. *J. Endourol.*, 12(3):273-277, 1998.

66. Kurooka, Y., Moriyama, N., Nasu, K., Kameyama, S., Fukasawa, R., Yano, J., and Kawabe, K.: Distribution of α_1-adrenoceptor subtype mRNAs in human renal cortex. *B.J.U. Int.*, 83(3):299-304, 1999.

67. Edwards, R.M. and Trizna, W.: Characterization of α-adrenoceptors on isolated rabbit renal arterioles. *Amer. J. Physiol.*, 254(2 Pt.2):F178-F183, 1988.

68. Blok, B.F., Sturms, L.M., and Holstege, G.: Brain activation during micturition in women. *Brain*, 121(Pt.11):2033-2042, 1998.

69. Blok, B.F., Sturms, L.M., and Holstege, G.: A PET study on cortical and subcortical control of pelvic floor musculature in women. *J. Comp. Neurol.*, 389(3):535-544, 1997.

Section IV

Diagnosis and Assessment

4.1

Diagnosis of Fibromyalgia and Evaluation of the Patient's Changing Status

A patient meets the American College of Rheumatology (ACR) diagnostic criteria for fibromyalgia when she has widespread pain of at least 3 months duration and 11 of 18 potential tender points. If the patient has associated symptoms typical of fibromyalgia, this supports the diagnosis. The appropriate ICD code is 729.0.

The patient should initially complete at least five measures of fibromyalgia status. The scores from the measures provide a baseline set against which subsequent sets scored during her metabolic rehabilitation can be compared. Changes in the scores through the course of treatment provide the clinician and patient with a record of the patient's changing fibromyalgia status. The five measures are (1) the mean pressure/pain threshold of tender points quantified by algometry, (2) pain distribution quantified by the percentage method, (3) symptom intensity quantified by visual analog scales, (4) depression assessed by a valid and reliable pencil and paper instrument such as Zung's Self-Rating Depression Scale or Beck's Depression Inventory, and (5) functional status measured by the Fibromyalgia Impact Questionnaire. Scores should be posted to line graphs so that the patient's changing status for each measure is obvious during visual in-spection, and in terms of the units peculiar to each measure.

For purposes of case management, the patient's scores on these tests are considered indices of tissue metabolic status: The worse the scores, the more extreme is the patient's hypometabolism. As the patient comes closer to eumetabolic status during treatment, her scores mirror her improvement. The objective is to bring the patient as close to eumetabolism as possible, as reflected in improved or normalized scores on the measures of fibromyalgia status. Clinical decisions, therefore, should be based on these scores and the changes in peripheral indices (see Chapter 4.3).

The clinician should differentiate fibromyalgia from other conditions whose features resemble those of fibromyalgia. These include chronic multi-muscle myofascial pain syndromes, myopathy, and polymyalgia rheumatica.

Fibromyalgia is diagnosed by a patient's report of widespread pain of at least 3 months duration and abnormal tenderness to pressure at a minimum of 11 of 18 potential tender point sites. The diagnosis is supported by the presence of symptoms that typically accompany fibromyalgia. At this time, the clinician should use the American College of Rheumatology (ACR) 1990 criteria for the diagnosis of fibromyalgia.[1] If the patient meets the criteria, this warrants use of the ICD code 729.0.

Table 4.1.1. American College of Rheumatology criteria for classifying patients as fibromyalgic.*

Criterion I. History (3 months) of widespread pain

Widespread pain means the patient meets three requirements:
1. She has pain on the right and left sides of her body (buttock *or* shoulder pain on one side of the body qualifies as pain on one side).
2. She has pain above and below the waist (low back pain qualifies as lower body pain).
3. She has axial skeletal pain. This means she must have: (a) cervical pain *or* (b) low back pain *or* (c) either thoracic spinal pain or anterior chest pain.

A patient meets this criterion, for example, when she has low back pain (axial pain), right gluteal pain (right-sided lower body pain), and left shoulder pain (left-sided upper body pain).[1,p.163]

Criterion II. Pain at 11 of 18 tender point sites upon digital palpation (Figure 4.1.1 shows the 18 tender point sites)

During digital palpation, the clinician should apply about 4 kg of pressure with the pulp of the thumb or the first two or three fingers. [Preferably, the clinician should use an algometer.] For a tender point to be considered "painful," the patient must state that the palpation is painful. "Tender" is not to be considered "painful."[1,p.171] The patient must have pain in at least 11 of the following 18 tender point sites:

1. *Occiput:* bilaterally, at the suboccipital muscle insertion.
2. *Lower cervical:* bilaterally, at the anterior aspects of the intertransverse spaces of C5-to-C7.†
3. *Trapezius:* bilaterally, at the midpoint of the upper border or crest.
4. *Supraspinatus:* bilaterally, at the origins (above the spine of the scapula near its medial border).
5. *Second rib:* bilaterally, at the second costochondral junction (on the anterior chest wall, on the upper surfaces, about 2 cm lateral to the junctions at the sternum).
6. *Lateral epicondyle:* bilaterally, 2 cm distal to the epicondyles.
7. *Gluteal:* bilaterally, in the upper outer quadrants of the buttocks in the anterior folds of the gluteal muscle.
8. *Greater trochanter:* bilaterally, about 2 cm posterior to the trochanteric prominence.
9. *Knee:* bilaterally, at the medial fat pad proximal to (about 2 cm above) the joint line.

* Wolfe, F., Smythe, H.A., Yunus, M.B., et al.: The American College of Rheumatology 1990 criteria for the classification of fibromyalgia: report of the multicenter criteria committee. *Arthritis Rheumatol.*, 33: 160-172, 1990.[1]

† I recommend that the lower cervical tender points be excluded from the tender point examination. These points are excruciatingly tender in many fibromyalgia patients, so much so that the patients report tenderness before the needle on the dial of the algometer registers 0.10 kg/cm². Also, in many stout patients with thick necks, it is difficult to locate the correct site even with a finger or thumb.

The ACR criteria, while useful for diagnosis, are severely limited for measuring changes in fibromyalgia status. Because of this, assessing changes in fibromyalgia status during treatment requires the use of methods that quantify a patient's status in a graded fashion.

The need for modifications of the ACR approach has been recognized by others. Bennett wrote in 1994, "Criteria for poorly defined diseases are not set in stone and it is already apparent that the 1990 ACR criteria [for diagnosing and assessing fibromyalgia] will need to be revised."[64] Littlejohn wrote in 1995, "New instruments to assess aspects of fibromyalgia are appearing all the time, and one needs to remain flexible in his choice of assessing instruments."[57]

The methods I describe below are modifications of the ACR criteria. They are more definitive and permit mathematical grading of a patient's status. I have found it necessary to develop and refine these methods for research purposes. Without them, it would be difficult to meaningfully evaluate treatment effects in studies of metabolic therapy (see Table 4.1.6). Of more concern to most readers, however, is the fact that these methods are immensely valuable in clinical practice. They enable the clinician to precisely assess the impact of metabolic therapy on a patient's fibromyalgia status. *Precise assessment provides the information necessary to make intelligent clinical decisions that maximize the patient's chances of recovery.*

These methods for grading changes in fibromyalgia status during therapy are as useful as measuring the Achilles reflex, resting pulse rate, or serum cholesterol. In most patients, the measures of fibromyalgia status can serve as indirect measures of tissue metabolism. As methods for quantitatively assessing patient status, they are all likely to remain useful to the clinician. It is my belief, though, that *as diagnostic criteria*, use of the ACR method and the more quantitative methods I describe will be short-lived.

The reason for this is simple: To say that a patient meets the diagnostic criteria for fibromyalgia is merely to say that she exhibits indirectly measurable manifestations of tissue hypometabolism. Other indirectly measurable manifestations of hypometabolism, such as hyperlipidemia,[29] mononeuropathies,[30] and endogenous depression,[31] lead to other diagnoses. But all these manifestations, resulting in different diagnoses, are bands of a spectrum emanating from the same pathophysiological source. It is likely that the features of hypometabolism we term fibromyalgia arise, as the other diagnostic categories do, from inadequate thyroid hormone regulation of gene transcription. If the weight of evidence comes to show this is true, then patients with the clinical features of fibromyalgia will be tested for mechanisms of inadequate thyroid hormone transcription regulation. Appropriate methods may include thyroid function tests, rapid gene sequencing to identify mutations of the β- and/or α-thyroid hormone receptor genes, and laboratory techniques for identifying thyroid hormone receptors competitively bound by chemicals with a higher receptor affinity than T_3. A diagnosis will be made on the basis of a demonstrable pathophysiology, and at that time, diagnostic criteria for fibromyalgia will no longer be needed. But for the present, we are constrained to use a combination of the ACR criteria (Table 4.1.1) and the modified methods I describe in this chapter.

● AMERICAN COLLEGE OF RHEUMATOLOGY 1990 CRITERIA FOR THE DIAGNOSIS OF FIBROMYALGIA

Publication of the ACR 1990 criteria for the diagnosis of fibromyalgia[1] provided a method, agreed upon by researchers, for deciding whether a patient has the condition. The ACR criteria (Table 4.1.1) provide a rationale for use of the ICD code 729.0 for fibromyalgia patients.

A MAJOR LIMITATION OF THE ACR CRITERIA

The development of the ACR criteria for diagnosing fibromyalgia was a boon to both fibromyalgia patients and their clinicians. Despite the benefits, however, the ACR criteria have at least one major limitation. Yunus wrote, "In clinical practice, not all patients will have 11 tender points or widespread pain . . . but may have otherwise characteristic fibromyalgia features. These patients may be diagnosed as having fibromyalgia for the practical purpose of case management."[23,p.12] This is advice, from one of the ACR committee members who established the criteria, *not* to adhere firmly to those criteria. The advice is necessary if many patients with lesser degrees of fibromyalgia are to receive the diagnosis. But clearly, if the criteria exclude some patients who have fibromyalgia, then they fail to serve their intended purpose—to sensitive-

ly and specifically distinguish patients with fibromyalgia from patients with other conditions that resemble fibromyalgia.

The main problem with the ACR criteria is that they constitute what in statistics is termed "discontinuous" variables. That is, the criteria are either/or; they are questions requiring a yes or no answer. If a patient with 11 of 18 tender points also has widespread pain according to the ACR criteria, then she has fibromyalgia. If she does not have widespread pain, she does not meet the criteria. At that point, strictly speaking, the possibility of her having fibromyalgia discontinues. She does or she does not have it. No shades of grey. And it is the same with the ACR tender point criterion. Fewer than 11 of 18 potential tender points and, again strictly speaking, the patient does not have fibromyalgia.

Using discontinuous variables to define the condition is incongruous with the "continuous" nature of fibromyalgia—the condition continues through a range from nonexistent to extremely severe, with all degrees in between. Measuring fibromyalgia with discontinuous criteria is like measuring the gasoline in a car's tank with a gauge that registers only yes or no. As a solution to this limitation, I converted the ACR criteria into "continuous" variables that can show quantified differences in intensity of each measure.

● MODIFICATIONS OF THE ACR CRITERIA IN ORDER TO ASSESS CHANGING FIBROMYALGIA STATUS

I use five measures to assess initial fibromyalgia status and changes in status during treatment: algometer measurements of tender points, pain distribution drawings, symptom intensity surveys using visual analog scales (FibroQuest questionnaires), the Fibromyalgia Impact Questionnaire (FIQ), and Zung's Self-Rating Depression Scale (Zung's).

MODIFICATIONS OF THREE FIBROMYALGIA MEASURES

In line with the effort to improve fibromyalgia assessment, I have modified three of the five standard assessment methods. The modifications enable greater precision at quantifying changes in patient status.

Modification 1: Algometry to Assess Tender Point Sensitivity

Tender point assessment according to the ACR entails applying 4 kg of pressure with a finger to 18 potential tender point sites. The patient meets the tender point criterion if she reports tenderness upon pressure at 11 or more of the 18 tender points.[1] Fischer demonstrated, however, that of 24 physicians experienced at diagnosing fibromyalgia by performing tender point exams, most could not reliably subjectively gauge 4 kg of pressure. Fischer stabilized an algometer to a holding stand. More than 90% (>22) of the physicians, when not observing the dial of the algometer, were not able to determine when they were applying 4 kg of pressure. When they were observing the dial, 62.5% (15) of the physicians believed that 4 kg of pressure was either too little or too much force to accurately identify fibromyalgia tender points. Fischer concluded that reliably diagnosing fibromyalgia by a tender point exam requires quantification of pressure by algometry.[60]

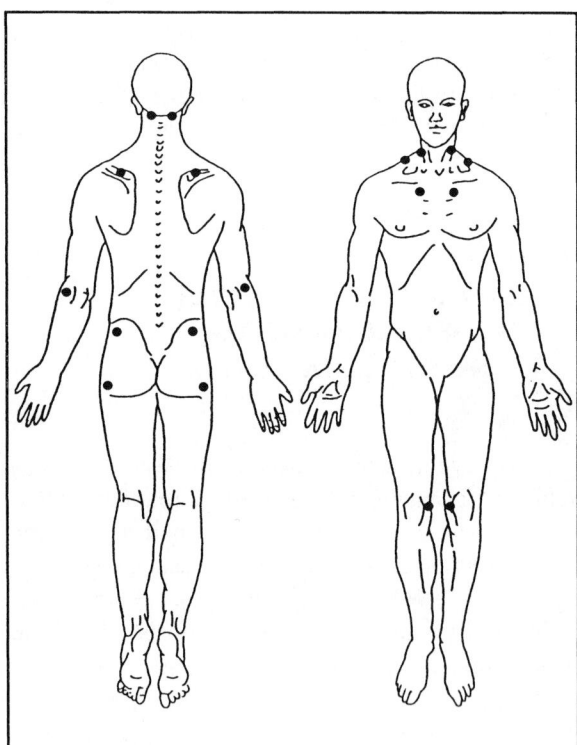

Figure 4.1.1. The 18 tender point sites specified in the ACR criteria.

Another study supports the value of algometry over manual palpation in differentiating degrees of tender point sensitivity.[79] The study involved 152 patients who had either rheumatoid arthritis, psoriatic arthritis, or HIV infection. In 102 patients, 842 anatomical sites were scored as having 0 (zero) tenderness when tested by manual palpation. But examination with algometry revealed widely different thresholds of tenderness. Variations in tenderness were significantly associated with sex and diagnosis.

The ACR criterion for the presence of tender points is an all-or-none requirement. By contrast, algometry makes possible precise quantification of tender point sensitivity and comparison of numerical differences on different exam dates. The algometer reliably measures the sensitivity of fibromyalgia tender points,[60][61] and its measurements correlate well with pain distribution reported by patients on body drawings.[19]

Modification 2: Percentage Method of Pain Distribution

The ACR diagnostic criterion of widespread pain is also an all-or-none requirement: either the patient meets the criterion (having pain above and below the waist, on the right and left sides of the body, and over an axial area) or not. My colleagues and I have quantified the ACR method, grading the patient's status by the number of the ACR's four stipulations she meets. This permits a pain distribution score of one-to-four units (0-1-2-3). According to this modified method, if the patient has pain above and below her waist, on the right and left sides of her body, and over an axial area, her pain distribution score is 3. If she has pain above and below her waist, on the right and left sides of her body, but no axial pain, her score is 2. If she has pain above and below her waist and on the right side of her body, but not on her left side or over an axial area, her score is 1. If she has no pain, or no pain other than regional pain related to a local structural or functional lesion, her score is 0 (zero).

We also use an alternate method that is far more definitive, adapted from the "rule of nines" for adult burn victims. (The rule of nines method gives a value for the percentage of body surface burned.[58][59]) This method was recommended to me by nurse practitioner Mervianna Thompson, and has been a boon to precision in documenting therapeutic changes in fibromyalgia pain distribution. My colleagues and I had reported the use of this method in two studies[8][63] when we learned that, almost simultaneously, a version of the method had been devised, employed, and reported by another research group in Norway.[81] Modified rule of nines methods for assessing the pain distribution of fibromyalgia patients had not been reported prior to 1997.

With our version of the method, termed the percentage method, we divide the body into 36 divisions (see Figure 4.1.3). Each division has a percentage value based on the amount of surface area it contains. A patient's percentage score at each reevaluation is based on the pain drawing she completes. The percentage values of all pain-containing divisions are totaled to derive the patient's pain percentage score for that evaluation date. (The body form on which the patient illustrates her pain pattern does *not* contain the 36 divisions. See below: "Scoring: the Percentage Method.")

Modification 3: Extended Symptom Intensity Scales

I have extended the number of visual analog scales (VASs) from the usual 1-to-4 used in fibromyalgia studies to include the 13 most commonly associated fibromyalgia symptoms.[1][53][54] These symptoms are: pain, fatigue, stiffness, headache, sleep disturbance, bowel disturbance, depression, cognitive dysfunction (poor memory and concentration), anxiety, coldness, paresthesias (numbness and tingling), Sicca symptoms, and difficulty with exercise.

FIBROMYALGIA IMPACT QUESTIONNAIRE AND ZUNG'S SELF-RATING DEPRESSION SCALE

In addition to the three modifications just described, we also use two other standard methods of fibromyalgia assessment: the Fibromyalgia Impact Questionnaire[66] and Zung's Self-Rating Depression Scale.[67] The Fibromyalgia Impact Questionnaire (FIQ) is a brief, self-administered pencil and paper instrument with demonstrated validity and reliability. It is widely used for assessing the impact fibromyalgia has on a patient's daily life. It measures physical function, work status, depression, anxiety, sleep, pain, stiffness, fatigue, and sense of well-being. Zung's is an easily self-administered, well-validated pencil and paper instrument for assessing the presence and severity of depression. It has acceptable sensitivity and specificity.[68] Zung's correlates significantly with other measures of depression including the Beck Depression Inventory.[69] We have patients complete the FIQ and Zung's at the initial and all subsequent evaluations.

GRAPHED SCORES FROM REPEATED MEASURES OF FIBROMYALGIA STATUS

After the patient has completed the forms required for an evaluation and we have performed an algometer exam of her tender points, we derive a single score for each measure (as I explain below). Next, we post each score to a separate line graph that allows, through visual inspection, a quick estimate of the patient's status (at the time of the initial exam) or her progress (at subsequent exams).

Visually inspecting a line graph (which has been described as "eye-balling" it) allows the clinician to see whether the trend of the data points indicates that the patient's fibromyalgia status, according to the particular fibromyalgia measure, has worsened, remained the same, or improved. One benefit of the visual inspection of graphs is that the method, compared to statistical analysis, is insensitive. Only substantial changes in patient status are likely to show up as changes in the progression of trend lines in the graphs. Subtle changes in patient status do not produce noteworthy changes in the progression of trend lines. As a result, noteworthy changes in the progression of trend lines reflect changes in patient status that are of a clinically significant magnitude.[33] (See Appendix B, paper titled "The Process of Change with T_3 Therapy for Euthyroid Fibromyalgia: A Double-Blind Placebo-Controlled Crossover Study.")

Positive changes in fibromyalgia status that are obvious upon visual inspection of the graphs are meaningful for practical purposes—the changes translate into objective measures documenting that the patient is improved or recovered, and corroborating the patient subjectively feeling improved or recovered. In contrast to the practical importance of improvements obvious from the inspection of line graphs, reports that patients taking amitriptyline or cyclobenzaprine had "statistically significant" improvement compared to patients taking placebos is meaningless for practical purposes. The "improvement" shown in studies of these medications has been so subtle that only supersensitive statistical methods have been able to detect a difference between the results from the use of these medications and placebos. Fibromyalgia patients treated with these medications have remained ill and functionally impaired despite their statistically significant differences from placebo-treated patients (see Chapter 5.1, abstract and subsections titled "Cyclobenzaprine" and "Amitriptyline").

Using continuous variables (those with a range of

possible scores) allows comparison of initial scores to subsequent ones from reevaluations. Clinical improvement is indicated when successive scores in the line graph form a trend line in a favorable direction.

A present limitation of this continuous method of assessing therapeutic effect is that we have not established cut-off points that distinguish normal from abnormal. In research, this is not an issue because we use statistics to determine whether the difference in measures between placebo and treatment phases is significant. In clinical practice, however, especially when the clinician has collected fewer than 6-to-8 baseline scores for a fibromyalgia measure, statistical analysis of a patient's graphs may not be possible. If two or more sets of scores can be obtained before treatment begins, however, this may provide a rough baseline against which to visually compare measurements taken after treatment begins. If the trend during treatment obviously varies in a favorable direction from the trend of pre-treatment measurements—especially if the favorable trend continues or is maintained over time—it is safe to infer that the treatment is having a beneficial impact on the patient's status.[32] In most cases, as the patient's metabolic rehabilitation progresses, data points in the graphs (representing the scores from the five fibromyalgia measures) all progress in a direction indicating improvement. In most cases, when the trend of data points in each of the five graphs indicates improvement, statistical analysis is not necessary to convince the clinician and patient.

● TENDER POINTS

The most characteristic feature of patients with a diagnosis of fibromyalgia is the report of tenderness at multiple body sites to amounts of pressure that do not cause tenderness in most people.[6][20][21][22] We call these sites "tender points." When measuring the pressure/pain thresholds of normal and abnormally tender body sites, Smythe found a distinct difference. Algometer values were about twice as high at control sites (such as the thumb nail) than at fibromyalgic tender points, indicating about 50% less tenderness at control sites. The investigators were able to differentiate well between control sites and tender points. They also found that fibromyalgia patients generally had lower pressure/pain thresholds (greater pressure sensitivity) than control subjects.[25] This finding corresponds to those of other investigators.[2][9]

In 1988, Quimby, Block, and Gratwick tested the pre-ACR criteria for fibromyalgia. Their study included 125 patients with generalized non-articular rheumatism, rheumatoid arthritis, or osteoarthritis. The investigators measured pain at tender point and control point sites using an algometer. They also assessed patients' responses to six standard psychological self-reports. Only pain at low amounts of pressure distinguished fibromyalgia patients from others with generalized non-articular rheumatism. The researchers concluded that except for having tender points, fibromyalgia patients probably do not differ in any important physical or psychological respects from other patients with generalized non-articular rheumatism. They wrote that the concept of fibromyalgia as an entity separate from the rest of generalized non-articular rheumatism may be an artifact of the physician's approach to a patient.[5]

Mikkelsson et al. measured pressure/pain thresholds and pressure/pain tolerances at non-trigger point muscle and bone. They used algometry to measure the thresholds and tolerances of two age-matched groups: 50 healthy women and 46 female patients with "primary" fibromyalgia. (Many researchers use the term "primary" fibromyalgia when they believe they have ruled out all well-documented diseases as the cause of the study patients' fibromyalgia symptoms.) Pressure/pain thresholds and pressure/pain tolerances of both muscle and bone were lower in fibromyalgia patients than in healthy controls. Although there was overlap between the thresholds and tolerances of patients and controls, the differences in the mean threshold and tolerance were highly significant statistically. The investigators concluded that the pain sensitivity (to pressure) of patients with "primary" fibromyalgia is generally amplified. Mikkelsson et al. suggested that the amplified pain is a sign that might be useful in diagnosing fibromyalgia.[9]

PAIN MODULATION IN FIBROMYALGIA AND THE USE OF TENDER POINTS

Granges and Littlejohn in Melbourne, Australia hypothesized that a change in pain threshold to pressure reflects a generalized change in the pain system affecting both tender and control points. Using an algometer, they assessed 18 tender points and 4 control points in 60 patients with fibromyalgia, 60 patients with localized (regional) chronic pain syndromes, and 60 pain-free subjects. They found a significant correlation between the low pressure/pain threshold (high sensitivity) at tender points and control points in the fibromyalgia patients. Granges and Littlejohn concluded that the correlation suggests a diffuse change in pain modulation in fibromyalgia and that the tender point is clinically useful.[4]

TIME OF DAY OF TENDER POINT EXAMS

Reilly and Littlejohn examined 17 female fibromyalgia patients twice on the same day, first at 9:00 am and then again at 7:00 pm. Fourteen patients reported that they felt best around mid-day, between 11:00 am and 2:00 pm, and 3 patients reported that

they felt best when they got up in the morning. None felt better at the end of the day than at the beginning.[6]

For the majority of patients, tender points became more numerous and more tender by evening. Ten patients had an increase in tender point sensitivity late in the day; 5 had a decrease. The mean change in tender point sensitivity for the whole group was a reduction in pressure/pain threshold of 2.9 kg/cm^2 by evening.

If these findings are born out by other studies, the time of day may be important in tracking changes in tender point scores over time. Therefore, repeated tender point measurements may be most reliable if performed at roughly the same time of day at each exam.

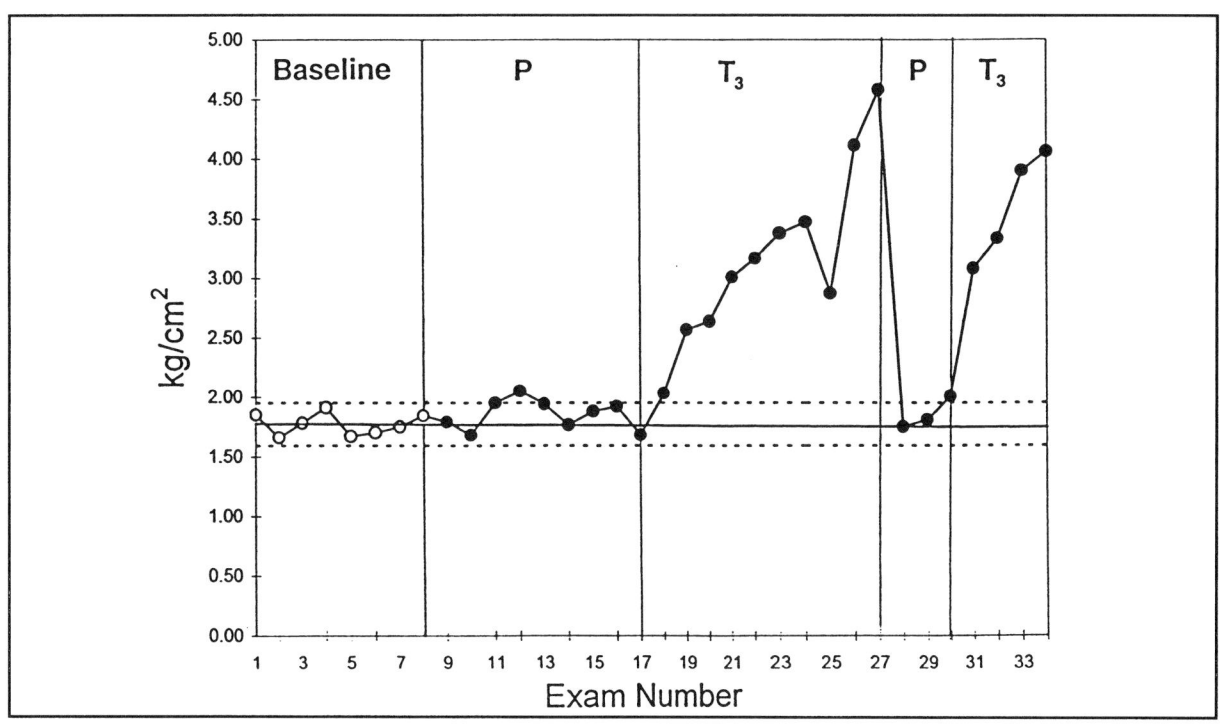

Figure 4.1.2. Variations in tender point scores in placebo and treatment phases.

TENDER POINT EXAMINATION

An examination for potential tender points may be performed manually or with an algometer. I believe that manual examination of tender points is unreliable. The procedure does not permit precise quantification of the pressure/pain thresholds of anatomical sites. For these reasons, I prefer the use of algometry to determine whether a patient's potential tender point sites are abnormally tender to pressure and to document the level of tenderness.

Manual vs Algometer Examinations

Some researchers have arrived at the erroneous conclusion that for the examination of tender points, manual palpation and algometry are equally useful. It is true that if the clinician is well-trained and experienced at performing palpatory tender point exams, he *may* be able to discern when a patient has fibromyalgia tender points. But with manual palpation, the clinician can only state after each exam that the patient has or does not have tender points. Manual palpation is at best a crude assessment of the presence or absence of tender points. It is useless, however, for grading changes in sensitivity. Can a clinician, even when trained and experienced in the palpatory examination of tender points, reliably detect a 0.5 kg change in the sensitivity of a tender point on successive examinations of a patient, spaced perhaps a week apart? Of course not, but he *can* do so with algometry.

It is interesting, nevertheless, to consider the studies upon which researchers equate manual palpation and algometry. Rasmussen and coworkers investigated the inter- and intra-observer agreements between the assessment of tender points with palpation and the assessment with algometry. The study had three components. First, two examiners assessed 25 female patients who had various rheumatic conditions. The examiners assessed 15 anatomical sites that are often tender in these conditions. They first used palpation, and followed immediately with algometry. There was acceptable agreement between the two methods *except at pressure thresholds under 5.0 kg/cm². (Since 4.0 kg/ cm² is the "normal" point for fibromyalgia measures, the results of this study *should* indicate that palpation is an unacceptable method for clinicians working with fibromyalgia patients.) Second, an examiner palpated the fat pads of the right knees of 25 female volunteers, after which he immediately tested the fat pads of the left knees with an algometer. Good agreement was found between both methods. Third, 65 consecutive patients admitted to Kong Christian X Hospital for Rheumatic Diseases were examined for tender points at 15 sites of predilection. Two examiners assessed the sites, one with palpation and the other immediately after with algometry. Agreement between the two methods was poor. The researchers concluded that using an algometer may be useful in research where quantifying the threshold of pain is desired. They stated, however, that in the daily clinical routine, palpatory examination for tender points is just as good or better than employment of an algometer.[10] Based on my experiences using both methods in clinical practice and experimental research, I adamantly disagree with this conclusion.

Cott and his coworkers evaluated the interrater reliability of digital (thumb) examination for tender points by comparison with algometer examination. They studied 15 patients with widespread pain and various rheumatological diagnoses. In an examiner-blind procedure, two rheumatologists determined the tender point count by digital examination of 18 sites. They also determined tender point threshold by using an algometer at 12 sites. A pressure/pain threshold of 4 kg/1.77 cm² or less defined the presence of tender points with both methods. The researchers reported

three findings. First, using pain complaints and digital examination for tender points was moderately reliable in distinguishing fibromyalgia patients from those with other diagnoses. Second, interrater agreement about the presence or absence of tenderness at individual points was not significantly lower for digital examination compared to algometry. However, analyses of the 12 anatomical sites measured by both methods showed that more sites were considered tender by digital examination as compared to algometry. The researchers concluded that digital and algometer measures are equally reliable.[3]

On the other hand, Fischer and colleagues demonstrated that experienced palpators could not accurately judge how much pressure they were applying with their fingers or thumbs to the tip of an algometer. They also could not accurately judge how much pressure was being applied to their fingers or thumbs through the tip of an algometer.[60] Smythe and coworkers found that tissue sites considered nontender by manual palpation had widely differing tenderness thresholds revealed by algometry.[79] These studies make it unlikely that digital palpation and algometry are equally accurate and reliable.

The algometer is an extremely precise and reliable instrument for assessing pressure/pain thresholds,[11][12][13][14][15][16][17] although examiner technique and patient responses can make repetitive measures vary somewhat. It is important to note, though, that the variations tend to be slight. When a patient undergoes a proper course of metabolic rehabilitation, the mean algometer score may change as much as 1-to-3 kg/cm². The variations in patients not treated metabolically seldom exceed 0.5 kg/cm². The minor variations in patients not treated metabolically are obvious from a comparison of patient scores (posted to line graphs) obtained during placebo phases of treatment as opposed to T_3 treatment phases[8] (see Figure 4.1.2).

Manual Tender Point Examination

Many clinicians and fibromyalgia researchers assess a patient's tender points by pressing into them with a finger or thumb. A point qualifies as "tender" according to a patient's response. If 11 of the 18 potential sites are tender, the clinician concludes that the patient meets the tender point criterion for fibromyalgia.[23,p.8]

Yunus described the procedure: "The pain thus elicited may be graded as mild, moderate, or severe; for moderate or greater pain, a visible physical sign (such as grimacing or withdrawal) should be present."[23,p.8] This procedure is subjective on the part of the clinician and the patient. It lacks the precision needed for both research and defense in courtroom testimony. The clinician is instructed to consider 4 kg of pressure the point at which his fingernail or thumbnail blanches,[6] yet blanching of different clinicians' nails must vary with pressures according to the principle of the bell curve. To use a patient's verbal report of pain, a grimace, and recoiling from the examiner's touch as a stepwise measure of pain intensity is to use behaviorally conditioned responses of biophysiologically protean individuals that vary considerably from person to person.

Algometer Tender Point Examination

Tender point assessment according to the ACR entails applying 4 kg of pressure with a finger to 18 potential tender point sites. The patient meets the tender point criterion if he or she reports tenderness upon pressure at 11 or more of the 18 tender points.[1] Recently, however, Fischer demonstrated that experienced clinicians could not accurately judge when they were applying 4 kg of pressure with a finger or thumb. Moreover, without watching a meter, they were not able to distinguish 4 kg of pressure when it was applied to a finger or thumb. Fischer concluded that quantifying applied pressure through algometry is required to reliably identify fibromyalgia patients.[60]

Tender point sensitivity objectively assessed with algometry is a sign. The clinician should measure this sign at each evaluation. The algometer reliably measures the sensitivity of fibromyalgia tender points,[10][61] and its measurements have been reported to correlate well with pain distribution reported by patients on body drawings.[19] The lower the pressure/pain thresholds of the 16 tender points (again, I exclude the lower cervical points), the more sensitive they are. Conversely, the higher the pressure/pain thresholds of the tender points, the less sensitive they are.

The therapeutic aim regarding tender point sensitivity is to raise the pressure/pain threshold to a normal level, presumed to be 4 kg/cm² or above. The problem with this objective is that for many patients, 4 kg/cm² or more does not appear to be normal. Table 4.1.2 shows the changes in mean pressure/pain threshold of 4 patients my colleagues and I treated with T_3 over a period of roughly one year. During the course of treatment, these patients were all in the process of recovering according to their subjective assessment and by other measures.[77]

In a single subject study using T_3, the mean threshold of a patient who thoroughly recovered from all features of fibromyalgia increased from 2.5 kg/cm² to

5.5 kg/cm².[78] The change in mean threshold was 3.0 kg/cm². In a blinded crossover group study, the mean threshold of one patient who completely recovered increased from a baseline value of 1.84 kg/cm² to a maximum in T_3 phases of 4.11 kg/cm². This was an increase in mean threshold of 2.27 kg/cm². The mean threshold of another patient who at the end of the study no longer met the criteria for fibromyalgia increased from a baseline of 2.36 kg/cm² to a maximum in T_3 phases of 3.91 kg/cm². This was an increase of 1.55 kg/cm². The mean threshold of a third patient who completely recovered increased from a baseline of 1.3 kg/cm² to a maximum T_3 value of 2.94 kg/cm², an increase of only 1.64 kg/cm². And the mean threshold of a fourth patient who totally recovered increased from a baseline of 2.08 kg/cm² to a maximum in T_3 phases of 2.16 kg/cm²—an increase of only 0.08 kg/cm²! Yet each of these patients who met the ACR criteria for fibromyalgia before the study began, and during two different placebo phases, no longer met the criteria during two separate T_3 phases, at a 2-month follow-up, and in one case, at a 2-year follow-up.[8] Simply having mean tender point thresholds lower than 4 kg/cm² did not classify them as having fibromyalgia because they no longer had widespread pain.

Table 4.1.2. Mean tender point pressure/pain thresholds (measured in kg/cm²) of 4 fibromyalgia patients treated with T_3 over the period of one year.*

PATIENT	INITIAL THRESHOLD	MAXIMUM THRESHOLD	FINAL THRESHOLD	DIFFERENCE BETWEEN INITIAL & FINAL THRESHOLD
#1	0.8	4.1	3.1	2.3
#2	2.5	5.3	4.4	1.9
#3	1.9	6.9	5.9	4.0
#4	2.5	3.7	3.7	1.2

*Lowe, J.C., Eichelberger, J., Manso, G., and Peterson, K.: Improvement in euthyroid fibromyalgia patients treated with T_3 (triiodothyronine). *J. Myofascial Ther.*, 1(2):16-29, 1994.[77]

Findings from these studies make the arbitrary cutoff point for normal of 4 kg/cm² highly dubious. Use of this criterion is rigid and unrealistic and would best be abandoned. A more practical criterion for improvement in patients undergoing treatment is to compare the mean thresholds of initial tender point exams with increases in mean thresholds at subsequent exams. Use of a line graph displaying mean value for each exam makes a favorable trend more obvious than the mere review of a list of algometer values.

Algometer. The algometer is a hand-held instrument that engineers call a "force gauge." The term force gauge describes the instrument's function—to quantify the amount of force (pressure) applied to a resistant surface by the instrument. Clinicians who use the instrument call it an algometer or dolorimeter. These terms are synonyms and literally mean "pain meter."

Clinicians use the algometer to determine the precise amount of pressure necessary to produce discomfort at a certain tissue site. Most clinicians use the algometer to determine the pressure sensitivity of trigger points and fibromyalgia tender points. They also use it to measure how much pressure causes pain over joints and paraspinal myofascial tissues.

One reason the algometer is useful is that when the clinician uses it properly, algometer measurements are highly reliable. That is, when the clinician measures the amount of pressure that induces discomfort at a potential tender point, subsequent measures taken in the same way (the same direction into the tender point at the same velocity) are likely to be within 0.10-to-0.20 kg/cm^2 of the previous measurement. Algometry measurements of tender point pressure/pain thresholds are also reproducible by different clinicians when they use the same technique.

Algometer Footplate. The plunger that extends from the cylindrical gauge has a rubber tip called the footplate. The 1 cm^2 tip is preferable to the 1.54 cm tip. The smaller tip permits the clinician to more precisely direct pressure into the anatomical site of choice. Including adjacent tissue in the measurement with a larger tip adds to the resistance to the pressure. More force may then be necessary to induce discomfort, increasing the pressure value according to the algometer.

This effect was shown by Smythe, who evaluated measurements performed with algometers with 1 cm^2 and 1.54 cm^2 tips. He found that the algometer with the 1 cm^2 footplate was more effective for detecting tender points and quantifying their sensitivity. The lower effectiveness of the algometer with the larger footplate was presumably due to the larger surface area of the footplate covering some normal as well as abnormal tissue.[24][25] Covering some normal tissue possibly obscured the measurement of the pressure/pain sensitivity of the abnormally tender tissue.[26,p.137] Use of the 1 cm^2 surface produced lower values at tender points and higher values at normally sensitive body sites. In addition, the algometer with the 1 cm^2 foot-

plate was more sensitive to differences between sites evaluated, and it was more sensitive to variations among subjects.[24][25] With a 1 cm^2 footplate, then, it is easier to show whether the pressure pain threshold of a tender point is abnormally sensitive.[26,p.136]

Algometer Technique. The clinician must use proper algometer technique to obtain accurate and reliable tender point measurements. First, the clinician applies pressure at a tender point site with the rubber tip of the algometer. Then, according to prior instructions, the patient signals the clinician with the word "now" when the pressure first becomes uncomfortable. The clinician stops increasing pressure at that moment and records the kg/cm^2 indicated by the point on the dial where the needle stopped moving. The value is recorded on the body form (Figure 4.1.4) at that tender point location.

The clinician should apply pressure with the algometer at the rate of about 0.5 kg per second.[23,p.8] List found a high correlation between the rate of pressure and the accuracy of the algometer measure. The slower the rate, the more reliable the repeated measures.[15]

Special Instructions for the Patient. Instructing the patient in how to cooperate in the tender point exam presents a semantic problem. During the exam, the patient must give a verbal signal when pressure into a tender point site first becomes noxious. Patients often are confused by the term "pressure/*pain*" threshold. Most patients interpret this to mean they should say "now" only when pressure from the algometer tip becomes almost intolerable. I explain to them that such a measurement would be the pressure/pain *tolerance*, but the distinction seems ambiguous to them. Because of this, I have abandoned the words "pressure/pain threshold" with fibromyalgia patients. Instead, I use terms such as the "discomfort threshold," or "the point where you just begin to feel slight discomfort."

The threshold is the point, while pressure is being increased, where the patient's perception of pressure takes on an unpleasant quality. In a tender point exam, we want to know the threshold of unpleasantness, not the threshold of intense pain. I explain this to patients with great care. "At first, you will feel only pressure," I say. "But at some point, the pressure will begin to take on an unpleasant quality. It is when you first feel this that I want you to say 'now.'" I also emphasize, repeatedly if necessary, that I do not want the patient to wait until she feels distinct pain. Males in general, however, have trouble accurately reporting the change of sensation early enough. They usually wait until they feel distinct pain, which is already beyond the point of slight unpleasantness. Extra instruction is sometimes necessary for male patients to understand exactly when to say "now."

Perceptually, the discomfort threshold is a grey area with no clear-cut boundary. This threshold is probably reached at the time when the rubber tip of the algometer, pressing into the tissue, initially arouses awareness of impending tissue damage. The awareness most likely occurs as the tip structurally distorts and activates a sufficient number of mechanoreceptors in the underlying tissue. Theoretically, the threshold is low in fibromyalgia patients because too little serotonin and norepinephrine are secreted by descending pain-inhibitory fibers in the dorsal horns of the spinal cord, and because fibromyalgia patients have higher than normal levels of substance P.

Normally, serotonin and norepinephrine stimulate the release of opioid chemicals from interneurons in the dorsal horns. The opioids hyperpolarize the endings of incoming "pain-transmitting" type C and A delta fibers from aroused tissue sites, such as those where we apply the algometer tip. With the deficient synthesis and secretion of serotonin and norepinephrine in fibromyalgia patients, the endings of the incoming afferent fibers are not properly hyperpolarized. In addition, increased exposure of the fibers to high levels of substance P facilitate transmission of the signals to secondary neurons in the spinal cord (see Chapter 3.19). Signals generated at the tender point site by the pressure from the algometer tip enter the dorsal horns, ascend through the spinothalamic tracts to the brain, and are perceived as unpleasant-to-painful, depending on the amount of pressure applied and the severity of the patient's serotonin and/or norepinephrine deficiency (see Chapter 3.15).

This impairment in pain modulation is corrected with metabolic therapy, and as a result, greater amounts of pressure can be applied before the patient begins to feel discomfort or pain. I simply explain to patients, however, that the therapy increases the chemicals in the spinal cord that prevent too many sensory nerve impulses from reaching the brain and causing pain perception.

Scoring. After performing the algometer exam of the patient's tender points, the clinician totals the kg/cm² for all the points measured, then divides by the total number of points to derive the mean value for that exam date. He then posts the mean kg/cm² to a graph similar to the one in Figure 4.1.2. With successive exams, increasing elevation of the line in the graph indicates improving mean tender point algometer scores.

Excluding Lower Cervical Tender Points from the Tender Point Exam

I recommend that the lower cervical tender points (bilaterally, at the anterior aspects of the intertransverse spaces of C5 to C7[1]) be excluded from the tender point examination. In many stout or muscular patients with thick necks, it is difficult to locate the correct sites with a finger or thumb and doubtful whether an algometer can be properly used to measure the pressure/pain threshold of these points. To examine these tender points, Smythe recommends having the patient lie supine and thoroughly relax. He wrote, "They learn from the way I start moving them," he stated, "that they can relax, and then I get in behind the sternomastoid with my thumb, or through it with the dolorimeter. The thumb is much better in this location."[70,p.38] Despite these suggestions, finger or thumb assessment may be inaccurate, and it is difficult at best to properly employ the algometer when examining these points.

In addition, the lower cervical points are excruciatingly tender to many fibromyalgia patients. Some patients report tenderness before the needle on the dial of the algometer registers 0.10 kg/cm². I ceased examining these points after many patients whom I had previously examined expressed dread at my doing so again. I therefore exclude these points from the exam, and measure the sensitivity of the remaining 16 points specified in the ACR criteria. This process protects my patients from unnecessary additional suffering, and still allows for an accurate quantification of their tenderness.

● PAIN DISTRIBUTION

Widespread pain is a requirement for the diagnosis of fibromyalgia. Because of this, measuring the patient's pain distribution is essential to establishing that diagnosis. It can also be a valuable method for assessing change in the patient's fibromyalgia status as treatment progresses.

We do use the ACR diagnostic criteria for widespread pain, which permits a pain distribution score of one-to-four units (0-1-2-3) to assess a patient's status. But we also use an alternate method I adapted from the "rule of nines" for adult burn victims (which describes the percentage of body surface burned).[58][59] With this method, the patient's pain distribution is expressed as a percentage, with a range of 0%-to-100% (see Figure 4.1.3).

A shortcoming of the percentage method, albeit one of little practical importance, is that we have not established what percentage constitutes widespread pain. After undergoing effective metabolic rehabilitation, most patients no longer meet the ACR criterion for widespread pain. However, it is common for a patient to still have pain in a small percentage of the 36 body divisions. In most cases, this small percentage reflects a regional musculoskeletal problem rather than systemic pain due to impaired pain modulation. (In most cases, effective physical treatment, most often involving therapy for the myofascial tissues and somatic joint dysfunction, eliminates the residual, regional pain. See Appendix B, paper titled "Facilitating the Decrease in Fibromyalgic Pain During Metabolic Rehabilitation: An Essential Role for Soft Tissue Therapies.") At present, the only way to distinguish the two is by use of the ACR criterion. We use the ACR criterion to classify a patient as having or not having widespread pain, and we use the percentage method to more definitively express how much of the patient's body contains pain. This dual method permits the clinician to diagnostically classify the patient and to precisely grade changes in her pain distribution during treatment.

CORRELATION OF THE PERCENTAGE METHOD WITH OTHER METHODS OF PAIN ASSESSMENT

In one blinded study, my colleagues and I found a high positive correlation between the ACR method and our percentage method for assessing pain distribution. During placebo phases, Spearman's correlation coefficient was 0.6008 (P=0.039). During T_3 phases, the coefficient was 0.6991 (P=0.01). During placebo phases, there was a positive correlation between our percentage method and the VAS for pain intensity, but the correlation did not reach significance (correlation coefficient was 0.4400 [P=0.15]). The positive correlation in T_3 phases, however, was highly significant. The coefficient was 0.6384 (P=0.025).[8]

MULTIPLE MEASURES OF PAIN

The patient's pain distribution, determined from her pain drawing, is valuable for assessing change during treatment. But combining this with the quantification of tender point sensitivity by algometry, and an estimate of pain intensity with a visual analog scale, provides a more useful gauge.

At the University Rheumatology Clinic in Basle, Switzerland, Lautenschlager and colleagues assessed pain in 47 fibromyalgia patients. They used three different assessment techniques: a simple visual analog scale, a body diagram on which patients could indicate pain separately in different regions of the body, and algometer measurements at 56 potential tender point sites. The investigators assessed pain at baseline and again after 4 weeks of therapy. Changes according to the three measures were compared via the Spearman correlation. Pain distribution on the body diagram correlated better with algometry measurements of tender points than it did with the simple visual analog scale. The investigators concluded that clinicians can more objectively assess the severity of fibromyalgia pain using all three techniques than with the visual analog pain scale alone. In particular, more objective therapeutic change may be best shown through use of the pain drawing and algometer measures of tender point sensitivity.[19] Jacobs et al., however, reported a lack of correlation between self-reported pain (via two self-assessment questionnaires) and mean tender point score for patients with fibromyalgia of shorter duration. They found a weak correlation for patients with fibromyalgia of longer duration.[65]

Croft found that in the general population, pain drawings showing the distribution of people's self-reported pain were directly correlated with the number and location of tender points found during exams. The actual number of tender points reflected the extent of pain a patient reported.[18]

EVALUATING PAIN DISTRIBUTION

At initial and subsequent evaluations, the patient should be given a drawing of the body such as that in Figure 4.1.4 (also see Appendix A). She can then complete what is termed a "pain drawing." The clinician should emphasize to the patient that although we call this a *pain* drawing, we use the term broadly. The patient should shade all body areas where she has perceived discomfort, aching, pain, soreness, or any other noxious perception she considers part of her fibromyalgia. She should use lighter shading to indicate less intensely painful areas, and darker shading to indicate more intensely painful areas.

It is best to provide the patient with a pencil and eraser so that she can make corrections to the drawing when necessary. On her initial visit, she should indicate her pain distribution over the past 3 months or so. On subsequent visits, she should indicate where she has had pain since her last evaluation.

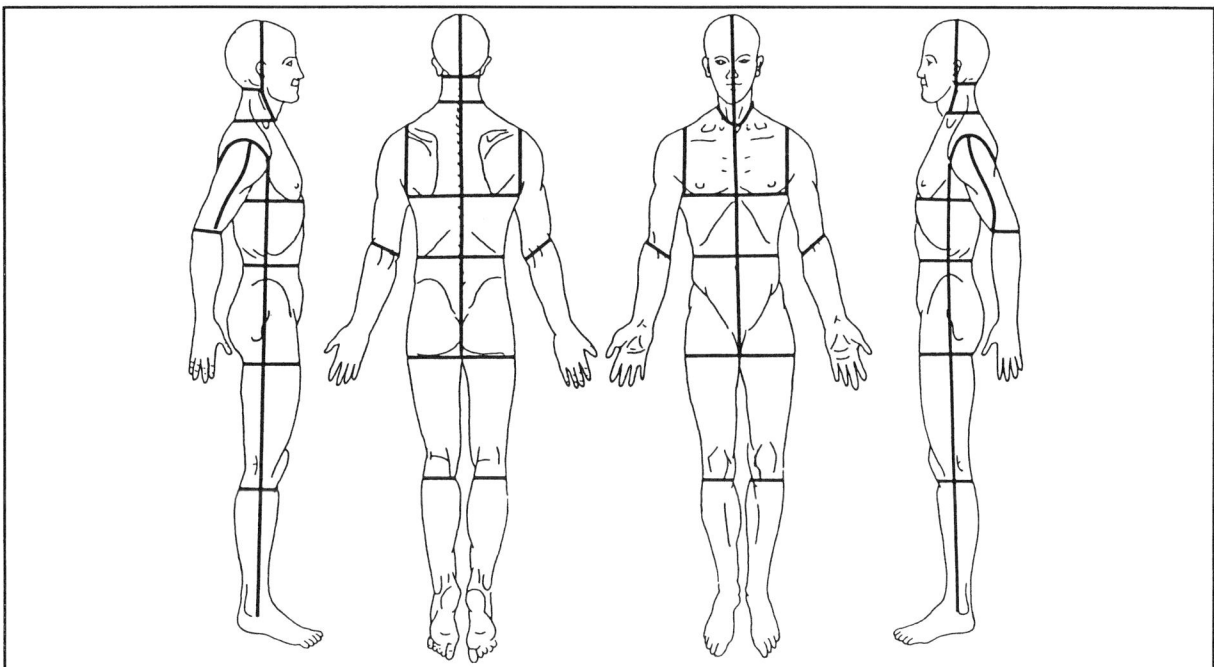

Figure 4.1.3. The 36 body divisions of the percentage method of measuring pain distribution.

Special Instructions for the Patient

An occasional patient has had an acute musculo-skeletal injury before her initial visit or between two evaluations. If this happens, the clinician should instruct the patient to either exclude the resulting painful body part from the drawing or include it in her pain drawing with a note on the sheet explaining that this area of pain is related to a specific event and is independent of her fibromyalgia. The clinician should exclude this from his calculation of her fibromyalgia pain distribution unless it is clear that her fibromyalgia-related pain typically includes this area.

It is important that the patient *shade* in the areas rather than *circle* body locations, as some are wont to do. With shading, the patient can provide a more thorough and precise representation of her pain distribution that can be scored more accurately.

Scoring: the ACR Method

Yunus wrote that the fibromyalgia patient usually complains of pain in all four extremities and the upper and lower back. He qualified, however, that pain in three widespread areas satisfies this symptom criterion.[23,p.5] This method (in which "widespread" means pain above and below the waist, on the right and left sides of the body, and axial pain), however, allows some patients with minimal pain distribution to meet the criterion for widespread pain, and other patients

with pain over large areas of the body not to meet the criterion. Figure 4.1.5A shows how a patient with pain over a small total portion of the body can meet this criterion. Figure 4.1.5B shows that a patient with pain over a substantial portion of the body can fail to meet the criterion (also see section above: "Modification 2: Percentage Method of Pain Distribution").

Scoring: the Percentage Method

With this method, pain distribution is expressed as a percentage. The value is based on the percentage of 36 body divisions that contain pain. The number of body areas included can be determined by placing a transparent template over the patient's pain drawing (Figure 4.1.3 reproduced on a transparency film). Since each body division has a percentage value, the values for those divisions that contain markings can be counted and a total percentage score for that evaluation date recorded. The score is posted to a line graph for pain distribution (Figure 4.1.6). Decline of the line over successive evaluations indicates that the percentage of the body containing pain is decreasing.

This method is more sensitive than the ACR method for assessing pain distribution. My colleagues and I found,[8] for example, that when using the ACR 0-1-2-3 scoring method, the difference between placebo and T_3 phases was significant at the 0.05 level. But with the percentage method, the difference was significant at the 0.015 level. The smaller P value for the percentage method shows that the likelihood of chance variation accounting for the difference between the scores of placebo and T_3 phases was much smaller using the percentage method.

The sensitivity of the percentage method compared to the ACR method is apparent by reviewing Figure 4.1.7 (constructed by overlaying a transparency of Figure 4.1.3 on top of Figure 4.1.5). In 4.1.7A, the patient meets the ACR criterion for widespread pain, yet she has pain in only 4.5% of the 36 body divisions. In 4.1.7B, the patient does not meet the ACR criterion, yet she has pain in a much larger proportion of her body, 49.5% of the 36 divisions.

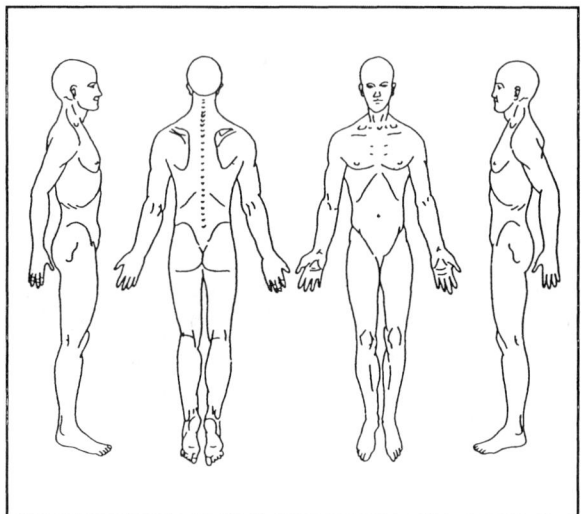

Figure 4.1.4. Body form.

For many patients who undergo metabolic rehabilitation, pain distribution decreases from widespread-to-none. Most patients, however, continue to report at least mild regional pain or discomfort. *If the pain or discomfort is due to a local structural or functional lesion, the clinician should not consider this a residual feature of fibromyalgia.*

● SYMPTOM INTENSITY

The ACR criteria do not require the presence of symptoms other than pain for the diagnosis of fibromyalgia.[1] But Table 4.1.3 lists the symptoms most often associated with fibromyalgia.[7] As shown in the table, the most common symptoms are widespread pain, fatigue, stiffness, and poor sleep.[23,p.5]

Quimby, Block, and Gratwick tested the pre-ACR criteria for fibromyalgia with 125 patients with generalized non-articular rheumatism, rheumatoid arthritis, or osteoarthritis. They found that fibromyalgia patients differed from other patients with generalized non-articular rheumatism in only one way: They experienced pain in response to amounts of pressures at potential tender point sites that did not induce pain perception in the other patients. Symptom criteria for fibromyalgia did not correlate significantly with the number of tender points. The researchers concluded that except for having tender points, fibromyalgia patients probably do not differ in any important physical or psychological respect from other patients with generalized nonarticular rheumatism, all of whom showed a high frequency of reporting manifold disagreeable symptoms.[5]

Nevertheless, in two blinded studies of T_3 therapy for euthyroid fibromyalgia patients, my colleagues and I found that intensities of 13 symptoms measured with visual analog scales significantly decreased during the treatment phases[8][63] (see Tables 4.1.4 and 4.1.5). In one study, for example, the mean intensity of 13 symptoms in placebo phases was 5.42 (0-to-10 point scale), and the mean in T_3 phases was 2.30. The difference was highly significant (P<0.0005). Despite this P value, a reduction of 3.12 points with a final mean symptom intensity of 2.30 may seem minimal. Bear in mind, however, that these figures come from a group study. Two of 7 patients did not markedly improve, and their unfavorable scores were averaged with the other 5 patients' favorable scores.[8] Table 4.1.4 shows the mean symptom intensities for the 2 patients who did not benefit from T_3 therapy, and those of the 5 who did. These results are typical of patients undergoing metabolic therapy.

EXTENDED SYMPTOM INTENSITY SCALES

I have extended the number of VASs from the usual 1-to-4 to include 13 of the most common associated fibromyalgia symptoms,[1][53][54] and have incorporated them into the FibroQuest forms (see Appendix A). These symptoms are pain, fatigue, stiffness, sleep disturbance, headache, bowel disturbance, coldness, paresthesias (numbness and tingling), Sicca symptoms, depression, cognitive dysfunction (poor memory and concentration), anxiety, and difficulty exercising.

Assessment of symptom intensities, especially pain, using VASs is customarily employed in fibromyalgia studies.[34][35][36][37] Scott and Huskisson reported that the VAS is the best available procedure for measuring pain.[55] VASs of pain have been shown to be reliable,[71] generalizable, [72] and comparatively sensitive measures of the effects of analgesic treatments.[73][74][75][76]

Special Instructions for the Patient

The visual analog scales on the FibroQuest long form, on which the patient estimates the intensities of her symptoms on the first visit, provide baseline values. Scores on the FibroQuest short form, used at subsequent reevaluations, can be contrasted with those from the baseline and previous reevaluations.

At the initial visit, the patient should estimate the intensity of each symptom over roughly the past 3 months. When she fills out the visual analog scales in the short version of the FibroQuest form at reevaluations, she should indicate the intensity of each symptom *since her last evaluation.* Each evaluation after the initial one is an assessment of her status since the time of the last evaluation. If she has not experienced a symptom, she should indicate this by marking or circling 0 (zero).

Scoring

At the initial visit, the values marked or circled on all visual analog scales should be totaled and divided by the number of symptoms the patient marked. At future evaluations, the *same number* of symptoms (as marked on the initial evaluation) should be divided into the total of the scales the patient marked. For example, if the patient rated 10 of the 13 symptoms on the initial visit, but after one month of treatment she indicates that she has experienced only 8, the total rating for the 8 symptoms should still be divided by 10. Otherwise, the total rating for the 8 symptoms, divided by 8, will fail to show the true reduction in the mean intensity of symptoms. In fact, dividing by 8 may actually indicate that the patient's symptoms are more severe. When the mean is obtained, it should be posted to a line graph for mean symptom intensity (similar to the graph for pain distribution in Figure 4.1.6.).

● FIBROMYALGIA IMPACT QUESTIONNAIRE (FIQ) AND ZUNG'S SELF-RATING DEPRESSION SCALE

The method for scoring the FIQ is provided with the questionnaire in Appendix A. The total score for each reevaluation should be posted to a line graph (also provided in Appendix A).

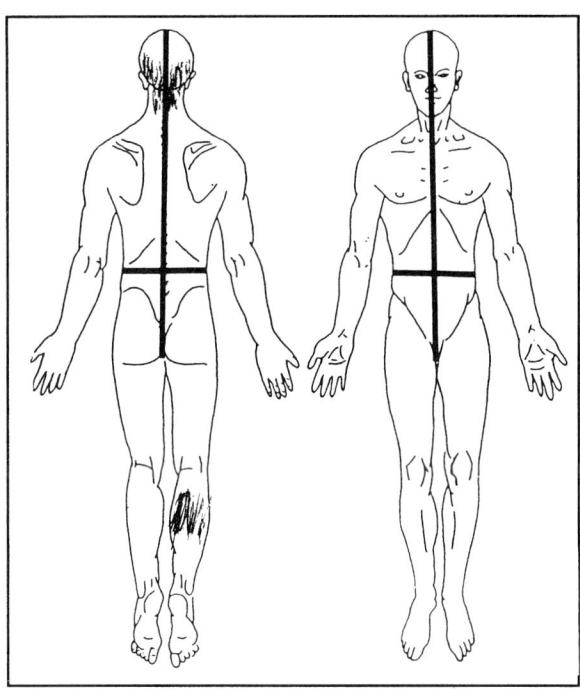

A.

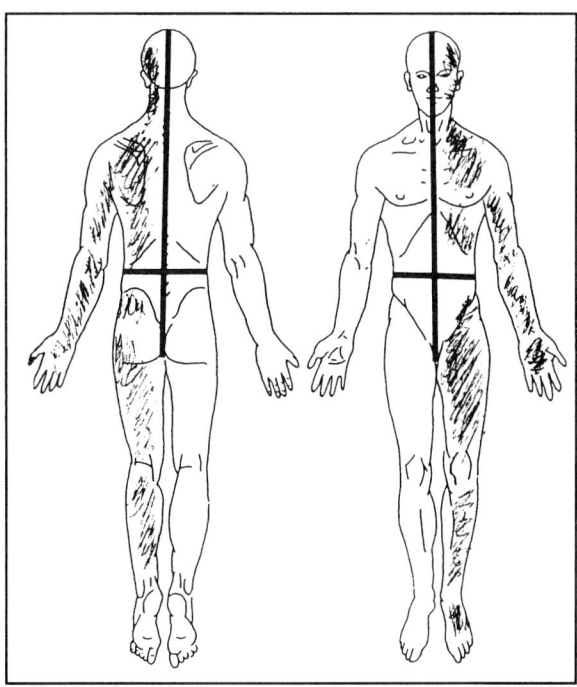

B.

Figure 4.1.5. Drawing A shows that a patient with body pain over a small proportion of her body can meet the ACR criterion for widespread pain. Drawing B shows that a patient with pain over a large total proportion of her body may not meet the ACR criterion.

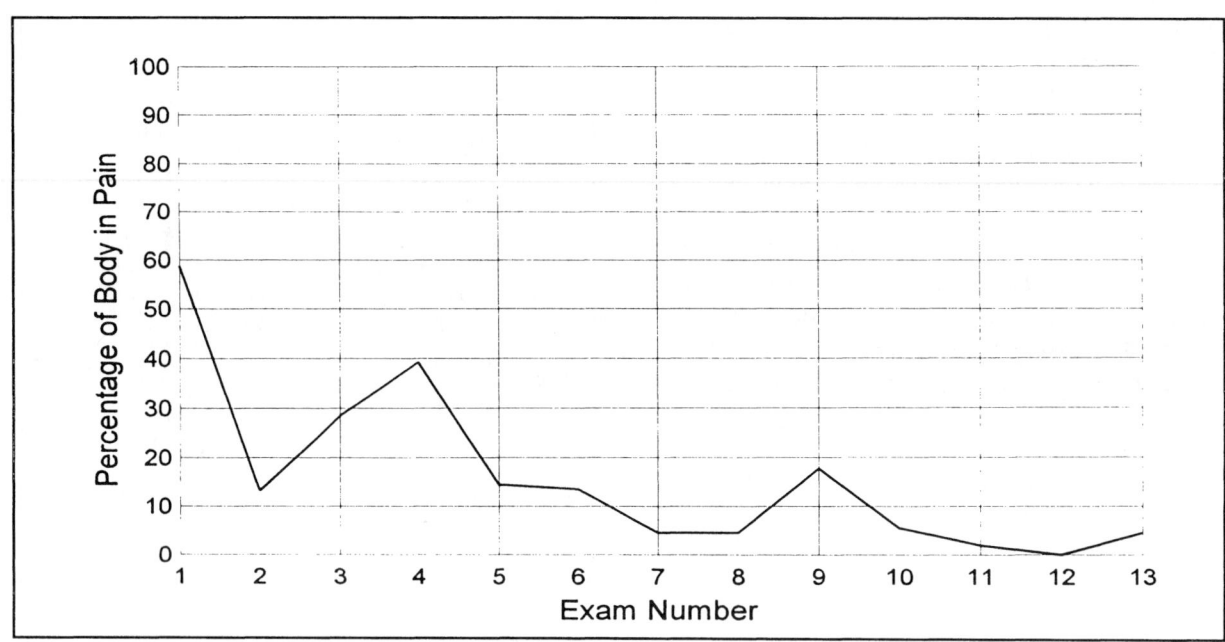

Figure 4.1.6. Line graph depicting the scores over time for pain distribution.

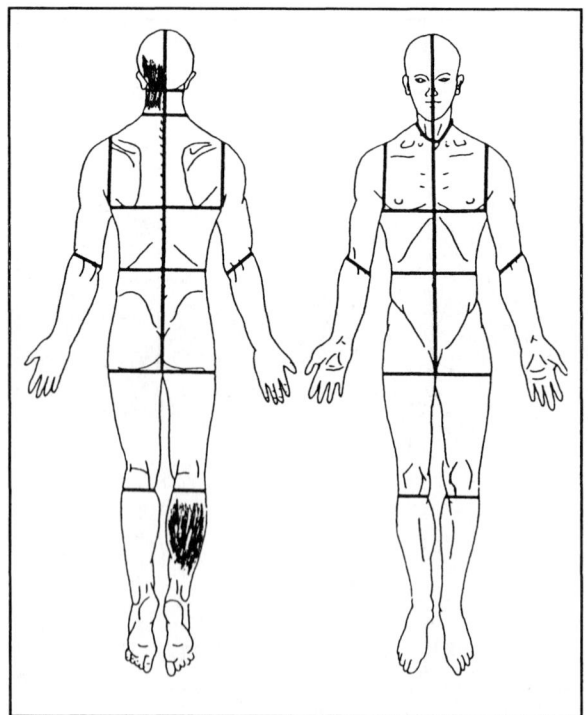

Figure 4.1.7A. Drawing shows how a patient can meet the ACR criterion for widespread pain, yet have pain in only 4.5% of the 36 body divisions.

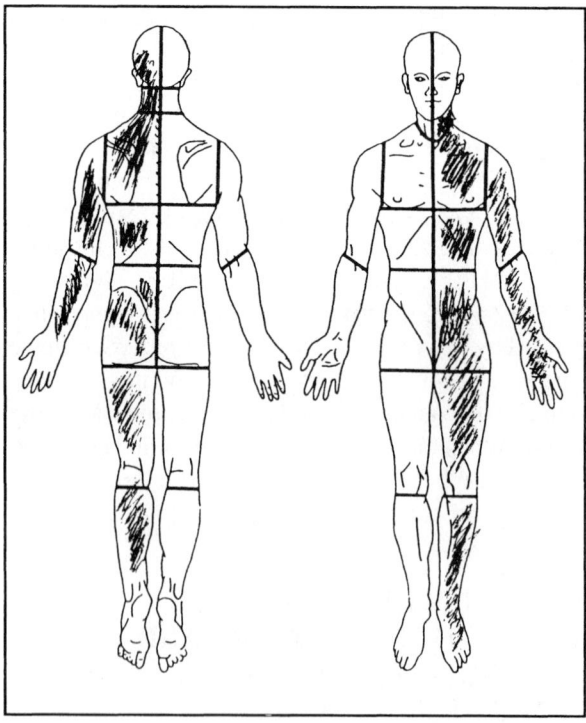

Figure 4.1.7B. The patient does not meet the ACR criterion, yet she has pain in a much larger proportion of her body, 49.5% of the 36 divisions.

● DIFFERENTIATING FIBROMYALGIA FROM OTHER CONDITIONS WITH SIMILAR CLINICAL FEATURES

The symptoms of several conditions can resemble those of fibromyalgia. These conditions include myofascial pain syndrome, arthritis, polymyalgia rheumatica, myopathy not related to hypothyroidism, diabetic polyneuropathies, ankylosing spondylitis, disk herniation, and cardiac or pleural pain. It is important to determine whether the patient's symptoms are caused by one or more of these other conditions so that the treatment the patient undergoes is appropriate to the condition. Many fibromyalgia researchers consider hypothyroidism a condition to be distinguished from fibromyalgia because the features of hypothyroidism appear to be those of fibromyalgia. The appearance of hypothyroidism in about half of fibromyalgia patients is in fact not merely appearance: the features termed fibromyalgia in these patients are a manifestation of thyroid hormone deficiency (see Appendix B, paper titled "Thyroid Status of 38 Fibromyalgia Patients: Implications for the Etiology of Fibromyalgia," and abstract titled "Thyroid Status of Fibromyalgia Patients").

MYOFASCIAL PAIN SYNDROME

Travell and Simons write that they agree with other authors[35][36][37][38][39][40][41][42] that myofascial pain syndrome and fibromyalgia are separate conditions clinically distinguishable from one another.[34,p.545] They also point out that an acute myofascial pain syndrome can easily be differentiated from fibromyalgia, but this is not always true of *chronic* myofascial pain syndrome.[34,p.546] This opinion applies especially to chronic *multi-muscle* syndromes. Table 4.1.7 shows the distinctions Travell and Simons made between chronic myofascial pain syndrome and fibromyalgia.

OTHER CONDITIONS TO DIFFERENTIATE FROM FIBROMYALGIA

Yunus listed seven conditions that might be confused with fibromyalgia.[23,pp.13,28] While the clinician can diagnose fibromyalgia by its own features, concomitant conditions should also be properly diagnosed and managed. Six of the conditions Yunus listed re-

quire only brief mention. But one, hypothyroidism, deserves more lengthy comment.

Arthritis
Yunus pointed out that a patient may complain of joint pain and subjective swelling. But when pain and subjective swelling are part of the patient's fibromyalgia, she will not have the objective joint swelling of true arthritis.

Table 4.1.3. The most common symptoms associated with fibromyalgia.*

SYMPTOM	% OF PATIENTS WITH THE SYMPTOM
Widespread pain	97.6
Fatigue	81.4
Morning stiffness >15 min.	77.0
Sleep disturbance	74.6
Paresthesias	62.8
Headache	52.8
Anxiety	47.8
Sensation of swelling	47.0
Dysmenorrhea history	40.6
Sicca symptoms	35.8
Prior depression	31.5
Irritable bowel syndrome	29.6
Urinary urgency	26.3
Raynaud's symptoms	16.7
Female urethral syndrome †	12.0
Cognitive dysfunction ‡	—

*After: Wolfe, F.: Diagnosis of fibromyalgia. *J. Musculoskeletal Med.*, 7:54, 1990.[7]
†Yunus, M.B. and Masi, A.T.: Fibromyalgia, restless legs syndrome, periodic limb movement disorder, and psychogenic pain. In *Arthritis and Allied Conditions: A Textbook of Rheumatology*. Edited by D.J. McCarty, Jr. and W.J. Koopman, Philadelphia, Lea & Febiger, 1992, pp.1383-1405.[28]
‡Nielson, W.R., Grace, G.M., Hopkins, M., and Berg, M.: Concentration and memory deficits in patients with fibromyalgia syndrome. *J. Musculoskeletal Pain*, 3(Suppl.1):123, 1995.[54]
NOTE: The reported frequency of different symptoms varies according to source.

Polymyalgia Rheumatica
A patient may report diffuse muscle aching and stiffness and general fatigue and weakness. When these symptoms are features of the patient's fibromyalgia, she will not have the elevated erythrocyte sedimentation rate, low hemoglobin, and weight loss characteristic of polymyalgia rheumatica.

Myopathy

The fibromyalgia patient typically perceives muscle weakness and fatigue. When these symptoms are due to myopathy, the patient will have elevated muscle enzymes and weakness that the clinician can objectively confirm.

Table 4.1.4. Differences in mean symptom intensity (0-to-10 point visual analog scale) between placebo and T_3 phases, and the amount of reduced intensity.*

PATIENT NUMBER	PLACEBO SCORE	T_3 SCORE	DIFFERENCE
Patients who did not significantly improve:			
1	6.39	4.08	2.31
2	0.77	1.62	0.85
Patients who did significantly improve:			
3	6.69	0.77	5.92
4	6.81	0.41	6.40
5	4.69	2.39	2.30
6	7.23	1.77	5.46
7	7.39	2.00	5.39

*Lowe, J.C., Garrison, R., Reichman, A., Yellin, J., Thompson, M., and Kaufman, D.: Effectiveness and safety of T_3 therapy for euthyroid fibromyalgia: a double-blind placebo-controlled crossover study. *Clin. Bull. Myofascial Ther.*, 2(2/3):31-57,1997.[8]

Some fibromyalgia patients, however, are likely to have myopathy due to inadequate thyroid hormone regulation of transcription. In many patients, abnormal muscle function is the predominant feature of hypothyroidism and is termed Hoffman's syndrome. The patient commonly complains of stiffness and slight discomfort in the large muscles, and movement is mildly painful. The patient may also have muscle cramping and aching.[43,p.1027] Hypothyroid myopathy can involve the respiratory muscles, thereby contributing to the dyspnea and easy fatigability seen in fibromyalgia patients. The myopathy can slow both muscle contraction and relaxation, causing the sluggish Achilles reflex common among fibromyalgia patients. The mechanism of hypothyroid myopathy has not been determined.[44,p.997]

Plasma creatine kinase is increased in hypothyroid patients whose muscles are significantly affected. In one study, creatine kinase levels for normal subjects ranged from 10-to-120 IU/L. For the entire group of hypothyroid patients, the mean was 679 IU/L, but for hypothyroid patients with serous effusions, myopathy, and abnormal biopsies, the mean was 1339 IU/L.[47]

Myopathic muscle abnormalities caused by hypothyroidism are relieved by proper thyroid hormone treatment.[45][46] Khaleeli and Edwards reported that patients' creatine kinase levels return to normal rapidly with thyroid hormone treatment, although muscle strength returns slowly.[48]

Diabetic Polyneuropathies

Peripheral nerves in the diabetic may become involved in polyneuropathy syndromes. The involvement is gradually progressive, diffuse, symmetric, and more distally than proximally distributed (consistent with the metabolic basis). Axonal degeneration is the underlying pathology. The mechanism appears to be poisoning of axons by the accumulation of sorbitol and fructose.[80,p.584]

Glucose enters most cells of the body only when plasma levels of insulin are normal. This is not true of nerve cells. Glucose enters nerve cells even when insulin levels are low. When glucose levels are high in nerve cells, the enzyme aldose reductase produces high concentrations of the sugar sorbitol. The osmotic pressure from the accumulating sorbitol causes nerve cells to swell and can cause nerve cell death.[27,p.684] The swelling can impede axoplasmic transport of substances vital for normal nerve cell function. Decreased provision of these substances can impair metabolic processes in the nerves that are dependent on the substances. Peripheral nerves, starting with their most distal branches, die in a distal-to-proximal direction. The process is diffuse, symmetric, slowly progressive, and most advanced in patients with poor glucose control.[80,pp.584-585]

Brown and Asbury describe five types of pain the patient may experience in diabetic polyneuropathy:

1. The most common type of pain is paresthesias, uncomfortable sensations that the patient may describe as "burning" or "raw" (as occurs in abrasions).
2. Dysesthesias are sensory discomforts that occur with contact and are especially common in the feet. The patient may complain that she feels like she is walking on glass.
3. The most severe form of pain is causalgia. This is pain similar to that of reflex sympathetic dystrophy. Reflex sympathetic dystrophy is a form of dysesthesia in which the slightest touch causes excruciating pain.

4. Deep aching pain may occur in paroxysms, as in neuralgia. The patient may describe it as "burning" or "stabbing."
5. The patient may have painful cramps of the calf or intrinsic foot muscles.[62]

When the patient's pain is especially widespread and chronic, she and the clinician may confuse it with the pain of fibromyalgia.

Foot pain is prominent in diabetic polyneuropathy when the unmyelinated type-C nerve fibers are more affected. The patient may complain of boring or burning pain that is felt deep in the bones.[80,p.585] Some fibromyalgia patients report similar symptoms. As a feature of fibromyalgia, the pain is worse when the patient tries to walk about after getting out of bed in the morning. For many fibromyalgia patients, the pain diminishes after they are up and about for 15-to-60 minutes. The diabetic patient may complain of diminished sensation in the feet and fingers, and paresthesias of the toes and soles. Examination may show that sensation to light touch, position, and vibration is out of proportion to any loss of temperature and pain sensation in the hands and feet (stocking-and-glove distribution). The Achilles reflex may be slowed to absent[80,pp.585-586] The slowed reflex in a diabetic patient with widespread pain, foot pain upon rising from bed, and hand or foot paresthesias, should raise the question of whether the patient has fibromyalgia. The clinician must bear in mind, however, that the symptoms and findings may also be features of diabetic polyneuropathy. Consultation with a diabetologist may be warranted.

Ankylosing Spondylitis

When back pain and spinal stiffness are associated with fibromyalgia, the patient does not have the sacroiliitis characteristic of ankylosing spondylitis unless the two conditions are concomitant.

Disc Herniation

The fibromyalgia patient may have the sciatic-like pain that can accompany a herniated disc, but the neurologic or imaging findings typical of disc herniation are not features of fibromyalgia.

Cardiac or Pleural Pain

Fibromyalgia patients often complain of chest pain. If the pain is a feature of fibromyalgia, the patients are not likely to have the typical history of true cardiac pain; pleural rub; or positive ECG, laboratory, or chest x-ray findings.

Hypothyroidism

Yunus's list of the conditions to be differentiated from fibromyalgia is generally accurate and potentially useful. With all due respect, however, his consideration of hypothyroidism suggests the same misunderstanding of thyroid function testing that has permitted the thyroid-related mechanisms of many patients' fibromyalgia to elude virtually all fibromyalgia researchers. Yunus correctly pointed out that the fatigue, sensitivity to cold, and muscle pain of fibromyalgia patients is well-known to occur in some hypothyroid patients. But he indicates that if the fibromyalgia patient does not have low T_4 and high TSH levels, she does not have hypothyroidism.[23,p.13]

Table 4.1.5. Symptoms assessed (VAS) and levels of significant difference in T_3 vs placebo phases (all patients).*

SYMPTOMS	SIGNIFICANCE LEVELS
Pain	p=0.002
Fatigue	p=0.001
Stiffness	p=0.002
Headache	p=0.006
Sleep disturbance	p=0.001
Bowel disturbance	p=0.006
Depression	p=0.004
Cognitive dysfunction	p=0.001
Anxiety	p=0.004
Coldness	p=0.011
Paresthesias	p=0.006
Sicca symptoms	p=0.043
Difficulty exercising	p<0.0005

*Lowe, J.C., Garrison, R., Reichman, A., Yellin, J., Thompson, M., and Kaufman, D.: Effectiveness and safety of T_3 therapy for euthyroid fibromyalgia: a double-blind placebo-controlled crossover study. *Clin. Bull. Myofascial Ther.*, 2(2/3):31-57, 1997.[8]

The absence of an elevated TSH level does rule out primary (thyroidal) hypothyroidism in most, although certainly not all, patients. As I have reported elsewhere, a patient may have low-normal T_4 and high-normal TSH, yet with further testing (TRH stimulation test, monitoring for nocturnal TSH surge, or antithyroid antibodies) be found to have primary hypothyroidism that responds dramatically well to thyroid hormone therapy.[49] In fact, in that there is an increase in the future incidence of thyroid disease among patients with TSH levels of 2.0 or more μU/mL,[82] it is contestable whether all fibromyalgia patients with

TSH levels 2.0 μU/mL or above can be pronounced euthyroid. If not—and I think not—the conclusions of researchers that their fibromyalgia study patients with TSH levels of 2.0 μU/mL or above were euthyroid are false.

In addition, basal T_4 and TSH levels do not reveal patients with central hypothyroidism due to pituitary or hypothalamic dysfunction (see Chapter 4.2). I found in a retrospective study of 38 consecutive fibromyalgia patients with complete thyroid function testing that 20 patients (52.6%) had laboratory test results consistent with central (hypothalamic or pituitary) hypothyroidism.[49] In a subsequent prospective study, my colleagues and I evaluated the thyroid status of an additional 54 patients. Results were consistent with euthyroidism in 26 patients (48.1%), primary hypothyroidism in 8 patients (14.8%), and central hypothyroidism in 20 patients (37.0%). We then combined the results of the two studies to determine percentages of the total of 92 patients within each classification of thyroid status. Results were consistent with euthyroidism in 40 patients (43.5%), primary hypothyroidism in 12 patients (13.0%), and central hypothyroidism in 40 patients (43.5%).[56] The laboratory thyroid function tests ordered today by most clinicians provide no indication that any of our patients might have central hypothyroidism. Without the benefit of the TRH stimulation test, these patients would have been considered to be euthyroid (see Chapter 4.2).

Neeck and Riedel reported TRH stimulation test results consistent with central hypothyroidism in all of the 17 fibromyalgia patients they tested. And Ferraccioli and coworkers reported blunted TSH responses to TRH in 5 of 24 fibromyalgia patients (20.8%).[51] Ferraccioli did not report what percentage of his patients had exaggerated TSH responses to TRH.[52] Had he done so, the percentage of patients with results consistent with central hypothyroidism might have been higher.

Bennett wrote of the "anecdotal observations that thyroid dysfunction is not common in patients with fibromyalgia."[50] But the laboratory findings cited above make it exceedingly unlikely that the anecdotal observations Bennett mentioned are correct. Ruling out hypothyroidism in fibromyalgia patients requires a knowledge of proper laboratory test result interpretation. But even when test results show that a patient is euthyroid, an etiological role of inadequate thyroid hormone regulation is not excluded. Most euthyroid fibromyalgia patients appear to have partial cellular resistance to thyroid hormone.

Table 4.1.6. Fibromyalgia measurement results.*

ALL PATIENTS	WORST	BEST	MEAN PLACEBO	MEAN T_3	SIGNIFICANCE
tender points	< 1	> 4	1.94 kg/cm²	3.31 kg/cm²	P<0.0005
pain distribution ACR method	3	0	3.00	1.75	P=0.019
pain distribution % method	100%	0%	48.34%	15.81%	P=0.002
symptom intensities (VASs)	10	0	5.81	1.54	P<0.0005
FIQ	80	0	54.97	13.71	P<0.0005
Zung's	80	20	43.75	31.75	P<0.0005

*Lowe, J.C., Reichman, A., Yellin, J.: The process of change during T_3 treatment for euthyroid fibromyalgia: a double-blind placebo-controlled crossover study. *Clin. Bull. Myofascial Ther.*, 2(2/3):91-124, 1997.[63]

Table 4.1.7. Differentiating between myofascial pain syndrome and fibromyalgia.*

CHARACTERISTIC	MYOFASCIAL PAIN SYNDROME	FIBROMYALGIA
Male/female ratio	Nearly equal.	73%-to-88% female.
Onset of condition	When *acute*, patient can identify time and place. Typically, muscle was subjected to momentary overload or vigorous movement. When *chronic*, patient may have difficulty identifying a precipitating event. More than one muscle is likely to be involved.	Usually develops insidiously.[†]
Palpatory findings	Involved muscles feel tense and is nontender, except at trigger point and in reference zone.	Muscles are diffusely tender, soft and doughy (except in areas of trigger points in taut bands).[‡]
Muscle fatigue	Muscle is weak without atrophy.	Weakness is severe and generalized.
Chronicity	Due to perpetuating factor(s) that are usually correctable.	Inherent to the disease.
Parts of body affected	A focal dysfunction of muscle.	A systemic disease.

*After Travell, J.G. and Simons, D.G.: *Myofascial Pain and Dysfunction: The Trigger Point Manual*, Vol.2. Baltimore, Williams and Wilkins, 1992, p.546. [34]

[†] About one third of fibromyalgia cases appear to be posttraumatic, although the onset of fibromyalgia symptoms may occur weeks after the inciting incident.

[‡] I have found a soft, doughy quality to the myofascial tissues only in patients who have been inactive for a prolonged time due to the severity of fibromyalgia symptoms, and in patients with myxedematous-like swelling that remits with thyroid hormone use (as in hypothyroid patients).

REFERENCES

1. Wolfe, F., Smythe, H.A., Yunus, M.B., et al.: The American College of Rheumatology 1990 criteria for the classification of fibromyalgia: report of the multicenter criteria committee. *Arthritis Rheumatol.*, 33:160-172, 1990.
2. Scudds, R.A.: A comparative study of pain, sleep quality and pain responsiveness in fibrositis and myofascial pain syndrome. *J. Rheumatol.*, 16 (Suppl.19):120-126, 1989.
3. Cott, A., Parkinson, W., Bell, M.J., Adachi, J., Bedard, M., Cividino, A., and Bensen, W.: Interrater reliability of the tender point criterion for fibromyalgia. *J. Rheumatol.*, 19(12):1955-1959, 1992.
4. Granges, G. and Littlejohn, G.: Pressure pain threshold in pain-free subjects, in patients with chronic regional pain syndromes, and in patients with fibromyalgia syndrome. Comment in: *Arthritis Rheum.*, 36(5):647-650, 1993.
5. Quimby, L.G., Block, S.R., and Gratwick, G.M.: Fibromyalgia: generalized pain intolerance and manifold symptom reporting. *J. Rheumatol.*, 15(8):264-270, 1988.
6. Reilly, P.A. and Littlejohn, G.O.: Diurnal variation in the symptoms and signs of the fibromyalgia syndrome (FS). *J. Musculoskel. Pain*, 1:237-243, 1993.
7. Wolfe, F.: Diagnosis of fibromyalgia. *J. Musculoskel. Med.*, 7:53-69, 1990.
8. Lowe, J.C., Garrison, R.L., Reichman, A.J., Yellin, J., Thompson, M., and Kaufman, D.: Effectiveness and safety of T₃ (triiodothyronine) therapy for euthyroid fibromyalgia: a double-blind, placebo-controlled response-driven crossover study. *Clin. Bull. Myofascial Ther.*, 2 (2/3):31-57, 1997.
9. Mikkelsson, M., Latikka, P., Kautiainen, H., Isomeri, R., and Isomaki. H.: Muscle and bone pressure pain threshold and pain tolerance in fibromyalgia patients and controls. *Arch. Phys. Med. Rehabil.*, 73(9):814-818, 1992.
10. Rasmussen, J.O., Smidth, M., and Hansen, T.M.: Examination of tender points in soft tissue. Palpation versus pressure-algometer. *Ugeskr. Laeger*, 152(21):1522-1526, 1990.
11. Vatine, J.J., Shapira, S.C., Magora, F., Adler, D., and Ma-

gora, A.: Electronic pressure algometry of deep pain in healthy volunteers. *Arch. Phys. Med. Rehabil.*, 74(5):526-530, 1993.

12. Antonaci, F., Bovim, G., Fasano, M.L., Bonamico, L., and Shen, J.M.: Pain threshold in humans: a study with the pressure algometer. *Funct. Neurol.*, 7(4):283-288, 1992.

13. Hogeweg, J.A., Langereis, M.J., Bernards, A.T., Faber, J.A., and Helders, P.J.: Algometry. Measuring pain threshold: method and characteristics in healthy subjects. *Scand. J. Rehabil. Med.*, 24(2):99-103, 1992.

14. Takala, E.P.: Pressure pain threshold on upper trapezius and levator scapulae muscles: repeatability and relation to subjective symptoms in a working population. *Scand. J. Rehabil. Med.*, 22(2):63-68, 1990.

15. List, T., Helkimo, M., and Karlsson, R.: Influence of pressure rates on the reliability of a pressure threshold meter. *J. Craniomandib. Disord.*, 5(3):173-178, 1991.

16. Chung, S.C., Um, B.Y., and Kim, H.S.: Evaluation of pressure pain threshold in head and neck muscles by electronic algometer: intrarater and interrater reliability. *Cranio*, 10(1):28-34, 1992.

17. Fischer, A.A.: Pressure algometry over normal muscles: Standard values, validity and reproducibility of pressure threshold. *Pain*, 30(1):115-126, 1987.

18. Croft, P., Burt, J., Scholium, J., and Silman, A.: Number of tender points and extent of reported pain: a linear relationship? Annual meeting: Am. Coll. Rheumatol. and Assoc. Rheumatol. Health Prof., Minneapolis, Oct. 23-27, 1994.

19. Lautenschlager, J., Seglias, J., Bruckle, W., and Muller, W.: Comparisons of spontaneous pain and tenderness in patients with primary fibromyalgia. *Clin. Rheumatol.*, 10 (2):168-173, 1991.

20. Yunus, M.B.: Primary fibromyalgia (fibrositis): clinical study of 50 patients with matched normal controls. *Semin. Arthritis Rheum.*, 11:151-171, 1981.

21. Smythe, H.A.: Non-articular rheumatism and fibrositis. In *Arthritis and Allied Conditions: A Textbook of Rheumatology.* Edited by D.J. McCarty, Philadelphia, Lea & Febiger, 1972, pp.874-884.

22. Smythe, H.A.: Non-articular rheumatism and psychogenic musculoskeletal syndromes. In *Arthritis and Allied Conditions: A Textbook of Rheumatology.* Edited by D.J. McCarty, Philadelphia, Lea & Febiger, 1979, pp.881-891.

23. Yunus, M.B.: Fibromyalgia syndrome and myofascial pain syndrome: clinical features, laboratory tests, diagnosis, and pathophysiologic mechanisms. In *Myofascial Pain and Fibromyalgia: Trigger Point Management.* Edited by E.S. Rachlin, St. Louis, Mosby, 1994, pp.3-29.

24. Smythe, H.A.: Relation between fibrositic and control tenderness: effects of dolorimeter scale length and footplate size. *J. Rheumatol.*, 19:284-289, 1992.

25. Smythe, H.A.: Control and fibrositic tenderness: comparison of two dolorimeters. *J. Rheumatol.*, 19:768-771, 1992.

26. Fischer, A.A.: Pressure algometry (dolorimetry) in the differential diagnosis of muscle pain. In *Myofascial Pain and Fibromyalgia: Trigger Point Management.* Edited by E.S. Rachlin, St. Louis, Mosby, 1994, pp.121-141.

27. Chandrasoma, P. and Taylor, C.R.: *Concise Pathology.* Norwalk, Appleton & Lange, 1991.

28. Yunus, M.B. and Masi, A.T.: Fibromyalgia, restless legs syndrome, periodic limb movement disorder, and psychogenic pain. In *Arthritis and Allied Conditions: A Textbook of Rheumatology.* Edited by D.J. McCarty, Jr. and W.J. Koopman, Philadelphia, Lea & Febiger, 1992, pp.1383-1405.

29. Althaus, B.U., Staub, J-J., De Leche, A.R., Oberhansli, A., and Stahelin, H.B.: LDL/HDL changes in subclinical hypothyroidism: possible risk factors for coronary heart disease. *Clin. Endocrinol.*, 28:157, 1988.

30. Phalen, G.S.: The carpal tunnel syndrome: 17 years experience in diagnosis and treatment of 654 hands. *J. Bone Joint Surg.*, (AM), 48:211, 1966.

31. Whybrow, P.C. and Prange, A.J.: A hypothesis of thyroid-catecholamine-receptor interaction: its relevance to affective illness. *Arch. Gen. Psychiatry*, 38:108, 1981.

32. Kazdan, A.E.: Methodological and interpretive problems of single case experimental designs. *J. Consult. Clin. Psychol.*, 46:629-642, 1978.

33. Parsonson, B.S. and Baer, D.M.: The analysis and presentation of graphic data. In *Single Subject Research: Strategies for Evaluating Change.* Edited by E.R. Kratochwill, New York, Academic Press, 1978.

34. Travell, J.G. and Simons, D.G.: *Myofascial Pain and Dysfunction: The Trigger Point Manual*, Vol.2. Baltimore, Williams and Wilkins, 1992.

35. Campbell, S.M.: Regional myofascial pain syndromes. In *The Fibromyalgia Syndrome: Rheumatic Clinics of North America*, Vol. 15. Edited by R.M. Bennett and D.L. Goldenberg, Philadelphia, W.B. Saunders, 1989, pp.31-44.

36. Bennett, R.M.: Myofascial pain syndromes and the fibromyalgia syndrome: a comparative analysis. In *Advances in Pain Research and Therapy: Myofascial Pain and Fibromyalgia*, Vol. 17. Edited by J.R. Fricton and E.A. Awad, New York, Raven Press, 1990, pp.43-65.

37. Hench, P.K.: Evaluation and differential diagnosis of fibromyalgia: approach to diagnosis and management. In *The Fibromyalgia Syndrome: Rheumatic Clinics of North America*, Vol. 15. Edited by R.M. Bennett and D.L. Goldenberg, Philadelphia, W.B. Saunders, 1989, pp.19-29.

38. Scudds, R.A., Trachsel, L.C., Luckhurst, B.J., and Percy, J.S.: A comparative study of pain, sleep quality, and pain responsiveness in fibrositis and myofascial pain syndrome. *J. Rheumatol.*, 19(Suppl.):120-126, 1989.

39. Sheon, R.P., Moskowitz, R.W., and Goldberg, D.M.: *Soft Tissue Rheumatic Pain*, 2nd edition. Philadelphia, Lea and Febiger, 1987.

40. Yunus, M.B., Kalyan-Raman, U.P., and Kalyan-Raman, K.: Primary fibromyalgia syndrome and myofascial pain syndrome: clinical features and muscle pathology. *Arch. Phys. Med. Rehabil.*, 69:451-454, 1988.

41. Wolfe, F.: Fibrositis, fibromyalgia, and musculoskeletal disease: the current status of the fibrositis syndrome. *Arch. Phys. Med. Rahabil.*, 69:527-531, 1988.

42. Wolfe, F., Simons, D.G., Fricton, J.R., et al.: The fibromyalgia and myofascial pain syndromes: a study of tender points and trigger points in persons with fibromyalgia, myofascial pain syndromes, and no disease. *Arthritis Rheum.*, 33(Suppl):S137, Abstract No. D22, 1990.

43. DeLong, G.R. and Adams, R.D.: The neuromuscular system and brain in hypothyroidism. In *The Thyroid: A Fundamental and Clinical Text*, 6th edition. Edited by L.E.

Braverman and R.D. Utiger, Philadelphia, J.B. Lippincott Co., 1991, pp.1027-1039.

44. Ingbar, D.H.: The respiratory system in hypothyroidism. In *The Thyroid: A Fundamental and Clinical Text*, 6th edition. Edited by L.E. Braverman and R.D. Utiger, Philadelphia, J.B. Lippincott Co., 1991, pp.993-1001.

45. Pearce, J. and Aziz, H.: The neuromyopathy of hypothyroidism: some new observations. *J. Neurol. Sci.*, 9:243, 1969.

46. Riggs, J.E.: Acute exertional rhabdomyolysis in hypothyroidism: the result of a reversible defect in glycogenolysis? *Milit. Med.*, 155:171, 1990.

47. Khaleeli, A.A., Griffith, D.G., and Edwards, R.H.: The clinical presentation of hypothyroid myopathy and its relationships to abnormalities in structure and function of skeletal muscle. *Clin. Endocrinol.* (Oxf), 19:365, 1983.

48. Khaleeli, A.A. and Edwards, R.H.: Effect of treatment on muscle dysfunction in hypothyroidism. *Clin. Sci.*, 66:63, 1984.

49. Lowe, J.C.: Thyroid status of 38 fibromyalgia patients: implications for the etiology of fibromyalgia. *Clin. Bull. Myofascial Ther.*, 2(1):47-64, 1997.

50. Bennett, R.M.: Literature reviews: fibromyalgia. *J. Musculoskel. Pain*, 2(2):101-112, 1994.

51. Neeck, G. and Riedel, W.: Thyroid function in patients with fibromyalgia syndrome. *J. Rheum.*, 19:1120-1122, 1992.

52. Ferraccioli, G., Cavalieri, F., Salaffi, F., Fontana, S., Scita, F., Nolli, M., and Maestri, D.: Neuroendocrinologic findings in primary fibromyalgia (soft tissue chronic pain syndrome) and in other chronic rheumatic conditions (rheumatoid arthritis, low back pain). *J. Rheum.*, 17:869-873, 1990.

53. Joos, E., Meeusen, R., and De Meirleir, K.: Measurement of physical capacity in fibromyalgia. *J. Musculoskel. Pain*, 3(Suppl.1):87, 1995.

54. Nielson, W.R., Grace, G.M., Hopkins, M., and Berg, M.: Concentration and memory deficits in patients with fibromyalgia syndrome. *J. Musculoskel. Pain*, 3(Suppl.1):123, 1995.

55. Scott, J. and Huskisson, E.C.: Graphic representation of pain. *Pain*, 2:175-184, 1976.

56. Lowe, J.C., Reichman, A., Honeyman, G.S., and Yellin, J.: Thyroid status of fibromyalgia patients (Abstract). *Clin. Bull. Myofascial Ther.*, 3(1):69-70, 1998.

57. Littlejohn, G.O.: A database for fibromyalgia. *Rheum. Dis. Clinics North Am.*, 21(2):527-557, 1995.

58. Wilkins, E.W., Dineen, J.J., Moncure, A.C., Gross, P.L., and Fitzgerald, C.P.: *MGH Textbook of Emergency Medicine*, 2nd edition. Baltimore, Williams & Wilkins, 1983, pp.624-627.

59. O'Boyle, C.M., Davis, D.K., Russo, B.A., Kraf, T.J., and Brick, P.D.: *Emergency Care: The First 24 Hours.* Norwalk, Appleton-Century-Crofts, 1985, pp.332-333.

60. Fischer, A.A., DeCosta, C., and Levy, H.: Diagnosis of fibromyalgia by manual pressure is unreliable: quantification of tender point sensitivity by algometer is necessary in clinical practice. *J. Musculoskel. Pain*, 3(1):139, 1995.

61. Putick, M., Schulzer, M., Klinkhoff, A., Koehler, B., Rangno, K., and Chalmers, A.: Reliability and reproducibility of fibromyalgic tenderness, measurement by electronic and mechanical dolorimeters. *J. Musculoskel. Pain*, 3(4):3-14, 1995.

62. Brown, M.J. and Asbury, A.K.: Diabetic neuropathy. *Ann. Neurol.*, 15:2-12, 1984.

63. Lowe, J.C., Reichman, A., and Yellin, J.: The process of change during T₃ treatment for euthyroid fibromyalgia: a double-blind placebo-controlled crossover study. *Clin. Bull. Myofascial Ther.*, 2(2/3):91-124, 1997.

64. Bennett, R.M.: Literature reviews. *J. Musculoskel. Pain*, 2(2):101-112, 1994.

65. Jacobs, J.W., Rasker, J.J., van der Heide, A., et al.: Lack of correlation between the mean tender point score and self-reported pain in fibromyalgia. *Arthritis Care Res.*, 9:105-111, 1996.

66. Burckhardt, C.S., Clark, S.R., and Bennett, R.M.: The fibromyalgia impact questionnaire: development and validation. *J. Rheumatol.*, 18(5):728-733, 1991.

67. Zung, W.W.K.: A self-rating depression scale. *Arch. Gen. Psychiatry*, 12:65-70, 1965.

68. Naughton, M.J. and Wiklund, I.: A critical review of dimension-specific measures of health-related quality of life in cross-cultural research. *Quality Life Res*, 2(6):397-432, 1993.

69. Rehm, L.P.: Assessment of depression. In *Behavioral Assessment: A Practical Handbook*. Edited by M. Hersen and A.S. Bellack, Oxford, Permagon Press, 1976, pp.246-295.

70. Smythe, H.A.: Discussion of tender points. *J. Musculoskel. Pain*, 2(3):37-39, 1994.

71. Wade, J.B., Price, D.D., Hamer, R.M., Schwartz, S.M., and Hart, R.P.: An emotional component analysis of chronic pain. *Pain*, 40:303-310, 1990.

72. Harkins, S.W., Price, D.D., and Braith, J.: Effects of extraversion and neuroticism on experimental pain, clinical pain, and illness behavior. *Pain*, 36:209-218, 1989.

73. Wallenstein, S.L., Heidrich, G., III, Kaiko, R., and Houde, R.W.: Clinical evaluation of mild analgesics: the measurement of clinical pain. *Brit. J. Clin. Pharm.*, 10:319S-327S, 1980.

74. Seymour, R.A.: The use of pain scales in assessing the efficacy of analgesics in post-operative dental pain. *Eur. J. Clin. Pharm. Therapeut.*, 34:441-444, 1982.

75. Price, D.D., von der Gruen, A., Miller, J., Rafii, A., and Price, C.: A psychophysical analysis of morphine analgesia. *Pain*, 22:261-269, 1985.

76. Price, D.D., Harkins, S.W., Rafii, A., and Price, C.: A simultaneous comparison of fentanyl's analgesic effects on experimental and clinical pain. *Pain*, 24:197-203, 1986.

77. Lowe, J.C., Eichelberger, J., Manso, G., and Peterson, K.: Improvement in euthyroid fibromyalgia patients treated with T₃ (triiodothyronine). *J. Myofascial Ther.*, 1(2):16-29, 1994.

78. Lowe, J.C.: T₃-induced recovery from fibromyalgia by a hypothyroid patient resistant to T₄ and desiccated thyroid. *J. Myofascial Ther.*, 1(4):26-31, 1995.

79. Smythe, H.A., Buskila, D., and Gladman, D.: Performance of scored palpation, a point count, and dolorimetry in assessing unsuspected nonarticular tenderness. *J. Rheumatol.*, 20(2):352-357, 1993.

80. Bernat, J.L. and Vincent, F.M.: *Neurology: Problems in Primary Care*, 2nd edition. Los Angeles, PMIC, 1993.

81. Wigers, S.H., Skrondal, A., Finset, A., and Götestam, K.G.: Measuring change in fibromyalgic pain: the relevance of pain distribution. *J. Musculoskel. Pain*, 5(2):29-41, 1997.

82. Weetman, A.P.: Hypothyroidism: screening and subclinical disease. *Brit. Med. J.*, 314:1175, 1997.

4.2

Laboratory Evaluation of Thyroid Status

Thyroid status refers to the functional adequacy of the thyroid gland. In clinical practice, thyroid status is most often inferred from the circulating thyroid hormone and TSH levels measured by laboratory tests. The TRH-stimulation test may be used to assess the functional status of the thyrotroph cells of the anterior pituitary, measured as changes in the circulating TSH level. Occasionally, the functional status of the thyroid gland is also assessed during the TRH-stimulating test by changes in circulating thyroid hormone levels.

Classifying the fibromyalgia patient according to thyroid status therefore depends on the results of laboratory thyroid function tests. In conventional practice, the patient's tissue metabolic status is inferred from the results of thyroid function laboratory tests. While in some cases the inference may be correct, thyroid status and metabolic status are not reliably correlated. Thus, the hypothesis that clinicians can generally infer metabolic status from thyroid status is false. It is imperative for humane purposes that clinicians abandon the use of such inferences in the care of their patients.

The clinician can generally establish the patient's thyroid status from the results of a profile of thyroid function tests. The clinician has the option of two commonly used profiles. One profile includes a T_4 RIA, T_3 uptake, T_7 (free thyroxine index), and a basal TSH. The second profile contains a free T_4 and basal TSH. With the results of the tests of either of these profiles, the clinician should be able to identify patients with probable primary (thyroidal) hypothyroidism. If the test results do not indicate primary hypothyroidism, the clinician should perform or order a TRH-stimulation test. The results of this test will be consistent with, but not prove, either euthyroidism or central hypothyroidism. A blunted or exaggerated TSH response is consistent with, but does not conclusively demonstrate, central hypothyroidism. Low free T_3 and free T_4 levels and the clinical features of hypothyroidism support the diagnosis of possible central hypothyroidism.

A mandate of conventional endocrinology (see abstract and introduction to Chapter 5.3) is that the patient whose TSH level is within the conventional normal range of around 0.4-to-5.0 µU/mL should not be permitted to use exogenous thyroid hormone. Many clinicians today, however, reject this mandate on clinical grounds—they have found that many patients benefit from the use of exogenous thyroid hormone despite having mid-range to high-normal TSH values before beginning thyroid hormone therapy. A recently published 20-year follow-up study provides scientific justification for these clinicians' rejection of the conventional TSH range of normal. The study showed that patients with TSH levels between 2.0 and 4.5 µU/mL had an increased risk of future hypothyroidism. This finding indicates that thyroid disease is so common that people predisposed to hypothyroidism or with incipient hypothyroidism are included in the reference populations of laboratories. As a result, these individuals' TSH values contaminate the upper half of the

95% reference interval, creating a falsely broad range of "normal." The finding also suggests that patients taking replacement dosages of thyroid hormone (those that permit patients' TSH levels to remain between 2.0 and 4.5 µU/mL) are being inadequately treated. These patients are also at risk for diseases of hypometabolism such as cardiovascular disease.

Among hypothyroid fibromyalgia patients, virtually none significantly improve or recover with thyroid hormone dosages that do not suppress patients' TSH levels. This finding necessitates that, after initially establishing the patient's thyroid status, the clinician titrate thyroid hormone dosage according to clinical indicators, not TSH levels (see Chapter 4.3). It is urgent and imperative that conventional endocrinology reassess its fundamental assumptions about the diagnosis and treatment of hypothyroid patients and revamp its standards of practice.

The TRH-stimulation test does not differentiate central hypothyroidism due to pituitary dysfunction from that due to hypothalamic dysfunction. A blunted TSH response (subnormal increase in TSH) following the injection of TRH suggests pituitary hypothyroidism. In most cases, the differentiation between hypothalamic and pituitary dysfunction—and in fact the diagnosis of central hypothyroidism—require further evidence. This evidence may include (1) a lesion detected upon imaging of the hypothalamus or pituitary, (2) hypothalamic or pituitary hormone abnormalities in addition to an abnormal TSH response to TRH, or (3) a molecular lesion such as a nucleotide substitution or deletion identified by gene sequencing. (Verification of such molecular lesions depends on gene testing not readily available to most practicing clinicians.) If the TRH-stimulation test is not available, the patient may have to undergo a trial of metabolic treatment with thyroid hormone without a differential diagnosis.

Thyroid antibody tests provide evidence of an autoimmune mechanism of abnormal thyroid gland function. These tests do not assess the functional status of the thyroid gland. For purposes of case management, however, functional status of the gland may in some cases be inferred from the test results.

The only cause of peripheral cellular resistance to thyroid hormone that can be determined by standard laboratory tests is decreased conversion of T_4 to T_3 (see Chapter 2.6 for laboratory results in other types of thyroid hormone resistance). The pattern of laboratory test values indicating decreased conversion are a high reverse-T_3, low or low-normal T_3, and high or high-normal T_4. If a high circulating or 24-hour urin-

ary cortisol level is present with this pattern, this may indicate cortisol-induced decreased T_4 to T_3 conversion. A normal cortisol level, however, does not decrease the likelihood of the diagnosis because decreased conversion may be a product of other mechanisms (such as a selenium deficiency or mercury toxicity). Impaired conversion, of T_4 to T_3, however, is rare. There is no scientific or clinical evidence that it ever occurs on a chronic basis.

Laboratory thyroid function tests enable clinicians to determine with considerable reliability the functional status of the thyroid gland. The functional status of the gland is referred to in abbreviated form as "thyroid status." The classifications of thyroid status refer to whether a patient's thyroid gland produces a normal, subnormal, or supranormal amount of thyroid hormone. That a patient has normal circulating levels of T_4 or T_3 does not mean, however, that she has enough of the hormones to insure normal tissue metabolism. Whether particular levels of circulating thyroid hormones are adequately maintaining tissue metabolic status can only be determined through assessing various metabolic indicators. The most useful indicators are symptoms, signs, and peripheral indices typical of altered thyroid status. Their absence indicates that tissue metabolism is sufficient, and their presence and severity indicate abnormal tissue metabolism. The symptoms, signs, and peripheral indices of value in the care of fibromyalgia patients are those that indicate inadequate thyroid hormone regulation of cell function (see Chapter 4.3).

● CLINICAL INDICATORS: INDISPENSABLE FOR ASSESSING THYROID STATUS

Before discussing individual laboratory thyroid function tests, it is important to put their use into proper clinical perspective. To do so, we must consider the advent of laboratory tests of thyroid function, extremist technocracy in medicine, the constituents of a more rational approach to diagnosis, and the advice of several medical authors.

ADVENT AND VALUE OF LABORATORY THYROID FUNCTION TESTS

From the time of the first successful treatment with

thyroid substance in 1891[13] until the early 1970s, most clinicians depended on clinical indicators (symptoms, signs, and peripheral indices thought to result from hypothyroidism) to decide which patients might benefit from the use of thyroid hormone. They also used these indicators to titrate the patients' dosages of thyroid hormone.

It was not possible, however, to actually determine which patients had low circulating thyroid hormone levels until the protein bound iodine test (PBI) came into use around 1940.[14,p.136] The PBI was the earliest test of circulating thyroid hormone levels.[15,p.763] The test is an estimate of the plasma level of thyroid hormones after the patient takes a dose of radioactive iodine 131I or 132I (measured by a directional scintillation counter), and by inference, of thyroid hormone transport proteins. The half-life of 131I is 8 days, and that of 132I is 2-to-3 days; the normal range 11%-to-33%. In thyrotoxicosis, about 90% of values are above normal, and in hypothyroidism, about 80% are below normal.[15,pp.762-763] Later, clinicians began testing the rate that the thyroid gland took up radioactive iodine (131I).

Until laboratory tests became available, it was simply impossible to determine whether a patient's hypothyroid-like symptoms, signs, and peripheral indices were actually due to low circulating thyroid hormone levels. Because of this, laboratory test results are essential in determining a patient's thyroid status. (See Chapter 2.5, subsections titled "Pursuit of Objective Confirmation That Non-specific Symptoms Are Thyroid-Related" and "Laboratory Thyroid Function Tests.")

EXTREMIST MEDICAL TECHNOCRACY AND THYROID FUNCTION TESTING

Of all endocrine radioimmunoassay tests done in 1983, 56% were for evaluation of thyroid function.[17] This led Mitchell to write, "The impressive volume of thyroid function tests indicates that physicians are placing increasingly more reliance on the laboratory to diagnose thyroid disease."[18,p.35] By the time Mitchell wrote this statement in 1986, clinicians were a good 10 years into a trend that undoubtedly has been detrimental to untold numbers of patients being evaluated and treated for thyroid hormone deficiencies. This pernicious trend entails clinicians abandoning evaluation of the patient's clinical status (symptoms, signs, and peripheral measures) and depending exclusively on thyroid function test results to prescribe, not to prescribe, or adjust thyroid hormone dosage.

Many conventional clinicians, particularly many endocrinologists, consider laboratory tests sufficient to determine both thyroid and metabolic status. Exemplifying this trend is Shlossberg's statement that he determines the "metabolic state" by measuring serum thyroid hormone levels.[20] Astonishingly, this is reiterated by some authorities of the highest echelon in thyroidology in such statements as: "Resin uptake tests done using labeled thyroxine automatically correct for this defect [abnormal protein binding of thyroid hormone] and *give a normal interpretation of the metabolic status*, as do assays of free T4 [italics mine]."[21,p.6]

It is important for clinicians to understand that thyroid function blood tests *do not* assess the patient's metabolism. (Some authorities might argue that thyroid hormone levels are a measure of the metabolic status of the thyroid gland and that the TSH level is a measure of the metabolic status of the thyrotroph cells of the anterior pituitary. However, since the levels may be influenced by other factors, such as the liver clearance of the hormones, the clinician must be cautious in making inferences about the metabolic status of the thyroid gland and pituitary based on hormone levels.) Neither Shlossberg nor the thyroidologist I referenced above mention using methods that actually assess tissue metabolic status. The practitioner who restricts himself solely to the results of laboratory tests in diagnosis and treatment is extremist; he practices as a pseudo-accountant and treats patients as quasi-spreadsheets.

Abandonment of Clinical Indicators and Clinical Judgment

Barnes wrote that after the PBI and other laboratory tests of thyroid function became available, ". . . the era of the laboratory had begun."[14,p.136] He described the extremist advocacy of these tests by many physicians. "The result was a pendulum-like swing to an extreme. Many physicians came to look upon the results of laboratory tests as absolutes. If a patient was hypothyroid, the laboratory was the place to determine so. If laboratory tests failed to indicate hypothyroidism, it could not be present—no matter the patient's symptoms or even if a patient was already on thyroid therapy and benefitting from it. Willy-nilly, if the lab report came back negative for low thyroid function, the patient got no thyroid therapy, and if the patient was already on it he or she was taken off it." Barnes also wrote that in 1967, Herbert Selenkow of Harvard began publicizing the unreliability of the PBI. The lack of reliability of the test prompts an ominous realization: For almost 30 years, some extremist technocratic physicians based their clinical decisions on undependable numbers on lab reports, and the "beneficiaries" of those decisions were the physicians' patients. The proper dosage of thyroid hormone has potent health-inducing effects; taking too little thyroid hormone when it is needed diminishes the potential benefits; taking no thyroid hormone when it is needed can have devastating consequences. Considering these three facts, how do we begin to calculate the cumulative harm done to the patients over that 30-year span by these technocratic physicians?

Irrelevance of the High Sensitivity of TSH Assays in Diagnosing and Treating Hypothyroidism

Today, conventional thyroidologists argue that all that is needed to diagnose hypothyroidism and titrate the thyroid hormone dosage of the hypothyroid patients is to measure the TSH. They buttress their opinion that the test is all that is needed by emphasizing the high sensitivity of the test. The value in the high sensitivity of modern TSH assays, however, is in measuring extremely *low* TSH levels in hyperthyroid patients,[86] not in identifying patients with hypothyroidism. For measuring high-normal or high TSH levels in hypothyroidism, the most recently developed TSH assays have no apparent advantage over the first generation assays used in the early 1970s.

According to the mandates of conventional endocrinology, a value of the highly sensitive TSH assays is in detecting low TSH levels due to the patient's use of excessive dosages of thyroid hormone so that the dosages can be reduced. It is debatable, though, whether the ability of TSH assays to detect low TSH levels is of any practical utility for titrating dosages. Referring to the use of older thyroid function tests, Moses et al. wrote in 1958, "It has been generally assumed that thyroid deficits do not exist if the usual indices such as serum protein bound iodine, iodine trapping, and protein bound iodine conversion ratios are normal." A slight degree of hypothyroidism might still exist, they wrote, even when lab values were normal. They hypothesized that hypothyroidism despite normal lab values might be responsible for some patients' elevated cholesterol and altered lipoprotein partition. To test the hypothesis, they gave full replacement doses of desiccated thyroid for up to 10 months to patients with high cholesterol. Dosages ranged from 2½-to-3 grains per day (TSH-suppressive dosages). Patients' total cholesterol and β-lipoprotein cholesterol dropped significantly. The investigators concluded: "The data indicate that even in subjects euthyroid by the usual indices, a thyroid deficit exerting considerable effect on the cholesterol-lipoprotein partition may be present."[24]

This conclusion is supported by more recent findings. Compared to replacement dosages of thyroid hormone, TSH-suppressive dosages produce significantly improved blood lipid measures, and there is reason to believe that higher-end dosages of thyroid hormone halt the progression of atherosclerosis (see Chapter 4.4, section titled "Improved Cardiovascular Status with Thyroid Hormone Therapy"). In addition, my clinical experience has shown that pain distribution, pain intensity, and the 13 associated fibromyalgia symptoms are relieved only when hypothyroid patients take TSH-suppressive dosages of thyroid hormone. Safety monitoring has shown that these TSH-suppressive dosages are not thyrotoxic. Therefore, I see no practical value in using TSH assays to learn that a hypothyroid patient's thyroid hormone dosage is TSH-suppressive. On the contrary, requiring a patient to reduce her dosage to relieve the TSH suppression typically results in her symptoms and signs reappearing. This demonstrates a practical disadvantage in using TSH assays to titrate dosage.

Crucial Role of Clinical Indicators and Clinical Judgment

Both before and since the development of highly sensitive laboratory thyroid function tests, medical authors have written of the crucial role of the use of clinical indicators and clinical judgment.

In 1959, Wilson and Walton wrote: "Diagnosis may depend on a 'high index of suspicion.' A low basal metabolic rate, high serum cholesterol level, reduced ^{131}I uptake, and low protein-bound iodine may afford confirmation of the diagnosis, but the results of these tests may be only slightly abnormal (*myxoedema frustes* of French writers); indeed they may even be normal . . . . In the last resort, diagnosis depends on the complete remission of symptoms with thyroid extract or more dramatically triiodothyronine."[25,pp.323-324]

In 1976, Barnes wisely explained that thyroid function tests are no substitute for ". . . a good physician's knowledge of what thyroid deficiency can bring about and his expert clinical impression of what it may be doing in a case of an individual patient."[14,pp.136-137] In that same year, Vagenakis and Braverman wrote that despite the value of laboratory tests of thyroid function, the tests "should not be used as a substitute for good clinical judgment or as the only factor in determining whether a given patient should be treated for suspected thyroid disease."[31,p.607]

DeGroot wrote in 1984 that the evaluation of thyroid status best begins with a careful clinical history and physical examination. The clinician should question, observe, and physically test the patient. It is at this point that an attentive clinician is likely to recognize most patients with thyroid hormone deficiencies.[30,p.311]

In their 1985 book on thyroid function testing, Mardell and Gamlen advised clinicians that "the quoted 'normal range' must be interpreted taking into account the clinical situation and the other available laboratory tests before diagnostic conclusions are drawn."[8,p.18]

In 1986, Mitchell wrote of thyroid function testing, "Until true metabolic activity can be easily quantified and free thyroid hormones estimated without a variety of factors confounding the results, thoughtful clinicians will have to continue to exercise their best judgment based on skill, knowledge, and experience."[18,p.43] In discussing the total T_4 test, he wrote: "In many instances, the true diagnosis will be revealed by additional laboratory procedures supported by a distinctive clinical picture. However, there will be occasions when because of the ambiguity of the test results and the lack of conspicuous clinical features, the decision to treat or not will be made on the basis of experience and judgment."[18,p.37] About the T_3 uptake, he wrote, ". . . there will be occasions when additional test procedures will be necessary to arrive at the functional state of the thyroid gland, and even then the diagnosis may still be in question."[18,p.39] As for the TSH, he wrote, ". . . the absence of an elevated TSH level in a patient with clinical manifestations of hypothyroidism should not discourage further investigation."[18,p.41]

In 1986, Fraser et al. conducted a study comparing the effectiveness of two methods for titrating hypothyroid patients' thyroxine dosages: (1) laboratory thyroid function tests, and (2) a questionnaire for assessing changes in hypothyroid signs and symptoms. As a result of the outcome, they wrote that tests of the total T_4, total T_3, free T_4, free T_3, and basal serum TSH were of *no* value in determining whether patients were taking enough, too little, or too much T_4. They concluded, "These [laboratory] measurements are therefore of little, if any, value in monitoring patients receiving thyroxine replacement."[16] Their results and conclusion were consistent with that of Johansen et al. in 1978.[32]

In 1996, Stockigt, in the major textbook of thyroidology *Werner's The Thyroid*, wrote, "In some situations (e.g., patients with ischemic heart disease and

hypothyroidism), the appropriate dose of T_4 should be based on clinical judgment rather than laboratory findings."[26,p.381] Also in 1996, LoPresti noted, "Currently available thyroid function tests have enhanced the diagnostic skills of the physician, but their effectiveness relies on clinical judgment rather than guidance from protocol or random application."[169]

Most recently, I have found that in treating hypothyroid and euthyroid hypometabolic fibromyalgia patients, clinical indicators and clinical judgment are crucial to a favorable therapeutic outcome. We have been able to provide virtually all hypothyroid fibromyalgia patients with complete relief from their symptoms without tissue thyrotoxicity by the use of nutritional supplementation, exercise to tolerance, and exogenous thyroid hormone. I state emphatically: *We have accomplished this therapeutic outcome by adjusting each patient's dosage according to indicators of clinical response—and without the further use of laboratory thyroid function testing after initially establishing the patient's thyroid status.*

INTEGRATION OF LABORATORY THYROID FUNCTION TESTING AND CLINICAL ASSESSMENT: A RATIONAL BASIS FOR DIAGNOSIS IN MEDICAL PRACTICE

It is common for extremist medical technocrats to express disdain for clinical assessment. Some have argued that favoring clinical assessment over the results of thyroid function tests is equivalent to tasting urine for sweetness as the gold standard against which to judge the plasma glucose concentration.[16] This statement implies that advocates of clinical medicine use only clinical indicators and reject the use of laboratory testing. By this implication, however, they set up and attack a straw man. Few practitioners of clinical medicine totally abstain from using laboratory testing. Instead, they integrate laboratory testing into a comprehensive approach to evaluation that also includes the patient's history, symptoms, signs, and peripheral indices.

The basis of the extremist technocratic position described in the above section may be a failure to define the diagnostic objective. The objective may be simply to compare the levels of circulating thyroid hormones or the TSH to accepted normal values. If so, the objective is to determine the patient's "thyroid status." To do so, there is no substitute for the use of laboratory thyroid function tests.

However, if the clinician's purpose is to determine

the patient's tissue metabolic status, thyroid function tests are useless. The tests only measure blood levels of TSH and thyroid hormones. The tests do not measure peripheral tissue metabolic status, and inferences about peripheral tissue metabolic status based on results of the tests are not reliable. Procedures other than thyroid function testing are necessary to assess the patient's tissue metabolic status (see Chapter 4.3). When not based on such procedures, conclusions about the patient's tissue metabolic status are unfounded. Assessing the patient's tissue metabolic status is necessary for determining the impact of hypothyroidism on the patient, and it is the quintessential method for determining the adequacy of thyroid hormone dosage.

The clinically-oriented practitioners I have communicated with appreciate the necessity of clinical indicators in assessing the patient's tissue metabolic status. They should also bear in mind, however, that we cannot accurately determine the patient's thyroid status on the basis of symptoms, signs, and peripheral indices. Laboratory test results are necessary for this purpose.

With the reasonably reliable blood tests available today, we would best consider symptoms, signs, and peripheral indices as only a part—although an essential part—of the initial diagnostic work up. This approach is consistent with other diagnostic protocols in medicine. In cardiology, for example, the clinician determines the significance of displacement of the ST segment on the ECG by considering the patient's clinical status.[22,p.29] Similarly, the diagnosis of subendocardial infarction is justified if (1) several of the limb and precordial leads show persistent ST depression and T wave inversions and (2) "the clinical picture justifies the diagnosis of infarction."[23,p.381]

Collins described the proper integration of laboratory testing and clinical assessment: "In summary," he advised, "listening to the patient, examining him with all the equipment that may be carried in the doctor's bag, and utilizing the best laboratory procedures available are all indispensable in clinical diagnosis. The importance of each must be determined separately in each case. The clinician must never underestimate the value of the laboratory in clinical diagnosis, but a healthy degree of skepticism is essential in interpreting laboratory results." He added: "Laboratory tests do not 'rule out' disease. A test giving a negative result in the face of strong clinical suspicion to the contrary should be repeated several times, and even then the clinical diagnosis often should prevail."[85,p.x] Medical technocrats will serve their patients best by adopting the orientation expressed by Collins.

● LABORATORY TESTS FOR EVALUATING THYROID FUNCTION

TESTING STRATEGY

We are in an era of advanced assay technology, and tests such as the supersensitive TSH are now available. Prominent authorities, however, express differences of opinion about the selection of tests and interpretation of the results.[80] With differences of opinion among leading authorities in thyroidology, it should be no surprise that other clinicians often find the choice and interpretation of tests uncertain or confusing. Moreover, some of the dazzling array of available blood tests are products of calculations of tests of uncertain reliability, and interpreting some of the tests may be an insurmountable task for some clinicians.[14,p.41] Because of this, the clinician should not necessarily question his knowledge and clinical competence when he has to use a copious quantity of clinical judgment in questions of patient care.

This is not to devalue the diligent efforts of investigators to develop sensitive and reliable tests of thyroid function. One cannot fail to appreciate the utility of highly sensitive TSH assays, the TRH-stimulation test, and other tests of pituitary-thyroid gland axis function for testing thyroid status. The clinician can use the TSH and the TRH-stimulation tests to assess the adequacy of hypothalamic/pituitary control of thyroid gland function. He can also use the tests to differentiate between primary hypothyroidism (due to thyroid gland dysfunction) and central hypothyroidism (due to pituitary or hypothalamic dysfunction). In addition, with these tests he can identify mild and subclinical forms of thyroid gland inadequacy[30,p.297] that are likely to respond well to treatment.[34]

In the late 1980s, the most widely used screening tests for thyroid dysfunction were the serum total T_4 and the free thyroxine index (FTI).[80][81] The supersensitive TSH is preferable to these two tests in that it is not affected by changes in thyroid hormone-binding proteins and is less affected by nonthyroidal illness.[84,pp.42-43] Toft wrote that in addition, the supersensitive TSH can identify subclinical hyperthyroidism and hypothyroidism.[82]

The thyroid function profiles I recommend in this chapter, in conjunction with the TRH-stimulation test, permit the clinician to classify patients according to thyroid status. This classification, combined with a thorough assessment of the patient's clinical status, can enable the clinician to make a justifiable decision about the initial course of treatment for the patient. (See the section below titled "Summary of Testing Strategy.")

I explain below those tests that are contained in the two optional thyroid screening profiles I recommend (see Table 4.2.1). The tests in the first profile are the total T_4 RIA assay, the T_3 uptake, the free thyroxine index (T_7), and a basal TSH. The second profile contains a serum free T_4 and the basal TSH. I also include the TRH-stimulation test in both profiles.

The reference ranges (ranges of normal) that I give for each test in the interpretation sections are from the laboratory I use or from standard texts on test result interpretation (see Table 4.2.2). Although most laboratories have similar ranges of normal, the clinician should check with the laboratory he uses for its adjusted ranges.

TOTAL T_4 OR T_4(RIA)

The total T_4 is a measurement of total T_4 concentration in the serum. All naturally occurring, iodine-containing compounds (which includes the total T_4) present in human serum are now measured by radioimmunoassay (RIA).[30,p.253] It is important to be familiar with the basic procedure involved in RIA.

RIA

In the 1950's, Berson and Yalow were studying the behavior of insulin tagged with radioactive iodine. Their observations during these studies led them to develop RIA for insulin in plasma. This work formed the basis of specific RIAs for other substances.[28] Berson and Yalow found that in patients treated with insulin, insulin-binding antibodies formed to the injected insulin. They also found that the antibodies would bind radioactive insulin. But when insulin that was not radioactively labeled was present in the medium, the unlabeled insulin displaced the labeled insulin—that is, the antibodies preferentially bound to the unlabeled insulin. The same phenomenon occurs with radioactively labeled and unlabeled T_4: T_4 antibodies preferentially bind the unlabeled T_4. It is this phenomenon that is the basis of the T_4(RIA).

To perform the T_4 assay, the technician uses two tubes that contain T_4 antibodies. He mixes the specimen taken from the patient (containing his untagged endogenous T_4) with the antibody-laden contents of one tube. He also adds the labeled T_4. The two forms of T_4 then compete to bind to the antibodies. The antibodies preferentially bind the unlabeled T_4. The great-

er the amount of unlabeled T_4 in the medium, the fewer antibodies bind to the labeled T_4. Next, the technician separates the two fractions of T_4, that bound to antibodies and that free or unbound. An instrument monitors the percentage of radioactive label bound to and unbound to antibodies. The instrument calculates the concentration of unlabeled T_4—that from the patient. It does so by comparing the amount of labeled T_4 in the sample to standard samples.[28] It is this quantity that the laboratory reports as a patient's T_4 (RIA) value. The reference interval of T_4 (RIA) in adults is about 4.5-to-12.5 µg/dL.[28,p.425]

T_4 by RIA is highly sensitive. It can detect levels of T_4 as low as 10-to-20 pg (a picogram is one trillionth of a gram). The test can detect serum volumes as low as 25 µg/L.[87,p.119]

Table 4.2.1. Optional laboratory profiles for evaluating thyroid status.

Profile I:

Total T_4 (RIA)
T_3 Uptake
Free T_4 Index (FTI or T_7)
TSH
TRH-Stimulation Test

Profile II:

Free T_4
TSH
TRH-Stimulation Test

Dynamics of the Serum Total T_4

In hypothyroidism, we expect the total T_4 level to be lower than optimal. If the hypothyroidism is severe enough, the level will be below the lower limit of the normal range. In hyperthyroidism, we expect the total T_4 level to be high-normal or high.

The total T_4 is a measure of the total amount of T_4 in the serum. Its level may not correlate with the concentration of free T_4, the fraction destined to soon enter cells, be monodeiodinated, and become metabolically active as T_3. The total T_4 concentration can change as a result of an increase or decrease of T_4 secretion as occurs in hyperthyroidism and hypothyroidism. It can also change in a number of other conditions. These include compensatory changes in the total T_4 due to high or low levels of serum T_3 and variations in the binding capacity of thyroid hormone transport proteins.[30,p.254] The T_4 level can also change at intervals of time after ingestion of the hormone.

T_4-Lowering Effect of Increased T_3 Levels. A decreased T_4 level is the compensatory change of most concern in the metabolic rehabilitation of fibromyalgia patients. Virtually all euthyroid fibromyalgia patients and many hypothyroid fibromyalgia patients improve or recover only when they use T_3 as part of their treatment regimen. Most require dosages of T_3 high enough to suppress TSH secretion. The reduced TSH secretion results in a secondary reduction in thyroid gland secretion of T_4 and a low-normal or low circulating T_4 level.

Measurements of thyroid hormone levels of fibromyalgia patients included in one of our studies illustrate the T_4-lowering effect of relatively high dosages of exogenous T_3. The patients were euthyroid; each patient's thyroid gland was fully capable of synthesizing and secreting normal amounts of T_4. We found that in patients taking between 87.5-and-150 µg of T_3, the free T_3 was elevated with a mean of 8.05 pg/mL (normal range: 2.3-to-4.2 pg/mL); the total T_4 was low with a mean of 3.05 µg/dL (normal range: 4.5-to-12.5 µg/dL). The TSH was also low with a mean of 0.05 µU/mL (normal range: 0.4-to-6.0 µU/mL). This pattern shows that the exogenous T_3 suppressed TSH secretion and secondarily reduced thyroid gland output of T_4.[88]

DeGroot wrote of this pattern of T_4 and T_3 values in patients taking T_3. He wrote that the clinician should not assume the low T_4 indicates that the patient is ingesting too little thyroid hormone and instruct her to increase her T_3 dosage.[21,p.11] This could result in hypermetabolism. The low T_4, typical low T_3-resin uptake, and the elevated serum T_3 of patients taking exogenous T_3 led DeGroot to state, "Fortunately, T_3 is used infrequently for therapy of hypothyroidism, since it certainly is prone to cause confusion in diagnosis and treatment."[21,p.11] As I indicated, however, practically all euthyroid and many hypothyroid fibromyalgia patients *must* take T_3 rather than T_4 if they are to acquire normal metabolism. Because of this requirement for the use of T_3, the clinician should familiarize himself with the pattern of laboratory values typical of the patient using T_3.

Alterations in Total T_4 Levels Due to Variations in the Binding Capacity of Thyroid Hormone Transport Proteins. Several extrathyroidal factors (such as exogenous estrogen, pregnancy, and acute liver disease) moderately increase the circulating thyroid hormone binding proteins, mainly thyroxine-binding globulin.[75] (For a description of the binding proteins, see Chapter 2.1, section titled "Thyroid Hormone Transport Proteins.") The increased number of binding proteins provides a greater total number of thyroid hormone binding sites. T_4 molecules bind to the sites on the proteins, resulting in an increase in the total serum T_4 level. The greater number of binding sites also results in a decrease of T_3 uptake. (See section below titled "T_3 Uptake.") This results because during the test, a higher than normal amount of T_3 is bound to transport proteins and less is available to bind to the test resin.

Other factors (such as testosterone or anabolic steroid administration) decrease the circulating binding proteins. This results in a reduction in the total number of thyroid hormone binding sites. Less T_4 binds to the proteins, and consequently, the total T_4 decreases. The T_3 uptake increases because less T_3 is bound to transport proteins and more is available to bind to the test resin.[87,p.119]

Drugs such as salicylates and diphenylhydantoin interfere with binding of hormones to proteins. Aspirin[90] and Dilantin,[91] for example, compete with T_4 for binding to thyroxine-binding globulin, reducing the total T_4 level. Under the influence of these drugs, the total T_4 level may not correspond to the functional state of the patient's pituitary/thyroid axis;[28,p.426] that is, thyroid gland secretion of T_4 may be normal despite a low-normal or low total T_4 level.

In contrast to the total T_4, the free T_4 level is not affected by abnormally high or low levels of T_4-binding proteins. In addition to this advantage of the free T_4, Hamburger speculated that the free T_4 assay correlates best with thyroid hormone activity at the tissue level.[33,p.119] This speculation, however, is not true[7][50] (see section below: "Free T_3"). The relatively high cost and time expenditure for assays that measure the actual free T_4 have created resistance to its use. However, the free thyroxine index (T_7) which estimates the free T_4 is also not affected by changes in binding protein levels. When the free T_4 index or the free T_4 are normal and the total T_4 is high or low, a high or low binding protein level may be responsible for the pattern. If the patient's history includes factors that are known to increase or decrease the binding protein level, the clinician should include a free T_4 index or the free T_4 in the patient's thyroid function test profile to accurately assess the T_4 binding protein level.

Variations in Serum T_4 Based on Time of Inges-

tion. When a patient is taking T_4 as a thyroid hormone supplement, it is preferable to have him abstain from taking his tablets on the day blood is drawn to measure the serum thyroxine level. Hamburger and members of his staff took 0.15 mg of Levothroid (a T_4 product) and measured the serum T_4 levels at baseline and 2, 4, and 6 hours later. At 2 and 4 hours, T_4 values increased 1-to-2 µg/dL.[21,p.16] Other studies have shown similar increases.[123][124][125]

Monitoring Thyroid Hormone Levels

Some medical writers have recommended that the clinician monitor patients taking T_4 by measuring the free T_3. Their justification for this view is that the free T_3 correlates better than the T_4 with the patient's clinical status.[45,p.88][48] (See the section on the free T_3 below.) However, the clinician should bear in mind that if his purpose is to determine how the patient is responding to thyroid hormone, monitoring measures of tissue response to thyroid hormone is the appropriate protocol (see Chapter 4.3). The responses of different tissues in the same individual, and those of the same tissues in different individuals, are variable. This variability makes it invalid to infer from circulating thyroid hormone levels how the tissues are responding to exogenous thyroid hormone.

Interpretation

The T_4 level may be elevated because the patient's thyroid hormone transport proteins are increased. This can result from the use of exogenous oral estrogen, pregnancy, or acute liver disease. The T_4 level may be low because of use of anabolic steroids, aspirin, Dilantin, or T_3. In the absence of such influences, a low T_4 level may indicate hypothyroidism, and a high level may indicate hyperthyroidism. The range of normal is 4.5-to-12.5 µg/dL.

FREE T_4

The free T_4 test is an RIA[8,p.13] (see section above titled "Total T_4 or T_4 (RIA): RIA"). The free T_4 comprises only a minute fraction of the total T_4. Because the free T_4 is not bound to thyroid hormone transport proteins, its circulating level is not affected by increases or decreases in the levels of these proteins.[18,p.39] The free T_4 may be elevated by amiodarone (a highly effective antianginal and antiarrhythmic drug) and radiopaque contrast media.[44] Nonetheless, Mitchell contended that the free T_4 more accurately assesses

thyroid function than the total T_4 or the T_3 uptake.[18,p.40]

For the initial test to identify hypothyroidism, Mardell and Gamlen recommended either the basal TSH or the free T_4. They explained that in the early stage of primary hypothyroidism (subclinical hypothyroidism), increased TSH secretion maintains thyroid hormone secretion.[8,p.55] The hypothyroidism is said to be "compensated." But as the ability of the thyroid gland to secrete normal amounts of thyroid hormone diminishes, even when exposed to high concentrations of TSH, the patient's status progresses from mild-to-severe hypothyroidism. During this time, the free T_4 decreases.

Table 4.2.2. Reference ranges for human serum TSH, thyroid hormone levels, and antithyroid antibodies.

NORMAL REFERENCE RANGE

Test	SI	Metric
Total T_4	60-140 nmol/L*	4.5-12.5 µg/dL†
Free T_4	10-25 pmol/L*	0.7-2.1 ng/dL*
Free T_3	3-8 pmol/L*	0.2-6.5 ng/dL†
Reverse-T_3	0.2-0.7 nmol/L*	15-45 ng/dL*
TSH‡ Conventional TSH‡		0.3-2.0 µU/mL 0.3-5.0 µU/mL*
Thyroglobulin antibodies		<200 mUI/mL^Y
Microsomal (peroxidase) antibodies		<150 mUI/mL^Y

*Stockigt, J.R.: Serum thyrotropin and thyroid hormone measurements and assessment of thyroid hormone transport. In *Werner and Ingbar's The Thyroid: A Fundamental and Clinical Text*, 6th edition. Edited by L.E. Braverman and R.D. Utiger, Philadelphia, J.B. Lippincott Co., 1991.[35,p.466]
†*Compendium of Services.* National Health Laboratories, Incorporated, 1050 N. Post Oak, #145, Houston, TX 77055.
‡Individuals with TSH values of 2.0 µU/mL or above appear to have an increased risk for future overt hypothyroidism.[154][155] This finding suggests that individuals with incipient thyroid disease are included in the reference populations of laboratories, resulting in a falsely broad range of normal (see section below titled "Thyrotropin (TSH)").
^{Y} Romaldini, J.H., Biancalana, M.M., Figueiredo, D.I., Farah, C.S., and Mathias, P.C.: Effect of L-thyroxine administration on antithyroid antibody levels, lipid profile, and thyroid volume in patients with Hashimoto's thyroiditis. *Thyroid*, 6(3):183-188, 1996.[167]

A low free T_4, however, is not necessary to the diagnosis of primary hypothyroidism. The clinician can make the diagnosis on the basis of (1) a clinical status that suggests it, (2) an elevated basal TSH, and possibly (3) other indicative evidence such as a goiter, antibodies indicating Hashimoto's thyroiditis, previous thyroidectomy, or previous ^{131}I therapy for hyperthyroidism.[45,p.103]

Interpretation. The free T_4 may be increased by amiodarone and radiopaque contrast media. The normal range for the free T_4 in adults has been reported as 0.7-to-2.1 ng/dL (10-to-25 pmol/L).[35,p.466] The current range for the laboratory I use is 0.69-to-1.38 ng/dL. The significance of the free T_4 test must be confirmed by a TSH level.[8,p.19]

FREE T_3

The serum free T_3 is based on the same principle as the free T_4 RIA[8,p.13] (see section above titled "Total T_4 or T_4 (RIA): RIA"). Some thyroidologists argue that the free T_3 is the fraction of the total T_3 that correlates best with thyroid hormone activity at the tissue level.[33,p.120] (This does not mean, however, that the metabolic status of tissues can be validly inferred from the free T_3 level.) An elevated free T_3 supports the conclusion that thyrotoxic-like signs and symptoms are a result of an excessive T_3 dosage. Sawin wrote that despite an elevated free T_3 value, a normal supersensitive TSH test result virtually excludes the possibility of thyroid hormone excess.[84,p.43] Actually, the normal TSH levels mean the anterior pituitary tissue is not being excessively inhibited by the elevated circulating free T_3 level. Inferences about the responses of other tissues to the T_3 should not be based on the response of the pituitary. Inferences about peripheral tissue response should be based on clinical assessment of the patient and the evaluation of measures that assess the responses of the peripheral tissues.

The free T_3 test is most useful as an indicator of hyperthyroidism.[39][40][41][82] Mardell and Gamlen wrote that the upper limit of the free T_3 is of use in identifying patients with thyroid gland overactivity or an excess dosage of exogenous thyroxine. They also wrote that the significance of the high free T_3 to the patient's thyroid status should be assessed by the use of a supersensitive TSH assay. They noted that the lower limit of the free T_3 is an insensitive indicator of hypothyroidism and is of little value in diagnosing this condition.[8,p.19] This concurs with the reports of other writers.[42] Hamburger stated that the free T_3 is as useless as the total T_3 assay for diagnosing hypothyroidism.[45,p.82]

In about 75% of patients with primary hypothyroidism, both the T_3 and T_4 are low, while the TSH is high. The other 25% of patients have normal T_3 levels. The normal levels result from continual TSH stimulation of the malfunctioning thyroid gland which preferentially incorporates trapped iodine into the T_3 synthesizing pathway.[92,p.1045] Investigators are not certain why the normal endogenous T_3 level does not suppress pituitary gland secretion of TSH. This is puzzling because studies show that equivalent exogenous doses of either T_4 or T_3 immediately suppress TSH secretion.[56]

When a patient uses T_3 as the sole thyroid hormone medication, the serum free T_3 value is typically elevated. This may occur even when the patient takes a physiologic dosage of T_3.[21,p.11] (a dosage that should maintain the circulating T_3 within the normal reference range).

An Elevated Free T_3 Level is Not Synonymous with Thyrotoxicosis

It is important to understand that an elevated free T_3 level is not synonymous with thyrotoxicosis. The clarification warrants emphasis because of confusion over terminology in the thyroidology literature. (See Chapter 4.4, Introduction.)

Hamburger mentioned the question of whether T_4-induced thyrotoxicosis is always associated with an elevated free T_3 level.[45,p.87] The answer, he stated, "depends upon whether one is inclined to accept or reject the evidence that there may be subclinical thyrotoxicosis without an elevated free T_3." His statement reflects the view that the free T_3 correlates better with tissue metabolism than does T_4; an elevated free T_3, more so than an elevated free T_4, is reason to *suspect* tissue thyrotoxicity. "Suspect" is the key word, for neither an elevated free T_4 nor free T_3 justifies a *conclusion* that the patient is thyrotoxic. A diagnosis of thyrotoxicity is justified only when (1) the patient exhibits the clinical syndrome of tissue overstimulation by thyroid hormone and (2) various tests of tissue metabolic status provide objective evidence that specific tissues are indeed thyrotoxic (see Chapter 4.3 and Chapter 4.4). Hamburger's reference to accepting that there "may be subclinical thyrotoxicosis without an elevated free T_3" illustrates extremist technocracy in clinical thyroidology—unjustifiable trust that the clinician can reliably infer that the patient has tissue thyrotoxicity from a serum thyroid hormone level rather than simply assessing whether in fact tissue thyrotoxicity exists. Thyroidologists define "subclinical thyrotoxicity" as a suppressed TSH despite normal T_3 and T_4 levels.[60,p.645] Many clinicians give the diagnosis to patients who have recovered from thyroid hormone deficiency symptoms by taking TSH-suppressive dosages of thyroid hormone. In that many of these patients have partial cellular resistance to thyroid hormone and require TSH-suppressive dosages to maintain normal metabolism, concluding that they have subclinical thyrotoxicity is simply wrong. The term thyrotoxicity implies tissue overstimulation, which these patients do not have. Clearly, clinicians cannot determine tissue overstimulation by thyroid hormone from elevated T_4 or T_3 levels or from a low TSH level. The clinician should consider whether the patient benefitting from T_3 is eumetabolic despite an elevated T_3 serum level. If so, this indicates that the patient is protected from hypermetabolism by partial cellular resistance to thyroid hormone, and that the exogenous T_3 effectively overrides the resistance and properly regulates metabolism.

Factors that Decrease Free T_3 Levels. Several conditions other than hypothyroidism can lower serum T_3 levels. These include various drugs, a low carbohydrate diet, starvation, acute illness, euthyroid sick syndrome in patients with chronic liver and kidney disease,[92,p.1045] and elevated cortisol during stress.[138] The T_3 level may be low in a chronically disabled or ill patient.[99] The low T_3 level in such a case is an adaptation of the patient's body so that, in the face of her reduced metabolic requirement, she is protected against catabolism by normal levels of T_3.[21,p.22]

Clinicians Should Use the Free T_3 (Or Total T_3) to Monitor Patients Taking T_4. The total T_3 or free T_3 are best for monitoring patients taking T_4.[46][47] Volpé wrote that in his view, serum T_3 levels correlate better with patients' clinical status than serum T_4 levels.[45,pp.87-88] Others concur.[48][74] According to Volpé, this is evident from comparing the severity of hyperthyroidism in two thyroid abnormalities, subacute thyroiditis and Graves disease. Typically, levels of T_4 are similar in the two diseases. But patients with Graves disease are clearly more ill, and this correlates with their higher levels of serum T_3 than in patients with subacute thyroiditis.[45,pp.87-88]

The TSH is not as useful for monitoring the patient taking T_4 because the effective dosage of T_4 may suppress the basal sensitive TSH and blunt the TSH response to TRH.[45,pp.87-88] (For more details about this, see the section on TSH below.)

Interpretation

The free T_3 is most useful for identifying patients who may have an excessively active thyroid gland or who are taking supraphysiologic amounts of exogenous thyroid hormone. The test is an insensitive indicator of hypothyroidism and should not be used in an attempt to identify patients with thyroid hormone deficiency. Patients taking exogenous T_3 are likely to have elevated free T_3 levels. Their dosage should not be reduced because of a high free T_3 unless symptoms, signs, and peripheral measures indicate that the patient has tissue hypermetabolism. The normal range for the free T_3 has been given as 0.2-to-6.5 ng/dL (3-to-8 pmol/L)[35,p.466] and 2.3-to-4.2 pg/mL.[136]

T_3 UPTAKE

The T_3 resin uptake is an estimate of the free fraction of T_4 and the total thyroid hormone-binding sites available on plasma proteins.[21,p.3] It does *not* estimate the circulating T_3,[18,p.38] and it is imperative to understand this distinction. In clinical parlance, as DeGroot pointed out, the "T_3 test" refers to the resin T_3 uptake test. And the "T_3" or "serum T_3 by RIA" refers to the assay for serum T_3 by radioimmune methods.[21,p.11]

One way to perform the T_3 uptake test is to add two items to the patient's plasma sample: (1) radioactively labeled T_3 and (2) a resin that absorbs T_3. When the technician adds the labeled T_3 to the sample, the T_3 distributes between the thyroid binding globulin and the resin. The T_3 binds preferentially to binding sites on the thyroid binding globulin. When the T_3 occupies all the available sites on the globulin, any T_3 not bound to it then binds to the absorbent resin. The number of binding sites available on the globulin therefore determines the amount of T_3 that will bind to the resin.[28,p.427] Thus, the T_3 uptake is a measure of the availability of T_4 globulin binding sites, and the uptake of T_3 by the resin is inversely proportional to the availability of the binding sites.[87,p.117]

The range of normal varies both with the substance used to absorb the labeled T_3[94] and the laboratory used.[28,p.427] The range of normal of the laboratory I use is 25%-to-35%.[136]

Dynamics. The uptake of T_3 is useful in distinguishing euthyroid patients from those with thyroid gland dysfunction.[57][58] In hypothyroidism, the low level of circulating T_4 leaves a relatively high percentage of binding sites unoccupied on circulating thyroid hormone binding proteins. The increased availability of binding sites enables more T_3 than normal to bind to the proteins. During the test procedure, more of the radioactive T_3 added to the patient's plasma sample binds to the proteins, leaving fewer radioactive T_3 molecules to bind to the test resin. As a result, in hypothyroidism the T_3 uptake (the amount of T_3 that binds to the resin) is lower than normal.[28,p.427]

In hyperthyroidism, the excess thyroid hormone molecules in the blood occupy more sites on the patient's thyroid hormone binding proteins. This leaves a lower than normal percentage of the binding sites unoccupied. Consequently, when radioactive T_3 is added to the patient's plasma during the test, a lower than normal amount of the radioactive T_3 binds to the proteins. This leaves more of the T_3 to bind to the test resin. The higher than normal binding of radioactive T_3 to the resin constitutes a high T_3 uptake.

Table 4.2.3. The relation of the total T_4 to the T_3 uptake: implications for thyroid hormone and binding protein abnormalities.

	Total T_4	T_3 uptake
Hypothyroidism	Low	Low
Hyperthyroidism	High	High
Decreased proteins	Low	High
Increased proteins	High	Low

In addition to hypothyroidism and hyperthyroidism, several other conditions can lower or raise the T_3 uptake in euthyroid patients. Estrogen can increase the binding proteins.[75] The increase in proteins provides a higher than normal amount of available binding sites. During the test, a greater than normal amount of the radioactive T_3 binds to the proteins. A lower than normal amount of T_3 is left to bind to the resin, resulting in a low T_3 uptake.

The most important factor that increases the levels of thyroid hormone binding proteins is an increased estrogen level during pregnancy and during the use of exogenous estrogens, as in oral contraceptives.[30,p.254] The estrogens increase the serum concentrations of thyroxine-binding globulin.[35,p.478][75] The greater amount of globulin provides additional sites for T_3 binding. Little T_3 binds to the resin, giving a low T_3 uptake, and suggesting possible hypothyroidism.[87,p.116] In such cases, the T_3 uptake does not accurately reflect thyroid status. Using only the T_3 uptake to test thyroid function could lead to the misdiagnosis of hypothyroidism.[31,p.607]

Anabolic steroids[95] and corticosteroids such as prednisone[108,p.813] can decrease the number of circulating thyroid hormone binding proteins. The decreased number of proteins provides a lower than normal num-

ber of binding sites. When the radioactive T_3 is added to the patient's plasma during the test, a lower than normal amount of the T_3 binds to proteins and more binds to the resin. The result is a high T_3 uptake.

Substances that compete for binding sites on the transport proteins, such as aspirin, displace thyroid hormones from the proteins.[95] During the test procedure, a lower than normal amount of the radioactive T_3 binds to the proteins and more binds to the resin, resulting in a high T_3 uptake.

Use of T_3 as the only thyroid hormone medication may also lower the value of the T_3 uptake. This tends to occur because the exogenous T_3 suppresses thyroid gland secretion of T_4.[21,p.11] As a result, fewer T_4 molecules are available in the blood to occupy binding sites on thyroxine-binding globulin. This leaves a relatively large percentage of binding sites on the globulin unoccupied. During the T_3 uptake test, when radioactive T_3 is added to the patient's plasma sample, a relatively large amount preferentially binds to the large number of available sites on the globulin. This leaves less than a normal amount of T_3 to bind to the test resin. Thus, the T_3 uptake by the resin is lower than normal. Consistent with this pattern, in one study of euthyroid fibromyalgia patients,[89] I found that use of T_3 as the sole thyroid hormone medication lowered the total and free T_4. Although all the patients' free T_3 levels were high, their mean T_3 uptake of 25.25% was at the lower end of the normal range of 25%-to-35%.

Distinguishing Abnormalities of Thyroid Hormone from Those of Transport Proteins. In general, by comparing the T_3 uptake and the total T_4, the clinician can differentiate abnormal levels of thyroid hormone from those of thyroid hormone transport proteins.[18,p.39] When the values of both the T_3 uptake and the total T_4 are in the same direction, either high or low, this indicates a thyroid hormone abnormality. When both values are low, the patient may be hypothyroid. Low T_4 levels in hypothyroidism leave increased numbers of protein binding sites available to bind T_3, reducing the amount of T_3 that is free to bind to the test resin. When both the total T_4 and T_3 uptake are high, the patient may be hyperthyroid. The increased number of T_4 molecules in hyperthyroidism occupies a high percentage of the binding sites on the transport proteins. Because a low percentage of binding sites are unoccupied and available for binding, more of the radioactive T_3 binds to the resin during the test.

If the total T_4 and T_3 uptake values are in opposite directions, the cause is more likely a protein-binding abnormality than a thyroid gland disorder. For example, if the total T$_4$ is high and the T$_3$ uptake low, this probably means there is a high quantity of binding proteins. The high number of proteins provides more hormone binding sites, and a greater than normal quantity of T$_4$ and T$_3$ binds to the sites. In addition, during the test, when radioactive T$_3$ is added to the patient's plasma, a greater than normal quantity binds to unoccupied sites on the proteins. As a result, fewer T$_3$ molecules bind to the resin. Thus, the T$_3$ uptake is low.

On the other hand, if the total T$_4$ is low and the T$_3$ uptake high, the quantity of binding proteins is most likely low. The low quantity provides fewer binding sites. As a result, the total T$_4$ level is low. When radioactive T$_3$ is added to the patient's plasma, the paucity of binding sites on the proteins leaves a greater than normal amount of the T$_3$ available to bind to the resin. As a result, T$_3$ uptake is high. (See Table 4.2.3)

Interpretation

The T$_3$ uptake does not measure the circulating T$_3$. Instead, it is an estimate of the binding sites available on circulating thyroid hormone transport proteins. The test value, expressed as a percentage, is inversely proportional to the quantity of available binding sites. The higher the T$_3$ uptake, the fewer the sites available on the carrier proteins; the lower the T$_3$ uptake, the more sites available on the proteins.

Exogenous T$_3$ and oral estrogen may lower the T$_3$ uptake. Corticosteroids such as prednisone and anabolic steroids may increase the T$_3$ uptake. In the absence of such factors, a low total T$_4$ and T$_3$ uptake indicate hypothyroidism. If the values of the total T$_4$ and T$_3$ uptake are in different directions, this indicates that the quantity of transport proteins is abnormal. Specifically, a low total T$_4$ and high T$_3$ uptake suggests a decrease in transport proteins with a decrease in the number of available binding sites. A high total T$_4$ and low T$_3$ indicates an increase in transport proteins with an increase in the number of available binding sites.[18,p.39] The normal range of the T$_3$ uptake is 25%-to-35%.[136]

FREE THYROXINE INDEX (FTI OR T$_7$)

The free thyroxine index is an estimate of the free T$_4$ concentration. When the concentration of thyroid hormone binding proteins changes, the total T$_4$ and the T$_3$ uptake also change (see section above titled "Distinguishing Abnormalities of Thyroid Hormone from Those of Transport Proteins"). The patient's clinical state, however, does not change. According to several

writers, when the patient has thyroid hormone binding protein abnormalities, the free or unbound T$_4$ more accurately correlates with both the patient's metabolic status and her tissue thyroid hormone levels.[28,p.427][30,p.264][87,p.122] To my knowledge, however, no one has established that the circulating T$_4$ level, free or total, correlates with metabolic status or tissue thyroid hormone levels. A less speculative statement is that when the patient has binding protein abnormalities, the free T$_4$ more accurately reflects the patient's thyroid status than does the total T$_4$ or the T$_3$ uptake. While the FTI can help clarify the patient's thyroid status despite increased or decreased binding proteins, the test is of no value in assessing her tissue metabolic status.

The FTI is the Product of the Total T$_4$ and the T$_3$ Uptake

An instrument derives the value of the FTI by multiplying the T$_3$ uptake by the total T$_4$.[18,p.40] The free hormone concentration is the diffusible fraction that can traverse cell membranes to exert metabolic effects. With rare exceptions, the free thyroid hormone concentration is high in hyperthyroidism, low in hypothyroidism, and normal in euthyroidism. The free thyroxine index correlates with thyroid status even when the thyroid binding globulin level is abnormal in some way.[28,p.427][30,pp.264-265] For example, a euthyroid patient who has a high thyroid binding globulin concentration will also have a high total T$_4$. But his FTI should be normal.[30,p.268]

The value of the FTI is controversial among thyroidologists. Regarding the FTI, Wellby admonished, ". . . it is a mathematical product of two assays and so any inaccuracy in either assay will be reflected in the FTI result."[87,p.123] Some thyroidologists claim that the FTI is obsolete.[21,p.3] DeGroot disagreed and stated, "This widely used test remains satisfactory for most purposes. Newer tests purporting to measure the 'free T$_4$' are in general as valuable as the FTI but do not uniformly exceed its discriminatory value."[21,p.3] Mitchell wrote that values calculated for the FTI agree with the free T$_4$.[18,p.40] Experiments have confirmed that when performed properly, the FTI is an accurate estimate of the absolute free T$_4$ concentration[30,pp.266-267] which is less than 0.1% (about 0.04%-to-0.05%).[87,p.107]

The Global Index. There are techniques for estimating the free T$_3$ index (FT$_3$I). Few laboratories use these in routine testing for thyroid function. The FT$_3$I correlates well with the free T$_3$ concentration, and it corrects for total T_3 concentration secondary to abnormalities of thyroid hormone binding proteins.[30,p.268] Some researchers have recommended that laboratories express the free T_4 index and the free T_3 index in a single value as a "global index." The combined thyroid hormone index includes measurements of total T_4, total T_3, and resin T_3 uptake. Preliminary tests showed the combined index to be more accurate in the diagnosis of hypothyroidism and hyperthyroidism than either the free T_4 index or the free T_3 index alone. Clinicians do not use the global index in clinical practice.[30,p.268]

Interpretation

With high reliability, the free T_4 concentration (indicated by the FTI) is high in hyperthyroidism, low in hypothyroidism, and normal in euthyroidism. The normal range is 0-25 pmol/L, or 0.7-2.1 ng/dL.[35,p.466]

REVERSE-T_3 (rT_3)

The compound 3,3',5'-triiodothyronine, also called reverse-T_3 (rT_3), was found in the blood and thyroglobulin of rats and reported in 1956.[149] In 1958, Dunn and Stanbury suggested that rT_3 is metabolized so quickly that the serum was not likely to contain detectable quantities.[150] Much later, researchers determined that rT_3 disappears from the body much more rapidly than does T_3: injected radioactively labeled rT_3 appears in the urine as iodine within 24-hours.[140,p.130] Clinicians began measuring their patients' rT_3, however, when in 1974 Chopra introduced a radioimmunoassay for measuring circulating levels[63] and studies showed that rT_3 levels varied in different disease states.[143]

The thyroid gland secretes about 1.2-to-4.2 μg of rT_3 per day. This is about 10% or less of the body's daily production of 40 μg of rT_3. Peripheral tissue deiodination of T_4 accounts for the remainder of the body's daily production of rT_3.[140,p.133] (For a description of the biochemistry and physiology of rT_3, see Chapter 2.1, section titled "Deiodinases That Convert T_4 to T_3 and Reverse-T_3.") Circulating rT_3 is practically all bound to proteins. Only about 0.3% of circulating rT_3 is free.[143]

Reverse-T_3 in Clinical Conditions

The serum rT_3 level is abnormal in starvation and an array of illnesses[140,p.134] (see Chapter 2.5, section titled "Disorders Involving Inhibition of T_4 to T_3 Conversion"). The rT_3 level is low in untreated hypothy-

roidism[148] but is practically normal in hypothyroid patients taking replacement dosages of T_4.[140,p.133] The level is also normal in euthyroid subjects using TSH-suppressive dosages of T_4. The level is increased in hyperthyroidism.[140,p.130]

In obese patients who are fasting, the T_3 level decreases and the rT_3 level increases no matter whether the patient has a normally functioning thyroid gland or is taking TSH-suppressive dosages of T_4.[146] During fasting, conversion of T_4 to T_3 decreases about 50% (from a rate of 35% down to 17%), and the conversion of T_4 to rT_3 increases nearly 50% (from a rate of 41% up to 61%).[144]

In conditions of catabolism, such as cirrhosis, starvation, and insulin-dependent diabetes mellitus, the daily production of T_3 decreases. The production rate of rT_3 remains normal, but the serum concentration increases because of a reduction in the catabolism of rT_3. The ratio of T_3 to T_4 production becomes subnormal, and the ratio of rT_3 to T_4 production remains normal or moderately increased.[140,p.133][147]

Rajkovic et al. found that in 11 normal women, abortion significantly reduced serum free and total T_3 levels, but the TSH and free and total rT_3 levels did not significantly change.[145] Juma et al., however, found that after major elective orthopedic surgery, the total and free T_3 significantly decreased, and the rT_3 significantly increased.[141] Legakis et al. studied changes in thyroid function test results in 22 patients who underwent laparoscopic cholecystectomy, a procedure the investigators considered mild surgical stress. TSH levels remained within the normal limits with transient changes during the study. Total T_4 levels varied within the normal range. The total T_3 decreased early during the induction of anesthesia. It remained low during the peri-operative period and decreased further at 24-hours after surgery. The rT_3 increased and reached its highest value—a statistically significant change—at 24-hours after surgery. The researchers noted the "asynchronous distribution" of rT_3 and total T_3.[137]

Comtois et al. described a 33-year-old woman treated for Cushing's disease, in which cortisol secretion is excessive. She underwent surgery to relieve the excess cortisol secretion, and she developed secondary adrenal insufficiency during the postoperative period. Her T_3 level was elevated and her rT_3 was low. These findings suggest that secondary adrenal deficiency may result in increased peripheral conversion of T_4 to T_3.[139]

Natori et al. found that patients with anorexia nervosa and patients with severe depression had impaired

T_4 to T_3 conversion due to increased cortisol secretion caused by emotional stress. The levels of T_3, T_4, free T_3, free T_4, and the ratio of T_3 to T_4 were all inversely related to disease severity.[138]

Wilson has proposed that T_4 to T_3 conversion can become "stuck," resulting in chronic symptoms of hypometabolism. His proposal is contrary to the available scientific evidence. My testing of fibromyalgia patients produced no laboratory evidence of impaired conversion. (See Chapter 2.5, section titled "Proposal of a Sustained Euthyroid Sick Syndrome Under the Expropriated Name 'Wilson's Syndrome.'") Treatment based on Wilson's proposed mechanism has become widespread. The clinician who proposes that his patient's symptoms are due to chronic impaired conversion of T_4 to T_3 should attempt to verify the mechanism by ordering the appropriate laboratory tests. It is unlikely, however, that laboratory testing will provide evidence for this mechanism in most fibromyalgia patients. This conclusion is based on my clinical experience. In my euthyroid fibromyalgia patients who improved or recovered only with the use of T_3, I did not find laboratory evidence of impaired T_4 to T_3 conversion. In 50 patients who responded to T_3 after failing to benefit from large dosages of T_4, I did not find the combination of elevated serum reverse-T_3, low-normal T_3, and elevated 24-hour urinary cortisol that would indicate cortisol-induced impairment of deiodination. A small percentage of the patients had slightly elevated 24-hour urinary cortisol, but none of these had elevated serum reverse-T_3 or low-normal T_3. These values indicate that impaired conversion of T_4 to T_3 is not the mechanism responsible for these fibromyalgia patients' failure to benefit from T_4.[66]

Confirming that the patient does not have impaired conversion may make obvious the merit of a treatment protocol different from that proposed by Wilson.

Interpretation

When evaluating the possibility that a patient has impaired conversion of T_4 to T_3, the clinician should consider possible mechanisms of impairment. These include elevated cortisol, mercury toxicity, and selenium deficiency. (See Chapter 2.6, section titled "Defects in the Conversion of T_4 to T_3.") The likelihood of impaired conversion is increased if in addition to an increased rT_3, the patient has low total and free T_3. Depending on the radioimmunoassay used for measurement, the serum concentration of rT_3 varies between 20 ng/dL and 40 ng/dL in normal adults.[140,p.130] Skovsted reported that the serum concentration in 36 nor-

mal subjects was 32±7 ng rT_3/100 mL.[142] Stockigt gives the normal values as 0.2-to-0.7 nmol/L or 15-to-45 ng/dL.[35,p.466]

THYROTROPIN (TSH)

According to classic physiology principle, when the hypothalamic-pituitary-thyroid axis functions normally, the serum TSH level hovers close to the middle of the range of normal. Thyroid hormone inhibits secretion of TSH by the thyrotroph cells of the pituitary gland. When the concentration of thyroid hormone reaching the thyrotroph cells increases, the cells decrease their secretion of TSH. When the thyroid hormone level decreases, the cells are disinhibited and increase their secretion of TSH. (See Chapter 2.1.)

Hay explained in his excellent history of TSH assays[84] that investigators demonstrated the action of pituitary extracts on the thyroid glands of live guinea pigs in 1929.[83] It was not until the 1950s that investigators developed bioassays for measuring the TSH in human plasma. Clinicians did not use these assays in practice because they were not sensitive, specific, or reliable enough.[80] Researchers published the initial report of the first radioimmunoassay (RIA) for TSH in human serum in 1965.[37] For the next 15 years, clinicians made widespread use of RIA TSH assays. These assays had detection limits of 1-to-2 μU/mL (mU/L). Clinicians used the assays to initially diagnose and thereafter monitor patients with primary hypothyroidism.[80] In 1980, Spencer introduced an RIA assay that had a sensitivity to TSH levels of 0.8 μU/mL.[38] However, the assay was too time-consuming to perform.[84,p.39]

Other TSH assays soon appeared on the market. From the mid-to-late 1980s, researchers developed immunometric assays that technicians could perform more rapidly.[81] These second generation tests are termed "supersensitive" TSH assays. Unlike their predecessors, these assays distinguish normal from lower-than-normal TSH levels.[39] Hay wrote of the assays, these supersensitive TSH assays "may soon be considered the single best indicator of abnormal thyroid function and potentially could become the best initial test of thyroid function in all situations of suspected thyroid dysfunction."[84,p.39]

Persisting Problems with the TSH Test

Despite Hay's and other researchers' enthusiastic judgments of the potential of immunometric TSH assays, the assays are not problem-free. In a 1993 report,

Laurberg noted that sensitive immunometric TSH assays have improved the clinician's ability to diagnose abnormalities of thyroid function. He also noted that the serum TSH is often used as the initial screening for assessing thyroid function. He wrote, however: "Shortly after the marketing of the first of these assays, it was discovered that some sera contained heterophilic antibodies leading to spuriously high TSH values. This problem is considered solved by modifications of the assays. We have, however, found that these assays may still give nonspecific results."[76]

Laurberg evaluated six different TSH assays: Beri-Lux, Spectria, London, Amerlite, Delfia, Delfia Ultra. He evaluated the assays using sera from 63 patients with untreated hyperthyroidism. Fifty-one of the patients had Graves' disease and 12 had Plummer's disease. He found several problems. Most important was a problem with specificity. According to at least one of the six assays, TSH levels were totally suppressed in all 63 serum samples. Despite this outcome, TSH levels in many samples were "clearly and reproducibly measurable" in one or more assays. According to at least one assay, TSH levels were higher than 0.10 μU/mL in 11 samples and higher than 0.40 μU/mL in 6 samples. The patterns of nonspecific values were different in all six assays. Laurberg also found that adding 10% mouse serum to the patients' sera resulted in unpredictable changes in lower TSH levels according to one assay. He concluded: "Hence a measurable serum TSH alone does not always exclude primary hyperfunction of the thyroid. Nonspecific TSH values are the most common cause of nonsuppressed TSH in hyperthyroidism and should be considered before other causes, such as pituitary TSH producing neoplasms or pituitary resistance to thyroid hormone."[76]

In 1996, researchers in Australia found that abnormal free T_4 levels were missed in 2.7% of cases because the patients' TSH levels were normal.[181] Also in 1996, Bauer and Brown reported that among 1835 patients with normal sensitive TSH results, the free T_4 level was low in 11 patients (0.6%) and high in 24 patients (1.3%).[134] Though these reports show that modern TSH assays are highly sensitive, they also show that the clinician will miss some patients with abnormal free T_4 levels if he orders only TSH assays.

Kraus et al. conducted a study in 1997 to learn the prevalence of exaggerated TRH-stimulation test results in a sample of depressed patients with "high-normal" screening TSH levels. The investigators performed TRH-stimulation tests on 60 depressed patients with TSH levels between 3.0 and 5.5 μU/mL. Of the 60 patients, 23 (38%) had exaggerated TSH response to

TRH. The investigators defined exaggerated as 25 μU/mL above the baseline value. They concluded, "Subtle thyroid underfunction may be contributing to depression in some patients with TSH in the upper half of the range usually considered normal. If so, then the TRH-stimulation test may be more sensitive in identifying this than measurement of TSH alone."[11] Kraus et al. also reported that an unexpected observation was a lack of correlation between TSH levels week-to-week (r = .17, non-significant). They also found a lack of correlation between screening TSH values and subsequent TRH-stimulation test results (r = .28, non-significant).[11]

Not all patients with elevated TSH and normal thyroid hormone levels have subclinical hypothyroidism and eventually develop overt hypothyroidism. Kabadi and Cech studied 17 patients who had elevated TSH and normal thyroid hormone levels. In 8 patients, the basal 24-hour ^{131}I uptake was low-normal. The increase in ^{131}I uptake following TSH administration, and the decrease in ^{131}I uptake following T_3 administration, were also low-normal. These patients developed overt hypothyroidism and required thyroid hormone treatment within 2 years. In the other 9 subjects, the 24-hour ^{131}I uptake was normal. The increase in ^{131}I uptake in response to TSH, and the decrease in ^{131}I uptake in response to T_3, were also normal. These patients did not develop overt hypothyroidism during a 16-year follow-up period. The researchers suggested that in the patient with an elevated TSH level, normal thyroid hormone levels, and a normally responsive thyroid gland, the elevated TSH represents a "reset thyrostat" at a higher TSH level for life.[160] This study brings into question categorical conclusions about patients with elevated TSH levels. It also brings into question the use of basal TSH level alone for diagnostic purposes.

Third-Generation TSH Assays

A common belief in conventional medicine is that third-generation TSH assays have made the TRH-stimulation test obsolete. The belief is patently false. The TRH-stimulation test remains valuable in the diagnosis of some cases of subclinical hypothyroidism[161] and in the diagnosis of central hypothyroidism (see section below titled "TRH-Stimulation Test"). The third-generation TSH chemiluminescent assay measures *low* TSH levels with extraordinary sensitivity (8-to-10 fold the sensitivity of the immunoradiometric assay).[136] However, as Ross et al. wrote, "The clinical utility of increasingly sensitive TSH assays will be to distinguish degrees of thyrotroph suppression in subclinical hyperthyroidism." The third-generation TSH assay is no more useful than the second-generation assay for identifying hypothyroid patients.[86]

Vanderpump et al. concluded from a cost-related study, "In financial terms, there is little justification for use of assays with sensitivity greater than the second generation (0.1 μU/mL)."[105]

Hyperthyroidism

Hyperthyroidism is sustained hyperfunction of the thyroid gland with continuing excess of thyroid hormone biosynthesis and secretion from the gland.[60,p.645] The clinician should be aware that hyperthyroidism and thyrotoxicosis are distinctly different conditions, although they may occur simultaneously. Hyperthyroidism is a description of thyroid gland activity and thyroid hormone levels—*not* a description of tissue metabolism. Rarely, for example, tissue metabolism is normal or abnormally slow despite the presence of hyperthyroidism. The term thyrotoxicosis, by contrast, refers to the clinical syndrome of hypermetabolism associated with elevated levels of free T_3 and T_4.[60,p.645] *In all of diagnostic practice, probably no other confusion of concepts likely results in more mistaken diagnoses and improper treatment of patients. I cannot overemphasize the importance of understanding the difference between hyperthyroidism and thyrotoxicosis.*

In hyperthyroidism, elevated T_3 and T_4 levels suppress TSH secretion by pituitary thyrotroph cells. Before highly sensitive TSH assays were available, as in the early 1980s,[130] the TRH-stimulation test was important in diagnosing hyperthyroidism. In the hyperthyroid patient, the excess thyroid hormone suppression of the thyrotroph cells caused a blunted TSH response to injected TRH. A normal rise in the TSH following a TRH injection excludes hyperthyroidism.[129]

The extremely sensitive TSH assays now available make the TRH-stimulation test unnecessary for diagnosing hyperthyroidism.[84] A low TSH; elevated total and free T_4; and clinical signs, symptoms, and peripheral indices of hypermetabolism are sufficient for the diagnosis.[64,p.655]

Primary Hypothyroidism

In primary hypothyroidism, the thyroid gland is impaired in its ability to synthesize and secrete thyroid hormone. As a result, the blood levels of T_3 and T_4 decrease to below normal. Because thyroid hormones inhibit the pituitary gland's secretion of TSH, dimin-

ishing levels of the hormones disinhibit the pituitary's secretion of TSH and the TSH level rises. But the level of elevation that indicates hypothyroidism is moot at this time. Regarding the diagnosis of primary hypothyroidism, the endocrinologist Ridgway recently wrote, "The most important diagnostic test is measurement of the serum thyrotropin (TSH) concentration, which will increase above the normal range in both mild and severe cases."[180] The diagnosis of hypothyroidism, however, is often not so cut-and-dried (see the subsection below titled "Interpretation" and the section titled "TRH-Stimulation Test: Primary Hypothyroidism").

Subclinical Hypothyroidism. Subclinical hypothyroidism is defined as an elevated TSH level and a low free T_4 level. Over time, the TSH level may decrease to within the normal range, or it may remain elevated despite the patient's free T_4 level remaining normal. In some patients, however, the free T_4 level may descend below the lower limit of normal. The diagnosis of overt hypothyroidism is then made. Among patients with subclinical hypothyroidism, those with the highest TSH levels and detectable antithyroid antibodies are more likely to develop overt hypothyroidism.[152] Because patients with subclinical hypothyroidism sometimes have subtle hypothyroid symptoms and may have mild abnormalities of serum lipoproteins and cardiac function, patients with definite and persistent TSH elevation should be considered for thyroid treatment.

One of the mandates of conventional endocrinology/thyroidology is that T_4 is the only thyroid hormone clinicians should prescribe for subclinical hypothyroidism. Another mandate is that patients should only use a dosage that keeps the TSH within the normal range. These mandates cannot be defended scientifically. Patients should use either a product such as desiccated thyroid that contains both T_4 and T_3, or T_3 alone.

Normally, an increased serum TSH level causes the thyroid gland to release more T_3 and T_4, increasing their serum levels. But when the thyroid gland is impaired, as the TSH level rises within its normal range, the gland can only slightly increase its secretion of T_3 and T_4. This modestly raises T_3 and T_4 levels in the blood. But to increase the serum T_3 and T_4 levels to the mid-normal range and maintain them there, the pituitary gland must secrete enough TSH to raise the TSH level beyond the upper limit of the normal range. The increase of TSH molecules binding to their receptors on the substrate-deprived or otherwise impaired thyroid gland drives it to secrete more hormones, raising their serum levels.

Thus, measurement of the TSH level is an evaluation of the pituitary-thyroid axis. Conventional thyroidologists believe this is true even without using thyroid hormone measures. According to Carlson and Hershman, a high serum TSH is the most sensitive laboratory index of primary hypothyroidism.[132] In fact, the pituitary gland's TSH-secreting thyrotroph cells are so sensitive to changes in T_4 levels that the TSH may elevate in a patient whose T_4 level is within the normal range but low for her normal "set point."[96,p.241]

"Owing to the local nature of the T_4 feedback at the pituitary," wrote LoPresti, "alterations in serum TSH values amplify small changes in circulating free T_4 values. The net result of these unique attributes of measuring TSH is the ability to detect thyroid dysfunction early in the course of thyroid disease."[169] Some clinicians suggest that the patient begin to use exogenous thyroid hormone when her TSH level is high, although she is "clinically euthyroid"—that is, when she appears to have normal metabolism. For example, some patients previously treated with radioactive iodine for hyperthyroidism (to decrease thyroid gland secretion of thyroid hormone) may show an elevated TSH while the T_4 is normal. This suggests a failing thyroid gland that is likely to result in hypothyroidism.[97] Taking a T_4 supplement is considered preemptive treatment for the patient.

. **Overt Hypothyroidism.** The clinician should make a tentative diagnosis of overt hypothyroidism when the patient's TSH is elevated and measures of thyroid hormones indicate low circulating levels. This criterion for the diagnosis conflicts with the recent finding that patients with basal TSH levels of 2.0 μU/mL or above within the normal reference range (high-normal) have an increased probability of future overt hypothyroidism.[154][155] The clinician must judge whether to make the diagnosis when the patient has low thyroid hormone levels and what is conventionally considered a high-normal TSH level.

Diagnosis of Primary Hypothyroidism: Tentative Without Supporting Evidence. A high TSH is not an absolute indicator of primary hypothyroidism. Hamburger advised that in addition to an elevated TSH, the clinician should support the conclusion that the patient has primary hypothyroidism with additional clinical and laboratory data.[33,p.121] The clinician should look for a cause for the suspected primary hypothyroidism. Hamburger noted that more than 95% of primary hypothyroidism in the United States results from Hashimoto's thyroiditis, previous thyroidectomy, or radioactive iodine therapy. "In the absence of these causes," he wrote, "one should make a diagnosis of

hypothyroidism reluctantly and only after careful documentation."[33,p.121] Such evidential data supports the conclusion that the patient is hypothyroid. But in its absence, a trial of exogenous thyroid hormone may nevertheless relieve the patient's hypothyroid-like signs and symptoms, suggesting (although not proving) that the patient was hypothyroid.

Incidence of Primary Hypothyroidism in Fibromyalgia Patients. Shiroky and coworkers found that of 34 fibromyalgia patients, 4 (12%) had primary hypothyroidism.[61] Eisinger reported that 6 of 62 fibromyalgia patients (10.3%) had primary hypothyroidism.[62] I found that of 38 fibromyalgia patients, 10.5% had primary hypothyroidism. The normal TSH range was 0.4-to-6.0 μU/mL. The range of my patients' high TSH levels was 6.5-to-9.08 μU/mL; the mean was 8.16 μU/mL.[36]

The results of these studies of the incidence of primary hypothyroidism in fibromyalgia indicate that primary hypothyroidism is far more common in fibromyalgia patients than in the general population.[93,p.40]

TSH Levels in Thyroid Hormone Resistance Syndromes

In general resistance and pituitary resistance to thyroid hormone, patients' TSH levels are inappropriately elevated for the patient's circulating thyroid hormone levels. For the classification of patients with thyroid hormone resistance, see Chapter 2.6, section titled "The Three Clinical Classifications of Thyroid Hormone Resistance."

Basal TSH Level: Not an Effective Basis for Titrating Thyroid Hormone Dosage

In the early 1970s, before the RIA was available for measuring TSH levels, most clinicians advised primary hypothyroid patients to use 200-to-400 μg (0.2-to-0.4 mg) of T_4 per day[45,p.91][51][52,p.456] or its equivalent of desiccated thyroid. The clinicians recommended this dosage range because their assessment of the tissue effects of thyroid hormone therapy showed that the dosage range was safe and effective. As Pearch and Himsworth wrote, in the long history of patients using such dosages, they had no apparent resulting adverse health effects.[158,p.695] Toft wrote that when TSH assays came into widespread use, it became clear that 100-to-200 μg (0.1-to-0.2 mg) of T_4 maintained normal thyroid hormone levels in 90% of patients. (Toft considered normal thyroid hormone levels to be those that maintained the TSH within the normal reference range.)[45]

When conventional medicine adopted thyroid hormone and TSH levels as the criteria by which to titrate dosages, clinicians generally came to ignore the tissue effects of thyroid hormone medication. The consequence is that legions of hypothyroid patients now bitterly complain about the incompetence of most clinicians treating them for the condition. The usual complaint is that conventional clinicians treat lab test results and not patients, obtaining the preferred laboratory test values but leaving the patients ill. The disenchantment of patients with conventional treatment has stimulated a substantial movement of patients from offices of conventional clinicians to those of alternative practitioners. The phenomenon is substantial enough to prompt complaints by some prominent conventional thyroidologists.[159] (See Chapter 2.5, section titled "Laboratory Thyroid Function Testing is of No Value in the Dosage Titration of Hypothyroid and Euthyroid Hypometabolic Patients.")

A dosage of 0.1-to-0.2 mg of T_4 may hold a patient's TSH in the middle of the normal range, but the dosage leaves many patients—perhaps most—hypometabolic and symptomatic. Use of such dosages subjects patients to serious health risks (see Chapter 4.4, section titled "Harm from Untreated and Undertreated Hypothyroidism"). The clinician should initially determine the patient's thyroid status through laboratory testing. During her treatment, however, he should titrate her thyroid hormone dosage according to changes in her symptoms, signs, and peripheral indices of tissue metabolism (see Chapter 4.3). The clinician has no scientific justification for ordering further tests of thyroid function, including the TSH.

Use of Thyroid Hormone Levels Rather Than TSH Levels to Titrate Thyroid Hormone Dosage

Hamburger contended that there can be no doubt that the supersensitive TSH test is the best for screening for abnormal thyroid function.[33,p.120] Hay wrote that the test is sensitive and specific for diagnosing thyroid disease *in patients with intact hypothalamic-pituitary function.*[84] In these patients, an abnormal supersensitive TSH strongly suggests clinical or subclinical thyroid hormone deficiency or excess. Upon finding the abnormal TSH level, the clinician can then confirm the deficiency with a free T_4 test or the excess with a free T_3 test. This is true. Nevertheless, TSH assays—no matter how sensitive—are useless for determining dosages that provide patients with normal tissue metabolism and freedom from symptoms.

Some writers have recommended that clinicians

use thyroid hormone levels rather than TSH levels to titrate thyroid hormone dosages. For example, some argued that the total T_3 or free T_3 are best for monitoring patients taking T_4.[46][47] Their reason was that the effective dosage of T_4 may suppress the basal TSH and blunt the TSH response to TRH. There is a two-point explanation for this.

First, as Volpé implied, exogenous T_4 and T_4 secreted by the thyroid gland exert a combined action in suppressing TSH secretion. The combined action suppresses TSH secretion so that the patient has a low basal TSH and a blunted TSH response to TRH. In a patient who has absolutely no thyroid gland secretion at the start of therapy, a replacement dosage of thyroid hormone does not have these TSH suppressive effects. In the typical patient beginning T_4 therapy, however, the thyroid gland secretes somewhere between a minute amount of thyroid hormone and a virtually normal amount. The exogenous T_4 combines with that secreted by the gland to suppress the basal TSH and blunt the TSH response to TRH. Volpé wrote, "If before treatment there is some degree of feedback, however minimal (with some TSH suppression, however minimal), then clearly less than a physiologic replacement dose is required to bring that particular person to a precisely 'normal' status—where the TSH response to TRH is perfectly normal and the sensitive TSH assay is in the middle of the normal range."[45,p.88]

The second point of the explanation is that if the clinician adjusts the patient's thyroid hormone dosage by monitoring thyroid hormone levels, he should monitor T_3 levels. Some researchers contend that serum T_3 levels correlate better with patients' clinical status than serum T_4 levels.[45,p.88][48] But to achieve a normal circulating level of T_3, the patient may have to take a large enough dosage of T_4 to suppress the basal TSH and blunt the TSH response to TRH. Bantle[49] and Larsen[45,p.90] essentially agreed with this view. About 18% of the total T_3 is secreted into the circulation by the thyroid gland. The other 82% derives from the peripheral conversion of T_4 to T_3. In the hypothyroid patient, the thyroid gland secretes a lower than normal amount of T_3. As a result, the total T_3 in the body is deficient by the amount the gland fails to secrete. The patient can maintain a normal serum T_3 level, however, by increasing her dosage of T_4; by doing so, she increases the amount of T_4 available to be deiodinated to T_3. "Practicing physicians should therefore not be surprised," wrote Volpé, "by moderately elevated T_4 concentrations in T_4-replaced patients and should not interpret such values as indicative of hyperthyroidism."[45,pp.88-89] Pearce and Himsworth agreed. They found that with replacement dosages of T_4, only modest increases in total and free T_3 accompanied large increases in total and free T_4 concentrations. They wrote that their "main practical conclusion is clear—namely, that supraphysiological free thyroxine concentrations are not necessarily accompanied by an increase in the free triiodothyronine concentration above the normal range."[74,p.693] They concluded, "The presence of total or free thyroxine concentrations above normal in patients taking thyroxine therefore are [sic] not necessarily of clinical consequence." Also, the TSH level will be below the much touted midrange value, and this, too, should not be misinterpreted as an indication of over-medication with thyroid hormone.[74,p.695]

The clinician should note, however, that T_4 and T_3 levels tell us no more than the TSH level about peripheral tissue metabolic status. Only the patient's symptoms, signs, and peripheral indices provide the clinician with an understanding of the effect of particular dosages on the patient's tissues.

Low Basal TSH Alone: Not Diagnostic of Hyperthyroidism

Baseline TSH levels in central hypothyroid patients vary. Some patents have elevated levels, some have normal levels, and others have low or undetectable levels.[93,p.46] The clinician should bear this in mind and not decide prematurely that a low or undetectable basal TSH level is diagnostic of hyperthyroidism. The patient may have central hypothyroidism.

When the patient's basal TSH level is low, a suspicion of hyperthyroidism is reasonable in that high thyroid hormone levels suppress TSH secretion. Still, the clinician should not diagnose hyperthyroidism unless the patient has a high free T_3 level and symptoms, signs, and peripheral indices indicative of tissue thyrotoxicosis. If the patient's clinical status suggests she is *hypo*metabolic rather than *hyper*metabolic, the clinician should not make a diagnosis of hyperthyroidism. A TRH-stimulation test may help the clinician determine the thyroid status of the patient with a low or undetectable basal TSH level.

Limitations of the Basal TSH

As indicated by the report by Laurberg that I described in the introduction to the TSH section, modern TSH assays are not failsafe.[76] Nonetheless, the assays are reasonably sensitive and reliable. The serious problems with the TSH test are inherent in some thyroidologists' exaggerated claims of the usefulness of the test. Notwithstanding their claims, the test has distinct

limitations. The failure of conventional medicine to heed the limitations has seriously compromised the effectiveness of the treatment of patients with inadequate thyroid hormone regulation of their tissues.

Braverman and Utiger wrote, "The term *hyperthyroidism* is used to mean sustained thyroid hyperfunction associated with sustained increases in thyroid hormone biosynthesis and release from the thyroid gland."[60,p.645] A low or suppressed TSH is not diagnostic of hyperthyroidism. This is true because the TSH level may be low or suppressed in pituitary hypothyroidism.

A low or suppressed TSH level is also not diagnostic of thyrotoxicosis. Ladenson pointed out that the free T_4 can be falsely elevated because of familial dysalbuminemic hyperthyroxinemia and certain nonthyroidal illnesses. Enigmatically, he then noted that the TSH is a "more sensitive way to screen for thyrotoxicosis." The clinician should note that he uses the words "screen for thyrotoxicosis." Many practicing endocrinologists, and other clinicians who subscribe to the endocrinologists' opinions, believe that a low or suppressed TSH level is synonymous with thyrotoxicosis. Ladenson wrote that "Low serum TSH values do not necessarily indicate clinically important thyrotoxicosis . . . ."[79,p.883] In fact, a low TSH only raises the *possibility* of thyrotoxicosis. Thyrotoxicity is possible because a high enough thyroid hormone level lowers or suppresses the TSH level. However, it is critical for patient welfare that the clinician understand that a low or suppressed TSH level does not demonstrate thyrotoxicosis. The clinician should bear in mind Braverman and Utiger's definition of thyrotoxicosis: "We use the term *thyrotoxicosis* to mean the clinical syndrome that results when the circulating concentration of free thyroxine (T_4) or triiodothyronine (T_3) is increased."[60,p.645] It is clearly false that a low TSH level is diagnostic of thyrotoxicosis. If the TSH is low, the clinician must examine the patient and perform other tests that can detect tissue effects of excessive thyroid hormone tissue stimulation (see Chapter 4.3).

Another limitation of the TSH test is that it does not provide the clinician with information on the metabolic status of tissues other than the pituitary. Some authors suggest that the clinician can infer from the patient's TSH level the status of peripheral tissues. In some cases, such an inference is potentially catastrophic. Perk and O'Neill wrote, for example, "With the help of modern, sensitive thyroid stimulating hormone assays, higher doses of L-thyroxine may be safer and more effective in the atherosclerosis management of this patient population."[128] This statement implies that the clinician can infer from the TSH how the patient's thyroid hormone dosage is affecting her heart. But the TSH level provides no information whatever about the patient's cardiac status. The level tells the clinician only how the pituitary thyrotrophs are responding to the thyroid hormone reaching and acting in these cells. To assume more from the TSH level—especially about how a patient's heart is responding to thyroid hormone—is to risk the patient's life.

Interpretation

Conventionally, the normal reference range for the TSH level is 0.4-to-6.0 µU/mL. However, some laboratories give 4.5, 5.0, or 5.5 µU/mL as the upper limit of normal. Despite this range, the clinician should consider possible thyroid gland hypofunction in the patient whose TSH level is 2.0 µU/mL or more. If the 30-minute TSH level of the patient with a basal TSH level of 2.0 µU/mL or more is exaggerated during a TRH-stimulation test, the patient probably has incipient hypothyroidism (see section below titled "TRH-Stimulation Test").

An elevated basal TSH in a clinically hypometabolic patient indicates primary hypothyroidism. When circulating thyroid hormone levels are normal, the conventional diagnosis is subclinical hypothyroidism. If circulating thyroid hormone levels are low, the conventional diagnosis is overt hypothyroidism. The diagnosis is more likely accurate if the patient has symptoms, signs, and peripheral indices characteristic of hypothyroidism. In fact, the diagnosis of primary hypothyroidism is tentative unless the patient has had a thyroidectomy, antithyroid drug therapy, has antithyroid antibodies, or has other evidence of thyroid gland damage. In the absence of these in fibromyalgia patients, however, a trial of thyroid hormone therapy is warranted.

The clinician should seek evidence of a cause for thyroid gland dysfunction. He should especially order tests for thyroid microsomal and thyroglobulin antibodies because autoimmune thyroiditis is the most common cause of subclinical and overt hypothyroidism (see section below titled "Thyroid Autoantibodies").

A low TSH *may* be due to hyperthyroidism. The diagnosis is confirmed if the patient has an elevated serum free T₃ and signs, symptoms, and peripheral indices characteristic of hypermetabolism. However, the TSH level may be low in central hypothyroidism due to anterior pituitary dysfunction. The clinician can best evaluate thyrotroph cell function with a TRH-stimulation test. In central hypothyroidism due to hypothala-

mic dysfunction, the basal TSH level is likely to be within the normal range. Nevertheless, the TSH may have low bioactivity and fail to maintain normal thyroid gland function.

TRH-STIMULATION TEST

The hypothalamus secretes thyrotropin releasing hormone (TRH). The TRH stimulates the thyrotroph cells of the anterior pituitary gland to secrete TSH (for physiology, see Chapter 2.1, section titled "Thyrotropin-Releasing Hormone"). In the TRH-stimulation test, the clinician injects TRH intravenously. Unless the function of the patient's pituitary thyrotroph cells is severely impaired, the injected TRH causes a rise in serum TSH.

Authors differ somewhat in their reports of the timing of the TSH response to TRH. Howanitz and Howanitz wrote that within 5 minutes or so after injecting 500 µg, the serum TSH level rises. The level peaks in 20-to-30 minutes and declines to the base level in 2-to-4 hours.[28,p.429] Carlson and Hershman wrote that the TSH level usually elevates within 10 minutes after the clinician injects the TRH. The TSH reaches a peak 15-to-30 minutes after the injection, followed by a decline to basal levels over the next 1-to-4 hours.[132] Utiger wrote that the TSH may peak between 15 and 45 minutes. For clinical purposes, he advised the clinician to take serum samples once or twice after injecting the TRH: once at 20 minutes, or once at 15 and 30 minutes.[100,p.512]

The increased TSH following a TRH injection temporarily stimulates the thyroid gland. In euthyroid patients, this increases the serum level of T₃ some 70% above its basal level 1-to-4 hours after the injection. The serum T₄ level increases about 15%-to-50%.[133] Utiger wrote that the increases in T₃ and T₄ are small and variable.[100,p.512] Because of this, he cautioned that the T₃ and T₄ levels not be substituted for the TSH in assessing the response to TRH.

Hyperthyroidism

For many clinicians, the most important use of the TRH-stimulation test is in ruling out hyperthyroidism. In hyperthyroidism, the elevated T₃ and T₄ levels suppress secretion of TSH by the thyrotrophs. So in hyperthyroid patients, the TSH response to injected TRH is blunted. In most hyperthyroid patients, the 30-minute TSH level is no higher than the baseline TSH level. A normal rise in the TSH following a TRH injection excludes hyperthyroidism.[129]

In 1984, sensitive TSH assays became available that could distinguish low basal levels of TSH in hyperthyroid patients.[130] Today, highly sensitive TSH assays detect TSH levels that were undetectable by all earlier assays. These highly sensitive assays make the TRH-stimulation test unnecessary only for diagnosing and monitoring hyperthyroid patients.[84] (See section above titled "Thyrotropin (TSH): Hyperthyroidism.")

Primary Hypothyroidism

Conventional medical clinicians used to use the TRH-stimulation test to diagnose hypothyroidism and to titrate thyroid hormone dosage. Most patients with incipient thyroid gland hypofunction have exaggerated TSH responses to TRH before they begin taking thyroid hormone. Before the basal TSH began being promoted as a "gold standard" of thyroid function, some clinicians also performed additional TRH-stimulation tests to help titrate the patients' thyroid hormone dosages. If a patient's TSH response to TRH was still exaggerated, this was considered evidence that her dosage was inadequate. The clinician continued to increase the patient's dosage and perform TRH-stimulation tests until the TSH response was within the normal range (see below, subsection titled "Interpretation").

Many patients with subnormal thyroid gland function do not have low T_3 and T_4 levels. This is often the case in patients with endemic goiter, thyroid damage from ^{131}I therapy, and autoimmune thyroiditis. When the basal TSH level is above the upper limit of the normal reference range, the conventional diagnosis is subclinical hypothyroidism. But many patients have basal TSH levels between the middle and the upper limit of the range. In these patients, the TRH- stimulation test is likely to result in an exaggerated 30-minute TSH level, suggesting thyroid gland hypofunction.[100,p.512] The exaggerated TSH response to TRH supports the diagnosis of hypothyroidism.[45,p.103] In addition to this pattern of lab values, and despite a high-sensitivity TSH within the normal range, the presence of clinical features of hypometabolism and a positive therapeutic response to thyroid hormone strongly support the diagnosis of primary hypothyroidism. In one recent study, patients with TSH levels of 2.0 or more μU/mL had a high risk of later developing overt hypothyroidism.[155] This suggests that patients with incipient hypothyroidism are among the population of individuals with basal TSH levels of 2.0 or more μU/mL.[154] It is probably justified to order a TRH-stimulation test on symptomatic patients with such TSH levels.

Utiger wrote, "An augmented TSH response to TRH is an even more sensitive indicator of thyroid deficiency than is an increased basal serum TSH concentration." He wrote that the patient will have an exaggerated TSH response to TRH even if she has only a small degree of thyroid hormone deficiency. He argued that the small degree of hormone deficiency seldom if ever produces symptoms and does not require the use of thyroid hormone.[100,p.516] The implication is that there is no need to use the TRH-stimulation test to identify such patients. Hamburger acknowledged at least a limited role for the test in identifying primary hypothyroid patients: "I find the test helpful in patients with evidence for Hashimoto's thyroiditis and borderline or slightly elevated TSH values, and for those with similarly borderline values, who are on thyroxine for *bona fide* primary hypothyroidism but still have persistent complaints that suggest (to them or to me) a need for a higher dose of thyroxine." He also stated, however, that it is arguable whether an exaggerated TSH response during the TRH-stimulation test has a role in the confirmation of mild primary hypothyroidism.[33,p.121]

Others, myself included, disagree with Utiger's and Hamburger's judgments that the TRH-stimulation test may be of no use. We disagree because we have found that many of our patients have troubling or debilitating symptoms associated with even incipient thyroid gland hypofunction.[104] In my clinical practice, the test has been useful in identifying patients with primary hypothyroidism not revealed by the standard profile of thyroid function tests and who subsequently markedly improved or recovered from their fibromyalgia with thyroid hormone therapy. I reported diagnosing a patient as primary hypothyroid despite 6 endocrinologists over an 8-year period pronouncing her euthyroid and denying her thyroid hormone therapy. I diagnosed this patient's condition as primary hypothyroidism even though her basal TSH levels on two occasions (5.3 and 5.54 μU/mL) were within the normal range of 0.4-to-6.0 μU/mL. I did so for two reasons. First, her total T_4 level was at the lower end of the normal range at 4.7 μg/dL (normal range: 4.5-to-12.5 μg/dL), and her high normal TSH was appropriately inversely proportional to the low-normal T_4. Second, a TRH-stimulation test in such cases often permits a definitive diagnosis, as in the case of this patient. Her 30-minute TSH response to TRH was 40.32 μU/mL, which was 34.78 μU/mL above the baseline value (normal range above baseline: 8.5-to-20 μU/mL). This post-TRH increase in TSH is also roughly proportionally appropriate to her basal TSH levels, as Seth and Beckett have shown.[9] Without the TRH-stimulation test results, some clinicians would have classified her as euthyroid and denied her thyroid hormone treatment. However, following a proper diagnosis, she dramatically recovered within 3 months from all features of fibromyalgia. Her metabolic rehabilitation included the use of non-TSH-suppressive dosages of T_4.[36] Many patients with subnormal thyroid function who benefit from thyroid hormone therapy can be identified *only* through the TRH-stimulation test. These patients' health and the quality of their lives critically depend on clinicians' use of the test.

Central Hypothyroidism

Central hypothyroidism is a deficiency of thyroid hormone secondary to hypothalamic or pituitary dysfunction. For distinguishing euthyroid patients from those with possible central hypothyroidism, the TRH-stimulation test is indispensable for most clinicians. Measurements taken to detect a subnormal "nocturnal TSH surge" in the late evening or early morning are also useful for identifying patients with central hypothyroidism.[65][67][68][69][70][71][72][73] Performing the test, however, requires hospitalization. This makes measuring the nocturnal TSH surge far more costly and inconvenient than the TRH-stimulation test.

Basal TSH: Not of Use in Diagnosing Central Hypothyroidism. The basal TSH test is useless for identifying patients with central hypothyroidism. I say this for two reasons. First, TSH levels are normal in most patients with central hypothyroidism, and second, the TSH of central hypothyroid patients may have low bioactivity.

Basal TSH Is Usually Normal in Central Hypothyroidism. Serum basal TSH concentrations are usually normal in patients with central hypothyroidism. Because of this, the basal TSH level does not accurately predict the TSH response to injected TRH. Some researchers have written that basal TSH levels are most often low-normal in patients with central hypothyroidism. They have reported such TSH values as 0.5-to-1.0 µU/mL or slightly lower.[5][6] However, Patel and Burger used an assay that met rigorous standards for sensitivity and specificity and found a normal or even slightly increased plasma TSH in 16 of 18 patients with confirmed hypothyroidism secondary to pituitary or hypothalamic lesions.[43]

Normally, when thyroid hormone levels are low, the pituitary thyrotroph cells become disinhibited. The cells then synthesize and secrete increased amounts of TSH, raising the circulating TSH level. But when low thyroid hormone levels are accompanied by a low-normal TSH level, it is possible that the patient's thyro-

trophs are not able to synthesize and secrete enough TSH to stimulate the thyroid gland to release an adequate amount of thyroid hormone to raise the circulating thyroid hormone level. If this in fact is the involved mechanism, a diagnosis of central hypothyroidism would be proper. Moreover, the finding of a low-normal TSH level and low-normal thyroid hormone levels would predict the outcome of the TRH-stimulation test and thus render the test unnecessary. However, my analysis of thyroid function test results in 38 patients indicates that the pattern of a low-normal TSH and low-normal thyroid hormone levels does not accurately predict the outcome of the TRH-stimulation test. Of 20 patients whose TRH-stimulation test results were consistent with central hypothyroidism, only 9 (45%) had low-normal T_4, free thyroxine index, and TSH levels. Of the 14 patients whose TRH-stimulation test results were consistent with euthyroidism, the same TSH and thyroid hormone pattern was present in the results of 7 (50%).[36]

Table 4.2.4 shows the percentage of 38 fibromyalgia patients in one study who were euthyroid, primary hypothyroid, and central hypothyroid, and the mean and range of basal TSH values for each. Of the patients with laboratory test results consistent with central hypothyroidism, those with blunted TSH responses to TRH had lower mean basal TSH values and a lower range of TSH levels than patients with exaggerated TSH responses. Euthyroid patients had basal TSH values between those of patients with blunted and exaggerated TSH responses to TRH.[36] Despite these differences, other than the elevated basal TSH value of primary hypothyroid patients, the basal TSH levels are not of practical importance in classifying patients according to thyroid status.

These findings do not support the view that clinicians can use this pattern of values from the thyroid profile to predict TRH-stimulation test results consistent with central hypothyroidism. The TRH-stimulation test, therefore, remains the most readily accessible and cost-effective tool for most clinicians. The TRH-stimulation test is definitely not obsolete.

Low Bioactivity of TSH in Central Hypothyroidism. The second reason I contend that the basal TSH is useless for diagnosing central hypothyroidism is the low bioactivity of TSH in some central hypothyroid patients. On principle, we would expect normal TSH levels to maintain normal thyroid hormone secretion by the thyroid gland. But despite normal basal TSH levels in central hypothyroidism due to hypothalamic dysfunction, the TSH molecules are apparently structurally altered, and the release of thyroid hormones by the thyroid gland in response to the altered TSH is suboptimal.[131] (See Chapter 2.1, section titled "Variations in TSH Bioactivity.") So despite having a normal basal TSH level, TSH stimulation of the patient's thyroid gland may be subnormal.

When completely deprived of TRH, the pituitary thyrotroph cells reduce their TSH secretion. But the cells continue to secrete at least small amounts of TSH. Secretion of these small amounts shows that the pituitary secretes TSH in response to low levels of T_3 and T_4 independently of TRH stimulation. This indicates that the hypothalamus and the TRH it secretes act as a fine control device that adjusts how sensitively the thyrotrophs respond to thyroid hormone.[102][127]

In hypothalamic hypothyroidism, TRH stimulates the pituitary thyrotrophs to synthesize and secrete structurally altered TSH. Even when TRH is deficient because of hypothalamic dysfunction, the thyrotrophs secrete normal amounts of TSH, but the TSH does not bind normally to TSH receptors on thyroid gland cells. Because of the lack of normal binding, we say that the TSH does not have normal "biologic activity"[131]— that is, it does not stimulate the thyroid gland to synthesize and secrete normal amounts of thyroid hormones. Hershman cited studies showing reduced biologic activity of the serum TSH of central hypothyroid patients.[93,pp.46-47] Beck-Peccoz and colleagues, for example, reported that in hypothalamic hypothyroidism, secreted TSH lacks normal biologic activity because it does not bind effectively to TSH receptors in the thyroid gland. Treatment with TRH corrects the problem, showing that the patients' endogenous TRH is somehow defective. They wrote, "These data suggest that TRH regulates not only the secretion of thyrotropin (TSH), but also its specific molecular and conformational features required for hormone action."[131,p.1085] Hershman wrote that in central hypothyroid patients, large increases in TSH following TRH injections usually result in subnormal T_3 increases. But the thyroid gland responds normally to exogenous TSH. Cytochemical bioassay has shown that the biologic activity of the endogenous TSH is below that expected based on immunologic activity. Hershman also stated that the molecular basis for the reduced activity is not known, but the altered TSH apparently fails to adequately prompt the thyroid gland to provide normal blood levels of thyroid hormone.[93,pp.46-47] This has created confusion in that many clinicians expect pituitary or hypothalamic dysfunction to result in diminished amounts of TSH rather than normal amounts of defective TSH. The circumstance is complicated, then, in that diagnosis cannot be made in a clear-cut fashion

based on a low TSH level (since the level is usually normal despite low thyroid hormone levels).

Another way of wording this is that we cannot predict from basal TSH and thyroid hormone levels the results of the TRH-stimulation test. Physiologically, if the total T_4 and free thyroxine index are in the lower half of the normal range, the expected finding would be that the TSH is, inversely, in the upper half of the normal range. But when all these measures are in the lower half of the normal range, this could indicate that because the pituitary thyrotroph cells are dysfunctional, they are not being properly disinhibited by lower levels of T_4. Thus, a diagnosis of central hypothyroidism could be made by simply looking for this pattern within the standard thyroid panel. If this were true, it would render the TRH-stimulation test unnecessary for diagnosis of central hypothyroidism. As I described in the previous section, however, I did not find this to be true in my analysis of the test results of 38 fibromyalgia patients who had complete thyroid function testing.

Incidence of Central Hypothyroidism in Fibromyalgia. The results of several studies indicate a high incidence of central hypothyroidism in fibromyalgia patients. Neeck and Riedel found that all of 13 female fibromyalgia patients had blunted TSH responses to TRH. This is consistent with pituitary hypothyroidism. The researchers definition of a blunted TSH was 8 µU/mL or less.[175] Ferraccioli and colleagues found that 5 of 24 female fibromyalgia patients (20.8%) had blunted TSH responses to TRH, defining a blunted response as 7 µU/mL or less.[176] I found that of 38 fibromyalgia patients, 20 patients (52.6%) had either a blunted or exaggerated TSH response to TRH.[36] Eleven of the 20 patients (55% of this category) had blunted TSH responses. This is 28.9% of the 38 patients in the study, which is close to Ferraccioli's finding of blunted TSH responses in 5 of 24 patients (20.8%).[176] The range of my patients' TSH levels above baseline was 0.00-to-8.5 µU/mL, and the mean was 4.74 µU/mL. Nine of my patients out of 20 (45% of this category) had abnormally high TSH responses. The range of their TSH levels above baseline was 20.70-to-33.0 µU/mL, with a mean of 25.85 µU/mL. My definition of a normal TSH level 30 minutes post-injection was 8.5-to-20 µU/mL above baseline. The incidence of possible central hypothyroidism among my 38 fibromyalgia patients was 250,476.19 times (52.6%/0.00021%) that in the general population.[93,p.40]

The TRH-stimulation test may also be of value in determining whether fibromyalgia patients are likely to benefit from EMG-biofeedback. In one study, 6 of 7 patients without endocrine abnormalities improved considerably with biofeedback. Two patients with blunted TSH responses to TRH failed to benefit from biofeedback. The researchers suggested that endocrine evaluation may help predict patients' potential for improvement through feedback.[156]

Because it is the most accessible test for identifying patients with possible central hypothyroidism, the clinician should make liberal use of the TRH-stimulation test when he suspects central hypothyroidism.

The TRH-Stimulation Test Does Not Distinguish Between Hypothalamic and Pituitary Hypothyroidism. The TRH-stimulation test does not reliably discriminate between pituitary and hypothalamic hypothyroidism.[3][10] When research with TRH-stimulation tests began, investigators believed the test could distinguish between hypothyroidism of pituitary

and hypothalamic origin. They thought that a normal or abnormally high TSH response delayed in time indicated hypothalamic disease. They wrote that the peak rise in TSH after a TRH injection was normal, but the peak was prolonged from 60-to-120 minutes.[126] Other researchers, however, later found that some patients with lesions within the sella turcica also had TSH responses previously thought typical of hypothalamic dysfunction. (The sella turcica is a concave space in the upper surface of the sphenoid bone. It houses the pituitary gland). This finding suggests that the TSH response thought unique to hypothalamic hypothyroidism is not definitive for that condition.[8,p.110] Researchers also thought that an abnormally low (blunted) response indicated pituitary disease. In general this is true, but a blunted response does not definitively distinguish hypothalamic from pituitary hypothyroidism.

Table 4.2.4. Basal TSH levels of euthyroid, primary hypothyroid, and central hypothyroid fibromyalgia patients.*

THYROID STATUS	NO. OF PATIENTS	% OF TOTAL	MEAN BASAL TSH LEVEL (μU/mL)	RANGE OF BASAL TSH VALUES (μU/mL)
Euthyroid	14	36.8	1.43	0.57-2.28
Primary hypothyroid	4	10.5	8.16	6.50-9.08
Central hypothyroid	20	52.6		
Blunted TSH response to TRH	11	28.9	0.61	0.03-1.34
Exaggerated TSH response to TRH	9	23.7	2.45	1.14-4.18

*Lowe, J.C.: Thyroid status of 38 fibromyalgia patients: implications for the etiology of fibromyalgia. *Clin. Bull. Myofascial Ther.*, 2(1):47-64, 1997.[36]

Snyder and colleagues argued that a low TSH response to TRH in a patient with central hypothyroidism is strong evidence of pituitary dysfunction caused by a lesion.[10] Nevertheless, they pointed out that only in idiopathic hypopituitarism might the magnitude of the TSH response to TRH differentiate between a pituitary and hypothalamic source of hypothyroidism.

Confidence in distinguishing between pituitary and hypothalamic hypothyroidism is further diminished by a study reported by Ferring Laboratories, manufacturer of one TRH product. Patients were given TRH-stimulation tests after they were diagnosed from

clinical history, physical examination, and other tests of thyroid and pituitary function. Of patients with hypothalamic hypothyroidism, the post-TRH injection TSH levels ranged from 2-to-38 μU/mL. Of patients with pituitary hypothyroidism, the post-TRH TSH levels in 59% were less than 2 μU/mL. However, in 41% of patients with pituitary hypothyroidism, the post-TRH TSH levels were above 2 μU/mL. Because of this, the authors of the study concluded that a TSH response to TRH of less than 2 μU/mL suggests pituitary hypothyroidism, but that a TSH response greater than this does not distinguish between hypothalamic and pituitary dysfunction.

Diagnosis of Central Hypothyroidism: Not Based Solely on the Outcome of the TRH-Stimulation Test. The diagnosis of central hypothyroidism should not be based on the result of the TRH-stimulation test alone nor in combination with the results of other tests of thyroid function. There should also be clinical, radiographic, or other imaging findings to support the diagnosis.[1,p.297]

Upon examination, most patients with central hypothyroidism show evidence of failure to secrete normal amounts of trophic hormones other than TSH; imaging of the pituitary fossa often shows abnormalities.[2] When the results of other diagnostic methods are not available, but the fibromyalgia patient's TRH-stimulation test result is typical of central hypothyroidism, it is proper to state that the result is _consistent with but not diagnostic of_ central hypothyroidism.

Lesions documentable through hormone assays and imaging are not the only causes of central hypothyroidism. TSH deficiencies may also result from mutations of the TSH gene, leaving other anterior pituitary hormone levels within the normal range.[29]

TRH-Stimulation Test Results in Patients Taking Thyroid Hormone

The TRH-stimulation test is not useful for deciding whether a hypothyroid fibromyalgia patient is taking an excessive dosage of thyroid hormone. Clearly, suppression of the TSH response of the pituitary to TRH can occur without thyrotoxic effects on other tissues. This is because the pituitary thyrotrophs are more sensitive to thyroid hormone than are the cells of other tissues.[55]

A dosage of T_3 too small to benefit the fibromyalgia patient is likely to blunt the TSH response to TRH. In one study, for example, only 25 µg of T_3 per day in divided doses for 2 days caused a 50% reduction in TRH-induced TSH secretion.[53] Many patients taking 0.1-to-0.2 mg of T_4 per day have no TSH increase after intravenous TRH.[45,p.91][54] Of patients taking T_4, the mean dosage of those with a normal TSH response to TRH was 0.127 mg (127 µg). The mean dosage of those who had a suppressed TSH response was 0.154 mg (154 µg).[135] Dosages this low virtually never improve fibromyalgia status. Some hypothyroid fibromyalgia patients improve or recover with higher dosages, especially with the equivalent of 0.2-to-0.4 mg of T_4 (see Appendix D). But these dosages suppress both the basal TSH level and the TSH response to TRH. The suppression renders the results of the TRH-stimulation test of no use for inferences about the patient's thyroid hormone dosage.

Can Highly Sensitive TSH Assays Replace The TRH-Stimulation Test?

Supersensitive TSH assays can now replace the use of the TRH-stimulation test for deciding whether a patient is hyperthyroid. These assays can detect TSH levels that were undetectable by previous generations of assays.[84] Supersensitive TSH assays sharply differentiate between subnormal and previously undetectable TSH levels. This has been confirmed by comparisons of TSH values (shown by supersensitive assays) with TRH-stimulation test results. When a supersensitive TSH assay showed a normal basal TSH, the TRH-stimulation test also did. Each patient with an undetectably low basal TSH level on a supersensitive TSH assay had no response or an abnormally low TSH response in the TRH-stimulation test.[8,p.109] For detecting hyperthyroidism, then, supersensitive TSH assays make the TRH-stimulation test unnecessary. This is convenient for the hyperthyroid patient in that the TSH is a single test that requires the drawing of only one blood sample.

Hamburger wrote, "Screening of ambulatory patients with clinical features suggestive of thyroid dysfunction with this single test would be highly cost effective."[33,p.120] This statement is appropriate when the dysfunction is hyperthyroidism; it is not true when the dysfunction is hypothyroidism.

Therefore, it is false to state, as some authors have, that modern TSH assays have made the TRH-stimulation test obsolete.[77,p.229][78] Many cases of central hypothyroidism would be missed without the use of the TRH-stimulation test.

Testing Procedure

It is important that the clinician perform the TRH-stimulation test using the appropriate materials and according to standard procedure.

Blood Samples During the TRH-Stimulation Test. When conducting the test, the clinician should take two or more blood samples from the patient so that the laboratory can measure the TSH concentrations in them. He should take the first sample just before injecting the TRH. Depending on the interests of the clinician, he may want to take additional samples at 15, 20, 30, 45, and 60 minutes. I usually order only a 30-minute sample because the TSH typically reaches its peak level 30 minutes after the TRH injection.

TRH-Stimulation Test Bolus. The amount of TRH injected is optional, but I prefer to follow the Ferring Laboratories recommendation of 500 µg.[101]

This bolus appears to be the optimum amount to provoke the maximum response in the largest percentage of patients. Larger doses are not likely to provoke a higher TSH response. For children 6-to-16 years old, Ferring Laboratories recommends a bolus of 7 μg/kg of body weight with a maximum of 500 μg.[101] Some clinicians administer as little as 200 μg and others 400 μg.[100,p.512]

Precaution in TRH Testing. Some patients have no symptoms upon receiving a TRH injection, and others have mild, transient symptoms. These symptoms occur within minutes after the injection and seldom last more than several minutes.[100,p.512]

Ratge et al. injected four groups of patients with TRH. The subjects included 14 normal volunteers, 23 with euthyroid goiter, 9 with hypothyroidism, and 17 with hyperthyroidism. Subjects in all four groups (86% of all subjects) had the same subjective symptoms: flushing, nausea, urinary urgency, dizziness, and headache. Shortly after the injection, systolic blood pressure increased by an average of 26±13 mm Hg; diastolic pressure increased an average of 14±6 mm Hg. The injections increased catecholamine levels in patients. Increases were higher in hypothyroid patients than in patients with euthyroid goiter and hyperthyroidism. These relative increases in catecholamine levels after the injections were proportional to the relative catecholamine levels in the groups of patients before the injections. The investigators concluded that TRH injections increase catecholamine levels by activating the sympathoadrenal system. The increased levels, however, were not high or quick enough to significantly increase blood pressure. Epinephrine increased 28%, and norepinephrine 21%. Maximum increases occurred between 2 and 4 minutes after the injections. At this point, subjective symptoms and increased blood pressure and heart rate were already subsiding. The symptoms therefore had a more rapid onset than the catecholamine increases. This finding suggests that injected TRH exerts its effects in the vascular or central nervous system, but not through increased catecholamine secretion. Since one patient's systolic blood pressure increased by 64 mm Hg, the researchers advised clinicians to remain cautious with patients who have risk factors such as compromised cardiac function.[19]

Interpretation

There are no rock-hard standards for interpreting the results of the TRH-stimulation test. Laboratories and authorities differ in what they consider a normal range. The variability in standards for interpretation

contributes to a rule of quality clinical practice—that the clinician interpret the results of all thyroid function tests, including the TRH-stimulation test, in light of other laboratory test results and the patient's symptoms, signs, and peripheral indices. Despite the medical technocrats' passion for objectifying every decision in practice, clinical judgment remains the *sine qua non* in quality care.

Ranges of Normal

Different writers have given different reference ranges for the results of the TRH-stimulation test. Howanitz and Howanitz considered a normal TSH rise above baseline to be about 16-to-26 μU/mL. They stated that the peak is slightly lower in men but did not give numerical values.[28,p.429] (The responses of TSH and prolactin to TRH are greater in most women than in men.[98] Responses in women are greater during their preovulatory phase than during the luteal phase of their menstrual cycle.[117]) Mardell and Gamlen gave the normal ranges for their laboratory for TSH levels 20 minutes after the TRH injection: men under 40 years old and women of any age, 4-to-20 mU/L (μU/mL) above the basal level; men over 40 years, 2-to-10 mU/L above the basal level.[8,p.107] Hamburger gave the normal range as an increase of 2-to-18 μU/mL over the baseline value.[45,p.65]

In studies of fibromyalgia patients, Ferraccioli and colleagues defined a blunted TSH response to TRH as 7 μU/mL or less.[176] Neeck and Riedel defined a blunted response as 8 μU/mL or less.[175]

The range of normal I use is a 30-minute post-injection TSH level of 8.5-to-20 μU/mL above the baseline TSH value.[36] I base my use of this range on two factors. The first factor is consideration of the ranges given by other researchers. The lower limit of this normal range is higher than that recommended by Mardell and Gamlen,[8,p.107] but it is close to the limit of 7 μU/mL specified by Ferraccioli[176] and 8 μU/mL indicated by Neeck and Riedel.[175] Yet the lower limit of 8.5 μU/mL is roughly mid-way between the lower limits recommended by Howanitz and Howanitz[28,p.429] and Mardell and Gamlen.[8,p.107] The second factor in my use of the range of 8.5-to-20 μU/mL is retrospective consideration of the post-TRH injection TSH levels of patients who improved or recovered from fibromyalgia with the use of T4. These patients' positive responses to the use of T4 indicate that their fibromyalgia was secondary to a thyroid hormone deficiency. In general, my patients whose TSH responses to TRH were below or above the normal range of 8.5-to-20.0 μU/mL over baseline (results which I consider consistent with central hypothyroidism) have benefitted from the therapy as do patients with thyroid hormone deficiencies.

I consider a 30-minute TSH response of more than 20.0 μU/mL above baseline an exaggerated TSH response and consistent with central hypothyroidism. Responses below 8.5 μU/mL above baseline are blunted and consistent with pituitary hypothyroidism.

There are gray areas in the interpretation of TRH-stimulation test results. According to Fitter, the predictive value of most laboratory tests gets lower when test values get closer to the outer limits of the normal reference range. The prevalence of the disease indicated by the test result tends to decrease closer to the outer limits of the range. In addition, the clinician should bear in mind that the likelihood of the disease is not spread evenly thoughout the reference range.[4] However, imperfect sensitivity and specificity of laboratory tests, including the TRH-stimulation test, do not negate the value of the tests if test results are considered as only one factor—albeit an important one—in the clinician's assessment of the patient's status. The range of normal is best considered a somewhat flexible guide to proper clinical decisions. Rather than rigidly adhering to any normal reference range, the clinician should exercise clinical judgment based on the patient's clinical status *and* laboratory test results.

De Rosa et al. described two methods for evaluating the 30-minute TSH response to TRH. The first is the absolute or delta TSH increase. This is determined by subtracting the 30-minute TSH value from the baseline value. The second is the relative increase. This is determined by dividing the baseline TSH value into the 30-minute value.[161]

THYROID AUTOANTIBODIES

Inflammatory thyroid gland disorders such as autoimmune thyroiditis are among the most common endocrine abnormalities.[168] The term autoimmune thyroid disease subsumes both autoimmune thyroiditis and Graves' disease. Similar genetic defects in the regulation of the immune system underlie the two diseases,[151,p.930] but their clinical manifestations are different (see Chapter 2.4, section titled "Autoimmune Thyroid Diseases"). In caring for fibromyalgia patients, the autoimmune thyroid disease of most concern is autoimmune thyroiditis or Hashimoto's thyroiditis. The reason for our concern is that in the Western world, autoimmune thyroiditis is the most common cause of subclinical and overt hypothyroid-

ism.[151,p.930][157]

According to Volpé, for each patient with autoimmune thyroiditis and overt hypothyroidism, there are several with subclinical hypothyroidism.[151,p.927] The patient is at risk for developing overt hypothyroidism if she has either subclinical hypothyroidism or thyroid microsomal antibodies; her risk is even greater if she has both.[154] Vanderpump et al. found in a 20-year follow-up that for women with subclinical hypothyroidism but no thyroid microsomal antibodies, the relative risk factor for acquiring overt hypothyroidism was 8. For women with normal thyroid function but thyroid antibodies, the risk factor was also 8. But for women with both subclinical hypothyroidism and thyroid antibodies, the risk factor for acquiring overt hypothyroidism was 36.[155] Thus, the presence of both subclinical hypothyroidism and thyroid microsomal antibodies has predictive value. Among patients with subclinical hypothyroidism, those with higher TSH values and detectable antithyroid antibodies are more likely to develop overt hypothyroidism.[152]

The clinical features of autoimmune thyroiditis differ widely among patients, and some patients have no symptoms or signs. The clinician may inadvertently be alerted to a patient's autoimmune thyroiditis in different circumstances: upon seeing the results of thyroid function or thyroid antibody tests, during surgery or at biopsy, or upon observing an enlarged thyroid gland. Some patients are overtly hypothyroid. These patients may or may not have goiters. (See Chapter 2.4, section titled "Autoimmune Thyroiditis: Clinical Features").

Antithyroid Antibodies. Most Graves', Hashimoto's, and idiopathic hypothyroid patients have thyroid microsomal antibodies. Titers of microsomal antibodies are correlated with the histologic lesions of Hashimoto's thyroiditis. The enzyme thyroid peroxidase is the microsomal antigen. The antigen is found in the apical cytoplasm and plasma membrane of follicular cells. Antibodies to thyroid peroxidase exert cytotoxic effects and can interfere with the enzymatic activity of thyroid peroxidase, reducing the production of thyroid hormones. Antibody levels usually decrease when the patient with autoimmune thyroiditis becomes hypothyroid or when she undergoes treatment with T_4. (See Chapter 2.4, section titled "Autoimmune Thyroiditis: Antithyroid Antibodies.") Kotani wrote that the clinician can use repeated measures of thyroid microsomal antibodies to judge the efficacy of thyroid hormone treatment.[172]

A study by Romaldini et al., however, suggests that treatment with T_4 may lower antithyroid antibodies in patients with overt but not subclinical hypothyroidism. The investigators used 2.0-to-2.5 μg T_4 to treat 23 patients with goiter due to Hashimoto's thyroiditis. Thirteen patients had subclinical hypothyroidism; 10 had overt hypothyroidism. At the end of the median treatment time of 6 months, TSH levels had decreased significantly in patients of both groups. Serum T_4 levels significantly increased only in overt hypothyroid patients. Serum levels of thyroglobulin antibodies and microsomal antibodies did not change in the subclinical hypothyroid patients, but levels of both types of antibodies decreased in the overt hypothyroid patients. The mean volume of goitrous thyroid gland tissue decreased in all overt hypothyroid patients and 77% of subclinical hypothyroid patients. The investigators proposed a mechanism by which the exogenous T_4 lowered thyroid autoantibody levels and reduced the thyroid gland volume in overt hypothyroid patients: Presumably, the T_4 reduced circulating TSH levels, thereby decreasing stimulation of thyroid tissue, and in turn lowering the levels of antigenic substances. The researchers wrote that benefits of T_4 replacement therapy in patients with subclinical hypothyroidism due to Hashimoto's thyroiditis have not yet been determined.[167]

Some researchers report that thyroglobulin antibody titers are more strongly associated with Hashimoto's thyroiditis than are titers of thyroid microsomal antibodies. Kasagi et al. compared the titers of thyroglobulin and microsomal antibodies with histological findings (following needle biopsy) in patients with Hashimoto's thyroiditis and diffuse goiter. The investigators reported that thyrogloblin antibody positivity was more closely associated with the histological diagnosis of Hashimoto's thyroiditis than was microsomal antibody positivity.[162] Volpé disagreed with this finding, stating that titers of thyroglobulin antibodies do not correlate with the histological findings of Hashimoto's as well as do titers of microsomal antibodies.[151,p.926] Based on their study results, Toldy et al. concurred with Volpé's view. They reported that measuring thyroid microsomal antibodies was the most sensitive method for identifying patients with Hashimoto's thyroiditis. Measurements of microsomal antibodies had more discriminative value than measurements of thyroglobulin antibodies. The researchers also found, however, that in subacute thyroiditis, antibody measurements were rarely informative.[170]

Within conventional medicine, the thyroid microsomal antibody titer and the serum TSH are considered the mainstays of modern thyroid testing strategies.[169] Senda et al. found that in Hashimoto's thyroiditis, di-

agnostic sensitivity increased when the thyroid microsomal antibody titer was used in combination with the thyroglobulin antibody titer.[166] LoPresti wrote that most thyroid diseases involve autoimmune processes of the thyroid gland. Because of this, he recommended that the clinician include a thyroid microsomal antibody titer in any approach to thyroid testing. Including the antibody titer, he suggested, "will enhance both the diagnostic and prognostic expertise of the physician."[169]

Many patients remain euthyroid for years despite having autoimmune thyroiditis.[151,p.927] Nevertheless, euthyroid patients may have symptoms due to suboptimal thyroid hormone regulation of tissue metabolism even though their thyroid function test results are normal. For some, the phenotypic expression is what we diagnosis as fibromyalgia. Aarflot and Bruusgaard, for example, tested a hypothesis based on their observations from general practice: that thyroid antibodies are associated with chronic widespread musculoskeletal complaints. They included 737 men and 771 women who ranged in age from 40-to-42 years. The researchers determined the prevalence of detected microsomal thyroid antibodies in subjects with and without chronic widespread musculoskeletal complaints. Those with chronic widespread musculoskeletal complaints had a significantly higher incidence of thyroid microsomal antibodies than did subjects without such complaints (16.0% versus 7.3%, p < 0.01). The prevalence of antibodies was significantly higher in women than men (20.4% versus 11.6%, p = 0.02). However, thyroid function test results did not differ significantly between the two groups. The investigators wrote, "The association between chronic widespread musculoskeletal pain complaints and thyroid antibodies in women may reflect a subgroup of patients in which thyroid autoimmunity, rather than thyroid function, is important." They discussed the possible relationship of thyroid antibodies to fibromyalgia.[12] The results of this study suggest that patients with microsomal thyroid antibodies may have symptoms due to suboptimal thyroid hormone tissue regulation before thyroid gland dysfunction is detectable by laboratory thyroid function tests.

Rodolico et al. reported the cases of 5 male and 5 female patients who were hypothyroid (atrophic variant) due to Hashimoto's thyroiditis. The patients did not have the lethargy, constipation, cold intolerance, myxedematous faces, or bradycardia that is typical of hypothyroidism. Instead, they had muscular fatigability, myalgia, cramps, or proximal weakness. An unusual finding among the patients was that thyroglobulin antibodies exceeded thyroid microsomal antibodies. The patients' muscle symptoms and signs ceased after they began to use T_4. *The researchers wrote that their observations of these patients indicate that isolated myopathy is not rare as the sole manifestation of hypothyroidism.* They concluded, "Thorough evaluation of thyroid function is appropriate in patients with myopathy of uncertain origin."[174]

Pies wrote that autoimmune thyroiditis, which can eventually lead to hypothyroidism, is often associated with depression, especially in postpartum patients.[171] Oomen et al. studied psychiatric patients to determine (1) the prevalence of thyroid function abnormalities on admission, and (2) whether thyroid abnormalities are associated with cognitive and affective disorders. The researchers found that 10% of patients (331 of 3316) were positive for thyroid peroxidase antibodies. Of this group, 5.9% (198 of 3316) had TSH levels below 4.0 μU/mL, and 4.1% (134 of 3316) had TSH levels above 4.0 μU/mL (high TSH levels). Of the patients with a TSH over 4.0 μU/mL, only 9.8% had low total T_4 levels. Thus, most of the patients with thyroid peroxidase antibodies had subclinical hypothyroidism. The investigators also found a significant association between rapid cycling bipolar disorders (18% compared to 0% in controls, P<0.001) and positive thyroid peroxidase antibodies. The association was particularly strong in patients with high antibody titers and/or TSH levels above 4.0 μU/mL. The researchers concluded, "Though causal relations cannot be determined from this cross-sectional study, this admission survey found early forms of autoimmune thyroid disease, sometimes characterized only by TPO-Abs [thyroid peroxidase antibodies], highly significantly associated with rapid cycles of a bipolar disorder."[153]

Michalopoulou et al. gave patients with high-normal TSH levels and elevated cholesterol levels 50 μg T_4. After beginning the thyroid hormone, patients who were positive for thyroid autoantibodies had a reduction in cholesterol; patients who were negative for autoantibodies did not have a reduction in cholesterol. The investigators concluded that patients with high-normal TSH levels and thyroid autoantibodies may have subclinical hypothyroidism and may benefit from the use of exogenous thyroid hormone.[27]

There are other such studies in the thyroidology literature. I cite these studies on widespread muscle pain,[12] other muscle symptoms and signs,[174] depression,[170] bipolar disorders,[153] and cholesterol,[154] only as examples to illustrate a point. The point is that the finding of thyroid microsomal antibodies—even in patients with what are conventionally considered normal thyroid function test results—may indicate that the patients' symptoms and signs are associated with suboptimal thyroid hormone regulation of tissue metabolism. In most cases, a trial of thyroid hormone is warranted in symptomatic patients who are positive for thyroid microsomal antibodies.

In a retrospective study of 218 patients with autoimmune thyroiditis, 13.7% had another autoimmune disease. The two most common autoimmune diseases were lupus and Sjögren's syndrome. The frequency of autoimmune diseases appears to be higher in patients with thyroid disorders than in the general population. A common underlying autoimmune process may be responsible for each of the autoimmune diseases. The authors of this retrospective study wrote that the frequency of the associated diseases suggests the need for a long-lasting survey of patients with thyroid disorders. They recommended an initial evaluation and regular reevaluations of patients suffering from autoimmune disease.[173]

Interpretation

Volpé noted that because low titers of thyroid antibodies accompany a variety of thyroid disorders (the antibodies are not exclusive to autoimmune thyroiditis), the presence of the antibodies is not diagnostic of autoimmune thyroiditis. On the other hand, the patient with autoimmune thyroiditis may not have detectable antithyroid antibodies.[151,p.929] Some patients with Hashimoto's thyroiditis have no laboratory evidence of antibodies,[163][164] and about a third of patients with autoimmune thyroiditis and hypothyroidism are negative for antibodies.[164][165]

According to Volpé, the diagnosis of autoimmune thyroiditis is usually based on the patient having hypothyroidism, a goiter (although in the atrophic type, there is no goiter), the finding of thyroid antibodies, or histologic findings characteristic of thyroiditis. Autoimmune thyroiditis is highly likely if the patient's titers of antithyroglobulin or antimicrosomal antibodies are 1:1000 or more. When some other cause of hypothyroidism is not obvious, a positive thyroid antibody test indicates autoimmune thyroiditis. Confirmation of the histological abnormalities characteristic of autoimmune thyroiditis is the conclusive method for diagnosing the condition. From the standpoint of clinical management, however, Volpé wrote that biopsy is rarely necessary to confirm the diagnosis.[151,pp.929-930]

The clinician should order tests for both thyroid microsomal and thyroglobulin antibodies. The normal serum concentration of thyroglobulin antibodies is < 200 mIU/mL; the normal concentration for thyroid microsomal (peroxidase) antibodies is < 150 mIU/mL.[167]

● DRUGS THAT MAY INTERFERE WITH THYROID TESTS

Several drugs may interfere with accurate laboratory testing of thyroid function (see Table 4.2.5). It is important that the clinician determine whether a patient he is testing for thyroid function is taking any of these common drugs.

Brent and Hershman[115] and Wenzel[116] provided lists of commonly used drugs that may affect thyroid function test results. Brent and Hershman listed the drugs by their mechanism of action.[115,p.97]

The drugs that in my experience most often interfere with thyroid function test results of fibromyalgia patients are estrogens, propranolol, benzodiazepines, and glucocorticoids.

ESTROGENS

Estrogens may alter thyroid function test results during pregnancy, oral contraceptive use, or oral estrogen replacement therapy in post-menopausal women. The total T_4 is usually elevated. The basal TSH may be normal in euthyroid patients and low in hypothyroid patients taking exogenous thyroid hormone (see Chapter 3.6). An elevated T_4 and low TSH is often found in hyperthyroid patients, but the clinician must not rush to this diagnosis when he finds this pattern of test values in a patient taking exogenous estrogen. If the patient is clinically hypometabolic, she most likely does not have hyperthyroidism. Her hypometabolic status should alert the clinician to the possibility that she may be pregnant or taking exogenous estrogen.

Estrogens May Increase Thyroid Hormone Transport Proteins and Elevate the Total T_4

When a woman takes estrogen orally, the estrogen clears from the blood rapidly during the first passage of the hormone through the liver. Compared to other target organs, the concentration of estrogen increases markedly in the liver. The high hepatic estrogen level increases the serum thyroxine-binding globulin[106] concentration 2-to-3-fold higher than normal. The increased globulin results not from increased synthesis but from decreased clearance of thyroxine-binding globulin. The globulin undergoes sialylation, which prolongs its half-life.[59]

Table 4.2.5. Drugs that interfere with thyroid function test results, listed by mechanism.*

I. Drugs that reduce thyroid hormone concentration
  A. Suppression of TSH
    1. Dopamine
    2. Glucocorticoids (for example, prednisone)
  B. Reduction of TBG level
    1. Androgens
    2. Glucocorticoids
  C. Impaired protein binding
    1. Salicylates
    2. Diphenylhydantoin
    3. Furosemide
  D. Impaired thyroid hormone production or secretion
    1. Propylthiouracil
    2. Methimazole
    3. Lithium
    4. Iodine

II. Drugs that raise T_4 concentration
  A. Increase in TBG level
    1. Estrogen
    2. Tamoxifen
  B. Impaired T_4 to T_3 conversion
    1. Amiodarone
    2. Ipodate sodium (Oragrafin)
    3. Iopanoic Acid (Telepague)
    4. Propranolol
    5. Glucocorticoids

*Brent, G.A. and Hershman, J.M.: Effects of nonthyroidal illness on thyroid function tests. In *The Thyroid Gland: A Practical Clinical Treatise.* Edited by Van Middlesworth, Chicago, Year Book Medical Publishers, Inc., 1986.[115]

Manufacturers have decreased the estrogen content of oral contraceptives in recent years. Nevertheless, the quantities of estrogen in today's contraceptives still slightly increase thyroxine-binding globulin levels. Burger wrote that only in an occasional woman does the serum total T_4 level exceed the upper limit of normal.[103,p.336] Stockigt noted that when moderate-to-large doses of estrogen increase serum thyroxine-binding globulin levels, the serum total T_4 typically increases also.[35,p.478] He added, though, that for many patients, the values remain in the upper normal range.

Elevated thyroxin-binding globulin increases serum levels of both total T_4 and total T_3. The increased number of binding sites provided by the additional thyroxine-binding globulin holds a larger than normal proportion of the serum T_3. As a result, fewer than normal T_3 molecules are available to attach to the resin in the T_3 uptake test. When the clinician orders a total T_4 and T_3 uptake, the values of the two test results will be shifted in opposite directions: the total T_4 will be increased and the T_3 uptake decreased. A change in opposite directions of the total T_4 and T_3 uptake values suggests an abnormality in thyroid hormone binding proteins: an increase in the total T_4 and a decrease in the T_3 uptake indicate an increase in thyroxine-binding globulin (see section above titled "T_3 Uptake"). In my clinical experience, 4-to-6 weeks after the patient stops taking oral contraceptives, the thyroxine-binding globulin has decreased and the T_3 uptake increased to normal.

With skin patches (transdermal estrogen therapy), the patient may avoid elevated liver estrogen concentrations and maintain normal serum thyroxine-binding globulin levels.[118]

Estrogen May Inhibit TSH Secretion

Gambert[120,p.352] noted that estrogens may inhibit TSH secretion.[121] "But any effect is transient," he adds, "because both men and women taking chronic estrogen therapy have normal serum free T_4, free T_3, and TSH levels." Other research suggests that this is true of euthyroid but not hypothyroid patients. The basal and TRH-stimulated TSH levels have been found not to decrease when *euthyroid* humans and other animals take exogenous estrogen. But in *hypothyroid* rats, pharmacologic doses of estradiol tend to increase the potency of exogenous thyroid hormone in suppressing TSH messenger RNA levels.[119] The thyrotrophs thus synthesize less TSH than if solely under the transcription-regulating influence of thyroid hormone. The reduced transcription for TSH messenger RNA occurs because of overlap in the control sequences on chromosomes that mediate transcription patterns dictated by thyroid hormone and estrogen.[122] (See Chapter 3.6.) Thus, in the hypothyroid patient, exogenous estrogen may potentiate the suppression of TSH production by exogenous thyroid hormone.

PROPRANOLOL

Propranolol interferes with the conversion of T_4 to T_3. Large doses may significantly elevate the serum T_4 and lower the serum T_3.[107] Propranolol is a β-adrenergic receptor blocker often prescribed for hypertension and anxiety attacks.

BENZODIAZEPINES

Several benzodiazepines inhibit TRH binding to brain tissue and the pituitary and consequently alter behavior.[109][110][111] Among the benzodiazepines are Valium (diazepam), Xanax (alprazolam), Librium, Libritabs (chlordiazepoxide), Dalmane (flurazepam), and Versed (midazolam).

To test the TRH antagonism of Xanax, Kozlowski induced drowsiness in animals by giving them barbiturates. First administering TRH or amphetamines, however, reduced how much drowsiness the barbiturate induced. But giving the animals Xanax before giving them TRH or amphetamines enabled the barbiturates to induce deeper levels of drowsiness.[109] A small dose of Xanax antagonized TRH, permitting the barbiturates to induce deep drowsiness. This finding agrees with some[110][111] but not all[112][113] reports of the effects of other benzodiazepines on TRH effects. The data suggest that benzodiazepines, by competitively binding to TRH receptors on the pituitary, may inhibit the TSH response during the TRH-stimulation test. In addition, patients medicated with benzodiazepines may not adapt normally to conditions that require increased thyroid function, such as exposure to cold.

GLUCOCORTICOIDS

When a euthyroid patient takes an exogenous glucocorticoid, her pituitary gland may become less sensitive to TRH. This may lower her basal level of TSH.[113] The diminished level of TSH may reduce serum T_3 and T_4 levels too low to maintain a normal metabolic rate.[113][114] The glucocorticoid may also lower T_4 to T_3 conversion. However, the antithyroid effects of glucocorticoids are transient, lasting only a few weeks.[177][178][179] It is possible, nonetheless, that the glucocorticoid, even when taken long-term, intermittently decreases TSH secretion and reduces T_4 to T_3 conversion. Because of this possibility, the patient should minimize her glucocorticoid dosage or stop it completely for thyroid function testing if she can.

● LIMITATIONS OF THYROID FUNCTION TESTING

There are definite limitations to accurately classifying patients according to thyroid status. Consider the "gray areas" of the normal reference ranges. These are spans of numerical values, in most cases at the upper and lower limits of normal ranges, where the clinician does not have definite criteria for "calling" the outcome. Instead, he must use clinical judgment. Fitter explained that with most laboratory tests, when the patient's test value is close to an outer limit of the normal reference range, the predictive value of the test gets lower. The prevalence of the disease being tested for tends to decrease as values get closer to the outer limits of the range. Also, the likelihood of the disease is not spread evenly throughout the reference range.[4]

There are also gray areas in the interpretation of TRH-stimulation test results. In a report by Ferring Laboratories, patients were diagnosed as having pituitary hypothyroidism or hypothalamic hypothyroidism through their clinical histories, physical examinations, and tests of thyroid and pituitary function. Then the patients underwent TRH-stimulation tests to determine whether a different TSH response pattern typified each form of central hypothyroidism. In patients with hypothalamic hypothyroidism, the post-TRH injection TSH levels ranged from 2-to-38 μU/mL. In patients with pituitary hypothyroidism, the post-TRH injection TSH levels in 59% of patients were less than 2 μU/mL. In 41% of pituitary hypothyroid patients, however, the post-TRH injection TSH levels increased from 2-to-40 μU/mL. The authors concluded that a TSH response to TRH of less than 2 μU/mL suggests pituitary hypothyroidism, but that a TSH response greater than this does not distinguish hypothalamic from pituitary hypothyroidism.[101] Other researchers have reported similar results.[3][10]

Notice that the TSH response levels of some of the patients in the Ferring study were within the normal range. Some hypothalamic hypothyroid patients' TSH values ranged between 2-to-38 μU/mL, and some pituitary hypothyroid patients' values ranged between 2-to-40 μU/mL. Some patients' values were within various ranges considered normal by one researcher or another. This means that some central hypothyroid patients have normal TSH responses in the TRH-stimulation test. Ferring researchers were testing to determine TSH response patterns that *in the majority of cases* are consistent with a hypothalamic or pituitary genesis of hypothyroidism.

When a patient with hypothalamic hypothyroidism has a 30-minute TSH response to TRH that is within the normal range, it is proper to conclude that the outcome is *consistent with but not diagnostic of* euthyroidism. But we cannot be certain that the patient is euthyroid. If the patient's clinical status and her other objective test results contradict the outcome of the

TRH-stimulation test, the discrepancy must be settled in some way. Clinical judgment should play a major role. In some cases, if the clinician believes the weight of the evidence indicates hypothyroidism, he must go with his suspicion and treat the patient "as if." This choice is of no harm in the vast majority of cases and stands the chance of tremendously benefitting the patient. Some technocrats will label this clinical approach as "guesswork"; others will vilify it as "bordering on malpractice." The first characterization is hyperbole; the second, Draconian. Both suggest an extremism that blinds one to the indispensable role of clinical judgment in all quality clinical care.

It is prudent to bear in mind that the phrase "in the majority of cases" applies to the ranges of values for most laboratory tests. One might argue that a low-normal free T_4 or free T_3 shows whether the patient has any form of hypothyroidism. But there are uncertainties with this approach, too. For some individuals, a low-normal free T_4 level is sufficient to maintain optimal cellular metabolism. In others, a mid-range or high-normal level is insufficient. Without prior free T_4 levels, taken when the patient had no clinical indicators of hypometabolism, we do not know for sure whether the present free T_4 value is actually adequate for her.

Then there are the patients who have partial resistance to thyroid hormone. The degree of resistance among individuals ranges from mild-to-severe (see Chapter 2.6). Many of these patients are euthyroid according to the results of thyroid function testing, yet they are distinctly hypometabolic and resemble hypothyroid patients in every way except for their normal thyroid function test results. Most of those patients diagnosable as euthyroid fibromyalgic become clinically normal after beginning the use of supraphysiologic doses of T_3. Identifying these patients and properly managing their treatment requires that the clinician rely on signs, symptoms, and peripheral indices (see Chapter 4.3). Laboratory thyroid function testing is useful with these patients only in distinguishing them from patients who are hypothyroid according to the tests. Laboratory thyroid function tests do not distinguish them from euthyroid patients who are not hypometabolic. We can differentiate hypometabolic euthyroid patients from eumetabolic euthyroid patients only through measures of tissue metabolic status.

These limitations leave us with an undeniable necessity—to use the clinical judgment that medical technocrats have maligned since the advent of modern laboratory thyroid function tests. The necessity for clinical judgment is likely to be repugnant to those who have expected too much from these laboratory tests. But to refuse to use a wholesome dose of such judgment in caring for fibromyalgia patients (and others with thyroid hormone-related health problems) is to forsake those who look to us for relief.

● SUMMARY OF TESTING STRATEGY

Fibromyalgia patients have a hypometabolic profile. Because of this, thyroid function testing is aimed at unearthing evidence of thyroid hormone deficiency. If testing indicates a deficiency from either primary or central hypothyroidism, the patient should begin the use of either desiccated thyroid or a combination of synthetic T_4 and T_3. If testing indicates that the patient is euthyroid, the clinician should try to determine whether the patient's apparent hypometabolism is a result of factors not related to inadequate thyroid hormone regulation of cell function. If such factors do not appear to be instrumental in the patient's hypometabolism, then he should have her begin therapy using T_3. Thyroid function laboratory testing, then, is of value in helping to distinguish hypothyroid from euthyroid fibromyalgia patients. The distinction enables the clinician to decide whether the patient might benefit from the use of exogenous thyroid hormone, and if so, which form it is preferable to begin with.

The clinician may order one of two profiles: (1) a second generation TSH and a serum free T_4, or (2) a second generation TSH, total T_4, T_3 uptake, and a free thyroxine index (T_7). To order only a TSH is inadequate thyroid function testing. The test result may identify patients with incipient, subclinical, or overt primary hypothyroidism, but only if the clinician is aware that basal TSH levels of 2.0 µU/mL or more may indicate incipient hypothyroidism.[154][155] To limit thyroid function testing to only the TSH because the patient's basal TSH level is between 2.0 µU/mL and the conventional upper limit of the reference range (between 4.5 and 6.0 µU/mL) is likely to leave many patients with subnormal thyroid hormone levels of varying degrees undetected and untreated. If the clinician uses only the basal TSH as a screening tool, finding a level of 2.0 µU/mL or above should prompt him to order either a serum free T_4 or a total T_4, T_3 uptake, and a free thyroxine index (T_7).

Primary Hypothyroidism

If the clinician suspects primary hypothyroidism, he should order one of the profiles I mentioned in the section above. He should also order tests for antithyroglobulin and antimicrosomal antibodies. The diagnosis of primary hypothyroidism is likely if the condition is suggested by the results of the laboratory thyroid function tests, the patient is clinically hypometabolic, and she has a history or physical evidence indicating thyroid gland dysfunction. Such evidence includes positive antithyroid antibodies, goiter, or a history indicating either thyroidectomy or previous ^{131}I therapy for hyperthyroidism.

Pituitary Hypothyroidism

A low TSH may indicate either hyperthyroidism or pituitary hypothyroidism. (In pituitary hypothyroidism, other hormones the pituitary secretes may also be low. In turn, so will their corresponding target tissue hormones.[92,p.1044]) A high free T_3 supports the diagnosis of hyperthyroidism. On the other hand, low thyroid hormone levels would theoretically support the diagnosis of pituitary hypothyroidism. In a clinically hypometabolic patient whose basal TSH and thyroid hormone levels are low, a blunted TSH response to a TRH injection supports the diagnosis of pituitary hypothyroidism.

Central Hypothyroidism

An exaggerated 30-minute TSH response to TRH supports the diagnosis of central hypothyroidism. The exaggerated response does not distinguish between hypothalamic and pituitary dysfunction. Unfortunately, the TRH-stimulation test may not be available to many clinicians. And many endocrinologists who are familiar with the test refuse to perform it because they erroneously believe that third generation TSH assays have made the TRH-stimulation test obsolete. Family physicians can perform the test, but at this time some third party payers may deny reimbursement because an endocrinologist did not perform the test. This necessitates direct payment by the patient. The knowledge of the patient's thyroid status provided by the test result, however, may well be worth the cost. With the test not available to many clinicians, the diagnosis may have to depend on the results of standard thyroid function tests, the patient's history, physical findings, and the patient's clinical response to a trial of thyroid hormone therapy.

Thyroid Hormone Resistance Syndromes

For the classification of patients with thyroid hormone resistance, see Chapter 2.6, section titled "The Three Clinical Classifications of Thyroid Hormone Resistance."

REFERENCES

1. Toft, A.D.: Thyrotropin: assay, secretory physiology, and testing of regulation. In *Werner's The Thyroid: A Fundamental and Clinical Text*, 5th edition. Edited by S.H. Ingbar and L.E. Braverman, Philadelphia, J.B. Lippincott Co., 1986, pp.287-305.

2. Klijn, J.G.M., Lamberts, S.W.J., and Doctor, R.: The function of the pituitary-thyroidal axis in acromegalic patients vs. patients with hyperprolactinaemia and a pituitary tumor. *Clin. Endocrinol.* (Oxf.), 13:577, 1980.

3. Faglia, G., Beck-Peccoz, P., and Ferrari, C.: Plasma thyrotropin response to thyrotropin-releasing hormone in patients with pituitary and hypothalamic disorders. *J. Clin, Endocrinol. Metab.*, 37:595, 1973.

4. Fitter, W.: Personal (verbal) communication, March 12, 1999.

5. Blunt, S., Woods, C.A., Joplin, G.F., and Burrin, J.M.: The role of a highly sensitive amplified enzyme immunoassay for thyrotrophin in the evaluation of thyrotroph function in hypopituitary patients. *Clin. Endocinol.* (Oxf.), 29:387, 1988.

6. Caron, P.J., Nieman, L.K., Rose, S.R., and Nisula, B.C.: Deficient nocturnal surge of thyrotropin in central hypothyroidism. *J. Clin. Endocrinol. Metab.*, 62:960, 1986.

7. Escobar-Morreale, H.F., del Rey, F.E., Obregón, M.J., and de Escobar, G.M.: Only the combined treatment with thyroxine and triiodothyronine ensures euthyroidism in all tissues of the thyroidectomized rat. *Endocrinology*, 137(6): 2490-2502, 1996.

8. Mardell, R.J. and Gamlen, T.R.: *Thyroid Function Tests in Clinical Practice*. Bristol, John Wright & Sons, Ltd., 1985.

9. Seth, J. and Becket, G.: Diagnosis of hyperthyroidism: the newer biochemical tests. *Clin. Endocrinol. Metab.*, 14: 373, 1985.

10. Snyder, P.J., Jacobs, S.L., Rabello, M.M., et al.: Diagnostic value of thyrotropin releasing hormone in pituitary and hypothalamic diseases. *Ann. Intern. Med.*, 81:751-757, 1974.

11. Kraus, R.P., Phoenix, E., Edmonds, M.W., Nicholson, I.R., Chandarana, P.C., and Tokmakejian, S.: Exaggerated TSH responses to TRH in depressed patients with "normal" baseline TSH. *J. Clin. Psychiatry*, 58(6):266-270, 1997.

12. Aarflot, T. and Bruusgaard D.: Association between chronic widespread musculoskeletal complaints and thyroid autoimmunity. Results from a community survey. *Scand. J. Prim. Health Care*, 14(2):1111-1115, 1996.

13. Murray, G.R.: Note on the treatment of myxoedema by hypodermic injections of an extract of the thyroid gland of a sheep. *Brit. Med. J.*, 2:796, 1891.

14. Barnes, B.O.: *Hypothyroidism: The Unsuspected Illness.* New York, Harper and Row, Publishers, 1976.

15. Maclagan, N.F.: Thyroid: tests of function. In *French's Index of Differential Diagnosis*, 10th edition. Edited by F.D. Hart, Chicago, Year Book Medical Publishers Inc., 1973, pp.762-764.

16. Fraser, W.D., Biggart, E.M., O'Reilly, D. St. J., Gray, H.W., and McKillop, J.H.: Are biochemical tests of thyroid function of any value in monitoring patients receiving thyroxine replacement? *Br. Med. J.*, 293:808-810, 1986.

17. Mayberry, W.E. and O'Sullivan, M.B.: The clinical utility of radioimmunoassays in the medical center and reference laboratory settings. In *Cost/Benefit and Predictive Value of Radioimmunoassay*. Edited by A. Albertini, R.P. Ekins, and R.S. Galen, Amsterdam, Elsevier and Science Publishers B.V., 1984, pp.217-223.

18. Mitchell, M.L.: Blood tests of thyroid function. In *The Thyroid Gland: A Practical Clincal Treatise*. Edited by Van Middlesworth, Chicago, Year Book Medical Publishers, Inc., 1986, pp.35-45.

19. Ratge, D., Barthels, U., Wisser, H., and Bode, J.C.: Adverse reactions and changes in norepinephrine and epinephrine in the plasma after intravenous thyroliberin in persons with normal and abnormal thyroid function. *J. Clin. Chem. Clin. Biochem.*, 25(7):393-400, 1987.

20. Shlossberg, A.H.: Thyroid tests: guide for primary care physicians. *Can. Fam. Physician*, 36:1807-1810, 1990.

21. DeGroot, L.J.: Abnormal thyroid function tests in euthyroid patients. In *Diagnostic Methods in Clinical Thyroidology*. Edited by J.I. Hamburger, New York, Springer-Verlag, 1989, pp.3-26.

22. *Electrocardiographic Rhythm Analysis Guide*. Plymouth, MN, EquiMed Corp., 1988.

23. Marriott, H.J.L.: *Practical Electrocardiography*, 7th edition. Baltimore, Willams & Wilkins, 1983.

24. Moses, C., Danowski, T.S., and Switkes, H.I.: Alterations in cholesterol and lipoprotein partition in euthyroid adults by replacement doses of desiccated thyroid. *Circulation*, 8:761, 1958.

25. Wilson, J. and Walton, J.N.: Some muscular manifestations of hypothyroidism. *J. Neurol. Neurosurg. Psychiat.*, 22:320-324, 1959.

26. Stockigt, J.R.: Serum thyrotropin and thyroid hormone measurements and assessment of thyroid hormone transport. In *Werner and Ingbar's The Thyroid: A Fundamental and Clinical Text*, 7th edition. Edited by L.P. Braverman and R.D. Utiger, Philadelphia, Lippincott-Raven Publishers, 1996, pp.377-396.

27. Michalopoulou, G., Alevizaki, M., Piperingos, G., Mitsibounas, D., Mantzos, E., Adamopoulos, P., and Koutras, D.A.: High serum cholesterol levels in persons with "high-normal" TSH levels: should one extend the definition of subclinical hypothyroidism? *Eur. J. Endocrinol.*, 138(2): 141-145, 1998.

28. Howanitz, P.J. and Howanitz, J.H.: Evaluation of endocrine function. In *Clinical Diagnosis and Management by Laboratory Methods*, Vol. 1. Edited by J.B. Henry, Philadelphia, W.B. Saunders Co., 1979, pp.402-476.

29. Mori, R., Sawai, T., Kinoshita, E., et al.: Rapid detection of a point mutation in thyroid-stimulating hormone beta-subunit gene causing congenital isolated thyroid-stimulating hormone deficiency. *Japan. J. Human Genetics*, 36 (4):313-316, 1991.

30. DeGroot, L.J., Larsen, P.R., Refetoff, S., and Stanbury, J.B.: *The Thyroid and Its Diseases*, 5th edition. New York, John Wiley & Sons, Inc., 1984.

31. Vagenakis, A.G. and Braverman, L.E.: Thyroid function tests—which one? *Ann. Intern. Med.*, 84(5):607-608, 1976.

32. Johansen, K., Hansen, J.M., and Skovsted, L.: Myxoede-

ma and thyrotoxicosis: relations between clinical state and concentrations of thyroxine and triiodothyronine in blood. *Acta Med. Scand.*, 204(5):361-364, 1978.

33. Hamburger, J.I.: Section summary: diagnosis of thyroid function. In *Diagnostic Methods in Clinical Thyroidology*. Edited by J.I. Hamburger, New York, Springer-Verlag, 1989, pp.112-123.

34. Sawin, C.T.: The development and use of thyroid preparations. In *The Thyroid Gland: A Practical Clinical Treatise*. Edited by Van Middlesworth, Chicago, Year Book Medical Publishers, Inc., 1986, pp.389-403.

35. Stockigt, J.R.: Serum thyrotropin and thyroid hormone measurements and assessment of thyroid hormone transport. In *Werner and Ingbar's The Thyroid: A Fundamental and Clinical Text*, 6th edition. Edited by L.E. Braverman and R.D. Utiger, Philadelphia, J.B. Lippincott Co., 1991, pp.463-485.

36. Lowe, J.C.: Thyroid statsus of 38 fibromyalgia patients: implications for the eitiology of fibromyalgia. *Clin. Bull. Myofascial Ther.*, 2(1):47-64, 1997.

37. Odell, W.D., Wilbur, J.F., and Paul, W.E.: Radioimmunoassay of human TSH in serum. *Metabolism*, 25:1179, 1965.

38. Spencer, C.A. and Nicoloff, J.T.: Improved radioimmunoassay for human TSH. *Clin. Chem. Acta*, 108:415, 1980.

39. Klee, G.G. and Hay, I.D.: Sensitive thyrotropin assays: analytic and clinical performance criteria. *Mayo Clin. Proc.*, 63:1123, 1988.

40. Caldwell, G., Kellett, H.A., and Gow, S.M.: A new strategy for thyroid function testing. *Lancet*, 1:1117, 1985.

41. Spencer, C.A.: Clinical utility and cost-effectiveness of sensitive thyrotrophin assays in ambulatory and hospitalized patients. *Mayo Clinic Proc.*, 63:1214, 1988.

42. Norman, R.J., Desai, R.K., Deppe, W.M., and Joubert, S.M.: Value of measuring free triiodothyronine and free thyroxine in serum in detection of hypothyroidism. *Clin. Chem.*, 30:169-170, 1984.

43. Patel, Y.C. and Burger, H.G.: Serum thyrotropin (TSH) in pituitary and/or hypothalamic hypothyroidism: normal or elevated basal levels and paradoxical responses to thyrotropin-releasing hormone. *J. Clin. Endocrinol. Metab.*, 37: 190-196, 1973.

44. Kaplan, M.M.: Interactions between drugs and thyroid hormones. *Clin. Chem.*, 29:2091, 1983.

45. Hamburger, J.I.: Strategies for cost-effective thyroid function testing with modern methods. In *Diagnostic Methods in Clinical Thyroidology*. Edited by J.I. Hamburger, New York, Springer-Verlag, 1989, pp.63-109.

46. Stock, J.M., Surks, M.I., and Oppenheimer, J.H.: Replacement dosage of L-thyroxine in hypothyroidism. *N. Engl. J. Med.*, 290:529, 1974.

47. Wong, M.M. and Volpé, R.: What is the best test for monitoring levothyroxine therapy? *Can. Med. Assn. J.*, 124: 1181, 1981.

48. Ingbar, J.C., Borges, M., and Iflah, S.: Evaluating serum thyroxine concentrations in patients receiving "replacement" doses of levothyroxine. *J. Endocrinol. Invest.*, 5:77, 1982.

49. Bantle, J.P.: Replacement therapy with levothyroxine: evolving concepts. *Thyroid Today*, 10:1, 1987.

50. Escobar-Morreale, H.F., Obregón, M.J., Escobar del Rey, F., and Morreale de Escobar, G.: Replacement therapy for hypothyroidism with thyroxine alone does not ensure euthyroidism in all tissues, as studied in thyroidectomized rats. *J. Clin. Invest.*, 96:2828-2838, 1995.

51. Salmon, D., Rendell, M., and Williams, J.: Chemical hyperthyroidism. *Arch. Intern. Med.*, 142:571, 1982.

52. Selenkow, H.A. and Ingbar, S.H.: In *Harrison's Principles of Internal Medicine*, 6th edition. Edited by J. Wintrobe, New York, McGraw-Hill, 1970.

53. Kleinmann, R.W., Vagenakis, A.G., and Braverman, L.E.: The effect of iopanoic acid on the regulation of thyrotropin secretion in euthyroid subjects. *J. Clin. Endocrinol. Metab.*, 51:399, 1980.

54. Evered, D., Young, E.T., and Ormston, B.J.: Treatment of hypothyroidism: a reappraisal of thyroxine therapy. *Brit. Med. J.*, 3:131, 1973.

55. Snyder, P.J. and Utiger, R.D.: Inhibition of thyrotropin response to thyrotropin-releasing hormone by small quantities of thyroid hormone. *J. Clin. Invest.*, 51:2077, 1972.

56. Fukuda, H., Yasuda, N., and Greer, M.A.: Acute effects of thyroxine, triiodothyronine and iodide on thyrotropin secretion. *Endocrinology*, 97:924-931, 1975.

57. Taylor, K., Winikoff, D., and Davies, W.: Resin uptake of ^{131}I-labelled triiodothyronine as a test of thyroid function. *Austral. Ann. Med.*, 13:240-246, 1964.

58. Sterling, K. and Tabachnick, M.: Resin uptake of I[131]-triiodothyronine as a test of thyroid function. *J. Clin. Endocrinol. Metab.*, 21:456-464, 1961.

59. Ain, K.B., Mori, Y., and Refetoff, S.: Reduced clearance rate of thyroxine-binding globulin (TBG) with increased sialylation: a mechanism for estrogen-induced elevation of serum TBG concentration. *J. Clin. Endocrinol. Metab.*, 65:689, 1987.

60. Braverman, L.E. and Utiger, R.D.: Introduction to thyrotoxicosis. In *Werner and Ingbar's The Thyroid: A Fundamental and Clinical Text*, 6th edition. Edited by L.E. Braverman and R.D. Utiger, Philadelphia, J.B. Lippincott Co., 1991, pp.645-647.

61. Shiroky, J.B., Cohen, M., Ballachey, M.L., and Neville, C.: Thyroid dysfunction in rheumatoid arthritis: a controlled prospective survey. *Ann. Rheumat. Dis.*, 52:454-456, 1993.

62. Eisinger, J., Arroyo, P., Calendini, C., Rinaldi, J.P., Combes, R., and Fontaine, G.: Anomalies biologiques au cours des fibromyalgies: III. Explorations endocriniennes. *Lyon Méditerranée Méd.*, 28:858-860, 1992.

63. Chopra, I.J.: A radioimmunoassay for measurement of 3,3',5'-triiodothyronine (reverse 3,3',5'-triiodothyronine). *J. Clin. Invest.*, 54:583, 1974.

64. Volpé, R.: Graves' disease. In *Werner and Ingbar's The Thyroid: A Fundamental and Clinical Text*, 6th edition. Edited by L.E. Braverman and R.D. Utiger, Philadelphia, J.B. Lippincott Co., 1991, pp.648-657.

65. Caron, P.J., Nieman, L.K., Rose, S.R., and Nisula, B.C.: Deficient nocturnal surge of thyrotropin in central hypothyroidism. *J. Clin. Endocrin. Metab.*, 62:960, 1986.

66. Lowe, J.C., Eichelberger, J., Manso, G., and Peterson, K.: Improvement in euthyroid fibromyalgia patients treated with T[3] (tri-iodothyronine). *J. Myofascial Ther.*, 1(2):16-29, 1994.

67. Patel, Y.C., Alford, F.P., and Burger, H.C.: The 24-hour

plasma thyrotrophin profile. *Clin. Sci.*, 43:71-77, 1972.

68. Vanhaelst, L., Van Cauter, E., Degaute, J.P., and Golstein, J.: Circadian variations in serum thyrotrophin levels in man. *J. Clin. Endocrinol. Metab.*, 35:479-484, 1972.

69. Evans, P.J., Weeks, I., Jones, M.K., Woodhead, J.S., and Scanlon, M.F.: The circadian variation of thyrotrophin in patients with primary thyroidal disease. *Clin. Endocrinol.* (Oxf.), 24:343-348, 1986.

70. Greenspan, S.L., Klibanski, A., Schoenfels, D., and Ridgway, E.C.: Pulsatile secretion of thyrotrophin in man. *J. Clin. Endocrinol Metab.*, 63:661-668, 1986.

71. Weeke, J. and Laurberg, P.: Diurnal TSH variations in hypothyroidism. *J. Clin. Endocrinol. Metab.*, 43:32-37, 1976.

72. Azukizawa, M., Pekary, A.E., Hershman, J.M., and Parker, D.C.: Plasma thyrotrophin, thyroxine, and triiodothyronine relationships in man. *J. Clin. Endocrinol. Metab.*, 43:533-542, 1976.

73. Brabant, G., Ranft, U., Ocran, K., Hesch, R.D., and Von zur Muhlen, A.: Thyrotrophin espisodically secreted hormone. *Acta Endocrinol.* (Copenh.), 112:315-322, 1986.

74. Pearce, C.J. and Himsworth, R.L.: Total and free thyroid hormone concentrations in patients receiving maintenance replacement treatment with thyroxine. *Brit. Med. J.*, 288:693-695, 1984.

75. Benencia, H., Ropelato, M.G., Rosales, M., et al.: Thyroid profile modifications during oral hormone replacement therapy in postmenopausal women. *Gynecol. Endocrinol.*, 12(3):179-184, 1998.

76. Laurberg, P.: Persistent problems with the specificity of immunometric TSH assays. *Thyroid*, 3(4):279-283, 1993.

77. Scanlon, M.F. and Toft, A.D.: Regulation of thyrotropin secretion. In *Werner and Ingbar's The Thyroid: A Fundamental and Clinical Text*, 7th edition. Edited by L.P. Braverman and R.D. Utiger, Philadelphia, Lippincott-Raven Publishers, 1996, pp.220-240.

78. Seth, J., Kellett, H.A., Caldwell, G., et al.: A sensitive immunoradiometric assay for serum thyroid stimulation hormone: a replacement for the thyrotropin-releasing hormone test? *Brit. Med. J.*, 289:1334, 1984.

79. Ladenson, P.W.: Diagnosis of thyrotoxicosis. In *Werner and Ingbar's The Thyroid: A Fundamental and Clinical Text*, 6th edition. Edited by L.E. Braverman and R.D. Utiger, Philadelphia, J.B. Lippincott Co., 1991, pp.880-886.

80. Gruhn, J.G., Barsano, C.P., and Kumar, Y.: The development of tests of thyroid function. *Arch. Pathol. Lab. Med.*, 111:84, 1987.

81. Larssen, P.R., Alexander, N.M., and Chopra, I.J.: Revised nomenclature for tests of thyroid hormones and thyroid-related proteins in serum. *Arch. Pathol. Lab. Med.*, 111:1141, 1987.

82. Toft, A.D.: Use of sensitive immunoradiometric assay for thyrotropin in clinical practice. *Mayo Clinic Proc.*, 63:1035, 1988.

83. Loeb, L. and Bassett, R.B.: Effect of hormones of anterior pituitary on thyroid gland in the guinea pig. *Proc. Soc. Exp. Biol. Med.*, 26:860, 1929.

84. Hay, I.D.: Supersensitive thyrotropin assays. In *Diagnostic Methods in Clinical Thyroidology*. Edited by J.I. Hamburger, New York, Springer-Verlag, 1989, pp.39-61.

85. Collins, R.D.: *Illustrated Manual of Laboratory Diag-*

nosis, 2nd edition. Philadelphia, J.B. Lippincott Co., 1975.

86. Ross, D.S., Ardisson, L.J., and Meskell, M.J.: Measurement of thyrotropin in clinical and subclinical hyperthyroidism using a new chemiluminescent assay. *J. Clin. Endocrinol. Metab.*, 69(3):684-688, 1989.

87. Wellby, M.L.: The laboratory diagnosis of thyroid disorders. *Ann. Rev. Med.*, 25:103-172, 1974.

88. Lowe, J.C., Garrison, R.L., Reichman, A.J., Yellin, J., Thompson, M., and Kaufman, D.: Effectiveness and safety of T₃ (triiodothyronine) therapy for euthyroid fibromyalgia: a double-blind placebo-controlled response-driven crossover study. *Clin. Bull. Myofascial Ther.*, 2(2/3):31-57, 1997.

89. Lowe, J.C., Reichman, A.J., and Yellin, J.: The process of change during T₃ treatment for euthyroid fibromyalgia: a double-blind placebo-controlled crossover study. *Clin. Bull. Myofascial Ther.*, 2(2/3):91-124, 1997.

90. Larsen, P.R.: Salicylate-induced increases in free triiodothyronine in human serum: evidence of inhibition of triiodothyronine binding to thyroxine-binding globulin and thyroxine-binding prealbumin. *J. Clin. Invest.*, 51:1125, 1972.

91. Suzuki, H., Yamazaki, N., and Suzuki, Y.: Lowering effect of diphenyldantoin on serum free thyroxine and thyroxine-binding globulin (TBG). *Acta Endocrinol.*, 105:477, 1984.

92. Davidson, I. and Henry, J.B.: *Clinical Diagnosis by Laboratory Methods*, 15th edition. Philadelphia, W.B. Saunders, 1974.

93. Hershman, J.M.: Hypothalamic and pituitary hypothyroidism. In *Recent Progress in Diagnosis and Treatment of Hypothyroid Conditions*. Edited by P.A. Bastenie, M. Bonnyns, and L. Vanhaelst, Amsterdam, *Excerpta Medica*, 1980, pp.40-50.

94. Wahner, H.W. and Walser, A.H.: Measurements of thyroxine-plasma protein interactions. *Med. Clin. North Amer.*, 56:849, 1972.

95. Clark, F.: The estimation of thyroid hormone binding by plasma proteins and of unbound levels of thyroxine in plasma. *J. Clin. Pathol.*, 20(Suppl.):344-352, 1967.

96. Tibaldi, J. and Barzel, U.S.: Thyroxine supplementation: method for the prevention of clinical hypothyroidism. *Amer. J. Med.*, 79:241-244, 1985.

97. Toft, A.D., Irvine, W.J., and Seth, J.: Thyroid function in the long term follow-up of patients treated with iodine-¹³¹ for thyrotoxicosis. *Lancet*, 2:576-578, 1975.

98. Noel, G.L., Dimond, R.C., Wartofsky, L., Earl, J.M., and Frantz, A.G.: Studies of prolactin and TSH secretion by continuous infusion of small amounts of thyrotropin-releasing hormone. *J. Clin. Endocrinol. Metab.*, 39:6, 1974.

99. Burrows, A.W., Shakespear, R.A., Hesch, R.D., Cooper, E., Aickin, C.M., and Burke, C.W.: Thyroid hormones in the elderly sick: "T₄ euthyroidism." *Brit. Med. J.*, 4:437-439, 1975.

100. Utiger, R.D.: Tests of thyroregulatory mechanisms. In *Werner's The Thyroid: A Fundamental and Clinical Text*, 5th edition. Edited by S.H. Ingbar and L.E. Braverman, Philadelphia, J.B. Lippincott Co., 1986, pp.511-523.

101. Ferring Laboratories, Inc., 400 Rella Blvd., Suite 201, Suffern, NY 10901. Phone 914-368-7916, Fax 914-368-1193. [Company markets injectable 500 µg boluses of Thyrel™ (TRH) to perform the TRH-stimulation test.]

102. Reichlin, S., Martin, J.B., Mitnick, M.A., et al.: The hypothalamus in pituitary thyroid regulation. *Rec. Prog. Horm. Res.*, 28:229-286, 1972.

103. Burger, A.G.: Effects of pharmacologic agents on thyroid hormone metabolism. In *Werner and Ingbar's The Thyroid: A Fundamental and Clinical Text*, 6th edition. Edited by L.E. Braverman and R.D. Utiger, Philadelphia, J.B. Lippincott Co., 1991, pp.335-346.

104. Gold, M.S., Pottash, A.L.C., and Extein, I.: Hypothyroidism and depression: evidence from complete thyroid function evaluation. *J.A.M.A.*, 245:1919, 1981.

105. Vanderpump, M.P., Neary, R.H., Manning, K., and Clayton, R.N.: Does an increase in the sensitivity of serum thyrotropin assays reduce diagnostic costs for thyroid disease in the community? *J. R. Soc. Med.*, 90(10):547-550, 1997.

106. Engbring, N.H. and Engstrom, W.W.: Effects of estrogen and testosterone on circulating thyroid hormone. *J. Clin. Endocrinol. Metab.*, 19:783, 1959.

107. Cooper, D.S., Daniels, G.H., and Ladenson, P.W.: Hyperthyroxinemia in patients treated with high-dose propranolol. *Amer. J. Med.*, 73:867, 1982.

108. Christy, N.P.: The adrenal cortex in thyrotoxicosis. In *Werner and Ingbar's The Thyroid: A Fundamental and Clinical Text*, 6th edition. Edited by L.E. Braverman and R.D. Utiger, Philadelphia, J.B. Lippincott Co., 1991, pp.806-815.

109. Kozlowski, M.R.: Inhibition of the binding and the behavioral effects of thyrotropin-releasing hormone (TRH) by the triazolobenzodiazepines. *Pharmacol. Biochem. Behav.*, 30:73-75, 1988.

110. Drummond, A.H.: Chlordiazepoxide is a competitive thyrotropin-releasing hormone receptor antagonist in GH3 pituitary tumour cells. *Biochem. Biophys. Res. Commun.*, 127:63-70, 1985.

111. Gershon, M.C. and Paul, M.E.: Chlordiazepoxide antagonized thyrotropin-releasing hormone (TRH)-receptor interaction in rat pituitary (GH3) cells. *Clin. Res.*, 33:533A, 1985.

112. Rinehart, R.K., Barbaz, B., Lyengars, S., et al.: Benzodiazepine interactions with central thyroid-releasing hormone binding sites: characterization and physiological significance. *J. Pharmacol. Exp. Ther.*, 238:178-185, 1986.

113. Otsuki, M., Dakoda, M., and Baba, S.: Influence of glucocorticoids on TRH-induced TSH response in man. *J. Clin. Endocrinol. Metab.*, 36:95-102, 1973.

114. Wilber, J.F. and Utiger, R.D.: The effect of glucocorticoids on thyrotropin secretion. *J. Clin. Invest.*, 48:2096-2103, 1969.

115. Brent, G.A. and Hershman, J.M.: Effects of nonthyroidal illness on thyroid function tests. In *The Thyroid Gland: A Practical Clincal Treatise*. Edited by Van Middlesworth, Chicago, Year Book Medical Publishers, Inc., 1986.

116. Wenzel, K.W.: Pharmacological interference with in vitro tests of thyroid function. *Metabolism*, 30:717, 1981.

117. Sanchez-Franco, F., Garcia, M.D., Cacicedo, L., et al.: Influence of sex phase of the menstrual cycle on thyrotrophin (TSH) response to thyrotropin-releasing hormone (TRH). *J. Clin. Endocrinol. Metab.*, 37:736, 1973.

118. Ryszard, J., Chetkowski, M.D., David, R., et al.: Biologic effects of transdermal estradiol. *N. Engl. J. Med.*, 314: 1615, 1986.

119. Ahlquist, J.A.O., Franklyn, J.A., Wood, D.F., et al.: Hormonal regulation of thyrotropin synthesis and secretion. *Horm. Metab. Res.*, 517:86, 1987.

120. Gambert, S.R.: Environmental effects and physiologic variables. In *Werner and Ingbar's The Thyroid: A Fundamental and Clinical Text*, 6th edition. Edited by L.E. Braverman and R.D. Utiger, Philadelphia, J.B. Lippincott Co., 1991, pp.347-357.

121. Gross, H.A., Appleman, M.D, Jr., and Nicoloff, J.T.: Effect of biologically active steroids on thyroid function in man. *J. Clin. Endocrinol. Metab.*, 33:242, 1975.

122. Glass, C.K., Holloway, J.M., Devary, O.V., and Rosenfeld, M.G.: The thyroid hormone receptor binds with opposite transcription effects to a common sequence motif in thyroid hormone and estrogen response elements. *Cell*, 54: 313, 1988.

123. Ingbar, J.C., Borges, M., and Iflah, S.: Elevated serum thyroxine concentration in patients receiving "replacement" doses of levothyroxine. *J. Endocrinol. Invest.*, 5:77, 1982.

124. Symons, R.G. and Murphy, L.J.: Acute changes in thyroid function tests following ingestion of thyroxine. *Clin. Endocrinol.*, 19:539, 1983.

125. Wennlund, A.: Variation in serum levels of T_3, T_4, FT_4 and TSH during thyroxine replacement therapy. *Acta Endocrinol.* (Copenh.), 113:47, 1986.

126. Costom, B.H., Grumbach, M.M., and Kaplan, S.L.: Effect of thyrotropin-releasing factor on serum thyroid stimulating hormone: an approach to distinguishing hypothalamic from pituitary forms of idiopathic hypopituitary dwarfism. *J. Clin. Invest.*, 50:2219, 1971.

127. Sterling, K. and Lazarus, J.H.: The thyroid and its control. *Ann. Rev. Physiol.*, 39:360, 1977.

128. Perk, M. and O'Neill, B.J.: The effect of thyroid hormone therapy on angiographic coronary artery disease progression. *Can. J. Cardiol.*, 13(3):273-276, 1997.

129. Jackson, I.M.D.: Thyrotropin-releasing hormone. *N. Engl. J. Med.*, 306:145-155, 1982.

130. Cobb, W.E., Lamberton, R.P., and Jackson, I.M.D.: Use of a rapid sensitive immunoradiometric assay for thyrotropin to distinguish normal from hyperthyroid subjects. *Clin. Chem.*, 30:1558-1560, 1984.

131. Beck-Peccoz, P., Amer, S., Menezes-Ferreira, M., Faglia, G., and Weintraub, B.D.: Decreased receptor binding of biologically inactive thyrotropin in central hypothyroidism. *N. Engl. J. Med.*, 312:1085-1090, 1985.

132. Carlson, H.E. and Hershman, J.M.: The hypothalamic-pituitary-thyroid axis. *Med. Clin. N. Amer.*, 59:1047, 1975.

133. Chopra, I.J., Ho, R.S., and Lam, R.: An improved radioimmunoassay of triiodothyronine in serum: its application to clinical and physiological studies. *J. Lab. Clin. Med.*, 80: 729-739, 1972.

134. Bauer, D.C. and Brown, A.N.: Sensitive thyrotropin and free thyroxine testing in outpatients. Are both necessary? *Arch. Intern. Med.*, 156(20):2333-2337, 1996.

135. Hennessey, J.V., Evaul, J.E., Tseng, Y.-Y., et al.: L-thyroxine dosage: a reevaluation of therapy with contemporary preparations. *Ann. Intern. Med.*, 105:11-15, 1986.

136. *Compendium of Services*. National Health Laboratories, Inc., 1050 N. Post Oak, #145, Houston, TX 77055.

137. Legakis, I.N., Golematis, B.C., Dourakis, N., Lymbero-

poulou, I., Mountokalakis, T., and Leandros, E.A.: Low T$_3$ syndrome with asynchronous changes of TT$_3$ and rT$_3$ values in laparoscopic cholecystectomy. *Endocr. Res.*, 24(2): 205-213, 1998.

138. Natori, Y., Yamaguchi, N., Koike, S., et al.: Thyroid function in patients with anorexia nervosa and depression. *Rinsho Byori*, 42(12):1268, 1994.

139. Comtois, R., Hebert, J., and Soucy, J.P.: Reversible hypertriiodothyroninaemia due to adrenal insufficiency. *J. Intern. Med.*, 230(1):79-82, 1991.

140. Chopra, I.J.: Nature, sources, and relative biologic significance of circulating thyroid hormones. In *Werner and Ingbar's The Thyroid: A Fundamental and Clinical Text*, 6th edition. Edited by L.E. Braverman and R.D. Utiger, Philadelphia, J.B. Lippincott Co., 1991, pp.126-143.

141. Juma, A.H., Ardawi, M.S., Baksh, T.M., and Serafi, A.A.: Alterations in thyroid hormones, cortisol, and catecholamine concentration in patients after orthopedic surgery *J. Surg. Res.*, 50(2):129-134, 1991.

142. Skovsted, L.: Radioimmunoassays of T$_3$, r-T$_3$ and r-T'$_2$ in human serum. *Acta Med. Scand. Suppl.*, 624:19-24, 1979.

143. Chopra, I.J., Solomon, D.H., Chopra, U., et al.: Reciprocal changes in serum reverse T$_3$ (rT$_3$) in systemic illness: evidence for independent pathways of T$_4$ metabolism in adults. *J. Clin. Endocrinol. Metab.*, 41:1043, 1975.

144. Suda, A.K., Pittman, C.S., Shimizu, T., et al.: The production and metabolism of 3,5,3'-triiodothyronine and 3,3',5'-triiodothyronine in normal and fasting subjects. *J. Clin. Endocrinol. Metab.*, 47:1311, 1978.

145. Rajkovic, D., Skreb, F., and Banovac, K.: Reduction of total and free triiodothyronine in serum after abortion. *Endokrinologie,* 79(1):44-48, 1982.

146. Vagenakis, A.G., Burger, A., Portnay, G.I., et al.: Diversion of peripheral thyroxine metabolism from activating to inactivating pathways during complete fasting. *J. Clin. Endocrinol. Metab.*, 41:191, 1975.

147. Chopra, I.J.: An assessment of daily turnover and significance of thyroidal secretion of reverse T$_3$. *J. Clin. Invest.*, 58:32, 1976.

148. Chopra, I.J., Solomon, D.H., Hepner, G.W., and Morgenstein, A.A.: Misleadingly low free thyroxine index and usefulness of reverse triiodothyronine measurement in nonthyroidal illness. *Ann. Intern. Med.*, 90:905, 1979.

149. Roche, J. Michael, R., and Nunez, J.: Sur la presence de la 3,3',5'-triiodothyronine dans le sang de rat. *C.R. Soc. Biol.* (Paris), 105:20, 1956.

150. Dunn, J.T. and Stanbury, J.B.: The metabolism of 3,3',5'-triiodothyronine in man. *J. Clin. Endocrinol. Metab.*, 18: 713, 1958.

151. Volpé, R.: Autoimmune thyroiditis. In *Werner and Ingbar's The Thyroid: A Fundamental and Clinical Text*, 6th edition. Edited by L.E. Braverman and R.D. Utiger, New York, J.B. Lippincott Co., 1991, pp.921-933.

152. Adlin, V.: Subclinical hypothyroidism: deciding when to treat. *Amer. Fam. Physician*, 57(4):776-780, 1998.

153. Oomen, H.A., Schipperijn, A.J., and Drexhage, H.A.: The prevalence of affective disorder and in particular of a rapid cycling of bipolar disorder in patients with abnormal thyroid function tests. *Clin. Endocrinol.* (Oxf.), 45(2):215-223, 1996.

154. Weetman, A.P.: Hypothyroidism: screening and subclini-

cal disease. *Brit. Med. J.*, 314:1175, 1997.

155. Vanderpump, M.P.J., Tunbridge, W.M.G., French, J.M., et al.: The development of ischemic heart disease in relation to autoimmune thyroid disease in a 20-year follow-up study of an English community. *Thyroid*, 6:155-156, 1996.

156. Ferraccioli, G., Chirelli, L., and Scita, F.: EMG-biofeedback training in fibromyalgia syndrome. *J. Rheumatol.*, 14:820-825, 1987.

157. Hallengren, B.: Hypothyroidism—clinical findings, diagnosis, therapy. Thyroid tests should be performed on broad indications. *Lakartidningen*, 95(38):4091-4096, 1998.

158. Pearch, C.J. and Himsworth, R.L.: Total and free thyroid hormone concentration in patients receiving maintenance replacement treatment with thyroxine. *Brit. Med. J.*, 288: 693-695, 1984.

159. Volpé, R.: Misinformation on diagnosis and treatment. *Thyroid Foundation of Canada Thyrobulletin*, 19(2):10, 1998.

160. Kabadi, U.M. and Cech, R.: Normal thyroxine and elevated thyrotropin concentrations: evolving hypothyroidism or persistent euthyroidism with reset thyrostat. *J. Endocrinol. Invest.*, 20(6):319-326, 1997.

161. De Rosa, G., Testa, A., Giacomini, D., et al.: Comparison between TRH-stimulated TSH and basal TSH measurement by a commercial immunoradiometric assay in the management of thyroid disease. *Q. J. Nucl. Med.*, 40(2): 182-187, 1996.

162. Kasagi, K., Kousaka, T., Higuchi, K., et al.: Clinical significance of measurements of antithyroid antibodies in the diagnosis of Hashimoto's thyroiditis: comparison with histological findings. *Thyroid*, 6(5):445-450, 1996.

163. Loeb, P.B., Drash, A.L., and Kenny, F.M.: Prevalence of low-titre and "negative" antithyroglobulin antibodies in biopsy-proved juvenile Hashimoto's thyroiditis. *J. Pediatr.*, 82(1):17-21, 1973.

164. Doniach, D., Dottazzo, G.F., and Russell, P.C.G.: Goitrous autoimmune thyroiditis (Hashimoto's disease). *J. Clin. Endocrinol. Metab.*, 8:63, 1979.

165. Doniach, D.: Humoral and genetic aspects of thyroid autoimmunity. *Clin. Endicrinol. Metab.*, 4:267, 1979.

166. Senda, Y., Nishibu, M., Kawai, K., Mizukami, Y., and Hashimoto, T.: Estimation of anti-thyroid peroxidase autoantibody (TPOAb) and anti-thyroglobulin autoantibody (TgAb) in patients with various thyroid disease—comparison between histopathological findings and serological results in patients with Hashimoto's thyroiditis. *Rinsho Byori*, 43(12):1243-1250, 1995.

167. Romaldini, J.H., Biancalana, M.M., Figueiredo, D.I., Farah, C.S., and Mathias, P.C.: Effect of L-thyroxine administration on antithyroid antibody levels, lipid profile, and thyroid volume in patients with Hashimoto's thyroiditis. *Thyroid*, 6(3):183-188, 1996.

168. Farwell, A.P. and Braverman, L.E.: Inflammatory thyroid disorders. *Otolaryngol. Clin. North Amer.*, 29(4):541-556, 1996.

169. LoPresti, J.S.: Laboratory tests for thyroid disorders. *Otolaryngol. Clin. North Amer.*, 29(4):557-575, 1996.

170. Toldy, E., Locsei, Z., Kalmar, I., Varga, L., and Kovacs, L.G.: Diagnostic value of thyroid antibodies. *Orv. Hetil.*, 137(38):2075-2080, 1996.

171. Pies, R.W.: The diagnosis and treatment of subclinical hy-

pothyroid states in depressed patients. *Gen. Hosp. Psychiatry*, 19(5):344-354, 1997.

172. Kotani, T.: Anti-TPO autoantibodies. *Rinsho Byori*, 46(4): 324-330, 1998.

173. Gaches, F., Delaire, L., Nadalon, S., Loustaud-Ratti, V., and Vidal, E.: Frequency of autoimmune diseases in 218 patients with autoimmune thyroid pathologies. *Rev. Med. Interne*, 19(3):173-179, 1998.

174. Rodolico, C., Toscano, A., Benvenga, S., et al.: Myopathy as the persistently isolated symptomatology of primary autoimmune hypothyroidism. *Thyroid*, 8(11):1033-1038, 1998.

175. Neeck, G. and Riedel, W.: Thyroid function in patients with fibromyalgia syndrome. *J. Rheum.*, 19:1120-1122, 1992.

176. Ferraccioli, G., Cavalieri, F., Salaffi, F., Fontana, S., Scita, F., Nolli, M., and Maestri, D.: Neuroendocrinologic findings in primary fibromyalgia (soft tissue chronic pain syndrome) and in other chronic rheumatic conditions (rheumatoid arthritis, low back pain). *J. Rheumatol.*, 17: 869-873, 1990.

177. Nicoloff, J.T., Fisher, D.A., and Appleman, M.D.: The role of glucocorticoids in the regulation of thyroid function in man. *J. Clin. Invest.*, 49:1922, 1970.

178. Alford, F.P., Baker, H.W.G., Burger, H.G., et al.: Temporal patterns of integrated plasma hormone levels during sleep and wakefulness. I. Thyroid-stimulating hormone, growth hormone and cortisol. *J. Clin. Endocrinol. Metab.*, 37:841, 1973.

179. Brabant, A., Brabant, G., Schuermeyer, T., et al.: The role of glucocorticoids in the regulation of thyrotropin. *Acta Endocrinol.* (Copenh.), 121:95, 1989.

180. Ridgway, E.C.: Modern concepts of primary thyroid gland failure. *Clin. Chem.*, 42(1):179-182, 1996.

181. Davey, R.X., Clarke, M.I., and Webster, A.R.: Thyroid function testing based on assay of thyroid-stimulating hormone: assessing an algorithm's reliability. *Med. J. Austral.*, 164(6):329-332, 1996.

4.3

Symptoms, Signs, and Peripheral Indices

In this chapter, the term "symptom" refers to a patient's perception of a variation from normal structure or function that indicates dysfunction or disease. The term "sign" refers to a manifestation of dysfunction or disease that the clinician can observe or measure. The term "index" refers to a sign that is measured and quantified against a fixed quantified standard. The term "peripheral tissue" refers to any tissue other than the pituitary, including central nervous system tissues that are usually considered "central" tissues. A "peripheral index" is an indirect measure of the metabolic status of a peripheral tissue. The term "clinical indicator" refers to indicators of peripheral tissue metabolic status; the indicators include the patient's symptoms, signs, and peripheral indices.

Fibromyalgia patients have symptoms, signs, and peripheral indices typical of the hypometabolism that results from inadequate thyroid hormone regulation of cell function. In some fibromyalgia patients, the symptoms, signs, and indices are manifestations of hypothyroidism. This is indicated by a suggestive history, clinical status, and laboratory thyroid function test results. In some other patients, the symptoms, signs, and indices result from partial cellular resistance to thyroid hormone. This is indicated by relief of the patient's symptoms with the use of supraphysiologic dosages of T_3, resulting in a sustained elevation of the serum free T_3 without thyrotoxicosis.

Because laboratory tests of thyroid function do not assess the response of the patient's peripheral tissues to thyroid hormone, these tests are of no use for determining the optimal dosage for the patient. Instead, objective evaluation of the patient's symptoms, signs, and peripheral indices are of most practical use. Periodic assessment of these clinical indicators enables the clinician to determine the impact that thyroid hormone, as part of the patient's more comprehensive metabolic rehabilitation regimen, is having on the tissues.

Objective assessment is critical because without it, evaluating the patient's response to metabolic rehabilitation is subject to wide subjective variation. The clinician can minimize subjective variability when working with the fibromyalgia patient by using the objective tools described in Chapters 4.1 and 5.2. However, the clinician can also make use of any of the symptoms, signs, and peripheral indices described in this chapter. Again, though, assessments must be objectified by quantification.

The patient's symptoms can be quantified with visual analog scales such as those contained in the long and short versions of the FibroQuest questionnaire. Clinical tools are not readily available for quantifying some signs such as dry skin and thin eyebrows. A fairly accurate assessment of changes in such signs as treatment progresses can be made by comparing the clinician's meticulous descriptions of the signs from the initial and each succeeding evaluation. Peripheral indices of tissue metabolism, such as *the Achilles reflex relaxation phase, pulse rate, serum cholesterol, and ECG tracings, provide highly objective measures of the patient's changing status.*

The conventional endocrinology paradigm decrees that the basal serum TSH level, possibly supplemented by other laboratory tests of thyroid function, is all that is needed to diagnose or rule out hypothyroidism. The paradigm also dictates that only patients diagnosed as hypothyroid by laboratory test results may undergo thyroid hormone therapy, and then only with T_4. The paradigm further rules that hypothyroid patients must restrict their T_4 dosage so as to keep the TSH level well within the "normal" reference range. These scientifically indefensible mandates leave many hypothyroid and euthyroid hypometabolic patients ill and dysfunctional. Fibromyalgia patients are among the much wider population afflicted by the mandates.

The main goal of those who subscribe to this conventional paradigm is normal thyroid function test results. For these practitioners, this goal must be achieved even if the patient must remain ill to achieve it. This is the opposite of a rational and humane objective: normal tissue metabolism with relief of symptoms and signs. For the patient's welfare, as long as there is no evidence of tissue overstimulation, this objective must be achieved regardless of the results of thyroid function test results.

To effectively accomplish this rational and humane goal, the clinician must take two steps. First, he must repeatedly and objectively assess the patient's symptoms, signs, and peripheral indices for tissue metabolic status. Second, he should use the results of the assessments to make adjustments to the patient's dosage of exogenous thyroid hormone. Within the context of a more comprehensive metabolic regimen, correct dosage adjustments should result in normal tissue metabolism (according to clinical indicators) and in turn, relief of the patient's suffering.

● THE GREATER USEFULNESS OF CLINICAL INDICATORS OF TISSUE METABOLIC STATUS

The basal serum TSH is touted as the "gold standard" for diagnosing or ruling out hypothyroidism and for adjusting exogenous thyroid hormone dosage. Among the reasons to reject this proposition is the difference in the sensitivity to thyroid hormone of the pituitary and peripheral tissues. Ribot et al. noted, ". . . there is some evidence that hypophyseal [pituitary] sensitivity to the administration of L-thyroxine may be different from that of other tissues, and a state of euthyroidism [eumetabolism] from the hypophyseal viewpoint does not completely rule out the possibility of hyperthyroidism [hypermetabolism] in other tissues."[90,p.151] Nor does normal sensitivity of the pituitary rule out *hypo*sensitivity to thyroid hormone of some or all peripheral tissues. The differential sensitivity of the pituitary and peripheral tissues to thyroid hormone renders the TSH completely useless as a gauge of peripheral tissue response to thyroid hormone. The patient's symptoms, signs, and peripheral indices are far more accurate and reliable indicators of her tissue metabolic status.[12][33,p.98] To use these indicators is to practice clinical medicine, a technique abandoned by many and perhaps most endocrinologists as well as the conventional medical practitioners who subscribe to the current endocrinological model.

The abandonment of clinical medicine in the care of hypothyroid patients today is based in part on published statements by thyroidologists such as Gow and coauthors. "Our findings indicate that TSH secretion can be used as a sensitive and representative test of peripheral tissue exposure to thyroid hormones in patients receiving T_4 replacement therapy."[91,p.369] Such statements were perhaps justified 30 years ago when the field of thyroidology was far shorter on scientific data than today. These authors might be correct if they altered their statement to say that the TSH level is a useful estimate of the amount of thyroid hormone that tissues are *likely* to be exposed to. But exposure of cells to thyroid hormone does not mean that T_4 is effectively converted to T_3 (the most metabolically active form of thyroid hormone) within the cells. Moreover, exposure does not mean that T_3-receptors in the nuclei of cells bind normally and interact properly with T_3. To accept today the mandates of the current endocrinology paradigm for the diagnosis and treatment of those who might benefit from exogenous thyroid hormone, we would have to ignore considerable scientific evidence contradicting that paradigm. Because this would be scientifically indefensible, it is proper to use laboratory thyroid function tests only as one indicator of metabolic problems related to inadequate thyroid hormone regulation of cell function. After the patient's thyroid status is initially determined, the use of laboratory thyroid function tests cannot be justified. Only clinical indicators are of practical use in the effort to normalize tissue metabolism.

In 1978, Johansen and coworkers reported that compared to the basal metabolic rate (BMR), clinical assessment (evaluation of the patient based on symptoms and signs) was a better indicator of the severity of both hyperthyroidism and hypothyroidism.[66] They had evaluated severity in both types of patients with an assessment instrument termed the "clinical diagnostic score index." The clinical status of hyperthyroid and hypothyroid patients significantly correlated with the free T_4 index and the free T_3 index. Moreover, the clinical diagnostic score index correlated better with the free T_4 and free T_3 than did the BMR. TSH levels, however, did *not* correlate with the patients' clinical status. Admittedly, the TSH used in this study was first-generation and thus less sensitive than those we use today. But little has changed: The more sensitive assays today are still less useful for gauging the severity of a patient's hyperthyroidism or hypothyroidism than an assessment of the patient's clinical status. And for patients who appear to have cellular resistance to thyroid hormone, the TSH and other thyroid hormone laboratory values are entirely useless except for initially establishing a patient's metabolic status.

The report by Johansen et al.[66] is consistent with the findings of Fraser et al. In 1986, Fraser and coworkers studied patients taking T_4. Four clinicians experienced in the use of T_4 evaluated the patients clinically and used the Wayne index. This index is a questionnaire used to indirectly evaluate metabolic status of patients through symptoms and signs. The clinicians classified patients as euthyroid, hypothyroid, or hyperthyroid. (It is obvious, by virtue of the form of assessment they used, that by these three terms, they meant, respectively, eumetabolic, hypometabolic, or hypermetabolic.) The clinicians' diagnoses were determined not to be biased by subjecting the Wayne index scores to the Kruskal-Wallis analysis of variance. There was no significant difference in the median scores of the four clinicians. By contrast, tests of the total T_4, total T_3, free T_4, free T_3, and basal serum TSH were of *no* value in determining whether patients were taking enough, too little, or too much T_4. The researchers wrote, "These [laboratory] measurements are therefore of little, if any, value in monitoring patients receiving thyroxine replacement."[12]

In a statement by Stockigt in the major textbook of thyroidology, *Werner's The Thyroid*, he agreed, perhaps inadvertently, with the above conclusions of Johansen et al.[66] and Fraser et al.[12] He wrote, "In some situations (e.g., patients with ischemic heart disease and hypothyroidism), the appropriate dose of T_4 should be based on clinical judgement rather than lab-

oratory findings."[5,p.381] This was a concession that titrating dosage by clinical indicators is superior to doing so on the basis of laboratory thyroid function test results. The implicit message in Stockigt's statement is that when adjusting the dosage of exogenous thyroid hormone is *really* important, as with cardiac patients, assessing the patient's symptoms and signs is more valuable than thyroid function test results. However, adjusting the thyroid hormone dosage of *all* hypothyroid and euthyroid hypometabolic patients is also *really* important. The quality of their lives is at stake, and for some, the continuation of life depends upon effective dosage adjustments. These patients deserve the greater efficacy of care allowed by the use of clinical factors (symptoms, signs, and indices) and denied by the exclusive use of laboratory tests results.

SYMPTOMS, SIGNS, AND PERIPHERAL INDICES ARE OF NO USE IN DETERMINING THE FUNCTIONAL STATUS OF THE PITUITARY-THYROID GLAND AXIS

The functional status of the pituitary-thyroid gland axis can only be determined by laboratory thyroid function testing. This form of testing, however, is not always definitive. Sonkin listed six conditions in which thyroid function laboratory tests are likely to give ambiguous values: low T_3 syndrome, inappropriate TSH secretion, incipient hypothyroidism, decreased thyroid hormone reserve of the thyroid gland, peripheral resistance to thyroid hormone, and symptomatic low metabolism that is responsive to thyroid hormone therapy. He stated, "Measurements of serum TSH and thyroid hormone levels in these conditions are unreliable indicators of peripheral metabolic function." Moreover, he wrote, "It appears that clinical trials [of thyroid medication] controlled by measurements of peripheral metabolic response, the BMR, and serum cholesterol levels should be revived when tests of thyroid hormone production are ambiguous or do not fit the clinical picture."[1,p.160]

Symptoms, signs, and peripheral indices are *not diagnostic* of hypothyroidism or cellular resistance to thyroid hormone. These clinical indicators of hypometabolism, however, do support the diagnosis of hypothyroidism when a suggestive history and laboratory test results indicate that the patient is hypothyroid. When laboratory test results indicate the patient is euthyroid, symptoms, signs, and peripheral indices indicative of hypometabolism justify a tentative diagnosis of thyroid hormone resistance. One reason for this is that presently it is only through a trial of thyroid hormone therapy that we can confidently infer that the patient has cellular resistance to thyroid hormone. The

Table 4.3.1. Symptoms of euthyroid hypometabolic patients listed by various authors.

WRITER	SYMPTOMS/SIGNS LISTED
Thompson & Thompson[2]	Headaches, dizziness, weakness, chronic fatigue, nervousness/low BMR
Thurmon & Thompson[3]	Lack of endurance, marked nervousness, marked tendency to worry and emotional upset at slight provocation, cold sensitivity, numbness and tingling of extremities, constipation, headache, vague pains, dizziness, palpitation, dyspnea on exertion/low pulse rate, delayed and scanty menstrual flow.
Sonkin[1]	A variety of symptoms suggesting hypothyroidism/slow Achilles reflex.
Goldberg[4]	Anxiety states, irritability and mood swings, easy fatigability, lethargy, decreased libido, premenstrual tension, GI disturbances, scalp seborrhea or hair loss, palpitations, muscle and joint pains, shortness of breath/prolonged contraction phase of Achilles reflex/low BMR

inference is justified when the patient has (1) a positive response to exogenous thyroid hormone (2) with high circulating thyroid hormone levels (3) but no tissue thyrotoxicosis. Symptoms, signs, and peripheral indices should serve as barometers of tissue metabolic change during a trial of thyroid hormone therapy, both for the hypothyroid patient and the patient with possible cellular resistance to thyroid hormone. The clinician can monitor these clinical indicators as a check on his impression that the patient's metabolic status is either remaining the same or changing under the influence of the patient's metabolic treatment regimen.

HYPOTHYROIDISM AND EUTHYROID HYPOMETABOLISM: SIMILAR SYMPTOMS, SIGNS, AND PERIPHERAL INDICES

The symptoms, signs, and peripheral indices of most patients' hypothyroidism and thyroid hormone-related euthyroid hypometabolism are similar. In fact, the clinical indicators are so similar that they allow no distinction between the two diagnostic classifications. Table 4.3.1 contains symptoms and signs of euthyroid hypometabolic patients listed by several authors.

Fibromyalgia is one clinical phenotype of inadequate thyroid hormone regulation of cell function in which central pain modulation is impaired. The impaired pain modulation results in widespread pain and tenderness to mechanical pressure. The widespread pain and tenderness are the only features that allow distinction from other clinical phenotypes of inadequate thyroid hormone regulation of cell function. The remainder of this chapter is devoted to an overview of clinical indicators of hypometabolism that the clinician should be aware of. He may wish to use any or all of these in the evaluation and treatment of fibromyalgia patients or other patients with hypothyroidism or euthyroid hypometabolism.

● SYMPTOMS OF HYPOMETABOLISM

The first suspicion of hypometabolism typically arises from the patient's symptoms. A clinician familiar with the symptoms of hypometabolism due to hypothyroidism, and who is also sensitive to his patient's report of the symptoms, will be alerted that thyroid function testing is warranted.

Whether the test results are positive or negative, the tentative hypothesis with each fibromyalgia patient should be that she is hypometabolic due to inadequate thyroid hormone regulation of cell function. Compiling a list of her symptoms makes it easier to decide whether cumulatively they suggest hypometabolism. Having her estimate the intensity of each symptom on a visual analog scale provides a baseline against which to compare subsequent estimates as treatment proceeds (see Chapters 4.1 and 5.2).

There is a wide variation in the sets of symptoms of hypometabolic patients. The variety probably results from the differences in the sets of tissues that are selectively involved in different patients. Those symptoms included in the remainder of this section are common symptoms of hypometabolic patients, particularly those whose phenotypical expression is fibromyalgia.

LISTS OF HYPOTHYROID SYMPTOMS

Each fibromyalgia patient will have only a subset of symptoms characteristic of hypothyroidism. Familiarity with the full range of hypothyroid symptoms prepares the clinician to recognize any subset reported by an individual fibromyalgia patient. To meet the ACR criteria for the diagnosis of fibromyalgia, the patient must have widespread pain and tender points (see Chapter 4.1). Typically, however, the patient also has numerous other symptoms characteristic of hypothyroidism.

Table 4.3.2. Hypothyroid symptoms listed by DeGowin & DeGowin*

1. *dry skin*	6. **constipation**
2. *hair loss*	7. *broken nails*
3. **slow thinking**	8. *weight gain with*
4. **cold intolerance**	*little food intake*
5. diminished libido	9. **excess menstrual flow**

*R.L. DeGowin and E.L. DeGowin, *Bedside Diagnostic Examination*, 3rd edition. New York, Macmillan Publishing Co., Inc., 1976.[30,p.860]

The symptoms listed by author vary. Table 4.3.2 lists the few symptoms reported by DeGowin and DeGowin[30,p.860] and Table 4.3.3. contains the more extensive list reported by DeGroot et al.[21,pp.577-578] (Table 4.3.3 lists the incidence in two studies of symptoms and signs of hypothyroidism in hypothyroid and control subjects.) In both tables, symptoms in bold print are generally considered to be associated with fibromyalgia. Symptoms in italics are not generally recognized as associated, but fibromyalgia patients commonly complain of them. The clinician will find that most patients have some or all of these before treatment. He will also find that as metabolic rehabilitation progresses, most fibromyalgia patients are relieved of the symptoms.

Table 4.3.3. Incidence of symptoms and signs of hypothyroidism.*

Symptoms & Signs	Study A % of 77 Cases	Study B % of 100 Cases	Normal Control Subjects % of 100
Weakness	99	98	21
Dry skin	97	79	26
Coarse skin	97	70	10
Lethargy	91	85	17
Slow speech	91	56	7
Edema of eyelids	90	86	28
Sensation of cold	89	95	39
Decreased sweating	89	68	17
Cold skin	83	80	33
Thick tongue	82	60	17
Edema of face	79	95	27
Coarseness of hair	76	73	43
Cardiac enlargement on x-ray	68	—**	—
Pallor of skin	67	50	14
Impaired memory	66	65	31
Constipation	61	54	10
Weight gain	59	76	36
Hair loss	57	41	21
Pallor of lips	57	50	—
Dyspnea	55	72	52
Peripheral edema	55	57	2
Hoarseness	52	74	18
Anorexia	45	40	15
Nervousness	35	51	42
Menorrhagia	32	33	—
Deafness	30	40	15
Palpitations	31	23	20
Poor heart sounds	30	—	—
Precordial pain	25	16	9
Poor vision	24	—	—
Fundus oculi changes	20	—	—
Dysmenorrhea	18	—	—
Weight loss	13	9	23
Atrophic tongue	13	9	—
Emotional instability	11	—	—
Choking sensation	9	—	—
Fineness of hair	9	—	—
Cyanosis	7	—	—
Dysphagia	3	—	—
Brittle nails	—	41	20
Depression	—	60	41
Muscle weakness	—	60	21
Muscle pain	—	36	17
Joint pain	—	29	24
Paresthesias	—	56	15
Heat intolerance	—	2	12
Slow cerebration	—	49	9
Exophthalmos	—	11	4
Sparse eyebrows	—	81	58

*L.J. DeGroot, P.R. Larsen, S. Refetoff, and J.B. Stanbury, *The Thyroid and Its Diseases*, 5th edition. New York, John Wiley & Sons, Inc., 1984.[21,pp.577-578]
**Dash indicates that the symptom or sign was not reported in the study.

PSYCHOLOGICAL STATUS

A patient may move slowly, appear lethargic, and say she is weak and unmotivated. In the absence of laboratory evidence of hypothyroidism, some clinicians are likely to have erroneously ascribed these symptoms to neurasthenia, psychoneurosis, or more recently, a somatoform disorder.

Depression

The patient may say she is despondent without apparent reason. The depressed patient may at first be reluctant to admit having this symptom. Typically though, the patient readily acknowledges depression when I broach the subject by saying something along the lines of: "Many people who have your symptoms are also depressed much of the time. You probably have hypometabolic brain tissues and depression is the main emotional or mood effect of this condition. Also, many fibromyalgia patients get depressed because they have suffered so long, have had little hope of recovery, and their loved ones and doctors have questioned their sincerity about their poor health. Have you felt this way recently?"

It is a smudge on the face of modern clinical practice that some clinicians coldly blame fibromyalgia patients' symptoms on "mental" problems and they recommend psychiatric care. The common result of this is a series of reactions by the patient. First, the patient gets angry at this "accusation." Then, she is tormented with self-doubt. Next, she takes on a defensive posture; and finally, she may resist openly discussing her depression with other clinicians. The iatrogenic defensiveness of these patients would best be remedied by sincere words of understanding and reassurance from clinicians. Otherwise, a favorable treatment outcome may be sabotaged by a lack of rapport between the clinician and patient.

The visual analog scale for depression on the FibroQuest form provides an estimate of the patient's depression. However, the clinician can use either Zung's Self-Rating Depression Scale[46] or Beck's Depression Inventory[47] for more reliable assessment of depression in fibromyalgia patients. These two instruments are easily administered, well-validated, and have acceptable sensitivity and specificity.[48][49] They measure the number and severity of depression symptoms, and researchers have used them extensively in fibromyalgia studies. These measures transmute depression as a symptom into depression as a sign.

Cognitive Dysfunction

Poor memory and concentration are the main cognitive effects of hypometabolism due to hypothyroidism. These two dysfunctions are common in fibromyalgia. The patient who is an accountant or bookkeeper may report that she can no longer hold numbers in her head or do simple mental calculations. A student may report not being able to remember what a professor said long enough to write it down. A patient may make statements such as, "I feel so stupid now— and I really used to be bright."

Comprehensive assessment of cognitive dysfunction requires evaluation by a neuropsychologist. For purposes of case management, however, the visual analog scales on the FibroQuest form provide a measure of the patient's subjective impression of the status of her memory and concentration. As with measures of depression, measures of cognitive dysfunction convert this symptom into a sign.

ALIMENTARY TRACT

The hypometabolic patient's weight may be increased or the same as in the past despite a minimal appetite and reduced food intake. The patient's tongue may be thick and affect her speech. She is likely to be constipated, although she may have diarrhea, or alternate between both.

REPRODUCTIVE SYSTEM

The typical male hypothyroid patient may have a decreased sex drive, although he is potent. The female is likely to be infertile and bleed excessively during her menstrual period. Her periods may also be irregular.[72,p.22]

SLEEP AND FATIGUE

Many hypothyroid patients report that they are sluggish and have a low energy level most of the time. Many also report that upon awakening, they lie in bed half asleep and do not feel they have the will or energy to get up. On the other hand, they may have trouble getting to sleep, and they tend to wake easily at night, often in pain. Only about 5% of hypothyroid patients report insomnia,[24,p.185] although most report disturbed, non-restorative sleep (see Chapter 3.18).

● SIGNS OF HYPOMETABOLISM (THE PHYSICAL EXAMINATION)

Signs indicating tissue hypometabolism are considered peripheral indices when they are measured and quantified against a fixed, quantified standard. The signs I list in this section are not easily quantified and therefore should not be listed under peripheral indices. Nevertheless, the clinician can observe these phenomena as opposed to the subjective experiences patients report.

When a patient's symptoms suggest hypothyroidism, the clinician should examine her for physical signs of the condition. When he finds characteristic signs, this supports the suspicion that the patient has thyroid-related hypometabolism. The clinician should bear in mind, however, that the absence of signs does not rule out hypometabolism.

LISTS OF HYPOTHYROID SIGNS

Like the symptoms of hypothyroidism, the signs listed by different authors vary. Table 4.3.4 lists, for example, the few signs reported by DeGowin and DeGowin.[30,p.860]

Table 4.3.3 contains a more extensive list of signs. Many fibromyalgia patients have several prominent signs characteristic of hypothyroidism. These usually include lethargy, prominent myxedema, drooping eyelids, and eyebrows thinning at their lateral ends. Other patients have only a few signs characteristic of hypothyroidism such as dry and thin skin. Other patients have no obvious signs although they are shown to be hypothyroid by laboratory thyroid function testing.[67] Some signs are so subtle that the clinician is certain of their presence only in retrospect, upon seeing their absence after a positive response to metabolic rehabilitation. An example is the listless appearance of some patients' eyes, replaced after metabolic rehabilitation with a radiant appearance.[53]

SKIN

The hypothyroid patient's skin may be cool, dry, rough, scaly, paper thin, and pale-to-yellowish in col-

or. A patient may complain of dry, rough, itching skin. The ear wax (cerumen) in the external auditory canal may be dry and compacted. The cerumen may interfere with hearing.[72,p.21]

Table 4.3.4. Hypothyroid signs listed by DeGowin & DeGowin.*

Round puffy face	Sluggish movement
Hoarseness	General muscle weakness
Cardiac enlargement	Delayed relaxation of knee
Pericardial effusion	or ankle jerk
Ankle edema	Normal or faint cardiac
Ascites	impulse
Dry, thick, scaling skin	Indistinct heart tones
Dry, coarse, brittle hair	Dry, longitudinally ridged
Bradycardia	nails
Slow speech	Periorbital edema

*R.L. DeGowin and E.L. DeGowin, *Bedside Diagnostic Examination*, 3rd edition. New York, MacMillan Publishing Co., Inc., 1976.[30,p.860]

EDEMA

During the first third of the 20th century, myxedema was the main sign by which clinicians diagnosed hypothyroidism.[9] Myxedema is the non-pitting edema at different skin tissue sites associated with hypothyroidism. The subcutaneous tissues of the myxedematous patient have been described as thick and "juicy."[72,p.21] As the data in Table 4.3.5 show, not all hypothyroid patients are myxedematous. Kimball argued in 1933 that recognition was long overdue that not all hypothyroid patients have myxedema.[104,p.488] A small percentage of the fibromyalgia patients I have examined and treated had myxedema. Some of the patients had primary or central hypothyroidism and some were euthyroid. I have also seen myxedema disappear from patients of all three classifications after they began taking exogenous thyroid hormone.

Myxedema may be most prominent over the forearms,[72,p.21] but I have seen it over the anterior thighs and back of the torso. In advanced cases, the patient's face may show distinct signs such as pale, yellowish, and puffy skin. The tissues around the eyes may be puffy with pouches of fluid beneath the eyes. In many patients, the eyes themselves are dull and lifeless. Eyebrows may be scanty, especially at their outer third. The fat pads just above the clavicle may bulge.

In the past, the edema associated with hypothyroidism was so prominent in some patients that it could be confused with the edema associated with nephrosis. Prankerd wrote in 1972, for example, that nephrosis was among the conditions confused with the swelling and associated symptoms and signs of myxedema.[105,p.52] Generalized myxedema rather than regional or localized myxedema may resemble the edema of nephrosis. Generalized myxedema typically develops in patients with longstanding and severe hypothyroidism[102,p.989] that has not been treated or has been undertreated. Other than this one resemblance—the swelling—the clinical features of nephrosis do not resemble those of hypothyroidism or cellular resistance to thyroid hormone. The trained and experienced clinician can usually distinguish the edema from either of these two thyroid hormone-related conditions from the edema associated with most other conditions.

Table 4.3.5. Percentage of patients in two studies with myxedematous swelling of different tissues, compared with percentages for controls with swelling in one study.*

Symptoms and Signs	Study A % of 77 Cases	Study B % of 100 Cases	Normal Control Subjects
Edema of eyelids	90	86	28
Thick tongue	82	60	17
Edema of face	79	95	27
Peripheral edema	55	57	2
Exophthalmosᵞ	—δ	11	4

*L.J. DeGroot, P.R. Larsen, S. Refetoff, and J.B. Stanbury, *The Thyroid and Its Diseases*, 5th edition. New York, John Wiley & Sons, Inc., 1984.[21,pp.577-578]

ᵞ Probably periorbital edema. (Smith, T.J.: Connective tissue in hypothyroidism. In *Werner's The Thyroid: A Fundamental and Clinical Text*, 6th edition. Edited by L.E. Braverman and R.D. Utiger, Philadelphia, J.B. Lippincott Co., 1991.[102,p.989])

δ—Dash means not reported in the study.

In untreated nephrotic syndrome, the patient loses a massive amount of protein into the urine. This diminishes the colloidal oncotic pressure of the circulation. The hypoalbuminemia that results from the protein loss in turn results in hypovolemia. Due to this, fluid and salt moves into the interstitial tissues and the tissues swell. This form of edema also occurs in other conditions that involve hypoalbuminemia. Examples are severe nutritional deficiency, protein-losing enteropathy, and chronic, severe liver disease.

During generalized edema in patients with these non-thyroid hormone-related conditions, the patient's face is puffy. The periorbital areas are especially puffy. Pressing a finger into the patient's skin causes a persistent indentation called "pitting." The tissue swelling is then termed pitting edema. Pressure during a tender point, trigger point, or spinal palpation exam may leave an indentation. Even lighter pressure, as from the rim of a stethoscope, may transiently indent the tissues.[101,p.179] In addition, the excess fluid in the tissues is said to "resorb" during recumbency; in effect, the fluid tends to submit to gravitational pressure and accordingly redistribute in the tissues.

The edema of myxedema, by contrast, is non-pitting: The edematous tissues do not "pit" upon pressure, and the edema does not rapidly resorb during recumbency.[102,p.989] Myxedematous swelling is underlain by the accumulation of hydrophilic mucopolysaccharides in the ground substance of the dermis and other tissues. The edema is nonpitting because the fluid in the connective tissues is anchored to mucopolysaccharides. As a result of this anchoring, the fluid cannot escape into adjacent interstitial spaces when pressure is applied. With the swelling associated with the binding of fluid by these mucopolysaccharide molecules, facial features are thickened and the skin in various body sites is doughy.[103,p.508] Periorbital swelling is often prominent, as in the edema of nephrosis.

MYOFASCIAL TISSUES

Some hypometabolic patients do not have taut myofascial bands and trigger points. Other hypometabolic patients' myofascial tissues appear to be the tissues primarily affected, and these tissues are riddled with taut bands and trigger points. Some of these latter patients have trigger points in virtually every muscle examined. Palpation is also likely to produce tenderness at most of the 18 fibromyalgia tender point sites, as well as at many other loci. The muscles of the head and neck are often heavily laden with trigger points. In some patients, even light pressure stimulates intense referral of pain or other sensations. Referral patterns may be classic, as described by Travell and Simons.[31][32] But some patients report that their pain is distributed in unusual patterns[8] and covers unusually large body areas. In many hypometabolic patients, trigger points do not submit to treatment techniques that are highly effective with eumetabolic patients. Continuous ultrasound, which is soothing to most patients, can cause referral from trigger points in some fibromyalgia patients even when the instrument is adjusted to low intensity.

The myofascial tissues of some hypometabolic patients are hypertonic, and some of the patients' muscles spasm easily. In contrast, some hypothyroid patients have lost considerable connective tissue tone. This may occur for several reasons. For example, inadequate thyroid hormone regulation of transcription of the growth hormone gene reduces growth hormone production. Also, inadequate thyroid hormone regulation of energy metabolism reduces energy production. In addition, inadequate regulation of dopaminergic neurons by thyroid hormone may reduce motor drive, making it prohibitively difficult for the patient to engage in tissue toning activities (see Chapter 3.4).

HAIR

Hair usually grows poorly in the hypothyroid pa tient. The patient is likely to complain that her hair is falling out, thinning, and becoming unmanageable.[72,p.21] The hair on the patient's head is typically dry and straw-like. The hair becomes oily only if the patient does not wash it for 2 or more days. There may be no surface luster, and each hair may stand distinctly away from others. The patient's pubic hair is usually normal. The hair over the rest of her body, including the arm pits, often has thinned out.[72,p.21]

GASTROINTESTINAL SYSTEM

Due to increased intestinal transit time and constipation, the hypothyroid patient's abdomen may distend. The clinician may be able to palpate masses of hard feces along her colon.[72,p.22]

● PERIPHERAL INDICES OF HYPOMETABOLISM

The clinician can use peripheral indices of metabolism to support his proposition that the patient is hypometabolic. Also, he should at intervals remeasure these indices to determine the impact metabolic therapy is having on the patient's status.

THE INDIRECT NATURE OF PERIPHERAL MEASURES

Barnes criticized the diagnostic strategy of purportedly assessing patients' metabolic status through blood tests. He wrote: "The efforts through the various tests to measure thyroid activity by determining the

amount of hormone stored in the gland or alternatively the amount present in the bloodstream fail to do what really counts: provide an indication of the amount of thyroid hormone available and being used within cells throughout the body. They are somewhat akin to trying to get an idea of a thrifty man's spending habits from the amount of money in his wallet or the size of his bank account. The amounts of money in the wallet or bank account, like tests for the amount of hormone in the gland or bloodstream, tell us nothing about how much is being spent."[71,pp.41-42]

Barnes' view highlights the fact that blood levels of thyroid hormones do not tell us anything about the metabolism of cells of peripheral tissues. Nor do the blood levels tell anything about the state of health or illness imposed by a patient's cellular metabolism. The two measures that come closest to permitting us to assess cell metabolism are the basal metabolic rate (BMR) and the basal body temperature (BBT). Today, it is difficult to find a facility with the necessary equipment and skilled personnel to measure the basal metabolic rate. Some BMR units cost $25,000 or more, and this amount is prohibitive for many clinicians in today's managed care environment. In addition, there are few technicians today skilled at running the BMR. Unfortunately, the basal body temperature does not reliably reflect changes in metabolic rate in some patients.[14]

There are other peripheral measures that can help us assess the metabolic status of our patients. These tests assess anatomical, physiological, and pathological effects of inadequate thyroid hormone regulation of cell function. The measures, however, are not *specific* barometers of the peripheral effects of thyroid hormone. Larsen writes that these tests *may or may not* reflect peripheral effects of thyroid hormone deficiency.[18,p.1072] Factors other than a thyroid deficiency may cause high serum cholesterol, for example, or a low BBT. These tests, nevertheless, *suggest* a patient's metabolic status, and they are useful if monitored regularly in a uniform manner with each patient. When several abnormal peripheral indices are considered together, they provide strong evidence that the patient is hypometabolic. This is especially so when the clinician rules out the influence of other factors that could account for the abnormal results of each peripheral index. When the patient's indices normalize upon repeated measurements during treatment, this indicates a positive response to her metabolic regimen.

The peripheral measures listed below are not exhaustive. With the exception of the BMR, however, they are those most accessible to the clinician.

● PERIPHERAL INDICES
OF METABOLIC STATUS

BASAL METABOLIC RATE

At the end of the last century, the pioneer clinician Magnus-Levy showed that a nurse consumed more oxygen after she ingested thyroid substance as a treatment for obesity. He referred to the oxygen consumption as the basal metabolic rate (BMR). He showed that hypothyroid patients have low BMRs and hyperthyroid patients have high BMRs.[69][70] Clinicians and researchers still use the term BMR today. Some writers suggest that lowering of the BMR is the most reliable deviation from normal in hypothyroidism.[21,p.578]

The normal range of the BMR is reported to be about -15% to +5%.[31,p.145] In patients with complete absence of thyroid function, the BMR may fall to -35% or -45%. The BMR in complete hypothyroidism is remarkably constant, differing less among hypothyroid patients than among normal individuals. The BMR in myxedematous patients usually falls between -35% and -45%, with an average of about -40%.[21,p.579]

Although changes in the BMR are striking in hypothyroidism, the BMR is not a clear-cut marker of hypothyroidism. Other conditions may lower the BMR.[11,p.168] In Addison's disease, the BMR may fall to -25% or -30%. In pituitary gland deficiency, it may decrease to below -50%.[21,p.578]

In 1975, Larsen pointed out that in the previous decade, the popularity of the BMR declined. With less demand, the expertise of technicians decreased, and this led to BMR test results of questionable reliability. This added to the demise of the BMR as a test of thyroid hormone impact on cells.[18,p.1072] The demise is unfortunate because the basal metabolic rate is a measure of *cellular function.* Unlike blood tests of thyroid function, the BMR, by measuring the rate of oxidation in the body's cells, actually assesses cellular function.

BASAL BODY TEMPERATURE

Another measure of cellular function is the basal body temperature (BBT). The first patient with myxedema treated with thyroid extract had a subnormal temperature of 95.6°-to-97.2° Fahrenheit (F). Dr. George Murray reported in 1891 that after he injected her with sheep's thyroid,[68] her temperature rose to 98.2°F.[17] Murray titrated a given preparation in each patient by checking the patient's pulse and temperature. So temperature has been important in the clinical care of hypothyroid patients from the start. More recently, some writers have reported that about 58% of hypothyroid patients tolerate cold poorly.[24,p.185] This shows that the rate of heat-releasing chemical reactions in their cells is relatively slow. But even in hypothyroid patients who feel hot when others about them feel cool, the average BBT is usually low.

Still, this measure of cellular energy-expending processes has never been popular with orthodox clinicians. Barnes was the major promoter of the BBT for assessing the peripheral effects of thyroid hormone.[71,pp.42-48] He performed a study in which 1000 college students used thermometers to determine their BBTs and underwent basal metabolism tests to determine their BMRs. Barnes concluded that the results showed that low body temperature is a better index of hypothyroidism than is the basal metabolic rate.[10]

Barnes promoted the test to the allopathic profession throughout his medical career, though largely without success. He wrote: "This simple technique of measuring basal body temperature as a guide to determining thyroid function and permitting proper treatment when necessary did not appeal to the medical profession. Apparently some physicians had reservations about a test that might permit patients to arrive at their own diagnoses. Perhaps some had reservations because the test involved no fee."[71,p.45]

Whatever may account for the indifference of the medical profession at-large, evidence underlies the tempered attitude of others toward use of the BBT. The renowned thyroidologist Samuel Refetoff, for example, believes the basal temperature is useful only with extreme changes in metabolism. He told me that in some humans whose hypothyroidism is confirmed through other tests, there is no significant change in the basal temperature. And in animals, the basal temperature does not change unless the thyroid gland is totally ablated and the animal is left for a time with no thyroid hormone. Refetoff pointed out that there are many factors that affect the basal body temperature, and he concludes that it is not a good criterion of mild degrees of hypothyroidism.[14]

Schmitz et al. noted that a clinically useful temperature measurement should strongly correlate with measurement of the body's core temperature. They compared peripheral and core temperatures in 13 febrile intensive care patients. Temperatures were taken in rapid sequence from an electronic thermometer for oral and axillary temperature, rectal probe, infrared ear thermometer on "core" setting, and pulmonary artery catheter. The temperatures were taken roughly every hour during the day and every 4 hours through the night. The patients had core temperatures of at least 37.8° Celcius (C) (100°F). Rectal temperatures correlated most strongly with the pulmonary artery blood temperature, and correlations were weaker respectively for oral, ear, and axillary temperatures. For detecting temperatures over 38.3°C (100.94°F), the rectal and ear temperatures were most sensitive. The researchers concluded that the rectal temperature is most sensitive, followed by the oral and then ear temperatures. They wrote that axillary temperatures did not correlate well with pulmonary artery blood temperature. They emphasized consistency of method is important in documenting temperature changes in patients.[125]

Henker and Coyne compared peripheral measures of body temperature with core temperature. They used nine methods at four sites to measure peripheral temperatures: (1) in the ear using two infrared thermometers, (2) in the mouth using a mercury in glass thermometer, electronic thermometer, and chemical indicator thermometer, (3) in the axilla using a mercury in glass thermometer, electronic thermometer, and chemical indicator thermometer, and (4) in the rectum using a mercury in glass thermometer and electronic thermometer. They found the differences between most peripheral temperatures and the core temperature were statistically significant. The only exception was the axillary chemical indicator temperature and both aural temperatures. The pulmonary artery temperatures correlated strongly with oral mercury, oral electronic, axillary electronic, rectal mercury, and rectal electronic temperatures (Pearson correlation coefficients of ≥ 0.79). The correlation between the pulmonary artery and aural temperatures was weak (correlation coefficients were < 0.20). Henker and Coyne wrote that the results showed that there is "no perfect instrument for approximating core temperature." Nonetheless, the correlation between measures of peripheral temperatures and the core temperature was strong. For example, the electronic thermometer used orally, compared to the pulmonary artery blood temperature, had a low mean difference of 0.18°C (0.32°F), a low standard deviation of the difference of 0.24°C (0.43°F), and a correlation coefficient of 0.79.[124] Thus, the lack of perfection in estimating the core temperature from peripheral temperature measures does not appear to be of practical importance in outpatient care.

Erickson and Kirklin studied the differences between ear, bladder, oral, and axillary temperature, and core body temperatures. The 38 critical care adult patients in the study had indwelling pulmonary artery thermistor catheters. Ear temperatures were taken with an infrared thermometer. Pulmonary artery, bladder, oral, and axillary temperatures were taken with thermistor-based instruments. Temperatures were taken every 20 minutes for 4 hours. The mean differences between the pulmonary artery temperature and the other temperatures were as follows: ear, 0.07°C (0.13°F); bladder, 0.03°C (0.05°F); oral, 0.05°C (0.09°F); and axillary, -0.68°C (-1.22°F). The researchers concluded that infrared ear thermometry provided a relatively close estimate of pulmonary artery core temperature. The ear method, however, was more variable than bladder or oral methods. Axillary readings were substantially lower than the pulmonary artery temperature and were highly variable.[34]

Fulbrook's conclusions provide some balance to those of other researchers. In his study, simultaneous recordings of pulmonary artery blood temperature and rectal and axillary temperatures of intensive care patients were taken every 4 hours for up to 7 days. Fulbrook reported that the mean difference in the rectal and axillary temperature was 0.32°C (0.58°F). The difference between the pulmonary artery blood and axillary temperatures was 0.19°C (0.34°F). The temperatures of the pulmonary artery blood, rectum, and axilla strongly correlated. Fulbrook wrote that the axilla is a highly accurate site for estimation of core body temperature. The axillary temperature was an accurate estimate of the core temperature regardless of the patient's age, number of samples taken, gender, and post and non-operative admissions to the intensive care unit. The author wrote that the axillary temperature is an accurate enough estimate under a variety of conditions that taking the temperature by mouth or rectum is not necessary."[123]

Hazama et al. investigated causative factors in senile dementia patients with low body temperatures (hypothermia). The mean age of the patients was 80.6 years. The researchers compared patients with a mean axillary temperature below 36°C (96.8°F) with those whose axillary temperature was higher. The group of patients whose mean temperature was lower than 36°C (96.8°F) had significantly higher serum total cholesterol, triglycerides, albumen, hemoglobin, and body weight than those with higher temperatures. More patients in the lower temperature group had diabetes mellitus and used major tranquilizers. Interestingly, the levels of the free T_3 and free T_4 did not differ between the two groups.[122] Barnes wrote that axillary temperatures below 97.8°F (36.55°C) indicate hypothyroidism, and those above 98.2°F (36.8°C) indicate hyperthyroidism.[71,p.46] If we can assume that the free T_3 and free T_4 levels were considered normal in the two groups, we must judge that the low body temperatures were caused by mechanisms not related to the sufficiency of circulating thyroid hormone. One possible mechanism is tissue resistance to thyroid hormone. Others are deconditioning in the elderly people, diabetes in some, and the use of tranquilizers in others. All of these are known to impede metabolism.

Based on the studies I site above, axillary temperature may vary more than temperatures of some other peripheral body sites. Also, it may not correlate as strongly with core temperature as the temperatures at some other body sites. However, there is only a small magnitude of difference between the axillary temperature, temperatures at other body sites, and core temperature. Results of the available studies do not disqualify the axillary temperature as a potentially useful tool in the outpatient setting, at least for some patients. If the BBT is responsive to thyroid hormone in a particular patient, the patient uses a consistent method to obtain the temperature, and the measures are posted to a line graph, the BBT can serve as a useful peripheral index. As with other peripheral indices, such as the Achilles reflex speed, the BBT should be only one of several peripheral indices used.

My clinical experiences cause me to doubt the usefulness of the BBT as the sole measure of cellular responsiveness to thyroid hormone. For example, I have had patients with subnormal BBTs who improved in every respect during metabolic rehabilitation without increases in their BBTs: their symptoms and signs were relieved, other abnormal peripheral indices of tissue metabolic status normalized, and the patients subjectively considered themselves well. But their BBTs changed little or none at all. These clinical experiences, and my personal experience with the BBT, compel me to agree with Refetoff. For all practical purposes, clinicians do not have ready access to the BMR. Because of this, I regret the failure of the BBT in some patients to reliably reflect changes in the metabolic status of tissues. Combined with other measures, however, the BBT is a useful indicator of metabolic change for *some* patients. Because of this, I include the information below on the BBT.

The False Proposition that Clinical Improvement with Use of T_3 Results from Increased Enzyme Activity Due to Increases in Temperature

Wilson proposed that various symptoms result from body temperature that is too low for body enzymes to function normally. Having usurped the name Wilson's syndrome (used for many years for another condition), he wrote, "The symptoms of Wilson's Syndrome are preeminently and foremost symptoms of Multiple Enzyme Dysfunction (MED) that are caused by aberrations in body temperature patterns."[92,p.17]

Wilson used this hypothetical mechanism to explain his clinical observations that a wide array of symptoms improve in many patients who use T_3. The available scientific evidence indicates that their improvement is mediated by quite another mechanism from temperature regulation by the T_3, and that his hypothetical explanation is based on misquotes and inaccurate interpretations of the available scientific data.

Wilson's line of thought is this: Enzymes are "at the very heart" of metabolism. How enzymes function depends upon their structure. They can change shape under various conditions, and this ability to change in typical ways is the basis of their function. Wilson specifically wrote, "The shape of an enzyme also depends on its temperature. When enzymes get too warm, they get too loose. And when they get too cold, then they get too tight. When they are just the right temperature, then they are just the right shape and the chemical reactions that they catalyze take place at the optimal rate and with the most ease. When the temperature is too hot, too cold, or unsteady, the enzymes will spend less time in their optimal shape which simply translates into having a less than optimal metabolism."[92,p.12]

Here, Wilson has not reported accurately how temperature affects enzymes. Over the range of 32°F to about 104°F (0°C-to-40°C), enzyme activity increases in a manner similar to that of all chemical reactions: the reaction rate roughly doubles with each 18°F (10°C) rise in temperature. The structure of enzymes, however, does not change under the influence of temperatures within this range. Their shape does change at temperatures above 104°F (40°C). At such temperatures, the kinetic motions of the amino acids and side groups that form the enzyme molecule increase. Also, the frequency and strength of collisions of the enzyme with surrounding molecules increase. As the collisions become violent enough, the hydrogen bonds of an enzyme break and the enzyme unfolds. The decrease in enzyme activity becomes extreme at 131°F (55°C), and enzyme activity decreases to zero only at 140°F (60°C).[93,p.96] So Wilson's explanation that changes in temperature within the human body alter the structure of enzymes is a stretch. Such changes only begin to occur above temperatures considered abnormally high for humans. Wilson himself notes that such temperatures produce headache, achiness, fatigue, and flu-like symptoms.[92,p.17] Substantial changes in the shape of enzymes occur only at temperatures that most humans could not survive.

Wilson also wrote, "And it just so happens that most of the important bodily enzymes function best at or near 98.6°F."[92,p.15] Wolfe pointed out that all enzymes have an optimal temperature. At the optimal temperature, there is maximum kinetic motion but no significant denaturing of the enzyme. For most enzymes, the optimum temperature lies between 104°F and 122°F (40°C-to-50°C).[93,p.96] The 98.6°F specified by Wilson does not fall within this range, yet he argues that this is the temperature at which enzymes function best.[92,p.13]

Wilson's stated clinical objective is to adjust the dosage of T_3 so that the body temperature increases to what he considers normal.[92,p.302] Purportedly, the increased temperature normalizes enzyme function and thereby relieves symptoms.[92,p.15] However, with the use of exogenous thyroid hormone, both enzyme activity and body temperature increase because the hormone alters gene transcription patterns. Thyroid hormone increases transcription of the protein constituents of many enzymes. It is the catalytic activities of these enzymes and the cleaving of the high-energy phosphate bonds of ATP to fuel the catalytic activities that secondarily increase body heat. In other words, the reverse of Wilson's argument is true: Thyroid hormone increases enzyme levels and activity, and the increased enzyme activity increases body heat.

The enzyme probably most responsible for increasing body heat is Na^+/K^+-ATPase. This enzyme uses cytoplasmic ATP and catalyzes activity of the Na^+/K^+ pump. The pump is one of the main energy-users of the cell. It accounts for 5%-to-40% of steady-state energy expenditure.[94] Heat is released as a by-product of the enzymatic activity. Thyroid hormone regulates genetic expression of this enzyme.[95] As more of the enzyme is synthesized under the influence of exogenous thyroid hormone, enzymatic activity increases, and body temperature rises as a result of the enzymatic activity. In addition, Na^+/K^+-ATPase has sweeping effects on cellular function, and some relief of symptoms of inadequate thyroid hormone regulation of gene transcription is mediated by a return to normal levels of this enzyme with thyroid hormone use. These symptoms do not remit because of a rise in body temperature, as Wilson has argued, but because of the increased Na^+/K^+-ATPase activity. Increased temperature is a product—not a cause—of the activity of the

enzyme. Thus, Wilson is wrong in stating that the resulting rise in body temperature increases activity of the enzyme; the reverse is true.

Thyroid hormone also regulates levels of another enzyme, α-glycerophosphate dehydrogenase, that contributes to control of body temperature (see Chapter 2.2). Most of the heat-producing effect from thyroid hormone action has been attributed to the combination of increased α-glycerophosphate dehydrogenase and Na^+/K^+-ATPase.[96,p.207] Again for the sake of emphasis, both these enzymes are decreased by low thyroid hormone levels and increased by high thyroid hormone levels. Body heat rises *secondarily* to the thyroid hormone-induced production of these enzymes.

Moreover, inadequate thyroid hormone regulation of gene transcription increases the production of three inhibitory molecules: α-adrenergic receptors, phosphodiesterase, and inhibitory G_i proteins. It is these molecules that account for virtually all the hypothyroid-like symptoms and signs of inadequate thyroid hormone regulation of transcription. These molecules slow cellular metabolism and secondarily contribute to a reduction in body temperature. Low body temperature, like the symptoms and other signs of too little thyroid hormone regulation of gene transcription, is a *consequence* of the action of these inhibitory molecules. And what improves symptoms and signs, including low body temperature, is providing sufficient exogenous thyroid hormone to properly regulate gene transcription. When the patient takes enough exogenous thyroid hormone, production of the inhibitory molecules decreases. As a result, cell metabolism increases and body temperature rises (see Chapter 2.2).

Wilson's proposed mechanism is, for practical purposes, a reiteration of a conjecture by Rene′ Descartes (published in 1637 in his *Discourse on Method*) that heat is the cause rather than the result of bodily motion.[114,p.xi] It is partly because of this mistaken idea that Lafleur judged Descartes' writings on physiology to be the least important of Descartes' scientific works, even though his descriptions of anatomy were accurate.[114,p.xi]

Clinically, the important matter to consider is that using body temperature to adjust thyroid hormone dosage is to use a gauge that for too many people is not snugly correlated with the desirable changes in tissue metabolic status. Some patients recover from fibromyalgia symptoms and signs with little if any change in body temperature despite taking supraphysiologic dosages of thyroid hormone. In these patients, it appears that thyroid hormone regulation of gene transcription increases the levels and activity of neurotransmitters, hormones, and enzymes other than those principally involved in heat generation. And it is these biochemical products of thyroid hormone regulation of gene transcription that improve the patient's status—all without the increases in body temperature that Wilson argues is the indispensable prerequisite to patient improvement.

Sympathetic Nervous System and Thermogenesis

One might argue that a patient in chronic pain, such as a fibromyalgia patient, develops a low body temperature because her sympathetic nervous system habituates and vegetative signs become prominent.[76][77,p.19] According to this argument, the patient may develop both a low BMR and a low BBT as a result of chronic pain. If by "sympathetic nervous system habituation" we mean reduced central nervous system activation of the sympathetic nervous system with a corresponding reduction in catecholamine secretion, then the habituation is certainly likely to reduce the rise in metabolic rate and body temperature *during stress*. However, as I explain below, the chronic pain patient's *basal* metabolic rate and *basal* body temperature are not likely to decrease solely because of habituation of her sympathetic nervous system.

Thyroid hormone interacts with the sympathetic nervous system to maintain metabolically-generated body heat.[74][75] To simplify somewhat, each of these two regulators (thyroid hormone and the sympathetic nervous system) of the metabolic rate and body temperature predominates under different conditions. The role of thyroid hormone is mainly to control the metabolic rate, and thus the body temperature, under basal (non-stressful, resting) conditions. The sympathetic system, on the other hand, adjusts heat production above basal rates in response to altered conditions (adaptation challenges). Examples of such conditions are environmental temperature changes, food intake,[75] emotional arousal, and intense physical activity.

If thyroid hormone regulation of the adrenergic genes is adequate, the chronic pain patient will have a normal ratio of β- to α-adrenergic receptors on cell membranes. Despite this normal ratio, if her sympathetic nervous system is habituated, her sympathetic neurons will secrete a subnormal amount of catecholamines during stress. As a result, the increase in her metabolic rate and body temperature *during stress* will also be subnormal. Under resting conditions, however, she will most likely continue to secrete her small basal quantity of catecholamines. Because thyroid hormone regulation of her adrenergic genes is normal, even this

small amount of catecholamines will bind at cell membranes to enough β-adrenergic receptors to continue her BMR apace, and in turn, her BBT will remain normal.

There is an exception to the above scenario. We would not expect the chronic pain patient's BMR and BBT to decrease *unless* her impaired ability to adapt to stress (due to sympathetic nervous system habituation) had markedly reduced her physical activity level and in turn her lean muscle mass. The reduction in the BBT in this case would result from her reduced physical activity level, not from sympathetic nervous system habituation (see Chapter 5.5, subsection titled "Resistance Training").

If thyroid hormone regulation of the adrenergic genes is inadequate, as in the hypothyroid patient, the individual is also likely to have impaired sympathetic nervous system responsiveness during stress. In this case, however, the impaired responsiveness occurs not because of sympathetic nervous system habituation; it occurs because the patient has too little thyroid hormone to adequately regulate the adrenergic receptor genes. The inadequate regulation results in a decrease in β-adrenergic receptors and an increase in α-adrenergic receptors on cell membranes. The normal increased quantity of catecholamines secreted during stress binds to the α-adrenergic receptors that are increased in density on cell membranes. This catecholamine/α-adrenergic receptor combination inhibits the adaptive cellular metabolic changes that would occur during stress if the cell membranes contained a normal density of β-adrenergic receptors. The inhibition of these adaptive metabolic changes prevents a sympathetic/catecholamine-driven increase in metabolic rate and body temperature. (Incidentally, interaction of increased catecholamines secreted during stress with a high density of α-adrenergic receptors on cell membranes tends to result in a metabolic crisis with related symptoms. This may be the basis of the worsening of fibromyalgia symptoms after the patient exercises at a level that increases catecholamine secretion. See Chapter 3.4, subsection titled "Increased Exercise Tolerance Due to a Thyroid Hormone-Induced Shift from α-Adrenergic Dominance.")

To summarize: Though a patient's impaired sympathetic nervous system may prevent a proper increase in body temperature under stressful conditions, if she has normal thyroid hormone regulation of adrenergic gene transcription, her *basal* metabolic rate and *basal* body temperature are not likely to be affected under normal resting conditions. With normal thyroid hormone regulation of her adrenergic genes, she will have a normal ratio of β- to α-adrenergic receptors on cell membranes. As long she has a normal ratio, the interaction of normal basal amounts of adrenaline and noradrenaline with the β-adrenergic receptors generated by normal thyroid hormone genomic activity is likely to maintain her BBT.

What is Normal Body Temperature?

Attempts to determine the "normal" body temperature have failed. One reason is the difficulty in correlating body temperature with the presence of disease processes. To help understand this, refer to Table 4.3.6., which lists the mean and range of body temperatures in "normal" subjects reported by early investigators.

Consider Ivy's study (last one in Table 4.3.6.). He took the oral temperatures of 276 medical students seated in class between 8 am and 9 am. He wrote that

Table 4.3.6. Temperature readings in "normal" subjects.*

	RESEARCHER(S) MEAN AND LOWER-TO-UPPER TEMPERATURES	
Investigator(s)*	Mean in °F	Range in °F
1. Wunderlich[78]	Average for well-closed axilla, same as oral: 98.6	"Really normal temperatures," axillary: 97.9-to-99.3 "Subfebrile temperature," axillary: 99.5-to-100.4 "Always very suspicious" when beyond, axillary: 97.7-to-99.5
2. Pembrey & Nicol[79]	343 recordings on Nicol, rectal: 98.7	96.8-to-100.6
3. Benedict & Carpenter[80]	8 men with food, 24 hrs, rectal: 98.3 4 men with no food, 24 hrs, rectal: 97.9 4 men, 72 days, 528 readings, 7 am-to-11 pm, oral: 98.1 46 men, 84 days, 252 readings 7 am-to-6 pm, oral: 98.3 "Well within range of physiological limits, lying quietly," rectal: 98.6	96.3-to-100.2 95.9-to-99.9 96.6-to-100.6
4. DuBois[81]	Men and women, 11 am-to-2 pm, in calorimeter, rectal: 98.5	97.2-to-99.7
5. Reimann[82]	Normal adults, oral: 98.6	97.0-to-100.2
6. Ivy[83]	276 medical students, 8 am-9 am, oral: 98.1	96.4-to-99.3

*After E.F. DuBois, *Fever and the Regulation of Body Temperature*. Springfield, Charles C. Thomas, 1948.[84,p.6]

95% of the students had temperatures that ranged between 97.3°F and 98.9°F.[83] About these temperatures, DuBois wrote: "Those whose temperatures fell toward the outward limits of this range could be considered normal but slightly suspicious. But even if an individual's temperature fell slightly outside the range, one could not categorically call the temperature abnormal."[84,p.5]

For a body temperature to be "abnormal" implies that it is somehow associated with pathophysiology.

To decide whether a particular low temperature or range of temperatures is abnormal in this respect, it must be established that a temperature or range of temperatures correlates significantly with a particular abnormal condition of health. Unfortunately, studies attempting to establish the "normal" range of temperatures have been confused by failure to show that the subjects were truly healthy. The medical students in Ivy's study may or may not have been healthy. The problem is in the definition of "healthy." If we define healthy as the absence of overt disease, they were healthy. If we define healthy as the absence of covert pathophysiological processes that would insidiously increase in magnitude to overt disease, then some of the students may not have been healthy. This line of thinking raises doubt that the temperatures reported in Table 4.3.6. were "normal." Insidious pathology and even physiological processes going awry may have accompanied the lower temperatures of some of the students. Later, the pathology or askew physiological processes may have seriously sabotaged the quality of the individuals' lives or even led to their deaths. As an example, the fat-metabolizing mechanisms of some students with low temperatures (if due to low metabolic rates) may have been impaired. This may have resulted in excess fat retention, atherosclerosis, and eventual death from heart attacks or strokes. Others with lower temperatures may have also had insufficient muscle energy metabolism, resulting in myofascial trigger point pain. In others, impaired central nervous system mechanisms may have led to general lowering of the pain threshold, resulting in diffuse aches and pains. Travell and Simons write about such myofascial effects of low body temperature: "We find that susceptibility of the muscles to TrPs is consistently increased when the mean basal temperature is as low as 36.1°C (97.0°F) or lower."[31,p.146] However, Ivy and his students may have dismissed the somatic symptoms as usual and ordinary and of no clinical significance.[85,pp.63-65] Some achy students may have avoided physical activities because of their discomfort; they may have eventually developed diseases associated with hypokinesis. Some may have suffered the long-range adverse effects of analgesic use such as GI ulceration[6] or nephrosis.[7]

My observations about Ivy's students are, of course, entirely conjectural. But the important point is that *slow metabolism* (possibly reflected in a low body temperature), *after exceeding some threshold, is likely to have deleterious effects on various body tissues.* Exactly what temperature indicates possibly harmful hypometabolism, however, remains to be determined. Barnes reported that normal values for the axillary temperature are 97.8°F-to-98.2°F. In general, this range can serve as a practical guide for patients who wish to control their BBTs. Barnes wrote that a temperature below 97.8°F indicates hypothyroidism, and that one above 98.2°F indicates hyperthyroidism.[71,p.46] I must emphasize, however, that in my clinical experience, for many patients the basal body temperature is *not* a reliable peripheral index of tissue metabolic status. For some patients, it is useful. For those patients for whom it is useful, I recommend that the temperature be used in combination with other peripheral indices.

Rectal, Oral, or Axillary Temperature

The axillary temperature may be a more reliable barometer of changing metabolic status than the rectal or oral temperatures. Oral temperature rises readily, and it may fluctuate when the patient has sinusitis or a subclinical infection of the mouth or throat.[71,p.45] As the metabolic rate increases during thyroid hormone therapy, cardiac output increases and more blood flows through the skin.[86][87,p.819] This increased cutaneous blood flow and increased heat production in cells increases the skin's warmth. The rectal temperature, however, does not increase as much as skin temperature. In studies by Stewart and Evans, when the oral intake of thyroid hormone increased metabolism to normal, skin temperature increased an average of 0.82°C (1.48°F). Rectal temperature, however, increased only 0.02°C[87,p.819] (0.036°F). If a patient takes her rectal temperature, she should inform her clinician of this. The rectal temperature averages 1°F-to-2°F higher than the oral and axillary temperatures.[84,p.5] Many patients' oral temperatures are roughly 1°F higher than their axillary temperatures.

Proper Procedure for Taking the Basal Temperature

The patient should shake the mercury in the thermometer all the way down into the bulb before going to sleep. She should put it on a nightstand where she can reach it easily from the bed. Upon waking after a restful sleep, she should stay in bed motionless except to put the thermometer deep into an armpit. She should leave it there for at least 10 minutes by the clock. During the 10-minute period, she must remain as still as possible. She may read, but to avoid raising her temperature, the subject matter should not arouse her physically or emotionally. For an accurate reading, the temperature of the room must be comfortable; cold air can markedly decrease the temperature of the skin.[84,p.7]

Fluctuations in Women's Temperatures

Men may take their temperatures on any day. Before menarche and after menopause, females may take their temperature on any day.[10][71,pp.47-48] Women of childbearing age, however, have temperature fluctuations that should not be included in their averages. A woman's temperature increases by about 0.5°F after ovulation due to secretion of progesterone by the corpus luteum. The increase in temperature occurs abruptly at ovulation.[106,p.913] Barnes wrote that in most cases the temperature is highest shortly before the start of the menstrual flow and lowest at the time of ovulation. He wrote that during a woman's menstrual years, her temperature is best taken on the 2nd and 3rd days of the period after the flow starts.[10][71,pp.47-48] At this time, the temperature will have come back down from the 0.5°F increase.[106,p.913]

CHOLESTEROL, TRIGLYCERIDES, AND LOW-DENSITY LIPOPROTEINS

Serum cholesterol is elevated in most hypothyroid patients.[16][36][37][38][39] The elevation is mainly due to an increased low density lipoprotein (LDL) fraction of cholesterol. Some authors recommend screening for subclinical hypothyroidism because it is a cause of elevated serum cholesterol.[45][107] Subclinical hypothyroidism is associated not only with high LDL cholesterol and low high density lipoprotein cholesterol (HDL), but also high lipoprotein(a) levels.[108] Vanderpump et al. conducted a 20-year follow-up study of ischemic heart disease and autoimmune thyroid disease in an English community. They concluded that among people with increased total plasma cholesterol, subclinical hypothyroidism was 2-to-3 times more common. Total cholesterol was 0%-to-30% above normal in subclinical hypothyroid patients. There was a small increase in the risk for cardiovascular disease among these patients. T_4 "replacement" had only a modest cholesterol lowering effect.[109] Some people will argue from this latter finding that T_4 is not particularly effective in lowering cholesterol associated with subclinical hypothyroidism. But it should be noted that it was T_4 "replacement" dosages that were not especially effective. I argue in this book that with most patients, replacement dosages are inadequate for relieving the symptoms, signs, and peripheral indices of inadequate thyroid hormone regulation of cell function. I have found in extensive clinical experience that non-thyrotoxic dosages of thyroid hormone that are larger than "replacement" dosages are highly effective in lowering cholesterol, triglycerides, and phospholipids. (See Chapter 4.4, section titled "Heart.")

Cholesterol, triglycerides, and phospholipids increase in hypothyroid patients because they break down at a slower rate than they form.[23][25][26] Decreased receptor-mediated catabolism of LDL cholesterol[40] and decreased biliary excretion and hepatic clearance of cholesterol[41] may be the mechanisms of the cholesterol elevation in hypothyroid patients.[42,p.488]

In the U.S.A., 25% of the adult population have elevated serum cholesterol.[35] By contrast, Watanakunakorn reported that more than 89% of myxedematous patients have hypercholesterolemia above 250 mg/dL.[24] Studies suggest that long-standing hypothyroidism is a risk factor for coronary artery disease and myocardial infarction.[13,p.239] For many years, clinicians considered the measure of cholesterol a valuable test for confirming hypothyroidism. The normal range is broad, however, and many other factors cause cholesterol to elevate. Thus, the test is not specifically diagnostic of hypothyroidism. It is proper to state that an elevated cholesterol,[22,p.417] triglycerides,[23] or LDL[21,p.579] is indicative of but not diagnostic of deficient thyroid hormone regulation of fat-metabolizing mechanisms. Diet can markedly compound the cholesterol- and triglyceride-elevating effects of thyroid hormone deficiency in myxedematous patients.[73] Serum triglycerides are less reliable than cholesterol as an indicator of hypothyroidism.

In hypothyroidism, cholesterol, triglyceride, and phospholipid levels promptly decrease into their normal ranges when the patient begins T_3 or T_4 therapy.[27][43][44] In my clinical experience, elevated cholesterol decreases into the normal range in virtually every fibromyalgia patient who undergoes treatment with thyroid hormone, whether the patient is hypothyroid or euthyroid before treatment.

WEIGHT GAIN

Most hypothyroid patients report difficulty in reducing excess weight. Contrary to popular belief, however, hypothyroid patients are not usually obese. About 2⁄3 of patients report weight gain. The gain is modest, however, and results more from fluid retention than from fat accumulation.[21,p.565] There is some fat retention, however. The carcasses of hypothyroid animals have relatively more fat than those of normal animals.[28] Fat retention persists even when the patient sticks to an austere, low-fat diet and exercises vigorously each day. The fat-retaining tendency shows an unbalanced metabolic ledger, with lipid synthesis in excess of lipid degradation.[29]

URINARY CORTISOL METABOLITES

Measurement of the ratio of two urinary cortisol metabolites, tetrahydrocortisone (THE) and tetrahydrocortisol (THF), appears to be a marker of thyroid hormone action in the suprarenal tissues. Taniyama, Honma, and Ban found that the THE/THF ratio was increased in hyperthyroidism (4.58±1.49) and decreased in hypothyroidism (1.31±0.55) compared to controls (1.93±0.35). They found a good correlation between the THE/THF ratio and serum thyroid hormone levels, especially in hypothyroidism. They concluded that the THE/THF ratio is a good biochemical indicator of deficient peripheral thyroid hormone action.[110]

These researchers also found that in patients with general thyroid hormone resistance, the THE/THF ratio was low despite the patients' elevated thyroid hormone levels. This finding indicates resistance of the adrenal cortices to normal and elevated thyroid hormone levels. The researchers concluded that the ratio of these cortisol metabolites is a good marker for peripheral thyroid hormone resistance. The ratio may be found to be low in patients suspected of having peripheral resistance to thyroid hormone. The test can be used to determine whether there is deficient thyroid hormone action at the tissue level even though the patient has normal thyroid function test results.

SERUM CAROTENE

Carotene is a class of yellow-red pigments called carotenoids. Carotenoids are widely distributed in plants and animals, particularly in carrots. They include precursors of vitamin A and are called provitamin A carotenoids.

The serum carotene level is elevated in some hypothyroid patients, especially those with long-term hypothyroidism.[117,p.986] The elevation appears to result from reduced intestinal conversion of carotene to vitamin A.[115] The reduced conversion results in hypercarotenemia.[116] Resulting elevations in the serum and tissue concentrations of carotene cause the patient's skin to have a yellowish tint. The tint is especially prominent in the skin of the palms, soles, and nasolabial folds.[117,p.986] The discolored skin may look sallow and may amplify the paleness of other skin regions if the patient is also anemic.[120,p.1072] The reduced visual adaptation to dark of some hypothyroid patients may be a result of diminished carotene conversion to vitamin A, resulting in low vitamin A levels.[119][121]

An Indicator of Elevated Lipoproteins
One of the most ominous results of untreated or undertreated hypothyroidism is increased levels of lipoproteins (see section above titled "Cholesterol, Triglycerides, and Low-Density Lipoproteins"). Lipoproteins are the sole transport compounds for carotene and lycopene.[118] (Lycopene is Ψ,Ψ-carotene, the red pigment of the tomato. It is considered the parent compound from which all natural carotenoid pigments are derived. Its chemical structure is similar to carotene.) When excess carotene is available in the blood, it binds to circulating lipoproteins. If the lipoprotein concentration is elevated, then the serum carotene level will also be elevated. Thus, an elevated serum carotene level is an indication that the patient's lipoprotein levels are elevated. "Replacement" dosages of thyroid hormone (dosages that keep the TSH within the normal range) are in many cases inadequate to reduce lipoproteins into the normal range. Thus, an elevated serum carotene level may indicate that the treated hypothyroid patient's thyroid hormone dosage is too low.

SERUM ENZYMES

The patient with primary hypothyroidism may have an elevated serum CPK and LDH. About 50% have high SGOT levels.[15] Aldolase levels may also be high.[1] Levels usually decrease to normal with treatment.[21,p.581]

ACHILLES REFLEX TIME

A slow relaxation phase of reflexes, especially the Achilles reflex, has long been considered a sign of hypothyroidism.[42,p.487] The Achilles reflex can be used in most patients to assess the metabolic effect of thyroid hormone on skeletal muscle.[88][89] About 75% of hypothyroid patients have slowed reflexes.[42,p.487] Soloman wrote that the most characteristic physical sign of hypothyroidism is a sluggish relaxation phase of the tendon reflexes.[72] Muscle studies have shown that the contraction phase is also delayed,[56][57] but clinically, a slow contraction phase usually is not as obvious as a slow relaxation phase. The amplitude of the reflex may be normal, increased, or decreased.[72,p.22]

I am aware of no studies (except mine) in which the speed of the Achilles reflex of fibromyalgia patients has been measured. However, in one study Elert et al. looked for differences in surface electromyography readings in fibromyalgia patients, myofascial pain syndrome patients, and healthy controls while they performed 100 repetitive shoulder flexions. There were no differences in mechanical performance or muscle composition. However, all fibromyalgia patients were unable to relax their muscles between contractions. The failure to relax muscles did not occur in healthy subjects. In myofascial pain syndrome patients, only myalgic muscles failed to relax between contractions.[99] Bennett commented that the inability of fibromyalgia patients' muscles to relax between contractions may indicate an important mechanism for the problem patients have in sustaining repetitive muscle contractions.[100,p.149] The finding certainly seems relevant to the slowed relaxation phase of the Achilles reflex found in the majority of hypothyroid and fibromyalgia patients. The failure of fibromyalgic muscles to relax between repetitive contractions (as occurs during reflex testing) suggests that, as in hypothyroidism, the muscles have low levels of ATP and Ca^{++}-ATPase—both of which are controlled by thyroid hormone (see Chapter 2.2).

There are limitations to the use of slowed reflexes as a peripheral index. First, reflex time is altered in a number of diseases not related to thyroid hormone. Among the diseases are protein-calorie malnutrition, anorexia nervosa, peripheral vascular disease, peripheral edema, diabetes mellitus, hypothermia,[42,p.487] and pernicious anemia.[16,p.530] Any of these could occur concomitantly with thyroid hormone abnormalities.[58]

Another limitation to the use of reflexes as a peripheral index is that normal values vary broadly. The relaxation half-time ranges from 240 ms-to-320 ms.[42,p.487] The time can be precisely measured with instruments such as the photomotograph.[59] Using a measure called Achilles Reflex Time (ART), Prange and his associates found that the Achilles reflex was toward the slow side in depressed patients. The investigators measured ART with a device that translates the reflex motion of the foot (caused by tapping the Achilles tendon) from mechanical energy to a recording on standard ECG paper. The clinician can analyze the tracings this creates.[19] Several drugs can influence ART,[20] but their effects are weak compared to the effect of changes in thyroid gland status. In the absence of neurological disease, slower than normal ART strongly suggests hypothyroidism. The depressed subjects in Prange's study had slow ART. For patients who took a thyroid supplement combined with the antidepressant imipramine, the speed increased.[19]

For the clinician experienced in the use of the Achilles reflex test, however, use of a device for measuring speed is not necessary. Sonkin uses the Achilles reflex without use of a measuring device. He wrote, "Among useful parameters were, first of all, the very clear-cut physical finding of a delayed ankle reflex,

which did not require any specialized equipment other than a neurological hammer for its demonstration."[1,p.165]

The clinician should, of course, record in his progress notes at each examination whether the relaxation phase of the reflex was slow, normal, or fast compared to the contraction phase. Little experience is needed to learn to differentiate a normal from an abnormal reflex in most fibromyalgia patients. The change from a slow reflex to a normal one after the patient begins using thyroid hormone is pronounced and obvious. The change in the speed of the relaxation phase is seldom equivocal.

The best sites for detecting a delayed recoil are the biceps and the Achilles tendons. From the finger pressing into the biceps tendon, the clinician may perceive the slowed relaxation phase even when he cannot see it. He should check both arms.[72,p.23] It is best to test the Achilles reflex with the patient kneeling on a chair, facing its back, with the ankles and feet hanging over the front of the seat. Some patients have trouble relaxing the muscles that control the ankle when sitting with the leg forward, heel touching the floor, and the examiner lightly dorsiflexing the foot to stretch the Achilles tendon. It is often easier to elicit the reflex by tapping the tendon when the foot is flat on the floor under the front edge of the chair so that the Achilles tendon is stretched slightly.

Before the patient begins using thyroid hormone, the reflex may be abnormal in a variety of ways. Most often, after a normal rapid contraction, the relaxation phase occurs slowly. Movement may be slow at the start of the relaxation phase, then begin a rapid return to the resting position, but pause briefly midway. Or the foot may briefly stop moving at the end of the contraction, jerk 1 or 2 times, and then return to the resting position at a rate somewhat slower than the contraction phase. Such movements contrast starkly with the brisk, virtually equal contraction and relaxation phases in patients whose calf muscle cell function is normally regulated by thyroid hormone.

I have found that most fibromyalgia patients' Achilles reflex is either slow or it stalls after the contraction phase before the relaxation phase commences. The reflex becomes normal in practically all patients early during their treatment with metabolic rehabilitation involving exogenous thyroid hormone.

Some authors such as Costin maintain that because Achilles reflex measurements correlate poorly with biochemical measures of thyroid function, it has limited use.[65] I retort, however, that the lack of correlation is evidence that thyroid function laboratory tests are poorly correlated with what really counts: peripheral indices of tissue metabolic status. The poor correlation makes laboratory tests a poor choice of gauge for adjusting the dosage of exogenous thyroid hormone. So, despite the lack of correlation between the Achilles reflex speed and laboratory test results, the reflex test is valuable.

The more severe a patient's hypothyroidism, the slower the Achilles reflex,[42,p.487] and the more detectable by the clinician. Refetoff[60,p.607] and Rives et al.,[59] however, contend that the test is of little value in patients with mild hypothyroidism. Ooi and coauthors do not concur. They found that in patients with subclinical hypothyroidism, the reflex was significantly prolonged, and it resumed normal speed upon treatment with T_3.[63] Patients with subclinical hypothyroidism have elevated TSH levels despite normal serum total T_4, and they are usually asymptomatic.[64,p.1256] Subclinical hypothyroidism is mild hypothyroidism, yet Ooi et al. report that the Achilles reflex is highly useful in caring for these patients.[63]

A sluggish Achilles reflex due to inadequate thyroid hormone regulation of muscle cell function may be compounded by a deficiency of vitamin B_{12} or B_1. In a vitamin B_{12} deficiency, reflex speed may be increased or impaired, depending on the stage of the deficiency.[31,p.128] In the dry (neuritic) form of beriberi, due to a severe thiamine deficiency the speed of deep tendon reflexes initially increases. With progression of the disease, the speed of the reflex may decrease and eventually may become absent.[111] Accelerated carbohydrate metabolism due to the use of exogenous thyroid hormone may create a thiamine deficiency in the patient who does not take B complex vitamin supplements. In such patients, the Achilles reflex may not become normal until they begin taking B complex vitamins.

Hyperreflexia (shortened duration of the Achilles reflex response) is a sign of neuromuscular thyrotoxicosis.[98] The value of the test during thyrotoxicosis is limited because the overlap with normal values is substantial. Investigators have reported that the sensitivity and specificity of the test for diagnosis is roughly only 35%.[61][62] Nonetheless, most experienced clinicians easily recognize hyperreflexia.

HEART FUNCTION

Heart rate is typically slow in the hypothyroid patient, but the blood pressure may be high, normal, or low.[72,p.22] The same is true of thyroid hormone-related euthyroid hypometabolic patients. The heart rate is usually slow for the patient's level of cardiovascular fitness. Changes in the pulse rate are an extremely useful index of metabolic status. I have observed many hypothyroid and euthyroid hypometabolic patients whose pulse rates at rest were from 50-to-60 bpm despite the patients having had no aerobic exercise for years. After taking as little as 0.15 mg of T_4 or 75 mcg of T_3 for a short time, still with no aerobic exercise, their pulse rates increased to as much as 80 bpm.

Changes in heart rate for most patients are probably the most sensitive indicator that exogenous thyroid hormone is taking effect in the body. Reflecting this high cardiac sensitivity to thyroid hormone, Dillman wrote, "The heart is a major target organ for thyroid hormone action, and cardiovascular symptoms frequently are the major manifestation of thyrotoxicosis."[50,p.763] Rapid heart rate is also an indication of the thyrotoxicosis associated with the general form of thyroid hormone resistance. In this form of resistance syndrome, the resistance of the pituitary gland to thyroid hormone results in a high level of secretion of TSH. The high TSH level causes an elevation of circulating thyroid hormone levels. Some of the patients' peripheral tissues are resistant to thyroid hormone and others respond normally. If the heart is among the normally responsive tissues, the patient exhibits the tachycardia typical of the thyrotoxicosis of hyperthyroidism. Refetoff, Weiss, and Usala write that tachycardia is the most common finding in thyrotoxicosis among general thyroid hormone resistance patients.[51,p.360]

At non-thyrotoxic dosages of exogenous thyroid hormone, the pulse rate is a useful peripheral index of changes in tissue metabolic status. In one study of T_3 therapy with euthyroid fibromyalgia patients,[52] my colleagues and I found that in placebo phases, patients' mean heart rate was 67.88 bpm. In T_3 phases, the mean rate increased to 83.96 bpm. The difference in the mean rates was highly significant (P=.003). In a second study of T_3 therapy with euthyroid patients,[53] the mean heart rate in placebo phases was 68.56 bpm and in T_3 phases was 83.94 bpm. The difference was significant (P=0.022). *Despite the patients' use of supraphysiologic T_3 dosages (ranging from 93.75 mcg-to-162.50 mcg), no patient in either study had tachycardia.*

Factors other than thyroid hormone dosage may influence heart rate. Other factors that the clinician should consider are underlying cardiac abnormalities, fitness level, and the use of medications such as β-adrenergic receptor blockers and tricyclic antidepressants.

Electrocardiography (ECG)

The hypothyroid patient may have low voltage deflections in the QRS complex of the ECG.[11,p.169][30,p.860] This is also true of the patient with thyroid hormone-related euthyroid hypometabolism. The patient may have flattened or shallow inversions of T waves in all or most leads without comparable ST displacement. The patient may also have sinus bradycardia. The QT interval may be prolonged, but this may be difficult to measure because of low or flat T waves.[54,p.465] In some fibromyalgia patients, the QT duration spans but does not exceed the range of normal (0.30-to-0.46 sec). (The duration is also often prolonged in patients with mitral value prolapse.[55]) Under the influence of exogenous thyroid hormone, the duration typically shortens within the normal range. Changes in these indices toward normal or median values indicate that thyroid hormone therapy is effectively impacting cardiac regulatory mechanisms.

In one study of the use of T₃ for euthyroid fibromyalgia, we found no statistically significant change in the mean values of the PR interval or the QRS complex. The mean QT interval, however, shortened from 0.40 sec in placebo phases to 0.36 sec in T₃ phases (normal range: 0.30-to-0.46 sec). This was a significant shortening (P=0.01) within the normal range, and indicates an increase in voltage of the ECG.[52] In a second study of T₃ treatment for euthyroid fibromyalgia, we also found no significant change in the values for the PR interval and the QRS complex. The QT interval, however, shortened significantly (P=0.027) from a mean of .39 sec in placebo phases to 0.35 sec in T₃ phases.[53] This shortening within the normal range again indicates an increase in voltage of the ECG.

These values, however, are *means*. The clinician should bear in mind that individual patients may show more extreme changes in PR, QRS, and QT intervals. For such patients, serial ECGs are extremely useful for determining that thyroid hormone is impacting heart function. Changes in this objective measure precede some patients' subjective awareness of any metabolic effect from thyroid hormone. Comparing ECG tracings with previous ones with longer intervals can be reassuring to the patient that metabolic changes are occurring. The heart, of course, is one of the most sensitive tissues to thyroid hormone.

If one or more intervals is shortened into the abnormal range, the patient should not increase the thyroid hormone dosage further. The patient may have to reduce the dosage slightly pending evaluation by a cardiologist. If a patient with abnormally shortened intervals has symptoms that may be cardiac in origin, use of small-to-moderate dosages of propranolol may be necessary. To avoid critically impairing cardiac contractility, large dosages of propranolol should not be used with patients whose cardiac function is compromised.[97,p.705] For electrocardiographic indications of cardiac overstimulation with thyroid hormone, see Chapter 4.4, subsection titled "Electrocardiographic Indications of Cardiac Thyrotoxicosis."

Echocardiography

Jennings et al. reported that systolic time intervals were reduced in T₄-treated patients who had high mean free T₄ and normal mean T₃ levels[112] In a similar study, Tseng and colleagues measured the systolic time intervals directly from echocardiographic tracings of normal subjects and hypothyroid and hyperthyroid patients. They reported that compared to normal subjects, patients with both subclinical and overt hyperthyroidism had a significantly shortened mean isovolumetric contraction time, preejection period, and left ventricular ejection time.[113] The values for subclinical hypothyroid patients were similar to those of normal subjects. Overt hypothyroid patients, however, had significantly increased mean values for the isovolumetric contraction time, preejection period, and left ventricular ejection time. The researchers concluded that in the absence of heart disease, echocardiography provides a rapid, reliable, and sensitive method for determining the systolic time interval. They also wrote that the method provides "direct" information on peripheral tissue thyroid functional status. More accurately stated, the method can be used as an *indirect* index of cardiac tissue response to thyroid gland status or thyroid hormone dosage.

ELECTROENCEPHALOGRAPHY (EEG)

In hypothyroidism, the electroencephalogram (EEG) may be abnormally flat with low voltage. In mild cases, the alpha rhythm may be slow. In severe cases, alpha waves may be completely blocked.[21,p.575]

REFERENCES

1. Sonkin, L.S.: Endocrine disorders and muscle dysfunction. In *Clinical Management of Head, Neck, and TMJ Pain and Dysfunction*. Edited by B. Gelb, Philadelphia, W.B. Saunders Co., 1985, pp.137-170.
2. Thompson, W.O. and Thompson, P.K.: Low basal metabolism following thyrotoxicosis. *J. Clin. Invest.*, 5:471-

501, 1928.

3. Thurmon, F.M. and Thompson, W.O.: Low basal metabolism with myxedema. *Arch. Intern. Med.*, 46:879-897, 1930.

4. Goldberg, M.: Diagnosis of euthyroid hypometabolism. *Am. J. Obst. Gynec.,* 81(5):1053-1058, 1961.

5. Stockigt, J.R.: Serum thyrotropin and thyroid hormone measurements and assessment of thyroid hormone transport. In *Werner and Ingbar's The Thyroid: A Fundamental and Clinical Text,* 7th edition. Edited by L.P. Braverman and R.D. Utiger, Philadelphia, Lippincott-Raven Publishers, 1996, pp.377-396.

6. Roth, S.H.: NSAIDs and gastropathy: a rheumatologist's view. *J. Rheumatol.,* 15:912-918, 1988.

7. Clive, D.M. and Stoff, J.S.: Renal syndromes associated with nonsteroidal antiinflammatory drugs. *New Engl. J. Med.,* 310:563-572, 1984.

8. Lowe, J. C.: Eccentric pain patterns. *Dyn. Chiro.*, June 6, 1990, pp.5,36.

9. Boothby, W.M. and Sandiford, I.: Summary of the basal metabolism data on 8614 subjects with especial reference to the normal standard for the estimation of the basal metabolic rate. *J. Biol. Chem.,* 54:783-803, 1922.

10. Barnes, B.: Basal temperature versus basal metabolism. *J.A.M.A.,* 119:1072-1074, 1942.

11. Tepperman, J. and Tepperman, H.M.: *Metabolic and Endocrine Physiology,* 5th edition. Chicago, Year Book Medical Publishers, Inc., 1987.

12. Fraser, W.D., Biggart, E.M., O'Reilly, D. S., Gray, H.W., and McKillop, J.H.: Are biochemical tests of thyroid function of any value in monitoring patients receiving thyroxine replacement? *Br. Med. J.,* 293:808-810, 1986.

13. Emerson, C.H., Liberman, C., and Braverman, L.E.: Hypothyroidism. In *The Thyroid.* Edited by W.L. Green, New York, Elsevier, 1987, pp.239-243.

14. Refetoff, S.: Personal communication. April 27, 1992.

15. Fleisher, G., McConahey, W., and Pankow, M.: Serum creatine kinase, lactic dehydrogenase, and glutamic-oxalacetic transaminase in thyroid diseases and pregnancy. *Mayo Clinic Proc.,* 40:300, 1965.

16. Ecker, D.V.: Metabolic indices. In *Werner's The Thyroid: A Fundamental and Clinical Text,* 5th edition. Edited by S.H. Ingbar and L.E. Braverman, New York, J.B. Lippincott Co., 1986, pp.524-533.

17. Murray, G.R.: The life history of the first case of myxedema treated by thyroid extract. *Brit. Med. J.,* Vol.1, March 13, 1920, p.359.

18. Larsen, P.R.: Tests of thyroid function. *Med. Clinics N. Amer.,* 59:1063-1074, 1975.

19. Prange, A.J. Jr., Ian, C.W., Rabon, A.M., and Lipton, M.A.: Enhancement of imipramine antidepressant activity by thyroid hormone. *Am. J. Psychiatry,* 126:463-464, 1969.

20. Nuttall, F.Q. and Doe, R.P.: The Achilles reflex in thyroid disorders: a critical evaluation. *Ann. Intern. Med.,* 61:269-288, 1964.

21. DeGroot, L.J., Larsen, P.R., Refetoff, S., and Stanbury, J.B.: *The Thyroid and Its Diseases,* 5th edition. New York, John Wiley & Sons, Inc., 1984.

22. Howanitz, P.J. and Howanitz, J.H.: Evaluation of endocrine function. In *Clinical Diagnosis and Management by Laboratory Methods,* 16th edition. Edited by J.B. Henry, Philadelphia, W.B. Saunders Co., 1979.

23. Nikkil, E.A. and Kekki, M.: Plasma triglyceride metabolism in thyroid disease. *J. Clin. Invest.,* 51:2103-2114, 1972.

24. Watanakunakorn, C., Hodges, R.E., and Evans, T.C.: Myxedema. *Arch. Intern. Med.,* 116:183-190, 1965.

25. Porte, D. Jr., O'Hara, D.D., and Williams, R.H.: The relation between postheparin lipolytic activity and plasma triglyceride in myxedema. *Metabolism,* 15:107, 1966.

26. Walton, K.W., Scott, P.J., Dykes, P.W., and Davies, J.W.L.: The significance of alterations in serum lipids in thyroid dysfunction. II. Alterations of the metabolism and turnover of ^{131}I-low-density lipoproteins in hypothyroidism and thyrotoxicosis. *Clin. Sci.,* 29:217, 1965.

27. Goodman, H.M. and Bray, S.O.: Role of thyroid hormones in lipolysis. *Am. J. Physiol.,* 210:1053, 1966.

28. Scow, R.O.: Development of obesity in force-fed young thyroidectomized rats. *Endocrinology,* 49:522, 1951.

29. Loeb, J.N.: Metabolic changes. In *The Thyroid,* 4th edition. Edited by S.C. Werner and S.H. Ingbar, New York, Harper and Row Publishers, 1987, pp.872.

30. DeGowin, R.L. and DeGowin, E.L.: *Bedside Diagnostic Examination,* 3rd edition. New York, Macmillan Publishing Co., Inc., 1976.

31. Travell, J.G. and Simons, D.G.: *Myofascial Pain and Dysfunction: The Trigger Point Manual, Vol. 1.* Baltimore, Williams & Wilkins, 1983.

32. Travell, J.G. and Simons, D.G.: *Myofascial Pain and Dysfunction: The Trigger Point Manual, Vol. 2, The Lower Extremities.* Baltimore, Williams & Wilkins, 1992.

33. Hamburger, J.I.: Strategies for cost-effective thyroid function testing with modern methods. In *Diagnostic Methods in Clinical Thyroidology.* Edited by J.I. Hamburger, New York, Springer-Verlag, 1989, pp.63-109.

34. Erickson, R.S. and Kirklin, S.K.: Comparison of ear-based, bladder, oral, and axillary methods for core temperature measurement. *Crit. Care Med.,* 21(10):1528-1534, 1993.

35. Report of the National Cholesterol Education Program Expert Panel on Detection, Evaluation, and Treatment of High Blood Cholesterol in Adults. *Arch. Intern. Med.,* 148:36, 1988.

36. Graninger, W., Pirich, K.R., Speiser, W., et al.: Effect of thyroid hormones on plasma protein concentrations in man. *J. Clin. Endocrinol. Metab.,* 63:407, 1986.

37. Klein, I.: Thyroid hormone and the cardiovascular system. *Am. J. Med.,* 88:631, 1990.

38. Singh, P.I., Sood, S., and Sood, A.K.: Left ventricular diastolic function in hyperthyroid and hypothyroid states. *J. Assoc. Physicians India,* 34:845, 1986.

39. Suko, J.: Alterations of Ca^{2+}-uptake and Ca^{2+}-activated ATPase of cardiac sarcoplasmic reticulum in hyper- and hypothyroidism. *Biochem. Biophys. Acta,* 252:324, 1971.

40. Thompson, G.R., Soutar, A.K., Spengel, F.A., et al.: Defects of receptor-mediated low density lipoprotein catabolism in homozygous familial hypercholesterolemia and hypothyroidism in vivo. *Proc. Natl. Acad. Sci.(USA),* 78:2591, 1981.

41. Day, R., Gebhard, R.L., Schwartz, H.C., et al.: Time course of hepatic 3-hydroxy-3-methyl glutaryl coenzyme: a reductase activity and messenger ribonucleic acid, biliary lipid

secretion and hepatic cholesterol content in methimazole-treated hypothyroid and hypophysectomized rats after T₃ administration—possible linkage of cholesterol synthesis to biliary secretion. *Endocrinology*, 125:459, 1989.

42. Klein, I.: Metabolic, physiologic, and clinical indices of thyroid function. In *The Thyroid: A Fundamental and Clinical Text*, 6th edition. Edited by L.E. Braverman and R.D.Utiger, Philadelphia, J.B. Lippincott Co., 1991, pp.486-492.

43. Ladenson, P., Goldenheim, P., and Ridgway, E.: Rapid pituitary and peripheral tissue responses to intravenous L-triiodothyronine in hypothyroidism. *J. Clin. Endocrinol. Metab.*, 56:1252, 1983.

44. Crowley, W.F., Ridgway, E.C., and Bough, E.W., et al.: Noninvasive evaluation of cardiac function in hypothyroidism. *N. Engl. J. Med.*, 298:1, 1977.

45. Roti, E., Minelli, R., Gardini, E., and Braverman, L.E.: The use and misuse of thyroid hormone. *Endocrin. Rev.*, 14: 401-423, 1993.

46. Zung, W.W.K.: A self-rating depression scale. *Arch. Gen. Psychiatry*, 12:65-70, 1965.

47. Beck, A.T., Ward, C.H., Mendelson, M., Mock, J., and Erbaugh, J.: Inventory for measuring depression. *Arch. Gen. Psychiat.*, 4:561-571, 1961.

48. Rehm, L.P.: Assessment of depression. In *Behavioral Assessment: A Practical Handbook*. Edited by M. Hersen and A.S. Bellack, Oxford, Pergamon Press, 1976, pp.246-295.

49. Naughton, M.J. and Wiklund, I.: A critical review of dimension-specific measures of health-related quality of life in cross-cultural research. *Quality Life Res.*, 2(6):397-432, 1993.

50. Dillman, W.H.: The cardiovascular system in thyrotoxicosis. In *The Thyroid: A Fundamental and Clinical Text*, 6th edition. Edited by L.E. Braverman and R.D. Utiger, Philadelphia, J.B. Lippincott Co., 1991, pp.759-770.

51. Refetoff, S., Weiss, R.E., and Usala, S.J.: The syndromes of resistance to thyroid hormone. *Endocrine Reviews*, 4(3): 348-399, 1993.

52. Lowe, J.C., Garrison, R., Reichman, A.J., Yellin, J., Thompson, M., and Kaufman, D.: Effectiveness and safety of T₃ (triiodothyronine) therapy for euthyroid fibromyalgia: a double-blind placebo-controlled response-driven crossover study. *Clin. Bull. Myofascial Ther.*, 2(2/3):31-57, 1997.

53. Lowe, J.C., Reichman, A.J., Yellin, J.: The process of change during T₃ treatment for euthyroid fibromyalgia: a double-blind placebo-controlled crossover study. *Clin. Bull. Myofascial Ther.*, 2(2/3):91-124, 1997.

54. Marriott, H.J.: *Practical Electrocardiography*, 7th edition. Baltimore, Williams & Wilkins, 1983.

55. Bekheit, S.G.: Analysis of QT interval in patients with idiopathic mitral valve prolapse. *Chest*, 81:620, 1982.

56. Klein, I., Parker, M., Mantel, P., and Levey, G.S.: Unusual manifestations of hypothyroidism. *Arch. Intern. Med.*, 144: 123, 1984.

57. Wiles, C.M., Young, A., Jones, D.A., and Rolt, E.: Muscle relaxation rate, fiber type composition and energy turnover in hyper- and hypothyroid patients. *Clin. Sci.*, 57:375, 1979.

58. Mier, A., Brophy, C., Wass, J.A.H., et al.: Reversible respiratory muscle weakness in hyperthyroidism. *Am. Rev.* *Respir. Dis.*, 139:529, 1989.

59. Rives, K.L., Furth, E.D., and Becker, D.V.: Limitations of the ankle jerks test: intercomparison with other tests of thyroid function. *Ann. Intern. Med.*, 62:1139, 1965.

60. Refetoff, S.: Thyroid function tests and effects of drugs on thyroid function. In *Endocrinology*, 2nd edition. Edited by L.J. DeGroot, New York, Grune and Stratton, 1988.

61. Becker, D.: Metabolic indices. In *Werner's The Thyroid: A Fundamental and Clinical Text*, 5th edition. Edited by S.H. Ingbar and L.E. Braverman, New York, J.B. Lippincott, 1986, p.524.

62. Olsen, B., Klein, I., Benner, R., et al.: Hyperthyroid myopathy and the response to treatment. *Thyroid*, 1:137, 1991.

63. Ooi, T.C., Whitlock, R.M.L., Frengley, P.A., and Ibbertson, H.K.: Systolic time intervals and ankle reflex time in patients with minimal serum TSH elevation: response to triiodothyronine therapy. *Clin. Endocrinol.* (Oxf), 13:621, 1980.

64. Ross, D.S.: Subclinical hypothyroidism. In *Werner and Ingbar's The Thyroid: A Fundamental and Clinical Text*, 6th edition. Edited by L.E. Braverman and R.D. Utiger, Philadelphia, J.B. Lippincott Co., 1991, pp.1256-1262.

65. Costin, G., Kaplan, S.A., and Ling, S.M.: The Achilles reflex time in thyroid disorders. *J. Pediatr.*, 76:277, 1970.

66. Johansen, K., Hansen, J.M., and Skovsted, L.: Myxedema and thyrotoxicosis: relations between clinical state and concentrations of thyroxine and triiodothyronine in blood. *Acta Med. Scandinav.*, 204(5):361-364, 1978.

67. Lowe, J.C.: A case of debilitating headache complicated by hypothyroidism: its relief through myofascial therapy. *Dig. Chiro. Econ.*, 31:73-75, Nov/Dec 1988.

68. Murray, G.R.: Note on the treatment of myxoedema by hypodermic injection of an extract of the thyroid gland of sheep. *Br. Med. J.*, 2:796, 1891.

69. Magnus-Levy, A.: Ueber den respiratorischen gaswechsel unter dem einfluss der thyreoidea sowie unter vreschiedenen pathologische. *Zustanden. Berl. Klin. Wochenschr.*, 32:650, 1895.

70. Magnus-Levy, A.: Energy metabolism in health and disease. *J. Hist. Med.*, 2:307, 1947.

71. Barnes, B.O.: *Hypothyroidism: The Unsuspected Illness.* New York, Harper and Row Publishers, 1976.

72. Soloman, D.H.: Clinical examination of the thyroid. In *The Thyroid Gland: A Practical Clinical Treatise*. Edited by R. Van Middlesworth, Chicago, Year Book Medical Publishers, Inc., 1986, pp.19-34.

73. O'Hara, D., Porte, D., Jr., and Williams, R.H.: The effect of diet and thyroxine on plasma lipids in myxedema. *Metabolism*, 15:123, 1966.

74. Himms-Hagen, J.: Thyroid hormones and thermogenesis. In *Mammalian Thermogenesis*. Edited by M.J. Stock and L. Girardier, London, Chapman and Hall, 1983.

75. Landsberg, L., Saville, M.E., and Young, J.B.: The sympathoadrenal system and regulation of thermogenesis. *Am. J. Physiol.*, 247:E181, 1984.

76. Sternback, R.A.: Chronic pain as a disease entity. *Triangle*, 20:27, 1981.

77. Bonica, J.J.: Definitions and taxonomy of pain. In *The Management of Pain, Vol 1*, 2nd edition. Philadelphia, Lea & Febiger, 1990.

78. Wunderlich, C.A.: *On the Temperature in Disease.* Trans-

lated from German by W.B. Woodman, London, New Sydenham Soc., 1871.

79. Pembrey, M.S. and Nicol, B.A.: Observations upon the deep and surface temperature of the human body. *J. Physiol.*, 23:386, 1898.

80. Benedict, F.G. and Carpenter, T.M.: The metabolism and energy transformation of healthy man during rest. Publ. No. 126, Carnegie Institute, Washington, 1910.

81. DuBois, E.F.: The temperature of the human body in health and disease. In *Temperature: Its Measurements and Control in Science and Industry.* American Institute of Physics, New York, Reinhold Corp., 1941.

82. Reimann, H.A.: The problem of long continued low grade fever. *J.A.M.A.*, 107:1089, 1936.

83. Ivy, A.C.: What is normal or normality? *Quart. Bull. Northwestern Univ. Med. School*, 18:22, 1944.

84. DuBois, E.F.: *Fever and the Regulation of Body Temperature.* Springfield, Charles C. Thomas, 1948.

85. Lowe, J.C.: *Spasm.* Houston, McDowell Publishing Co., 1983.

86. Steward, H.J., Deitrick, J.E., and Crane, N.F.: Studies of the circulation in patients suffering from spontaneous myxedema. *J. Clin. Investig.*, 17:247, 1938.

87. Stewart, H.J. and Evans, W.F.: Peripheral blood flow in myxedema. *Arch. Intern. Med.*, 69:808-821, 1942.

88. Chaney, W.C.: Tendon reflexes in myxedema: a valuable aid in diagnosis. *J. Am. Med. Assoc.*, 82:2013-2016, 1924.

89. Lambert, E.H., Underdahl, L.O., Beckett, S., and Mederos, L.O.: A study of the ankle jerk in myxedema. *J. Clin. Endocrinology*, 11:1186-1205, 1951.

90. Ribot, C., Tremollieres, F., Pouilles, J.M., and Louvet, J.P.: Bone mineral density and thyroid hormone therapy. *Clin. Endocrinol.*, 33:143-155, 1990.

91. Gow, S.M., Caldwell, G., Toft, A.D., et al.: Relationship between pituitary and other target organ responsiveness in hypothyroid patients receiving thyroxine replacement. *J. Clin. Endocrinol. Metab.*, 64:364-369, 1987.

92. Wilson, E.D.: *Wilson's Syndrome.* Orlando, Cornerstone Publishing Co., 1991.

93. Wolfe, S.L.: *Molecular and Cellular Biology.* Belmont, Wadsworth Publishing Co., 1993.

94. Ismail-Beigi, F. and Edelman, I.S.: The mechanism of the calorigenic action of thyroid hormone: stimulation of Na^+-K^+-activated adenosinetriphosphatase activity. *J. Gen. Physiol.*, 57:710-722, 1971.

95. Ismail-Beigi, F.: Thyroid horomone regulation of Na^+-K^+-ATPase expression. *Trends Endocrinol. Metab.*, 4:152-155, 1993.

96. Shambaugh, III, G.E.: Biologic and cellular effects. In *The Thyroid: A Fundamental and Clinical Text*, 5th edition. Edited by S.C. Werner and S.H. Ingbar, New York, Harper and Row, Publishers, 1986.

97. Wartofsky, L.: Thyrotoxic storm. In *Werner and Ingbar's The Thyroid: A Fundamental and Clinical Text*, 7th edition. Edited by L.P. Braverman and R.D. Utiger, Philadelphia, Lippincott-Raven Publishers, 1996, pp.701-712.

98. DeLong, G.R.: The neuromuscular system and brain in thyrotoxicosis. In *Werner and Ingbar's The Thyroid: A Fundamental and Clinical Text*, 7th edition. Edited by L.P. Braverman and R.D. Utiger, Philadelphia, Lippincott-Raven Publishers, 1996, pp.645-652.

99. Elert, J.E., Rantaäa-Dahlqvist, S.B., Henriksson-Larsën, K., Lorentzon, R., and Gerdlë: Muscle performance, electromyography and fibre type composition in fibromyalgia and work-related myalgia. *Scand. J. Rheumatol.*, 21:28-34, 1992.

100. Bennett, R.M.: Exercise and exercise testing in fibromyalgia patients: lessons learned and suggestions for future studies. *J. Musculoskel. Pain*, 2(3):143-152, 1994.

101. Braunwald, E.: Edema. In *Harrison's Principles of Internal Medicine*, 8th edition. Edited by G.W. Thorn, R.D. Adams, E. Braunwald, K.J. Isselbacher, and R.G. Petersdorf, New York, McGraw-Hill Book Co., 1977, pp.176-182.

102. Smith, T.J.: Connective tissue in hypothyroidism. In *Werner's The Thyroid: A Fundamental and Clinical Text*, 6th edition. Edited by L.E. Braverman and R.D. Utiger, Philadelphia, J.B. Lippincott Co., 1991, pp.989-992.

103. Ingbar, S.H. and Woeber, K.A.: Diseases of the thyroid. In *Harrison's Principles of Internal Medicine*, 8th edition. Edited by G.W. Thorn, R.D. Adams, E. Braunwald, K.J. Isselbacher, and R.G. Petersdorf, New York, McGraw-Hill Book Co., 1977, pp.501-519.

104. Kimball, O.P.: Clinical hypothyroidism. *Kentucky Med. J.*, 31:488-495, 1933.

105. Prankerd, T.A.J.: Anaemia. In *French's Index of Differential Diagnosis*, 10th edition. Edited by F.D. Hart, Chicago, Year Book Medical Publishers Inc., 1973, pp.28-62.

106. Guyton, A.C.: *Textbook of Medical Physiology*, 8th edition. Philadelphia, W.B. Saunders Co., 1991.

107. Danese, M.D., Powe, N.R., Sawin, C.T., and Ladenson, P.W.: Screening for mild thyroid failure at the periodic health examination: a decision and cost-effectiveness analysis. *J.A.M.A.*, 276:285-292, 1996.

108. Kung, A.W.C., Pang, R.W.C., and Janus, E.D.: Elevated serum lipoprotein(a) in subclinical hypothyroidism. *Clin. Endocrinol.*, 43:445-449, 1995.

109. Vanderpump, M.P.J., Tunbridge, W.M.G., French, J.M., et al.: The development of ischemic heart disease in relation to autoimmune thyroid disease in a 20-year follow-up study of an English community. *Thyroid*, 6:155-156, 1996.

110. Taniyama, M., Honma, K., and Ban, Y.: Urinary cortisol metabolites in the assessment of peripheral thyroid hormone action: application for diagnosis of resistance to thyroid hormone. *Thyroid*, 3(3):229-233, 1993.

111. Williams, R.D., Mason, H.L., Power, M.H., et al.: Induced thiamine (vitamin B_1) deficiency in man. *Arch. Intern. Med.*, 71:38-53, 1943.

112. Jennings, P.E., O'Malley, B.P., and Griffin, K.E.: Relevance of increased serum thyroxine concentrations associated with normal serum triiodothyronine values in hypothyroid patients receiving thyroxine: a case for "tissue thyrotoxicosis." *Br. Med. J.*, 289:1645, 1984.

113. Tseng, K.H., Walfish, P.G., Persaud, J.A., and Gilbert, B.W.: Concurrent aortic and mitral value echocardiography permits measurement of systolic time intervals as an index of peripheral tissue thyroid functional status. *J. Clin. Endocrinol. Metab.*, 69(3):633-638, 1989.

114. Lafleur, L.J.: Translation of *Rules for the Direction of the Mind* by Rene' Descartes. Indianapolis, The Bobbs-Merrill Company, Inc., 1961.

115. Drill, V.A.: Interrelations between thyroid function and vitamin metabolism. *Physiol. Rev.*, 23:355, 1943.

116. Escamilla, R.F.: Carotenemia in myxedema: explanation of the typical slightly icteric tint. *J. Clin. Endocrinol. Metab.*, 2:33, 1942.

117. Freedberg, I.M. and Vogel, L.N.: The skin in hypothyroidism. In *Werner's The Thyroid: A Fundamental and Clinical Text*, 6th edition. Edited by L.E. Braverman and R.D. Utiger, Philadelphia, J.B. Lippincott Co., 1991, pp.985-988.

118. Marrocco, W., Adonencecchi, L., Suraci, C., et al.: Comporetamento dela vitamin A, del β-carotene, della proteina leganta il retinol e della prealbumina nel plasma di sogetta ipo ed ipertiroidei. *Boll. Soc. Ital. Biol. Sper.*, 60: 769, 1984.

119. Walton, K.W., Campbell, D.A., and Tonks, E.L.: The significance of alterations in serum lipids in thyroid dysfunction. I. The relation between serum lipoproteins, carotenoid, and vitamin A in hypothyroidism and thyrotoxicosis. *Clin. Sci.*, 29:199, 1965.

120. Rivlin, R.S.: Vitamin metabolism in hypothyroidism. In *Werner's The Thyroid: A Fundamental and Clinical Text*, 6th edition. Edited by L.E. Braverman and R.D. Utiger, Philadelphia, J.B. Lippincott Co., 1991, pp.1072-1077.

121. Smith, F.R. and Goodman, D.S.: The effects of diseases of the liver, thyroid and kidneys on the transport of vitamin A in human plasma. *J. Clin. Invest.*, 50:2426, 1971.

122. Hazama, S., Takahata, T., Kaneshiro, E., Kadoya, Y., and Tagami, S.: Mild hypothermia in patients with senile dementia. *Nippon Ronen Igakkai Zasshi*, 29(1):47-53, 1992.

123. Fulbrook, P.: Core temperature measurement: a comparison of rectal, axillary and pulmonary artery blood temperature. *Intensive Crit. Care Nurs.*, 9(4):217-225, 1993.

124. Henker, R. and Coyne, C.: Comparison of peripheral temperature measurements with core temperature. *AACN Clin. Issues*, 6(1):21-30, 1995.

125. Schmitz, T., Bair, N., Falk, M., and Levine, C.: A comparison of five methods of temperature measurement in febrile intensive care patients. *Am. J. Crit. Care*, 4(4): 286-292, 1995.

4.4

Adverse Effects of Excessive and Inadequate Thyroid Hormone

A clinician's beliefs regarding thyroid hormone overstimulation are likely to significantly impact the outcome of his care of patients who use exogenous thyroid hormone. It is imperative then that he clearly understand the concepts and terminology regarding this subject. The word hyperthyroidism refers to excessive biosynthesis of thyroid hormones by the thyroid gland, with resulting elevated serum levels of T_3 and T_4 and/or a low serum TSH. This term is not synonymous with thyrotoxicosis, which refers to the clinical syndrome resulting from cellular overstimulation associated with elevated levels of T_4 and/or T_3.

In clinical practice, these terms are often confused. As a result, when laboratory tests show a low-normal or low TSH level, the clinician assumes the patient's peripheral tissues are being adversely affected. For some patients, this is true, but for many others, it is not. Some fibromyalgia patients, especially those who are euthyroid, can use an exogenous thyroid hormone dosage sufficient to suppress the TSH level and still be hypometabolic because their tissues are partially resistant to thyroid hormone. Thus, when a clinician reduces the thyroid hormone dosages of these patients, their hypometabolism may worsen. This can adversely affect the patients' health and quality of life.

The hypothyroid fibromyalgia patient may be hypometabolic and symptomatic when she is required to limit her thyroid hormone dosage to an amount that keeps her serum T_4 within the normal range. Many hypothyroid fibromyalgia patients are eumetabolic only when using large enough T_4 dosages to provide mid-range free T_3 levels. The T_4 dosage that produces a mid-range T_3 level may cause high-normal T_4 and low TSH levels. With these patients, clinicians should not infer the high-normal T_4 and low TSH values are indicative of tissue thyrotoxicity. It is possible that some tissues in some patients may be thyrotoxic with such dosages, but this is a rare occurrence and can only be determined by tests that reveal evidence of thyroid hormone overstimulation of specific tissues.*

The clinician should assess each patient as an individual when considering the possibilities of critically reduced bone density and adverse cardiac effects in patients using exogenous thyroid hormone. However, the potential for these effects has been exaggerated. Clinicians today commonly believe that TSH-suppressive dosages of exogenous thyroid hormone generally cause osteoporosis. This belief, based on early flawed studies, is false. Considerable evidence now indicates that the risk of decreased bone mineral density with thyroid hormone therapy has been overstated, and the risk of osteoporosis has been exaggerated in the extreme. Fractures are not a feature of the natural history of treated hypothyroid patients. An increased fracture rate has never been documented even in patients treated long-term with thyroid hor-

mone. Post-menopausal women taking exogenous thyroid hormone, especially women who previously had thyrotoxicosis due to thyroid gland disease, have been found to have reduced bone density. However, those taking TSH-suppressive dosages of T_4 were not found to have statistically significant lower bone density than those taking replacement dosages.

The use of even a small dosage of exogenous thyroid hormone may induce transient osteoclastic hyperresorption in trabecular and cortical bone. The hyperresorption tends to occur in patients taking dosages small enough that the patients exhibit no obvious clinical or biological signs of thyrotoxicosis. The hyperresorption, with a reduction in bone mineral density, may begin in as few as 7 days and persist from 1-to-2 years. Increases in biochemical markers such as urinary calcium and hydroxyproline suggest bone hyperresorption. However, the increases are insignificant except in the case of the patient who was osteoporotic before beginning the use of thyroid hormone and may be at risk for fractures.

Some researchers have reported an increased bone mineral density in patients taking exogenous thyroid hormone. The increased density most likely results from the patients' increased physical activity levels made possible by the use of thyroid hormone.

Many clinicians today believe that the patient taking TSH-suppressive dosages of thyroid hormone risks cardiac arrest. Elderly patients with low levels of cardiovascular conditioning are at risk, especially when they make large increases in their thyroid hormone dosages. The clinician should take proper steps to protect the health of these patients when they use thyroid hormone (see Chapter 5.2).

Evidence indicates that the increase in the incidence of death from ischemic heart disease in patients taking T_4 is no greater in patients taking TSH-suppressive dosages than in those taking only replacement dosages.

Many patients are predisposed to cardiovascular disease because their clinicians restrict their dosages of thyroid hormone to "replacement" amounts. For the past 30 years, conventional clinicians have restricted patients' thyroid hormone dosages in an attempt to prevent osteoporosis and adverse cardiac effects. Patients' whose dosages of thyroid hormone have been kept too low by this strategy have been subjected to an increased risk of cardiovascular disease. The outcome in terms of resulting pathology and premature death is undetermined, but may be of colossal proportions. Erring on the side of safety with some patients may mean allowing them to use a higher,

rather than a lower than average, dosage of thyroid hormone.

The clinician must protect the patient from peripheral tissue overstimulation. For a safe (and effective) therapeutic outcome, the clinician must base decisions regarding thyroid hormone dosage on the individual patient's health status and tissue responses to the hormone. Thyroid function laboratory test results provide information only about the response of the pituitary and thyroid glands to the current thyroid hormone dosage; they provide no information whatsoever about the responses of other tissues to the dosage. A loss of the patient's health and well-being is often the cost of the clinician inferring peripheral tissue responses from the circulating levels of TSH and thyroid hormones. At most, the clinician should consider circulating thyroid hormone and TSH levels typical of hyperthyroidism to only raise the possibility of tissue overstimulation; the results are not prima facie *evidence for tissue thyrotoxicosis. The clinician should not assume that a suppressed TSH level is evidence of tissue thyrotoxicosis, even when the T_3 or T_4 level is high. The tissues of the patient with these test results may be hyporesponsive to thyroid hormone. As a result, restricting the patient to a dosage of thyroid hormone that keeps the TSH and thyroid hormone levels within the normal range may subject the patient to tissue hypometabolism that predisposes her to cardiovascular disease. Whether thyroid hormone overstimulation of tissues is occurring can only be determined by the presence of a clinical syndrome of thyrotoxicosis and positive biochemical, electrophysiological, or imaging tests for tissue thyrotoxicosis.*

To avoid over- and understimulation of tissues, the clinician should progressively increase the thyroid hormone dosage until the patient reaches the desired state, indicated by her clinical status and measures of therapeutic change. While increasing the dosage, any adverse cardiac effects should be detected by the use of serial ECGs and should be properly managed. After reaching the patient's optimal dosage, assessments should be made to insure that the patient's heart, bone, muscle, and liver are not being adversely affected. Assessments should involve testing that is specific to each tissue of concern. Adverse effects should be alleviated by thyroid hormone dosage titration and any other appropriate procedures.

Accumulating studies indicate that the safe dosage range for T_4 is wider than previously believed. For most patients, the use of 0.2-to-0.4 mg of T_4 or its equivalent of desiccated thyroid hormone appears to *be safe. This is attested to by the lack of evidence of harmful effects during the long history of patients taking such dosages, which are much higher than the currently approved replacement dosages. Fewer studies are available from which to judge the breadth of the safe dosage range for T_3. Many euthyroid fibromyalgia patients with apparent partial cellular resistance to thyroid hormone improve or recover with the use of supraphysiologic dosages of T_3 with no evidence of tissue thyrotoxicity. Hopefully, additional studies of these patients will contribute to a reprieve from the prejudicial judgments of T_3 by conventional endocrinology; a reprieve will hopefully result in the use of the hormone in more human studies. Regardless, disapproval of the sole use of T_3 is an* a priori *denouncement by conventional endocrinology, and it is clear at this time that when the hormone is properly used, it has no adverse effects. Aside from the question of safety, T_3 is far more effective than T_4 with most euthyroid hypometabolic and hypothyroid fibromyalgia patients.*

In 1989, Hamburger wrote: ". . . no matter how unconvincing to some authorities, low-level overdosage of thyroxine may be harmful. Finally, it is consistent with the practical reality that there is no reason to think it necessary to give enough thyroxine to produce an undetectable sensitive-TSH value in the treatment of hypothyroidism."[1,p.122] At the same time, Toft wrote,[5,p.92] "There is increasing evidence that doses of thyroxine sufficient to suppress thyrotroph secretion cause tissue hyperthyroidism in other organs such as heart, kidney, bone, and liver despite the lack of clinical evidence of thyrotoxicosis." Tepperman and Tepperman wrote, "The patient with Graves' disease literally burns up his own substance."[6,p.168] Tepperman and Tepperman are correct that in severe, untreated Graves' disease, the patient undergoes tissue catabolism. But the judgments of Hamburger and Toft quoted above are quite another matter: The judgments were dubious when these thyroidologists made them, and today they are scientifically indefensible. The proposition that TSH-suppressive dosages of thyroid hormone invariably cause adverse tissue effects is simply false.

Nonetheless, judgments such as those above by Hamburger and Toft heavily influence the decisions of practicing physicians regarding the treatment of their hypothyroid patients. The consequences of those judgments for many hypothyroid patients have been devastating, and the toll in human suffering is incalculable.

Virtually every hypothyroid patient I have seen who was diagnosed and treated for the condition prior to consulting me has made the same complaint: Their physicians denied their requests for symptom relief through an increase in their dosages of thyroid hormone. Many of the patients had good reason for making the request. Some had been permitted by previous physicians to take higher dosages, and some had taken higher dosages for a time without the consent of their physicians; they knew from first-hand experience the symptom relief provided by higher dosages. The reflex refusal of the typical physician to prescribe higher dosages is virtually always accompanied by the same assertion—that an increase in dosage will suppress the TSH and is likely to cause osteoporosis, a heart attack, or other adverse effects. In my experience, most physicians do not know that their refusals cannot be justified scientifically, and they do not know that the refusals are far more likely to harm their patients than would the requested increases in thyroid hormone dosage. To understand how this bizarre circumstance came about, see the more detailed account of the advent and misuse of the TSH in Chapter 2.5, subsection titled "Advent of the TSH Assay" and Chapter 5.3, subsection: "Basis of the Problem of Replacement Dosages."

In practicing responsibly, the physician must determine a dosage of exogenous thyroid hormone that is both effective and safe for each hypothyroid patient. A common misbelief of physicians is that effectiveness and safety can be determined by keeping the patient's circulating TSH level within the normal reference range. The inference made is that the TSH level corresponds to the metabolic status of tissues. The belief is that if the TSH level is normal, then invariably, the tissues are eumetabolic; if the TSH level is high, then invariably, the tissues are hypometabolic; and if the TSH is low, then invariably, the tissues are hypermetabolic (thyrotoxic). The belief that the TSH level is an accurate gauge of tissue metabolic status is so ingrained in the minds of most physicians today that they sternly warn patients of the horrors that are to follow if their dosages of thyroid hormone are not maintained exactly as the TSH dictates. It matters not that the patients exhibit classic symptoms and signs of hypothyroidism. Both physicians and patients must yield to the dictates of the TSH level—a policy that I term the tyranny of the TSH. I use the word tyranny for two specific reasons: First, control of the behavior of physicians and patients through the TSH test is an unmerciful exercise of power through fear. And second, the way in which behavior is controlled leaves patients undertreated and subjected to possible insidious patho-genesis and a diminished quality of life. The tyranny of the TSH issues from the reigning thyroidology para-digm and constitutes a form of extremist technocracy.

Mandates of the current thyroidology paradigm often result in patients developing signs and symptoms of inadequate thyroid hormone regulation of cell func-tion that we diagnose as fibromyalgia. Consider the following published case of a patient with iatrogenic pituitary hypothyroidism. The phenotypic expression of her hypothyroidism was diagnosed as fibromyalgia. In 1991, Disdier et al. reported the case of the 54-year-old woman. She underwent surgery for the removal of a pituitary microadenoma. Because of excess bleeding during surgery, the surgeon removed her entire anteri-or pituitary gland. This left her with pituitary hypothy-roidism since she no longer had thyrotroph cells to secrete TSH. Seven days after surgery, she began taking 0.05 mg of T_4. Within a month, because her plasma T_4 level was low, her dosage was increased to 0.1 mg, and this brought her plasma T_4 level to nor-mal.[33] Usually, an effective dosage of thyroid hor-mone cannot be reliably calculated based on body weight, but when we consider that this woman weighed 202.4 lbs, it is obvious that for her, 0.1 mg was a paltry dose. The authors wrote, ". . . diffuse musculoskeletal pains occurred. The patient was aching all over, particularly in the spine, shoulders, and arms. These pains occurred mainly at night and prevented the patient from sleeping." One year later, she was depressed, more anxious, and often had in-somnia. Declofenac, amitriptyline, and cyamemazine proved ineffective for her. The authors also wrote, "a relationship between transient post-operative hypothy-roidism and fibromyalgia in the patient described here is unlikely." They then noted that her fibromyalgia symptoms appeared before her replacement dosage of hydrocortisone was adequate, but that her symptoms became more severe in spite of increases in her daily hydrocortisone dosage. It is likely that increases in the dosage of hydrocortisone blocked the conversion of her meager quantity of exogenous T_4 to T_3. If conver-sion was blocked by the hydrocortisone, a sufficient dosage of T_3 most likely would have proven highly effective for her. Were T_4 to have worked at all, how-ever, the effective dosage would most likely have been 2-to-4 times the 0.1 mg she was allowed to take. As well as relieving her symptoms, this would have result-ed in a high-normal level of T_4—a laboratory value prohibited by the dictates of the current thyroidology paradigm.

Let me emphasize here that a patient can have harmful tissue effects from dosages of thyroid hor-mone that *for her* are excessive. Because of this po-tential for harm, the clinician must determine whether a particular dosage is both effective and safe for the patient. The effectiveness and safety of a particular dosage of thyroid hormone can be determined *only* by assessing how the individual patient's tissues are responding to the hormone. The TSH test is an as-sessment of how only one group of cells, the TSH-secreting anterior pituitary thyrotrophs, is responding to circulating thyroid hormone. The TSH test measures nothing more, period. Inferring the metabolic status of tissues other than the anterior pituitary from the TSH level cannot be justified scientifically. (For a detailed argument against the use of the TSH to infer the status of peripheral tissues, see Chapter 5.3, subsection titled "Mandates of the Conventional Medical Hypothyroid-ism Paradigm.")

● SIGNS AND SYMPTOMS OF THYROID HORMONE OVERSTIMULATION

Table 4.4.1 lists 11 symptoms and 8 signs that commonly occur during thyrotoxicity due to hyperthy-roidism.[153] It is important for the clinician to be as familiar with the symptoms and signs of overstimula-tion from thyroid hormone as he is with those of un-derstimulation. This is especially true because the effective dosage for some patients is just short of an overstimulating dosage (see Chapter 5.2). When a patient reports one or more of the symptoms listed in Table 4.4.1 and the clinician finds one or more of the signs, he should consider that the patient's thyroid hor-mone dosage is excessive. The clinician should order or perform an ECG to screen for nonspecific changes indicative of cardiac thyrotoxicosis (see Table 4.4.2).

Whether a thyroid hormone dosage that generates symptoms and signs of tissue overstimulation is harm-ful depends on the general health and susceptibility of the individual patient. With the patient who has cardi-ac fragility, low adrenal reserve, or osteoporosis, the clinician should insure that the patient's dosage is kept well below the amount likely to exacerbate the ab-normality. Even with the robustly healthy patient, however, the clinician and patient would best be knowledgeable of the symptoms and signs of over-stimulation and take appropriate steps at the first recognition that they are occurring.

To insure the patient's safety, the clinician must carefully monitor any and all objective and subjective responses to exogenous thyroid hormone. This is especially important because some patients subjectively feel they need dosages of thyroid hormone that are mildly thyrotoxic. In fact, some patients tolerate distinct thyrotoxicity well[154] and are not aware of the tissue overstimulation until it is brought to their attention. In patients with apparent cellular resistance to thyroid hormone, objective measures typically indicate that only supraphysiologic dosages are effective. Since different tissues in the same individual may have variable responses to the same amount of thyroid hormone, a dosage that produces objective and subjective improvement in one tissue may have adverse effects on others. For patients who appear to have markedly differential tissue effects, a compromise dosage may be required. The dosage should provide the maximum symptom relief without overstimulating tissues that are normally or excessively responsive to thyroid hormone.

Table 4.4.1. Common symptoms and signs of thyroid hormone overstimulation.*

SYMPTOMS	SIGNS
Appetite change (typically increase)	Hyperactivity
Fatigue	Hyperreflexia
Heat intolerance	Muscle weakness
Hyperactivity	Stare and eyelid retraction
Increased perspiration	Systolic hypertension
Menstrual disturbances	Tachycardia or cardiac arrhythmia
Nervousness	Tremor
Palpations	Warm, moist, smooth skin
Tremor	
Weakness	
Weight change (usually decrease)	

*From Braverman, L.E. and Utiger, R.D.: Introduction to thyrotoxicosis. In *The Thyroid: A Fundamental and Clinical Text*, 6th edition. Edited by L.E. Braverman and R.D. Utiger, Philadelphia, J.B. Lippincott Co., 1991, p.646.[153]

On theoretical and practical grounds, then, it is not likely that the clinician can use TSH and thyroid hormone levels to determine the effective and safe dosage of exogenous thyroid hormone for the individual patient. The clinician would best gauge whether the dosage is effective and safe through the use of various indicators of tissue responses to the hormone. To insure safety, the clinician should be highly sensitized to indications of thyrotoxicity. At the same time, he should acquire a realistic awareness of the potential risks from excessive dosages of thyroid hormone. This is critically important for two reasons: the potential adverse effects from the use of exogenous thyroid hormone have been exaggerated,[163] and there are potential adverse effects from restricting patients to insufficient dosages of thyroid hormone (see section below titled "Harm from Untreated and Undertreated Hypothyroidism").

● STUDIES OF POSSIBLE ADVERSE EFFECTS OF THYROID HORMONE ON VARIOUS TISSUES

Researchers have investigated the possible adverse effects of exogenous thyroid hormone on joints, muscle proteins, bone, heart, liver, psychiatric status, and the pituitary and thyroid glands.

MUSCULOSKELETAL SYMPTOMS AFTER THE INITIATION OF THYROID HORMONE THERAPY

Delamere and his colleagues wrote that changing thyroid status during treatment may initiate or worsen musculoskeletal symptoms. They report 2 cases in which such symptoms occurred when the hypothyroid patients became euthyroid. One of the patients was a 64-year-old woman. After taking T_4 for 3 months, she developed early morning stiffness that lasted some 90 minutes. She also experienced bilateral shoulder girdle pain and weakness. The stiffness, pain, and weakness later spread to the proximal muscles of her arms and legs. The authors reported that her symptoms resolved within several days after she began taking 10 mg daily of prednisolone (a corticosteroid).[147]

The other patient was a 76-year-old woman. She became euthyroid after 8 weeks of treatment with 0.1 mg T_4 daily. Then she suddenly developed severe pain and weakness in her shoulder and pelvic girdle regions. She was also tender and stiff on both sides of her body for several hours in the mornings. She could not raise her arms above her head, and she could not walk more than a few yards. Her symptoms improved within 48 hours after beginning treatment with 7.5 mg/day of prednisolone. Within 3 weeks, she regained full power and movement.[147]

There are at least three possible mechanisms of the occurrence of musculoskeletal symptoms at the initiation of thyroid hormone therapy. First, in some cases, musculoskeletal symptoms may be coincidental and not causatively related to the exogenous thyroid hormone. Second, the 2 patients reported by Delamere et al.[147] may have had decreased adrenocortical reserve that transformed into an adrenocortical deficiency under the influence of thyroid hormone (see Chapter 5.2, subsection titled "Decreased Adrenal Reserve"). This may happen in patients who have both central hypothyroidism and deficient secretion of ACTH due to pituitary dysfunction. In these cases, too little ACTH is secreted to stimulate production of normal amounts of adrenocortical hormones. Increasing the demand for cortisol by exogenous thyroid hormone may unmask a subclinical adrenocortical deficiency and in fact induce an adrenal crisis.[164] If the patients of Delamere et al. developed a frank adrenal insufficiency under the influence of exogenous thyroid hormone, then the prednisolone may have relieved the deficiency.

The third possible mechanism of musculoskeletal symptoms during the initial phase of thyroid hormone therapy is a dosage that is too low to adequately drive the metabolism of peripheral tissues. For patients affected by this mechanism, musculoskeletal symptoms are the phenotypic expression of inadequate thyroid hormone regulation of cell function. In general, transcription regulation in cells is dependent upon the percentage of nuclear T_3-receptors occupied by T_3. The differential hypersensitivity of the thyrotrophs to thyroid hormone may be due to the high average occupancy of their T_3-receptors by T_3 in the anterior pituitary. In the rat pituitary, 78% of nuclear T_3-receptors were occupied. Other rat tissues differed in that only 50% of their T_3-receptors were occupied.[17] If human mechanisms correspond to those of the rat, then thyroid hormone levels sufficient to suppress thyrotroph secretion of TSH are not adequate to stimulate other target tissues.[5,p.92] Since the pituitary T_3-receptors have a high T_3 occupancy, little additional thyroid hormone is needed to repress transcription of TSH mRNA. Pituitary thyrotroph cells, then, are highly sensitive to thyroid hormone, especially T_4 (converted in the pituitary to T_3). TSH secretion can be suppressed by dosages that may be inadequate to properly regulate the metabolism of peripheral tissues. The reduced amounts of TSH reaching and stimulating the thyroid gland lowers the serum thyroid hormone level even more, leaving peripheral cells metabolically understimulated. In such cases, increasing the thyroid hormone dosage enough to adequately regulate metabolism of peripheral tissues usually relieves the patient's symptoms. The TSH level should be ignored. Restricting the patient's thyroid hormone dosage so as to keep the TSH within the normal reference range is likely to maintain the metabolic insufficiency of peripheral tissues. For most patients using T_4, the dosage must be increased enough to suppress the TSH and raise the T_4 level into the high-normal range. This should produce a normal T_3 level and increase the likelihood of a normal peripheral tissue metabolic rate.[5,p.88][166][167] (See Chapter 5.3, subsection titled "Synthetic T_4.")

Regardless of the mechanism of musculoskeletal symptoms during the initial phase of thyroid hormone therapy, such symptoms occur only in a small percentage of patients.

PROTEIN CATABOLISM AND LOSS OF MUSCLE MASS

Inducing tissue thyrotoxicity with excessive dosages of thyroid hormone increases synthesis and degradation of protein; degradation predominates. The patient typically has a net protein catabolism and reduced muscle mass. When thyrotoxicity is extreme, the patient usually has rapid tissue wasting. She has negative nitrogen balance, meaning that she excretes more nitrogen than she takes in. The urinary creatine elevates, and concentrations of creatinine and phosphocreatine decrease in muscle.[6,p.170][168,p.848] In addition, the circulating albumin and low-density lipoproteins are mildly reduced.[171]

Sandler et al. found that administering a high enough dosage of T₃ to humans increased the release of the amino acid alanine through gluconeogenesis. This demonstrates protein catabolism.[169] However, concurring with Du Bois,[170,p.333] Loeb wrote, "Although an increase in protein degradation thus accompanies the increased catabolism of fat and carbohydrate, it can be minimized, and indeed in some instances positive nitrogen balance can be achieved, if the thyrotoxic state is accompanied by adequate protein in the diet and a sufficient increase in caloric intake."[168,p.848]

BONE

Bone Turnover

Bone synthesis increases in hyperthyroidism due to thyroid gland disease.[91][92] Despite this, when bone is catabolic due to exposure to excess thyroid hormone, the patient's bone degrades at a faster rate than it is synthesized.[93,p.1193] Resorption by osteoclasts during hyperthyroidism due to thyroid gland disease may cause increased cortical porosity.[49] In hyperthyroidism, thyroid activity is positively correlated with osteoclastic resorption and inversely correlated with bone formation.[51] Bone minerals are mobilized, and the amount of cancellous bone and the length of osteoid seams may be decreased.[52] Because bone degradation exceeds bone synthesis, some writers have judged hyperthyroidism to be a risk factor for osteoporosis.[82] Hyperthyroidism from thyroid disease has been reported to induce osteoporosis,[141][142] and some studies have suggested that exogenous thyroid therapy in high enough dosages does the same,[113][141] at least in post-menopausal women taking too little or no exogenous estrogen.[143] Ross claimed that many patients take too much T₄, consequently have subclinical hyperthyroidism, and as a result are predisposed to osteoporosis.[146]

Increased Bone Turnover and Lost Density in Thyrotoxicosis

Overt hyperthyroidism can increase bone turnover and decrease bone density. There are exceptions, however. The hyperthyroid patient may also have osseous resistance to thyroid hormone. Korsic et al., for example, proposed that the magnitude of bone loss depends on both the serum level of thyroid hormones and the

functional state of thyroid hormone receptors in bone tissue.[185] If the patient does have osseous resistance, her bones can be expected to be less susceptible to decreases in mineral density under the influence of abnormally high circulating levels of thyroid hormone. Although a patient may not have clinically significant osseous thyroid hormone resistance, she may be on the lower end of the bell curve for thyroid hormone receptors in bone cells. This may render her less susceptible to decreases in bone mineral density with high circulating levels of thyroid hormone.

For most individuals, however, hyperthyroidism due to thyroid gland disease is a risk factor for reduced bone mineral density, especially when other factors that lower mineral density also impinge on the patient. Other factors include extremely low physical activity level and low calcium intake. A combination of these other factors and excessive thyroid hormone stimulation of bone are likely to place the patient at a significant risk for osteoporosis.

Shirota assessed biochemical markers of excess stimulation of bone and muscle in 16 patients with hyperthyroidism due to untreated Graves' disease. He compared them with 16 normal controls. The blood urea nitrogen (BUN) was significantly elevated and creatinine was significantly low in these untreated patients. As a result, the BUN/creatinine ratio was significantly elevated. Renal excretion of urea was increased by 117% and excretion of creatinine was decreased by 77%. These differences, however, were not statistically significant. After antithyroid drug therapy, levels of T₄, T₃, BUN, and creatinine, and the BUN/creatinine ratio normalized.[67]

Popelier et al. compared laboratory markers of bone turnover in 13 normal controls to 13 patients who were hyperthyroid due to Graves' disease. Hyperthyroid patients had significantly elevated serum calcium, phosphorus, alkaline phosphatase, osteocalcin, urinary calcium, and hydroxyproline. Their serum creatinine was significantly low.[43] Wakasugi et al. compared vertebral and femoral bone density with markers of bone turnover in 52 patients (20 males and 32 females) hyperthyroid due to Graves' disease. The researchers used the bone density of control subjects as the normative standard and compared the bone density of hyperthyroid patients as a percentage of the mean value. By this method, patients' vertebral bone mineral density was 92.6% of that of controls. This represents a 7.4% decrease in density. In this study, bone density inversely correlated with the levels of osteocalcin, alkaline phosphatase, and serum TSH receptor antibodies.[44]

Garnero and coworkers compared 30 control subjects to 27 hyperthyroid patients (20 women and 7 men). Twenty-four of the patients had Graves' disease, 2 had toxic multinodular goiter, and 1 had amiodarone-associated hyperthyroidism. Biochemical markers of bone formation and resorption (serum osteocalcin and bone-specific alkaline phosphatase, and urinary pyridinoline cross-link excretion) were elevated. The markers returned to normal within about a month after the hyperthyroidism was corrected.[61]

Women with active, overt hyperthyroidism had low bone mineral density of the lumbar spine, the femoral neck, and Ward's triangle. In pre-menopausal women who had been treated for hyperthyroidism or who took T_4 in dosages that did not suppress TSH levels, there was no significant decrease in bone density when compared with normal reference standards. In post-menopausal women with previous hyperthyroidism and in those taking T_4, there was a significant decrease in bone density. The greatest decrease in density was in tissues made up predominantly of trabecular bone: the lumbar spine and Ward's triangle.[19]

Studies Reporting That TSH-Suppressive Dosages of Thyroid Hormone Reduce Bone Density

Many clinicians firmly believe that even slightly TSH-suppressive dosages of exogenous thyroid hormone insure that the patient is thyrotoxic and will lose bone mineral density. Their belief is based on studies from the 1980s suggesting that TSH-suppressive dosages reduce bone density, especially in post-menopausal women.

A 1998 study by Korsic et al. provides data that falsifies the hypothesis that TSH-suppressive dosages induce significantly more bone mineral loss than do replacement dosages in post-menopausal women. The researchers' purpose was to determine whether there was a differential effect of replacement dosages and TSH-suppressive dosages of T_4 on the bone mineral density of post-menopausal women. The study included 30 post-menopausal women. Nineteen of the women had taken replacement dosages (1.22 ± 0.35 µg/kg) for 11.4 ± 7.2 years. Eleven patients had taken TSH-suppressive dosages (1.45 ± 0.71 µg/kg) for 9.5 ± 7.2 years. The investigators included 60 healthy women matched for age and menopausal status as controls. Dual-energy absorptiometry was used to measure bone mineral density at the lumbar spine (L2-L4), femoral neck, Ward's triangle and trochanter. Single-photon absorptiometry was used to measure the bone density

of the distal forearm. In women using replacement dosages, the mean TSH and thyroid hormone levels were within normal limits; in women using TSH-suppressive dosages, the mean T_3 level was significantly higher (p<0.05) than those using replacement dosages. Compared to controls, the bone mineral density at each site was significantly lower in patients taking replacement dosages. Compared to controls, density was lower in patients taking TSH-suppressive dosages, but the difference was not statistically significant. *Thus, patients taking replacement dosages had a statistically significant lower bone density than patients taking TSH-suppressive dosages.* The investigators suggested that although the use of exogenous thyroid hormone by post-menopausal women may lower bone density, the magnitude of bone loss depends on both the serum level of thyroid hormones and the functional state of thyroid hormone receptors in bone tissue. It is possible that selection bias included an imbalance of women with lower bone T_3-receptor status in the group taking TSH-suppressive dosages.[185] Regardless of the responsible mechanism, however, these results falsify the proposition that TSH-suppressive dosages of T_4 induce lower bone mineral density than replacement dosages, at least in post-menopausal women.

In 1989, whether TSH-suppressive dosages of thyroid hormone cause more loss of bone mineral density than replacement dosages was still a controversial issue.[5,p.89] More recent studies, however, have demonstrated that T_4 does not cause substantial changes in bone mass, except in post-menopausal women. In fact, some newer studies show *increased* bone mass in patients using T_4.[18] Before reviewing these new studies, I will review some of the reports typical of those showing lost bone density with TSH-suppressive thyroid hormone dosages.

In 1983, Fallon and coworkers reported osteopenia in 3 post-menopausal women taking exogenous thyroid hormone.[143] Each had elevated total T_4 levels: 12.1, 11.9, and 17.8 µg/dl (normal: 5-to-11 µg/dl). They also had low parathyroid hormone levels, suggesting decreased mobilization of calcium from bone. All had elevated serum phosphate levels and generalized demineralization of bone. In 2 patients, bone density was below 3 standard deviations from the mean. One patient had taken 0.4 mg of T_4 for 4 years, another had taken 300 mg of desiccated thyroid for 5 years, and the third had taken 240 mg of desiccated thyroid for 2 years. Only the third patient was taking estrogen. She had taken it for 12 years at 2.5 mg per day. The investigators allowed, as other authors have,[103] that estrogen deficiency may have contributed to the osteopenia, but they considered the patients' use of exogenous thyroid hormone to be the main cause of the osteopenia. Fallon did not report the patients' serum TSH levels, but it is safe to assume the levels were largely suppressed because the T_4 levels were above the upper limit of normal reference range. Fallon and his coworkers did not have the benefit of later studies showing the critical interactive role of estrogen deficiency in osteopenia-associated use of upper end dosages of thyroid hormone. They concluded, "These accumulated findings emphasize the need for careful monitoring of thyroid status in patients receiving replacement medication and adequate patient awareness, particularly in peri-menopausal and post-menopausal women, of the risk of osteopenia in conjunction with hyperthyroidism."[143,p.444]

Paul studied 31 pre-menopausal women whose TSH levels were suppressed for 5 years by T_4 therapy. He used dual-photon absorptiometry to measure the bone density in the lumbar spine, femoral trochanter, and femoral neck. He then compared the measures to those of age- and weight-matched controls. There was no difference between the two groups in lumbar vertebral density, which was normal. On the other hand, compared to control subjects, the mean bone density of the patients' femoral necks was 12.8% lower. The mean density of their femoral trochanters was lower by 10.1%. The patients also had lower TSH levels than the controls. Seventeen (55%) of the 31 patients had serum TSH values below 0.3 µU/mL. The authors stated that the TSH levels were consistent with excessive T_4 dosages. However, patients' serum T_4 and FTI levels were somewhat elevated and T_3 levels were normal.[94,p.3137] Because the T_3 measure correlates better with metabolic status, and high normal T_4 levels do not indicate thyrotoxicosis, it is questionable whether the patients were taking excessive T_4 dosages. The likelihood of selection bias in this study is high because the number of patients and controls was small. Larger selections of patients and controls may have eliminated the differences between the two groups in trochanter measures.

Ross and his colleagues studied pre-menopausal women treated with T_4 for more than 10 years. (T_4 was prescribed to shrink goitrous thyroid tissues or to prevent growth of abnormal thyroid tissue.) The researchers compared the patients with age-matched controls. The basal TSH was below 0.08 µU/mL in 23 patients. The TSH response to TRH was undetectable in 13 patients and subnormal in 10. Bone density measurements were taken with direct photon absorptiometry at the junction of the proximal ⅔ and distal ⅓ of the

nondominant radius. Patients who had taken T_4 for 10 or more years had a 9% lower bone density compared to controls.[113] The lower bone density, however, may have been due to selection bias. These patients may normally have had bone densities on the lower end of the normal bell curve. In this case, if controls had a mean bone density in the middle of the bell curve, the patients' mean bone density would have been lower even before they began using thyroid hormone.

In a later paper, Ross wrote that clearly, an asymptomatic patient with an elevated serum T_4 and T_3 and an undetectable sensitive TSH has "subclinical hyperthyroidism" and is at risk for developing physiological abnormalities. Yet he also wrote, "Because the clinical consequences of the physiologic changes associated with subclinical hyperthyroidism may be minimal or perhaps inconsequential, one should not withhold suppressive therapy from a patient with a clear indication for suppression of serum TSH (as in a patient with abnormal thyroid gland tissue growth)."[146,p.1228]

Taelman reported that compared to controls, the forearm bones of pre-menopausal euthyroid (meaning normal thyroid function tests) goitrous women had a 5% lower bone density. The patients had undergone long-term T_3 therapy.[114] Taelman did not assess hip and vertebral bone density, and he did not compare the bone densities of the patients to either homologous controls or to their own pre-treatment densities.

It would have been helpful if these investigators had classified pre-menopausal women according to types of activities they engaged in and their activity levels. Inactivity may predispose to bone loss, and sufficient activity of the right types may protect against bone loss. A low intake or absorption of calcium may also result in reduced bone density in pre-menopausal women, just as low estrogen levels may in post-menopausal women. Paul et al. were the only researchers in the above studies who matched patients and controls for non-use of calcium supplements.[94]

Studies Reporting No Adverse Bone Density Effects

Considerable evidence has accumulated indicating that the risk of decreased bone mineral density with thyroid hormone therapy has been exaggerated. The risk of osteoporosis has been exaggerated in the extreme.

In a review of the literature, Bartalena and Pinchera noted that overt hyperthyroidism, as in untreated Graves' disease, is a well-known risk factor for osteoporosis. They also noted that studies in the late 1980s suggested that T_4-treated patients have reduced bone density, especially of cortical bone in post-menopausal women. "More recent studies," the authors continued, "have failed to show any substantial T_4-related change in bone mass. Taken together, the evidence from the literature suggests that TSH-suppressive therapy with T_4 is, if well-controlled, probably not associated with significant loss of bone mass, at least in pre-menopausal women.[18]

In 1990, Chabert-Orsini tested 37 women ages 40-to-62 who had very slight subclinical hyperthyroidism (suppressed TSH levels with normal thyroid hormone levels) for a prolonged time. The aim was to determine whether the women had suffered adverse bone effects. The women had been slightly hyperthyroid from 3.2-to-12.8 years. Thirty-six of the 37 women showed normal vertebral bone density.[140]

In 1991, Greenspan et al. reported testing the hypothesis that long-term T_4 use in which the free T_4 index was maintained within physiologic limits has minimal impact on vertebral and femoral bone mineral density in both pre-menopausal and post-menopausal women. The researchers measured hip integral and spinal trabecular and integral bone densities in 28 premenopausal and 28 post-menopausal women. The women had been taking T_4 for a median of 12 and 15 years, respectively. The T_4 dosage had been titrated to keep the free T_4 index within the normal range. Premenopausal and post-menopausal women had slightly lower hip bone density than expected for their ages. However, when the researchers excluded women with previously treated Graves' disease (4 in each group), differences in hip bone density compared to age-matched controls were no longer seen. Greenspan et al. noted that there was only a weak and generally insignificant relationship between thyroid hormone status and bone density. Age was more significantly correlated with bone density at the spine and hip than thyroid status. The researchers wrote, "These data provide the first supportive evidence that long-term L-thyroxine therapy that maintains the [free T_4 index] in the physiologic range is associated with a statistically significant, but clinically minimal, decrement in spinal and hip bone density in both pre-menopausal and post-menopausal women. The decrement at the hip was entirely due to the inclusion of patients with treated Graves' disease. Thus, the changes in bone density in women receiving long-term L-thyroxine therapy are minimal at most and should not be a contraindication to therapy."[152]

In a well-controlled follow-up study, researchers found no adverse effect on bone mineral density even with doses of T_4 that suppressed TSH levels.[8] Salmon,[9] Fish,[10] Pearce,[11] Bayer,[12] and their coauthors reported that T_4 dosages formerly thought to be harmful (those that raise the T_4 level or suppress the TSH level) actually are not. Salmon and coauthors wrote that a wider margin of safety exists in using T_4 than previously believed.[9,p.573]

Volpé, in 1989, evaluated 100 patients taking T_4 and 100 healthy control subjects for clinical evidence of bone disease. The patients had taken 0.2 mg of T_4 per day for 20 years and had suppressed TSH levels. Volpé found no difference between the two groups.[5,p.89]

Whybrow conducted an open psychiatric study of 11 patients (1 man and 10 women, 9 of whom were pre-menopausal) with rapid cyclic psychiatric disorders (meaning more than four episodes a year). Patients took TSH-suppressive dosages of T_4. The dosages were about 150% of those usually permitted. Patients experienced a reduction in the amplitude and frequency of manic and depressive episodes. Whybrow wrote, "Careful evaluation of possible side effects like osteoporosis revealed surprisingly an even higher bone density in treated patients."[23]

Leb and colleagues published a review of the effects on bone of TSH-suppressive and non-suppressive thyroid hormone doses. They wrote that some risk factors for thyroid hormone-induced osteopenia are generally accepted. These include long-standing, clinically-manifested hyperthyroidism (a condition that early diagnosis and proper treatment have made very rare today), old age, menopause, and total thyroidectomy. The researchers concluded, however, "Thyroid hormone therapy (whether TSH-suppressive or not) has not been proven so far to lead to manifest osteoporosis."[151]

One of the most sophisticated studies dealing with the question of bone loss and fracture risk with TSH-suppressive doses of T_4 was conducted by De Rosa et al. They studied 50 Caucasian women, 25 premenopausal and 25 post-menopausal. The researchers matched the patients with 50 control subjects according to age, sex, body mass index, menopausal status, and thyroid diseases. Patients and controls were also evaluated for minor contributions to bone loss such as heredity and lifestyle factors. All the women had nontoxic goiters and were treated with slightly TSH-suppressive doses of T_4. Dosages ranged from 50-to-200 µg/day. Patients had subnormal serum TSH levels and normal thyroid hormone levels. De Rosa wrote, "No difference in bone mineral density or biochemical markers was found between patients and controls." The researchers found no relationship between bone density or turnover and T_4 usage. Bone density and turnover, however, were significantly influenced by menopausal status. They concluded, "Our study suggests that slightly suppressive L-thyroxine administration in nontoxic goitre can activate bone turnover but constitutes neither an actual risk factor for bone loss nor, consequently, for osteoporotic fractures."[27,p.503] They added, ". . . in clinical practice, L-T_4 administration in slightly suppressive doses does not significantly affect bone mineral density and, consequently, should not involve the risk of osteoporotic fractures either in pre- or post-menopausal women with nontoxic goitre."[27,p.507]

Schneider and colleagues compared 33 elderly men (ages 50-to-98) who had taken a thyroxine-equivalent dose of 130 µg for an average of 15.5 years with men who did not use thyroid hormone. The authors reported, "Bone density . . . did not differ according to thyroid hormone type, duration of use, or use of suppressive doses adjusted for body weight. Long-term thyroid hormone use was not associated with adverse effects on bone mineral density in men."[21]

Faber and Galloe noted the reported association of T_4 treatment with reduced serum TSH levels and reduced bone mass and a potential for premature development of osteoporosis. They also noted that several recent studies failed to document detrimental osseous effects. To further assess the possible adverse effects, they performed a meta-analysis based on 13 published reports. Women using T_4 and having suppressed TSH levels were compared with control subjects. In the studies, researchers obtained cross-sectional measures of bone mass in the distal forearm, femoral neck, or lumbar spine. Because estrogen protects against bone loss, the women were categorized as pre- and post-menopausal. Based on the meta-analysis, the researchers concluded that a pre-menopausal woman 39.6 years old taking 164 µg of T_4 per day for 8.5 years, resulting in a suppressed TSH level, had 2.67% less bone mass than matched controls. This percentage corresponds to an excess annual bone loss of 0.31% after 8.5 years of treatment.[183] This is not a clinically significant reduction in bone mass.

Franklyn et al., noting the conflicting reports of the effects of T_4 on bone mineral density, hypothesized that the results were in part due to researchers including in studies patients who have a variety of thyroid disorders. To test the hypothesis, they studied the influence of previous thyroid history and long-term T_4 treatment on the bone density of 148 females. They

included patients who had undergone radioiodine therapy for thyrotoxicosis and those who had not. They also included formerly thyrotoxic patients who had not subsequently used T_4. No significant differences were found in femoral or lumbar spine bone density between matched controls and (1) pre-menopausal and post-menopausal patients with a history of thyrotoxicosis and subsequent use of T_4 or (2) post-menopausal patients with a history of thyrotoxicosis but no subsequent use of T_4. Post-menopausal patients had the lowest bone density at all sites. Bone density at all anatomical sites was lower in post-menopausal patients who previously had thyrotoxicosis and did or did not take T_4. In those post-menopausal patients who did take T_4, the density of the femoral trochanter was reduced 3.9% (P<0.05) and of the lumbar spine was reduced 5.6%-to-8.5% (P=0.01). In post-menopausal patients who did not take T_4, the density of the femoral trochanter was reduced 3.9% (P<0.01), of the lumbar spine was reduced 8.5% (P=0.01), and of Ward's triangle was reduced 5.6% (P<0.05). No relationship was found between normal and reduced TSH levels and bone mineral density. In addition, in none of the patient groups was there a correlation between bone density and duration of T_4 therapy, dosage of T_4, or serum free T_4 or TSH level. Franklyn et al. concluded, "Thyroxine therapy alone does not represent a significant risk factor for loss of bone mineral density but there is a risk of bone loss in post-menopausal (but not pre-menopausal) females with a previous history of thyrotoxicosis treated with radioiodine."[184]

Fowler et al. assessed the effect of TSH-suppressive dosages of T_4 on the bone mineral density of 31 treated hypothyroid women. An average of 22.7 months after the initial measurements, the researchers repeated the measurements of bone density of the lumbar spines and femoral necks of the 7 patients with the lowest value. The patients' T_4 dosages were based on clinical assessment. Serum T_3 levels were kept within the normal range; TSH levels were kept within the normal range or suppressed. The patients had taken replacement dosages of T_4 for a mean of 12.7 years. TSH levels were normal in 10 patients (⅓) and suppressed in 21 (⅔). Fifteen patients had formerly had thyrotoxicosis. The investigators compared the bone density of patients with normal TSH levels with that of patients with suppressed TSH levels. They also compared the density of those with and without a past history of thyrotoxicosis. None of the patients had pathological fractures. The investigators wrote, "One had a Z value for the femoral neck of -1.6, denoting early but definite osteoporosis, and five had borderline osteoporosis with Z values for one or another site between -1.1 and -1.5." However, none of the 7 patients with the lowest bone densities had had a significant change in density when the researchers repeated the measurements. The difference in Z values between patients with normal and suppressed TSH levels was not significant for the femoral neck (p = 0.28) or the lumbar spine (p = 0.68). The investigators wrote, "A past history of thyrotoxicosis had a greater effect on [bone mineral density] for both sites than thyrotrophin suppression, but again the difference between those with and without a past history of thyrotoxicosis was significant neither for the lumbar spine (p = 0.18) nor for the femoral neck (p = 0.34)." They concluded that compared to patients with normal TSH levels and no history of thyrotoxicosis, the combination of TSH suppression and a history of thyrotoxicosis did not significantly reduce the bone density of the lumbar spine (p = 0.38) or femoral neck (p = 0.30).[157]

Use of Exogenous Thyroid Hormone Not Correlated with an Increase in Fracture Risk

In a 1994 review, Ross stated that women with subclinical hyperthyroidism due to the use of exogenous T_4 had reduced density of trabecular bone and, even more so, of cortical bone. Even so, he noted that subclinical hyperthyroidism has not been shown to increase the risk of fractures.[22] In fact, an increase in osteoporotic fractures in patients using T_4 has not been reported, either in pre- or post-menopausal women[108] or in patients with normal or suppressed TSH levels.[109] It is clear at this time that fractures are not a feature of the natural history of treated hypothyroid patients.[157]

Assessment for Adverse Effects of Exogenous Thyroid Hormone on Bone

In assessing the effects of exogenous thyroid hormone on the bone density of fibromyalgia patients, it is important to understand the significance of various forms of assessment and the proper strategy for their use. Many patients undergoing thyroid hormone therapy have slightly abnormal levels of biochemical markers of bone turnover. The relevant question in these cases is whether these markers have any practical clinical significance. Except for patients who have densitometry results showing bone density near or within the fracture risk range, the answer is usually no. Abnormal biochemical markers indicate bone turnover

that is typically not reflected in abnormal densitometry results. The clinician should remember that even with reports of lowered bone density in patients taking thyroid hormone, there are *no* reports of reduced bone density in exogenous thyroid hormone users resulting in an increase in osteoporotic fractures. This is true of both pre- and post-menopausal women[108] and patients with normal and suppressed TSH levels.[109] If reduced bone density in such patients does not appear to result in an increase in fractures, it is highly improbable that the oft-found slightly abnormal biochemical markers[63] are of any clinical significance.

Except in women at risk of osteoporotic fracture, bone densitometry results showing lower than normal bone mineral density compared to age-matched controls should not necessarily prompt a reduction in thyroid hormone dosage. Lower than normal density for a patient may be genetically normal for that patient, or the patient may never have acquired peak bone mineral density earlier in life.[111][112]

Patients who show low bone mineral density should undergo densitometry at intervals to determine whether density is progressively decreasing. *Worsening of biochemical markers with repeated testing may indicate progressively decreasing bone density, but only with densitometry can the clinician determine a patient's probable risk for fractures.* Densitometry is of major value in predicting fractures of the proximal femur and vertebrae. Orwoll and colleagues report, for example, that in women 65 and older, each decrease in density of the femoral neck by one standard deviation increases the age-adjusted risk for hip fracture by 2.6 times.[38]

Faber conducted a study of pre-menopausal women with nontoxic goiter and low TSH levels. According to convention, these lab test results classify the women as having spontaneous subclinical hyperthyroidism. Markers of bone turnover were within normal limits. During follow-up (from 8-to-108 months), serum alkaline phosphatase and urinary hydroxyproline levels were increased. However, bone mass was not decreased in the distal forearm or lumbar spine.[60] The finding of normal bone density highlights the importance of using multiple tests, especially bone densitometry, to assess the possible adverse osseous effects of exogenous thyroid hormone. Bone densitometry may not confirm the turnover indicated by the biochemical markers.[60] The negative densitometry result renders the positive biochemical markers clinically insignificant except for patients who were osteoporotic and at risk for fractures *before* beginning the use of thyroid hormone.

Timing of Testing for Bone Turnover

The timing of bone densitometry testing is important; the time of testing may give variable results. Evidence suggests that in hypothyroid women treated with appropriate dosages of T_4, bone mineral density may decrease during the first 12 months. Ribot and coauthors wrote, however, ". . . the fact that an increased fracture rate has not been documented in long-term treated patients, and the results of our cross-sectional study, suggest that this bone mass reduction could be transient and reversible due to new bone formation at the end of the resorptive sequence."[138,p.143]

Coindre et al. performed a histomorphometric study on biopsied undecalcified bone specimens from primary hypothyroid patients treated with a thyroid hormone formulation that contained 20 μg of T_3 and 100 μg (0.1 mg) of T_4. In the first month of hormone replacement, the patients had osteoclastic hyperresorption in trabecular and cortical bone, despite the small doses of thyroid hormone. At 6 months, the bone resorption persisted, and there was a loss of trabecular and cortical bone. Increases in urinary calcium and hydroxyproline were insignificant but suggested bone hyperresorption. The researchers stated that bone hyperremodeling was the cause of the bone loss and was similar to the hyperremodeling of hyperthyroidism. They pointed out, however, that "our patients did not exhibit obvious clinical or biological signs of excessive thyroid replacement."[7,p.53]

Coindre and his associates suggested that one mechanism underlying the bone hyperremodeling is hypersensitivity to thyroid hormone in hypothyroid patients. They wrote, "Trabecular hyperresorption from as early as the seventh day of replacement with small doses of thyroid hormone would suggest this, at least at the beginning of treatment." They continued by writing that this hypersensitivity would disappear or diminish after a time.[7,p.53]

A study by Tremollieres and colleagues indicates that transient hyperresorption may persist from 1-to-2 years. They assessed changes in femoral and vertebral bone density over 2 years in 4 men and 5 women taking thyroid hormone for hypothyroidism. Clinically, none of the patients appeared to be overdosed, and the free T_4, total and free T_3, and ultrasensitive TSH were within normal range. In the first year, dual photon absorptiometry showed significantly reduced bone density of the lumbar vertebrae (-5.4%), femoral neck (-7%), and trochanter (-7.3%). Accompanying the bone loss was an early increase in osteocalcin, the urinary calcium/creatinine ratio, and sex hormone-binding globulin, indicating increased bone turnover.

In the second year, however, patients completely recovered their initial values of vertebral and trochanteric bone density. Density of the neck of the femur, however, remained significantly lower than initial density. The authors wrote that the patients' "transitory" bone loss might result from tissue hyperthyroidism and/or temporary "hypersensitivity" of hypothyroid bone to thyroid hormone.[64] The influence of this transitory bone loss on the subsequent risk of fracture is not known.

The result of this study indicates that other studies showing that the use of exogenous thyroid hormone causes bone loss may reflect a temporary state rather than a static osteopenia. Certainly, intermittent monitoring with densitometry and possibly laboratory markers is warranted. All things considered, however, each patient should be assessed on an individual basis in view of the risk-to-benefit ratio for her.

Preventing Bone Loss

The possibility of osteoporosis in post-menopausal women should not be neglected. Osteoporosis is a widespread public health problem resulting in some 1.2 million fractures each year. The bones fractured are the vertebrae (538,000 cases), hip (227,000 cases), the distal forearm (172,000 cases), and bones in other limbs (283,000).[82,p.1676] Orwoll and associates wrote that in older women, osteoporotic fractures are a major cause of illness and death.[38,p.187] The spine and proximal femur are the most common sites of fracture, and the fracture rate exponentially increases in later life.[90] Riggs and Melton estimated that 1/3 of women over 65 will have vertebral fractures,[82,p.1676] and by extreme old age, 1/3 of women and 1/6 of men will have had a hip fracture.[83]

In women, normal plasma estrogens play a physiological role in preventing osteoporosis.[24] In post-menopausal women, estrogen use is associated with increased bone mineral density.[38] Special consideration should be given to post-menopausal women with previous hyperthyroidism who were treated with radioiodine therapy. Their bone densities tend to be lower whether they have used T_4 or not. Periodic densitometry is advisable, and estrogen supplementation should be considered. Post-menopausal women with previous hyperthyroidism treated with surgery appear to be at less risk for bone loss.[56]

Several lifestyle factors are associated with increased bone mineral density, and may militate against lost density in patients who must use high thyroid hormone dosages to remain symptom-free. These factors include dietary and supplemental calcium, adequate estrogen exposure in women, sufficient activity level, and muscle strength.[38]

Orwoll and coworkers studied 7963 ambulatory non-black women ages 65 years or older. They reported the following regarding factors that were negatively (inversely) associated with bone density: advancing age was negatively associated at all sites measured; tobacco use was inversely associated with femoral neck density; and a history of hip fracture in a mother, sister, or brother was associated with lower density of the spine and femoral neck. The use of glucocorticoids was associated with lowered spine but not femoral neck density.[38,p.187] This corresponds to the report of bone loss with the prolonged use of only 5 mg of prednisone daily.[110]

Patients can manipulate some of these risk factors for their benefit. For example, they can stop smoking cigarettes. In the Orwoll study, the amount of reduced density associated with smoking was only -0.1-to- -0.2% of the mean adjusted for age and weight. This is a small percentage, but the cumulative impact may be critical for some women who, because of involutional osteoporosis, are already close to or within the fracture risk range.

Several factors were positively associated with bone density, some of which can be used to the advantage of women who will actively take part in preemptive protection of bone density.[38] The strongest association with density at all sites was weight. This was true regardless of age, estrogen status, or any other variable. Weight accounted for 9%-to-21% of the difference between subjects. A 10-kg increase in weight (weight *per se* and not body size) was associated with a 6% higher density of the spine and femoral neck. Other researchers have reported this association.[97][98][99] The proposed mechanisms relating higher bone density to higher body weight are mechanical loading,[100] the metabolic concomitants of higher-weight bodies, and the diet necessary to maintain the weight in pre-menopausal women but not men.[101][102] The investigators recommended that patients avoid excessive thinness.[38,p.193]

Also positively associated with high density were early menarche, late menopause, past and current use of oral estrogen and oral contraceptives, current calcium intake from all dietary sources or supplements, vitamin D intake, and use of diuretics, especially thiazides. Muscle strength and bone density were anatomically related. Grip strength, for example, was positively associated with higher radial density, and quadriceps strength was positively associated with femoral density. Bone density may increase directly by

loading (weight bearing and impact) during exercise,[137] and indirectly through muscle tension.[38,pp.193-194] Higher activity level during the preceding year was associated with higher density at all sites. Walking speed was positively associated with the density at the femoral neck. And though heavy alcohol intake has adverse effects on bone,[95][96] these researchers found that moderate alcohol consumption was positively associated with higher bone density.

The relative impact of these different positive factors is uncertain. Interestingly, Orwoll and colleagues[38,p.192] found that factors not associated with spine or femoral bone density included progestin use, antacid use, childbirth, history of breast feeding, and past hyperthyroidism. *Also, past or present use of thyroid hormone was not negatively associated with bone density.*[38,p.190]

Measures to Recover Lost Bone Density

In addition to lifestyle measures patients can take to militate against lost bone density, such as exercise and maintenance of adequate weight, patients can use a number of agents to stop loss of bone density. A new series of drugs, calcium, calcitonin, and estrogen can inhibit osteoclasts. Sodium fluoride, low dosage I-34 synthetic fragment of parathyroid hormone, combined calcitonin and oral phosphase, and anabolic steroids all stimulate osteoblasts.

Use of Drugs That Inhibit Bone Resorption. Riggs and Melton wrote that antiresorptive agents do not substantially increase bone mass. They do, however, stop bone loss and weakening by stabilizing bone structure. Through this mechanism, the agents decrease the incidence of fractures.[82,p.1683] Studies have shown that the vertebral fracture rate is reduced some 50% with calcium use, 69% with vitamin D or $1,25(OH)_2D$ use, and 78% by use of calcium and estrogen.[105][106]

In one study, hypothyroid patients using thyroid hormone showed a temporary bone loss during the first year. In the second year, vertebrae and trochanters but not femor necks recovered normal density. The researchers wrote that because of this transitory loss, detection of demineralization prior to treatment may justify the patient's temporary use of an antiosteoclastic agent.[64]

Kung and Ng found that in rats, the antiresorptive agent cyclical sodium etidronate prevents bone loss induced by high dosages of exogenous T_4. They proposed that etiodronate may prevent osteoporosis in patients using TSH-suppressive doses of T_4.[25]

Alendronate has been shown to inhibit osteoclastic bone resorption in late post-menopausal osteoporotic women.[53] The drug reduced markers to the normal pre-menopausal range. Pamidronate also suppressed bone resorption in normal men taking 100 μg of T_3 per day. By contrast, a marker showed bone resorption in men taking placebos with the T_3.[54] Britto reported that salmon calcitonin inhibited osteoclast activity stimulated by T_3.[57]

Calcium. Calcium decreases bone resorption. Like estrogen, it acts primarily by decreasing activation of new bone-remodeling units, probably by decreasing secretion of parathyroid hormone.[84] Treatment with calcium is safe except in patients with hypercalcemia or nephrolithiasis.[85]

One research group reported that calcium carbonate increased radial shaft bone density in post-menopausal osteoporosis patients.[116] Another reported that only calcium citrate stabilized the condition.[117,p.407][118]

Blumsohn found that taking 1000 mg of calcium at 8 am had no significant effect in decreasing bone resorption, but taking it at 11 pm did have a significant effect.[55] Evening calcium supplementation suppressed the nocturnal increase in parathyroid hormone and markers of bone resorption. This indicates that evening calcium supplementation suppresses the circadian rhythm of bone loss which occurs during bed rest.[59]

Calcitonin. Calcitonin inhibits bone resorption upon attaching to calcitonin receptors on osteoclasts, thus directly affecting the cells. Patients tolerate calcitonin well, but it is expensive, must be administered parenterally, and some patients become resistant to it.[104]

Estrogen. Coindre and coauthors indicate that the role of thyroid hormone in the genesis of osteoporosis is of concern in post-menopausal women.[7,p.53] The reason is that these women are more affected by involutional osteoporosis, and as Meunier has pointed out,[81] their vertebrae may not be far from the fracture threshold.[7,p.53]

Harvey and his coworkers found that many pre-menopausal women use enough exogenous T_4 to cause subnormal TSH levels. But the investigators found no evidence of bone collagen breakdown in their study subjects. They suggested that pre-menopausal women's endogenous estrogen protects their bones from degrading.[93,p.1193]

Limanova studied men and pre- and post-menopausal women using TSH-suppressive doses of thyroid hormone. Vertebral bone density and biochemical markers of bone formation were elevated only in post-menopausal women. He indicated that biochemical markers for bone formation and resorption negatively

correlated with TSH levels. He concluded that there is no safe suppressive dose of thyroid hormone for post-menopausal women.[58]

Taelman and colleagues reported that pre-menopausal women taking thyroid hormone had 5% lower forearm bone density than controls. Post-menopausal women taking thyroid hormone, however, had a 20% lower density. Although there were methodological problems with this study, the large difference between the bone densities of pre- and post-menopausal women suggests that it is prudent for post-menopausal women taking thyroid hormone to also take some form of estrogen and for their clinicians to monitor for changes in bone density.[114]

Stall and associates studied post-menopausal women who, over a 2-year period, took T_4 for hypothyroidism but did not take estrogen or other steroids. The dosages of T_4 were enough to reduce the women's serum TSH to subnormal levels. The researchers found that the patients' rates of vertebral bone loss increased. They concluded, "When compared with women without known thyroid disease, post-menopausal women who receive thyroid hormone replacement therapy and have low TSH levels have an accelerated rate of loss of bone mineral density from the spine and a trend toward greater bone loss at the radius and hip."[139,p.269]

Harvey and colleagues tested post-menopausal women taking enough T_4 to reduce their serum TSH to subnormal levels but who were not taking estrogen supplements.[93,p.1194] These women's urine contained an increased amount of bone collagen breakdown products. The investigators concluded that bone collagen breakdown is increased in post-menopausal women using TSH-suppressive dosages of T_4 but not taking supplemental estrogen.

Schneider and coworkers conducted a study of the effect of long-term use of thyroid hormone on bone density and the protective effects of estrogen involving women ages 50-to-98. The researchers compared the bone density of 196 women who had taken thyroxine for an average of 20.4 years with 795 women not using thyroxine. They reported that women taking 200 μg (0.2 mg) or more per day had significantly lower density at the midshaft radius and hip compared to woman taking less than 200 μg. Women who took 1.6 μg/kg (for a 120 lb woman, this is 87.27 μg or 0.087 mg of thyroxine) or more had more bone loss than women who took less than 1.6 μg/kg. These findings were independent of age, body mass, smoking status, and use of thiazides, corticosteroids, and estrogen. Women who took thyroxine (1.6 μg/kg or more) and estrogen had a higher bone density at all bone sites measured than women taking thyroxine without estrogen. Women who took thyroxine and estrogen had bone densities equivalent to women who took only estrogen. The authors wrote, "Long-term thyroid hormone use at thyroxine-equivalent doses of 1.6 μg/kg or greater was associated with significant osteopenia at the ultradistal radius, midshaft radius, hip, and lumbar spine. Estrogen use appears to negate thyroid hormone-associated loss of bone density in post-menopausal women."[20]

Bone Formation Stimulation

Agents that stimulate osteoblastic proliferation and new bone formation, thereby reducing fracture risk, include sodium fluoride,[86][115][116] low dosage I-34 synthetic fragment of parathyroid hormone,[87] combined calcitonin and oral phosphase,[88] and anabolic steroids.[89]

Riggs and Melton wrote that sodium fluoride, which directly stimulates osteoblasts, has been studied most. Dosages of 40-to-80 mg per day increase the density of the trabecular bone of the axial skeleton. They do not, however, increase density of cortical bone in the appendicular bones. The patient should simultaneously take calcium while taking sodium fluoride to minimize defects in mineralization that occur with the sole use of sodium fluoride. The use of these two agents together strengthens bone and reduces fractures by 64%. When estrogen is also used, the fracture rate decreases by 94%.[82,p.1683]

The minimal effective dosage of sodium fluoride should be used because excessive exposure may cause abnormal bone formation, microfractures, and gastric bleeding.[115][116] A high dosage of plain sodium fluoride significantly increased the vertebral bone density, but the spinal fracture rate remained the same. Microfractures and fractures of the appendicular bone increased.[116]

To avoid this outcome with plain sodium fluoride, Pak and coworkers used a cyclic, intermittent lower dose of less bioavailable, slow-release sodium fluoride and continuous calcium citrate supplementation. They compared the effects of these agents (25 mg sodium fluoride and 400 mg bid calcium citrate) with those of a placebo in women with post-menopausal osteoporosis. The fluoride and calcium group had a lower individual vertebral fracture rate than the placebo group (0.064±0.182 compared to 0.205±0.297; P=0.002), and a higher fracture-free rate (85.4% compared with 56.9%; P=0.001). The fluoride group had no change in radial shaft bone density, and recurrent spinal fracture rate did not differ between groups. But femoral neck

density of the fluoride group increased by 2.38%-to-3.33% per year. L2-L4 bone mass substantially increased in the fluoride group by 4%-to-5% per year for 4 years. Neither group had microfractures nor gastric ulcers, and the frequency of minor side effects were similar in the two groups. Of the fluoride group, 9.3% of patients had minor gastrointestinal symptoms, as did 7.1% of placebo patients. Minor musculoskeletal symptoms were experienced by 11.1% of fluoride patients and 14.3% of placebo patients.[117]

Pak et al. wrote that the benefits from slow-release sodium fluoride resulted from both the delayed release of fluoride, its intermittent withdrawal, and supplementation with calcium citrate. The calcium citrate apparently accommodated the increased need for calcium during fluoride-induced stimulation of bone formation. The overall effects of the treatment were sustained formation of new, normally mineralized bone stimulated by sodium fluoride, and reduction of bone resorption by calcium citrate through its inhibition of parathyroid hormone secretion.[117,p.406]

Use of T₃ in Combination with Osteoclast Inhibitors to Stimulate Bone Remodeling in Osteoporosis

T_3 can be used as an activator of bone remodeling in osteoporosis. Hasling and coworkers had patients take 100-to-160 μg of T_3 for 1 week and monitored various measures for 10 weeks. Bone resorption by osteoclasts increased during the first week. This was evident from the increase in serum calcium and osteocalcin, and from the renal excretion of calcium, phosphate, and hydroxyproline. From weeks 6-to-8, serum alkaline phosphatase also increased. This pattern indicates that the T_3 activates bone remodeling and initiates bone resorption by osteoclasts that is followed by bone formation by osteoblasts. The sequence of events is in accordance with the timing shown by bone histomorphometry. The authors argued that osteopenic states, as in osteoporosis, may be treated by using T_3 combined with osteoclast-inhibiting agents such as calcitonin and diphosphates to selectively suppress bone resorption.[107]

Potential Adverse Osseous Effects of Ibuprofen

The female patient at risk for osteoporosis should be aware that ibuprofen intake may have adverse osseous effects. Sibonga et al. found that in female rats, ovariectomy increased radial bone growth, lowered the serum 17β-estradiol level, reduced uterine weight, and decreased the cancellous bone area of the tibial metaphysis. In both ovariectomized and sham-operated rats, ibuprofen did not change the 17β-estradiol level or uterine weight, but it reduced radial bone growth and cancellous bone area of the tibial metaphysis. Tamoxifen (a tissue-selective estrogen agonist) and 17β-estradiol prevent cancellous osteopenia. Ibuprofen completely blocked this preventive effect of tamoxifen and partially blocked the effect of 17β-estradiol. Ibuprofen also inhibited uterine growth in response to estrogen. The researchers concluded that in the female rat, ibuprofen blocks selective estrogen receptor-mediated activities.[181]

HEART

Excessive thyroid hormone stimulation of the cardiovascular regulatory system can have disastrous consequences. The rare patient may have severe adverse cardiovascular effects from dosages that are innocuous to most patients. Because of the possibility of idiosyncratic susceptibility to adverse cardiovascular effects from relatively small dosages, the clinician should be ever vigilant for indications of adverse effects. However, the evidence indicates that common warnings of the potential risks to the average patient have been exaggerated.

Some thyroidologists, for example, presume without substantiating evidence that cardiac physiological variations associated with subclinical or overt hyperthyroidism are harmful to patients. Some of the reported variations are dubious because the studies in which they occurred were methodologically faulty. Jennings et al. reported that systolic time intervals were reduced in T_4-treated patients who had high mean free T_4 and normal mean T_3 levels.[2] Franklyn and Sheppard challenged the conclusions of Jennings et al., pointing out inconsistencies and inadequate controls.[3] Volpé also criticized the conclusions. He wrote that the Jennings et al. study did not have adequate controls. He also pointed out that the researchers incorrectly discussed metabolic disturbance in terms of systolic time intervals. Of most importance, Volpé added that even if study patients' systolic time intervals were reduced, this does not appear to have any clinical correlation.[5,p.89] This last criticism also applies to the results reported by Tseng and colleagues. They measured systolic time intervals directly from aortic and mitral valve echocardiographic tracings. They reported that patients with both subclinical and overt hyperthyroidism had a significantly shortened mean isovolu-

metric contraction time, pre-ejection period, and left ventricular ejection time.[155]

Do these variations forebode disastrous cardiovascular consequences? When a patient's well-being is at stake, we should err on the side of caution. This does not necessarily mean, however, that we should restrict the patient's dosage of thyroid hormone so as to avoid cardiac physiological variations that appear to have no adverse consequences. In some cases, restricting patients on this basis may mean subjecting them to adverse cardiovascular effects from inadequate thyroid hormone regulation of lipid-metabolizing and cardiovascular-regulating systems (see subsection below titled "Harm from Untreated and Undertreated Hypothyroidism: Heart"). For an effective and safe therapeutic outcome, the clinician must base decisions regarding thyroid hormone dosage on the *individual* patient's health status and tissue responses. After initially establishing the patient's thyroid status, the clinician should not base dosage decisions on thyroid function laboratory test results. Such results provide information only about the response of the pituitary and thyroid glands to the current thyroid hormone dosage, but they provide no information whatsoever about the response of cardiac tissue to the dosage.

Adverse Cardiovascular Effects Potentially Induced by Thyrotoxicosis

The potential cardiovascular symptoms of hyperthyroidism include palpitations, angina pectoris, and dyspnea on exertion; and orthopnea or paroxysmal nocturnal dyspnea.[29] Some patients with overt hyperthyroidism have associated tachyarrhythmias[30] or dysrhythmias.[34,p.142] In elderly patients with apathetic hyperthyroidism, the only clinical manifestation of hyperthyroidism may be atrial fibrillation or congestive heart failure.[29] Among the potential adverse cardiac effects of thyrotoxicosis, Klein and Levey listed 8 that occur with high frequency[190] (see Table 4.4.2).

One group reported a significantly increased mean nocturnal heart rate and a lesser daytime increase in patients taking T_4. The patients' thyroid hormone levels were within the normal range, but their TSH levels did not respond to TRH injections.[4] The reduced TSH response to TRH indicates some degree of thyrotroph suppression. This study deserves closer evaluation; I have read one-sentence references to it that potentially leave the reader with the assumption that the statistically significant increase in nocturnal heart rate was clinically significant. Patients' heart rates were recorded continuously throughout the 24-

hour cycle both before and during their use of T_4. Patients weighing less than 137.5 lbs (62.5 kg) took 0.15 mg (150 μg) of T_4, and patients weighing more than this amount took 0.20 mg (200 μg). According to the investigators, the increased heart rate was recognition by the heart that thyroid hormone levels were inappropriately high.[4,p.515] It is arguable, however, whether the increases in heart rate were of any clinical importance. The mean increase in nocturnal heart rate was 7.1±0.7 bpm (mean maximum increase was 9±2.1 and mean minimum was 5±0.9). The mean increase in the daytime rate was 4.0±0.8 bpm (mean maximum was 4±1.3, and mean minimum was 2.4±0.7).[4,p.514] From the graphed data in the published paper, it appears that at 12:00 pm and 7:30 am the mean heart rate reached 90 bpm, but never reached tachycardia (100 bpm). The pattern of changes in mean heart rate throughout the 24-hour cycle before and during the patients' use of T_4 was virtually identical.

Table 4.4.2. Eight high-frequency cardiac effects of thyrotoxicosis.*

CARDIAC EFFECT	FREQUENCY
Tachycardia	95%
Palpitations	85%
Widened pulse pressure	75%
Hyperdynamic precordium	75%
Exercise intolerance	65%
Cardiac flow murmurs	50%
Dyspnea on exertion	45%
Atrial fibrillation	10%-15%

*After Klein, I. and Levey, G.S.: The cardiovascular system in thyrotoxicosis. In *Werner and Ingbar's The Thyroid: A Fundamental and Clinical Text*, 7th edition. Edited by L.P. Braverman and R.D. Utiger, Philadelphia, Lippincott-Raven Publishers, 1996.[190,p.609]

Patients under my care have typically shown similar increases in heart rate after beginning thyroid hormone therapy. The heart rate in many of these patients has tended to be highest for a period of days or weeks after they begin the use of thyroid hormone therapy; after this period, the rate has tended to decrease between 5 bpm and 10 bpm. This phenomenon may be an example of transient tissue hyper-responsiveness in patients just beginning to use thyroid hormone after prolonged understimulation by thyroid hormone. (Tremollieres et al. reported this apparent phenomenon in

bone.[64]) Rather than harming the patients, however, it is likely that the increased heart rate contributed to their improved health status.[72][73]

That such increases in heart rate are innocuous is indicated by the lack of evidence of harmful effects during the long history of patients taking dosages much higher than the currently approved replacement dosages.[11] Volpé tested 100 patients who had taken 0.2 mg of T_4 per day for 20 years and had suppressed TSH levels. He compared them to an age- and sex-matched healthy control group of 100. There was no difference between the groups regarding clinical evidence for heart disease.[5,p.89]

Bartalena and Pinchera commented on a study of the effects of TSH-suppressive doses of T_4 on the heart. Cross-sectional echocardiographic examination showed increased left ventricular contractility and mild myocardial hypertrophy. They wrote, "Whether the latter represents a risk for the patients remains a matter of debate. Clinically it does not seem to be important." They added: "The long-term evaluation of T_4 therapy has provided controversial results. Some have reported that T_4-treated patients under the age of 65 have an increased risk of ischemic heart disease, whereas others were unable to find any change in morbidity, mortality, and quality of life, including cardiovascular events."[18]

Many practicing physicians, including endocrinologists, restrict their patients' thyroid hormone dosages to amounts insufficient to provide relief from distinct hypothyroid symptoms and signs. Many have expressed to me that they do so because they believe that amounts of exogenous thyroid hormone larger than replacement dosages are likely to cause death from ischemic heart disease. Leese et al., over the period of a year, evaluated 1180 patients who were taking T_4. Of these patients, TSH levels were suppressed in 59% and 'normal' in 38%. Patients under 65 years of age on T_4 had an increased risk of ischemic heart disease compared to the general population (female 2.7 vs 0.7%, P<0.001; male 6.4 vs 1.7%, P<0.01). However, the risk was no different between those with normal and suppressed TSH levels.[158] This study indicates that the belief is not warranted that TSH-suppressive dosages of T_4 represent a greater risk than do replacement dosages for death due to ischemic heart disease. (Incidentally, it was not clear from this study whether the use of T_4 at any dosage level was responsible for the increased rate of death from ischemic heart disease. I do not know whether the investigators controlled for the use of cardioprotective measures such as aerobic exercise, diet, and nutritional supplementation.)

None of the euthyroid patients in two blinded studies my colleagues and I conducted had any detectable adverse cardiac effects from supraphysiologic dosages of exogenous T$_3$. All ECGs were normal throughout the 8-month study and at 2-month follow-up, despite follow-up thyroid profiles that are customarily considered typical of "T$_3$-thyrotoxicosis."[72][73] This finding suggests that the cardiovascular regulatory systems of the fibromyalgia patients in these studies were partially resistant to thyroid hormone. ECGs of some of our patients who have taken supraphysiologic dosages of T$_3$ for 1-to-10 years have been normal. The only exceptions have occurred in patients who have of their own accord raised their dosages to thyrotoxic amounts.

Worsening of the Manifestations of Coronary Heart Disease

Thyroid hormone therapy is potentially hazardous to people with compromised cardiovascular status. This is especially likely if the dosage is high enough to cause tissue thyrotoxicosis. The Teppermans wrote illustratively, "If hyperthyroidism occurs in a middle-aged or elderly person and the peremptory demands of a racing metabolic motor are made on a heart that is supplied by narrowed, atherosclerotic vessels, cardiac decompensation may occur."[6,p.169] Geriatric patients or patients with underlying valvular or ischemic heart disease are generally the victims of congestive heart failure induced by thyrotoxicosis. Except among these patients, congestive heart failure induced by thyrotoxicosis is unusual.[119][120] Only rarely does thyrotoxicosis induce ventricular dysrhythmias and sudden death.[121]

In principle, the lower the individual's level of cardiovascular fitness, the more susceptible she is to adverse cardiovascular effects during thyrotoxicosis.[144,p.2653] In fact, for people with severe cardiovascular deconditioning, even a replacement dose may be hazardous. Haynes, acknowledging the potential harm, recommended the patient build up to full thyroid replacement with graduated doses. This approach is more likely to avoid excessively taxing the heart and inducing adverse cardiac effects. He also pointed out that long-standing hypothyroidism predisposes the patient to atherosclerosis. Resuming a normal metabolic rate may benefit these patients by reversing atherosclerosis. Haynes therefore recommended that a full replacement dose be the ultimate aim if possible.[145,p.1372] Similar to the protocol advised by Haynes, Aronow recommended that elderly hypothyroid patients with coronary artery disease use replacement thyroid hormone with caution. Caution should avert precipitating or exacerbating angina pectoris, acute myocardial infarction, and precipitating or aggravating ventricular arrhythmias or congestive heart failure.[29]

Sawin et al. studied whether low serum TSH levels in clinically euthyroid elderly people are a risk factor for subsequent atrial fibrillation. The researchers included 2007 individuals (814 men and 1193 women) who were age 60 or older and who did not have atrial fibrillation. The incidence of arrhythmia was assessed during a 10-year follow-up period. At follow-up, among the 61 subjects with low serum TSH values (< or = 0.1 mU/L), 13 had atrial fibrillation. Among the 187 subjects with slightly low values (> 0.1-to-0.4 mU/L), 23 had atrial fibrillation. Among the 1576 subjects with normal TSH values (> 0.4 to 5.0 mU/L), 133 had fibrillation. And among the 183 subjects with high TSH values (> 5.0 mU/L), 23 had fibrillation. Cumulatively, 28% of subjects with low TSH levels had atrial fibrillation at 10 years compared to 11% of subjects with normal levels. The investigators concluded that over the 10 years, there was a threefold increase in the risk of atrial fibrillation among subjects 60 years or older.[182] It is not clear what cardiac risk factors the investigators controlled for in this study. It is possible that maintaining cardiovascular conditioning through physical exercise and consuming cardio-protective nutrients may have reduced the incidence of fibrillation in patients with low TSH levels. Nonetheless, the results of this study should encourage the clinician to be cautious in the treatment of elderly patients with thyroid hormone.

I recommend that the clinician evaluate the patient's cardiac status before she begins metabolic rehabilitation. Before the patient begins thyroid hormone therapy, the clinician should insure that any abnormality detected does not contraindicate the therapy. If he has any doubt, he should refer the patient for an evaluation by a cardiologist. I also recommend serial ECGs on all fibromyalgia patients undergoing thyroid hormone therapy. ECGs should be performed most often on patients with significant risk factors for cardiovascular disease such as obesity, diabetes, detrimental dietary habits, or physical deconditioning. Using this protocol in my practice, I have occasionally found indications of abnormalities that necessitated cardiology consults after the patient began metabolic rehabilitation. In some patients, cardiac stimulation by thyroid hormone unearths on the ECG tracing underlying cardiac abnormalities that were not detectable before they began treatment. Evidence of valvular or ischemic heart disease should prompt extreme caution.[119][120]

Adverse Cardiac Manifestations of Thyrotoxicosis Due to Thyroid Gland Disease. Cardiac abnormalities that occur during thyrotoxicosis due to thyroid gland disease can be severe.

Vlase and coworkers studied 403 patients with different forms of thyroid hormone overstimulation: toxic multilocular goiter (36.70%); toxic adenoma (4.90%); Graves' thyroiditis, painless thyroiditis, and Hashitoxicosis (21.09%); thyrotoxicosis factitia (0.74%); and T$_3$-thyrotoxicosis (9.42%). Eighty-seven patients (21.50%) had disturbed cardiac function. Of arrhythmias, the following were most common: atrial fibrillation (4.0%), ventricular premature beats (2.77%), paroxysmal supraventricular tachycardia (2.23%), and atrial flutter (1.00%). Of the 403 patients, 42 (10.42%) had congestive heart failure.[36]

Vlase converted paroxysmal tachyarrhythmias to normal sinus rhythms in 90% of patients with the use of sustained treatment with DC cardioversion, cardiac glycosides (deslanosid), β-adrenergic blockers (propranolol, 60-to-120 mg per 24 hours), calcium channel blockers (verapamil, 40-to-60 mg per 24 hours), carbimazole (30-to-40 mg per day), and Lugol solution (10-to-15 drops per day). Patients underwent thyroidectomy or radioactive iodine (^{131}I) to prevent recurrences or complications from thyrotoxicosis. The authors wrote, "Thus, we succeeded in maintaining the patients in a euthyroid state, in sinus rhythm and with an adequate cardiovascular function in 95.4% of cases."[36]

Umpierrez and coworkers described 7 patients admitted to the hospital with congestive heart failure. All patients had hyperthyroidism, dilated cardiomyopathy, and low-output cardiac failure. Hyperthyroidism in 6 patients was due to Graves' disease and in 1 was due to toxic multinodular goiter. The means of the patients' thyroid function tests were: T$_4$, 21 μg/dL; T$_3$, 411 ng/mL; and TSH, <0.03 μU/mL. Two-dimensional echocardiograms showed dilation of both ventricles or all four chambers and impaired performance of left ventricles. The patients' hyperthyroidism and heart failure improved rapidly with therapy. At follow-ups of 5 months-to-9 years, left ventricular ejection fraction improved from a mean of 28% to a mean of 55%. Dilated cardiomyopathy resolved and the systolic function normalized in 5 patients. The other 2 patients' left ventricular dysfunction improved from severe to mild. The investigators wrote, "We conclude that some patients with hyperthyroidism may have a reversible form of dilated cardiomyopathy and low-output failure. Assessment of thyroid hormone status in patients with heart failure might permit the identification of pa-

tients with dilated cardiomyopathy and thyrotoxicosis who are likely to have reversible cardiac dysfunction."[37]

Wilson and Hamilton reported a case of an obese (288.2 lbs) 43-year-old man with increasing fatigue, lightheadedness, and dyspnea upon ambulating 20 feet. ECGs showed that he had atrial fibrillation with a ventricular rate of 106 bpm and dilated cardiomyopathy. He had no significant underlying cardiac disease. The physicians determined that he had subclinical thyrotoxicosis and initially treated him with 40 mg of propranolol daily. His TSH level was <0.1 μU/mL, his total T$_4$ was 117 nmol/L (normal: 65-to-168 nmol/L), his T$_3$ uptake was 46% (normal: 25%-to-35%), and his free T$_4$ was 38.7 pmol/L (normal: 10.3-to-22.3 pmol/L). After admission he was treated with digoxin and quinidine for the fibrillation. Endomyocardial biopsy showed generalized myocyte hypertrophy and moderate interstitial fibrosis. On the 3rd day of hospitalization, he began 10 mg of propranolol 3 times daily, and 200 mg of propylthiouracil 3 times per day. After 3 days of this treatment, his cardiac rhythm converted to a normal sinus rhythm. On the 6th day, he again had ventricular tachycardia with no pulse and was electrically converted to a normal sinus rhythm. On the 8th day, he was discharged with no cardiac complications. He continued the propylthiouracil for 10 months. As his thyrotoxicosis was relieved, his cardiac function improved with reversal of chamber dilatation.[122]

Need for Cautious and Gradual Increases in Thyroid Hormone Dosage

Angina pectoris may cease to occur after hypothyroid patients begin taking thyroid hormone. However, angina may appear for the first time, or pre-existing angina may worsen, after a patient begins using thyroid hormone. The dosage of thyroid hormone should be increased very gradually by these patients to avoid myocardial infarction.[32,pp.118-120]

A gradual increase in thyroid hormone dosage is especially important in elderly patients. Locker et al. reported the case of a 71-year-old woman who had a myocardial infarction associated with an abruptly increased dosage of thyroid hormone. The patient had undergone a total thyroidectomy. Three years before the infarction, she had undergone thyroid gland irradiation because of follicular carcinoma. After the irradiation, she alternated between a daily T$_4$ replacement dosage of 0.15 mg and 0.2 mg. Because she was still hypometabolic despite these dosages, her dosage was increased to 0.3 mg per day. Three weeks after increasing the dosage, the patient had an acute posterior myocardial infarction. She had had no prior history of coronary artery disease. Coronary arteriograms did not reveal evidence of disease of the major vessels. Three weeks after the infarction, a persistent perfusion defect was still obvious by myocardial scintigraphy. Locker et al. noted that thyroid hormone increases tissue oxygen demand. They conjectured that a rapid increase in oxygen use due to the patient's abrupt increase in T_4 dosage was responsible for her myocardial infarction. They cautioned clinicians to avoid such sudden increases in dosage.[161]

Bergeron et al. reported a similar case in which a dosage of thyroid hormone that was thyrotoxic for a patient induced acute reversible myocardial ischemia. They wrote that acute myocardial ischemia and/or infarction are rare in thyrotoxicosis when patients do not have coronary artery disease. Some patients, however, who were thyrotoxic from the use of thyroid hormone have had acute myocardial infarctions although they did not have fixed coronary artery stenosis or coronary artery spasm. The researchers reported the case of a 68-year-old woman who was clinically thyrotoxic from taking 0.30 mg/day of exogenous thyroid hormone. She had severe, reversible myocardial ischemia. She was found to have a large apical dyskinetic region through echocardiography and scintigraphy. When the patient's dosage was decreased to 0.15 mg, she became clinically euthyroid. Echocardiography, scintigraphy, and cardiac catheterization then showed normal left ventricular contractility and normal coronary anatomy. The investigators wrote that exogenous thyroid hormone may directly alter myocardial oxygen supply and demand, even in the absence of coronary artery disease and coronary spasm. The increased demand may then induce acute myocardial ischemia and reversible left ventricular segmental wall motion abnormalities.[162]

Caution is therefore necessary in adjusting each patient's thyroid hormone dosage. *Until he is confident that the contrary is the case, the clinician should consider that each patient may have the potential for idiosyncratic adverse cardiovascular reactions to dosages of thyroid hormone that are safe for most other patients.*

Nonspecific Electrocardiographic Changes in Cardiac Thyrotoxicosis. In thyrotoxicosis, there are no specific identifiable electrocardiographic changes.[71] There are, however, nonspecific changes. These are listed in Table 4.4.3.

In contrast to the bradycardia (<50 bpm) found in

some hypothyroid patients,[123,p.465] half of thyrotoxic patients have *sinus tachycardia* (>100 bpm).[126][127] One tenth of hyperthyroid patients have persistent atrial fibrillation.[126][127] The fibrillation is a thyrotoxic cardiac effect. In fact, thyrotoxicosis is among the "big four" causes of fibrillation. (The other three causes are mitral diseases, ischemic disease, and hypertension.)[123,p.187] If a patient under the age of 40 has fibrillation and right axis deviation, this is virtually diagnostic of mitral stenosis. But the combination is also occasionally found in atrial septal defect and in thyrotoxicosis.[123,p.457]

Table 4.4.3. Nonspecific ECG changes associated with thyrotoxicosis.

Complete or 3° right bundle block
Increased U wave amplitude
Persistent atrial fibrillation
PR interval prolongation
Right axis deviation with atrial fibrillation
Shortened QT interval
Sinus tachycardia
ST segment elevation
Wolff-Parkinson-White syndrome

The *PR interval* may be prolonged in rheumatic or coronary disease. The PR interval is the time from the beginning of the P wave to the beginning of the PQR complex (normally 0.12-to-0.20 sec). It measures the period taken for the impulse to travel from the sino-atrial node to the ventricular muscle fibers. The measurement is prolonged when the conducting system is diseased or affected by digitalis. The prolongation may be a normal variation.[71,p.764] The interval varies with the heart rate, being shorter at faster rates.[123,p.17] Because of this, as exogenous thyroid hormone increases the heart rate, as it customarily does, the PR interval is likely to shorten to within the normal range.

It is important, as Marriott has emphasized,[123,p.16] that prolongation of the PR interval does not necessarily indicate cardiac abnormality. "At relatively slow rates, a few apparently normal people, with no evidence of heart disease, have been found to have intervals ranging considerably above 0.20 sec."[123,p.16] Of 67,000 apparently healthy airmen, 52% had prolonged PR intervals. Eighty percent ranged from 0.21-to-0.24 sec, with the remainder ranging to 0.39 sec.[148] Among 19,000 men, 59 (0.31%) had PR intervals 0.24 sec or above.[133] Marriot wrote of the prolonged PR interval,"Obviously it is a signal for a thorough search to exclude cardiac abnormality, but if none is found, the heart should be acquitted without reservation."[123,p.16]

When transmission of the impulse to the ventricles is faster than normal, the PR interval will be abnormally short. This often occurs in hypertension[134] and when there is a tendency toward paroxysms of tachycardia.[135] It also occurs as Wolff-Parkinson-White syndrome in thyrotoxicosis.[71,p.764] The classic pattern on the ECG is a short PR interval (<0.12 sec) and a wide QRS complex, preceded and merging with a premature and sharply ascending component called the "delta" wave.[123,p.257] The delta wave represents premature ventricular depolarization.[128,p.148]

Muggia reported complete or 3° right bundle block in thyrotoxic myocarditis.[125] In complete block, no atrial impulses reach the AV node and there is no ventricular response. It is in this circumstance that an ectopic pacemaker in either the AV node or a ventrical becomes active. The pacemaker generates an atrial rate and an independent ventricular rate.[128,p.135] This change may be caused by inflammation of the conduction system in the thyrotoxic heart.[125] When the right bundle branch is blocked, depolarization creeps around the blocked branch and spreads to the right ventricle. The left ventricle fires first, and after a delay, the right fires. This is shown on the ECG tracing as a widened QRS complex (>0.12 sec) and two R waves (R and R') in leads V_1 and V_2.[128,p.139] The bundle branch block is diagnosed primarily from the widened QRS complex. Commonly, sudden appearance of bundle branch block indicates impending myocardial infarction.[128,p.146]

The *QT interval* may be shortened by digitalis, calcium excess, potassium intoxication, and by thyrotoxicosis.[123,p.24][124]

Substantial displacement of the *ST segment* is found in any of the syndromes of coronary artery disease, and it is the hallmark of myocardial ischemia or injury.[123,p.21] The ST segment may also be elevated in thyrotoxicosis.[124] Exogenous thyroid hormone usually increases metabolic demand in cardiac muscle. This may put at risk a patient with marginally sufficient coronary artery flow. Because of this, monitoring of the ST segment is particularly important. ST elevation is not likely to indicate myocardial infarction when there are no T-wave inversions, and especially when there are no new Q waves or increased prominence of pre-existing ones.[123,p.374]

The *U wave*, a small low voltage wave that sometimes follows the T wave, may indicate thyrotoxicosis.

It is usually best observed in the V_3 lead. The polarity of the U wave is generally the same as that of the T wave and changes from negative to positive as the T wave does.[123,p.24] The U wave may indicate one of numerous conditions such as myocardial ischemia and left ventricular overload due to hypertension,[129][130] but its amplitude may be increased by epinephrine, digitalis, quinidine, hypercalcemia, exercise, and thyrotoxicosis.[131][132]

Mechanisms and illustrations of the ECG patterns I describe in this section can be found in standard texts on ECG interpretation.[123][128]

Proper Procedure When Electrocardiography Indicates Cardiac Thyrotoxicosis. For treatment and management of patients with cardiac thyrotoxicosis, see Chapter 5.2, subsections titled "Precautions in the Use of Exogenous Thyroid Hormone: Cardiac Disease" and "Managing Thyrotoxic Reactions to Excessive Intake of Exogenous Thyroid Hormone."

Adverse Cardiac Effects of Untreated Hypothyroidism. Adverse cardiac effects of untreated hypothyroidism vary. Some people will live unscathed, while others will die long before they would have if they had used exogenous thyroid hormone (see section below: "Harm from Untreated and Undertreated Hypothyroidism").

LIVER

Hamburger wrote, "Suggestive of subclinical liver damage from inappropriately high T_4 doses is the finding of an increase in glutathione *S*-transferase levels."[5,p.86] Volpé countered that the study in which patients had increased glutathione *S*-transferase levels had inadequate controls. He also noted that the finding, if factual, does not appear to have clinical significance.[5,p.89]

The question of clinical significance that Volpé noted is critically important to the debate over proper dosages of exogenous thyroid hormone. Clearly, thyroidologists such as Hamburger have presumed that findings such as an increased glutathione *S*-transferase indicate tissue damage. This is falsified by reports such as that by Pearch and Himsworth. They noted that in the long history of patients taking dosages of thyroid hormone higher than the currently recommended replacement dosages, the patients have had no apparent resulting adverse health effects.[74,p.695] It is incumbent upon thyroidologists such as Hamburger to provide evidence that such findings as the glutathione *S*-transferase are of clinical significance.

Bartalena and Pinchera pointed out that in patients taking TSH-suppressive T$_4$ dosages, elevations of hepatic enzymes (glutathione-*S*-transferase, gamma glutamyltransferase, and angiotensin-converting enzyme) are mild.[18] In my studies of euthyroid fibromyalgia patients taking supraphysiologic dosages of T$_3$, I found no abnormal test results related to the liver.[72][73]

TREMORS, IRRITABILITY, RESTLESSNESS AND HEAT INTOLERANCE

Among the most common symptoms of excessive thyroid hormone stimulation are tremors, restlessness, emotional irritability, and the perception of being too hot when others are comfortable or cool. Fibrillary twitching and tremors, caused by the relentless bombardment of the patient's muscles by motor signals, are particularly bothersome to patients.[6,p.170] Symptoms such as these provide barometers of thyroid hormone overdosage. The patient who is knowledgeable about these symptoms can help monitor her own condition and provide information that may be critical to properly titrating her thyroid hormone dosage.

PSYCHIATRIC REACTIONS

Adverse Reactions in Psychotic Patients

The clinician should be cautious while treating the psychotic patient with exogenous thyroid; the treatment may worsen the psychosis.[28] In some patients who are not actively psychotic, thyroid replacement therapy may cause psychotic delirium. This reaction may be instigated by too large an initial dose.

Whybrow wrote that in susceptible individuals, T$_4$ therapy can precipitate dysphoric manic-like symptoms. The patient with this condition may require treatment with neuroleptics. Chlorpromazine (thorazine) may be helpful in reducing dangerous excitatory behavior or assaults by the patient.[23]

PITUITARY AND THYROID GLANDS: REVERSIBILITY OF SUPPRESSED FUNCTION BY EXOGENOUS THYROID HORMONE

Some clinicians and patients hold the misconception that once a person takes exogenous thyroid hormone, she will have to do so forever. They state the belief that the suppression of anterior pituitary and thyroid gland function caused by exogenous thyroid hormone is permanent.

The experiences of thousands of people for scores of years show this idea to be wrong in general. Incalculable numbers of people who have taken exogenous thyroid for years have stopped taking the hormone and resumed an acceptable level of pituitary and thyroid function. This phenomenon is similar to the resumption of pituitary and ovarian function after a woman stops taking exogenous estrogen.

Pinchera et al. wrote that when a patient abruptly stops taking exogenous thyroid hormone, a laboratory test pattern typical of pituitary hypothyroidism results (low thyroid hormone and TSH levels, and a subnormal or absent TSH response to injected TRH).[189,p.973] The pattern of lab values indicative of pituitary hypothyroidism is short-lived in patients with normal thyroid gland function.[149][165] According to Guyton, permanent suppression of the hypothalamus-pituitary-thyroid axis is not likely. "When a complete replacement dose of thyroid hormone is continued for many years," he said, "a very small percentage of patients may have permanent suppression."[16]

Greer found that after stopping exogenous thyroid hormones, the pre-treatment output of the hypothalamic-pituitary-thyroid axis resumed after approximately 11 weeks.[69] Pinchera et al. wrote that TSH secretion and circulating thyroid hormone levels return to normal in 3-to-5 weeks.[189,p.973]

● ALTERNATE CONCEPTS OF "FINE TUNING"

To conventional thyroidologists, "fine tuning" refers to adjusting the patient's thyroid hormone dosage so that the TSH is maintained within the normal reference range—regardless of how the patient's tissues are responding to the thyroid hormone. This view of "fine tuning" dosage is an extremist technocratic orientation. A more humane and rational orientation is to "fine tune" the patient's dosage according to tissue responses to the hormone, with optimal clinical status as the foremost aim.

The extremist technocratic orientation has been justified by thyroidologists with statements that are logically and scientifically indefensible. Toft stated, for example, that a suppressed TSH level is a "thyrotoxic" level, and that a normal TSH is a "euthyroid" level.[5,p.91] He defined "subclinical hyperthyroidism" as a normal or raised free T_4 or total T_4, normal or raised free T_3 or total T_3, and an absent TSH response to TRH or undetectable basal TSH.[5,p.92] Through these operational definitions, Toft redefined the clinical syndrome of tissue overstimulation by excessive amounts of thyroid hormone (thyrotoxicity) as hormone blood levels. He did so in the absence of evidence that tissue metabolic status reliably correlates with the hormone blood levels. Some patients with the blood levels he specified will have tissue thyrotoxicity. But many individuals who have the same blood levels will nonetheless have perfectly normal tissue metabolic status. Practitioners who learn protocol from Toft will diagnose these latter patients as thyrotoxic despite their having no thyrotoxicity whatsoever! The practitioners will reduce their patients' dosages of thyroid hormone (to "fine tune" the dosage) and thereby induce tissue hypometabolism with associated symptoms and signs.

Practitioners have also been encouraged to adopt the extremist technocratic orientation by careless statements by some thyroidologists. For example, Hamburger stated, "Hyperthyroidism clearly causes loss of bone mineral density."[5,p.86] In this statement, Hamburger implies that hyperthyroidism is synonymous with reduced bone density, a manifestation of osseous thyrotoxicity. But hyperthyroidism and thyrotoxicosis are not one and the same phenomenon. *Hyperthyroidism refers only to elevated thyroid hormone levels due to hyperactivity of the thyroid gland; thyrotoxicity refers to the adverse effects of tissue hypermetabolism due to excess thyroid hormone stimulation.*[150] We cannot logically conclude that blood hormone levels consistent with a hyperactive thyroid gland are invariably accompanied by tissue thyrotoxicity. To do so is to ignore the fact that there is variability in tissue responsiveness to thyroid hormone in the same individual and between individuals. Thyroid hormone levels that induce thyrotoxicity in one patient will leave another with symptom-generating hypometabolism and yet another with optimal tissue metabolism. Realizing this should make it clear that metabolic status cannot be determined by blood levels of these hormones. Only by evaluating indications of the patient's tissue responses to thyroid hormone (through changes in symptoms, signs, and peripheral indices) can the clinician intelligently assess the degree of success or failure of the patient's thyroid hormone therapy.

To conventional thyroidologists, deciding how to adjust the patient's thyroid hormone dosage is strictly a matter of reading laboratory thyroid function test values. Discussion of thyrotoxicity is almost exclusively a discussion of thyroid function test values and is virtually devoid of mention of other tests that are capable of detecting adverse tissue effects of excess thyroid hormone. Consider the following discussion between Hamburger and Volpé.[5,pp.85-87]

According to Hamburger, we should expect that "thyrotoxicosis" in patients with lesser degrees of T_4 overdosage will be hard to prove, even with sophisticated tests. The prudent physician in clinical practice will have two options. First, follow the advice of those who argue that unless data confirms that a T_4 dosage is harmful, the clinician can disregard lab findings that suggest it (such as a supersensitive TSH).[13] Or second, act according to the belief that current thyroid function tests are more reliable than the clinician's assessment.[14] "In my opinion," he stated, "the burden of proof lies with those who advise ignoring the T_4 overdose implications of a subnormal supersensitive TSH. Unless they can provide compelling data suggesting the need for (of course excepting treatment of thyroid cancer, when full suppression of TSH may be desirable) and long-term safety of overdosage, it might be preferable to prescribe the lower doses of T_4 that produce clinical euthyroidism and normal supersensitive TSH values as well."[5,p.87]

Hamburger's use of the word "overdosage" presupposes what he is trying to prove—that the patient's TSH-suppressive T_4 dosage is necessarily "excessive" and harmful. I doubt that Hamburger intended the word to mean this, but his use of the term is a reminder of the quagmire of confused terminology in thyroidology that the clinician must struggle with to understand current concepts and procedures.

Volpé replied to Hamburger: "My, how this controversy does go on! I will be pleased to respond to the point you have raised: namely, does thyroxine overdosage-induced thyrotoxicosis occur without an elevated serum T_3 (or free T_3) level?" He pointed out that in the treatment of hypothyroidism, precise T_4 replacement consistent with optimal good health is the final aim. "It is indeed clear," he wrote, "that the best current arbiter of normal replacement of thyroxine in hypothyroidism would be a TSH value (performed by a 'sensitive' assay) that is in the middle of the normal range. That would mean that the patient is completely finely tuned as far as it is humanly possible to accomplish this. The big question is," he asked, "is there any harm to a patient when the TSH is suppressed, providing that the total serum triiodothyronine (or free T_3) is in the middle of the normal range? That is, does a somewhat elevated serum thyroxine have deleterious implications, in the face of a completely normal serum T_3 level?" He answered this question by stating, "My current view is that it does not, and that it is not worth the manipulation and individual attention to thyroxine dosage that some have claimed are necessary for 'fine tuning.'"[5,pp.87-88]

This view is supported by Pearch and Himsworth. Regarding fine tuning with the TSH, they wrote: "It is the common experience that no characteristic pathology develops in patients treated for hypothyroidism even after many years, nor is life expectancy diminished. Moreover, this knowledge is derived from a period when larger doses of thyroid hormones were given than are now customary. It seems, therefore, that although physiological measurements [lab values] in such patients can show evidence of overexposure to thyroid hormone, there are no deleterious biological consequences of this lack of fine tuning of dosage."[74,p.695]

Volpé explained that serum T_3 levels correlate better with clinical status than do serum T_4 levels. He pointed out, in agreement with Bantle,[15] that to achieve a normal serum T_3 level in a hypothyroid patient, the T_4 dosage may have to be sufficient to cause an elevated T_4 level and a suppressed TSH level. He concluded, ". . . one would not obtain an over-replacement dosage merely by suppressing TSH. Thus an elevated T_4 with a normal serum T_3 and a suppressed TSH value is not an indicator of overdosage, under these circumstances."[5,p.88]

If Volpé and these authors are correct that T_3 levels correspond more closely to tissue metabolic status than T_4 levels, then maintaining normal T_4 and TSH levels at the cost of a low T_3 will leave the patient hypometabolic and symptomatic. This is the status of most fibromyalgia patients I see who already take T_4 for hypothyroidism. In most cases, the fibromyalgia dramatically improves or is completely relieved merely by raising the T_4 level high enough to suppress the TSH.

There may be two reasons for the necessity to raise the thyroid hormone dosage high enough to suppress the TSH level before most patients improve. First, as Volpé wrote, the free T_3 correlates better with tissue metabolism. Raising the T_3 high enough to insure normal metabolism may require that the patient's T_4 dosage be high enough to elevate the T_4 level[74] and possibly suppress the TSH level. The T_3 level, however, may return to the normal range before the TSH is suppressed. Fish et al., for example, evaluated the replacement dose of T_4 in 19 patients with hypothyroidism. The dose was adjusted at monthly intervals

until TSH levels were within the normal range. The mean T_4 replacement dose was 112($\pm$19) μg per day. The TSH levels of patients on replacement therapy returned to normal when serum T_3 levels were essentially the same as in normal subjects. Although TSH levels were within the normal range, serum T_4 levels were significantly above those of normal subjects (11.3 μg/dL vs 8.7 μg/dL).[10] In my experience, however, the hypothyroid symptoms and signs of many hypothyroid fibromyalgia patients who take T_4 are improved or relieved only when their TSH levels are suppressed, resulting in high-normal T_3 and extremely high normal T_4 levels. These hormone levels have not been associated with tissue thyrotoxicity in these patients.

The second reason TSH-suppressive dosages of thyroid hormone may be necessary is that many patients appear to have some degree of cellular resistance to thyroid hormone. Unless the thyroid dosage is sufficient to override the cellular resistance, the patient remains hypometabolic and symptomatic. In virtually all patients, dosages that are "sufficient" cause "abnormal" thyroid hormone and TSH levels. Tragically, this prompts many well-intended but misguided clinicians to lower a patient's dosage and return her to a symptomatic state that is often debilitating. In no such case that I have seen to date did the clinician base his decision to lower the patient's dosage on objective evidence that the higher dosage was adversely affecting the patient's tissues. The decision was based instead on the erroneous view that blood levels of thyroid hormone and TSH are measures of the metabolic status of tissues.

The caution not to overstimulate patients with thyroid hormone expresses concern based on a real possibility. Many thyroidologists, however, exaggerate the possibility due to their false assumption that thyroid hormone and TSH levels are accurate gauges of tissue metabolic status. My position is that the thyroid hormone dosage should be tailored to each patient's personal needs: high enough to relieve signs and symptoms but low enough that the patient has no symptoms, signs, or peripheral indices indicative of tissue thyrotoxicity. With this approach, therapy can meet the needs even of the patient with a seemingly exorbitant requirement for thyroid hormone. And for the patient who is more sensitive to thyroid hormone, well-being can be insured by keeping her dosage low enough to avoid tissue thyrotoxicity. Clinicians cannot achieve these outcomes by adjusting dosages according to thyroid hormone or TSH blood levels. Individual requirements are simply too variable. The clinician would best "fine tune" the patient's dosage according to peripheral tissue effects. The available methods of assessing tissue effects are not perfect, but they are far more meaningful indicators of the metabolic response to thyroid hormone dosage than are circulating thyroid hormone and TSH levels.

Volpé stated that to him the matter is one of long experience. He wrote: ". . . it is difficult for me to agree that 'fine tuning' is really necessary. It is also true that there are patients who do have complaints when they feel they are being overmedicated. What is required to determine whether they are truly complaints secondary to the medication itself, or whether the complaints are functional, is to study this question with an appropriate control group. This control group should also be taking some placebo and the exhortations must be entirely similar. Such a study is yet to be done. Until such a study is complete and indicates with certainty that the medication is causing clinical symptoms, I remain unmoved. 'Fine tuning' is, for me, logistically enabling, expensive, and in the final analysis, probably unappealing."[5,p.89]

● **HARM FROM UNTREATED AND UNDERTREATED HYPOTHYROIDISM**

Unlike distinct hyperthyroidism, untreated hypothyroidism apparently has minimal if any direct adverse effects on bone. The most probable indirect adverse effect associated with hypothyroidism in regard to bone is the disinclination of untreated individuals to perform weight-bearing exercises (see section below).

The cardiovascular effects of untreated hypothyroidism, however, constitute a potentially serious risk to health. The cardiovascular risks make it imperative that the hypothyroid patient be treated with sufficiently large dosages of thyroid hormone. Hypothyroid patients are at greater risk for complications such as heart failure during surgery. Patients with untreated thyroid hormone resistance syndromes probably share the risks. The partial hormone resistance of these latter patients should be therapeutically overridden with exogenous T_3, since T_4 is usually ineffective for the purpose.

It is not known whether hypothyroidism is associated with adverse effects on liver. There is, however, an association between untreated primary hypothyroidism and primary biliary cirrhosis.

Bastenie stated that hypothyroidism is a "destructive process." He concluded, "In view of the general physical, vascular, and neurological damage induced by thyroid deficiency, there is clearly an urgent need for screening the general population, especially in the age group over 50 years, for early recognition of thyroid pathology."[35] It is clear that the adverse consequences of hypothyroid patients taking too little exogenous thyroid hormone are likely to be as detrimental to their health as severe excess stimulation with thyroid hormone. The conventional protocol for treating hypothyroid patients imposes these risks on patients. On behalf of their patients, therefore, I encourage clinicians to reject the dictates of the conventional protocol for treatment with thyroid hormone and treat patients according to the protocol outlined in Chapter 5.2.

BONE

Thevenon and colleagues assessed bone changes in 20 hypothyroid patients. They found normal levels of urinary and blood calcium, phosphorus, parathyroid hormone, and vitamin D as dihydroxycholecalciferols. Histological examination of biopsied and tetracycline-labeled iliac crest bone showed normal trabeculation volume and rates of resorption and calcification. The relative osteoid volume and the osteoid thickness index, however, were increased. The authors conjectured that these latter changes were probably due to the general slowing of bone cell metabolism in hypothyroidism.[42]

However, the disinclination of hypometabolic individuals to perform weight-bearing exercises highlights an indirect adverse effect of hypothyroidism on bone density. The mechanical loading of weight-bearing exercise is associated with higher bone density,[100][137] and the lack of such exercise can be a risk factor for decreased bone density.

HEART

La Brocca recently wrote that the clinician should consider the possibility of hypothyroidism during an initial evaluation of the patient who has hypercholesterolemia, cardiac ischemia, and hypertension (especially diastolic). He noted that it should make no difference whether the patient has clinical symptoms and signs of hormonal deficiency. Particular attention should be paid to female patients because they have a higher incidence of hypothyroidism than males. The patient with these findings may be found to be hypothyroid and thyroid hormone therapy may be essential to improvement or recovery.[160]

A case recently reported by Fujimoto and colleagues shows the potentially severe cardiac effects of untreated hypothyroidism. The patient was a middle-aged woman with "myxedema heart." She was admitted to the hospital because of dyspnea and facial and peripheral edema. Chest x-rays showed severe cardiomegaly and bilateral pleural effusion. A coronary arteriogram did not show significant stenosis. She had raised TC, CPK, and LDH values. Immunological tests showed a high antithyroid antibody and microsome titer. Her low T_3 and T_4 and high TSH levels indicated overt primary hypothyroidism. She had congestive heart failure due to myocardial damage caused by "myoedema." Serial endomyocardial biopsy showed reversible and irreversible myocardial abnormalities. She received thyroid hormone replacement, digitalis, and diuretics. After 7 months of treatment her clinical status had dramatically improved. At hospital admission, transvenous right ventricular endomyocardial biopsy showed vacuolated degeneration. After treatment, the same test showed slight fibrosis. The authors wrote, "This pathological finding suggests that 'myxedema heart' is able to produce both reversible and irreversible myocardial damage."[31]

Cardiac abnormalities are expected from some risk factors associated with hypothyroidism. Hypertension and elevated cholesterol and triglycerides are common.[32,p.117] Bastenie wrote that in full-blown hypothyroidism, three cardiac conditions may arise: enlarged "myxedema heart," cardiac ischemia, and cardiac failure.[35] Table 4.4.4 lists ECG findings in 56 hypothyroid patients and 56 matched controls.

Bernstein et al. pointed out that in some patients with severe hypothyroidism, replacement dosages of T_4 induce or worsen angina pectoris, but in other hypothyroid patients, the dosages stop or reduce angina. The researchers conducted a study to determine the basis of this paradoxical phenomenon. Other investigators had proposed that the mechanism is either asymmetric septal hypertrophy as a form of reversible endocrine cardiomyopathy or reversible anatomical narrowing of the coronary arteries. In another study, researchers used radionuclide ventriculography to assess myocardial performance in severely hypothyroid patients just beginning to use replacement dosages of T_4. The results indicated that the patients had reversible coronary dysfunction rather than asymmetric septal

hypertrophy. Bernstein et al. replicated the study. They found that 6 severely hypothyroid patients did not have echocardiographic evidence of asymmetric septal hypertrophy or coronary artery disease. The researchers had patients exercise and used redistribution tomographic myocardial thallium-201 imaging (SPECT) to measure blood flow. Measurements were done before the patients began replacement dosages of T_4 and at 10 days and 2 months after they began replacement therapy. Four patients had "substantial regional perfusion defects" after exercising. Perfusion became normal when the patients were at rest. In 1 patient, perfusion became normal during exercise after 10 days of T_4 use. The researchers wrote, "With restoration of euthyroidism, exercise and redistribution SPECT were normal in every patient." They also wrote that the confidence limits revealed that the incidence of myocardial perfusion defects in hypothyroid patients, indicating myocardial ischemia, will be at least 22% with 95% probability. They concluded, "Despite the relatively low specificity of SPECT, it seems pertinent to conclude that impaired myocardial perfusion as assessed by SPECT probably is due to reversible coronary dysfunction inherent in the hypothyroid state, and that this is not an infrequent manifestation of severe hypothyroidism."[186]

Improved Cardiovascular Status with Thyroid Hormone Therapy

Cardiac abnormalities tend to disappear when hypothyroid patients undergo adequate thyroid hormone therapy.[160] Electrocardiograms of untreated hypothyroid patients during exercise often show an "ischemic" pattern, but the pattern disappears after patients begin thyroid therapy.

Perk and O'Neill studied the effect of adequacy of T_4 replacement therapy on coronary atherosclerosis. Ten elderly hypothyroid patients who had coronary angiography more than once during 1992 and 1993 were included. Each of 5 patients inadequately treated for hypothyroidism had angiographic evidence that their coronary atherosclerosis had progressed. In 5 of 7 patients who were treated adequately, atherosclerosis did not progress (P = 0.02). In all of 6 patients whose dosages were reduced to or maintained at 100 µg or less, coronary atherosclerosis progressed. But in 5 of 6 patients whose dosages were increased to or fixed at 150 µg or more, the disease had not progressed (P=0.015). The investigators concluded that the progression of coronary artery disease in hypothyroid patients may be prevented by adequate thyroid replacement. They wrote, "Thyroid hormones can protect against athero-sclerosis, presumably due to their metabolic effects on plaque progression."[187]

During cardiac surgery, hypothyroid patients have a higher incidence of heart failure than euthyroid patients (29% vs 6%).[180] Accumulating evidence indicates that such complications can be prevented by the use of thyroid hormone. Researchers have reported that thyroid hormone has a spectrum of therapeutic uses with stroke[176] and heart transplant patients.[175] T_4 was found to be effective medium-term in the treatment of idiopathic dilated cardiomyopathy.[174]

Table 4.4.4. ECGs from 56 hypothyroid patients and 56 matched controls*

	Hypothyroid patients	Controls
Normal	3	16
Nonspecific myocardial changes	24	27
Low voltage	18	4
Bradycardia	11	0
Disturbed atrioventricular conduction	10	1
Disturbed intraventricular conduction	5	4
Ischemia	6	0
Myocardial infarct	9	8
Left ventricular strain	9	6

*After Vanhaelst, L.: Hypothyroidism and coronary heart disease. In *Recent Progress in Diagnosis and Treatment of Hypothyroid Conditions*. Edited by P.A. Bastenie, M. Bonnyns, and L. Vanhaelst, Amsterdam, *Excerpta Medica*, 1980.[32,p.118]

T_3 in particular is useful for a variety of purposes with patients who have cardiovascular abnormalities. Administering T_3 intravenously improves the cardiac index during cardiac surgery and causes a paradoxical decrease in the incidence of atrial fibrillation.[163] Researchers have recently reported that T_3 improved left ventricular function after ischemic injury,[172] enhanced left ventricular function after hypothermic ischemia,[173] had positive hemodynamic effects during coronary artery bypass surgery[177] and with stunned myocardium,[178] and reversed acute severe post-ischemic myocardial depression.[179]

Hamilton et al. noted that a low T_3 level, as occurs in severe illness, results in impaired hemodynamics and is a predictor of poor survival. Patients with advanced congestive heart failure have low T_3 levels.

The researchers studied the safety and hemodynamic effects of short-term intravenously administered T_3 in 23 patients with advanced heart failure. The mean left ventricular ejection fraction was 0.22 ± 0.01. Patients received an intravenous bolus dose of T_3. Some patients were also given a 6-to-12-hour infusion of T_3. The cumulative dose was 0.15-to-2.7 µg/kg. The researchers monitored cardiac rhythm and hemodynamic status for 12 hours, assessed basal metabolic rate with indirect calorimetry, used echocardiographic parameters of systolic function and valvular regurgitation, and measured thyroid hormone and catecholamine levels at baseline and at 4-to-6 hours. There were no episodes of ischemia or arrhythmia, and heart rates and metabolic rates did not significantly change. Core temperature increased minimally. Cardiac output increased and systemic vascular resistance decreased in patients receiving the largest dose. The decreased resistance is consistent with the expected peripheral vasodilatory effect from the administration of T_3. The researchers wrote, "Acute intravenous administration of triiodothyronine is well tolerated in patients with advanced heart failure, establishing the basis for further investigation into the safety and potential hemodynamic benefits of longer infusions, combined infusion with inotropic agents, oral triiodothyronine replacement therapy, and new triiodothyronine analogs."[188]

In one study, a researcher found that T_3 levels were significantly lower in 42 of 65 stroke patients.[176] It is certainly possible that the low levels of T_3 were partly responsible for the strokes. It is well-known that low thyroid hormone levels result in high blood fat levels, and high blood fat levels predispose patients to heart attacks and strokes. By lowering blood fat levels, the use of T_3 is likely to help prevent strokes.

The use of T_3 can be beneficial in patients with the most frail heart conditions. Vavouranakis et al. wrote, "Triiodothyronine [T_3] administration in patients undergoing cardiopulmonary bypass surgery is safe, may lessen the need for pharmacological (vasodilator) therapy, but may increase heart rate."[177] In rabbits recovering from post-ischemic heart damage, T_3 enhanced recovery without adverse effects such as excessively forceful heart contractions.[178]

Salter induced severe ischemic heart injury in rats. They then administered T_3 to some of the injured rats but not to others. They wrote, "We conclude that administration of T_3 in a severe left ventricular injury model significantly augments rapid ventricular recovery."[179]

Research reports that some patients' cardiovascular status is improved by the use of thyroid hormone confirm some clinicians' anecdotal observations of such benefits. These reports will hopefully temper the common exaggerated warnings of the risks of thyroid hormone therapy so that they become consistent with the available scientific evidence. At the same time, the reported cardiovascular benefits of thyroid hormone therapy would best not diminish the clinician's resolve to safeguard each individual patient from potential adverse cardiovascular effects from the use of thyroid hormone (see subsection above titled "Need for Cautious and Gradual Increases in Thyroid Hormone Dosage").

Inadequacy of Conventional T₄ Replacement Therapy for Elevated Blood Lipids

Elevated cholesterol, triglycerides, and phospholipids; elevated low-density lipoproteins; and low high-density lipoproteins are risk factors for cardiovascular disease. There is a high incidence of these lipid findings in hypothyroidism, including the subclinical form. (For a description of the abnormal blood lipids in untreated or undertreated hypothyroid patients, see Chapter 4.3, subsection titled "Cholesterol, Triglycerides, and Low-Density Lipoproteins.")

Yildirimkaya et al. reported that replacement dosages of T_4 lowered the levels of athrogenic lipids in patients with subclinical hypothyroidism.[159] Weetman wrote, however, that "The effects of thyroxine *replacement* on cholesterol lowering alone are modest [italics mine]."[156] The key to the modest reduction of cholesterol with T_4 treatment is the word "replacement." This term means the restriction of the patient to a dosage that keeps the TSH level well within the normal reference range. However, dosages of T_4 greater than replacement dosages—that is, TSH-suppressive dosages—decrease cholesterol levels even further.

Fowler et al. assessed the relative effects of replacement dosages of T_4 to those of larger dosages that suppressed the TSH level. They compared the cholesterol concentrations of 31 hypothyroid women before they began using T_4 with concentrations after using T_4. The patients had taken thyroxine replacement for a mean of 12.7 years. Ten of the women had normal TSH levels and 21 had suppressed levels. Women whose TSH levels were not suppressed were taking a mean daily T_4 dosage of 140 µg (0.14 mg). Their mean decrease in cholesterol was 0.89 mmol/L. Women with TSH suppression were taking a mean T_4 dosage of 171 µg (0.171 mg). Their mean decrease in cholesterol was 2.1 mmol/L. Thus, patients with a higher mean intake of T_4 (31 µg or 0.031 mg) had a greater mean decrease

in cholesterol (1.21 mmol/L). No patient, including those with TSH suppression, had atrial fibrillation or cardiographic evidence of coronary artery disease. The investigators' concluding remarks are enlightening. They noted that because of the fear of osteoporosis, physicians generally restrict their hypothyroid patients' thyroid hormone dosages; yet fractures are not a feature of the natural history of treated hypothyroid patients. By contrast, they pointed out that "cardiovascular disease is a common cause of death in these patients," and because of this, "the serum cholesterol concentration should play at least as important a part in influencing the dose of thyroxine as a fear of osteoporosis."[157] For many patients with hypothyroidism and thyroid hormone-related euthyroid hypometabolism, treatment with dosages of thyroid hormone high enough to largely or completely rectify lipid abnormalities is a matter of survival. The conventional use of replacement dosages is not adequate for this purpose.

LIVER

Untreated primary hypothyroidism is associated with primary biliary cirrhosis. These two conditions share an autoimmune relation;[26] effectively treating the hypothyroidism may not alter the hepatic condition. This view is based on observations of patients treated with "replacement" dosages of T_4. Replacement dosages, however, are inadequate for effectively treating hypothyroidism. Whether effectively treating hypothyroid patients with higher than replacement dosages improves biliary cirrhosis must be determined through new studies. In hypothyroidism, aspartate aminotransferase is likely to be elevated, but if there are clinical implications to this finding, they are not clear.[26] Slowed liver metabolism may decrease clearance of various medications. For example, even small doses of cortisone may induce symptoms and signs of Cushing's syndrome (see Chapter 5.1, subsection titled "Corticosteroids"). The slowed clearance should be considered when calculating the proper dosages of medications.

COMPLICATIONS FROM SURGERY

Ladenson et al. reported that hypothyroid patients are susceptible to an increased risk of several minor complications from surgery. Their group of 40 hypothyroid patients did not differ from control surgery patients in perioperative infection. However, fever was less frequent in hypothyroid patients: 35% of hypothyroid patients and 79% of controls had fever. During noncardiac surgery, hypothyroid patients had a higher incidence of hypotension than controls (61% vs 30%). During cardiac surgery, there was a higher incidence of heart failure among hypothyroid patients than euthyroid patients (29% vs 6%). After surgery, hypothyroid patients had more gastrointestinal complaints than controls (19% vs 1%). Hypothyroid patients also had more neuropsychiatric complications than controls (38% vs 18%).[180]

Ladenson et al. wrote that such potential adverse effects for hypothyroid patients undergoing anesthesia and surgery should be anticipated and preemptively managed.[180] In line with the mandates of the current endocrinology paradigm, hypothyroid patients with clearly elevated basal serum TSH levels are likely to be identified and hopefully protected through the use of exogenous thyroid hormone.

There is reason to believe, however, that some undetermined percentage of individuals with TSH levels above 2.0 μU/mL (normal reference range: approximately 0.4-to-6.0 μU/mL) have undetected thyroid disease. This is indicated by the increased incidence of frank thyroid disease among individuals who have previously had high-normal TSH levels.[156] Some of these patients may have cardiovascular abnormalities associated with incipient suboptimal thyroid hormone levels.

In addition, some undetermined percentage of the population has various degrees of cellular resistance to thyroid hormone (see next section). These individuals may also be susceptible to the same complications during surgery as hypothyroid patients. In that surgeons are likely to subscribe to the current endocrinology paradigm for the diagnosis of thyroid disease, these patients are not likely to be detected and properly protected during surgery.

● HARMFUL EFFECTS OF THYROID HORMONE RESISTANCE

The adverse effects of resistance to thyroid hormone by different tissues are not as well documented as the effects of thyroid hormone deficiency. Also, the effects of thyroid hormone resistance are more variable. The variability is a product of normal responses of some tissues of some patients to thyroid hormone, blunted responses in other tissues, and exaggerated responses in still others.

This variability is most often seen in patients with the general form of thyroid hormone resistance. In these patients, the pituitary is among the resistant tissues. As a result, the thyrotrophs are not properly inhibited by thyroid hormone and they secrete enough TSH to raise the thyroid hormone level. Only when the elevated thyroid hormone level overrides the resistance of the pituitary are TSH synthesis and secretion inhibited. The high thyroid hormone levels compensate for the resistance of some tissues, maintaining a normal metabolic rate in them. But the high levels fail to override the resistance of other tissues, leaving them hypometabolic. Moreover, the high levels overstimulate tissues with no resistance, rendering them thyrotoxic. Thus, the patient may simultaneously exhibit clinical features typical of euthyroidism, hypothyroidism, and hyperthyroidism. Patients may seek medical attention for signs and symptoms of a variety of seemingly unrelated conditions.[70,p.359]

In the peripheral form of resistance, the pituitary gland is spared and is normally responsive to thyroid hormone; thyroid hormone properly suppresses TSH synthesis and secretion. As a result, thyroid hormone levels remain normal. This leaves tissues that are partially resistant to thyroid hormone hypometabolic. The clinical features resulting from the hypometabolism are typical of hypothyroidism, although the patient has normal thyroid hormone levels. The features found in different patients that are hypothyroid-like include muscle pain due to a hypothyroid-like myopathy, retarded growth, delayed dentition or skeletal maturation, hyperbilirubinemia, hypofibrinogenemia, hypercholesterolemia, myocardial infarction, adrenal insufficiency, recurrent syncopy, headaches, chronic back pain, congenital deafness, congenital nystagmus, neonatal jaundice, hypotonia in infants, delayed speech, learning disabilities or mental retardation in children, fatigue, somnolence, weight gain, and facial puffiness in adults.[70,p.361] When a patient's peripheral resistance is not overcome with the proper form and dosage of exogenous thyroid hormone, her idiosyncratic clinical manifestations of hypometabolism are likely to progress to their logical extremes. The possible extremes range from a poor quality of life to death.

Studies of fibromyalgia patients by my research group indicate that roughly half of these patients have partial cellular resistance to thyroid hormone. As with other thyroid hormone resistance patients, the consequences of not overriding partial cellular resistance in these patients with the proper form and dosage of thyroid hormone may well be lethal.

● RECOMMENDED "SAFETY" TESTS

Whether a particular dosage of thyroid hormone is having adverse tissue effects can be determined only by assessing the patient's symptoms, signs, and peripheral indices of tissue metabolic status. The objective tests most useful for determining whether tissues are thyrotoxic are the electrocardiogram, bone densitometry, and various blood and urine biochemical tests.

DETERMINING THE EFFECTIVE THYROID HORMONE DOSAGE TO MAINTAIN NORMAL TISSUE METABOLISM

It is not possible—by monitoring the TSH level—to determine the dosage of thyroid hormone that is effective and safe in maintaining normal tissue metabolism. Basing judgment on the TSH level infers that the TSH level accurately reflects metabolic status of tissues other than the anterior pituitary gland. This inference is false. The TSH level may correlate poorly with the metabolic status of various tissues. *The closest we can come to assessing the metabolic effects of a particular thyroid hormone dosage on the patient's tissues is to measure changes in symptoms, signs, and peripheral indices of tissue metabolic status.* These measures are indirect, but they provide a more accurate assessment of peripheral tissue metabolic status than does the TSH level.

During the process of adjusting thyroid hormone dosage and after the effective dosage is determined, the clinician should perform or order tests capable of showing whether the dosage is having adverse effects on tissues that are at risk from excessive thyroid hormone. Bone, heart, muscle, and liver are the tissues most susceptible to adverse effects. Accordingly, the clinician should make use of tests that assess possible adverse effects on these tissues. Possible adverse cardiac effects can be detected in ECG tracings; bone effects through densitometry; and muscle, hepatic, and osseus effects through blood and urine laboratory tests.

ELECTROCARDIOGRAPHY

Of foremost concern in the treatment of patients with thyroid hormone is the possibility of adverse cardiac effects. The clinician should spare no effort or expense in insuring that the patient does not have ad-

verse cardiac effects, and the overriding principle must be to err on the side of safety. Both the clinician and patient should be familiar with the indications of cardiac overstimulation by thyroid hormone and be keenly watchful for the occurrence of any of these.

The patient who before beginning the use of exogenous thyroid hormone had no symptoms, signs, or ECG indications of abnormal cardiac function may exhibit some of these when using a hormone dosage that is excessive for her. Symptoms are typically the first indication of thyrotoxicosis of the cardioregulatory system. Symptoms may include palpitations, angina pectoris, and dyspnea on exertion; and orthopnea or paroxysmal nocturnal dyspnea.[29] Signs may include tachycardia, widened pulse pressure, and cardiac flow murmurs.[161] The clinician should also examine the patient for indications of thyrotoxicity of other tissues. Two neuromuscular indications that typically are present in patients with cardiac thyrotoxicity are muscle weakness and hyperreflexia. Evidence of these phenomena, respectively, are strained inspiration and an Achilles reflex that is too brisk in both contraction and relaxation phases. (See subsection above titled "Adverse Cardiac Effects of Thyrotoxicosis.")

If symptoms and signs indicate overstimulation, an ECG should be performed. In the elderly patient, the only clinical manifestation of overstimulation of cardioregulatory mechanisms may be atrial fibrillation or congestive heart failure.[29] Because of this, I recommend screening ECGs at intervals, depending on the individual patient's estimated risk for adverse cardiac effects. I also recommend screening ECGs in patients taking supraphysiologic dosages of thyroid hormone.

For abnormal ECG findings characteristic of thyrotoxicosis, see subsection above titled "Electrocardiographic Indications of Cardiac Thyrotoxicosis." (For related information, see Chapter 4.3, subsection titled "Electrocardiography.")

BONE DENSITOMETRY

Bone densitometry provides measurements of bone mineral density. As a standard, the patient's results are compared with that of age-matched controls. It is valuable, if feasible, to obtain a baseline densitometry measurement before the patient begins taking thyroid hormone. Subsequent densitometry results can then be compared with the baseline values. The importance in baseline densitometry is that some patients before beginning the use of thyroid hormone have extreme low-normal bone mineral density compared to age-matched controls. If the extreme low-normal density is found upon densitometry only after the patient begins using thyroid hormone, the relatively low value may mistakenly be attributed to the patient's dosage of thyroid hormone. Out of concern, the clinician may then unnecessarily lower the patient's dosage to an ineffective amount. This is especially likely to happen if the patient is post-menopausal and the clinician is concerned that this risk factor may compound low-normal bone density mistakenly attributed to the patient's dosage of thyroid hormone.

If a patient who has found an effective thyroid hormone dosage turns out to have a low bone mineral density compared to age-matched controls, the clinician and patient should consult a radiologist knowledgeable about the effects of thyroid hormone on bone density. A radiologist's advice, based on the risk factors involved in the patient's case, is often helpful in clarifying the risk/benefit ratio.

I have found that many female fibromyalgia patients, after taking TSH-suppressive dosages of thyroid hormone for several years, have bone mineral densities above that of age-matched controls. The most likely explanation is the patient's increased physical activity level made possible by her use of exogenous thyroid hormone. However, it is poor procedure to make clinical decisions based on assumptions about the probability of the effects of exogenous thyroid hormone on a patient's bone mineral density. The clinician should assess each patient individually by ordering bone densitometry at baseline and appropriate intervals.

LABORATORY TESTS AND THEIR INTERPRETATION

Several blood and urine laboratory tests are useful in determining whether the patient's dosage of thyroid hormone is adversely affecting various tissues. The tests include serum calcium, phosphorus, creatinine, BUN, and alkaline phosphatase, and urinary calcium, phosphorus, creatinine, and N-telopeptides.

Serum alkaline phosphatase, calcium, phosphorus, and creatinine are available for little expense in the conventional automated chemistry profile or ACP (formerly termed SMAC). Urinary calcium, phosphorus, and creatinine must be measured from a 24-hour urine sample collected in a container with HCL. A separate urine sample (other than a first morning sample) must be taken for measurement of N-telopeptides. Cross-linked N-telopeptides are a marker of bone resorption

that is specific to the type I collagen found in bone.[39][40] They are a direct degradation product of bone resorption: they directly reflect the amount of bone collagen undergoing resorption. They are stable and are excreted in urine. Unlike hydroxyproline, they are not affected by diet and are solely related to bone resorption.[41] At present, the N-telopeptides test is also preferable to the hydroxyproline because of the difference in cost. At present, the physician's cost at some commercial laboratories for the hydroxyproline is $175.00, while the cost for N-telopeptides is $55.00.

Serum Alkaline Phosphatase

Bone is rich in the enzyme alkaline phosphatase. In patients with bone diseases involving increased osteoblastic activity, resulting in increased bone synthesis, blood levels of alkaline phosphatase rise.[65,pp.357-358] Hyperthyroidism is one such disease,[26][43][44][45][48][51][63] although thyrotoxic bone also has an increased osteoclastic breakdown of bone. Wakasugi assessed the correlation of alkaline phosphatase values with bone mineral density in hyperthyroid patients measured by dual energy x-ray absorptiometry. He found an inverse relationship and concluded that an increased level of alkaline phosphatase is a sensitive marker of altered bone metabolism in hyperthyroidism.[44]

Alkaline phosphatase levels are lower in malnourished individuals.[65,p.358] The clinician should consider this when testing patients who have severely restricted their diets to lose weight. Liver diseases can cause elevated serum alkaline phosphatase, but other abnormal lab values and clinical features usually provide a clear distinction between liver and bone involvement. If necessary, the clinician can order alkaline phosphatase isoforms to distinguish the source of alkaline phosphatase as liver, bone, spleen, kidney, or intestine.[65,p.358] *Normal range:* 25-to-140 U/L.

Calcium

Calcium is the body's most abundant mineral. Some 95% of body calcium is a constituent of bone, mainly as hydroxyapatite (a crystal lattice of calcium, phosphorus, and hydroxide). Of the remainder of body calcium, about half is in extracellular fluids. The blood level is maintained within narrow limits, and the major route of excretion is urine. The skeleton plays an important role in maintaining calcium homeostasis through the interaction of various hormones, primarily parathyroid and those derived from the renal metabolism of vitamin D_3.

Thyroid hormone can affect the concentrations of

calcium in bone, serum, and urine.[65,pp.277-278] In hyperthyroidism, serum concentrations and urinary excretion of calcium are increased.[43][47][50] Elevated levels correlate with bone resorption by osteoclasts.[51] *Normal serum range:* 8.5-to-10.8 mg/dL. *Normal urine range:* 100-to-300 mg/24 hrs.

Phosphorus

Phosphorus is the most abundant element in the body. It is present in all cellular and extracellular locations. Some 85% of phosphorus is present in bone hydroxyapatite as inorganic phosphorus. Most of the phosphorus in serum is also inorganic.[65,pp.278-279] Serum phosphorus levels vary considerably in health and have a circadian rhythm.[66] In hyperthyroidism, serum levels and urinary excretion of phosphorus are elevated.[50] Elevated levels correlate with osteoclastic resorption of bone.[51]

Diet can significantly affect phosphorus levels. Practically all foods contain phosphorus, and ingesting phosphorus rich foods can increase levels. For this reason, before laboratory samples are taken, patients should be asked to abstain from consuming foods with a high phosphorus content. High phosphorus foods include almonds, beans, barley, bran, cheese, cocoa, chocolate, eggs, lentils, liver, milk, oatmeal, peanuts, peas, walnuts, whole wheat, rye, beef, asparagus, cabbage, carrots, celery, cauliflower, chard, chicken, clams, corn, cream, cucumbers, eggplant, fish, figs, meat, prunes, pineapple, pumpkin, raisins, and string beans. A high carbohydrate diet can significantly lower phosphorus levels.[65,p.279] *Normal serum range:* 2.5-to-4.5 mg/dL. *Normal urine range:* 340-to-1000 mg/24 hrs.

Creatinine

Creatinine is an index of lean body mass and is useful for evaluating body composition.[136] Creatinine derives from creatine, which is important in muscle metabolism. Creatine participates in the storage of high-energy phosphates in the form of phosphocreatine. Creatine is synthesized in the liver and is distributed widely throughout the body but mainly to muscle cells. In fact, the body content of creatine is proportional to muscle mass.

Creatinine is formed from creatine in a spontaneous, irreversible reaction. Some 2% of the body's creatine is converted to creatinine every 24 hours. The body does not reuse free creatinine but excretes it in the urine as a waste product of creatine. Thus, creatinine formation is directly related to muscle mass.[65,pp.262-263] Creatinine excretion is fairly constant

in a given individual, but severe exercise and a high meat diet cause a markedly increased excretion of creatinine.[65,p.263] The patient should not exercise vigorously or consume meals with a high meat content for several days before being tested for the serum or urinary creatinine level.

Serum and urine creatinine are lower than normal in hyperthyroidism.[43][62][63][67] Ford et al. discuss two mechanisms for the decreased levels. They measured levels of various constituents of venous plasma and urine in 21 patients who were hyperthyroid due to Graves' disease and 2 hyperthyroid due to Plummer's disease. The researchers tested the patients before antithyroid treatment and again after they had been euthyroid for at least 4 months. While still hyperthyroid, the mean ratio of total protein, albumin, and N-acetylglucosaminidase to creatinine increased. The ratios decreased when the patients became euthyroid. The investigators stated, however, that most measures, although different before and after treatment, were within their normal ranges throughout the study time. Ford et al. pointed out that most thyrotoxic patients have mild proteinuria that is not due to glomerular or tubular renal injury. After becoming euthyroid, urate and chloride significantly decreased and creatinine significantly increased.[68,p.298]

Ford et al. wrote that it is probable that low levels of plasma creatinine in hyperthyroidism result from an increased glomerular filtration rate[68,p.298] which others have found.[75][76] In a short-term study, Moses gave patients dosages of desiccated thyroid large enough to induce thyrotoxicosis. During the use of the desiccated thyroid, the patients' serum creatinine levels decreased too quickly to have resulted from substantial loss of muscle mass.[77] The mean 24-hour urinary creatinine of long-term thyrotoxic patients is significantly lower than after treatment renders them euthyroid. The lowered levels, by contrast, probably result from reduced production of creatinine from creatine, reflecting reduced muscle mass.[78][79][80]

Normal serum range: 0.6-to-1.5 mg/dL. *Normal urinary range:* 1000-to-2000 mg/24 hrs.

BUN

Urea is the major end product of amino acid and protein catabolism. In the U.S., the urea level is expressed as the blood urea nitrogen (BUN) content. It derives from the urea cycle in the liver. Most is excreted in the urine. Excess thyroid hormone has a catabolic effect on protein, and the protein catabolism raises the BUN.[65,pp.259-260][67] The BUN is elevated in hyperthyroidism, and the BUN/creatinine ratio is increased.[62][65,p.261][67] The clinician should bear in mind that in patients with reduced muscle mass (such as patients deconditioned because of severe fibromyalgia) creatinine is subnormal to begin with. The low creatinine level results in a high BUN/creatinine ratio.

Serum urea is influenced by dietary intake of protein and the patient's state of hydration. Because of this, the clinician should consider the patient's protein intake and state of hydration when interpreting the BUN level or the BUN/creatinine ratio.[65,p.260] *Normal range:* BUN/creatinine ratio is about 10:1.[65,p.261] *Normal serum BUN:* 5-to-25 mg/dL.

Hydroxyproline

Urine hydroxyproline levels are increased in hyperthyroidism.[43][46][47][63] But clinicians should be aware that hydroxyproline levels are affected by diet. *Normal free urinary range:* 0.2-to-1.8 mg/24 hrs. *Normal total urinary range:* 20-to-77 mg/24 hrs.

Cross-linked N-telopeptides

N-telopeptides are elevated in hyperthyroidism. This test is extremely sensitive to increases in bone turnover. In my fibromyalgia patients treated with supraphysiologic dosages of thyroid hormone, increased bone turnover indicated by N-teleopeptides has generally not been reflected in decreased bone mineral density according to bone mineral densitometry.

Normal urinary levels (measured in nmol bone collagen equivalents/nmol creatinine): in men, <65; pre-menopausal women, 5-to-65 with a mean of 35; and post-menopausal women, 0-to-135 with a mean of 57.

REFERENCES

1. Hamburger, J.I.: Section summary: diagnosis of thyroid function. In *Diagnostic Methods in Clinical Thyroidology.* Edited by J.I. Hamburger, New York, Springer-Verlag, 1989, pp.112-123.
2. Jennings, P.E., O'Malley, B.P., and Griffin, K.E.: Relevance of increased serum thyroxine concentrations associated with normal serum triiodothyronine values in hypothyroid patients receiving thyroxine: a case for "tissue thyrotoxicosis." *Br. Med. J.,* 289:1645, 1984.
3. Franklyn, J.A. and Sheppard, M.C.: Tissue thyrotoxicosis. *Br. Med. J.,* 290:393, 1985.
4. Bell, G.M., Sawers, J.S.A., Forfar, J.C., Doing, A., and Toft, A.D.: The effect of minor increments in plasma thyroxine on heart rate and urinary sodium excretion. *Clin. Endocrinol.* (Oxf.), 18:511-516, 1983.
5. Hamburger, J.I.: Strategies for cost-effective thyroid function testing with modern methods. In *Diagnostic Methods in Clinical Thyroidology.* Edited by J.I. Hamburger, New York, Springer-Verlag, 1989, pp.63-109.
6. Tepperman, J. and Tepperman, H.M.: *Metabolic and Endocrine Physiology*, 5th edition. Chicago, Year Book Medical Publishers, Inc., 1987.
7. Coindre, J.-M., David, J.-P., and Riviere, L.: Bone loss in hypothyroidism with hormone replacement. *Arch. Intern. Med.,* 146:48-53, 1986.
8. Ahmann, A.J., Solomon, B., Duncan, W.I., and Wortofsky, L.: Normal bone mineral density (BMD) in premenopausal women on suppressive doses of L-thyroxine. *Abstract 41, American Thyroid Association 62nd Meeting,* Washington, 1987.
9. Salmon, D., Rendell, M., and Williams, J.: Chemical hyperthyroidism: serum triiodothyronine levels in clinically euthyroid individuals treated with levothyroxine. *Arch. Intern. Med.,* 142:571-573, 1982.
10. Fish, L.H., Schwartz, H.L., Cavanaugh, J., et al.: Replacement dose, metabolism, and bioavailability of levothyroxine in the treatment of hypothyroidism: role of triiodothyronine in pituitary feedback in humans. *N. Engl. J. Med.,* 316(13):764-770, 1987.
11. Pearce, C.J. and Himsworth, R.L.: Total and free thyroid hormone concentrations in patients receiving maintenance replacement treatment with thyroxine. *Br. Med. J.,* 288:693, 1984.
12. Bayer, M.F., Kriss, J.P., and McDougall, I.R.: Clinical experience with sensitive thyrotropin measurements: diagnostic and therapeutic implications. *J. Nucl. Med.,* 26:1248, 1985.
13. Hennessey, J.V., Evaul, J.E., and Tseng, Y.C.: L-thyroxine dosage: a reevaluation of therapy with contemporary preparations. *Ann. Intern. Med.,* 105:11, 1986.
14. Toft, A.D.: Thyroxine replacement treatment: clinical judgment or biochemical control? *Br. Med. J.,* 291:233, 1985.
15. Bantle, J.P.: Replacement therapy with levothyroxine: evolving concepts. *Thyroid Today,* 10:1, 1987.
16. Guyton, A.C.: Personal communication, Oct.9, 1990.
17. Larsen, P.R.: Thyroid-pituitary interaction. *N. Engl. J. Med.,* 306:23, 1982.
18. Bartalena, L. and Pinchera, A.: Effects of thyroxine excess on peripheral organs. *Acta Med. Austriaca,* 21(2):60-65, 1994.
19. Campos-Pastor, M.M., Munoz-Torres, M., Escobar-Jimenez, F., Ruiz de Almodovar, M., and Jodar-Gimeno, E.: Bone mass in females with different thyroid disorders: influence of menopausal status. *Bone and Mineral,* 21(1):1-8, 1993.
20. Schneider, D.L., Barrett-Connor, E.L., and Morton, D.J.: Thyroid hormone use and bone mineral density in elderly women: effects of estrogen. *J.A.M.A.,* 271(16):1245-1249, 1994.
21. Schneider, D.L., Barrett-Connor, E.L., and Morton, D.J.: Thyroid hormone use and bone mineral density in elderly men. *Arch. Intern. Med.,* 115(18):2005-2007, 1995.
22. Ross, D.S.: Hyperthyroidism, thyroid hormone therapy, and bone. *Thyroid,* 4(3):319-326, 1994.
23. Whybrow, P.C.: The therapeutic use of triiodothyronine and high dose thyroxine in psychiatric disorders. *Acta Med. Austriaca,* 21(2):47-52, 1994.
24. Vermeulen, A.: Environment, human reproduction, menopause, and andropause. *Environ. Health Perspect.,* 2

(Suppl.101):91-100, 1993.

25. Kung, A.W. and Ng., F.: A rate model of thyroid hormone-induced bone loss: effect of antiresorptive agents on regional bone density and osteocalcin gene expression. *Thyroid*, 4(1):93-98, 1994.

26. Huang, M.J. and Liaw, Y.F.: Clinical associations between thyroid and liver diseases. *J. Gastroenterol. and Hepatol.*, 10(3):344-350, 1995.

27. De Rosa, G., Testa, A., Maussier, M.L., Calla, C., Astazi, P., and Albanese, C.: A slightly suppressive dose of L-thyroxine does not affect bone turnover and bone mineral density in pre- and post-menopausal women with nontoxic goitre. *Hormone and Metab. Res.*, 27(11):503-507, 1995.

28. Bernstein, R.S. and Robbins, J.: Intermittent therapy with L-thyroxine. *N. Engl. J. Med.*, 281:1444, 1969.

29. Aronow, W.S.: The heart and thyroid disease. *Clin. Geriatric Med.*, 11(2):219-229, 1995.

30. Unger, J., Mavroudakis, N., Lipski, A., and van Coeverden, A.: Treatment of supraventricular tachyarrhythmias associated with hyperthyroidism by radioiodine, amiodarone, and propylthiouracil. *Thyroidology*, 3(2):85-88, 1991.

31. Fujimoto, K., Tagata, M., Nagao, M., et al.: A case of myxedema heart with serial endomyocardial biopsy. *Kokyu to Junkan: Respiration and Circulation*, 40(10):1019-1023, 1992.

32. Vanhaelst, L.: Hypothyroidism and coronary heart disease. In *Recent Progress in Diagnosis and Treatment of Hypothyroid Conditions*. Edited by P.A. Bastenie, M. Bonnyns, and L. Vanhaelst, Amsterdam, *Excerpta Medica*, 1980, pp.117-121.

33. Disdier, P., Harle, J.-R., Brue, T., Jaquet, P., Chambourlier, P., Grisoli, F., and Weiller, P.-J.: Severe fibromyalgia after hypophysectomy for Cushing's disease. *Arthritis Rheumatol.*, 34(4):493-495, 1991.

34. Symons, C. and Colquhoun, M.C.: Asymptomatic thyroiditis and atrial dysrhythmias. In *Recent Progress in Diagnosis and Treatment of Hypothyroid Conditions*. Edited by P.A. Bastenie, M. Bonnyns, and L. Vanhaelst, Amsterdam, *Excerpta Medica*, 1980, pp.137-143.

35. Bastenie, P.A.: Problems for the future. In *Recent Progress in Diagnosis and Treatment of Hypothyroid Conditions*. Edited by P.A. Bastenie, M. Bonnyns, and L. Vanhaelst, Amsterdam, *Excerpta Medica*, 1980, pp.156-157.

36. Vlase, H., Lungu, G., and Vlase, L.: Cardiac disturbances in thyrotoxicosis: diagnosis, incidence, clinical features, and management. *Endocrinologie*, 29(3-4):155-160, 1991.

37. Umpierrez, G.E., Challapalli, S., and Patterson, C.: Congestive heart failure due to reversible cardiomyopathy in patients with hyperthyroidism. *Am. J. Med. Sci.*, 310(3):99-102, 1995.

38. Orwoll, E.S., Bauer, D.C., Vogt, T.M., and Fox, K.M.: Axial bone mass in older women. *Ann. Intern. Med.*, 124(2):187-194, 1996.

39. Rosen, N.M. and Dresner-Pollak, R.: Specificity of urinary excretion of cross-linked N-telopeptides of type I collagen as a marker of bone turnover. *Calcification Tissue International*, 54:26-29, 1994.

40. Hanson, D.A., Weis, M.A.E., Bollen, A.K., et al.: A specific immunoassay for monitoring human bone resorption: quantitation of type I collagen cross-linked N-telopeptides

in urine. *J. Bone Mineral Res.*, 7:1251-1258, 1992.

41. Bone loss detection through a simple urine test. Product description: Center for Molecular Biology and Pathology, Research Triangle Park, North Carolina 27709. (800) 533-0567.

42. Thevenon, A., Hardouin, P., Wemeau, J.L., et al.: Bone involvement in hypothyroidism in adults: apropos of 20 patients. *Ann. de Med. Intern.*, 137(3):212-215, 1986.

43. Popelier, M., Jollivet, B., Fouquet, B., et al.: Phosphorus-calcium metabolism in hyperthyroidism. *Presse Med.*, 19(15):705-708, 1990.

44. Wakasugi, M., Wakao, R. Tawata, M., et al.: Bone mineral density in patients with hyperthyroidism measured by dual energy x-ray absorptiometry. *Clin. Endocrinol. (Oxf.)*, 38(3):283-286, 1993.

45. Price, C.P., Mitchell, C.A., Moriarty, J., Gray, M., and Noonan, K.: Mass versus activity: validation of an immunometric assay for bone alkaline phosphatase in serum. *Ann. Clin. Biochem.*, 32(part 4):405-441, 1995.

46. Gasinska, T., Drozdz, M., Izbicka, M., and Szydlo, E.: Effect of various beta-adrenolytic drugs and calcium channel blocker (nifedipine) on selected indicators of calcium-phosphorus metabolism in patients with hyperthyroidism and simple goiter. *Endokrynologia Polska*, 39(6):327-337, 1988.

47. Gasinka, T., Wawrzyniak, L., and Widala, E.: Acetylation phenotype and the changes in selected indicators of calcium-phosphate metabolism in patients with hyperthyroidism treated with propranolol. *Endokrynologia Polska*, 40(6):291-300, 1989.

48. Leger, J., Czernichow, P., Garabedian, M., Brauner, R., and Rappaport, R.: Severe osteopenia in young children with hyperthyroidism. *Arch. Francaises de Ped.*, 43(2):123-125, 1986.

49. Mosekilde, L. and Melsen, F.: Effect of antithyroid treatment on calcium-phosphorus metabolism in hyperthyroidism. II: bone histomorphometry. *Acta Endocrinol.*, 87(4):751-758, 1978.

50. Mosekilde, L., Christensen, M.S., Melsen, F., and Sorensen, N.S.: Effect of antithyroid treatment on calcium-phosphorus metabolism in hyperthyroidism. I: chemical quantities in serum and urine. *Acta Endocrinol.*, 87(4):743-750, 1978.

51. Mosekilde, L., Melsen, F., Bagger, J.P., Myhre-Jensen, O., and Sorensen, N.: Bone changes in hyperthyroidism: interrelationships between bone morphometry, thyroid function, and calcium-phosphorus metabolism. *Acta Endocrinol.*, 85(3):515-525, 1977.

52. Melsen, F. and Mosekilde, L.: Morphometric and dynamic studies of bone changes in hyperthyroidism. *Acta Pathologica et Microbiologica Scandinavica*: Section A, Pathology, 85A(2):141-150, 1977.

53. Garero, P., Shih, W.J., Gineyts, E., Karpf, D.B., and Delmas, P.D.: Comparison of new biochemical markers of bone turnover in late post-menopausal osteoporotic women in response to alendronate treatment. *J. Clin. Endocrinol. Metab.*, 79(6):1693-1700, 1994.

54. Rosen, H.N., Dresner-Pollak, R., Moses, A.C., et al.: Specificity of urinary excretion of cross-linked N-telopeptides of type I collagen as a marker of bone turnover. *Calcif. Tissue Internat.*, 54(1):26-29, 1994.

55. Blumsohn, A., Herrington, K., Hannon, R.A., Shao, P., Eyre, D.R., and Eastell, R.: The effect of calcium supplementation on the circadian rhythm of bone resorption. *J. Clin. Endocrinol. Metab.*, 79(3):730-735, 1994.

56. Grant, D.J., McMurdo, M.E.T., Mole, P.A., and Paterson, C.R.: Is previous hyperthyroidism still a risk factor for osteoporosis in post-menopausal women? *Clin. Endocrinol.*, 43(3):339-345, 1995.

57. Britto, J.M., Fenton, A.J., Holloway, W.R., and Nicholson, G.C.: Osteoblasts mediate thyroid hormone stimulation of osteoclastic bone resorption. *Endocrinol.*, 134(1): 169-176, 1994.

58. Limanova, Z. and Stepan, J.: The risk for osteoporosis in persons treated with thyroid hormones. *Vnitrni Lekarstvi*, 38(9):860-867, 1992.

59. Schmidt-Gayk, H., Roth, H.J., Becker, S., Reichel, H., Boneth, H.G., and Knuth, U.A.: Noninvasive parameters of bone metabolism. *Curr. Opinion Nephrol. Hyperten.*, 4(4): 334-338, 1995.

60. Faber, J., Overgaard, K., Jarlov, A.E., and Christiansen, C.: Bone metabolism in pre-menopausal women with non-toxic goiter and reduced serum thyrotropin levels. *Thyroidology*, 6(1):27-32, 1994.

61. Garnero, P., Vassy, V., Bertholin, A., Riou, J.P., and Delmas, P.D.: Markers of bone turnover in hyperthyroidism and the effects of treatment. *J. Clin. Endocrinol. Metab.*, 78(4):955-959, 1994.

62. Shirota, T., Shinoda, T., Yamada, T., and Aizawa, T.: Alteration of renal function in hyperthyroidism: increased tubular secretion of creatinine and decreased distal tubule delivery of chloride. *Metabolism: Clin. Exper.*, 41(4):402-405, 1992.

63. Krakauer, J.C. and Kleerekoper, M.: Borderline-low serum thyrotropin level is correlated with increased fasting urinary hydroxyproline excretion. *Arch. Intern. Med.*, 152(2): 360-364, 1992.

64. Tremollieres, F., Pouilles, J.M., Louvet, J.P., and Ribot, C.: Transitory bone loss during substitution treatment for hypothyroidism: results of a two-year prospective study. *Revue du Rhumatisme et des Maladies Osteo-Articulaires*, 58(12):869-875, 1991.

65. Woo, J., Treuting, J.J., and Cannon, D.C.: Metabolic intermediates and inorganic ions. In *Clinical Diagnosis and Management by Laboratory Methods*, 16th edition. Edited by J.B. Henry, Philadelphia, W.B. Saunders Co., 1979.

66. Goldsmith, R.S.: Laboratory aids in the diagnosis of metabolic bone disease. *Orthop. Clin. North Am.*, 3:545, 1972.

67. Shirota, T.: Studies on the renal handling of urea nitrogen, creatinine, water, and electrolytes in hyperthyroid patients with Graves' disease. *Nippon Naibunpi Gakkai Zasshi: Folia Endocrinologica Japonica*, 67(5):611-621, 1991.

68. Ford, H.C., Lim, W.C., Chisnall, W.N., and Pearce, J.M.: Renal function and electrolyte levels in hyperthyroidism: urinary protein excretion and the plasma concentrations of urea, creatinine, uric acid, hydrogen ion, and electrolytes. *Clin. Endocrinol.*, 30(3):293-301, 1989.

69. Greer, M.A.: Effects on endogenous thyroid activity of feeding desiccated thyroid to normal human subjects. *N. Engl. J. Med.*, 244:385, 1951.

70. Refetoff, S., Weiss, R.E., and Usala, S.J.: The syndromes of resistance to thyroid hormone. *Endocrine Rev.*, 14(3):

348-399, 1993.

71. Dillman, W.H.: The cardiovascular system in thyrotoxicosis. In *The Thyroid: A Fundamental and Clinical Text*, 6th edition. Edited by L.E. Braverman and R.D. Utiger, Philadelphia, J.B. Lippincott Co., 1991, pp.759-770.

72. Lowe, J.C., Garrison, R., Reichman, A.J., Yellin, J., Thompson, M., and Kaufman, D.: Effectiveness and safety of T_3 (triiodothyronine) therapy for euthyroid fibromyalgia: a double-blind placebo-controlled response-driven crossover study. *Clin. Bull. Myofascial Ther.*, 2(2/3):31-57, 1997.

73. Lowe, J.C., Reichman, A.J., and Yellin, J.: The process of change during T_3 treatment for euthyroid fibromyalgia: a double-blind placebo-controlled crossover study. *Clin. Bull. Myofascial Ther.*, 2(2/3):91-124, 1997.

74. Pearch, C.J. and Himsworth, R.L.: Total and free thyroid hormone concentration in patients receiving maintenance replacement treatment with thyroxine. *Brit. Med. J.*, 288: 693-695, 1984.

75. Bardley, S.E.: Renal function—body water and electrolytes. In *The Thyroid*, 4th edition. Edited by S.C. Werner and S.H. Ingbar, Hagerstown, Harper & Row, 1976, pp.720-726.

76. Vaamonde, C.A. and Michael, U.F.: The kidney in thyroid dysfunction. In *The Kidney in Systemic Disease*. Edited by W.N. Suki and G. Eknoyan, New York, John Wiley & Sons, 1981, pp.361-415.

77. Moses, C., Sunder, G.H., Vester, V.W., and Danowski, T.S.: Hydrocortisone and/or desiccated thyroid in physiologic dosage. XI. Effects of thyroid hormone excesses on lipids and other blood and serum solutes. *Metabolism*, 13:717-728, 1964.

78. Beylot, S.M., Riou, J.P., Sautot, G., and Mornex, R.: Absence d'effet du propranolol du l'elimination urinaire de la 3-methylhistidine dans l'hyperthyroidie. *La Presse Medicale*, 13:1829-1831, 1984.

79. Rodier, M., Richard, J.L., Bringer, J., Cavalie, G., Bellet, H., and Mirouze, J.: Thyroid status and muscle protein breakdown as assessed by urinary 3-methylhistidine excretion: study in thyrotoxic patients before and after treatment. *Metabolism*, 33:97-100, 1984.

80. Adlerberth, A., Angeras, U., Jagenburg, R., Lindstedt, G., Stenstrom, G., and Hasselgren, P.O.: Urinary excretion of 3-methylhistidine and creatinine and plasma concentrations of amino acids in hyperthyroid patients following preoperative treatment with antithyroid drug or β-blocking agent: results from a prospective, randomized study. *Metabolism*, 36:637-642, 1987.

81. Meunier, P.J., Edouard, C., Coupron, P., et al.: Morphometric analysis of osteroid in iliac trabecular bone: methodology: dynamical significance of the osteoid parameters. In *Vitamin D and Problems Related to Uremic Bone Disease*. Edited by A.W. Normal, K. Schaeffer, H.G. Grigoleit, et al., Berlin, Walter de Gruyter, 1975, pp.149-155.

82. Riggs, B.L. and Melton, L.J.: Involutional osteoporosis. *N. Engl. J. Med.*, 314:1676-1684, 1986.

83. Melton, L.J. and Riggs, B.L.: Epidemiology of age-related fractures. In *Osteoporotic Syndrome*. Edited by A.V. Avioli, New York, Grune and Stratton, 1983, pp.45-72.

84. Riggs, B.L., Jowsey, J., Kelly, P.J., Hoffman, D.L., and

Arnaud, C.D.: Effects of oral therapy with calcium and vitamin D in primary osteoporosis. *J. Clin. Endocrinol. Metab.*, 42:1139-1144, 1976.

85. Health, H., III. and Callaway, C.W.: Calcium tablets for hypertension? *Ann. Intern. Med.*, 10:946-947, 1985.

86. Riggs, B.L.: Treatment of osteoporosis with sodium fluoride: an appraisal. In *Bone and Mineral Research, Annual 2: A Yearly Survey of Developments in the Field of Bone and Mineral*, New York: Elsevier, 1984, pp.366-393.

87. Slovik, D.M., Neer, R.M., and Potts, J.T., Jr.: Short-term effects of synthetic human parathyroid hormone-(I-34) administration on bone mineral metabolism in osteoporotic patients. *J. Clin. Invest.*, 68:1261-1271, 1981.

88. Rasmussen, H., Bordier, P., Marie, P., et al.: Effects of combined therapy with phosphate and calcitonin on bone volume in osteoporosis. *Metab. Bone Dis. Relat. Res.*, 2: 107-111, 1980.

89. Chesnut, C.H., III, Ivey, J.L., Gruber, H.E., et al.: Stanozolol in post-menopausal osteoporosis: therapeutic efficacy and possible mechanisms of action. *Metabolism*, 32: 571-580, 1983.

90. Cooper, C. and Melton, L.J.: Epidemiology of osteoporosis. *Trends Endocrinol. Metab.*, 3:224-229, 1992.

91. Lukert, B.P., Higgins, J.C., and Stoskopf, M.M.: Serum osteocalcin is increased in patients with hyperthyroidism and decreased in patients receiving glucocorticoids. *J. Clin. Endocrinol. Metab.*, 62:1056-1058, 1986.

92. Hyldstrup, L., Clemmesen, I., Jensen, B.A., and Transbl, I.: Non-invasive evaluation of bone formation: measurement of serum alkaline phosphatase, whole body retention of diphosphonate and serum osteocalcin in metabolic bone disorders and thyroid disease. *Scand. J. Clin. Lab. Invest.*, 48:611-619, 1988.

93. Harvey, R.D., McHardy, K.C., Reid, I.W., Paterson, F., Bewsher, P.D., Duncan, A., and Robins, S.P.: Measurement of bone collagen degradation in hyperthyroidism and during thyroxine replacement therapy using pyridium cross-links as specific urinary markers. *J. Clin. Endocrinol. Metab.*, 72:1189-1194, 1991.

94. Paul, T.L., Kerrigan, J., Kelly, A.M., Braverman, L.E. and Baran, D.T.: Long term L-thyroxine therapy is associated with decreased hip bone density in pre-menopausal women. *J.A.M.A.*, 259:3137-3141, 1988.

95. Laitinen, K. and Valimaki, M.: Alcohol and bone. *Calcif. Tissue Int.*, 49:570-573, 1991.

96. Schapira, D.: Alcohol abuse and osteoporosis. *Sem. Arthritis Rheum.*, 19:371-376, 1990.

97. Bauer, D.C., Browner, W.S., Cauley, J.A., et al.: Factors associated with appendicular bone mass in older women. The Study of Osteoporotic Fractures Research Group, *Ann. Intern. Med.*, 118:657-665, 1993.

98. Slemenda, C.W., Hui, S.L., Longcope, C., Wellman, H., and Johnson, C.C., Jr.: Predictors of bone mass in perimenopausal women. A prospective study of clinical data using photon absorptiometry. *Ann. Intern. Med.*, 112:96-101, 1990.

99. Liel, Y., Edwards, J., Shary, J., Spicer, K.M., Gordon, L., and Bell, N.H.: The effects of race and body habits on bone mineral density of the radius, hip, and spine in pre-menopausal women. *J. Clin. Endocrinol. Metab.*, 66:1247-1250, 1988.

100. Glauber, H.S., Vollmer, W.M., Nevitt, M.C., Ensrud, K.E., and Orwoll, E.S.: Body weight versus body fat distribution, adiposity, and frame size as predictors of bone density. *J. Clin. Endocrinol. Metab.*, 80:1118-1123, 1995.

101. Reid, I.R., Ames, R., Evans, M.C., et al.: Determinants of total body and regional bone mineral density in normal post-menopausal women—a key role for fat mass. *J. Clin. Endocrinol. Metab.*, 75:45-51, 1992.

102. Reid, I.R., Plank, L.D., and Evans, M.C.: Fat mass is an important determinant of whole body bone density in pre-menopausal women but not in men. *J. Clin. Endocrinol. Metab.*, 75:779-782, 1992.

103. Riggs, B.., Jowsey, J., Goldsmith, R.S., Kelly, P.J., Hoffman, D.L., and Arnaud, C.D.: Short- and long-term effects of estrogen and synthetic anabolic hormone in post-menopausal osteoporosis. *J. Clin. Invest.*, 51:1659-1663, 1972.

104. Austin, L.A. and Heath, H.H., III.: Calcitonin physiology and pathophysiology. *N. Engl. J. Med.*, 304:269-278, 1981.

105. Riggs, B.L., Seeman, E., Hodgson, S.F., Taves, D.R., and O'Fallon, W.M.: Effect of the fluoride/calcium regimen on vertebral fracture occurence in post-menopausal osteoporosis: comparison with conventional therapy. *N. Engl. J. Med.*, 306:446-450, 1982.

106. Gallagher, J.C., Jerpbak, C.M., Jee, W.S.S., Johnson, K.A., DeLuca, H.F., and Riggs, B.L.: 1,25-Dihydroxyvitamin D_3: short- and long-term effects on bone and calcium metabolism in patients with post-menopausal osteoporosis. *Proc. Natl. Acad. Sci.*, 79:3325-3329, 1982.

107. Hasling, C., Eriksen, E.F., Charles, P., and Mosekilde, L.: Exogenous triiodothyronine activates bone remodeling. *Bone*, 8:65-69, 1987.

108. Soloman, B.L., Wartofsky, L., and Burman, K.D.: Prevalence of fractures in post-menopausal women with thyroid disease. *Thyroid*, 3:17-23, 1993.

109. Leese, G.P., Jung, R.T., Guthrie, C., Waugh, N., and Browning, M.C.K.: Morbidity in patients on L-thyroxine: a comparison of those with a normal TSH to those with a suppressed TSH. *Clin. Endocrinol.*, 37:500-503, 1992.

110. Hajerousson, V.J. and Webley, M.: Prolonged low-dose corticosteroid therapy and osteoporosis in rheumatoid arthritis. *Ann. Rheum. Dis.*, 43:24, 1984.

111. Seeman, E.: The dilemma of osteoporosis in men. *Am. J. Med.*, 98(2A):76-88, 1995.

112. Kelepouris, N., Harper, K.D., Gannon, F., Kaplan, F.S., and Haddad, J.G.: Severe osteoporosis in men. *Am. Coll. Physicians*, 123(6):452-460, 1995.

113. Ross, D.S., Neer, R.M., Ridgeway, E.C., and Daniels, G.H.: Subclinical hyperthyroidism and reduced bone density as a possible result of prolonged suppression of the pituitary-thyroid axis with L-thyroxine. *Am. J. Med.*, 82:1167-1170, 1987.

114. Taelman, P., Kaufman, J.M., Jansenns, X., Vandecauter, H., and Vermeulen, A.: Reduced forearm bone mineral content and biochemical evidence of increased bone turnover in women with euthyroid goitre treated with thyroid hormone. *Clin. Endocrinol. (Oxf.)*, 33:107-117, 1990.

115. Faccini, J.M. and Teotia, S.P.: Histopathological assess-

ment of endemic skeletal fluorosis. *Calcif. Tissue Res.*, 16:45-57, 1974.

116. Riggs, B.L., Hodgson, S.F., O'Fallon, W.M., et al.: Effect of fluoride treatment on the fracture rate in postmenopausal women with osteoporosis. *N. Engl. J. Med.*, 322:802-809, 1990.

117. Pak, C.Y.C., Khashayar, S., Adams-Huet, B., Piziak, V., Peterson, R.D., and Poindexter, J.R.: Treatment of postmenopausal osteoporosis with slow-release sodium fluoride: final report of a randomized controlled trial. *Ann. Intern. Med.*, 123(6):401-409, 1995.

118. Harvey, J.A., Zobitz, M.M., and Pak, C.Y.: Dose dependency of calcium absorption: a comparison of sodium carbonate and calcium citrate. *J. Bone Miner. Res.*, 3: 253-258, 1988.

119. Ikram, H.: The nature and prognosis of thyrotoxic heart disease. *Q.J. Med.*, 54:19, 1985.

120. Sandler, G. and Wilson, G.M.: The nature and prognosis of heart disease in thyrotoxicosis: a review of 150 patients treated with 131I. *Q.J. Med.*, 28:347, 1959.

121. Magner, J.A., Clark, W., and Allenby, P.: Congestive heart failure and sudden death in a young woman with thyrotoxicosis. *West J. Med.*, 149:86, 1988.

122. Wilson, B.E. and Hamilton, E.C.: Significant reversal of thyrotoxicosis-associated dilated cardiomyopathy with induction of the euthyroid state. *J. Endocrinol. Invest.*, 19:54-58, 1996.

123. Marriott, H.J.: *Practical Electrocardiography*, 7th edition. Baltimore, Williams and Wilkins, 1983.

124. Hoffman, I. and Lowrey, R.D.: The electrocardiogram in thyrotoxicosis. *Am. J. Cardiol.*, 8:893, 1960.

125. Muggia, A.L., Stjernholm, M., and Houle, T.: Complete heart block with thyrotoxic myocarditis. *N. Engl. J. Med.*, 283:1099, 1970.

126. Agner, T., Almdal, T., Thorsteinsson, B., and Agner, E.: A reevaluation of atrial fibrillation in thyrotoxicosis. *Dan. Med. Bull.*, 31:157, 1984.

127. Ciaccheri, M., Cecchi, F., Arcangeli, C., et al.: Occult thyrotoxicosis in patients with chronic and paroxysmal isolated atrial fibrillation. *Clin. Cardiol.*, 7:413, 1984.

128. Dubin, D.: *Rapid Interpretation of EKGs*, 3rd edition. Tampa, Cover Publishing Co., 1974.

129. Gerson, M.C. and McHenry, P.L.: Resting U wave inversion as a marker of stenosis of the left anterior descending coronary artery. *Am. J. Med.*, 69:545, 1980.

130. Kishida, H.: Negative U wave: a highly specific but poorly understood sign of heart disease. *Am. J. Cardiol.*, 49: 2030, 1982.

131. Palmer, J.H.: Isolated U wave negativity. *Circulation*, 7:205, 1953.

132. Lepeschkin, E.: The U wave of the electrocardiogram. *Arch. Intern. Med.*, 96:600, 1955.

133. Manning, G.W. and Sears, G.A.: Postural heart block. *Am. J. Cardiol.*, 9:558, 1962.

134. Scherf, D. and Dix, J.H.: Short P-R interval and its occurrence in hypertension. *Bull. N.Y. Coll. Med.*, 43:116, 1941.

135. Lown, B., Ganong, W.B., and Levine, S.A.: The syndrome of short P-R interval, normal QRS complex, and paroxysmal rapid heart action. *Circulation*, 5:693, 1952.

136. Welle, S., Thornton, C., Totterman, S., and Forbes, G.:

Utility of creatinine excretion in body-composition studies of healthy men and women older than 60 years. *Am. J. Clin. Nutri.*, 63(2):151-156, 1996.

137. Shangold, M.M.: Exercise in menopausal women. *Obstet. Gyn.*, 75(Suppl.4):53S-58S, 1990.

138. Ribot, C., Tremollieres, F., Pouilles, J.M., and Louvet, J.P.: Bone mineral density and thyroid hormone therapy. *Clin. Endocrinol.* (Oxf.), 33:143-153, 1990.

139. Stall, G.M., Harris, S., Siokoll, L.J., and Dawson-Hughes, B.: Accelerated bone loss in hypothyroid patients overtreated with L-thyroxine. *Ann. Intern. Med.*, 113:265-269, 1990.

140. Chabert-Orsini, V., Conte-Devolx, B., Thiers-Bautrant, D., et al.: Bone density after iatrogenic subclinical long-term thyrotoxicosis: measurement by dual photon absorptiometry. *Presse Med.*, 19:1709-1711, 1990.

141. Krolner, B., Vesterdal-Jorgensen, J., and Pors-Nielsen, S.: Spinal bone mineral content in myxoedema and thyrotoxicosis: effects of thyroid hormone(s) and antithyroid treatment. *Clin. Endocrinol.*, 18:439-446, 1983.

142. Seeman, E., Wahner, H.W., and Offord, K.P.: Differential effects of endocrine dysfunction on the axial and appendicular skeleton. *J. Clin. Invest.*, 69:1302-1309, 1982.

143. Fallon, M.D., Perry, H.M., Bergfeld, M., Droke, D., Teitelbaum, S.L., and Avioli, L.V.: Exogenous hyperthyroidism with osteoporosis. *Arch. Intern. Med.*, 143:442-444, 1983.

144. Sawin, C.T., Geller, A., Hershman, J.M., Castelli, W., and Bacharach, P.: The aging thyroid: the use of thyroid hormone in older persons. *J.A.M.A.*, 261:2653-2655, 1989.

145. Haynes, R.C., Jr.: Thyroid and antithyroid drugs. In *Goodman and Gilman's The Pharmacological Basis of Therapeutics*, 8th edition. New York, Pergamon Press, 1990, pp.1361-1383.

146. Ross, D.S.: Subclinical hyperthyroidism: possible danger of overzealous thyroxine replacement therapy. *Mayo Clin. Proc.*, 63:1223-1229, 1988.

147. Delamere, J.P., Scott, D.L., and Felix-Davies, D.D.: Thyroid dysfunction and rheumatic diseases. *J. Royal Society Med.*, 75:102, 1982.

148. Johnson, R.L.: Electrocardiographic findings in 67,375 asymptomatic individuals, part VII. A-V block. *Am. J. Ccardiol.*, 6:153, 1960.

149. Vagenakis, A.G., Braverman, L.E., Azizi, F., Portnay, G.I., and Ingbar, S.H.: Recovery of pituitary thyrotropic function after withdrawal of prolonged thyroid-suppression therapy. *N. Engl. J. Med.*, 293:681, 1975.

150. Refetoff, S.: Personal communication (letter) to J. Yellin, July 10, 1996.

151. Leb, G., Warnkross, H., and Obermayer-Pietsch, B.: Thyroid hormone excess and osteoporosis. *Acta Med. Austriaca*, 21(2):65-67, 1994.

152. Greenspan, S.L., Greenspan, F.S., Resnick, N.M., Block, J.E., Friedlander, A.L., and Genant, H.K.: Skeletal integrity in pre-menopausal and post-menopausal women receiving long-term L-thyroxine therapy. *Am. J. Med.*, 91: 5-14, 1991.

153. Braverman, L.E. and Utiger, R.D.: Introduction to thyrotoxicosis. In *The Thyroid: A Fundamental and Clinical*

Text, 6th edition. Edited by L.E. Braverman and R.D. Utiger, Philadelphia, J.B. Lippincott Co., 1991, pp.645-647.

154. Refetoff, S.: Thyroid hormone resistance syndromes. In *Werner's The Thyroid: A Fundamental and Clinical Text*, 5th edition. Edited by S.H. Ingbar and L.E. Braverman, Philadelphia, J.B. Lippincott Co., 1986, pp.1292-1293.

155. Tseng, K.H., Walfish, P.G., Persaud, J.A., and Gilbert, B.W.: Concurrent aortic and mitral valve echocardiography permits measurement of systolic time intervals as an index of peripheral tissue thyroid functional status. *J. Clin. Endocrinol. Metab.*, 69(3):633-638, 1989.

156. Weetman, A.P.: Hypothyroidism: screening and subclinical disease. *Brit. Med. J.*, 314:1175, 1997.

157. Fowler, P.B., McIvor, J., Sykes, L., and Macrae, K.D.: The effect of long-term thyroxine on bone mineral density and serum cholesterol. *J. R. Coll. Physicians Lond.*, 30(6):527-532, 1996.

158. Leese, G.P., Jung, R.T., Guthrie, C., Waugh, N., and Browning, M.C.: Morbidity in patients on L-thyroxine: a comparison of those with a normal TSH to those with a suppressed TSH. *Clin Endocrinol (Oxf.)*, 37(6):500-503, 1992.

159. Yildirimkaya, M., Ozata, M., Yilmaz, K., Kilinc, C., Gundogan, M.A., and Kutluay, T.: Lipoprotein(a) concentration in subclinical hypothyroidism before and after levothyroxine therapy. *Endocr. J.*, 43(6):731-736, 1996.

160. La Brocca, A.: Hypothyroidism with pseudo-ischemic and hypertensive clinical presentation: physiopathological and diagnostic considerations. *Ann. Ital. Med. Int.*, 12(2):94-97, 1997.

161. Locker, G.J., Kotzmann, H., Frey, B., et al.: Factitious hyperthyroidism causing acute myocardial infarction. *Thyroid*, 5(6):465-467, 1995.

162. Bergeron, G.A., Goldsmith, R., and Schiller, N.B.: Myocardial infarction, severe reversible ischemia, and shock following excess thyroid administration in a woman with normal coronary arteries. *Arch. Intern. Med.*, 148(6):1450-1453, 1988.

163. Goichot, B. and Schlienger, J.L.: Les indications extra-thyroïdiennes des traitements par hormones thyroïdiennes. *Rev. Méd. Interne*, 19:720-725, 1998.

164. Means, J.H., Hertz, S., and Lerman, J.: The pituitary type of myxedema of Simmonds' disease masquerading as myxedema. *Trans. Assoc. Am. Physicians*, 55:32, 1940.

165. Krugman, L.C., Hershman, J.M., Chopra, I.J., et al.: Patterns of recovery of the hypothalamic-pituitary-thyroid axis in patients taken off chronic thyroid therapy. *J. Clin. Endocrinol. Metab.*, 41:70, 1975.

166. Bantle, J.P.: Replacement therapy with levothyroxine: evolving concepts. *Thyroid Today*, 10:1, 1987.

167. Sonkin, L.S.: Myofascial pain due to metabolic disorders: diagnosis and treatment. In *Myofascial Pain and Fibromyalgia: Trigger Point Management*. Edited by E.S. Rachlin, St. Louis, Mosby, 1994, pp.45-60.

168. Loeb, J.N.: Metabolic changes in thyrotoxicosis. In *Werner and Ingbar's The Thyroid: A Fundamental and Clinical Text*, 6th edition. Edited by L.E. Braverman and R.D. Utiger, New York, J.B. Lippincott Co., 1991, pp.845-853.

169. Sandler, M.P., Robinson, R.P., Rabin, D., et al.: The effect of thyroid hormones on gluconeogenesis and forearm metabolism in man. *J. Clin. Endocrinol. Metab.*, 56:479, 1983.

170. Du Bois, E.F.: *Basal Metabolism in Health and Disease*, 3rd edition. Philadelphia, Lea & Febiger, 1936.

171. Walton, K.W., Scott, P.J., Dykes, P.W., and Davies, J.W.L.: The significance of alterations in serum lipids in thyroid dysfunction. II. Alterations of the metabolism and turnover of ^{131}I-low-density lipoproteins in hypothyroidism and hyperthyroidism. *Clin. Sci.*, 29:217, 1965.

172. Dyke, C.M., Yeh, T., Jr., Lehman, J.D., et al.: Triiodo-thyronine-enhanced left ventricular function after ischemic injury. *Ann. Thorac. Surg.*, 52:14-19, 1991.

173. Klemperer, J.D., Zelano, J., and Helm, R.E.: Triiodothyronine improves left ventricular function without oxygen wasting effects after global hypothermic ischemia. *J. Thorac. Cardiovasc. Surg.*, 109:457-465, 1995.

174. Moruzzi, P., Doria, E., and Agostoni, P.G.: Medium-term effectiveness of L-thyroxine treatment in idiopathic dilated cardiomyopathy. *Am. J. Med.*, 101:461-467, 1996.

175. Jeevanandam, V.: Triiodothyronine: spectrum of use in heart transplantation. *Thyroid*, 1:139-145, 1997.

176. Liang, D.S.: Stroke and thyroid hormones. *Chinese J. Neurol. Psychiat.*, 24(6):352-354, 384, 1991.

177. Vavouranakis, I., Sanoudos, G., Manios, A., Kalogeropoulou, K., Sitaras, K., and Kokkinos, C.: Triiodothyronine administration in coronary artery bypass surgery: effect on hemodynamics. *J. Cardiovasc. Surg.* (Torino), 35(5):383-389, Oct., 1994.

178. Wechsler, A.S., Kadletz, M., Ding, M., Abd-Elfattah, A., and Dyke, C.: Effects of triiodothyronine on stunned myocardium. *J. Card. Surg.*, 8(Suppl.2):338-341, Mar., 1993.

179. Salter, D.R.: Acute severe post-ischemic myocardial depression reversed by triiodothyronine. *Ann. Thorac. Surg.*, 54(2):301-305, Aug., 1992.

180. Ladenson, P.W., Levin, A.A., Ridgway, E.C., and Daniels, G.H.: Complications of surgery in hypothyroid patients. *Am. J. Med.*, 77(2):261-266, 1984.

181. Sibonga, J.D., Bell, N.H., and Turner, R.T.: Evidence that ibuprofen antagonizes selective actions of estrogen and tamoxifen on rat bone. *J. Bone Miner. Res.*, 13(5):863-870, 1998.

182. Sawin, C.T., Geller, A., Wolf, P.A., et al.: Low serum thyrotropin concentrations as a risk factor for atrial fibrillation in older persons. *New Engl. J. Med.*, 331(19):1249-1252, 1994.

183. Faber, J. and Galloe, A.M.: Changes in bone mass during prolonged subclinical hyperthyroidism due to L-thyroxine treatment: a meta-analysis. *Eur. J. Endocrinol.*, 130(4):350-356, 1994.

184. Franklyn, J., Betteridge, J., Holder, R., Daykin, J., Lilley, J., and Sheppard, M.: Bone mineral density in thyroxine-treated females with or without a previous history of thyrotoxicosis. *Clin. Endocrinol.* (Oxf.), 41(4):425-432, 1994.

185. Korsic, M., Cvijetic, S., Dekanic-Ozegovic, D., Bolanca, S., and Kozic, B.: Bone mineral density in patients on long-term therapy with levothyroxine. *Lijec Vjesn*, 120(5):103-105, 1998.

186. Bernstein, R., Muller, C., Midtbo, K., Smith, G., Haug, E., and Hertzenberg, L.: Silent myocardial ischemia in hypothyroidism. *Thyroid*, 5(6):443-447, 1995.

187. Perk, M. and O'Neill, B.J.: The effect of thyroid hormone therapy on angiographic coronary artery disease progression. *Can. J. Cardiol.*, 13(3):273-276, 1997.

188. Hamilton, M.A., Stevenson, L.W., Fonarow, G.C., et al.: Safety and hemodynamic effects of intravenous triiodothyronine in advanced congestive heart failure. *J. Cardiol.*, 81(4):443-447, 1998.

189. Pinchera, A., Martino, E., and Faglia, G.: Central hypothyroidism. In *Werner and Ingbar's The Thyroid: A Fundamental and Clinical Text*, 6th edition. Edited by L.E. Braverman and R.D. Utiger, New York, J.B. Lippincott Co., 1991, pp.968-984.

190. Klein, I. and Levey, G.S.: The cardiovascular system in thyrotoxicosis. In *Werner and Ingbar's The Thyroid: A Fundamental and Clinical Text*, 7th edition. Edited by L.P. Braverman and R.D. Utiger, Philadelphia, Lippincott-Raven Publishers, 1996, pp.607-615.

Section V

Treatment:
Metabolic Rehabilitation

5.1

Review of Studies: Fibromyalgia Treatments

Some fibromyalgia patients markedly improve or recover from fibromyalgia by obtaining a sustained increase in their metabolism through the use of thyroid hormone, nutritional supplementation, and exercise to tolerance. These three forms of treatment are the core procedures of metabolic rehabilitation. Many patients, to improve or recover, must also undergo one or more other forms of treatment as adjuncts to their regimen of metabolic rehabilitation. The purpose of this chapter is to review the available information on current treatments that may serve as adjuncts during the patients' rehabilitation. Familiarizing himself with the results of tests of the various treatments should enable the clinician to select treatments that may help optimize an individual patient's treatment outcome.

Using appropriate adjunctive treatments in the care of fibromyalgia patients is in line with the insights of physicians such as Leon Chaitow and Paul White. Their opinion is that improvement or recovery from fibromyalgia will not come solely through the use of any "magic bullet" treatment. Instead, improvement or recovery is likely only when the patient undergoes the combination of interventions that are requisite to optimizing that individual's health. With most every patient, the combination includes improved diet, nutritional supplementation, exercise to tolerance, sufficient rest and recreation, improved biomechanical function, stress reduction, and minimized exposure to endogenous and exogenous pollutants. Paltry few fibromyalgia patients improve or recover when they only use thyroid hormone. But most do when they conform to the holistic concept expressed by authors such as Chaitow and White and take up a variety of other health-inducing practices to supplement their metabolic rehabilitation.

Practices such as exercise to tolerance and nutritional supplementation are indispensable components of metabolic rehabilitation. Physical treatments such as myofascial trigger point therapy and spinal manipulation are also essential for many patients, particularly for optimal pain relief. Investigators have conducted a number of studies on the fibromyalgia treatment effects of physical exercise. But nutritional and physical therapies for fibromyalgia patients have undergone precious little testing.

Some patients do not improve with metabolic rehabilitation, not even when various other treatments are used as adjuncts. These patients would best not be consigned by default to the long-term use of medications that have been proven ineffective and potentially hazardous, such as amitriptyline and cyclobenzaprine. It is to these patients' advantage that their clinicians work with them to assemble a combination of noninvasive and nontoxic treatments that provide them at least palliative relief until a truly effective treatment enables them to recover from their symptoms.

No treatment other than the metabolic rehabilitation described in this book has been shown to enable some patients to completely recover and remain recovered from fibromyalgia. However, a range of other chemical, physical, and psychological treatments for fibromyalgia have been subjected to clinical scrutiny. The clinician should be aware of the results of the studies of the various treatments so that he can decide which may or may not be of help with individual fibromyalgia patients.

Some of the tested treatments are not intended to relieve fibromyalgia by correcting an underlying pathological mechanism. The treatments are instead offered by researchers only as interventions to provide palliative relief from some symptoms. The use of antidepressant medications as a fibromyalgia treatment is an exception. At least originally, these medications were used based on the hypothesis that fibromyalgia is a clinical manifestation of a serotonin deficiency. The hypothesis was based on evidence that some fibromyalgia patients had low peripheral serotonin levels. It was thus reasonable to test the hypothesis that increasing serotonin levels with antidepressant medications would relieve fibromyalgia symptoms. The failure of these medications to provide significant relief from symptoms contributes to the falsification of the serotonin deficiency hypothesis of fibromyalgia. Despite the negative results from antidepressant trials, however, some researchers and authors of review papers continue to falsely report that the medications are "effective" as a treatment for fibromyalgia. To understand the falsity of the claim that antidepressant medications are effective in the treatment of fibromyalgia, the clinician should familiarize himself with the information on the use of antidepressant medication in this chapter and in Chapters 1.1 and 1.2.

Inaccurate reports that antidepressant medications are effective in the treatment of fibromyalgia may have seriously adverse consequences for fibromyalgia patients and their treating physicians. Many patients begin using the medications with the belief that studies have shown the medications to be effective fibromyalgia treatments. When these patients continue to suffer from fibromyalgia, the poor outcome of their own treatment may, at minimum, be confusing. For some patients, failure to obtain relief with these medications may be disheartening and even lead to a sense of hopelessness. In addition, in my experience, reports that these medications are effective have resulted in practicing physicians maintaining false expectations of the potential of the medications to relieve fibromyalgia symptoms. It is conceivable that therapeutic failure involving the medications leads to a credibility gap between some of these physicians and their patients. Unfortunately, the gap is based on false assumptions. The patient may come to doubt the competence of her physician who offers assurances based on research reports; the physician may come to suspect that the treatment failure indicates some underlying psychological motive overriding the patient's desire to improve.

The clinician should be vigilant of two faults in the conclusions of some fibromyalgia researchers. One fault is reaching the conclusion that a treatment is "effective" when this may be true statistically but not clinically. The other fault is the use of outcome measures that are of questionable value in determining whether a treatment is truly effective with some patients.

The usual practice in the rheumatology fibromyalgia research literature is to report a treatment to be effective if there is a statistical difference between the outcome for the experimental treatment (such as amitriptyline) and that for the placebo. "Statistical significance," however, is not necessarily tantamount to "clinical significance." In most studies of amitriptyline and cyclobenzaprine, researchers reported that these drugs were "effective." A careful reading of the results, however, shows that patients had only the most modest improvement and that improvement lasted only a brief time, even though patients continued to use the medications. In contrast, as found in one case-control study, some fibromyalgia patients recovered through metabolic rehabilitation and remained recovered for up to 5 years. In clinical practice, other fibromyalgia patients have maintained their full recovery, attained through metabolic rehabilitation, for more than 10 years. There are no comparable records of treatment outcomes from the use of antidepressant medications in the treatment of fibromyalgia. In fact, while referring to antidepressant medications as "effective" fibromyalgia treatments, the same researchers have publically conceded that they cannot get fibromyalgia patients significantly improved or well. Therefore, the term "effective" is a misnomer when used as an adjective to describe the "antidepressant treatment of fibromyalgia."

And in some studies, researchers used only a few gauges of patients' fibromyalgia status, usually visual analog scales. These alone do not provide sufficient documentation that the status of patients has actually changed during treatment.

Recognizing the faults of linguistic carelessness and inadequate outcome measures in fibromyalgia research, my research group has made extensive efforts not to repeat such faults in our studies and in clinical practice. To our group, "effective" means that after undergoing the treatment the patient no longer meets the ACR criteria for fibromyalgia and no longer meets our more stringent research criteria. According to our definition of effective, the patient is free from symptoms and signs and regains full function. And the patient's improved status continues as long as she continues the procedures necessary to sustain her newly normalized metabolism. Without such a definition for "effective," a study conclusion that a treatment is effective is for all practical purposes meaningless.

Metabolic rehabilitation as described in this book is the only fibromyalgia treatment protocol that meets a stringent definition of effective. Nonetheless, a few other treatments improve some features of some patients' fibromyalgia. Unfortunately, the limited improvement has led some clinicians to illogically conclude that the therapeutically affected mechanism is the underlying mechanism of fibromyalgia as a whole. An example of this is the limited beneficial effect of growth hormone injections for some patients. The improvement led to the conclusion that a growth hormone deficiency must underlie all fibromyalgia and that relieving the deficiency is the treatment of choice. Growth hormone deficiency, however, does not explain all the documented features of fibromyalgia. Thus, defining fibromyalgia as the manifestation of a growth hormone deficiency is an ad hoc hypothesis. It is not offered as an extension of a more comprehensive hypothesis but only to account for the finding of low growth hormone or somatomedin C levels. The growth hormone deficiency hypothesis is, therefore, scientifically inadequate. The example serves to illustrate why some treatments have provided patients with some degree of relief.

Inadequate thyroid hormone regulation of cell function does explain all the documented features of fibromyalgia, including the growth hormone deficiency. (Transcription of the growth hormone gene is directly regulated by thyroid hormone. This has been shown repeatedly by the most extensive group of studies ever done on a single gene regulated by thyroid hormone.) Also, our studies show that the proper form and dosage of exogenous thyroid hormone not only relieves the features of fibromyalgia that can be attributed to a growth hormone deficiency, but the hormone also relieves all other features as well.

Since I reviewed fibromyalgia treatment studies in 1995,[114] the availability of effective treatments has changed only in one way: metabolic rehabilitation has been shown to be the only completely effective treatment providing relief that lasts long term.

In this chapter, I review published studies of chemical, psychological, and physical treatments for fibromyalgia. Some of the treatments are reported to provide patients with a measure of improvement, but in general, the treatments are at best palliative. Gold-

enberg wrote in 1989, "Most physicians treating patients with fibromyalgia know that current therapeutic programs are not very effective." He added, "Thus patients have usually tried multiple therapies and none seem to be very effective."[1,pp.61-62] Neither drug nor non-drug therapies reported in the literature seem particularly beneficial.[1][2][3][4] As Schmidt noted in 1991, medical, physical, and psychological therapies are at best about 50% effective.[5] Schmidt's assessment was liberal in the extreme considering my thorough 1995 review of published studies of fibromyalgia treatments in the *Journal of Myofascial Therapy*. This updated review of studies indicates that aside from the studies of metabolic therapy by my research group, nothing has changed.

In a 1993 review of fibromyalgia treatment programs, Goldenberg wrote that before 1986, most studies of fibromyalgia treatment were not controlled. Controlled studies have accumulated, but most of these have major methodological problems. In this review, I do not point out methodological flaws in studies. In fact, in most of the studies I review here, I also do not note whether the researchers included control groups, placebos, or other experimental measures that help determine whether a particular therapy is effective in itself. Most studies did use controls, although as Goldenberg pointed out, some controls were not adequate.[6,p.72] For the most part, I mention methodological issues only when they must temper the conclusions drawn from a study.

● **THE FOCUS OF RESEARCH IN FIBROMYALGIA TREATMENTS**

Chemical treatments have been tested far more extensively than psychological or physical treatments. This is a result of rheumatologists spearheading research into fibromyalgia treatment. These specialists traditionally have treated patients with allopathic drug therapies, and it is understandable that they have largely tested the form of treatment they are accustomed to. Other specialists have been comparatively inactive in fibromyalgia research, and consequently, there are comparatively few studies of therapies peculiar to these other specialties.

Despite this, McCain wrote in 1989 that most rheumatologists would argue that one or another non-drug multidisciplinary intervention helps most fibromyalgia patients.[10,p.73] He maintained that drug therapies alone often do not significantly improve the fibromyalgia patient's condition.[11,p.34] Many clinicians typically use other forms of treatment and assign drug therapies to an adjunctive role. Still, researchers had evaluated few of these therapies with acceptable scientific methods. McCain pointed out that practitioners typically use such therapies "with little rationale, often haphazardly, and rarely in conjunction with pharmacologic therapies."

The comparative usefulness of common fibromyalgia treatments was illustrated by the results of a study by Goldenberg in 1989. He surveyed 87 fibromyalgia patients, asking about their assessment of how well various therapies had worked for them during a 2-year period. The most effective medication was amitriptyline. There was little difference in the effectiveness of any other medications, and patients rated non-drug treatments as effective as medications.[1,p.62] As I wrote above, the available studies indicate that little has changed save for the metabolic therapy described in this book. Table 5.1.1 lists the treatments included in this review.

● **CHEMICAL THERAPIES**

Among chemical therapies, allopathic medications, hormones, nutritional agents, and one homeopathic remedy have been tested.

ANTIDEPRESSANT DRUGS

Tertiary amine tricyclic drugs, including amitriptyline, imipramine, clomipramine, and doxepin, inhibit neuronal reuptake of serotonin. They also inhibit reuptake of secondary demethylated amine metabolites, including desipramine and nortriptyline.[164] Deficient serotonin was a plausible mechanism for the pain and sleep disturbance of fibromyalgia. Because of this, in the 1980s several studies were conducted to determine whether amitriptyline was of benefit. There was reason to tentatively believe it was of benefit in that it was reported to suppress rapid eye movement (REM) and to prolong stage 3 and stage 4 non-REM sleep.[164] The results of several uncontrolled studies published in 1981 raised the possibility that the medication provided fibromyalgia patients with some improvement.[165][166][167]

Some controlled studies in the 1980s indicated that cyclobenzaprine and amitriptyline, at least over the short term, were somewhat effective.[7][43][44] The drugs were believed to work via several possible me-

chanisms. These include (1) increased brain levels of serotonin and endogenous opioids, (2) increased stage 4 sleep, (3) reduced motor (muscle) activity through the brain stem, (4) anticholinergic effects, and (5) decreased depression.[1,p.63]

The minimal improvement occurred within the first 2-to-4 weeks.[7][43] Beyond that time, there appeared to be no further improvement.[45][46] Felson and coworkers, for example, followed 39 patients for 3 years. More than 60% had persistent symptoms that were moderate-to-severe. Twenty percent of the patients reported feeling well or very well at the end of the 3 years. More than 60% were still moderately or extremely tired upon awakening. Nonetheless, 83% were still taking one or more drugs for fibromyalgia. Only 5% of patients were symptom-free throughout the 3 years.[45][1,p.68]

In 1992, Carette and his colleagues published preliminary results from the first long-term trial of the two most often prescribed tricyclic antidepressants, amitriptyline and cyclobenzaprine. The results indicated that at 3 and 6 months, these drugs were no more effective than placebos. The final report was published in 1994, confirming the preliminary results.[9] Despite these reports, various writers, in 1994,[102] 1995,[98] and 1996,[103][173] wrote that tricyclic antidepressants are effective.

"It is obvious," Goldenberg wrote, "that medications are not the only answer in the treatment of fibromyalgia." Some patients stop taking such medications because of adverse effects. In general, though, patients appear to tolerate well and benefit from the use of some drugs, including low doses of tricyclics.[1,p.68]

Goldenberg recently wrote, however, that uncontrolled observations over time indicate that patients perceive the effectiveness of tricyclic drugs waning as time passes.[1][6,p.75] He also wrote that preliminary results from the first long-term clinical trial of tricyclic drugs suggest that the drugs' short-term benefits regress to the mean over time.[6]

In a 1997 study, Jung et al. searched for randomized, controlled trials of the use of selective serotonin reuptake inhibiting drugs (SSRIs) for chronic pain. They searched Medline indexing from 1966-to-1997 and contacted manufacturers of the drugs in the United States. They reported that it is unclear from the available evidence whether these drugs are beneficial for migraine headaches, tension headaches, diabetic neuropathy, or fibromyalgia. They wrote, "For those patients, it may be reasonable to reserve SSRIs for those who fail to respond to other medications or who are intolerant of their side effects."[162]

Cyclobenzaprine (Flexeril)

Cyclobenzaprine is a tricyclic drug, the structure of which is similar to that of amitriptyline. It has been advertised to have muscle relaxant properties by reducing brain stem noradrenergic activity and motor neurone activity.[171] Campbell et al., based on a short-term study, reported that cyclobenzaprine was effective in the treatment of fibromyalgia.[68] But in a later study, cyclobenzaprine caused no statistically significant reduction in pain severity for the whole population of patients. The drug did, however, improve their sleep.[4] Gatter wrote that cyclobenzaprine often provides restorative sleep after one or two days of treatment.[44,p.65] EMGs showed that cyclobenzaprine relaxes skeletal muscle spasms.[1,p.63] It does so by acting at the brain stem level to reduce tonic somatic motor activity.[47]

Bennett and colleagues treated 120 fibromyalgia patients with cyclobenzaprine or a placebo for 3 months. The dosage range was 10-to-40 mg. Patients receiving cyclobenzaprine experienced overall improvement and a reduction not only in muscle spasm, but also in pain, tenderness, disturbed sleep, and morning fatigue. Muscle stiffness did not improve.[48] Cyclobenzaprine, like other tricyclics, may cause morning lethargy. This tends to diminish as the patient continues to use the drug or reduce her dosage. Taking the night dose earlier before bed may also decrease morning lethargy.[44,p.64] In addition to drowsiness, a common adverse effect of cyclobenzaprine use by fibromyalgia patients is dry mouth.[48]

Researchers have reported finding significantly low levels of the metabolite of norepinephrine, homovanillic acid, in the cerebrospinal fluid of fibromyalgia patients compared to rheumatoid arthritis and control subjects.[168] If fibromyalgia patients already have low levels of homovanillic acid in their cerebrospinal fluid, indicating low norepinephrine levels, with resulting central nervous system changes that may mediate some features of fibromyalgia, it does not seem advisable to possibly accentuate the low levels by decreasing adrenergic drive with cyclobenzaprine.[171]

Amitriptyline (Elavil)

Some controlled studies in the 1980s indicated that amitriptyline, at least over the short term, is somewhat effective in the treatment of fibromyalgia.[7][43][44]

Table 5.1.1. Classifications of treatment included in this chapter.

CHEMICAL THERAPIES
Antidepressants
　　Cyclobenzaprine
　　Amitriptyline
　　Trazodone (Desyrel)
　　Fluoxetine (Prozac)
　　Citalopram
　　5-Hydroxytryptophan
Hypnotics and sedatives
　　Benzodiazepines
　　　　Xanax (Alprazolam)
　　　　Bromazepan
　　Ambien
　　Zopiclone
　　Phenothiazines
　　　　Thorazine
NSAIDS
　　Naproxen
　　Tenoxicam
　　S-Adenosylmethionine
Milder analgesics
　　Acetaminophen
　　Ibuprofen (also an NSAID)
Hormones
　　Corticosteroids
　　Growth hormone
Nutritional Agents
　　Malic acid and magnesium
　　Sodium
Homeopathic agent: Rhus toxicodendron

PHYSICAL THERAPIES
Exercise
　　Cardiovascular training
　　Physical conditioning
Chiropractic manipulation
Soft tissue manipulation
Acupuncture
Balneotherapy

ELECTROTHERAPY
Electrical stimulation and TENS

TREATMENT REGIMENS
General
Conditioning
Multimodal
Metabolic

PSYCHOLOGICAL THERAPIES
Placebo
Biofeedback
Cognitive-behavioral therapy
Hypnosis
Marital counseling and psychomotor therapy
Meditation-based stress reduction
Patient education

Isomeri and coworkers conducted a study involving amitriptyline. They divided 45 patients into three groups. One group took 25 mg of amitriptyline in the evenings and performed light stretching exercises. The second group underwent physical fitness training that was progressively more strenuous. The third group engaged in the same physical fitness program as group two did, but they also took 25 mg of amitriptyline.[18]

The researchers evaluated the status of patients at the beginning of the trial and after 15 weeks. They used a 100-mm visual analog scale and measured the patients' pain thresholds and tolerances with a dolorimeter (algometer). The investigators wrote that their results were disappointing: ". . . pressure pain experience did not decrease during the therapy. On the contrary, the pressure pain threshold and tolerance deteriorated in patients receiving [amitriptyline] treatment alone, and an improvement was seen only in patients receiving the combination therapy" (amitriptyline and physical fitness training).[18, p.257]

Table 5.1.2. Improvement in fibromyalgia patients after 1, 3, and 6 months of treatment with amitriptyline, cyclobenzaprine, and placebo.

% OF PATIENTS SIGNIFICANTLY IMPROVED[*]

	Amitriptyline (n=84)	Cyclobenzaprine (n=82)	Placebo (n=42)
Month 1	20.7	11.7	0.00
Month 3	18.4	19.4	13.5
Month 6	35.9	32.9	19.4

[*]After Carette, S., Bell, M., Reynolds, J., et al.: A controlled trial of amitriptyline, cyclobenzaprine, and placebo in fibromyalgia. *Arthritis Rheum.*, 35(Suppl 9):112, 1992.[9]

In a longer-term evaluation (6 months), Carette and colleagues treated patients with amitriptyline and cyclobenzaprine. About 30% of the patients improved on 11 of 13 outcome measures during the first month. The measures they did not improve on were tender point scores and the Stanford Health Assessment Questionnaire.[9]

After 1 month of treatment, patients taking either of these two drugs had improved more than patients taking placebos. At 3- and 6-month reevaluations, however, patients taking placebos had improved about as much as those taking the drugs. As a result, the study tends to confirm a 30% short-term improvement rate in patients taking amitriptyline or cyclobenza-

prine. The study did not confirm long-term effectiveness, though, due to the improvement in patients taking placebos.[9] See Table 5.1.2.

The majority of patients in this study by Carette did not improve. Of the placebo patients at 1 month, 100% failed to benefit. Of the amitriptyline patients, 79%, and of cyclobenzaprine patients, 88% failed to benefit. Put another way, 21% of amitriptyline patients and 12% of cyclobenzaprine patients improved. The superiority of the drugs over placebos, slight as it was, was only evident during the first month of the study. At 3 and 6 months, placebo patients had improved as much as the drug patients.[105]

Carette speculated that with more subjects in his study groups he might have shown a real superiority of the drugs over the placebo.[105] It would be questionable, however, whether a treatment effect detected only by means of a large number of subjects, although statistically significant, is of any practical clinical importance. Of patients taking cyclobenzaprine, 98% of patients had adverse effects, and 13% of patients stopped the drug because of adverse effects. This means more patients had bad side effects than improved: 13% compared to 12%.[101]

In another study, Carette et al. found that neither a placebo nor amitriptyline improved the alpha non-rapid eye movement sleep anomaly in fibromyalgia patients. Of 22 patients in the study, only 6 (27%) had some benefit from amitriptyline.[121]

In 1995, Goldenberg et al. tested fibromyalgia patients for the effects of amitriptyline and fluoxetine (Prozac) separately and in combination. The randomized double-blind placebo-controlled study consisted of four 6-week trials. Before each phase of the study, patients underwent a 2-week washout period. The investigators reported that for each of the drug trials, the drugs improved scores on the Fibromyalgia Impact Questionnaire and visual analog scales for pain, global well-being, and sleep disturbance. Scores did not show significant improvement for the Beck depression scale, fatigue, feeling refreshed upon awakening, and tender point score. They concluded that both drugs are effective treatments for fibromyalgia and work better in combination.[124] The results of this study should be considered in light of the reports by Carette et al. in 1992 and 1994.[9][105] These studies showed that short term, amitriptyline compared to a placebo provided slight improvement on some fibromyalgia measures. But long term, the drug was no more effective than placebos. Assessment of amitriptyline and fluoxetine in this study, using four 6-week trials, was equivalent to Carette's short-term assessment showing more effectiveness than the placebo. But had the assessment continued longer, the drugs may have proven no more effective than the placebo.

Ginsberg et al. studied the effects of 25 mg of sustained-release amitriptyline as a fibromyalgia treatment. Twenty-four patients took the medication once per day. Conventional amitriptyline reaches a peak plasma concentration at 4 hours, but the sustained-release form peaks at 7 hours. The peak for sustained-release amitriptyline was 50% lower than that of the conventional form. The level of the sustained-release form also declined more slowly with fewer fluctuations and less pronounced adverse effects. To evaluate the effects of the drug and the placebo, the researchers used a set of "clinically meaningful" response criteria. Assessment of effectiveness involved tender point evaluation by digital palpation, and visual analog scales for pain, sleep disturbance, fatigue, duration of morning stiffness, and global evaluation by patient and clinician. A patient was considered a "responder" when he or she met three of four criteria: 50% improvement in patient global assessment or clinician global assessment, 50% improvement in pain, and 25% reduction in tender point score. At 4 weeks, 5 of the 24 patients (21%) taking amitriptyline were responders. None of the placebo patients were. At 8 weeks, 14 of the patients taking amitriptyline (58%) were responders. The investigators reported that most measures of the drug-treated group improved by about 50%, but number of tender points improved by 31%, tender point score by 42%, and duration of morning stiffness by 70%. Patients taking the drug had adverse effects that included dry mouth, digestive symptoms, vertigo, and "neuro-psychic symptoms." One patient discontinued treatment because of digestive and neuro-psychic symptoms. The investigators concluded that this form of amitriptyline ". . . may be beneficial in the treatment of some FS patients."[125] As with the Goldenberg study,[124] this study is repetitious of other short-term evaluations of amitriptyline. Differences in measures between the drug-treated group and the placebo group may have disappeared in a longer-term evaluation.

Reports continue to appear in which amitriptyline is claimed to have been effective in the treatment of fibromyalgia. Trojan and Cashman, for example, reported that 50% of postpoliomyelitis patients with fibromyalgia responded to low-dose, night-time amitriptyline therapy.[122] This is an anecdotal report that is inconsistent with the outcome of the control assessment of this form of treatment.

Some fibromyalgia researchers have continued to advocate the use of amitriptyline despite experimental studies showing that it is ineffective as a fibromyalgia treatment. The justification usually given for continued use of the drug with fibromyalgia patients is that it helps them sleep.[172] This claim is contradicted by study results showing that amitriptyline did not improve the stage 4 (slow wave sleep) of fibromyalgia patients.[121]

Trazodone (Desyrel)

Trazodone is a triazolopyridine derivative. It is a chemical unrelated to tricyclic drugs, but like them, it inhibits the reuptake of serotonin from the synapses. Saccomani and colleagues published a report of the cases of two juveniles with fibromyalgia treated with trazodone. The female was 11 years old and the male was 7. The diagnoses were based on the presence of musculoskeletal pain, tender points, and associated symptoms with the exclusion of any other known etiology. The authors reported anecdotally that both patients improved after treatment with the antidepressant serotonergic drugs trazodone and amitriptyline.[20]

Fluoxetine (Prozac)

Wolfe and coworkers compared the effects of fluoxetine (20 mg) with a placebo in the treatment of 42 fibromyalgic women. According to standard fibromyalgia assessment methods, there was no significant improvement in the fluoxetine-treated patients at 3 and 6 weeks. Patients taking fluoxetine did improve at 6 weeks on the AIMS Depression and Beck Depression Scales. They also had some improvement in quality of sleep.[152]

Goldenberg et al. tested the effects on fibromyalgia patients of fluoxetine and amitriptyline separately and in combination (see section on amitriptyline). They concluded that both drugs are effective treatments for fibromyalgia and work better in combination.[124] Evaluations were short-term, however. Had long-term assessments been performed, the drugs may have proven no more effective than the placebo, as Carette et al. found with amitriptyline and cyclobenzaprine.[9][105]

Citalopram

Nørregaard et al. tested the serotonin reuptake inhibitor citalopram as a treatment for fibromyalgia. They included 22 patients in a randomized, double-blind, placebo-controlled study. For 4 weeks, 22 patients took 20 mg citalopram and 21 patients took a placebo. Patients increased the dosage after 4 weeks to 40 mg and continued this dosage for another 4 weeks.

At the end of the 8 weeks of treatment, no changes had occurred in five measures: self-assessment of symptoms, clinicians' global assessment, tender points, Beck depression score, and voluntary muscle strength. Measures for the drug and placebo groups were not significantly different. The investigators concluded that citalopram had no demonstrable effect on fibromyalgia status.[120]

5-Hydroxytryptophan

5-Hydroxytryptophan is the immediate precursor of serotonin (5-hydroxytryptamine). Caruso et al. conducted a double-blind assessment of the effects of 5-hydroxytryptophan and a placebo on fibromyalgia symptoms. In contrast to the male/female ratio of patients in most fibromyalgia studies, the majority of patients were males (43 males and 7 females). Twenty-five patients used placebos and 25 used 5-hydroxytryptophan, 100 mg three times per day. The researchers evaluated fibromyalgia status at baseline, 15 days, and 30 days. At baseline, the two groups did not differ on measures of fibromyalgia status. In the placebo group, at 15 days but not at 30 days, patients had a decrease in stiffness and the number of tender points. At 30 days, they had a decrease in pain perception and improved sleep. By contrast, at 30 days, patients using 5-hydroxytryptophan had a statistically significant decrease in pain perception and the number of tender points. They also had reduced anxiety, fatigue, and morning stiffness, and improved sleep. Adverse effects were reported by 24.0% of patients taking 5-hydroxytryptophan and 12.0% of patients taking placebos.[176]

One problem with this study is that it ended after 30 days. Whether the benefits from the use of 5-hydroxytryptophan would have persisted long term cannot be determined from this study. As I point out in Chapter 1.5, the serotonin deficiency hypothesis of fibromyalgia is falsified by its failure to account for all the features of fibromyalgia. Using medication that is expected to increase serotonin levels, such as 5-hydroxytryptophan, can be predicted to improve or relieve features of fibromyalgia that are underlain by a serotonin deficiency. This would account for some degree of improvement with the use of 5-hydroxytryptophan. However, in that inadequate thyroid hormone regulation of cell function can account both for a serotonin deficiency and all other features of fibromyalgia, and that 5-hydroxytryptophan does not correct inadequate thyroid hormone regulation, it is predictable that treatment with 5-hydroxytryptophan will be limited. For example, the mean changes in

symptom intensity in the Caruso study were limited. The percentage of improvement in perceived pain was 45%, morning stiffness was 38%, sleep disturbance was 40%, anxiety was 40%, and fatigue was 43%. The mean percentage of improvement for these five symptoms was 41.2%. Thus, while the mean intensity of symptoms favorably changed, the results indicate that the patients were still symptomatic following treatment.[176]

Sarzi Puttini and Caruso conducted a 90-day open trial of 5-hydroxytryptophan with fibromyalgia patients. As with the Caruso et al.[176] study described above, the results indicate that patients improved but were still symptomatic during the course of treatment. The authors wrote that nearly 50% of the patients experienced good clinical improvement.[133,p.184]

The results of these two studies indicate that 5-hydroxytryptophan may be useful in reducing the intensity of some fibromyalgia symptoms in some patients.

Potential Adverse Effects of Antidepressant Drugs

Hypotension. Le Feuvre and coauthors pointed out that tricyclic antidepressant drugs can induce orthostatic hypotension,[75] a phenomenon many already-hypotensive fibromyalgia patients would best avoid.

Ischemic Heart Disease and Heart Attacks. See Chapter 1.1, subsection titled "Possible Harm in Antidepressants Used as a Fibromyalgia Treatment."

Female Cancers. See Chapter 1.1, subsection titled "Possible Harm in Antidepressants Used as a Fibromyalgia Treatment."

Slowing of the Metabolic Rate. Riley and coworkers reported that administering fluoxetine (Prozac) to adult rats decreased the levels of TRH mRNA by 48±4%.[76,p.254] This finding raises the possibility that Prozac may have adverse metabolic effects that resemble those of hypothalamic hypothyroidism.

Two antidepressants, imipramine and tranylcypromine, have been shown to profoundly decrease resting metabolic rate (17% to 24%) and to increase weight.[77] And another, carbamazepine, while not producing "frank hypothyroidism," causes a significant fall in thyroid hormone levels.[78] Puech pointed out that "co-prescriptions" of noradrenergic antidepressants and various other drugs can render the patient resistant to noradrenergic antidepressants.[100] These antidepressants work by increasing activity of β-adrenergic receptors. Yet some patients also simultaneously use β-blocking drugs that nullify the β-adrenergic-activating effect of the antidepressants. In addition, some patients also take benzodiazepines and these also tend to decrease noradrenergic neuronal activity. Because untreated hypothyroid patients have reduced numbers of β-adrenergic receptors, they too may be resistant to noradrenergic antidepressants.[100]

The issue of concern from studies showing slowed resting metabolic rate is whether the effect is lasting, even after the patient stops the antidepressant medication. Does a longer and higher dose exposure to tricyclics and monoamine oxidases (MAOs) render an individual hypometabolic even after she ceases the medication?[78,p.785] Herman et al. reported that repeated and lengthy use of tricyclic and MAO antidepressants appear to sustain hypometabolism. They found that the more months patients took antidepressants in the previous 5 years, the lower their resting metabolic rate tended to be.[78,p.785]

Suicidal Depression. Although antidepressants that selectively increase norepinephrine levels have not been tested under blinded conditions as a fibromyalgia treatment, they are often prescribed for fibromyalgia patients. When patients begin using antidepressants that increase central nervous system norepinephrine levels, a risk is suicidal depression. Antidepressants such as imipramine and its metabolite desipramine serve this function selectively. Such drugs increase norepinephrine concentration at synapses by preventing its reuptake. Underlying the risk is the upregulation of α_2-adrenergic receptors in the cortex when there is a deficiency of norepinephrine.[160][161]

α_2-Adrenergic receptors are presynaptic inhibitory receptors on serotonin-releasing neurons. Secretion of serotonin by serotonergic neurons is tonically regulated by exposure to normal amounts of norepinephrine.[160][161] When norepinephrine is deficient, α_2-adrenergic receptors upregulate and tonically inhibit serotonin release despite minimal exposure to norepinephrine (see Chapter 2.3, section titled "Other Molecular products of Thyroid Hormone Regulation of Transcription: Serotonin").

When a patient takes a drug that blocks norepinephrine reuptake, the concentration of norepinephrine at synapses increases. When a patient begins taking a norepinephrine reuptake inhibiting drug, her serotonergic neurons may have a high density of α_2-adrenergic receptors due to the previous norepinephrine deficiency. Binding of the increased amounts of norepinephrine to the high density of α_2-adrenergic receptors may excessively inhibit serotonin secretion. This may lower her serotonin levels low enough to induce attempts at suicide. Nordström and Åsberg proposed this mechanism as a biological correlate of suicide during

the initial phase of patients taking norepinephrine reuptake inhibitors.[69][79] Rouillon and colleagues found support for the mechanism in a large clinical study of patients who took maprotiline, a norepinephrine reuptake inhibitor.[70] Until the α_2-adrenergic receptors on serotonergic neurons downregulate under the influence of the therapeutically-increased norepinephrine levels, as the receptors have been found to do,[161] patients taking norepinephrine reuptake inhibitors should be cautiously observed during treatment.

Assessments of Antidepressant Treatment of Fibromyalgia

Russell in 1994[102] and 1996[173] and McCain [103] in 1996 reported that antidepressant medications are effective in treating fibromyalgia. Other researchers have given more properly tempered endorsements of the putative effectiveness of amitriptyline and cyclobenzaprine, stating that the drugs have been shown to have "some efficacy"[120] and that amitriptyline has been found to be "modestly" effective.[124] Endorsements of such drugs, when not properly qualified, have an unfortunate effect. That effect is that reviewers, such as Godfrey,[119] disseminate the unqualified conclusion to other clinicians through medical journals. Russell and McCain referenced older short-term studies and failed to mention the long-term trial by Carette et al. that showed the drugs to be slightly effective at 1 month, but having effects no different from the effects of a placebo at 3 and 6 months.[9][105]

In the face of such evidence, some rheumatology fibromyalgia researchers justify the continued use of antidepressants by asserting that they improve patients' sleep.[172] But such claims are dubious. For example, Carette et al. published experimental findings showing that amitriptyline did not improve stage 4 (slow wave sleep) of fibromyalgia patients.[121]

In assessing the value of a treatment, it is important to bear in mind the difference between statistical and practical significance. If a large enough group of patients is used in a drug trial, sensitive statistical tests can detect a difference in the drug effect compared to that of a placebo. But the difference may be of no practical importance. This is the case with the results of efficacy studies of antidepressant medications for fibromyalgia. The changes in measures are so minimal that, although they show statistical significance, they are virtually useless to patients. Arguably their use is not worth the risk of adverse drug effects. An argument can be made that if a therapeutic effect is not obvious from a small N trial, then the effect probably is of no practical importance.

Others, such as one neurologist, have expressed resentment: "The absence of good studies confirming the efficacy of conventional allopathic treatment engenders therapeutic nihilism, opening the door to 'alternative' medical approaches and leaving too many patients unhelped."[93,p.122] This writer's use of the term "therapeutic nihilism" makes no apparent sense, but his objection to the door being open to "alternative medical approaches" appears to me to be a whining resentment of the success of such practitioners. His reference in the same breath to ". . . leaving too many patients unhelped" is a pejorative denouncement of alternative practitioners' abilities to help fibromyalgia patients.

Bennett wrote, "Fibromyalgia syndrome is remarkably persistent and chronic and it is not surprising that patients seek other modalities considering the poor results of standard medical therapies."[92,p.104] Wolfe has also expressed dissatisfaction with the results of conventional rheumatology treatment for fibromyalgia.[106]

Comment. Antidepressant medications continue to be endorsed by some researchers as efficacious in the treatment of fibromyalgia. As a result, practicing clinicians tend to prescribe these medications for fibromyalgia patients.[101] This practice cannot be condoned logically or scientifically for three reasons: (1) the negative results of experimental long-term assessment of antidepressant treatment for fibromyalgia, (2) the absence of credible evidence that anyone has ever recovered from fibromyalgia with this treatment, and (3) the likelihood of adverse effects in patients taking the medications long term. Statistically significant short-term "improvements," as reported in some studies, are not clinically important. Considering these points, it seems important to circumvent further dissemination through general medical journals the erroneous statement that antidepressant medications are effective in the treatment of fibromyalgia.

Reviewers such as Godfrey[119] only reiterate what is reported by fibromyalgia researchers. Other reviewers such as Goodnick and Sandoval studied the published reports (such as the early amitriptyline trials) and based on them, have formulated rules for probable effective antidepressants for different fibromyalgia/chronic fatigue syndrome symptoms. They reached the tentative conclusion that serotonergic drugs (such as clomipramine) are more effective for alleviating pain than depression, and catecholaminergic drugs (such as maprotiline and bupropion) are effective for relieving depression.[123] Such therapeutic rules founded on highly dubious study conclusions can lead to confu-

sion, poor clinical outcomes, patient disappointment, and problems in patient/clinician interactions. To avoid such problems, it is incumbent on those researchers who report that antidepressants are effective to revise their conclusions to accurately reflect the results of recent treatment studies. Their revised conclusions should include explanations that their former statements about the effectiveness of antidepressant treatment were based on statistical rather than clinical significance.

Hypnotics and Sedatives

Benzodiazepines. Benzodiazepines, such as Valium (diazepam) and Xanax (alprazolam), may benefit some patients initially by enabling them to sleep better. Electroencephalograms, however, showed that Valium did not stop alpha-wave intrusion into stage 4 (delta) sleep. In fact, benzodiazepines may reduce stage 4 slow sleep waves.[49,p.288] During long-term use, benzodiazepines may intensify depression and cause nightmares.[44,p.64] In addition, the drugs may impede the activity of most antidepressants. They were found to decrease serotonergic and noradrenergic activity.[100] This suggests that if used regularly, benzodiazepines may worsen fibromyalgia symptoms mediated by low serotonin levels and may worsen the patient's hypometabolic status by impairing adrenergic responsiveness.

Xanax. Kravitz and his coworkers evaluated the effects of alprazolam, ibuprofen, alprazolam-ibuprofen combined, and a placebo on fibromyalgia patients over a 5-week period. Patients obtained some benefit from the combination of the two drugs. Results from the use of neither drug alone were significantly better than results from the other. Neither drug alone was more effective than the placebo. Although the combination of the two drugs was more effective than either alone, the combination of the two drugs provided little benefit. For example, no group of patients taking one or a combination of the drugs showed a significant improvement in number of tender points during treatment.[71,p.16]

Bromazepan. In an 8-week study, Quijada-Carrera et al. tested bromazepan (a benzodiazepine) and tenoxicam (an NSAID) as fibromyalgia treatments. Of the patients who used a combination of the two drugs, 29% had significant improvement. Only 17% of placebo patients improved. Improvement occurred in 10% of patients taking only tenoxicam, and in 12% of patients taking only bromazepan. The combination was only slightly more effective than the placebo.[137]

Other Hypnotics and Sedatives. Other hypnotics

and sedatives that have been tested are Ambien, zopiclone, and chlorpromazine.

Ambien (Zolpidem). Ambien is a hypnotic drug that in the central nervous system selectively binds benzodiazepine receptors. The drug is short-acting, having a 2½-hour half-life. Moldofsky and coworkers studied the effects of Ambien on the fibromyalgia status of 1 male and 18 female patients. All patients had alpha EEG non-REM sleep anomaly. The study lasted 16 days. This time was divided into four periods of 4 days each. During one period, patients received a placebo. In the other three periods, patients took one of three doses of Ambien: 5 mg, 10 mg, or 15 mg. Each patient completed all four phases in random order. Patients progressed from one period to the next without a washout period. Patients taking the drug woke fewer times during sleep. They reported that their daytime energy was higher and their quality of sleep improved. There was no improvement during drug periods in sleepiness and fatigue in the mornings, pain rating, number of tender points, concentration, or mood.[85]

This study showed some improvement in some measures of sleep but no improvement in other fibromyalgia measures.[85] It might be argued that the study was too short-term to show improvement in other measures, but this conflicts with clinical observation and evidence from other studies that a good night's sleep can rapidly improve other fibromyalgia measures. We would expect Ambien to improve sleep in fibromyalgia patients, however, in that it is a sleep-inducing medication. Ambien is especially effective for relieving transient insomnia such as that induced by stress, jet lag, or an unfamiliar environment.[86] Ambien is a strong sedative, but it has only minor anxiety-reducing, muscle-relaxing, and anticonvulsant effects.[87]

The fibromyalgia patient with memory impairment should be made aware that this symptom may be worsened temporarily while Ambien is actively affecting the patient. This "amnesic" effect is similar to that of Halcion (triazolam), a medication that has somewhat stronger memory-impairing and sedative effects than Ambien. When a patient takes both of these two sleep-inducing drugs, the hypnotic and memory-impairing effects are coupled: the higher the dosage, the greater the sedative and amnesic effects.[88] When compared with the effects of Halcion and Restoril (temazepam), two benzodiazepines, Ambien produced the same dose-related impairment of learning, recall, and performance. But the time to maximum drug effect was faster with Ambien than with Halcion and Restoril.[89]

Zopiclone. Investigators evaluated the effects of zopiclone, a hypnotic drug, on the clinical status and brain wave patterns (using polysomnography) of fibromyalgia patients in a double-blind controlled study. Patients reported that they were not as tired during the day while taking the drug, and they had fewer subjective sleep complaints. There were no improvements, however, in pain, stiffness, muscle fatigue, pressure at tender points, or in overall assessment of symptoms. Severity of symptoms, with the exception of sleep complaints, remained constant over time. Patients continued to take the same amounts of analgesics throughout the study.[49]

Patients went to sleep sooner after beginning zopiclone. Sleep quality and the total time they slept also increased. They awoke fewer times during the night, and their conditions were improved in the mornings after beginning the drug. Their overall evaluation of sleep significantly improved.

On the other hand, sleep brain wave patterns, demonstrated by polysomnography, did not change. Treatment produced no significant changes in sleep states. Particularly, there was no quantitative improvement in the deeper sleep stages.

The researchers reported that patients taking zopiclone judged the drug to improve the quality of their sleep and to diminish their tiredness through the day. The authors concluded that the drug may benefit patients for whom sleep complaints are a major feature of their fibromyalgia syndromes.[49]

Chlorpromazine (thorazine). Chlorpromazine is a phenothiazine that has been reported to improve some fibromyalgia symptoms. Its usefulness is limited, however, because of its toxicity and by reports from patients that it causes unpleasant morning drowsiness.[49][51]

Non-steroidal Anti-inflammatory Drugs (NSAIDs)

Naproxen. Naproxen is a non-steroidal aspirin-like agent with anti-inflammatory, analgesic, and antipyretic activity.[62,p.664] Schmidt reported that in most cases of fibromyalgia, NSAIDs, as well as steroid anti-inflammatory drugs, completely fail.[5] Conversely, Gatter reported that in his experience, naproxen taken twice daily, in combination with cyclobenzaprine at bedtime, is effective with some fibromyalgia patients.[44,p.65]

Goldenberg and coworkers gave 500 mg of naproxen twice a day to fibromyalgia patients in a well-controlled study. The researchers reported that there was no significant improvement in any of the outcome variables (tender point score, pain, fatigue, sleep, global assessment) in any of the patients.[7]

Tenoxicam. In a study by Quijada-Carrera et al., improvement occurred in only 10% of fibromyalgia patients who took tenoxicam alone. (see section above: "Bromazepan").[137]

S-Adenosylmethionine. S-adenosylmethionine takes part in many metabolic processes in the body as a methyl donor. When used as an oral agent, it has anti-inflammatory, analgesic, and antidepressant effects. Studies have shown that it is as effective as ibuprofen and naproxen in the treatment of osteoarthritis. Its main adverse effects are gastrointestinal symptoms.[63,p.294]

In one study, 200 mg of the drug taken daily was more effective than a placebo in improving fibromyalgia patients' muscle tenderness and mood.[64] In a follow-up double-blind study, fibromyalgia patients took 800 mg daily for 6 weeks. They each took one tablet in the morning and one in the evening, preferably 30 minutes before meals to avoid interference from food absorption. The investigators wrote that patients experienced a reduction in morning stiffness. Tender point scores decreased slightly, but the decrease was not statistically significant. Isokinetic muscle strength did not change. Pain while resting (assessed by visual analog scale) and fatigue improved. However, pain during physical activity, depression, quality of sleep, and overall well-being did not change significantly. The investigators concluded that there was some beneficial effect from S-adenosylmethionine. They wrote that it may be an important treatment option, especially since there are few other effective treatments.[63]

In another study, researchers tested the efficacy of S-adenosylmethionine administered intravenously as a fibromyalgia treatment. In a crossover trial, they administered the medication (600 mg IV) or a placebo each day to 34 fibromyalgia patients for 10 days. There was no significant difference in improvement in tender points status between the two groups. In patients who received the medication, there was a trend toward statistically significant improvement in subjective perception of pain at rest (p=0.08), pain on movement (p=0.11), and overall well-being (p=0.17). There was slight improvement only in fatigue, quality of sleep, morning stiffness, and scores on the Fibromyalgia Impact Questionnaire for pain. No benefit was found for isokinetic muscle strength, Zerrsen self-assessment questionnaire, and the face scale. The authors concluded that in this short-term study, they found no effect of the medication on fibromyalgia patients.[169]

When recommending NSAIDs, the clinician should consider the possible adverse effects. NSAIDs are often harmful to the stomach and intestines,[96] and they may cause kidney damage.[97] Fowler reported that there is a 10% incidence of adverse gastrointestinal effects in patients taking over-the-counter NSAIDs.[94]

Mild Analgesics

For some patients, Goldenberg wrote, no therapy other than simple analgesics is necessary.[1,p.69] Cathey et al. agreed with this view. They wrote that their data suggested that fibromyalgia patients can manage their symptoms with simple and limited analgesics.[22]

Yunus cautioned that in treating fibromyalgia patients, clinicians should avoid addictive and narcotic drugs. He suggested that some patients benefit from non-steroidal anti-inflammatory drugs (NSAIDs), although his double-blind study indicated that ibuprofen is not effective (see below, this section). He advised, "In view of the high cost and general inefficacy of the NSAIDs, cheaper, simple analgesics, such as acetaminophen, should be prescribed first. Medications should always be taken on regular dose schedules, and not as needed, in fibromyalgia."[21,p.18]

Acetaminophen. In some studies, such as that of Jacobsen and coworkers, acetaminophen served as the only "rescue medication." This term means that patients used acetaminophen only when they needed pain relief during the study. Only 13% of their 81 patients reported using narcotics at any time during the year of the study. Only 11% used analgesics other than aspirin and acetaminophen.[63,p.297] Use of acetaminophen is not without risks; it is associated with some 4,000-to-5,000 kidney failures per year.[95]

Ibuprofen. Yunus et al. found in a blinded 6-week study of fibromyalgia treatment that ibuprofen was no more effective than a placebo. Patients taking ibuprofen and patients taking the placebo all improved slightly. Patients had less fatigue, swelling, and paresthesias, and fewer total pain sites and total tender points. The authors wrote that their data suggested that the interaction of physicians with patients and a "study effect" (as opposed to any inherent effect of ibuprofen) may have helped relieve the pain of fibromyalgia.[8]

Kravitz and colleagues evaluated fibromyalgia patients' responses to taking ibuprofen and alprazolam (Xanax) separately and in combination. They compared these responses with the effects of a placebo. Neither drug nor the combination of the two was more effective than the placebo.[71]

Goldenberg et al.[7] and Le Gallez et al. [72] also found in randomized, double-blind clinical trials that non-steroidal anti-inflammatory drugs have little efficacy as a fibromyalgia treatment. Goldenberg's group tested naproxen; Le Gallez's group tested ibuprofen.

HORMONES

Besides thyroid hormones, which my colleagues and I have tested, only corticosteroids and growth hormone have been tested as fibromyalgia treatments.

Corticosteroids

Some authors recommend injecting corticosteroids into trigger points. They admit, however, that symptom relief is short-lived.[52][53] Others report that the drugs completely fail.[54] With other therapies available, one must question the wisdom of injecting patients with these drugs in light of the risks that have been cited. Gottlieb and Riskin wrote, ". . . this approach remains controversial; soft-tissue corticosteroid injections commonly afford only symptomatic relief, and may be associated with a spectrum of local complications."[53] Some of these complications include septic arthritis or tenosynovitis; skin, subcutaneous, and periarticular soft-tissue atrophy; tendon and cartilage attrition; crystal-induced arthritis, and pericapsular calcification.[55][56][57] Other authors point out that long-acting steroids may destroy muscle fibers when injected into them.[58]

A few authors claim that adverse systemic effects of local corticosteroid injections are not common. Nevertheless, some authors point out that hypothalamic-pituitary-adrenal axis suppression may occur. This is indicated by several days of lowered plasma cortisol levels and depressed response to insulin-induced hypoglycemia following corticosteroid injections into joints.[59]

In a 2-week trial with 20 fibromyalgia patients, 20 mg of prednisone was no more effective than a placebo. Patients showed a trend toward deterioration in most measured variables.[60] This finding warrants the caution two authors expressed in their text: The possible benefits of these drugs "must be carefully weighed in each patient against the widespread effects on every part of the organism."[61,p.349] If fibromyalgia in the patients in this study were a manifestation of inadequate thyroid hormone regulation of cell function, the deterioration in clinical status would be a predictable outcome. In primary and central hypothyroid patients, even small replacement dosages of cortisone or

other corticosteroids may induce signs of glucocorticoid excess, as in Cushing's syndrome.[80][178,p.1048][179] This effect tends to occur because inadequate thyroid hormone regulation of liver function results in a delayed clearance of corticosteroids from the body.[81]

Growth Hormone Injections

Bennett et al. carried out a double-blind placebo-controlled study of growth hormone injections with 55 female fibromyalgia patients. The purpose was to determine how effective growth hormone injections (with Nutropin, marketed by Genentech, Inc.) were with patients with low somatomedin C levels (<160ng/mL).[107]

After being randomly assigned, patients were given injections either of a placebo or growth hormone for 9 months. The starting dose of growth hormone was 0.0125 mg/kg/day. Patients were reevaluated at 3, 6, and 9 months. Measures included the Fibromyalgia Impact Questionnaire (FIQ), number of tender points, and the myalgic score. The difference between groups was significant: FIQ, p=0.05; tender points, p=0.016, and myalgic scores, p=0.011. The researchers reported that 25% of the patients had a dramatic improvement. Among the adverse effects were fluid retention (growth hormone, 24%; placebo, 24%), arthralgias (growth hormone, 60%; placebo, 43%), and carpal tunnel syndrome (growth hormone, 28%; placebo, 4%).[107]

The researchers concluded that impaired growth hormone secretion is a part of the fibromyalgia complex that can be treated with replacement therapy. They also wrote that the therapy provides symptom relief for many patients with low somatomedin C levels.[107]

Possible Adverse Effect of Growth Hormone Treatment on Thyroid Status. When low growth hormone levels result from inadequate thyroid hormone regulation, it is important to treat the patient with the proper form and dosage of thyroid hormone, not growth hormone. When exogenous growth hormone is used to increase growth hormone and somatomedin C levels in the body, other effects of the inadequate thyroid hormone regulation may go untreated—with long-range adverse effects. Also, injections of exogenous growth hormone may themselves adversely affect the patient. Antibodies to growth hormone have been reported in 30%-to-40% of children treated with injected somatrem (recombinant methionyl-growth hormone) and 7%-to-20% treated with somatropin (recombinant growth hormone).[110] These preparations, derived from recombinant DNA, are intramuscular injectables. The injections are minimally painful, but may lead to local lipoatrophy.[111,p.1342]

Of most concern is the possibility of malignancy from growth hormone-induced tissue hyperplasia.[112] In one study with children, there was a twofold increase in the size of melanocytic naevi during therapy with biosynthetic human growth hormone.[113] However, there was no evidence of neoplasms or premalignant changes. The increase in the size of the naevi was not correlated with growth, dose of growth hormone, or duration of therapy. In one patient who stopped taking growth hormone, the changes were fully reversed. Slyder wrote, "This study is a cogent reminder that growth hormone is a potent biological agent inducing widespread tissue hyperplasia. Pediatricians need no reminder that malignancy is a feature of hyperplastic syndromes."[112,p.524]

Moreover, treatment with growth hormone was found to inhibit the thyroid gland from taking up iodine,[108] possibly antagonizing formation of thyroid hormone. In addition, growth hormone may cause important impeding changes in thyroid hormone metabolism.[109,p.E192] Some children treated with growth hormone developed hypothyroidism.[111,p.1342] If a fibromyalgia patient is hypothyroid, taking growth hormone may worsen the thyroid hormone deficiency. If a patient is not hypothyroid, inhibition of iodine uptake by the gland may cause a thyroid hormone deficiency.

Improvement in Fibromyalgia Status with Use of Growth Hormone May Result from Increased Deiodination of T_4 to T_3. Studies referenced in the section above indicate a possible adverse effect of exogenous growth hormone on thyroid gland function. Despite this possible antagonistic effect of growth hormone on thyroid gland function, growth hormone may at least transiently increase availability of T_3.

In one study, patients not taking exogenous T_4 and patients taking T_4 were treated with biosynthetic human growth hormone (Norditropin). Serum total and free T_4 levels decreased and serum total and free T_3 levels increased in both groups of patients. In both groups, the reverse T_3 levels after growth hormone therapy were lower than during use of placebos. These laboratory values suggest that growth hormone temporarily increased peripheral deiodination of T_4 to T_3. They researchers concluded that their results were consistent with a growth hormone-induced enhancement of peripheral deiodination of T_4 to T_3.[128] This finding raises the possibility that growth hormone-induced deiodination, with an increase in the metabolically active thyroid hormone, may have accounted for the temporary improvement in Bennett's fibromyalgia patients.

This is likely in that there is a high incidence of both primary[32][129]130][131][132][134] and central hypothyroidism in fibromyalgia.[131][135] Hypothyroid fibromyalgia patients would be expected to have some benefit from a growth hormone-induced increase in T_3. In addition, some euthyroid fibromyalgia patients with cellular resistance to thyroid hormone would also be expected to benefit from an increase in T_3 while using growth hormone. To my knowledge, Bennett et al. did not attempt to identify hypothyroid patients in his study or monitor for changes in T_4 or T_3 levels.[107]

NUTRITIONAL THERAPIES

Unfortunately, few studies of nutritional therapies have been reported.

Malic Acid and Magnesium

Abraham and Flechas carried out an open trial using malic acid and magnesium and reported favorable results.[83] In another study, researchers tested a proprietary formulation, tablets which contained 200 mg of malic acid and 50 mg of magnesium. Twenty-four sequential fibromyalgia patients were randomly assigned to either a placebo group or an experimental group for 4 weeks. The experimental group took a fixed dose of three tablets twice per day. After the 4 weeks, they continued in an open label trial for 6 months. During this time, they increased their dosages up to six tablets twice per day. Researchers assessed patients for changes in pain and tenderness, and functional and psychological indices. After the 4-week blinded phase, the researchers found no treatment effect they could attribute to the product. During the open phase, with patients aware of what they were taking and the escalating dosages, the researchers reported significant reductions in the severity of pain and tenderness. They concluded that the data suggest that the product is safe and beneficial in the treatment of fibromyalgia patients.[84] It is possible that the improvement reportedly found during the open phase of the study may have been a product of the expectations of the researchers and patients rather than the product.

A serious limitation of studies of this nature is the failure of the researchers to determine which of the participating patients have thyroid hormone deficiencies. Malic enzyme is under the genetic control of thyroid hormone (see Chapter 2.2, subsection titled "Malate in the Citric Acid Cycle."). Inadequate regulation of the malic acid gene by thyroid hormone would be expected to lesion the point in the citric acid cycle where malic enzyme acts. We would expect a thyroid hormone deficient patient to benefit from the use of a malic acid supplement in that the supplement might, despite a malic enzyme deficiency, enable enough oxaloacetate to be produced so that the citric acid cycle could proceed normally.

Sodium

Bou-Holaigah et al. compared the clinical symptoms and responses evoked by upright tilt-table testing of 23 chronic fatigue syndrome patients and 14 normal controls. After participants completed a symptom questionnaire, they were subjected to a three-stage, upright tilt-table test. The authors reported that 22 of the patients and 4 of the controls had abnormal responses to tilt. Seventy-five percent of patients but no controls had abnormal responses to 45 minutes at 70° tilt.[136]

Patients were offered treatment for neurally mediated hypotension. Options involved fludrocortisone acetate (Florinef), β-adrenergic blocking drugs, and disopyramide, alone or in combination. Patients were instructed to increase their intake of dietary salt, which 61% reported that they usually or always tried to avoid. Outcome measures were responses to upright tilt and scores on symptom questionnaires before and during follow-up. The authors reported that nearly half of the treated patients reported complete or nearly complete relief of symptoms within 1 month of starting treatment.[136]

It is interesting that the contents of this paper were so widely publicized in the popular press. The paper essentially consists of patients' responses to various paper and pencil tests, and patients' subjective estimates of their response to treatment under completely open conditions. There were no controls to prevent the authors from coloring the reported results according to their desires and expectations. The authors did only a short-term follow-up and used no randomization, blinding, or placebo control. The observations suggest an area for controlled study but must be viewed as suggestive at best.

The Homeopathic Agent
Rhus toxicodendron

Fisher et al. reported that use of the 6C dilution of Rhus toxicodendron (Rhus tox) improved fibromyalgia status.[115] In a second study, the 3 fibromyalgia patients using the 6X dilution of Rhus tox showed no improvement.[116] Selecting the homeopathic remedy that is most likely to benefit the patient must be based on the symptoms as well as the "constitutional profile," temperament, and personality of the patient. The homeopathic remedy selected is the one most likely to produce the symptoms of concern in individuals not suffering from the symptoms. Also, a patient's personality and temperament must match those of individuals who in past testing have been most responsive to the remedy. According to Chaitow, "This means that while two people might have the *same* named condition—say asthma—they might require *different* remedies if they have different personalities, likes and dislikes, and were affected differently by particular factors."[117,p.202] (These criteria distinguish homeopathic practice from allopathic practice. In allopathy, a medication is usually selected based on the patient's diagnosis—the prediction that a particular drug will alleviate one or a set of symptoms—or ideally, an understanding of the underlying pathophysiological process.) Presumably, these principles were observed in the two studies of the effects of Rhus tox on fibromyalgia patients.

In critiquing these studies, Chaitow explained that there is an enormous difference in 6X and 6C dilutions of a homeopathic remedy. He wrote, "With one study using Rhus tox 6C and claiming marked benefits for fibromyalgia sufferers and one using Rhus tox 6X showing no benefit, the jury is still out." He also advised that with the total absence of adverse effects with homeopathy, there is little to lose in trying Rhus tox. But patients should use the 6C rather than the 6X dilution.[117,p.203]

It is not certain, however, that the difference in dosage was responsible for the disparity between the results of the two studies. Selection of the particular remedy is of supreme importance in homeopathy, according to Vithoulkas,[118,p.213] and the choice of potency is merely an accessory factor. He wrote regarding potency, "There is a tendency, particularly among beginning prescribers, to pay a lot of attention to potency selection. Strangely enough, it is more common for a homeopathic instructor to be asked why a particular potency is selected in a given case than why a particular remedy is selected. In actual fact, potency selection is secondary in importance to remedy selection." Vithoulkas concluded, "If the correct remedy is selected, then it will act curatively in any potency, even though a correct potency will act more gently for the comfort of the patient; conversely, an *incorrect* remedy can be either inactive or disruptive to a case, regardless of what potency is given."[118,p.213] From this, it would appear that if Rhus tox were the proper homeopathic remedy for the patients in the study, some therapeutic effect would have been found in each study. It seems more likely that rather than an ineffective potency of Rhus tox in the second study, the remedy was not the proper selection for each individual patient studied. According to classical homeopathy, it is the fact that the therapy is based on the individual patient that renders homeopathy effective. To ignore this in a test of the therapy may nullify the test.

● PHYSICAL TREATMENTS

Physical forms of treatment that have been systematically studied include cardiovascular and general physical conditioning exercise, physical therapies such as soft tissue and spinal manipulation, acupuncture, balneotherapy, and high-frequency transcutaneous electrotherapy.

EXERCISE

Some clinicians and researchers purporting to have expertise in fibromyalgia/chronic fatigue syndrome espouse that the solution to these conditions is for patients to exercise. Steven Straus, in his comments on chronic fatigue syndrome patients, is one example. According to him, a significant portion of the symptoms results from "poor sleep hygiene" and abstinence from exercise.[104,p.685] Statements such as this from Straus and others raise serious questions about their responsibility as researchers. The available studies indicate that in general, fibromyalgia patients may benefit from low-level exercise with an increase in fitness level. But as Mengshoel concluded from the available studies, training has shown little benefit with regard to pain.[142] Table 5.1.3 contains the outcome of fibromyalgia patients' responses to questions about the effectiveness of treatments they have undergone. Although 86.8% reported engaging in exercise, 40.9% reported no improvement from it, and only 25.0% reported marked-to-greater improvement.[2][23]

Rather than benefitting, many patients experience an exacerbation of their symptoms with exercise. Hillary Johnson, in *Osler's Web*, described the circumstance: "Exercise, of course, was the great pillar of the Mayo Clinic's prescribed regime for sufferers. Those doctors who maintained a consistent relationship with their CFS patients, however, knew exercise to be among the most predictably devastating events—second only, perhaps, to the physical trauma of a car accident or surgery, in the lives of such patients; in-

creased severity of symptoms usually began 24-to-48 hours after even a minor workout. Vigorous exercise, in fact, frequently moved people who were only partially disabled into the category of fully disabled for an indefinite period of time."[104,p.491] According to Table 5.1.3, exercise was one of the three treatments tried by the highest percentage of patients. But it is little wonder that of the twelve treatments listed in Table 5.1.3, exercise benefitted the lowest percentage of patients.

Nonetheless, for some patients, although certainly not all, regular exercise of low enough intensity has been shown to provide limited improvement in fibromyalgia status.

Cardiovascular Fitness Training: Aerobic Exercise

Women with Fibromyalgia Typically have Poor Physical Fitness. Clark evaluated 95 fibromyalgic women for fitness level, exercise patterns, and perceived exertion during exercise. While the women exercised on a treadmill, researchers measured their oxygen consumption and carbon dioxide production. During the testing, the incline of the treadmill increased 2.5% every 2 minutes. Researchers monitored each patient's heart rate, workload, and minutes of exercise. They also assessed each patient's perceived exertion by her verbal statements. They did this both when her workload increased and at the end of testing.[12]

Clark concluded from the study that many fibromyalgic women do not engage in regular endurance exercises and that they have poor physical fitness.[12] This is consistent with the conclusions of other studies.[13][14] Clark found that only 11% of the women in her study engaged in exercise at a level adequate to increase or sustain endurance. She pointed out that this is consistent with data for the general adult population in the United States.[15] In addition, she stated that this is "unacceptable" since endurance exercises are important to reducing the physical limitations associated with fibromyalgia.[12,p.195] She also found that most of the women perceived their levels of exertion as normal.

Studies of the Effects of Cardiovascular Fitness Training on Fibromyalgia Patients' Pain. Moldofsky and Scarisbrick pointed out that a high level of physical fitness may be important in preventing fibromyalgia.[16] Physical fitness may also be important for recovering from the condition.

McCain and his coworkers reported the effects of cardiovascular fitness training on some features of fibromyalgia. Forty-two fibromyalgia patients took part in a 20-week exercise program. They engaged in either of two conditions: (1) cardiovascular fitness training or (2) a flexibility program. The investigators found that 83% of patients in the cardiovascular fitness training program improved their cardiovascular fitness. By contrast, as one might expect, none of the patients in the flexibility program improved their cardiovascular fitness.[17]

The patients in the cardiovascular fitness training group and their physicians considered the patients' overall well-being improved. Despite the significant distinction in overall fitness between the two groups, there was no difference in a number of specific measures: (1) present pain intensity (measured by visual analog scale), (2) percent total body involved in fibromyalgia, (3) hours per night or nights per week of disturbed sleep, and (4) psychological profiles. The investigators concluded that cardiovascular fitness training improved some objective and subjective features of fibromyalgia.[10,p.85][17]

In another study by Isomeri and colleagues, cardiovascular fitness training did not measure up as well. They compared the effects of three treatment conditions: (1) amitriptyline alone, (2) cardiovascular fitness training alone, and (3) amitriptyline and cardiovascular fitness training combined. Researchers assessed changes in three factors: (1) pressure pain thresholds, (2) pressure pain tolerances, and (3) patients' subjective evaluations of changes in their pain (via visual analog scale). Pressure pain thresholds did not increase during the therapy. The only patients who significantly improved were those receiving the combination of amitriptyline and cardiovascular fitness training. The improvement from the combined therapy, however, was minimal.[18] (See the section on amitriptyline above for the results of treatment with amitriptyline alone.)

Sixty-six chronic fatigue syndrome patients underwent 12 weeks of either graded aerobic exercise or flexibility exercises and relaxation therapy. Patients who completed the flexibility exercises were then given an opportunity to undergo exercise therapy. The researchers used the self-rate clinical global impression as the measure of improvement. The ratings "very much better" or "much better" indicated clinically important therapeutic change.[163]

In the exercise group, 4 patients dropped out; 3 of those in the flexibility group dropped out. After finishing the exercise program, 16 of 29 patients rated themselves as better. Of those who completed the flexibility program, 8 of 30 patients considered themselves

better. There was greater improvement in energy level (less fatigue), functional capacity, and fitness in patients who took part in the exercise program. After patients who first participated in the flexibility program switched over to and completed the exercise program, 12 of the 22 rated themselves as better. Three months after completing the exercise program, 32 of 47 patients rated themselves as better. One year after completing the exercise program, 35 of 47 patients considered themselves better. The researchers concluded, "These findings support the use of appropriately prescribed graded aerobic exercise in the management of patients with the chronic fatigue syndrome."[163]

Physical Conditioning Programs

In one study, patients had significant improvements in tenderness, global assessment, and physical capacity. But the trend of improvement on pain scores was not significant.[143] In another study,[144] physical training did not improve fibromyalgia symptoms. An evaluation of the effects of physical training in the form of aerobic walking was inconclusive.[145]

Mengshoel and Førre had 11 female fibromyalgia patients participate in low-intensity endurance training. The researchers were looking for changes in pain and fatigue in the patients. Twice per week for 20 weeks, the patients engaged in a modified low-impact aerobic dance program. During the activities, continuous dynamic exercises activated their large muscle groups. Each patient maintained a training intensity so that her heart rate did not exceed 150 beats per minute. The researchers evaluated the patients' pain through the McGill Pain Questionnaire.[19]

All patients reported a general feeling of well-being after exercising. Nine of them also reported feeling that their muscle tension diminished. In addition, their capacity for endurance increased and pain in their upper extremities upon exercising decreased. Their overall pain and fatigue, however, did not change significantly. Mengshoel and Førre concluded that fibromyalgia patients can take part in low-intensity endurance training without it worsening their pain and fatigue.[19]

Nørregaard et al. randomly assigned fibromyalgia patients to one of three forms of treatment: an aerobic dance program three times per week that slowly increased patients' exertion (15 patients), a 50-minute steady exercise program two times per week (15 patients), or hot packs twice per week (8 patients). The researchers tested these forms of physical conditioning because the ergometer exercise training typically employed tends to be boring for patients.[139]

Treatment was continued for 12 weeks. There was a high attrition rate. Completing the program were 5 in the aerobic group, 11 in the steady exercise group, and 7 in the hot pack group. For those who completed the program, there was no improvement in pain, fatigue, general condition, sleep, Beck's depression score, functional status, muscle strength, or aerobic capacity, regardless of the group.[139]

The investigators wrote, "There were no significant improvements in any of the parameters in any of the groups nor were there any differences between the groups. All muscle strength parameters were unchanged in all groups after training." They noted the low percentage of volunteers for the study, the high dropout rate, and the failure of improvement in aerobic capacity. These findings, they wrote, illustrate the difficulty in treating patients with physical modalities.[139]

Some observations in the study are worth highlighting. The investigators pointed out that many patients declined to participate because they feared exacerbating their fibromyalgia symptoms. Many from the exercise groups reported that they wanted to drop out of the study because the aerobic training worsened their fibromyalgia symptoms. Because of this, the researchers were not able to increase the training load as had been planned.[139] This corresponds to the finding of Verstappen et al.[153] that fibromyalgia patients may avoid potentially beneficial physical exercise because of the muscle soreness it may cause.

Wigers et al. studied the comparative effects on fibromyalgia patients of aerobic exercise, stress management (cognitive therapy), and treatment as usual. Sixty patients were randomly assigned to one of the three groups for 14 weeks of treatment. Measures were taken at baseline, half way through treatment, at the end of treatment, and 4 years later. Measures included a pain drawing, algometer measurements of tender point sensitivity, ergometer cycle test, global subjective improvement, and visual analog scales for pain, disturbed sleep, low energy, and depression. Patients who did aerobic exercise or stress management had some short-term improvement. Aerobic exercise was most effective, despite patients' initial scepticism toward this possibility. Symptom severities, however, did not differ significantly at 4-year follow-up. The lack of difference for the aerobic exercise group resulted partly from a compliance problem.[149]

Burkhardt et al. tested the effects on fibromyalgia patients of physical training at 12 weeks and 4-to-8 months after patients started the program. Every week for 6 weeks, patients underwent an hour of training. The training included stretching, pool therapy

sessions, range of motion activities, and aerobic conditioning by walking, swimming, or cycling. The patients also attended a 90-minute self-management education class. Another group of patients only attended the education class, and another group was on a waiting list and started treatment after the earlier patients had completed 12 weeks of participation in the program. The group who had physical training and education classes showed the most improvement, but there was no improvement on the Fibromyalgia Impact Questionnaire, the quality of life questionnaire, 6-minute walk time, tender point score, and myalgic score. Benefits were only modest.[151]

● PHYSICAL THERAPIES

Schmidt wrote in 1991 that physical therapies are not very effective in fibromyalgia cases.[5] Researchers have not rigorously evaluated physical forms of treatment, but Schmidt's statement corresponds to my extensive clinical experience using various forms of physiotherapy with fibromyalgia patients.

Yunus remarked in 1988 that no one had published controlled studies of physical treatments of fibromyalgia patients. He pointed out, however, that such treatments may benefit patients. He stated that the therapy may improve mobility, enable patients to engage in physical exercise soon after the therapy, improve sleep quality, and decrease patients' fixation on their pain. He wrote that the overall goal with physical treatment is to get patients to participate in functional activities throughout the day. This is preferable to permitting "the patient to spend an inordinate amount of time in steam baths and the like, which would encourage shirking of such daily responsibilities."[21,p.17]

Yunus noted that in difficult cases, the clinician should consult a physiatrist. The physiatrist can set up a well-defined program of physical therapy.[21,p.17] The term "physiatrist" refers to a physician who specializes in physical medicine and rehabilitation. Although some naturopathic, allopathic, osteopathic, chiropractic, and naprapathic physicians provide physiatrics care, occupational and physical therapists and trigger point myotherapists may provide equivalent services.

Spinal Manipulative Therapy
Goldenberg recently pointed out that manual therapy and chiropractic are among the non-medicinal treatments for fibromyalgia that no one had yet adequately studied.[6]

In 1985, Wolfe and his colleagues interviewed 81 fibromyalgia patients and 81 control subjects using a structured questionnaire.[2][23] He wrote, "In our current series, we asked patients to indicate if a drug or treatment had reduced their pain . . . . Of interest is that patients reported more benefit from 'lifestyle' modifications such as rest and relaxation than from other interventions. Chiropractic treatment also scored among the most effective measures."[2,p.13] Table 5.1.3 shows the treatments patients reported undergoing, the percentage of patients who underwent each form of treatment, and the percentage of patients who reported either no improvement or moderate-to-great improvement.

Wolfe emphasized that the data in Table 5.1.3 came from patient responses to questionnaires. He did not know what treatment the patients received from chiropractic physicians. He commented, however, that fibromyalgia patients often reported that chiropractic treatment gave them relief.[3][23] Because spinal manipulative therapy is the therapeutic mainstay of most chiropractic physicians, it is likely that the patients underwent this form of treatment. Wolfe also commented in 1991 that since his 1985 study, he had seen nothing to change his mind about the effectiveness of chiropractic treatment.[23]

Rubin conducted a study at the Texas College of Osteopathic Medicine. He evaluated the effects of spinal manipulation, drugs, and placebos on fibromyalgia patients. He reported his results in a book for the general public that he coauthored with a fibromyalgia patient. He and his coauthor describe the study as follows.[24]

Patients received one of four forms of treatment:
(1) placebo and no manipulation,
(2) placebo and manipulation,
(3) alprazolam (a benzodiazepine drug that is also called Xanax), ibuprofen, and no manipulation, or
(4) alprazolam and ibuprofen with manipulation.

Rubin wrote that the drugs were effective, but he did not say in what respect. Manipulation, which involved massaging the paraspinal soft tissues and manipulating the spine, improved the patients' overall sense of well-being. Rubin wrote that the two procedures were used to remove muscular or bony impediments to normal nerve conduction and blood and lymph flow.[24,p.45]

Two studies have reported that chiropractic physicians are prominent among the "alternative" practitioners fibromyalgia patients use. At a university-based

chronic fatigue clinic, 388 patients completed a follow-up questionnaire 1.7 years after their initial assessments. The results showed that those with chronic fatigue, chronic fatigue syndrome, and fibromyalgia were significantly more likely to use more chiropractic and other alternative provider services.[90]

Table 5.1.3. Percentages of fibromyalgia patients in interviews reporting improvement from different forms of treatment.*

| | | IMPROVEMENT | |
TREATMENT	% OF PATIENTS WHO RECEIVED	NONE	MODERATE-TO-GREAT
Rest	97.3	15.1	65.7
Relaxation	84.2	21.8	46.8
Chiropractic	48.7	16.2	45.9
Analgesics	88.2	46.3	45.8
Narcotics	61.5	45.8	45.8
Physical therapy	37.5	31.5	37.5
Antidepressants	51.5	51.5	36.3
Steroid injections	52.6	45.0	36.0
Amitriptyline (only)	51.0	56.6	30.2
Vacation	76.3	53.4	29.3
Exercise	86.8	40.9	25.0
Tranquilizers	28.6	28.6	23.8

*Wolfe, F.: The clinical syndrome of fibrositis. *Am. J. Med.*, 81 (Suppl.3A):7-14, 1986.[2]
NOTE: Table 5.1.3 is modeled after another summarizing these data in Chaitow, L.: *Fibromyalgia & Muscle Pain*, Hammersmith, Thorsons, 1995.[117,p.191]

Blunt et al. assessed the effectiveness of chiropractic management of 21 fibromyalgia patients. As outcome measures, the investigators used reported pain levels, cervical and lumbar ranges of motion, strength, flexibility, tender points, myalgic score and perceived functional ability. They used randomized crossover trial and assessed patient status before and after the treatment. Patients underwent treatment for 1 month. Treatment consisted of spinal manipulation, soft tissue therapy, and passive stretching. Treatment at each visit was at the chiropractors' discretion. Favorable changes occurred according to scores on the Oswestry Pain Disability Index, Neck Disability Index, and Visual Analog Scale, and according to the results of the straight leg raise test and lumbar and cervical ranges of motion. The investigators wrote that chiropractic management improved cervical and lumbar ranges of motion, straight leg raise, and pain levels reported by the patients. They judged the treatment to be "clinically important" to the patients in the study.[99]

Pioro-Boisset and coworkers interviewed 280 fibromyalgia patients through a questionnaire regarding the use of alternative medicine and compared the results with 222 consecutive rheumatology control patients. Among the fibromyalgia patients, 91% used alternative medicine as opposed to 63% of the controls. The most common alternative practitioners used were chiropractic physicians and massage therapists.[91]

Bennett, commenting on this study, correctly pointed out that the clinical effects of these alternative therapies were not assessed in the study. He also wrote, "Fibromyalgia syndrome is remarkably persistent and chronic and it is not surprising that patients seek other modalities considering the poor results of standard medical therapies."[92,p.104] It is unfortunate that other conventional medical practitioners do not address the use of alternative treatments with similar nonprejudicial commentary. The comments of an Internet neurologist[93] who claims he treats "large numbers of fibromyalgia patients" is a contrast to those of Bennett. The neurologist Nye wrote, "The absence of good studies confirming the efficacy of conventional [allopathic] treatment engenders therapeutic nihilism, opening the door to 'alternative' medical approaches and leaving too many patients unhelped."[93,p.122] Nye's use of the term "therapeutic nihilism" makes no sense. His objection to the door being open to "alternative medical approaches" seems to be a pejorative denouncement of these treatment methods. That fibromyalgia patients may use alternative treatments because they provide some measure of relief appears to have escaped Nye or is irrelevant to him.

Fibromyalgia patients undoubtedly continue seeking relief through different practitioners until they find one whose treatment provides sufficient relief to eliminate the motivation to continue searching. If chiropractic physicians and massage therapists did not provide sufficient relief, the patients would certainly decrease their use of such services. A 1996 Belgium study indicated that fibromyalgia patients using complementary therapies were of a higher socioeconomic group. Some patients did not use complementary therapies because of the comparatively high costs and lack of information on the therapies. These results were derived from a questionnaire sent to 90 fibromyalgia patients who had attended a Belgian outpatient rheumatology clinic.[150]

Soft Tissue Manipulation

As I mention above, massage therapists, along with chiropractic physicians, are the "alternative" practitioners most commonly used by fibromyalgia patients.[91] Occasionally, authors of a publication mention that a patient has benefitted from physical soft tissue treatment. Disdier and coauthors, for example, wrote of a woman who developed fibromyalgia after her anterior pituitary gland was surgically removed. They stated in passing, without details, that her pain was reduced by thermal baths and massage.[73]

Other than the brief mention of massage by Rubin, I have found only two studies in which investigators evaluated the effectiveness of soft tissue manipulation with fibromyalgia patients.[24,p.45] In one study, Danneskiold-Samsøe et al. massaged firm, tender, palpable foci in 13 patients' muscles. After 10 massage treatments, patients reported that they were free from pain. Their muscle nodules had softened so that palpatory findings such as firmness were less distinct, and the nodules were no longer tender. In this study, Danneskiold-Samsøe and coworkers found an interesting effect of massage when applied to the taut, painful nodules characteristic of myofascial pain syndromes. (In their first study, these investigators used the old term "fibrositis" in referring to the nodules. It is not clear whether the researchers were massaging these nodules in fibromyalgia patients or in patients with myofascial pain syndromes.) They compared the effects of the massage on myoglobin levels in the patients' serum. Myoglobin is located inside muscle cells and helps transport the oxygen required for aerobic metabolism inside the cell. The researchers took blood samples from the patients before massage, and for each hour after the first sample for 6 hours. Mean myoglobin levels increased after massage and decreased from the 3rd through the 6th hour after massage.[25][26]

The results of the study suggest that the cell membranes of patients' noduled muscles are friable—they rupture easily when mechanically distorted with manual manipulation. This may have occurred because reduced blood flow through the nodules delivered too little antioxidant nutrients and cortisol (membrane stabilizers) to the muscle cell membranes. The result of this study may have implications for the effects of massage on fibromyalgia patients in light of their abnormal diurnal variations of growth hormone[27] and cortisol levels.[27][146][177]

Growth hormone and somatomedin C, the compound through which it mediates its effects, are essential for repair of damaged tissues. Low levels indicate that these patients' tissues did not repair well.

Since the Danneskiold-Samsøe study suggests friability of noduled muscle, fibromyalgia patients may not recover well from excessively deep soft tissue massage. Clinicians should thus temper the pressure they apply during this form of therapy. Low cortisol levels may result in a low threshold for inflammation during manual manipulation of myofascial tissues.

In the other study of massage, Sunshine et al. compared the effects of massage with those of transcutaneous electrical stimulation (TENS) and sham TENS. Patients were treated twice per week for 30 minutes over a 5-week period. Patient status was assessed before and after treatment. Those who underwent massage had lowered depression scores, state anxiety, and salivary cortisol levels. There was no improvement in visual analog scales, stiffness, fatigue, or tender point sensitivity measured with algometry.[141] (See below for results of the TENS group.)

ACUPUNCTURE

Sprott et al. found that the serum serotonin level was lower in fibromyalgia patients (146 ng/ml) than in controls (250 ng/ml), and that the platelet serotonin level was high-normal ($\bar{x} = 0.525 \mu g/10^9$ cells). Following acupuncture treatment, the serum serotonin level increased to 177 ng/ml (P=0.001), and the platelet serotonin level decreased slightly ($\bar{x} = 0.422 \mu g/10^9$ cells).[170] The investigators did not report whether these changes were reflected in changes in the clinical status of fibromyalgia patients.

Sprott also tested acupuncture as a treatment for fibromyalgia under controlled conditions. He assigned 30 patients to either an acupuncture group, a placebo group "treated" with a disconnected laser device, or a no-treatment group. Those in the acupuncture and placebo groups each had 6 treatments. Changes in patient status were measured with a visual analog scale, a pain score, dolorimetry, and a questionnaire. The questionnaire provided information about a patient's psychological status, perception of his motor apparatus, and vegetative symptoms. Acupuncture patients had a decrease in the number of tender points and an increase in pain threshold. The increased pain threshold, however, was not significantly different between acupuncture and placebo patients. No changes were obvious according to the visual analog scales. There was a trend toward reduced pain in all groups. Acupuncture patients had a non-significant reduction in pain scores after an acupuncture treatment, but there was no improvement at a 2-month follow-up. Sprott concluded

that acupuncture is useful only when used as an adjunct within a comprehensive therapeutic program. He wrote, "The clinician is cautioned not to use acupuncture as the only remedy."[174]

BALNEOTHERAPY

Nicollet noted that medical publications that describe the use of water in the treatment of fibromyalgia are rare. Nonetheless, he indicates that it may be useful as a "secondary" therapy to provide patients with some comfort and to diminish physicians' embarrassment for not having an effective treatment. He also noted that it is commonly believed that hydrotherapy provides some fibromyalgia patients with temporary pain relief.[175,p.46] He performed a retrospective study of the results of the use of a device for intensive water-air pressure therapy. He explained that balneotherapy strictly means the use of baths in the treatment of disease, but treatment with the device he used was best described as a hydrodynamic blood pressure therapy. The device employs water-air jets that operate continuously or alternately. In the study, 22 fibromyalgia patients underwent two series of 10 whole-body treatments in hot water (28°-to-29°C) with a 15-day interval between the two series. Treatments, in which the jets were preferentially focused on particularly painful body parts, lasted 15-to-20 minutes according to patient tolerance. The patients' sleep improved. They also had improved pain for 1 day in 37% of patients, for 1-to-4 weeks in 30%, and 1 month for 33%. Nicollet concluded that the hydraulic pressure therapy provided better results than other forms of ordinary balneotherapy, but the results with these patients were not as good as with patients with rheumatic diseases.

ELECTROTHERAPY

In one study, 75 fibromyalgia patients were treated for treatment-resistant headaches with a cranial electrical therapy unit. The unit was battery-powered and imparted an extremely low level, high frequency current (0-4mA, 15-15,000 Hz) through the skin covering the cranium. The researcher noted that FDA guidelines contraindicate the cranial use of TENS units. TENS units transmit high amounts of low-frequency electricity (some 40-80 mA), while the unit tested in this study used a high frequency current of 4 mA.[28] The modality reportedly has virtually no adverse effects, and in other studies, it was more effective than placebos for tension headaches.[29]

All 75 patients rated the effects of the treatment on their chronic headaches. While 8 patients reported no improvement, 6 reported that they were entirely free from headaches. Twenty percent of the patients (15 of the 75) rated their improvement, or effectiveness of the therapy, as 7 on a 1-to-10 point scale. This represented moderate improvement in both frequency and severity of headache. About 50% of the patients (38 of the 75) rated their improvement as greater than 7.[28]

The research measured the pressure/pain thresholds of 6 tender sites and 3 control sites (typically less tender) both before and at 1-to-2 months after beginning use of the electrotherapy unit. The tenderness of control points did not change with treatment. According to the researchers, of the tender points, 42% were improved, 19% were worse, and 39% were unchanged. There were significant improvements in tender points above the waist. Tender points in the occipital and trapezius areas improved most.[28]

Sunshine et al. compared the effects on fibromyalgia status of transcutaneous electrical nerve stimulation (TENS), sham TENS, and massage (see above). Patients were treated for 30 minutes twice per week over a 5-week period. Patient status was assessed before and after treatment. Those who received TENS had reduced state anxiety and lowered depressed mood scores. Those who underwent massage, however, had lowered depression scores, state anxiety, and salivary cortisol levels. There was no improvement in visual analog scales, stiffness, fatigue, or tender point sensitivity measured with algometry.[141]

● TREATMENT REGIMENS

PROGRAMS RECOMMENDED IN THE FIBROMYALGIA LITERATURE

General

In addition to patient education, Goldenberg recommended discussion about exercise, posture, recreation, the patient's workplace, and stress. Some patients, he said, require no treatment other than simple analgesics. He started patients on 10 mg of amitriptyline at bedtime. If a patient did not improve but did not have adverse reactions to the drug, he increased the dose to 20-to-35 mg. He pointed out that some 10%-to-20% of patients cannot tolerate the adverse effects (drowsiness, dry mouth and eyes, constipation,

and weight gain). He may switch these patients to cyclobenzaprine or some other tricyclic drug. He also recommended individually tailored measures. These included relaxation, heat, massage, vapocoolant sprays, analgesic injections of tender points, biofeedback, and exercise programs.[1,pp.69-70]

Littlejohn recommended the following program to manage "localized fibromyalgia": (1) make an accurate diagnosis and assess and treat occult tissue damage, (2) dissociate the patient's belief of injury when his symptoms do not indicate injury, (3) remove postural and ergonomic triggers for pain, (4) increase aerobic fitness, (5) have the patient stay at work and use the symptomatic body part, (6) relieve sleep disturbance, (7) reduce stress with behavior modification, and finally, (8) encourage the patient to avoid adversarial compensation litigation.[41,p.171]

Yunus and his colleagues reported that the following program lessened the severity of symptoms in juvenile fibromyalgia patients: a firm diagnosis, reassurance that the condition is benign (perhaps by comparing it to juvenile rheumatoid arthritis), stress management, moderation of physical activity, physical therapy (heat and stretching exercises), and nonaddictive analgesics such as NSAIDs.[65]

Yunus also wrote that there are several important features (similar to those above) for effective management of patients with fibromyalgia: (1) firmly diagnosing the condition, (2) reassuring the patient that the condition is benign, (3) helping the patient accept the pain, (4) encouraging the patient to increase functional activities and exercise tolerance, and (5) prescribing tricyclic drugs.[21]

Conditioning

In 1991 Laywood described the treatment program for fibromyalgia he observed at the Oregon Health Science University in Portland.[66] Fundamental to this program are two assumptions: first, that generalized deconditioning and physical inactivity are major components in the pathogenesis of fibromyalgia; and second, that as some studies show, aerobic exercise reduces pain and point tenderness, alleviates associated symptoms, increases the patient's sense of well-being, improves sleep, and relieves fatigue.

Laywood noted that first, staff members confirm the diagnosis of fibromyalgia. The patient fills out a series of questionnaires that provide a general overview of the patient. The patient's coping strategies are assessed, along with her mental state and some of the ways she perceives and manages her discomfort. A psychologist analyzes the patient's responses to determine whether she is likely to benefit from the program.

Next, staff members of the University Human Performance Laboratory assess the patient's level of physical fitness. The assessment involves aerobic exercise using a treadmill walk. The treadmill is set at a speed of 3.0 km/hour for a period of 10 minutes. The treadmill elevates so that the patient essentially begins climbing a gradient that increases at a rate of 1% per minute. While on the treadmill, the patient breathes through a spirometer. The spirometer calculates the highest volume of oxygen taken up by the patient. In healthy persons, this is 30-to-70 liters per minute. In fibromyalgia patients, it is 20 or fewer liters per minute. The patient's level of fitness is measured by the point at which she reaches the anaerobic threshold.

A physical examination assesses the patient's flexibility, triceps, biceps, and digital grip strength, range of spinal flexion, and endurance while walking. An exercise physiologist works with the patient to design a muscular flexibility program (according to the American College of Sports Medicine recommendations) and a general anatomical stretching program. The exercises are tailored to the individual's abilities and are periodically modified to assure maximum benefit.

At regular meetings, treatment coordinators provide psychological support or counseling and help patients resolve any stress-related problems. Physicians may also prescribe mild antidepressants to facilitate restorative sleep. Patients participate in the program for 1 year and undergo assessment at 3-to-6-month intervals.

Laywood pointed out, "Although there is no cure for this disorder, it is believed that by following this treatment programme, there is a great deal that can be done to alleviate pain."[66,p.236]

Multimodal

Bennett et al. studied the effects on 104 fibromyalgia patients of a 6-month multidisciplinary outpatient program. Patients underwent education, exercise therapy, cognitive restructuring, trigger point injections, myofascial spray and stretch, and treatment with tricyclic medications including cyclobenzaprine. The authors reported that after 6 months, 70% of patients had fewer than 11 tender points, and there was a 25% improvement in scores on the Fibromyalgia Impact Questionnaire. The training index and the reduced catastrophizing on the subscale of the coping strategies questionnaire were the best predictors of improvement. At 2-year follow-up, 33 of the patients still were im-

proved and had maintained the improved quality of life according to the Fibromyalgia Impact Questionnaire.[140] A control group showed no improvement.

Teitelbaum and Bird reported the results of an open trial multimodal treatment of 64 patients with severe fatigue that markedly curtailed normal activities. Of these patients, 44 met the ACR criteria for fibromyalgia. The treatment protocol a patient used was based on the diagnosis. Patients were treated accordingly after being diagnosed as having subclinical hypothyroidism; underactive adrenal cortices; chronic infections; depression, anxiety, and episodes of hyperventilation; or deficiencies of micronutrients. Forty-six patients had at least three or more diagnoses. Patients were treated for a median of 7 weeks. The clinicians felt that treating coexisting problems at the same time would improve the effectiveness of the treatment, but they found that it was difficult to assess how effective any one treatment was. Table 5.1.4 shows the treatment(s) administered for each diagnosis. They reported complete resolution of fatigue in 57% of patients and incomplete improvement in 39%.[154]

Metabolic Rehabilitation

For most patients, my colleagues and I recommend T_3 or a combination of T_4 and T_3 as the basis of the treatment regimen, the dosage carefully adjusted to individual requirements. We use other methods to help produce a sustained increase in metabolism and still others to decrease metabolic demand. We *require* patients to take therapeutic doses of nutritional supplements, particularly B complex vitamins, because of the critical roles of the supplements in metabolic processes.[54][67] We have patients use aerobic and toning exercises and possibly caffeine to help increase their energy metabolism. We may have patients use meditation, myofascial stretching exercises, progressive relaxation training, and cognitive-behavioral therapy to decrease the metabolic demand. With most patients, we also use physical methods such as myofascial and spinal manipulative therapies to provide palliative relief through desensitizing pain-mediating myofascial and joint lesions (see Appendix B, paper titled "Facilitating the Decrease in Fibromyalgic Pain During Metabolic Rehabilitation: An Essential Role for Soft Tissue Therapies").

● PSYCHOLOGICAL TREATMENTS

Treatments of a psychological nature that have

been studied are placebos, biofeedback, cognitive-behavioral therapy, hypnotherapy, marriage and family counseling, mediation, and patient education.

PLACEBO RESPONSE

Placebo Response in Clinical Practice

Some clinicians may argue that giving patients placebos is not a true treatment. Instead, it is a bogus or fake procedure that has no real therapeutic value. This view disregards the relief that belief and expectation can provide many patients (albeit seldom lasting). In diminishing or relieving pain, placebos can invoke potent biochemical mechanisms. For example, evidence indicates that placebo analgesia is mediated by endogenous opiates.[50] In day-to-day patient care, the clinician may value *any* influence, physical or psychological, that contributes to a patient's improvement. For example, a clinician may intentionally display confidence in the outcome of a therapy solely to psychologically potentiate the inherent effectiveness of the therapy. In most cases, both the clinician's and the patient's objectives are served by such efforts. The placebo response wanes over time, however, and the patient is likely to lose the portion of improvement attributable to psychological effect.

There is at least one major downside to indulgence in the placebo response: the patient may fail to pursue and undergo treatment that is more likely to provide lasting relief by affecting the underlying pathophysiological mechanism. I have communicated with many fibromyalgia patients who expended their personal funds and insurance benefits for drug treatments recommended by rheumatology fibromyalgia researchers after the drugs were shown experimentally to be ineffective. They began these treatments with trust in their effectiveness. The trust was instilled by the treating clinicians who also had trust that the drugs were effective.[101] My questioning of some clinicians indicated that their trust was based on published statements by a few rheumatology fibromyalgia researchers that the drugs were effective.[102][103] These statements were published after studies had been available showing that in fact the drugs were not effective.

For practical reasons, practicing clinicians tend to trust the judgment of high-profile investigators known to be doing research into various health conditions. Considering the current information deluge, this is understandable, although a far better system would be for clinicians to evaluate evidence themselves rather than trusting authoritative opinion. Nonetheless, for better

or worse, trust by clinicians in reports by researchers often translates into expressions of confidence by clinicians and consequent placebo responses in patients. The clinician must judge on an individual basis whether a placebo response is an appropriate therapeutic aim with a patient. Unfortunately, there is no reason to believe that conventional rheumatology treatments for fibromyalgia such as antidepressant medications have any value other than placebo potential. It is questionable whether their potential adverse effects are worth brief psychologically-based relief. (In many cases in my experience, patients tend to continue taking tricyclic drugs because they are afraid they will be worse if they stop.) In light of the ineffectiveness of these medications and their potential risks, treatments such as chiropractic care, massage therapy, balneotherapy, and cognitive-behavioral therapy are preferable to the medications in three important respects: they are non-invasive, nontoxic, and many fibromyalgia patients report that these treatment methods provide palliative relief.

Placebo Response in Research

In the research setting, investigators usually want to measure the precise effect of a chemical, psychological, or physical treatment on a symptom, sign, or some other measure of a disease. To accomplish this, they must separate the actual effect of the treatment from the effect of researchers' and patients' beliefs that the remedy is effective. To make this differentiation, especially with drug trials, investigators often design studies through which it is possible to evaluate the effect of the treatment compared to the effect of an inert substance (the placebo). In efficacy studies of fibromyalgia treatment, placebo responses have been minimal-to-substantial.

Goldenberg, Felson, and Dinerman reported that in a randomized, controlled study, only a few fibromyalgia patients improved with oral placebos. Patients who took placebos did not significantly improve on any of the outcome variables (tender point score, pain, fatigue, sleep, global assessment).[7,p.1375]

Yunus et al. reported results that indicate placebos may benefit fibromyalgia patients. They gave one group of patients ibuprofen and another a placebo. Both groups improved slightly, but neither did better than the other. The researchers speculated that physician interaction, the effects of participating in a study, or a patient's belief that the placebo was effective accounted for patient improvement.[8]

Carette and colleagues conducted a 6-month, double-blind, controlled trial of amitriptyline, cyclobenzaprine, and placebo with 208 patients. The researchers evaluated 13 different outcome measures after 1, 3, and 6 months of treatment. After 1 month, patients on either drug significantly improved on all measures except tender point score and the Stanford Health Assessment Questionnaire. Patients taking placebos had improved on only 1 measure. At the 6-month evaluation, however, patients taking placebos had improved on 9 of the 13 measures. According to the authors, at 1 month, the patients taking drugs showed the most improvement. At 6 months, there was no significant difference in improvement between medicated and placebo-treated patients.[9] Goldenberg wrote of these results, "Thus, although this study confirms the short-term efficacy of amitriptyline and cyclobenzaprine in fibromyalgia, long-term efficacy could not be demonstrated because of a significant placebo response over time." The placebo response rate in the Carette study was as high as 50%. It should be noted that what is termed "short-term efficacy" was very slight improvement.[6,p.75] The efficacy should not be construed to mean that amitriptyline and cyclobenzaprine are clinically useful (see section on antidepressant drugs).

BEHAVIORAL TREATMENTS

Biofeedback Training

In a study of the effects of biofeedback training, Ferraccioli gave 15 fibromyalgia patients 15 sessions of EMG biofeedback over 5 weeks. Nine patients improved with a decrease in three measures: (1) number of tender points, (2) present pain intensity (according to visual analog scale), and (3) morning stiffness.[30]

The improvements lasted up to 6 months after the biofeedback training. A follow-up study by the same investigators produced similar results. Benefits from the training lasted through 5-week and 6-month evaluations. The researchers noted that EMG-biofeedback appears to reduce plasma ACTH and β-endorphin levels during treatment, and this raises the possibility that neuroendocrine and opioid mechanisms were responsible for the improvements in their fibromyalgia patients.[31]

In another study, Ferraccioli et al. gave EMG-biofeedback training to two groups of fibromyalgia patients. One group consisted of 7 patients who had no detectable endocrine abnormalities. At the end of 15 sessions, 6 of the 7 patients had improved. The researchers defined improvement as 50% better scores on tender point exams, the McGill Pain Questionnaire, and a visual analog scale.[32,p.871]

The other group in the Ferraccioli study consisted

of 3 patients who had endocrine abnormalities. Two of them had a blunted TSH response to TRH injections. The 3rd had non-suppression of cortisol blood levels after taking dexamethasone. (Dexamethasone is a synthetic cortisol that normally suppresses blood cortisol levels.) None of these 3 patients benefitted from biofeedback training. Six months after the first assessment, 2 of these patients had severe exacerbations of their aches and pains. The researchers evaluated them for endocrine dysfunction again at that time. The endocrine abnormalities revealed on their first evaluation were still clearly present during this second testing.

Table 5.1.4. Diagnoses of and treatments for 64 patients with severe fatigue.*

DIAGNOSIS	TREATMENT(S)	DOSAGE
Subclinical hypothyroidism	T$_4$	25-50 µg (0.025-0.050 mg)
Hypoadrenocortical function	Cortef	5-7.5 mg qd-qid
Fibromyalgia	Amitriptyline Cyclobenzaprine	10-50 mg 5-20 mg
Chronic infections Bacterial Bowel parasites Fungal	Not given Not given Itraconazole Nystatin	200 mg qd 500,000 units
Depression, anxiety, and hypertension	Tricyclic antidepressants Selective serotonin reuptake inhibitors	Not given Not given
Micronutrient deficiencies	Vitamin B complex Minerals Mg chloride	25 mg Not given Not given

*Teitelbaum, J. and Bird, B.: Effective treatment of severe chronic fatigue: a report of a series of 64 patients. *J. Musculoskel. Pain*, 3(4):91-110, 1995.[154]

Ferraccioli et al. wrote that these results support the point of view that neuroendocrine evaluation may be important in devising a therapeutic regimen for fibromyalgia patients. At least such testing may help identify patients (those without neuroendocrine abnormalities) likely to benefit from EMG-biofeedback.[32,p.872][33][34]

Cognitive-Behavioral Therapy

In a pilot study, cognitive-behavioral therapy improved the status of 5 of 7 juveniles with fibromyalgia. The 7 patients ranged in age from 8.6-to-17.7 years. Those who completed treatment underwent 4-to-9 sessions. At the end of treatment, they reported that their pain was absent or negligible. Parents reported that the patients' school attendance, participation in family activities, and peer interaction returned to normal. At 4-month and 24-month follow-ups, 4 patients reported having no pain. The 5th patient said she had intermittent mild pain that she easily controlled with the techniques she learned in cognitive-behavioral therapy. The patients said they were free from their former sleep difficulties and mood problems.[35]

The 2 patients who did not improve were older and had pain longer than the other patients. One of these patients did not return for treatment after the initial meeting. The other attended 4 sessions, was displeased with the intervention, and dropped out.

Treatment procedures involved progressive relaxation training and guided imagery. The researchers tried this regimen partly because of its success with juveniles with rheumatoid arthritis.[36] The aim of the regimen was self-regulation of pain, and involved the following sequence:

1) Patients learned progressive relaxation of major muscle groups. They associated the relaxed state with cues they could later use to help elicit relaxation when they needed it. They used the cues, for example, when trying to initiate or maintain sleep.

2) Patients practiced guided imagery with two purposes. A first type of imagery distracted them from their pain. The scenes they chose to imagine were ones in which they had previously been pain-free. They imaged themselves actually in the scenes rather than observing themselves there. The therapist gave the patients detailed multisensory descriptions to help them form effective images. Patients later repeated the descriptions aloud. The therapist also used a variety of scenes to stimulate the patients' interest and attention.

A second type of imagery represented a metaphor for the patients' pain. By changing the metaphor, they were able to change their pain perceptions. The therapist and patients discussed the patients' metaphoric images to help concretize them. The investigators wrote, "If the pain was labeled as 'pressing,' a metaphoric image might be that 'there is a vise gripping my leg.' An image is then generated in which the vise is opened and the pain relieved."[35,p.1618] Another technique involved the use of color. Patients imaged their painful body parts as a particular color. They contrast-

ed this color with one for non-painful tissues. Next, they imaged the painful color shrinking and disappearing.

The cognitive-behavioral intervention was individualized, based on each patient's level of development, comfort, and interest. Patients had audio tapes of the techniques to use at home. They also had discussions with the therapist that focused on their personal effectiveness in mastering their pain. These talks were to help reduce anxiety and depression.[35]

In another study, Nielson and colleagues assessed 30 consecutive patients on three occasions at a rheumatic diseases facility. The first assessment took place 5 months before admission of subjects as inpatients to a 3-week cognitive-behavioral treatment program. The second assessment took place at the time of admission, and the third was upon discharge from the program. The program involved cognitive-behavioral interventions by members of six disciplines: medicine, psychology, social work, physiotherapy, occupational therapy, and nursing. These practitioners intended to help patients become more active, resourceful, and self-managing in coping with their fibromyalgia. Toward this aim, they used relaxation, biofeedback, physiotherapy, and aerobic exercises.[37]

Vlaeyen et al. studied fibromyalgia patients' responses over a 6-week period to one of three different conditions: combined cognitive/educational intervention, group education, or a wait-list control group. Psychological measures were used, but other measures of fibromyalgia status were not. The researchers evaluated patients' status 2 weeks before treatment, at the initiation of treatment, immediately after treatment, and at 6-month and 12-month follow-ups. Compared to patients on the waiting list, patients who underwent cognitive training were better able to cope with pain and had a better understanding of fibromyalgia. Patients who underwent education were better able to cope with pain, controlled pain better, and had less fear than patients who were on the waiting list or who had cognitive training.[138] Education produced better results than cognitive-behavioral therapy. Compared to the effects of education, cognitive-behavioral therapy was of minimal benefit.

Researchers assessed the outcome of the program mainly with psychological measures. These showed that patients improved in several respects: (1) the severity of their pain, (2) affective distress (tension, irritability, mood, depression), and (3) the interference their pain caused during their daily activities. Patients also enhanced their sense of control and mastery over their life circumstances. Short-term assessment showed these improvements. The researchers provided no long-term follow-up data.[138]

These investigators did not assess changes in fibromyalgia measures such as morning stiffness and pressure/pain threshold at tender points. Functional abilities, however, did improve. For example, the patients were able to spend longer times out of bed and they became more active. The researchers concluded that cognitive-behavioral therapy, when administered by qualified clinicians, can benefit some patients. As noted above, however, education was more effective than cognitive-behavioral therapy.[138]

In another study that compared the effects of education with behavioral intervention, both groups showed some improvement in depression, self-reported pain behaviors, observed pain behaviors, and myalgia scores. However, the outcome between the two forms of treatment did not differ significantly.[82]

Mengshoel and coworkers conducted a study of a multidisciplinary treatment program for fibromyalgia patients. The program focused on helping patients solve difficulties associated with their everyday activities. Sixteen females completed the 10-week program which entailed both exercise and cognitive restructuring. After 10 weeks, patients had more general pain, but pain intensity was decreased. At 6-month follow-up, pain intensity remained improved.[127]

White and Nilson conducted a long-term follow-up of cognitive-behavioral therapy for fibromyalgia and compared the results with pre-treatment values. The investigators evaluated the status of 22 subjects 30 months after the end of treatment. At follow-up, only 3 of 10 values were improved. These included observed pain behavior and control over pain. There was an insignificant trend toward improvement for all 10 measures.[126]

Major depression was the most important predictor of failed response to cognitive-behavioral treatment for patients with post-viral fatigue syndrome.[74]

Researchers have conducted several studies of cognitive-behavioral therapy for chronic fatigue patients. Of 32 patients treated in an open uncontrolled trial, 22 (69%) were considered clinically improved in symptoms and function. Treatment emphasized a gradual increase in activity and challenged the belief that patients had an organic disease. The researchers wrote that improvements persisted at a 3-month follow-up.[156]

In a controlled study, 22 chronic fatigue syndrome patients underwent group cognitive-behavioral therapy for 6-to-9 weeks. At the end of the study, measures of fatigue and other symptoms for the patients who went through the therapy were no different from those of patients who had declined to undergo the treatment.[157]

In another controlled trial with 68 patients, the effects of cognitive-behavioral therapy were compared with those of standard medical treatment. During the 6 biweekly treatments, gradual increases in activity were emphasized, but beliefs that patients suffered from an organic disease were not challenged. Both at the end of treatment and 7 months after the end, there was no difference in the measures of distress and disability between the two groups of patients. However, at 7-month follow-up, fatigue and depression were lower for both groups.[158]

Sharpe suggested that the reason improvement was greater in the open trial[156] than in the two controlled studies[157][158] was that the therapist in the open trial, unlike those in the other studies, challenged patients' beliefs that their symptoms were a product of organic disease. Thus, Sharpe speculated, treatment in the controlled studies was more acceptable to patients but less effective.[155,p.145]

Sharpe conducted another study with chronic fatigue syndrome patients in which beliefs about the organic etiology of the condition were challenged. An effort was made to avoid the faults in the other studies. Sixty patients whose symptom duration was fewer than 10 years were treated. Each had 16 1-hour individual treatments over a 4-month period. Treatment objectives included establishing a collaboration with the patient, negotiating a formulation of the illness that was acceptable to both patient and therapist, overcoming avoidance of activity, and ". . . helping them re-evaluate the accuracy and helpfulness of their attribution of symptoms to organic disease." With some patients, unrealistic expectations and criticism of themselves were addressed, and problem-solving methods were used to help with social difficulties. Treatment was compared with standard hospital care and that of a primary care physician. Results were evaluated at 1, 3, and 8 months post-treatment. Patients rated the status of their symptoms and functional abilities, and an independent evaluator assessed overall status. Sharpe concluded that patients who had cognitive-behavioral therapy had made substantial gains.[159]

Comment on the Use of Cognitive-Behavioral Therapy. Cognitive-behavioral therapy may help patients avoid or correct compounding their troubles with exaggerated assessments of their plight and prognosis. Using behavioral techniques as a therapy to control manifestations of a metabolic disorder can be helpful, as by counteracting the tendency to worsen a bad circumstance through catastrophizing or by countering the tendency toward less and less physical activity. But the outcome of using these techniques with fibromyalgia/chronic fatigue syndrome patients will, in general, be minimal at best. The result is akin to using reasoning to improve the symptoms during an episode of hypoglycemia or diabetic hyperglycemia. Symptoms in most cases will relentlessly recur until the underlying metabolic disorder is corrected.

HYPNOTHERAPY

Haanen et al. included 40 fibromyalgia patients in a study that assessed the effects of hypnotherapy compared to physical therapy. Patients underwent treatment and were evaluated for outcome at 12 weeks and at a 24-week follow-up. The outcome for patients treated with hypnotherapy was better according to several measures: pain experience, fatigue on awakening, sleep pattern, and global assessment. Patients who underwent hypnotherapy had a greater improvement in feelings of somatic and psychological discomfort, but some continued to have strong discomfort. Patients in neither group had a significant improvement in total myalgic score derived through algometry measurements. The investigators concluded that hypnotherapy may provide fibromyalgia patients symptom relief.[38]

MARITAL COUNSELING AND PSYCHOMOTOR THERAPY

De Voogd and coworkers used marriage counseling and psychomotor therapy with fibromyalgia patients. They explained that psychomotor therapy "is a behavioral therapy that refers to body-experience and awareness. It consists of relaxation combined with visualization techniques and stimulation of social activities. It aims to break through the preoccupation circle with pain and other physical complaints."[39]

The investigators included 50 patients in their study. Their aims were fourfold: to help patients (1) learn to cope with their disabilities, (2) improve their ability to relax, (3) increase their assertiveness, and (4) learn how to better differentiate between body signals associated with fibromyalgia and those associated with other body cues and emotions. Fifty other fibromyalgia patients acted as controls by not taking part in the therapy.[39]

The first effort in the program was to diminish patients' preoccupation with their unpleasant physical

sensations. They used focusing techniques to shift attention to pleasant body sensations and to relax their bodies. Therapists advised patients to balance their activities to accommodate their compromised conditions and to allow them to relax. Patients were also encouraged to engage in various activities that would expand their social involvement and their sources of social reinforcement. Therapists attempted to teach patients to cope with their disabilities by assertively declining to do other people favors that might exacerbate their symptoms. Some patients were not able to comply with this measure. Patients also had marriage counseling with a social worker.[39]

After the therapy, 70% percent of the patients were satisfied with their improved ability to relax and their heightened self-confidence. Sixty-six percent reported that they were better able to deal with their disabilities. The investigators' assessment procedures, however, did not confirm these positive evaluations by participating patients. At the end of the study, patients who underwent treatment exhibited no significant differences from control patients. None of the treated patients experienced any reduction of pain or improvement in other physical complaints.[39]

The researchers concluded that their treatment program did not induce significant or enduring improvements in fibromyalgia patients. In fact, the investigators stated that they were going to modify their treatment program and use cognitive-behavioral therapy because it offered more structure to patients. During the study, 24% of the patients had asked for a more structured approach.[39]

MEDITATION-BASED STRESS REDUCTION

Kaplan, Goldenberg, and Galvin-Nadeau assessed the effectiveness of a meditation-based stress reduction program with fibromyalgia patients. The patients took part in a 10-week program. Therapists followed a carefully defined treatment protocol and met weekly to promote uniformity.

The researchers evaluated the patients before and after the program. The initial evaluation included a psychiatric-structured clinical interview. Researchers used visual analog scales to assess global well-being, pain, sleep, fatigue, and feelings of being restored after sleep. Patients completed several questionnaires to help assess the outcome of therapy.

The mean scores of all patients completing the program showed improvement. Fifty-one percent showed moderate-to-marked improvement. The researchers included only this 51% as "responders" to the therapeutic intervention. The conclusion reached was that these findings indicate that a meditation-based stress reduction program is effective for fibromyalgia patients.[40]

PATIENT EDUCATION

Goldenberg wrote that the cornerstone of treatment for fibromyalgia is patient education. He wrote that most physicians find an initial discussion with the fibromyalgia patient and her family the most valuable therapeutic modality. Patients usually feel relieved to learn that fibromyalgia is a common condition and that it is not life-threatening.[1,p.69]

Littlejohn proposed that when fibromyalgia is associated with a repetitive motion injury, education is an indispensable part of treatment. He wrote, "If the patient can let go of the belief that they [sic] are injured and that something 'has done this to me,' then they [sic] have made a major step toward improvement. The changing of this fixed belief about injury is the key point in management." He added, "If the belief cannot be changed, then all other treatment measures have little impact on the symptoms."[41,p.171]

The 81 fibromyalgia patients studied by Cathey and her associates had a high hospitalization rate prior to clinicians giving them the diagnosis of fibromyalgia. The patients were hospitalized mainly for general pain; skeletal, neck, back, and joint symptoms; and depression. For the year following the patients' diagnoses of fibromyalgia, their hospitalization rate dropped. Cathey and her coauthors wrote, ". . . it seems possible that diagnosis leads to a reduction in hospitalization and hence to a significant reduction in the lifetime cost of the disease."[22,p.83]

Kogstad and Hintringer had 71 fibromyalgia patients participate in "pain school." The school consisted of education, group therapy, and psychomotoric physiotherapy. (Psychomotoric physiotherapy is a subspecialty in Norwegian physiotherapy education.) In this study, psychomotoric physiotherapy involved training in relaxation techniques, guided imagery, vivid imagery, self-talk, and distraction techniques. The intention was "to activate patients' own positive powers in fighting the pain, managing chronic pain consequences, and improving life quality."[42,p.261] Patients attended 2-hour sessons once a week for 6 weeks. The sessions involved education, exercise/physical training, and relaxation. Patients also took part in group discussions. The educators discussed communication

difficulties and problem-solving with patients, and they attempted to teach patients self-help principles and methods for coping with chronic pain. At 1-year follow-up, patients reported having a better global outcome than control subjects did. Patients and control subjects did not differ, however, in depression, physical activity, medication use, sleep disturbance, and fatigue. There was no significant improvement in pain scores. Patients considered group therapy more important to them than either the psychomotoric physiotherapy or the academic part of the education.[42]

Patients in this study had reduced their use of health services by 10% at follow-up compared to controls. The difference, however, was not statistically significant. More patients (up from 5 to 13) than control subjects (down from 23 to 12) had found paying jobs. The investigators suggested that it was difficult to determine whether this might be a result of the program. They concluded that structured pain school is a useful supplement to other treatments for fibromyalgia. Pain "consequences" (though not pain itself) and life quality improved.[42]

The question of the value of education must be balanced by other findings. Based on other publications regarding musculoskeletal pain patients,[147][148] Nørregaard et al. conjectured that diagnostic labeling has a negative impact on prognosis in pain patients who do not have a specific known peripheral pathology.[139,p.77]

POSSIBLE MECHANISM OF IMPROVEMENT IN FIBROMYALGIA WITH PSYCHOLOGICAL THERAPIES

Biofeedback, cognitive-behavioral therapy, hypnosis, and other methods that incorporate mental calming, relaxation, and imagery may benefit fibromyalgia patients by several mechanisms. First, such treatments probably reduce the activity level of the gamma motor nerve pathway to skeletal muscles. The resulting lengthening muscle spindles would relax skeletal muscles, reducing their metabolic demand. Considering the size of the skeletal muscle system, the reduced metabolic demand could relieve symptoms caused by a sustained metabolic crisis. Such a crisis in fibromyalgia patients may result from reduced blood flow and impaired ATP production. Also, reducing patients' general arousal levels with psychological therapies might lower their basal catecholamine levels and the frequency or extremity of catecholamine surges. If a patient, in accordance with the hypothesis I posit in this book, has an increased density of α_2-adrenergic receptors on cell membranes, then reducing the exposure of the cells to catecholamines will reduce the severity of her symptoms. Binding of catecholamines predominantly to α_2-adrenergic receptors on cell membranes inhibits the metabolic processes within the cells.

In addition, inadequate thyroid hormone regulation of cells of the hypothalamic-pituitary-adrenal axis may account for the abnormalities of this axis in fibromyalgia patients. The abnormalities may account for some fibromyalgia symptoms, including worsening status subsequent to stress. Psychological therapies, by raising the threshold of sympathetic activation, may minimize the demand for a vigorous hypothalamic-pituitary-adrenal axis response to stress, resulting in generally improved fibromyalgia status.

REFERENCES

1. Goldenberg, D.L.: Treatment of fibromyalgia syndrome. *Rheum. Dis. Clin. North Am.*, 15:61-71, 1989.
2. Wolfe, F.: The clinical syndrome of fibrositis. *Am. J. Med.*, 81(Suppl.3A):7-14, 1986.
3. Lowe, J.C.: Fibromyalgia: are chiropractic adjustments appropriate? *Dyn. Chiro.*, Dec. 1992, p.23.
4. Hamaty, D., Valentine, J.L., Howard, R., Howard, C.W., Wakefield, V., and Patten, M.S.: The plasma endorphin, prostaglandin and catecholamine profile of patients with fibrositis treated with cyclobenzaprine and placebo: a 5-month study. *J. Rheum.*, 16:164-168, 1989.
5. Schmidt, K.L.: Generalized tendomyopathy (fibromyalgia): differential diagnosis, therapy, and prognosis. *Z. Gesamte. Inn. Med.*, 46:370-374, 1991.
6. Goldenberg, D.L.: Fibromyalgia: treatment programs. *J. Musculoskel. Pain*, 1:71-81, 1993.
7. Goldenberg, D.L., Felson, D.T., and Dinerman, H.: A randomized controlled trial of amitriptyline and naproxen in the treatment of patients with fibromyalgia. *Arthritis Rheum.*, 29:1371-1377, 1986.
8. Yunus, B.M.B., Masi, A.T., and Aldag, J.C.: Short term effects of ibuprofen in primary fibromyalgia syndrome: a double-blind, placebo-controlled trial. *J. Rheumatol.*, 16: 527-532, 1989.
9. Carette, S., Bell, M., Reynolds, W.J., et al.: A controlled trial of amitriptyline, cyclobenzaprine, and placebo in fibromyalgia. *Arthritis Rheum.*, 35(Suppl.9):112, 1992.
10. McCain, G.A.: Nonmedicinal treatments in primary fibromyalgia. *Rheumat. Dis. Clin. North Am.*, 15:73-89, 1989.
11. McCain, G.A.: Treatment of fibromyalgia and myofascial pain syndrome. In *Myofascial Pain and Fibromyalgia: Trigger Point Management*. Edited by E. S. Rachlin, St. Louis, Mosby, 1994, pp.31-44.
12. Clark, S.R.: Fitness characteristics and perceived exertion in women with fibromyalgia. *J. Musculoskel. Pain*, 1:191-197, 1993.
13. Bennett, R.M., Clark, S.R., Goldberg, L., Nelson, D., Bonafede, R.P., Porter, J., and Specht, D.: Aerobic fitness in the fibrositis syndrome: a controlled study of respiratory gas exchange and ^{133}xenon clearance from exercising muscle. *Arthritis Rheum.*, 32:454-460, 1989.
14. Klug, G.A., McAuley, E., and Clark, S.R.: Factors influencing the development and maintenance of aerobic fitness: lessons applicable to the fibrositis syndrome. *J. Rheumatol.*, 16(Suppl.19):30-39, 1989.
15. Center for Disease Control: Progress toward achieving the 1990 national objectives for physical fitness and exercise. *Morbidity and Mortality Weekly Report*, 38:451-453, 1989.
16. Moldofsky, H. and Scarisbrick, P.: Induction of neurasthenic musculoskeletal pain syndrome by selective sleep stage deprivation. *Psychosom. Med.*, 38:35-44, 1976.
17. McCain, G.A., Bell, D.A., Mai, F.M., and Halliday, P.D.: A controlled study of the effects of a supervised cardiovascular fitness training program on the manifestations of primary fibromyalgia. *Arthritis Rheum.*, 31:1135-1141, 1988.
18. Isomeri, R., Mikkelsson, M., Latikka, P., and Kammonen, K.: Effects of amitriptyline and cardiovascular fitness training on pain in patients with primary fibromyalgia. *J. Musculoskel. Pain*, 1(3/4):253-265, 1993.
19. Mengshoel, A.M. and Førre, O.: Physical fitness training in patients with fibromyalgia. *J. Musculoskel. Pain*, 1: 267-272, 1993.
20. Saccomani, L., Vigliarolo, M.A., Sbolgi, P., Ruffa, G., and Doria-Lamba, L.: Juvenile fibromyalgia syndrome: two clinical cases. *Pediatr. Med. Chir.*, 15:99-101, 1993.
21. Yunus, M.B.: Diagnosis, etiology, and management of fibromyalgia syndrome: an update. *Comprehensive Ther.*, 14:8-20, 1988.
22. Cathey, M.A., Wolfe, F., Kleinheksel, S.M., and Hawley, D.J.: Socioeconomic impact of fibrositis: a study of 81 patients with primary fibrositis. *Am. J. Med.*, 81:78-84, 1986.
23. Wolfe, F.: Personal communication, March 8, 1991.
24. Backstrom, G. and Rubin, B.R.: *When Muscle Pain Won't Go Away*. Dallas, Taylor Publishing Company, 1992 (study scheduled for journal publication).
25. Danneskiold-Samsøe, B., Christiansen, E., Lund, B., and Bach-Andersen, R.: Regional muscle tension and pain (fibrositis). *Scand. J. Rehab. Med.*, 15:17-20, 1982.
26. Danneskiold-Samsøe, B., Christiansen, E., and Bach-Andersen, R.: Myofascial pain and the role of myoglobin. *Scand. J. Rehab. Med.*, 15:174-178, 1986.
27. Tilbe, K., Bell, D.A., and McCain, G.A.: Loss of diurnal variation in serum cortisol, growth hormone, and prolactin in patients with primary fibromyalgia. *Arthritis Rheum.*, 31:4, 1988.
28. Romano, T.J.: The usefulness of cranial electrotherapy in the treatment of headache in fibromyalgia patients. *Am. J. Pain Manag.*, 3:15-19, 1993.
29. Solomon, S., Elkind, A., Freitag, G., Gallagher, R.M., Moore, K., Swedlow, B., and Malkin, S.: Safety and effectiveness of cranial electrotherapy in the treatment of tension headache. *Headache*, 29:445-450, 1989.
30. Ferraccioli, G., Chirelli, L., and Scita, F.: EMG-biofeedback training in fibromyalgia syndrome. *J. Rheumatol.*, 14:820-825, 1987.
31. Molina, E., Cecchettin, M., and Fontana, S.: Failure of

EMG-BF after sham BF training in fibromyalgia. *Fed. Proc.*, 46:A1357, 1987.

32. Ferraccioli, G., Cavalieri, F., Salaffi, F., Fontana, S., Scita, F., Nolli, M., and Maestri, D.: Neuroendocrinologic findings in primary fibromyalgia (soft tissue chronic pain syndrome) and in other chronic rheumatic conditions (rheumatoid arthritis, low back pain). *J. Rheumatol.*, 17:869-873, 1990.

33. Langer, G., Koinig, G., and Hatzinger, R.: Response of thyrotropin to thyrotropin-releasing hormone as a predictor of treatment outcome. *Arch. Gen. Psychiatry*, 43:861-868, 1986.

34. Blumer, Z., Zorik, F., Heilbronn, M., and Roth, T.: Biological markers for depression in chronic pain. *J. Behav. Med.*, 4:1-39, 1981.

35. Walco, G.A. and Ilowite, N.T.: Cognitive-behavioral intervention for juvenile primary fibromyalgia syndrome. *J. Rheumatol.*, 19:1617-1619, 1992.

36. Walco, G.A., Varni, J.W., and Howite, N.T.: Cognitive-behavioral pain management in child with juvenile rheumatoid arthritis. *Pediatrics*, 89:1075-1079, 1992.

37. Nielson, W.R., Walker, C., and McCain, G.A.: Cognitive behavioral treatment of fibromyalgia syndrome: preliminary findings. *J. Rheumatol.*, 19:98-103, 1992.

38. Haanen, H.C., Hoenderos, H.T., van Romunde, L.K., et al.: Controlled trial of hypnotherapy in the treatment of refractory fibromyalgia. *Rheumatol.*, 18:72-75, 1991.

39. de Voogd, J.N., Knipping, A.A., de Blécourt, and van Rijswijk, M.H.: Treatment of fibromyalgia syndrome with psychomotor therapy and marital counselling. *J. Musculoskel. Pain*, 1:273-281, 1993.

40. Kaplan, K.H., Goldenberg, D.L., and Galvin-Nadeau, M.: The impact of a meditation-based stress reduction program on fibromyalgia. *Gen. Hosp. Psychiatry*, 15:284-289, 1993.

41. Littlejohn G.: Medicolegal aspects of fibrositis syndrome. *J. Rheum.*, 16:169-173, 1989.

42. Kogstad, O. and Hintringer, F.: Patients with fibromyalgia in pain school. *J. Musculoskel. Pain*, 1:261-265, 1993.

43. Carette, S., McCain, G.A., Bell, D.A., and Fam, A.G.: Evaluation of amitriptyline in primary fibrositis. *Arthritis Rheum.*, 29:655-659, 1986.

44. Gatter, R.A.: Pharmacotherapeutics in fibrositis. *Am. J. Med.*, 81:63-66, 1986.

45. Felson, D.T. and Goldenberg, D.L.: The natural history of fibromyalgia. *Arthritis Rheum.*, 29:1522-1526, 1986.

46. Hawley, D.J., Cathey, M.A., and Wolfe, A.: A study of fibrositis symptoms over 12 months. *Arthritis Rheum.*, 30:196, 1987.

47. Share, N.N. and McFarlane, C.S.: Cyclobenzaprine: a novel centrally-acting skeletal muscle relaxant. *Neuropharmacol.*, 14:675-684, 1975.

48. Bennett, R.M., Gatter, R.A., Campbell, S.M., Andrews, R.P., Clark, S., and Scarola, J.A.: A double-blind study of cyclobenzaprine versus placebo in patients with fibrositis. *Arthritis Rheum.*, 27:S76, 1984.

49. Drewes, A.M., Andreasen, A., Jennum, P., and Nielsen, K.D.: Zopiclone in the treatment of sleep abnormalities in fibromyalgia. *Scand. J. Rheumatol.*, 20:288-293, 1991.

50. ter Riet, G., de Craen, A.J.M., de Boer, A., and Kessels, A.G.H.: Is placebo analgesia mediated by endogenous opioids? A systematic review. *Pain*, 76:273-275, 1998.

51. Moldofsky, H. and Lue, F.A.: The relationship of alpha and delta EEG frequencies to pain and mood in "fibrositis" patients treated with chlorpromazine and L-tryptophan. *Electroencephalogr. Clin. Neurophysiol.*, 50(1-2):71-80, 1980.

52. Kraus, H.: Trigger points. *N.Y. State J. Med.*, 1973, pp.1310-1314.

53. Gottlieb, N.L. and Riskin, W.G.: Complications of local corticosteroid injections. *J. Am. Med. Assoc.*, 243(15):1547, April 18, 1980.

54. Lowe, J.C., Eichelberger, J., Manso, G., and Peterson, K.: Improvement in euthyroid fibromyalgia patients treated with T₃ (tri-iodothyronine). *J. Myofascial Ther.*, 1(2):16-29, 1994.

55. Hollander, J.L.: Intrasynovial corticosteroid therapy. In *Arthritis and Allied Conditions*, 8th edition. Edited by J.L. Hollander and D.J. McCarty, Philadelphia, Lea and Febiger Publishers, 1972, pp.517-534.

56. Steinbrocker, O. and Neustadt, D.H.: *Aspiration and Injection Therapy in Musculoskeletal Disorders*, New York, Harper and Row Publishers, 1972.

57. McCarty, D.J.: Treatment of rheumatoid joint inflammation with triamcinolone hexacetonide. *Arthritis and Rheumatism*, 15:157-173, 1972.

58. Pizzolato, P. and Mannheimer, W.: *Histopathologic Effects of Local Anesthetic Drugs and Related Substances*. Springfield, IL, Charles C. Thomas, 1961, pp.40,41,60,71.

59. Koehler, B.E., Urowitz, M.B., and Killinger, D.W.: The systemic effects of intra-articular corticosteroid. *J. Rheum.*, 1:117-125, 1974.

60. Clark, S., Tindall, E., and Bennett, R.M.: A double-blind crossover trial of prednisone versus placebo in the treatment of fibrositis. *J. Rhuematol.*, 12:980-983, 1985.

61. Meyers, F.H., Jawetz, E., and Golfein, A.: *Review of Medical Pharmacology*, 4th edition. Los Altos, Lange Medical Publications, 1974.

62. Gilman, A.G., Rall, T.W., Nies, A.S., and Taylor, P.: *The Pharmacological Basis of Therapeutics*, 8th edition. New York, Pergamon Press, 1990.

63. Jacobsen, S., Danneskiold-Samsøe, B., and Andersen, R.B.: Oral S-adenosylmethionine in primary fibromyalgia: double-blind clinical evaluation. *Scand. J. Rheumatol.*, 20:294-302, 1991.

64. Tavoni, A., Vitali, C., Bombardieri, S., and Pasero, G.: Evaluation of S-adenosylmethionine in primary fibromyalgia: a double-blind crossover study. *Am. J. Med.*, 83 (Suppl.5A):107-110, 1987.

65. Yunus, M.B. and Masi, A.T.: Juvenile primary fibromyalgia syndrome: a clinical study of thirty-three patients and matched normal controls. *Arthritis Rheum.*, 28:138-145, 1985.

66. Laywood, A.A.: Letter to the Editor: fibromyalgia. *Brit. J. Rheum.*, 30:235-236, 1991.

67. Lowe, J.C.: Results of an open trial of T₃ therapy with 77 euthyroid female fibromyalgia patients. *Clin. Bull. Myofascial Ther.*, 2(1):35-37, 1997.

68. Campbell, S.M., Gatter, R.A., and Clark, S.: A double-blind study of cyclobenzaprine versus placebo in patients with fibrositis. *Arthritis Rheum.*, S76:D3, 1984.

69. Nordström, P., and Åsberg, M.: Suicide risk and serotonin. *Int. Clin. Psychopharmacol*, 6(Suppl.6):12-21, 1992.

70. Rouillon, F., Serrurier, D., Miller, H.D., and Gerard, M.J.: Prophylactic efficacy of maprotiline on unipolar depression relapse. *J. Clin. Psychiatry*, 52(10):423-431, 1991.

71. Kravitz, H.M., Katz, R.S., Helmke, N., Jeffries, H., Bukovsky, J., and Fawcett, J.: Alprazolam and ibuprofen in the treatment of fibromyalgia—report of a double-blind placebo-controlled study. *J. Musculoskel. Pain*, 2(1):3-27, 1994.

72. Le Gallez, P., Reeve, F.B.A., Crawley, M.A., and Bird, H.A.: A double-blind comparison of ibuprofen, placebo, and ibuprofen with meptazinol in soft tissue rheumatism. *Curr. Med. Res. Opin.*, 10:1371-1377, 1986.

73. Disdier, P., Harle, J.-R., Brue, T., Jaquet, P., Chambourlier, P., Grisoli, F., and Weiller, P.-J.: Severe fibromyalgia after hypophysectomy for Cushing's disease. *Arthritis Rheum.*, 34(4):493-495, 1991.

74. Wessely, S., Butler, S., Chalder, T., and David, A.: *The Cognitive Behavioral Management of the Post-viral Fatigue Syndrome: Post-viral Fatigue Syndrome.* Edited by R. Jenkins, J. Mowbray, Chichester, John Wiley & Sons, 1991, pp.305-334.

75. Le Feuvre, C., Baubion, N., Berdah, J., Heulin, A., and Vacheron, A.: Drug-induced cardiovascular complications. *Ann. de Med. Intern.*, 140(7):597-599, 1989.

76. Riley, L.A., Jonakait, G.M., and Hart, R.P.: Serotonin modulates the levels of mRNAs coding for thyrotropin-releasing hormone and preprotachykinin by different mechanisms in medullary raphe neurons. *Mol. Brain Res.*, 17:251-257, 1993.

77. Fernstrom, M., Epstein, L., Spiker, D., and Kupfer, D.: Resting metabolic rate is reduced in patients treated with antidepressants. *Biol. Psychiatry*, 20:688-692, 1985.

78. Herman, R., Obrzanek, E., Mikalauskas, K.M., Post, R.M., and Jimerson, D.C.: The effects of carbamazepine on resting metabolic rate and thyroid function in depressed patients. *Biol. Psychiatry*, 29:779-788, 1991.

79. Åsberg, M.: Neurotransmitters and suicidal behavior. The evidence from cerebrospinal fluid studies. *Ann. N. Y. Acad. Sci.*, 836:158-181, 1997.

80. Parfitt, A.M.: Cushing's syndrome with normal replacement dose of cortisone in pituitary hypothyroidism. *J. Clin. Endocrinol. Metab.*, 24:560, 1964.

81. Peterson, R.E.: The influence of the thyroid on adrenal cortical function. *J. Clin. Invest.*, 37:736, 1958.

82. Nicassio, P.M., Radojevic, V., Weisman, M.H., Schuman, C., Kim, J., Schoenfeld-Smith, K., and Krall, T.: A comparison of behavioral and educational interventions for fibromyalgia. *J. Rheumatol.*, 24(10):2000-2007, 1997.

83. Abraham, G.E. and Flechas, J.D.: Management of fibromyalgia: rationale for the use of magnesium and malic acid. *J. Nutri. Med.*, 3:49-59, 1992.

84. Russell, I.J., Michalek, J.E., Flechas, J.D., and Abraham, G.E.: Treatment of fibromyalgia syndrome with Super Malic: a randomized, double-blind, placebo-controlled, crossover pilot study. *J. Rheumatol.*, 22:953-958, 1995.

85. Moldofsky, H., Lue, F.A., Mously, C., Roth-Schechterb, W.J., and Reynolds, W.J.: Zolpidem in patients with fibromyalgia: a dose range, double-blind, placebo-con-

trolled, modified crossover study. *J. Rheumatol.*, 23:529-533, 1996.

86. Roth, T., Roehrs, T., and Vogel, G.: Zolpidem in the treatment of transient insomnia: a double-blind, randomized comparison with placebo. *Sleep*, 18(4):246-251, 1995.

87. Salva, P. and Costa, J.: Clinical pharmacokinetics and pharmacodynamics of zolpidem. *Clin. Pharmacokinetics*, 29(3):142-153, 1995.

88. Wesensten, N.J., Balkin, T.J., and Belenky, G.L.: Effects of daytime administration of zolpidem versus triazolam on memory. *Eur. J. Clin. Pharmacol.*, 48(2):115-122, 1995.

89. Rush, C.R. and Griffiths, R.R.: Zolpidem, triazolam, and temazepam: behavioral and subject-rated effects in normal volunteers. *J. Clin. Psychopharmacol.*, 16(2):146-157, 1996.

90. Bombardier, C.H. and Bachwald, D.: Chronic fatigue, chronic fatigue syndrome, and fibromyalgia: disability and health care use. *Med. Care*, 34(9):924-930, 1996.

91. Pioro-Boisset, M., Esdaile, J.M., and Fitzcharles, M.S.: Alternative medicine use in fibromyalgia syndrome. *Arthritis Care and Res.*, 9:13-17, 1996.

92. Bennett, R.M.: Fibromyalgia review. *J. Musculoskel. Pain*, 5(1):91-104, 1997.

93. Nye, D.A.: Unproven treatments for fibromyalgia. In "Letters to the Editor," *J. Musculoskel. Pain*, 5(1):121-122, 1997.

94. Fowler, P.D.: Aspirin, paracetamol, and non-steroidal anti-inflammatory drugs: a comparative review of side effects. *Med. Tox.*, 2:338-366, 1987.

95. Perneger, T.V., Whelton, P.K., and Klag, M.J.: Risk of kidney failure associated with the use of acetaminophen, aspirin, and non-steroidal anti-inflammatory. *N. Engl. J. Med.*, 331:1675-1678, 1994.

96. Roth, S.H.: NSAIDs and gastropathy: a rheumatologist's view. *J. Rheumatol.*, 15:912-918, 1988.

97. Clive, D.M. and Stoff, J.S.: Renal syndromes associated with non-steroidal anti-inflammatory drugs. *N. Engl. J. Med.*, 310:563-572, 1984.

98. Clauw, D.J.: The pathogenesis of chronic pain and fatigue syndromes, with special reference to fibromyalgia. *Med. Hypotheses*, 44:369-378, 1995.

99. Blunt, K.L., Rajwani, M.H., and Guerriero, R.C.: The effectiveness of chiropractic management of fibromyalgia patients: a pilot study. *J. Manipul. Physiol. Ther.*, 20(6): 389-399, 1997.

100. Puech, A.: Contributions of pharmacology in the treatment of resistance to antidepressive agents. *Encephale*, 19 Spec.(2):407-412, 1993.

101. Lowe, J.C.: Reliable scientific reporting. "Editorial." *J. Myofascial Ther.*, 1(4):3, 1995.

102. Russell, I.J.: Pathogenesis of fibromyalgia: the neurohormonal hypothesis. *J. Muscloskel. Pain*, 2(1):73-86, 1994.

103. McCain, G.A.: A clinical overview of the fibromyalgia syndrome. *J. Muscloskel. Pain*, 4(1/2):9-34, 1996.

104. Johnson, H.: *Osler's Web*. New York, Penguin Books, 1996.

105. Carette, S., Bell, M., Reynolds, W.J., et al.: Comparison of amitriptyline, cyclobenzaprine, and placebo in the treatment of fibromyalgia. *Arthritis Rheum.*, 37(1):32-40, 1994.

106. Wolfe, F.: Personal written communication, November,

1997.

107. Bennett, R.M., Clark, S.R., Burckhardt, C.S., and Walczyk, J.: A double-blind placebo controlled study of growth hormone therapy in fibromyalgia. (Abstract) *J. Musculoskel. Pain*, 3(Suppl.1):110, 1995.

108. Root, A.W., Bongiovanni, A.M., and Eberlein, W.R.: Inhibition of thyroidal radioiodine uptake by human growth hormone. *J. Pediatr.*, 76:422-429, 1970.

109. Dratman, M.B., Crutchfield, F.L., Gordon, J.T., and Jennings, A.S.: Iodothyronine homeostasis in rat brain during hypo- and hyperthyroidism. *Am. J. Physiol.*, 245:E185-E193, 1983.

110. Marshak, D.R. and Liu, D.T. (Editors): *Banbury Report 29: Therapeutic Peptides and Proteins: Assessing the New Technologies.* New York, Cold Spring Harbor Laboratory, 1988.

111. Kuret, J.A. and Murad, F.: Adenohypophyseal hormones and related substances. In *The Pharmacologic Basis of Therapeutics*, 8th edition. Edited by A.G. Gilman, T.W. Rall, A.S. Nies, and P. Taylor, New York, Pergamon Press, 1990, pp.1334-1360.

112. Slyper, A.: The safety and effectiveness of human growth hormone using pharmacological dosing. *Med. Hypotheses*, 48:523-528, 1995.

113. Bourguignon, J.-P., Pierard, G.E., Ernould, C., et al.: Effects of human growth hormone therapy on melanocytic naevi. *Lancet*, 341:1505-1506, 1993.

114. Lowe, J.C.: The treatment of fibromyalgia patients: a review of studies. *J. Myofascial Ther.*, 1(2):37-49, 1994.

115. Fisher, P.: Effect of homeopathic treatment of fibrositis (primary fibromyalgia). *Brit. Med. J.*, 32:365-366, 1989.

116. Gemmell, H.: Homeopathic Rhus toxicodendron in the treatment of fibromyalgia. *Chiro. J. Austral.*, 21(1):2-6, 1991.

117. Chaitow, L.: *Fibromyalgia & Muscle Pain*, Hammersmith, Thorsons, 1995.

118. Vithoulkas, G.: *The Science of Homeopathy*. New York, Grove Weidenfeld, 1980.

119. Godfrey, R.G.: A guide to the understanding and use of tricyclic antidepressants in the overall management of fibromyalgia and other chronic pain syndromes. *Arch. Intern. Med.*, 156(10):1047-1052, 1996.

120. Nørregaard, J., Volkmann, H., and Danneskiold-Samsøe, B.: A randomized controlled trial of citalopram in the treatment of fibromyalgia. *Pain*, 61(3):445-449, 1995.

121. Carette, S., Oakson, G., Guimont, C., and Steriade, M.: Sleep electroencephalography and the clinical response to amitriptyline in patients with fibromyalgia. *Arthritis Rheumatol.*, 38(9):1211-1217, 1995.

122. Trojan, D.A. and Cashman, N.R.: Fibromyalgia is common in a postpoliomyelitis clinic. *Arch. Neurol.*, 52(6):620-624, 1995.

123. Goodnick, P.J. and Sandoval, R.: Psychotropic treatment of chronic fatigue syndrome and related disorders. *J. Clin. Psychiatry*, 54(1):13-20, 1993.

124. Goldenberg, D.L., Manisky, M., Mossey, C., Ruthazer, R., and Schmid, C.: The independent and combined efficacy of fluoxetine and amitriptyline in the treatment of fibromyalgia. *Arthritis Rheum.*, 38(Suppl.):S229, 1995.

125. Ginsberg, F., Mancaux, A., Joos, E., Vanhove, P., and Famaey, J-P.: A randomized placebo-controlled trial of sustained-release amitriptyline in primary fibromyalgia. *J. Musculoskel. Pain*, 4(3):37-47, 1996.

126. White, K.P. and Nilson, W.R.: Cognitive behavioral treatment of fibromyalgia syndrome: a follow-up assessment. *J. Rheumatol.*, 122:717-721, 1995.

127. Mengshoel, A.N., Forseth, K.L., Haugen, M., Walle-Hansen, R., and Førre, O.: Multidisciplinary approach to fibromyalgia pilot study. *Clin. Rheumatol.*, 14:165-170, 1995.

128. Jorgensen, J.O., Pedersen, S.A., Laurberg, P., Weeke, J., Skakkebaek, N.E., and Christiansen, J.S.: Effects of growth hormone therapy on thyroid function of growth hormone-deficient adults with and without concomitant thyroxine-substituted central hypothyroidism. *J. Clin. Endocrinol. Metab.*, 69(6):1127-1132, 1989.

129. Eisinger, J., Arroyo, P., Calendini, C., Rinaldi, .JP., Combes, R., and Fontaine, G.: Anomalies biologiques au cours des fibromyalgies: III. Explorations endocriniennes. *Lyon Méditerranée Méd.*, 28:858-860, 1992.

130. Gerwin, R.: A study of 96 subjects examined both for fibromyalgia and myofascial pain. *J. Musculoskel. Pain*, 3 (Suppl.1):121, 1995.

131. Lowe, J.C.: Thyroid status of 38 fibromyalgia patients: implications for the etiology of fibromyalgia. *Clin. Bull. Myofascial Ther.*, 2(1):47-64, 1997.

132. Shiroky, J.B., Cohen, M., Ballachey, M-L., and Neville, C.: Thyroid dysfunction in rheumatoid arthritis: a controlled prospective survey. *Ann .Rheumat. Dis.*, 52:454-456, 1993.

133. Sarzi Puttini, P. and Caruso, I.: Primary fibromyalgia syndrome and 5-hydroxytryptophan: a 90-day open study. *J. Intern. Med. Res.*, 20:182-189, 1992.

134. Neeck, G. and Riedel, W.: Thyroid function in patients with fibromyalgia syndrome. *J. Rheumatol.*, 19:1120-1122, 1992.

135. Lowe, J.C., Reichman, A.J., Honeyman, G.S., Yellin, J.: Thyroid status of fibromyalgia patients. (Abstract) *Clin. Bull. Myofascial Ther.*, 3(1):69-70, 1998.

136. Bou-Holaigah, I., Rowe, P.C., Kan, J., and Calkins, H.: The relationship between neurally mediated hypotension and the chronic fatigue syndrome. *J.A.M.A.*, 274(12):961-967, 1995.

137. Quijada-Carrera, J., Valenzuela-Castano, A., Povedano-Gomez, J., el al.: Comparison of tenoxicam and bromazepan in the treatment of fibromyalgia: a randomized, double-blind, placebo-controlled trial. *Pain*, 65(2-3):221-225, 1996.

138. Vlaeyen, J.W.S., Teeken-Gruben, N.G., Goossens, M.E.J.B., Rutten, M.P.M.H., Pelt, H., vanEek, H., and Heut, P.H.G.T.: Cognitive-educational treatment of fibromyalgia-randomized clinical trials. *J. Rheumatol.*, 23: 1237-1245, 1996.

139. Nørregaard, J., Lykkegaard, J.J., Mehlsen, J., and Danneskiold-Samsøe, B.: Exercise training in treatment of fibromyalgia. *J. Musculoskel. Pain*, 5(1):71-79, 1997.

140. Bennett, R.M., Burckhardt, C.S., Clark, S.R., O'Reilly, C.A., Wiens, S.M., and Campbell, S.M.: Group treatment of fibromyalgia six-month outpatient program. *J. Rheumatol.*, 23:521-528, 1996.

141. Sunshine, W., Field, T.M., Quintino, O., et al.: Fibromyalgia benefits from massage therapy and transcutaneous

electrical stimulation. *J. Clin. Rheumatol.*, 2:18-22, 1996.

142. Mengshoel, A.M.: Effect of physical exercise in fibromyalgia. *Tidsskr Nor Laegeforen*, 116:746-748, 1996.

143. McCain, G.A.: Role of physical fitness training in the fibrositis/fibromyalgia syndrome. *Am. J. Med.*, 81:73-77, 1986.

144. Mengshoel, A.M., Komnæ, H.B., and Førre, O.: The effects of 20 weeks of physical fitness training in female patients with fibromyalgia. *Clin. Exp. Rheumatol.*, 10:345-349, 1992.

145. Nichols, D.S. and Glen, T.M.: Effects of aerobic exercise on pain perception, affect, and level of disability in individuals with fibromyalgia. *Phys. Ther.*, 74:327-332, 1994.

146. Crofford, L.J., Pillemer, S.R., Kalogeras, K.T., et al.: Hypothalamic-pituitary-adrenal axis perturbations in patients with fibromyalgia. *Arthritis Rheum.*, 37:1583-1592, 1994.

147. Hadler, N.M.: *Occupational Musculoskeletal Disorders.* New York, Raven Press, 1993.

148. Fordyce, W.E. (Editor): *Back Pain in the Workplace.* Seattle, IASP Press, 1995.

149. Wigers, S.H., Stiles, T.C., and Vogel, P.A.: Effects of aerobic exercise versus stress management treatment in fibromyalgia. *Scand. J. Rheumatol.*, 25:77-86, 1996.

150. Dimmock, S., Troughton, P.R., and Bird, H.A.: Factors predisposing to the result of complementary therapies in patients with fibromyalgia. *Clin. Rheumatol.*, 15:478-482, 1996.

151. Burkhardt, C.S., Mannerkorpi, K., Hedenberg, L., and Bjelle, A.: A randomized common control clinical trial of education and physical training for women with fibromyalgia. *J. Rheumatol.*, 21:714-720, 1994.

152. Wolfe, F., Cathey, M.A., and Hawley, D.J.: A double blind placebo controlled trial of fluoxetine in fibromyalgia. *Scand. J. Rheumatol.*, 23:255-259, 1994.

153. Verstappen, F.T.J., van Santen-Hoeufft, H.M.S., van Sloun, S., Bolwijn, P.H., and van der Linden, S.: Fitness characteristics of female patients with fibromyalgia. *J. Musculoskel. Pain*, 3(3):45-58, 1995.

154. Teitelbaum, J. and Bird, B.: Effective treatment of severe chronic fatigue: a report of a series of 64 patients. *J. Musculoskel. Pain*, 3(4):91-110, 1995.

155. Sharpe, M.: Cognitive behavior therapy and the treatment of chronic fatigue syndrome. *J. Musculoskel. Pain*, 3(2):141-147, 1995.

156. Butler, S., Chalder, T., Ron, M., and Wessely, S.: Cognitive behavior therapy in chronic fatigue syndrome. *J. Neurol. Neurosurg. Psychiatry*, 54:153-158, 1991.

157. Friedberg, F. and Krupp, L.B.: A comparison of cognitive behavioral treatment for chronic fatigue syndrome and primary depression. *Clin. Infect. Dis.*, 18(Suppl.):S105-S109, 1994.

158. Lloy, A.R., Hickie, I., Brockman, A., et al.: Immunologic and psychologic therapy for patients with chronic fatigue syndrome: a double-blind placebo-controlled trial. *Am. J. Med.*, 94:197-203, 1993.

159. Sharpe, M.C.: Non-pharmacological approaches to treatment: chronic fatigue syndrome. *CIBA Foundation Symposium 173.* Edited by G.R. Brock and J. Whelan, Toronto, John Wiley & Sons, 1993, pp.298-317.

160. Clement, H-W., Gemsa, D., and Wesemann, W.: The effect of adrenergic drugs on serotonin metabolism in the nucleus raphe dorsalis of the rat, studied by *in vivo* voltammetry. *Eur. J. Pharmacol.*, 217:43-48, 1992.

161. Feuerstein, T.J., Mutschler, A., Lupp, A., Van Velthoven, V., Schlicker, E., and Göthert, M.: Endogenous noradrenaline activates α_2-adrenoceptors on serotonergic nerve endings in human and rat neocortex. *J. Neurochem.*, 61(2):474-480, 1993.

162. Jung, A.C., Staiger, T., and Sullivan, M.: The efficacy of selective serotonin reuptake inhibitors for the management of chronic pain. *J. Gen. Intern. Med.*, 12(6):384-389, 1997.

163. Fulcher, K.Y. and White, P.D.: Randomized controlled trial of graded exercise in patients with the chronic fatigue syndrome. *Brit. Med. J.*, 314(7095):1647-1652, 1997.

164. Potter, W.Z., Rudoffer, M.V., and Manji, H.: The pharmacologic treatment of depression. *N. Engl. J. Med.*, 325:633-642, 1991.

165. Connally, R.G.: Treatment of fibromyositis with fluphenazine and amitriptyline: a preliminary report. *Delaware Med. J.*, 53:189-191, 1981.

166. Smythe, H.A.: Fibrositis and other diffuse musculoskeletal syndromes. In *Textbook of Rheumatology*. Edited by W.N. Kelly, E.D. Harris, S. Ruddy, and C.B. Sledge, Philadelphia, W.B. Saunders, pp.485-493, 1981.

167. Yunus, M.B., Masi, A.T., Calabro, J.J., et al.: Primary fibromyalgia (fibrositis): clinical study of 50 patients with matched normal controls. *Seminars in Arthritis Rheum.*, 11:151-171, 1981.

168. Russell, I.J., Vaeroy, M., Jabors, M., and Nyberg, F.: Cerebrospinal fluid biogenic metabolites in fibromyalgia/fibrositis syndrome in rheumatoid arthritis. *Arthritis Rheumat.*, 35:550-556, 1992.

169. Volkmann, H., Nørregaard, J., Jacobsen, S., Danneskiold-Samsøe, B., Knoke, G., and Nehrdich, D.: Double-blind, placebo-controlled cross-over study of intravenous S-adenosyl-L-methionine in patients with fibromyalgia. *Scand. J. Rheumatol.*, 26(3):206-211, 1997.

170. Sprott, H., Kluge, H., Franke, S., and Hein, G.: Altered serotonin-levels in patients with fibromyalgia. *J. Musculoskel. Pain*, 3(Suppl.1):65, 1995.

171. Barnes, C.D., Fung, S.J., and Gintautus, J.: Brainstem noradrenergic system depression by cyclobenzaprine. *Neuropharmacol.*, 19:221-224, 1980.

172. Russell, I.J.: Personal written communication, June, 1995.

173. Fransen, J. and Russell, I.J.: *The Fibromyalgia Help Book: Practical Guide to Living Better with Fibromyalgia.* Saint Paul, Smith House Press, 1996.

174. Sprott, H.: Efficiency of acupuncture in patients with fibromyalgia. *Clin. Bull. Myofascial Ther.*, 3(1):37-43, 1998.

175. Nicollet, M.: Point pressure biphasic balneotherapy (with special blood circulation activator) for fibromyalgia and myofascial syndromes: preliminary results. *Clin. Bull. Myofascial Ther.*, 3(1):45-59, 1998.

176. Caruso, P., Sarzi Puttini, P., Cazzola, M., and Azzolini, V.: Double-blind study of 5-hydroxytryptophan versus placebo in the treatment of primary fibromyalgia syndrome. *J. Intern. Med. Res.*, 18:201-209, 1990.

177. McCain, G.A. and Tilbe, K.S.: Diurnal hormone variation in fibromyalgia syndrome: a comparison with rheumatoid arthritis. *J. Rheumatol.*, 16(Suppl.):154-157, 1989.

178. Christy, N.P.: The adrenal cortex in hypothyroidism. In *Werner and Ingbar's The Thyroid: A Fundamental and Clinical Text*, 6th edition. Edited by L.E. Braverman and R.D. Utiger, New York, J.B. Lippincott Co., 1991, pp.1045-1049.

179. Howard, J.E. and Migeon, C.J.: Cushing's syndrome produced by normal replacement doses of cortisone in a patient with defective mechanism for steroid degradation. *Am. J. Med. Sci.*, 235:387, 1958.

5.2

Treatment Protocol

This chapter is merely a digest, a recipe, to be carefully and exactly followed if the clinician is to match the successful clinical results that have made it an ethical necessity for me to publish this book. The contents of this chapter are the essence of the treatment regimen for helping fibromyalgia patients improve and recover through metabolic rehabilitation. The clinician definitely should not, however, neglect studying and making use of the information in other parts of this book. To do so will be to compromise his ability to successfully use the protocol described in this chapter. The clinician determined to use the protocol with maximum effectiveness simply cannot ignore the other parts of this book, as the contents of the other parts are essential to utmost efficacy.

To guide the fibromyalgia patient to marked improvement or recovery, the clinician must understand metabolism and its relation to thyroid hormone and other metabolism-regulating agents and procedures. The more the clinician understands, the better he will be able to preserve the integrity of the protocol while adapting it to each patient's individual needs. The clinician can acquire the requisite understanding by studying the other parts of this book and, over time, attain higher levels of competence in administering the protocol by integrating what he learns into his clinical interaction with successive patients.

Some patients recover from their fibromyalgia signs and symptoms after beginning to take nutritional supplements and engage in exercise. Others do so only after eliminating the use of or exposure to metabolism-impeding agents such as β-blocking drugs and other medications such as muscle relaxants, anxiolytics, tranquilizers, and narcotics that disincline the patient

to engage in sufficient physical activity. When patients improve as a result of such actions, they either do not have inadequate thyroid hormone tissue regulation, or they have such a slight degree of inadequate regulation that the previously-mentioned actions override its metabolism-impairing effects. This chapter addresses fibromyalgia patients who have inadequate thyroid hormone regulation of tissues, due either to hypothyroidism or partial cellular resistance to thyroid hormone. For these patients, the use of exogenous thyroid hormone, combined with nutritional supplementation and exercise to tolerance, are the sine qua non *of the metabolic rehabilitation this chapter describes.*

Thyroid Status

Before beginning treatment, the clinician should determine the patient's thyroid status with laboratory thyroid function tests. If the patient's standard thyroid profile does not indicate primary hypothyroidism, the patient should undergo a TRH stimulation test to rule out possible central hypothyroidism. In most cases, the initial choice of T_4 (or desiccated thyroid) or T_3 is based on the patient's thyroid status. Most hypothyroid patients start treatment with T_4 or desiccated thyroid; euthyroid patients begin with T_3.

Objective of Treatment

The treatment goal is to improve as much as possible all objective measures of fibromyalgia status and all signs, symptoms, and peripheral indices of inadequate thyroid hormone tissue regulation (see Chapter 4.3). There are five standard measures of fibromyalgia status: (1) tender point sensitivity (measured by algometry), (2) pain distribution (quantified by the percentage method), (3) symptom intensity (measured with visual analog scales), (4) assessment of function abilities (via the Fibromyalgia Impact Questionnaire), and (5) a measure of depression (by Beck's or Zung's Self-Rating Depression Scale). Measures of peripheral tissue response to metabolic therapy include the Achilles reflex, pulse rate, body temperature, blood pressure, and electrocardiography.

The scores of the five fibromyalgia measures establish quantitatively the patient's baseline fibromyalgia status. The patient's changing fibromyalgia status during treatment, determined by use of the five measures on successive evaluation dates, will be compared with this baseline. The five measures are taken at each evaluation so that current scores can be compared with previous ones. These comparisons are the primary source of decisions about thyroid hormone dosage, nutritional supplements, and exercise.

Measures of Clinical Status

During a therapeutic trial, the fibromyalgia patient's clinical response to thyroid hormone must be judged by changes in her fibromyalgia measures and one or more of the physical indices. Optimizing the patient's dosage critically depends on carefully evaluating her responses to treatment and repeatedly adjusting her dosage with the aim of improving her scores.

Improvement in the patient's symptom intensities is reflected in decreases in the mean intensity of the 13 symptoms on the visual analog scales. Improvement in functional status is shown by decreases in the scores of the Fibromyalgia Impact Questionnaire, and improvements in depression are shown by decreases in the scores from the Zung's Self-Rating Depression Scale (or a similar instrument). The aim with pain distribution is to reduce as close to 0 (zero) as possible the percentage of the 36 body divisions containing pain. The objective with tender point sensitivity is to raise the mean pressure/pain threshold as high as possible above the patient's baseline mean score. The smallest effective dosage of exogenous thyroid hormone should be used.

The scores from the five measures must each be posted to a different line graph (i.e., one for each measure). The clinician can usually obtain a clear impression of the patient's status and progress by inspecting the graphs after each evaluation. Typically, the five measures change in concert, either in a direction of "improvement," "no improvement," or "worse."

The aim with the Achilles reflex is to increase the speed of the relaxation phase until it is approximately equal to the contraction phase. The speed can be measured, but a slow speed is visibly obvious to the observant clinician. The patient's resting pulse rate should be increased to a rate appropriate for her level of cardiovascular conditioning. The objective in serial ECGs is to observe an increase in voltage and a slight degree of shortening of the intervals within normal ranges.

In a small percentage of patients, some of these measures are normal at the initial evaluation despite inadequate thyroid hormone tissue regulation. When this is true, the normal measures are not useful for assessing the patient's response to thyroid hormone and can be eliminated from the assessment.(ECGs nevertheless are necessary at intervals for insuring patient safety.)

Repeat Measures at Intervals

Measurements should be made at each evaluation. For the patient to improve or recover at a maximum rate, the clinician can reevaluate the patient's status at 1-to-2-week intervals. Reevaluations at monthly intervals, however, may be preferable for some patients. Reevaluations at wider intervals may cost some degree of coherency in the patient's treatment regimen and are not advisable. Without scores from measures at reevaluations, the clinician does not have quantifiable gauges of the patient's fibromyalgia status, and he can exercise little control over the patient's condition. In this case, the probability of clinical failure is high. According to Refetoff, in the treatment of patients with peripheral cellular resistance to thyroid hormone, ". . . judgment rests with less reliable tests of peripheral tissue action and subjective response to therapy." This is true of both euthyroid and hypothyroid fibromyalgia patients treated with metabolic rehabilitation. But with the deliberate and conscientious use of the measures described, the clinician can guide most euthyroid and hypothyroid fibromyalgia patients to marked improvement or complete recovery. Laboratory thyroid function test results are of no value in guiding patients to improvement or recovery; reliance on such test results in conventional medical practice constitutes an obstacle to a favorable therapeutic outcome.

Changes in the patient's subjective status typically correspond closely to changing scores for the fibromyalgia measures. Small, subtle changes in scores—subjectively undetectable to the patient—may occur first, however. The diligent clinician will be able to see these small changes by reviewing the graphs of the patient's assessment scores.

Nutrition and Exercise

In addition to taking the proper form of thyroid hormone, the patient must actively participate in the other parts of the treatment regimen. She must engage in procedures and lifestyle changes that enable her to capitalize on the increased metabolic capacity provided by the exogenous thyroid hormone. In general, these procedures and changes contribute to a sustained increase in metabolism and/or a decrease in metabolic demand. The patient must engage in some procedures, such as taking nutritional supplements, from the very beginning of her metabolic rehabilitation. She should begin exercising as soon as her metabolic capacity is sufficiently increased. Few patients will significantly improve or recover if they do not take nutritional supplements and exercise to tolerance. Using exogenous thyroid hormone may prove hazardous to some of these patients who do not follow these other aspects of the protocol.

Full Protocol

I emphatically urge the clinician to observe a caveat. Each step in the protocol has been determined to be indispensable for patient safety and for a maximally favorable clinical outcome. Only by the clinician and the patient properly employing each step of the protocol is it likely that the patient will safely improve or recover.

Other Procedures

Some patients may benefit further from various health care measures such as the use of other nutritional agents, herbs, and hormones or hormone-precursors. These agents, in combination with the protocol described in this chapter, may optimize the patient's health. However, for the patient whose fibromyalgia is a result of inadequate thyroid hormone tissue regulation, these other agents alone are not likely to generally improve the patient's fibromyalgia status. The other agents should not be used as a substitute for exogenous thyroid hormone; prolonged inadequate thyroid hormone tissue regulation may have life-threatening pathological consequences (see Chapter 4.4). These agents should also not be used in such a way that they obscure the clinician's view of the effects of exogenous thyroid hormone on the patient's status.

Physical Treatment

Most patients benefit substantially from physical treatments such as myofascial trigger point and spinal manipulative therapies. The benefit is especially reflected in the measures of pain distribution and intensity and in the pressure/pain thresholds of tender points. Failure of some patients to undergo physical treatment during metabolic rehabilitation may seriously compromise the level of improvement they attain (see Appendix B, paper titled "Facilitating the Decrease in Fibromyalgic Pain During Metabolic Rehabilitation: An Essential Role for Soft Tissue Therapies").

I describe below the steps we take to diagnose fibromyalgia, monitor for changes in the patient's status, and make treatment decisions. Some patients who meet the criteria for fibromyalgia do so via mechanisms other than inadequate thyroid hormone regulation of tissues. Typically, there is a combination of etiological factors, none of which alone would produce fibromyalgia. The factors may include nutritional deficiencies, deconditioning, biomechanical faults, use of β-blocking drugs, and various other medications and conditions that impede the metabolism of tissues that are capable of giving rise to the signs and symptoms of fibromyalgia. When such etiological factors are responsible and they are effectively eliminated or compensated for, the patient is likely to recover from the syndrome. It is in the spirit of clinical medicine for the practitioner to study the patient's history, signs, symptoms, and test results to determine the combination of contributing factors and to work with the patient to eliminate or control the factors so that she improves or recovers. Today, this approach is best exemplified by Travell and Simons in their trigger point manuals.[21][137] Only through clinical detective work, based on a knowledge of putative mechanisms, can the clinician determine the combination of factors responsible for sustaining fibromyalgia symptoms in the individual patient so that they can be eliminated or controlled.

In particular, it is wise for the euthyroid patient who has not used nutritional supplements or exercised to tolerance to begin doing so before embarking on a course of thyroid hormone therapy. The reason for this is that the signs and symptoms diagnosed as fibromyalgia in some patients are products of nutritional deficiencies and/or deconditioning. These patients should use the nutritional supplements I recommend below, or an equivalent regimen, and engage daily in aerobic, resistance, and stretching exercises to tolerance. (Exercise should be kept below a level that exacerbates the patient's fibromyalgia, even if this means, as it does for a small minority, not exercising at all.) If these efforts do not, over the period of several weeks, improve fibromyalgia status according to the objective fibromyalgia measures I describe below, the patient's fibromyalgia may be a manifestation of inadequate thyroid hormone regulation of transcription. A trial of thyroid hormone therapy is then in order. Other factors may be contributing to the patient's signs and symptoms. If so, her improvement with metabolic rehabilitation is not likely to be complete. The clinician should try to identify other contributing factors and eliminate or correct them.

For many other patients, nutritional supplementation and other methods will have less than satisfactory or no beneficial effects until the patients use the proper form and dosage of exogenous thyroid hormone. I intend the protocol I explain in this chapter to be for these patients—those whose fibromyalgia is a product of inadequate thyroid hormone regulation of cell function, resulting either from a thyroid hormone deficiency or cellular resistance to thyroid hormone.

An Emphatic *Caveat*. Each of the steps of the protocol I describe here is included for one reason: Extensive clinical experience, systematic observation, trial and error, and rigorous, controlled experimentation over 10 years have shown that each step is essential to providing the patient with the highest probability of safely improving or recovering from fibromyalgia. To make the protocol as parsimonious as possible, each step has been systematically scrutinized and determined to be requisite to the effectiveness of the protocol.

To exclude portions of the protocol during the patient's care will diminish the safety and effectiveness of the protocol. *Optimal improvement requires use of the full protocol exactly as I describe it below.*

● ASSESSMENT

The initial assessment of the patient includes paper and pencil tests, a history, physical examination, an ECG, thyroid function tests, a CBC, SMAC, and urinalysis. The clinician should use the procedures I describe below for assessing tender point sensitivity, pain distribution, and symptom intensity. These are more advanced modifications of the procedures described in the 1990 American College of Rheumatology diagnostic criteria,[145] and they provide greater pre-

cision and quantification.[138][139][140] They enable the clinician to make evidence-based, data-driven decisions in patient care.

PAPER AND PENCIL TESTS

The patient should complete four forms at the initial visit and at all subsequent evaluations.

FibroQuest Questionnaire (long form) and FibroQuest Symptoms Survey (short form)

The FibroQuest Questionnaire form (see Appendix A) is used only for the initial assessment. It furnishes the clinician with historical and current fibromyalgia-related information about the patient. The patient's responses can provide a jumping off point during history-taking for discussion of her complaints. The Questionnaire contains 100 mm visual analog scales for the 13 most common fibromyalgia symptoms. The patient indicates with a mark on the scale her perception of the intensity of each symptom. A lower value indicates that the symptom is less severe, with a higher value indicating greater severity. She should, for example, mark 0 if she does not have the symptom, or 10 if the symptom is as severe as possible. The clinician or an assistant should total the ratings of symptom severity, divide by the number of symptoms with ratings above 0, and post the mean score to Graph 1 (see Appendix A).

At subsequent evaluations, the patient should complete the *FibroQuest Symptoms Survey* (short form). This is a shortened version of the initial *FibroQuest Questionnaire*. It contains only the 13 visual analog scales from the long form. At all assessments subsequent to the initial one, the patient should fill out the short form. When scoring this form, the total for the visual analog scales should be calculated. Rather than dividing by the total number of symptoms (indicated by the number of visual analog scales the patient marks), *the total should be divided by the same number of scales as the patient marked on the initial visit.* This is necessary to avoid mean values at reassessments that incorrectly equal the baseline mean value, despite increases or decreases in the number of symptoms at the reassessments. (At a reassessment, a decrease in the number of symptoms, but of higher total intensity than at the initial assessment, might give a mean value close to that of the baseline. Consider the example of a patient who on the first visit marks 10 of the 13 VASs, each with an intensity of 8. The total score will be 80, and dividing by 10 gives a mean of 8. On her twelfth visit, she marks only 2 VASs, each with an intensity of 8. This totals to 16, which divided by the 2 symptoms gives a mean of 8—the same mean as at her initial evaluation. Improvement is indicated by the reduction from 10 to 2 symptoms, but the equivalent means completely conceal the improvement. Similarly, an increase in the number of symptoms—if the symptoms at reassessment are of lower intensity than those at the initial assessment—may also calculate to a mean that closely approximates the baseline mean.)

The mean of the symptom intensities generally provides a more sensitive index of change than the number of symptoms. However, the number of symptoms is relevant to assessing the patient's progress and should be taken into consideration in the clinician's overall assessment.

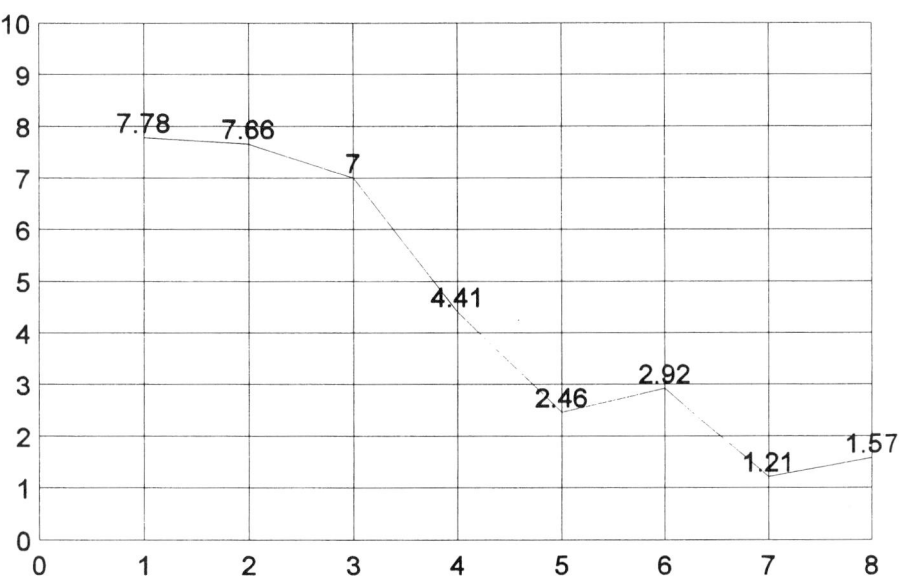

Figure 5.2.1. Mean symptom intensity of a euthyroid patient during metabolic rehabilitation. Horizontal axis shows the number of the patient's evaluations (1-to-8). Vertical axis shows potential mean symptom intensity ranging from 0-to-10.

As at the initial evaluation, the patient's mean score for symptom intensity at each reevaluation should be posted to Graph 1 (see Appendix A). A line should be drawn to connect the new score to the score from the last evaluation. This running graph gives a quantified visual depiction of changes in the patient's mean symptom intensity. Figure 5.2.1 contains the line graph for a euthyroid fibromyalgia patient treated by Dr. Gina S. Honeyman.[142] (See also Appendix B, Figure 3 in the paper titled "The Process of Change During T_3 Treatment for Euthyroid Fibromyalgia: A Double-Blind Placebo-Controlled Crossover Study."[139])

The line graph allows the clinician to see the direction and pattern of change. The clinician should use progression of this line with successive evaluations, and those of Graphs 2, 3, 4, and 5 (see Appendix A)—examples of which I describe below—to make decisions about the patient's management such as adjustments in thyroid hormone dosage.

For details on assessing symptom intensities, see Chapter 4.1, section: "Symptom Intensity."

Pain Distribution Body Form

There are four drawings of the human body on the pain drawing form in Appendix A. At the initial evaluation, the patient should shade the parts of the body as accurately as possible where she has in general experienced aching, pain, soreness, or tenderness over the past 3 months. She should indicate with darker shading areas of more intense pain. At each subsequent evaluation, she should shade in where she has experienced these sensations *since her last evaluation*. It is important to ask the patient to be precise in depicting the distribution of her pain. This will enable more accurate quantification of her pain distribution.

To score the pain drawing, the clinician or an assistant can place the transparent template over the patient's drawing (see Appendix A). The template is a copy of the body drawing with the body divided into 36 divisions. These divisions are based on the rule of nines for assessing the burned surface area of burn victims. At the suggestion of a member of my research team, nurse practitioner Mervianna Thompson, I developed this percentage method for quantifying pain distribution for fibromyalgia patients.[138][139][140] Wigers et al. in Norway apparently simultaneously adapted the rule of nines method for the same purpose.[141]

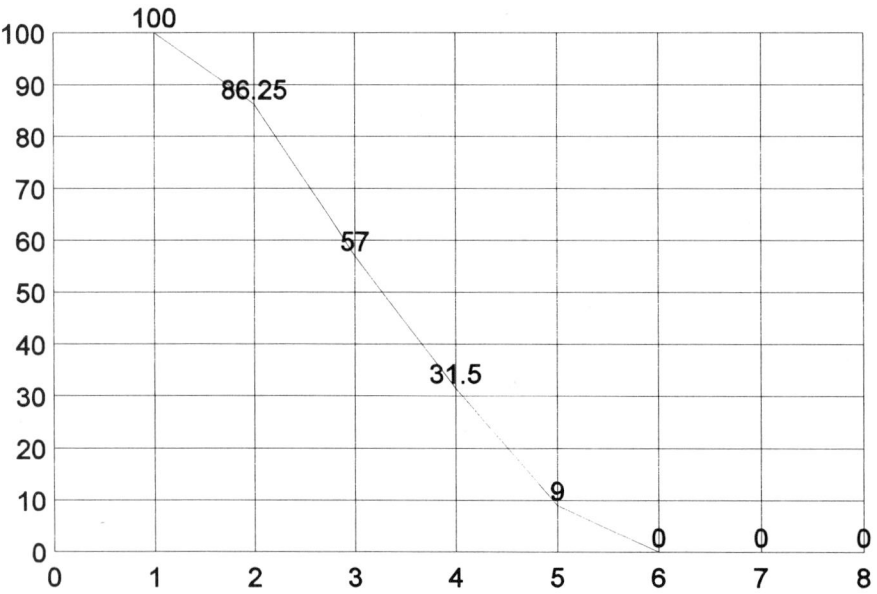

Figure 5.2.2. Pain distribution of a euthyroid patient during metabolic rehabilitation. The horizontal axis shows the number of evaluations (1-to-8). The vertical axis shows the percentage of 36 body divisions containing pain, ranging from 0%-to-100%.

According to my adaptation, the pain distribution is expressed as the percentage of the 36 body divisions that contain pain. The percentage is placed on Graph 2 (see Appendix A) from each evaluation. Figure 5.2.2 contains the line graph for a euthyroid fibromyalgia patient treated by Honeyman.[142] (See also Appendix B, Figure 2 in "The Process of Change During T_3 Treatment for Euthyroid Fibromyalgia: A Double-Blind Placebo-Controlled Crossover Study."[139])

Based on my clinical and research experience, I must agree with Wigers et al. that this method of measuring pain distribution is a more useful indicator of changing fibromyalgia status than are tender point measures with algometry.[141] For the typical patient who improves with metabolic therapy, the magnitude of change in pain distribution (expressed as the percentage of the body in pain) is greater than the change in tender point measures. It appears, then, that pain distribution, quantified by this method, is a more sensitive gauge of change in fibromyalgia status than is tender point sensitivity.

For more details on assessing pain distribution, see Chapter 4.1, section: "Pain Distribution."

Fibromyalgia Impact Questionnaire (FIQ)

The patient should complete the FIQ form and her total score should be posted to Graph 3 (Appendix A). A component of this instrument assesses the impact the patient's fibromyalgia is presently having on her functional abilities. The patient's total FIQ score is posted to Graph 3 (see Appendix A) at each evaluation. Figure 5.2.3 contains the line graph for a euthyroid fibromyalgia patient treated by Honeyman.[142] (See also Appendix B, Figures 4 and 9 in the paper "Metabolic Therapy for Hypothyroid and Euthyroid Fibromyalgia: Two Case Reports."[142]) For details on the use and scoring of this questionnaire, see the instructions that accompany the FIQ in Appendix A.

Zung's Self-Rating Depression Scale

This form allows the clinician to assess the presence and severity of depression. (If the patient has no depression, then it is not necessary to continue with this form at subsequent evaluations.) There are four classifications: (1) no depression, (2) mild, (3) moderate, and (4) severe. The classification is derived from a raw score that is converted to an SDS score. The SDS score should be posted to Graph 4 (see Appendix A). Other depression inventories such as Beck's may be used instead of Zung's. The patient's converted

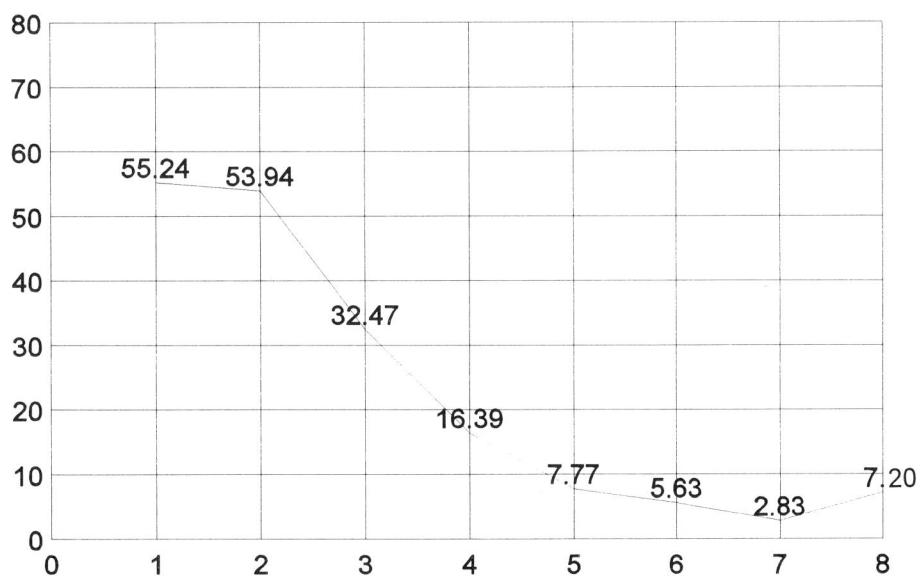

Figure 5.2.3. Fibromyalgia Impact Questionnaire scores of a euthyroid patient during metabolic rehabilitation treated by Honeyman. The horizontal axis shows the number of evaluations (1-to-8). The vertical axis shows the trend of changing scores ranging from 0%-to-80%. A decreasing line shows reduction of fibromyalgia's impact on daily life (an increase in functional abilities).

SDS score should be Graph 4 (see Appendix A) at each evaluation. Figure 5.2.4 contains the line graph for a euthyroid fibromyalgia patient treated by Honeyman.[142] (See also Appendix B, Figures 5 and 10 in the paper "Metabolic Therapy for Hypothyroid and Euthyroid Fibromyalgia: Two Case Reports."[142]) For details on the use and scoring of this depression scale, see the instructions that accompany the Zung's form in Appendix A.

TESTS AND PHYSICAL EXAMINATION

Before the patient begins metabolic treatment with thyroid hormone, the clinician should order or perform a baseline ECG. ECGs should also be performed at other times during the patient's treatment (see below). The clinician should also order thyroid function tests to determine the patient's thyroid status, but such tests are of *no* value in titrating the dosage of exogenous thyroid hormone or in evaluating for thyrotoxicity (see Chapter 4.4).

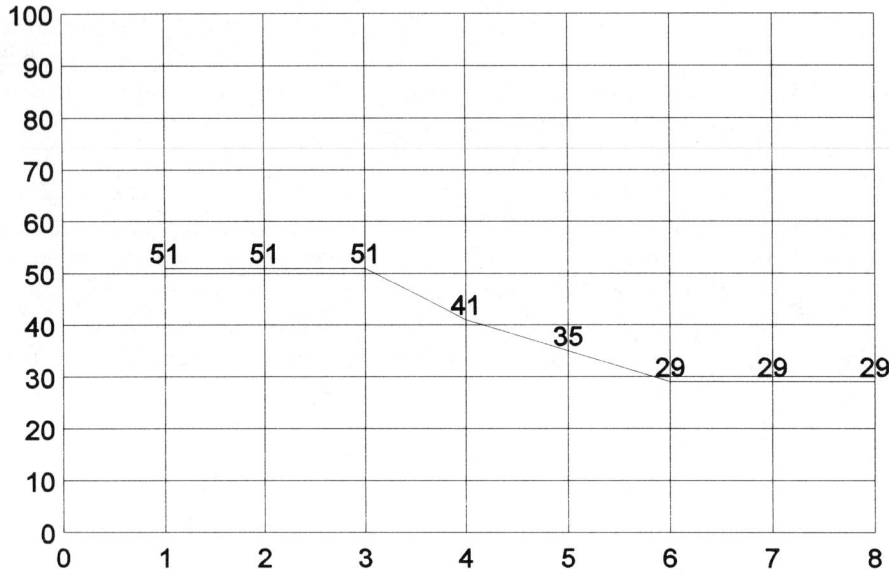

Figure 5.2.4. Zung's Self-Rating Depression Scale scores of a euthyroid patient during metabolic rehabilitation treated by Honeyman. The horizontal axis shows the number of evaluations (1-to-8). The vertical axis shows percentage SDS scores. (Less than 50 = normal; 50-59 = mild depression; 60-69 = moderate depression; 70 or > = severe depression.)

NOTE: After the euthyroid patient has improved or recovered with a supraphysiologic dosage of T_3 with no evidence of thyrotoxicosis, thyroid function tests may support the hypothesis that she has partial cellular resistance to thyroid hormone. This is indicated by a pattern of high free and total T_3 levels, and low free and total T_4 and TSH levels. If instead, the T_3 levels are normal despite supraphysiologic dosages and no thyrotoxicosis, the patient may have abnormally rapid clearance of T_3 rather than cellular resistance.

If the clinician orders laboratory thyroid function tests for academic or defensive purposes after a patient begins treatment, he should know that since the euthyroid fibromyalgia patient is taking a supraphysiologic dosage of thyroid hormone, she would be expected to have suppressed TSH, low T_4, and high T_3 levels. *This pattern of values is not synonymous with tissue thyrotoxicosis. The clinician should evaluate the patient for thyrotoxicosis by assessing for symptoms, signs, and peripheral indices of tissue overstimulation (see Chapter 4.3). If a thorough evaluation reveals no evidence of tissue thyrotoxicity, the clinician should consider the patient eumetabolic regardless of the results of thyroid function laboratory test results.*

Examinations to Perform Initially

Thyroid Function Testing. Before the patient begins treatment, the clinician should determine her thyroid status (see Chapter 4.2). The clinician can identify many patients—although certainly not all—with primary hypothyroidism (thyroid hormone deficiency due to thyroid gland hypofunction) through the results of a standard thyroid profile containing a T_4, T_3 uptake, T_7, and TSH. In untreated primary hypothyroidism, either the TSH is elevated or the TSH is in the upper half of the normal range and the thyroid hormone levels are low-normal or low (see Chapter 4.2).

There is a common belief among practicing clinicians that for identifying hypothyroid patients, the third-generation TSH assay has made the TRH stimulation test obsolete. This is patently false. The third-generation TSH chemiluminescent assay measures *low* TSH levels with extraordinary sensitivity (8-to-10-fold the sensitivity of the immunoradiometric assay). The clinician should bear in mind a statement by Ross et al.: "The clinical utility of increasingly sensitive TSH assays will be to distinguish degrees of thyrotroph suppression in subclinical *hyperthyroidism* [italics mine]."[136] Third generation TSH assays are thus useful in assessing hyperthyroidism, but they are no more useful than second-generation assays for identifying hypothyroid patients.

The diagnosis of primary hypothyroidism by the results of laboratory tests is tentative unless the patient has had a thyroidectomy, antithyroid drug therapy, or evidence of antithyroid antibodies. But even in the absence of such supportive historical data, a trial of thyroid hormone therapy is warranted for fibromyalgia patients with suggestive laboratory test results.

We can identify euthyroidism (normal function of the hypothalamic-pituitary-thyroid gland axis) and central hypothyroidism (thyroid hormone deficiency due to pituitary or hypothalamic dysfunction) in only two ways: (1) by monitoring for the normal nocturnal TSH surge that usually occurs roughly between 12:00 am and 2:00 am, or (2) with a TRH stimulation test.[63] The TRH stimulation test is more readily available since hospitalization may be necessary to assess the nocturnal TSH surge.

In the TRH stimulation test, a blood sample is taken to measure the basal TSH level. TRH is injected and 30 minutes later another blood sample is taken to again measure the TSH level. (Most patients' TSH levels peak approximately 30 minutes into a response to the TRH injection.) The test result is obtained by subtracting the baseline TSH level from the 30-minute level. A result between 8.5μU/mL and 20.0μU/mL is consistent with normal thyroid function. A result below 8.5μU/mL is consistent with pituitary hypothyroidism. A result above 20.0μU/mL is consistent with central hypothyroidism. (An exaggerated TSH response to TRH does not distinguish between pituitary and hypothalamic hypothyroidism.) The diagnosis of pituitary or central hypothyroidism is tentative without other evidence of pituitary and/or hypothalamic dysfunction. The other evidence may consist of other pituitary or hypothalamic hormone abnormalities (shown by assays), pituitary or hypothalamic structural abnormalities (revealed by imaging), or mutations of the TRH or TSH gene (identified through nucleotide sequencing). In the absence of such confirmatory evidence, when the patient's TRH stimulation test result is blunted or exaggerated, it is proper to state that *the patient's test result is consistent with, although not definitive for, pituitary or central hypothyroidism.* It is also proper for the patient with a positive test result to undergo a trial of thyroid hormone therapy. At 6-month intervals, the clinician should reevaluate the patient with a test result consistent with pituitary or central hypothyroidism for evidence of other pituitary or hypothalamic abnormalities.[193,p.979]

Examinations to Perform Initially and Intermittently

Electrocardiography. A baseline ECG should be obtained before the patient begins thyroid hormone therapy. ECGs should also be performed in two other cases: any time the patient's cardiac status is in question, and before increasing the patient's thyroid hormone dosage to, or substantially within, the supraphysiologic range—and at intervals afterward.

The heart is particularly sensitive to exogenous thyroid hormone.[104,p.763] Because of this, for some patients changes in the ECG are sensitive signs of treatment response. For example, some patients initially have low voltage ECGs. The PR, QRS, or QT interval may be of maximum normal width or greater. As the thyroid hormone dosage reaches the threshold at which β-adrenergic receptor density on heart muscle cell membranes increases, the intervals may shorten. The amplitude of the deflections may also increase. The most common change, however, is an increase in heart rate.

If there is any question as to whether the patient is having an adverse cardiac effect from exogenous thyroid hormone, the clinician should obtain another ECG. In an occasional patient, increased heart rate and contractility may amplify the effects of underlying cardiac abnormalities such as mitral valve prolapse. When this occurs, the patient's thyroid hormone dosage should be adjusted to insure safety. The patient should also consult a cardiologist for evaluation. Thus, the purpose of periodic ECGs is twofold: to assess cardiac status in response to thyroid hormone therapy, and to monitor for cardiac abnormalities that may be revealed.

Examinations to Perform at the Initial and All Subsequent Evaluations

At each examination, the clinician should perform three physical exam procedures. These include an algometer exam of the patient's tender points, assessment of the relaxation phase of the Achilles reflex, and measurement of the patient's resting pulse rate and blood pressure.

Algometer (Force Gauge) Exam of Tender Points. The clinician should use an algometer to examine the 16 tender points represented by dots on the body drawing (see Appendix A). Using the same form the patient has shaded, the clinician should record for each point the pressure (in kg/cm²) at which the patient first experiences discomfort. [*Note that the body drawing the patient is to shade should not contain dots (see*

Appendix A). I have found that some patients, when provided with a form with dots, do not shade all body areas where they have experienced pain. Instead, they circle or shade over only some of the dots—those at which they have experienced pain. They do this repeatedly at reassessments, even after I have instructed them that I do not want them to indicate at which dots they have had pain.]

What is measured with the algometer is the pain *threshold*, not the tolerance. The patient should be taught to distinguish the threshold at which she first senses a noxious quality to the slowly increasing pressure (see Chapter 4.1, section: "Tender Points: Manual vs Algometer Examinations"). Many patients say they are not sure they are reporting discomfort at the correct time. If the clinician performs the algometer exam in a uniform fashion, however, measurements are likely to be highly reliable. (See Chapter 4.1, section: "Algometer Tender Point Examination: Special Instructions for the Patient" and "Scoring"). The mean kg/cm² for the 16 tender points is to be posted to Graph 5 (see Appendix A and Chapter 4.1, section: "Scoring"). Figure 5.2.5 contains the line graph for a euthyroid fibromyalgia patient treated by Honeyman.[142] (See also Appendix B, Figure 1 in the paper titled "The Process of Change During T_3 Treatment for Euthyroid Fibromyalgia: A Double-Blind Placebo-Controlled Crossover Study."[139])

Achilles Reflex. The Achilles reflex is abnormal in most fibromyalgia patients before they begin taking thyroid hormone. Either the relaxation phase is slower than the contraction phase, or the foot stalls briefly and possibly wobbles or jerks before beginning a slow or normally rapid relaxation phase. As the patient increases her dosage of thyroid hormone, the relaxation phase normalizes: It shortens and eventually equals the contraction phase.

The speed of the relaxation phase may be slow because calf muscle energy metabolism is impeded and/or the levels and activity of calcium ATPase are low (see Chapter 4.3, section titled "Achilles Reflex Time"). In hypothyroidism, muscle energy metabolism is decreased and Ca^{++}-ATPase levels and activity may be reduced. When energy metabolism is low in the calf muscles, a longer time is require to muster enough energy to fuel separation of the actin and myosin filaments with consequent lengthening of the muscle fibers. With decreased Ca^{++}-ATPase activity, calcium ions are transferred from the sarcoplasm to the sarcoplasmic reticulum more slowly than normal. The prolonged presence of calcium ions in the sarcoplasm slows separation of actin and myosin, thus slowing

relaxation of skeletal muscle. When subnormal muscle energy metabolism and reduced Ca^{++}-ATPase activity are corrected with thyroid hormone, the contraction and relaxation phases of the reflex occur at a fairly equal, brisk speed.

On the other hand, excess metabolic stimulation with thyroid hormone causes most patients to have hyperreflexia (abnormally shortened duration of the Achilles reflex[153]). Until the patient has found her optimal thyroid hormone dosage, the clinician should have her stand or sit and lift her heels while her metatarsophalangeal joints and toes remain on the floor. If her legs and ankles quiver in this position, it indicates, just as a hyperreactive Achilles reflex does, excessive thyroid hormone stimulation. (See Chapter 4.3, section titled "Achilles Reflex Time.")

Resting Pulse Rate and Blood Pressure. The typical fibromyalgia patient has low blood pressure. Her pulse rate may be normal, but is more likely to be slow for her level of cardiovascular conditioning. Some have bradycardia. Recently, some researchers have come to refer to low blood pressure in fibromyalgia/chronic fatigue syndrome patients by terms such as "neurogenic hypotension." They use the term to refer to a fall in blood pressure upon rising from a recumbent position, a phenomenon traditionally termed orthostatic hypotension.

Thyroid hormone therapy normalizes the resting pulse rate and blood pressure of the typical fibromyalgia patient. The pulse rate is far more responsive to thyroid hormone than is the blood pressure, which responds only minimally in some patients.

Obtaining True Resting Values for the Heart Rate and Blood Pressure. For monitoring the heart rate and blood pressure, the clinician should obtain true *resting* values. In attempting to do so, the clinician should bear in mind that thyroid hormone accentuates the cardiovascular response to catecholamines. Pulse rate and blood pressure vary considerably as people move from situation to situation throughout the day. Physical exertion, such as walking up a short flight of stairs or moving quickly from the reception room to an exam room, accelerates the pulse rate and raises blood pressure. Also, different social situations have variable potency in producing sympathetic-cardiovascular responses. For many patients, the presence of a clinician produces particularly strong responses. Measurement of the patient's pulse rate and blood pressure under such circumstances are likely to produce values that vary considerably from resting values. This phenomenon, in which a patient's blood pressure is normal at home but high in the presence of clinicians, is termed

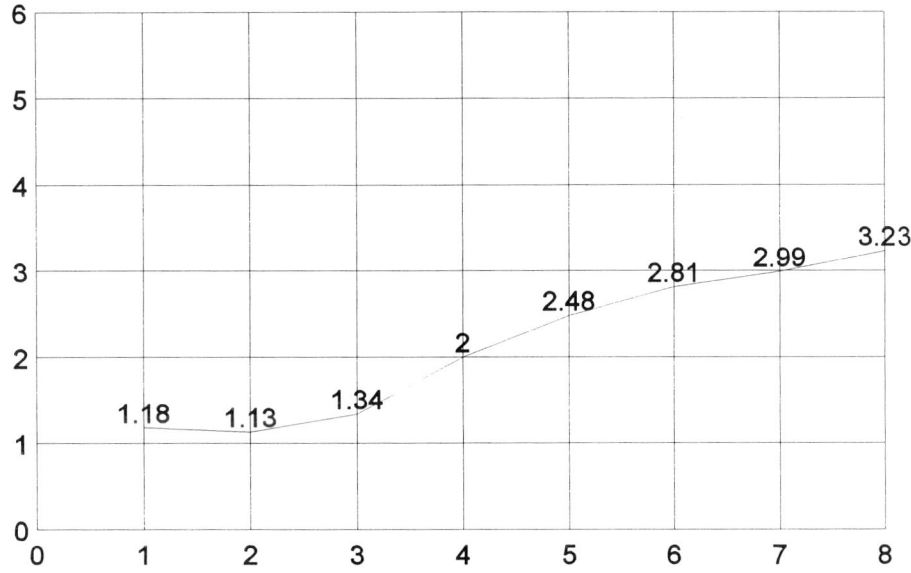

Figure 5.2.5. Mean tender point pressure/pain thresholds of a euthyroid patient during metabolic rehabilitation treated by Honeyman. The horizontal axis shows the number of evaluations (1-to-8). The vertical axis shows the mean pressure in kg/cm² that was necessary to induce perception of discomfort at the potential tender point sites. The higher the value, the more improved the patient.

"white coat" hypertension[190]and by extension, "white coat" tachycardia.

For these reasons, to obtain a measure in the clinical milieu that is as close as possible to the patient's resting heart rate and blood pressure, it is essential to have the patient relax. It is helpful to ask the patient to close her eyes and image a scene that is particularly comforting and calming to her. Before taking the measurement, the clinician should allow a short time for the pulse rate and blood pressure to decrease to a resting level.

The resting value at each reevaluation should be compared with the baseline value and with those for other exam dates preceding the present examination. This will contribute to the clinician's overall appreciation of the patient's clinical status and her responsiveness to exogenous thyroid hormone.

The Patient Should be Able to Take and Record Her Resting Pulse Rate. The clinician should also teach the patient the proper method for taking her own pulse rate. It is preferable to show the patient how to palpate the carotid artery with the palmar aspects of the ipsilateral fingers. The pulsing of this artery is more obvious to most patients than that of other arteries.

The patient should take her pulse and record it at least once per day *while relaxed*. The patient is more likely to get a true resting pulse rate when alone in a room where she is free from distractions. *She should not lie down to take the rate.* The rate may increase during recumbency, especially in patients with low blood pressure.

It is important that the patient be able to take her own pulse rate at home. With this ability, she can help the clinician determine whether any thyrotoxic-like symptoms are due to excessive thyroid hormone stimulation. The patient should familiarize herself with the symptoms of cardiovascular overstimulation from thyroid hormone, such as rapid heart rate. If the patient phones the clinician, reports that she has developed a rapid heart rate, and expresses concern that it may indicate overstimulation, it is important to know what her resting pulse rate is. If the rapid heart rate the patient reports is, for example, 120, but her resting pulse rate is 86, this may indicate that the rate of 120 is due to some other factor. The clinician should ask whether the patient's heart rate has been steadily rapid, even when the patient has not exerted herself, as during sitting. A steadily rapid rate would suggest that she has thyroid hormone overstimulation. But if the rate decreases considerably during non-exertion, and especially when taking the resting rate by the procedure I described above, then the rapid rate may not be due to thyroid hormone. The rapidity may be a result of caffeine consumption (from coffee, soft drinks, or pain medications), hypoglycemia, or emotional arousal. While these factors are likely to sustain a rapid heart rate during non-exertion, their effects last only briefly compared to the continuous influence of thyroid hormone. Caffeine, for example, has a half-life of 5 hours, and its stimulatory effects usually subside well before the half-life has elapsed. Caffeine is a particularly important factor to consider because thyroid hormone typically renders the patient more sensitive to sympathomimetic substances. As a result, smaller amounts than previously can be excessively stimulating (see section on caffeine below). Most patients, when questioned about such factors, can recall whether another factor is temporarily related to the delimited period during which she has experienced rapid heart rate.

Tissues vary in their responsiveness to thyroid hormone. Because the heart is particularly sensitive to thyroid hormone,[104,p.763] some patients must settle for a heart rate more rapid than what is considered ideal for the sake of adequately stimulating apparently less sensitive tissues. With these patients, it is particularly important to assure cardiac safety with serial ECGs and in appropriate cases, an evaluation by a cardiologist. Patients must engage in regular cardiovascular exercise and use cardio-protective nutrients (see section on cardio-protective nutrients below) including B complex vitamins and antioxidants. (See Chapter 4.3, subsection titled "Heart Function," and Chapter 4.4, subsection titled "Electrocardiography.")

● BIOCHEMICAL TREATMENT

First and foremost, the biochemical treatments necessary for improvement or recovery for most patients' thyroid hormone-related fibromyalgia involves the use of exogenous thyroid hormone and nutritional supplements. However, other biochemical agents may be necessary during the initial phase of treatment to modulate troublesome symptoms.

Biochemical treatment involves four indispensable components: (1) selecting the proper form of thyroid hormone, (2) properly titrating the dosage, (3) inducing patients to take nutritional supplements, and (4) encouraging patients to engage in exercise to tolerance. While exercise is not *per se* a biochemical treatment, it determines to a profound degree the biochemical status of the patient and her response to biochemical agents, and it cannot be neglected if most patients are to improve or recover.

PROPER FORM OF THYROID HORMONE

If the patient is euthyroid, she should be treated with T_3. In my experience, few euthyroid fibromyalgia patients have benefitted from the use of T_4 or desiccated thyroid. Most have improved or recovered, however, with T_3 as part of their metabolic treatment regimen.

In the past, I have recommended that the patient with primary or central hypothyroidism begin treatment with T_4. My preference for T_4 over desiccated thyroid was that I had far more experience with patients taking only T_4. My more extensive experience with T_4 resulted from the preference for Synthroid by physicians who prescribed for my patients early in my study of fibromyalgia. Desiccated thyroid had been in widespread use,[114] but progressively more physicians were declining to prescribe it and instead would prescribe only Synthroid. It has become clear to me in recent years, however, that the widespread preference for Synthroid among conventional practitioners resulted from two phenomena: (1) a powerful marketing campaign to promote Synthroid sales and (2) the tendency of conventional medical practitioners' to mistake marketing hype for scientific knowledge.

During my years of recommending T_4 for the hypothyroid fibromyalgia patient, if the patient did not improve after reaching a dosage of 0.4 mg of T_4, or if the patient developed symptoms or signs of overstimulation at a lower dosage, I recommended switching her to T_3. Virtually all patients switched to T_3 benefitted more than they did from T_4. Most improved or recovered with the use of T_3 after having failed to improve with T_4. The cumulative clinical experiences of Honeyman-Lowe and myself have led us to rethink the protocol of beginning hypothyroid patients with T_4. In that we can find no good scientific reasons to object to patients taking T_3 from the start, we now question whether it is humane to force patients to begin treatment with T_4 or desiccated thyroid. A minority of hypothyroid patients do improve satisfactorily or recover with the use of T_4. But several months to a year may be required to determine whether a patient is going to respond satisfactorily to T_4. Some of our patients have lamented that they continued to suffer for this length of time before quickly recovering upon being switched to T_3. We are entirely sympathetic with their feelings.

I am aware of some hypothyroid fibromyalgia patients who have improved or recovered with the use of desiccated thyroid after failing to benefit from the use of T_4 alone. The presence of T_3 in this medication undoubtedly accounts for its superiority over the sole use of T_4 with some patients. This presumption is supported by the recent finding of Bunevicius et al. that substituting 12.5 µg T_3 for 50 mg of each patients' daily T_4 dosage significantly improved mood and neuropsychological functioning compared to patients taking only T_4.[103] However, I have had some hypothyroid fibromyalgia patients who did not improve with the use of desiccated thyroid but subsequently improved or recovered with the use of T_3. Some patients who did not improve became thyrotoxic with 4-to-6 grains of desiccated thyroid. Most of these patients subsequently improved or recovered without thyrotoxicity with supraphysiologic dosages of T_3. Generally, I recommend switching the hypothyroid fibromyalgia patient from desiccated thyroid to T_3 under two circumstances: (1) if she fails to improve with 4 grains of desiccated thyroid or (2) if she develops symptoms or signs of overstimulation at a lower dosage.

As I explain in greater detail in Chapter 5.3, the studies of Escobar-Morreale et al. have shown that in rats, T_4 alone did not provide normal concentrations of T_3 in the cells of all tissues. When both T_4 and T_3 (in proportions normally secreted by the rat thyroid gland) were infused, intracellular T_3 concentrations became normal. The investigators noted that the dosages of T_4 necessary to normalize the cellular concentrations of T_3 were lower than when T_4 was used alone. If these findings are generalizable to the human being, and the recent report of Bunevicius et al. indicates that they are,[103] they explain why most hypothyroid fibromyalgia patients do not benefit from the use of T_4 alone.[33][34] They do not, however, explain why researchers in the 1950s found that some patients with low BMRs and symptoms characteristic of hypothyroidism failed to improve with T_4 or desiccated thyroid but improved or recovered when switched to T_3 (see Chapter 2.5, subsections titled "Thyroid Hormone-Related Euthyroid Hypometabolism" and "Recognition of Euthyroid Hypometabolism and the Advent of T_3"). The reports of these mid-twentieth century researchers are consistent with the findings of

my research team.[35][36][125]

Presently, on experiential and theoretical grounds, I believe that if the hypothyroid patient is to use a preparation containing T_4, it should be either desiccated thyroid or another product containing both synthetic T_4 and T_3. I do not believe the use of synthetic T_4 alone can be justified scientifically. Although a minority of hypothyroid fibromyalgia patients respond satisfactorily to T_4 alone, it is relatively or completely ineffective with most.

The individual clinician, hopefully in collaboration with the hypothyroid fibromyalgia patient, must make a judgment as to which form of thyroid hormone to begin using. If a patient does respond to T_4, there is one practical advantage. Upon coming under the care of a new conventional physician, the physician is more likely to renew the prescription for T_4 than for desiccated thyroid, a product containing synthetic T_4 and T_3, or T_3 alone. The argument that most conventional physicians will prescribe only T_4 (in most cases the product Synthroid), however, has no bearing on the logical and scientific issues involved. The difficulty in patients obtaining prescriptions for desiccated thyroid, products containing both synthetic T_4 and T_3, or T_3 alone is a social and practical problem, not a scientific one. (It is important that the clinician read Chapter 5.3 for an elaboration of the ideas I have expressed in this section.)

Regardless of the thyroid hormone product the patient uses, the clinician should provide most patients with 20 mg propranolol tablets to use *only* in case of overstimulation that is bothersome or threatening. Propranolol is contraindicated for asthmatic patients and should not be prescribed for them. Propranolol preferentially binds β-adrenergic receptors. In the bronchial tubes, the binding increases bronchial secretions, can result in bronchial constrictions, and thereby predisposes the patient to asthmatic episodes.

PROPERLY ADJUSTING DOSAGE

Main Objective of Dosage Adjustments

The main objective of dosage adjustments is maximum improvement on all measures of fibromyalgia status. Typically, improvement in the measures corresponds to the patient subjectively feeling improved. There may be a lag, however, between objective and subjective improvement; in some cases either objective or subjective improvement precedes the other.

Rarely does a patient improve solely through the

use of thyroid hormone. In the vast majority of cases, complete recovery depends on the patient engaging in exercise to tolerance and taking nutritional supplements. Other forms of treatment may also be necessary. The use of nutritional supplements and exercise to tolerance enable the patient to capitalize on the improved metabolic capacity conferred by exogenous thyroid hormone. *The patient should use the smallest effective and non-thyrotoxic dosage of exogenous thyroid hormone.*

Adjusting Dosage

The starting dosage is an individual matter. For the patient without contraindications due to cardiac or adrenal conditions, the dosage can be any amount that the clinician roughly calculates to be a replacement dosage for the patient. With most fibromyalgia patients, 75 µg of T_3, 0.15 mg of T_4, or approximately 1.5 grains of desiccated thyroid is a good starting point. (If the clinician uses synthetic T_3 with synthetic T_4, he should use roughly the same equivalent as in desiccated thyroid: 4 parts T_4 to 1 part T_3. For conversions, see the equivalency chart in Appendix D. Use of synthetic T_4/T_3 combination drugs is not recommended, as some of these contain only 1 part T_3 to 10 parts T_4.) If this starting dosage is excessive, as it is in a small percentage of cases, the patient should *not* stop the thyroid hormone but should decrease the dosage just far enough to stop any indication of overstimulation. A small percentage of patients benefit fully from this initial dosage and do not have to increase it further. Most patients, however, benefit only after increasing the dosage according to the protocol I describe in this chapter. Most euthyroid fibromyalgia patients benefit only from dosages considerably higher than the recommended starting dosage.

For the typical patient, T_3 can be increased at 1-to-2-week intervals, and T_4 or desiccated thyroid at 3-to-4-week intervals. In general, dosage increases at these intervals are 12.5-to-25 µg of T_3, 0.05-to-0.075 mg of T_4, and ½-to-¾ grain of desiccated thyroid. As patients approach what appears to be an effective dosage, increases should be more modest: 6.25 µg of T_3, 0.025 mg of T_4, or ¼ grain of desiccated thyroid. This way, patients avoid "over-shooting" and having to reduce the dosage.

The clinician can increase the dosage of T_3 more aggressively than the dosage of T_4. This is because the effects of T_3 have a faster onset with increased dosages and offset with decreased dosages. Finding the effective T_4 dosage usually requires more patience, as the effects of an increase may not be apparent for 2-to-4

weeks. Some therapeutic effects of T_4 occur only after months have passed.

Cookbook guidance is of limited help in properly adjusting dosages. Only experience with patients, in the spirit of clinical medicine, will teach the clinician how to properly adjust a patient's dosage to meet individual needs. This knowledge and skill comes by closely observing, examining, and communicating with patients as their dosages are adjusted. With sufficient experience, the clinician is likely to become comfortable fine-tuning a patient's clinical status with thyroid hormone as a part of her metabolic treatment regimen.

With most patients, an ECG before each dosage adjustment in the supraphysiologic (or TSH-suppressive) range can rule out most possible effects of cardiac thyrotoxicity. This is of foremost concern. *If* they have any overstimulation, most fibromyalgia patients experience it as rapid heart rate, tremors, or excess body heat. These effects do not usually signal dangerous overstimulation, although some patients may be bothered by them. If a rapid or "pounding" heart with minimal exertion is the predominant symptom indicating overstimulation, the patient should have an ECG. The clinician should make sure that the tracing is free from indications of cardiac thyrotoxicity (see Chapter 4.3, section titled "Heart," and Chapter 4.4, section titled "The Heart").

Up to a point, a rapid heart rate alone does not portend adverse cardiac consequences. But if an abnormal ECG warrants it, the patient should reduce her dosage by a proper amount indicated by her unique need. The amount is a highly individual issue. If tachycardia at rest and during activity is the only cardiac sign of overstimulation, and there are no apparent impending adverse effects on cardiac function, a dosage reduction of 6.25-to-12.5 µg of T_3 may be sufficient. The clinician's aim should be to reduce the dosage enough to slow the resting heart rate but not so much as to induce rebound hypometabolism. (For the patient whose clinical phenotype is the syndrome of fibromyalgia, rebound will entail reactivation or intensification of fibromyalgia symptoms and signs.)

This issue of possible rebound also applies to the patient who takes T_4. But it requires even more careful calculation by the clinician. With T_3, rebound from miscalculation and too great a reduction in dosage can be relieved within 1-to-2 days by a carefully calculated increase in dosage. But the patient taking T_4 may not experience rebound for 1-to-2 weeks after reducing the dosage, and rebound symptoms and signs may persist for 1-to-2 weeks after the patient increases the dosage again. To avoid rebound, it may be prudent for the patient with tachycardia (but otherwise normal cardiac status) who takes T_4 to reduce her dosage by 0.025-to-0.050 mg and use propranolol (unless she is asthmatic) to control the rapid heart rate when it is bothersome to her.

For patients at risk for adverse cardiac effects, the dosage reduction should be sufficient to safeguard the patient, regardless of possible rebound. Again, unless the patient is asthmatic, she may use propranolol to avert dangerous cardiac effects until the dosage reduction ceases the overstimulation. In most cases, 20-to-60 mg of propranolol effectively stops β-adrenergic-mediated abnormalities of cardiac function within 30 minutes. The clinician should keep in mind, however, that for patients with severely compromised cardiac function, too large a dosage of propranolol may dangerously reduce cardiac output. The clinician should tailor the dosage to the patient's individual needs should the drug be necessary. It seldom is, however, when patients follow the proper protocol.

Middle-aged and elderly patients who are severely deconditioned should begin thyroid hormone at a *very low dosage* and increase it *very gradually* at greater intervals than I recommend above. At the same time, these patients *must* engage in cardiovascular conditioning activities to tolerance, progressively increasing the intensity as tolerance increases. They should also take nutrients scientifically shown to protect the cardiovascular system (see section on cardio-protective nutrients below).

If persistent tremors are the predominant symptom of overstimulation, reducing the thyroid hormone dosage will stop them. As with tachycardia, this may take 1-to-2 days with T_3 or 1-to-2 weeks with T_4. Some patients may find tremors bothersome in business or social situations. Propranolol, 20-to-60 mg taken 30 minutes to an hour before an anticipated situation, will stop the tremors. (Some public speakers, musicians, and other entertainers use propranolol before performances to control nervousness and anxiety.)

Dosage Adjustments within the Non-Thyrotoxic Range Should Be Tissue Response-Driven

Decisions to change thyroid hormone dosages within the non-overstimulating range should be response-driven; that is, a patient's response to the previous dosage should be the basis of further dosage changes. The patient's "response" consists of changes in the objective fibromyalgia measures, the patient's subjective estimate of her status, results of a physical examination, and non-quantified changes in the patient observed by the clinician (see below).

During treatment, objective fibromyalgia measures may show favorable trends in fibromyalgia status before the patient is subjectively aware of improvement and before improvement in the patient is obvious to the clinician. On the other hand, subjective changes may precede those of objective measures. The pattern for any particular patient becomes apparent only as therapy progresses. In any case, there is little temporal discrepancy between objective data and subjective impressions, and therapeutic decisions are best made by considering both.

The clinician *must* use line graphs to observe trends in data points that represent mean scores from fibromyalgia measures. These provide objective data to calculate into therapeutic decisions. Although clinical judgment of a patient's status should influence clinical decisions, decisions should primarily be data-driven by the scores on the objective measures. The empirical feedback from graphed data provides a high level of control in patient management, and the feedback aids judgment regarding alterations in the patient's regimen. By referring to established patterns of therapeutic response shown in line graphs, such as those my colleagues and I have reported (see Appendix B, paper titled "The Process of Change During T_3 Treatment for Euthyroid Fibromyalgia: A Double-Blind Placebo-Controlled Crossover Study"[139]), the clinician can formulate proper expectations regarding clinical outcome. The graphs can help determine whether a particular patient is responding with a pattern that represents therapeutic change.

Non-Quantified Patient Responses. I cannot emphasize too strongly the importance of subjective clinical judgment based on the non-quantified patient responses to treatment, combined with the use of objective data. Today, clinician-based medicine is not esteemed by most medical practitioners. Instead, most clinicians pride themselves on their participation in what is rightfully termed extremist technological medicine, an orientation in which subjective judgment by the clinician is viewed with disdain. Regardless, to assure the most favorable therapeutic outcome, the clinician using metabolic therapy must base his decisions in part on unmitigated subjective judgment. It might be clinical utopia for the assessment of patient status to be reduced entirely to easily measurable criteria. Long-term clinical use of our treatment protocol, however, has shown that this is not possible. As most fibromyalgia patients undergo treatment with thyroid hormone, some changes that are difficult to quantify are obvious in varying degrees to the experienced clinician who is familiar with the individual patient. The changes typically signify improving patient status, and their failure to occur may indicate the need to adjust the hormone dosage. When considered with the outcome of the objective measures, these phenomena may contribute substantially to proper clinical decisions.

The speed of the Achilles reflex is quantifiable, but in clinical practice, quantification is not necessary with most patients. The clinician can learn with minimal experience the difference between a slow and a normal Achilles reflex relaxation phase[152] (see Chapter 4.3). There are other, more difficult to define responses the clinician should watch for. *One is a change from a torpid and pensive facial expression to a zestful expression, and a distinct change in the eyes from a dull, listless appearance to an energetic alertness.*

Some clinicians are likely to imprudently ignore or reject a pronouncement by the patient that she is well, even after she has been symptom-free for months. The main reason for this posture is that the clinician has failed from the beginning of the patient's care to closely observe her. Consequently, he has little baseline knowledge about her with which to compare her changed status. For virtually all fibromyalgia patients who make the pronouncement of improvement or recovery after undergoing metabolic therapy, objective measures verify the assertion. The clinician must, of course, have used the objective measures to be able to check for concurrence with the patient's subjective judgment. With close observation and repeated objective measures, the clinician will find that such changes occur and persist in most fibromyalgia patients who benefit from thyroid hormone therapy.

Therefore, during the course of the patient's care, it is judicious for the clinician to note and record nonquantified but observable changes in the patient. He should calculate these into judgment of the patient's fibromyalgia status. To ignore or otherwise exclude such phenomena from patient assessment is to forfeit one of the richest sources of information upon which to base sound clinical judgment.

Serum TSH Levels vs Peripheral Measures in Dosage Decisions

It is critical that the patient's thyroid hormone dosage *not* be adjusted based on any theoretically "ideal" serum TSH level. There is today a common false belief among conventional clinicians that TSH levels correlate with tissue metabolic rate. The TSH level and metabolic rate, however, are out of sync in many and perhaps most patients. I have found no studies documenting a correlation between TSH levels and tissue metabolic rate. There is, however, considerable evidence to indicate that the two do not correlate snugly.[49] As an example, the relaxation phase of the Achilles reflex, which is slow in most hypothyroid patients, does not correlate with biochemical measures of thyroid function.[151] Also, in primary hypothyroid patients, dosages of T_3 (20-to-25 µg per day) that normalized the basal metabolic rate, cardiac systolic time, serum cholesterol, and creatine phosphokinase activity, did not lower basal serum TSH levels and peak TSH responses to TRH. These values remained high until the patient used higher dosages of T_3 (20-to-50 µg per day) or T_4.[171] The higher dosages did not cause further changes in peripheral tissue measures. This shows a discordance between pituitary and peripheral tissue responses to thyroid hormone.

Fibromyalgia patients improve when their dosage is adjusted based on indirect "peripheral" measures of metabolic status. These measures, such as the Achilles reflex, serum cholesterol, resting heart rate, and increased voltage of the ECG, are more directly related to tissue metabolic status than is the TSH or thyroid hormone levels. We have spent a considerable amount of time discerning whether a fibromyalgia patient's subjective recovery and increased functional abilities correlate with improvement on objective measures of fibromyalgia status. They generally do. Certainly, these measures enable the clinician to make far more judicious dosage decisions than does the serum TSH, even when serum thyroid hormone levels are also used. The objective fibromyalgia measures can also be considered indirect indices of peripheral tissue metabolic status. These, added to the physiological phenomena such as the Achilles reflex, constitute the barometers by which the clinician should adjust dosage.

PROPERLY IDENTIFYING THYROTOXICOSIS

The clinician must distinguish between the serum TSH and thyroid hormone levels on the one hand, and tissue metabolic status on the other. They are *not* one and the same. Clinicians are taught today to adjust thyroid hormone dosage according to TSH levels. The assumption is that the TSH level is an accurate gauge of tissue metabolic status. There is no scientific basis to this belief. Moreover, arguments that TSH-suppressive dosages have adverse tissue effects are a matter of highly debatable opinion rather than fact (see Chapter 4.4). Unbeknownst to most clinicians, even research thyroidologists who favor thyroid function laboratory testing debate the issue. Some say that when the TSH level is in the middle of the range, the T_4 blood level is perfect for maintaining normal tissue metabolism. Others point out that the free T_3 level best correlates with tissue metabolic status.[30,p.88][81] But to maintain a normal free T_3 level, the T_4 dosage must be high enough to suppress the TSH level. The suppressed TSH level alarms many clinicians who falsely believe that TSH-suppression is synonymous with thyrotoxicosis.

Few fibromyalgia patients derive any benefit from thyroid hormone when the dosage is adjusted so as to avoid TSH suppression. These patients are among those for whom TSH-suppressive dosages typically provide substantial and often complete relief. Without such doses, these patients continue to suffer from fibromyalgia. And their risk for diseases such as atherosclerosis increases. Though these dosages suppress the TSH, they do not induce tissue thyrotoxicity.

It is critical for the clinician to realize that *the blood levels of TSH and thyroid hormones do not in general correlate with the patient's tissue metabolic status.* Hence, a suppressed TSH level does not necessarily mean that the patient's tissues are thyrotoxic. It is far more reasonable to use various tests for tissue overstimulation than to make inferences based on the values of laboratory tests of thyroid function[49] (see Chapter 4.3). Our protocol is to use, among other things, serial ECGs, laboratory tests (serum calcium, phosphorus, creatinine, and alkaline phosphatase; and urinary calcium, phosphorus, creatinine, and type I collagen), and bone density tests. If a particular dosage relieves symptoms but also induces some tissue overstimulation, the patient must find a compromise dosage that minimizes symptoms and relieves the thyrotoxicosis.

In my view, a clinician forsakes responsibility for providing humane care when he dictates a patient's thyroid hormone dosage based strictly on TSH levels. The results of ECGs, lab tests, and bone densitometry can answer definitively whether a given dosage is potentially harmful to an individual patient. The TSH level does not do so.

PRECAUTIONS IN THE USE OF EXOGENOUS THYROID HORMONE

Patients with cardiac disease or adrenal insufficiency may have adverse reactions to exogenous thy-

roid hormone unless proper precautions are taken. With a few exceptions, which I discuss below, the same precautions should be exercised with patients taking T_4, T_3, or both (see Chapter 4.4).

Cardiac Disease

The clinician who first treated human beings with thyroid substance[31] reported later that 4 of his patients in 1891 and 1892 died of heart disease after starting treatment.[51] The dosages he administered, however, were crudely adjusted and may have overloaded the cardiac systems of vulnerable patients. The Coronary Drug Project found that D-thyroxine, administered to lower patients' cholesterol, increased the death rate in men who had previously had heart attacks.[50] This was reported in 1972, a time when many medical physicians vigorously denounced as valueless practices now known to protect the cardiovascular system—practices such as the use of aerobic exercise, vitamins C and E, and other nutritional supplements. The increased heart attack rate among the men using T_4 must be considered in light of this. Increasing inotropic and chronotropic effects on the heart by exogenous thyroid hormone can be detrimental to the patient with an unhealthy heart, but may have no adverse effects in the patient who engages in cardio-protective practices.

Even for patients with ischemic heart disease due to atherosclerosis, if managed properly, exogenous thyroid hormone can improve cardiovascular status. In this regard, Sawin wrote that most clinicians are aware that exogenous thyroid hormone may worsen the cardiac condition of a hypothyroid patient. He went on to say, "Not as many know, however, that there is as good a chance of improving angina as of worsening it."[85,p.397] Keating et al. concurred.[52] Recent studies confirm their view (See Chapter 4.4, subsection titled "Improved Cardiovascular Status with Thyroid Hormone Therapy"). Before initiating thyroid hormone therapy and before each dosage increase, the clinician should exercise great care with patients whose cardiac health is questionable. The patient should *gradually* increase his or her dosage of exogenous thyroid hormone to avoid coronary insufficiency.[53]

Precautions with the Patient Whose Cardiac Function Is Compromised. Bastenie wrote that changing a patient's status from hypothyroid to euthyroid (meaning thyroid function test results in the normal range) with replacement doses of thyroid hormone subjects the patient in general, and particularly his heart, to severe stress.[1,p.124] So, with a patient more than 50 years old (even with a normal ECG), the clinician should err on the side of safety and consider that the patient may have atherosclerosis. The patient's treatment should be planned accordingly. If the patient has compromised heart function, the initial dosage of thyroid hormone should be low enough to avoid aggravating the heart condition. Vanhaelst stresses the importance of very gradual increases in the dose of thyroid hormone to avoid myocardial infarction.[3,p.120]

Bastenie advised that the clinician avoid T_3 because of its rapid and intensive action.[1,pp.124-125] However, some hypothyroid fibromyalgia patients and most euthyroid fibromyalgia patients benefit only from the use of T_3. Most of these patients can safely use T_3 when both clinician and patient observe necessary precautions.

For the patient of average size, the starting dosage should in most cases be 12.5 μg of T_3 or 0.025 mg of T_4 (0.25 grain of desiccated thyroid). If the patient tolerates this dosage well, a safe dosage increase is 12.5 μg of T_3 every 2-to-3 weeks, or 0.0125 mg of T_4 (0.125 grain of desiccated thyroid) once per month. (For conversions, see the equivalency chart in Appendix D.)

Before the patient increases her dosage, she should have an ECG to confirm that no adverse cardiac effects have occurred from the previous dosage. If adverse effects have occurred, the patient should reduce her dosage sufficiently to assure safety. If the patient appears to be at risk, she may have to take 20-to-60 mg of propranolol several times per day for 24-to-48 hours if she is taking T_3, or for 1-to-2 weeks if she is taking T_4 or desiccated thyroid. The patient's cardiac status should be determined by a cardiologist.

Views differ on how best to manage the patient who has adverse cardiac effects from exogenous thyroid hormone. Haynes wrote that if the patient taking T_4 has angina pectoris, the clinician should exercise care, but stopping the hormone may not be necessary.[84,p.1372] DeGroot and his coauthors wrote that it is of great importance to watch for precordial distress, definite angina, or indications of congestive heart failure. If the patient experiences these, they advise that she stop taking the hormone until the symptoms subside, then resume the hormone with a smaller dose. They caution that the cardiac patient may have to content herself with a dosage that leaves her slightly below normal metabolically (they suggest a free thyroxine index of 4 or 5 and a slightly elevated TSH level). They wrote that the dosage should be low enough to avoid angina yet high enough so that the patient does not become intolerably hypometabolic.[2,p.564] They also suggested that the hormone may be tolerated better if taken in several divided doses

through the day rather than in a single dose.[2,p.564]

If the patient has adverse cardiac effects from the lowest dosage that improves her fibromyalgia status, she and her clinician must resign themselves to a dosage low enough to relieve the adverse effects until she can improve her cardiac fitness with exercise and the use of cardio-protective nutritional supplements (see section on nutritional supplementation below).

Patients Who Do Not Comply with the Dosage Schedule. Some patients will not follow the dosage schedule the clinician recommends. In such cases, Sawin recommended that the clinician educate the patient about the importance of taking the right dosage on schedule. He also suggests that the clinician enlist the help of family or friends to induce the patient to comply.[85,p.397] With patients who are incorrigible in this respect, T_4 can be administered as an injection once each week.[86] This is certainly not the preferable schedule for taking T_4, but it may be better than the patient not taking the hormone at all. (T_4 binds tightly to plasma proteins and releases only slowly. The binding constitutes a hormone reserve that gradually expends itself. Because T_3 releases from circulating proteins more easily and is cleared more rapidly, this injection method is impractical with T_3.)

Special Considerations for Patients Taking T_3. Bastenie and others advised that the clinician not prescribe T_3 because of its rapid and intense action.[1,pp.124-125] The belief underlying this advice is that because T_3 is absorbed rapidly and the serum level peaks rapidly, the heart may be adversely impacted. The timing of effect of thyroid hormone on cardiac tissue is rapid. Nuclear effects (with increases in transcription and synthesis of enzyme and contractile proteins) occur within 30 minutes to an hour after thyroid hormone is administered to cardiac tissue. Extranuclear effects (such as transport of calcium, sugar, and amino acids across cell membranes, and increased mitochondrial activity) occur within minutes after the administration of thyroid hormone.[87]

It is not established, however, that single daily dosages of T_3 have adverse cardiac effects. During years of extensive electrocardiographic monitoring of euthyroid and hypothyroid fibromyalgia patients using single daily doses of T_3, I have not found the cardiac arrhythmias that some writers have expressed concern about. It is possible, of course, that fibromyalgia patients differ from the general population of hypothyroid patients Bastenie and others referred to and are not prone to adverse cardiac effects from single daily dosages of T_3. I think this is unlikely, however, in that hypothyroid fibromyalgia patients apparently differ from other hypothyroid patients only in their pheno-typic expression of the hormone deficiency. Nonetheless, the clinician should evaluate each patient as an individual. He should exercise extreme caution with the patient whose cardiac status is dubious. Such patients include those who are elderly, deconditioned, or who do not take nutritional supplements known to have cardio-protective effects. If a patient's cardiac status is questionable, she should undergo an evaluation by a cardiologist.

Adrenal Insufficiency

The hypothyroid patient may have hypofunction of the adrenal cortices. The adrenal cortices of some hypothyroid patients secrete a lower-than-normal amount of cortisol, and the patients' urinary excretion of 17-hydroxycorticosteroids[54,p.811] and 17-ketosteroids[57] is abnormally low. Treatment with thyroid hormone normalizes the values.[54,p.811] Autopsies of hypothyroid patients without pituitary lesions have shown that their adrenal cortices were normal, but one autopsy of a patient with advanced primary hypothyroidism revealed adrenal atrophy.[56] However, animals made hypothyroid by antithyroid drugs typically have adrenocortical atrophy.[32,p.1045]

Although adrenocortical production of cortisol may be reduced in hypothyroidism, the peripheral tissues may be exposed to normal amounts of cortisol. The reason for the normal exposure is that clearance of cortisol from the body is decreased in the hypothyroid patient.[54,p.811] In fact, the 24-hour serum cortisol concentration may be slightly elevated.[55]

The hypothyroid patient with adrenocortical hypofunction appears to have relative adrenal insufficiency. Under basal conditions, her adrenocortical output is usually sufficient to meet the requirement of her tissues for cortisol. Even during stress, her tissues may have sufficient exposure to cortisol because of her slowed hepatic cortisol clearance.[32,p.1046][57][58] Because of this, the patient may not have symptoms of cortisol deficiency until she is exposed to stressful conditions that substantially increase her tissue requirements for cortisol.

Thyroid hormone deficiency is not the only cause of relative adrenal insufficiency. When adrenal insufficiency is acute and severe, it justifies the diagnosis of Addison's disease. But adrenal insufficiency may also be chronic and mild, manifesting as a failure of the adrenal cortices to secrete enough cortisol to meet increased need during stress. The diagnosis in this case should be "decreased adrenal reserve." In either case, the use of exogenous thyroid hormone may exacerbate

the adrenal condition. The clinician should exercise extreme caution to rule out or properly treat any form of adrenal insufficiency before or at the time the patient begins thyroid hormone therapy.

Severe Adrenal Insufficiency. Primary adrenal insufficiency is rare, but it is associated with high morbidity and mortality if it is permitted to progress. Early recognition and intervention are vital in altering the course of acute adrenal insufficiency. Typical features include a constellation of nonspecific symptoms such as weakness, easy fatigability, nausea, anorexia, and weight loss.[88] The clinician should be especially suspicious if the patient has hyper-pigmentation of the skin and hypotension,[89] hypoglycemia,[90] low sodium and/or high potassium levels, a history of autoimmune diseases such as hypothyroidism or diabetes, recent prior use of exogenous steroids, or current use of anticoagulants. If the patient's status deteriorates (hypotension, fever, diminished mental status), especially when suffering from an acute illness, she should undergo aggressive treatment with synthetic corticosteroids even before laboratory testing confirms the diagnosis.[88][91]

Decreased Adrenal Reserve. In decreased adrenal reserve, normal amounts of glucocorticoids are secreted under non-stressful conditions, but during stress, the adrenal cortices are not able to secrete the additional amounts necessary to adapt to the stress. Theoretically, the patient's symptoms worsen during or following severely stressful experiences. In such patients, serum and urinary cortisol levels may be normal, but during the ACTH stimulation test, the cortisol level does not rise appropriately above the baseline value.

Testing for Adrenal Insufficiency. Diagnosis of adrenal insufficiency is best made with the use of the classic and well-established ACTH stimulation test for adrenocortical function. It is the cortisol-secreting fasciculata cells of the adrenal cortex that are tested with the procedure. In the test, the adrenal cortex is challenged with pure synthetic 1-24 ACTH, and the adrenocortical response is measured by an increase in the plasma level of cortisol. The test is quick, reliable, and safe.[173,p.319] Compared to the effects of porcine ACTH, adverse effects from synthetic ACTH are rare.[174][176]

In one study, adrenocortical response was not significantly different when 250 µg of ACTH was given by bolus injection versus ACTH given intravenously over a 2-hour period.[177] Longer exposure of the adrenal cortex to exogenous ACTH should generate progressively more hyperresponsiveness. The adrenal gland was hyperresponsive for as long as 3 days after an 8-hour infusion of ACTH, although the basal cortisol level had become normal again.[178]

ACTH Stimulation Test. Wood et al. introduced the ACTH test in 1965 after synthetic ACTH became available.[174] A baseline blood sample is taken for measuring the plasma cortisol level. ACTH (250 μg) is injected, and after 30 minutes, another blood sample is taken. (The 250 μg of synthetic ACTH is bioequivalent to 25 units of natural ACTH.) A variation, in which the second sample is taken at 60 minutes,[175] probably offers no advantage. The plasma cortisol response is more reproducible at 30 minutes than at 60 minutes.[173,p.320]

Time of Day. Some researchers have speculated that the normal decrease in basal levels of plasma cortisol during the day might be reflected in an alteration in responsiveness of the adrenal gland to exogenous ACTH.[173,p.321] However, ACTH stimulation tests of subjects at 8:00 am and at 4:00 pm showed no difference in the 30-minute adrenocortical response.[179] This was true even when subjects were given dexamethasone to cause lower basal cortisol levels. This finding confirms those of other researchers.[180][181] Nevertheless, most investigators prefer to perform the test between 6:00 am and 9:00 am, when the basal cortisol level in most patients is higher than it will be for the rest of the day.[173,p.322]

Adrenal Response Criteria. The debatable aspect of testing for adrenal insufficiency is in the interpretation of the results. Arguable issues involve what exactly constitutes an insufficient adrenocortical response to ACTH, and what the response means in terms of the integrity of the hypothalamic-pituitary-adrenal axis. In the United Kingdom, there has been little agreement on how to interpret the test among endocrinologists who use it.[182]

In interpreting the test result, the clinician may consider (1) the basal cortisol level, (2) the maximum cortisol level reached, and (3) the difference between the two, termed the incremental response.[173,p.322] The basal cortisol level may be increased significantly by circumstances such as apprehension, the pain of venipuncture, or illness at the time. Or, the cortex of the normal adrenal gland may be hypertrophied from prolonged exposure to ACTH during long-term stress. The incremental response can also vary, especially in patients experiencing acute stress. This appears as an increased basal level but without adrenocortical hypertrophy.

There is, however, some correlation between the three variables. The baseline cortisol level is positively correlated with the maximum post-injection level. The baseline level is also negatively correlated with the incremental response.[183][184] James[173,p.323] concluded that the maximum level at 30 minutes is the most definitive indicator of adrenocortical reserve. She wrote that for a patient with a high basal level and minimal peak response, it is not necessary that the patient have a normal increment. "Indeed," she wrote, "such a high resting level is in itself an indication of adequate adrenocortical responsiveness."[173,p.323]

According to Teitelbaum and Bird, during the ACTH stimulation test, the baseline serum cortisol level should be measured first. Then a 25-unit dose of cortrosyn (ACTH) should be injected intramuscularly. Again at 30 and 60 minutes post-injection, the serum cortisol levels should be checked. These authors consider a low baseline to be less than 6 μg/dL. They qualify, however, that some of their chronic fatigue patients have benefitted from glucocorticoid therapy even if the baseline was as high as 11 μg/dL. They consider a normal response to the injection to be doubling of the cortisol level at 1 hour or an increase of 7 μg/dL at 30 minutes and 11 μg/dL at 1 hour.[93,p.93]

Basal Cortisol Level. Hagg and coauthors reported a high positive correlation between the basal cortisol level and the peak response during the insulin-induced hypoglycemia test. They concluded that a basal level below 100 nmol/L strongly suggests dysfunction, and a level above 300 nmol/L virtually excludes ACTH insufficiency.[68]

Insulin-Induced Hypoglycemia Test. The ability of the pituitary gland to secrete ACTH in response to stress is best measured by the insulin-induced hypoglycemia test. The response is measured in terms of the plasma cortisol level. The test can reveal impaired pituitary secretion of ACTH, whereas the ACTH stimulation test *theoretically* could show normal adrenocortical reserve despite impaired ACTH secretion. However, impaired function of the hypothalamic-pituitary-adrenal axis, with reduced exposure of the adrenal cortex to ACTH, is likely to be accompanied by some degree of adrenocortical atrophy. If so, then the result of the ACTH stimulation test is likely to show impaired function of the hypothalamic-pituitary-adrenal axis.[173,p.323] The available evidence supports this proposition.

A number of studies have shown a highly significant correlation between the cortisol response to the insulin-induced hypoglycemia test and the ACTH stimulation test.[128][129][144][182] The studies indicate that in most cases the ACTH test can replace the insulin-induced hypoglycemia test.[83] Advantages of the

ACTH stimulation test are that it is less difficult to perform, is more pleasant for the patient, and is potentially less harmful than the insulin-induced hypoglycemia test.[173,p.323]

Low Dose Hydrocortisone Treatment for Adrenal Insufficiency. Jefferies recommended as low dose hydrocortisone, 5 mg qid.[95][96] Teitelbaum and Bird, however, report that most patients with low adrenocortical reserve respond well to 5 mg Cortef (hydrocortisone) in the morning and, if necessary, 2.5-to-5 mg at lunchtime. Some of their patients have required 5-to-7.5 mg tid or qid.[93,pp.93-94] The object of this regimen is to approximate the levels of cortisol that result from the circadian rhythm of the endogenous hormone.[94,p.254] In most people, the levels are maximum at 8 am. Levels decrease through the day and reach the lowest point about 1 am. If it is effective for the patient, she should take a lower dose in the evening in an attempt to approximate the normal circadian rhythm of the endogenous hormone.

Low Dose Hydrocortisone Therapy and the Question of Suppression of Adrenocortical Function. The prolonged use of large dosages of hydrocortisol may result in permanent suppression of adrenocortical function. A full replacement dose of hydrocortisone is roughly 40 mg/day taken in 4 divided doses of 10 mg each. Jefferies defined low dosage hydrocortisone therapy as a total of 20 mg or less per day, in divided doses at maximum intervals of 8 hours. This dosage usually partially inhibits ACTH secretion by the pituitary gland as a compensatory reaction and suppresses adrenocortical function to about 50% of the normal level.[96,p.267] According to Jefferies, this leaves sufficient adrenal function to allow adequate responses to stress. It also avoids the complete suppression of endogenous androgen synthesis. Complete suppression of the synthesis of androgen may be responsible for the higher incidence of adverse effects in women than in men.[96,p.276]

Jefferies wrote that low dosage hydrocortisone therapy only partially suppresses adrenocortical function, and it does not cause hypercorticism (as a summation effect of endogenous and exogenous cortisol) except for the first few days of treatment while the hypothalamic-pituitary-adrenal axis adjusts. Thus, it does not lower resistance to stress. He concluded, "It is consequently not accompanied by the hazards that attend the use of larger doses."[96,p.271]

Essentially, low dose hydrocortisone therapy appears to be effective and safe, even for prolonged use, and provides therapeutic effects without causing an excess of glucocorticoids in the body. Jefferies' view is supported by a study reporting no adverse effects in 38 male volunteers who took low dose (20 mg) hydrocortisone therapy for 3 years. Thirteen of the subjects underwent 15 major surgical procedures without additional glucocorticoid therapy with no indication of adrenal insufficiency.[172] Similarly, Jefferies found no signs of hypercorticism in 339 women using low dose glucocorticoids for periods ranging from 6 months-to-9 years.[96,p.277] He also reported that a search of the literature failed to produce any reports of the signs or symptoms of hypercorticism in patients taking low dose glucocorticoids. There were also no reports of such patients failing to respond properly to stress. This suggests that low dose hydrocortisone therapy corrects decreased adrenal reserve.[96,p.276]

Adrenal Insufficiency in Pituitary Hypothyroidism. The possibility of adrenal insufficiency should always be considered in the patient with pituitary hypothyroidism.[92,p.380] Pituitary hypothyroidism is diagnosed by either a low serum free T_4 and a normal or low basal TSH, or by a blunted 30-minute TSH response to a TRH injection (see Chapter 4.2, section titled "TRH-Stimulation Test"). These test results indicate an impairment in the synthesis and secretion of TSH by the anterior pituitary gland. When the anterior pituitary produces too little TSH, it may also produce too little ACTH. ACTH stimulates the cortices of the adrenal glands to release adrenocortical hormones (see Chapter 3.5). Under-stimulation of the cortices by ACTH may be sufficient to constitute decreased adrenal reserve or, more seriously, frank adrenal insufficiency. When a cortisol-deficient patient takes exogenous thyroid hormone and her metabolism is accelerated, the lowered amount of cortisol will be catabolized rapidly, provoking an adrenal crisis. Because of this, thyroid hormone therapy is contraindicated during adrenal insufficiency. The clinician should correct the patient's adrenal insufficiency first or simultaneously with thyroid therapy.[89] Severe adrenal insufficiency should be corrected *before* the patient begins thyroid hormone therapy.

Estrogen and Progesterone Deficiency

According to Travell, to avoid estrogen deficiency symptoms, women who begin taking exogenous thyroid hormone may have to increase their estrogen intake slightly.[185] I have found this to be true of some fibromyalgic women. For example, some post-menopausal women, subsequent to beginning exogenous thyroid hormone, begin experiencing hot flushes until their estrogen doses are increased. Episodes of excess body heat due to estrogen deficiency are distinguishable from the heat intolerance from excessive thyroid hormone. While the latter is steady and lasts continually until the thyroid hormone dosage is reduced, the former tends to occur as episodic surges of extreme heat, interspersed with episodes of normal body temperature.

Osteoporosis

The osteoporotic patient should have a baseline bone density study and repeat studies at 6-month intervals after beginning the use of exogenous thyroid hormone. With the dosages that most fibromyalgia patients require for improvement or recovery, biochemical tests for bone turnover may be temporarily positive. Serum and urinary calcium, phosphorus, and alkaline phosphatase are usually normal. More sensitive tests, such as the urinary cross-linked N-telopeptides (a specific marker for bone resorption), may be positive although clinically insignificant (see Chapter 4.4, section titled "Bone Density").

The clinician must evaluate each patient individually. Some patients occupy a wing of the bell curve for progressively exaggerated impact of exogenous thyroid hormone on bone. Generally, though, while overt hyperthyroidism with osseous thyrotoxicosis is a risk factor for bone turnover and for decreases in bone density, recent studies have not shown substantial T_4-related changes in bone mass. The available evidence suggests that TSH-suppressive therapy with T_4 does not induce significant loss of bone mass, at least in premenopausal women.[146] And TSH-suppressive thyroid hormone therapy has not been proven to lead to manifest osteoporosis (see Chapter 4.4, section titled "Bone Density").

Normal plasma estrogens help prevent osteoporosis in women.[148] In postmenopausal women, estrogen use is associated with increased bone mineral density.[149] The clinician should carefully monitor postmenopausal women with previous hyperthyroidism who were treated with radioiodine therapy. Their bone densities tend to be lower whether they have used T_4 or not. Periodic densitometry is advisable, and estrogen supplementation should be considered. Postmenopausal women with previous hyperthyroidism treated with surgery appear to be at less risk for bone loss.[150]

If bone density is decreased significantly, the patient may be treated with an osteoblast stimulant such as sodium fluoride or an osteoclast inhibitor such as calcitonin or diphosphate (see Chapter 4.4, section titled "Bone Formation Stimulation"). The patient should also use mineral supplements (including 1-to-2 gm of calcium), "bone-jerking" or weight-bearing types of exercises calibrated to tolerance, and possibly female sex hormone replacement if she is post-menopausal. The osteoporotic patient may have to settle for a thyroid hormone dosage calculated to favor reinstitution of bone density. (See Chapter 4.4, section titled "Bone Density.")

Catabolism and Weight Loss

Some patients may experience catabolism with loss of lean tissue mass and weight after their metabolism is increased to normal with thyroid hormone simply because they are accustomed to consuming small quantities of food each day. In most cases, the lost lean tissue and weight are recovered when the patient begins consuming a sufficient amount of food each day. In these cases, the problem is not an excessive dosage of thyroid hormone but a deficient consumption of food.

In one case under my care, the patient's debilitating pain was mitigated only with a T_3 dosage that induced moderate catabolism. When taking a high enough dosage of T_3 to satisfactorily reduce her pain, she experienced loss of lean tissue mass and weight. Her pain had been so severe and debilitating that she previously had been hospitalized several times for as long as a week to be treated with intravenous narcotics. She objected to reducing her T_3 dosage to a level that would allow the debilitating pain to return. Other than the loss of lean tissue and weight, she had no other indications of tissue thyrotoxicity. Because of this, and because she had customarily consumed only a small amount of food each day, she continued her pain-reducing T_3 dosage. However, she increased her consumption of food each day to a level that allowed her to recover and maintain normal lean tissue mass and weight despite continuing the same T_3 dosage.

The approach taken with this patient was based on recommendations in the thyroidology literature for dealing with thyrotoxic catabolism (though my patient had no other evidence of thyrotoxicity). When a thyrotoxic patient is catabolic and losing weight, she can counterbalance the catabolism by "adequate protein in the diet and a sufficient increase in caloric intake."[97,p.333] In fact, despite the increased catabolism of fats, carbohydrates, and proteins in thyrotoxicosis, the catabolism ". . . can be minimized, and indeed in some instances positive nitrogen balance can be achieved, if the thyrotoxic state is accompanied by sufficient protein and carbohydrate intake."[98,pp.845-853] In regard to patients with severe illness taking T_3, DeGroot stated, "We recommend full nutritional support to avoid starvation because that is a far more important cause of tissue catabolism than a T_3 supplement."[99,p.23]

The key concern of the clinician should be that the patient's dosage is not inducing thyrotoxicosis of tissues such as bone and heart. Whether or not this is occurring can be determined through bone density and cardiac evaluations. However, inferences about possible tissue thyrotoxicosis based on circulating levels of TSH or thyroid hormones are not valid and have no clinical value.

Ideally, the patient and clinician should find a compromise dosage of thyroid hormone low enough to avoid catabolism but high enough to minimize or relieve fibromyalgia symptoms and signs.

COMPLIANCE: INSISTING THE PATIENT COOPERATE WITH PROPER PROTOCOL

As a precaution, I encourage clinicians to be vigilant for patients who do not cooperate in the proper use of exogenous thyroid hormone. Some patients find exercising "too hard" or obnoxious and refuse to engage in it. Other patients will not take nutritional supplements. Some complain that taking B complex vitamins on an empty stomach nauseates them, yet they decline to take the vitamins with food. Some of these patients expect exogenous thyroid hormone to relieve symptoms that are partly a product of inactivity and nutritional insufficiencies. Typically, such patients' symptoms improve somewhat with thyroid hormone. But without exercise and nutritional supplements, most of these patients remain symptomatic to some degree. Many of them state that they expect to improve further if they can progressively increase their thyroid hormone dosage. Some will increase it against the clinician's advice. Many such patients already have an increased probability of lifestyle-related cardiac abnormalities. Such abnormalities may be exacerbated by the increase in heart rate and force of contraction induced by thyroid hormone. Beyond some dosage threshold unique to each such patient, further increases are potentially hazardous. *Unless this type of patient can be induced to cooperate, it is in the patient's and the clinician's best interests that the patient's prescription for thyroid hormone be discontinued.*

Stopping the Use of Medications that Interfere with Metabolic Treatment. Some patients are not able to muster the drive to exercise because of their use of medications such as Vicodin, Xanax, or Soma Compound. These drugs may have previously made

life tolerable, but they can limit the benefits the patient derives from a metabolically-based therapeutic regimen. It is judicious of the clinician to obtain a commitment from new patients to stop these medications in the proper way as early into their metabolic treatment as possible. Patients should be required to abide by their commitment. Unfortunately, some patients are not willing to forfeit the use of such medications.

Other medications that may interfere with metabolic treatment are antidepressant medications. These alone may cause tachycardia and ischemic heart disease. Thyroid hormone typically increases the heart rate as it increases the density of β-adrenergic receptors on cardiac muscle. In some patients, the simultaneous use of antidepressants and thyroid hormone causes a greater increase in heart rate than does either medication alone. Patients should therefore stop the use of the antidepressants as early as possible during metabolic therapy. There is little point in taking them anyway. The only long-term study of their effects with fibromyalgia patients showed that other than a faint improvement in roughly a third of patients during the first month of use, the drugs are no more effective than placebos. (See Chapter 5.1, section titled "Antidepressant Drugs.") Some patients report that they are not able to sleep without these drugs, but it is possible that this is a placebo effect. Most of my patients sleep quite well by taking 50 mg of diphenhydramine HCL 30 minutes before bedtime if necessary. Diphenhydramine has a short half-life, and some patients must take another 50 mg after 4 or 5 hours of sleep.

If they are to improve, it is critical that patients stop the long-term use of β-blocking medications. β-Blockers nullify the β-adrenergic effects of thyroid hormone, and it is largely these effects that mediate the metabolism acceleration from thyroid hormone. Some patients take β-blockers for mild hypertension. But the hypertension is often a result of inadequate thyroid hormone regulation of transcription, and the proper form and dosage of thyroid hormone can reduce the blood pressure to normal. The tendency of β-blockers to cause disturbed sleep, fatigue, and depression highlights the molecular pathway that leads from inadequate thyroid hormone to fibromyalgia symptoms.

MANAGING THYROTOXIC REACTIONS TO EXCESSIVE INTAKE OF EXOGENOUS THYROID HORMONE

If the patient takes an excess of T_4, she can take the β-blocker propranolol to stop thyrotoxic symptoms such as tachycardia and tremors.[100][101] Thyrotoxic symptoms such as tremors are relieved in most fibromyalgia patients within 20-to-30 minutes after taking 20-to-60 mg. The prescription should be for 20 mg plain tablets. Much higher dosages of sustained-release propranolol may be required to stop acute thyrotoxic symptoms.[113,p.234] But this form of the medication is not as useful for prompt management of thyrotoxicity. And, the risks for reactivating fibromyalgia symptoms are greater with the higher dosage of the more slowly-acting, sustained-release propranolol.

Peak effects of propranolol occur within 1-to-2 hours after ingestion. The half-life of propranolol is 3 hours,[104,p.766] but the relief it provides may last from 2-to-10 hours. Some effects, such as anti-hypertension, last sufficiently long so that the patient may have to take tablets only once or twice per day.[113,p.234] I have seen some fibromyalgia patients whose cardiac and neuromuscular overstimulation was blocked effectively for a full day by one 40 mg dose of propranolol. Most patients, however, require two or more dosages during a day to alleviate acute thyrotoxic symptoms.

Patients taking T_3 may have to use propranolol only 1-to-2 days because the excess T_3 is depleted from the body rapidly. By contrast, overdosage with T_4 may require that the patient take propranolol for a longer time, perhaps for 1-to-2 weeks. The excess T_4 may take that long to be depleted.

The preferential binding of propranolol to β-adrenergic receptors effectively blocks the receptors' from binding to epinephrine and norepinephrine. Since cAMP in cells is formed when β-adrenergic receptors are exposed to epinephrine and norepinephrine, propranolol indirectly lowers formation of cAMP.[107][108] Propranolol also lowers elevated serum and urine calcium and decreases the excess urinary hydroxyproline that can result from thyroid hormone excess.[105][106]

Rarely, the drug may enhance hypoglycemia after meals in a patient with alimentary or idiopathic hypoglycemia.[110] Alimentary hypoglycemia occurs after meals in patients who have had surgery that removed part of the stomach or small intestine.[109,pp.1191-1192] Normally, circulating epinephrine has an inhibiting effect on insulin. When propranolol exerts its β-adrenergic blocking effect, removal of this normal insulin restrainer may result in cellular hypersensitivity to insulin so that glucose is removed from the circulation too rapidly, inducing hypoglycemia. The effect is more likely in insulin-treated diabetics during bouts of exercise.[109,p.1195]

Patients for whom β-blocking drugs are contra-indicated, such as those with asthma, may be able to control cardiac thyrotoxicosis with calcium channel-blocking drugs.[102] These drugs have α-adrenergic but not β-adrenergic blocking properties.[127,p.869] The calcium channel blockers verapamil and diltiazim, used as anti-arrhythmic drugs, impede cardiac impulse formation. *In vitro*, they slow the spontaneous firing of pacemaker cells in the sinus node. *In vivo*, however, the heart rate may decrease only minimally. This is because the effect of the medication is countered by an increase in reflex sympathetic nervous system activity due to the dilation of arteries.[127,p.869]

Choice of β-Blocking Drugs

β-Blocking drugs are not considered antithyroid drugs *per se* (they do not inhibit synthesis or secretion of thyroid hormones by the thyroid gland). They are, however, an important part of the armamentarium for treatment of hyperthyroidism.[111,p.900][112] Propranolol, a β_1 and β_2 antagonist, tends to inhibit conversion by deiodinase of T_4 to T_3, and in this sense it may be considered an antithyroid drug. This blocking effect may be desirable when treating hyperthyroidism. But when attempting to block acute tissue overstimulation from excessive doses of exogenous thyroid hormone, the clinician may prefer not to block deiodination. Refetoff, Weiss, and Usala recommend atenolol, a β_1 antagonist that inhibits T_4 to T_3 conversion less than propranolol[115,p.390] and has the benefit of a longer duration of action.[111,p.900] Very little atenolol penetrates the blood/brain barrier.[113,p.237] As a result, its use over prolonged periods may have fewer adverse central nervous system effects than propranolol, which readily passes the blood/brain barrier[113,p.233] (see below).

When the sole aim is to stop the cardiac effects of excess thyroid hormone intake, esmolol, a cardio-selective β_1-blocker, may be used. Unfortunately, it must be administered by intravenous infusion and has a rapid onset (6-to-10 minutes) and offset (20 minutes).[113,p.237] Although not of practical value for most fibromyalgia patients, this drug may be appropriate for patients whose pain is relieved only with dosages of exogenous thyroid hormone that induce undesirable inotropic and chronotropic cardiac effects. Theoretically, the cardiac overstimulation can be blocked while the patient takes a dosage of thyroid hormone that effectively reduces or relieves pain. But the drug may have a profound hypotensive effect[113,p.237] and should be used with caution in fibromyalgia/chronic fatigue syndrome patients, many of whom are already hypotensive.

Precautions in the Use of β-Blocking Drugs

β-Blocking drugs are valuable as adjuncts to be used only sparingly during the course of metabolic treatment of *some* fibromyalgia patients. It is critical, however, that the clinician and patient understand the function of these drugs and take proper and necessary precaution in their use.

Caution with Patients with Cardiac Abnormalities. Of the body systems, it is the cardiovascular system that responds most profoundly to β-blocking drugs. Heart rate and cardiac output are rapidly decreased by these drugs. They also may nullify the sympathetic drive of the myocardium. Because of this, β-blockers may be used with caution with patients who have minor cardiac compromise associated with thyrotoxicosis, but they should not be used with patients who have moderate-to-severe congestive heart failure.[117,p.705][118] Large dosages of propranolol should not be used with patients whose cardiac function is compromised.[117,p.703]

Atherosclerosis may improve in hypothyroid patients who take exogenous thyroid hormone. However, patients with angina pectoris constitute a dilemma in that the thyroid hormone may worsen the symptom. The patient may take β-blockers, but these can cause angina because they increase norepinephrine secretion. The norepinephrine binds to α-adrenergic receptors, which are increased in hypothyroidism,[143] decreasing heart rate and increasing peripheral vascular resistance, including the coronary arteries.

Ellyin et al. pointed out that management of patients with chest pain and hypothyroidism is a clinical dilemma. Thyroid replacement therapy may exacerbate angina pectoris. Administration of a β-blocker such as propranolol (Inderal) concomitantly with thyroid replacement therapy is useful in treatment of angina. The β-blockers, however, may also induce angina. This may occur because of an increase in norepinephrine secretion and interaction of the norepinephrine with α-adrenergic receptors (the density of which is increased in cardiac cell membranes in hypothyroidism).[143] The clinician must take care, then, in the use of β-blocking medications.

Patients taking medications that impair sinus-node function (such as the calcium-channel blocker varapamil and various anti-arrhythmic drugs[113,p.238]) should be especially cautious in using β-blocking drugs.

Asthmatic Patients Should Not Use β-Blocking Drugs. β-Blocking drugs are contraindicated for patients with asthma or a history of bronchospasm. Blockade of $β_2$-adrenergic receptors, which mediate brochodilation, may induce life-threatening resistance to airflow in asthmatic patients.[113,p.239]

Fibromyalgia Patients Must Not Use a β-Blocking Drug as Maintenance Medication. I must emphasize that the fibromyalgia patient should *not* use any β-blocking drug except for *acute* management of thyrotoxicosis due to *excess* intake of thyroid hormone. Most patients do not have adverse consequences under two conditions: when they use the drug only in small doses to control acute thyrotoxic reactions, and when they stop the drug after the reduced thyroid hormone dosage takes effect.

All clinicians should bear in mind that the use of a β-blocking drug over a prolonged time or in moderate-to-large doses may induce or intensify fibromyalgia symptoms in many patients. I have had some patients—who had apparently been marginally hypometabolic—whose fibromyalgia began shortly after they began taking a β-blocking drug. For most of these patients, fibromyalgia symptoms ceased after (as part of their metabolic therapy) they stopped taking the drug. This observation warrants repetition and elaboration because of the potential of β-blocking drugs for inducing fibromyalgia. Some patients' fibromyalgia begins when they begin taking a β-blocking medication to control symptoms of mitral valve prolapse. This iatrogenic form of fibromyalgia is fairly common, probably because there is a high incidence of mitral valve prolapse among fibromyalgia patients (Pelligrino et al. reported a 75% incidence[192]), and β-blockers are commonly prescribed to control symptoms of mitral valve prolapse. In these patients, use of the medication appears to create an α-adrenergic dominance that mediates the fibromyalgia symptoms and signs. In some cases, the symptoms and signs of α-adrenergic dominance, which clinicians diagnose as fibromyalgia, cease when the patient stops the medication. In most cases, however, the patient must also undergo metabolic rehabilitation to fully recover metabolic sufficiency. (For more on mitral valve prolapse in fibromyalgia patients, see Chapter 3.3.)

One of the theses of this book is that fibromyalgia results in part from the inhibitory cellular effects of a shift away from α-adrenoceptor/β-adrenoceptor balance toward α-adrenoceptor dominance. The therapeutic effect of the exogenous thyroid hormone used by fibromyalgia patients partly involves correction of this imbalance. β-Blocking drugs, by competitively binding to β-adrenergic receptors, prevent catecholamines from binding to the receptors and block the metabolism-stimulating effects of the catecholamines. Knowledge of this pharmacologic phenomenon permits prediction of the development of fibromyalgia symptoms with the daily use of β-blocking drugs by individuals who already have marginally sufficient cellular metabolism. Adverse central nervous system effects from β-blocking drugs include fatigue, sleep disturbances (insomnia and nightmares), and depression.[113,p.239][116] Peripheral effects include cold extremities,[113,p.238] impaired cardiovascular adjustment to submaximal exercise,[113,p.232] and bradycardia.[117,p.705] Such adverse effects are especially likely with the prolonged use of propranolol because, in contrast to atenolol, it readily passes the blood/brain barrier.[113,p.233]

Corticosteroids

Corticosteroids, such as prednisone or dexamethasone, prevent conversion of T_4 to T_3. They will stop endogenous or T_4-exogenous thyrotoxic symptoms.[2,p.188][119][120] Such drugs quickly reduce the T_4 and T_3 levels in thyrotoxic patients with Graves' disease.[119] Rather than corticosteroids, however, the use of β-blockers is preferable with fibromyalgia patients.

SOME PATIENTS DO NOT IMPROVE WITH T_4 OR DESICCATED THYROID BUT DO RESPOND TO T_3

If the patient's laboratory test results originally (pre-treatment with thyroid hormone) confirmed hypothyroidism, she should not cease using exogenous thyroid hormone even though she may not have shown much symptom improvement. There are distinct health hazards from inadequate cell regulation by thyroid hormone due to untreated hypothyroidism. These include general physical, hepatic, cardiovascular, and neurological damage (see Chapter 4.4, section titled "Harm from Untreated and Undertreated Hypothyroidism").

For some hypothyroid fibromyalgia patients, T_4 and desiccated thyroid are simply not effective (even at dosages as high as 0.40 mg and 4 grains, respectively). Some hypothyroid patients do not absorb T_4 at a normal rate. As a result, despite taking relatively large dosages, their serum TSH levels may remain elevated. There are several possible reasons for inadequate absorption. The patient may have an intestinal mucosal disease such as sprue, or a short bowel from post-jejunoileal bypass. The rate of absorption may be decreased because of the use of sucralfate, aluminum hydroxide, ferrous sulfate, or cholestyramine. Or the intestinal clearance rate may be increased by the use of rifampin, carbamazepine, or phenytoin.[121,p.886]

Another cause of inadequate absorption may be the brand of T_4. All brands have the same hormone content, but different brands of tablets are broken down at different rates in the GI tract. With a brand that breaks down more slowly, the patient with short transit time may not absorb enough of the T_4.[122][123] In such cases, changing brands may relieve the problem. But some patients must change the form of thyroid hormone to T_3 because it is more easily absorbed.[121,p.886] For other patients, something besides inadequate absorption accounts for a failure to benefit from T_4.

This was a subject of consideration in 1943. Winkler studied patients who failed to respond to desiccated thyroid or T_4 except in very large dosages. He wrote that deficient absorption could not be entirely eliminated as an explanation, but "there are weighty arguments against it." First, as far as he could determine, his patients had no other defect in absorption and no gastrointestinal lesions. Second, he was aware of no case in which a hypothyroid patient did not respond to oral desiccated thyroid or T_4 but did respond to injected thyroid hormone. This suggested to him that malabsorption of desiccated thyroid and T_4 was not common. And third, failure to absorb desiccated thyroid or T_4 did not explain these patients' measurably reduced responses to injected T_4. He had to inject some patients with large dosages of T_4 intravenously to increase their BMRs. He tentatively concluded that the hormone is inactivated after absorption or injection. The amount of T_4 in the injection exceeded the rate at which the hormone was being inactivated, while hormones being absorbed and entering the system more slowly were inactivated before being able to exert metabolic effects.[124,pp.542-543] In a small percentage of my hypothyroid fibromyalgia patients and most euthyroid hypometabolic fibromyalgia patients, it is clear from their suppressed third-generation serum TSH levels that they have absorbed large dosages of T_4. Yet these dosages are not of benefit, although the patients subsequently improve or recover with the use of T_3.

In 1995, I published the case history of a hypothyroid fibromyalgia patient who failed to respond to large dosages of either desiccated thyroid or T_4, but she promptly recovered from all fibromyalgia symptoms when, at my request, her psychiatrist switched her to T_3.[125] Other authors have described similar cases. In 1959, for example, Wilson and Walton reported the case of a woman whose only hypothyroid symptoms were muscle aches and pains, fatigue that began an hour after she got out of bed, weakness when climbing stairs, and an "after-tennis feeling" of her muscles. She had antibodies to thyroglobulin, suggesting hypothyroidism due to thyroiditis (Hashimoto's disease). The patient was given lactose tablets as a placebo but did not improve. However, 40 µg of T_3 daily resulted in prompt remission of symptoms and a feeling of well-being. "During the succeeding weeks, all muscular pain and weakness vanished, the patient became energetic and symptom-free, and was able to return to her previous occupation. After six months' treatment with triiodothyronine [T_3], dried thyroid extract [desiccated thyroid], 3 grains daily, was begun, and two weeks later, tri-iodothyronine was withdrawn. In another two weeks the muscular pain and aching had returned. Owing to increasingly severe symptoms, tri-iodothyronine was again given, with prompt and sustained remission and the patient has remained well for one year, taking 40 µg of this drug daily."[126,p.321]

Wilson and Walton also reported that other hypothyroid patients with muscle symptoms responded rapidly to T_3. One patient had generalized aches and pains. She took 40 µg of T_3, and "when next seen one week later she was asymptomatic and composed. All the muscular pain and stiffness had disappeared."[126,p.321] About another patient who began taking 20 µg of T_3 bid, they said, "Within a few days, all muscular pain and stiffness had disappeared and the carpopedal spasms were greatly reduced in frequency and severity."[126,p.322] When rapid improvement is a therapeutic goal with hypothyroid patients, T_3 is preferable.

Determining Whether the Patient Taking T_4 or Desiccated Thyroid Is Improving

Whether or not the hypothyroid fibromyalgia patient is benefitting from T_4 or desiccated thyroid should be determined by the use of repeated fibromyalgia assessments. These should involve mean symptom intensity using the VAS, pain distribution measured by the percentage method, tender point pressure/pain threshold measured with algometry, the Fibromyalgia Impact Questionnaire, and a paper-and-pencil depression test such as Zung's or Beck's. The single mathematical score for each of these measures should be posted to a line graph for each measure (see earlier in this chapter). From these, over sequential assessments, it should be clear whether the patient's fibromyalgia status is changing in a positive direction.

For most patients, if they are responding to progressively increased dosages of T_4 or desiccated thyroid, the speed of the relaxation phase of the Achilles reflex will increase gradually over repeated exams.

The resting pulse rate usually increases as well. (In the presence of the clinician, the pulse rate may be substantially increased over the resting rate, and the pulse may be increased to highly variable rates. Because of this, it is usually best for the patient to take the resting pulse rate at home after relaxing in a comfortable sitting position and after imaging some scene that for her is pleasant and calming.) The patient's ECG may also show alterations indicating a positive cardiovascular response to the thyroid hormone (see Chapter 4.3, section titled "Heart Function").

I cannot emphasize enough, however, that none of these physiological indices of response to exogenous thyroid hormone is entirely reliable alone. We are not necessarily concerned with "improvement" in these indices, but rather with improvement in the five fibromyalgia measures combined with positive changes in the indices. Within a short time frame, the patient's subjective status usually reflects her status according to the fibromyalgia measures. The aim is to improve the patient's fibromyalgia status by manipulating these measures through metabolic therapy.

Indications of Excessive Tissue Stimulation Without Improvement in Fibromyalgia Measures

For patients who do not respond to T_4 or desiccated thyroid, scores on the fibromyalgia measures and the physical indices of metabolic status may not change at all (or only to an insignificant degree) in a favorable direction. For some patients, however, while scores on the fibromyalgia measures do not change, physical indices may indicate overstimulation of target tissues. The tissues most often affected are the neuromuscular system (tremors and restlessness), the cardiovascular system (almost constant palpitations), the thermogenic systems (constant excess body heat), or the central nervous system (irritability). It is a paradox that these patients appear to be overstimulated, yet their fibromyalgia measures do not change. In some patients, however, in concert with physical indices of overstimulation, the fibromyalgia measures worsen.

With this outcome, the clinician should question the patient to determine whether she is taking nutritional supplements, particularly B complex vitamins. Failing to do so may account for the poor therapeutic response. Accelerating cellular metabolism with thyroid hormone may induce frank vitamin deficiencies in patients who do not take supplemental B vitamins (or who take supplements containing nothing more than the RDAs).

The clinician should also inquire about the patient's level of physical activity. Regular exercise can improve and hasten the patient's response to exogenous thyroid hormone.

Switching the Patient from T₄ or Desiccated Thyroid Hormone to T₃

Some patients will not benefit from the use of T_4 or desiccated thyroid despite high dosages. Some will have some indication(s) of tissue thyrotoxicosis. Typically, if a patient is not benefitting by the time she reaches a dosage of either 0.4 mg of T_4 or 4 grains of desiccated thyroid, we switch her to T_3. (This assumes that the patient also did not show signs of overstimulation on a lower dose, in which case we would have switched her to T_3 before reaching this dosage level.) Virtually all hypothyroid fibromyalgia patients who do not improve with T_4 or desiccated thyroid improve or recover with the use of T_3. In most cases, the improvement occurs with supraphysiologic dosages but without evidence of thyrotoxicosis.

T_4 binds tightly to transport proteins in the blood and releases gradually over 10 days-to-2 weeks. As a result, the T_4 (including the T_4 contained in desiccated thyroid hormone) a patient took up to 2 weeks before may currently be driving her metabolism to some degree. So when switching a non-responding patient from T_4 to T_3, the clinician should have the patient completely eliminate her dose of T_4 and introduce T_3 in gradually increased daily doses over a 2-week period. This gradual increase in dosage should culminate at the full (but minimum) dose the patient is likely to respond to. If this calculated dose is 75 µg, for example, the patient might abstain from taking T_3 (and T_4) for the first week, then begin with 6.25 µg (¼ of a 25 µg tablet) of T_3 on the 8th day. From the 9th day through the 14th day, the patient may increase the dose to, respectively, 12.5 µg, 25 µg, 37.5 µg, 50 µg, 62.5 µg, and 75 µg.

These doses, however, are somewhat arbitrary. The clinician should communicate with the patient to make sure the combination of T_3 and the T_4 remaining in his or her system does not cause overstimulation. This usually manifests as tremors, palpitations, excess body heat, diarrhea, irritability, or other such symptoms (see Chapter 4.4). If these become bothersome or threaten the patient's welfare, reduce the T_3 dosage slightly and have the patient take 20-to-40 mg of propranolol every 6 hours or so. This will control the symptoms until the reduced thyroid hormone dosage relieves the overstimulation without propranolol.

STOPPING AN UNSUCCESSFUL TRIAL OF THYROID HORMONE THERAPY

In rare cases, a patient may have to stop taking exogenous thyroid hormone, although she has benefitted from it. For example, an underlying cardiac abnormality may be discovered that would best be managed or corrected in the absence of cardiac stimulation by exogenous thyroid hormone.

When the patient ceases taking exogenous thyroid hormone, her former symptoms and signs of hypometabolism will resume. However, reducing the dosage of thyroid hormone gradually may prevent or minimize additional symptoms and signs due to rebound hypometabolism. If safety considerations permit such a gradual retrograding of dosage, the patient may avoid a rebound by reducing her dosage by ¼ every 1-to-2 weeks. The gradual reduction in dosage may allow enough time for her pituitary and thyroid glands to increase, according to their capabilities, the secretion of their respective hormones. The gradually increased secretion of thyroid hormone by the thyroid gland may avert a precipitous decrease of the circulating thyroid hormone level due to the patient's decreased consumption of exogenous thyroid hormone.

When the patient stops taking exogenous thyroid hormone, she is likely to go through an adaptation period of hypometabolism. During this time, she is likely to experience a recurrence or intensification of the symptoms and signs the exogenous thyroid hormone had relieved. After stopping the hormone, it may take 4-to-6 weeks, or longer in some individuals, before the TSH rises to its pre-treatment level. (Exogenous thyroid hormone is likely to suppress TSH secretion.) If the patient's thyroid function was normal before treatment, after the adaptation period has passed, the T_3, T_4, and TSH levels should return to some point within the normal range. If the patient's thyroid function was deficient, however, the values will assume a pattern that reflects the status of the patient's hypothalamic-pituitary-thyroid axis. (The ability to make this type of comparison is another reason why baseline determination of the patient's thyroid status is essential.)

The clinician should inform the patient about this period of hypometabolism. Experiencing this without prior warning can be unnecessarily distressing to the patient.

OTHER BIOCHEMICAL AGENTS THAT MAY BE USEFUL DURING THE INITIAL PHASE OF METABOLIC TREATMENT

The agents I discuss in this section have proven useful to me in treating some patients, and I recommend that the clinician use the agents selectively as appropriate in individual cases. However, it is critically important that the clinician not use these agents or others to attain some degree of control over the patient's symptoms and then neglect to correct the underlying mechanism of the patient's fibromyalgia through comprehensive metabolic rehabilitation. Metabolic rehabilitation is the *sine qua non* of effective fibromyalgia treatment; the other agents are merely ancillary.

Somniferous Agents

Several antihistamines are likely to help prolong sleep in patients who wake too easily. For many patients, 25-to-50 mg diphenhydramine hydrochloride before sleep appears to facilitate more restful and prolonged sleep. As Travell and Simons noted, diphenhydramine (Benadryl is one brand name) has a short half-life, and most patients need to take another 25-to-50 mg after 4 hours sleep to continue the benefits. Some patients report, however, that a 12.5-to-25 mg dosage is sufficient to prolong sleep for 6-to-8 hours. Travell and Simons point out that 50 mg of diphenhydrinate (Dramamine) is a more potent soporific than diphenhydramine. They also recommend Phenergan (promethazine), 12.5 mg at bedtime, for patients who fall asleep easily but wake too easily and often. This medication also has an anxiolytic effect.[21,p.91]

Although diphenhydramine is useful for deeper and more prolonged sleep, it does not facilitate the initiation of sleep in many patients. Another medication, Ambien (zolpidem), a medication presently in widespread use by fibromyalgia patients, is effective for most patients in initiating sleep. Ambien is a hypnotic drug that selectively binds in the central nervous system to benzodiazepine receptors. (Benzodiazepine drugs that also attach to these receptors include Valium, Xanax, Librium, Halcion, and Ativan.) Ambien is short-acting, having a 2.5 hour half-life.

Ambien is especially effective for relieving transient insomnia, such as that induced by stress, jet lag, and attempting to sleep in an unfamiliar environment.[160] Ambien is a strong sedative, but it has only minor anxiety-reducing, muscle-relaxing, and anticonvulsant effects.[161] Fibromyalgia patients with memory impairment should be made aware that this symptom may be worsened temporarily when using Ambien. The "amnesic" effect of the drug is similar to that of Halcion (triazolam), which has somewhat stronger memory-impairing and sedative effects than Ambien. The hypnotic and memory-impairing effects of each of these two sleep-inducing drugs are coupled: the higher the dosage, the greater the sedative and amnesic effects.[162] When compared with the effects of Halcion and Restoril (temazepam), two benzodiazepines, Ambien produced the same dose-related impairment of learning, recall, and performance. But the time to maximum drug effect was faster with Ambien than with Halcion or Restoril.[163]

Ambien is Not Effective as a Fibromyalgia Treatment. While Ambien does induce sleep, it is not effective as a treatment for fibromyalgia. Moldofsky and coauthors studied the effects of Ambien on the fibromyalgia status of 1 male and 18 female patients. All patients had alpha EEG non-REM sleep anomaly. The study lasted 16 days. This time was divided into 4 periods of 4 days each. During 1 period, patients received a placebo. In the other 3 periods, patients took one of these doses of Ambien: 5 mg, 10 mg, or 15 mg. Each patient completed all 4 phases in random order. Patients progressed from one period to the next without a washout period between. Patients taking the drug woke fewer times during sleep. They reported that their daytime energy was higher and the quality of their sleep improved. In drug periods, however, there was no improvement in sleepiness and fatigue in the mornings, pain rating, number of tender points, concentration, or mood.[164]

Patients in this study showed some improvement in some fibromyalgia measures of sleep, but no improvement in other measures. It might be argued that the study was too short-term to show improvement in other measures, but this conflicts with clinical observation and evidence from other studies that a good night's sleep can rapidly improve other fibromyalgia measures.[37][59][60][61] We would expect Ambien to improve sleep in fibromyalgia patients in that it is a sleep-inducing medication. [See Chapter 5.1, section titled "Other Hypnotics and Sedatives: Ambien (Zolpidem)."]

For patients undergoing metabolic therapy including the use of thyroid hormone, Ambien is a preferable alternative to the use of antidepressant medications. Antidepressants prevent the reuptake of neurotransmitters such as serotonin and norepinephrine, and the improvement in mood and cognitive function with thyroid hormone is mediated in part by increasing secretion of these same neurotransmitters. Thus, many patients who take both appear to have symptoms related to the combined effects of the antidepressants and thyroid hormone. This can be avoided by the use of Ambien rather than antidepressants.

Antidepressant Medication

Some patients with biochemical depression can maintain a normal mood only by the use of antidepressant medication. I recommend the use of St. John's Wort (extracts of hypericum perforatum). My reason for doing so is that this product has been reported to have fewer and less severe adverse effects than other antidepressants currently available. Lende et al. reported the results of a meta-analysis of randomized clinical trials that involved the use of hypericum extracts for depression. The researchers reported that hypericum extracts were significantly superior to placebos. The effectiveness of the extracts was similar to that of standard antidepressants. Moreover, in the studies, 2 patients (0.8%) using Hypericum extracts dropped out because of adverse side effects while 7 patients (3.0%) taking standard antidepressant drugs dropped out for the same reason. Side effects occurred in 50 patients (19.8%) taking hypericum and 84 patients (52.8%) taking standard antidepressants.[186]

Most fibromyalgia patients, however, after normalizing thyroid hormone regulation of transcription, are depression-free without the use of antidepressants. Patients are able to gradually decrease their dosages of antidepressant medication as improvement in fibromyalgia status increases (seen in improved scores on the fibromyalgia measures, especially the Zung's Self-Rating Depression Scale and the depression visual analog scale). Most patients are able to stop the antidepressants without consequent depression.

A Precaution. St. John's Wort can apparently effectively relieve depression with fewer adverse effects than other antidepressants. However, this finding should not obviate the use of exogenous thyroid hormone by patients whose fibromyalgia is a manifestation of inadequate thyroid hormone regulation of cell function. If depression is the predominant symptom of inadequate thyroid hormone regulation, relief with hypericum extracts may eliminate motivation to continue thyroid hormone therapy. This could result in adverse long-term effects from hypometabolism such as cardiovascular disease (see Chapter 4.4, section titled "Harm from Untreated Hypometabolism").

As I point out elsewhere in this book, all fibromyalgia patients taking thyroid hormone should also take nutritional supplements. A patient's depression may be partially or completely a result of the patient's intake of inadequate quantities of some B complex vitamins. A folic acid deficiency, for example, may cause depression.[188][189][190] Until the nutritional deficiency is corrected, the patient's depression may persist despite her use of antidepressant medication and thyroid hormone. Minimizing or relieving the patient's depression with antidepressant medication and/or thyroid hormone will not prevent the neurological complications of the folic acid deficiency.[147]

METHODS TO BE USED BY THE PATIENT TO CAPITALIZE ON THE INCREASED METABOLIC CAPACITY

A small percentage of fibromyalgia patients improve only minimally or not at all from the use of exogenous thyroid hormone. In a very few cases, we have not been able to determine why. Most often, however, patients have failed to make the lifestyle changes that are essential components of metabolic therapy for fibromyalgia. The most important changes are regular exercise to tolerance and the use of nutritional supplements. Engaging in exercise and taking nutritional supplements *substantially* increase the probability of a successful outcome.

Exercise

It is critical that the patient regularly engage in toning and aerobic exercise *to tolerance*. The qualification of "to tolerance" means that at the beginning of treatment, some patients cannot exercise at all. After their metabolic capacity is increased to some degree, however, most patients are able to begin exercising.

As I pointed out in two published reviews, vigorous physical activity in the form of exercise is potent for improving psychological status in normal individuals.[39][40][48] Thayer found in several studies that even moderate exercise significantly raised energy feelings.[41][42][44] As with increases in energy feelings from caffeine intake, Thayer believes that with exercise, one's perception of problems may also change.[19,p.9] If this is true, it may have implications for helping fibromyalgia patients deal more constructively with the frustrations and uncertainties associated with their condition.

Fibromyalgia patients who have low physical fitness levels and those with psychological troubles may stand to gain the most from exercise. I say this because investigators have found that the psychological benefits from exercise are most pronounced in those with the lowest physical fitness scores before beginning exercise training.[45][46] Morgan conducted a 6-week study during which college professors engaged in various types of exercise. He found that the professors who were not depressed before the program reported that they nevertheless felt better psychologically. However, professors who had been depressed before the study experienced a significant reduction in their depression by the end of the 6 weeks.[48]

DeVries conducted a study in which he looked for a tranquilizing effect from exercise. He measured muscle relaxation in 18 male college professors. The men participated in 17 one-hour vigorous workouts involving weight training and running. Compared to 7 control subjects who did not train, EMGs showed that the exercisers underwent a 25% reduction in muscle tension. DeVries noted that the muscle relaxation occurred soon after brief exercise, and it also persisted as a "chronic" or "long-term" effect following the more extensive exercise program. He reported that muscle exercise reduces anxiety in "both normal *and* high anxiety subjects." His subjects with the greatest muscle tension to begin with derived the greatest benefits from the exercise.[47] Folkin wrote, "The present study suggests that those who are in the poorest physical and/or psychological condition will show the greatest improvement, both physically and psychologically."[46,p.507]

Exercising to Tolerance. Clinical experience and theoretical considerations indicate that the intensity of the exercise should be below the level that induces an increase in circulating catecholamines. The worsening of symptoms after patients exercise too vigorously may result from increased concentrations of catecholamines binding to the α-adrenergic receptors that predominate over β-adrenergic receptors on cell membranes. The catecholamine/α-adrenoceptor binding results in a decrease in the very sequence of metabolic events that are essential for the body to adapt to vigorous activity. (See Chapter 3.4.) The consequent worsening of symptoms following exercise causes some fibromyalgia patients to instinctively avoid exercise.[38] *It is important, therefore, that exercise be calibrated so as to avoid a substantial increase in catecholamine secretion.*

An exercise program must be graded so as not to exacerbate the fibromyalgia patient's symptoms. Exercise should be within the limits of the patient's tolerance, yet be sufficient to induce a training effect. This means that the benefits from exercise are likely to come only after thyroid hormone has increased the metabolic capacity of the patient. When this happens,

she can engage in regular exercise of greater exertion than she could have before she began to use the hormone. Without this "training effect," the patient may not benefit psychologically from the activity. One study using junior college students who did not have fibromyalgia suggests this. Students who engaged in archery and golf, which involve little physical exertion, did not improve at all on psychological measures. Students who took a jogging course, however, improved significantly. The researchers wrote, "The greater the improvement (for women) in the time of the 1.75-mile run, the more likely it is that the subject will become less depressed, more confident, more personally adjusted, more efficient at work, and experience more restful sleep."[46] (See Chapter 5.5, sections titled "Effects of Aerobic Exercise on Resting Metabolic Rate" and "Resistance Training.")

Nutritional Supplementation

It is important to read the section on nutritional supplements in Chapter 5.5 (titled "Nutritional Supplementation"). The increased rate of glycolysis stimulated by exogenous thyroid hormone can be expected to increase the amount of nutrients expended in the pathway of reactions (see Chapter 2.2). Thus, it is critical that patients take increased amounts of the nutrients used in energy metabolism to avoid inducing insufficiencies or deficiencies of the nutrients.

It is essential that the patient take high potency B complex vitamins daily. Patients stand the best chance of recovery, though, when they take the full array of supplemental nutrients. They should dispense with the "one-per-day" mentality and make use of modern scientific nutritional information as reported by scientists such as Linus Pauling and Roger Williams.

If patients have an aversion to swallowing tablets and capsules, they might try wafer nutritional supplements that dissolve in the mouth. The list of supplements in Table 5.2.1 is the one that I have fibromyalgia patients take while undergoing metabolic therapy. The supplements should include B complex vitamins, antioxidants, minerals, and trace elements.

Patients who are able to take only a minimum of tablets and capsules may take a product such as the Therapeutic Vitamin & Mineral Formula (product #2) marketed by Bronson Pharmaceuticals.[166] The patients should take a minimum of 3 tablets per day with food. This product contains B complex vitamins, antioxidants, and minerals. But patients should also take a separate product containing calcium and especially magnesium (see Chapter 5.5, section titled "Nutritional Supplements: Magnesium"), and another containing a far-higher dosage of vitamin C. The multivitamin recommended by Teitelbaum, TwinLab Daily One Caps™, is also an excellent product available in most health food stores.[43,p.18]

For patients who have never taken nutritional supplements or who have not done so in a long time, I customarily recommend an injection of B complex vitamins and a separate one of vitamin B_{12}, usually 3 times per week for several weeks.

Fortunately, many long-suffering fibromyalgia patients, in their quest for relief, have already acquired a high quality, wholesome diet supplemented by most every vitamin, mineral, and trace element even before they begin metabolic therapy. Many have also adopted other measures considered to induce and sustain health. These patients have the highest probability of therapeutic success from the use of thyroid hormone. (They also usually respond the quickest, especially those patients who are already exercisers.)

Table 5.2.1. Nutritional supplements for fibromyalgia patients.

Supplement	Dosage
B complex	50-100 mg of most
Vitamin C	2000-10,000 mg
Calcium	2000 mg
Magnesium	1000 mg
Multi-minerals	
Iron	5-20 mg
Phosphorus	83.4-333.6 mg
Iodine	50-200 µg
Zinc	5-20 mg
Selenium	6.7 µg
Copper	0.67-2.68 mg
Manganese	1.67-6.68 mg
Chromium	66.7-266.8 µg
Molybdenum	33.3-133.2 µg
Vitamin E complex	200-800 IU
Beta carotene	15-60 mg

Cardio-Protective Nutrients. The nutrients with cardio-protective properties are contained in the list of nutrients I recommend for all patients (Table 5.2.1). However, for select patients with cardiac abnormalities, the clinician may elect to have the patient take specially-prepared products such as Cardio Formula™ (product #370) by Bronson Pharmaceuticals.[166] Table 5.2.2 contains the list of nutrients in each tablet of this product. Patients should take a minimum of one tablet

bid, or as the clinician directs. *It is important to remember that this product is not a complete nutritional supplement regimen in itself.* The patient should also take at least substantially more vitamin C and a vitamin B complex formulation that provides the B vitamins not contained in this product.

Nutrient Dosage. In 1989, I wrote, "The dosages I recommend here are practical target amounts rather than scientific quantifications. Our base of scientific information in nutrition is not sufficient to specify exact dosages that are scientifically defensible. Therefore, practical targets are my present aim. Treatment cannot be determined on the basis of statistics; rather, it remains uniquely individual and empirical. Your clinical judgment, based on scrutiny of your patients, is the ultimate determinant of the dosages you specify."[156,p.4] This view was consistent with my advice to clinicians in a previous publication on nutritional therapy.[165,p.A] Except for the fat-soluble vitamins D and A, there is virtually no risk of overdosage with other vitamins. For most patients, it is best to err on the side of wastefully high dosage than to use dosages that are too low.

Table 5.2.2. Nutrients contained in Bronson's Cardio Formula.™

Nutrient	Amount
Vitamin A (as mixed carotenoids)	6,250 IU
Vitamin C (EsterC®)	500 mg
Vitamin E (d-alpha tocopheryl succinate)	200 IU
Vitamin B_6 (pyridoxine HCL)	50 mg
Folate	400 µg
B_{12} (cyanocobalamin)	100 µg
Zinc (OptiZinc®)	15 mg
Selenium (L-methionate)	25 µg
Copper (a.a. chelate)	250 µg
Citrus bioflavonoids	50 mg

The only water soluble vitamin that is toxic in some individuals when taken regularly in very high dosages is vitamin B_6. In one report, 6 patients who took 2000-to-5000 mg per day developed a peripheral neuropathy (loss of sensation of the toes and a tendency to stumble). The condition was reversible, with relief of the neuropathy with no residual nervous system damage.[167]

The toxic level in these patients was 1000-to-3000 times the RDA. Pauling wrote, "We may conclude that there is an upper limit, one thousand times the RDA, to the daily intake of vitamin B_6. The authors of the report were far more cautious, however; they recommended that no one take more than the RDA of this vitamin, 1.8-to-2.2 mg per day. To follow this recommendation would deprive many people of a means for improving their health by taking 50 or 100 mg or more every day . . . ." He also pointed out that many orthomolecular psychiatrists recommend that their patients take 200 mg per day, and some recommend as much as 600 mg per day.[169] He and Hawkins reported, "In more than 5,000 patients we have not observed a single side effect from pyridoxine administration of 200 mg of vitamin B_6 daily."[170] I urge clinicians to suspend acceptance of the conclusions in medical journals about the toxicity of vitamins until they read Pauling's discussion of this subject.[168,pp.334-360] I also urge clinicians to read his chapter titled "Organized Medicine and the Vitamins"[168,pp.300-316] (see Chapter 5.5, section titled "Nutritional Supplementation").

Caffeine

One drug I encourage patients to use, *if* they have no adverse effects from it, is caffeine. Caffeine is an undeserving victim of reflex denouncement. Health care professionals and members of the general public alike contribute to the condemnation. Why do so many people denounce the use of caffeine? My communications with many of its denouncers, and my familiarity with the scientific literature on caffeine, lead me to conclude that with few exceptions denouncers hold pejorative beliefs about caffeine use and defend them without examining the relevant evidence. Their conclusion is therefore prejudicial. Despite the prejudice, this maligned methylxanthine can be of enormous help to fibromyalgia patients before, during, and as a continuing component of their metabolic therapy.

Caffeine increases the resting metabolic rate, internal and skin temperature,[4][5][6][7][8] and mitochondrial oxygen consumption;[9][10] produces physiological arousal;[11][12] improves perception of problems;[13] and mitigates pain.[131][132][133][134][135] Even small doses can improve mood[11][12][22] and decrease the risk of suicide progressively as dosage increases.[130]

Dosage. *When used in proper dosages for the individual*, caffeine accelerates metabolism without the neuromuscular overstimulation that manifests as tremors, anxiety, and irritability. Most of my fibromyalgia patients who have benefitted from caffeine intake have used between 50 mg and 200 mg 2-to-3 times each day. In general, the last dose is best taken 5 or 6 hours before bedtime. When taken closer to bedtime, the caffeine may make it difficult to drop off to sleep.

Carefully controlled studies confirm that caffeine,

while active in the body, interferes with [ ]. Reducing consumption of coffee, tea, and [ ] relieve insomnia.[16][17] There are significar[ ] ces between people in the amount and qual[ ] [ ]eep they get while taking caffeine. I should note, however, that caffeine disturbs sleep more significantly in some individuals than in others. Moreover, the amount of disturbance can vary for the same individual.[18] This is also true of other behavior effects of caffeine. Because of this, each patient must learn how she responds to varying schedules of different doses of caffeine. She can then use this knowledge to benefit from taking the chemical.

Table 5.2.3. Estimates of the caffeine content of beverages.*

	Ground Coffee	Instant Coffee	Decaf. Coffee	Tea	Colas
Mg per cup	88-190	30-99	1-75	19-150	19-55

*Adapted from R.M. Gilbert: Caffeine as a drug of abuse. In *Research Advances in Alcohol and Drug Problems*, Vol. 3. Edited by J.R. Gibbins, Y. Israel, H. Kalant, R.E. Popham, W. Schmidt, and R.G. Smart, New York, John Wiley & Sons, 1976, p.126.

Adverse Effects and Precautions. Travell and Simons note that while small-to-moderate dosages of caffeine may help relieve trigger points by stimulating vasodilation in skeletal muscles, larger amounts of caffeine may aggravate trigger points.[21,p.92] Large amounts also may cause restlessness and irritability that exacerbate the fibromyalgia patient's general sense of discomfort. After drinking a cup of strong coffee containing about 100 mg of caffeine, some subjects report marked subjective tension, with "tension" connoting an unpleasant state. Subjects may also experience increases in energy mixed with the tension.[19,p.159][20] Gilliland and Andress reported that subjects who drank an average of 2.5 cups-to-8.1 cups of coffee per day had elevated trait anxiety and more self-rated depression. (These measures were normal in subjects who drank less than 1 cup per day and those who drank none.)[22]

Because of potential adverse effects, the patient should try various dosages of caffeine and find the one most suited to her. She should also monitor her intake through other sources, such as cola drinks, coffee, tea, and various over-the-counter and prescription drugs.

Table 5.2.3 shows the caffeine content of 5 beverages. For each beverage, the low and high caffeine content reported are given. These data were taken from 9 published reports, only 3 of which are based on laboratory determinations.

Caffeine's half-life in humans is 5.2 hours. That is, the body disposes of 50% of a dose of caffeine in this time.[23,pp.48-56] The clinician should inform the patient of this when he orders laboratory tests affected by caffeine. Norepinephrine secretion, for example, may be elevated in fibromyalgia patients who use caffeine.[24][25] Increased norepinephrine secretion may alter fasting glucose. When a patient consumes caffeine within a couple of hours before testing, measurements of catecholamine secretion and blood glucose level may reflect the caffeine intake.

In addition, understanding this may prevent the patient from misinterpreting the source of the increased psychophysiological arousal she experiences from an overdose of caffeine. There is evidence that the human tends to explain his chemically-induced general psychophysiological arousal as a reaction to the social circumstance he or she is in.[26][27][28] In several studies, researchers gave groups of people chemical sympathetic stimulants to generally arouse them. The subjects' resulting emotions were as diverse as anger and euphoria. What determined a subject's description of his emotional reaction was not the arousing stimulus—the chemical. Instead, it was the suggestive influence of a particular emotional behavior exhibited by other people serving as experimental "plants" in the same situation at the same time. For example, if the plant convincingly described the situation as offensive and expressed anger, subjects also expressed anger. Bandura reviewed the relevant studies and wrote, "Results of both physiological and psychological studies support the conclusion that a common diffuse state of physiological arousal mediates diverse forms of emotional behavior and that different emotional states are identified and discriminated primarily in terms of external stimuli rather than internal somatic cues."[29,p.488]

The arousing effect of caffeine is prolonged in some patients. Due to this, a patient may lose sight of the connection between his caffeine consumption and his arousal. He may then attribute the arousal to a social interaction that ordinarily would be emotionally inert to him. This can obviously lead to adverse social and personal consequences.

Why Caffeine Helps Fibromyalgia Patients. The biochemical mechanism of caffeine's metabolic effect is its inhibition of two enzymes: phosphodiesterase and adenosine. When caffeine inhibits these in-

hibitory enzymes, the effect is sustained metabolic acceleration. Because of caffeine's 5.2-hour half-life, a dose of 50-to-150 mg every 3-to-4 hours increases energy level for many patients, improves their cognitive function, and relieves their depression. (See Chapter 5.5, section titled "Caffeine.") Once thyroid hormone supplementation sufficiently increases β-adrenergic density, patients benefit from lower doses of caffeine.

● PHYSICAL TREATMENT

NEED FOR SPECIFIC MUSCULOSKELETAL THERAPY

In his discussion of euthyroid hypometabolism, Sonkin pointed out, "A cycle of muscle pain, trigger points, and spasm occurring in hypothyroidism often requires rehabilitation therapy in conjunction with hormone replacement."[152,p.160] "Rehabilitation therapy" refers, of course, to specific physical treatment. This form of care is necessary for perhaps most hypothyroid and euthyroid fibromyalgia patients, even after they have benefitted substantially from systemic metabolic therapy.

Normalizing Metabolism Typically Relieves Mild-to-Moderate, Pain-Generating Musculoskeletal Lesions

When the patient's metabolic state normalizes with therapy, mild-to-moderate muscle hypertonicity usually subsides. In addition, mildly active trigger points usually become inactive (latent) without specific treatment and latent trigger points may spontaneously cease to exist.[156] But in most patients, intense hypermyotonia and moderately or highly irritable trigger points desensitize only with specific myofascial therapy. Therapy is typically necessary for total pain relief even though the patient's metabolism has completely normalized and most fibromyalgia symptoms are gone.

Severe Pain-Generating Musculoskeletal Lesions Tend to Persist Despite Normalized Metabolism; This is Reflected as Higher Scores on Measures of Fibromyalgic Pain

Some patients who respond well to metabolic therapy but who do not undergo physical treatment are left with regional musculoskeletal pain that they may misinterpret as persisting fibromyalgia. (Some clinicians and patients misname this residual pain "regional fibromyalgia.") In patients whose metabolism has normalized, persisting regional pain is usually reflected in the pain measures used to assess fibromyalgia status. The patient with regional pain is likely to have a higher pain distribution according to the percentage method, higher pain intensity on the visual analog scale, and a higher mean tender point sensitivity (lower mean pressure/pain threshold) measured by algometry. For these patients, the scores on fibromyalgia pain measures do not accurately show the benefits they have derived from metabolic therapy.

Sources of regional pain that worsen fibromyalgia pain scores include acute and chronic injuries; chronic inflammatory musculoskeletal disease such as arthritis; articular lesions, especially of spinal joints (termed vertebral subluxations by chiropractic physicians); fascial adhesions; hypertonic muscle; and particularly myofascial trigger points.

Myofascial trigger points are common causes of regional pain in fibromyalgia patients. The taut bands that house trigger points appear to involve contractile filaments that are contractured due to an energy deficiency. The energy deficiency can be caused or exacerbated by inadequate thyroid hormone regulation of muscle cell processes. Thus, reduced energy metabolism due to thyroid hormone deficiency or cellular resistance to thyroid hormone can increase the irritability of myofascial trigger points. This contributes to the trigger points' sustained symptom-referring activity and renders them resistant to specific myofascial therapy.

The cycle of reduced blood flow and low threshold nerve endings in the taut bands of muscle housing trigger points persists in some patients even after their general metabolism has been normalized. Expertly applied physical treatment techniques may be necessary to inactivate these trigger points and help return the involved muscle to a normal state. For these reasons, I recommend, in agreement with Starlanyl,[154][155] that all fibromyalgia patients be evaluated for myofascial trigger points and, if necessary, undergo trigger point therapy.

The clinician should suspect that regional pain is adversely affecting fibromyalgia pain measures when other measures of fibromyalgia status (such as the Zung's or Beck's depression score, the Fibromyalgia Impact Questionnaire score, and the visual analog scales for symptoms other than pain) show positive changes that are out of proportion or contrary to the pain measures. Effective myofascial treatment that targets the sources of regional pain is virtually always reflected in improved fibromyalgia pain measures. The patient's positive response to regional treatment, especially myofascial trigger point therapy, is further evidence that the patient's metabolism has improved or normalized.

Before fibromyalgia status improves from metabolic therapy, patients' tissues tend to be resistant to physical treatment. In the early 1980s, this is what interested me in patients I would later learn had fibromyalgia—their resistance to otherwise highly effective myofascial therapy. I suspected (in line with the approach taken by Travell and Simons[21]) that these patients were treatment-resistant because of some underlying factor(s). It is now clear that after improving with metabolic therapy, most patients respond as successfully to myofascial therapy as do non-fibromyalgic patients. The first-line approach to improving the status of most fibromyalgia patients is metabolic therapy, but treatment of the sources of regional pain is necessary in many patients before their pain measures normalize.

MANIPULATIVE THERAPIES

Spinal and Myofascial Manipulation

While myofascial techniques are valuable for most fibromyalgia patients, so is spinal manipulation. Manipulation relieves segmental facilitation. Facilitation lowers resistance to transmission of nociceptive signals from the periphery into the brain stem and brain through the spinothalamic tracts. It also lowers the threshold for activation of preganglionic sympathetic neurons and alpha motor neurons of an involved segment, inducing peripheral vasoconstriction and shortening muscle fibers of the motor unit.[156] Two controlled studies have shown that spinal manipulation (combined with paraspinal soft tissue manipulation) increased the "global well-being" of fibromyalgia patients.[157] Fibromyalgia patients indicated on questionnaires the value of chiropractic care for them—they ranked it among the most effective treatment measures.[158][159] Spinal manipulation, *carefully calibrated* to a fibromyalgia patient's tolerance, should be included in most patients' treatment regimens.

In discussing musculoskeletal manipulative therapy for thyroid disorders, Weinberg pointed out that the clinician has two goals: first, to manipulate the spine to improve intervertebral motion, and second, to manipulate the posterior cervical muscles to reduce their tone. These procedures are expected to reduce reflex feedback that may impair vasomotor activity of the blood vessels that supply the thyroid gland.[71,p.252] The clinician may also manipulate the anterior cervical muscles to reduce residual tension that may hamper the venous and lymphatic drainage of the gland. Johnson also recommended "springing the clavicles forward with the thumbs."[191,p.261]

The studies of Melander et al. indicate that the sympathetic adrenergic system is important in the control of thyroid function.[62][64][66] Sympathetic adrenergic fibers are abundant in the human thyroid gland. The anatomy of the fibers suggests that they influence both thyroid follicle cells and the blood vessels that course through the gland. Mouse studies indicate that sympathetic stimulation may cause prompt, short-term changes in the rate that the gland secretes hormones. Manipulative therapy, therefore, may improve the sympathetic nerve supply of the thyroid gland.

The thyroid gland has a profuse blood supply. Flow to the gland constitutes about 1% of cardiac output.[67] Branches of the cervical sympathetic trunk course through the gland adjacent to arteries. Parasympathetic fibers travel with the superior laryngeal and recurrent laryngeal nerves. Both types of autonomic fibers, which appear to regulate blood flow, terminate at blood vessels and thyroid gland follicles.[2,p.142]

There are a number of studies of the effects of nerve stimulation on thyroid gland function. Soderberg found that blood flow through the rabbit thyroid gland is significantly altered by stimulation of nerves. Stimulation of the cervical sympathetic nerves or injection of epinephrine into veins decreased blood flow and uptake of iodide in the gland. Both stimulation of the cervical sympathetic nerves and injection of small amounts of epinephrine increased iodine secretion slightly. These effects occurred only when TSH was present.[69] In contrast to stimulation of sympathetic nerves, parasympathetic stimulation (by excitation of the superior laryngeal nerves or the vagus nerve, or by injection of acetylcholine) increased blood flow and iodide uptake. Although these studies had some faults,[2,p.142] they indicate that: (1) the nerves in the gland are not secretory, and (2) the recorded effects of nerve stimulation were a facilitation of the response of the gland to TSH.[69]

Stimulation of the vagus nerves (their ganglion nodosum) increased within 15 minutes the quantity of radioactive protein bound iodine in the thyroid vein.[65] This effect may have been caused directly by the nerve stimulation or by increased blood flow mediated by the stimulated nerves.[2] Administering epinephrine to dogs systemically reduced thyroid gland blood but did not change iodide clearance or thyroid hormone release from the gland.[70]

The monoamines may be mediators by which TSH activates the thyroid gland.[72][73] TSH stimulates mast cells in the gland, causing the gland to release amines into the thyroid tissue. The monoamines norepinephrine and dopamine stimulate adrenergic receptors in thyroid follicle cells. This causes the cells to synthesize thyroid hormones.

Confusion about the role of nerve stimulation and catecholamine exposure arises from numerous observations. Under some experimental conditions, for example, epinephrine and norepinephrine induce vasoconstriction in the thyroid gland and inhibit its secretion of hormones.[74] Conversely, catecholamines cause *release* of thyroid hormones in dogs[75] and mice.[76] Yet thyroid function is normal in humans with an adrenal tumor (pheochromocytoma) that releases abnormally large amounts of catecholamines into the blood.[2,p.143] It may be that normal autonomic innervation does not directly affect thyroid hormone synthesis and secretion, but by favoring thyroid tissue homeostasis, normal autonomic innervation facilitates the responsiveness of the gland to TSH.

Physiological effects of neural stimulation of the thyroid gland suggest that manipulation, by optimizing the autonomic innervation of the gland, can influence to some degree the response of the gland to TSH. But as DeGroot and coauthors[2,p.143] cautioned, we cannot yet draw firm conclusions about the effects of the sympathetic nervous system and the catecholamines on human thyroid function. According to these researchers: (1) autonomic nerve stimulation or administration of catecholamines does not appear to play a significant regulatory role in human thyroid gland function, and (2) most likely, circulating TSH is the only physiologically significant stimulus to thyroid hormone secretion.

Chiropractic studies comparing somato-visceral effects with symptom-related outcome studies[77,pp.1,30] may provide data on the effects of manipulative therapy on thyroid gland function. But at present, I am aware of no studies testing the relationship.

Manipulating the Thyroid Gland

Most clinicians warn against manipulating the delicate thyroid gland itself. One reason for caution is that manipulation of the gland may cause release of calcitonin.[78][79] The released calcitonin could decrease the efflux of calcium from bones to the extracellular fluid, potentially resulting in spasm and tetany.[80][81]

But in patients with thyroid glands injured in auto accidents, gently manipulating the gland itself (as well as the cervical spine and the neck's myofascia) may be therapeutic. Schutt and Dohan wrote that whiplash-type injuries of the neck may cause thyroid hemorrhage.[82] Impaired thyroid function from this type of injury might account for some patients' sustained low energy level and the onset of fibromyalgia following this type of trauma. The clinician must exercise astute judgment regarding manipulative therapy in these cases.

Johnson described a procedure for manipulating the thyroid gland. "Get the fingers underneath the mass," he wrote, "and stretch the tissues upward so that there will be an increased drainage, loosening up all the muscles and ligaments in relation to the gland." He cautioned the clinician not to overtreat the gland, warning that overtreatment may cause excess secretion of hormones, leaving the patient tremulous.[191,p.262] He also advised the clinician, as part of the treatment, to relax all the muscles of the patient's neck and shoulders down to the 7th thoracic vertebra. He recommended that the patient participate by leaning back and extending the head up and back for 3 minutes to drain the gland.[191,p.261]

● ROLES OF CLINICIANS OF VARIOUS DISCIPLINES

PRESCRIBING CLINICIANS

In the United States, clinicians who are permitted to prescribe thyroid hormone and propranolol are medical, osteopathic, and naturopathic physicians. Family physicians, naturopathic physicians, biologically-oriented psychiatrists, and preventive medicine practitioners have been most cooperative. I believe their willingness to participate is due to a high level of open-mindedness and an interest in innovative and investigational treatments for fibromyalgia. Some gynecologists, neurologists, and rheumatologists have also cooperated in using our protocol.

NON-PRESCRIBING CLINICIANS

Most prescribing clinicians are oriented toward internal disorders and infectious diseases. Many prefer not to assess patients through procedures such as algometry. Instead, because of fast-paced practices, they leave the more time-consuming assessment procedures

to neuromusculoskeletally-oriented clinicians. (Medical and osteopathic physiatrists and naturopathic physicians are prescribing clinicians who often are exceptions to this.) But any willing prescribing clinician can, of course, both perform the assessments and adjust thyroid hormone dosages.

The orientation of physical therapists, naprapaths, and some massage therapists enables them to incorporate assessment into their practices. Naturopathic physicians who are graduates of accredited naturopathic medical schools are well qualified to include assessment in their practices because of their training in physical medicine and manipulative therapies. Chiropractic physicians are also suited to assess patients because of their advanced training in neuromusculoskeletal diagnosis and treatment, including manual manipulation. Physical therapists, physiatrists, and naturopathic and chiropractic physicians may also be trained and experienced in the use of physical treatment modalities (such as ultrasound) that can increase the comfort level of many fibromyalgia patients. As Honeyman-Lowe and I described, for many fibromyalgia patients such physical treatment is essential to the complete and long-lasting relief of pain.[187]

REFERENCES

1. Bastenie, P.A.: Treatment of myxoedema associated with coronary heart disease. In *Recent Progress in Diagnosis and Treatment of Hypothyroid Conditions.* Edited by P.A. Bastenie, M. Bonnyns, and L. Vanhaelst, Amsterdam, *Excerpta Medica*, 1980, pp.122-125.
2. DeGroot, L.J., Larsen, P.R., Refetoff, S., and Stanbury, J.B.: *The Thyroid and Its Diseases*, 5th edition. New York, John Wiley & Sons, Inc., 1984.
3. Vanhaelst, L.: Hypothyroidism and coronary heart disease. In *Recent Progress in Diagnosis and Treatment of Hypothyroid Conditions.* Edited by P.A. Bastenie, M. Bonnyns, and L. Vanhaelst, Amsterdam, *Excerpta Medica*, 1980.
4. Koot, P. and Deurenberg, P.: Comparison of changes in energy expenditure and body temperatures after caffeine consumption. *Ann. Nutri. Metab.*, 39(3):135-142, 1995.
5. Yoshioka, K., Yoshida, T., Kamanaru, K., Hiraoka, N., and Kondo, M.: Caffeine activates brown adipose tissue thermogenesis and metabolic rate in mice. *J. Nutri. Sci. Vitaminology*, 36(2):173-178, 1990.
6. Dulloo, A.G., Geissler, C.A., Horton, T., Collins, A., and Miller, D.S.: Normal caffeine consumption: influences on thermogenesis and daily energy expenditure in lean and postobese human volunteers. *Am. J. Clin. Nutri.*, 49(1):44-50, 1989.
7. Tulp, O.L. and Buck, C.L.: Caffeine and ephedrine stimulated thermogenesis in LA-corpulent rats. *Pharmacol. Toxicol.*, 85(1):17-19, 1986.
8. Poehlman, E.T., LaChance, P., Tremblay, A., et al.: The effect of prior exercise and caffeine ingestion on metabolic

rate and hormones in young adult males. *Canadian J. Physiol. Pharmacol.*, 67(1):10-16, 1989.

9. LeBlanc, J., Jobin, M., Cote, J., Samson, P., and Labrie, A.: Enhanced metabolic response to caffeine in exercise-trained human subjects. *J. Appl. Physiol.*, 59(3):832-837, 1985.

10. Jung, R.T., Shetty, P.S., James, W.P., Barrand, M.A., and Callingham, B.A.: Caffeine: its effect on catecholamines and metabolism in lean and obese humans. *Clin. Sci.*, 60 (5):527-535, 1981.

11. Gilliland, K. and Bullock, W.: Caffeine: a potential drug of abuse. *Adv. Alcohol Subst. Abuse*, 3:53-73, 1983-1984.

12. Sawyer, D.A., Julia, H.L., and Turin, A.C.: Caffeine and human behavior: arousal, anxiety, and performance effects. *J. Behav. Med.*, 5:415-439, 1982.

13. Thayer, R.E.: Problem perception, optimism, and related states as a function of time of day (diurnal rhythm) and moderate exercise: two arousal systems in interaction. *Motiv. Emotion*, 11:19-36, 1987.

14. Goldstein, A. and Kaizer, S.: Psychotropic effects of caffeine in man. III. A questionnaire survey of coffee drinking and its effects on a group of housewives. *Clin. Pharmacol. Ther.*, 10:477-488, 1969.

15. Goldstein, A., Kaizer, S., and Whitby, O.: Psychotropic effects of caffeine in man. IV. Quantitative and qualitative differences associated with habituation to coffee. *Clin. Pharmacol. Ther.*, 10:489-497, 1969.

16. Silver, W.: Insomnia, tachycardia, and cola drinks. *Pediatrics*, 47:635, 1971.

17. Greden, J.F.: Anxiety or caffeinism: a diagnostic dilemma. *Am. J. Psychiatry*, 131:1089-1093, 1974.

18. Goldstein, A., Warren, R., and Daizer, S.: Psychotropic effects of caffeine in man. I. Individual differences in sensitivity to caffeine-induced wakefulness. *J. Pharmacol. Exp. Ther.*, 149:156-159, 1965.

19. Thayer, R.E.: *The Biopsychology of Mood and Arousal.* New York, Oxford University Press, 1989.

20. Anderson, K.: Impulsivity and caffeine: a within and between subjects test of the Yerkes-Dodson Law. Paper presented at the annual meeting of the International Society for the Study of Individual Differences, Toronto, Canada, 1987.

21. Travell, J.G. and Simons, D.G.: *Myofascial Pain and Dysfunction: The Trigger Point Manual,* Vol. 1. Baltimore, Williams and Wilkins, 1983.

22. Gilliland, K. and Andress, D.: Ad lib caffeine consumption, symptoms of caffeinism, and academic performance. *Am. J. Psychiat.*, 138:512-514, 1981.

23. Bonati, M., and Garattini, S.: Interspecies comparison of caffeine disposition. In *Caffeine.* Edited by P.B. Dews, New York, Springer-Verlag, 1984.

24. Russell, I.J., Vipraio, G.A., and Morgan, W.W.: Is there a metabolic basis for the fibrositis syndrome? *Amer. Journal of Medicine*, 81(3A):50-56, 1986.

25. Russell, I.J., Vipraio, G.A., Morgan, W.W., et al.: Catecholamine excretion in fibromyalgia syndrome. (unpublished material, 1988).

26. Ax, A.F.: The physiological differentiation between fear and anger in humans. *Psychosomatic Med.,* 15:433-442, 1953.

27. Schachter, J.: Pain, fear and anger in hypertensives and normotensives: a psychophysiological study. *Psychoso-*

matic Med., 19:17-29, 1957.

28. Schachter, S. and Singer, J.E.: Cognitive, social and physiological determinants of emotional states. *Psychol. Rev.*, 69:379-399, 1962.

29. Bandura, A. *Principles of Behavior Modification.* New York, Holt, Rinehart and Winston, Inc., 1969.

30. Hamburger, J.I.: Strategies for cost-effective thyroid function testing with modern methods. In *Diagnostic Methods in Clinical Thyroidology.* Edited by J.I. Hamburger, New York, Springer-Verlag, 1989, pp.63-109.

31. Murray, G.R.: Note on the treatment of myxoedema by hypodermic injections of an extract of the thyroid gland of a sheep. *Br. Med. J.*, 2:796, 1891.

32. Christy, N.P.: The adrenal cortex in hypothyroidism. In *Werner's The Thyroid: A Fundamental and Clinical Text,* 6th edition. Edited by L.E. Braverman and R.D. Utiger, Philadelphia, J.B. Lippincott Co., 1991, pp.1045-1049.

33. Escobar-Morreale, H.F., Obregón, M.J., Escobar del Rey, F., and Morreale de Escobar, G.: Replacement therapy for hypothyroidism with thyroxine alone does not ensure euthyroidism in all tissues, as studied in thyroidectomized rats. *J. Clin. Invest.*, 96:2828-2838, 1995.

34. Escobar-Morreale, H.F., del Rey, F.E., Obregon, M.J., and de Escobar, G.M.: Only the combined treatment with thyroxine and triiodothyronine ensures euthyroidism in all tissues of the thyroidectomized rat. *Endocrinology,* 137(6): 2490-2502, 1996.

35. Lowe, J.C., Eichelberger, J., Manso, G., and Peterson, K.: Improvement in euthyroid fibromyalgia patients treated with T$_3$ (tri-iodothyronine). *J. Myofascial Ther.*, 1(2):16-29, 1994.

36. Lowe, J.C., Cullum, M.E., Graf, L.H., and Yellin, J.: Mutations in the c-erbAβ$_1$ gene: do they underlie euthyroid fibromyalgia? *Med. Hypotheses*, 48:125-135, 1997.

37. Agnew, H.W., Webb, W.B., and Williams, R.L.: Comparison of stage four and 1-REM sleep deprivation. *Percept. Mot. Skills*, 24:851-8, 1967.

38. Nørregaard, J., Lykkegaard, J.J., Mehlsen, J., and Danneskiold-Samsøe, B.: Exercise training in treatment of fibromyalgia. *J. Musculoskel. Pain*, 5(1):71-79, 1997.

39. Lowe, J.C.: Physical activity: a form of physiopsychotherapy. *Dig. Chiro. Econ.*, 21:33-37, 1978.

40. Lowe, J.C.: Psychological benefits of physical activity. *ACA J. Chiro.*, 13:S-1-6, 1979.

41. Thayer, R.E.: Energy, tiredness, and tension effects of a sugar snack versus moderate exercise. *J. Personal. Soc. Psychol.*, 52:119-125, 1987.

42. Thayer, R.E.: Problem perception, optimism, and related states as a function of time of day (diurnal rhythm) and moderate exercise: two arousal systems in interaction. *Motiv. Emotion*, 11:19-36, 1987.

43. Teitelbaum, J.: *From Fatigued to Fantastic!* New York, Avery Publishing Group, 1996.

44. Thayer, R.E.: Toward a psychological theory of multidimensional activation (arousal). *Motiv. Emotion*, 2:1-34, 1978.

45. Gutin, B.: Effects of increase in physical fitness on mental ability following physical and mental stress. *Res. Quart.*, 37:211-220, 1966.

46. Folkin, C.H., Lynch, S., and Gardner, M.M.: Psychological fitness as a function of physical fitness. *Arch. Phys. Med.*

Rehabil., 53:503-508, 1972.

47. deVries, H.A.: Immediate and long term effects of exercise upon resting muscle action potential level. *J. Sports Med. Phys. Fitness*, 8:1-11, 1968.

48. Morgan, W.P., Roberts, J.A., Brand, F.R., and Feinerman, A.D.: Psychological effect of chronic physical activity. *Med. Sci. Sports*, 2:213-217, 1970.

49. Fraser, W.D., Biggart, E.M., O'Reilly, D.St. J., Gray, H.W., and McKillop, J.H.: Are biochemical tests of thyroid function of any value in monitoring patients receiving thyroxine replacement? *Br. Med. J.*, 293:808-810, 1986.

50. Stamler, J.S.: The coronary drug project: findings leading to further modifications of its protocol with respect to dextrothyroxine. *J.A.M.A.*, 220:996, 1972.

51. Murray, G.R.: The pathology and treatment of myxoedema: remarks on the treatment of myxoedema with thyroid juice, with notes of four cases. *Br. Med. J.*, 2:449, 1892.

52. Keating, F.R., Jr., Parkin, T.W., and Selby, J.B.: Treatment of heart disease associated with myxedema. *Prog. Cardiovasc. Dis.*, 3:364,1961.

53. Le Feuvre, C., Baubion, N., Berdah, J., Heulin, A., and Vacheron, A.: Drug-induced cardiovascular complications. *Ann. de Med. Intern.*, 140(7):597-599, 1989.

54. Christy, N.P.: The adrenal cortex in thyrotoxicosis. In *Werner's The Thyroid: A Fundamental and Clinical Text*, 6th edition. Edited by L.E. Braverman and R.D.Utiger, Philadelphia, J.B. Lippincott Co., 1991, pp.806-815.

55. Iranmanesh, A., Lizarralde, G., Johnson, M.L., and Veldhuis, J.D.: Dynamics of 24-hour endogenous cortisol secretion and clearance in primary hypothyroidism assessed before and after partial thyroid hormone replacement. *J. Clin. Endocrinol. Metab.*, 70:155, 1990.

56. Berkheiser, S.W.: Adult hypothyroidism: report of an advanced case with autopsy study. *J. Clin. Endocrinol. Metab.*, 15:44, 1955.

57. Peterson, R.E.: The influence of the thyroid on adrenal cortical function. *J. Clin. Invest.*, 37:736, 1958.

58. Peterson, R.E.: The miscible pool and turnover rate of adrenocortical steroids in man. *Recent Prog. Horm. Res.*, 15:231, 1959.

59. Moldofsky, H., Scarisbrick, P., England, R., and Smythe, H.: Musculoskeletal symptoms and non-REM sleep disturbance in patients with "fibrositis syndrome" and healthy subjects. *Psychosomatic Med.*, 37(4):341-51, 1975.

60. Moldofsky, H. and Scarisbrick, P.: Induction of neurasthenic musculoskeletal pain syndrome by selective sleep stage deprivation. *Psychosomatic Med.*, 38:35-44, 1976.

61. Moldofsky, H.: Fibromyalgia, sleep disorder and chronic fatigue syndrome. *Ciba Found. Sympos.*, 173:262-271, 1993.

62. Melander, A., Ericson, L.E., Sundler, F. and Ingbar, S.H.: Sympathetic innervation of the mouse thyroid and its significance in thyroid hormone secretion. *Endocrinology*, 94: 959-966, 1974.

63. To obtain injectable 500 µg boluses of Thyrel™ (TRH) to perform the TRH stimulation test, contact Ferring Laboratories, 400 Rella Blvd., Ste 201, Suffern, NY 10901 Tel. (914) 368-7916 FAX (914) 368-1193.

64. Melander, A., Ericson, L.E., and Sundler, F.: Sympathetic regulation of thyroid hormone secretion. *Life Sci.*, 14:237-245, 1974.

65. Ishie, J.: Effect of stimulation of the vagal nerve on the thyroidal release of 131I-labelled hormones. *Folia Endocrinol. Japan.*, 35:1433, 1960.

66. Melander, A., Ericson, L.E., Ljunggren, et al.: Sympathetic innervation of the normal human thyroid. *J. Clin. Endocrinol. Metab.*, 39:713-718, 1974.

67. Soderberg, U.: Temporal characteristics of thyroid activity. *Physiol. Rev.*, 39:777, 1959.

68. Hagg, E., Asplund, K., and Lithner, F.: Value of basal plasma cortisol assays in the assessment of pituitary-adrenal insufficiency. *Clin. Endocrinol.*(Oxf.), 26:221-226, 1987.

69. Soderberg, U.: Short-term reactions in the thyroid gland. *Acta Physiol. Scand.*, 42(suppl):147, 1958.

70. Ahn, C.S., Athans, J.C., and Rosenberg, I.N.: Effects of epinephrine and of alterations in glandular blood flow upon thyroid function: studies using thyroid vein cannulation in dogs. *Endocrinology*, 84:501, 1969.

71. Weinberg, T.: Disorders of the thyroid gland. In *Osteopathic Medicine*. Edited by J.M. Hoag, W.V. Cole and S.G. Bradford, New York, McGraw-Hill Book Co., Inc., 1969.

72. Melander, A., Hakanson, R., Westgren, U., Ownman, C. and Sundler, F.: Significance of thyroid mast cells in the regulation of thyroid activity. *Agents Actions*, 3:186, 1973.

73. Melander, A., Sundler, F. and Westgren, U.: Intrathyroidal amines and the synthesis of thyroid hormone. *Endocrinology*, 93:193-200, 1973.

74. Melander, A. and Sundler, F.: Interactions between catecholamines, 5-hydroxytryptamine and TSH on the secretion of thyroid hormone. *Endocrinology*, 90:188, 1972.

75. Ackerman, N.B. and Arons, W.L.: The effect of epinephrine and norepinephrine on acute thyroid release of thyroid hormones. *Endocrinology*, 62:723, 1958.

76. Melander, A.: Amines and mouse thyroid activity: release of thyroid hormone by catecholamines and indoleamines and its inhibition by adrenergic blocking drugs. *Acta Endocrinol.*, 65:371, 1970.

77. Wilk, C.: AMA dollars will fund chiro research. *Dyn. Chiro.*, Feb. 12, 1993.

78. Rasmusson, B., Borgestov, S., and Holme-Hanson, B.: Changes in serum calcitonin in patients undergoing thyroid surgery. *Acta Chiro. Scand.*, 146:15-17, 1980.

79. Watson, C.G., Steed, D.I., Robinson, A.G., and Deftos, L.J.: The role of calcitonin and parathyroid hormone in the pathogenesis of post-thyroidectomy hypocalcemia. *Metabolism*, 30:588-589, 1981.

80. Percival, R.C., Hargreaves, A.W., and Kanis, J.A.: The mechanism of hypocalcaemia following thyroidectomy. *Acta Endocrinologica*, 109:220-226, 1985.

81. Sonkin, L.S.: Myofascial pain due to metabolic disorders: diagnosis and treatment. In *Myofascial Pain and Fibromyalgia: Trigger Point Management*. Edited by E.S. Rachlin, St. Louis, Mosby, 1994, pp.45-60.

82. Schutt, C.H. and Dohan, F.C.: Neck injury to women in auto accidents: a metropolitan plague. *J.A.M.A.*, 206:2692, 1968.

83. Clayton, R.N.: Diagnosis of adrenal insufficiency. *Lancet*, i:271-272, 1989.

84. Haynes, R.C., Jr.: Thyroid and antithyroid drugs. In *Goodman and Gilman's The Pharmacological Basis of Therapeutics*, 8th edition. New York, Pergamon Press, 1990, pp.1361-1383.

85. Sawin, C.T.: The development and use of thyroid preparations. In *The Thyroid Gland: A Practical Clinical Treatise*. Edited by Van Middlesworth, Chicago, Year Book Medical Publishers, Inc., 1986, pp.389-403.

86. Bernstein, R.S. and Robbins, J.: Intermittent therapy with L-thyroxine. *N. Engl. J. Med.*, 281:1444, 1969.

87. Dillmann, W.H.: Cardiac function in thyroid disease: clinical features and management considerations. *Ann. Thorac. Surg.*, 56(Suppl.1):S9-S14, 1993.

88. Werbel, S..S. and Ober, K.P.: Acute adrenal insufficiency. *Endocrinol. Metab. Clinics North Am.*, 22(2):303-328, 1993.

89. Stojsic, D.: Addison's disease. *Medicinski Pregled*, 47(3-4):134-136, 1994.

90. Gao, T.S., Shi, Y.F., and Gao, S.M.: Evaluation of adult idiopathic growth hormone deficiency with other pituitary hormones deficiency. *Chinese J. Intern. Med.*, 29(4):205-209, 1990.

91. Herren, T.: Hypotensive crisis. *J. Suisse de Med.*, 123(17): 853-867, 1993.

92. Stockigt, J.R.: Serum thyrotropin and thyroid hormone measurements and assessment of thyroid hormone transport. In *Werner and Ingbar's The Thyroid: A Fundamental and Clinical Text*, 7th edition. Edited by L.P. Braverman and R.D. Utiger, Philadelphia, Lippincott-Raven Publishers, 1996, pp.377-396.

93. Teitelbaum, J. and Bird, B.: Effective treatment of severe chronic fatigue: a report of a series of 64 patients. *J. Musculoskel. Pain*, 3(4):91-110, 1995.

94. Harvey, R.A. and Champe, P.C.: *Pharmacology*. Philadelphia, J.B. Lippincott Co., 1992.

95. Jefferies, W.: *Safe Uses of Cortisone*. Springfield, Charles C. Thomas, 1981.

96. Jefferies, W.: Low dose glucocorticoid therapy: an appraisal of its safety and mode of action in clinical disorders, including rheumatoid arthritis. *Arch. Intern. Med.*, 119:265-278, 1967.

97. Du Bois, E.F.: *Basal Metabolism in Health and Disease*, 3rd edition. Philadelphia, Lea & Febiger, 1936.

98. Loeb, J.N.: Metabolic changes in thyrotoxicosis. In *The Thyroid*, 6th edition. Edited by L.E. Braverman and R.D. Utiger, Philadelphia, J.B. Lippincott Co., 1991, pp.845-853.

99. DeGroot, L.J.: Abnormal thyroid function tests in euthyroid patients. In *Diagnostic Methods in Clinical Thyroidology*. Edited by J.I. Hamburger, New York, Springer-Verlag, 1989, pp.3-26.

100. Mackin, J.F., Canary, J.J., and Pittman, C.S.: Thyroid storm and its management. *N. Engl. J. Med.*, 291:1396, 1974.

101. Mazzaferri, E.L., Reynolds, J.C., Young, R.L., Thomas, C.N., and Parisi, A.F.: Propranolol as primary therapy for thyrotoxicosis. *Arch. Intern. Med.*, 136:50, 1976.

102. Roti, E., Montermini, M., Roti, S., et al.: The effects of diltiazem, a calcium channel-blocking drug, on cardiac rate and rhythm in hyperthyroid patients. *Arch. Intern. Med.*, 148:1919, 1988.

103. Bunevicius, B., Kazanavicius, G., Zalinkevicius, R., and Prange, A.J. Jr.: Effects of thyroxine as compared with thyroxine plus triiodothyronine in patients with hypothyroidism. *N. Engl. J. Med.*, 340(6):424-429, 1999.

104. Dillmann, W.H.: The cardiovascular system in thyrotoxicosis. In *Werner and Ingbar's The Thyroid: A Fundamental and Clinical Text*, 6th edition. Edited by L.E. Braverman and R.D. Utiger, New York, J.B. Lippincott Co., 1991, pp.759-770.

105. Gasinska, T., Drozdz, M., Izbicka, M., and Szydlo, E.: Effect of various β-adrenolytic drugs and calcium channel blocker (nifedipine) on selected indicators of calcium-phosphorus metabolism in patients with hyperthyroidism and simple goiter. *Endokrynologia Polska*, 39(6):327-337, 1988.

106. Gasinka, T., Wawrzyniak, L., and Widala, E.: Acetylation phenotype and the changes in selected indicators of calcium-phosphate metabolism in patients with hyperthyroidism treated with propranolol. *Endokrynologia Polska*, 40 (6):291-300, 1989.

107. Melander, A.: Interactions of adrenergic blocking drugs with the *in vivo* release of thyroid hormone induced by thyrotrophin and long-acting thyroid stimulator. *Acta Endocrinol.*, 66:151, 1971.

108. Gilman, A.G. and Rall, T.W.: Factors influencing adenosine 3',5'-phosphate accumulation in bovine thyroid slices. *Endocrinology*, 243:5867, 1968.

109. Sherwin, R.S. and Felig, P.: Hypoglycemia. In *Endocrinology and Metabolism*, 2nd edition. Edited by P. Felig, J.D. Baxter, A. Broadus, and L.A. Frohman, New York, McGraw-Hill Book Co., 1987, pp.1179-1202.

110. Abramson, E.A., Arky, R.A., and Woeber, K.A.: Effects of propranolol on the hormonal and metabolic response to insulin-induced hypoglycemia. *Lancet*, 2:1386, 1966.

111. Cooper, D.S.: Treatment of thyrotoxicosis. In *Werner and Ingbar's The Thyroid: A Fundamental and Clinical Text*, 6th edition. Edited by L.E. Braverman and R.D. Utiger, New York, J.B. Lippincott Co., 1991, pp.887-916.

112. Feely, J. and Peden, N.: Use of β-adrenoceptor blocking drugs in hyperthyroidism. *Drugs*, 27:425, 1984.

113. Hoffman, B.B. and Lefkowitz, R.J.: Adrenergic receptor antagonists. In *The Pharmacologic Basis of Therapeutics*, 8th edition. Edited by A. G. Gilman, T.W. Rall, A.S. Nies, and P. Taylor, New York, Pergamon Press, 1985, pp.221-243.

114. Sawin, C.T., Geller, A., Hershman, J.M., Castelli, W., and Bacharach, P.: The aging thyroid: the use of thyroid hormone in older persons. *J.A.M.A.*, 261:2653, 1989.

115. Refetoff, S., Weiss, R.E., and Usala, S.J.: The syndromes of resistance to thyroid hormone. *Endocrine Reviews*, 14: 348-399, 1993.

116. Drayer, D.E.: Lipophilicity, hydrophilicity, and the central nervous system side effects of beta blockers. *Pharmacotherapy*, 7:87-91, 1987.

117. Wartofsky, L.: Thyrotoxic storm. In *Werner and Ingbar's The Thyroid: A Fundamental and Clinical Text*, 7th edition. Edited by L.P. Braverman and R.D. Utiger, Philadelphia, Lippincott-Raven Publishers, 1996, pp.701-712.

118. Ikram, H.: Hemodynamic effect of β-adrenergic blockade in hyperthyroid patients with and without heart failure. *Br. Med. J.*, 1:1505, 1977.

119. Chopra, I.J., Williams, D.E., Orgiazzi, J., and Soloman, D.H.: Opposite effects of dexamethasone or serum concentration of 3,3',5'-triiodothyronine (reverse T_3) and 3,5,3'-triiodothyronine (T_3). *J. Clin. Endocrinol. Metab.*, 41:911,

1975.

120. Duick, D.S., Warren, D.W., Nicoloff, J.T., Otis, C.L., and Croxson, M.S.: Effect of a single dose of dexa-methasone on the concentration of serum triiodothyronine in man. *J. Clin. Endocrinol. Metab.*, 39:1151, 1974.

121. Brent, G.A. and Larsen, P.R.: Treatment of hypothyroidism. In *Werner and Ingbar's The Thyroid: A Fundamental and Clinical Text*, 7th edition. Edited by L.P. Braverman and R.D. Utiger, Philadelphia, Lippincott-Raven Publishers, 1996, pp.883-887.

122. LeBoff, M.S., Kaplan, M.M., Silva, J.E., and Larsen, P.R.: Bioavailability of thyroid hormones from oral replacement preparations. *Metabolism*, 31:900, 1982.

123. Fish, L.H., Schwartz, H.L., Cavanaugh, J., Steffes, M.W., Bantle, J.P., and Oppenheimer, J.H.: Replacement dose, metabolism, and bioavailability of levothyroxine in the treatment of hypothyroidism. *N. Engl. J. Med.*, 316:764, 1987.

124. Winkler, A.W., Lavietes, P.H., Robbins, C.L., and Man, E.B.: Tolerance to oral thyroid and reaction to intravenous thyroxine in subjects without myxedema. *J. Clin. Invest.*, 22:535-544, 1943.

125. Lowe, J.C.: T₃-induced recovery from fibromyalgia by a hypothyroid patient resistant to T₄ and desiccated thyroid. *J. Myofascial Ther.*, 1(4):26-31, 1995.

126. Wilson, J. and Walton, J.N.: Some muscular manifestations of hypothyroidism. *J. Neurol. Neurosurg. Psychiat.*, 22:320-324, 1959.

127. Bigger, J. and Hoffman, B.F.: Anti-arrhythmic drugs. In *Goodman and Gilman's The Pharmacological Basis of Therapeutics*, 8th edition. New York, Pergamon Press, 1990, pp.840-873.

128. Kehlet, H., Bichert-Toft, M., Lindholm, J., and Rasmussen, P.: Short ACTH test in assessing hypothalamic- pituitary-adrencortical function. *Br. Med. J.*, 1:249-251, 1976.

129. Lindholm, J. and Kehlet, H.: Re-evaluation of the clinical value of the 30-minute ACTH test in assessing the hypothalamic-pituitary-adrenocortical function. *Clin. Endocrinol.*(Oxf.), 26:53-59, 1987.

130. Kawachi, I., Willett, W.C., Colditz, G.A., Stampfer, M.J., and Speizer, F.E.: A prospective study of coffee drinking and suicide in women. *Arch. Intern. Med.*, 156(5):521-525, 1996.

131. Aicher, B. and Kraupp, O.: The value of fixed combination analgesics as exemplified by Thomapyrine. *Wiener Klinische Wochenschrift*, 108(8):219-233, 1996.

132. Currier, S.R., Wilson, K.G., and Gautheir, S.T.: Caffeine and chronic low back pain. *Clin. J. Pain*, 11(3):214-219, 1995.

133. Hoyovadillo, C., Perezurizar, J., and Lopezmunoz, F.J.: Usefulness of the pain-induced functional impairment model to relate plasma levels of analgesics to their efficacy in rats. *J. Pharm. Pharmcol.*, 47(6):462-465, 1995.

134. Ward, N., Whitney, C., Avery, D., and Dunner, D.: The analgesic effects of caffeine in headache. *Pain*, 44:151-155, 1991.

135. Laska, E.M., Sunshine, A., Mueller, G., et al.: Caffeine as an analgesic adjuvant. *J.A.M.A.*, 251:1711-1718, 1984.

136. Ross, D.S., Ardisson, L.J., and Meskell, M.J.: Measurement of thyrotropin in clinical and subclinical hyperthyroidism using a new chemiluminescent assay. *J. Clin. Endocrinol. Metab.*, 69(3):684-688, 1989.

137. Travell, J.G. and Simons, D.G.: *Myofascial Pain and Dysfunction: The Trigger Point Manual*, Vol. 2. Baltimore, Williams and Wilkins, 1992.

138. Lowe, J.C., Garrison, R., Reichman, A.J., Yellin, J., Thompson, M., and Kaufman, D.: Effectiveness and safety of T₃ (triiodothyronine) therapy for euthyroid fibromyalgia: a double-blind placebo-controlled response-driven crossover study. *Clin. Bull. Myofascial Ther.*, 2(2/3):31-57, 1997.

139. Lowe, J.C., Reichman, A.J., and Yellin, J.: The process of change during T₃ treatment for euthyroid fibromyalgia: a double-blind placebo-controlled crossover study. *Clin. Bull. Myofascial Ther.*, 2(2/3):91-124, 1997.

140. Lowe, J.C., Garrison, R.L., Reichman, A.J., and Yellin, J.: Triiodothyronine (T₃) treatment of euthyroid fibromyalgia: a small-N replication of a double-blind placebo-controlled crossover study. *Clin. Bull. Myofascial Ther.*, 2(4):71-88, 1997.

141. Wigers, S.H., Skrondal, A., Finset, A., and Götestam, K.G.: Measuring change in fibromyalgic pain: the relevance of pain distribution. *J. Musculoskel. Pain*, 5(2):29-41, 1997.

142. Honeyman, G.S.: Metabolic therapy for hypothyroid and euthyroid fibromyalgia: two case reports. *Clin. Bull. Myofascial Ther.*, 2(4):19-49, 1997.

143. Ellyin, F., Fuh, C.Y., Singh, S.P., and Kumar, Y.: Hypothyroidism with angina pectoris: a clinical dilemma. *Postgrad. Med.*, 79(7):93-98, 1986.

144. Kehlet, H. and Binder, C.: Value of an ACTH test in assessing hypothalamic-pituitary-adrencortical function in glucocorticoid-treated patients. *Br. Med. J.*, 1:147-149, 1973.

145. Wolfe, F., Smythe, H.A., Yunus, M.B., et al.: The American College of Rheumatology 1990 criteria for the classification of fibromyalgia: report of the multicenter criteria committee. *Arthritis Rheumatol.*, 33:160-172, 1990.

146. Bartalena, L. and Pinchera, A.: Effects of thyroxine excess on peripheral organs. *Acta Medica Austriaca*, 21(2):60-65, 1994.

147. Reynolds, E.H.: Interrelationships between the neurology of folate and vitamin B12 deficiency. In *Folic Acid in Neurology, Psychiatry and Internal Medicine*. Edited by M.I. Botez and E.H. Reynolds, New York, Raven Press, 1979.

148. Vermeulen, A.: Environment, human reproduction, menopause, and andropause. *Environ. Health Perspect.*, 2 (Suppl.101):91-100, 1993.

149. Orwoll, E.S., Bauer, D.C., Vogt, T.M., and Fox, K.M.: Axial bone mass in older women. *Ann. Intern. Med.*, 124 (2):187, 1996.

150. Grant, D.J., McMurdo, M.E.T., Mole, P.A., and Paterson, C.R.: Is previous hyperthyroidism still a risk factor for osteoporosis in post-menopausal women? *Clin. Endocrinol.*, 43(3):339-345, 1995.

151. Costin, G., Kaplan, S.A., and Ling, S.M.: The Achilles reflex time in thyroid disorders. *J. Pediatr.*, 76:277, 1970.

152. Sonkin, L.S.: Endocrine disorders and muscle dysfunction. In *Clinical Management of Head, Neck and TMJ Pain and Dysfunction*. Edited by B. Gelb, Philadelphia, W.B. Saunders Co., 1985, pp.137-170.

153. DeLong, G.R.: The neuromuscular system and brain in thyrotoxicosis. In *Werner and Ingbar's The Thyroid: A Fundamental and Clinical Text*, 7ᵗʰ edition. Edited by L.P. Braverman and R.D. Utiger, Philadelphia, Lippincott-Raven Publishers, 1996, pp.645-652.

154. Starlanyl, D. and Copeland, M.E.: *Fibromyalgia and Myofascial Pain Syndrome: A Survival Manual.* Oakland CA, New Harbinger Publications, 1996.

155. Starlanyl, D.: Fibromyalgia and myofascial pain syndrome: a special challenge, *Clin. Bull. Myofascial Ther.*, 2(2/3):75-89, 1997.

156. Lowe, J.C.: *The Purpose and Practice of Myofascial Therapy* (Audiocassette program with manual). Houston, McDowell Publishing Co., 1989.

157. Backstrom, G. and Rubin, B.R.: *When Muscle Pain Won't Go Away* (study scheduled for journal publication). Dallas, Taylor Publishing Company, 1992 .

158. Wolfe, F.: The clinical syndrome of fibrositis. *Am. J. Medicine*, 81(suppl 3A):7-14, 1986.

159. Wolfe, F.: Personal communication, March 8, 1991.

160. Roth, T., Roehrs, T., and Vogel, G.: Zolpidem in the treatment of transient insomnia: a double-blind, randomized comparison with placebo. *Sleep*, 18(4):246-251, 1995.

161. Salva, P. and Costa, J.: Clinical pharmacokinetics and pharmacodynamics of zolpidem. *Clinical Pharmacokinetics*, 29(3):142-153, 1995.

162. Wesensten, N.J., Balkin, T.J., and Belenky, G.L.: Effects of daytime administration of zolpidem versus triazolam on memory. *Eur. J. Clin. Pharmacol.*, 48(2):115-122, 1995.

163. Rush, C.R. and Griffiths, R.R.: Zolpidem, triazolam, and temazepam: behavioral and subject-rated effects in normal volunteers. *J. Clin. Psychopharmacol.*, 16(2):146-157, 1996.

164. Moldofsky, H., Lue, F.A., Mously, C., Roth-Schechterb, W.J., and Reynolds, W.J.: Zolpidem in patients with fibromyalgia: a dose range, double-blind, placebo-controlled, modified crossover study. *J. Rheumatology*, 23:529-533, 1996.

165. Lowe, J.C.: *Nutritional Therapy: A Desk Manual.* Houston, Gulf Coast Publishing, 1982.

166. Bronson Pharmaceuticals: Product Reference Guide. P.O. Box 46903, St. Louis, MO 63146. Phone: 800-610-4848; Fax: 800-722-3821.

167. Schaumberg, H., Caplan, J., and Windebrank, A.: Sensory neuropathy from pyridoxine use: a new megavitamin syndrome. *N. Engl. J. Med.*, 309:445-448, 1983.

168. Pauling, L.: *How to Live Longer and Feel Better.* New York, Avon Books, 1987.

169. Pauling, L.: Sensory neuropathy from pyridoxine abuse. *N. Engl. J. Med.*, 310:197, 1984.

170. Hawkins, D. and Pauling, L.: *Orthomolecular Psychiatry.* San Francisco, W.H. Freeman and Co., 1973.

171. Ridgway, E.C., Cooper, D.S., Walker, H., et al.: Therapy of primary hypothyroidism with L-triiodothyronine: discordant cardiac and pituitary responses. *Clin. Endocrinol.*, 13(5):479-488, 1980.

172. Danowski, T.S.: Hydrocortisone and/or desiccated thyroid in physiologic dosage: VII. Pituitary-adrenocortical and thyroidal function. *Metabolism*, 11:705, 1962.

173. James, V.H.T.: Testing adrenocortical function. In *The Adrenal Gland*, 2ⁿᵈ edition. Edited by V.H.T. James, New York, Raven Press, Ltd., 1992, pp.319-326.

174. Wood, J.B., Frankland, A.W., James, V.H.T., and Landon, J.: A rapid test of adrenocortical function. *Lancet*, i:243-245, 1965.

175. Speckart, P.F., Nicoloff, J.T., and Bethune, J.E.: Screening for adrenocortical insufficiency with cosynthropin (synthetic ACTH). *Arch. Intern. Med.*, 128:761-763, 1971.

176. Landon, J., James, V.H.T., Cryer, R.J., Wynn, V., and Franklin, A.W.: Adrenocorticotrophic effects of a synthetic polypeptide-1-24 corticotrophin in man. *J. Clin. Endocrinol. Metab.*, 24:1206-1213, 1964.

177. Munabi, A.K., Fevillan, P., Staton, R.C., et al.: Adrenal steroid responses to continuous intravenous adrenocorticotropin infusion compared to bolus injection in normal volunteers. *J. Clin. Endocrinol. Metab.*, 63:1036-1040, 1986.

178. Kolanowski, J., Pizarro, M., and Crabbe, J.: Potentiation of adrenocortical response upon intermittent stimulation with corticotropin in normal subjects. *J. Clin. Endocrinol. Metab.*, 41:453-465, 1975.

179. Dickstein, G., Schechner, C., Nicholson, D., et al.: Adrenocortical stimulation test: effects of basal cortisol level, time of day, and suggested new sensitive low dose test. *J. Clin. Endocrinol. Metab.*, 72:773-778, 1991.

180. McGill, P.E., Greig, W.R., Browning, M.C.K., and Boyle, J.A.: Plasma cortisol response to Synacthen (1-24 ACTH) at different times of day in patients with rheumatic disease. *Ann. Rheum. Dis.*, 26:123-126, 1967.

181. Azziz, R., Bradley, E., Hugh, J., Boots, L.R., Parker, R.C., and Zacur, H.A.: Acute adrenocorticotropin (1-24) (ACTH) adrenal stimulation in eumenorrheic women: reproducibility and effect of ACTH dose, subject weight, and sampling time. *J. Clin. Endocrinol.*, 70:1273-1279, 1990.

182. Stewart, P.M., Corrie, J., Seckl, J.R., Edwards, C.R.W., and Padfield, P.L.: A rational approach for assessing the hypothalamic-pituitary-adrenal axis. *Lancet*, i:1208-1210, 1988.

183. May, E. and Carey, R.M.: Rapid adrenocorticotrophic hormone test in practice. *Am. J. Med.*, 79:679-684, 1985.

184. Kukreja, S.C. and Williams, G.A.: Corticotrophin stimulation test: inverse correlation between basal serum cortisol and its response to corticotrophin. *Acta Endocrinol. (Copenh)*, 97:522-524, 1981.

185. Travell, J.G.: Personal communication, July 9, 1992.

186. Linde, K., Ramirez, G., Mulrow, C.D., Pauls, A., Weidenhammer, W., and Melchart, D.: St John's wort for depression: an overview and meta-analysis of randomised clinical trials. *Brit. Med. J.*, 313(7052):253-258, 1996.

187. Lowe, J.C. and Honeyman-Lowe, G.: Facilitating the decrease in fibromyalgic pain during metabolic rehabilitation: an essential role for soft tissue therapies. *J. Bodywork Movem. Ther.*, 2(4):208-217, 1998.

188. Kariks, J. and Perry, S.W.: Folic acid deficiency in psychiatric patients. *Med. J. Aust.*, 1:1192-1195, 1970.

189. Thornton, W.E. and Thornton, B.P.: Folic acid, mental function, and dietary habits. *J. Clin. Psychiat.*, 39:315-322, 1978.

190. Carney, M.W.P.: Psychiatric aspects of folate deficiency. In *Folic Acid in Neurology, Psychiatry and Internal Medicine*. Edited by M.I. Botez and E.H. Reynolds, New York, Raven Press, 1979.

191. Johnson, A.C.: *Chiropractic Physiological Therapeutics*, 5th edition. Palm Springs, self published, 1977.

192. Pelligrino, M.J., Fossen, D.V., Gordon, C., et al: Prevalence of mitral valve prolapse in primary fibromyalgia: a pilot investigation. *Arch. Phys. Med. Rehabil.*, 70:541-543, 1989.

193. Pinchera, A., Martino, E., and Faglia, G.: Central hypothyroidism. In *Werner and Ingbar's The Thyroid: A Fundamental and Clinical Text*, 6th edition. Edited by L.E. Braverman and R.D. Utiger, New York, J.B. Lippincott Co., 1991, pp.968-984.

5.3

T_4 (Thyroxine) and Combined T_4 /T_3 Preparations: Considerations for the Treatment of Hypothyroid Fibromyalgia

In 1973, the objective for conventional clinicians in treating hypothyroid patients changed. Before this time, the objective had been to induce normal tissue metabolism and relieve patients' symptoms. The objective changed to providing "replacement dosages" of T_4, amounts that keep the thyroid hormone and/or TSH levels within their respective "normal" reference ranges. Thyroidologists recommended this because some patients taking TSH-suppressive dosages of thyroid hormone had variations from normal biochemical and physiological measures. The thyroidologists conjectured that these variations portended adverse effects on various tissues in these patients. However, the scientific evidence now shows that these variations were of no clinical importance. Nevertheless, most clinicians still argue that a dosage of thyroid hormone that keeps the patient's TSH within the normal range is the only "safe" dosage. Some thyroidologists encouraged this belief by falsely defining TSH-suppres-

sive dosages of thyroid hormone as "thyrotoxic."

Beliefs of conventional clinicians regarding hypothyroidism have been profoundly influenced by two factors: (1) the misinterpretation of biochemical and physiological variations in patients taking TSH-suppressive dosages and (2) the acceptance of too broad a range of normal for the TSH. These factors have led to four prevailing propositions of the reigning endocrinology/thyroidology paradigm: (1) the only cause of thyroid hormone deficiency symptoms and signs is hypothyroidism, (2) clinicians should not permit patients with normal thyroid function test results to use thyroid hormone, (3) hypothyroid patients should use only "replacement" dosages of thyroid hormone, and (4) hypothyroid patients should use only T_4. Each of these propositions is false: (1) Patients with partial cellular thyroid hormone resistance have normal thyroid function test results although their symptoms and signs are usually identical to those of patients with

981

hypothyroidism. (2) Patients with cellular resistance to thyroid hormone, despite having normal thyroid function test results, improve or recover without thyrotoxicity when they use high enough dosages of exogenous thyroid hormone. (3) A replacement dosage is an amount that keeps thyroid hormone and/or TSH levels within their respective ranges of normal. TSH-suppressive dosages of thyroid hormone, however, do not harm most hypothyroid patients when they keep their dosages low enough to avoid tissue overstimulation. Replacement dosages of T_4 are inadequate for properly regulating metabolism in many, and perhaps most, tissues. Typically, replacement dosages do not produce normal circulating T_3 levels, normal cellular thyroid hormone concentrations, or normal measures of tissue metabolic status. Replacement dosages are likely to harm patients who require greater amounts to maintain normal metabolic status. (4) Recent studies showed that in hypothyroid animals, T_4 alone does not normalize cellular concentrations of thyroid hormone or tissue metabolism; treatment with T_4 and T_3 combined, however, normalizes both. This finding corresponds to the greater improvement of hypothyroid humans using a combination of T_4 and T_3 compared to those using only T_4. Hypothyroid fibromyalgia patients usually improve or recover under only one condition: when their clinicians abandon the current conventional endocrinology/thyroidology protocol for one similar to the protocol generally used before 1973.

In general, conventional clinicians misbelieve that researchers have established the four propositions of the endocrinology/thyroidology paradigm as true. They therefore believe the propositions to be mandates for clinical practice. Their need to justify clinical decisions in malpractice suits has favored belief in the four propositions and the trend toward extremist medical technocracy. Consequently, conventional clinicians do not, for the most part, effectively and safely treat hypothyroid patients. Clinicians either deny patients the use of exogenous thyroid hormone or restrict them to dosages too low to maintain normal tissue metabolism. As a result, the patients remain symptomatic, suffer reduced quality of life, and risk pathological processes such as cardiovascular disease that may cause premature death. The Internet has made it obvious that patients across the world are dissatisfied with the conventional treatment for hypothyroidism; their dissatisfaction has led to widespread contempt for the endocrinology/thyroidology specialty.

The clinician should initially establish a patient's thyroid status with laboratory thyroid function tests. The clinician should not use these tests, however, to ti-

trate the patient's thyroid hormone dosage; research has shown the tests to be useless for this purpose. To properly adjust the patient's dosage, the clinician should use instead a multi-modal assessment of the patient's tissue metabolic status. Measures should include the patient's symptoms, signs, and peripheral indices (see Chapter 4.3). In addition, the five fibromyalgia measures described in Chapter 4.1 are essential to optimizing the hypothyroid fibromyalgia patient's response to therapy.

Some hypothyroid patients obtain satisfactory therapeutic benefits from the use of T_4 alone. These patients, however, are exceptions. The therapeutic outcome is virtually always superior when patients use desiccated thyroid or preparations containing both synthetic T_4 and T_3. Some researchers favor a T_4/T_3 ratio similar to the ratio of T_4 to T_3 secreted by the thyroid gland (10:1-to-14:1). The lower T_4/T_3 ratio of desiccated thyroid, however, is preferable. The larger relative amount of T_3 in desiccated thyroid may benefit patients who have some degree of cellular thyroid hormone resistance. In addition, no credible scientific evidence shows that the use of T_3, even in supraphysiologic dosages, adversely affects patients when they use non-thyrotoxic dosages.

Some hypothyroid patients do not benefit from the use of T_4 alone, desiccated thyroid, or synthetic T_4/T_3 combinations, no matter how high the dosage. Most of these patients markedly improve or recover from their symptoms when they switch to T_3 alone. Patients obtain best therapeutic results when they use T_3 as part of a more comprehensive metabolic rehabilitation regimen (see Chapters 5.2 and 5.4).

No matter which thyroid hormone preparation they take, most patients maximally improve when they use TSH-suppressive—but non-thyrotoxic—dosages. In fact, most patients remain symptomatic until they begin using amounts of thyroid hormone greater than "replacement" dosages. The clinician should progressively increase the patient's dosage until it produces the desired subjective and objective state.

The clinician should take several precautions by evaluating patients before, during, and after they begin the use of thyroid hormone. (1) He should evaluate patients with central hypothyroidism for possible deficiency of pituitary hormones other than TSH. Particularly important to watch for is a possible ACTH deficiency causing adrenal insufficiency. The clinician should correct the patient's adrenal insufficiency before the patient begins thyroid hormone therapy. Occasionally, after the patient begins thyroid hormone therapy, the appearance or worsening of symptoms *such as muscle weakness suggests decreased adrenal reserve (see Chapter 5.2, section: "Precautions in the Use of Exogenous Thyroid Hormone: Adrenal Insufficiency"). (2) The clinician should closely monitor patients at risk for adverse cardiac effects (see Chapter 4.4). (3) If the patient is post-menopausal or has significantly low bone mineral density before beginning thyroid hormone therapy, the clinician should order bone densitometry at intervals. The results of densitometry should be used within a collaborative professional interaction to insure the patient's safety. Patients taking exogenous estrogen and benefitting from it may have to increase their estrogen dosages after beginning thyroid hormone therapy to maintain the benefits. Overall, the risks of adverse cardiac and osseous effects have been exaggerated. The exaggeration has induced fear-based adherence by clinicians to the four propositions of the current endocrinology/thyroidology paradigm. The exaggeration has also resulted in an enormous expenditure of health care dollars for useless laboratory thyroid function testing during the treatment of hypothyroid patients.*

The conventional treatment of hypothyroid patients since 1973 has been one of the most tragic disasters in the history of medicine. Today, conventional endocrinology/thyroidology is tenaciously resisting the mounting pressure to change the paradigm that is responsible for this disaster. Four propositions articulate the reigning endocrinology/thyroidology hypothyroidism paradigm. The grounds for the method of treating hypothyroidism I recommend in this chapter should be clear upon considering the falsehood of the four propositions.

● **MANDATES OF THE CONVENTIONAL MEDICAL HYPOTHYROIDISM PARADIGM**

I began studying the relation of fibromyalgia to hypothyroidism some 14 years ago. Since then, my co-treating physicians and I have treated hypothyroid patients with either T₄ (usually Synthroid) alone or desiccated thyroid. The choice depended on the co-treating prescribing physician for each patient: conventional physicians preferred T₄ and alternative physicians preferred Armour desiccated thyroid. Some hypothyroid fibromyalgia patients markedly improved or recovered with the use of these forms of thyroid hormone; others derived no benefit whatsoever from them. In 1990, I

discovered the thyroid hormone resistance literature. Soon after, I discussed with thyroidologists studying thyroid hormone resistance the possibility that euthyroid fibromyalgia was a phenotypic expression of cellular resistance to thyroid hormone. These researchers concurred that the possibility was worth pursuing. A physician in my clinic and I then began co-treating euthyroid fibromyalgia patients with T₃ according to the protocol used for patients with proven thyroid hormone resistance. The outcome was largely successful (see Chapter 5.4 and Appendix B, paper titled "Results of an Open Trial of T₃ Therapy with 77 Euthyroid Female Fibromyalgia Patients"[104]).

We also used T₃ in our treatment of hypothyroid fibromyalgia patients who failed to benefit from T₄ or desiccated thyroid. Again, the outcome in virtually every case was successful. Appendix B contains a published case that clearly illustrates this phenomenon (see paper titled "T₃-Induced Recovery from Fibromyalgia by a Hypothyroid Patient Resistant to T₄ and Desiccated Thyroid"[78]). Until recently, my colleagues and I continued to initially treat hypothyroid patients with T₄. If a patient did not satisfactorily respond to T₄, we switched her to T₃. T₃ has practically always been effective when used as a component of the patient's metabolic rehabilitation, enabling the patient to markedly improve or completely recover.

In retrospect, had some of my more conventional co-treating physicians ignored the propositions of the conventional hypothyroidism paradigm, more of the patients we treated with T₄ would have benefitted from its use. Even more of these patients would have benefitted from desiccated thyroid. In the section below, I provide reasons for rejecting the four propositions. I do so because those reasons are the basis for the positions I take in the remainder of this chapter.

(1) HYPOTHYROIDISM IS THE EXCLUSIVE CAUSE OF THYROID DEFICIENCY SYMPTOMS

The first proposition of conventional endocrinology/thyroidology is that hypothyroidism is the exclusive cause of symptoms characteristic of thyroid hormone deficiency.[48,p.49] The well-substantiated phenomenon of thyroid hormone resistance syndromes (see Chapters 2.5, 2.6, and 5.4) conclusively falsifies this proposition. Those who propound the first proposition ignore the massive published research literature on thyroid hormone resistance. Mutations in the c-*erb*Aβ gene are at this time the only unequivocally proven cause of thyroid hormone resistance. Research evidence for other causes is minimal right now. Despite this, cellular resistance to thyroid hormone is common, especially among fibromyalgia patients.

My research has documented cellular resistance to thyroid hormone in euthyroid fibromyalgia patients through three related findings: (1) the typical euthyroid fibromyalgia patient recovers (no longer meets the criteria for fibromyalgia) with the proper use of supraphysiologic dosages of T_3; (2) the recovered patient has extremely high serum free T_3 levels; and (3) despite the patient's use of supraphysiologic dosages of T_3 and high circulating free T_3 levels, she does not have tissue thyrotoxicity. The high serum free T_3 levels show that the patient is not clearing the hormone from her body at an accelerated rate. The high T_3 levels suggest that her cells are exposed to extraordinarily large amounts of the hormone. If her cells were normally responsive to T_3, she would have indications of tissue thyrotoxicity. But she does not.[154][155][156]

These findings in recovered euthyroid fibromyalgia patients engender two deductions. The first is that the patients have partial cellular resistance to thyroid hormone. The second is that the cellular resistance mediates the thyroid hormone deficiency-like signs and symptoms these patients have before undergoing proper treatment with supraphysiologic dosages of T_3. Ergo, the proposition is false that hypothyroidism is the only cause of symptoms characteristic of thyroid hormone deficiency.

(2) PATIENTS WITH NORMAL THYROID FUNCTION TEST RESULTS SHOULD NOT BE PERMITTED TO USE THYROID HORMONE THERAPY

The second proposition of conventional endocrinology/thyroidology is that clinicians should not permit patients with normal thyroid function test results to undergo therapeutic trials of thyroid hormone.[48,p.49] The proposition has two implications: (1) thyroid hormone therapy will not benefit patients whose thyroid function test results are normal, or (2) their use of thyroid hormone will harm them. Ample evidence negates this second proposition through falsifying its underpinning implications.

Patients With Peripheral Resistance to Thyroid Hormone: Improvement or Recovery with Thyroid Hormone Therapy Despite Normal Thyroid Function Test Results

Patients with peripheral resistance to thyroid

hormone have normal circulating levels of TSH and thyroid hormones (see Chapter 2.6, section titled "Peripheral Tissue Resistance to Thyroid Hormone"). My colleagues and I learned from two studies that about 44% of fibromyalgia patients were euthyroid.[95][157] We can accurately classify these patients as having peripheral cellular resistance to thyroid hormone. We also found in systematic open trials,[77][78][158][159] double-blind trials,[154][155][156] and extensive clinical experience that most of these patients improve or recover when permitted to use enough thyroid hormone as part of a more comprehensive regimen of metabolic rehabilitation. Yet conventional clinicians have often attempted to intervene with one of two objectives: first, to get recovered patients to stop using T_3 altogether, or second, to get the patients to reduce the thyroid hormone dosages that enabled them to get well. The main argument of these practitioners has been that the patients' use of T_3 would lead to disastrous health consequences. The practitioners have apparently been unaware of the leaflet pharmacists give patients when they fill their prescriptions for Cytomel (a brand of T_3). *Verbatim et literatim*, the leaflet says: "NO COMMON SIDE EFFECTS HAVE BEEN REPORTED with the proper use of this medicine."[105]

Lack of Harm from Thyroid Hormone Use by Patients with Normal Thyroid Function Test Results

Several observations contradict the implication that exogenous thyroid hormone will harm patients who have normal thyroid function test results. First, the published studies by my research group show that when euthyroid fibromyalgia patients follow the protocol I describe in Chapter 5.2, they improve or recover without evidence of tissue thyrotoxicity (see subsection above titled "(1) Hypothyroidism is the Exclusive Cause of Thyroid Deficiency Symptoms").[154][155][156] This means that the patients' use of thyroid hormone did not harm them. We have not found thyrotoxicity in properly treated patients in both experimental and clinical settings. The patients were indubitably euthyroid (they had normal thyroid gland function) according to laboratory thyroid function testing including the TRH-stimulation test (see Chapter 4.2).

The findings of my research group are not unique. In recent years, a growing number of physicians have rejected the second proposition of conventional endocrinology/thyroidology and treated euthyroid patients with exogenous thyroid hormone. The results have been satisfactory enough so that the trend of treating euthyroid patients with thyroid hormone is growing. Unfortunately, physicians' apprehension of using TSH-suppressive dosages of thyroid hormone has mitigated their patients' benefits from this unconventional practice. Most physicians I have communicated with who treat euthyroid patients with thyroid hormone titrate dosages according to patients' TSH levels; they restrict patients to dosages that hold TSH levels within the normal range. The belief that TSH-suppressive dosages of thyroid hormone are harmful is true for some patients; it is false, however, for most (see subsections below titled "(3) The Patient Should Only be Permitted to Use Replacement Dosages of Thyroid Hormone"). Morever, it is the replacement dosages that are potentially harmful to many patients. Unfortunately, patients around the world are systematically deprived of TSH-suppressive dosages by conventional clinicians who believe the third proposition (see next section).

(3) THE PATIENT SHOULD ONLY BE PERMITTED TO USE REPLACEMENT DOSAGES OF THYROID HORMONE

The third proposition of the conventional endocrinology/thyroidology paradigm is that the clinician should treat the hypothyroid patient only with a "replacement" dosage of T_4. Demonstrating the falsehood of this proposition is extremely important. A recently published statement of the well-known chronic fatigue syndrome researcher David Bell shows why. Bell expressed the belief that conventional medical physicians commonly hold: "If thyroid function is impaired, it should be treated." And, "Any patient with abnormal thyroid hormone levels should be treated in the *standard* manner [italics mine]."[114,p.87] And what is the "standard" manner? Bell explained. First, he noted that the majority of chronic fatigue syndrome patients have normal thyroid hormone levels. Then he wrote: ". . . it has been suggested that in illnesses with excess levels of cytokines, the function of thyroid hormone is blocked. If this were the case, treatment with thyroid preparations might improve symptoms. I would like to say that thyroid *replacement* is the solution to the problem of CFIDS [italics mine]. It would be a wonderful, safe, and simple treatment. Unfortunately, I have not found it to be effective."[114,p.207] Had Bell used TSH-suppressive dosages instead of the "standard" replacement dosages, his report would be quite different. His statements in the quote above are predictable in that he apparently subscribes to the third false

proposition of the endocrinology/thyroidology paradigm.

The term "replacement dosage" has broad and narrow senses. In its broadest sense, a replacement dosage is an amount of T_4 that keeps thyroid hormone and TSH levels within their respective normal reference ranges. In the narrow sense, a replacement dosage is an amount that keeps the TSH within its normal range[48,p.53] without consideration of thyroid hormone levels. Within this definition, thyroid function test results other than that of the TSH are irrelevant in the clinical care of the hypothyroid patient, just as the patient's clinical status is immaterial. Some thyroidologists now extol this narrow definition of replacement dosage, and many conventional clinicians use it to titrate patients' thyroid hormone dosages. This narrow definition, however, ushers its proponents into the realm of the most preposterous extremity of medical technocracy. The definition is ludicrous if the clinician's aim is to provide patients with normal tissue metabolism, health, and well-being. Treatment of hypothyroidism based on this definition has devastated the health and life-quality of incalculable numbers of patients. Many hypothyroid patients are outspoken, especially on the Internet, about their dissatisfaction with treatment based on the narrow definition of replacement dosage. They scoff, jeer at, and hold in contempt the researchers and clinicians who promote or subscribe to the definition. Their derision is understandable. Other patients dissatisfied with the definition, and the prescribing of only T_4, have been articulate in denouncing the definition and clinical practice derived from it. In support of their denunciation, I recently published the following statement to my Web site (http://www.drlowe.com); I quote it here because of its relevance to proposition number three:

Physicist John Ziman wrote an excellent book on the grounds for belief in science. In it, he said: "The experts in a particular field can become so indoctrinated and so committed to the current paradigm that their critical and imaginative powers are inhibited, and they cannot 'see beyond their own noses.'"[51,p.134] When the experts can no longer see beyond their noses, the public has grounds for not believing in their science. In recent years, steadily growing numbers of people have expressed the belief that the experts in conventional endocrinology can't "see beyond their noses." Why do people express this belief about the experts? Mainly for one reason: The experts' beliefs about thyroid hormone treatment keep many people sick.

And these people remain sick until they undergo treatment by practitioners who don't share the experts' beliefs. Obviously, the expert's beliefs are wrong. Yet despite the continuing illness of patients and their subsequent recovery under the care of other practitioners, the experts hold tenaciously to their false beliefs. It is little wonder then that patients question the credibility of conventional endocrinology "experts."

Professor Ziman also wrote, "In these circumstances, scientific progress may come to a halt—knowledge may even regress—until intellectual intruders come through the interdisciplinary frontiers and look at the field without preconceptions."[51,p.134]

Scientific progress in the treatment of hypothyroid patients *has* regressed. Before the early 1970s, most hypothyroid patients were satisfied with the safe and effective treatment doctors provided. But in the early 70s, the TSH and other modern thyroid tests came into widespread use. With the advent of these tests, endocrinologists agreed among themselves to permit patients to take only half the dosage of thyroid hormone previously used. In addition, one powerful pharmaceutical company purchased the allegiance of conventional endocrinology. In accord with the implicit financial deal, conventional endocrinology used its authority for the good of the company. The "experts" influenced patients and their doctors to believe that the only legitimate thyroid product to use was that company's brand—a brand we now know often provides patients with inferior treatment results.

In recent years, out of this sorry state of affairs, examples of the "intellectual intruders" Ziman referred to have come forth. Some of these "intruders" are doctors outside the endocrinology fraternity. They are dedicated foremost to the welfare of patients, and they couldn't care less for the affluence and prestige derived through allegiance to the interests of powerful pharmaceutical companies.

Also among the "intellectual intruders" are some patients forsaken by conventional endocrinology. The beliefs of the experts in conventional endocrinology are partly a product of financial manipulations by pharmaceutical companies. But the beliefs of these intruding patients are a product of personal experience with the miseries caused by the beliefs of the endocrinology experts. These intruding pa-

tients are the salvation of other patients who have remained ill because of the beliefs of the experts.

Recently, two such patients, Mary Shomon[149] in the U.S. and Karen Goodfellow[150] in England, have publicly spoken out. These "intruders," with intelligence and eloquence, have taken conventional endocrinology to task. In that most patients' fibromyalgia is a product of too little thyroid hormone regulation of tissues, I urge fibromyalgia patients to read what Mary and Karen have written. I also recommend that physicians—especially endocrinologists—read with an open mind what these two patients have to say. Their views may help melt away the cognitive shackles buckled into place by vested corporate interests through conventional medical education.

Basis of the Problem of Replacement Dosages

The concept of replacement dosages calculated from laboratory test results is based on two factors: (1) misinterpretation of investigative data in the early 1970s and, over time, gradual transformation of the misinterpretation into scientific "fact" within the belief system of conventional medicine; and (2) the dubious TSH range of normal.

Misinterpretation of Investigative Data and Its Gradual Acceptance as Scientific Fact. Since 1973, conventional clinicians treating hypothyroid patients have practiced based on an odd assumption. They have assumed that the function of thyroid hormone therapy is to maintain "normal" circulating thyroid hormone or TSH levels. Sawin wrote, for example, that the main goal of thyroid hormone therapy is to assure a constant supply of thyroid hormone to the body's tissues. The supply should mimic the normal person's constant levels of T_3 and T_4.[13,p.394] Volpé wrote: "It is indeed clear that the best current arbiter of normal replacement of thyroxine in hypothyroidism would be a TSH value (performed by a 'sensitive' assay) that is in the middle of the normal range. That would mean that the patient is completely finely tuned as far as it is humanly possible to accomplish."[21,p.87] Stockigt stated, "A serum TSH value in the low-normal range is probably the best single indicator of appropriate dosage . . . ."[63,p.381] According to Hamburger, normal serum basal TSH levels exclude thyroid dysfunction.[21,p.70] For conventional clinicians treating hypothyroid patients, achieving a "normal" basal TSH level has become the emblem of success.

Before 1973, clinicians based their treatment of hypothyroid patients on a different assumption about thyroid gland function and thyroid hormone therapy. The assumption was rational and generally led to successful treatment results. Published statements by Kimball and Whorton in the 1930s exemplified the objective of these pre-1973 clinicians. According to Kimball in 1933, the major function of the thyroid gland is to maintain the rate of cellular oxidation above a certain level, allowing for individual variations.[42,p.495] Whorton wrote in 1939, "The chief function of the thyroid gland is to regulate the speed of the metabolic processes of the body."[44,p.371] The ultimate biological function of the thyroid gland has not changed since then. If thyroid hormone therapy is to be effective, it must share this ultimate function—to maintain a sufficient cellular metabolic rate. Yet since 1973, the patient's metabolic status has become virtually irrelevant to clinicians. The only consideration of conventional clinicians is whether TSH levels are within the "normal range."

Researchers developed useful TSH radioimmunoassays in the early 1970s. Until the advent of these assays, clinicians usually treated primary hypothyroid patients with 200-to-400 µg (0.2-to-0.4 mg) of T_4 daily or the equivalent in desiccated thyroid.[23,p.456][135] Clinicians based this range on clinical grounds,[152,p.91] that is, clinicians titrated patients' dosages upward until the clinicians and patients judged that the dosage produced the desired effect on symptoms, signs, the basal metabolic rate, and other peripheral indices (see Chapter 4.3). This protocol was both effective and safe. The 200-to-400 µg dosages used before the early 1970s generally suppress patients' TSH levels below the lower limit of the normal reference range. Because the dosages are TSH-suppressive, they by definition exceed today's "replacement dosages."

Some thyroidologists such as Toft have used the terms "suppressed TSH" and "thyrotoxic" as synonyms. This use of these words implies that the thyroidologists believe that TSH-suppressive dosages of thyroid hormone guarantee thyrotoxicity. This belief, however, is patently false, as shown by evidence I present in Chapter 4.4. The available scientific evidence supports what Pearch and Himsworth wrote of the clinical approach to titrating thyroid hormone dosage: "It is the common experience that no characteristic pathology develops in patients treated for hypothyroidism even after many years, nor is life expectancy diminished. Moreover, this knowledge is derived from a period when larger doses of thyroid hormones were given than are now customary."[153,p.695]

Dubious Conventional TSH Range of Normal. The conventional normal reference range for the TSH varies. For some laboratories it is 0.45-to-4.5 µU/mL; for other laboratories it is 0.4-to-6.0 µU/mL. The validity of such ranges of normal is dubious. Doubt is based on the results of the recently published Whickham survey study. This study involved a randomly selected population of 2779 adults living in Whickham, Tyne, and Wear, England. Thyroid function tests were available at baseline and at a 20-year follow-up. Of the 1877 survivors, 96% took part in the follow-up and 91% underwent further testing. The researchers reported that people with a baseline TSH level of 2.0 µU/mL or higher had an increased risk of future hypothyroidism compared to those with TSH levels below that level.[132] Weetman wrote of this finding, "The simplest explanation is that thyroid disease is so common that many people predisposed to thyroid failure are included in a laboratory's reference population . . . ."[134] In other words, when laboratories calculated the range of normal for the TSH, they include in the calculation the TSH values of patients predisposed to hypothyroidism or with incipient hypothyroidism. If laboratories excluded these patients, the range of normal for the TSH would probably be 0.4-to-2.0 µU/mL or close to it.

TSH-Suppressive Dosages of Thyroid Hormone are Not Ipso Facto Harmful

Many conventional clinicians assume that TSH-suppressive dosages of thyroid hormone are invariably thyrotoxic. However, studies peppered through the recent thyroidology literature falsify this proposition. True, TSH-suppressive dosages are potentially harmful to some patients, but they are essential to health for others.

The clinician should keep the dosage of the patient with cardiac fragility, low adrenal reserve, or osteoporosis below the amount likely to exacerbate the abnormality. However, TSH-suppressive dosages do not cause osteoporosis and do not increase the risk for fracture. Although post-menopausal women may have reduced bone density, those taking TSH-suppressive dosages do not have lower bone density than those taking replacement dosages (see Chapter 4.4, section titled "Bone Density"). My testing of patients has shown that those taking TSH-suppressive dosages tend to have higher bone density than patients taking replacement dosages. The higher density most likely results from the patients' increased levels of physical activity mediated by the TSH-suppressive dosages.

The clinician should exercise reasonable precaution regarding cardiac safety by considering each patient individually. However, the incidence of death from ischemic heart disease in patients taking T_4 is no greater in those taking TSH-suppressive dosages than in those taking replacement dosages. TSH-suppressive dosages of thyroid hormone lower circulating lipid levels more than replacement dosages. In addition, higher-end dosages of the hormone are capable of halting progression of coronary artery disease. When patients do not have coronary artery disease, myocardial ischemia and/or infarction are rare even in thyrotoxic patients. Moreover, restricting many patients to replacement dosages predisposes them to cardiovascular disease and premature death. With these patients, erring on the side of safety means their using higher-end rather than lower-end dosages of thyroid hormone. (see Chapter 4.4, section titled "The Heart"). The cardiac risks are so minimal with TSH-suppressive dosages that Shapiro et al. reported in 1997, "In the absence of symptoms of thyrotoxicosis, patients treated with TSH-suppressive doses of L-T_4 may be followed clinically without specific cardiac laboratory studies."[52]

Skinner et al. recently advocated trials of thyroid hormone therapy for patients who are clinically hypothyroid but euthyroid according to thyroid function test results. Regarding objections, they wrote, "The dangers of osteoporosis and cardiac catastrophe—particularly during a three-month trial—are sometimes quoted, but these worries are unfounded and condemn many patients to years of hypothyroidism with its pathological complications and poor quality of life."[55]

Inadequacy of Replacement Dosages for the Treatment of Hypothyroid Patients

The results of the Whickham study suggest that the "normal" reference range may be 2-to-3 times broader than it should be: A range of 0.4-to-2.0 μU/mL rather than 0.4-to-5.5 or so μU/mL may more accurately represent normal pituitary-thyroid axis function. If this is true, then patients with TSH levels in what conventional clinicians view as the high-normal range (from 2.0-to-4.5 or 6.0 μU/mL) may benefit from the use of thyroid hormone. Yet according to the second proposition of the conventional endocrinology/thyroidology paradigm, clinicians must deny patients with TSH levels within the conventional normal range the use of exogenous thyroid hormone. Clinicians are thus likely to deny patients with "high-normal" TSH levels the opportunity to use thyroid hormone due to the falsely broad TSH reference range. For many patients, the denial is likely to lead to a diminished quali-

ty of life; for others, it is likely to result in pathogenic processes, such as atherosclerosis, that lead to diminished mental and physical abilities and premature death. (See Chapter 4.4, section titled "The Harm from Untreated and Undertreated Hypothyroidism").

Completely denying patients thyroid hormone they may benefit from is not the only problem with the dubious normal TSH range. Clinicians who depend on the conventional range of normal may also restrict patients using thyroid hormone to dosages that are too low to be effective. Weetman raised this possibility in commenting on the Whickham survey. He wrote that the finding of a higher incidence of future overt hypothyroidism in patients with TSH levels 2.0 μU/mL or above raises a question: Is T_4 replacement adequate in patients with TSH levels above 2.0 μU/mL?[134] The available evidence indicates that it is not.

Many hypothyroid patients have consulted me for symptoms that lowered the quality of their lives. These symptoms had debilitated some patients. Typically, when my co-treating physicians and I increased the patients' thyroid hormone dosages to TSH-suppressive amounts, the patients' symptoms improved or were completely relieved. It is worth emphasizing again that these patients' improvement or recovery occurred without tissue thyrotoxicity. At this point, I am convinced that restricting most hypothyroid patients to replacement dosages consigns them to suffer from continuing symptoms and signs of inadequate thyroid hormone regulation of tissue metabolism. Recent research findings explain these clinical experiences and my conclusion. The research findings lead to four main propositions: Typically, replacement dosages 1) do not produce normal circulating free T_3 levels, 2) do not produce normal cellular thyroid hormone concentrations, 3) do not normalize measures of tissue metabolic status, and 4) harm some patients by depriving them of enough thyroid hormone to maintain normal tissue metabolism. (Note that I have qualified each of these propositions as "typically" true; the propositions are therefore not categorically, invariably true. The propositions are based on studies that used group statistics. The outcomes reported statistical significance levels based on comparison of group measures. For some individuals, the propositions are false, but on average, they are true.)

1) Replacement dosages do not produce normal circulating free T_3 levels. Some writers have argued that hypothyroid patients can achieve normal tissue metabolism by taking enough T_4 to produce a normal circulating free T_3 level. A high enough dosage of T_4 to do so results in a moderately elevated T_4 level and a low-normal TSH level.[21,pp.88-89] The results of rat experiments conducted by Escobar-Morreale et al. provide some support for this line of thought. These researchers found that inducing supraphysiologic plasma T_4 levels with infused T_4 was necessary to normalize plasma T_3 levels.[142,p.2833] But the conjecture that producing a normal circulating T_3 level produces normal tissue metabolism in all tissues is doubtful. Escobar-Morreale et al. reported that in several rat tissues, T_3 concentrations became normal only under one condition—when the rats received high enough infusions of T_4 to produce supraphysiologic circulating T_3 levels.[142,p.2832] Producing supraphysiologic circulating T_3 levels in hypothyroid patients requires T_4 dosages that conventional clinicians do not allow because the dosages suppress TSH levels. Korsic et al., for example, found that patients taking replacement dosages of T_4 had normal-range T_3 and TSH levels. Patients with significantly higher T_3 levels, however, were taking TSH-suppressive dosages of T_4.[119] Conventional clinicians are likely to deny patients high enough T_4 dosages to achieve normal circulating free T_3 levels; they are even more likely to deny patients high enough dosages to produce supraphysiologic T_3 levels. Consequently, some tissues of the patient using T_4 replacement dosages are likely to have abnormally low T_3 concentrations and hypometabolism.

2) Replacement dosages do not produce normal cellular thyroid hormone concentrations. Escobar-Morreale et al. studied the relationships between circulating and tissue concentrations of T_4 and T_3 in thyroidectomized rats. The researchers looked at these relationships with respect to different amounts of infused T_4. They found that infusing rats with T_4 did not produce a linear increase in circulating T_4 and T_3: The highest infused amounts of T_4 increased plasma T_4 levels to a range of 14%-to-352% of the mean T_4 level for control (non-thyroidectomized) rats. In comparison, the infused T_4 increased plasma T_3 levels to a range of 16%-to-245% of the mean of control rats. From this finding, the researchers reported, "Plasma T_3 increases less than T_4 in the hypothyroid range, and supraphysiologic plasma T_4 levels have to be reached for normalization of plasma T_3."[142,p.2833]

Escobar-Morreale et al. were not able to predict the change in tissue concentrations of T_4 or T_3 from the plasma T_4 or T_3 levels alone. The ratio of plasma T_4 and T_3 to tissue T_4 and T_3 differed for different tissues. Moreover, changes in plasma T_4 and T_3 levels changed the ratios of T_4 to T_3 in some tissues but not others.[142,p.2833]

The investigators reported that a normal plasma T_3 level did not ensure a normal T_3 concentration in all tissues. In some tissues, T_3 concentrations were low despite normal plasma T_3 levels following T_4 infusions. Exceptions included the cerebral cortex and cerebellum, and less reliably, kidney, skeletal muscle, and spleen. T_3 concentrations were normal in these tissues. They also reported that normal plasma T_4 levels did not ensure normal T_4 concentrations in all tissues. When plasma T_4 levels were normal, concentrations of T_4 were high in skeletal muscle and cerebellum cells, low in heart cells, and less reliably low in kidney and liver cells.[142,pp.2833-2834]

Escobar-Morreale et al. also calculated the circulating T_4 and T_3 levels that ensured that T_4 and T_3 concentrations in each tissue were comparable to those in control rats. Cerebral concentration of T_3 remained normal even when plasma T_4 and T_3 levels were low, confirming tight homeostatic control of cerebral T_3 concentrations. Normal T_3 concentrations in lung cells occurred only when T_4 infusions produced supraphysiologic plasma T_3 levels. (These T_3 levels are TSH-suppressive.) The concentration of T_3 in brown adipose tissue cells did not increase above normal; concentrations remained within the normal range even when the plasma T_4 level was 3.5 times normal and the plasma T_3 level was 2.5 times normal.[142,p.2834]

The researchers wrote that their findings raise questions about the current practice of treating hypothyroid patients with replacement dosages of T_4 alone. Referring to another study,[129] they noted that peripheral compensatory mechanisms do not provide sufficient circulating levels of T_4 and T_3 in hypothyroid patients taking T_4 alone. To induce normal circulating T_3 levels, patients must take enough T_4 to produce higher than normal circulating levels of T_4. Escobar-Morreale et al. pointed out that this corresponds to their findings in studying rats. They concluded, "Euthyroidism is not restored in plasma and all tissues of thyroidectomized rats on T_4 alone." They also concluded, "If our results are shown to be pertinent to humans, the current replacement therapy of hypothyroidism should no longer be considered adequate, and might possibly lead to the development of new strategies of therapy combining administration of both T_4 and T_3, albeit at a much higher T_4 to T_3 molar ratio (possibly 14:1) than previously used clinically (4:1[76])."[142,p.2837] In a second study, Escobar-Morreale et al. found that infusing rats with a combination of T_4 and T_3 restored normal tissue concentrations of T_3. The amount of infused T_4 needed to produce this effect was much lower than the amount required when only T_4 was infused.[121]

3) Replacement dosages do not normalize measures of tissue metabolic status. Replacement dosages of T_4 are not likely to produce normal peripheral tissue metabolism. As I described in the two sections above, replacement dosages of T_4 do not normalize the circulating free T_3 level; they also do not normalize the concentration of T_3 within the cells of some tissues. Moreover, evidence suggests that only supraphysiologic circulating T_3 levels result in normal T_3 concentrations in some tissues. The mandate that clinicians permit patients to use only replacement dosages of T_4 insures that most patients will have hypometabolism of at least some peripheral tissues. This is almost certain because replacement dosages of T_4 result in low-normal circulating T_3 levels. Studies of patients with anorexia nervosa show that low or low-normal circulating free T_3 levels are associated with low peripheral tissue metabolism. Bannai et al. studied 16 female anorexia patients during self-induced starvation. Thyroid function testing showed the expected reduced T_3 levels (see Chapter 4.2, subsection titled "Factors that Increase or Decrease Free T_3 Levels"). The patients had several clinical indications of hypothyroidism: cold intolerance, constipation, bradycardia, hypothermia, hypercholesterolemia, and decreased serum total T_3 and T_4 levels. Markedly decreased T_3 levels correlated positively with mean heart rate and negatively with total cholesterol level. The researchers concluded: "This result may suggest that the peripheral metabolic state of the underweight anorexics depends considerably upon the serum T_3 concentration. Despite decreased total thyroid hormones, free T_4 assayed by radioimmunoassay was normal in all five cases examined and the free T_4 index in fifteen cases was normal except in one case. Basal TSH was not increased and TSH response to exogenous TRH was not exaggerated in any. These results may be compatible with a theory that free T_4 has a dominant influence on pituitary TSH secretion." They also concluded, "It is suggested that normal sensitivity of peripheral tissues and pituitary thyrotrophs to different circulating thyroid hormones is maintained in anorexia nervosa patients even during severe self-induced starvation, and that the metabolic state in these patients is considerably under the influence of circulating T_3."[110] This study suggests that normal T_4 levels are likely to maintain normal TSH levels, but a simultaneously low-normal T_3 level is likely to result in peripheral tissue hypometabolism. Dosages of T_4 that keep the TSH level within the normal range (replacement dosages) typically result in low-normal circulating T_3 levels. As a result, these dosages are likely to keep peripheral tissues hypometabolic.

The reaction of a thyroidology researcher to the lack of correlation between thyroid function test results and indicators of peripheral tissue metabolic status is revealing: It shows the irrationality inherent in extremist medical technocracy. For example, the Achilles reflex speed is valuable for titrating dosage even with most patients who have mild hypothyroidism.[111] The relaxation phase of the reflex is abnormally slow in most hypothyroid patients, but the speed becomes normal when they use TSH-suppressive dosages of thyroid hormone. At the same time, most other measures of peripheral tissue metabolism also become normal. Costin argued that because Achilles reflex measurements correlate poorly with laboratory thyroid function test results, the reflex has limited use in the treatment of hypothyroidism.[112] The poor correlation, however, is evidence that it is the thyroid function laboratory tests that do not accurately gauge what really counts in thyroid hormone therapy—peripheral tissue metabolic status.

Using several indicators of peripheral tissue metabolic status is essential to quality treatment of the hypothyroid patient. Only by using them can we know how the patient's thyroid hormone dosage is affecting her various tissues. Thyroid function test results do not correlate well with most indicators of tissue metabolism. Because of this, the thyroid test results are of no value in fine-tuning the metabolism of peripheral tissues (see Chapter 4.3, section titled "Achilles Reflex Time").

Lack of Evidence of Correlation Between Thyroid Hormone and TSH Levels, and Tissue Metabolism. Underlying the transition in the early 1970s from the use of peripheral indices of metabolism to laboratory tests of thyroid function was an implicit hypothesis. It asserts that by permitting the hypothyroid patient to use only amounts of thyroid hormone that keep the circulating thyroid hormone levels and/or TSH level within the normal range, the patient's cellular metabolism will be normal. The assumption to conventional medicine is that this is established scientific fact. The proposition that normal thyroid hormone and TSH levels correlate with normal tissue metabolism distills to pure conjecture by thyroidologists.

For example, DeGroot stated, "Current evidence supports the idea that maintenance doses of thyroxine that keep the patient's TSH in the normal range are probably providing a normal metabolic status for the patient's whole body." (He did not cite the "current evidence," and I have not been able to find it despite diligent searching.) After this statement, he referenced Gow,[2] who published similar statements. DeGroot continued, "Obviously, one is in fact measuring the apparent metabolic status of the pituitary alone, but it is also probable that the metabolic status of other organs more or less falls in line with that of the pituitary."[1,p.9] This statement is false. The metabolic status of the pituitary is far more responsive to changes in circulating thyroid hormone levels than that of peripheral tissues. In fact, the extreme sensitivity of the pituitary compared to other tissues to changes in thyroid hormone levels is the basis of the diagnosis of subclinical hypothyroidism. In this condition, increased pituitary metabolism (increased synthesis and secretion of TSH by the pituitary thyrotroph cells) occurs before (1) laboratory testing detects changes in circulating thyroid hormone levels and (2) symptoms or signs of peripheral tissue hypometabolism occur. (See Chapter 4.2, subsection titled "Thyrotropin (TSH): Subclinical Hypothyroidism.")

A 1989 discussion of thyroid function tests by prominent thyroidologists is an unintentional repudiation of the view these researchers have promulgated to conventional clinicians. The thyroidologists expressed the speculative nature of a relation between thyroid hormone levels and metabolism. Wartofsky commented to Hamburger, "You say that unbound hormone fraction correlates well with thyroid function, but the correlation is with 'metabolic state.'" Hamburger responded, "Dr. Wartofsky is correct . . . . However, the suggested 'metabolic status' seems somewhat imprecise. Perhaps we could agree that free hormone levels correlate more reliably than total hormone levels with thyroid hormone activity in tissues."[21,pp.80-81] The fact is, they had no evidence to justify their belief that thyroid hormone levels correlate with either cellular thyroid hormone concentrations or cellular metabolism. Their belief that serum basal TSH levels reliably correlate with cellular metabolic status was, and still is, an investigational idea. Some studies indicate a correlation between TSH levels and metabolic status. In 1997, al-Adsani et al. reported finding a negative correlation between TSH levels and resting energy expenditure: decreased TSH resulted in increased energy expenditure; normal TSH resulted in normal expenditure; and increased TSH resulted in decreased expenditure.[53] In other studies, however, TSH levels and measures of tissue metabolism did not correlate, contradicting the thyroidologists I quoted above. Wolf et al., for example, reported in 1996 that basal energy expenditure was significantly lower in hypothyroid patients not taking T₄ than in controls. When using T₄, their energy expenditure increased but was not significantly different from controls. Energy expenditure was

still not significantly different in a subgroup of T₄-treated patients whose free T₃ and T₄ levels were above the upper limits of normal. The researchers reached two conclusions: (1) that energy expenditure significantly decreased in patients deprived of thyroid hormone, but (2) "no evidence of excess metabolic effects of thyroid hormone during thyrotropin [TSH]-suppressive thyroxine therapy was found."[54]

Clearly, the belief that the TSH of hypothyroid patients would best be kept within the "normal" reference range is speculative. The available evidence shows that the speculation is false.

Superiority of Clinical Indicators and Clinical Judgment Over Replacement Dosages Based on Thyroid Function Test Results. Replacement dosages of thyroid hormone do not insure normal tissue metabolism. In fact, these dosages deprive many patients of normal metabolism, sustaining their hypothyroid symptoms and signs. To benefit from the use of thyroid hormone, some patients must take dosages that produce borderline-low TSH levels; others must use TSH-suppressive dosages of thyroid hormone. This is clear when the clinician ignores laboratory thyroid function test results and titrates patients' dosages according to clinical indicators. By doing so, I have found that most hypothyroid patients with the fibromyalgia phenotypic expression become normal in every respect only with TSH-suppressive dosages of thyroid hormone. (I emphasize, however, that a successful therapeutic outcome depends on the patient using thyroid hormone *within the context* of a more comprehensive metabolic rehabilitation regimen). Other medical writers have similarly, although hedgingly, reported that titrating dosage by clinical indicators is preferable to the use of laboratory thyroid function test results. And still others have frankly concluded that laboratory thyroid function tests, including TSH levels, are useless for adjusting dosage.

Stockigt wrote a chapter on the TSH in the 1996 revision of *Werner's The Thyroid*. In it, he wrote, "In evaluating patients receiving T₄ therapy, some have suggested that hormone measurements add little to a clinical assessment made by experts . . . ." He leaned toward a rational view when he wrote, "In some situations (e.g., patients with ischemic heart disease and hypothyroidism), the appropriate dose of T₄ should be based on clinical judgment rather than laboratory findings."[63,p.381] Essentially, Stockigt argued that for these patients, the clinician can best determine proper dosage by assessing clinical indicators of the peripheral tissue effects of thyroid hormone. This was a concession, although probably inadvertent, that this method is superior to the use of laboratory thyroid function test results. He then hedged, however, expressing the conventional view: ". . . but there is justification for periodic serum TSH assessment to avoid subtle tissue effects of thyroid hormone excess or deficiency."[63,p.381]

Other medical writers have not hedged as Stockigt did. In 1986, for example, Fraser et al., reported that their study showed laboratory thyroid function tests to be of no value in adjusting the T_4 dosages of hypothyroid patients. These investigators studied patients taking T_4. Four clinicians experienced in the use of T_4 evaluated the patients clinically. The clinicians used the Wayne index,[69] a tool for scoring patient symptoms and signs, to classify the patients as euthyroid, hypothyroid, or hyperthyroid. By subjecting the Wayne index scores to Kruskal-Wallis analysis of variance, the diagnoses were determined not to be biased. There was no significant difference in the 4 median scores of the 4 clinicians. By contrast, tests of the total T_4, total T_3, free T_4, free T_3, and basal TSH were of *no* value in determining whether patients were taking enough, too much, or too little T_4. The researchers wrote, "These measurements are therefore of little, if any, value in monitoring patients receiving thyroxine replacement."[56,p.810]

A granite-hard conclusion of conventional endocrinology/thyroidology is that replacement dosages assure normal tissue metabolism and that patients should be confined to them. My clinical and research experiences and published statements by medical writers, such as those of Stockigt[63] and Fraser et al.[56] in the three paragraphs above, repudiate this conclusion.

4) Replacement dosages harm some patients by depriving them of enough thyroid hormone to maintain normal tissue metabolism. TSH-suppressive dosages of thyroid hormone are not *ipso facto* harmful to patients. In fact, some patients require TSH-suppressive dosages of thyroid hormone to have normal tissue metabolism and freedom from symptoms and signs of hypometabolism. For these patients, TSH-suppressive dosages are harmless; failure to use TSH-suppressive dosage is harmful. Thus, for such patients, replacement dosages are potentially harmful because the dosages sustain tissue hypometabolism.

Inadequate Treatment Based on the Dubious Normal TSH Reference Range. Certain knowledge of the ideal normal-range TSH level is a prevailing myth in conventional medicine. Even leading thyroidologists merely guess about the ideal level with no credible scientific justification for the opinions they hold. So, some thyroidologists such as Volpé advise that

replacement dosages should hold the TSH level in the "middle of the normal range."[21,p.87] At the same time, others such as Stockigt counsel that proper dosages hold the TSH level in the "low-normal range."[63,p.381] (See section above titled "Basis of the Problem of Replacement Dosages: Misinterpretation of Investigative Data and Its Gradual Acceptance as Scientific Fact.") It is little wonder, then, that many conventional clinicians restrict their patients to replacement dosages that keep TSH levels in the upper half of the "normal range." My communications with many of these clinicians suggest that they do so partly to keep the patient well away from a "thyrotoxic dosage." As a result, the dosages sustain tissue hypometabolism and the patients' symptoms and signs. Weetman recently implied that holding the TSH level in the upper half of the "normal range" (2.0 µU/mL or higher) with replacement dosages is probably inadequate treatment.[134] (See section above titled "Basis of the Problem of Replacement Dosages: Dubious Conventional TSH Range of Normal.")

Creating "New Diseases" by Defining Away Continuing Indicators of Hypometabolism. That replacement dosages, especially those that hold the TSH level in the upper half of the normal range, are inadequate is obvious to clinicians who titrate dosage according to patients' symptoms, signs, and peripheral indices. In most patients, replacement dosages simply do not satisfactorily change these clinical indicators. But TSH-suppressive dosages do. Clinicians who subscribe to the mandates of the reining endocrinology/thyroidology paradigm typically have not had the benefit of an important clinical experience—seeing patients' symptoms, signs, and peripheral indices eliminated by treatment based on clinical indicators (after treatment based on replacement dosages had failed). By their definition, these continuing symptoms, signs, and peripheral indices cannot possibly be products of inadequate thyroid hormone treatment. These clinicians adamantly believe that replacement dosages guarantee that the patient's metabolism in all tissues is normal. They therefore infer that some other disease must be the cause of the symptoms, signs, and peripheral indices. This pattern of thought, generated by the notion of replacement dosages of thyroid hormone, has led to an enormous amount of fruitless medical testing for other diseases. This pattern of thought has also contributed substantially to the birth and development of entire new fields of clinical research—a different one for each phenotypic expression of inadequate thyroid hormone regulation of tissue function. It is staggering to consider the amount of time, energy, and money invested in the search for non-existent mechanisms to explain these symptoms and signs resulting from inadequate treatment of hypothyroid patients with replacement dosages of thyroid hormone.

Treatment of Residual Symptoms, Signs, and Peripheral Indices with Medications Other Than Thyroid Hormone. The belief of conventional clinicians that continuing hypometabolism-like symptoms, signs, and peripheral indices in patients using replacement dosages must be caused by some other disease has had another unfortunate result. The result is the use by these patients of various medications to control the symptoms, signs, and peripheral indices. This is a serious public health problem. Health care costs are increased by patients using medications that would be unnecessary if they were treated with adequate dosages of thyroid hormone. Also, patients are exposed to potential adverse effects from the prolonged use of the medications, most of which are non-orthomolecular substances.

In my clinical and research experiences, practically every fibromyalgia patient with primary or central hypothyroidism completely recovers from their signs and symptoms under two conditions: when we (1) ignore thyroid function test results and (2) give these patients high enough dosages of thyroid hormone to produce normalization of measures of peripheral tissue response. Many patients previously used replacement dosages of thyroid hormone without benefit. Conventional clinicians virtually always treat these patients with antidepressant medications rather than thyroid hormone. Some clinicians assume these medications are innocuous, but the assumption is risky. The medications may cause: (1) orthostatic hypotension (which many patients already have), (2) ischemic heart disease and heart attacks (a potential the patients should avoid because reduced cardiovascular fitness accompanies their low fitness levels), (3) slowing of the metabolic rate (a worsening of the underlying mechanism of the fibromyalgia), and (4) an increased risk of suicidal depression. (See Chapter 5.1, section titled "Antidepressant Drugs: Potential Adverse Effects of Antidepressant Drugs.")

Problems and Limitations with TSH Assays

Conventional endocrinology/thyroidology touts the basal TSH test as the "gold standard" for deciding who might and might not benefit from the use of exogenous thyroid hormone. The main argument given for the use of modern TSH assays is their high sensitivity.[160] The high sensitivity of the assays, however, is only of value in more precisely measuring *low* TSH levels. In primary hypothyroidism, *high* TSH levels are of concern. Low TSH levels may be of concern in diagnosing central hypothyroidism, but the TRH-stimulation test is of most value for this diagnosis. And in the TRH-stimulation test, the high sensitivity of third-generation TSH assays has no advantage over the lower sensitivity of second-generation assays. The high sensitivity of third-generation assays is of most value when measuring extremely low TSH levels in *hyper*thyroid patients. One tenet of this book is that inadequate thyroid hormone regulation of cell function underlies most patients' fibromyalgia. A corollary to this tenet is that excessive thyroid hormone regulation of cell function is incompatible with fibromyalgia. If this is true, the high sensitivity of TSH assays is irrelevant to the care of fibromyalgia patients. In fact, the high sensitivity is irrelevant to all hypothyroid patients, whatever the phenotypic expression of their thyroid hormone deficiency.

The sensitivity of TSH assays is not the only important issue regarding their use. Studies I included in Chapter 4.2 (section titled "Thyrotropin (TSH): Persisting Problems with the TSH Test") show that clinicians should consider other issues. The studies show that the TSH test alone does not identify all patients with primary hypothyroidism. The basal TSH is of no use in identifying patients with central hypothyroidism (see Chapter 4.2, section titled "TRH-Stimulation Test: Central Hypothyroidism: Basal TSH: Not of Use in Diagnosing Central Hypothyroidism"). TSH test results are within the normal range in a small percentage of patients with low free T₄ levels. This is of concern because most patients with low free T₄ levels presumably have inadequate thyroid hormone regulation of their tissues. In addition, researchers have found that TSH values vary from week-to-week. This finding puts the reliability of TSH test results in doubt. The finding also suggests that whether clinicians permit some patients to use thyroid hormone or not depends arbitrarily on the time when laboratories perform the patients' TSH tests.

The TSH is not the impeccable test some researchers and clinicians tout it to be. The test, in fact, has noteworthy limitations and problems. And still, it is the basis of T₄ replacement therapy. The limitations of and problems with the test add to the reasons clinicians should not use the TSH in titrating thyroid hormone dosages of hypothyroid patients.

(4) HYPOTHYROID PATIENTS SHOULD BE PERMITTED TO USE ONLY T₄

For an extended time during my study of fibromyalgia, my colleagues and I treated hypothyroid fibromyalgia patients initially with T_4. Many of these patients continued their use of T_4 because the hormone provided them some benefit. However, I now believe—from the advantage of hindsight—that I minimized the potential improvement of some of them. In a 1-to-5-year follow-up study, the group means of hypothyroid fibromyalgia patients for all measures showed that their improvement with T_4 lasted long term.[141] Nevertheless, I suspect they would have improved more had they been using desiccated thyroid, other preparations that contained both synthetic T_4 and T_3, or synthetic T_3 alone. Several recent studies show that treatment with combined T_4/T_3 is more effective than T_4 alone. Escobar-Morreale et al. reported that they could normalize the thyroid hormone content of all tissue cells studied only by including both T_3 and T_4 in the infusion they gave rats.[121][142] Bunevicius et al. recently reported that compared to hypothyroid patients taking T_4 alone, patients taking a combination of T_3 and T_4 had improved mood and neurocognitive function.[166]

I also realize that I prolonged the suffering of some patients whom my co-treating clinicians and I eventually switched to T_3, which was effective in virtually every case. We switched some patients to T_3 because high dosages of T_4 alone or desiccated thyroid produced thyrotoxicity without any obvious therapeutic benefit. This corresponds to reports by other researchers in the 1950s and 1960s (see Chapters 2.5 and 5.4). We switched most patients to T_3 because dosages of 400 µg of T_4 were ineffective although not thyrotoxic. Garrison, however, recently progressively increased 25 hypothyroid fibromyalgia patients' T_4 dosages to between 600 and 800 µg of T_4. He increased the dosages until the patients had improved. He assessed improvement by clinical response rather than TSH levels. Some patients' fibromyalgia improved or was relieved by less than 500 µg. Four patients improved or recovered from their fibromyalgia symptoms only with dosages between 600 and 800 µg. Two of the patients, however, soon developed what appeared to be a hyper-reverse-T_3 syndrome. The patients had high free T_4 levels (> 6.0 ng/dL), low TSH levels (0.0 µU/mL), and low free T_3 levels (below or

at the lower end of the normal range). Their reverse T_3 levels were high (>1000 ng/dL). Garrison described the condition as a distinctive syndrome involving nausea, gastroesophageal reflux, heartburn, and esophageal spasm. The patients had blurred vision and premature ventricular contractions without a fast heart rate or palpitations. We need further studies of the use of such high T_4 dosages, but Garrison's findings suggest that the use of high T_4 dosages are less safe than high T_3 dosages.[106]

Past and recent experiences with my patients are interesting academically and scientifically. Desiccated thyroid did not benefit some of my hypothyroid fibromyalgia patients who subsequently recovered from their signs and symptoms dramatically and completely with T_3. I specifically reported the case of one such patient[78] and included another in a long-term follow-up study that showed her recovery continued with T_3.[141] To this time, I have found no scientifically sound reason that these hypothyroid patients should stop their sole use of T_3. These hypothyroid patients with the fibromyalgia phenotypic expression correspond to other patients in the 1950s and 1960s who recovered from their symptoms with T_3 after failing to benefit from high dosages of T_4 or desiccated thyroid (see Chapters 2.5 and 5.4). Reports of such patients confirm that a subset of hypothyroid patients improve or recover only with the sole use of T_3. Another subset improves or recovers only with a combined T_4/T_3 preparation.

The findings I cite in this section falsify the fourth sweeping proposition of the current endocrinology/thyroidology paradigm: that clinicians should only prescribe T_4 for hypothyroid patients. They also falsify this proposition's corollary: that all hypothyroid patients benefit sufficiently from the use of T_4. Clinicians should recognize these falsifications and accordingly adapt their prescribing practices for hypothyroid patients.

● IMPROPER TREATMENT OF HYPOTHYROID FIBROMYALGIA PATIENTS

Few clinicians today treat hypothyroid patients so that the patients attain normal metabolism and freedom from their symptoms and signs. The clinician should understand how this deplorable circumstance came about and how to remedy it. I provide a detailed account of the development of the circumstance in Chapter 2.5 (see especially the section titled "Thyroid

Hormone-Related Euthyroid Hypometabolism").

In 1996, Ridgway described the conventional approach to hypothyroidism: "Therapy of hypothyroidism is easy, inexpensive, and precise, involving pure L-thyroxine and measuring dose requirements and efficacy by monitoring serum TSH concentrations."[11] In 1999, Toft wrote of this conventional approach, "... it should not be forgotten that the majority of patients taking a dose of thyroxine that satisfies the recommendations of the American Thyroid Association have no complaints about their medication."[151] Despite Toft's belief, a multitude of hypothyroid patients bitterly complain about the ineffectiveness of the treatment approach Ridgway described for hypothyroidism. The patients' complaints directly contradict Toft's assurance that most patients have no complaints about conventional hypothyroid treatment.

DISSATISFACTION OF HYPOTHYROID PATIENTS TREATED WITH CONVENTIONAL THYROID HORMONE THERAPY

The belief that normal thyroid hormone and/or TSH levels correspond to normal tissue metabolic status cannot be justified scientifically. Yet since 1973, the belief has dictated conventional clinicians' decisions regarding the diagnosis and treatment of hypothyroidism.[38,p.810][181][182] There is ample reason to believe that the opinion has substantially lowered the quality of life for incalculable numbers of people and has shortened the lives of many (see Chapter 4.4, section titled "Harm from Untreated and Undertreated Hypothyroidism"). Any clinician who doubts that replacement dosages of T₄ leave a multitude of patients sick and dissatisfied has only to spend time monitoring the Internet "thyroid newsgroups." Mary Shomon's thyroid Web site[149] and the International Thyroid Group Web site[150] are particularly convincing. Mary Shomon's Web site has had up to 500,000 "hits" per month. ("Hits" are visits to the site by Internet users.) Such numbers suggest that Toft has misjudged hypothyroid patients' presumed satisfaction with replacement dosages of T₄. Through these newsgroups, individuals around the world learn that others share the same problem caused by the current endocrinology/thyroidology paradigm for the diagnosis and treatment of hypothyroidism. The shared problem is sustained suffering from hypothyroid symptoms despite the use of replacement dosages of T₄. Without access to the newsgroups, many—perhaps most—of these individuals would suffer in isolation, unaware that their suf-

fering is the result of a failed clinical paradigm. The newsgroups thus serve a humanitarian purpose, and I encourage patients and clinicians to visit them. Some clinicians, however, outspokenly detest such newsgroups. Such clinicians find it threatening that patients can learn through the Internet as much or more than the clinicians know about the patients' diseases. Regardless, clinicians must now face the fact that they no longer have exclusive access to information about patients' diseases. This availability of information to patients appears to be forcing clinicians into a more collaborative interaction with patients. Many clinicians encourage this type of interaction and enjoy it. Others prefer to exert authoritative control over submissive patients. Patients' access to the Internet, however, will prevail over these clinicians' preferences.

A common complaint of dissatisfied hypothyroid patients on the Internet is that their clinicians blame their continuing hypothyroid symptoms on other undetermined diseases. According to the clinicians, the patients' replacement dosages of T₄ insure that deficient thyroid hormone is not the cause of the symptoms. If the patient's predominant symptom is fatigue, the clinician decides she has chronic fatigue syndrome; if her predominant symptom is pain, he decides she has fibromyalgia. An occasional patient will write on the Internet that she inadvertently took more than her prescribed dosage of T₄ for a time. The higher dosage markedly improved or completely alleviated her symptoms—until her clinician, often an endocrinologist, coerced her to reduce the dosage, at which time her symptoms returned or intensified. The clinicians contend that the higher dosage of thyroid hormone will cause adverse effects. Many patients then write that they prefer to risk the effects for the relief they experienced with the higher dosages. While I do not advocate that patients increase their dosages on their own without professional guidance, these Internet reports, nevertheless, seem to justify patients' dissatisfaction with conventional care.

Admittedly, patients who participate in the newsgroups constitute a select patient sample. It is not likely that hypothyroid patients satisfied with the results of their T₄ dosages are accurately represented in thyroid newsgroup postings. Still, the common complaint of undertreatment with T₄ corresponds to that of many previously diagnosed and treated hypothyroid patients I have seen in my practice over the years. The percentage of patients undertreated is not established. I am confident, however, that the phenomenon is widespread. Underdosing has resulted in incalculable iatrogenic human suffering. And the suffering will continue until clinicians who unquestioningly subscribe to the assumptions of conventional endocrinology/thyroidology revise their thinking and rectify their methods of practice.

ADVERSE EFFECTS OF THE CURRENT ENDOCRINOLOGY PARADIGM ON PATIENT/CLINICIAN RELATIONS

My conversations with older hypothyroid patients suggest that their interactions with clinicians were more collaborative before 1973. The more collaborative interactions were necessary for a mutual effort by the patient and clinician—to find a dosage of thyroid hormone that optimized the patient's clinical status. The clinician asked questions about how the patient had responded to the present dosage. He also examined her for changes in her signs of thyroid hormone deficiency.

Conventional clinicians began reducing patients' dosages in the early 1970s. When patients became dissatisfied with the results, a wedge began to form between patients and their prescribing clinicians. The consequences have been detrimental to both parties. Clinicians were misled by endocrinologists/thyroidologists to believe that only the reduced dosages were safe for patients. Faced with patient dissatisfaction, the clinicians tended to become more dictatorial in specifying dosages. The patients, whom clinicians began holding at arms-distance, complained about the ineffectiveness of the treatment. Pressure from patients led to clinicians believing that patients, if left to make their own choices, might harm themselves. The desire of clinicians to protect patients plus avoid malpractice suits seemed to justify a paternalistic, authoritarian stance by the clinician "on the patient's behalf." This attitude, perceived as smug condescension, led some patients to resent their treating clinicians and hold them in contempt. Some patients refused to tolerate unpalatable relationships with conventional clinicians and began seeking care from more open-minded, rational, and collaborative "alternative" clinicians. Conventional clinicians intimidated less fortunate patients who obsequiously complied with the clinicians' dictates. An undeterminable number of such patients must have paid for holding their tongues when they remained ill with conventional thyroid hormone therapy. The likely price was slowly developing cardiovascular pathology and a diminished quality of life. Many of these patients, suffering from hypothyroid symptoms despite conventional treatment, are now the victims of

hypothesized new diseases. Medical researchers have not and will not find causes for the patients' symptoms other than untreated or undertreated hypometabolism. Many patients will continue to suffer from the imagined new diseases sustained by their continuation of replacement dosages of thyroid hormone. That they continue the therapy will provide thyroidologists such as Toft reason for concluding that patients do not complain about conventional hypothyroid treatment.[151]

The 1970s and 1980s were a span of time when patients and their attorneys were filing record numbers of malpractice suits against clinicians. Many suits were warranted. Conventional medicine had reached the zenith of its sense of aristocracy and flagrant arrogance. Public resentment of conventional physicians appears to have driven the filing of malpractice suits to a draconian level in the form of nuisance suits. The expectancy of suits contributed further to clinicians restricting their clinical decisions to those justifiable by objective measures, such as laboratory thyroid function tests.[21,p.102] The tendency of clinicians to use clinical judgment diminished even further. Thus, a progressive altering of the practice of medicine and deterioration of patient/doctor interaction galvanized the strain, mutual distrust, and poor communication between conventional clinicians and their patients.

These dynamics may have been the final force that brought to an end for many clinicians the practice of clinical medicine merely complemented by technology. Clinicians largely abandoned this rational, humane approach to clinical practice exemplified by Drs. William Osler and Janet G. Travell. Clinical medicine has now given way to extremist medical technocracy. In this approach to practice, the patient is at most a secondary consideration to the results of establishment-condoned objective measures. The consequence for the hypothyroid patient is that most clinicians only "treat" her serum TSH levels. Many clinicians, especially endocrinologists, now totally disregard the patient's clinical status. The continuation of fibromyalgia symptoms in many hypothyroid patients taking replacement doses of T_4 is a product of the current endocrinology/thyroidology paradigm which encourages extremist medical technocracy. My impression is that progressively more conventional clinicians are turning away from extremist medical technocracy. They are in an awkward circumstance, however. Their style of practice is largely a product of some 30 years of unseemly changes in conventional medicine. Yet they know instinctively that treatment decisions based on extremist medical technocracy are often not in the best interest of their patients.

● **GENERAL TREATMENT STRATEGY FOR HYPOTHYROID FIBROMYALGIA PATIENTS**

Barnes wrote, "In thousands of patients, use of the basal temperature test to detect hypothyroidism and then to correct it—starting with very small doses of thyroid medication and increasing them, if necessary, until retesting has shown the temperature rising—has led to gratifying results."[88,p.6] The basal body temperature Barnes suggested patients use is but one index of tissue metabolic status. I recommend that the clinician and patient use several clinical indicators of peripheral tissue response to thyroid hormone (see Chapter 4.3). Nonetheless, Barnes' statement encapsulates the essence of a rational approach to correcting hypothyroidism: (1) select objective and subjective measures of the effects of tissue hypometabolism that suggest hypothyroidism; (2) begin metabolic therapy that includes thyroid hormone, starting with a dosage the clinician calculates will increase the patient's metabolism; (3) monitor for changes in the measures; (4) gradually increase the hormone dosage until the patient reaches maximum improvement or achieves optimal metabolic status; and (5) if the measures suggest the patient's metabolic rate is excessive, gradually reduce the dosage until the patient has maximum improvement without tissue thyrotoxicity.

The clinician should not titrate the patient's thyroid hormone dosage according to the results of laboratory thyroid function tests, including the TSH test. Despite clinicians' widespread use of such tests to titrate thyroid hormone dosage, they are of no value in finding an effective dosage.[56] I give extensive reasons for this opinion in Chapter 4.3 (see the introduction and the section titled "The Greater Usefulness of Clinical Indicators of Tissue Metabolic Status"). After the patient begins therapy with thyroid hormone, the clinician can optimize her clinical status in only one way—by adjusting her dosage according to peripheral measures of tissue metabolic status.

Some clinicians recognize that normal thyroid function test results do not show that the patient's dosage is effective. For example, Teitelbaum wrote in his book for fibromyalgia and chronic fatigue syndrome patients, "If your temperature is routinely under 97.4° F, consider a trial of thyroid hormone regardless of what your blood test shows." Whitaker advised patients with normal thyroid test results, "If your doctor resists giving you a trial of low doses of thyroid hormone, I would strongly recommend you seek another

physician who will."[96,p.29]

I suggest that clinicians ignore Teitelbaum's qualification that the patient should ". . . follow up with a blood test to make sure that your thyroid levels are in a safe range."[87,pp.34-35] "Safe" ranges, according to convention, are defined as "normal" range TSH and thyroid hormone levels. A suppressed TSH level or a high-normal thyroid hormone level merely raises the *possibility* that the patient's dosage is adversely affecting her peripheral tissues. The TSH level measures only the response of the pituitary thyrotroph cells to circulating thyroid hormone levels. But the TSH level provides no information whatsoever about the response of other tissues to thyroid hormone. Serum levels of thyroid hormones, in turn, tell us nothing about whether metabolism in peripheral cells is being adequately regulated by those levels. Blood tests no more measure the metabolic rate of peripheral tissues than a car's gas gauge measures how fast the car is traveling. The clinician can determine in only one way that a patient's TSH-suppressive dosage is adversely affecting her peripheral tissues—by finding positive results on tests that assess metabolic overstimulation of particular peripheral tissues. Such positive results might include symptoms, signs, and peripheral indices suggesting tissue thyrotoxicosis (see Chapters 4.3 and 4.4).

Conventional clinicians can quickly improve the quality of their care of hypothyroid patients. They can do so by (1) abandoning their current use of thyroid function tests for titrating patients' thyroid hormone dosages, and by (2) using instead indicators of peripheral tissue response to the hormone.

THERAPEUTIC CONSIDERATIONS IN PRIMARY AND CENTRAL HYPOTHYROIDISM

The treatment of primary and central hypothyroidism is usually the same. Thyroid hormone therapy is safe and most patients tolerate it well.[74,p.883] Precautions are warranted with both types of patients, especially with those who have central hypothyroidism.

Initial Dosage for the Patient with Primary Hypothyroidism

Our clinical objectives in using thyroid hormone with the hypothyroid fibromyalgia patient are clear. We must find a dosage that relieves the patient's symptoms, normalizes all measures of peripheral tissue metabolic status, and does so without producing indications of tissue thyrotoxicity. We cannot predict on a scientific basis the exact dosages that will accomplish these objectives for different patients. The most productive approach is to calculate an initial dosage that is low enough not to overstimulate the patient's tissues but close to what might be an effective dosage for her. As I have propounded in this book, the clinician can determine whether a particular thyroid hormone dosage is safe and effective for the patient. He can do so only by repeatedly measuring clinical indicators of tissue metabolic status, comparing the results with the outcomes of previous measurements, and striving to normalize all clinical indicators.

A Safe and Nearly Effective Initial Dosage. I have found that the safe and effective thyroid hormone dosage for most hypothyroid patients is between the equivalent of 200-to-400 µg of T_4. (I make recommendations in equivalents of T_4 because most clinicians are accustomed to using this form of thyroid hormone.) The equivalent in desiccated thyroid or combined synthetic T_4/T_3 is 2-to-4 grains (120-to-240 mg). Some patients simply do not benefit from T_4-containing preparations, even those that contain T_3. Two grains of desiccated thyroid contain 76 µg of T_4 and 18 µg of T_3. In changing the patient from a T_4-containing preparation to synthetic T_3, the clinician should bear in mind that the equivalent to 2-to-4 grains of desiccated thyroid is 50-to-100 µg of T_3. (See Appendix D for dosage equivalents.)

The clinician should aim to start the patient with a dosage that is not overstimulating to any tissue. To accomplish this, he should start the patient with some amount less than these typically safe and effective dosages. How much less? The answer depends on the robustness or frailty of the patient, particularly her cardiovascular status. Several writers have made recommendations that are useful for starting dosages. The clinician should keep in mind, however, that most writers have had one main objective: to lower an elevated TSH level to within the normal reference range. For example, Brent and Larsen wrote, agreeing with Gow et al.:[2] "Since it is difficult to measure accurately thyroid hormone action in many tissues, the usual approach is to normalize the serum TSH concentration. By this means, the clinician can identify patients who are receiving too much T_4 (serum TSH concentration below the normal range) and those who are receiving too little (serum TSH concentration above the normal range)."[74] But merely lowering the TSH within the normal range, even the low-normal range, seldom produces normal tissue metabolism and

practically never leaves the patient clinically normal. So the clinician would best consider the recommended dosages of these authors only as starting points. And he should completely ignore laboratory thyroid function test results after the patient begins thyroid hormone therapy.

Brent and Larsen stated that the healthy patient less than 60 years old, with no history of cardiac or respiratory disease, can start T_4 therapy with a full replacement dose: from 1.6-to-1.8 µg/kg of ideal body weight/day. (To calculate the dosage, divide the patient's body weight by 2.2 and multiply the quotient by 1.6, 1.7, or 1.8 µg.) The daily dosage they recommended thus ranges from 75-to-125 µg (0.075-to-0.125 mg) for women and 125-to-200 µg (0.125-to-0.200 mg) for men.[101] The patient should continue these dosages from 4-to-8 weeks. This is the time, they say, necessary for tissue effects and TSH levels to reach a steady state.[74,p.884] (From my point of view, of course, TSH levels should be of no concern in deciding dosage adjustments.)

Rosenbaum et al.[102] and Sawin et al.[103] pointed out that the dosage of T_4 for "elderly" patients is 20%-to-30% less than that for younger adults. (I do not know their definition of "elderly.") The recommended starting dosage is no more than 50 µg (0.05 mg) per day, with 25 µg (0.025 mg) increases at intervals no shorter than 6 weeks apart.[74,p.884]

During treatment, some patients may experience mild symptoms of thyroid hormone overstimulation (see Chapter 4.3 and the section titled "Properly Identifying Thyrotoxicosis" in Chapter 5.2). I have described the protocol for properly dealing with overstimulation in Chapter 5.2, section titled "Managing Thyrotoxic Reactions to Excessive Intake of Exogenous Thyroid Hormone."

Monitoring for Adequacy of T_4 Therapy. According to the current endocrinology paradigm, after the patient begins using thyroid hormone, the clinician should reevaluate within about 8 weeks. The reevaluation entails measuring the serum basal TSH level. If the TSH is elevated, the patient should increase her T_4 dosage; if the TSH is low, she should decrease her dosage. Brent and Larsen recommended dosage changes of 12-to-25 µg (0.012-to-0.025 mg), depending on the desired effect on the TSH level.[74,p.885] (For equivalent amounts of desiccated thyroid and T_3, see Appendix D.)

Brent and Larsen's recommendation that the clinician use the TSH level to assess the adequacy of treatment ignores the clinical status of the patient. They make no use whatever of the most valuable indices of metabolic status—the patient's clinical status and indirect measures of the responses of peripheral tissues to thyroid hormone. The clinician using their protocol only manipulates the patient's serum TSH level. The TSH level is a tiny part of the patient, and it is a part that is thoroughly irrelevant to the metabolic status and health of the hypothyroid patient using thyroid hormone. Adjusting the patient's thyroid hormone dosage by her TSH level while ignoring the hormone's effect on her tissue metabolism is like adjusting the flame under a pot on the stove by a pre-determined setting on the burner's dial, while ignoring the effects of the heat on the food in the pot. The outcome of this approach to cooking is likely to be as unpalatable as the outcome of Brent and Larsen's approach to thyroid hormone dosage adjustments.

Special Considerations in Central Hypothyroidism

Thyroid Hormone Preparation. Brent and Larsen[74,p.885] and Martino et al.[37,p.787] wrote that the clinician should treat patients with central hypothyroidism with T_4. The patient is likely to obtain faster and superior therapeutic effects, however, by beginning treatment with desiccated thyroid or a preparation that contains synthetic T_4 and T_3. If the patient does not benefit satisfactorily from the desiccated thyroid or combined synthetic T_4 and T_3, she may have partial cellular resistance to thyroid hormone. In this case, the clinician should switch her to synthetic T_3.

Method of Determining Proper Dosage for the Patient with Central Hypothyroidism. Brent and Larsen wrote that the serum TSH is not as useful for titrating dosage in central hypothyroidism as it is in primary hypothyroidism. Instead, they recommended the clinician use the serum free T_4 or the serum free T_4 index. They suggested that he adjust the patient's dosage to keep the test values in the middle or upper end of the normal range.[74,p.885] The clinician should disregard this recommendation, however, and titrate the central hypothyroid patient's thyroid hormone dosage according to peripheral tissue responses to the hormone. Laboratory thyroid function tests are of value to the clinician only in establishing that the patient has central hypothyroidism. They are of no value in adjusting the patient's dosage of thyroid hormone.

Initial Thyroid Hormone Dosage. Martino et al. wrote that patients who do not have an ACTH deficiency may begin T_4 at a dosage of 1.4-to-1.6 µg/kg of body weight for 4-to-6 weeks.[37,p.788] (To calculate the dosage, divide the patient's body weight by 2.2 and multiply the quotient by 1.4, 1.5, or 1.6 µg.) Accord-

ing to this recommendation, a woman of 120 lbs should begin with a dosage equivalent to roughly 76-to-87 µg (0.076-to-0.087 mg) of T_4. This amount is roughly equivalent to ¾-to-1 grain (45-to-60 mg) of desiccated thyroid and 19.00-to-21.75 µg of T_3. (See Appendix D for equivalent dosages of desiccated thyroid and T_3).

For elderly patients, those with an ACTH deficiency, or cardiovascular disease, Martino et al. advised an initial dosage of 0.3-to-0.7 µg/kg for 3-to-4 weeks. After that time, they suggested the clinician gradually increase the dosage to achieve the desired effect.

Martino et al. wrote that the clinician cannot use TSH measurements to decide thyroid hormone dosages for central hypothyroid patients (though they believe clinicians can use the TSH for primary hypothyroid patients). These researchers wrote that after the patient begins to use thyroid hormone, the clinician should titrate the dosage according to its peripheral effects and by serum total and free T_4 levels.[37,p.788] Despite their advice and that of Brent and Larsen[74,p.885] regarding thyroid function test results, the results are of no value for determining the central hypothyroid patient's effective and safe dosage of thyroid hormone.

Diagnosing Central Hypothyroidism. The clinical effects of primary and central hypothyroidism may be indistinguishable from one another.[37,p.785] Because of this, the clinician must make the diagnosis of central hypothyroidism mainly on four bases: (1) symptoms, signs, and peripheral indices characteristic of hypothyroidism, (2) laboratory thyroid function test results, (3) pituitary hormone assays, and possibly (4) imaging procedures (see Chapter 4.2).

Martino et al. wrote that the clinician should suspect central hypothyroidism when the patient has signs and symptoms typical of hypothyroidism, but she has a low TSH level despite a low free T_4 or low serum free T_4 index.[37,p.785] Other medical writers have reiterated this belief. To wit: "When the TSH is low, low T_4 levels will identify pituitary failure."[70,p.228]

Some clinicians assume that the results of the standard thyroid test profile thus enables them to predict the outcome of the TRH-stimulation test, making the stimulation test unnecessary. Physiologically, if the total T_4 and free T_4 index are in the lower half of the normal range, the expected finding would be that the TSH is, inversely, in the upper half of the normal range. But when all these measures are in the lower half of the normal range, this could indicate that the pituitary thyrotroph cells are not being properly disinhibited by lower levels of T_4. Thus, the clinician could make a diagnosis of central hypothyroidism simply by looking for this pattern within the standard thyroid panel, as Martino et al. suggested. If this were true, it would render the TRH-stimulation test unnecessary.

Contrary to the conventional view, I did not find that this pattern of laboratory values was predictive of central hypothyroidism in fibromyalgia patients based on the TRH-stimulation test.[95] I studied this issue with 38 consecutive fibromyalgia patients. Of 20 patients whose TRH-stimulation test results were consistent with central hypothyroidism, the pattern described above—low normal T_4, free thyroxine index, and TSH—was present in the results of only 9 (45%). Of 14 patients whose TRH-stimulation test results were consistent with euthyroidism, the same pattern (low normal T_4, free thyroxine index, and TSH) was present in the results of 7 (50%).[95] These findings falsify the proposition that this pattern of values from the standard profile reliably predicts the results of the TRH-stimulation test. Thus, contrary to the conventional view, the TRH-stimulation test *is* necessary for the identification of patients with possible central hypothyroidism.

To diagnose central hypothyroidism, the clinician should order or perform one of two tests other than the standard thyroid profile: the nocturnal TSH surge or the TRH-stimulation test. Researchers reported that the nocturnal TSH surge was more reliable than the TRH-stimulation test for diagnosing central hypothyroidism.[92] Nevertheless, the inconvenience of the recommended drawing of blood samples every 30 minutes between 11:00 pm and 2:00 am[37,p.786] makes the TRH-stimulation test more practical for most clinicians. A low or absent nocturnal TSH surge or a blunted or exaggerated TSH response to injected TRH supports the diagnosis of central hypothyroidism[37,p.786] (see Chapter 4.2).

Second-generation TSH assays detect basal TSH levels of 0.3 µU/mL or higher. Third-generation assays (variously termed "highly sensitive," "super-sensitive," or "ultra-sensitive")[93,p.229] detect TSH levels below 0.3 µU/mL. Some writers falsely believe that these sensitive assays have made the TRH-stimulation test obsolete.[94] The tests are useful *only* when the clinician wants to learn the precise level of the TSH below 0.3 µU/mL. Such levels are of interest only when identifying or treating hyperthyroid patients. The test is useful, for example, in deciding whether a patient's muscle weakness is due to hyperthyroidism. In general, when the fibromyalgia patient's second-generation TSH assay level is 0.3 µU/mL (the lowest level the assay is capable of detecting) or lower, the clin-

cian gets no further benefit from the use of a more sensitive third-generation TSH assay. Our hypothesis is that fibromyalgia symptoms and objective findings are manifestations of inadequate thyroid hormone regulation of cell function. The inadequate regulation may result from hypothyroidism but not hyperthyroidism. Second-generation TSH assays adequately detect the high-normal or high TSH levels in hypothyroidism.

Identifying Deficiencies of Other Pituitary Hormones. In the patient who has a blunted TSH response to TRH, pituitary hormones other than TSH may also be deficient. The clinician can identify other hormone deficiencies by using specific laboratory basal and stimulation tests. Martino et al. recommended basal and stimulation tests to evaluate growth hormone and prolactin secretion. They also recommended tests of the pituitary-adrenal and pituitary-gonadal axes. Abnormal results of these tests are common for patients with central hypothyroidism. However, the thyroid hormone deficiency may cause deficiencies of other pituitary, adrenal, and gonadal hormones (see section below on adrenal insufficiency). Treatment with thyroid hormone may restore normal growth hormone and adrenal hormone levels.[37,p.787]

Adrenal Insufficiency. Some patients who have deficient pituitary secretion of TSH also have deficient pituitary secretion of ACTH. These patients are also likely to have deficient secretion of adrenocortical hormones. But although cortisol secretion may be subnormal, hepatic clearance of the hormone in hypothyroid patients is usually decreased. The slowed hepatic clearance may leave the blood cortisol level normal. Brent and Larsen pointed out that such patients may have symptoms of hypothyroidism but not of hypocortisolism until they begin treatment with thyroid hormone. When the exogenous thyroid hormone increases liver cell metabolism, hepatic clearance of cortisol accelerates. The increased clearance decreases the blood cortisol level because of the inability of the adrenal cortices to secrete normal quantities of cortisol. Brent and Larsen stated that if the clinician has any doubt about a patient's adrenocortical reserve, he should have her use both thyroid hormone and hydrocortisone until he can evaluate her hypothalamic-pituitary-adrenal function.[74,p.885] (See Chapter 5.2, section titled "Decreased Adrenal Reserve").

The patient's adrenocortical deficiency may be secondary to thyroid hormone deficiency because thyroid hormone regulates transcription of corticotropin-releasing hormone in the hypothalamus (see Chapter 3.5, section titled "Corticotropin-Releasing Hormone"). In the patient with decreased corticotropin-releasing hormone secretion due to hypothyroidism, correcting the thyroid hormone deficiency should increase corticotropin-releasing hormone secretion. In tandem, increased corticotropin-releasing hormone secretion should normalize ACTH and cortisol secretion. This is a theoretical consideration, however, and the clinician should proceed with caution when he suspects hypocortisolism.

Imaging Procedures for Locating Hypothalamic or Pituitary Lesions. Computed tomography and magnetic resonance imaging are highly sensitive procedures for identifying hypothalamic and pituitary lesions responsible for abnormal laboratory test results. The clinician may make use of these procedures to identify several abnormalities: enlargement of the sella turcica, erosion of the sella floor, elevation or erosion of the anterior clinoid processes, extrasellar extension of a pituitary tumor, suprasellar calcification that suggests craniopharyngioma, or small sella indicative of nontumorous lesions. Angiography is largely outdated by computed tomography and magnetic resonance imaging. However, the procedure may be useful for identifying aneurysms of the internal carotid artery that are responsible for hypopituitarism.[37,p.787]

Further Evaluations of Pituitary Function. Martino et al. recommended that the clinician carefully evaluate patients with isolated TSH deficiency at least twice per year to detect further loss of pituitary function.[37,p.788]

● **T₄/T₃-CONTAINING PREPARATIONS**

DESICCATED THYROID

In 1983, desiccated thyroid accounted for about 40% of the thyroid preparations sold in the U.S.[103,p.2655] In 1983, an author titled his paper "No further use of desiccated thyroid gland."[116] In 1984, another author titled a paper "Desiccated thyroid preparations: obsolete therapy."[117] These titles reflect the anti-desiccated thyroid attitude in conventional medicine about that time.

In 1991, 30% of patients taking exogenous thyroid hormone were taking thyroid gland extracts or combinations of synthetic T₄ and T₃.[100] Most clinicians now prefer their patients to take synthetic T₄, particularly the brand Synthroid, rather than desiccated thyroid. Over the past 30 years, a larger percentage of patients taking exogenous thyroid have taken T₄.[100]

The growing preference among physicians for Synthroid in the 1990s was not based on scientific justification but on intense marketing. Nevertheless, desiccated thyroid is still in widespread use. Its use is particularly widespread among two groups of patients: (1) elderly people who began treatment at what some medical writers consider "a time of less specific indications,"[103,p.2655] and (2) the new wave of Internet-educated hypothyroid patients who are now demanding that their physicians prescribe desiccated thyroid. In recent years, many hypothyroid patients frustrated with the ineffectiveness of T₄ alone have attained symptom relief with desiccated thyroid or combined synthetic T₄ and T₃.

The 38 µg of T₄ and 9 µg of T₃ contained in Armour Thyroid is not synthetic but is derived from pig thyroid glands. (Pigs have a higher T₃\T₄ ratio than sheep or cows.[163] Nittler wrote that he preferred pork thyroid because it is closer to the hormone composition of the human thyroid gland.[165,p.352]) The Armour laboratory analyzes the T₄ and T₃ content of the full strength thyroid powder when it arrives. The laboratory blends 2-to-5 different lots of thyroid powder to create the exact T₄/T₃ ratio for each lot of Armour Thyroid tablets. Technicians then assay a representative sample of the final product to assure it contains the correct ratio. The laboratory uses the same type of assay with the natural pig T₄ and T₃ as it does with Levothyroid, the company's product containing synthetic T₄ and T₃. Both products meet the same USP standards.[68]

Arguments Against the Use of Desiccated Thyroid

Medical writers have proffered a variety of arguments against the use of desiccated thyroid. Most are poor arguments; none should dissuade the clinician from using desiccated thyroid to treat hypothyroid patients.

Putative Variations in the Potency of Desiccated Thyroid Tablets. Despite propaganda from the manufacturers of competitive products and the views of some medical writers, desiccated thyroid is a reliable product.

In 1970, Mangieri reported that the biological activity of desiccated thyroid may vary even when it meets the USP criterion for organic iodine content.[162] He wrote that the reason for the variable biologic activity is that the T₃\T₄ ratios of animal thyroid glands differ. According to this view, consistent biological activity of the product is more likely if the pharmacist fills the patient's prescription with tablets from the same animal source. However, in producing Armour Thyroid tablets, the laboratory blends 2-to-5 different lots of thyroid powder to create the exact T_4/T_3 ratio for each lot of tablets.[68] This current production method should resolve the problem of variable biological activity of lots of desiccated thyroid tablets.

Sawin wrote that the biological activity of desiccated thyroid may also vary because of the traditional method of estimating potency. The USP method estimates hormonal content of a product by its iodine content. As a result, inspectors may classify tablets as potent even after the hormones in the tablets have deteriorated. The tablets still contain measurable amounts of iodine, but a decreased percentage of it is a constituent of thyroid hormone molecules. Depending on the degree of deterioration, the tablets may be less potent than indicated by the label, or they may be totally inert.[164] Patients can easily avoid this potential problem by only using tablets from bottles with expiration dates that have not passed.

Putative Problems with the T_3 in Desiccated Thyroid. Brent and Larsen wrote that thyroid extracts containing both T_4 and T_3 were used for treatment before companies began formulating and marketing synthetic combination products.[74,p.883] Subsequently, animal[97] and human[98] studies showed that about 80% of circulating T_3 derives from conversion of T_4 to T_3 in the peripheral tissues. Brent and Larsen concluded that the sole use of exogenous T_4 generates sufficient serum and tissue concentrations of T_3 and that this replicates normal physiology.[74,p.883]

Not surprisingly, Brent and Larsen reported that some patients taking thyroid extracts or synthetic combination preparations were reluctant to change to T_4. They wrote that if the patient continues with the other products, then the clinician should determine dosage by using the serum TSH and not T_4 and T_3 levels.[74,p.884] No one who has read much of this book will be surprised when I adjudge Brent and Larsen's advice misguiding. One of my tenets in this book, of course, is that except in rare cares, neither the TSH nor thyroid hormone levels are of any value in determining thyroid hormone dosage, regardless of the form of thyroid hormone the patient is using.

Manufacturers formulated the T_4 to T_3 ratio in desiccated thyroid mixtures based on the T_4 to T_3 ratio in the circulation of humans. This was before researchers learned that conversion of T_4 in cells other than those of the thyroid gland is the source of most extrathyroidal T_3 in the body. "Hence," Sawin wrote, arguing for treatment of hypothyroidism with T_4 alone, "one gives T_3 simply by giving T_4."[13,p.393] Theoreti-

cally, when a patient takes exogenous T_4, she effectively converts it to T_3. Presumably, according to conventional thyroidology, this provides the proper circulating and cellular ratio of T_3 to T_4. Therefore, desiccated thyroid or products containing synthetic T_4 and T_3 were not necessary to normal metabolism.

An argument of conventional thyroidology against the use of desiccated thyroid (and by extension, products containing synthetic T_4 and T_3) is that the T_3 it contains increases the circulating and cellular ratio of T_3 to T_4. Presumably, this was somehow harmful to patients. Yet I have found no evidence in the thyroidology literature to support the presumption. Conversely, during my 14 years of observing patients taking desiccated thyroid, I have witnessed no adverse effects from products *per se.* The only exception is the few patients taking dosages that were thyrotoxic for them. I discerned no adverse effects, however, when we titrated their dosages to effective yet non-thyrotoxic amounts.

Another argument of conventional thyroidology against the use of desiccated thyroid (and by extension, products containing synthetic T_4 and T_3) is the postabsorptive peak in the serum T_3 concentration following ingestion.[128,p.1099][129] One author called this peak "part-of-the-day hypertriiodothyroninemia caused by desiccated thyroid."[14] LeBoff et al. reported that the time to peak serum T_3 levels after ingestion did not significantly differ when patients ingested 75 μg synthetic T_3 (Cytomel), 6 grains of desiccated thyroid (Armour Thyroid, containing 99 μg T_3), or 5 grains of thyroglobulin (Proloid, containing 90 μg T_3). The mean time to peak T_3 level was 2 hours.[115]

The postabsorptive peak is of concern only with the patient who has an extremely fragile cardiac status. On principle, the clinician prescribing thyroid hormone is ethically responsible for carefully considering each patient's individual responsiveness to the hormone. For most patients, however, high peak serum T_3 levels are clinically inconsequential. In performing serial electrocardiograms on many patients taking high dosages of synthetic T_3, I did not find the arrhythmias some clinicians and researchers conjecture will result from T_3 therapy.

The high peak serum T_3 levels may be beneficial for patients with euthyroid fibromyalgia. If the patient has peripheral cellular resistance to thyroid hormone due to mutated T_3 receptors, then only a high concentration of T_3 in the nucleus may override the resistance of the mutant receptors. Mutant T_3 receptors do not regulate transcription in the presence of physiologic concentrations of T_3. They do so, however, when exposed to supraphysiologic dosages (see Chapter 2.6, section subtitled "Mutations in the c-erbAβ Gene: Mechanism of Most Cases of General Thyroid Hormone Resistance"). In one study, for example, fibroblasts from patients with thyroid hormone resistance responded only to a concentration of T_3 50 times that of the normal (physiological) free T_3.[161] *In vitro* studies have shown that only high-saturation concentrations of T_3 induce gene transcription regulation by mutant T_3-receptors (see Chapter 2.6). These research findings suggest that surges in the cellular concentration of T_3 following peaks in the serum T_3 level may provide surges in transcription regulation. Such surges in transcription regulation may be the basis of some fibromyalgia patients with thyroid hormone resistance improving or recovering with the use of supraphysiologic dosages of T_3. The T_3 in desiccated thyroid may similarly benefit patients with milder resistance to thyroid hormone. This is more likely to occur in patients taking desiccated thyroid which has a 4:1 T_4 to T_3 ratio than in patients taking synthetic products that have a 10:1 ratio.

Dosages of Desiccated Thyroid

Medical writers have recommended a variety of dosages for hypothyroid patients. In 1933, Kimball wrote that his only recommendation was to begin with a small dose and to gradually increase it to patient tolerance. He wrote that a 150-lb man with no thyroid function requires 6 grains (USP) of thyroid extract daily to keep his basal metabolic rate at the average normal level. A child of 50 lbs, however, could tolerate at most 2 grains per day. He wrote that the clinician should start the child on about ¼ that amount (½ grain). The child should then increase dosage gradually to tolerance over an 8-week period. "These are the theoretical averages," he cautioned, "but you will find considerable variation."[42,p495]

In 1939, Wharton wrote that patients often benefit from small doses of desiccated thyroid, about ½ grain twice per day. He reported finding no ill effects from this dosage when he kept patients under observation.[44,p.373]

In 1942, Barnes recommended an initial dose of 1 grain (0.065 gm) of USP thyroid. He used Armour thyroid. He had the patient take the entire dose at breakfast for the sole purpose of forming a habit. After the patient had taken 1 grain for 4 weeks, she took her basal body temperature on 2 or 3 mornings. If the temperature had not risen enough, the patient increased her daily dosage by another grain. After a month on this dosage, she took her basal temperature again. If it

had not increased enough, she increased her dosage by another grain. Of 1000 patients using this regimen that he tested, the majority had normal temperatures within 6 months. He wrote, "Patients will be encountered requiring more, but if the dose is raised gradually, as here outlined, and the temperature followed closely at monthly intervals, probably no great harm will be done."[89,p.1073]

The 1990 PDR recommended a starting dosage of desiccated thyroid of 30 mg (roughly ½ grain) with increments of 15 mg every 2-to-3 weeks.[43,p.1889] When the patient reaches the correct dosage, according to the PDR her TSH and T_4 levels should be within their respective normal ranges after 2-to-3 weeks. The authors of the PDR recommended that the clinician check the patient's status through clinical and laboratory methods and then adjust the dosage after about 1 month. The optimal dosage for most patients, according to this source, is between 60 and 120 mg.[43,p.1889] But this does not hold true for the many hypothyroid patients my colleagues and I have enabled to recover from fibromyalgia. We have found that the equivalent of about 200-to-400 µg of T_4 has been effective and safe for many patients. (Bear in mind, however, that we now use desiccated thyroid or T_3 rather than T_4 with hypothyroid patients.) The 60-to-120 mg of desiccated thyroid the PDR considered optimal is equivalent only to 100-to-200 µg of T_4. In my experience, this dosage will not benefit most hypothyroid fibromyalgia patients. Nor will it satisfy extremist technocratic clinicians: Taking the equivalent of approximately 145-to-171 µg T_4 (2½-to-2¾ grains, or 150-to-165 mg, desiccated thyroid) is likely to suppress patients' TSH levels and distress the technocrats as they warn of impending thyrotoxicosis. Despite this ludicrousness, for most hypothyroid patients the equivalent of 200-to-400 µg of T_4 (2-to-4 grains, or 120-to-240 mg, desiccated thyroid) is harmless and usually effective in relieving the patient's fibromyalgia—but only when she uses the thyroid hormone within the context of a more comprehensive metabolic rehabilitation program (see Chapter 5.2).

Greater Effectiveness of Desiccated Thyroid Compared to T_4 on a µg by µg Basis. Desiccated thyroid, on a µg by µg basis, is more effective than T_4 in the treatment of hypothyroidism. The greater effectiveness of desiccated thyroid is due to its T_3 content. In line with the USP standard, desiccated thyroid contains 38 µg of T_4 and 9 µg of T_3.[99] The T_4/T_3 ratio is 4:1.

A recent blinded trial showed benefits of hypothyroid patients taking T_3 in addition to T_4. Bunevicius et al. compared the effects of T_4 alone with those of T_4 plus 12.5 µg of T_3. Compared to patients who used T_4 alone, those who used T_4 plus T_3 had significantly improved mood and neuropsychological function. They improved on 6 of 17 scores on tests of cognitive performance and assessments of mood. They also improved on 10 of 15 visual analog scales that assessed mood and physical status. The T_4/T_3 ratio in daily medicine intake varied among the patients. The variations occurred because the researchers substituted 12.5 µg of T_3 for 50 µg of each patient's usual T_4. The mean of the participating patients' usual T_4 dosages was 175±53 µg (0.175±0.053 mg) per day; the range of their usual dosages was 100-to-300 µg (0.1-to-0.3 mg) per day. Thus, the mean T_4/T_3 ratio was 14:1; the range of T_4/T_3 ratios of the daily dosages was 8:1-to-24:1.[166]

Based on clinical and research experiences and familiarity with the current thyroidology literature, I conjecture that the patients in this study would have had significantly more improvement without thyrotoxicity had their medication contained more T_3 (a lower T_4/T_3 ratio). Contrary to my view, however, was the response of Toft to the Bunevicius et al. study. Toft commented that "Most, if not all, of the currently available combined preparations of thyroid hormones contain *an excess of triiodothyronine* as compared with thyroxine." Then he wrote, "*The ideal medication would contain approximately 100 µg of thyroxine and 10 µg of triiodothyronine, the latter in slow-release form to avoid adverse cardiac effects*[italics mine]."[151] It is my view that these statements by Toft are potentially damaging to the quality of treatment hypothyroid patients are likely to receive in the near future. In the italicized parts of the two statements, by using the adjective "excess," he presumes that the amount of T_3 in current combined T_4/T_3 medications is harmful in some way. Some practicing physicians will consider Toft's opinion authoritative; they will assume his opinion is based on sound scientific reasons and is scientifically factual. As a result, these physicians will tend to be prejudiced against the T_4/T_3 ratio in current medications such as desiccated thyroid.

Yet Toft's defining the ratio as "excess" is *a priori* thinking. He cannot scientifically justify his sweeping judgment. In addition, we can easily show it to be false. His statements are similar in their potential harm to his 1989 statements in which he called suppressed TSH levels "thyrotoxic."[113,p.91] Clearly, a suppressed TSH is not synonymous with thyrotoxicity. But careless use of terminology by thyroidologists such as Toft, implying that they are synonymous, has adversely impacted clinical care of the hypothyroid patient. Their careless terminology has contributed to the apprehension of practitioners when they find a suppressed TSH level in a hypothyroid patient using thyroid hormone.

The term "thyrotoxicosis" refers to the *clinical* syndrome resulting from increased circulating free T_4 and T_3 levels.[82] At least two classes of patients may have suppressed TSH levels without tissue thyrotoxicity: (1) some with pituitary hypothyroidism and (2) those with peripheral resistance to thyroid hormone who maintain normal metabolism by taking supraphysiologic dosages of thyroid hormone. Patients in the first class are hypometabolic and those in the second, when their thyroid hormone dosages are properly titrated, are eumetabolic. Yet I know of patients in both classes whose physicians interpreted their suppressed TSH levels as "thyrotoxic." The clinicians denied patients of the first class the use of thyroid hormone they needed. Clinicians urged patients in the second class to reduce their dosages to amounts that would have left them hypometabolic and symptomatic. The second class of patients, those with cellular resistance to thyroid hormone, are metabolically normal only with a high T_3 content in their thyroid medication; they may require far higher T_3 dosages than desiccated thyroid provides. To be normal metabolically and healthy, these patients require amounts of T_3 that Toft presumes and pronounces to be "excessive."

My point is that Toft's defining the amount of T_3 in combined T_4/T_3 preparations as an "excess" is an unjustified presumption. Clinicians should sensitize themselves to this type of careless and problem-causing misuse of terminology by some thyroidologists. Toft may be unaware that the "excess" implies that the dosage is overstimulating. Yet tissue overstimulation is relative to the individual patient. As I have shown experimentally and observed in clinical practice, some fibromyalgia patients with peripheral cellular resistance to thyroid hormone must use 20-to-33 times the amount of T_3 in a grain of desiccated thyroid to maintain normal metabolism and obtain symptom relief. Yet these dosages are thoroughly non-toxic for these patients (see section above titled "Putative Problems with the T_3 in Desiccated Thyroid").[154][155][156] In one well-documented case of peripheral cellular resistance to thyroid hormone, a patient had normal metabolism and freedom from symptoms when she took 56 times the amount of T_3 in a grain of desiccated thyroid.[120] For her, this large amount of T_3 was not thyrotoxic.

Such high dosages are excessive for most individuals, but they are not excessive for some patients. This illustrates that Toft's sweeping presumption that the T_3 in most combined T_4/T_3 medications is excessive is wrong. If companies subscribed to his presumption that the "ideal medication" would contain a T_4/T_3 ratio of 10:1, many patients who use combined medications would suffer adverse consequences. Using medication with the T_4/T_3 ratio he recommended would subject them to chronic tissue hypometabolism, sustained suffering from symptoms of hypometabolism, and an increased risk of cardiovascular disease and premature death (see Chapter 4.4, section titled "Harm from Untreated and Undertreated Hypothyroidism").

Proper Method of Determining Dosage. The clinician's purpose in reevaluating the patient taking thyroid hormone should be to learn how her peripheral tissues have responded to a particular dosage. He can assess her peripheral tissue responses only through symptoms, signs, and indices of peripheral tissue metabolic status. Laboratory thyroid function test results are without value for this purpose. (See Chapters 4.2, 4.3, and 5.2.)

The clinician must determine what dosage is safe and effective for each patient as an individual. Dosage *must* be individually determined. As Kimball wrote in 1933, dosage recommendations are only "theoretical averages"; patients' requirements vary substantially.[42,p495] Restricting the patient to a predetermined, cookbook dosage usually results in therapeutic failure.

PREPARATIONS CONTAINING SYNTHETIC T₄ AND T₃

Most of the information on desiccated thyroid in the section above also apples to preparations that contain a combination of synthetic T_4 and T_3. I suggest that clinicians select a product that contains the ratio of T_4 to T_3 in desiccated thyroid (4:1) rather than the 10:1 ratio recommended by Toft (see section above titled "Greater Effectiveness of Desiccated Thyroid Compared to T_4 on a μg by μg Basis"). Synthetic preparations are an alternative to desiccated thyroid for at least two groups of patients: vegetarians who do not consume animal products, and those who do not consume pig products for religious reasons.

Another alternative for the clinician is to have the patient take synthetic T_3 along with separate synthetic T_4. Ratios can then be manipulated to benefit each individual patient.

● SYNTHETIC T₄

For many years, my co-treating physicians and I began hypothyroid fibromyalgia patients' treatment with T_4 as part of their metabolic rehabilitation. Some patients completely recovered with the use of T_4. Others improved satisfactorily, but for many, improvement was unacceptably paltry. Still others did not improve at all, even after reaching dosages that were thyrotoxic for them. Most patients who improved or recovered did so only when they took TSH-suppressive dosages of T_4. For most hypothyroid patients, replacement dosages of T_4 were ineffective. Of patients who did not improve with T_4, however, virtually everyone significantly improved or completely recovered when we switched them to T_3.

Some recently published research provides potential explanations for our results in treating hypothyroid patients with T_4. First, in 1995 Escobar-Morreale et al. found that in hypothyroid rats, no single dosage of T_4 simultaneously restored normal plasma levels of TSH, T_4, and T_3, and normal levels of T_4 and T_3 in all tissues. Administering enough T_4 to produce a normal plasma T_4 level did not result in normal tissue T_3 levels. In most tissues the researchers examined, the dosage of T_4 required to provide normal T_3 levels resulted in supraphysiologic T_4 concentrations. The researchers concluded that their findings suggest that current T_4 replacement therapy is not adequate.[142,p.2837]

Escobar-Morreale et al. reported another significant finding: that infusing rats with enough T_4 to produce normal circulating T_3 levels did not normalize T_3 levels in all tissues. Some thyroidologists have pointed out that a normal circulating free T_3 correlates best with tissue metabolism. Volpé wrote, for example, that the serum T_3 level correlates better with a patient's clinical status than does the serum T_4 level.[21,p.88][48] He wrote that to achieve a normal circulating level of T_3, the patient may have to take a high enough dosage of T_4 to suppress the basal TSH and blunt the TSH response to TRH. Bantle[24] and Larsen[21,p.90] essentially concurred with this view. The thyroid gland secretes about 18% of the total T_3 into the circulation. Peripheral cellular conversion of T_4 to T_3 contributes the other 82%. In the hypothyroid patient, the thyroid gland secretes a lower-than-normal amount of T_3. As a result, the total T_3 in the body is deficient by the amount the gland fails to secrete. (Since the thyroid gland in hypothyroidism also secretes a lower-than-normal amount of T_4, the body's total T_3 deficiency may be compounded by a reduction in the total amount of T_4 converted to T_3.) According to the view of these writers, the patient can maintain a normal serum T_3 level by increasing her T_4 dosage. The increased dosage makes more T_4 available for cells to deiodinate. "Practicing physicians should therefore not be surprised," wrote Volpé, "by moderately elevated T_4 concentrations in T_4-replaced patients and should not interpret such values as indicative of hyperthyroidism."[21,pp.88-89] The recommendation is that the patient using T_4 as her sole thyroid medication should increase the dosage until her circulating free T_3 is normal. Presumably, reaching a normal circulating free T_3 level results in normal tissue metabolism. The presumption of these writers, however, is doubtful. Doubt is raised by a finding of Escobar-Morreale et al.: that normalizing the circulating free T_3 level does not ensure normal tissue T_3 concentrations.[142]

In 1996, Escobar-Morreale et al. wrote that it is not possible to restore normal thyroid hormone concentrations in all tissue of hypothyroid rats with T_4 alone. They conducted another study to determine whether a combination of T_4 and T_3 would restore normal tissue thyroid hormone concentration. In reporting their findings, they wrote: "Circulating and tissue T_4 levels were normal in all the groups infused with thyroid hormones. On the contrary, T_3 in plasma and most tissues and plasma TSH only reached normal levels when T_3 was added to the T_4 infusion. The combination of 0.9 µg T_4 and 0.15 µg T_3/100 g bodyweight per day resulted in normal T_4 and T_3 concentrations in plasma and all tissues as well as normal circulating TSH and normal or near-normal 5'-deiodinase activities." They also wrote: "Combined replacement therapy with T_4 and T_3 (in proportions similar to those secreted by the normal rat thyroid) completely restored euthyroidism in thyroidectomized rats at much lower doses of T_4 than those needed to normalize T_3 in most tissues when T_4 alone was used. If pertinent to man, these results might well justify a change in the current therapy for hypothyroidism."[121]

Results of the recently published report by Bunevicius et al. are consistent with those of the rat studies reported by Escobar-Morreale et al. Bunevicius et al. had hypothyroid patients replace 50 µg of their usual T_4 dosages with 12.5 µg of T_3. Other hypothyroid patients took their usual dosages of T_4 without T_3. Compared to these latter patients, those who took both T_4 and T_3 had significantly improved mood and neuropsychological scores.[166]

The reports of Escobar-Morreale et al.[121][142] and Bunevicius et al.[166] have necessitated reassessment of our initial use of T_4 alone for hypothyroid fibromyal-

gia patients. I now believe that some of our hypothyroid fibromyalgia patients in the past who did not improve sufficiently or at all with T_4 alone would have done so had we treated them with desiccated thyroid. Still, though, I would predict that some hypothyroid patients would not improve sufficiently even with the use of desiccated thyroid. In fact, in my early years of treating hypothyroid fibromyalgia patients, I observed some who did not improve with desiccated thyroid. They did not improve although they took dosages high enough to induce tissue thyrotoxicosis. The patients subsequently improved or recovered with the use of T_3 alone. This finding is consistent with the reports of researchers in the 1950s and 1960s (see Chapters 2.5 and 5.4).

Some patients will improve enough with T_4 alone and will not further benefit from the use of desiccated thyroid or synthetic T_3 alone. Honeyman-Lowe and I have treated many patients, however, who recovered with the use of T_3 after failing to benefit from the use of T_4. The prolonged time necessary to determine whether T_4 alone will be effective for patients subjects too many of them to prolonged suffering. I have in mind a recent case under the care of Honeyman-Lowe who completely recovered with T_3 within a couple of months after obtaining minimal improvement with T_4 during a year-long effort to find an effective dosage. We believe that subjecting more patients to such extended suffering is inhumane. For this reason, we now use desiccated thyroid in the initial treatment of hypothyroid fibromyalgia patients. We switch those patients who do not benefit sufficiently from its use to T_3. We are not opposed to patients and their physicians trying T_4 alone first—if the decision to do so is a collaborative one between the two parties. However, we now believe that with most hypothyroid fibromyalgia patients, the chance of successful therapeutic outcomes with T_4 alone is minimal. We base this belief on both pragmatic and theoretical grounds.

Conventional T_4 Dosage Recommendations

I do not agree with the dosage recommendations contained in this section. I present them only so that clinicians will be aware of conventional recommendations. The clinician should consider the statements of the authors I include in this section in view of the findings I included in the section above.

Toft wrote that before the RIA for TSH (in the early 1970s),[21,p.91] clinicians advised patients with primary hypothyroidism to use 200-to-400 µg (0.2-to-0.4 mg) of T_4 per day.[22][23,p.456] Clinical assessment was used to determine the appropriate dose. With the advent of TSH assays, Toft wrote further, it became clear that normal thyroid hormone levels (based on reducing the TSH into the normal range) were accomplished in 90% of patients with 100-to-200 µg (0.1-to-0.2 mg). Refetoff, Weiss, and Usala wrote that hypothyroidism requires replacement with physiologic doses of thyroid hormone, which they specified as 100-to-150 µg (0.10-to-0.15 mg) T_4.[50,p.391] Sonkin wrote that a physiologic dosage of about 0.112 mg of T_4 may control hypothyroidism due to failure of some point in the hypothalamic-pituitary-thyroid axis.[48,p.48]

Haynes wrote that a reasonable therapeutic regimen for adults is 50 µg of T_4 daily for 2 weeks followed by 100 µg per day for the next 2 weeks. He also wrote that the patient can make any refinements to this dosage after this 4-week period. According to Haynes, the optimal dose is usually between 100 µg and 150 µg. The patient has reached her optimal dosage when her clinical state is normal and her plasma TSH level is within the normal range. The optimal dosage varies considerably; some patients require as little as 50 µg, others as much as 400 µg.[133,p.1372] The TSH may not fall into the normal range with the usual dosage of T_4. If not, Haynes wrote, the clinician should repeatedly measure the TSH while raising the dose by 25 µg or 50 µg per day every 1-to-2 months. When the patient's TSH is within the normal range, and her metabolic state is normal, she should maintain the present dosage. Switching to a single tablet of the correct dosage may be less expensive and more convenient for the patient.[133,p.1372]

Larsen wrote that for patients with primary hypothyroidism, he prescribed about 0.8 µg (0.0008 mg) of Synthroid or Levothyroid per pound of body weight.[21,p.90] For a 120-lb person, the dosage would be 96 µg (0.096 mg). He considered this "a rough approximation for replacement." With this dosage, he wrote, the patient is likely to have the following laboratory values: TSH of 0.10-to-0.15 µU/mL (normal range = 0.5-to-5.0 µU/mL), serum T_3 of 100-to-120 ng/dL (normal = 75-to-175 ng/dL), and serum T_4 of about 8.0-to-11.0 µg/dL (normal = 4.5-to-12.5 µg/dL). He stated that the free T_3 is usually slightly subnormal and the TSH low-normal. If the TSH fell below 0.5 µU/mL, he reduced the patient's T_4 dosage.[21,p.91]

Effective T_4 *Dosage*

The oft recommended replacement dosage range of 100-to-200 µg of T_4 is based on false assumptions: that reliably, a "normal" TSH corresponds to normal tissue metabolism, an elevated TSH corresponds to tissue hypometabolism, and a low TSH corresponds to

tissue hypermetabolism. These assumptions are conjectures that are falsified by experimental studies. (See section above titled "Lack of Evidence of Correlation Between Thyroid Hormone and TSH Levels, and Tissue Metabolism.") Careful observations of hypothyroid patients treated with replacement dosages show that if such relationships exist, they are rare. Most hypothyroid patients using such dosages remain hypometabolic and symptomatic. The clinician must keep in mind that a normal TSH level does not necessarily correspond to normal tissue metabolism.

For most hypothyroid patients, an effective dosage of T_4 will suppress the TSH level. The clinician's therapeutic aim should be to alleviate the patient's symptoms and signs, and to normalize peripheral indices of tissue metabolic status. Thyroid function test results are useless for this purpose.[56] In my experience, most patients who improve or recover with the use of T_4 do so only with dosages between 200 µg and 400 µg.

Sawin wrote that we cannot predict the right dose of T_4 for an individual because patients vary in the amount they require.[13,p.396] There are several reasons for this. First, the human gut absorbs only part of ingested T_4 (70%-to-80% of T_4, compared to almost 100% of T_3[74,p.883]). The amount absorbed varies in the same person, from 40%-to-90%.[15] Older patients may require less T_4 than younger ones.[102] Patients may require more T_4 when taking drugs such as phenytoin[16] (the anticonvulsant drug Dilantin) or cholestyramine[18] (a drug that lowers cholesterol). Patients who have had intestinal bypass surgery for obesity also may require more because the absorptive surface may be too small.[131] Patients should take T_4 on an empty stomach; otherwise, food may interfere with its absorption.

Clinicians usually recommend that the patient take T_4 as a single dose before breakfast. Mardell and Gamlen wrote that this is "unphysiological" and may raise free T_4 levels 10%-to-25% above normal 4-to-6 hours after the patient takes 200 µg.[19] This raised µg level, however, does not appear to adversely affect the patient.[20]

The half-life of T_4 is 6-to-7 days. This time span is indicated by observations of patients who have undergone thyroidectomy for hyperthyroidism. They may remain thyrotoxic and require propranolol therapy for more than a week until their circulating T_4 is expended.[41,p.905] Because of the long half-life of T_4, failing to take her dose for a few days is not likely to alter the patient's metabolic status.[74,p.884] The serum variation in T_4 levels is less than 15% between single daily doses.[74,p.883] LeBoff et al. found that the peak serum free T_3 level after 75 μg T_3 occurred at 2 hours. By comparison, the peak after 3 mg of T_4 occurred at 2 days. The mean peak free T_3 (500) after 75 μg T_3 was much higher than the mean peak free T_3 (290) after 3 mg of T_4 .[115]

Some patients are not capable of caring for themselves. Writers have recommended that if such a patient has not taken her oral dose for a period longer than a few days, the clinician may want to inject her with T_4. The injection should contain 20%-to-25% of her oral dose.[128,p.1101][129][130]

Choice of T_4 Brand

Manufacturers standardize the content of synthetic T_4 tablets. The method they use is supposed to assure that the content of T_4 stated on a label is consistent with the amount in the tablets, [13,p.394] give or take 10%. Thus, the T_4 content, standardized by high-pressure liquid chromatography, must be between 90% and 110% of the amount stated on the label.[74,p.883] Dong et al. determined that Synthroid, Levoxyl, and two generic brands of T_4 were bioequivalent by FDA criteria. They concluded that the brands are interchangeable for the majority of patients using T_4 replacement therapy.[118] (See the Glossary for specific brand names.)

● EXOGENOUS THYROID HORMONE: AN ORTHO-MOLECULAR SUBSTANCE

Many individuals today enthusiastically turn away from medications with high potential for toxicity used by conventional physicians. Some are disinclined to take any medication prescribed by a conventional physician, including thyroid hormone. These individuals would likely benefit from making an important distinction between classes of medications—those that are foreign to the body and those that are not. We term medications that are not foreign to the body "orthomolecular substances."

Linus Pauling defined an orthomolecular substance as one normally present in the body and essential to health.[143,p.252] Pauling was the honorary father of orthomolecular medicine. This form of practice is the preservation of good health and the treatment of disease by varying the concentrations in the human body of substances normally present in the body and necessary for health.[144] Examples of orthomolecular medicine are the use of exogenous thyroid hormone

for hypothyroidism, insulin injections for diabetes mellitus, and megadoses of vitamin C to boost resistance to infection.[143,p.118] Pauling noted that just as supplemental vitamins, minerals, and trace elements are orthomolecular substances, so is thyroid hormone.

In contrast, Rimland described conventional allopathic practice, which has traditionally employed chemicals alien to the body, as toximolecular medicine.[145] Many orthomolecular substances can produce toxic effects when taken in extreme excess for the individual. This is true of thyroid hormone. But altering the concentrations of orthomolecular substances within nontoxic limits in the body can have distinctly beneficial effects.

● OTHER FORMS OF THERAPY FOR THE HYPOTHYROID FIBROMYALGIA PATIENT

Nutritional therapy, and possibly thyroid gland manipulative therapy, may normalize some patients' subnormal thyroid gland function. Some clinicians believe that these treatment methods are preferable to the use of exogenous thyroid hormone. Inducing and maintaining normal thyroid gland function without the use of exogenous thyroid hormone can free patients from expense and inconvenience. These methods are of no use, however, for some patients—those whose hypothyroidism stems from autoimmune thyroiditis, thyroid surgery, antithyroid drugs, thyroid gland trauma, or thyrotroph-destroying pituitary adenomas. These hypothyroid patients must take exogenous thyroid hormone. The hormone compensates for the impaired part of the hypothalamic-pituitary-thyroid axis by providing sufficient thyroid hormone to maintain normal metabolism and health. Some patients simply have irreparably damaged links in their hypothalamic-pituitary-thyroid axes. Trying to induce these patients' thyroid glands to secrete normal amounts of thyroid hormone through nutritional or manipulative treatment will prove futile. Such treatment may also needlessly prolong the patient's suffering. Exogenous thyroid hormone in proper dosages can relieve her hormone deficiency and provide normal metabolism.

Nutritional inadequacies or neurovascular dysfunctions may cause an extremely low percentage of patients' thyroid gland hypofunction in the U.S. For some patients, the resulting subjective experience is tolerable. These patients and their clinicians may prefer to collaborate in trying to recover normal thyroid gland function. If they succeed, the patient will have no need to use exogenous thyroid hormone. (For manipulative methods, see Chapter 5.2, "Manipulative Therapies: Manipulating the Thyroid Gland.")

However, the extremely severe symptoms of many hypothyroid fibromyalgia patients should compel the clinician to promptly provide appropriate symptom-abating dosages of thyroid hormone. The symptoms of some patients are so severe that beginning treatment with T_3 rather than a T_4/T_3 combination is more humane. When the patient takes a high enough dosage, metabolic effects of T_3 begin within days. By contrast, the effects of T_4 and products that contain more T_4 than T_3 may take from 10 days-to-2 weeks.

REFERENCES

1. DeGroot, L.J.: Abnormal thyroid function tests in euthyroid patients. In *Diagnostic Methods in Clinical Thyroidology*. Edited by J.I. Hamburger, New York, Springer-Verlag, 1989, pp.3-26.

2. Gow, S.M., Caldwell, G., Toft, A.D., Seth, J., Hussey, A.J., and Sweeting, V.M.: Relationship between pituitary and other target organ responsiveness in hypothyroid patients receiving thyroxine replacement. *J. Clin. Endocrinol. Metab.*, 64:364, 1987.

3. Melander, A., Ericson, L.E., Sundler, F., and Ingbar, S.H.: Sympathetic innervation of the mouse thyroid and its significance in thyroid hormone secretion. *Endocrinology*, 94:959-966, 1974.

4. Johnson, A.C.: *Chiropractic Physiological Therapeutics*, 5ᵗʰ edition. Palm Springs, self-published, 1977.

5. Melander, A., Ericson, L.E., and Sundler, F.: Sympathetic regulation of thyroid hormone secretion. *Life Sci.*, 14:237-245, 1974.

6. Ishie, J.: Effect of stimulation of the vagal nerve on the thyroidal release of ¹³¹I-labeled hormones. *Folia Endocrinol. Japan.*, 35:1433, 1960.

7. Melander, A., Ericson, L.E., Ljunggren, J.G., et al.: Sympathetic innervation of the normal human thyroid. *J. Clin. Endocrinol. Metab.*, 39:713-718, 1974.

8. Soderberg, U.: Temporal characteristics of thyroid activity. *Physiol. Rev.*, 39:777, 1959.

9. DeGroot, L.J., Larsen, P.R., Refetoff, S., and Stanbury, J.B.: *The Thyroid and Its Diseases*, 5ᵗʰ edition. New York, John Wiley & Sons, Inc., 1984.

10. Soderberg, U.: Short-term reactions in the thyroid gland. *Acta Physiol. Scand.*, 42(Suppl):147, 1958.

11. Ridgway, E.C.: Modern concepts of primary thyroid gland failure. *Clin. Chem.*, 42(1):179-182, 1996.

12. Ahn, C.S., Athans, J.C., and Rosenberg, I.N.: Effects of epinephrine and of alterations in glandular blood flow upon thyroid function: studies using thyroid vein cannulation in dogs. *Endocrinology*, 84:501, 1969.

13. Sawin, C.T.: The development and use of thyroid preparations. In *The Thyroid Gland: A Practical Clinical Treatise*. Edited by L. Van Middlesworth, Jr., Chicago, Year

Book Medical Publishers, Inc., 1986, pp.389-403.

14. Lev-Ran, A.: Part-of-the-day hypertriiodothyroninemia caused by desiccated thyroid. *J.A.M.A.* 250(20):2790-2791, 1983.

15. Wenzel, K.W. and Kirschsieper, H.E.: Aspects of the absorption of oral L-thyroxine in normal man. *Metabolism*, 26:1, 1977.

16. Blackshear, J.L., Schultz, A.L., and Napier, J.S.: Thyroxine replacement requirements in hypothyroid patients receiving phenytoin. *Ann. Intern. Med.*, 99:341, 1983.

17. Melander, A., Sundler, F., and Westgren, U.: Intrathyroidal amines and the synthesis of thyroid hormone. *Endocrinology*, 93:193-200, 1973.

18. Northcutt, R.C., Stiel, J.N., and Hollifield, J.W.: The influence of cholestyramine on thyroxine absorption. *J.A.M.A.*, 208:1857, 1969.

19. Mardell, R.J. and Gamlen, T.R.: *Thyroid Function Tests in Clinical Practice*. Bristol, John Wright & Sons, Ltd., 1985.

20. Symons, R.G. and Murphy, L.J.: Acute changes in thyroid function tests following ingestion of thyroxine. *Clin. Endocrinol.*, 19:539-546, 1983.

21. Hamburger, J.I.: Strategies for cost-effective thyroid function testing with modern methods. In *Diagnostic Methods in Clinical Thyroidology*. Edited by J.I. Hamburger, New York, Springer-Verlag, 1989, pp.63-109.

22. Salmon, D., Rendell, M., and Williams, J.: Chemical hyperthyroidism. *Arch. Intern. Med.*, 142:571, 1982.

23. Selenkow, H.A. and Ingbar, S.H.: In *Harrison's Principles of Internal Medicine*, 6ᵗʰ edition. Edited by J. Wintrobe, New York, McGraw-Hill, 1970.

24. Bantle, J.P.: Replacement therapy with levothyroxine: evolving concepts. *Thyroid Today*, 10:1, 1987.

25. Vanhaelst, L.: Hypothyroidism and coronary heart disease. In *Recent Progress in Diagnosis and Treatment of Hypothyroid Conditions*. Edited by P.A. Bastenie, M. Bonnyns, and L. Vanhaelst, Amsterdam, *Excerpta Medica*, 1980. pp.112-118.

26. Bastenie, P.A.: Treatment of myxoedema associated with coronary heart disease. In *Recent Progress in Diagnosis and Treatment of Hypothyroid Conditions*. Edited by P.A. Bastenie, M. Bonnyns, and L. Vanhaelst, Amsterdam, *Excerpta Medica*, 1980, pp.122-125.

27. Gasinska, T., Drozdz, M., Izbicka, M., and Szydlo, E.: Effect of various beta-adrenolytic drugs and calcium channel blocker (nifedipine) on selected indicators of calcium-phosphorus metabolism in patients with hyperthyroidism and simple goiter. *Endokrynologia Polska*, 39(6):327-337, 1988.

28. Gasinka, T., Wawrzyniak, L., and Widala, E.: Acetylation phenotype and the changes in selected indicators of calcium-phosphate metabolism in patients with hyperthyroidism treated with propranolol. *Endokrynologia Polska*, 40 (6):291-300, 1989.

29. Surks, M.I., Schadlow, A.R., and Oppenheimer, J.H.: A new radioimmunoassay for plasma L-triiodothyronine: measurements in thyroid disease and in patients maintained on hormonal replacement. *J. Clin. Invest.*, 51:3140, 1972.

30. Werbel, S..S. and Ober, K.P.: Acute adrenal insufficiency. *Endocrinol. Metab. Clinics North Am.*, 22(2):303-328,

1993.

31. Herren, T.: Hypotensive crisis. *J. Suisse de Med.*, 123(17): 853-867, 1993.

32. Stojsic, D.: Addison's disease. *Medicinski Pregled*, 47(3-4):134-136, 1994.

33. Gao, T.S., Shi, Y.F., and Gao, S.M.: Evaluation of adult idiopathic growth hormone deficiency with other pituitary hormones deficiency. *Chinese J. Intern. Med.*, 29(4):205-209,252, 1990.

34. Le Feuvre, C., Baubion, N., Berdah, J., Heulin, A., and Vacheron, A.: Drug-induced cardiovascular complications. *Ann. Med. Intern.*, 140(7):597-599, 1989.

35. Beck-Peccoz, P. and Persani, L.: Variable biological activity of thyroid-stimulating hormone. *Eur. J. Endocrinol.*, 131:331, 1994.

36. Faglia, G., Bitensky, I., Pinchera, A., et al.: Thyrotropin secretion in patients with central hypothyroidism: evidence for reduced biological activity of immunoreactive thyrotropin. *J. Clin. Endocrinol. Metab.*, 48:989, 1979.

37. Martino, E., Bartalena, L., Faglia, G., and Pinchera, A.: Central hypothyroidism. In *Werner and Ingbar's The Thyroid: A Fundamental and Clinical Text*, 7th edition. Edited by L.P. Braverman and R.D. Utiger, Philadelphia, Lippincott-Raven Publishers, 1996, pp.779-791.

38. Åsbert, M. and Nordström, P.: Biological correlates of suicidal behavior. In *Current Issues of Suicidology*. Edited by H.J. Möller, A. Schmidtke, and R. Weltz, Berlin, Springer, 1988, pp.221-241.

39. Rouillonm, F., Phillips, R., Serrurier, E., Ansart, E., and Gerard, M.J.: Prophylactic efficacy of maprotiline on relapses of unipolar depression. *Encéphale*, XV:527-534, 1989.

40. Fisher, D.A.: Physiological variations in thyroid hormones: physiological and pathophysiological considerations. *Clin. Chem.*, 42(1):135-139, 1996.

41. Cooper, D.S.: Treatment of thyrotoxicosis. In *Werner and Ingbar's The Thyroid: A Fundamental and Clinical Text*, 6th edition. Edited by L.E. Braverman and R.D. Utiger, New York, J.B. Lippincott Co., 1991, pp.887-916.

42. Kimball, O.P.: Clinical hypothyroidism. *Kentucky Med. J.*, 31:488-495, 1933.

43. *Physicians Desk Reference*, 44th edition. Oradell, Medical Economics Company, Inc., 1990.

44. Wharton, G.B.: Unrecognized hypothyroidism. *Canadian Med. Assoc. J.*, 40:371-376, 1939.

45. Rasmusson, B., Borgestov, S., and Holme-Hanson, B.: Changes in serum calcitonin in patients undergoing thyroid surgery. *Acta Chiro. Scand.*, 146:15-17, 1980.

46. Watson, C.G., Steed, D.I., Robinson, A.G., and Deftos, L.J.: The role of calcitonin and parathyroid hormone in the pathogenesis of post-thyroidectomy hypocalcemia. *Metabolism*, 30:588-589, 1981.

47. Percival, R.C., Hargreaves, A.W., and Kanis, J.A.: The mechanism of hypocalcaemia following thyroidectomy. *Acta Endocrinol.*, 109:220-226, 1985.

48. Sonkin, L.S.: Myofascial pain due to metabolic disorders: diagnosis and treatment. In *Myofascial Pain and Fibromyalgia: Trigger Point Management*. Edited by E.S. Rachlin, St. Louis, Mosby, 1994, pp.45-60.

49. Gentile, F. and Aloj, S.M.: Congenital hypothyroidism: etiology and pathogenesis. *Annali del Instituto Superiore di Sanita*, 30(3):299-308, 1994.

50. Refetoff, S., Weiss, R.E., and Usala, S.J.: The syndromes of resistance to thyroid hormone. *Endocrine Reviews*, 14: 348-399, 1993.

51. Ziman, J.: *Reliable Knowledge: An Exploration of the Grounds for Belief in Science.* Cambridge, Cambridge University Press, 1978.

52. Shapiro, L.E., Sievert, R., Ong, L., et al.: Minimal cardiac effects in asymptomatic athyreotic patients chronically treated with thyrotropin-suppressive doses of L-thyroxine. *J. Clin Endocrinol. Metab.*, 82(8):2592-2595, 1997.

53. al-Adsani, H., Hoffer, L.J., and Silva, J.E.: Resting energy expenditure is sensitive to small dose changes in patients on chronic thyroid hormone replacement. *J. Clin. Endocrinol. Metab.*, 82(4):1118-1125, 1997.

54. Wolf, M., Weigert, A., and Kreymann, G.: Body composition and energy expenditure in thyroidectomized patients during short-term hypothyroidism and thyrotropin-suppressive thyroxine therapy. *Eur. J. Endocrinol.*, 134(2):168-173, 1996.

55. Skinner, G.R.B., Thomas, R., Taylor, M., et al.: Thyroxine should be tried in clinically hypothyroid but biochemically euthyroid patients (Letter). *Brit. Med. J.*, 314:1764, 1997.

56. Fraser, W.D., Biggart, E.M., O'Reilly, D.St.J., Gray, H.W., and McKillop, J.H.: Are biochemical tests of thyroid function of any value in monitoring patients receiving thyroxine replacement? *Br. Med. J.*, 293:808-810, 1986.

57. Melander, A. and Sundler, F.: Interactions between catecholamines, 5-hydroxytryptamine and TSH on the secretion of thyroid hormone. *Endocrinology*, 90:188, 1972.

58. Ackerman, N.B. and Arons, W.L.: The effect of epinephrine and norepinephrine on acute thyroid release of thyroid hormones. *Endocrinology*, 62:723, 1958.

59. Melander, A.: Amines and mouse thyroid activity: release of thyroid hormone by catecholamines and indoleamines and its inhibition by adrenergic blocking drugs. *Acta Endocrinol.*, 65:371, 1970.

60. Wilk, C.: AMA dollars will fund chiro research. *Dyn. Chiro.*, Feb. 12, 1993.

61. Schutt, C.H. and Dohan, F.C.: Neck injury to women in auto accidents: a metropolitan plague. *J.A.M.A.*, 206: 2692, 1968.

62. Tepperman, J. and Tepperman, H.M.: *Metabolic and Endocrine Physiology*, 5th edition. Chicago, Year Book Medical Publishers, Inc., 1987.

63. Stockigt, J.R.: Serum thyrotropin and thyroid hormone measurements and assessment of thyroid hormone transport. In *Werner and Ingbar's The Thyroid: A Fundamental and Clinical Text*, 7th edition. Edited by L.P. Braverman and R.D. Utiger, Philadelphia, Lippincott-Raven Publishers, 1996, pp.377-396.

64. Jefferies, W.: *Safe Uses of Cortisone.* Springfield, Charles C. Thomas, 1981.

65. Jefferies, W.: Low dose glucocorticoid therapy. *Arch. Intern. Med.*, 119:265-278, 1967.

66. Teitelbaum, J. and Bird, B.: Effective treatment of severe chronic fatigue: a report of a series of 64 patients. *J. Musculoskel. Pain*, 3(4):91-110, 1995.

67. Harvey, R.A. and Champe, P.C.: *Pharmacology.* Philadelphia, J.B. Lippincott Co., 1992.

68. Wesche, D.: Drug Information Associate, Professional Affairs Department, Forest Pharmaceuticals, Inc., personal communication, Dec.1, 1998.

69. Wayne, E.J.: Clinical and metabolic studies in thyroid disease. *Br. Med. J.*, i:1-11, 78-90, 1960.

70. Simons, D.G., Travell, J.G., and Simons, L.S.: *Travell & Simons Myofascial Pain and Dysfunction: The Trigger Point Manual, Vol. 1, Upper Half of Body*, 2nd edition. Baltimore, Williams & Wilkins, 1999.

71. Murray, G.R.: The pathology and treatment of myxoedema: remarks on the treatment of myxoedema with thyroid juice, with notes of four cases. *Br. Med. J.*, 2:449, 1892.

72. Stamler, J.S.: The coronary drug project: findings leading to further modifications of its protocol with respect to dextrothyroxine. *J.A.M.A.*, 220:996, 1972.

73. Keating, F.R., Jr., Parkin, T.W., and Selby, J.B.: Treatment of heart disease associated with myxedema. *Prog. Cardiovasc. Dis.*, 3:364,1961.

74. Brent, G.A. and Larsen, P.R.: Treatment of hypothyroidism. In *Werner and Ingbar's The Thyroid: A Fundamental and Clinical Text*, 7th edition. Edited by L.P. Braverman and R.D. Utiger, Philadelphia, Lippincott-Raven Publishers, 1996, pp.883-887.

75. LeBoff, M.S., Kaplan, M.M., Silva, J.E., and Larsen, P.R.: Bioavailability of thyroid hormones from oral replacement preparations. *Metabolism*, 31:900, 1982.

76. Hershman, J.M.: Hypothyroidism and hyperthyroidism. In *Manual of Endocrinology and Metabolism*. Edited by N. Lavin, Boston, Brown and Company, 1986, pp.365-378.

77. Winkler, A.W., Lavietes, P.H., Robbins, C.L., and Man, E.B.: Tolerance to oral thyroid and reaction to intravenous thyroxine in subjects without myxedema. *J. Clin. Invest.*, 22:535-544, 1943.

78. Lowe, J.C.: T₃-induced recovery from fibromyalgia by a hypothyroid patient resistant to T₄ and desiccated thyroid. *J. Myofascial Ther.*, 1(4):26-31, 1995.

79. Wilson, J. and Walton, J.N.: Some muscular manifestations of hypothyroidism. *J. Neurol. Neurosurg. Psychiat.*, 22:320-324, 1959.

80. Cooper, D.S.: Treatment of thyrotoxicosis. In *Werner and Ingbar's The Thyroid: A Fundamental and Clinical Text*, 6th edition. Edited by L.E. Braverman and R.D. Utiger, New York, J.B. Lippincott Co., 1991, pp.887-916.

81. Feely, J. and Peden, N.: Use of β-adrenoceptor blocking drugs in hyperthyroidism. *Drugs*, 27:425, 1984.

82. Braverman, L.E. and Utiger, R.D.: Introduction to hyperthyroidism. In *Werner and Ingbar's The Thyroid: A Fundamental and Clinical Text*, 6th edition. Edited by L.E. Braverman and R.D. Utiger, New York, J.B. Lippincott Co., 1991, pp.645-647.

83. Drayer, D.E.: Lipophilicity, hydrophilicity, and the central nervous system side effects of beta blockers. *Pharmacotherapy*, 7:87-91, 1987.

84. Hoffman, B.B. and Lefkowitz, R.J.: Adrenergic receptor antagonists. In *The Pharmacologic Basis of Therapeutics*, 8th edition. Edited by A.G. Gilman, T.W. Rall, A.S. Nies, and P. Taylor, New York, Pergamon Press, 1985, pp.221-243.

85. Wartofsky, L.: Thyrotoxic storm. In *Werner and Ingbar's The Thyroid: A Fundamental and Clinical Text*, 7th edi-

tion. Edited by L.P. Braverman and R.D. Utiger, Philadelphia, Lippincott-Raven Publishers, 1996, pp.701-712.

86. Ikram, H.: Hemodynamic effect of β-adrenergic blockade in hyperthyroid patients with and without heart failure. *Br. Med. J.*, 1:1505, 1977.

87. Teitelbaum, J.: *From Fatigued to Fantastic: A Manual for Moving Beyond Chronic Fatigue & Fibromyalgia*. Garden City Park, Avery Publishing Group, 1996.

88. Barnes, B.O.: *Hypothyroidism: The Unsuspected Illness*. New York, Harper and Row Publishers, 1976.

89. Barnes, B.: Basal temperature versus basal metabolism. *J.A.M.A.*, 119:1072-1074, 1942.

90. Mackin, J.F., Canary, J.J., and Pittman, C.S.: Thyroid storm and its management. *N. Engl. J. Med.*, 291:1396, 1974.

91. Mazzaferri, E.L., Reynolds, J.C., Young, R.L., Thomas, C.N., and Parisi, A.F.: Propranolol as primary therapy for thyrotoxicosis. *Arch. Intern. Med.*, 136:50, 1976.

92. Bartalena, I., Martino, E., Falcone, M., et al.: Evaluation of the nocturnal serum thyrotropin (TSH) surge, as assessed by TSH ultrasensitive assay, in patients receiving long term L-thyroxine suppression therapy and in patients with various thyroid disorders. *J. Clin. Endocrinol. Metab.*, 65:1265, 1987.

93. Scanlon, M.F. and Toft, A.D.: Regulation of thyrotropin secretion. In *Werner and Ingbar's The Thyroid: A Fundamental and Clinical Text*, 7th edition. Edited by L.P. Braverman and R.D. Utiger, Philadelphia, Lippincott-Raven Publishers, 1996, pp.220-240.

94. Seth, J., Kellett, H.A., Caldwell, G., et al.: A sensitive immunoradiometric assay for serum thyroid stimulation hormone: a replacement for the thyrotropin-releasing hormone test? *Brit. Med. J.*, 289:1334, 1984.

95. Lowe, J.C.: Thyroid status of 38 fibromyalgia patients: implications for the etiology of fibromyalgia. *Clin. Bull. Myofascial Ther.*, 2(1):47-64, 1996.

96. Whitaker, J.: *Dr. Whitaker's Guide to Natural Hormone Replacement*. Potomac, Phillips Publishing, Inc., 1996.

97. Oppenheimer, J.H., Schwartz, H.L., and Surks, M.I.: Propylthiouracil inhibits the conversion of L-thyroxine to L-triiodothyronine: an explanation of the antithyroxine effect of propylthiouracil and evidence supporting the concept that triiodothyronine is the active thyroid hormone. *J. Clin. Invest.*, 51:2493, 1972.

98. Braverman, L.E., Ingbar, S.H., and Sterling, K.: Conversion of thyroxine (T₄) to triiodothyronine (T₃) in athyreotic subjects. *J. Clin. Invest.*, 49:855, 1970.

99. Blumberg, K.R., Mayer, W.J., Parikh, D.K., and Schnell, L.A.: Liothyronine and levothyroxine in Armour thyroid. *J. Pharm. Sci.*, 76:346, 1993.

100. Kaufman, S.C., Gross, T.P., and Kennedy, D.L.: Thyroid hormone use: trends in the United States from 1960 through 1988. *Thyroid*, 1:285, 1991.

101. Mandel, S.J., Brent, G.A., and Larsen, P.R.: Levothyroxine therapy in patients with thyroid disease. *Ann. Intern. Med.*, 119:492, 1993.

102. Rosenbaum, R.L. and Barzel, U.S.: Levothyroxine replacement dose for primary hypothyroidism decreases with age. *Ann. Intern. Med.*, 96:53, 1982.

103. Sawin, C.T., Geller, A., Hershman, J.M., Castelli, W., and Bacharach, P.: The aging thyroid: the use of thyroid hor-

mone in older persons. *J.A.M.A.*, 261:2653-2655, 1989.

104. Lowe, J.C.: Results of an open trial of T₃ therapy with 77 euthyroid female fibromyalgia patients. *Clin. Bull. Myofascial Ther.*, 2(1):35-37, 1997.

105. Medi-Span, Inc.: Database Version 97.2. Data © 1997.

106. Garrison, R.: Personal communication, January 15, 1999.

107. Magnus-Levy, A.: Ueber den respiratorischen Gaswechsel unter den Einfluss der Thyreoidea sowie unter vreschiedenen pathologische. *Zustanden. Berl. Klin. Wochenschr.*, 32:650, 1895.

108. Magnus-Levy, A.: Energy metabolism in health and disease. *J. Hist. Med.*, 2:307, 1947.

109. Cooper, D.S.: Subclinical hypothyroidism. *J.A.M.A.*, 258:246-247, 1987.

110. Bannai, C., Kuzuya, N., Koide, Y., et al.: Assessment of the relationship between serum thyroid hormone levels and peripheral metabolism in patients with anorexia nervosa. *Endocrinol. Jpn.*, 35(3):455-462, 1988.

111. Ooi, T.C., Whitlock, R.M.L., Frengley, P.A., and Ibbertson, H.K.: Systolic time intervals and ankle reflex time in patients with minimal serum TSH elevation: response to triiodothyronine therapy. *Clin. Endocrinol.* (Oxf), 13:621, 1980.

112. Costin, G., Kaplan, S.A., and Ling, S.M.: The Achilles reflex time in thyroid disorders. *J. Pediatr.*, 76:277, 1970.

113. Hamburger, J.I.: Strategies for cost-effective thyroid function testing with modern methods: comments by Dr. Anthony D. Toft. In *Diagnostic Methods in Clinical Thyroidology.* Edited by J.I. Hamburger, New York, Springer-Verlag, 1989, pp.91-98.

114. Bell, David S.: *The Doctor's Guide to Chronic Fatigue Syndrome: Understanding, Treating, and Living with CFIDS.* Redding, Perseus Books, 1995.

115. LeBoff, M.S., Kaplan, M.M., Silva, J.E., and Larsen, P.R.: Bioavailability of thyroid hormones from oral replacement preparations. *Metabolism*, 31(9):900-905, 1982.

116. Hennemann, G.: No further use of desiccated thyroid gland. *Ned. Tijdschr. Geneeskd.*, 127(14):602-603, 1983.

117. Smith, S.R..: Desiccated thyroid preparations. Obsolete therapy. *Arch. Intern. Med.*, 144(5):926-927, 1984.

118. Dong, B.J., Hauck, W.W., Gambertoglio, J.G., Gee, L., White, J.R., Bubp, J.L., and Greenspan, F.S.: Bioequivalence of generic and brand-name levothyroxine products in the treatment of hypothyroidism. *J.A.M.A.*, 277 (15):1205-1213, 1997.

119. Korsic, M., Cvijetic, S., Dekanic-Ozegovic, D., Bolanca, S., and Kozic, B.: Bone mineral density in patients on long-term therapy with levothyroxine. *Lijec Vjesn*, 120(5):103-105, 1998.

120. Kaplan, M.M., Swartz, S.L., and Larsen, P.R.: Partial peripheral resistance to thyroid hormone. *Am. J. Med.*, 70:1115-1121, 1981.

121. Escobar-Morreale, H.F., del Rey, F.E., Obregón, M.J., and de Escobar, G.M.: Only the combined treatment with thyroxine and triiodothyronine ensures euthyroidism in all tissues of the thyroidectomized rat. *Endocrinology*, 137 (6):2490-2502, 1996.

122. Ain, K.B., Pucino, F., Shiver, T.M., and Banks, S.M.: Thyroid hormone levels affected by time of blood sampling in thyroxine-treated patients. *Thyroid*, 3:81, 1993.

123. Melander, A.: Interactions of adrenergic blocking drugs with the *in vivo* release of thyroid hormone induced by thyrotrophin and long-acting thyroid stimulator. *Acta Endocrinol.*, 66:151, 1971.

124. Gilman, A.G. and Rall, T.W.: Factors influencing adenosine 3',5'-phosphate accumulation in bovine thyroid slices. *Endocrinology*, 243:5867, 1968.

125. Sherwin, R.S. and Felig, P.: Hypoglycemia. In *Endocrinology and Metabolism*, 2ⁿᵈ edition. Edited by P. Felig, J.D. Baxter, A. Broadus, and L.A. Frohman, New York, McGraw-Hill Book Co., 1987, pp.1179-1202.

126. Abramson, E.A., Arky, R.A., and Woeber, K.A.: Effects of propranolol on the hormonal and metabolic response to insulin-induced hypoglycemia. *Lancet*, 2:1386, 1966.

127. Weinberg, T.: Disorders of the thyroid gland. In *Osteopathic Medicine.* Edited by J.M. Hoag, W.V. Cole, and S.G. Bradford, New York, McGraw-Hill Book Co., Inc., 1969, p.252.

128. Surks, M.I.: Treatment of hypothyroidism. In *The Thyroid: A Fundamental and Clinical Text*, 6ᵗʰ edition. Edited by L.E. Braverman and R.D. Utiger, New York, J. M. Lippincott Co., 1991, pp.1099-1103.

129. Fish, L.H., Schwartz, H.L., and Cavanaugh, J.: Replacement dose, metabolism, and bioavailability of levothyroxine in the treatment of hypothyroidism. *N. Engl. J. Med.*, 316:764-770, 1987.

130. Hays, J.T.: Absorption of oral thyroxine in man. *J. Clin. Endocrinol. Metab.*, 28:749, 1968.

131. Guyton, A.C.: Personal communication, Oct. 9, 1990.

132. Vanderpump, M.P.J., Tunbridge, W.M.G., French, J.M., et al.: The incidence of thyroid disorders in the community: a twenty-year follow-up of the Whickham survey. *Clin. Endocrinol.*, 43:55-68, 1995.

133. Haynes, R.C., Jr.: Thyroid and antithyroid drugs. In *Goodman and Gilman's The Pharmacological Basis of Therapeutics*, 8ᵗʰ edition. New York, Pergamon Press, 1990, pp.1361-1383.

134. Weetman, A.P.: Fortnightly review: hypothyroidism, screening, and subclinical disease. *Brit. Med. J.*, 314:1175, 1997.

135. Salmon, D., Rendell, M., Williams, J., et al.: Chemical hyperthyroidism. *Arch. Intern. Med.*, 142:571, 1982.

136. Du Bois, E.F.: *Basal Metabolism in Health and Disease*, 3ʳᵈ edition. Philadelphia, Lea & Febiger, 1936.

137. Loeb, J.N.: Metabolic changes in thyrotoxicosis. In *The Thyroid*, 6ᵗʰ edition. Edited by L.E. Braverman and R.D. Utiger, Philadelphia, J.B. Lippincott Co., 1991, pp.845-853.

138. Dillmann, W.H.: Cardiac function in thyroid disease: clinical features and management considerations. *Ann. Thorac. Surg.*, 56(Suppl.1):S9-S14, 1993.

139. Dillmann, W.H.: The cardiovascular system in thyrotoxicosis. In *Werner and Ingbar's The Thyroid: A Fundamental and Clinical Text*, 6ᵗʰ edition. Edited by L.E. Braverman and R.D. Utiger, New York, J.B. Lippincott Co., 1991, pp.759-770.

140. Roti, E., Montermini, M., Roti, S., et al.: The effects of diltiazem, a calcium channel-blocking drug, on cardiac rate and rhythm in hyperthyroid patients. *Arch. Intern. Med.*, 148:1919, 1988.

141. Lowe, J.C., Reichman, A., Yellin, J.: A case-control study

of metabolic therapy for fibromyalgia: long-term follow-up comparison of treated and untreated patients (Abstract). *Clin. Bull. Myofascial Ther.*, 3(1):23-24, 1998.

142. Escobar-Morreale, H.F., Obregón, M.J., Escobar del Rey, F., and Morreale de Escobar, G.: Replacement therapy for hypothyroidism with thyroxine alone does not ensure euthyroidism in all tissues, as studied in thyroidectomized rats. *J. Clin. Invest.*, 96:2828-2838, 1995.

143. Pauling, L.: *How to Live Longer and Feel Better.* New York, Avon Books, 1987.

144. Pauling, L.: Orthomolecular somatic and psychiatric medicine. *J. Vital Subst. Dis. Civiliz.*, 14:1-3, 1968.

145. Rimland, B.: High-dosage levels of certain vitamins in the treatment of children with severe mental disorders. In *Orthomolecular Psychiatry: Treatment of Schizophrenia.* Edited by D. Hawkins and L. Pauling, San Francisco, W.H. Freeman, 1973, pp.513-539.

146. Davis, F.B., Cody, V., Davis, P.J., Borzynski, L.J., and Blas, S.D.: Stimulation by thyroid hormone analogs of red blood cells Ca²⁺-ATPase activity *in vitro. J. Biol. Chem.*, 258:12373, 1983.

147. Oppenheimer, J.H., Schwartz, H.L., and Strait, K.A.: The molecular basis of thyroid hormone actions. In *Werner and Ingbar's The Thyroid: A Fundamental and Clinical Text*, 7th edition. Edited by L.P. Braverman and R.D. Utiger, Philadelphia, Lippincott-Raven Publishers, 1996, pp.162-184.

148. Travell, J.G. and Simons, D.G.: *Myofascial Pain and Dysfunction: The Trigger Point Manual, Vol 1.* Baltimore, Williams and Wilkins, 1983.

149. Mary Shomon's Thyroid Web site: < http://www.thyroid-info.com/ >

150. International Thyroid Group Web site: < http://www.my4tune.u-net.com/itg.htm >

151. Toft, A.D.: Thyroid hormone replacement: one hormone or two? *N. Engl. J. Med.*, 340(6):469-470, 1999.

152. Toft, A.D.: Comments: Cost-effective thyroid function testing. *Diagnostic Methods in Clinical Thyroidology.* New York, Springer-Verlag, 1989, pp.91-98.

153. Pearch, C.J. and Himsworth, R.L.: Total and free thyroid hormone concentration in patients receiving maintenance replacement treatment with thyroxine. *Brit. Med. J.*, 288:693-695, 1984.

154. Lowe, J.C., Garrison, R.L., Reichman, A.J., Yellin, J., Thompson, M., and Kaufman, D.: Effectiveness and safety of T₃ (triiodothyronine) therapy for euthyroid fibromyal-gia: a double-blind placebo-controlled response-driven crossover study. *Clin. Bull. Myofascial Ther.*, 2(2/3):31-57, 1997.

155. Lowe, J.C., Reichman, A.J., and Yellin, J.: The process of change during T₃ treatment for euthyroid fibromyalgia: a double-blind placebo-controlled crossover study. *Clin. Bull. Myofascial Ther.*, 2(2/3):91-124, 1997.

156. Lowe, J.C., Garrison, R.L., Reichman, A.J., and Yellin, J.: Triiodothyronine (T₃) treatment of euthyroid fibromyalgia: a small-N replication of a double-blind placebo-controlled crossover study. *Clin. Bull. Myofascial Ther.*, 2(4):71-88, 1997.

157. Lowe, J.C., Reichman, A., Honeyman, G.S., Yellin, J.: Thyroid status of fibromyalgia patients (Abstract). *Clin. Bull. Myofascial Ther.*, 3(1):69-70, 1998.

158. Honeyman, G.S.: Metabolic therapy for hypothyroid and euthyroid fibromyalgia: two case reports. *Clin. Bull. Myofascial Ther.*, 2(4):19-49, 1997.

159. Lowe, J.C., Eichelberger, J., Manso, G., and Peterson, K.: Improvement in euthyroid fibromyalgia patients treated with T₃ (tri-iodothyronine). *J. Myofascial Ther.*,1(2):16-29, 1994.

160. Volpé, R.: Misinformation on diagnosis and treatment. *Thyroid Foundation of Canada Thyrobulletin*, 19(2):10, 1998.

161. Chait, A., Kanter, R., Green, W., and Kenny, M.: Defective thyroid hormone action in fibroblasts cultured from subjects with a syndrome of resistance to thyroid hormone. *J. Clin. Endocrinol. Metab.*, 54:767-772, 1982.

162. Mangieri, C.N. and Lund, M.H.: Potency of United States Pharmacopeia desiccated thyroid tablets as determined by the antigoitrogenic assay in rats. *J. Clin. Endocrinol. Metab.*, 30:102, 1970.

163. Wiberg, G.S., Devlin, W.F. and Stephenson, N.R.: A comparison of the thyroxine:tri-iodothyronine content and biological activity of thyroid from various species. *J. Pharm. Pharmacol.*, 14:777, 1962.

164. Sawin, C.T., Surks, M.I., and London, M.: Oral thyroxine: variation in biologic action and tablet content. *Ann. Intern. Med.*, 100:641, 1984.

165. Nittler, A.H.: *Health Questions & Answers.* New York, Pyramid Publications, 1976.

166. Bunevicius, B., Kazanavicius, G., Zalinkevicius, R., and Prange, A.J. Jr.: Effects of thyroxine as compared with thyroxine plus triiodothyronine in patients with hypothyroidism. *N. Engl. J. Med.*, 340(6):424-429, 1999.

5.4

T_3 (triiodothyronine): Considerations for the Treatment of Fibromyalgia

A small percentage of hypothyroid fibromyalgia patients, and most euthyroid fibromyalgia patients, do not benefit from the use of synthetic T_4 or desiccated thyroid. Most do benefit, however, from the use of synthetic T_3. This is especially true when patients take the full daily dosage at one time. To improve or recover, most of these patients require supraphysiologic dosages of T_3. Compared to T_4, T_3 has a speedy therapeutic effect that quickly dissipates when the hormone is withdrawn. T_3 is rapidly absorbed and reaches its peak circulating concentration 2-to-4 hours after ingestion. Serum concentrations are elevated for 6-to-8 hours after a dose as low as 25 µg. Serum concentrations vary widely based on the time when T_3 is ingested. The circulating half-life of T_3 is 1 day; that of T_4 is 7 days.

The current endocrinology/thyroidology paradigm stipulates that: (1) only the hypothyroid patient should be permitted to use exogenous thyroid hormone, (2) the hypothyroid patient should be allowed to use only T_4, and (3) the patient should only use dosages of T_4 that keep the serum basal TSH level well within the normal range. In line with this model, most conventional clinicians oppose the use of exogenous thyroid hormone by the euthyroid patient. Moreover, these clinicians oppose the use of T_3 by anyone, even hypothyroid patients. Since the mid-1960s, many conventional clinicians, including many endocrinologists, have held the misbelief that there is a high risk of harm to patients who use exogenous T_3. This belief is patently false, as long as reasonable precautions are exercised. No adverse effects have been documented in patients properly using T_3. T_3 and T_4 are extraordinarily safe among prescription medications because they are orthomolecular substances. Orthomolecular substances are natural to the body and essential to health. Adverse reactions to such substances would be incompatible with life.

Most euthyroid fibromyalgia patients, presumably those with cellular resistance to thyroid hormone, benefit from the use of exogenous T_3—but only when dosage adjustments are based on repeated assessments of tissue metabolic status. Laboratory thyroid function tests assess nothing more than the functional status of the thyroid gland and the TSH-secreting thyrotroph cells of the anterior pituitary. These tests are of no value in adjusting the T_3 dosage of the euthyroid fibromyalgia patient.

In my clinical and research experience, the safe and effective dosage range for most euthyroid fibromyalgia patients has been 75 µg-to-162.5 µg. In general, dosages within this range have improved or alleviated patients' fibromyalgia symptoms and signs without thyrotoxicosis. Most hypothyroid fibromyalgia *patients who do not benefit from T₄ or desiccated thyroid improve or recover with the use of T₃—but only when used as part of a more complete metabolic rehabilitation regimen. Most of these hypothyroid patients, like euthyroid fibromyalgia patients, require higher-end dosages of T₃. This suggests that the hypothyroid patients have some degree of cellular resistance to thyroid hormone.*

Many hypothyroid fibromyalgia patients improve or recover with the use of desiccated thyroid or synthetic T_4. A minority of these patients do not benefit from these forms of thyroid hormone. They improve or recover only with the use of synthetic T_3. In my clinical experience, the circumstance is reversed for euthyroid fibromyalgia patients. A small minority of them benefit from the use of desiccated thyroid hormone or T_4. The majority, however, improve or recover only with the use of synthetic T_3 as the exogenous thyroid hormone in their metabolic regimen. A relatively high daily dosage of T_3 is usually required. For most euthyroid patients, the effective dosage is considerably higher than the "total replacement dosage" that conventional endocrinologists/thyroidologists mistakenly consider adequate for the hypothyroid patient.

The extraordinary effectiveness of T_3 in relieving symptoms and signs typical of fibromyalgia has been acknowledged by numerous researchers since the middle of the 20th century (see Chapter 2.5). In my experience, the relief from fibromyalgia symptoms and signs typically lasts as long as the patient continues use of the hormone— but only if she also continues a more complete metabolic regimen that includes nutritional supplements and exercise (see Chapter 5.5). This point of view now has the support of considerable clinical and experimental evidence. Nevertheless, this approach is rejected and opposed today by most conventional clinicians. The source of the opposition, as Sonkin argued[10,p.49] and as I described in Chapter 2.5, is the current endocrinology/thyroidology paradigm.

According to this paradigm, symptomatic patients are permitted treatment with thyroid hormone only if thyroid function laboratory test results indicate hypothyroidism. Sonkin wrote that according to this model, (1) the single cause of symptoms of thyroid hormone insufficiency is hypothyroidism, (2) patients with normal thyroid function test results should not be permitted to undergo therapeutic trials with thyroid hormone, and (3) patients should not be treated with thyroid hormone dosages that lower the TSH below the lower limit of the normal reference range.[10,p.53]

Most euthyroid fibromyalgia patients, however, benefit only from TSH-suppressive dosages of T_3. During the patient's metabolic treatment with T_3, the clinician must disregard the serum basal TSH level and adjust the dosage according to the patient's symptoms, signs, and peripheral indices (see Chapter 4.3). In the assessment and treatment of fibromyalgia, the relevant question for clinician and patient is the same as in the treatment of all forms of cellular hormone resistance: "Does the target organ respond properly to the hormone in question?"[23,p.746]

The patient with thyroid hormone-related euthyroid fibromyalgia exhibits signs, symptoms, and peripheral indices typical of hypothyroidism despite having normal thyroid hormone and TSH levels. This suggests that the patient has partial cellular resistance to thyroid hormone. Whether this patient is responding therapeutically to exogenous thyroid hormone can be determined only by repeated reassessments of the status of her symptoms, signs, and peripheral indices. The specific indices I described in Chapter 4.3 are indicators of peripheral tissue responses to thyroid hormone.

TSH AND THYROID HORMONE LEVELS ARE IRRELEVANT TO ASSESSING THE RESPONSE OF PERIPHERAL TISSUES TO THYROID HORMONE

If the clinician is to effectively treat euthyroid fibromyalgia patients, it is critical that he understand one major point: Thyroid hormone and TSH levels are *not* an assessment of the response of most body tissues to thyroid hormone. The TSH level is a measure solely of the pituitary's response to circulating thyroid hormone, and thyroid hormone levels are a measure only of the thyroid gland's response to TSH. Neither TSH nor thyroid hormone levels provide any information whatsoever about the metabolic status of other tissues. That the metabolic status of peripheral tissues can be accurately inferred from TSH and thyroid hormone levels is an assumption that cannot be logically or scientifically defended.

● T₃ (TRIIODOTHYRONINE)

T_3 (triiodothyronine) is a crystalline thyroid hormone compound that contains 3 iodine atoms.[26] It is available under the trade names Trionine and Cytomel.

Compared to T_4, this preparation has a speedy therapeutic effect and a quick dissipation of action when withdrawn. T_3 is rapidly absorbed and reaches its peak circulating concentration 2-to-4 hours after ingestion. Serum concentrations are elevated for 6-to-8 hours after a dose as low as 25 μg. Serum concentrations vary widely based on the time when T_3 is ingested. The circulating half-life of T_3 is 1 day, compared to 7 days for T_4.[12,p.883]

These features of T_3 make it particularly useful when a rapid therapeutic effect is needed with the hypothyroid[2,p.147] or euthyroid patient. T_3 is especially useful compared to T_4 for two reasons. First, T_3 releases from plasma proteins more easily than does T_4. This provides cells with a more rapid influx of thyroid hormone. Second, T_3 in high enough dosages effectively overrides cellular resistance to thyroid hormone and rapidly exerts cellular effects. Either or both of these features may account for some patients benefitting from T_3 after failing to respond to T_4. (Exogenous T_3 also bypasses any possible faults in T_4 to T_3 conversion. Laboratory testing in my clinic, however, indicates that conversion problems are not common in euthyroid fibromyalgia patients.)

● **THERAPEUTIC TRIALS OF T_3 ARE INNOCUOUS WHEN REASONABLE PRECAUTIONS ARE TAKEN**

Many clinicians believe there is a high risk of harm to the patient who uses exogenous T_3. This is not true, however. The leaflet given to patients by pharmacists who dispense Cytomel (T_3) makes the safety of T_3 abundantly clear. *Verbatim et literatim*, it says: "NO COMMON SIDE EFFECTS HAVE BEEN REPORTED with the proper use of this medicine."[1]

The fact is, there is virtually no risk of harm in the use of T_3 and there is the potential for great benefit, provided reasonable precautions are taken. Thus, I concur with Sonkin's view: "It seems reasonable in the face of current evidence and uncertainty to give the patient the benefit of the doubt and offer a therapeutic trial with thyroid, which is innocuous and frequently effective."[10,p.49] He made this statement in regard to T_4, but it applies equally well to T_3.

The proper use of T_3 mainly involves two precautions. First, the clinician should insure before the patient begins use of the hormone that she does not have a cardiac, adrenal, osseous, or other condition that

contraindicates the use of T_3. Second, the clinician should monitor and quantitatively document changes in the metabolic status of tissues during treatment (see Chapter 4.3).

● **T_3 DOSAGE**

For two purposes, I include several case reports and studies below. The first purpose is to show that other authors have reported in the medical literature that some patients fail to respond therapeutically to desiccated thyroid and T_4 but subsequently respond to T_3. My second purpose is to review the range of dosages that authors have reported to be effective for these patients. The mechanism(s) that prevented these patients from responding to desiccated thyroid or T_4 is not known.

DOSAGES OF T_3 REPORTED TO BE EFFECTIVE

Wiener and Lindeboom treated a woman with longstanding hypothyroid complaints. She was not cretinous and did not have a goiter. Her basal metabolism was low, and her serum cholesterol and body weight were high. Her thyroid gland functioned normally, yet clinically she displayed features of hypothyroidism. Her hypothyroid-like symptoms dated from 1944. It was not until 1957, though, that clinicians proposed that she suffered from partial peripheral cellular resistance to her endogenous thyroid hormones. She did not improve with 500 mg daily of desiccated thyroid nor with daily injections of T_4. She reached a eumetabolic state with a daily T_3 dosage of 200 μg.[24]

After a 4-year-old cretinous girl failed to improve with desiccated thyroid, Hutchison and Arneil treated her effectively with 100 μg of T_3. She improved dramatically within an 82-day period. After 3 months, her dosage was reduced to 80 μg. Two years later, her dosage was reduced to 40 μg because she had begun to experience tachycardia, tremulousness, and sweating. After maintaining this dosage for a year, she was completely normal physically and mentally.[27]

Frawley described a patient with postoperative hypothyroidism who did not respond to doses of desiccated thyroid as high as 12 grains (0.8 Gm) per day. This patient improved dramatically, however, with 50 μg of T_3. The patient maintained improvement when switched to a daily T_4 dosage of 0.2 mg.[3] The researchers did not determine why the patient was able to respond to T_4 only after responding to T_3.

Morton administered T_3 to 51 euthyroid hypometabolic patients. Forty-six (90%) of the patients had good to excellent responses to T_3. Only 3 (6%) of the 51 patients had previously responded well to desiccated thyroid, thyroglobulin, or thyroxine. Morton started each patient with 5-to-25 µg daily and gradually increased the dosage at weekly intervals. Maximum doses ranged from 10 µg-to-100 µg. When an occasional patient experienced jitteriness, tachycardia, or nervousness, the reactions disappeared completely within 5 days after reducing the T_3 dosage.[29,p.126]

Fields administered T_3 to euthyroid hypometabolic children who ranged in age from 1-to-17 years. He used 5 µg daily during the 1st week. If the patient's tolerance permitted, he increased the dosage to 10 µg daily for the 2nd week and then to 15 µg daily for the 3rd week. The 4th week, he withheld treatment. For the 1st week of the 2nd month, each patient took 25 µg. If the patient tolerated this well, Fields increased the dosage to 50 µg. Patients continued this dosage through the 3rd week. He raised the dosage of 10 patients to 100 µg in an attempt to produce an optimum response. A small percentage of patients reacted with irritability, headache, insomnia, and palpitations; the reactions subsided when Fields lowered their dosages.[30,p.818]

Goldberg disagreed with Morton's and Fields' approaches of starting with a low dosage and gradually increasing it. He observed that when using this protocol, some patients' hypometabolism worsened in the early days of treatment. He proposed a three point mechanism for the worsened hypometabolism: (1) the small amount of exogenous T_3 depressed TSH secretion, (3) the reduced TSH decreased thyroid hormone secretion by the thyroid gland, and (3) the small amounts of T_3 failed to maintain the pre-treatment metabolic rate that had been maintained by the greater amount of thyroid hormone secreted by the thyroid gland. He recommended that younger patients initially take 25 µg three times per day, increasing the dosage within 1-to-2 weeks to 50 µg two times a day. He argued that higher initial dosages of T_3 maintained or increased the metabolic rate despite suppression of TSH secretion.[5]

The average effective daily dosage for Goldberg's adult patients was 100 µg-to-125 µg. The range was 75 µg-to-150 µg. He examined patients at 2-week intervals and adjusted their dosages. (He determined optimum dosage by a reflex timing device. His objective was an Achilles reflex contraction speed of approximately 200 msec.[5,p.1056])

Goldberg[5,p.1056] reported a difference between the responses of hypothyroid patients and euthyroid hypometabolic patients to T_3 therapy. Hypothyroid patients improved rapidly in the first 3-to-4 days. Euthyroid hypometabolic patients, however, required 2-to-4 weeks. For most euthyroid hypometabolic patients, a high dosage of T_3 was necessary for symptomatic relief (or for an increase in the speed of the Achilles reflex).

Kurland, Hamolsky, and Freedberg published reports of patients who did not improve with T_4 but did with T_3.[31][32] They wrote that the euthyroid hypometabolic patient requires a higher dosage of thyroid hormone than the hypothyroid patient to restore normal metabolism.[31,p.1355] They reported a striking clinical and metabolic response to T_3 (and to a combination of T_3 and T_4 in 2 patients) after patients had failed to respond to desiccated thyroid or T_4. The optimal dosage of T_3 when used alone was 105 µg; 70 µg of T_3 alone was not effective in elevating the patients' metabolic rates. The optimal dosage of combined therapy was 25 µg-to-35 µg of T_3 and 0.2-to-0.3 mg of T_4 (200 µg-to-300 µg).[32,p.59]

Kurland, Hamolsky, and Freedberg also reported that a previously ineffective dosage of T_4 may raise the metabolic rate when administered immediately after a large dose of T_3. For example, 0.4 mg (400 µg) of T_4 daily did not raise the BMR of one patient nor improve his clinical condition. After 15 days of taking 105 µg of T_3, however, 0.3 mg (300 µg) of T_4 raised his BMR from -20% to -1%. In such cases, T_4 may not remain effective. For one patient, after taking 210 µg of T_3 for 4 weeks, 4 grains of desiccated thyroid raised the BMR from -30% to -5%. This BMR remained higher for 6 months, then gradually declined to -22%. The decrease occurred even though the patient took the same dosage of desiccated thyroid that had been effective for 6 months.[31,pp.1364-1365]

Jefferies remarked that the patients of Kurland et al. who were resistant to T_4 were also relatively resistant to T_3. One required 105 µg and another 210 µg of T_3 to increase the metabolic rate. These dosages are equivalent to 3 and 6 grains of desiccated thyroid, respectively.[21,p.586]

I reported the case of a woman with fibromyalgia who had been previously diagnosed as hypothyroid. When she first consulted me, she was taking 2 grains of desiccated thyroid without benefit except a slight reduction in cold sensitivity. She had failed to improve significantly with as much as 4 grains. She completely and dramatically recovered from hypothyroid fibromyalgia with 82.5 µg of T_3.[13]

Clinicians have used T_3 extensively to overcome

thyroid hormone resistance of the pituitary and/or peripheral tissues, and to relieve the clinical manifestations of the resistance.[6][9][28][37][38] The highest dosage of T_4 reported to be necessary to produce beneficial effects in a patient resistant to thyroid hormone has been 1.0 mg (1000 µg).[18,p.390] Kaplan et al. reported the case of a woman with peripheral resistance to thyroid hormone who did not improve with desiccated thyroid. Her symptoms were relieved and objective measures of metabolism normalized only when she took 500 µg of T_3.[19]

The dosage range that has alleviated fibromyalgia symptoms and signs without thyrotoxicosis in patients treated by my research group is 75-to-162.5 µg.[14][15][16][17] Among private patients I have cotreated, the highest effective dosage has been 300 µg. Both patients who initially responded to this dosage eventually reduced their dosage after developing mild symptoms of overstimulation. Their optimal effective dosages were 250 µg each.

Most patients with thyroid hormone resistance have been reported to improve with supraphysiologic dosages of T_3. I have found that a small percentage of hypothyroid, and most euthyroid, fibromyalgia patients respond only to T_3. In one report, however, investigators describe a patient whose tissue resistance to thyroid hormone was more effectively overcome with T_4 than with T_3.[11]

In my euthyroid fibromyalgia patients who improved or recovered only with T_3, I did *not* find laboratory evidence of impaired T_4 to T_3 conversion. In 50 patients who responded to T_3 after failing to benefit from large dosages of T_4, I did not find the combination of elevated serum reverse-T_3, low T_3, and elevated 24-hour urinary cortisol that would indicate cortisol-induced impairment of deiodination. A small percentage of the patients had slightly elevated 24-hour urinary cortisol, but none of these had elevated serum reverse-T_3 or low T_3. These values indicate that impaired conversion of T_4 to T_3 was not the mechanism responsible for these fibromyalgia patients' failure to benefit from T_4.

PUTATIVE DISADVANTAGES OF T₃: GRADUAL IMPACT OF T₄ VS ABRUPT IMPACT OF T₃

Sawin wrote that the main goal of the use of exogenous thyroid hormone is to insure a constant supply of the hormone to tissues. According to this view, the supply should mimic the normal person's presumed constant levels of T_3 and T_4.[34,p.394] He then pointed out that T_4 achieves this goal better than T_3.[34,p.394] After T_4 is absorbed, the serum level of T_4 rises only slightly, and when deiodinase functions normally, cells constantly convert the T_4 to T_3.[35]

It may be, however, that it is in part this slower constant supply of hormone to the cells that prevents a therapeutic effect in some patients who use exogenous T_4. If a patient has cellular resistance to thyroid hormone due to mutant T_3-receptors that have low affinity for T_3, exposing those receptors to large amounts of T_3 may be necessary to stimulate normal transcription regulation. This may also be the reason time- or sustained-release T_3 is not effective with some patients.

In contrast to T_4, a preparation containing T_3 (including desiccated thyroid and thyroid extracts such as Proloid) causes a distinct rise in serum T_3 shortly after the patient ingests it. No such rise occurs with endogenously-produced T_3.[35] Sawin points out that the rise would be of little consequence except that it may cause symptoms such as angina pectoris in some patients.[36] He concluded, "The symptoms are unnecessary because T_3 has no advantage over T_4."[34,p.394] This may be true when treating a hypothyroid patient whose cells are able to effectively convert T_4 to T_3, and when that patient does not have cellular resistance. It certainly is not true, however, for patients with cellular resistance to thyroid hormone, including patients who concurrently are hypothyroid. These patients improve or recover only with the use of T_3 and usually only with supraphysiologic dosages.

I should emphasize that my monitoring and follow-up of euthyroid fibromyalgia patients has shown that large single doses of T_3 have *not* caused adverse cardiac reactions. I refer here for the most part to patients who before beginning treatment did not have cardiac conditions susceptible to exacerbation by the inotropic and chronotropic cardiac effects of T_3. Increasing the heart rate or contractile force with T_3 has unearthed in a few patients some underlying cardiac abnormalities that were not detected before the patients began treatment. These patients have been in a minority, however. The clinician should carefully monitor all patients to assure their safety.

Supranormal T₃ Concentrations in Cells from Exogenous T₃ Use

In 1983, Larsen and Silva speculated about one potential disadvantage of T_3 therapy—supranormal concentrations of T_3 in cells.[33,pp.382-383] They wrote that T_3 in the brain may be derived mainly from conversion of T_4 to T_3. This implies that not providing T_4 in thyroid hormone preparations may result in a deficiency in some brain cells. Yet in a seeming contradiction, they cautioned that preparations that contain T_3 may cause abnormally high concentrations of T_3 in cells. They pointed out that we cannot infer from the amount of T_3 in serum what is inside the cell and we cannot monitor intracellular T_3. Because of this, they reasoned, normal serum T_3 and T_4 levels are our best evidence of normal intracellular T_3 concentration. The ideal replacement therapy, they wrote, must duplicate the normal physiological state (referring to the ratio of circulating T_4 to T_3) if abnormalities in intracellular T_3 are to be avoided. They also wrote that a strong case can be made for using T_4 exclusively for thyroid hormone replacement.[33,pp.382-383]

Larsen and Silva did not specify what if any adverse effects might be anticipated from abnormal concentrations of T_3 in brain cells. But indeed, thyrotoxicity may be accompanied by a range of brain-related disorders. Neuropsychiatric syndromes can include nervousness, irritability, tremulousness, and mild deficits in memory, concentration, and problem-solving ability. Worse neuropsychiatric conditions include major depression, anxiety disorder, mania or hypomania, and schizophreniform disorder.[39]

However, brain cells appear to be protected from excess T_3 exposure, up to a point, by a buffering system that involves the down regulation of brain cell type II 5'-deiodinase. Ordinarily, 50% or more of brain cell T_3 is generated from T_4 by the action of 5'-deiodinase. But the activity of the enzyme undergoes a rapid 3-to-5-fold change with alterations of thyroid status.[25] Thus, during hyperthyroidism, more T_3 in the rat cerebral cortex and cerebellum cells is derived from the circulation than from the conversion of T_4.[40] The rat cerebral cortex, for example, has shown a remarkably efficient homeostasis of its T_3 concentrations, providing metabolic protection of this tissue against wide changes in thyroid hormone availability.[4][20,p.2835] Nevertheless, the neuropsychiatric disorders associated with thyrotoxicosis that are mentioned in the previous paragraph show that the capacity of the buffering can be exceeded, with adverse central nervous system effects, at least in patients free from cellular resistance to thyroid hormone.

Implicit in Larsen and Silva's precaution is the conjecture that supranormal intracellular concentrations of T_3 in brain cells will be harmful to the patient. They did not allow, however, for patients with cellular resistance to thyroid hormone. Paradoxically, supraphysiologic intracellular concentrations of T_3 are ne-

cessary for many patients to improve or recover from the symptoms and signs of inadequate thyroid hormone regulation of cell function (see Chapter 2.6). A patient's hypothyroid-like symptoms and signs, for example, may be the result of mutant T_3-receptors that do not normally bind normal concentrations of T_3. If so, it is likely that exposure of the mutant receptors to high concentrations of T_3 may be the only way to induce them to properly regulate transcription. Such mutations may be the cause of some hypothyroid patients failing to benefit from forms of thyroid hormone that result in exposure of cell nuclei to only normal concentrations of T_3. T_4 and desiccated thyroid, especially in replacement (non-TSH-suppressive) dosages, may permit only a normal concentration of T_3 to reach the nuclei as the T_3 is released by deiodination. Timed-release T_3 may also allow only a normal concentration of T_3 in cell nuclei because of gradual release of the hormone from the ingested product. None of these products may provide the surge in T_3 concentration necessary to saturate T_3-receptors and override their T_3 resistance.

In 1983 when Larsen and Silva wrote their precaution, evidence was not available that supported or denied their conjecture. A policy of erring on the side of patient safety rendered the conjecture tentatively acceptable. In the interim, however, to my knowledge no evidence has come to light that justifies the precaution for all patients. Of far greater importance is the substantial evidence that some patients require supraphysiologic dosages of T_3 for normal function but have no tissue thyrotoxicity from the dosages. This finding falsifies the precaution of Larsen and Silva if it is considered a general proposition, and necessitates that the precaution be properly qualified to exclude patients with thyroid hormone resistance.

It is prudent for the clinician and patient to consider the possibility of adverse effects from the use of any exogenous medicinal agent. When there is a likely possibility of harm, the clinician and patient should collaboratively evaluate the risk/benefit ratio. With the extraordinarily good safety record of T_3, the risk/benefit ratio is extremely low. In contrast, the risk/benefit ratio of some patients not using T_3 is extremely high. Such patients, for example, include some at risk of suicide from depression and some at risk of strokes or heart attacks due to severe atherosclerosis related to inadequate thyroid hormone regulation of cell function (see Chapter 4.4, section titled "Harm from Untreated or Undertreated Hypothyroidism"). Even the question of simply a lower quality of life must be calculated into any benefit-to-risk ratio in *not* using T_3.

Distinctive Laboratory Thyroid Test Values

DeGroot wrote that in the "proper" dosage range, T_3 provides both normal metabolism and a normal TSH level. If the dosage is higher, however, T_3 suppresses activity of the thyroid gland (the gland reduces its secretion of thyroid hormones) and suppresses the TSH level. DeGroot also pointed out that with the use of T_3, the resin T_3-uptake is usually in the lower end of the normal range and the serum T_3 is typically highly elevated. He wrote that even "physiological replacement doses" produce these T_3 and T_3-uptake values.[22,p.11]

DeGroot's problem with the use of T_3 appears to be the distinctive laboratory test values that result and the confusion it may cause clinicians. He wrote that to understand these relationships, it is imperative for the physician to comprehend the difference between the T_3-uptake and the serum T_3. He then concluded, "Fortunately, T_3 is used infrequently for therapy of hypothyroidism since it certainly is prone to cause confusion in diagnosis and treatment."[22,p.11]

Confusion over the distinctive laboratory test pattern is not a major drawback to the use of T_3. Granted, it is not easy to master the interpretation of laboratory thyroid function test values. But once the clinician does so, he is likely to find it an easy chore to also learn the peculiar pattern of values of most patients taking physiologic or supraphysiologic dosages of T_3. Table 5.4.1 shows the typical patterns of values for patients taking physiologic or supraphysiologic dosages of T_3. In contrast to these values, the patient whose liver clears T_3 at an unusually rapid rate is likely to have normal thyroid function test result values.

As I have argued elsewhere in this book, in terms of guiding the euthyroid fibromyalgia patient to an optimal clinical state, thyroid function test results are only of academic value. The results are of no value in making decisions about dosage adjustments, and the values do not assess whether or not the exogenous hormone is beneficially or adversely affecting peripheral tissues.

● OVERDOSAGE

Patients with cellular resistance to thyroid hormone usually tolerate high dosages of T_3 well. Sonkin notes Refetoff's observation that effective treatment of patients with peripheral resistance to thyroid hormone requires supraphysiologic dosages of thyroid hormone,

and that clinical evaluations show that these dosages do not induce an iatrogenic subclinical thyrotoxic "high."[10,p.52] Nevertheless, the clinician should carefully monitor each individual patient's responses to thyroid hormone to determine if tissue overstimulation is occurring.

Table 5.4.1. Typical patterns of values of thyroid function test results in a patient taking a physiologic dosage of T_3 and a patient taking a supraphysiologic dosage.

	Physiologic dosage*	Supraphysiologic dosage†
TSH	Normal	Low
Total and free T_4	Normal	Low
Free T_4 Index	Normal	Low
Total and free T_3	High	High‡
T_3-uptake	Low normal	Normal

*DeGroot, L.J.: Abnormal thyroid function tests in euthyroid patients. In *Diagnostic Methods in Clinical Thyroidology.* Edited by J.I. Hamburger, New York, Springer-Verlag, 1989, p.11.
†The mean pattern for 7 euthyroid fibromyalgia patients using supraphysiologic dosages of T_3: Lowe, J.C., Garrison, R.L., Reichman, A.J., Yellin, J., Thompson, M., and Kaufman, D.: Effectiveness and Safety of T_3 (Triiodothyronine) Therapy for Euthyroid Fibromyalgia: A Double-Blind Placebo-Controlled Response-Driven Crossover Study. *Clinical Bulletin of Myofascial Therapy,* 2(2/3):31-58, 1997.
‡In the study by my research group,† we did not measure total T_3.

THE POSSIBILITY OF ADVERSE EFFECTS FROM EXOGENOUS T₃ IS BEST ASSESSED BY MONITORING FOR SIGNS OF TISSUE HYPERMETABOLISM

Terms such as "thyroid hormone overdosage," "excessive thyroid hormone intake," and "thyrotoxicosis" are meaningful and relevant only when used in reference to tests that indicate thyroid hormone-induced hypermetabolism of tissues (see Chapter 4.3). These tests do not include laboratory thyroid function tests such as those detecting the levels of TSH and thyroid hormones. Using symptoms, signs, and peripheral indices of tissue metabolic status is the only reasonable approach to identifying excess thyroid hormone stimulation because it is adverse tissue effects—not circulating hormone levels—that are of concern. There are distinctive patterns of thyroid function test values typically found in patients taking amounts of thyroid hormone that induce tissue toxicity (see Chapter 4.2). But *defining* overdosage or excess *as* these patterns of laboratory test values is fraught with problems. Of most concern is the problem of restricting a patient to a dosage that for some theoretical "average" patients maintains laboratory test values within the normal range, is sufficient to maintain normal metabolism, and is non-toxic. For the particular patient in question, however, this "average" dosage may not be enough to maintain normal metabolism. Using normal laboratory test results as the objective in titrating dosage would leave virtually all patients with cellular resistance to thyroid hormone hypometabolic.

Adjusting dosage according to the patient's symptoms, signs, and peripheral indices (see Chapter 4.3) may result in the patient briefly experiencing indications of mild tissue thyrotoxicity. The presence of these indications should prompt the clinician to titrate the patient's dosage of thyroid hormone down to an appropriate level.

The clinician should bear in mind that after tissues have been hypometabolic for a time, they tend to initially respond with excess vigor to exogenous thyroid hormone. During this time, the tissue may show signs of thyrotoxicosis, but these signs typically subside and disappear. The clinician should monitor the hyper-responsive tissues to make sure the signs subside.

If deemed necessary, the patient can stop tissue hypermetabolism within 20-to-30 minutes with oral propranolol.[8,p.766] She can also slow her metabolic rate, although more gradually, by decreasing her dosage of thyroid hormone.[34,p.394-395] After decreasing the dosage, hypermetabolism from T_3 decreases within 1-to-2 days and from T_4 within 10-to-14 days. In some cases, however, the offset of hypermetabolism is even more rapid with reductions in the T_3 dosage. The reports of variable lengths of time for symptoms of overstimulation to subside are consistent with my clinical experiences. Tittle wrote that when his patients had adverse reactions to T_3, the reactions disappeared within several days after the patients discontinued or reduced their dosages of T_3.[7,p.273] In contrast, Wiener and Lindeboom reported that they gave a patient a dose of 300 µg of T_3 per day for 2 weeks. "The patient grew restless and nervous, her eyes gleamed, and she complained of headache, cold perspiration, and palpitation. Her pulse rate was 120." Her symptoms of overdosage disappeared in the course of the same day when they reduced her dosage to 150 µg (50 µg tid).[24]

REFERENCES

1. Medi-Span, Inc.: Database Version 97.2. Data © 1997.
2. Travell, J.G. and Simons, D.G.: *Myofascial Pain and Dysfunction: The Trigger Point Manual*. Baltimore, Williams and Wilkins, 1983.
3. Frawley, T.G., McClintock, J.C., and Beebe, R.T.: Metabolic and therapeutic effects of triiodothyronine. *J.A.M.A.*, 160:646, 1956.
4. Dartman, M.B., Crutchfield, F.L., Gordan, J.T., and Jennings, A.S.: Iodothyronine homeostasis in rat brain during hypothyroidism and hyperthyroidism. *Am. J. Physiol.*, 245:E185-E193, 1983.
5. Goldberg, M.: Diagnosis of euthyroid hypometabolism. *Am. J. Obst. & Gynec.*, 81(5):1056-1058, 1961.
6. Linde, R., Alexander, N., Island, D.P., and Rabin, D.: Familial insensitivity of the pituitary and periphery to thyroid hormone: a case report in two generations and a review of the literature. *Metabolism*, 31(5):510-513, 1982.
7. Tittle, C.R.: Effects of 3,5,3' l-triiodothyronine in patients with metabolic insufficiency. *J.A.M.A.*, 162:271-273, 1956.
8. Dillmann, W.H.: The cardiovascular system in thyrotoxicosis. In *Werner and Ingbar's The Thyroid: A Fundamental and Clinical Text*, 6th edition. Edited by L.E. Braverman and R.D. Utiger, New York, J.B. Lippincott Co., 1991, pp.759-770.
9. Cooper, D.S., Ladenson, P.W., Nisula, B.C., Dunn, J.F., Chapman, E.M., and Ridgway, E.C.: Familial thyroid hormone resistance. *Metabolism*, 31(5):504-509, 1982.
10. Sonkin, L.S.: Myofascial pain due to metabolic disorders: diagnosis and treatment. In *Myofascial Pain and Fibromyalgia: Trigger Point Management*. Edited by E.S. Rachlin, St. Louis, Mosby, 1994, pp.45-60.
11. Seif, F.J., Scherbaum, W., and Klingler, W.: Syndrome of elevated thyroid hormone and TSH blood levels: a case report (Abstract). *Ann. d'Endocrinol.*, 87(215 suppl):81-82, 1978.
12. Brent, G.A. and Larsen, P.R.: Treatment of hypothyroidism. In *Werner and Ingbar's The Thyroid: A Fundamental and Clinical Text*, 7th edition. Edited by L.P. Braverman and R.D. Utiger, Philadelphia, Lippincott-Raven Publishers, 1996, pp.883-887.
13. Lowe, J.C.: T_3-induced recovery from fibromyalgia by a hypothyroid patient resistant to T_4 and desiccated thyroid. *J. Myofascial Ther.*, 1(4):26-31, 1995.
14. Lowe, J.C., Eichelberger, J., Manso, G., and Peterson, K.: Improvement in euthyroid fibromyalgia patients treated with T_3 (tri-iodothyronine). *J. Myofascial Ther.*, 1(2):16-29, 1994.
15. Lowe, J.C., Garrison, R., Reichman, A.J., Yellin, J., Thompson, M., and Kaufman, D.: Effectiveness and safety of T_3 therapy for euthyroid fibromyalgia: a double-blind placebo-controlled crossover study. *Clin. Bull. Myofascial Ther.*, 2(2/3):31-57, 1997.
16. Lowe, J.C., Reichman, A.J., and Yellin, J.: The process of change during T_3 treatment for euthyroid fibromyalgia: a double-blind placebo-controlled crossover study. *Clin. Bul. Myofascial Ther.*, 2(2/3):91-124, 1997.
17. Lowe, J.C., Reichman, A.J., Garrison, R.L., and Yellin, J.: Triiodothyronine (T_3) treatment for euthyroid fibromyalgia: a small-N replication of a double-blind placebo-controlled crossover study. *Clin. Bull. Myofascial Ther.*, 2(4):71-88, 1998.
18. Refetoff, S., Weiss, R.E., and Usala, S.J.: The syndromes of resistance to thyroid hormone. *Endocrine Reviews*, 14:

348-399, 1993.

19. Kaplan, M.M., Swartz, S.L., and Larsen, P.R.: Partial peripheral resistance to thyroid hormones. *Am. J. Med.*, 70: 1115-1121, 1981.

20. Escobar-Morreale, H.F., Obregón, M.J., Escobar del Rey, F., and Morreale de Escobar, G.: Replacement therapy for hypothyroidism with thyroxine alone does not ensure euthyroidism in all tissues, as studied in thyroidectomized rats. *J. Clin. Invest.*, 96:2828-2838, 1995.

21. Jefferies, W. McK.: Occult hypothyroidism and "metabolic insufficiency." *J. Chronic Dis.*, 14:582-592, 1961.

22. DeGroot, L.J.: Abnormal thyroid function tests in euthyroid patients. In *Diagnostic Methods in Clinical Thyroidology*. Edited by J.I. Hamburger, New York, Springer-Verlag, pp.3-26, 1989.

23. Davidsohn, I. and Henry, J.B.: *Clinical Diagnosis by Laboratory Methods*, 15th edition. Philadelphia, W.B. Saunders, 1974.

24. Wiener, J.D. and Lindeboom, G.A.: Observations on an unusual case of myxoedema. *Acta Endocrinol.*, 39:439-456, 1962.

25. Leonard, J.L., Silva, J.E., Kaplan, M.M., et al.: Acute post-transcriptional regulation of cerebrocortical and pituitary iodothyronine 5'-deiodinases by thyroid hormone. *Endocrinology*, 92:998, 1984.

26. Gross, J. and Pitt-Rivers, R.: The identification of 3:5:3'-triiodothyronine in human plasma. *Lancet*, 1:439, 1952.

27. Hutchison, J.H. and Arneil, G.C.: Deficiency of an extrathyroid enzyme in sporadic cretinism. *Lancet*, 2:314-315, 1957.

28. Elewaut, A., Mussche, M., and Vermeulen, A.: Familial partial target organ resistance to thyroid hormones. *J. Clin. Endocrinol. Metab.*, 43:575-581, 1976.

29. Morton, J.H.: Sodium liothyronine in metabolic insufficiency syndrome and associated disorders: preliminary report. *J.A.M.A.*, 65(2):124-129, 1957.

30. Fields, E.M.: Treatment of metabolic insufficiency and hypothyroidism with sodium liothyronine. *J.A.M.A.*, 163: 817, 1957.

31. Kurland, G.S., Hamolsky, M.W., and Freedberg, A.S.: Studies in non-myxedematous hypometabolism: I. the clinical syndrome and the effects of triiodothyronine, alone or combined with thyroxine. *J. Clin. Endocrinol.*, 15:1354-1365, 1955.

32. Freedberg, A.S., Kurland, G.S., and Hamolsky, M.W.: Effect of l-tri-iodothyronine alone and combined with l-thyroxine in nonmyxedematous hypometabolism. *N. Engl. J. Med.*, 253:57-60, 1955.

33. Larsen, P.R. and Silva, J.E.: Intrapituitary mechanisms in the control of TSH secretion. In *Molecular Basis of Thyroid Hormone Action*. Edited by J.H. Oppenheimer and H.H. Samuels, New York, Academic Press, 1983, pp.351-385.

34. Sawin, C.T.: The development and use of thyroid preparations. In *The Thyroid Gland: A Practical Clinical Treatise*. Edited by Van Middlesworth, Chicago, Year Book Medical Publishers, Inc., 1986, pp.389-403.

35. Surks, M.I., Schadlow, A.R., and Oppenheimer, J.H.: A new radioimmunoassay for plasma L-triiodothyronine: measurement in thyroid disease and in patients maintained on hormonal replacement. *J. Clin. Invest.*, 51:3104, 1972.

36. Lev-Ran, A.: Part-of-the-day hypertriiodothyroninemia caused by desiccated thyroid (letter). *J.A.M.A.*, 250:2790, 1983.

37. Gershengorn, M.C. and Weintraub, B.D.: Thyrotropin-induced hyperthyroidism caused by selective pituitary resistance to thyroid hormone: a new syndrome of "inappropriate secretion of TSH." *J. Clin. Invest.*, 56:633-642, 1975.

38. Novogroder, M., Utiger, R., and Boyar, R.: Juvenile hyperthyroidism with elevated thyrotropin (TSH) and normal 24-hour FSH, LH, GH, and prolactin secretory patterns. *J. Clin. Endocrinol. Metab.*, 45:1053-1059, 1977.

39. DeLong, G.R. and Adams, R.D.: The neuromuscular system and brain in thyrotoxicosis. In *Werner and Ingbar's The Thyroid: A Fundamental and Clinical Text*, 6th edition. Edited by L.E. Braverman and R.D. Utiger, New York, J.B. Lippincott Co., 1991, pp.793-802.

40. Raskind, P.N., Kolodny, J.M., and Larsen, P.R.: The regional hypothalamic distribution of type II 5'-monodeiodinase in euthyroid and hypothyroid rats. *Brain Res.*, 420:194, 1987.

5.5

Complementary Methods: Increasing Metabolic Capacity and Decreasing Metabolic Demand

To significantly improve or recover, the patient whose fibromyalgia is caused by inadequate thyroid hormone regulation of cell function must use exogenous thyroid hormone. The patient's improvement or recovery, however, is critically dependent on her also engaging in other metabolism-regulating methods. These other methods are "complementary" in that they are indispensable if thyroid hormone is to help the patient completely normalize her metabolism. Other practices are not necessary for the patient's improvement or recovery but may contribute to maximum improvement.

Some complementary methods increase the resting metabolic rate. Aerobic exercise contributes most importantly by increasing VO_2 max. Resistance exercises contribute to an increased metabolic rate mainly by increasing the ratio of lean-to-fat body tissue; lean tissue has a higher resting metabolic rate. Before being able to exercise without adverse effects, many fibromyalgia patients must first begin using exogenous thyroid hormone to shift the balance of α- and β-adrenergic receptors away from α-isoform dominance. This enables cells to adapt to the increased demand for energy during exercise.

Patients should avoid restriction of food intake because it slows the metabolic rate. A vegetarian diet may increase the metabolic rate. Nutritional supplementation is essential if the patient is to improve. Some patients recover from their symptoms with nutritional supplementation alone, but most do not. Nutritional supplementation, however, is essential to the safe and effective use of exogenous thyroid hormone. No patient should take thyroid hormone unless she also takes nutritional supplements, especially B complex vitamins.

The resting metabolic rate of most pregnant women is increased. This undoubtedly accounts in part for the improvement of fibromyalgia symptoms during pregnancy.

Caffeine causes a transient increase in resting metabolic rate by sustaining the effects of catecholamines on cellular metabolic processes. Some patients have adverse effects from caffeine and should abstain from using it. Others experience variable degrees of temporary relief from their fibromyalgia symptoms. Use of the chemical is safe for most patients when used judiciously.

Other practices appear to benefit fibromyalgia patients by reducing metabolic demand. These include rest, progressive relaxation, biofeedback, hypnosis, *meditation, cognitive-behavioral techniques, and physical exercise.*

The word "complementary" means something that fills up, completes, or makes perfect—something that supplies a lacking or a missing ingredient. This is precisely what the methods in this chapter do for the fibromyalgia patient: They help to provide the portion of improvement that exogenous thyroid hormone cannot. For some patients, fibromyalgia results simply from a failure to use these methods in the first place, and making use of the methods is sufficient to relieve their symptoms and signs. Conversely, a patient is rarely freed from fibromyalgia merely by taking thyroid hormone. Most patients, however, if they are to significantly improve or recover, use the methods in this chapter combined with thyroid hormone. Thus, for most patients, the methods I describe here are not mere extras that the patient can ignore while thyroid hormone does the entire therapeutic job. They are, for the fibromyalgia patient as for most other human beings, essential to health and well-being.

Of 77 fibromyalgia patients my medical colleagues and I treated with metabolic therapy in 1990, 25% did not improve sufficiently to justify continuing to take T_3. Analysis of case records made it clear that this 25% was heavily weighted with patients who declined to make lifestyle changes, such as exercising and taking nutritional supplements.[54] In the years since, my observations in clinical practice and in conducting clinical studies have convinced me: whether or not a patient engages in methods such as those I discuss in this chapter is a fairly reliable predictor of whether she will benefit from exogenous thyroid hormone.

I have had many patients who were initially uncooperative about using these methods, despite having responded poorly to thyroid hormone alone. Of those who have finally relented to my insistence that they cooperate, most improved in their fibromyalgia status. Such observations have led me to a conclusion that I now staunchly maintain: The measures in this chapter are not extras to be used only if needed—they are *essential* if most patients are to significantly improve.

A number of methods can accelerate metabolism and benefit fibromyalgia patients to some degree. When used as the sole therapeutic method, however, they are likely to provide minimal relief at best. When they do help a patient, some of the methods can be used while waiting for a more profound and sustained

acceleration through thyroid hormone therapy. The measures in this chapter, then, are not curative, but may provide some measure of palliative relief. When used in conjunction with the proper form and dosage of thyroid hormone, these methods are likely to contribute substantially to a patient's response to thyroid hormone.

● INDICATIONS OF THE ROLE OF SUBOPTIMAL METABOLISM IN FIBROMYALGIA

Two studies by Moldofsky and his colleagues in the late 1970s suggested that aerobic fitness provides protection against fibromyalgia. These studies suggested that metabolic efficiency was a factor in someone's susceptibility to fibromyalgia. The investigators intentionally woke sleeping study subjects when their EEGs showed they were entering slow-wave (stage 4) sleep. Sedentary subjects developed fibromyalgia-like symptoms, but subjects who were aerobically fit, such as athletes, were resistant to developing such symptoms, even though they too had been deprived of slow wave sleep. This result raised the possibility that the relative hypometabolism of people with low levels of aerobic fitness predisposed them to fibromyalgia-like symptoms when deprived of sleep as a precipitating factor.[28][29] (This study did not show that athletes do not get fibromyalgia. Even highly conditioned athletes, if metabolically predisposed, can develop symptoms and signs of hypometabolism when stressors are great enough.)

An etiologic role for metabolic efficiency was also suggested by studies showing that regular aerobic activity can improve fibromyalgia status of some patients. Many fibromyalgic women have poor physical fitness. Several studies suggest that fibromyalgic women do not engage in regular endurance exercise and have poor physical fitness as a result.[30][31][32] Clark reported that only 11% of the fibromyalgic women in her study engaged in regular activity at a level necessary to increase or sustain endurance.[30] That other metabolism-impeding factors are involved in some of my patients' fibromyalgia is indicated by the fact that they were physically fit when they developed the condition, and have continued to be fibromyalgic despite valiant efforts to maintain fitness.

The benefits of exercise to the health and feeling of well-being of humans are clearly established. I have summarized elsewhere extensive evidence that physical activity has beneficial psychological and emotional effects.[3][4] Exercise tends to relieve depression, a common symptom in fibromyalgia. Researchers found that brief exercise significantly reduced depression[13] and that ten weeks of jogging significantly improved various depressive disorders.[17] A positive relationship has been shown between fitness level and emotional stability in middle-aged men.[18] Also, daily exercise improved both the physical and psychiatric status of institutionalized elderly mental patients.[19] According to deVries, "The wisdom of the ages that suggested that vigorous exercise makes you feel good is now supported by laboratory evidence."[2, p.249]

Thayer has shown that even moderate exercise significantly raises energy feelings. Such benefits result from both aerobic and resistance exercise.[93][94][95] (People with fibromyalgia should exercise only to tolerance, as overdoing is as harmful as underdoing. Thyroid hormone therapy can increase exercise tolerance, but until a patient's tolerance is increased, exercising only to tolerance is essential.)

● INCREASING RESTING METABOLIC RATE

The resting metabolic rate can be increased through aerobic and resistance exercise. To avoid a reduction in the metabolic rate, patients should avoid taking in less energy than expended through daily activities. A vegetarian diet and the use of nutritional supplements tend to increase the resting metabolic rate. Resting metabolic rate also increases during pregnancy and after caffeine intake.

EFFECTS OF AEROBIC EXERCISE ON RESTING METABOLIC RATE

Acute Aerobic Exercise and Resting Metabolic Rate

Shah, Geissler, and Miller had 16 previously obese women and 16 lean women use a bicycle ergometer for four minute periods at 60%-to-80% of VO_2 max. The researchers monitored the women's resting metabolism for up to 24 hours after the exercise. The aerobic exercise did not significantly increase the 24-hour resting metabolic rate. During waking hours, the rate was increased by 5%. This was not a statistically significant change. Post-obese women had a 3% increase (50 kcal), and lean women a 2% increase (30

kcal). During sleep, the metabolic rate of post-obese women remained the same, and that of the lean women decreased by 2%.[83]

Elliot and coauthors reported that the majority of caloric expenditure in aerobic exercisers occurs while they are exercising. The energy expended during the recovery phases after exercise accounted for only a minor portion of total energy use from aerobic exercise. The researchers had measured the metabolic rates of 6 healthy individuals for 90 minutes after they had exercised on a bicycle at 80% maximal intensity. Cycling for 10 minutes had induced a 37% increase in metabolic rate, and for 30 minutes, a 32% increase. By 30 minutes after the exercise, metabolic rates were no different from controls who had not exerted themselves. The average energy expended during recovery, above the mean baseline metabolic rate, was 11.4 kcal.[82]

Other researchers found no difference in resting metabolic rate between young men who did not exercise before a metabolic test, those who exercised 24 hours before, and others who exercised 48 hours before. The investigators concluded that acute exercise did not exert a detectable effect on resting metabolic rate.[62]

Long-Term Aerobic Exercise and Resting Metabolic Rate

Regular aerobic exercise over a period of weeks appears to increase the metabolic activity of lean tissue, thereby increasing the resting metabolic rate. Shinkai and colleagues had mildly obese middle-aged women use a diet that was calculated to be energy-restrictive for each. For 12 weeks, they engaged in aerobic exercise 45-to-60 minutes per day, at 50%-to-60% aerobic capacity (VO_2 max). After 12 weeks, subjects' body mass had decreased by a mean of 4.5 kg. The decrease was largely due to fat loss with little loss of fat-free mass. Compared to control subjects, the women had a 10% increase in resting metabolic rate per unit of body mass, and a 4% increase per unit of fat-free mass. There was no change in resting heat production per unit of fat tissue mass. However, heat did increase an average of 21% per unit of essential body mass.[44]

Shah and coauthors measured energy expenditure after previously obese women and lean women exercised by stepping for four 30-minute periods at 12 steps per minute. The researchers termed the exercise "prolonged mild activity." The net energy expenditure was considerably greater than that expended when the women exercised with a bicycle. The expenditure for post-obese women from cycling was 180 kcal; the expenditure from stepping was 250 kcal. The expenditure for lean women from cycling was 220 kcal and from stepping was 290 kcal. The researchers suggested that the prolonged mild activity of walking often is more effective than bicycling in increasing energy expenditure for the purpose of controlling obesity.[83]

Svendsen and coauthors studied overweight postmenopausal women consuming a 4200 kj/day (approximately 1,017 kc/day) diet who were taking part in aerobic and anaerobic exercise. The resting metabolic rate of control subjects increased by 4%, and that of the exercising women increased by 11%.[43]

Poehlman et al. questioned the cause of the negative relationship between age and resting metabolic rate in men over 40. They determined that the relationship results from factors such as a decrease in the muscle-to-fat tissue ratio and a decrease in aerobic capacity (VO$_2$ max).[55] Aerobic exercise, by increasing VO$_2$ max, has been shown to increase the resting metabolic rate independent of men's fat-free weight. Compared to aerobically untrained men, endurance-trained younger and older men had a 6% higher resting metabolic rate.[56]

Ballor and Poehlman studied physical characteristics, cardiovascular risk factors, and resting metabolic rate in 82 young non-obese women. They divided the women into three groups: sedentary, resistance-trained, or aerobically-trained. There was no difference between the groups for blood pressure and blood lipids. The women in all the groups were similar in body mass and fat-free (lean) mass. Compared to women in the sedentary group, the percent body fat was lower for those in the aerobically-trained group (mean=16.2%); the percent body fat was even lower for those in the resistance-trained group (mean= 14.7%). The mean resting metabolic rate (kj/min) for the sedentary group was 3.99, for the resistance-trained group was 4.25, and for the aerobically-trained group was 4.31. When adjusted for differences in fat-free mass, mean metabolic rates were not significantly different between the sedentary (4.05) and resistance-trained groups (4.13). But the mean rate for the aerobically-trained group (4.24) was significantly different from the other two groups.[67]

Toth and coauthors measured the resting metabolic rates of 86 men between the ages of 36 and 59. The men were divided into three groups, depending on whether by habit they did not exercise or they engaged in aerobic or resistance exercises. When differences in metabolic rate were adjusted for fat-free mass, there was no significant difference between the rates of men who did not exercise and those who did resistance exercises. The mean metabolic rate of aerobic exercisers was somewhat higher than that of resistance exercisers, but the difference was not significant (P=0.09). However, the difference between men who did not exercise and those who did aerobic exercise was significant (P=0.05).[81]

Poehlman and coauthors found that whole body fat oxidation decreases with advancing age. The decrease results mainly from an age-related decrease in fat-free tissue mass. They found that endurance training shifted disposal of fatty acids from nonoxidative to oxidative biochemical pathways. The increase in fat oxidation with training was related to an increased norepinephrine appearance rate during endurance exercise. The researchers wrote that endurance exercise induces a sympathetically-mediated rise in resting metabolic rate in both elderly men and women. During the non-exercising portion of the day, however, there may be a compensatory decline in energy expenditure, suggesting that vigorous endurance exercise could be counterproductive if fat loss is the patient's objective.[39]

Herring et al. found that when 9 highly trained women runners ceased training, urinary norepinephrine and epinephrine excretion decreased. The women's mean resting metabolic rate decreased from 274 kj/hr while they were still training to 252 kj/hr upon ceasing. When they stopped running, the higher metabolic rate lasted between 15 and 39 hours. The researchers speculated that the drop in catecholamine levels accounted for the lower metabolic rate.[40]

For fibromyalgia patients who can engage in aerobic exercise, the decrease in fat tissue, increase in VO$_2$ max, and increase in metabolic activity of muscle should raise resting metabolic rate. As a component of their metabolic regimen, aerobic exercise can contribute substantially to patients' recovery.

RESISTANCE TRAINING

Some researchers have reported that resistance training does not increase resting metabolic rate.[67][81] It is more often reported that resistance training builds lean muscle mass. Increases in muscle mass, however, are correlated with an increased resting metabolic rate.[49][50][85][86]

The hypothesis that the resting metabolic rate is positively related to higher lean-to-fatty body tissue has strong support. A typical study is that by Lawrence and coauthors. They measured the basal metabolic rate of women from Scotland, Gambia, and Thailand. They found no difference related to race, climate, diet or nutritional status. Differences in the metabolic rate were explained by differences in body fat content and fat-free muscle. The researchers pointed out that adipose tissue has a low metabolic rate compared to muscle.[73]

Pratley and coauthors tested the hypothesis that a strength training program designed to increase fat-free mass would increase the resting metabolic rate in older men. During a 16-week period, 13 "healthy" men (ages 50-to-65) engaged in a heavy resistance strength training program. The investigators measured the resting metabolic rate, body composition, and plasma concentrations of hormones known to affect resting metabolic rate. Strength increased by 40%. Body weight did not change, but body fat decreased and fat-free mass increased. Resting metabolic rate, measured with indirect calorimetry, increased 7.7%. Also, plasma norepinephrine increased. Fasting glucose, insulin, and thyroid hormone levels did not change. The investigators concluded, "These results indicate that a heavy resistance strength training program increases resting metabolic rate in healthy older men, perhaps by increasing fat-free mass and sympathetic nervous system activity."[85]

Is There a Lower Resting Metabolic Rate Associated with Gender and Aging?

Some researchers argue that women and older people in general have lower resting metabolic rates. Whether one believes this argument or not is important because the belief is likely to affect one's expectations of therapeutic outcome.

Cunningham wrote that we may view the resting metabolic rate in adults from two perspectives. From the clinical perspective, the resting metabolic rate is indexed through body surface area. The rate is sex-specific and lower in women. From the physiological perspective, the rate varies based on the mass of metabolically active cells. This view is asexual, and while the rate is usually lower in females, this is due to their smaller muscle mass. Cunningham argues that the metabolic rate is proportionately reduced and that athletic training equalizes body compensation (fat and fat-free tissue ratio) and metabolic rate between men and women.[52]

Sanborn and Jankowski argued that the difference in resting metabolic rate between women and men is not due to gender. They noted that women have a larger surface area-to-mass ratio, which may be advantageous in dry heat. Compared to men, women gen-

erally have more body fat and less lean muscle mass. Because fat is less metabolically active than muscle, women have lower resting metabolic rate. But the researchers stated, "The lower resting metabolic rate is not related to gender *per se*."[46] If these authors are correct, actions to increase the lean-to-fat tissue ratio and to increase VO_2 max are likely to provide women with the increased resting metabolic rate thought to provide men with a metabolic advantage.

There is some evidence, though, for a gender difference in resting metabolic rate independent of metabolism-impacting factors such as lean muscle mass. Arciero and coauthors studied gender differences in resting metabolic rate. They controlled for differences due to body composition and aerobic fitness. They tested 328 men (ages 17-to-80 years), and 194 women (ages 18-to-81 years). The mean resting metabolic rate of men was 23% higher than that of women. The investigators used multiple regression analysis to determine that 84% of individual variation in the resting metabolic rate resulted from fat-free mass, fat mass, peak VO_2 max, and gender. When they controlled for fat-free mass, fat mass, and peak VO_2 max, women still had a 3% lower resting metabolic rate. The mean adjusted resting metabolic rate for women was 1,563 kcal/day and for men was 1,613 kcal/day. The adjusted resting metabolic rate of premenopausal and post-menopausal women was also lower than men of roughly the same age.[47]

Poehlman and coauthors tested the hypothesis that the lower resting metabolic rate in older men is related to reduced maximal aerobic capacity (VO_2 max). Three hundred healthy men (ages 17-to-78) took part in the study. The researchers found no reduction in resting metabolic rate in men younger than 40. In men older than 40, however, the metabolic rate was negatively related to age. This negative relationship was still present with statistical control for fat-free weight and fat weight. But with statistical control for fat-free weight, fat weight, *and* VO_2 max, there was no association between age and resting metabolic rate. Thus, while a decrease in lean tissue mass can account for a lower resting metabolic rate in older men, this study suggests that deteriorating aerobic capacity may be a more decisive factor.[55]

Increasing Resting Metabolic Rate Through Resistance Training

Gillette and colleagues tested the effects of strenuous resistance exercise, stationary cycling, and quiet sitting on energy expenditure. They obtained the resting metabolic rate the morning of each trial and the morning after. Compared to those who cycled and those who sat quietly, resistance exercisers had a significantly elevated resting metabolic rate measured 14.5 hours after exercise. The investigators wrote, "These results suggest that strenuous resistive exercise results in a greater excess post-exercise oxygen consumption compared to steady-state endurance exercise [cycling] of similar estimated energy cost."[188]

In a study of 12 men and women (ages 56-to-80) before and after 12 weeks of resistance training, researchers measured body composition and energy metabolism. The subjects maintained a protein and energy dietary intake calculated to maintain body weight. Fat mass decreased by a mean of 1.8 kg. There was also a mean increase in total body water content of 1.6 kg, but neither the protein-plus-mineral mass nor the body cell mass changed significantly. The average energy intake required to maintain body weight increased by 15%. The increased expenditure of energy involved both the cost of doing resistance exercises and the increase in resting metabolic rate. The researchers concluded, "Resistance training is an effective way to increase energy requirements, decrease body fat mass, and maintain metabolically active tissue mass in healthy older people, and it may be useful as an adjunct to weight-control programs for older adults."[66]

Toth and Poehlman studied 54 healthy middle-aged women who by habit did not exercise or who did either aerobic or resistance exercise. The mean resting metabolic rate of women who engaged in aerobic or resistance exercise was significantly higher than that of those who did not exercise. There was not a significant difference between the mean metabolic rates of the women in the two exercise groups.[80]

Lemons et al. found that in combination with a 16-week very low calorie diet, isotonic resistance exercises were more beneficial than bicycle ergometry. They concluded that exercise with the diet, particularly isotonic resistance training, improved muscular efficiency and resting metabolic rate.[69] Poehlman and coauthors reviewed the available data and concluded that resistance exercise in older individuals increases the resting metabolic rate and basal sympathetic nervous activity.[39]

Some of the researchers referenced above found that resistance training increased the metabolic rate more than aerobic exercise; other researchers found the opposite. Both forms of exercise provide unique benefits in addition to possible increased metabolism. Because of this, it is prudent for the fibromyalgia patient to engage in both forms of exercise. The patient

who does so is likely to achieve a sustained increase in metabolic rate regardless of which form of exercise is primarily responsible.

DIET

Restricted Food Intake

Many hypometabolic patients maintain a moderate excess of body fat, even when they restrict their food intake and engage in moderate exercise. As a result, they restrict their food intake even further. Typically, this produces minimal returns or is completely counterproductive.

Dietary restriction can reduce the resting metabolic rate up to 20% within 14 days. After 5 weeks on an 800 kcal/day liquid formula diet, eight obese women had a 20% drop in resting metabolic rate. Five of these women had taken part in a supervised aerobic exercise program.[84] Exercise, then, does not seem to compensate for the lowered metabolic rate that results from dietary restriction.

Exercise that increases the muscle-to-fat tissue ratio, as with resistance training, can counteract this reduction by raising the resting metabolic rate.[57] This was shown in a study by Broeder and coworkers. They had 47 males (ages 18-to-35) either remain sedentary or engage in 12 weeks of high-intensity endurance or resistance training. Both exercise groups had a significant drop in relative body fat by decreasing their total fat weight and maintaining or increasing their fat-free weight. Resting metabolic rate did not change for any group. There was a small decline, however, in energy intake and an increase in energy expenditure (650 kcal per training day) for both groups. The researchers wrote, "These results suggest that both endurance and resistance training may help prevent an attenuation in resting metabolic rate normally observed during extended periods of negative energy balance (energy intake less than expenditure) by either preserving or increasing a person's fat-free weight."[68]

In a study by Racette and colleagues, resting metabolic rate decreased (-0.54 mj/d) in moderately obese women who used either a low carbohydrate diet or a low fat reducing diet for 12 weeks. Despite the reduced metabolic rate, aerobic exercise maintained the total daily expenditure of energy so that the women lost weight. Those using the low carbohydrate diet lost more weight than those on the low fat diet (a mean of -10.6 versus -8.1 kg).[42] In contrast to the reduction in resting metabolic rate during reduced food intake, feasting on a balanced carbohydrate, fat, and protein meal can raise body temperature and increase resting metabolic rate.[53] These increases are transient, and the rise in body temperature is referred to as "postprandial thermogenesis."

Wadden and coauthors assessed changes in weight, mood, and T_3 and reverse T_3 levels in 15 obese women over an 18-week period. After 4 weeks on a 1200 kcal/day diet, patients were divided into two groups. One consumed a very low calorie diet (400 kcal/day), and the other consumed a balanced-deficit diet (1200 kcal/day). Both groups continued these diets for 12 more weeks. Patients in the very low calorie group lost significantly more weight but had a 66% decrease in T_3 and a 27% increase in reverse T_3. Their T_3 levels increased after they increased their calories to 1000 kcal/day, but the hormone remained 22% below normal at the end of the study. The group of patients on the balanced-deficit diet had a 40% decrease in T_3. Mood improved in patients in both groups, and depression was not associated with alterations in T_3 levels.[124]

Vegetarian Diet

Toth and Poehlman studied the resting metabolic rate and sympathetic nervous activity of young male vegetarians and nonvegetarians. The mean carbohydrate intake by the vegetarians was 62%, and that of the nonvegetarians was 51%. The mean fat intake of vegetarians was 25%, and that of the nonvegetarians was 33%. There was no difference between the two groups of men, however, in total daily energy intake, body composition (determined by underwater weighing), or VO_2 max (maximal aerobic capacity).[41] Vegetarians had an 11% higher absolute resting metabolic rate (a mean of 1.29 compared to 1.16 kcal/min). They had a higher mean plasma concentration of norepinephrine (216 pg/mL versus 165 pg/mL) and a higher appearance rate of norepinephrine (0.50 μg/min compared to 0.36 μg/min). These differences were all statistically significant. When the investigators controlled statistically for differences in carbohydrate and fat intake and for norepinephrine levels, there was no statistical difference in the adjusted resting metabolic rate between the groups. This indicates that the higher resting metabolic rate of the vegetarians was partly due to the difference in micronutrient content of their diet and partly to increased sympathetic nervous activity.[41]

The higher sympathetic nervous activity has implications for those who tend to retain fat, like many fibromyalgia patients. In Caucasians at least,[48] activity of the sympathetic nervous system determines energy expenditure to a considerable extent. Individuals with a lower metabolic rate because of lower muscle content and activity, and lower sympathetic nervous activity, may be at risk for gain and retention of body weight from fat accumulation.

It is likely that many fibromyalgia patients have a slowed metabolic rate due in part to an increase in α-adrenergic receptor density on cell membranes. The increased density of these receptors reduces the amount of energy expended by the patient's cells. This reduction, combined with a low activity level, can result in an increase in fat retention. Some patients attempt to limit fat retention by restricting their food intake. Restricted food intake, however, can reduce the resting metabolic rate even further. This may worsen the patient's status. As part of the patient's metabolic rehabilitation, she should strive to consume enough food so that her energy intake is roughly equivalent to her energy expenditure. A diet that is exclusively or predominantly vegetarian may facilitate a sustained increase in metabolic rate.

NUTRITIONAL SUPPLEMENTATION

Fundamental to the spirit of science is the open-minded pursuit of truth. Prejudice—holding an emotionally-laden conclusion without rational consideration of the available evidence relevant to that conclusion—is the direct antithesis of this spirit. It is due to the predominance of prejudicial decision-making in conventional medicine today that I must begin this section with an appeal to reason. Most practicing medical clinicians today have been victimized by some medical editors' and medical educators' outright prejudice against nutritional supplementation. Linus Pauling, two-time Nobel Prize winner and officially recognized as one of the 20 greatest scientists in history, explained this as well as anyone can. His point of reference was personal experience as he detailed accounts of medical clinicians being deprived of accurate information on nutrition by publications such as Harvard's *Medical Letter* and *J.A.M.A.* He described some of his exasperating experiences, especially regarding vitamin C, and he described the fraudulent misrepresentation of research findings about the vitamin by Mayo Clinic researchers, representatives from the National Cancer Institute, and the editor of the *New England Journal of Medicine*.[182,pp.233-240] He wrote: "These actions suggest that the A.M.A. works to protect American physicians from information that runs counter to its own prejudices. The evidence indicates that the A.M.A. is prejudiced against vitamin C."[182,p.310]

For the sake of fibromyalgia patients, I implore the medical clinicians who use the information in this book to obtain a copy of Professor Pauling's book, *How to Live Longer and Feel Better*. The clinician should read the chapter titled "Organized Medicine and the Vitamins."[182,pp.300-316] The commercially-oriented title should not deter the clinician from obtaining this extremely important book. Pauling addressed the book to the general public, which accounts for the title, although some of the contents may be difficult for readers without some education in biochemistry. The book was Pauling's effort to impart to the general public information of vital importance to their health. He felt this action was necessary because some members of the medical establishment who control the dissemination of information to physicians systematically obstructed his efforts. The A.M.A. was instrumental in depriving medical physicians of evidence vital to arriving at scientifically-based conclusions about nutrition and health. In the book, Pauling wrote, ". . . I have given space in this book to the arguments against its thesis that come from many physicians and from old-fashioned nutritionists. I have had to do so because I have not always been able to answer them in their publications and other forums where they have made their criticisms. It is more likely that you have heard from them than from me. In these pages, you have heard both sides."[182,p.364]

When Pauling wrote *Vitamin C and the Common Cold*,[183] he wanted to share the information because it could help relieve the suffering of millions of human beings. The public was receptive, but many in organized medicine were not. They prejudged the issue, argued their bias as if it were truth, and attacked Pauling personally. He pointed out that the American Orthomolecular Medical Association, of which he was honorary President, had some 500 members. These physicians make recommendations about optimum nutritional intake along with their conventional medical procedures. Orthomolecular medicine, however, has been considered a threat to conventional medicine, and orthomolecular physicians are harassed by officials of the medical establishment.

The tide is changing, however, and physicians should take note. Hoffer wrote of recent evidence of victory over the medical establishment's prejudicial conclusions and manipulation of the thinking of medical physicians. He mentioned the early vitamin E research of physicians Wilfred and Evan Shute. Then he wrote, "However, the medical profession, instead of doing its duty which is to investigate claims made by reputable physicians and scientists, persisted in down-grading their work. In fact, one of the publications with the Harvard name on it, *The Medical Letter*, did a hatchet job on the Shutes' work many years ago. By doing so, it effectively killed interest for many decades. In this *Medical Letter*, they reviewed four studies published between 1940 and 1950 which they claimed were final definitive studies which proved that vitamin E had no therapeutic value for treating heart disease. I examined the four original papers, something which few doctors seem to have done. I found them to be inept, and so badly done that even journals willing to publish vitamin papers would have rejected them. They did not follow the directions described by the Drs. Shute, using too little vitamin E for too short periods of time." Hoffer estimated conservatively that had the public not been diverted from using vitamin E, about 200 patients per day (over several decades) might have avoided death from heart attacks. He went on to point out that in 1992, scientists from Harvard reported a 35%-to-50% reduction in heart disease in people who take vitamin E. In conclusion, he wrote, "The recent Harvard findings illustrate again the rapid advance of the orthomolecular paradigm in overthrowing the anti-vitamin paradigm—which has done so much harm in the past twenty years."[184]

Nutritional Supplements are Necessary but Not Sufficient if Most Fibromyalgia Patients are to Improve or Recover

Some patients have symptoms caused by nutritional inadequacies or deficiencies that are diagnosed as fibromyalgia. Teitelbaum wrote that many chronic fatigue syndrome patients' fatigue resolves with nutritional supplementation, indicating that they had increased nutritional needs.[178,p.132] I also have observed some patients—although a distinct minority—who met the criteria for fibromyalgia and whose symptoms were completely relieved after beginning a broad scope program of nutritional supplementation. I have observed far more patients, however, who have had full-fledged fibromyalgia despite a superb diet and long history of using nutritional supplements. Most of these patients improved or recovered from their fibromyalgia symptoms after beginning the use of exogenous thyroid hormone as part of a more comprehensive metabolic rehabilitation program. So while a few fibromyalgia patients improve or recover from the use of nutritional supplements alone, most do not without the simultaneous use of thyroid hormone.

On the other side of the ledger, few fibromyalgia patients using exogenous thyroid hormone significantly improve or recover if they are not concurrently taking nutritional supplements. I have had numerous patients who had fully recovered from severe fibromyalgia but whose symptoms returned at about 50% of their previous intensity within weeks after they ceased taking nutritional supplements, particularly B complex vitamins. These patients' symptoms again remitted within a couple of weeks after they resumed taking nutritional supplements. I insist that fibromyalgia patients using exogenous thyroid hormone take nutritional supplements because of possible adverse effects from not doing so while taking thyroid hormone.

Thus, while nutritional supplements appear curative for a minority of fibromyalgia patients, supplements are at best mildly palliative for others, and for a few others are of no benefit at all for the relief of fibromyalgia symptoms. Nevertheless, patients who take thyroid hormone improve far more and maintain the improvement indefinitely *only* if they also take nutritional supplements. Nutritional supplements are indispensable if the typical fibromyalgia patient is to significantly improve or recover from fibromyalgia with the use of exogenous thyroid hormone.

Vitamins

Although some enzymes are pure protein, most are a combination of a protein (called the apoenzyme) and a metal or vitamin, each of which is called a coenzyme. With the exception of vitamin C, all vitamins serve as coenzymes. Not all the apoenzyme in the body is converted to active enzymes. *Increased amounts of vitamins in the body that serve as coenzymes increase the percentage of apoenzyme that is converted to active enzymes.* The increased metabolism induced by exogenous thyroid hormone must be facilitated by greater quantities of active enzymes made available by higher vitamin intake. Thus, *optimum* vitamin intake[182,pp.87-88] must be considered in the effort to increase metabolism. Optimum intake can be considered the amounts of vitamins needed so that essential biochemical reactions in the human body proceed at rates that lead to the best of health.[182,p.340] Optimum intake must be distinguished from the RDAs, which are the minimum amounts of vitamins (plus 50% more) necessary to ward off deficiency diseases.

B Complex Vitamins. Energy metabolism is critically dependent on vitamin B_1. Depression may be the major symptom of patients who are deficient in vitamins B_6,[179] B_{12},[180] and folic acid.[181,pp.480-482] Folic acid deficiency is an especially important consideration. Travell and Simons wrote that patients with low-normal (lowest quartile) or subnormal serum folic acid levels have a number of symptoms and signs typical of patients with thyroid hypofunction (see folic acid section below).[1,p.132]

Vitamin B_1. Vitamin B_1 (thiamine) is essential to normal energy metabolism. An inadequacy, then, may increase the susceptibility to trigger points.[1,pp.116-117] According to Travell and Simons, vitamin B_1 potentiates the effectiveness of thyroid hormones. Vitamin B_1 may alleviate symptoms of hypothyroidism and even normalize thyroid laboratory values. The patient taking exogenous thyroid hormone who then begins to take a vitamin B_1 supplement may have to reduce her dosages of thyroid hormone to prevent hyperthyroid symptoms.[1,p.120]

Tepperman and Tepperman wrote that extremely hypermetabolic individuals are susceptible to vitamin deficiencies. The hypermetabolic individual with a vitamin B_1 deficiency may develop a beriberi-type heart syndrome that may lead to cardiac failure.[185,p.169] Travell and Simons pointed out that a vitamin B_1 deficiency may make a patient intolerant of even low-dose thyroid therapy. As the patient's metabolism accelerates, B_1 deficiency symptoms may intensify. After correcting the vitamin deficiency, the patient tolerates well the same or a larger dose of thyroid hormone.[1,p.147]

To summarize the interactions of vitamin B_1 and thyroid hormone: Vitamin B_1, by accelerating metabolism, may partially compensate for a thyroid hormone deficiency. When the patient taking vitamin B_1 begins to also take exogenous thyroid hormone, she may require a smaller dosage of the hormone than if she were not taking vitamin B_1. (Vitamin B_1 may affect thyroid hormone laboratory values by increasing metabolism in the thyroid gland.) On the other hand, for the patient with a vitamin B_1 deficiency, exogenous thyroid hormone, by accelerating metabolism, may worsen the adverse effects of the deficiency. The adverse effects of the vitamin B_1 deficiency are said to make the patient "intolerant" of thyroid hormone. When the patient begins taking vitamin B_1, the adverse effects of the deficiency are relieved. The patient is then said to have an increased tolerance of the same dosage of thyroid hormone. She may in fact tolerate an even higher dosage than during the vitamin deficiency.

Folic Acid. Travell and Simons wrote that folic acid inadequacy depresses the patient's basal temperature.[1,p.146] The patient tires easily, sleeps poorly, and feels discouraged and depressed. They wrote, "In our experience, these patients also frequently feel cold and have a reduced basal temperature, as do patients with thyroid hypofunction; their symptoms are often relieved by multivitamin therapy including folic acid."[1,p.132]

A high percentage of psychiatric patients are folic acid deficient,[186][187] and their diagnosis is usually depression.[181,pp.480-482] This is predictable in that folic acid deficiency tends to adversely affect cognitive and emotional function.[189,pp.504-514]

Table 5.5.1. Minimum supplemental nutrients I recommend fibromyalgia patients take each day.

SUPPLEMENT	DOSAGE
B Complex formulation (Providing at least 50 mg B₁ per tablet)	1 bid
Vitamin C	1-5 gm bid
Vitamin E	800-1600 IU
Carotenoids	15 gm
Multi-mineral formulation	bid
Calcium	2000 mg per day
Magnesium	1000 mg per day

Minerals. *Iodine.* Ingesting subthreshold amounts of iodine can increase iodine uptake by the thyroid gland, decrease thyroxine synthesis, increase the ratio of T_3/T_4 secretion, increase the ratio of circulating T_3/T_4 concentrations, increase TSH secretion, and lead to goiter formation. Conversely, ingesting excess iodine can also inhibit thyroid hormone synthesis by blocking biosynthetic enzymes in the thyroid gland. This results in decreased secretion of T_4, increased TSH levels, goiter, and if the iodine excess is chronic, hypothyroidism.[190]

Ancient Egyptian physicians treated goiter patients with dried seaweed and sea sponges. It was in this century, however, when the researcher named Marine demonstrated the relationship between iodine deficiency and goiter. He documented the high incidence of goiter in inland populations, and he showed that people could prevent the condition by taking as little as two grams of potassium iodide twice yearly. One effective method for avoiding goiter is to consume table salt to which manufacturers have added iodide.[185,pp.157-158]

Larsen pointed out that in the U.S., iodine restricted diets (used to limit salt intake) may critically reduce the body's iodine pool. A patient may also take a potent diuretic drug that increases the renal clearance of iodide. This further decreases the iodine pool.[192,pp.1070-1071] In the patient whose thyroid gland is sensitive to decreases in iodine, this factor may be critical in initiating thyroid inadequacy. Pregnant women require a higher amount of iodine than non-pregnant women. It has been recommended that when a pregnant woman restricts her salt intake, she should take an iodine supplement.[196,p.141] (The same applies to anyone who restricts his or her salt intake because of cardiovascular disease. The disease may be secondary to hypothyroidism, and restricting iodine intake may worsen cardiovascular status.) Excess iodine intake by pregnant women, however, may result in transient congenital hypothyroidism in the infant.[191]

Nettler[193,p.353] and Johnson[194,p.261] recommended kelp and seaweed as iodine supplements. As an alternative, they recommended taking one drop daily of a mixture of ½ water and ½ tincture of iodine.[193,p.353]

Human adults need between 100 μg and 200 μg of iodine each day. Seafood contains a considerable amount, but other vegetable sources vary widely because of soil content. The average foods eaten by Americans do not provide the daily requirement. People make up the deficit by consuming iodized table salt. Salt is the main dietary source of iodine. Every 10 grams of salt provides 1 mg of iodine. Between the late 1950s and late 1970s, agricultural and technological practices resulted in more iodine in drugs and foods such as milk and bread. People ingest about 5-to-10 times the RDA of iodine, but moderate amounts in excess of the RDA are not considered harmful.[195,p.155]

Magnesium. The red blood cells of fibromyalgia patients have been found to have low magnesium levels.[197] A magnesium loading test also showed low magnesium levels in fibromyalgia patients.[198] The lower the magnesium levels, the more pain experienced by the patients.[170] Patients with myofascial pain syndrome were also reported to have low red cell and plasma magnesium levels.[200]

Magnesium oxide is an inexpensive preparation. Absorption of magnesium oxide may be poor, however, necessitating that the patient take higher dosages. At the same time, magnesium oxide may be irritating to the GI tract. Lower dosage preparations such as Slow-Mag® (magnesium chloride) and Mag-Tab®SR (magnesium l-lactate dihydride) may be better tolerated.[200,p.12]

It is likely that most fibromyalgia patients do not obtain enough magnesium in their diets. Because of this, I recommend that they take a magnesium supplement. The nutrients I recommend patients take, at a minimum, are included in Table 5.5.1.

PREGNANCY AND RESTING METABOLIC RATE

The resting metabolic rate increases in pregnancy. The increase can explain the improvements in fibromyalgia status that many patients have reported to me after becoming pregnant.

The increase in resting metabolic rate in pregnancy is well documented.[74][75][76][77] Blackburn and Calloway reported that metabolic rate increased more than body weight during pregnancy. There was a small drop in the basal rate per unit of body mass near term. The small fall, however, was not due to a shift in body composition toward increased fat or water. They pointed out that the prolonged rate of recovery after hard work indicates that oxygen uptake is increased in the pregnant woman for a longer period after work.[79]

Van Raaij and colleagues reported that in 57 healthy Dutch women, the cumulative increment in basal metabolism during pregnancy was a mean of 34,350 kcal.[71] Nagy and King measured the basal metabolic rate in nonpregnant women, women in early pregnancy, and others in late pregnancy. Metabolic rate in early pregnancy was 13% higher than in the nonpregnant state. The rate in late pregnancy was 28% higher than in early pregnancy. However, when energy expenditure at rest was expressed as kcal/kg body weight, there was no significant difference in metabolic rate between early and late pregnancy.[78]

Energy expenditure increases in pregnancy because of greater maternal and fetal tissue energy requirements and more rapid resting metabolic rate. The extra energy requirement is roughly 250-to-300 kcal/day. Durnin[70] studied energy intake, basal metabolic rate, body weight and fatness, physical activity, and mechanical efficiency of movement in 162 Scottish women at 2-to-4-week intervals throughout pregnancy. He compared his data with that from a similar study in the Netherlands and calculated the normal expected cost-of-pregnancy expenditure energy (250-300 kcal/day). But increases in energy intake by the women were equivalent to only 100 kcal/day. He attributed the lack of adverse effects from the deficit of 150-to-200 kcal/day to a diminished energy requirement due to relatively small decreases in physical activity by the pregnant women.[70][76] Van Raaij and colleagues argued that a diminished metabolic (thermogenic) response to food intake also partially compensates for a potential energy deficit.[75]

Based on such findings, it is prudent for the pregnant fibromyalgic woman who intends to increase her physical activity level (to accelerate her metabolic rate above that conferred by pregnancy) to consult an obstetrician knowledgeable about balancing energy intake and expenditure. She should insure that she has no individual problem that must be allowed for in her exercise regimen. It is advisable that she also maximize her structural/biomechanical integrity through the assistance of a qualified musculoskeletal specialist. This implies the use of procedures such as postural training and possibly orthotics rather than mere passive submission to spinal manipulation. Manipulation can be helpful, but usually only when employed within the context of a more sophisticated program of care.

Van Raaij et al. reported that no allowance for increased energy requirements in pregnancy need be made for physical activity. Based on their study of the absolute and net energy costs in 39 women at 12, 24, and 36 weeks gestation, they specified no additional energy allowance is needed "... even if a woman's activity pattern includes a substantial amount of externally paced work."[72]

It might be advantageous to inform pregnant women of the findings of Nagy and King. In their study, women in late pregnancy walked 400 meters 20% more slowly than women in early pregnancy. But when the women in early pregnancy at the beginning of the study were in late pregnancy, their pace was only 4.5% slower than their early pregnancy pace. The investigators wrote, "These data suggest that individual behavioral differences have a greater effect on pace than stage of gestation." While a woman's weight was the major determinant of energy expended during walking, an increased walking pace increased the rate of energy expenditure per kilogram of body weight.[78] In terms of maximizing the increase in metabolic rate, women should be encouraged to exercise at their maximum, well-tolerated level.

CAFFEINE

Because it is the most commonly used drug today, caffeine has been subjected to extensive clinical and experimental study.[160] Caffeine reduces, and in rare cases appears to temporarily relieve, some fibromyalgia patients' pain, fatigue, weakness, cognitive dysfunction, and depression. Caffeine increases the resting metabolic rate, internal and skin temperatures,[58][59][60][61][62] and mitochondrial oxygen consumption.[63][65] It produces physiological arousal,[87][88] can improve mood[87][88][91] and perception of problems,[90,p.9] and mitigates pain.[1,p.92][101][103][104][105][106][108][109][110][111][112] The long-term use of caffeine, however, produces tolerance to some of its pharmacological effects.[171]

For instructions on the judicious use of caffeine to facilitate a sustained increase in metabolism, see Chapter 5.2, subsection titled "Caffeine: Dosage."

I am aware of only one controlled study that involved caffeine in the treatment of fibromyalgia. Vaeroy and colleagues compared the effects of carisoprodol (a muscle relaxant analgesic whose active metabolite is meprobamate[99]), paracetamol (acetaminophen), and caffeine with that of a placebo. Patients were treated for 8 weeks. The investigators reported that the pain, sleep quality, and general feeling of sickness of those taking the "active" therapy significantly improved. The pressure/pain thresholds of patients in the active treatment group increased (improved) at 70% of the sites assessed, compared to increases at 30% of sites in placebo patients. Pain and sleep quality, however, also improved in placebo patients. The researchers reported that improvement in the placebo group may have resulted from "the large amount of extra medications in this group." Of the 23 placebo patients, 56.5% also took analgesics or nonsteroidal anti-inflammatory drugs, as did 20% of the 20 active treatment patients. In addition, 43% of the placebo patients, but none of the treatment patients, used tricyclic antidepressants, anxiolytics, or sedatives. The multiple medications used by both active treatment and placebo patients confuse the outcome of this study. Nevertheless, the researchers concluded that the active treatment, containing caffeine, was comparatively effective in the treatment of fibromyalgia.[98]

Effects of Caffeine

Effects of Caffeine on Resting Metabolic Rate. Koot and Deurenberg had young men consume 150 ml of "decaffeinated" coffee. The coffee half the men consumed contained 200 mg of caffeine. Measures were taken before coffee consumption (the fasting state) and up to 3 hours later. After the men consumed caffeine-containing coffee, their mean resting metabolic rate increased immediately (0.2 kj/min). The rate remained increased for the 3 hours that measurements were taken. Mean caffeine-induced thermogenesis was 0.3 kj/min. This converts to a mean increase in metabolic rate of 7% during the 3 hours of measurements. Internal temperature began increasing after the men consumed coffee with or without caffeine. But at 2 hours, the temperatures of subjects drinking caffeine-laced coffee were significantly increased compared to the temperatures of those consuming only decaffeinated coffee. The mean skin temperature increased after coffee consumption; at 90 minutes post-consumption, those with caffeine in their coffee had a significantly elevated temperature compared to those without. The authors wrote that after caffeine consumption, energy expenditure increases first, and after some delay, internal and skin temperatures also increase.[58]

In mice, intraperitoneal injections of caffeine (60 mg/kg) significantly elevated brown adipose tissue temperature. There was a smaller rise in core temperature. Oxygen consumption increased in the mitochondria of brown adipose tissue, and resting metabolic rate increased. The investigators concluded that caffeine increases brown adipose tissue thermogenesis, and this may contribute to increases in metabolic rate.[59]

A single-dose oral intake of 100 mg of caffeine was shown to increase the resting metabolic rate of both lean and previously obese individuals. There was a 3%-to-4% increase in rate over 150 minutes. *The post-obese subjects had defective, diet-induced thermogenesis that was improved by the caffeine-induced increase in metabolic rate.* Repeated intake of 100 mg of caffeine at 2-hour intervals over a 12-hour period during the day increased energy expenditure of both lean and previously obese subjects by 8%-to-11% during that time. The subsequent nighttime 12-hour resting metabolic rate was not influenced by the prior caffeine consumption. Lean subjects had a 150 kcal increase in daily energy expenditure, and previously obese subjects had a 79 kcal increase. The investigators wrote, "Caffeine at commonly consumed doses can have a significant influence on energy balance and may promote thermogenesis in the treatment of obesity."[60]

In young, lean rats, resting metabolic rate was greater than in corpulent rats. In both phenotypes of rats, ephedrine increased thermogenesis (measured as VO₂ max) by a mean of 32%, caffeine by 48%, and ephedrine and caffeine combined by 50%. VO₂ max increased at the same rate in both phenotypes, but the duration of the increase was longer in corpulent rats: 50% for ephedrine, 26% for caffeine, and 42% for both chemicals combined. Corpulent rats lost more weight acutely with administration of one or more of the sympathomimetic chemicals (corresponding to the longer period of VO₂ max), and a normal end-organ sympathomimetic receptor system.[61]

No difference in resting metabolic rate was found between (1) young men who did not exercise before the metabolic test, (2) those who exercised 24 hours before, and (3) others who exercised 48 hours before. Acute exercise *per se* did not exert a detectable effect on resting metabolic rate. The men took caffeine to determine its effects under the three conditions. The resting metabolic rate increased by an average of 7%, but it was about the same for men in each of the three groups. Caffeine increased the resting metabolic rate of all the men, but acute exercise did not, regardless of whether or not the men had taken caffeine.[62]

LeBlanc and his fellow researchers studied the effects of caffeine on the resting metabolic rate of 8 young men who were exercise-trained and 8 who were not. After ingesting 4 mg of caffeine per kg of body weight (280 mg for a 154 lb man), the trained men had a greater increase in metabolic rate. They also had a higher increase in plasma free fatty acids and a greater fall in respiratory quotient. This indicates that the trained men had a larger increase in lipid oxidation in response to caffeine. Both groups of men had a decrease in plasma norepinephrine and an increase in plasma epinephrine, but the effects were significantly greater in trained men. "It is suggested," the researchers wrote, "that the greater increase in resting metabolic rate in trained subjects following caffeine ingestion is related to an enhanced lipid mobilization, possibly produced by a greater epinephrine secretion, and by subsequent increased lipid oxidation."[63]

In one study, men with and without endurance exercise training ingested 300 mg of caffeine and underwent measurement of their resting metabolic rates for 90 minutes. Before taking caffeine, there were no significant differences between the metabolic rates of the men. In response to the caffeine, the untrained men had a greater increase in metabolic rate than the trained men. There was no significant difference in response between men who regularly used caffeine and those who did not. The researchers concluded that endurance training reduces the metabolic response to a caffeine challenge.[64]

Jung and coworkers measured changes in the resting metabolic rates of lean, obese, and previously obese women in response to ingested caffeine. The rise in metabolic rate in lean and obese women was similar, but previously obese women had a less pronounced rise in rate. β-Adrenoceptor blockade did not diminish the response to caffeine, indicating that the increase in metabolic rate was independent of the adrenergic system. The increase in metabolic rate corresponded to increases in plasma levels of free fatty acids. The authors suggested that the metabolic effects of caffeine appear to be mediated by increases in adi-

pocyte lipolysis rather than action of the adrenergic system.[65]

Thermogenic Effect of Caffeine. Caffeine is thermogenic and increases body temperature.[58][59][60][61][62] Koot and Deurenberg reported that after young healthy males consumed 200 mg of caffeine, their metabolic rates increased immediately and remained increased for 3 hours. Their internal (rectal) temperatures increased. Skin temperatures increased significantly compared to controls after 90 minutes. The researchers wrote that increases in skin and internal temperature were delayed compared to the increase in metabolism (energy expenditure measured as indirect calorimetry).[156]

Bracco and colleagues studied the thermogenic effects of caffeine on lean and obese women. The magnitude of thermogenesis in obese women was significantly smaller than in lean women. In lean women, the thermogenesis was prolonged into the night. The effects were gone the next day. There was a significant increase in lipid oxidation in both groups, but it was blunted in obese women. Lipid oxidation increased in lean women by 29% and in obese women by 10%.[154]

Effects of Caffeine on Physiological Arousal and Energy. Caffeine increases physiological arousal[87][88] and wakefulness.[148] A significant arousal reaction to caffeine is evident in changes in the spontaneous EEG.[172] Within minutes of consumption, the consumer senses an increase in energy.[146][147] Thayer wrote that when it works optimally, caffeine increases alertness and energy while decreasing tension.[90,p.8] Others have reached the same conclusion.[88] *Optimal use implies taking a sufficiently large dosage of caffeine, but less than the amount that excessively stimulates the neuromuscular system.* Because of its potential ergogenic effects, several governing bodies of sports have prohibited the use of caffeine during competition.[161]

Effects of Caffeine on Mood, Depression, and Problem Perception. Caffeine can improve mood, relieve depression, and improve an individual's perception of problems.

Mood and Depression. Caffeine, even in small doses,[87][88][91] improves mood.[107] The chemical is referred to as a nootropic (mind-stimulating) agent.[158] One study showed that among hospitalized psychiatric patients, those with depression had the highest consumption of caffeine.[141] This indicates that depressed patients are reinforced for caffeine consumption by the rewarding emotional effects. (An increased tendency to consume caffeine because of its reinforcing properties is to be *distinguished* from physical addiction.)

Thayer explained the conditioning process involving agents such as caffeine: "The uncomfortable feeling that initiates the use of the substance—most likely tense-tiredness—is repeatedly paired with at least temporary cessation following consumption of the substance. In each case, the uncomfortable feeling and the thoughts about the substance would represent the vague craving that motivates the use."[90,p.162]

Perception of Problems. Thayer wrote that caffeine (as well as sugar consumption and exercise) changes one's perception of problems. According to him, "*Interpretations* of personal problems at any one time appear to be only partly influenced by what is actually happening in the external environment [he determined this in a previous study[89]]. Also important is how energetic or tired one is at the moment, together with the degree of tension or calmness. While these differences are not large, over time they can be important." He indicated that as one's energy increases, ". . . important elements of perceptual reality . . ." improve.[90,pp.8-9]

The potential benefits of this phenomenon for fibromyalgia patients faced with fatigue and an uncertain prognosis should be obvious. This is evident in another statement by Thayer, reflecting the views of Blaney[96] and Bower[97]: "The immediate theoretical extensions of the ideas regarding moods, personal problems, and even optimism are quite important, and the implications arising from this viewpoint are wide-ranging indeed. For example, one can consider mood-cognition relationships as similar to the memory associations that occur with drug conditions. In this state-dependency paradigm, learned responses seem to be closely associated with artificially induced states. Thus, each time those states are reintroduced, the same learned responses are consciously produced."[90]

Thayer also wrote that there may be similar cognitive-emotional states associated with moods that occur naturally: "For example, when an individual feels highly energetic, and at the same time is relatively calm, his or her perceptions of both self and the world are distinctly different from when that person is tired and at the same time tense. Not only are memories of past successes and failures likely to be different, but perceived likelihoods of future successes and failures are also probably different. In one case, self-esteem is high, and in the other, it is low."[90,p.9]

Kawachi and coauthors,[123] noting the improvement in mood with caffeine use, conducted a 10-year follow-up study to determine the relation between coffee/caffeine consumption and the risk of suicide. The researchers used a food frequency questionnaire to de-termine coffee and caffeine consumption, and physician review of death certificates determined deaths from suicide. During 832,704 person years of observation, there were 56 cases of suicide. The researchers concluded that there is a strong inverse relationship between caffeine intake and the risk of suicide. The conclusion was justified even after adjusting for a broad range of possibly confounding factors. These included self-reported stress, smoking habit, alcohol intake, concurrent diseases, marital status, and medication (such as diazepam and phenothiazine).

Effects of Caffeine on Cognitive Function. For people in general, caffeine improves cognitive function. My clinical experience has shown that this is especially likely if a patient's cognitive abilities are impaired as a feature of fibromyalgia.

There are many published studies on the beneficial effects of caffeine on cognitive function. It fact, caffeine is listed as a mild brain stimulant and "cognitive enhancer."[5] Caffeine has been reported to improve performance on tests of sustained attention,[201] semantic memory, logical reasoning, free recall, and recognition memory tasks.[33] In one study, caffeine improved attention, delayed recall (but not immediate recall), and problem-solving. Even small amounts induced users to feel more "clearheaded," happier, calmer, and less tense.[199] When 9003 British adults were tested, researchers found that cognitive performance was improved with caffeine use on tests of simple reaction time, choice reaction time, incidental verbal memory, and visuo-spatial reasoning. The researchers also reported that there was little if any "tolerance" to the performance-enhancing effects of caffeine.[35] Mitchell and Redman reported that caffeine improved performance on all mental speed-related tasks, but compared to low and moderate dosage caffeine users, high dosage users performed more poorly on the verbal reasoning task.[36]

Battig and coauthors reported that caffeine consumption increased the regularity of letter cancellation performance, showing improvement in behavioral routine and speed.[92] Children using caffeine have been reported to have slightly increased anxiety, significantly less sluggishness, and improved attention on some tests.[34]

(In contrast to the beneficial effects of caffeine on cognitive function, Galduroz and Carlini reported finding no cognitive improvement with long-term use of the Brazilian plant guarana (paulinia cupana) by normal elderly people.[51])

Effects of Caffeine on Pain. Caffeine is an antinociceptive chemical.[149][152][153] Travell and Simons noted that clinically, small-to-moderate amounts of caffeine dilate blood vessels in skeletal muscles, and that this may help eliminate trigger points.[1,p.92] Such dosages may also reduce pain in fibromyalgia patients by increasing blood flow in their myofascial tissues. This is especially likely when caffeine is used in conjunction with other analgesics.

Hoyovadillo and coauthors, for example, found that motor impairment (decreased time of contact with a rotating cylinder) from induced pain (intra-articular administration of uric acid) in Wistar rats was not reduced by caffeine alone. However, caffeine increased the reduction of pain-induced impairment by naproxen.[104] In a review of the available scientific evidence, Aicher and Kraupp reported that the analgesic action of over-the-counter painkillers containing caffeine is increased 1.4-fold. They concluded that combination analgesics are proper and effective for self-medication for pain of different kinds.[101] Other studies have also shown that the analgesic effects of aspirin and acetaminophen are significantly greater with the simultaneous use of caffeine.[106]

Kuntz and Brossel found that caffeine potentiated pain relief by the analgesic paracetamol. The combined effect was equivalent to that of paracetamol and the centrally-activating dextropoxyphen, but without the centrally-mediated effects of the latter drug such as drowsiness and constipation.[173]

In a controlled study, Kraetsch and coauthors tested the ability of the analgesic propyphenazone to reduce the amplitude of chemo-somatosensory event-related potentials elicited by stimulation of the nasal mucosa. This drug at 400 mg did not reduce the amplitude when compared with the effect of a placebo. Six-hundred mg was required to reduce the amplitude. However, adding either 100 mg or 150 mg of caffeine significantly increased the antinociceptive effects of propyphenazone so that it more effectively reduced amplification of the potentials.[172]

In 1991, Ward and coauthors used a double-blind placebo-controlled multiple crossover experimental design to determine whether caffeine used without other medications affected pain. They found that in 53 patients with non-migrainous headaches, caffeine had an independent analgesic effect. The effect was equivalent to that of acetaminophen. Caffeine was effective even when the investigators made statistical adjustments for prior consumption of caffeine and the drug's mood effects.[151]

Currier and colleagues noted that although caffeine modulates pain perception in a number of acute pain states, its effects on the experience of chronic pain were not determined. They performed a retrospective chart review of 131 chronic low back pain patients to assess self-reported daily caffeine consumption. The researchers classified patients' caffeine consumption as low (< 100 mg), moderate (100-to-400 mg), and high (> 400 mg). (Such classifications are arbitrary. For example, other researchers consider 250-to-600 mg caffeine per day moderate consumption.[155]) They reported no differences between the classes of patients in self-reported measures of pain severity, affective distress, anxiety-related symptoms, sleep behavior, and the amount of caffeine use. They wrote that their findings did not indicate that caffeine consumption was related to the global experience of pain and disability in patients with chronic low back pain.[103]

Analgesia. Positive mood can influence people to report less pain.[108][109][110][111] Since caffeine improves mood, there has been some question as to whether this improvement accounts for the apparent pain relief from caffeine. Caffeine also relieves headaches due to caffeine withdrawal.[112] Ward et al. conducted a study that factored out the effects of both mood and caffeine withdrawal. They concluded that caffeine (65 mg and 130 mg) has a direct analgesic effect not mediated by mood or withdrawal.[105]

Possible Analgesic Effects of Diuresis. Coffee consumption (6 cups containing 642 mg caffeine) increased 24-hour urine excretion with a reduction in total body water and a concomitant decrease in body weight. Urinary excretion of sodium, and to a lesser extent potassium, was increased.[125] This diuretic effect of caffeine may alleviate pain due to sodium and fluid retention in some women, as I explain below.

Headaches due to fluid retention are common among women, especially during the premenstrual phase and in women taking birth control pills or other drugs with similar pharmacologic ingredients.[134] The probable mechanism is sodium and water retention. Estrogen is purported to cause only slight fluid retention, and progestogens, a decrease in fluid retention.[126,p.906] Fluid retention, however, is considered a precaution when oral contraceptives are prescribed.[127,p.2189] Some authors consider fluid retention one of the main adverse effects of oral estrogen therapy, causing swelling, breast tenderness, and diffuse edema.[128,p.645]

Among the factors that may interact with fluid retention to induce headaches is fibrous adhesions of the upper cervical myofascia. Fascia is made up of a glue-like ground substance with collagen and elastin fibers embedded in it. When a muscle is subjected to high-frequency work overload, fibroblasts in the muscle's investing fascia become more active and deposit more collagen fibers.[129] Progressively more collagen deposits in the fascia, reinforcing its tensile strength. This shows fascia to be a dynamic tissue that adapts to stresses imposed upon it.

When fascia is relatively immobile, its collagen fibers knit together with cross-bindings.[130] This is expected to occur when a patient habitually holds her neck in hyperextension, keeping the upper cervical myofascia relatively immobile. When the myofascia is not stretched sufficiently, as in this posture, its collagen fibers tend to coil in on themselves and shorten.[131] As a result, the fascia progressively contracts and compresses whatever is contained within it, including blood vessels and nerves.[132] Under these conditions, fascia becomes a shrinking straightjacket of fibrotic tissue.

In healthy, non-fibrotic fascia, collagen fibers are not significantly cross-linked. Fascial sheets are able to slide past one another, and the tissues of which they are constituents are flexible and expansible. When the tissue spaces collect an abnormally high content of fluid (as occurs during sodium retention), the fascia adapts: the distance between collagen fibers increases and the elastin fibers stretch to permit the expansion required by the high fluid content. But when the ground substance contains an overabundance of collagen fibers that have cross-linked and coiled in on themselves, the fascia is less able to adapt. The inelastic fascial meshwork is relatively unyielding and expands poorly. When fluid is retained, tremendous tension may mount inside the tissue spaces. As the tension mounts, veins and lymphatics collapse, resulting in retention of nerve-irritating metabolites.[135,pp.36-37][136] These lower the threshold for noxious signal transmission when receptors are subjected to slight mechanical pressure. At some threshold point, mechanoreceptors will begin reacting to the intramuscular pressure much as they respond to a palpating digit that compresses them. The nerves will conduct noxious signals into the central nervous system and stimulate referred pain that is described as a headache.

After a woman ovulates, she begins releasing progestogen. This may add to the sodium and fluid retention stimulated by the estrogen she began releasing after her last period. The puffiness this causes in some women may disturb them, especially when they retain more than 10 pounds of fluid.[133,p.330] At this point, a woman's swollen skin may markedly obscure underlying bony landmarks and visibly alter her usual appearance.

Caffeine consumption induces urinary sodium and fluid excretion. This may counteract in some women the pain-inducing effects I have just described.

Mechanisms of the Clinical Effects of Caffeine

Inhibition of Phosphodiesterase. Methylxanthines, such as caffeine, are best known as inhibitors of phosphodiesterase, the intracellular enzyme that inactivates cAMP. By inhibiting phosphodiesterase, caffeine increases cAMP concentration[150][157][163] and prolongs the cellular effects of catecholamines.

Inhibition of Adenosine. Adenosine activates an inhibitory GTP-binding protein (G_i) that decreases cAMP formation. The result is a decrease in the firing of neurons and decreased secretion of neurotransmitters. Caffeine overcomes these inhibitory effects of adenosine and increases central nervous system activity.[159][162]

Caffeine, theophylline, and theobromine are adenosine receptor antagonists.[146] Adenosine receptor antagonists have motor-activating effects; adenosine receptor agonists have motor-depressant and sedative-hypnogenic effects.[145]

Adenosine Receptors. It has been experimentally demonstrated that adenosine receptors have inhibitory effects in rats. Activation of the A_1 isoform decreases anxiety and the A_2 form decreases locomotor activity. Jain and coauthors[142] reported that the A_1 adenosine receptor agonist (N-6-cyclopentyladenosine) mediated anxiolytic-like activity in mice. An A_1 adenosine antagonist (1,3-diprophyl-8-cyclopentyl-xanthine) blocked the anxiolytic-like activity of the selective A_1 adenosine agonist. The A_2 adenosine receptor agonist had no effect on anxiety behavior, but depressed locomotor activity. Caffeine administration had anxiogenic-like effects on the rats, presumably by acting as an A_1 adenosine receptor antagonist. Sawynok and Reid[149] reported that in rats, antinociception and locomotor activation is mediated by interaction of xanthines such as caffeine with A_1 adenosine receptors.

Continuous, heavy consumption of caffeine leads to upregulation of adenosine receptors. Caffeine then ceases to produce the effects that result from its inhibition of adenosine receptors. This is called caffeine tolerance.[159]

Other Receptors Affected by Caffeine. Caffeine may also directly inhibit ryanodine receptors (Ca^{++} release channel in the membrane of the sarcoplasmic reticulum). The inhibition probably potentiates calcium release from the sarcoplasmic reticulum of skeletal muscle cells. Inhibition of receptors by caffeine causes increased lipolysis, facilitation of central nervous system signal transmission, decreased potassium levels during exercise, and sparing of glycogen (largely due to increased fatty acid oxidation).[137]

Adenosine antagonists such as caffeine are capable of increasing the activity of central nervous system dopamine[113][114] and norepinephrine.[115][116][117][154] Stimulating D-2 (dopamine) receptors[118][119] or α_2-adrenergic receptors[120][121] enhances analgesia. These findings raise the possibility that these two receptors mediate caffeine analgesia.[105,p.154] Other possible mechanisms of analgesia include anti-inflammatory, antipyretic, and vasoconstrictive effects[122] (see Chapter 3.2).

Other Mechanisms of the Effects of Caffeine

Caffeine may have beneficial clinical effects through other mechanisms.

Catecholamine, Adipose, and Vascular Effects. Many of the effects of caffeine occur because it increases circulating levels of epinephrine and norepinephrine, and it sustains the processes mediated by adrenergic receptors and catecholamines. But there are also specific tissue effects that occur independently of the adrenergic system. Thus, caffeine directly affects adipose tissue with an increase in circulating free fatty acids and glycerol. It also affects vascular tissue, with an increase in blood pressure during the first hour post-ingestion.[147] Its effects on vasculature counteract postprandial hypotension.[171]

Adverse Effects of Caffeine

There are some precautions to be taken in the use of caffeine, and some individuals clearly should abstain from its use. But, most of the adverse effects hypothesized over the years have not been found to occur.

Adverse Effects from Caffeine Withdrawal. For some people, withdrawal from even moderate dosages results in transient symptoms such as headache,[112] fatigue, and anxiety.[171]

Adverse Effects from Caffeine Use. According to Tarnopolsky, long-term ingestion of caffeine in amounts less than 5 cups/day does not appear to increase the risk of a number of diseases, such as cardiac arrhythmias, peptic ulcers, cardiovascular disease, or cancer. Nonetheless, he wrote, "The short-term consumption of caffeine may result in increased urination, gastrointestinal distress, tremors, decreased sleep, and anxiety symptoms in certain individuals."[137] Most people, however, have these adverse effects only when

they ingest too much caffeine. For example, many institutionalized elderly people have insomnia and poor sleep quality from drinking coffee or tea close to bedtime.[144] This is a problem of self- or institutional mismanagement. In general, individuals can avoid adverse reactions by finding for them what is a useful but less than adverse dosage. Some individuals, however, are so sensitive to caffeine that they have adverse reactions even to small dosages.

Why some patients are extraordinarily prone to adverse effects from caffeine is not certain. Several hormonal and neurotransmitter interactions are implicated. Increasing the ratio of β-adrenergic receptors to α-adrenergic receptors by exogenous thyroid hormone potentiates responsiveness to caffeine. For this reason, when patients begin taking thyroid hormone, they should be cautioned that they are likely to have both positive and negative reactions to lower dosages of caffeine.

Lamarine reviewed the available evidence for possible adverse effects on behavior and health from acute and chronic caffeine use. He concluded that the relationship between caffeine ingestion and illnesses such as cardiovascular disease and cancer are equivocal. He wrote, "Prudence might dictate that pregnant women and chronically ill individuals exercise restraint in their use of caffeine, although research suggests relatively low or nonexistent levels of risk associated with moderate caffeine consumption."[164]

Osteoporosis. Blaauw and coauthors studied the risk factors that appear to predispose men and women to osteoporosis. They obtained data from 56 patients with confirmed osteoporosis and 125 controls without osteoporosis. Table 5.5.2 shows the risk factors that these researchers reported to predispose the men and women to osteoporosis. The researchers also reported that the intake of caffeine, calcium, phosphorus, and protein was essentially the same among osteoporotic and normal groups, and that these agents are therefore not related to osteoporosis.[165]

Breast Disease. In some studies of rats and mice, caffeine administration influenced normal, hyperplastic, and carcinomatous mammae development. But studies of a possible relationship between caffeine consumption and breast disease have been inconsistent and inconclusive.[160]

Folsom et al. studied the association of caffeine intake to post-menopausal breast cancer in 34,388 women. The women ranged in age from 55-to-69 years. Caffeine intake was assessed by a food frequency questionnaire, and the study spanned from 1986 to 1990. The researchers reported that there was no apparent association between caffeine intake and breast cancer. This was true even when adjustments were made for age or multiple breast cancer risk factors, despite the consumption of regular coffee or other caffeine-containing foods.[167]

Table 5.5.2. Risk factors that predispose men and women to osteoporosis.

	Men	Women
Positive family history of osteoporosis		X
Fair complexion		X
Lower body mass	X	X
Lower height	X	X
No breast-feeding of babies	X	X
Fat distribution around waist	X	X
Lack of exercise	X	X
History of smoking	X	
Preference for salty foods	X	
High alcohol consumption	X	X

Although breast tenderness has been attributed to caffeine consumption, Reynolds and coauthors[168] did not find that caffeine intake contributed to pain experienced by 89 women undergoing needle localization in the breast (indicated by the women's use of a visual analog scale). Premenopausal women in the second half of the menstrual cycle had a significantly higher score than those in the first half (3.54 vs 1.70, P=0.05).

Over the years of my professional practice, women patients have repeatedly told me that they have eliminated fibrocystic lesions by taking high dosages of vitamin E despite continuing their intake of caffeine.

Serotonin. Caffeine may increase the production and breakdown of serotonin. In one study, when subjects took caffeine orally, their urine contained a higher than normal concentration of 5-hydroxyindoleacetic acid, the metabolite of serotonin.[140] (See Table 5.5.3.)

Large dosages of caffeine (20 mg, 40 mg, and 80 mg/kg) increased rat brain levels of tryptophan, 5-hydroxytryptamine (serotonin), and 5-hydroxyindoleacetic acid. When rats given saline for 5 days were given caffeine (80 mg/kg) on the 6th day, brain levels of tryptophan, serotonin, and 5-hydroxyindoleacetic acid increased. When rats given caffeine for 5 days were given saline on the 6th day, brain tryptophan levels remained the same, but serotonin and 5-hydroxy-

indoleacetic acid decreased.[143]

P-cholorophenylalanine, a drug that depletes serotonin, reduces the excitatory effects of caffeine. Conversely, drugs that prevent the breakdown of serotonin (monoamine oxidase inhibitors) substantially increase toxic effects of extremely high quantities of caffeine.[138][139]

Fibromyalgia patients with low serotonin levels may require higher dosages of caffeine to produce beneficial effects. After beginning the use of thyroid hormone, a resulting increase in the secretion of serotonin may result in the patient perceiving an increased sensitivity to caffeine. She may then find that a smaller caffeine dosage produces the same benefits as a higher dosage previously did.

Abdominal Pain. Georges and Heitkemper had 20 mid-life women use a symptom diary and food record. The record showed that distressing abdominal pain was not related to caffeine consumption. Low fiber intake was related to abdominal pain, awakening with abdominal pain, nausea, awakening with nausea, and awakening with rectal pain.[100]

Pruritus Ani. Metcalf advised abstention from caffeine and other dietary items to help patients recover from pruritus ani.[102]

Harm to Newborns. Nehlig and Debry reviewed the available evidence for adverse effects on newborns of caffeine consumption by pregnant women. The researchers wrote, "We conclude in this review that maternal caffeine consumption in moderate amounts during gestation and lactation has no measurable consequences on the fetus and newborn infant." Nevertheless, they cautioned pregnant women to moderate their ingestion of caffeine because the half-life of the chemical is prolonged during the last trimester of pregnancy and in the newborn infant.[166]

Prostate Cancer. Slattery and coauthors studied men newly diagnosed with prostate cancer to determine whether the disease was correlated with various factors considered to be risks. They found that cigarette smoking, alcohol intake, coffee, tea, and other forms of caffeine consumption were not associated with prostate cancer risk. Theobromine, another xanthine chemical, was associated with prostate cancer in older men who consumed more than 11 mg of theobromine per day.[169]

● **REDUCING METABOLIC DEMAND**

Under the corrugated, newly-evolved upper layers

of the human brain is the older, more primitive brain. This older part of the brain, called the limbic system, controls motivation and emotions. When we are emotionally aroused, efferent signals descend from the limbic system to the skeletal muscles via the gamma motor system of efferent fibers. The signals reach the muscle spindles and shorten them. When a muscle begins to lengthen, receptors in the shortened spindles respond by transmitting afferent signals to the spinal cord. Through reflex connections in the cord, the afferent signals activate alpha motor neurons. These neurons transmit signals to the lengthening skeletal muscle fibers, inducing them to cease lengthening or to shorten. Thus, when impulses from the limbic system shorten skeletal muscle spindle-sensors, the net effect is that the muscles remain shortened. The shortened state is synonymous with increased muscle tone.

Increased skeletal muscle tone has survival value. When we anticipate the need for emergency action, as when we suspect that we might slip and fall, the limbic system activates. Gamma motor signals are transmitted to skeletal muscle spindle-sensors, inducing them to tighten muscles in preparation for self-preserving action. The same limbic system/muscle shortening phenomenon presumably is operative in shortened (hypertonic) skeletal muscles due to cognitive activation. The muscle tightening might occur when a fibromyalgia patient fears that her symptoms are actually a life-threatening disease such as lupus.

This protective mechanism can worsen fibromyalgia symptoms for a specific reason: When nerve impulses cause muscles to remain tightened, the muscles expend more energy. Energy metabolism in the fibromyalgia patient is already compromised, and if sustained muscle tension increases the demand for energy, the ability of the muscle cells to provide sufficient energy may be critically exceeded.

Chronic fatigue syndrome patients are often described as "overachieving, duty-driven"[24,p.113] and "pedantic and having great needs for order, perfectionism, planning, and cleanliness . . . ."[23,p.249] Studies do not support this generalization, certainly not as a description of a predisposing personality for the development of chronic fatigue syndrome or fibromyalgia. But after illness befalls a victim, worries, concerns, uncertainties, and fears are the typical patient's lot. These are cognitive/emotional states that are capable of maintaining gamma motor nerve input to the skeletal muscles, resulting in generalized hypertonicity. Consequently, the patient's energy demands may further exceed her metabolic capacity. For the patient with inadequate thyroid hormone regulation of cell function,

taking exogenous thyroid hormone can increase her metabolic capacity to the point that energy demand no longer exceeds capacity and energy expenditure no longer results in fatigue or other symptoms. Until this therapeutic potential is fulfilled, moderate or even mild activity that engages skeletal muscles may exceed metabolic capacity and induce or worsen symptoms.

Table 5.5.3. Steps in serotonin synthesis and catabolism.

tryptophan
↓
5-hydroxytryptophan
↓
serotonin (5-hydroxytryptamine)
↓
5-hydroxyindoleacetaldehyde
↓
5-hydroxyindoleacetic acid

To counter this process, the patient may derive some improvement from practices that reduce metabolic demand by decreasing limbic system gamma motoneuron efferent activity. Such methods include rest, relaxation exercises, meditation, and somatic therapies such as myofascial therapy, massage, and spinal manipulation. These practices reduce skeletal muscle tension and thereby appear to decrease metabolic demand on muscle. The reduced metabolic demand may diminish fibromyalgia symptoms associated with heightened muscle tone.

REST

Rest is possibly the most often recommended treatment for chronic fatigue syndrome at this time. Wessely cited some of the self-help literature that advises "Rest, rest, and more rest,"[25] and "Aggressive rest therapy."[26] "Rest is an effective short-term strategy for dealing with acute fatigue, particularly after acute infection, which is so often the trigger for chronic fatigue syndrome. For most subjects, such rest is only used as a short-term coping strategy, and the majority are able to resume normal activity."[24,p.117]

Wessely cautioned, however, that rest that is too prolonged is not wise, concluding, "Rest as a coping strategy is thus of short-term benefit to those with acute fatigue syndromes, but in the long term is harmful."[24,p.118] Shepherd warned that the patient who has prolonged bed rest ". . . may then become trapped in a vicious circle of immobility and weakness, and become almost bedridden."[27]

One of the problems of prolonged rest is progressive deconditioning. Wessley noted that many chronic fatigue syndrome sufferers engage in a vigorous exercise program. Some are especially athletic and fit, and they are prone to aggressively resume their pre-illness level of activity. These patients are likely to cause themselves to relapse, possibly with more severe symptoms than before.[24]

Deconditioned patients who exercise beyond their tolerance are likely to suffer adverse consequences for doing so, such as muscle soreness. However, simple deconditioning cannot account for the severe and often debilitating exacerbation of chronic fatigue syndrome and fibromyalgia symptoms that results from even mild exercise. A more likely mechanism is α-adrenergic receptor dominance in these patients. As long as this isoform dominance persists, activity to a degree sufficient to increase catecholamine levels is likely to impede the very cellular metabolic processes that are vital for the patient to adapt to the metabolic demands of the exercise. When α-adrenergic receptor dominance is due to inadequate thyroid hormone regulation of transcription of the adrenergic genes, the proper form and dosage of exogenous thyroid hormone will induce a shift toward a normal balance of α- and β-adrenergic receptors. Mediation of adaptive cellular processes by catecholamine/β-adrenergic receptor interaction will then eliminate the adverse effects of vigorous exercise. The patient may then be able to engage in more vigorous conditioning activities without the previous adverse effects. (See Chapters 3.1 and 3.4.)

PROGRESSIVE RELAXATION

Edmund Jacobson, who developed progressive relaxation training, wrote that resting by a person not trained to relax his muscles does not really result in muscle relaxation. The person still has measurable levels of muscle contraction. Centripetal signals generated by the person's contracted muscles sustain central nervous system activity that is incompatible with rest. Undoubtedly, the central activity involves centrifugal flow of gamma motor signals back to skeletal muscles, increasing their resting tone and metabolic demand.[6]

People who are physically fit, such as athletes, are able to relax their muscles more quickly and completely than those who are not. Yet people who have undergone training to relax their muscles can relax more

quickly and completely than athletes who have not been similarly trained.[10]

Most patients can teach themselves to use progressive relaxation training with guidance from Jacobson's book, *Progressive Relaxation*.[6] Some health care professionals, especially behavior therapists and biofeedback trainers, have formal training in progressive relaxation techniques and can quickly teach patients how to properly use the techniques.

BIOFEEDBACK

Fibromyalgia patients have shown some improvement with the use of EMG-biofeedback.[175][176] Biofeedback trainers have traditionally used progressive relaxation training to enable patients to regulate their own physiological stress responses. As I stated above, use of relaxation training can reduce gamma motor nerve activity. In addition, the use of feedback devices can facilitate the patient's acquisition of the ability to reduce mental and physical activity. Combined use of these methods may enhance the effectiveness of metabolic therapy for fibromyalgia patients by significantly reducing skeletal muscle metabolic demand.

MEDITATION

In one study, 51% of fibromyalgia patients improved somewhat in a meditation-based program. Meditation can be highly effective in reducing neuromuscular activity—at least in part by reducing gamma motor activity.[177]

COGNITIVE-BEHAVIORAL THERAPY

Some fibromyalgia patients have benefitted from cognitive-behavioral therapy.[20][21] This form of therapy can be quite pleasant. In one study with fibromyalgia patients, the treatment involved progressive relaxation training and guided imagery.[20] The aim of the regimen was to teach the patients how to regulate their pain. These were the steps in their training:

(1) Patients learned progressive relaxation of major muscle groups. They associated the relaxed state with cues they could later use to help elicit relaxation when they needed it. They used the cues, for example, when trying to initiate or maintain sleep.

(2) Patients practiced guided imagery with two purposes:

(a) The imagery distracted them from their pain. The scenes they chose to imagine were ones in which they had previously been pain-free. They imaged themselves actually in the scenes rather than observing themselves there. The therapist gave the patients detailed multi-sensory descriptions to help them form effective images. Patients later repeated the descriptions aloud. The therapist also used a variety of scenes to stimulate the patients' interest and attention.

(b) The images represented a metaphor for the patients' pain. So, by changing the metaphor, they were able to change their pain perceptions. The therapist and patients discussed the patients' metaphoric images to help concretize them. The investigators wrote, "If the pain was labeled as 'pressing,' a metaphoric image might be that 'there is a vise gripping my leg.' An image is then generated in which the vise is opened and the pain relieved."

Another technique involved the use of color. Patients imaged their painful body parts as a particular color. They then contrasted this color with one for non-painful tissues. They next imaged the painful color shrinking and disappearing.

It is worth noting that this cognitive-behavioral intervention was individualized, based on each patient's level of development, comfort, and interest. Patients had audio tapes of the techniques to use at home. They also had discussions with the therapist focusing on their personal effectiveness in mastering their pain. These talks were to help reduce anxiety and depression.[20]

HYPNOSIS

Undergoing hypnosis can also reduce gamma motor activity and reduce metabolic demand. The mental focus distracts the patient from other stimuli that can be psychophysiologically arousing. The practice has the added benefit, through posthypnotic suggestion, of sustaining the reduced arousal through selective attention.

PHYSICAL EXERCISE

In addition to increasing metabolic capacity, physical exercise also has a "tranquilizer effect." The evidence for this is substantial, as I summarized in two previous publications.[3][4]

Muscle Tension

In a study of fibromyalgia patients, Tavares et al.

found a positive correlation between the tender point count and the patients' subjective feelings of muscle tension when going to sleep.[37] If relaxation is effective, research has not yet confirmed it. While weak evidence indicates that relaxation can diminish acute pain,[45] studies do not support a similar beneficial effect with chronic pain.[21][22]

During anxiety and other such emotions, skeletal muscles become more active.[2,p.248] The muscles contract more and this expends energy (energy that is in short supply in the muscles of fibromyalgia patients). Edmund Jacobson showed this with electromyography in the early part of this century.[6][7][10] Later Sainsbury and Gibson[8] and Nidever[9] showed that even when a person is resting, emotional states such as anxiety are reflected in increased muscle activity of one or two muscles.

Those who are more physically fit are able to relax their muscles more quickly and completely than those who are not.[10] In one study, 5 minutes of bench-stepping exercise substantially reduced subjects' nervous and muscle tension. One hour after the exercise, muscle tension (measured as electrical activity) was 58% lower than before the exercise. As subjects performed the exercise regularly and became conditioned, their reduced muscle activity became long-lasting.[11]

In another study, the muscle-relaxing effect of exercise was compared with the effect of the tranquilizer meprobamate. Study subjects who walked at a heart rate of 100 bpm showed reduced muscle tension (measured as electrical activity). Immediately after the exercise, muscle activity was lower by 20%; at thirty minutes, by 23%; and one hour later, by 20%. By contrast, the tranquilizer meprobamate did not reduce muscle tension.[12]

Other researchers have found similar tranquilizing effects of exercise.[13][14][15][16] Again, though, I caution fibromyalgia and chronic fatigue syndrome patients to exercise to tolerance and *not* overdo.

● A WORD ABOUT THE HOLISTIC APPROACH

HOLISTIC OR PREVENTIVE MEDICINE

In their book *Solving the Puzzle of Chronic Fatigue Syndrome*, Rosenbaum and Susser stated to medical physicians that "the striking similarity between fibromyalgia and chronic fatigue syndrome cannot be ignored," and that in some studies, 80% of chronic fatigue syndrome patients also have fibromyalgia. These authors, who are preventive medicine physicians, wrote, "Our credo has been to shore up the body's own defenses against disease with proper diet, exercise, a healthy lifestyle, and the judicious use of nutritional supplements." They use nutritional and hormone therapies, stress management, specific medications, allergy treatments, immune system bolstering, and psychological support.[174,p.76] This approach is the *raison d'être* of naturopathic medicine. Naturopathy, as practiced in states such as Washington and Oregon where these physicians combined the use of conventional and natural medicine, should serve as the standard for holistic medical care.

I, too, subscribe to this theoretical orientation, as does Chaitow.[38] Directly or indirectly, I provide my patients with a similar array of preventive and therapeutic measures. A small percentage of fibromyalgia patients respond superbly to these methods with significant improvement or complete relief of their symptoms. Teitelbaum reported that mild-to-moderate fatigue has been relieved in many of his patients merely by their beginning nutritional supplementation.[178,p.132] This is also true of the mild hypometabolic symptoms of some of my fibromyalgia patients. This indicates, as Teitelbaum stated, that these patients' symptoms were related to increased nutritional needs.[178,p.132] For most fibromyalgia patients, however, these holistic, preventive methods alone provide minimal improvement. The majority of patients significantly improve or recover from their symptoms while using these practices only when they are also using the proper form and dosage of exogenous thyroid hormone.

Most of my fibromyalgia patients, through their persistent pursuit of relief, became health enthusiasts long before they consulted me. Many of them have gone through "detox" regimens, and used regular protective doses of antioxidant nutrients, minerals, trace elements, and megadoses of various vitamins. They have done aerobic, toning, stretching, and relaxation exercises. Some have used guided imagery, programming in the alpha brain wave state, and meditation. Yet after engaging in all these practices, most still suffered from severe fibromyalgia symptoms.

This is not to negate the value of the holistic approach. In fact, this approach is the foundation of good health and should be a first line of attack against any disease. In addition, this approach gives the fibromyalgia patient the edge in improving with metabolic rehabilitation. I have worked with recovered fibromyalgia patients who, upon stopping nutrient supplementation, resumed having fibromyalgia symptoms at about 50% of their previous intensity, even though the patients were still using thyroid hormone therapy. Holistic, preventive methods are indispensable for insuring the recovery of fibromyalgia patients. But fibromyalgia patients in general do not have sufficient metabolic capacity to fully benefit from the holistic, preventive approach. After beginning to use thyroid hormone, however, most patients gain the capacity to benefit. Because most patients improve or recover only after beginning the proper use of exogenous thyroid hormone, I do not believe the molecular lesion responsible for most patients' fibromyalgia is directly amenable to the methods of the holistic approach—unless, of course, the use of thyroid hormone is considered an integral part of that approach. Holistic methods do appear to compensate to some degree for the effects of the lesion, but in general, they alone do not rectify it.

REFERENCES

1. Travell, J.G. and Simons, D.G.: *Myofascial Pain and Dysfunction: The Trigger Point Manual*, Vol. 1. Baltimore, Williams and Wilkins, 1983.
2. deVries, H.A.: *Physiology of Exercise*, 4th edition. Dubuque, Wm. C. Brown Publishers, 1986.
3. Lowe, J.C.: Physical activity: a form of physiopsychotherapy. *Digest Chiro. Econom.*, 21(2):33-37, Sept-Oct, 1978.
4. Lowe, J.C.: Psychological benefits of physical activity. *ACA J. Chiro.*, 13(1):S1-S6, 1979.
5. Riedel, W.J. and Jolles, J.: Cognition enhancers in age-related cognitive decline. *Drugs & Aging*, 8(4):245-274, 1996.
6. Jacobson, E.: *Progressive Relaxation*. Chicago, Univ. of Chicago Press, 1938.
7. Jacobson, E.: The cultivation of physiological relaxation. *Ann. Intern. Med.*, 19:965-972, 1943.
8. Sainsbury, P. and Gibson, J.G.: Symptoms of anxiety and the accompanying physiological changes in the muscular system. *J. Neurol. Neurosurg. Psychiatry*, 17:216-224, 1954.
9. Nidever, J.E.: A factor analytic study of general muscular tension. Ph.D. dissertation, University of California at Los Angeles, 1959.
10. Jacobson, E.: The course of relaxation of muscles of athletes. *Am. J. Psychol.*, 48:98-108, 1936.
11. deVries, H.A.: Immediate and long-term effects of exercise upon resting muscle action potential level. *J. Sports Med. Phys. Fitness*, 8:1-11, 1968.
12. deVries, H.A.: Tranquilizer effect of exercise: A critical review. *Physician and Sports Med.*, Nov. 1981, pp.46-55.
13. Morgan, W.P. and Horstman, D.H.: Anxiety reduction following acute physical activity (Abstract). *Med. Sci. Sports*, 8:62, 1976.

14. Sime, W.E.: A comparison of exercise and meditation in reducing physiological response to stress. *Med. Sci. Sports*, 9:55, 1977.

15. deVries, H.A., Wiswell, R.A., Bulbulian, R., and Moritani, T.: Tranquilizer effect of exercise: acute effects of moderate aerobic exercise on spinal reflex activation level. *Am. J. Phys. Med.*, 60:57-66, 1981.

16. deVries, H.A., Simard, C., Wiswell, R.A., Heckathorne, E., and Caragetta, V.: Fusimotor system involvement in the tranquilizer effect of exercise. *Am. J. Phys. Med.*, 61: 111-112, 1982.

17. Brown, R.S., Ramirez, D.E., and Taub, J.M.: The prescription of exercise for depression. Paper read at ACSM meeting, Washington, D.C., May 24, 1978.

18. Young, R.J. and Ismael, A.H.: Relationship between anthropometric, physiological, biochemical and personality variables before and after a four-month conditioning program for middle-aged men. *J. Sports Med. Phys. Fitness*, 16:267-276, 1976.

19. Stamford, B.A., Hambacher, W., and Fallica, A.: Effects of daily physical exercise on the psychiatric state of institutionalized geriatric mental patients. *Res. Quart.*, 45:34-41, 1974.

20. Walco, G.A. and Ilowite, N.T.: Cognitive-behavioral intervention for juvenile primary fibromyalgia syndrome. *J. Rheumatol.*, 19:1617-1619, 1992.

21. Nielson, W.R., Walker, C., and McCain, G.A.: Cognitive behavioral treatment of fibromyalgia syndrome: preliminary findings. *J. Rheumatol.*, 19:98-103, 1992.

22. Carroll, D. and Seers, K.: Relaxation for the relief of chronic pain: a systematic review. *J. Adv. Nursing*, 27: 476-487, 1998.

23. Johannsson, V.: Does a fibromyalgia personality exist? *J. Musculoskel. Pain*, 1(3/4):245-252, 1993.

24. Wessely, S.: Social and cultural aspects of chronic fatigue syndrome. *J. Musculoskel. Pain*, 3(2):111-122, 1995.

25. Feiden, K.: *Hope and Help for Chronic Fatigue Syndrome*. New York, Prentice Hall, 1990.

26. Franklin, M. and Sullivan, J.: *The New Mystery Fatigue Epidemic. ME. What Is It? Have You Got It? How To Get Better*. London, Century, 1989.

27. Shepherd, C.: *Living with ME: A Self-Help Guide*. London, Heinemann, 1989.

28. Moldofsky, H. and Scarisbrick, P.: Induction of neurasthenic musculoskeletal pain syndrome by selective sleep stage deprivation. *Psychosom. Med.*, 38:35-44, 1976.

29. Moldofsky, H., Scarisbrick, P., England, R., and Smythe, H.: Musculoskeletal symptoms and non-REM sleep disturbance in patients with "fibrositis syndrome" and healthy subjects. *Psychosom. Med.*, 37:341-351, 1975.

30. Clark, S.R.: Fitness characteristics and perceived exertion in women with fibromyalgia. *J. Musculoskel. Pain*, 1:191-197, 1993.

31. Bennett, R.M., Clark, S.R., Goldberg, L., Nelson, D., Bonafede, R.P., Porter, J., and Specht, D.: Aerobic fitness in the fibrositis syndrome: a controlled study of respiratory gas exchange and [133]xenon clearance from exercising muscle. *Arthritis Rheum.*, 32:454-460, 1989.

32. Klug, G.A., McAuley, E., and Clark, S.R.: Factors influencing the development and maintenance of aerobic fitness: lessons applicable to the fibrositis syndrome. *J.*

Rheumatol., 19(Suppl.):30-39, 1989.

33. Smith, A., Kendrick, A., Maben, A., and Salmon, J.: Effects of breakfast and caffeine on cognitive performance, mood, and cardiovascular functioning. *Appetite*, 22(1):39-55, 1994.

34. Bernstein, G.A., Carroll, M.E., Crosby, R.D., et al.: Caffeine effects on learning, performance, and anxiety in normal school-aged children. *J. Am. Acad. Child Adoles. Psychia.*, 33(3):407-415, 1994.

35. Jarvis, M.J.: Does caffeine intake enhance absolute levels of cognitive performance? *Psychopharmacology*, 110(1-2):45-52, 1993.

36. Mitchell, P.J. and Redman, J.R.: Effects of caffeine, time of day, and user history on study-related performance. *Psychopharmacology*, 109(1-2):121-126, 1992.

37. Tavares, V. and Branco, J.: Relation of sleep related complaints with tender points and pain intensity in fibromyalgia syndrome. *J. Musculoskel. Pain*, 3(Suppl.1):138, 1995.

38. Chaitow, L.: *Fibromyalgia & Muscle Pain*. London, Thorsons, 1995.

39. Poehlman, E.T., Toth, M.J., and Fonong, T.: Exercise, substrate utilization, and energy requirements in the elderly. *Intern. J. Obesity Related Metab. Disord.*, 19(Suppl.4): S93-S96, 1995.

40. Herring, J.L., Mole, P.A., Meredith, C.N., and Stern, J.S.: Effect of suspending exercise training on resting metabolic rate in women. *Med. Sci. Sport Exer.*, 24(1):59-65, 1992.

41. Toth, M.J. and Poehlman, E.T.: Sympathetic nervous system activity and resting metabolic rate in vegetarians. *Metab.: Clin. Exper.*, 43(5):621-625, 1994.

42. Racette, S.B., Schoeller, D.A., Kushner, R.F., and Neil, K.M.: Effects of aerobic exercise and dietary carbohydrate on energy expenditure and body composition during weight reduction in obese women. *Am. J. Clin. Nutri.*, 61 (3):486-494, 1995.

43. Svendsen, O.L., Hassager, C., and Christiansen, C.: Physical exercise as a supplement to diet: effects on body composition, resting metabolic rate, and cardiovascular risk factors in postmenopausal overweight women. *Ugeskrift for Laeger*, 156(41):6035-6038, 1994.

44. Shinkai, S., Watanabe, S., Kurokawa, Y., Torii, J., Asai, H., and Shephard, R.J.: Effects of 12 weeks of aerobic exercise plus dietary restriction on body composition, resting energy expenditure, and aerobic fitness in mildly obese middle-aged women. *Eur. J. Appl. Physiol. Occup. Physiol.*, 68(3):258-265, 1994.

45. Seers, K. and Carroll, D.: Relaxation techniques for acute pain management: a systematic review. *J. Adv. Nursing*, 27:466-475, 1998.

46. Sanborn, C.F. and Jankowski, C.M.: Physiologic considerations for women in sports. *Clin. North Am.*, 13(2):315-327, 1994.

47. Arciero, P.J., Goran, M.I., and Poehlman, E.T.: Resting metabolic rate is lower in women than in men. *J. Appl. Physiol.*, 75(6):2514-2520, 1993.

48. Spraul, M., Ravussin, E., Fontvieille, A.M., Rising, R., Larson, D.E., and Anderson, E.A.: Reduced sympathetic nervous activity: a potential mechanism predisposing to body weight gain. *J. Clin. Invest.*, 92(4):1730-1735, 1993.

49. Deriaz, O., Fournier, G., Tremblay, A., Despres, J.P., and Bouchard, C.: Lean-body-mass composition and resting energy expenditure before and after long-term overfeeding. *Am. J. Clin. Nutri.*, 56(5):840-847, 1992.

50. Shangold, M.M.: Exercise in menopausal women. *Obstet. Gyn.*, 75(Suppl.4):53S-58S, 1990.

51. Galduroz, J.C. and Carlini, E.A.: The effects of long-term administration of guarana on the cognition of normal, elderly volunteers. *Revista Paulista de Medicina*, 114(1):1073-1078, 1996.

52. Cunningham, J.J.: Body composition and resting metabolic rate: the myth of feminine metabolism. *Am. J. Clin. Nutri.*, 36(4):721-726, 1982.

53. Owen, O.E., Reichard, G.A., Jr., Patel, M.S., and Boden, G.: Energy metabolism in feasting and fasting. *Adv. Exper. Med. Biol.*, 111:169-188, 1979.

54. Lowe, J.C.: Results of an open trial of T_3 therapy with 77 euthyroid female fibromyalgia patients. *Clin. Bull. Myofascial Ther.*, 2(1):35-37, 1997.

55. Poehlman, E.T., Berke, E.M., Joseph, J.R., Gardner, A.W., Katzman-Rooks, S.M., and Goran, M.I.: Influence of aerobic capacity, body composition, and thyroid hormones on the age-related decline in resting metabolic rate. *Metab.: Clin. Exper.*, 41(8):915-921, 1992.

56. Poehlman, E.T., McAuliffe, T.L., Van Houten, D.R., and Danforth, E., Jr.: Influence of age and endurance training on metabolic rate and hormones in healthy men. *Am. J. Physiol.*, 259(1 Pt.1):E66-E72, 1990.

57. Korsten-Reck, U., Muller, H., Pokan, R., et al.: Prevention and therapy of obesity with diet and sports: an ambulatory therapy program for overweight children. *Wiener Medizinische Wochenschrift*, 140(9):232-240, 1990.

58. Koot, P. and Deurenberg, P.: Comparison of changes in energy expenditure and body temperatures after caffeine consumption. *Ann. Nutri. Metab.*, 39(3):135-142, 1995.

59. Yoshioka, K., Yoshida, T., Kamanaru, K., Hiraoka, N., and Kondo, M.: Caffeine activates brown adipose tissue thermogenesis and metabolic rate in mice. *J. Nutri. Sci. Vitaminology*, 36(2):173-178, 1990.

60. Dulloo, A.G., Geissler, C.A., Horton, T., Collins, A., and Miller, D.S.: Normal caffeine consumption: influences on thermogenesis and daily energy expenditure in lean and postobese human volunteers. *Am. J. Clin. Nutri.*, 49(1):44-50, 1989.

61. Tulp, O.L. and Buck, C.L.: Caffeine and ephedrine stimulated thermogenesis in LA-corpulent rats. *Pharmacol. Toxicol.*, 85(1):17-19, 1986.

62. Poehlman, E.T., LaChance, P., Tremblay, A., et al.: The effect of prior exercise and caffeine ingestion on metabolic rate and hormones in young adult males. *Can. J. Physiol. Pharmacol.*, 67(1):10-16, 1989.

63. LeBlanc, J., Jobin, M., Cote, J., Samson, P., and Labrie, A.: Enhanced metabolic response to caffeine in exercise-trained human subjects. *J. Appl. Physiol.*, 59(3):832-837, 1985.

64. Poehlman, E.T., Despres, J.P., Bessette, H., Fontaine, E., Tremblay, A., and Bouchard, C.: Influence of caffeine on the resting metabolic rate of exercise-trained and inactive subjects. *Med. Sci. Sports Exerc.*, 17(6):689-694, 1985.

65. Jung, R.T., Shetty, P.S., James, W.P., Barrand, M.A., and Callingham, B.A.: Caffeine: its effect on catecholamines and metabolism in lean and obese humans. *Clin. Sci.*, 60(5):527-535, 1981.

66. Campbell, W.W., Crim, M.C., Young, V.R., and Evans, W.J.: Increased energy requirements and changes in body composition with resistance training in older adults. *Am. J. Clin. Nutri.*, 60(2):167-175, 1994.

67. Ballor, D.L. and Poehlman, E.T.: Resting metabolic rate and coronary-heart-disease risk factors in aerobically and resistance-trained women. *Am. J. Clin. Nutri.*, 56(6):968-974, 1992.

68. Broeder, C.E., Burrhus, K.A., Svanevik, L.S., and Wilmore, J.H.: The effects of either high-intensity resistance or endurance training on resting metabolic rate. *Am. J. Clin. Nutri.*, 55(4):802-810, 1992.

69. Lemons, A.D., Kreitzman, S.N., Coxon, A., and Howard, A.: Selection of appropriate exercise regimens for weight reduction during VLCD and maintenance. *Intern. J. Obes.*, 13(Suppl.2):119-123, 1989.

70. Durnin, J.V.: Energy requirements of pregnancy. *Diabetes*, 40(Suppl.2):152-156, 1991.

71. van Raaij, J.M., Schonk, C.M., Vermaat-Miedema, S.H., Peek, M.E., and Hautvast, J.G.: Body fat mass and basal metabolic rate in Dutch women before, during, and after pregnancy: a reappraisal of the energy cost of pregnancy. *Am. J. Clin. Nutri.*, 49(5):765-772, 1989.

72. van Raaij, J.M., Schonk, C.M., Vermaat-Miedema, S.H., Peek, M.E., and Hautvast, J.G.: Energy cost of walking at a fixed pace and self-paced rate before, during, and after pregnancy. *Am. J. Clin. Nutri.*, 51(2):158-161, 1990.

73. Lawrence, M., Thongprasert, K., and Durnin, J.V.: Between-group differences in basal metabolic rates: an analysis of data collected in Scotland, Gambia, and Thailand. *Euro. J. Clin. Nutri.*, 42(10):877-891, 1988.

74. Thongprasert, K., Tanphaichitre, V., Valyasevi, A., Kittigool, J., and Durnin, J.V.: Energy requirements of pregnancy in rural Thailand. *Lancet*, 2(8566):1010-1012, 1987.

75. van Raaij, J.M., Schonk, C.M., Vermaat-Miedema, S.H., Peek, M.E., and Hautvast, J.G.: Energy requirements of pregnancy in the Netherlands. *Lancet*, 2(8565):953-955, 1987.

76. Durnin, J.V., McKillop, F.M., Grant, S., and Fitzgerald, G.: Energy requirements of pregnancy in Scotland. *Lancet*, 2(8564):897-900, 1987.

77. Contaldo, F., Scalfi, L., Coltorti, A., Di Palo, M.R., Martinelli, P., and Guerritore, T.: Reduced regulatory thermogenesis in pregnancy and overiectomized women. *Intern. J. Vit. Nutri. Res.*, 57(3):299-304, 1987.

78. Nagy, L.E. and King, J.C.: Energy expenditure of pregnant women at rest and walking self-paced. *Am. J. Clin. Nutri.*, 38(3):369-376, 1983.

79. Blackburn, M.W. and Calloway, D.H.: Basal metabolic rate and work energy expenditure of mature pregnant women. *J. Am. Dietet. Assoc.*, 69(1):24-28, 1976.

80. Toth, M.J. and Poehlman, E.T.: Resting metabolic rate and cardiovascular disease risk in resistance- and aerobic-trained middle-aged women. *Intern. J. Obesity Relat. Metab. Dis.*, 19(10):691-698, 1995.

81. Toth, M.J., Garner, A.W., and Poehlman, E.T.: Training status, resting metabolic rate, and cardiovascular disease risk in middle-aged men. *Metab.: Clin. Experi.*, 44(3):

340-347, 1995.

82. Elliot, D.L., Goldberg, L., and Kuehl, K.S.: Does aerobic conditioning cause a sustained increase in the metabolic rate? *Am. J. Med. Sci.*, 296(4):249-251, 1988.

83. Shah, M., Geissler, C.A., and Miller, D.S.: Metabolic rate during and after aerobic exercise in post-obese and lean women. *Euro. J. Clin. Nutri.*, 42(6):455-464, 1988.

84. Hill, J.O., Sparling, P.B., Shields, T.W., and Heller, P.A.: Effects of exercise and food restriction on body composition and metabolic rate in obese women. *Am. J. Clin. Nutri.*, 46(4):622-630, 1987.

85. Pratley, R., Nicklas, B., Rubin, M., et al.: Strength training increases resting metabolic rate and norepinephrine levels in healthy 50-to-65-year-old men. *J. Applied Physiol.*, 76(1):133-137, 1994.

86. Tzankoff, S.P. and Norris, A.H.: Effect of muscle mass decrease on age-related BMR changes. *J. Appl Physiol.*, 43:1001, 1977.

87. Gilliland, K. and Bullock, W.: Caffeine: a potential drug of abuse. *Advances in Alcohol and Substance Abuse*, 3: 53-73, 1983-1984.

88. Sawyer, D.A., Julia, H.L., and Turin, A.C.: Caffeine and human behavior: arousal, anxiety, and performance effects. *J. Behav. Med.*, 5:415-439, 1982.

89. Thayer, R.E.: Problem perception, optimism, and related states as a function of time of day (diurnal rhythm) and moderate exercise: two arousal systems in interaction. *Motiv. Emotion*, 11:19-36, 1987.

90. Thayer, R.E.: *The Biopsychology of Mood and Arousal.* New York, Oxford University Press, 1989.

91. Gilliland, K. and Bullock, W.: Ad lib caffeine consumption, symptoms of caffeinism and academic performance. *Am. J. Psychiat.*, 138:512-514, 1981.

92. Battig, K., Buzzi, R., Martin, J.R., and Feierabend, J.M.: The effects of caffeine on physiological functions and mental performance. *Experientia*, 40(11):1218-1223, 1984.

93. Thayer, R.E.: Toward a psychological theory of multidimensional activation (arousal). *Motivation and Emotion*, 2:1-34, 1978.

94. Thayer, R.E., Cook, M.W., Hooe, E.S., and Lotts, D.J.: Exercise-induced arousal change as a function of extraversion, neuroticism, and psychoticism. Paper presented at the International Conference on Personality and Individual Differences, Toronto, Canada, 1987.

95. Thayer, R.E. and Peters, D.P.: Smoking reduction, mood, and short brisk walks. Long Beach, California State University, unpublished manuscript, 1987.

96. Blaney, P.H.: Affect and memory: a review. *Psychol. Bull.*, 99:229-246, 1986.

97. Bower, G.H.: A history of introspection. *Psychol. Bull.*, 36:129-148, 1981.

98. Vaeroy, H., Abrahamsen, A., Førre, O., and Kass, E.: Treatment of fibromyalgia (fibrositis syndrome): a parallel double-blind trial with carisoprodol, paracetamol and caffeine (Domadril comp.) versus placebo. *Clin. Rheumatol.*, 8(2):245-250, 1989.

99. Dalen, P., Alvan, G., Wakelkamp, M., and Olsen, H.: Formation of meprobamate from carisoprodol is catalysed by CYP2C19. *Pharmacogenics*, 6(5):387-394, 1996.

100. Georges, J.M. and Heitkemper, M.M.: Dietary fiber and distressing gastrointestinal symptoms in mid-life women. *Nursing Res.*, 43(6):357-361, 1994.

101. Aicher, B. and Kraupp, O.: The value of fixed combination analgesics as exemplified by Thomapyrine. *Wiener Klinische Wochenschrift*, 108(8):219-233, 1996.

102. Metcalf, A.: Anorectal disorders: five common causes of pain, itching, and bleeding. *Postgrad. Med.*, 98(5):81ff, 1995.

103. Currier, S.R., Wilson, K.G., and Gautheir, S.T.: Caffeine and chronic low back pain. *Clin. J. Pain*, 11(3):214-219, 1995.

104. Hoyovadillo, C., Perezurizar, J., and Lopezmunoz, F.J.: Usefulness of the pain-induced functional impairment model to relate plasma levels of analgesics to their efficacy in rats. *J. Pharm. Pharmcol.*, 47(6):462-465, 1995.

105. Ward, N., Whitney, C., Avery, D., and Dunner, D.: The analgesic effects of caffeine in headache. *Pain*, 44:151-155, 1991.

106. Laska, E.M., Sunshine, A., Mueller, G., et al.: Caffeine as an analgesic adjuvant. *J.A.M.A.*, 251:1711-1718, 1984.

107. Lieberman, H.R., Wurtman, R.J., Emde, G.G., et al.: The effects of caffeine and aspirin on mood and performance. *J. Clin. Psychopharmacol.*, 7:315-319, 1987.

108. Kaiko, R.F., Wallensstein, S.L., Rogers, A.G., et al.: Analgesic and mood effects of heroin and morphine in cancer patients. *N. Engl. J. Med.*, 304:1501-1504, 1981.

109. Taenzer, P., Melzack, R., and Jeans, M.E.: Influence of psychological factors on postoperative pain, mood, and analgesic requirements. *Pain*, 24:331-342, 1986.

110. Ward, N., Bokan, J.A., Phillips, M., et al.: Antidepressants in concomitant chronic back pain and depression: doxepin and desipramine compared. *J. Clin. Psychiat.*, 45: 54-57, 1984.

111. Ward, N., Bokan, J., Ang, J., et al.: Differential effects of fenfluramine and dextroamphetamine on acute and chronic pain. In *Advances in Pain Research and Therapy*, Vol. 9. Edited by H.L. Fields, New York, Raven Press, 1985, pp.753-760.

112. Greden, J.F., Victor, B.S., Fontaine, P., et al.: Caffeine-withdrawal headache: a clinical profile. *Psychosomatics*, 21:411-418, 1980.

113. Erinoff, L., Kelly, P.H., Basura, M., et al.: Six-hydroxy-dopamine induced hyperactivity: neither sex differences nor caffeine stimulation are found. *Pharmacol. Biochem. Behav.*, 20:707-713, 1984.

114. Snyder, S.H. and Sklar, P.: Behavioral and molecular actions of caffeine: focus on adenosine. *J. Psychiat. Res.*, 18:91-106, 1984.

115. Galloway, M.P. and Roth, R.H.: Neuropharmacology of 3-isobutylmethylxanthine: effects on central noradrenergic systems *in vivo. J. Pharmacol. Exp. Ther.*, 227:1-8, 1983.

116. Harms, H.H., Wardch, G., and Mulder, A.H.: Adenosine modulates depolarization-induced release of ^{3}H-noradrenaline from slices of rat brain neocortex. *Eur. J. Pharmacol.*, 49:305-308, 1978.

117. Olpe, H.R., Jones, R.S.G., and Steinmann, M.W.: The locus coeruleus: actions of psychoactive drugs. *Experientia*, 39:242-249, 1983.

118. Gonzlez, J.P., Swell, R.D.E., and Spencer, P.S.J.: Evidence for central selective dopamine receptor stimulation in the mediation of nomifensine-induced hyperalgesia and

the effects of opiate antagonists. *Neuropharmacology*, 29: 1039-1045, 1981.

119. Robertson, J., Weston, R., Lewis, M.J., et al.: Evidence for the potentiation of the antinociceptive action of morphine by bromocriptine. *Neuropharmacology*, 20:1029-1032, 1981.

120. Misra, A.L., Pontani, R.B., and Vadlamani, N.L.: Stereospecific potentiation of opiate analgesia by cocaine: predominant role of noradrenaline. *Pain*, 28:129-138, 1987.

121. Yaksh, T.L., Durant, P.A.C., Gaumann, D.M., et al.: The use of receptor-selective agents as analgesics in the spinal cord: trends and possibilities. *J. Pain Sympt. Manag.*, 2: 129-138, 1987.

122. Seegers, A.J.M., Jager, L.P., Zandberg, P., et al.: The anti-inflammatory, analgesic, and antipyretic activities of non-narcotic analgesic drug mixtures in rats. *Arch. Int. Pharmacodyn.*, 251:237-254, 1981.

123. Kawachi, I., Willett, W.C., Colditz, G.A., Stampfer, M.J., and Speizer, F.E.: A prospective study of coffee drinking and suicide in women. *Arch. Intern. Med.*, 156(5):521-525, 1996.

124. Wadden, T.A., Mason, G., Foster, G.D., Stunkard, A.J., and Prange, A.J.: Effects of a very low calorie diet on weight, thyroid hormones, and mood. *Intern. J. Obesity*, 14(3):249-258, 1990.

125. Neuhauserberthold, M., Beine, S., Verwied, S.D., and Luhrmann, P.M.: Coffee consumption and total body water homeostasis as measured by fluid balance and bioelectrical impedance analysis. *Ann. Nutri. Metab.*, 41(1):29-36, 1997.

126. Guyton, A.C.: *Textbook of Medical Physiology*, 8th edition. Philadelphia, W.B. Saunders Co., 1991.

127. *Physician's Desk Reference*. Oradell, Medical Economics Company, Inc., 1990.

128. Willson, J.R., Beecham, C.T., and Carrington, E.R.: *Obstetrics and Gynecology*. Saint Louis, C.V. Mosby Co., 1975.

129. Chamberlain, G.J.: Cyriax's friction massage: a review. *J. Orthopaeic. Sports Physi. Ther.*, 4:(1)20,1982.

130. Akeson, W.H., Amiel, D., and LaViolette, D.: The connective tissue response to immobility: an accelerated aging response? *Experi. Geront.*, 3:289-301, 1968.

131. Guyton, A.C.: Personal communication, 1990.

132. Lowe, J.C.: Hypertonic fascia. *Dyn. Chiro.*, 8:28, 1990.

133. DeGowin, R.L. and DeGowin, E.L.: *Bedside Diagnostic Examination*, 3rd edition. New York, Macmillan Publishing Co., Inc., 1976.

134. Lowe, J.C.: Fascia and pre-menstrual headaches. *Mass. Ther. J.*, 30(2):21-24, Spring, 1991.

135. Lowe, J.C.: *Spasm*. Houston, McDowell Publishing Co., 1983.

136. Lowe, J.C.: *The Purpose and Practice of Myofascial Therapy* (Audio album). Houston, McDowell Publishing Co., 1989, tape 1.

137. Tarnopolsky, M.A.: Caffeine and endurance performance. *Sports Med.*, 18(2):109-125, 1994.

138. Berkowitz, B.A., Spector, S., and Pool, W.: The interaction of caffeine, theophylline, and theobromine with monoamine oxidase inhibitors. *Eur. J. Pharmacol.*, 16: 315-321, 1971.

139. Estler, C.-J.: Effects of alpha- and beta-adrenergic blocking agents and para-chlorphenylalanine on morphine- and caffeine-stimulated locomotor activity in mice. *Psychopharmacologia*, 28:261-268, 1973.

140. Degkwitz, R. and Sieroslawsky, H.: Erhohung der 5-hydroxyindolessogsaure-(HIES-): ausscheidung im harn nach coffein, pervitin und preludin. *Klin. Wochenschr*, 41: 902-905, 1963.

141. Rihs, M., Muller, C., and Baumann, P.: Caffeine consumption in hospitalized psychiatric patients. *Eur. Arch. Psychiat. Clin. Neurosci.*, 246(2):83-92, 1996.

142. Jain, N., Kemp, N., Adeyemo, O., Ruchanan, P., and Stone, T.W.: Anxiolytic activity of adenosine receptor activation in mice. *Brit. J. Pharmcol.*, 116(3):2127-2133, 1995.

143. Haleem, D.J., Yasmeen, A., Haleem, M.A., and Zafar, A.: 24-Hour withdrawal following repeated administration of caffeine attenuates brain serotonin but not tryptophan in rat brain—implications for caffeine-induced depression. *Life Sci.*, 57(19):PL285-PL292, 1995.

144. Naranjo, C.A., Hermann, N., Ozdemir, V., and Bremner, K.E.: Abuse of prescription and licit psychoactive substances by the elderly: issues and recommendations. *Cns Drugs*, 4(3):207-211, 1995.

145. Ferre, S., Popoli, P., Tinnerstaines, B., and Fuxe, K.: Adenosine A_1 receptor-dopamine D_1 receptor interaction in rat limbic system: modulation of dopamine D_1 receptor antagonist binding sites. *Neurosci. Lett.*, 208(2):109-112, 1996.

146. Jacobson, K.A., Vonlubitz, D.K.J.E., Daly, J.W, and Fredholm, B.B.: Adenosine receptor ligands: differences with acute versus chronic treatment. *Trends Pharmcol. Sci.*, 17(3):108-113, 1996.

147. Vansoeren, M., Mohr, T., Kjaer, M., and Graham, T.E.: Acute effects of caffeine ingestion at rest in humans with impaired epinephrine responses. *J. Appl. Physiol.*, 80(3): 999-1005, 1996.

148. Bertorelli, R., Ferri, N., Adami, M., and Ongini, E.: Effects of selective agonists and antagonists for A_1 or A_2 adenosine receptors on sleep-waking patterns in rats. *Drug Develop. Res.*, 37(2):65-72, 1996.

149. Sawynok, J. and Reid, A.: Caffeine antinociception: role of formalin concentration and adenosine A_1 and A_2 receptors. *Eur. J. Pharmcol.*, 298(2):105-111, 1996.

150. Sullivan, G.W., Luong, L.S., Carper, H.T., Barnes, R.C., and Mandell, G.L.: Methylxanthines with adenosine alter TNF-alpha-primed PMN activation. *Immunopharmacol.*, 31(1):19-29, 1995.

151. Ward, N., Whitney, C., Avery, D., and Dunner, D.: The analgesic effects of caffeine in headache. *Pain*, 44:151-155, 1991.

152. Schachtel, B.P., Fillingham, J.M., Lane, A.C., Thoden, W.R., and Baybutt, R.I.: Caffeine as an analgesic adjuvant: a double-blind study comparing aspirin with caffeine to aspirin and placebo in patients with sore throat. *Arch. Intern. Med.*, 151(4):733-737, 1991.

153. Migliardi, J.R., Armellino, J.J., Friedman, M., Gillings, D.B., and Beaver, W.T.: Caffeine as an analgesic adjuvant in tension headache. *Clin. Pharmacol. Therapeu.*, 56(5): 576-586, 1994.

154. Bracco, D., Ferrara, J.M., Arnaud, M.J., Jequier, E., and Schultz, Y.: Effects of caffeine on energy metabolism,

heart rate, and methylxanthine metabolism in lean and obese women. *Am. J. Physiol. Metab.*, 32(4):E671-E678, 1995.

155. Lorist, M.M., Snel, J., Mulder, G., and Kok, A.: Aging, caffeine, and information processing: an event-related potential analysis. *Electroencephalography Clin. Neurophysiol.: Evoked Potent.*, 96(5):453-467, 1995.

156. Koot, P. and Deurenberg, P.: Comparison of changes in energy expenditure and body temperatures after caffeine consumption. *Ann. Nutri. Metab.*, 39(3):135-142, 1995.

157. Hatano, Y., Mizumoto, K., Yoshiyama, T., Yamamoto, M., Iranami, H.: Endothelium-dependent and -independent vasodilation of isolated rat aorta induced by caffeine. *Am. J. Physiol.: Heart Circu.*, 38(5):H1678-H1684, 1995.

158. Williams, M. and Jarvis, M.F.: Adenosine antagonists as potential therapeutic agents. *Pharmacol. Biochem. Behav.*, 29(2):433-444, 1988.

159. Ammon, H.P.: Biochemical mechanism of caffeine tolerance. *Archiv. der Pharmazie*, 324(5):261-267, 1991.

160. Wolfrom, D. and Welsch, C.W.: Caffeine and the development of normal, benign, and carcinomatous human breast tissues: a relationship? *J. Med.*, 21(Suppl.5):225-250, 1990.

161. Powers, S.K. and Dodd, S.: Caffeine and endurance performance. *Sports Med.*, 2(3):165-174, 1985.

162. White, T.D.: Characteristics of neuronal release of ATP. *Prog. Neuro-Psychopharmol. Biol.*, 8(4-6):487-493, 1984.

163. Morse, E.E.: Effects of drugs on platelet function. *Ann. Clin. Lab. Sci.*, 7(1):68-71, 1977.

164. Lamarine, R.J.: Selected health and behavioral effects related to the use of caffeine. *J. Commun. Health*, 19(6):449-466, 1994.

165. Blaauw, R., Albertse, E.C., Beneke, T., Lombard, C.J., Laubscher, R., and Hough, F.S.: Risk factors for the development of osteoporosis in a South African population: a prospective analysis. *S. African Med. J.*, 84(6):328-332, 1994.

166. Nehlig, A. and Debry, G.: Consequences on the newborn of chronic maternal consumption of coffee during gestation and lactation: a review. *J. Am. Coll. Nutri.*, 13(1):6-21, 1994.

167. Folsom, A.R., McKenzie, D.R., Bisgard, K.M., Kushi, L.H., and Sellers, T.A.: No association between caffeine intake and postmenopausal breast cancer incidence in the Iowa Women's Health Study. *Am. J. Epidemiol.*, 138(6):380-383, 1993.

168. Reynolds, H.E., Jackson, V.F., and Musick, B.S.: Preoperative needle localization in the breast: utility of local anesthesia. *Radiology*, 187(2):503-505, 1993.

169. Slattery, M.L. and West, D.W.: Smoking, alcohol, coffee, tea, caffeine, and theobromine: risk of prostate cancer in Utah. *Cancer Cause Control*, 4(6):559-563, 1993.

170. Clauw, D.J., Ward, K., Katz, P., and Rajan, S.: Muscle intracellular magnesium levels correlated with pain tolerance in fibromyalgia (Abstract). *Arthritis Rheum.*, 37(51):R29, 1994.

171. Sawynok, J.: Pharmacological rationale for the clinical use of caffeine. *Drugs*, 49:37-50, 1995.

172. Kraetsch, H.G., Hummel, T., Lotsch, J., Kussat, R., and Kobal, G.: Analgesic effects of propyphenazone in comparison to its combination with caffeine. *Eur. J. Clin. Pharmacol.*, 49:377-382, 1996.

173. Kuntz, D. and Brossel, R.: Analgesic effect and clinical tolerability of the combination of paracetamol 500 mg and caffeine 50 mg versus paracetamol 400 mg and dextropropoxyphene 30 mg in back pain. *Presse Med.*, 25:1171-1174, 1996.

174. Rosenbaum, M. and Susser, M.: *Solving the Puzzle of Chronic Fatigue Syndrome.* Tacoma, Life Sciences Press, 1992.

175. Ferraccioli, G., Chirelli, L., and Scita, F.: EMG-biofeedback training in fibromyalgia syndrome. *J. Rheumatol.*, 14:820-825, 1987.

176. Ferraccioli, G., Cavalieri, F., Salaffi, F., Fontana, S., Scita, F., Nolli, M., and Maestri, D.: Neuroendocrinologic findings in primary fibromyalgia (soft tissue chronic pain syndrome) and in other chronic rheumatic conditions (rheumatoid arthritis, low back pain). *J. Rheumatol.*, 17:869-873, 1990.

177. Kaplan, K.H., Goldenberg, D.L., and Galvin-Nadeau, M.: The impact of a meditation-based stress reduction program on fibromyalgia. *Gen. Hosp. Psychiatry*, 15:284-289, 1993.

178. Teitelbaum, J.: *From Fatigued to Fantastic!* Garden City Park, Avery Publishing Group, 1996.

179. Sauberlich, H.E. and Canham, J.E.: Vitamin B_6. In *Modern Nutrition in Health and Disease*, 6th edition. Edited by R.S. Goodhart and M.E. Shils, Philadelphia, Lea & Febiger, 1980, pp.219-225.

180. Roe, D.A.: *Drug-Induced Nutritional Deficiencies.* AVI Publishing, 1976, pp.72, 83, 120, 217.

181. Carney, M.W.P.: Psychiatric aspects of folate deficiency. In *Folic Acid in Neurology, Psychiatry, and Internal Medicine.* Edited by M.I. Botez and E.H. Reynolds, New York, Raven Press, 1979.

182. Pauling, L.: *How to Live Longer and Feel Better.* New York, Avon Books, 1987.

183. Pauling, L.: *Vitamin C and the Common Cold.* New York, Bantam Books, 1971.

184. Hoffer, A.: Editorial: The true cost of cynicism. *J. Orthomolec. Med.*, 7(4):1-2, 1992.

185. Tepperman, J. and Tepperman, H.M.: *Metabolic and Endocrine Physiology*, 5th edition. Chicago, Year Book Medical Publishers, Inc., 1987.

186. Kariks, J. and Perry, S.W.: Folic acid deficiency in psychiatric patients. *Med. J. Aust.*, 1:1192-1195, 1970.

187. Thornton, W.E. and Thornton, B.P.: Folic acid, mental function, and dietary habits. *J. Clin. Psychiat.*, 39:315-322, 1978.

188. Gillette, C.A., Bullough, R.C., and Melby, C.L.: Postexercise energy expenditure in response to acute aerobic or resistive exercise. *Int. J. Sport Nutr.*, 4(4):347-360, 1994.

189. Reynolds, E.H.: Interrelationships between the neurology of folate and vitamin B_{12} deficiency. In *Folic Acid in Neurology, Psychiatry and Internal Medicine.* Edited by M.I. Botez and E.H. Reynolds, New York, Raven Press, 1979.

190. Fisher, D.A.: Physiological variations in thyroid hormones: physiological and pathophysiological considerations. *Clin. Chem.*, 42(1):135-139, 1996.

191. Gentile, F. and Aloj, S.M.: Congenital hypothyroidism: etiology and pathogenesis. *Annali dell Instituto Superiore di Sanita*, 30(3):299-308, 1994.

192. Larsen, P.R.: Tests of thyroid function. *Med. Clin. N. Am.*, 59:1063-1074, 1975.

193. Nettler, A.H.: *Health Questions & Answers.* New York, Pyramid Publications, 1976.

194. Johnson, A.C.: *Chiropractic Physiological Therapeutics*, 5th edition. Palm Springs, self published, 1977.

195. Williams, S.R.: *Nutrition and Diet Therapy,* 3rd edition. Saint Louis, C.V. Mosby Co., 1977.

196. Burton, B.T.: *Human Nutrition*, 3rd edition. New York, McGraw-Hill Book Co., 1976.

197. Romano, T.J. and Stiller, J.W.: Magnesium deficiency in fibromyalgia syndrome. *J. Nutr. Med.*, 4:165-167, 1994.

198. Clauw, D.J., Wilson, K., Phadia, S., Radulovic, D., and Katz, P.: Low tissue levels of magnesium in fibromyalgia (Abstract). *Arthritis Rheum.*, 37(52):R29, 1994.

199. Warburton, D.M.: Effects of caffeine on cognition and mood without caffeine abstinence. *Psychopharmocology*, 119(1):66-70, 1995.

200. Romano, T.J.: Magnesium deficiency in patients with myofascial pain. *J. Myofascial Ther.*, 1(3):11-12, 1994.

201. Smith, A., Maben, A., and Brockman, P.: Effects of evening meals and caffeine on cognitive performance, mood, and cardiovascular functioning. *Appetite*, 22(1):57-65, 1994.

Appendices

Appendix A

**FIBROMYALGIA ASSESSMENT FORMS
AND BLANK LINE GRAPHS**

Appendix B

**PUBLISHED PAPERS ON FIBROMYALGIA BY
DR. JOHN C. LOWE AND COLLEAGUES**

Appendix C

DEBATE WITH MICHAEL WEINTRAUB, M.D.

Appendix D

**CONVERSIONS:
T_4, T_3, AND DESICCATED THYROID**

Appendix A

**FIBROMYALGIA ASSESSMENT FORMS
AND BLANK LINE GRAPHS**

Assessment Instruments

Appendix A contains the forms needed to properly monitor and record the status of the fibromyalgia patient. Included are the following:

FibroQuest Questionnaire (long form)
FibroQuest Symptoms Survey (short form)
Fibromyalgia Impact Questionnaire (FIQ)
    Scoring Instructions for the FIQ
Body Drawings
    Blank Body Drawing
    Body Drawing with Tender Points
    Body Drawing with 36 Divisions
    Body Drawing with 36 Divisions (and
        percentage value of each division)
    Sample of Form Completed by Patient
        and Clinician
Blank Line Graphs
    Graph for Mean Symptom Intensity
    Graph for Pain Distribution
    Graph for Mean Tender Point Scores
        (pressure/pain threshold)
    Graph for FIQ Scores
    Graph for Zung's or Beck Depression Scores

The forms in this appendix should be copied and used to assess and record patient status. For instructions on the use of the forms, refer to Chapters 4.1 and 5.2.

METHODS FOR ASSESSING FIBROMYALGIA STATUS

We use five methods, described below, to evaluate fibromyalgia status. The forms needed to employ the methods and record the results are included in this appendix.

FibroQuest Questionnaire (long form)

The FibroQuest Questionnaire is the initial history form we use. The answers elicited from the patient by the questions in the form usually serve as jumping off points for further inquiry during history taking and the initial examination. The FibroQuest Questionnaire contains the visual analog scales for the 13 most common fibromyalgia symptoms that are also contained in the FibroQuest Symptoms Survey used for subsequent evaluations of fibromyalgia status (see next section).

FibroQuest Symptoms Survey (short form)

The FibroQuest Symptoms Survey consists of visual analog scales for 13 of the most common fibromyalgia symptoms. After the patient rates the intensity of all the symptoms she has on that date, the values should be added, and the sum divided by the number of symptoms the patient had *at the first evaluation*. The mean of the values should be posted as a data point to the Mean Symptom Intensity line graph.

Pain Distribution: Percentage Method

To determine the patient's pain distribution according to the percentage method, the clinician needs the body drawing and a transparency template that contains the 36 body divisions and the percentage value of each division. The template can be made by copying the Body Drawing with 36 Divisions (and percentage value of each division) onto a transparency sheet. The patient should shade in her pain distribution as accurately as possible. By placing the transparency template over the shaded drawing, the percentage value of each painful body region can be determined. The percentages for all of the body divisions containing shading should be totaled to arrive at the percentage of the patient's body in pain. The percentage should be posted as a data point to the Pain Distribution line graph.

Mean Tender Point Scores

The clinician should use an algometer to measure the pressure/pain threshold of each of the 16 possible tender points. (I have excluded the upper cervical tender points because of the intense discomfort most patients experience when pressure is applied to these points.) The value for each tender point should be posted at the appropriate site on the body drawing the patient has shaded to show her pain distribution. The pressure/pain thresholds of the 16 points should be totaled and then divided by 16. The result is the mean of the 16 tender point pressure/pain thresholds. The clinician should next post the mean value as a data point to the line graph for Mean Tender Point Scores.

FIQ

The standard instrument for assessing the functional status of fibromyalgia patients is the Fibromyalgia Impact Questionnaire (FIQ). With the kind permission of Carol Burckhardt, Ph.D., we have provided the latest updated version of the FIQ questionnaire and scoring instructions. The grand score for the FIQ should be posted as a data point to the FIQ line graph.

Depression Assessment

The score from the depression instrument should be posted as a data point to the Depression Scores line graph. Although I have always used Zung's Self-Rating Depression Scale, the Beck Depression Inventory is equivalent. It does not matter which instrument is used. Any other instrument for assessing depression that studies have shown to be valid and reliable will also serve the intended purpose.

Zung's Self-Rating Depression Scale. Clini-cians can obtain a manual on the instrument and copies of assessment forms from Eli Lilly & Company. Contact information:

Eli Lilly & Company
Lilly Corporate Center
Indianapolis, Indiana 46285
Customer Service number: (800) 545-5979

Qualifications for obtaining the form: Must be a doctoral level "health care provider" (D.C., D.D.S., D.M.D., D.O., D.P.M., M.D., N.D., O.D., Ph.D.), pharmacist, nurse practitioner, or physician's assistant.

Beck Depression Inventory. Clinicians can obtain a manual on the instrument and copies of assessment forms from The Psychological Corporation. Contact information:

The Psychological Corporation
Post Office Box 839954
San Antonio, TX 78283-3954
Customer Service number: (800) 211-8378

Qualifications for obtaining the form: Health care provider must have (1) doctorate (D.C., D.D.S., D.M.D., D.O., D.P.M., M.D., N.D., O.D., Ph.D.) or (2) a Master's degree with training in psychological assessment (M.A., M.S., M.S.W., etc.). Request a "qualification form" from Customer Service. The form must be completed and returned.

FIBROQUEST
Questionnaire

Answer the questions below as best you can. I know symptoms tend to vary over time, so answer the questions in light of your symptoms over the past month or so. For example, you may have been in pain for several years. If you want to make a note about this, please do so. But in answering the questions about pain, reflect back over how you've felt over the past month or so. If you're not certain about some option I've given you, use your best judgment at the moment. Just pick the option that seems more correct than the others. If you want to say something about a question, please feel free to write your comment. Thank you in advance for completing this form. © 1995 John C. Lowe

Name:_____ Today's Date:_____ Occupation:_____

Phone:_____Are you still working? ☐ Yes ☐ No   If not, about how long has it been since you worked?

_____ Years & ____ Months Why did you stop work?_____ How do you spend most of your day?

☐ standing   ☐ walking   ☐ sitting   ☐ lying   ☐ lifting

☐ typing   ☐ using phone   ☐ computer work   ☐ driving   ☐ other:_____

What is your **main** complaint?_____ What was the initial cause?_____

_____ When did it begin?_____ What seems to aggravate it?_____

_____ What do you think causes your pain?_____

_____ Has anything given you relief ? _____

Is it getting worse?_____ Does it interfere with your: ☐ work ☐ sleep ☐ recreational or leisure activities

☐ family or marital responsibilities   ☐ other aspects of your life? (Please specify)_____

I suffer from this ☐ when I wake up ☐ later in the day ____% of my waking hours.

"Your main complaint." (Marking "0" means the symptom doesn't bother you. "10" is as severe as possible.)

0	1	2	3	4	5	6	7	8	9	10

Check the appropriate boxes: I'm pregnant. ☐ Yes ☐ No   I wear a pacemaker. ☐ Yes ☐ No

I take anticoagulant drugs. ☐ Yes ☐ No   I'm allergic to the following drugs or foods:_____

I've been diagnosed as having cancer. ☐ Yes ☐ No   I have problems with my blood circulation. ☐ Yes ☐ No

If you smoke tobacco, how many packs per day?___ __   If you drink alcoholic beverages, about how much and how often?_____

Do you wear orthotics?_____ How often do you have headaches?_____

Do you use caffeine tablets such as NoDoz or Vivarin?_____If so, how much and how often?_____

If you are sexually active, are there any problems?_____I live: ☐ with my spouse alone ☐ with my family

☐ with a friend ☐ alone. I'm ☐ satisfied ☐ dissatisfied with this arrangement. Are you aware of having any heart problem ? ☐ Yes ☐ No   or adrenal gland problem ? ☐ Yes ☐ No

Please list medical conditions (other accidents, illnesses, infections, pain, or disabilities) within the past 10 years:

Condition	Date	Condition	Date

PREVIOUS TREATMENT

Please list the other health care providers you have seen for your present condition.

Name	Type of Practitioner	Date	Results (Diagnosis if you recall)

1060

MEDICATIONS

List all medications you are presently (or have recently been) taking:

Medication	Dosage	Medication	Dosage
_____	_____	_____	_____
_____	_____	_____	_____
_____	_____	_____	_____
_____	_____	_____	_____

Have you ever taken oral contraceptives? If so, for how long?_____ Are you still taking them? ☐ Yes ☐ No If not, when did you stop?_____ Do you still have menstrual periods? ☐ Yes ☐ No If no, check either of the following: (1) I became menopausal naturally ☐ (2) I had a hysterectomy ☐ (what year?): _____. If you still have menstrual periods, are they ☐ normal ☐ irregular ☐ painful ☐ short ☐ prolonged? Do you have ☐ heavy or ☐ light flow? Are you peri-menopausal? ☐ Yes ☐ No Do you use any form of female sex hormone replacement? Please describe:_____

VITAMINS, MINERALS, & HERBS List any vitamins, mineral, and/or herbs you take:

Vitamin, Mineral, Herb	How often	Vitamin, Mineral, Herb	How Often
_____	_____	_____	_____
_____	_____	_____	_____
_____	_____	_____	_____
_____	_____	_____	_____
_____	_____	_____	_____
_____	_____	_____	_____

DIET Please describe your eating habits (time of day and foods you usually consume): _____

Are you vegetarian? ☐ Yes ☐ No Do you eat sugary foods each day? ☐ Yes ☐ No When you don't eat at regular intervals, do you feel (check all that apply) ☐ dizzy ☐ faint ☐ clammy ☐ headachy ☐ shaky ☐ pounding heart? Does eating relieve these feelings? ☐ Yes ☐ No What foods relieve the feelings?_____

If you restrict your food intake for weight control, do you do so ☐ regularly or ☐ at intervals? About how many glasses of liquids do you drink each day?_____ Of the following caffeinated drinks, how many cups, cans, or bottles do you usually consume each day? coffee____ tea____ soft drinks ____.
List any symptoms the caffeine improves:_____

PAIN Would you describe your pain as (check all that apply) ☐ mild ☐ moderate ☐ severe? ☐ sharp ☐ dull ☐ burning ☐ aching ☐ throbbing? ☐ having clear-cut boundaries (you could specifically outline its margins with your finger) or ☐ hazy boundaries (fades as it spreads from the most intense area)?

How intense has your pain been? (Marking "0" means you have no pain. "10" is as severe as possible.)

0   1   2   3   4   5   6   7   8   9   10

How tired have you felt? ("0" means you have no fatigue. "10" means you have the worse fatigue possible.)

0   1   2   3   4   5   6   7   8   9   10

STIFFNESS When I get up in the morning, I am ☐ not stiff ☐ mildly stiff ☐ moderately stiff ☐ severely stiff.
It takes _____ hours and/or _____minutes to loosen up.
Describe:_____

How stiff have you felt? (Marking "0" means you haven't felt stiff. "10" means you've felt severely stiff.)
0   1   2   3   4   5   6   7   8   9   10

HEADACHES Please describe:_____

How intense have your headaches been? (Marking "0" means no headaches. "10" means as severe as possible.)
0   1   2   3   4   5   6   7   8   9   10

SLEEP (check appropriate boxes) ☐ I have no trouble sleeping. ☐ I often have trouble sleeping. ☐ I sometimes have trouble sleeping. ☐ I always have insomnia. ☐ My pain wakes me during the night.
I usually wake up feeling: ☐ refreshed ☐ better ☐ as tired as when I went to bed ☐ mentally and physically sluggish.
What position(s) do you usually sleep in? ☐ Face down ☐ On my back ☐ Left side ☐ Right side. How old is your mattress?_____

How disturbed has your sleep been? ("0" means you've had no sleep disturbance. "10" means severely disturbed.)
0   1   2   3   4   5   6   7   8   9   10

STOMACH, INTESTINAL, AND URINARY SYSTEM
I usually have:

	Mild	Moderate	Severe
1) diarrhea or watery stools:	☐	☐	☐
2) constipation (need to strain/hard stool):	☐	☐	☐
3) bloating (intestinal gas):	☐	☐	☐
4) abdominal cramps:	☐	☐	☐
5) abdominal pain:	☐	☐	☐

How many times do you usually urinate each day?_____

How disturbed has your bowel function been? ("0" means your bowel function is fine. "10" means severely disturbed.)
0   1   2   3   4   5   6   7   8   9   10

EMOTIONS
Most of the time lately I feel: ☐ happy ☐ relaxed ☐ worried ☐ depressed ☐ sad ☐ anxious ☐ contented ☐ enthusiastic ☐ irritable ☐ calm ☐ angry ☐ pleasant ☐ restless ☐ friendly

How depressed have you felt? (Marking "0" means no depression. "10" means the worse depression possible.)
0   1   2   3   4   5   6   7   8   9   10

THINKING AND ATTENTION Do you have problems with ☐ memory ☐ concentration? Further description:_____
_____

How bad have your concentration and/or memory been? ("0" means fine. "10" means as bad as possible.)

0   1   2   3   4   5   6   7   8   9   10

If you experience anxiety, it is: ☐ often ☐ seldom ☐ brief ☐ long-lasting ☐ mild ☐ moderate ☐ severe

How anxious have you felt? (Marking "0" means no anxiety. "10" means the worse anxiety possible.)

0   1   2   3   4   5   6   7   8   9   10

I'm usually cold ☐ or hot ☐ when others around me are comfortable. Which body parts are too cold or hot? ☐ hands
☐ feet ☐ most of my body   Further description?_____

How cold have you felt? (Marking "0" means you haven't been too cold. "10" means severely cold.)

0   1   2   3   4   5   6   7   8   9   10

I have abnormal sensations (such as tingling or numbness) in my: ☐ hands ☐ feet ☐ other body parts:_____
Please describe your abnormal sensation(s):_____

How much numbness or tingling have you felt? (Marking "0" means none. "10" means severe numbness or tingling.)

0   1   2   3   4   5   6   7   8   9   10

I have dryness of my: ☐ eyes ☐ mouth ☐ hair ☐ other:_____

How dry have your mucous membranes, skin, or hair been? ("0" means not dry. "10" means the worst possible.)

0   1   2   3   4   5   6   7   8   9   10

EXERCISE AND ACTIVITY I have trouble exercising. ☐ Yes ☐ No I have the energy and endurance I need to exercise.
☐ Yes ☐ No   My symptoms worsen after I exercise. ☐ Yes ☐ No   Which symptoms worsen?_____
_____ How long do the worsened symptoms last?_____
How many days per week do you engage in the following?
1) aerobic exercise:_____   Mark which aerobic activities you engage in: ☐ walking ☐ running ☐ aerobics
                                                          ☐ other: _____
2) stretching exercises:_____   Mark which stretching activities: ☐ yoga ☐ martial arts
                                                          ☐ others:_____
3) toning exercises:_____   Mark which toning activities: ☐ weights at a gym or home ☐ calisthenics
                                                          ☐ other:_____

How difficult is it for you to exercise? (Marking "0" means exercise is not difficult. "10" means severe difficulty.)

0   1   2   3   4   5   6   7   8   9   10

FIBROQUEST
Symptoms Survey

Name..**Date**..............................
    The symptoms of fibromyalgia are listed in large, bold print below. The shaded boxes below the symptom names contain numbers 0 through 10 along a line. Indicate the level of your experience *since your last evaluation* by marking an "X" at the appropriate spot along the line. "0" means you have *not* experienced the symptom. "10" means the symptom has been as bad as possible. © 1995 John C. Lowe

Pain   How *intense* has your pain been?

0	1	2	3	4	5	6	7	8	9	10

Fatigue   How tired have you felt?

0	1	2	3	4	5	6	7	8	9	10

Stiffness   How stiff have you felt?

0	1	2	3	4	5	6	7	8	9	10

Headaches   How intense have your headaches been?

0	1	2	3	4	5	6	7	8	9	10

Sleep Disturbance   How disturbed has your sleep been?

0	1	2	3	4	5	6	7	8	9	10

Bowel Disturbance   How disturbed has your bowel function been?

0	1	2	3	4	5	6	7	8	9	10

Depression   How depressed have you felt?

0	1	2	3	4	5	6	7	8	9	10

(Please complete the opposite side of this sheet.)

Memory & Concentration   How bad have your memory and concentration been?

0	1	2	3	4	5	6	7	8	9	10

Anxiety   How anxious have you been?

0	1	2	3	4	5	6	7	8	9	10

Coldness   How cold have you been (whether your hands, feet, or whole body)?

0	1	2	3	4	5	6	7	8	9	10

Numbness or Tingling   How much of these sensations have you experienced?

0	1	2	3	4	5	6	7	8	9	10

Dry Tissues   How dry have your mucous membranes, skin, or hair been?

0	1	2	3	4	5	6	7	8	9	10

ADDITIONAL QUESTIONS Please answer the following questions about your status since your last evaluation.

1. Approximately how many times per day do you urinate? _____

2. If you have exercised, check below what type, and indicate how long or how intensely:
   - ☐ Aerobic exercise
      How many days per week:_____
      How long each time:_____(minutes)
   - ☐ Toning exercise
      How many days per week:_____
      How intensely: ☐ mildly ☐ moderately ☐ severely
   - ☐ Stretching exercise
      How many days per week:_____
      How intensely: ☐ mildly ☐ moderately ☐ severely

Exercise   How difficult is it for you to exercise?

0	1	2	3	4	5	6	7	8	9	10

Fibromyalgia Impact Questionnaire (FIQ)

Date _____

Name _____

Directions: For questions 1 through 11, please circle the number that best describes how you did overall for the past week. If you don't normally do something that is asked, cross out the question.

Have you been able to:	Always	Most times	Occasionally	Never
1. Do shopping?	0	1	2	3
2. Do laundry with a washer and dryer?	0	1	2	3
3. Prepare meals?	0	1	2	3
4. Wash dishes/cooking utensils by hand?	0	1	2	3
5. Vacuum a rug?	0	1	2	3
6. Make beds?	0	1	2	3
7. Walk several blocks?	0	1	2	3
8. Visit friends or relatives?	0	1	2	3
9. Do yard work?	0	1	2	3
10. Drive a car?	0	1	2	3
11. Climb stairs?	0	1	2	3

12. Of the 7 days in the past week, how many days did you feel good?   0 1 2 3 4 5 6 7 (circle one)

13. How many days last week did you miss work, including housework, because of fibromyalgia?
     0 1 2 3 4 5 6 7 (circle one)

Directions: For the remaining items, mark the point on the line that best indicates how you felt *overall* for the past week. (**Note:** Marking the extreme left end of the line means you had *no* difficulty with a problem or symptom. Marking the extreme right end means that you had *great* difficulty with the problem or symptom.)

14. When you worked, how much did pain or other symptoms of your fibromyalgia interfere with your ability to do your work, including housework?

     0   1   2   3   4   5   6   7   8   9   10

15. How bad has your pain been?

     0   1   2   3   4   5   6   7   8   9   10

16. How tired have you been?

     0   1   2   3   4   5   6   7   8   9   10

17. How have you felt when you got up in the morning?

     0   1   2   3   4   5   6   7   8   9   10

18. How bad has your stiffness been?

     0   1   2   3   4   5   6   7   8   9   10

19. How tense, nervous, or anxious have you felt?

     0   1   2   3   4   5   6   7   8   9   10

20. How depressed or blue have you felt?

     0   1   2   3   4   5   6   7   8   9   10

Fibromyalgia Impact Questionnaire (FIQ)

PURPOSE
The FIQ is an assessment and evaluation instrument developed to measure fibromyalgia (FM) patient status, progress, and outcomes. It has been designed to measure the components of health status that are believed to be most affected by FM.

CONTENTS
The FIQ is composed of 20 items. The first 11 items make up a physical functioning scale. Each item is rated on a 4 point likert-type scale. Items 12 and 13 ask patients to mark the number of days they felt well and number of days they were unable to work because of FM symptoms. Items 14 through 20 are 10 centimeter visual analog scales marked in 1 centimeter increments on which the patient rates work difficulty, pain, fatigue, morning stiffness, anxiety, and depression.

ADMINISTRATION
The FIQ is a brief, self-administered instrument that takes approximately 5 minutes to complete. The directions are simple and self-explanatory.

SCORING
The FIQ is scored in such a way that a higher score indicates a greater impact of the syndrome on the person. The questionnaire is scored in the following manner:

1. Items 1 through 11 are scored and summed to yield one physical impairment score. Raw scores on each item can range from 0 (always) to 3 (never). Because some patients may not do some of the tasks listed, they are given the option of deleting the items from scoring. In order to obtain a valid summed score for items 1 through 11, the scores for the items that the patient has rated are summed and divided by the number of items rated. An average raw score between 0 and 3 is obtained in this manner.

2. Item 12 is recoded so that a higher number indicates impairment (i.e., 0 = 7, 7 = 0, etc.). Raw scores can range from 0 to 7.

3. Item 13 is scored as number of days the patient was unable to do regular work activities. Raw scores can range from 0 to 7.

4. Items 14 through 20 are scored in 1 centimeter increments. Raw scores can range from 0 to 10. If the patient marks the space between two vertical lines on any item, that item is given a score that includes .5.

5. Once the initial scoring has been completed, the resulting scores are subjected to a normalization procedure so that all scores are expressed in similar units. The range of normalized scores is 0 to 10 with 0 indicating no impairment and 10 indicating maximum impairment.

SCALE	ITEMS	RECODE	SCORE	RANGE NORMALIZATION
*Physical Impairment	1-11	No	0-3	S x 3.33 (S = raw or summed score)
*Feel Good	12	Yes	0-7	S x 1.43
Work Missed	13	No	0-7	S x 1.43
Do Job	14	No	0-10	None
*Pain	15	No	0-10	None
*Fatigue	16	No	0-10	None
*Rested	17	No	0-10	None
*Stiffness	18	No	0-10	None
*Anxiety	19	No	0-10	None
*Depression	20	No	0-10	None

6. Starred (*) items may be combined into a total score of fibromyalgia impact which ranges from 0 to 80.

Citation: Burckhardt, C.S., Clark, S.R., and Bennett, R.M.: The Fibromyalgia Impact Questionnaire: Development and validation. *J. Rheumatol.*, 18:728-734, 1991.

Address for copies

Carol S. Burckhardt, Ph.D.
School of Nursing, SN-4S
Oregon Health Sciences University
Portland, OR 97201-3098

Phone: (503) 494-3895
Fax: (503) 494-3691
E-mail: burckhac@ohsu.edu

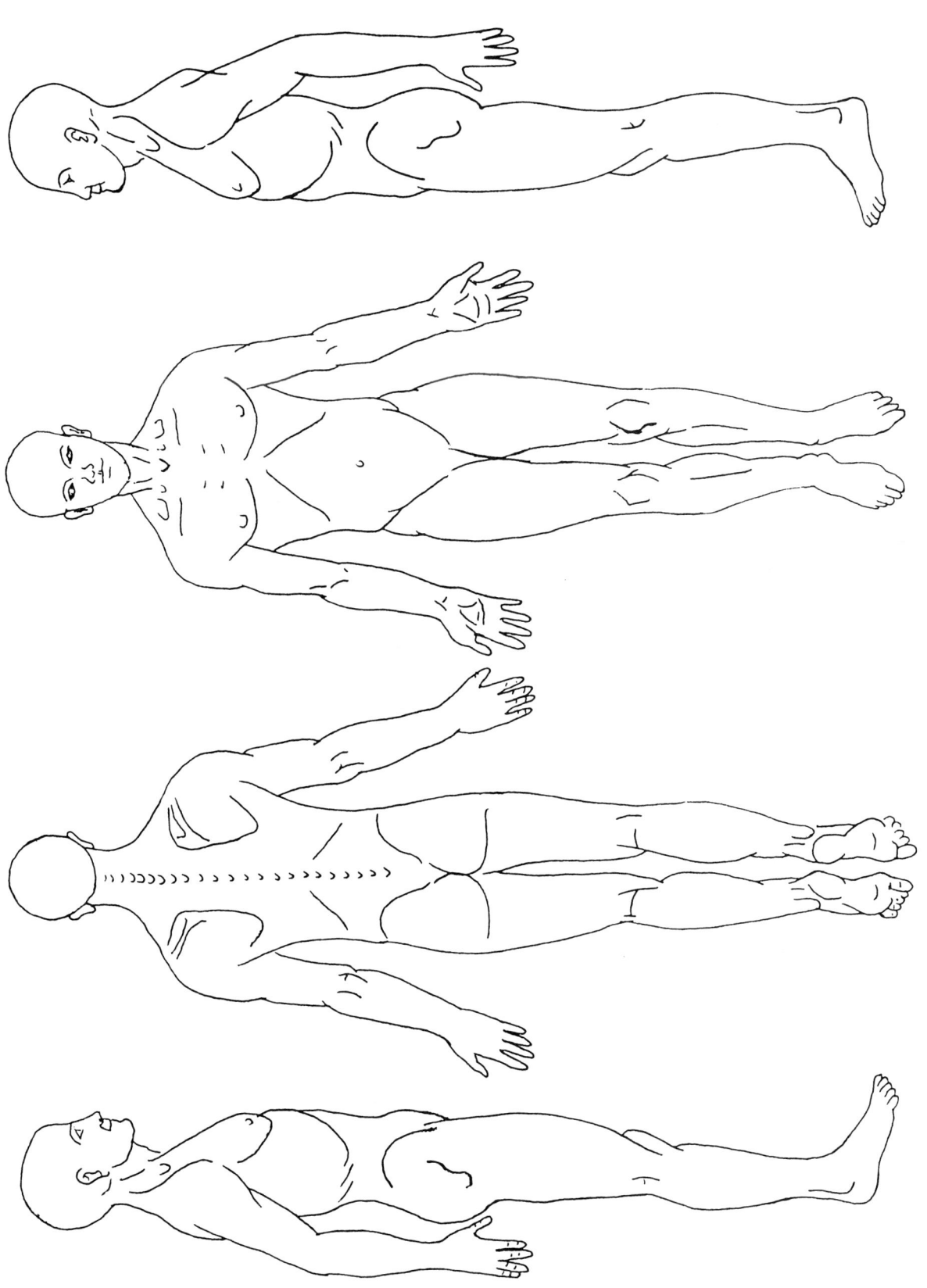

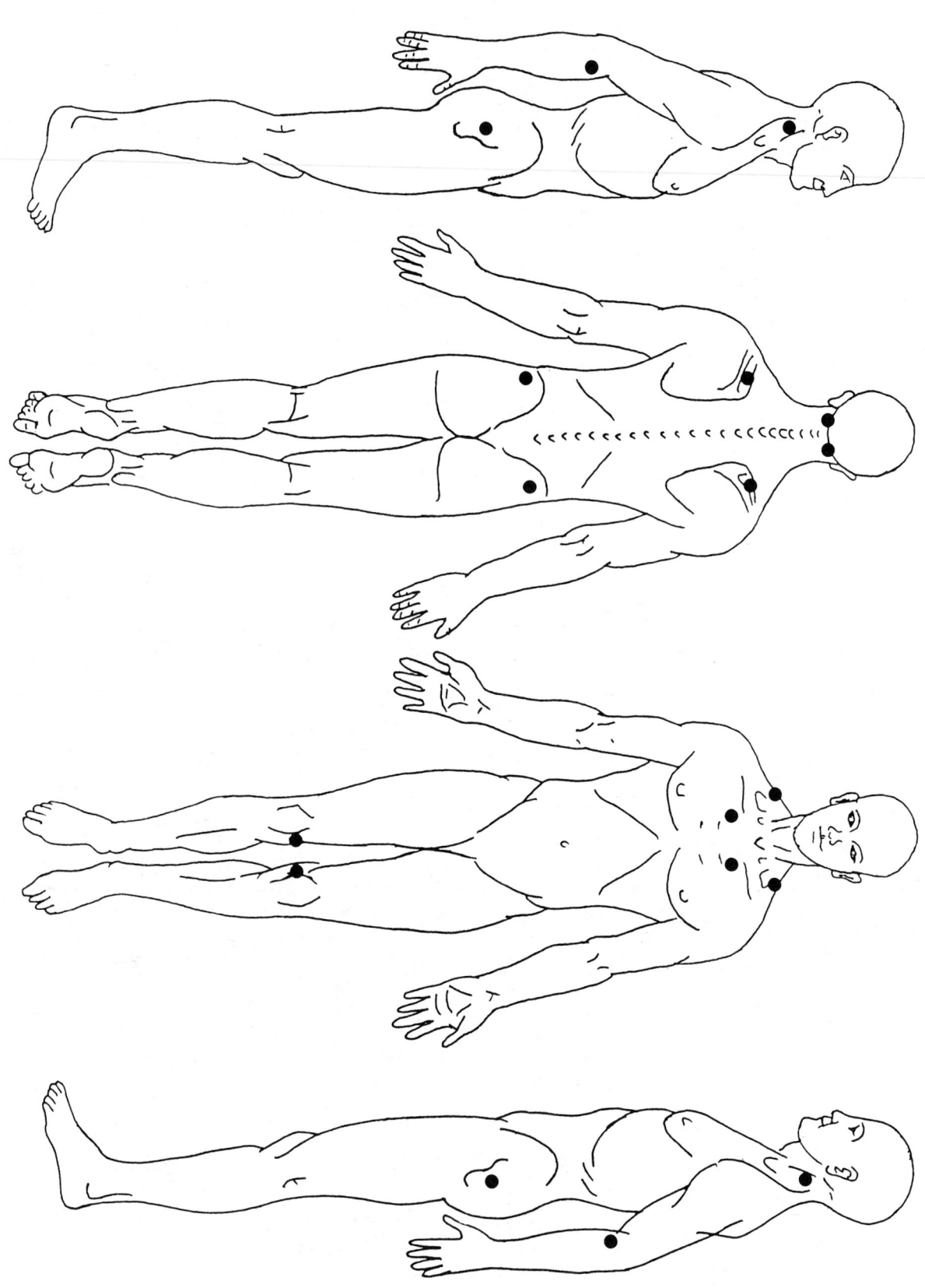

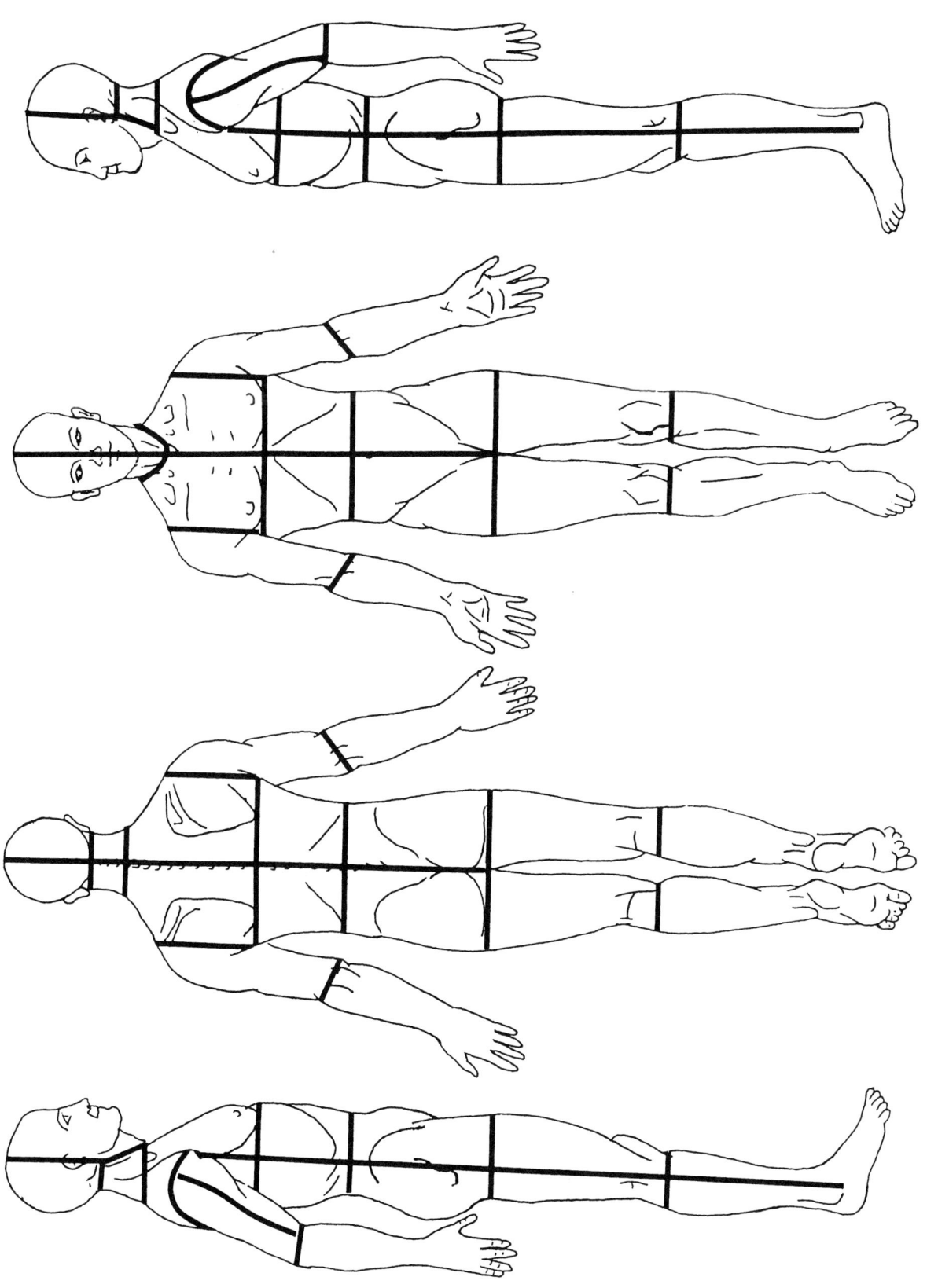

1070

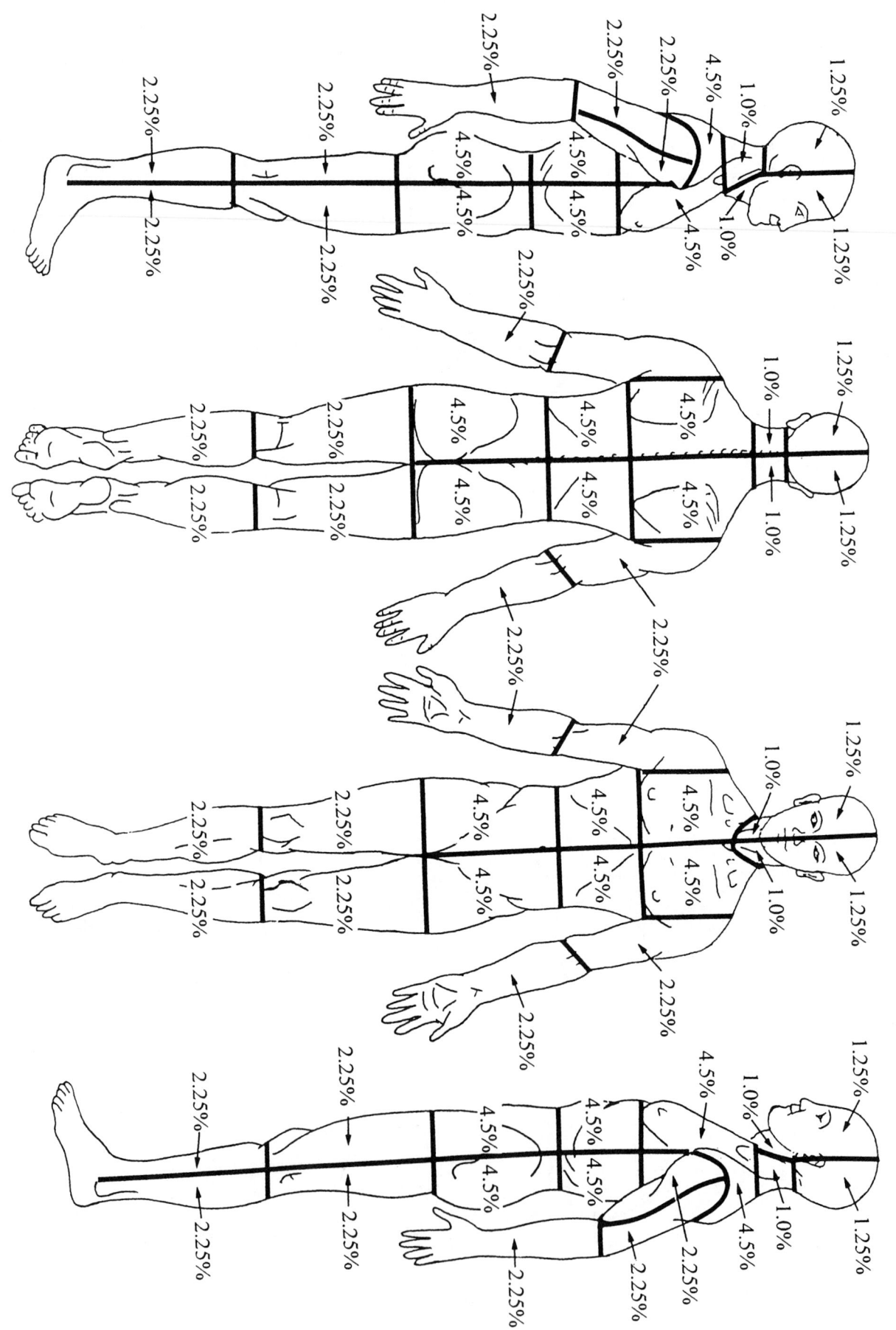

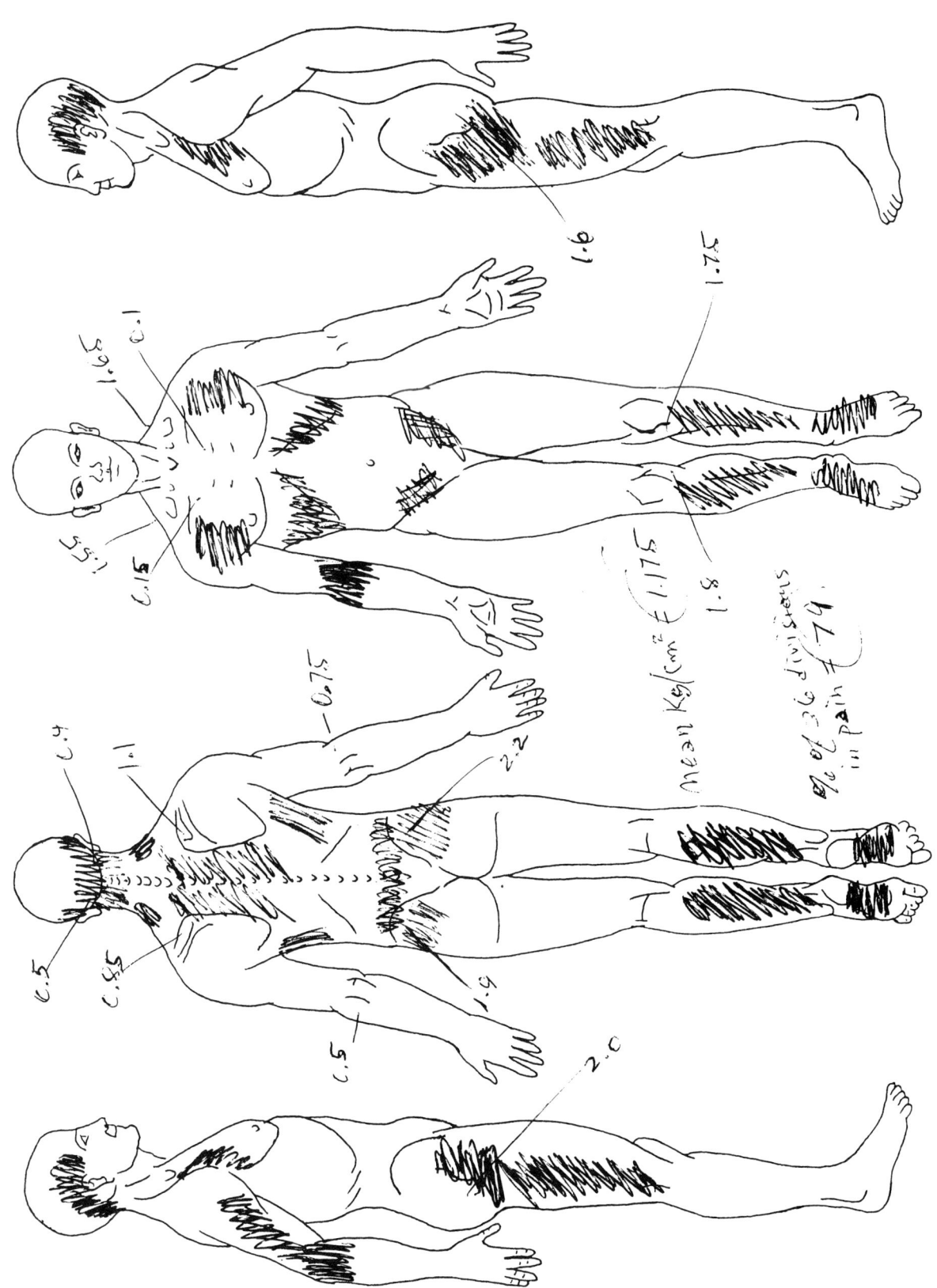

mean kg/cm² = 1.175

% of 36 individuals in pain = 74

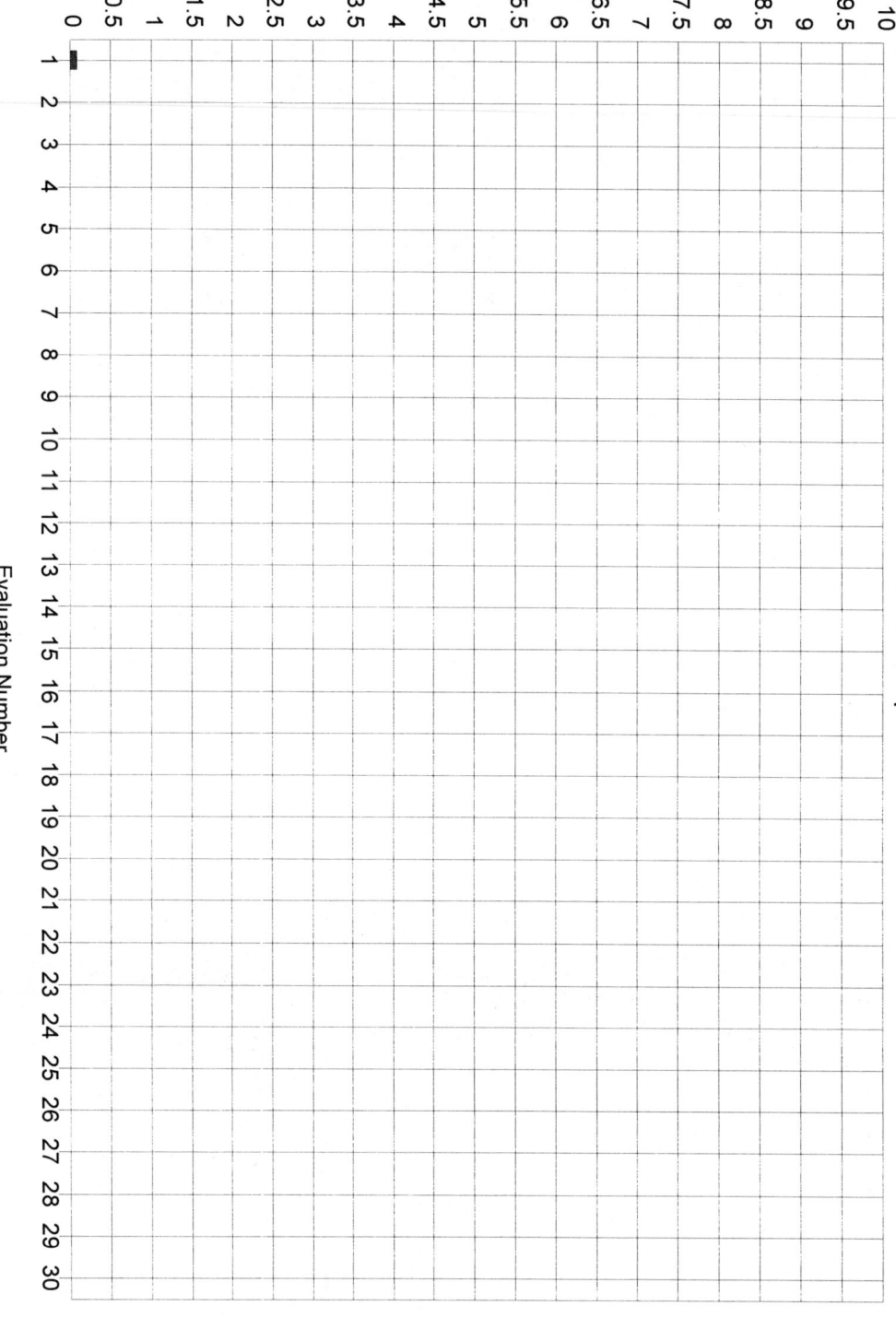

Mean Symptoms Intensity
Line Graph

Mean Intensity

Evaluation Number

Pain Distribution
Line Graph

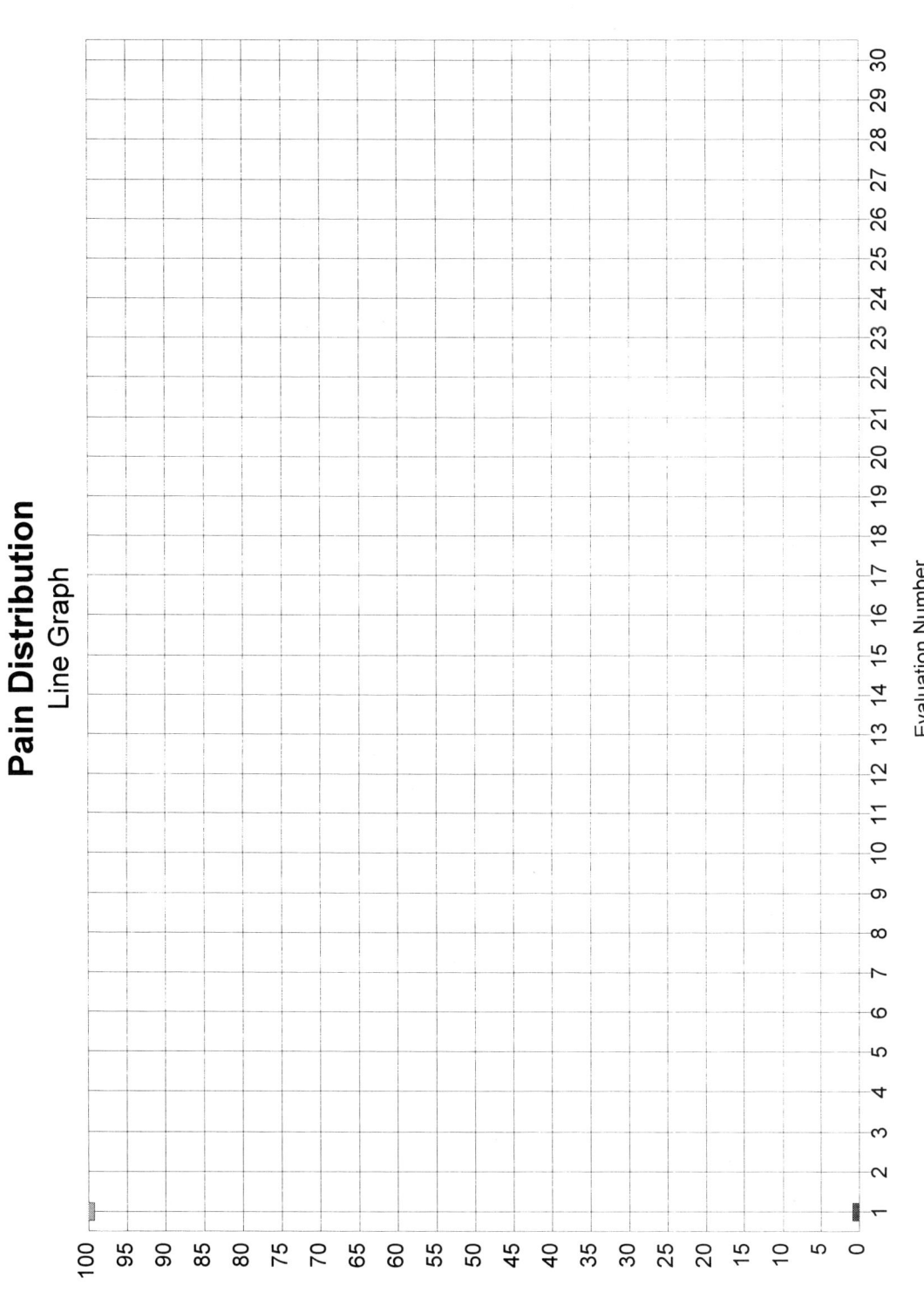

Mean Tender Point Scores
Line Graph

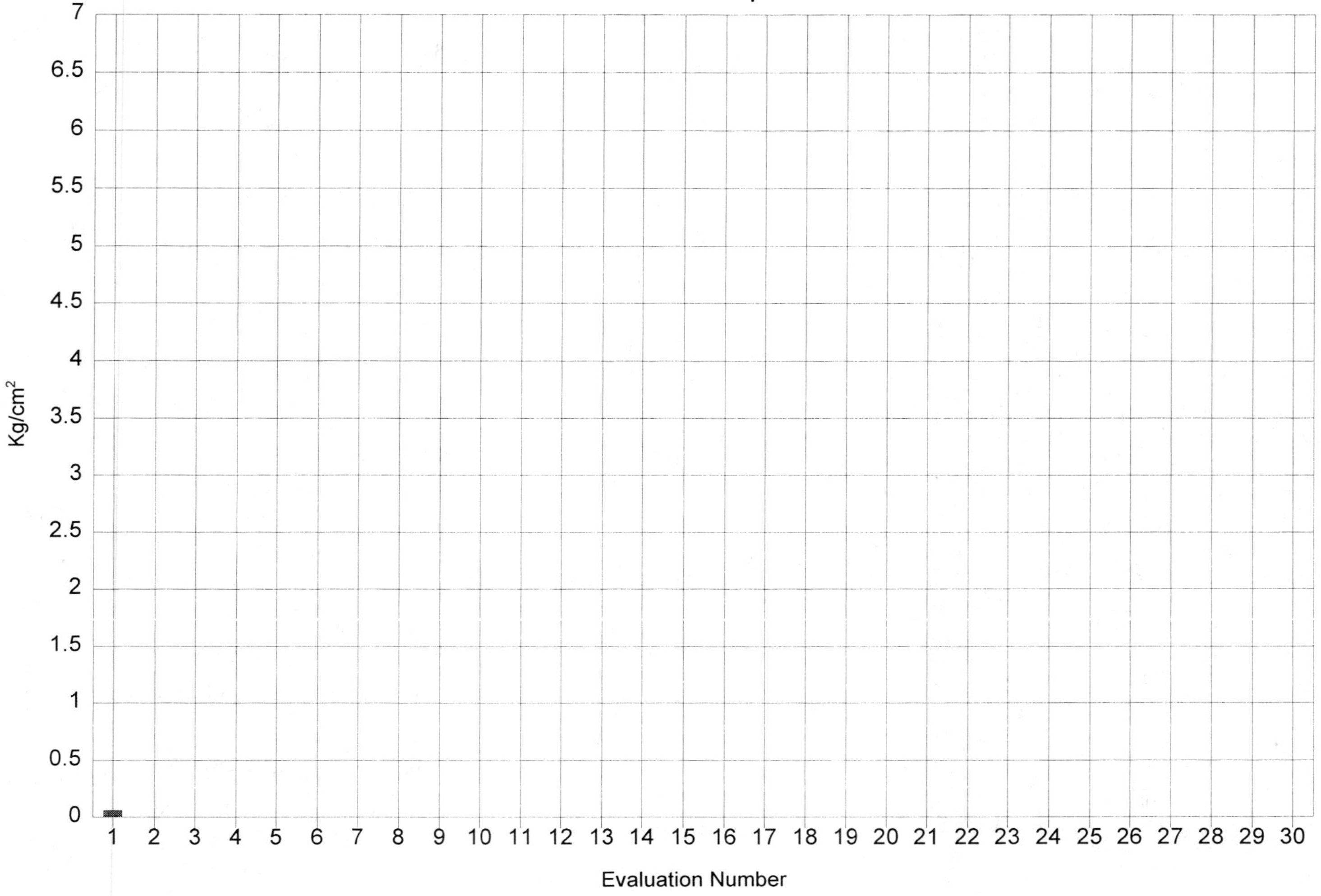

Kg/cm²

7
6.5
6
5.5
5
4.5
4
3.5
3
2.5
2
1.5
1
0.5
0

0 1 2 3 4 5 6 7 8 9 10 11 12 13 14 15 16 17 18 19 20 21 22 23 24 25 26 27 28 29 30

Evaluation Number

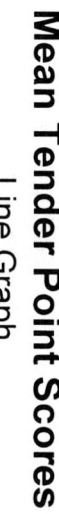

Fibromyalia Impact Questionnaire
Line Graph

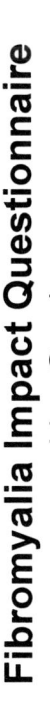
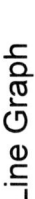

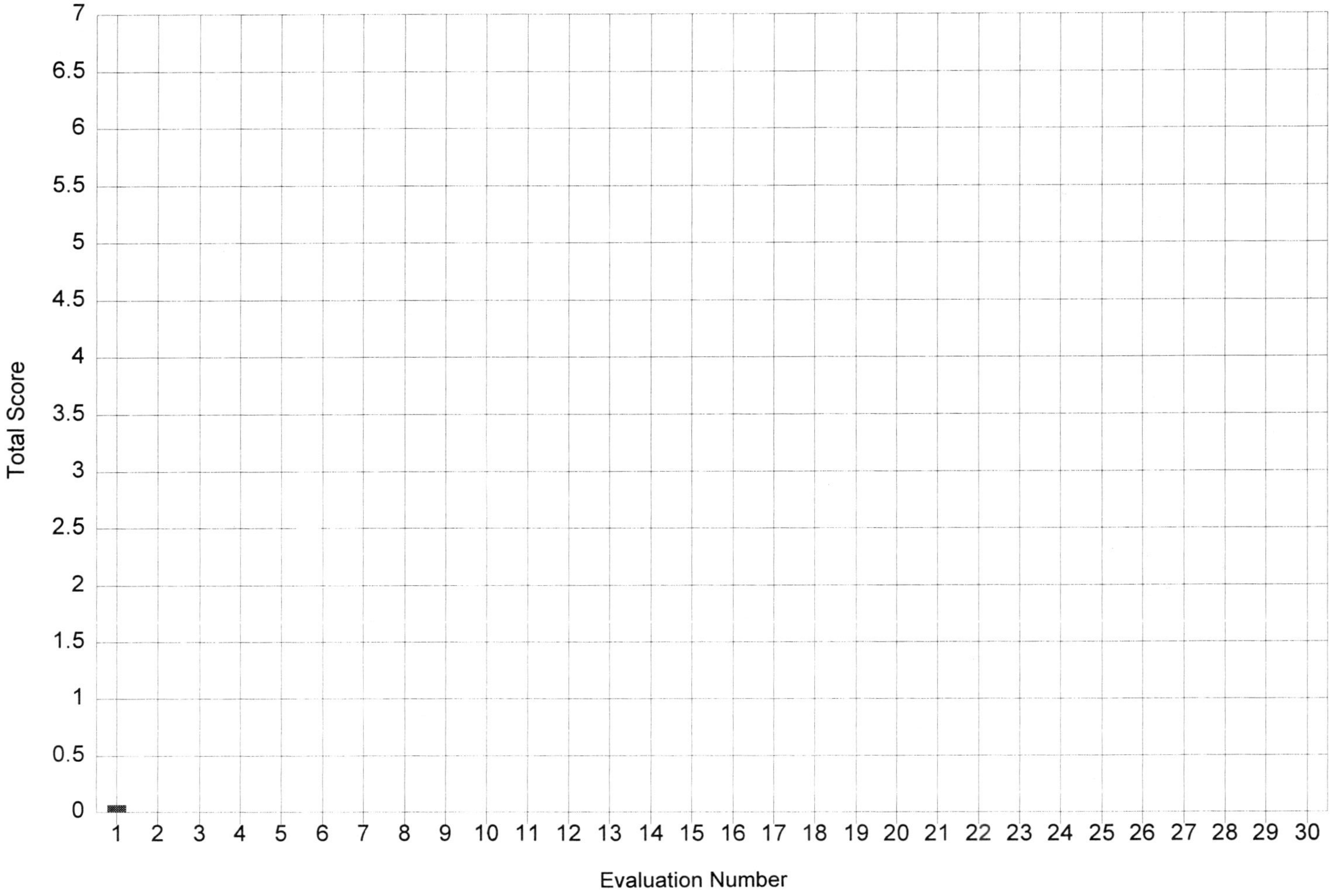

Total Score

Evaluation Number

Depression Scores
Line Graph

Self-Rating Depression Scale Index

Evaluation Number

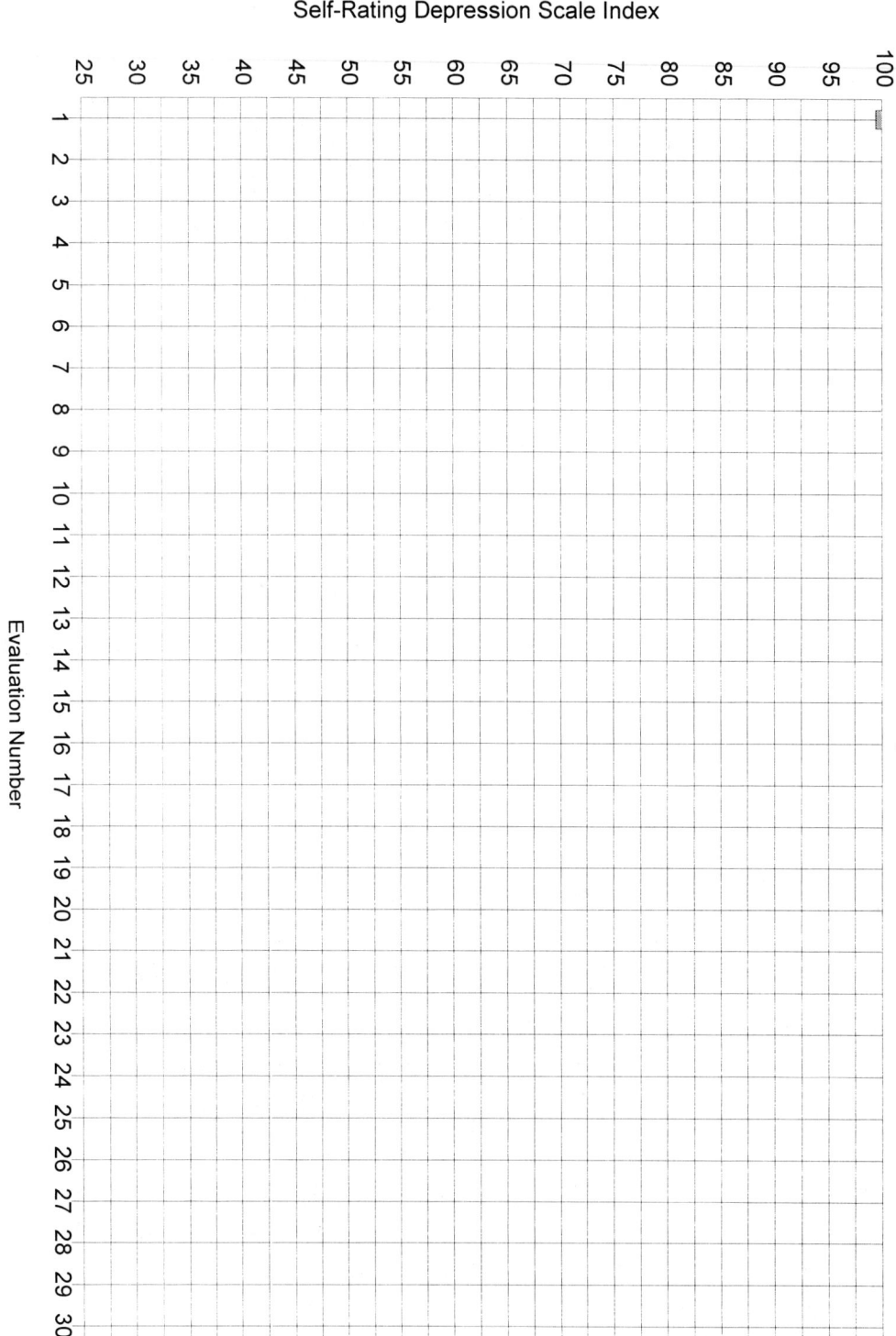

Appendix B

PUBLISHED PAPERS ON FIBROMYALGIA BY DR. JOHN C. LOWE AND COLLEAGUES

IMPROVEMENT IN EUTHYROID FIBROMYALGIA PATIENTS TREATED WITH T₃ (TRI-IODOTHYRONINE)

John C. Lowe, MA, DC
John Eichelberger, MD
Gilbert Manso, MD
Kit Peterson, MD

This article originally appeared in the *Journal of Myofascial Therapy*, 1(2):16-29, 1994.
It is reprinted with permission of McDowell Publishing Company.

Abstract. *Four fibromyalgia patients were treated on a case study basis with T_3 (Cytomel) and a physical regimen. Three patients took supraphysiologic doses of T_3 and another took a replacement dose. Each patient's mean algometer score—the mean of the quantified pressure/pain thresholds of her 18 tender point sites—improved significantly. Two patients' algometer scores reached and remained well within the normal range. One other patient's scores reached normal and then remained slightly subnormal although markedly higher than her baseline score. The other patient's scores approached normal. Each patient's symptoms significantly improved. Two patients had almost complete relief of symptoms, one retained some mild symptoms, and another patient, after some symptom relief, began experiencing severe symptoms including widespread pain. Our uncontrolled observations suggest that supraphysiologic doses of T_3 override an underlying neuromuscular molecular abnormality in some fibromyalgia patients.*

Key Words: *Fibromyalgia, T_3, α-Adrenergic receptors, Hypometabolism, Algometer score, Algometry.*

INTRODUCTION

Fibromyalgia is the most common condition of chronic, widespread musculoskeletal pain with a poor prognosis.[75,pp.297& 301] In 1990, a committee of the American College of Rheumatology[1] established specific diagnostic criteria for the condition. The criteria include widespread pain and tenderness at 11 of 18 specific anatomical sites. Widespread pain is pain above and below the waist, on the right and left sides of the body, and at some axial portion of the body such as the chest or low back. Tenderness is defined as pain upon pressure of fewer than 4 kg/cm² at 11 of 18 specific anatomical sites.[63,p.136] Fibromyalgia patients also tend to have numerous associated symptoms in common, but these are not essential to the diagnosis. There is no agreement at this point as to the etiology of fibromyalgia, and no one has provided evidence of a highly effective treatment.[2]

Numerous authors have suggested that there is a relationship between fibromyalgia and hypothyroidism.[6][7][8][9][10][11][12][13][14][15][17][18][49][61] Some clinical researchers state that hypothyroidism is the most common systemic condition underlying fibromyalgia.[4][5] Some researchers exclude hypothyroid patients from their fibromyalgia studies, thereby implying a similarity between the symptoms of the two conditions.

Many fibromyalgia patients, however, are euthyroid; that is, they have no hypothalamic, pituitary, or thyroid abnormalities that result in low synthesis or release of thyroid hormone. Fibromyalgia, then, exists in the absence of hypothyroidism. Partly because of this, the consensus committee of the American College of Rheumatology[1] and the Copenhagen committee members[2] have implied that fibromyalgia is *not* secondary to hypothyroidism, although the two conditions may occur concomitantly.

Nevertheless, most features of fibromyalgia bear a striking resemblance to features of hypothyroid myofascial and nervous system tissues. Some of these features include: 1) biochemical, histological, and spectroscopic findings that indicate impaired muscle energy metabolism;[23][24][35][36][37][38][39][40][41][42][43] 2) reduced muscle strength and easily fatigued muscles;[19,p.269-270] 3) muscle symptoms and abnormalities typical of the hypometabolic effects of deconditioning;[4] and 4) in biopsy samples, high concentrations of mucopoly-saccharides, suggesting inadequate inhibition of fibroblasts by thyroid hormone.[17][18] In addition, subjects with high levels of aerobic fitness (and thus high metabolic capacity) were resistant to developing fibromyalgia symptoms when deprived of slow-wave sleep, but people with low levels of aerobic fitness (diminished metabolic capacity) were susceptible.[44] Aerobic training has improved the status of fibromyalgia patients,[45][46] indicating that enhanced metabolic efficiency favorably affects the mechanism underlying fibromyalgia. Also, cognitive-behavior therapy has improved the status of fibromyalgia patients,[47][48] possibly by reducing metabolic demand through decreasing gamma motor activity and relaxing skeletal muscles.

Noting such features in euthyroid fibromyalgia patients who improved with supraphysiologic doses of T_3, Lowe proposed the hypometabolism hypothesis of fibromyalgia.[112] According to this hypothesis, fibromyalgia in most patients results from an impaired ability of thyroid hormone to exert its transcription-regulating effects at chromosomes, possibly due to a thyroid hormone receptor defect. The defect may be one or more amino acid substitutions in the T_3-binding domain of the receptor molecule. The defect occurs selectively in myofascial and nervous system tissues. Because of this tissue selectivity, the clinical features of fibromyalgia resemble those arising from hypothyroid myofascial and nervous system tissues.

Researchers have precisely determined the genetic and molecular nature of mutated thyroid hormone receptors in many patients who have partial resistance to their endogenous thyroid hormones.[16][109][110][111] In these patients, the thyroid hormone receptors of some tissues but not others are mutated.[109][110] In other words, any one patient may have some tissues whose thyroid hormone receptors are highly resistant to thyroid hormone and other tissues whose receptors are normally responsive to thyroid hormone. Lowe[112] proposes that fibromyalgia is a form of the least-studied classification of thyroid hormone resistance—the "peripheral" form in which tissues other than the pituitary gland contain resistant thyroid hormone receptors, but the pituitary gland's TSH-secreting thyrotrophic cells contain normal thyroid hormone receptors.[16,pp.1304-1305][111,pp.3823]

According to this hypothesis, mutated thyroid hormone receptors diminish the stimulatory effect of thyroid hormone on myofascial and nervous system tissues, rendering these tissues hypometabolic. The hypometabolism of neuromuscular tissues causes euthyroid patients to have multiple symptoms characteristic of hypothyroidism. When the symptoms include widespread pain and multiple tender anatomical sites, a clinician may diagnose the condition as fibromyalgia. As occurs with many patients with euthyroid hypometabolism of undetermined etiology,[26][27][28][29][30][31][32][33] and those with thyroid hormone resistance syndromes,[34][53][54][55][56][57][115] some patients' fibromyalgia symptoms significantly improve or completely cease when they take oral supraphysiologic doses of T_3.[25]

During a clinical observation of 77 fibromyalgia patients treated with T_3, Lowe and Poo noted that 58 (roughly 75%) benefited to varying degrees.[25] Unfortunately, because these results were not entirely expected, these clinicians did not make the patients' records uniform enough to quantify degrees of improvement.

Of the 58 patients who benefited, most of those who continued to take supraphysiologic doses of T_3 had only mild to moderate symptoms intermittently. Some remained completely free from symptoms. The pressure/pain thresholds of their tender points increased (improved) significantly. In every case, tenderness of trigger points or their numbers either decreased or disappeared altogether. Some patients' irritable trigger points that were previously treatment-resistant disappeared without direct physical treatment. In other patients, physical treatment neutralized formerly recalcitrant trigger points with fewer than 10 treatments.

The dosages of T_3 that were effective for patients ranged from 75 mcg to 150 mcg. Most patients required between 81.25 mcg and 100 mcg. Few patients had symptoms of excess thyroid hormone stimulation. In most who did have such symptoms, progressively reducing the T_3 dosage by 6.25 mcg relieved the symptoms. Based on experience with previous patients,[25] Lowe and Poo cautioned patients not to reduce their dosages more than 6.25 mcg during any two-to-four week period. Rapid decreases in dosage usually reactivated fibromyalgia symptoms. As little as 20 mg of propranolol stopped symptoms of excess metabolic stimulation and so was preferred over large T_3 dosage reductions. Few patients had to reduce their dosages more than 6.25 mcg to stop the symptoms. After reducing the dosage by even this small an amount, some fibromyalgia symptoms reappeared in mild form. These reactions tended to subside, however, within a week or two. As a result, patients retained the levels of improvement they had obtained at the higher dosages.[25]

Lowe based the hypometabolism hypothesis of fibromyalgia[112] on two observations: 1) hypothyroid-like features of fibromyalgia in euthyroid patients, and 2) the favorable response of euthyroid fibromyalgia patients to supraphysiologic doses of T_3. In line with these observations, the four case studies reported in this paper test a null hypothesis: that euthyroid fibromyalgia patients formerly unresponsive to treatment would not improve during the oral use of supraphysiologic doses of T_3 as part of their treatment regimen. Careful records were kept in three forms: 1) frequent algometer exams by J.C.L. to quantify patients' *algometer scores* (the mean of the pressure/pain thresholds of their 18 tender point sites), 2) patients regularly verbally reporting their experiences with symptoms, and 3) patients completing and submitting at exam times a "symptoms questionnaire."

METHODS

Patients. Patients taking part in these case studies gave informed consent. Four female patients who met the 1990 ACR criteria for fibromyalgia[1] took part.

Clinicians had previously diagnosed patient #1 as having fibromyalgia. This patient, who was 37 years old, had extremely severe fibromyalgia for 10 years. She had been hospitalized for debilitating pain.

J.C.L. diagnosed the other three patients as having fibromyalgia. Patient #2, aged 46, had fibromyalgia symptoms for six years. Patient #3, 21 years old, reported having fibromyalgia symptoms for two years. Patient #4, aged 45, said she had suffered from fibromyalgia symptoms her entire life.

None of the patients were taking drugs such as β-adrenergic inhibitors (propranolol), estrogen, or progestins that might generate fibromyalgia-like symptoms. None of them had health conditions such as lupus erythematosus whose symptoms can mimic fibromyalgia.

None of the patients were hospitalized, on disability, or involved in litigation. All patients were either working or engaged in major daily activities. No control subjects were included in the study.

Procedure. After establishing that patients met the ACR criteria for fibromyalgia, laboratory profiles were run. Patients whose thyroid function tests confirmed hypothyroidism, cardiac abnormalities contraindicating T₃ treatment, or adrenal insufficiency would have been excluded from the study, but none met these criteria.

The patients were subjected to a battery of laboratory tests. These included a 24-hour urinary cortisol, calcitonin, parathyroid hormone, total and ionized calcium, a SMAC with CBC, and a thyroid profile. The thyroid profile contained a T₄ (RIA), T₃-uptake, T₇ (free thyroxine index), TSH, and reverse-T₃.

J.E. performed a TRH-stimulation test on patients #1, #2, and #3 to eliminate the possibility of subclinical hypothyroidism—that is, to assure euthyroidism. Another internist performed the same test on patient #4.

EKGs confirmed that no cardiac abnormalities contraindicated the use of T₃. EKG exams were available in case cardiac symptoms appeared, but these were seldom necessary.

G.M. or K.P. prescribed T₃ (Cytomel)[114] for the patients. Patients underwent regular treatments by J.C.L. with a physical protocol. This consisted of continuous ultrasound, soft tissue manipulation, moist heat, and stretching. The patients agreed to complete symptoms questionnaires and return them at the time of weekly exams.

The experimentally manipulated variable was the dosage of T₃ taken daily by each patient. The variable monitored for therapeutic change was the algometer score. A baseline mean algometer score was determined for each patient. To derive the algometer score, J.C.L. used an algometer[113] to quantify the pressure/pain threshold of each of the 18 tender point sites. The mean of the 18 algometer scores was calculated and recorded.

After each patient started oral T₃, her algometer scores were derived by algometer measurements once per week. During the latter part of the study, intervals between algometer exams were somewhat wider for patient #2. They were also wider on a few occasions for the other patients.

With the algometer, J.C.L. applied pressure to tender point sites at the rate of approximately 1 kg per second.[72,p.8] With rare exceptions, he examined patients in the late afternoon and early evening, between 4 pm and 7 pm. (The time of day may influence the status of a fibromyalgia patient's condition.[74] Consistency in exam times decreases the likelihood that changes in the algometer scores over time are due to diurnal variations.) Patients' pain distributions were also recorded.

Patients were instructed to continue any treatment regimen they had engaged in that provided them with palliative relief. Previous fitness activities had failed to improve their fibromyalgia status. They agreed, however, that to the extent they were able to tolerate it, they would engage in some form of aerobic exercise at least three days per week.

T₃ Dosage. One assumption underlying the protocol in this study was that improvement in patients was critically dependent on carefully individualized T₃ dosages. The clinical experiences of Lowe and Poo[25] indicate that the fibromyalgia patient benefits from T₃ only when the clinician follows a specific procedure: careful monitoring of the patient's reactions or absence of reactions to T₃, followed by responsive, appropriate dosage adjustments.

Patients #2, #3, and #4 began T₃ with the standard replacement dose, 75 mcg per day. Patient #1, who had previously taken desiccated thyroid and was currently taking synthetic T₄ (Synthroid) without apparent benefit, began with 50 mcg.

All patients were evaluated to determine whether cardiac or other indications of toxicity had developed. If a patient's status had not improved after one month, she increased the dosage initially by 12.5 mcg and later by 6.5 mcg every two weeks.

Patients continued these progressive increases until (a) their algometer scores began increasing, or (b) the first indication of excess metabolic stimulation developed. Patients were taught possible symptoms of excess metabolic stimulation due to use of exogenous thyroid hormone and instructed in self-monitoring for such symptoms. The symptoms questionnaire they were required to complete contained a list of thyrotoxic symptoms. Each patient was required to check off any of these she experienced.

All four patients had regularly taken nutrient supplements prior to participating in the study. Because various nutrients are essential to normal metabolism,[60] they were all instructed to continue taking supplements containing the B complex vitamins, vitamin C, the antioxidant nutrients, and multiple minerals including calcium and magnesium.

RESULTS

We have presented the rounded mean algometer scores in line form in graphs #1, #2, #3, and #4. The number of each graph corresponds to the patient number. Graph #1, for example, represents the algometer scores for patient #1. The graphs show on each exam date, the average amount of pressure necessary to induce the perception of pain (the pressure/pain threshold) at the 18 tender point sites. *Pain upon pressure of 4 kg/cm^2 or more is considered normal. Pain upon pressure of fewer than 4 kg/cm^2 is considered abnormal.*[63,p.136] Using this criterion, all four patients had initial algometer scores that were abnormally low. The graphs show that each patient's algometer scores increased substantially over time. By the end of the study, two patients no longer met the diagnostic criteria for fibromyalgia.

Patient #1. Patient #1 had fibromyalgia for approximately ten years. Her symptoms included migraines, irritable bowel syndrome, sleep disturbance, stiffness, generalized pain, fatigue, and suboptimal mood. She was treated by numerous physicians—including pain management specialists, holistic physicians, and a rheumatologist—all without significant relief. Two and a half years before consulting J.C.L., she had been hospitalized once for pain and twice for procedures related to pain control. J.C.L. also treated her for almost one year with physical treatment procedures before she began using T$_3$. During that time, her condition did not improve. She participated in this study for almost one year (from August 11, 1993 to August 8, 1994).

Her baseline algometer score on August 11, 1993 was 0.8 kg/cm^2. At the 22nd weekly algometer exam after she began taking T$_3$, her algometer score reached 4.1 kg/cm^2. As the curve in Graph #1 shows, during the period between baseline and the 22nd week, her mean algometer scores progressed in a zigzag pattern: they increased variably over a period of three to five weeks, then deceased for one to three weeks before

ascending again. The overall pattern, however, was ascension.

At the 23rd week, her algometer score dropped to 3.5 kg/cm^2, and at the 24th week, her score rose again to 4.1 kg/cm^2. The following two weeks, her algometer scores decreased to 3.5 and 3.3 kg/cm^2. The next week the score increased to 3.5 kg/cm^2 and the next, the 28th week, to 4.0 kg/cm^2. The 29th week, the algometer score decreased to 3.9 kg/cm^2. After that date and for the remainder of the study, the algometer scores varied between 3.8 and 2.7 kg/cm^2.

According to her questionnaire, the only symptom that markedly changed during the course of the study was her degree of disturbed sleep. During her baseline period, her disturbed sleep rating was 4.9 (0-to-10 point scale) and her algometer score was extremely low–0.8 kg/cm^2. Her most disturbed sleep (5.5) was during the 29th, 30th, and 31st weeks of the study. The 29th week, her algometer score was 4.0 kg/cm^2. The 30th week, her algometer score dropped to 3.2 kg/cm^2. The 31st week, her algometer score rose to 3.8 kg/cm^2 and her degree of disturbed sleep decreased (improved) to 2.8.

It is clear that her questionnaire did not accurately reflect this patient's improved status. Between the 10th and 31st weeks of her participation in the study, her status was remarkably improved compared to the year prior to her starting T$_3$. She reported to J.C.L. that she felt well, and his evaluation was that she appeared energetic and happy with a distinctly improved appearance of well-being. After the 31st week, however, she was subjected to considerably increased physical stress at her place of employment. This appears to have adversely affected her symptom status.

Late in the study, she began using an NSAID, Daypro. She did so because her pain level and stiffness (mainly in her legs) had substantially increased. The Daypro relieved much of her stiffness, but she had to stop the drug twice because of adverse gastrointestinal effects. Although these symptoms were troubling, she maintained that she was far better off than before starting to take T$_3$. By the end of the study, for example, her pain was far more limited in distribution than before. In August of 1993, just before she entered the study, her pain was 9 on a 0-to-10 point scale. On August 8, 1994, although some of her other symptoms had reappeared, her pain was 5 to 6. She said that during her participation in the study, when her pain would periodically worsen, she could control or stop it by taking higher doses of T$_3$. But when she increased the dosage to 125 mcg, symptoms of excess thyroid hormone stimulation developed. These symptoms—heart palpitations, extremity tremors, and uncomfortable body heat—became the factor limiting her ability to

MEAN ALGOMETER SCORES
GRAPH #1

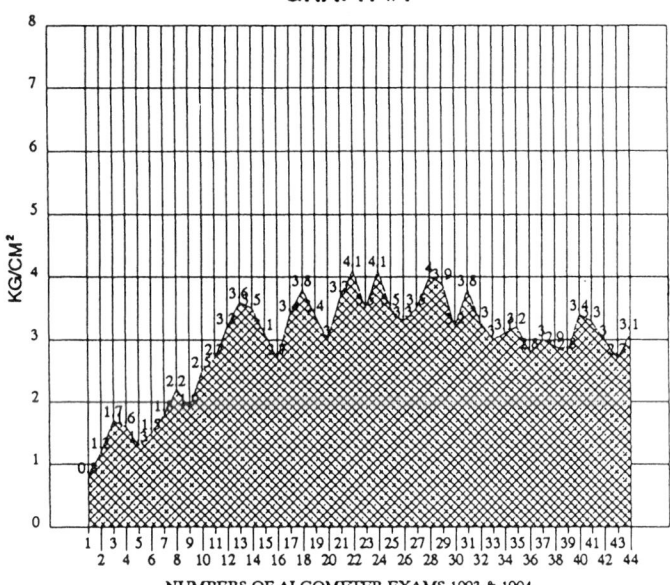

NUMBERS OF ALGOMETER EXAMS 1993 & 1994

control her pain. She had to tolerate some measure of pain, then, to minimize thyrotoxic symptoms from the higher dosages of T_3.

She stated that her energy level was low regardless of her dosage of T_3. When she increased her dosage to control periodic increased pain, her energy level was better for a week or two. The level would fall again, however. A low energy level remained her most troubling symptom.

Patient #1 emphasized at the close of the study that she had experienced substantial improvements from taking T_3. Before this therapy, she had severe migraine headaches. As her T_3 treatment progressed, her migraines decreased in frequency until she was completely free from them. By the end of the study, she only had headaches when her upper cervical spinal segments needed adjusting, about once per week. She described these headaches as "nagging." She empha-sized their tolerable nature compared to the nausea and "blinding in one eye" that had accompanied the migraines.

After one month on T_3, her irritable bowel syndrome with lower abdominal pain completely stopped. Before starting T_3, she was not able to tolerate the cold and stiffness she experienced while wearing sandals in an air conditioned room that was comfortable to other people. After one to two months of taking T_3, however, her "terribly cold and stiff fingers and toes" and bluish discoloration of her toes and fingers completely stopped. She can now wear sandals in air conditioned environments.

Before starting T_3, she had a blood pressure history of 90/58 to 90/60. Measurements throughout the study showed that her blood pressure increased to 110/70 to 120/70. Her heart rate increased from typically 54 to 60 before starting T_3 to 74 to 88. For years before participating in this study, her cholesterol had been 212 mg/dl. When she began the study, it was 195 mg/dl. Six months into the study, G.M. tested her cholesterol and the value was 160 mg/dl.

Patient #2. Patient #2 had symptoms of fibromyalgia for six years. J.C.L. was the first to assign the diagnosis. Because her pain caused her to stop running regularly, she had been treated by an orthopedic surgeon and a podiatrist, both of whom specialized in sports injuries. An internist had also treated her.

Her algometer score reached 4 kg/cm² between the 9th and 10th weeks after she began taking T_3 (see Graph 2). Her algometer scores remained considerably above 4 kg/cm² for some eight months of subsequent algometer exams. During the last five months of her participation in the study, J.C.L. performed exams at intervals greater than one week. Because of this, there may have been some unrecorded variation in her mean algometer scores. Nonetheless, the recorded algometer values show that her normal algometer scores persisted over the months.

After the patient's baseline algometer score of 2.5 kg/cm², the score the following week decreased to 1.5 kg/cm². Over the next four weeks, the algometer scores gradually rose back to 2.5 kg/cm². Thereafter, the scores increased and remained above the normal value of 4 kg/cm^2.

The patient's symptoms questionnaire indicated noteworthy improvements. Her pain distribution, anxiety, and stress levels decreased. Thus, her symptom changes corresponded to her increased algometer scores.

At the end of the study, however, she still had some mild symptoms. She was significantly stiff after remaining still for five minutes or more, but this was a marked improvement over her pre-T₃ experiences. The stiffness was limited to her knees and hips. Previously, she felt stiff "all over" and "felt like I could hardly move."

She stated that her symptoms were worse during the month after her father's death when she had just begun taking T₃. During this time, she felt as though she had myalgia typical of the flu. At the end of the study, she still had neck and upper thoracic pain, but she did not "hurt all over" as she had before taking T₃. She said she had experienced numerous generalized improvements in her health. These included absence of three phenomena: 1) orthostatic hypotension, 2) swelling after consuming sodium, and 3) wide fluctuations in "water-weight." She also cited an increased intestinal tolerance of meat and dairy products. And, she was able to resume her previous regimen of more strenuous aerobic exercise.

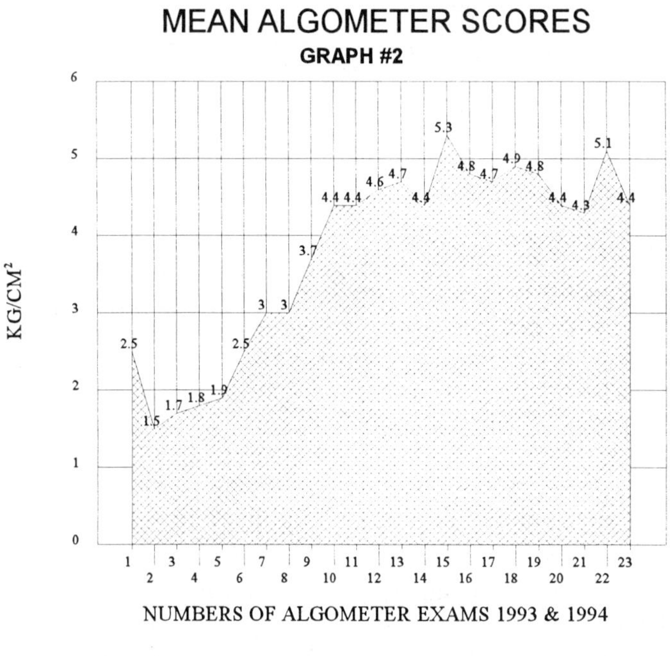

MEAN ALGOMETER SCORES
GRAPH #2

NUMBERS OF ALGOMETER EXAMS 1993 & 1994

Patient #3. Patient #3 had symptoms of fibromyalgia for two years before consulting J.C.L., who diagnosed the condition. Before she consulted J.C.L., she received treatment by one DC, an MD who practiced homeopathy, two general practice MDs, and one psychiatrist. Her baseline algometer score was 1.9 kg/cm^2. The score reached 4 kg/cm^2 between the 7th and 8th weeks after she began T₃. Her mean algometer scores remained well above normal for her remaining five months in the study.

Her pain was so intense before beginning the treatment program that she spent hours in bed on some days and was not able to perform her duties as a missionary. Her pain was widespread. By her second month of T₃ treatment, her only remaining tendency

toward pain was across her lower thoracic region just below her bra strap and at her suboccipital region. At most, the pain was mild and intermittent.

At the time of her participation in the study, this patient lived and worked in close contact with other missionaries. During her last six weeks in the study, she and most of her immediate coworkers became ill with what appeared to be a viral infection. They were somewhat fatigued and had recurrent gastrointestinal symptoms. The patient reported gastrointestinal symptoms at this time, whereas she did not have these symptoms prior to this point in the study. These symptoms did not indicate a reaction to an excessive dose of T₃ (this patient did not have to increase her T₃ dosage above the initial 75 mcg). The viral infection did not affect her algometer scores. They remained at an average of 5.9 kg/cm² with a range of 5.7 to 6.1 kg/cm².

During the second month after she began taking T_3, she reported her status was 70% to 80% improved. Her symptoms questionnaire also indicated this improvement.

Her estimate of disturbed sleep decreased from the initial 10 (0-to-10 point scale) the first month after beginning T_3 to 0.5 the second month. The subsequent months' ratings were 0.7, 0.4, 1.6, and 0.7. Her estimate of feeling rested in the mornings increased from 1 the first month to 4.2, 4.6, 3.75, 3.7, and 4.3 in the following months.

Her estimate of pain decreased from 9 to 4.1, but 4.1 did not correspond to the virtual absence of pain that patient #3 reported to J.C.L. during most examinations. Her energy level increased from 1.5 the first month to 5 or higher during most of the following months. Her headaches decreased from constant and intense (rating of 10) at the beginning of her participation in the study to 3.6, 3.4, 2, 2.7, and 3.6 throughout the remainder of the study. Her cold sensitivity decreased from 5 the first month to 0.4, 0.1, 0, 0, and 0 the following months.

Her overall assessment of her emotional and physical well-being decreased during the last two months of

MEAN ALGOMETER SCORES

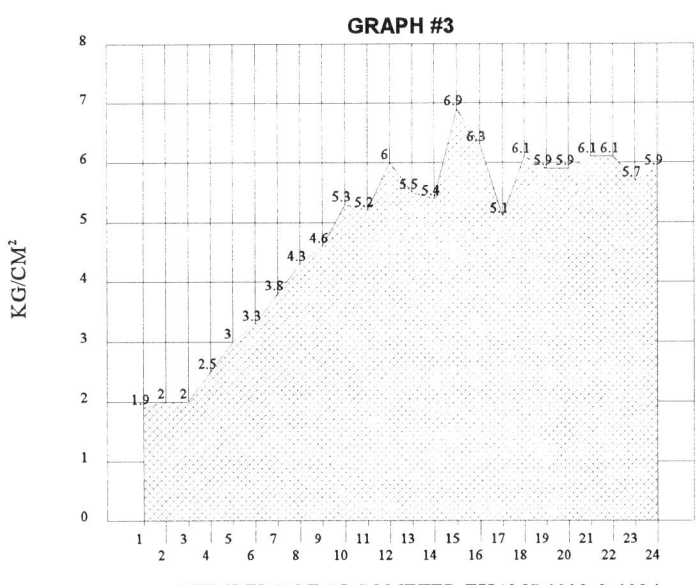

GRAPH #3

NUMBERS OF ALGOMETER EXAMS 1993 & 1994

the study. The patient attributed this to her growing disenchantment with some aspects of her mission in Houston and her persisting viral illness. She terminated her mission and returned home at the end of this two-month period. Overall, this patient reported that she felt recovered from her fibromyalgia symptoms.

Patient #4. Patient #4 reported having had symptoms characteristic of fibromyalgia (especially chronic fatigue and widespread aching and pain) her entire life. J.C.L. diagnosed her condition as fibromyalgia and treated her with a physical protocol for approximately one year prior to the patient beginning T_3 therapy. During this time, the physical treatment provided her with relief only briefly after each visit. She began taking T_3 only about 18 weeks before the

end of the study and may not have had time to achieve maximum benefit from T_3 before preparation of this paper. During her participation in the study, her algometer scores rose significantly from a baseline of 2.5 kg/cm². During the last three weeks, her algometer scores approached normal (Graph #4).

During her 6th week in the study, because she felt no relief, patient #4 increased her dosage of T_3 from 75 to 87.5 mcg. By the 9th algometer exam, when her algometer score was 2.9 kg/cm², she told J.C.L. she had days of complete pain relief with a strong sense of well-being. At her 10th algometer exam, her algometer score increased to 3.1 kg/cm². She indicated that relief of pain and other symptoms was substantial at this point.

Between her 10th and 12th exams, she reported that her status had worsened somewhat. She increased her dosage of T_3 to 94 mcg. Over the next three weeks, her algometer scores increased significantly.

Initially, patient #4 had widespread pain. Eight weeks after starting T_3, her only remaining pain was at one location: an area about the circumference of a half dollar, located in her left thoracic region at the attachment of the iliocostalis thoracis muscle. This pain appeared to be related to her sitting posture. Due to her short legs, she sat on the edges of chairs flexed slightly forward at the waist. This induced sustained paraspinal erector muscle contractions for postural support.

This patient's symptoms questionnaire indicated a decrease in several symptoms. These included disturbed sleep, times awakened at night, pain during the day, stiffness upon awakening, and headaches. She was more rested upon awakening, her energy level and overall emotional/physical rating increased, and her cognitive function seemed improved.

DISCUSSION

Results. In this study, three fibromyalgia patients took supraphysiologic doses of T_3 (patients #1, #2, and #4). Patient #3 took a replacement dose. The mean algometer scores of all patients significantly improved. This means that the average amount of pain at their 18 tender point sites decreased (the pressure/pain thresholds increased). This is noteworthy because the mean algometer score of the 18 tender point sites is a highly objective measure of fibromyalgia status. Symptoms in all patients improved significantly. The symptoms of patient #1, however, did not keep pace with her increased algometer scores. During the later months of her participation in the study, her symptoms became severe again, although not as severe as before she began taking T_3.

In some studies of fibromyalgia patients, such as one by Romano, a change (for better or worse) in algometer score was defined as a change in value of >1 kg/1.54 cm^2.[85] (Romano used a larger circumference algometer in his study—one that covered an area of 1.54 cm^2 instead of 1 cm^2.)

The least-improved algometer scores in this study were those of patient #4. This was perhaps due to her shorter time of participation. The maximum improvement over baseline in her scores was 1.2 kg/cm^2 at the 15th and 16th weeks. The maximum for patient #1 was 3.3 kg/cm^2, for patient #2 was 2.8 kg/cm^2, and for patient #3 was 5 kg/cm^2.

T_3 Dosage. Goldenberg recently mentioned the need to evaluate individualized drug dose schedules.[70,p.78] Our view is that without individualizing the dosage of T_3, most patients are not likely to improve.

According to Lowe and Poo,[25] patients benefit only when the clinician does two things: 1) carefully monitors the fibromyalgia patient's reactions or absence of reactions to T_3, and 2) increases or decreases the dosage as many times as necessary to fine-tune the patient's improved status.

In this study, patients increased their dosages at two times: 1) when no improvement occurred after two or three weeks of a particular dosage, and 2) when symptoms that had been relieved by a particular dosage of T_3 reappeared. Patients decreased their T_3 intake when a particular dosage was followed by symptoms of excess metabolic stimulation.

The maximum T_3 dosage of patient #1 was 125 mcg. With this dosage, her pain was decreased or gone altogether. After two weeks at 125 mcg, however, she had to reduce this to a maintenance dosage of 100 mcg because of heart palpitations, tremors of her extremities (shakiness), and heat intolerance. In seeking her optimal dosage, she gradually reduced her T_3 dosage to 87.5 mcg and then gradually increased it to 106 mcg. At the direction of the prescribing physician, when a test showed that her TSH level was below the lower end of the normal range, she reduced the dosage to 100 mcg. The maximum dosage of patient #2 was 125 mcg but she reduced it gradually to 87.5 mcg to stop heart palpations and extremity tremors. At one point, she reduced the dosage to 80 mcg, but she began experiencing pain again and increased the dosage to 87.5 mcg.

The maximum (and maintenance) dosage for patient #3 was 75 mcg, and the maximum (and maintenance) dosage for patient #4 was 94 mcg.

The Symptoms Questionnaire. The questionnaire used in this study has not been validated as an instrument for assessing symptom changes. The data we derived from it therefore is of questionable value. Except for patient #3, each patients' verbal report of her symptoms during exams and at the end of the study did not correlate tightly with the symptoms ratings on the questionnaire. Also, improvements in symptoms usually did not correlate well with increases in algometer scores. One possible explanation for the discrepancy is that the questionnaire did not allow flexible enough answers to show the variability in symptoms reflected in patients' verbal reports. It is also possible that when a patient focused on her symptoms to report them on the questionnaire, the symptoms magnified in her perception. If perceptual magnification was cumulative through the course of the study, the questionnaire would not reflect a patient's symptoms under natural conditions—that is, when she is not monitoring and reporting her symptoms.

Laboratory Test Results. One objective of the laboratory tests performed before patients began taking T_3 was retrospective—to determine after the study whether those who improved on T_3 differed according to lab results from those who did not improve. In contrast to the results of similar tests in other studies,[7][24] test results were normal for all our patients. Thus, there was no possibility of differentiating the patients on the basis of laboratory test results.

A number of normal test results (the 24 hour urinary cortisol, reverse-T_3, TSH, and T_3-uptake) were important diagnostically. They ruled out one explanation for the patients' positive responses to T_3. That explanation is hypometabolism due to subtle cortisol-induced (or autogenetic) hypothyroidism. In this

phenomenon, elevated cortisol (as during periods of stress) inhibits TSH secretion by the pituitary gland and inhibits the monodeiodinating enzyme that converts T_4 to T_3. Because T_3 is the metabolically active thyroid hormone, this results in hypothyroidism that usually lasts about one week.[64] Some clinicians assume this is the underlying mechanism of fibromyalgia, referring to it as "Wilson's syndrome." Cortisol-induced hypothyroidism is, of course, a long-recognized phenomenon.[65][66][67] Oddly, however, Wilson recently named the phenomenon after himself based on his accurate observation that T_3 supplements relieve many patients' health problems.[68] Regardless, this was not a causative factor in our four patients.

MEAN ALGOMETER SCORES

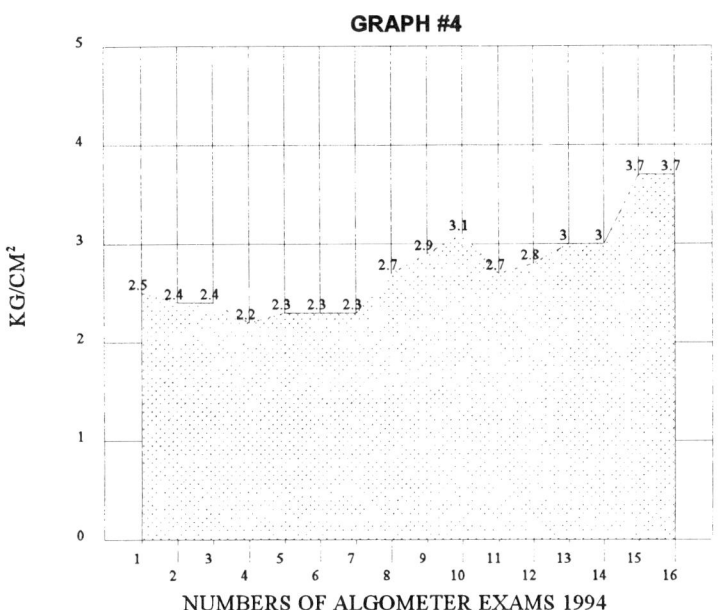

GRAPH #4

NUMBERS OF ALGOMETER EXAMS 1994

One research group found low calcium levels in fibromyalgia patients.[7] Normal calcium levels in our patients eliminated the possibility that their fibromyalgia symptoms were related to hypocalcemia. This, too, is important because low calcium levels can adversely affect myofascial[50,pp.141-142] and neuromusculoskeletal tissues.[51][52]

Suppressive Effects of Stress on Algometer Scores. The baseline algometer score for patient #2 was 2.5 kg/cm². The following week, an algometer exam showed that her mean algometer score had decreased to 1.5 kg/cm². Over the next four weeks, the mean algometer scores were, seriatim, 1.7, 1.8, 1.9, and 2.5 kg/cm². Afterward, her algometer scores steadily rose to and remained above the normal value of 4 kg/cm². The precipitous drop in her algometer score (the week

after baseline) occurred when her father died. The drop during psychological stress may have resulted from a predominance of α-adrenergic receptors in her neuromuscular tissues (see below: *Physiological Changes Induced by T_3*). She began taking T_3 during the period of stress. She may not have been taking it long enough at that time, however, to override thyroid hormone receptor resistance and shift transcription to increase β-adrenergic receptor production and decrease α-adrenergic receptor production. As a result, increased catecholamine levels associated with her stress may have interacted with predominant α-adrenergic receptors to accentuate her neuromuscular hypometabolism and her fibromyalgia symptoms. Increased catecholamine-α-adrenergic receptor activity, for example, would be expected to inhibit serotonin release in the central nervous system.[91] This would impede pain modulation by the descending serotonergic spinal cord pathways.

Patient #1 improved considerably for months after starting T₃ supplements. This suggests, according to the hypometabolism hypothesis, that her nervous and myofascial tissues had become more properly balanced in terms of α-adrenergic and β-adrenergic function. When her algometer scores were briefly above normal, her symptoms were minimal. But when the scores were slightly below normal, she often had severe symptoms. She stated that what limited her pain relief was her adverse reaction to doses of T₃ above 106 mcg. When she took 125 mcg for two weeks, she was for all practical purposes pain-free, but she had to decrease the dosage because of tremors, heart palpitations, and heat intolerance. This observation may indicate that the dosage of T₃ necessary to shift the balance of adrenergic receptors on her serotonergic cells significantly toward the β form (with the result of triggering serotonin release) caused too great a shift toward β-adrenergic dominance in other tissues (with symptoms of excess metabolic stimulation). This suggests that differential tissue sensitivity to T₃, due to normal thyroid hormone receptors in some tissues and faulty ones in others, may limit patients' abilities to benefit from this therapy. In other words, a tissue with *extreme* thyroid hormone receptor resistance (and thus α-adrenergic receptor dominance) will require a very high dosage of T₃. The receptors in this tissue, however, may be therapeutically inaccessible because tissues with normal thyroid hormone receptors (and thus a normal balance of α- and β-adrenergic receptors) are in the line of fire. In these tissues, T₃ will cause a predominance of β-adrenergic receptors with resulting symptoms of thyrotoxicosis. This will limit the T₃ dosage for this patient to an amount insufficient to completely override resistance in the tissue with extreme thyroid hormone resistance.

One other factor was probably instrumental in the severe symptoms of patient #1. Eighteen weeks after beginning T₃, her mean algometer score approached normal (3.8 kg/cm²). Over the next 13 weeks, the scores remained close to normal. The range of scores over this period was 3 to 4.1 kg/cm², and the mean score was 3.6 kg/cm². On the 10th week of this 13-week period, she reported to J.C.L. that because of layoffs at her place of employment, her physical work load had become intense. Her symptoms had become more severe because of this. After the 13th week of sustained relatively high values, her mean algometer scores decreased to a range of 2.7 to 3.4 kg/cm² with an average of 3.0 kg/cm². Her symptoms became more severe. This turn of events for patient #1 indicates that

her increased work load exceeded her tolerance for biomechanical stress.

Lack of Control Subjects in this Study. No formal control subjects were included in this study. In a sense, though, three of these subjects, and possibly all four, served as their own controls. Before they entered this study, J.C.L. had treated three of the patients (patients #1, #2, #4) and G.M. had treated one (patient #1) for fibromyalgia for prolonged periods of time without symptomatic relief or increases in algometer scores. Prior to being included in this study, patient #3 had been treated by a chiropractic physician and numerous other practitioners for a period of two years before consulting J.C.L.

None of the patients significantly improved until they began taking T₃. Subsequent to the addition of this agent to their treatment regimen, their algometer scores began significantly increasing at one week (patient #1), five weeks (patient #2), three weeks (patient #3), and seven weeks (patient #4).

Sonkin has commented on the difficulty in performing double-blind studies of hypothyroid treatment. He writes that the character of the response of hypothyroidism to treatment does not lend itself to such methodology for at least eight reasons. These reasons also apply to studies of patients with euthyroid forms of hypometabolism. Sonkin writes:[49,p.159-160]

1. Hypothyroid patients may have to take a thyroid supplement for months before a therapeutic response is clear-cut.

2. A patient's subjective responses to thyroid therapy may be obscured for long periods by personal, mental or emotional problems. Depression may persist, for example, and its symptoms may cover up clinical evidence of the patient's improved metabolic state.

3. The hypothyroid patient may have persistent physical and mental discomfort. Because of this, he may require support and encouragement from a clinician who knows what therapy is being prescribed.

4. When non-hypothyroid patients are switched in a study from a thyroid supplement to a placebo, they may be hypothyroid for a period as long as 11 weeks.

5. The ethics of subjecting normal controls to thyroid withdrawal symptoms is open to question.

6. Identifying controls may be difficult. A substantial number of patients taking a thyroid supplement learn of their hypothyroid symptoms only when they stop the supplement. They realize retrospectively the benefits from the supplement. In other words, there may be res-

ponders in the control groups.

7. The number of control subjects required for a suitable study greatly increases the cost of the study.
8. A cycle of muscle pain, trigger points, and spasm may accompany hypothyroidism. These phenomena require proper treatment in conjunction with a thyroid supplement, and this introduces another variable into an already complicated experiment.

To these reasons, we add that the dosage of thyroid supplement may have to be adjusted repeatedly to find a dose that is therapeutic for a particular patient. As dosages are adjusted into the higher range, the clinician familiar with the effects of high doses of T₃ may readily distinguish the patients taking T₃ from those taking placebos. As a result, unless substantial resources are available, an effective blinded study with control subjects is highly inconvenient.

Improvement Rates in other Studies. Felson and Goldenberg conducted a 3-year follow-up study of fibromyalgia patients.[79] Although 85% had used medication during the three years, only 5% of patients had sustained remission of all their symptoms. In spite of therapy, two thirds of the patients still had marked or moderate pain. Over 60% of patients still complained of substantial fatigue and non-restorative sleep.[79]

Isomeri and coauthors wrote[80,p.254] "Complete and long-lasting cure of symptoms has not been reported with any of the therapies used, although some benefits have been achieved with tricyclic antidepressants, analgesic drugs, biofeedback, hypnosis, and physical fitness training strenuous enough to increase oxygen intake capacity." In their study, however, the pain thresholds of patients receiving only amitriptyline as a therapy decreased (worsened). The pressure pain thresholds also decreased (worsened) in patients who underwent physical fitness training of increasing strenuousness as their only therapy. The only patients whose pressure pain thresholds increased (improved) were those receiving both amitriptyline and physical fitness training. The average increase in pressure pain threshold for these 45 patients was 0.125 (the difference between 1.75 kg/cm² before treatment and 1.875 kg/cm² after treatment). This small increase does not compare favorably with the results presented in this paper.

Schmidt noted that medical, physical, and psychological therapies are at best about 50% effective.[73] According to panel members of the Copenhagen consensus committee, a sparsity of data makes the natural history of the condition uncertain. Some follow-up studies, however, indicate that fibromyalgia is a chronic condition with a poor social prognosis.[75,p.301]

Hazleman,[76] for example, cited the report of the Nottingham group on the outcome and functional impairment of 72 fibromyalgia patients treated in a single clinic. After four years, 97% of the patients still had symptoms. Many were significantly disabled. The patients had undergone a variety of treatments, yet more than half of the patients received no benefit from the therapy. The investigators concluded that their study demonstrated a poor prognosis, and that many patients had functional impairments with anxiety and depression. Fibromyalgia patients in most longitudinal studies have continued to suffer significant pain and other symptoms, in spite of ongoing treatment.

There has been little evidence of remissions and these few remissions have been short-term. Cathey and colleagues surveyed 81 fibromyalgia patients' medication use during the previous year.[78] The average patient had used 4.7 drugs during the year and at year's end was taking 3.8 drugs. Fifty percent of the patients were taking amitriptyline or cyclobenzaprine, and only one third had enough relief to report that they had moderate or great improvement. Patients reported that analgesics were as effective as either amitriptyline or cyclobenzaprine.

Goldenberg and coworkers[81][82] showed results similar to Cathey's. They followed 87 patients undergoing treatment for three years. Over 50% of the patients failed to benefit from numerous pharmacological and non-pharmacological therapies. Goldenberg's results prompted McCain to conclude, "This indicates that fibromyalgia patients present difficult treatment problems, and that the average patient will require multiple methods of treatment over the natural course of the disease, often with limited success."[83,p.33]

Jacobsen and colleagues[84] used tender points as one of their assessments of the effects of S-adenosylmethionine, an oral anti-inflammatory, an anti-depressant, and an analgesic agent. Patients took a particular drug for six weeks. One person performed the tender point exams using the 14 sites suggested by Smythe. The investigators calculated the tender point score as the sum of values from the 14 sites palpated. If there was no pain at a point, the value was 0. If the patient agreed that the point was tender when the examiner asked him, the value was 1. If the patient responded with a spontaneous verbal report, the value was 2. If the patient reacted with withdrawal, the value was 3. The tender point scores decreased (improved) from 31 to 19.3 for patients taking the drug and 30 to 24.3 for subjects taking a placebo. The researchers wrote that the number of tender points showed a tendency toward reduction, but the change was not statistically significant.

As Goldenberg pointed out, most studies of fibromyalgia treatments have been short-term, lasting only 6 to 12 weeks.[70,p.72] Examinations of patients taking part in our study lasted considerably longer. J.C.L. examined patient #1 from August 11, 1993 to August 8, 1994; patient #2 from August 31, 1993 through July 8, 1994; patient #3 from September 4, 1993 through March 18, 1994; and patient #4 from February 9, 1994 through July 15, 1994.

McCain stated that although researchers have evaluated some therapies with scientific rigor, no definitive treatment strategy has emerged.[83,p.32] If the results from our case studies are later reflected in controlled studies, T_3 supplementation will be a definitive treatment based on a coherent theoretical basis. The case studies we report here, though, do not conclusively validate the treatment protocol we used with our four fibromyalgia patients. Validity can be firmly established only with randomized controlled trials. We intended only to show changes in the quantified mean algometer scores of each patient's 18 tender point sites over periods that would make placebo effects unlikely.

Possible Mechanisms of Changes in Patients.
Suggestion. This study involved management of patients with severe and distressing symptoms. Guiding instructions and adjustments in their dosages of T_3 were based on their individual clinical responses. This made it impossible to avoid close communication with the patients. In studies of this type, the possibility of suggestion affecting the variable being measured (in this case, mean algometer scores) is always likely.

Goldenberg and coworkers found that few fibromyalgia patients improved with oral placebos.[81] There were no beneficial changes in tender point scores, pain, fatigue, sleep, or global assessment.

In contrast, Yunus and colleagues,[87] found that fibromyalgia patients taking placebos improved slightly, as did patients taking ibuprofen. The researchers conjectured that the improvement in patients taking ibuprofen may also have been a placebo effect. They reasoned that the patients' improvement may have resulted from interaction with physicians in the study, or from psychological effects of being involved in a study.

Carette and colleagues[71] found in a longitudinal study that after one month of treatment, 30% of their fibromyalgia patients had improved most on amitriptyline or cyclobenzaprine. After six months of treatment, however, these patients' improvement was not significantly greater than that of patients taking placebos.

These reports of the beneficial effects of placebos with fibromyalgia patients highlight the possibility that improvements in our four patients were due to a placebo or other purely psychological effect. We propose,

however, that this is not highly likely. Three of our patients had only brief, palliative, and incomplete symptom relief from numerous forms of treatment given by J.C.L. They began significantly improving only after they began taking T_3, and their improvements persisted for prolonged periods. These three facts indicate that a real therapeutic effect occurred.

Nevertheless, Haanen and coworkers[89] found in a controlled study that patients who underwent hypnotherapy experienced less pain and less physical and psychological discomfort. This indicates that hypnosis or less ceremonial forms of suggestion may improve the status of fibromyalgia patients. If this is true in the general population of fibromyalgia patients, these patients may have a high degree of suggestibility. We recognize that a high degree of suggestibility may have enabled our patients to improve merely through the suggestion that they could do so.

On the other hand, suggestion, by inducing a more confident and relaxed state of mind, may reduce gamma motor nerve activity, allowing skeletal muscle spindles to lengthen, resulting in decreased muscle tone. This could feasibly reduce the metabolic demand of the patients' skeletal muscles, thereby diminishing muscle symptoms. If this decreased the chronic tension of musculotendinous junctions (where most tender point sites are located),[62] algometer scores may have increased (improved) through suggestion-based psychophysiological mechanisms.

Physiological Changes Induced by T_3. It is possible that increases in the algometer scores of patients in this study were due to physiological changes induced by T_3. These putative effects are best considered through the propositions of the hypometabolism hypothesis of fibromyalgia.[112]

Many fibromyalgia patients who seem to have hypothyroidism have no thyroid hormone deficiency. Despite this, some of these patients improve with T_3 treatment. They resemble patients with thyroid hormone resistance syndromes in at least two respects: 1) they have some hypothyroid-like symptoms, and 2) these symptoms can often be relieved with supraphysiologic doses of T_3 without significant symptoms of thyrotoxicosis.

These observations led Lowe to propose the hypometabolism hypothesis of fibromyalgia.[112] This hypothesis posits that fibromyalgia symptoms arise from hypometabolic myofascial and nervous system tissues due to inadequate thyroid hormone stimulation.

According to this hypothesis, in hypothyroid fibromyalgia patients, the inadequate thyroid hormone stimulation giving rise to fibromyalgia symptoms results from a frank deficiency of the hormones. This may be due to thyroid, pituitary, or hypothalamic dysfunction.

In most euthyroid fibromyalgia patients, thyroid hormone does not fully exert its transcription-regulating effects at chromosomes, despite sufficient quantities of circulating thyroid hormone. This is possibly due to mutations of thyroid hormone receptors stationed on the chromosomes.

Effects of Inadequate T_3 Stimulation on the Adrenergic System. The result of inadequate exposure of chromosomes to thyroid hormone (whether due to hypothyroidism or thyroid hormone receptor defects) is a shift in transcription patterns. There is a shift away from transcription of the code for β-adrenergic receptors, and an increase in transcription of the code for α-adrenergic receptors.[98][102]

As the hypothesis states, when the membranes of nervous system and myofascial cells acquire an abnormal predominance of α-adrenergic receptors, the individual becomes susceptible to developing fibromyalgia. The only available research data that supports this contention is the finding of increased α_2-adrenergic receptors on the platelets of fibromyalgia patients.[99]

When the normal basal level of circulating epinephrine and norepinephrine reach cell membranes, the cellular and physiological effects are those mediated by the predominance of α-adrenergic receptors. A review of the cellular and physiological effects of α-adrenergic dominance shows that these effects in neuromuscular tissues can explain the findings in fibromyalgia patients. This makes it clear why the findings in fibromyalgia are not characteristic of any specific disease. Instead, they are characteristic of aberrant physiology due to sustained α-adrenergic dominance in neuromuscular tissues.

For example, hypothyroid patients (who all have inadequate thyroid hormone expression at the chromosomes) have the same pattern of disrupted stage four (slow-wave) sleep as fibromyalgia patients.[59] This disruption may be due to a relatively low serotonin level. This is indicated by two findings: 1) serotonin mediates sleep, and 2) parachlorophenylalanine, an inhibitor of serotonin synthesis, disrupts sleep.[69,p799] In both hypothyroid and fibromyalgia patients (whether associated with hypothyroidism or euthyroid hypometabolism) the basis of the loss of slow-wave sleep may be the inhibitory effect of a high density of α_1-adrenergic receptors on serotonin secreting cells in the brain.[91] When catecholamines in the brain[106][107][108] attach to α_1-adrenergic receptors on serotonergic cells, the catecholamine-receptor combination inhibits the release of serotonin from the cells.[91] By inhibiting serotonin release, α_1-adrenergic receptors mimic the sleep-disrupting effects of parachlorophenylalanine.

The benefits from amitriptyline and cyclobenza-prine for fibromyalgia patients probably result from the drugs inhibiting the reuptake of serotonin from synapses in the brain. As expected, this facilitates restful sleep in some patients. The benefits, however, seem to be temporary, attenuating over time.[70,p.75][71][82]

The benefits of amitriptyline and cyclobenzaprine may be temporary because their effects are eventually overridden by a more widespread and persistent inhibition of serotonin secretion by α-adrenergic receptors on serotonergic neurons. Supraphysiologic doses of T_3, by decreasing the density of α-adrenergic receptors on serotonergic neurons, may disinhibit these neurons so that they secrete more serotonin. In psychiatry,[105] researchers have found that thyroid hormone potentiates the effects of drugs that inhibit neurotransmitter uptake. In a similar vein, T_3 and uptake-inhibiting drugs may have some beneficial synergistic effects in fibromyalgia patients.

Normal brain blood flow and function are dependent on activation of the high concentration of β-adrenergic receptors in many brain regions.[100][101] A shift away from β-adrenergic receptor synthesis, such as when chromosomes are inadequately exposed to thyroid hormone, would result in relative α-adrenergic dominance and vasoconstriction. This may well explain the diminished blood flow in both the brain[95][96] and peripheral tissues[19] of fibromyalgia patients. α_2-Adrenergic activation results in hyperpolarization of the sympathetic ganglia, reducing sympathetic tone.[92][93] This reduces peripheral blood flow, and it would explain why stellate ganglion blocks[21] decrease pain and tender point counts in fibromyalgia patients. The block would temporarily stop the circulation-impeding effects of α_2-adrenergic receptors in the ganglia.

Hyperpolarization of sympathetic ganglia by α_2-adrenergic receptor dominance also impairs the ability of the cardiovascular system to adapt to vigorous activity and may reduce vascular flow to the brain.[94,p.206] This would explain a number of fibromyalgia features, such as patients' muscle weakness, low skeletal muscle work capacity,[41] and cold sensitivity.[4] It would also explain the detraining effects Bennett emphasizes.[4]

Of particular interest, it also explains why fibromyalgia patients may experience a worsening of their symptoms after vigorous exercise. Such activity increases the amount of circulating catecholamines. When these interact with α-adrenergic receptors, the predicted effect would be an intensification of cellular and physiologic slow-down. The tissues most affected, and thus those from which symptoms arise, are those most sensitive to catecholamine-α-adrenergic receptor mediation. In individuals susceptible to fibromyalgia, these tissues are primarily the myofascial and nervous system tissues.

The Hypometabolic Profile. Effects such as these, when viewed as the general functioning and appearance of an individual, are known as an α-adrenergic or hypometabolic profile. As opposed to the speed-up typical of β-adrenergic dominance, α-adrenergic dominance is characterized as a general slow-down of body processes. Certain features are predictable, such as the increased count of α_2-adrenergic receptors found on platelets[99] and the elevated urinary norepinephrine levels reported by Russell.[116] These are both compensatory reactions of the sympathetic nervous system. They induce peripheral vasoconstriction to preserve core body heat during hypometabolic states such as hypothyroidism.[58][117][118][119][120][121]

Other predictable phenomena have no apparent compensatory function. An example is the skin discoloration Yunus termed "cutaneous hyperemia,"[72,p.9] Travell and Simons called "dermatographia,"[50,p.57] and others reported.[77] Travell and Simons state that regular use of antihistamines may be indicated.[50,p.58] A phenomenon that is probably related to those reported by Yunus and Travell and Simons is the "livedo reticularis" (a bluish skin mottling that worsens with cold exposure) that Caro found in fibromyalgia patients.[86] Caro wrote that this appears to result from vascular permeability.[104,pp.46-47] Vascular permeability is a classic reaction to histamine.[88,p.580] It is probable that α_2-adrenergic receptors mediate histamine release in the skeletal muscle[103] and skin of fibromyalgia patients, and induce these skin reactions.

This reaction also may account for both the reduced blood flow through muscles and relative hypotension seen in fibromyalgia patients. This occurs because activation of α_2-adrenergic receptors constitutes a chemical sympathetic blockade, and as a result, vascular tone lowers. It may be that the improvement seen in many fibromyalgia patients who use antihistamines results from these drugs countering the histamine release induced by α-adrenergic receptor activation.

Many individuals temporarily experience the hypometabolic profile when they take β-blocking drugs such as propranolol.[90,p.239] These drugs competitively bind β-adrenergic receptors and essentially temporarily take them out of operation. This produces a relative α-adrenergic dominance. Central nervous system effects include disturbed sleep, fatigue, and depression.[90,p.239]

Peripheral effects of β-adrenergic blockers include a fall in peripheral vascular resistance with reduced blood flow through skeletal muscles[90,p.232] and skin, cold extremities, development of Raynaud's phenomenon,[90,p.238] and attenuation of normal cardiovascular

adaptation to exercise.[90,p.231]

It is likely that we can deduce all features of fibromyalgia from our knowledge of the tissue effects of decreased β-adrenergic mediation and increased α-adrenergic mediation—if we keep in mind that individuals vary in their tissue sensitivities to adrenergic responsiveness. Idiosyncratic tissue sensitivities may account for the variations of associated symptoms between patients. In fact, idiosyncratic patterns of tissue sensitivity to various peptides and hormones, including adrenergic receptors, account in part for the uniqueness of human beings.[97]

Increased Metabolic Capacity. The potency of T_3 in increasing the metabolic rate of cells makes it likely that the improved status of patients in this study was due to such an increase. Moldofsky performed a study that showed subjects who had a high level of aerobic fitness were more resistant to developing fibromyalgia symptoms when deprived of sleep.[44] Since that early study, fitness has been considered a determining factor in the status of fibromyalgia patients. There is good reason to believe, however, that fibromyalgia patients are not able to benefit from aerobic activities as other people do. First, while such fitness activities benefit fibromyalgia patients, it is not curative for them. It appears that they lack the metabolic capacity to fully benefit from aerobic activities.

Questions arise from these observations. First, why do some individuals but not others who have poor physical fitness develop fibromyalgia symptoms when deprived of sleep? Also, why does a lack of aerobic activity worsen the status of fibromyalgia patients but not many sedentary individuals who do not have fibromyalgia? Obviously, something is different about the effects of inadequate aerobic activity in fibromyalgia patients. It is possible that individuals susceptible to fibromyalgia have borderline low metabolic capacity. If so, the added metabolic slow-down from inadequate aerobic activity would be sufficient to induce symptoms of neuromuscular hypometabolism.

The mechanism of low metabolic capacity in euthyroid fibromyalgia patients may be thyroid hormone receptor defects. Perhaps abnormal nucleotide sequences in chromosomes 3 and 17 result in improper amino acid sequences in the protein that constitutes the thyroid hormone receptor. These mutated receptors would have a low affinity for T_3. If this is the mechanism, most patients should improve by taking doses of supplemental T_3 that would be sufficient to induce thyrotoxicosis in euthyroid subjects and hypothyroid patients. The results of the four case studies reported here suggest that this is true.

Further Study. The patients in this study will be asked to participate in follow-up genetic testing. From those who agree, erythrocytes, leukocytes, or skin fibroblasts will be used to obtain chromosomes. In these specimens, chromosome 3 and possibly chromosome 17 will be analyzed. The nucleotides that are coded for synthesis of thyroid hormone receptors will be sequenced. The objective will be to identify any sequence irregularities that would account for T_3 resistance of the patients' thyroid hormone receptors. Researchers have identified such abnormal nucleotide sequences in many patients with thyroid hormone resistance syndromes.[16][109][110][111]

If nucleotide sequences are mutated in our patients, the sequence of amino acids in the protein that constitutes the thyroid hormone receptor should reflect the mutation. A mutated amino acid sequence may create low affinity of the receptor for T_3. This abnormality in the neuromuscular system may be the molecular basis of fibromyalgia.

Goldenberg writes that currently the best approach to treatment involves three components: medications that decrease pain and promote sleep, combined with physical and psychosocial management.[70,p.71] If the results of our case studies represent those from eventual randomized controlled trials with T_3, then this agent will most effectively decrease pain and promote sleep. It will accomplish this by inducing a sustained acceleration of neuromuscular metabolism and by relieving the hypometabolic symptoms that give rise to the diagnosis of fibromyalgia.

ACKNOWLEDGMENTS

The authors would like to thank Thomas Romano, MD, PhD for his critical comments on the contents of this article, particularly on nomenclature. They would also like to thank Jackie Yellin, BA, Diana Deel, and Mervianna Thompson, RN, MSN for their editorial comments.

REFERENCES

1. Wolfe, F., Smythe, H.A., Yunus, M.B., Bennett, R.M., Bombardier, C., Goldenberg, D.L., Tugwell, P., Campbell, S.M., Abeles, M., Clark, P., Fam, A.G., Farber, S.J., Fiechtner, J.J., Franklin, C.M., Gatter, R.A., Mamaty, D., Lessard, J., Lichtbroun, A.S., Masi, A.T., McCain, G.A., Reynolds, W.J., Romano, T.J., Russell, I.J., and Sheon, R.P.: The American College of Rheumatology 1990 criteria for the classification of fibromyalgia: report of the multicenter criteria committee. *Arthritis Rheumatol.*, 33:160-172, 1990.

2. Consensus Document on Fibromyalgia: The Copenhagen Declaration. *Myopain '92*, August 17-20, 1992, pp.15-16.

3. Tilbe, K., Bell, D.A., and McCain, G.A.: Loss of diurnal variation in serum cortisol, growth hormone and prolactin in patients with primary fibromyalgia. *Arthritis Rheum.*, 31:4, 1988.

4. Bennett, R.M.: Muscle physiology and cold reactivity in the fibromyalgia syndrome. *Rheum. Dis. Clin. North Am.*, 15:135-147, 1989.

5. Bennett, R.M., Goldenberg, D., Simons, D.G., and Travell, J.G.: Panel discussion on definitions and diagnostic criteria for muscular pain syndromes. *First International Symposium on Myofascial Pain and Fibromyalgia*, Minneapolis, Minnesota., May 8, 1989.

6. Beetham, W.P., Jr.: Diagnosis and management of fibrositis syndrome and psychogenic rheumatism. *Med. Clin. North Am.*, 63:433-439, 1979.

7. Neeck, G. and Riedel, W.: Thyroid function in patients with fibromyalgia syndrome. *J. Rheumatol.*, 19:1120-1122, 1992.

8. Golding, D.N.: Hypothyroidism presenting with musculoskeletal symptoms. *Ann. Rheum. Dis.*, 29:10-14, 1970.

9. Bland, J.H. and Frymoyer, J.W.: Rheumatic syndromes of myxedema. *New Eng. J. Med.*, 282:1171-1174, 1970.

10. Wilke, W.S., Sheeler, L.R., and Makarowski, W.S.: Hypothyroidism with presenting symptoms of fibrositis. *J. Rheum.*, 8:627-630, 1981.

11. Becker, K.I., Ferguson, R.H., and McConahey, W.M.: *New Eng. J. Med.*, 268:177-280, 1963.

12. Hochberg, M.C., Koppes, G.M., Edwards, C.Q., Barnes, H.V., and Arnett, F.C., Jr.: Hypothyroidism presenting as a polymyositis-like syndrome: report of two cases. *Arthritis Rheum.*, 19:1363-1366, 1976.

13. Delamere, J.P., Scott, D.L., and Felix-Davies, D.D.: Thyroid dysfunction and rheumatic diseases. *J. Royal Soc. Med.*, 75:102,1982.

14. Fessel, W.J.: Myopathy of hypothyroidism. *Ann. Rheum. Dis.*, 27:590-596, 1968.

15. Wilson, J. and Walton, J.N.: Some muscular manifestations of hypothyroidism. *J. Neurol. Neurosurg. Psychiat.*, 22:320-324, 1959.

16. Refetoff, S.: Thyroid hormone resistance syndromes. In *Werner's The Thyroid: A Fundamental and Clinical Text*, 5th edition. Edited by S.H. Ingbar and L.E. Braverman, Philadelphia, J.B. Lippincott Co., 1986, pp.1292-1293.

17. Awad, E.A.: Pathological changes in fibromyalgia. *First International Symposium on Myofascial Pain and Fibromyalgia*. Minneapolis, Minnesota, May 9, 1989.

18. Awad, E.A.: Histopathological changes in fibrositis. In *Advances in Pain Research and Therapy*, Vol.17. Edited by J.R. Fricton and E.A. Awad, New York, Raven Press, Ltd., 1990, pp.249-258.

19. Bach-Andersen, R., Jacobsen, S., Danneskiold-Samsøe, B., Bartels, E., Jensen, K.E., Thomsen, C., Henriksen, O., and Arlien-Søborg, P.: New diagnostic tools in primary fibromyalgia: findings from the Copenhagen Research Group on fibromyalgia. In *Advances in Pain Research and*

Therapy, Vol.17. Edited by J.R. Fricton and E.A. Awad, New York, Raven Press, pp.269-276.

20. Duick, D.W., Warren, D.W., Nicoloff, J.T., Otis, C.L., and Croxson, M.S.: Effect of a single dose of dexamethasone on the concentration of serum triiodothyronine in man. *J. Clin. Endocrinol. Metab.*, 39:1151, 1974.

21. Backman, E., Bengtsson, A., Bengtsson, M., Lennmarken, C., and Henriksson, K.G.: Skeletal muscle function in primary fibromyalgia: effect of regional sympathetic blockade with guanethidine. *Acta Neurol. Scand.*, 77:187-191, 1988.

22. Clark, S., Tindall, E., and Bennett, R.: A double-blind crossover study of prednisone in the treatment of fibrositis (Abstr). *Arthritis Rheum.*, 27:S76,1984.

23. Henriksson, K.G., Bengtsson, A., Larsson, J., et al.: Muscle biopsy findings of possible diagnostic importance in primary fibromyalgia (fibrositis, myofascial syndrome). *Lancet*, ii:1395, 1982.

24. Kalyan-Raman, U.P., Kalyan-Raman, K., Yunus, M.B., et al.: Muscle pathology in primary fibromyalgia syndrome: a light microscopic, histologic and ultrastructure study. *J. Rheumatol.*, 11:808-814, 1984.

25. Lowe, J.C. and Poo, I.: Tri-iodothyronine treatment of euthyroid fibromyalgia patients: clinical observations. Unpublished paper, 1991.

26. Morton, J.H.: Sodium liothyronine in metabolic insufficiency syndrome and associated disorders: preliminary report. *J.A.M.A.*, 165(2):124-128.

27. Freedberg, A.S., Kurland, G.S., and Hamolsky, M.W.: Effect of l-tri-iodothyronine alone and combined with l-thyroxine in nonmyxedematous hypometabolism. *New Eng. J. Med.*, 253: 57-60, 1955.

28. Morton, J.H.: Sodium liothyronine in metabolic insufficiency syndrome and associated disorders. *J.A.M.A.*, 165: 124-129, 1957.

29. Fields, E.M.: Treatment of metabolic insufficiency and hypothyroidism with sodium liothyronine. *J.A.M.A.*, 163: 817, 1957.

30. Kurland, G.S., Hamolsky, M.W., and Freedberg, A.S.: Studies in non-myxedematous hypometabolism: I. the clinical syndrome and the effects of triiodothyronine, alone or combined with thyroxine. *J. Clin. Endocrinol.*, 15:1354, 1955.

31. Tittle, C.R.: Effects of 3,5,3' l-triiodothyronine in patients with metabolic insufficiency. *J.A.M.A.*, 162:271, 1956.

32. Goldberg, M.: Diagnosis of euthyroid hypometabolism. *Amer. J. Obst. & Gynec.*, 81:(5)1057-1058, May, 1961.

33. Frawley, T.G., McClintock, J.C., and Beebe, R.T.: Metabolic and therapeutic effects of triiodothyronine. *J.A.M.A.*, 160:646, 1956.

34. Refetoff, S.: Personal communication. April 27, 1992.

35. Bengtsson, A., Bengtsson, M., and Jorfeldt, L.: Diagnostic epidural opioid blockade in primary fibromyalgia at rest and during exercise. *Pain*, 39:171-180, 1989.

36. Bengtsson, A., Henriksson, K.G., and Larsson, J.: Muscle biopsy in primary fibromyalgia: light-microscopical and histochemical findings. *Scand. J. Rheumatol.*, 15:1-6, 1986.

37. Bengtsson, A., Henriksson, K.G., and Larsson, J.: Reduced high-energy phosphate levels in the painful muscles of patients with primary fibromyalgia. *Arthritis Rheum.*, 29:817-821, 1986.

38. Matthews, P.M., Allair, C., Shoubridge, E.A., Karpati, G., Carpenter, S., and Arnold, D.L.: In vivo muscle magnetic resonance spectroscopy in the clinical investigation of mitochondrial disease. *Neurology*, 41:114-120, 1991.

39. Mattur, A.K., Gatter, R.A., Bank, W.J., and Schumacher, H.R.: Abnormal 31P-NMR spectroscopy of painful muscles of patients with fibromyalgia (Abstr). *Arthritis Rheum.*, 31:S23, 1988.

40. Wolfe, R.F., Kamman, R.L., Mooyaart, E.L., de Blecourt, A.C., and van Rijswijk, M.H.(eds): 31P MR spectroscopy of muscle in patients with fibromyalgia. In *Society of Magnetic Resonance in Medicine*. Ninth Annual Meeting and Exhibition, Book of Abstracts, Vol. 1, New York, 1990, p.887.

41. Jacobsen, S., Jensen, K.E., Thomsen, C., Danneskiold-Samsøe, B., and Henriksen, O.: 31P magnetic resonance spectroscopy of skeletal muscle in patients with fibromyalgia. *J. Rheum.*, 19:1600-1603, 1992.

42. Backman, E., Bengtsson, A., Bengtsson, M., Lennmarken, C., and Henriksson, K.G.: Skeletal muscle function in primary fibromyalgia: effect of regional sympathetic blockade with guanethidine. *Acta Neurol. Scand.*, 77:187-191, 1988.

43. Jacobsen, S., Wildschiodtz, C.G., and Danneskiold-Samsøe, B.: Isokinetic and isometric muscle strength combined with transcutaneous electrical muscle stimulation in primary fibromyalgia syndrome. *J. Rheumatol.*, 18:1390-1393, 1991.

44. Moldofsky, H. and Scarisbrick, P.: Induction of neurasthenic musculoskeletal pain syndrome by selective sleep stage deprivation. *Psychosom. Med.*, 38:35-44, 1976.

45. McCain, G.A., Bell, D.A., Mai, F.M., and Halliday, P.D.: A controlled study of the effects of a supervised cardiovascular fitness training program on the manifestations of primary fibromyalgia. *Arthritis Rheum.*, 31:1135-1141, 1988.

46. Klug, G.A., McAauley, E., and Clark, S.: Factors influencing the development and maintenance of aerobic fitness: lessions applicable to the fibrositis syndrome. *J. Rheum.*, 16:30-39, 1989.

47. Walco, G.A. and Ilowite, N.T.: Cognitive-behavioral intervention for juvenile primary fibromyalgia syndrome. *J. Rheumatol.*, 19:1617-1619, 1992.

48. Nielson, W.R., Walker, C., and McCain, G.A.: Cognitive behavioral treatment of fibromyalgia syndrome: preliminary findings. *J. Rheumatol.*, 19:98-103, 1992.

49. Sonkin, L.S.: Endocrine disorders and muscle dysfunction. In *Clinical Management of Head, Neck and TMJ Pain and Dysfunction.* Edited by B. Gelb, Philadelphia, W.B. Saunders Co., 1985, pp.137-170.

50. Travell, J.G. and Simons, D.G.: *Myofascial Pain and Dysfunction: The Trigger Point Manual,* Vol. 1. Williams and Wilkins, Baltimore, 1983.

51. Lowe, J.C.: Calcium and magnesium deficiencies and the vertebral subluxation. *A.C.A. Journal Chiro.,* IX:S128-S129, 1975.

52. Lowe, J.C.: Calcium, magnesium, and muscle spasms, *Chiro. Family Physician.,* 3:18-21, 1981.

53. Kaplan, M.M., Swartz, S.L., and Larsen, P.R.: Partial peripheral resistance to thyroid hormone. *Am. J. Med.,* 70: 1115-1121, 1981.

54. Linde, R., Alexander, N., Island, D.P., and Rabin, D.: Familial insensitivity of the pituitary and periphery to thyroid hormone: a case report in two generations and a review of the literature. *Metabolism,* 31(5):510-513, 1982.

55. Gershengorn, M.C. and Weintraub, B.D.: Thyrotropin-induced hyperthyroidism caused by selective pituitary resistance to thyroid hormone: a new syndrome of "inappropriate secretion of TSH." *J. Clin. Invest.,* 56:633-642, 1975.

56. Novogroder, M., Utiger, R., and Boyar, R.: Juvenile hyperthyroidism with elevated thyrotropin (TSH) and normal 24-hour FSH, LH, GH, and prolactin secretory patterns. *J. Clin. Endocrinol. Metab.,* 45:1053-1059, 1977.

57. Elewaut, A., Mussche, M., and Vermeulen, A.: Familial partial target organ resistance to thyroid hormones. *J. Clin. Endocrinol. Metab.,* 43:575-581, 1976.

58. Williams, R. S. and Lefkowitz, R.J.: The effects of thyroid hormone on adrenergic receptors. In *Molecular Basis of Thyroid Hormone Action.* Edited by J.H. Oppenheimer and H.H. Samuels, New York, Academic Press, Inc., 1983, pp.325-349.

59. Kales, A., Heuser, G., Jacobsen, A., Kales, J.D., Hanley, J., Zweizig, J.R., and Paulson, M.J.: All night sleep studies in hypothyroidism patients, before and after treatment. *J. Clin. Endocrinol.,* 27:1593-1599, 1967.

60. Lowe, J.C.: The need for nutritional supplementation in myofascial pain syndromes. *Anabolism: J. Preventive Med.,* 13:5, 1988.

61. Lowe, J.C.: A case of debilitating headache complicated by hypothyroidism: its relief through myofascial therapy. *Digest Chiro. Econ.,* Nov/Dec:73-75, 1988.

62. Romano, T.: Fibromyalgia syndrome criteria: what they are and why they're important. *J. Myofascial Ther.,* 2:36-37, 1994.

63. Fischer, A.A.: Pressure algometry (dolorimetry) in the differential diagnosis of muscle pain. In *Myofascial Pain and Fibromyalgia: Trigger Point Management.* Edited by E.S. Rachlin, St. Louis, Mosby, 1994, pp.121-141.

64. Bartalena, L., Martino, E., and Brandi, L.S.: Lack of nocturnal serum thyrotropin surge after surgery. *J. Clin. Endocrinol. Metab.,* 70:293, 1990.

65. Christy, N.P.: The adrenal cortex in thyrotoxicosis. In *Werner and Ingbar's The Thyroid: A Fundamental and Clinical Text,* 6th edition. Edited by L.E. Braverman and R.D. Utiger, Philadelphia, J.B. Lippincott Co., 1991, pp.806-815.

66. Nicoloff, J.T., Fisher, D.A., and Appleman, M.D.: The role of glucocorticoids in the regulation of thyroid function in man. *J. Clin. Invest.,* 49:1922, 1970.

67. Brabant, A., Brabant, G, and Schuermeyer, T.: The role of glucocorticoids in the regulation of thyrotropin. *Acta Endocrinol* (Copenhagen), 121:95, 1989.

68. Wilson, E.D.: *Wilson's Syndrome.* Orlando, Cornerstone Publishing Co., 1991.

69. Kelly, D.D.: Sleep and dreaming. In *Principles of Neural Science,* 3rd edition. Edited by E.R. Kandel, J.H. Schwartz, and T.M. Jessell, Norwalk, Appleton & Lange, 1991, pp.792-804.

70. Goldenberg, D.L.: Fibromyalgia: treatment programs. *J. Musculoskel. Pain,* 1:71-81, 1993.

71. Carette, S., Bell, M., Reynolds, J., Haraoui, B., McCain, G., Bykerk, V., Edworthy, S., Baron, M., Koehler, B., Fam, A., Bellany, N., and Gulmont, C.: A controlled trial of amitriptyline, cyclobenzaprine, and placebo in fibromyalgia. *Arthritis Rheum.,* 35(Suppl 9):112, 1992.

72. Yunus, M.B.: Fibromyalgia syndrome and myofascial pain syndrome: clinical features, laboratory tests, diagnosis, and pathophysiologic mechanisms. In *Myofascial Pain and Fibromyalgia: Trigger Point Management.* Edited by E.S. Rachlin, St. Louis, Mosby, 1994, pp.3-29.

73. Schmidt, K.L.: Generalized tendomyopathy (fibromyalgia): differential diagnosis, therapy, and prognosis. *Z. Gesamte. Inn. Med.,* 46:370-374, 1991.

74. Reilly, P.A. and Littlejohn, G.O.: Diurnal variation in the symptoms and signs of the fibromyalgia syndrome (FS). *J. Musculoskel. Pain,* 1:237-243, 1993.

75. Consensus Document on Fibromyalgia: The Copenhagen Declaration. *J. Musculoskel. Pain,* 1:295-312, 1993.

76. Hazleman, B.: Soft tissue rheumatism. *Brit. J. Rheumat.,* 31:135, 1992.

77. Kraft, G.H., Johnson, E.W., and LeBan, M.M.: The fibrositis syndrome. *Arch. Phys. Med.,* 49:155-162, 1968.

78. Cathey, M.A., Wolfe, F., Kleinheksel, S.M., and Hawley, D.J.: Socioeconomic impact of fibrositis: a study of 81 patients with primary fibrositis. *Amer. J. Med.,* 81:78-84, 1986.

79. Felson, D.T. and Goldenberg, D.L.: The natural history of fibromyalgia. *Arthritis Rheum.,* 29:1522-1526, 1986.

80. Isomeri, R., Mikkelsson, M., Latikka, P., and Kammonen, K.: Effects of amitriptyline and cardiovascular fitness training on pain in patients with primary fibromyalgia. *J. Musculoskel. Pain,* 1:253-260, 1993.

81. Goldenberg, D.L., Felson, D.T., and Dinerman, H.: A randomized, controlled clinical trial of amitriptyline and naproxen in the treatment of patients with fibromyalgia. *Arthritis Rheum.*, 29:1371-1377, 1986.

82. Goldenberg, D.L.: Treatment of fibromyalgia syndrome. *Rheum. Dis. Clin. North Am.*, 15:61-67, 1989.

83. McCain, G.A.: Treatment of fibromyalgia and myofascial pain syndrome. In *Myofascial Pain and Fibromyalgia: Trigger Point Management*. Edited by E. S. Rachlin, St. Louis, Mosby, 1994, pp.31-44.

84. Jacobsen, S., Danneskiold-Samsøe, B., and Andersen, R.B.: Oral S-adenosyl-methionine in primary fibromyalgia: double-blind clinical evaluation. *Scand. J. Rheumatol.*, 20:294-302, 1991.

85. Romano, T.J.: The usefulness of cranial electrotherapy in the treatment of headache in fibromyalgia patients. *Am. J. Pain Manag.*, 3:15-19, 1993.

86. Caro, X.J.: Immunofluorescent detection of IgG at the dermal-epidermal junction in patients with apparent primary fibrositis syndrome. *Arthritis Rheum.*, 27:1174, 1984.

87. Yunus, B.M.B., Masi, A.T., and Aldag, J.C.: Short term effects of ibuprofen in primary fibromyalgia syndrome: a double-blind, placebo-controlled trial. *J. Rheumatol.*, 16:527-532, 1989.

88. Garrison, J.C.: Histamine, bradykinin, 5-hydroxytryptamine, and their antagonists. In *The Pharmacological Basis of Therapeutics*, 8th edition. Edited by A.G. Gilman, T.W. Rall, A.S. Nies, and P. Taylor, New York, Pergamon Press, 1990, pp.574-599.

89. Haanen, H.C., Hoenderos, H.T., and van Romunde, L.K.: Controlled trial of hypnotherapy in the treatment of refractory fibromyalgia. *Rheumatol.* 18:72-75, 1991.

90. Hoffman, B.B. and Lefkowitz, R.J.: Adrenergic receptor antagonists. In *The Pharmacological Basis of Therapeutics*, 8th edition. Edited by A.G. Gilman, T.W. Rall, A.S. Nies, and P. Taylor, New York, Pergamon Press, 1990.

91. Frankhyzen, A. and Muller, A.: In vitro studies on the inhibition of serotonin release through α-adrenoreceptor activity in various regions of the rat CNS. *Abstract of 5th Catecholamine Symposium*, 1983, p.137.

92. Smith, P.A., Rafuse, P.E., and Zidichouski, J.A.: Mechanisms of alpha₂-adrenergic hyperpolarization in sympathetic ganglia. In *Pharmacology of Adrenoceptors*. Edited by E. Szabadi, C.M. Bradshaw, and S.R. Nahorski, Weinheim (Feberal Republic of Germany), Verlagsgesellschaft, 1985, pp.325-326.

93. Ramage, A.G. and Wilkinson, S.J.: Evidence to suggest that central alpha₁- and alpha₂-adrenoceptors have opposing actions on sympathetic tone. In *Pharmacology of Adrenoceptors*. Edited by E. Szabadi, C.M. Bradshaw, and S.R. Nahorski, Weinheim (Feberal Republic of Germany), Verlagsgesell-schaft, 1985, pp.323-324.

94. Homewood, A.E.: *Neurodynamics of the Vertebral Subluxation*. St. Petersburg, Valkyrie Press, Inc., 1962.

95. Romano, T. and Govindan, S.: Brain SPECT findings in fibromyalgia patients with headache. *Arthritis Rheum.*, 36:R23, 1993.

96. Mountz, J.M., Bradley, L., Modell, J.G., Triana, M., Alexander, R., and Mountz, J.D.: Limbic system dysregulation in fibromyalgia measured by regional cerebral blood flow. *Arthritis Rheum.*, 36:R23, 1993.

97. Pert, C.B., Ruff, M.R., Weber, R.J., and Herkenham, M.: Neuropeptides and their receptors: a psychosomatic network. *J. Immunology*, 135:820s-826s, 1985.

98. Kunos, G., Vermes-Kunos, I., and Nickerson, M.: Effects of thyroid state on adrenoceptor properties. *Nature*, 250:779-781, 1974.

99. Bennett, R.M., Clark, S.M., and Campbell, S.M.: Symptoms of Raynaud's syndrome in patients with fibromyalgia: a study utilizing the Nielsen test, digital photoplethysmography and measurements of platelet α₂-adrenergic receptors. *Arthritis Rheum.*, 34:264-269, 1991.

100. De Paermentier, F., Cheetham, S.C., Crompton, M.R., and Horton, R.W.: Beta-adrenoceptor binding sites in post-mortem human brain. *Brit. J. Pharmacology*, 97:383P, 1989.

101. Janig, W.: The autonomic nervous system. In Schmidt, R.F.: Integrative functions of the central nervous system. In *Fundamentals of Neurophysiology*, 3rd edition. Edited by R.F. Schmidt, New York: Springer-Verlag, 1985, pp.216-269.

102. Williams, L.T. and Lefkowitz, R.J.: Molecular pharmacology of alpha adrenergic receptors: utilization of [3H] dihydroergocryptine binding in the study of pharmacological receptor alterations. *Molecular Pharm.*, 13:304-313, 1977.

103. Camazine, B., Shannon, R.P., Guerrero, J.L., Graham, R.M., Powell, W.J., Jr.: Neurogenic histaminergic vasodilation in canine skeletal muscle: mediation by alpha₂-adrenoceptor stimulation. *Circ. Res.*, 62:871-883, 1988.

104. Caro, X.J.: Immunofluorescent studies of skin in primary fibrositis syndrome. *Am. J. Med.*, 81(suppl 3A):43-49, 1986.

105. Prange, A.J., Wilson, I.C., Rabon, A.M., and Lipton, M.A.: Enhancement of imipramine antidepressant activity by thyroid hormone. *Am. J. Psychiatry*, 126:464, 1969.

106. Pearson, J., Goldstein, M., Kitahama, K., Sakamoto, N., and Michel, J.-P.: Catecholaminergic neurons of the human central nervous system. In *An Introduction to Neurotransmission in Health and Disease*. Edited by P. Riederer, N. Kopp, and J. Pearson, Oxford, Oxford University Press, 1990.

107. Kopp, N., Denoroy, L., Renaud, B., Pujol, J.F., Tabib, A., and Tommasi, M.: Distribution of adrenaline-synthesizing enzyme activity in the human brain. *J. Neurol. Sci.*, 41:379-409, 1979.

108. Hortnagl, H., Schlogl, E., Sperk, G., and Hornykiewicz, O.: The topographical distribution of the monoaminergic innervation in the basal ganglia of the human brain. In *Molecular and Cellular Interaction Underlying Higher Brain Functions: Progress in Brain Research*, Vol. 58. Edited by J.-P. Changeux, J. Glowinski, M. Imbert, and F.E. Bloom, 1983, pp.269-274.

109. Usala, S. J., Bercu, B.B., and Refetoff, S.: Diverse abnormalities of the c-erbAβ thyroid hormone receptor gene in generalized thyroid hormone resistance. In *Advances in Perinatal Thyroidology*. Edited by B.B. Bercu and D.I. Shulman, New York, Plenum Press, 1991.

110. Usala, S. and Weintraub, B.D.: Familial thyroid hormone resistance: clinical and molecular studies. *Endocrin. Metab.*, 2:59-76, 1991.

111. Refetoff, S., Weiss, R.E., and Usala, S.J.: The syndromes of resistance to thyroid hormone. *Endocrine Rev.*,14:348-399, 1993.

112. Lowe, J.C.: *Fibromyalgia: The Hypometabolism Hypothesis (Diagnosis and Treatment)*. Houston, McDowell Publishing Co., 1994, in press.

113. Algometer. JMT, P.O. Box 980005, Houston, TX 77098 (713-621-2522).

114. Smith, Kline & Beecham, 1500 Spring Garden St., Philadelphia, PA 19101.

115. Bantle, J.P., Seeling, S., Mariash, C.N., Ulstrom, R.A., and Oppenheimer, J.H.: Resistance to thyroid hormones: a disorder frequently confused with Graves disease. *Arch. Intern. Med.*, 142:1867-1871, 1982.

116. Russell, I.J., Vipraio, G.A., and Morgan, W.W.: Is there a metabolic basis for the fibrositis syndrome? *Amer. J. Med.*, 81(3A):50-56, 1986.

117. Wahi, R.S., Chansouria, J.P.N., and Udupa, K.N.: Normal levels of norepinephrine in short term hypothyroidism. *J. Clin. Endocrinol. Metab.*, 51:934-935, 1980.

118. Lipton, M.A., Prange, A.J., and Dairman, W.: Increased rate of norepinephrine biosynthesis in hypothyroid rats. *Fed. Proc.*, 27:399, 1968.

119. Prange, A.J., Jr., Meed, J.L., and Lipton, M.A.: Catecholamines: diminished rate of norepinephrine biosynthesis in rat brain and heart after thyroxine pretreatment. *Life Sci.*, 9:901, 1970.

120. Harrison, T.S.: Adrenal medullary and thyroid relationships. *Physiol. Rev.*, 44:161, 1964.

121. McConnaughey, M.M., Jones, L.R., Watanabe, A.M., Besch, H.R., Jr., Williams, L.T., and Lefkowitz, R.J.: Thyroxine and propylthiouracil effects on alpha- and beta-adrenergic receptor number, ATPase activities, and sialic acid content of rat cardiac membrane vesicles. *J. Cardiovasc. Pharmacol.*, 1:609-623, 1979.

T3-INDUCED RECOVERY FROM FIBROMYALGIA
BY A HYPOTHYROID PATIENT
RESISTANT TO T4 AND DESICCATED THYROID

John C. Lowe, MA, DC

This article originally appeared in the *Journal of Myofascial Therapy*, 1(4):26-31, 1995.
It is reprinted with permission of McDowell Publishing Company.

Abstract: The main purpose of this case report is to illustrate a clinical observation common to me: that fibromyalgia patients with central hypothyroidism who fail to benefit from T4 or desiccated thyroid completely recover when they switch to T3. Changing status in the patient was evaluated in three ways: a psychiatrist used a depression inventory, a physical therapist performed functional musculoskeletal assessments, and I performed algometer tender point exams and monitored symptoms. I hope the description of the management of this case provides a protocol that other clinicians will use with fibromyalgia patients similar to the one who is the subject of this report.

Key Words. Fibromyalgia, Hypothyroidism, T3, T4, TSH, Desiccated thyroid, Algometry.

INTRODUCTION

A number of researchers in the 1950s and 1960s reported that hypothyroid patients responded to T_3, the metabolically active thyroid hormone, after failing to benefit from T_4, desiccated thyroid, or thyroglobulin.[8][9,p.13][10,p.274][11][12][13][14] Many of the symptoms the patients in these reports recovered from are remarkably similar to those characteristic of fibromyalgia. The symptoms are listed in Table 1.

The fibromyalgia patient whose case I report here resembles the patients in the 1950s and 1960s case reports in two respects: first, she shares with them the same general symptoms; and second, she responded to T_3 afer failing to benefit from desiccated thyroid. The patient discussed in this report and other fibromyalgia patients may be modern day examples of those 1950s and 1960s patients.

Like fibromyalgia patients studied by Ferraccioli and coworkers[18] and Neeck and Riedel,[19] this patient had a blunted TSH response to TRH, and this, combined with her thyroid hormone profiles, indicates that she had central (probably pituitary) hypothyroidism. Her complete recovery from fibromyalgia may point the way to relief for other fibromyalgia patients with central hypothyroidism.

METHODS

Patient. The patient in this case study was a 41-year old Caucasian female. She was a homemaker and mother of two children.

On March 2, 1993 the patient's automobile, traveling at 20 miles per hour, struck another that came into her path. Immediately after the impact, she experienced neck and left shoulder pain. Subsequently, she underwent treatment, seriatim, by a chiropractic physician, a medical physician, a physical therapist, two additional chiropractic physicians, and myself. I concurred with the other practitioners that the patient had a traumatically-induced regional cervical injury but also diagnosed her as having fibromyalgia. Apparently she had had fibromyalgia symptoms for many years.

At the beginning of the study, she indicated on body drawings that she had widespread pain according to the American College of Rheumatology 1990 criteria:[23] pain above and below the waist and on the left and right sides of her body. The body areas she shaded on the drawings included the anterior, posterior, and lateral neck, the upper posterior thoracic area, the supraspinatus muscles, the interscapular region down to about the T6 level, and the low back and gluteal muscles. She described her pain as "throbbing, aching, burning, and sometimes shooting and stabbing." she stated that her muscles felt too tense. She also reported the symptoms listed in Table 2.

Previous Treatment. On March 25, 1988 her psychiatrist prescribed desiccated thyroid. The supplement was intended to increase her energy level and serve as an adjunct to the antidepressant Desyrel®. She also took the antidepressant Wellbutrin®. She continued the thyroid supplement until we began this study although it benefitted her only in one way: her coldness decreased in distribution. Before taking desiccated thyroid, her whole body was cold. After beginning the supplement, only her hands and feet were cold–the Raynaud's-like symptom of fibromyalgia.

After delivering a baby in March 1990, she experienced severe post-partum depression and started an estrogen supplement.

Table 1. Symptoms reportedly relieved by T₃ after T₄, desiccated thyroid, or thyroglobulin failed to do so.

- Aching in both knees, skin pallor, facial puffiness, a dull feeling, and tiredness.[8]
- Lethargy, easy fatigue, nervousness, irritability, sensitivity to cold, headache, musculoskeletal pain, diminished sexual potency, and menstrual irregularities.[9]
- Chronic fatigue, muscle and joint aches, excess weight, bowel dysfunction, cold intolerance.[10]
- Muscle aches, stiffness, chronic fatigue, excess weight, menstrual disturbances, dry hair and skin, brittle fingernails, nervousness, irritability, depression, mental apathy, puffiness of the face.[11]
- In school children, poor school records, short attention span, lack of ability to concentrate, "don't care attitude," anxiety, restlessness, poor appetite, constipation.[12]
- Muscle and joint pains, fatigue, irritability and mood swings, lethargy, decreased libido, premenstrual tension, GI disturbances, scalp seborrhea or hair loss, palpitations, and shortness of breath.[13]

Methods of Assessment. There were several forms of evaluation.

Musculoskeletal Functional Evaluation. A physical therapist performed functional musculoskeletal assessments of the patient on three occasions.

Psychiatric Evaluation. The patient filled out a Zung's Depression Inventory on July 23, 1994 at the beginning of treatment and on January 13, 1995 at the end.

Fibromyalgia Evaluation. The patient's fibromyalgia status was assessed through three methods: weekly pain drawings, mean algometer scores (the average of the pressure/pain thresholds of the 18 tender points), and diaries of symptoms. Between July

2 and August 8, 1994, I performed five baseline algometer exams. Between August 14, 1994 and January 27, 1995, I performed 19 treatment-phase algometer exams.

Laboratory Evaluation. The patient's laboratory profiles were available dating back to 1988. Each included a CBC, SMAC, lipid profile, and thyroid profile. At my request, on July 6, 1994, an internist performed a TRH-stimulation test to evaluate the patient's TSH response to TRH, the hypothalamic hormone. Between July 19 and 20, 1994, he also performed a dexamethasone suppression test to assess adrenal cortical function.

In the TRH-stimulation test, the internist drew a blood sample to establish the patient's TSH serum baseline level. Thirty minutes after injecting TRH, he drew a second blood sample to measure the change in the TSH level. The baseline level was 0.88 IU/ml; the second TSH level was 7.83 IU/ml. This was a blunted TSH response to TRH.

The internist also measured the patient's serum cortisol on July 19, 1994 which was 16.65 ug/dl. After he injected the patient with the synthetic glucocorticoid dexamethasone, he again measured the cortisol level on July 20, 1994. The value was 0.84 ug/dl. This constituted proper adrenocortical suppression.

Imaging Procedures. The patient had cervical plain film x-rays that were taken on April 7, 1993. She had a cervical MRI on May 26, 1994. In the radiology report, dated May 27, 1994, the radiologist noted that the patient had a "small central disc bulge and small posterior osteophytes at C5-C6." The MRI study was otherwise unremarkable.

Treatment. After her automobile accident on March 2, 1993, the patient had treatment at intervals by two other chiropractors. Each performed directional non-force technique (a gentle manual spinal treatment procedure). She also received treatment several times by a physical therapist. The treatment involved exercise therapy and manual cervical traction. This treatment continued during the case study.

The patient took Armour® desiccated thyroid from 1988 until the beginning of this case study. She was taking 2 grains when she first consulted me. Throughout the treatment phase of the study, she took various doses of T₃ prescribed by her psychiatrist. After the baseline period (the first five exams), she abruptly stopped her desiccated thyroid hormone intake and immediately began taking T₃. Her starting dose was 67 mcg of T₃. On November 15, 1994, she increased her dosage to 82.5 mcg. She did so because of a brief reappearance of her symptoms and a drop in her mean algometer score.

Throughout the study, the patient held constant her intake of Ciba Estraderm® patch, containing 4 mg of estradiol. On November 17, 1995 she stopped her previous 100 mg of Wellbutrin®. She continued to take Desyrel® on occasion. During the study, she received in my office treatment with ultrasound, soft tissue manipulation, moist heat, stretch and spray, and manual cervical traction.

RESULTS

Changes in Musculoskeletal Function. The patient's physical therapist performed three functional exams. On April 13, 1994, the therapist wrote: The patient "has two children, ages 4 and 13. She is unable to play games with them because of her symptoms. She has a housekeeper full-time and has not done significant housework, gardened, swum, or exercised since her accident. Sleeping is uncomfortable."

On June 10, 1994, the therapist wrote that the burning sensation in the patient's neck and shoulders had improved 75%. She still had dysfunction and trouble sleeping.

On September 23, 1994, the therapist wrote: The patient "has been seen weekly for chiropractic treatment and began taking T_3. She reports a dramatic improvement in her energy level. Now she has periods when she is pain-free. She states she is able to exercise now up to 1½ hours without feeling extreme fatigue as in the past." The patient's grip strength and shoulder flexor strength had improved bilaterally. She was able to sleep through the night most nights, and she had a marked increase in all ranges of cervical motion. Flexion and retraction were no longer painful. The patient did, however, still have regional pain and cervical spinal dysfunction associated with her cervical traumatic injury.

Changes in Psychiatric Status. On July 23, 1994, the patient's raw score on the Zung's Depression Inventory was 43. This converts to an SDS index of 54. The equivalent clinical global impression for the index is "presence of minimal-to-mild depression." On January 13, 1995, some six months later, her raw score on Zung's was 28. This converts to an SDS index of 35. The equivalent clinical global impression for this index is "within normal range: no psychopathology."

Changes in Fibromyalgia Status. By October 4, 1994–about two months after beginning T_3–the patient no longer met the 1990 criteria for fibromyalgia.[23]

Pain Drawings. By September 21, the patient's pain decreased from widespread (according to the

ACR 1990[23] criteria). She continued, however, to have regional pain related to her cervical injury.

Algometer Scores. On October 4, 1994, the patient's mean algometer score exceeded 4 kg/cm², the cut off point for normal.

Figure 1 shows the weekly mean algometer scores graphically plotted to show the change over a six-month period. The horizontal axis shows the number of each weekly measurement, and the vertical axis shows the pressure (applied with an algometer, registered in kg/cm²) she could tolerate before experiencing discomfort at the tender point sites. When viewing the graph in Figure 1, keep in mind that the patient began taking 67 mcg of T_3 on August 8, 1994. On this date, I performed her 5th algometer exam and recorded the result on the graph. Because her symptoms briefly worsened and her mean algometer score dropped, she increased the dosage to 82.5 mcg on November 11, 1994 (the date of her 20th algometer exam).

Table 2. Symptoms reported by the patient at the beginning of the case study.

1. Sleep disturbance.
2. Prolonged morning stiffness (requiring 2-to-12 hours to loosen).
3. Occasional irritable bowel syndrome.
4. Daily headaches.
5. Depression.
6. Poor memory and concentration.
7. Cold hands and feet.
8. Chronic fatigue and sluggishness.
9. Husky voice.
10. Coarse, rough skin.
11. Puffy face and eyes.
12. Not sufficiently alert and attentive.
13. Difficulty losing weight.
14. Dry hair that fell out easily.

Visual inspection reveals an increase in the patient's mean algometer scores beginning the 13th week of the study. In the 19th week, the scores fell but not to baseline. But within three and a half weeks, they ascended again reaching and exceeding the normal value of 4 kg/cm². The scores remained above normal for the rest of the study and throughout follow-up.

Symptoms. At the end of the case study, the patient was completely free from all the symptoms listed in Table 2. Her pain was intermittent and limited to her posterior cervical and left upper thoracic regions.

She reported during several post-study follow-up contacts that her status had continued to improve. At follow-up on April 1, 1995, she maintained that she had remained free from all aspects of fibromyalgia for six months and thus considered herself completely recovered.

Table 3. Four thyroid panels available on patient.

Date	Test	Value	Normal Range
03-28-88:	T_4 (RIA)	8.0	(5.5-11.5 μg/dl)
	T_3 (RIA)	133	(90-200 ng/dl)
	TSH	1.7	(0.4-4.3 μg/dl)
07-06-94:	T_4 (RIA)	6.4	(4.5-12.5 μg/dl)
	T_3 Uptake	25%	25% - 35%
	T_7	1.6	1.0-4.0 Units
	TSH	0.7	(0.4-6.0 μg/dl)
09-07-94:	T_4 (RIA)	1.8	(4.5-10.9 μg/dl)
	T_3 (RIA)	154	(60-181 ng/dl)
	TSH	0.89	(0.35-5.5 μg/dl)
01-19-95:	T_4 (RIA)	1.6	(4.5-10.9 μg/dl)
	T_3 (RIA)	199	(60-181 ng/dl)
	TSH	0.43	(0.35-5.5 μg/dl)

Changes in Laboratory Values. Four thyroid panels were available and are listed in Table 3. The profile performed in March 1988 shows that the patient's TSH, T_4 (RIA) and T_3 (RIA) were low normal. In July 1994, this same pattern prevailed, and the TRH-stimulation test performed on the same day shows a blunted TSH response. This indicated that she had central (probably pituitary) hypothyroidism.

The September 1994 and January 1995 profiles show that the TSH level decreased and the T_4 (RIA) decreased. In contrast to the March 1988 profile, however, the T_3 (RIA) increased above normal. This pattern indicates that her supplemental T_3 was inhibiting the pituitary glands's thyrotrophs so that they secreted a lower quantity of TSH. The lower exposure of thyroid gland cells to TSH apparently resulted in a reduced secretion of T_4.

DISCUSSION

Study Design. The format of this study was a single-subject design, also called a "functional design." Chiropractic and medical researchers currently most value another study design–one that tests hypotheses by comparing the responses of groups of subjects to therapeutic interventions. Such comparisons of groups are excellent for testing hypotheses. But investigators who use functional or single-subject designs are not so much concerned with hypothesis testing. Instead, they are concerned with quantifying a patient's response to a therapeutic intervention and measuring it repeatedly through the course of treatment. It is the *functional relationship* between the two variables (the therapy and the response) that interests them. Behavioral scientists–who typically are far better grounded in logic and the philosophy of science–make an argument that other clinical researchers could (were they to listen) profit from: meaningful hypotheses seldom if ever derive from studies that compare differences between groups. By contrast, such hypotheses *do* tend to emerge inductively from the data derived from functional or single-subject studies.[24]

Most medical researchers measure groups of subjects' responses once before and once afer the therapy. By contrast, investigators conducting single-subject studies measure the subject's responses repeatedly throughout the course of the study. These repetitive measures provide a more detailed account of changes in the subject's responses over time. They show the *process* of therapeutic change plotted against the amount or intensity of therapeutic stimulus. This can reveal with clarity the functional relationship between the therapy and the patient's responses to it.[4,pp.29-37] We should use a functional design with single subjects when we aim for greater precision than group studies allow in determining the relationship between the independent variable (treatment) and the dependent variable (the patient's measured response).[4,p.14] I posit that the thorough failure of other fibromyalgia researchers to unearth the nature of or effective treatment for fibromyalgia is a direct outgrowth of their naive distrust of clinical observation and single-subject case studies.

Changes in Zung's Depression Inventory. The change in the patient's Zung's Depression Inventory indicates that she experienced a decrease from "minimal-to-mild" depression to "within the range of normal." This might be interpreted as reflecting an increase in serotonin secretion. The increase can be predicted to result from thyroid hormone stimulation decreasing the number of inhibitory α-adrenergic receptors and increasing the number of stimulatory β-adrenergic receptors on her CNS serotonergic cells. This would disinhibit their secretion of serotonin.[25,p.137] Also, increased numbers of β-adrenergic receptors in her CNS due to transcription regulation by T_3-thyroid hormone receptor complex may have increased the metabolism of CNS neuronal pathways that mediate a non-depressed mental state.

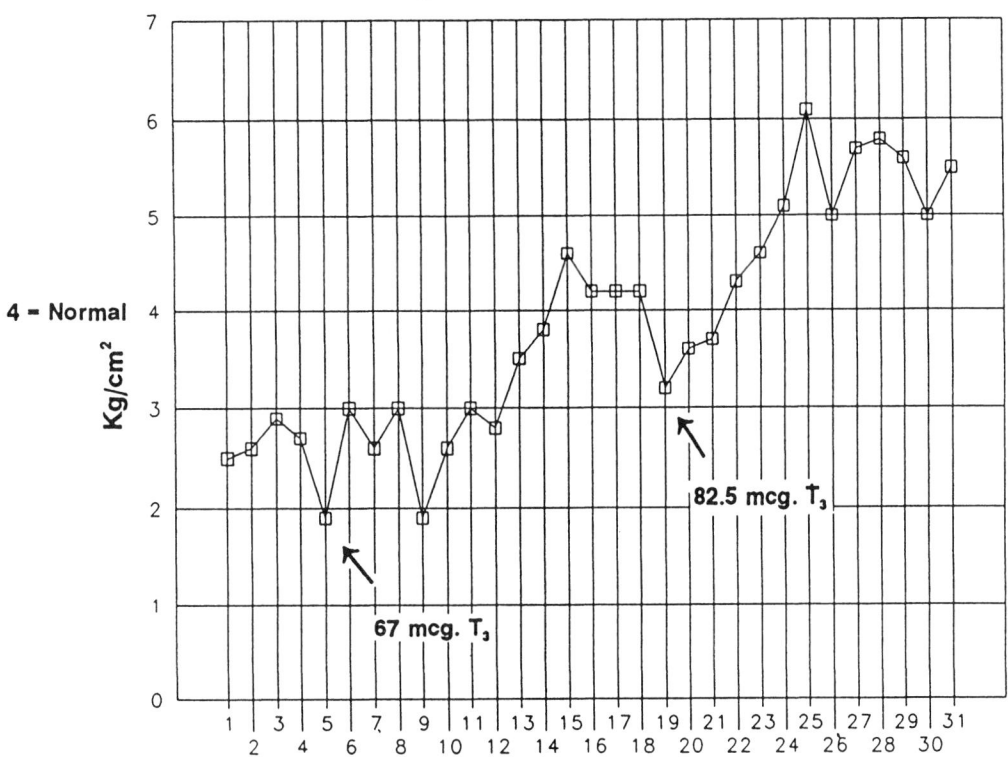

Mean Algometer Scores of Tender Points

Numbers of Weekly Algometer Exams

Figure 1

Interpretation of Laboratory Tests Results. In the TRH-stimulation test, the internist drew a blood sample to establish the patient's TSH serum baseline level. After injecting TRH, he drew a second sample after 30 minutes. The change from the baseline TSH level of 0.88 IU/ml to the 30-minute post-injection level of 7.83 IU/ml indicated a suppression of TSH response to TRH. There are several possible mechanisms for this blunted TSH response.

Was the patient's T_4 elevated and her TSH low because of her estrogen supplement? The patient used a transdermal estrogen patch. It is not likely that this accounted for her low TSH values. Oral estrogen supplements tend to increase the concentration of thyroid-binding globulin (TBG) in the blood. They do so by increasing sialylation of TBG, prolonging its biologic half-life.[1] This occurs because the liver clears a large percentage of the estrogen during its first passage through the liver, resulting in high liver estrogen concentrations. Even the low-dose estrogens in today's oral contraceptives increase TBG concentrations slightly. Only in occasional patients, however, does the serum total T_4 exceed normal limits.[2,p.336] Transdermal estrogen therapy allows the hormone to enter the circulation gradually rather than in the bursts characteristic of oral estrogen therapy. Because of this, estrogen does not accumulate in high concentrations in the liver. As a result, TBG levels may increase only a little.[3] It is unlikely, then, that suppression of TSH secretion by elevated thyroid hormone levels due to increased TBG levels would account for the patient's suppressed TSH response to TRH.

Was the patient's blunted TSH response due to hyperadrenocortical secretion? During the dexamethasone suppression test, the patient's serum cortisol level decreased from 16.65 ug/dl on July 19, 1994 to 0.84 ug/dl on July 20, 1994 after an injection of the synthetic corticosteroid dexamethasone. This was an adequate suppression of adrenocortical secretion of endogenous cortisol indicating that the patient did not have hypersecretion of endogenous cortisol. From this result, I concluded that the patient's blunted TSH response to TRH was not likely due to suppression of the pituitary thyrotrophs and obstruction of T_4-to-T_3 conversion by excess concentrations of cortisol. The result of this test is also inconsistent with the previous findings of failed adrenocortical suppression in some fibromyalgia patients.[18][20]

Comparative Doses of Desiccated Thyroid and T_3. When various investigators reported benefits from T_3 after patients had failed to improve with desiccated thyroid,[8][9,p.13][10,p.274][11][12][13][14] Jefferies objected that the doses of T_3 were higher than those of desiccated thyroid, and that the higher doses were responsible for the benefits rather than the form of thyroid hormone.[6] This is incompatible with many of my clinical observations. Many patients under Poo's and my care[22] took doses of T_4 and desiccated thyroid high enough to produce distinct thyrotoxicosis. When the patients stopped taking desiccated thyroid and switched to T_3, however, fibromyalgia symptoms dramatically improved or ceased completely without toxicity on doses that were proportionately lower than the thyrotoxic doses of T_4 and desiccated thyroid.

This indicates that in some way, T_3 corrects or overrides the underlying mechanisms of fibromyalgia symptoms when T_4 or desiccated thyroid does not do so. One possible explanation for this difference is that T_4 (in desiccated thyroid and products such as Synthroid® and Levothroid®) is not effectively converted to T_3, the metabolically active thyroid hormone. If this were true, laboratory tests would show high cortisol output, low TSH, and high reverse T_3. Laboratory profiles I ordered have not shown this pattern in some two hundred of my patients who failed to respond to T_4 or desiccated thyroid but later, after the lab tests, responded to T_3. It is not likely, therefore, that a conversion problem is responsible for this therapeutic outcome.

Patient's Blunted TSH Response to TRH. Neeck and Reidel[19] found that 17 female fibromyalgia patients had a blunted TSH response to injected TRH. My patient also had a blunted TSH response. A blunted TSH response implies a deficiency of TSH, and secondarily, yet without certainty, a thyroid hormone insufficiency. The insufficiency can produce

fibromyalgia symptoms.[15] Correcting the thyroid hormone insufficiency can relieve the fibromyalgia symptoms. If the patient's fibromyalgia symptoms were due solely to a thyroid hormone deficiency, conventional medical thought would be that T_4 or desiccated thyroid would relieve the symptoms. My patient, however, failed to respond for some seven years to two grains of desiccated thyroid (equivalent to 0.2 mg of T_4), a considerable dose.

The purpose of this case study was to determine whether my patient would respond to T_3 after failing to respond to T_4. She did, and this suggests that her symptoms were not due solely to a thyroid hormone deficiency. An alternate mechanism for her failure to respond to desiccated thyroid or T_4 is mutated thyroid hormone receptors.[21] It is possible that such mutations require that she take 86 mcg of T_3 to recover from fibromyalgia. T_3 probably was required at the cellular level to relieve her symptoms.

Possible Placebo Response of Patient. After numerous clinicians reported that patients improved on T_3 after failing to benefit from desiccated thyroid or T_4, Jefferies in 1961 argued that T_3 was probably a placebo and referred to the "suggestibility of many patients."[6,p.533] He wrote: "The practicing physician is, of course, often in a poor position from which to exercise critical judgement as to the relative efficacy of drugs in his patient. The patient consults a physician because he wishes to feel better, and the physician treats the patient with a sincere desire to oblige. Hence, the two together unconsciously conspire to produce a result pleasing to both."[6,p.534]

In the way of an answer, one must concede that double-blind studies are nonpareil in clinical science. When data from blinded studies are not available, however, it is clearly unreasonable to ignore other forms of evidence, although they are less rigorously derived than data from blinded studies. The issue brings to mind Carlton Fredericks' response to opponents of orthomolecular therapy.[7,p.97] Calling clinical observations "unblinded" is justified. But calling them "uncontrolled" is logically incorrect. In other published studies mentioned above and in this one, patients improved with T_3 *after they had failed to improve over a period of months or even years with desiccated thyroid or T_4.* Because of this, each patient was her own control. Patients' lack of response to desiccated thyroid and T_4 over a prolonged period provided a baseline against which to plot their degree of response to T_3.

The patient who is the subject of this report took substantial doses of desiccated thyroid for seven years without benefit, but she responded dramatically to T_3. Critics such as Jefferies warn that the response may be a placebo reaction. This is to say that the patient would have responded just as well if tablets contained an inert substance rather than T_3. The obvious reply is: Where was the placebo effect when she was taking desiccated thyroid or T_4? Why does T_3 cause a placebo response when other forms of thyroid hormone fail to do so? The likelihood that T_3 acted in this case report and other reports as a placebo is infinitesimally small.

Studies have shown no other therapies for fibromyalgia to be significantly effective,[16] while millions of fibromyalgia patients suffer non-remitting symptoms.[17] Because of this, clinicians and researchers should not ignore the possible benefits of T_3 therapy for their fibromyalgia patients.

REFERENCES

1. Ain, K.B., Mori, Y., and Refetoff, S.: Reduced clearance rate of thyroxine-binding globulin (TBG) with increased sialylation: a mechanism for estrogen-induced elevation of serum TBG concentrations. *J. Clin. Endocrinol. Metab.*, 65:689, 1987.

2. Burger, A.G.: Effects of pharmacologic agents on thyroid hormone metabolism. In *The Thyroid: A Fundamental and Clinical Text*, 6th edition. Edited by L.E. Braverman and R.D. Utiger, New York, J.B. Lippincott Co., 1991, pp.335-346.

3. Baranetsky, N.G., Chertow, B.S., Webb, M.D., Leonard, R.F., and Sivitz, W.I.: Combined phenytoin and salicylate effects on thyroid function tests. *Arch. Int. Pharmacodyn.*, 284:166, 1986.

4. Johnson, H.H. and Solso, R.L.: *An Introduction to Experimental Design in Psychology: A Case Approach.* New York, Harper & Row, Publishers, 1971.

5. Ottenbacher, K.J.: Analysis of data in idiographic research. *Am. J. Phys. Med. Rehabil.*, 71:202-208, 1992.

6. Jefferies, W.Mck.: Occult hypothyroidism and "metabolic insufficiency." *J. Chron. Dis.*, 14:582-592, 1961.

7. Fredericks, C.: *Psycho-Nutrition.* New York, Crosset & Dunlap, 1976.

8. Freedberg, A.S., Kurland, G.S., and Hamolsky, M.W.: Effect of l-triiodothyronine alone and combined with l-thyroxine in nonmyxedematous hypometabolism. *New Engl. J. Med.*, 253:57-60, 1955.

9. Kurland, G.S., Hamolsky, M.W., and Freedberg, A.S.: Studies in non-myxedematous hypometabolism: I. The clinical syndrome and the effects of triiodothyronine, alone or combined with thyroxine. *J. Clin. Endocrinol.*, 15:1354, 1955.

10. Tittle, C.R.: Effects of 3,5,3' l-triiodothyronine in patients with metabolic insufficiency. *J.A.M.A.*, 162:271, 1956.

11. Morton, J.H.: Sodium liothyronine in metabolic insufficiency syndrome and associated disorders. *J.A.M.A.*, 165:124-129, 1957.

12. Fields, E.M.: Treatment of metabolic insufficiency and hypothyroidism with sodium liothyronine. *J.A.M.A.*, 163:817, 1957.

13. Goldberg, M.: The case for euthyroid hypometabolism. *Am. J. Med. Sc.*, 240:479-493, 1960.

14. Goldberg, M.: Diagnosis of euthyroid hypometabolism. *Am. J. Obst. & Gynec.*, 81(5):1053-1058, May, 1961.

15. Lowe, J.C.: *The Metabolic Treatment of Fibromyalgia.* Houston, McDowell Publishing Company, in press.

16. Lowe, J.C.: The treatment of fibromyalgia patients: a review of studies. *J. Myofascial Ther.*, 1(2):37-49, 1994.

17. Henriksson, C.M.: Long-term effects of fibromyalgia in everyday life: a study of 56 patients. *J. Rheumatol.*, 23(1):36-41, 1994.

18. Ferraccioli, G., Cavalieri, F., Salaffi, F., et al.: Neuroendocrinologic findings in primary fibromyalgia (soft tissue chronic pain syndrome) and in other chronic rheumatic conditions (rheumatoid arthritis, low back pain). *J. Rheumatol.*, 17:869-873, 1990.

19. Neeck, G. and Riedel, W.: Thyroid function in patients with fibromyalgia syndrome. *J. Rheumatol.*, 19:1120-1122, 1992.

20. McCain, G.A.: Nonmedicinal treatments in primary fibromyalgia. *Rheuma. Dis. Clin. North Am.*, 15:73-89, 1989.

21. Lowe, J.C., Eichelberger, J., Manso, G., and Peterson, K.: Improvement in euthyroid fibromyalgia patients treated with T_3 (tri-iodothyronine). *J. Myofascial Ther.*, 1(2):16-29, 1994.

22. Lowe, J.C. and Poo, I.: Tri-iodothyronine treatment of euthyroid fibromyalgia patients: clinical observations. Unpublished paper, 1991.

23. Wolfe, F., Smythe, H.A., Yunus, M.B., et al.: The American College of Rheumatology 1990 criteria for the classification of fibromyalgia: report of the multicenter criteria committee. *Arthritis Rheumatol.*, 33:160-172, 1990.

24. Scott, J.P.: The place of observation in biological and psychological science. *Amer. Psychologist*, 10:61-64, 1955.

25. Frankhyzen, A. and Muller, A.: In vivo studies on the inhibition of serotonin release through alpha-adrenoceptor activity in various regions of the rat CNS. Abstract of 5th Catecholamine Symposium, 1983.

Results of an Open Trial of T_3 Therapy with 77 Euthyroid Female Fibromyalgia Patients

John C. Lowe, M.A., D.C.

This article originally appeared in the *Clinical Bulletin of Myofascial Therapy*, 2(1):35-37, 1997.
It is reprinted with permission of Haworth Medical Press.

INTRODUCTION

Lowe and coworkers[1] reported a 1990-1991 open trial by Lowe and Poo of 77 female fibromyalgia syndrome (FS) patients treated with a regimen based on the use of T_3. Data from that trial are quantified in this abstract.

SUBJECTS

None of the 77 patients had thyroid function test results indicating hypothyroidism. Therefore, they were considered euthyroid (normal thyroid function). No patient had cardiac, adrenal, or bone abnormalities that contraindicated thyroid hormone supplementation. Patients ranged in age from 21-to-49.

TREATMENT

Dosages of T_3 that patients and clinicians considered effective ranged from 75 mcg to 150 mcg. (normal replacement doses range from 25-to-75 mcg). Most patients required between 81.25 mcg and 100 mcg. Patients, in addition to taking T_3, were instructed to follow a treatment regimen that included lifestyle changes (see 1. below).

The few patients who had symptoms of excess metabolic stimulation (most often tremors, tachycardia, and excess body heat) relieved the symptoms by reducing their T_3 dosages by 6.25 mcg. This effectively stopped most patients' overstimulation. (A few patients used 20 mg of propranolol on one or more occasions to stop symptoms of excess stimulation.) After reducing the dosage, some patients experienced mild recurrence of FS symptoms. These reactions tended to subside in a week or two, and patients retained the levels of improvement they had obtained at the higher dosages.

ALGOMETRY

Average pressure/pain thresholds of the 18 tender points were measured with algometry before and after treatment. Post-treatment increases in algometer scores were considered to signify improvement only if they equaled or exceeded 1 kg/cm². Also, patients were asked to rate recurrent experiences with FS symptoms after variable lengths of treatment.

Of the 77 patients, 58 (75.32%) had post-treatment increases in algometer scores of 1 kg/cm² or more. They reported that they benefitted from treatment to varying degrees. Nineteen patients (24.67%) had scores that increased less than 1 kg/cm² after treatment.

STATISTICS

Quantification of the data collected from these 77 cases was performed. A *t*-test for paired samples was performed on the algometer scores of the 19 patients whose scores had increased less than 1 kg/cm² after treatment. The difference between pre- and post-treatment scores was significant (p: 0.01).

The difference between pre- and post-treatment scores of the remaining 58 patients was highly significant (p < 0.0005). When all 77 sets of pre- and post-algometer scores were combined and tested, the difference was still highly significant (p: < 0.0005). The pressure/pain thresholds of the 18 tender points sites of the group of 77 patients, therefore, were significantly higher (improved) after T_3 treatment.

OUTCOME

The 19 patients who did not judge that T_3 had improved their status were withdrawn from the hormone and no data were collected on recurrences of FS symptoms. The remaining 58 patients were asked to estimate any recurring FS symptoms as none, mild, moderate, or severe. Outcome: none, 23 patients (39.66% of the 58); mild, 21 (36.20% of 58); moderate, 11 (18.97% of 58); and severe, 3 (5.17% of 58).

IMPLICATIONS

The most important lessons of protocol gleaned from this trial are that the FS patient benefits most when:

1. she makes lifestyle changes (increased aerobic activities, wholesome diet, and nutrient supplementation) that enable her to capitalize on the

increased metabolic capacity conferred by T$_3$,

2. the clinician carefully monitors the patient's reactions or absence of reactions to T$_3$, and

3. she increases or decreases her dosage as many times as necessary to fine-tune her improved clinical status. The factors most common to patients who did not benefit from T$_3$ were abstention from aerobic activities and lack of B complex vitamin supplementation.

Data from this and other open trials[1][2] suggest that a treatment regimen based on T$_3$ use may be effective with euthyroid FS patients. These trials have also led to a double-blind placebo-controlled crossover study of T$_3$ with euthyroid fibromyalgia patients that is presently being conducted.

REFERENCES

1. Lowe, J.C., Eichelberger, J., Manso, G., and Peterson, K.: Improvement in euthyroid fibromyalgia patients treated with T$_3$ (tri-iodothyronine). *J. Myofascial Ther.*, 1(2):16-29, 1994.

2. Lowe, J.C.: T$_3$-induced recovery from fibromyalgia by a hypothyroid patient resistant to T$_4$ and desiccated thyroid. *J. Myofascial Ther.*, 1(4):26-31, 1995.

Thyroid Status of 38 Fibromyalgia Patients: Implications for the Etiology of Fibromyalgia

John C. Lowe, M.A., D.C.

This article originally appeared in the *Clinical Bulletin of Myofascial Therapy*, 2(1):47-64, 1997.
It is reprinted with permission of Haworth Medical Press.

Abstract.   Thyroid function tests were used to classify 38 fibromyalgia patients according to thyroid status. Results were consistent with euthyroidism (normal thyroid status) in 14 patients (36.8%), primary (thyroidal) hypothyroidism in 4 patients (10.5%), and central (hypothalamic or pituitary) hypothyroidism in 20 patients (52.6%). The percentages of primary and central hypothyroidism in this group of fibromyalgia patients are extremely higher than those in the general population. There was no statistical difference for the mean intensity of fibromyalgia symptoms (measured by visual analogue scales) and the mean tender point scores (measured with algometry) between any of the categories of patients. The mean algometer scores and symptom intensities being essentially the same for all three categories of patients may show that the mechanisms involved were due to the same abnormal process—inadequate thyroid hormone regulation of gene transcription. In primary and central hypothyroid patients, this would result from a frank hormone deficiency, and in euthyroid patients, possibly from cellular resistance to thyroid hormone due to mutations in the c-erbAβ₁ gene.

Key Words: Fibromyalgia, Hypothyroidism, Euthyroid, TSH, TRH stimulation test, Thyroid hormone resistance

INTRODUCTION

Carette and Lefrancois[1] studied 100 hypothyroid patients to determine the percentage who had fibromyalgia. Nineteen (19%) reported that they had pain and stiffness. These patients were likely candidates for the diagnosis of fibromyalgia according to their responses to a questionnaire. Only five of these patients, however, had seven or more tender points when examined. The investigators concluded that only 5% of the hypothyroid patients had fibromyalgia.[1,p.1420] The incidence of fibromyalgia among hypothyroid patients, then, appears to be low.

The incidence of hypothyroidism among fibromyalgia patients, however, has not yet been determined. Some researchers have attempted to identify hypothyroid patients (to exclude them from their fibromyalgia studies) through testing with the T_4 and T_3 resin uptake.[2] Other researchers have included a basal TSH.[3] The T_4 and T_3 resin uptake are no longer the preferable tests for identifying patients with abnormal thyroid function,[4,p.120] and the basal TSH level can identify only patients with primary (thyroidal) hypothyroidism. Even combining the T_4 and T_3 resin uptake with the basal TSH does not distinguish patients who may have thyroid hormone deficiency of pituitary or hypothalamic origin, termed central hypothyroidism.

To date, the only researchers who have provided quantitative figures on the incidence of primary hypothyroidism among fibromyalgia patients are Shiroky and coworkers[82] and Eisinger and colleagues.[85] The former group reported that of 34 fibromyalgia patients, 4 (12%) had primary hypothyroidism. The latter group reported that 6 of 62 patients (10.3%) had primary hypothyroidism. There have been two reports concerning fibromyalgia patients with possible central hypothyroidism,[5][6] although the researchers did not use this term. They did use, however, the most readily available procedure that distinguishes patients with possible central hypothyroidism: the TRH stimulation test.

Neeck and Riedel compared TSH responses to TRH injections in 13 female "primary" fibromyalgia patients to responses in 10 control subjects.[5] All the fibromyalgia patients had blunted TSH responses at 30 minutes. The average TSH response for patients was 8 µU/ml and for controls was 16 µU/ml. The authors did not specify their cut-off point for normal, but considered the average of 8 µU/ml blunted. Patients also had lower free T_3 and free T_4 levels in response to TRH injections.

Ferraccioli and colleagues found that of 24 female fibromyalgia patients, five (20.8%) had blunted TSH responses to TRH (defined in their study as a post-TRH injection rise in TSH level of less than 7 µU/ml).[6] These researchers reported that blunted TSH responses were the most common hormone finding in their fibromyalgia patients.[6,p.871]

The investigators in these two studies did not classify their patients according to thyroid status. To estimate the incidence of euthyroidism (normal thyroid status), primary hypothyroidism, and possible central hypothyroidism in fibromyalgia patients, I performed a retrospective analysis of 38 case records.

METHODS

Subjects. For this analysis, I included 1 male and 37 female patients, all Caucasian, ranging in age from 21-to-71. Patients were consecutive, and seen between January and June, 1995. All patients met the 1990 American College of Rheumatology diagnostic criteria for fibromyalgia.[7] Each had chronic widespread pain and a mean pressure/pain threshold of the 18 tender point sites of less than 4 kg/cm². Each patient underwent testing that was sufficient to categorize him or her according to thyroid status. None were taking drugs such as corticosteroids or L-dopa that tend to blunt the TSH response to TRH.[8,p.430]

Laboratory Procedures. A profile of thyroid function tests was ordered for each patient. The profile contained a T_3 uptake, total T_4 RIA, T_7 (free thyroxine index), and a basal serum TSH. The TSH test employed second generation assays that detected TSH levels of 0.3 µU/ml and above.[9,p.108]

With one exception, patients with elevated basal TSH levels (and therefore diagnoses of primary hypothyroidism) did not undergo TRH stimulation tests. Patients with normal basal TSH levels were given TRH stimulation tests. TSH levels were measured for baseline and at 30 minutes after intravenous injection of 500 µg of TRH (Thyrel® TRH, protirelin).[10]

NOTE: Neeck and Riedel recorded their *research* patients' thyroid hormone levels in response to TRH stimulation.[5] My patients, however, were initially evaluated as *clinical* cases. So I followed the typical procedure of not measuring thyroid hormone levels during TRH stimulation tests.[8,p.429]

Classification. From the profile of thyroid function tests, I diagnosed a patient as having **primary hypothyroidism** if his or her basal TSH level was above the upper limit of the normal range of 0.4-6.0 µU/ml.[11] From the TRH stimulation test, I considered a TSH response consistent with **euthyroidism** to be within the range of 8.5-to-20.0 µU/ml (above baseline). A TSH response consistent with **central hypothyroidism** was a value that, minus the baseline value, was either below the lower limit of 8.5 µU/ml or above the upper limit of 20.0 µU/ml.[12][13][14][8]

Statistics. For this retrospective analysis, I divided patients into 3 groups according to thyroid status (see bold above). Groups were then compared to each other with regard to: 1) the intensity of the patients' fibromyalgia symptoms according to visual analogue scales, and 2) the mean pressure/pain thresholds of patients' tender points (measured by algometry). Comparison of means was performed with the ANOVA and with the *t*-test for a difference between two independent means.

RESULTS

Primary hypothyroidism. Of the 38 patients included in the analysis, 4 (10.5%) had primary hypothyroidism. I diagnosed 3 patients as having primary hypothyroidism because of high basal TSH levels. The range of high TSH values was 6.5-to- 9.08 µU/ml, with a mean of 8.16 µU/ml.

I diagnosed a fourth patient as being in this same category because of the pattern of her thyroid function test results. Her total T_4 level was at the lower end of the normal range at 4.7 µg/dl, and her basal TSH level was at the upper end of the normal range at 5.3 µU/ml. At the time of her TRH test, her baseline TSH level was 5.54 µU/ml. Her 30-minute TSH response to TRH was 40.32 µU/ml, which was 34.78 µU/ml above the baseline value.

Euthyroidism. I diagnosed 14 patients (36.8%) as euthyroid because 1) their basal TSH levels were not elevated, and 2) their 30-minute TSH responses to TRH were within a range considered consistent with normal thyroid function (8.5-to-20.0 µU/ml above baseline). The range of these patients' TSH responses above baseline was 9.12-to-18.56 µU/ml. The mean was 13.29 µU/ml.

Central Hypothyroidism. I classified the 30-minute TSH responses (above baseline) to TRH in 20 patients (52.6%) as consistent with (but not diagnostic of) central hypothyroidism. A TSH response was considered abnormal when its value, minus the baseline value, was either below or above the range of 8.5-to-20.0 µU/ml.

According to these criteria, 11 patients of the 20 (55% of this category) had blunted TSH responses. The range of their TSH levels above baseline was 0.00-to-8.5 µU/ml, and the mean was 4.74 µU/ml. Nine patients out of 20 (45% of this category) had abnormally high TSH responses. The range of their TSH levels above baseline was 20.70 to 33.0 µU/ml, with a mean of 25.85 µU/ml.

Statistical Analysis. Comparison of means of the algometer scores (tender point pressure/pain thresholds) for the three categories of thyroid status was performed with the ANOVA. The F value of 1.40 with df equal to 2 and 34 was not significant at the 0.05 level. This indicates that there was no significant difference with regard to mean algometer scores between the three categories of patients.

Comparisons with ANOVA were also performed for the mean symptom intensities of the three categories. The F value of 0.48 with df equal to 2 and 28 was also not significant at the 0.05 level. Again, this indicates that the means did not significantly differ.

The t-test for a difference between two independent means was performed for the means of the euthyroid, primary hypothyroid, and possible central hypothyroid patient categories, both for mean algometer scores and for mean symptom intensities. There was no statistical difference between the patient categories for the means of algometer scores or symptom intensities.

DISCUSSION

Bennett wrote of the ". . . anecdotal observations that thyroid dysfunction is not common in patients with fibromyalgia."[84] Such anecdotal observations, according to the results of this retrospective analysis, are not correct. Of 38 case records, test results suggest that: 14 patients (36.8%) were euthyroid, 4 patients (10.5%) had primary hypothyroidism, and 20 patients (52.6%) had patterns consistent with central hypothyroidism (suggesting hypothalamic or pituitary dysfunction). Eleven patients in this last category had blunted TSH responses to TRH. This is 28.9% of the 38 patients in the study, which is close to Ferraccioli's finding of blunted TSH responses in 5 of 24 patients (20.8%).[6] My finding of 4 patients with primary hypothyroidism (10.5%) is close to the 4 (12%) of 34 fibromyalgia patients reported by Shiroky and colleagues[82] and the 6 (10.3%) of 62 patients reported by Eisinger and coworkers.[85]

Hershman[83, p.40] reported that the incidence of primary hypothyroidism is 1% of the general adult population and 3% of geriatrics. Central hypothyroidism, however, occurs in only 0.00021% of the population. According to Hershman's figures, then, central hypothyroidism is about 1/4,800 (0.00021%/1%) as frequent as primary hypothyroidism.

The incidence of primary hypothyroidism (4 patients) among this report's 38 patients is 10.5 times (10.5%/1%) the incidence in the general population. The incidence of possible central hypothyroidism in these 38 patients is 250,476.19 times (52.6%/0.00021%) that in the general population. The inci-

dence, therefore, of the two forms of hypothyroidism in these 38 fibromyalgia patients is exponentially inversely proportional to incidences in the general population.

The means of the 38 patients' algometer tender point scores and the means of their symptom intensities were compared for the three categories of thyroid status. There was no significant difference between the means of these three categories.

Diagnosis of Primary Hypothyroidism. Second generation TSH assays are sensitive enough to detect elevated TSH levels in most patients, supporting the diagnosis of primary hypothyroidism.[15] Of the 4 primary hypothyroid patients reported in this analysis, 3 had elevated TSH levels. The normal TSH range was 0.4-to-6.0 µU/ml.[11] Their range of high TSH levels was 6.5-to-9.08 µU/ml; the mean was 8.16 µU/ml.

I diagnosed a fourth patient as being primary hypothyroid even though her basal TSH levels on two occasions (5.3 µU/ml and 5.54 µU/ml) were within the normal range of 0.4-to-6.0 µU/ml. I did so for the following reasons. Her total T_4 level was at the lower end of the normal range at 4.7 µg/dl, and her TSH was at the high normal end. This pattern—an inversely proportional relationship between total T_4 and TSH, with both measures being close to the cut-off points for normal—is suggestive of primary hypothyroidism when combined with her other test results. Her 30-minute TSH response to TRH was 40.32 µU/ml, which was 34.78 µU/ml above her baseline value of 5.54 µU/ml. Seth and Beckett showed[15] that, as a rule, patients with high normal basal TSH levels have exponential increases in TSH following a TRH injection. This patient's post-TRH increase in TSH was just such a response. This is, again, suggestive of primary hypothyroidism.

Many clinicians often misdiagnose patients with high normal TSH levels as being euthyroid. Understanding the relevant physiology, and combining that with a review of the pattern of a patient's laboratory test results, can help a clinician decide whether or not to diagnose a patient as hypothyroid. As in this patient's case, the TRH stimulation test may permit a definitive diagnosis. Cases such as this one illustrate the importance of several researchers' prudent advice: use clinical judgement in evaluating patients' thyroid status rather than solely the results of standard thyroid function tests.[16][17][18]

Importance of the TRH Stimulation Test. The TRH stimulation test is a sensitive method for identifying small changes in TSH secretion that are not detected by measuring basal serum TSH levels.[19,p.512] During this test, a blood sample is taken to use for measuring the basal TSH level. TRH is then injected. A second blood sample is taken, preferably 30 minutes post-injection, to use for measuring the patient's TSH response to the injected TRH. The TSH response is the second TSH value above the baseline TSH value in μU/ml (or mU/l).

Some clinicians state that the TRH-stimulation test is now unnecessary, since second and third generation assays of TSH are highly sensitive. Without the TRH stimulation test, however, a definitive diagnosis may not be possible in many cases. There are several reasons for this.

THE SERUM TSH. Some patients with central hypothyroidism have normal basal serum TSH. Levels in these patients are most often low normal: 0.5-to-1.0 μU/ml, or slightly lower.[20][21] If central hypothyroidism means that the hypothalamus is not able to secrete normal amounts of TRH to stimulate pituitary thyrotroph secretion of TSH, or that the pituitary thyrotroph cells are not able to secrete sufficient TSH, why would the basal TSH levels be normal in these patients?

One reason could be that, for a particular patient, what seems to be a normal level is actually low for that patient.[11,p.297] Another reason is that in central hypothyroidism (especially hypothalamic hypothyroidism), the TSH molecule secreted by the pituitary may have abnormal molecular structure and low bioactivity.[22] Structurally faulty TSH does not bind normally to thyroid gland TSH receptors. As a result, normal levels of this faulty TSH do not adequately stimulate the thyroid gland to secrete normal amounts of thyroid hormones. So though the patient's blood levels of TSH seem normal enough to maintain adequate thyroid hormone secretion, the patient is hypothyroid. The clinician, then, cannot diagnose central hypothyroidism based on basal TSH levels alone, no matter how sensitive the assay. A supersensitive assay may only show a normal level of structurally faulty TSH.

THE STANDARD THYROID PROFILE. It might be assumed that the results of the standard thyroid profile enable the clinician to predict the outcome of the TRH stimulation test, making the stimulation test unnecessary. Physiologically, if the total T_4 and free thyroxine index are in the lower half of the normal range, the expected finding would be that the TSH is, inversely, in the upper half of the normal range. But when all these measures are in the lower half of the normal range, this could indicate that the pituitary thyrotroph cells are not being properly disinhibited by lower

levels of T_4. Thus, a diagnosis of central hypothyroidism could be made by simply looking for this pattern within the standard thyroid panel. If this were true, it would render the TRH stimulation test unnecessary.

But of my 20 patients whose test results were consistent with central hypothyroidism, the pattern described above—low normal T_4, free thyroxine index, and TSH—was present in the results of only 9 (45%). Of the 14 patients who were euthyroid, the same pattern was present in the results of 7 (50%). These findings do not support the view that clinicians can use this pattern of values to predict TRH stimulation test results consistent with central hypothyroidism. While a deficient nocturnal surge in TSH may identify patients with possible central hypothyroidism,[21] testing for this nocturnal response requires hospitalization of the patient. The TRH stimulation test, therefore, remains the most readily accessible tool for many clinicians.

NOTE: A blunted TSH response to TRH suggests pituitary hypothyroidism, but an exaggerated TSH response does not distinguish between hypothalamic and pituitary hypothyroidism. In a report by Ferring Laboratories,[23] patients were diagnosed as having pituitary hypothyroidism or hypothalamic hypothyroidism by clinical history, physical examination, and tests of thyroid and pituitary function. Then, the patients underwent TRH stimulation tests to determine whether a different TSH response pattern typified each form of central hypothyroidism. In patients with hypothalamic hypothyroidism, the post-TRH injection TSH levels ranged from 2-to-38 μU/ml. In patients with pituitary hypothyroidism, the post-TRH TSH levels in 59% of patients were less than 2 μU/ml. In 41% of pituitary hypothyroid patients, however, the post-TRH TSH levels increased from 2-to-40 μU/ml. The authors concluded that a TSH response to TRH of less than 2 μU/ml suggests pituitary hypothyroidism, but that a TSH response greater than this does not distinguish hypothalamic from pituitary hypothyroidism.

Notice that the TSH response levels of some of these patients were within the normal range. Some central hypothyroid patients have normal responses to TRH stimulation tests. This illustrates that the TRH stimulation test must be interpreted in light of clinical and other test data indicating pituitary or hypothalamic dysfunction. Ferring researchers were trying to determine TSH response patterns that *in the majority of cases* are consistent with hypothalamic or pituitary genesis of hypothyroidism. The conclusions of the Ferring report are supported by the findings of other researchers.[12][13]

Diagnosis of Central Hypothyroidism. I classified patients with normal basal TSH levels but blunted or exaggerated TSH responses to TRH as having test result patterns *consistent* with central hypothyroidism. This terminology is necessary because the diagnosis of central hypothyroidism should not be made solely on the basis of thyroid function test results. In most cases, the diagnosis is firm only when there are also clinical, radiographic, and other imaging findings to support the diagnosis.[11,p.297] Most patients with central hypothyroidism show evidence of failure to secrete normal amounts of other trophic hormones, and imaging of the pituitary fossa often shows abnormalities.[24] In some cases, a TSH deficiency may result from a mutation in the TSH gene. In these patients, levels of anterior pituitary hormones other than the TSH are within their normal ranges,[25] and there are no associated abnormalities capable of being imaged.

Complete endocrinological workups and hypothalamic and pituitary imaging were not available for most of the patients in this study. Therefore, the history, clinical status, and laboratory test results of 20 patients (52.6%) were consistent with, but not diagnostic of, central hypothyroidism.

Thyroid Hormone Deficiency. The results of the analysis reported here are important. They suggest that 24 of 38 fibromyalgia patients (63.2%) had thyroid hormone deficiencies. Thyroid hormone in normal concentrations at the chromosomes exerts powerful regulatory effects on the transcription of genes. It activates some genes and inhibits others. In thyroid hormone deficiency, transcription patterns normally inhibited by the hormone are disinhibited. There is an increase in transcription of mRNAs for inhibitory molecules. These include phosphodiesterase,[26] inhibitory G proteins,[27][28][29] and α-adrenergic receptors.[30][31][32][33][34] Other effects include a decrease in serotonin[35][36][37] and growth hormone levels,[38][39][40][41][42][43] and an increase in substance P.[44][45][46]

In addition to these molecular, hormonal, and neurotransmitter changes, a number of objective phenomena and symptoms can occur. These include: alpha intrusion into slow wave sleep,[47] decreased brain blood flow,[48] impeded carbohydrate metabolism,[49] fatigue,[50] aches and pains,[51][52][53][54] cold sensitivity,[55][50] dysmenorrhea,[56,p.577][55,p.19] depression,[56] and cognitive dysfunction.[48][57][58,p.170]

These symptoms and hormone, neurotransmitter, and other objective findings in thyroid hormone deficient patients are also typical of fibromyalgia

patients.[7][48][59][60][61][62][63][64][65][66][67][68][69][70][71] And although I will not list them here (as I do in a recent publication[72]), every other objective finding and symptom of fibromyalgia is well accounted for by the effects of inadequate transcription regulation by thyroid hormone.

Euthyroid Fibromyalgia: One Clinical Phenotype of Partial Resistance to Thyroid Hormone? Euthyroid fibromyalgia patients do not have a thyroid hormone deficiency. Yet, this analysis shows that they share in intensity the hypothyroid-like symptoms and objective findings (lower pressure/pain thresholds of tender points) of hypothyroid fibromyalgia patients. This suggests that euthyroid fibromyalgia patients' symptoms and objective findings result from the same mechanism that affects hypothyroid fibromyalgia patients: inadequate thyroid hormone regulation of gene transcription.

In general, euthyroid fibromyalgia patients benefit from T_3 just as most hypothyroid fibromyalgia patients do from T_4 (blinded efficacy studies have been completed but have not yet been published). One mechanism that could account for this therapeutic response to T_3 in euthyroid fibromyalgia patients is partial cellular resistance to thyroid hormone. As my coauthors and I have pointed out,[73][74][75][76] euthyroid fibromyalgia patients resemble patients with thyroid hormone resistance syndromes in three ways: 1) both types of patients have some hypothyroid-like clinical features but clearly are not hypothyroid, 2) effective doses of T_3 for them are typically supraphysiologic, yet 3) these doses usually do not induce hypermetabolism. It is possible, then, that euthyroid fibromyalgia is a clinical phenotype of partial resistance to thyroid hormone.

Investigators have pinpointed mutations in the c-erbAβ_1 gene on chromosome 3 that are responsible for many patients' partial resistance to thyroid hormone.[77][78][79][80] These mutations result in thyroid hormone receptors with a low affinity for T_3. This low affinity effectively blocks gene transcription normally regulated by thyroid hormone. This allows alternate transcription patterns, those that would occur when thyroid hormone is deficient. In affected tissues, then, the transcriptional effects of mutant thyroid hormone receptors would be the same as those of thyroid hormone deficiency.

If euthyroid fibromyalgia is a clinical phenotype of partial resistance to thyroid hormone (involving the same tissues as hypothyroid fibromyalgia), this would explain the statistically similar algometer tender point scores and symptom intensities of the three categories of patients. We would predict this if the tender points and symptoms of all the patients—those with primary hypothyroidism, possible central hypothyroidism, and even euthyroidism—are a clinical manifestation of the same molecular lesion: inadequate thyroid hormone transcription regulation.

If euthyroid fibromyalgia patients are shown to have mutant thyroid hormone receptors, it will be a formidable task indeed to resist the working hypothesis that *all fibromyalgia is a manifestation of inadequate thyroid hormone regulation of gene transcription.* Forslind and colleagues[81] will have been correct to challenge the proposition that fibromyalgia is a "primary" condition. Clinicians will then use the term fibromyalgia only as a convenient label for a particular pattern of symptoms of hypometabolism due to too little thyroid hormone control of transcription. And correct diagnosis and treatment will depend on the patient's history, clinical status, thyroid function testing including the TRH stimulation test, and for euthyroid patients, rapid detection methods for pinpointing mutations.[25]

ACKNOWLEDGEMENT

I would like to thank Jackie Yellin, my medical editor, for assuring that this paper is expressed clearly and in proper English, and also for her tireless help at honing the contents to logical consistence. I would also like to thank David G. Simons, M.D. and Steve Usala, M.D., Ph.D. for their valuable comments on the contents of this paper.

REFERENCES

1. Carette, S. and Lefrancois, L.: Fibrositis and primary hypothyroidism. *J. Rheum.*, 15:1418-21, 1988.
2. Kravitz, H.M., Katz, R.S., Helmke, N., Jeffriess, H., Bukovsky, J., and Fawcett, J.: Alprazolam and ibuprofen in the treatment of fibromyalgia: report of a double-blind placebo-controlled study. *J. Musculoskeletal Pain*, 2(1):3-27, 1994.
3. Jacobsen, S., Danneskiold-Samse,B., and Andersen, R.B.: Oral S-adenosylmethionine in primary fibromyalgia: double-blind clinical evaluation. *Scand. J. Rheum.*, 20:294-302, 1991.
4. Hamburger,J.I.: Use of modern thyroid tests in illustrative ambulatory patients.In *Diagnostic Methods in Clinical Thyroidology*. Edited by J.I. Hamburger, N.Y., Springer-Verlag, 1989, pp.111-123.
5. Neeck, G. and Riedel, W.: Thyroid function in patients with fibromyalgia syndrome. *J. Rheum.*, 1992, 19:1120-1122.
6. Ferraccioli, G., Cavalieri, F., Salaffi, F.,Fontana, S., Scita, F., Nolli, M., and Maestri, D.: Neuroendocrinologic findings in primary fibromyalgia (soft tissue chronic pain syndrome) and in other chronic rheumatic conditions (rheumatoid arthritis, low back pain). *J. Rheum.*, 17:869-73, 1990.
7. Wolfe, F., Smythe, H.A., Yunus, M.B., Bennett, R.M., Bombardier, C., Goldenberg, D.L., Tugwell, P., Campbell, S.M., Abeles, M., Clark, P., Fam, A.G., Farber, S.J., Fiechtner, J.J., Franklin, C.M., Gatter, R.A., Mamaty, D., Lessard, J., Lichtbroun, A.S., Masi, A.T., McCain, G.A., Reynolds, W.J., Romano, T.J., Russell, I.J., and Sheon, R.P.: The American College of Rheumatology 1990 criteria for the classification of fibromyalgia: report of the multicenter criteria committee. *Arthr. Rheum.*, 33:160-172, 1990.
8. Howanitz, P.J. and Howanitz, J.H.: Evaluation of endocrine function. In pp.402-476. In *Clinical Diagnosis and Management by Laboratory Methods*, Vol. 1. Edited by J.B. Henry, Philadelphia, W.B. Saunders Co., 1979.
9. *Compendium of Service.* National Health Laboratories, Incorporated, 1050 N. Post Oak, #145, Houston, TX 77055.
10. Ferring Laboratories, Suffem, NY 10901 by Taylor Pharmacal Co., Decatur, IL 62525.
11. Toft, A.D.: Thyrotropin: assay, secretory physiology, and testing of regulation. In *Werner's The Thyroid: A Fundamental and Clinical Text*, 5th edition. Edited by S.H. Ingbar and L.E. Braverman, Philadelphia, J.B. Lippincott Co., 1986, pp.287-305.
12. Faglia, G., Beck-Peccoz, P., and Ferrari, C.: Plasma thyrotropin response to thyrotropin-releasing hormone in patients with pituitary and hypothalamic disorders. *J. Clin. Endocrin. Metab.*, 37:595, 1973.
13. Snyder, P.J., Jacobs, L.S., and Rabello, M.M.: Diagnostic value of thyrotropin-releasing hormone in pituitary and hypothalamic diseases: assessment of thyrotrophin and prolactin secretion in 100 patients. *Ann. Intern. Med.*, 81:751, 1974.
14. Snyder, P.J., Jacobs, S.L., Rabello, M.M., Sterling, F.H., Shore, R.H., Uitger, R.D. and Daughaday, W.H.: Diagnostic value of thyrotropin releasing hormone in pituitary and hypothalamic diseases. *Ann. Int. Med.*, 81:751-757, 1974.
15. Seth, J. and Beckett, G.: Diagnosis of hyperthyroidism: the newer biochemical tests. *Clin. Endocrin. Metab.*, 14:373, 1985.
16. Wilson, J. and Walton, J.N.: Some muscular manifestations of hypothyroidism. *J. Neurol. Neurosurg. Psychiat.*, 22:320-324, 1959.
17. Mitchell, M.L.: Blood tests of thyroid function. In *The Thyroid Gland: A Practical Clincal Treatise*. Edited by Van Middlesworth, Chicago, Year Book Medical Publishers, Inc., 1986, pp.35-45.
18. Vagenakis, A.G. and Braverman, L.E.: Thyroid function tests—which one? *Ann. of Int. Med.*, 84(5):607-608, 1976.
19. Utiger, R.D.:Tests of thyroregulatory mechanisms. In *Werner's The Thyroid: A Fundamental and Clinical Text*, 5th edition. Edited by S.H. Ingbar and L.E. Braverman, Philadelphia, J.B. Lippincott Co., 1986, pp.511-523.
20. Blunt, S., Woods, C.A., Joplin, G.F., and Burrin,J.M.: The role of a highly sensitive amplified enzyme immunoassay for thyrotropin in the evaluation of thyrotroph function in hypopituitary patients. *Clin. Endocrin.* (Oxf.), 29:387, 1988.
21. Caron, P.J., Nieman, L.K., Rose, S.R., and Nisula, B.C.:

Deficient nocturnal surge of thyrotropin in central hypothyroidism. *J. Clin. Endocrin. Metab.*, 62:960, 1986.

22. Beck-Peccoz, P., Amr. S., Menezes-Ferreira, M., Faglia, G., and Weintraub, B.: Decreased receptor binding of biologically inactive thyrotropin in central hypothyroidism. *N. Engl. J. Med.*, 312:1085, 1985.

23. *Thyrel® TRH (protirelin) for Intravenous Administration.* Ferring Laboratories, Suffern, NY, 10901 by Taylor Pharmacal Co., Decatur, IL 62525.

24. Klijn, J.G.M., Lamberts, S.W.J., and Doctor, R.: The function of the pituitary-thyroidal axis in acromegalic patients v. patients with hyperprolactinaemia and a pituitary tumor. *Clin. Endocrin.* (Oxf.), 13:577, 1980.

25. Mori, R., Sawai, T., Kinoshita, E., Baba, T., Matsumoto, T., Yoshimoto, M., Tsuji, Y., Satake, Y., and Sawada, K.: Rapid detection of a point mutation in thyroid-stimulating hormone beta-subunit gene causing congenital isolated thyroid-stimulating hormone deficiency. *Japanese J. Human Genetics*, 36(4):313-6, 1991.

26. Goswami, A. and Rosenberg, I.N.: Effects of thyroid status on membrane-bound low K_m cyclic nucleotide phosphodiesterase activity in rat adipocytes. *J. Biol. Chem.*, 260: 82-85, 1985.

27. Milligan, G., Spiegel, A.M., Unson, C.G., and Saggerson, E.D.: Chemically induced hypothyroidism produces elevated amounts of the α subunit of the inhibitory guanine nucleotide binding protein (G_i) and the β subunit common to all G-proteins. *Biochem. J.*, 247:223-227, 1987.

28. Rapiejko, P.J., Watkins, D.C., Ros, M., and Malbon, C.C.: Thyroid hormones regulate G-protein β-subunit mRNA expression in vivo. *J. Biol. Chem.*, 264:16183-16189, 1989.

29. Ros, M., Northup, J.K., and Malbon, C.C.: Steady-state levels of G-proteins and β-adrenergic receptors in rat fat cells. *J. Biol. Chem.*, 263:4362-4368, 1988.

30. Bilezikian, J.P. and Loeb, J.N.: The influence of hyperthyroidism and hypothyroidism on α- and β-adrenergic receptor systems and adrenergic responsiveness. *Endoc. Rev.*, 4:378-388, 1983.

31. Kunos, G.: Thyroid hormone-dependent interconversion of myocardial α- and β-adrenoceptors in the rat. *Brit. J. Pharmacol.*, 59:177-189, 1977.

32. Kunos, G., Mucci, L., and O'Regan, S.: The influence of hormonal and neuronal factors on rat heart adrenoceptors. *Brit. J. Pharmaco.*, 71:371-386, 1980.

33. Isac, E.J.N., Pennefather, J.N., and Handberg, G.M.: Effect of changes in thyroid state on atrial α- and β-adrenoceptors, adenylate cyclase activity, and catecholamine levels in the rat. *J. Cardiovasc. Pharmacol.*, 5:396-405, 1983.

34. Lazar-Wesley, E., Hadcock, J.R., Malbon, C.C., Kunos, G., and Ishac, E.J.N.: Tissue-specific regulation of α_{1B}- and β_2-adrenergic receptor mRNAs by thyroid state in the rat. *Endocrinology*, 129(2):1116-1118, 1991.

35. Mason, G.A., Bondy, S.C., Nemeroff, C.B., Walker, C.H., and Prange, A.J., Jr.: The effects of thyroid state on beta-adrenergic and serotonergic receptors in rat brain. *Psychoneuroendocrinology*, 12:261-270, 1987.

36. Tóth, S. and Csaba, B.: The effect of thyroid gland on 5-hydroxytryptamine (5-HT) level of brain stem and blood in rabbits. *Experientia*, 22:755-756, 1966.

37. Frankhyzen, A. and Muller, A.: In vitro studies on the inhibition of serotonin release through α-adrenoreceptor activity in various regions of the rat CNS. *Abstract of 5th Catecholamine Symposium*, 1983, p.137.

38. Seo, H., Vassart, G., Brocas, H. and Refetoff, S.: Triiodothyronine stimulates specifically growth hormone mRNA in rat pituitary tumor cells. *Proc. Natl. Acad. Sci.*, USA 74:2054, 1977.

39. Seo, H., Refetoff, S., Martino, E., Vassart, G. and Brocas, H.: The differential stimulatory effect of thyroid hormone on growth hormone synthesis and estrogen on prolactin synthesis due to accumulation of specific messenger ribonucleic acid. *Endocrinology*, 104:1083, 1979.

40. Martial, J.A., Baxter, J.D. and Goodman, H.M.: Regulation of growth hormone messenger RNA by thyroid and glucocorticoid hormones. *Proc. Natl. Acad. Sci.*, 74:1816, 1977.

41. Shapiro, L.E., Samuels, H.H. and Yaffe, B.M.: Thyroid and glucocorticoid hormones synergistically control growth hormone mRNA in cultured GH-1 cells. *Proc. Natl. Acad. Sci.*, 75:45, 1978.

42. Valcavi, R., Dieguez, C., Preece, M., Taylor, A., Portioli, I., and Scanlon, M.F.: Effect of thyroxine replacement therapy on plasma insulin-like growth hormone releasing factor in hypothyroid patients. *Clin. Endocrin.*, 27:85, 1987.

43. Williams, T., Maxon, H., Thorner, M.O., and Frohman, L.A.: Blunted growth hormone (GH) response to GH-releasing hormone in hypothyroidism resolves in the euthyroid state. *J. Clin. Endocrin. Metab.*, 61:454, 1985.

44. Jones, P.M., Ghatei, M.A., Wallis, S.C., and Bloom, S.R.: Differential response to neuropeptide Y, substance P, and vasoactive intestinal polypeptide in the rat anterior pituitary gland to alterations in thyroid hormone status. *J. Endocrin.*, 143:393-397, 1994.

45. Jonassen, J.A., Mullikin-Kirkpatrick, D., McAdam, A., and Leeman, S.E.: Thyroid hormone status regulates preprotachykinin-A gene expression in male rat anterior pituitary. *Endocrinology*, 121:1555-1561.

46. Lam, K.S., Lechan, R.M., Minamitani, N., Segerson, T.P., and Reichlin, S.: Vasoactive intestinal peptide in the anterior pituitary is increased in hypothyroidism. *Endocrinology*, 124:1077-1084, 1989.

47. Kales, A., Heuser, G., Jacobsen, A., Kales, J.D., Hanley, J., Zweizig, J.R. and Paulson, M.J.: All night sleep studies in hypothyroidism patients, before and after treatment. *J. Clin. Endocrin.*, 27:1593-9, 1967.

48. Scheinberg, P., Stead, E.A. Jr., Brannon, E.S. and Warren, J.V.: Correlative observations on cerebral metabolism and cardiac output in myxedema. *J. Clin. Invest.*, 29:1139, 1950.

49. Ensinger, J., Plantamura, A., and Ayavou, T.: Glycolysis abnormalities in fibromyalgia. *J. Am Coll. Nutr.*, 13:144-148, 1994.

50. Watanakunakorn, C., Hodges, R.E., and Evans, T.C.: Myxedema: a study of 400 cases. *Arch. Intern. Med.*, 116:185, 1965.

51. Fessel, W.J.: Myopathy of hypothyroidism. *Ann. Rheumatic Dis.*, 27:590-596, 1968.

52. Bergouignan, M., Vital, C. and Bataille, J.M.: Les myopathies hypothyroidiennes: aspects cliniques et histopathologiques, *Presse Med.*, 75:1551, 1967.

53. Alajouanine, T. and Nick, J.: De l'existence d'une myopathie d'origine hypothyroïdienne. *Paris Med.*, 35:346, 1945.
54. Golding, D.N.: Hypothyroidism presenting with musculoskeletal symptoms. *Ann. Rheum. Dis.*, 29:10-4, 1970.
55. Kirk, E. and Kvorning, S.A.: *Hypometabolism: A Clinical Study of 308 Consecutive Cases.* Copenhagen, Einar Munksgaard, Publisher, 1946, pp.11 & 20.
56. DeGroot, L.J., Larsen, P.R., Refetoff, S. and Stanbury, J.B.: *The Thyroid and its Disease*, 5th edition. New York, John Wiley & Sons, 1984.
57. Browning, T.B., Atkins, R.W. and Weiner, H.: Cerebral metabolic disturbances in hypothyroidism: clinical and electroencephalographic studies in the psychosis of myxoedema and hypothyroidism. *A.M.A. Arch. Intern. Med.*, 93:938, 1954.
58. Tepperman, J. and Tepperman, H.M.: *Metabolic and Endocrine Physiology*, 5th edition. Chicago, Year Book Medical Publishers, Inc., 1987.
59. Moldofsky, H.: Sleep mechanisms and fibromyalgia. *First International Symposium on Myofascial Pain and Fibromyalgia.* Minneapolis, Minnesota, May 9, 1989.
60. Goldenberg, D.L.: Psychologic studies in fibrositis. *Am. J. Med.*, 81(suppl 3A):67-70, 1986.
61. Bennett, R.M.: Muscle physiology and cold reactivity in the fibromyalgia syndrome. *Rheu. Dis. Clinics North Am.*, 15:135-147, 1989.
62. Clauw, D.J., Morris, S., Starbuck, V., Blank, C., and Kay, G.: Impairment in cognitive function in individuals with fibromyalgia. Abstract No. 1119, Annual Meeting: Am. Coll. of Rheumatol. and Ass.Rheumatol.Health Prof., Oct. 23-27, 1994.
63. Mountz, J.M., Bradley, L., Modell, J.G., Triana, M., Alexander, R., and Mountz, J.D.: Limbic system dysregulation in fibromyalgia measured by regional cerebral blood flow. *Arthritis Rheum.*, 36:R23, 1993.
64. Moldofsky, H. and Warsh, J.J.: Plasma tryptophan and musculoskeletal pain in non-articular rheumatism ("fibrositis syndrome"). *Pain*, 5:65-71, 1978.
65. Russell, I.J.: Neurohormonal aspects of fibromyalgia syndrome. *Rheum. Dis. Clin. North Am.*, 15:149-168, 1989.
66. Russell, I.J., Michalek, J.E., Vipraio, G.A., Fletcher, E.M., and Wall, K.: Serum amino acids in fibrositis/fibromyalgia syndrome. *J. Rheumatol.*, (16 suppl.),19:158-163, 1989.
67. Russell, I.J., Michalek, J.E., Vipraio, J.A., Fletcher, E.M., Javors, M.A., and Bowden, C.A.: Platelet 3H-imipramine uptake receptor density and serum serotonin levels in patients with fibromyalgia/fibrositis syndromes. *J. Rheumatol.*, 19:104-9, 1992.
68. Houvenagel, E., Forzy, G., Cortet, B., and Vincent, G.: 5-Hydroxyindoleacetic acid in cerebrospinal fluid in fibromyalgia. *Arthritis Rheum.*, 33:S55, 1990.
69. Russell, I.J., Vaeroy, H., Javors, M., and Nyberg, F.: Cerebrospinal fluid biogenic amine metabolites in fibromyalgia/fibrositis syndrome and rheumatoid arthritis. *Arthritis Rheum.*, 35:550-556, 1992.
70. Bennett, R.M., Clark, S.R., Campbell, S.M., and Burckhardt, C.S.: Low levels of somatomedin C in patients with the fibromyalgia syndrome. *Arthr. Rheumat.*, 35(10):1113-1116, 1992.
71. Vaerøy, H., Helle, R., Øystein, F., Kåss, E., and Terenius, L.: Elevated CSF levels of substance P and high incidence of Raynaud phenomenon in patients with fibromyalgia: new features for diagosis. *Pain*, 32:21-26, 1988.
72. Lowe, J.C.: *The Metabolic Treatment of Fibromyalgia.* Houston, McDowell Publishing Company, 1999.
73. Lowe, J.C., Cullum, M., Graff, L., and Yellin, J.: Mutations in the c-erbAβ₁ gene: do they underlie euthyroid fibromyalgia? Paper in preparation, 1996.
74. Lowe, J.C. and Poo, I.: Tri-iodothyronine treatment of euthyroid fibromyalgia patients: clinical observations. Unpublished paper, 1991.
75. Lowe, J.C., Eichelberger, J., Manso, G., and Peterson, K.: Improvement in euthyroid fibromyalgia patients treated with T₃ (tri-iodothyronine). *J. Myofascial Ther.*, 1(2):16-29, 1994.
76. Lowe, J.C.: T₃-induced recovery from fibromyalgia by a hypothyroid patient resistant to T₄ and dessicated thyroid. *J. Myofascial Ther.*, 1(4):26-31, 1995.
77. Usala, S.J., Tennyson, G.E., Bale, A.E., Lash, R.W., Gesundheit, N., Wondisford, F.E., Accili, D., Hauser, P., and Weintraub, B.D.: A base mutation of the c-erbAβ thyroid hormone receptor in a kindred with generalized thyroid hormone resistance: molecular heterogeneity in two other kindreds. *J. Clin. Invest.*, 85:93-100, 1990.
78. Sakurai, A., Takeda, K., Ain, K., Ceccarelli, P., Kakai, A., Seino, S., Be, G.I., Refetoff, S., and DeGroot, L.J.: Generalized resistance to thyroid hormone associated with a mutation in the ligand-binding domain of the human thyroid hormone receptor β. *Proc. Natl. Acad. Sci. (USA)*, 86:8977-8981, 1989.
79. Takeda, K., Sakurai, A., DeGroot, L.J., and Refetoff, S.: Recessive inheritance of thyroid hormone resistance caused by complete deletion of the protein-coding region of the thyroid hormone receptor-β gene. *J. Clin. Endocrin. Metab.*, 74:49-55, 1992.
80. Refetoff, S., Weiss, R.E., and Usala, S.J.: The syndromes of resistance to thyroid hormone. *Endocrine Reviews*, 14: 348-399,1993.
81. Forslind,K.,Fredricksson, E., and Nived, O.: Does primary fibromyalgia exist? *Brit. J. Rheumatol.*, 29:368-70, 1990.
82. Shiroky, J.B., Cohen, M., Ballachey, M.L., and Neville, C.: Thyroid dysfunction in rheumatoid arthritis: a controlled prospective survey. *Ann. Rheumat. Dis.*, 52:454-456, 1993.
83. Hershman, J.M.: Hypothalamic and pituitary hypothyroidism. In *Progress in the Diagnosis and Treatment of Hypothyroid Conditions.* Edited by P.A. Bastenie, M. Bonnyns, and L.VanHaelst, Amsterdam, Excepta Medica, 1980, pp.41-50.
84. Bennett, R.M.: Literature reviews: fibromyalgia. *J. Musculoskel. Pain*, 2(2):101-112, 1994.
85. Eisinger, J., Arroyo, Ph., Calendini, C., Rinaldi, J.P., Combes, R., Fontaine, G.: Anomalies biologiques au cours des fibromyalgies: III. Explorations endocriniennes. *Lyon Méditerranée Méd.*, 28:858-860, 1992.

Mutations in the c-erbA β_1 Gene: Do They Underlie Euthyroid Fibromyalgia?

J.C. Lowe, DC
M.E. Cullum, PhD
L.H. Graf, Jr., PhD
J. Yellin, BA

This article originally appeared in *Medical Hypotheses*, 48(2):125-135, 1997.
It is reprinted with permission of Churchill-Livingstone (Pearson Professional Ltd).

Date received 3 May 1996
Date accepted 16 May 1996

Abstract: Fibromyalgia, a chronic condition of widespread pain, stiffness, and fatigue, has proven unresponsive to drugs the use of which is based on the "serotonin deficiency hypothesis." An alternate hypothesis, failed transcription regulation by thyroid hormone, can explain the serotonin deficiency and other objective findings and symptoms of euthyroid fibromyalgia. Virtually every feature of fibromyalgia corresponds to signs or symptoms associated with failed transcription regulation by thyroid hormone. In hypothyroid fibromyalgia, failed transcription regulation would result from thyroid hormone deficiency. In euthyroid fibromyalgia, failed transcription regulation may result from low affinity thyroid hormone receptors coded by a mutated c-erbAβ_1 gene, yielding partial peripheral resistance to thyroid hormone. The hypothesis of this paper is that in euthyroid fibromyalgia, a mutant c-erbAβ_1 gene (or alternately, the c-erbAα_1 gene) results in low affinity thyroid hormone receptors that prevent normal thyroid hormone regulation of transcription. As in hypothyroidism, this would cause a shift toward α-adrenergic dominance and increases in both cAMP phosphodiesterase and inhibitory G$_i$ proteins. The result would be tissue specific hypothyroid-like symptoms despite normal circulating thyroid hormone levels.

DEFINITION OF FIBROMYALGIA

Fibromyalgia syndrome (FS) is the most common condition of chronic, widespread musculoskeletal pain with a poor physical, psychological, and social prognosis.[1][2][3][4][5][6] The incidence in the U.S. is 2%, and more than 90% of patients are female.[7] Diagnostic criteria include widespread pain and quantifiable tenderness.[8] Associated symptoms include stiffness, chronic fatigue, sleep disturbance, headaches, dysmenorrhea, dry mucous membranes, depression, poor memory and concentration, urinary frequency, cold intolerance, irritable bowel syndrome, and paresthesias.

SEROTONIN HYPOTHESIS AND DRUG STUDIES

The "serotonin hypothesis" of the etiology of FS resulted from evidence of low serotonin levels in the serum[9][10][11][12] and CNS[13][14] of FS patients. These findings led to the proposition that tricyclic antidepressants and selective serotonin reuptake inhibitors (SSRI), by increasing synaptic content of serotonin, would relieve patients' symptoms. Drug treatments based on the serotonin hypothesis have provided slight, brief improvement, but otherwise have proven no more effective than placebos (which were slightly effective).[15][16][17][18]

These negative drug study results suggest that a more fundamental and influential underlying mechanism may account for low serotonin levels in FS patients. A possible mechanism is partial failure of thyroid hormone to regulate transcription in serotonergic cells.

AN ALTERNATE MECHANISM: FAILURE OF THYROID HORMONE TO REGULATE TRANSCRIPTION

In a variety of physiological and pathological conditions, the functional expression of α-adrenoceptors and β-adrenoceptors is inversely regulated.[19][20][21][22][23] In general, alterations in mRNA levels for these two receptor types correlate with changes in cell adrenoceptor density and reactivity.[22][23][24][25][26][27][28][29][30][31] Hypothyroidism reduces β-adrenoceptor density and reactivity in a number of tissues including the heart[22][23][24][25][26][27][31] and lungs.[32] Increases in α_{1B}-adrenoceptor mRNA in hypothyroid rat heart correlates with the potentiation of inotropic and chronotropic heart responsiveness mediated by α_{1B}-adrenoceptors.[22][25][31] Conversely, administration of thyroid hormone increases β-adrenoceptor mRNA and the membranous population of β-adrenoceptors,[33][34][35] and decreases α-adrenoceptor density in most tissues.[26][31][36] Because both α- and β-adrenoceptor genes contain thyroid hormone response elements, the inverse relationship between α- and β-adrenoceptor mRNA and adrenoceptor subtypes suggests that in various tissues, thyroid hormone activates the β-adrenoceptor gene and represses the α-adrenoceptor gene.[37] (In the liver, however, this relationship is reversed.)

T_3 attached to the ligand-binding domain of the thyroid hormone receptor stimulates transcription of some target genes such as the growth hormone gene,[38] and inhibits others such as the pituitary TSH gene.[39] When T_3 is absent, the unliganded thyroid hormone receptor bound to a thyroid hormone response element (TRE) induces expression of target genes opposite from those induced by T_3-activated thyroid hormone receptors.[40][41] Thus, when thyroid hormone is deficient, α-adrenoceptor count increases and β-adrenoceptor count decreases in various tissues. FS patients have increased α_2-adrenoceptors on platelets.[42]

α_2-Adrenoceptors located presynaptically on serotonergic nerve terminals inhibit secretion of serotonin[43] in the rat hippocampus,[44] rat medullary nucleus tractus solitarii,[45] rat and rabbit brain cortex,[45] and human neocortex when activated by norepinephrine secreted by neighboring noradrenergic neurons.[46] This inhibitory effect of α_2-adrenoceptors on serotonin secretion,[43] added to evidence of a probable shift toward α-dominance[42] in FS, makes plausible the hypothesis that inadequate transcription regulation by thyroid hormone mediates the low serotonin levels in FS patients.

Similarities between FS and Hypothyroidism. The shift toward α-adrenergic dominance accounts for many of the metabolic and physiological changes characteristic of thyroid hormone deficiency and, we hypothesize, of FS as well. The effects are similar to common experiences of patients who take β-blocking drugs such as propranolol.[47] These drugs competitively bind β-adrenergic receptors so that they are not available for catecholamine/adrenoceptor-triggered cellular actions. This produces a relative α-adrenergic dominance. Central nervous system effects include disturbed sleep, fatigue, and depression, symptoms also experienced by FS patients.[8] Peripheral effects of

β-adrenergic blockers include a fall in peripheral vascular resistance with reduced blood flow through skeletal muscles and skin, cold extremities, development of Raynaud's phenomenon, and attenuation of cardiovascular adaptation to exercise.[47] These same phenomena have been documented in FS patients.[48][49][50][51][52][53]

Virtually all FS symptoms and objective findings resemble features of hypothyroidism. Abnormalities in the carbohydrate metabolism of FS patients are similar to those of hypothyroid patients.[54][55][56] Eisinger reported that glycolysis findings in hypothyroidism and fibromyalgia are similar, with increased pyruvate/lactate ratio and decreased lactate production.[57] FS patients have biochemical, histological, and spectroscopic findings characteristic of impaired muscle energy metabolism.[48][49][50][51][52] Their muscles have the fatigue and reduced strength[58] typical of hypometabolic muscle.[59] Biopsy samples show that some patients have high concentrations of mucopolysaccharides,[60] suggesting inadequate inhibition of fibroblasts by thyroid hormone.[61][62]

In one study, subjects with high levels of aerobic fitness (and thus high metabolic capacity) were resistant to developing FS symptoms when deprived of slow-wave sleep, but people with low levels of aerobic fitness (diminished metabolic capacity) were susceptible.[63] Mild aerobic training slightly improves the status of FS patients,[53][64] indicating that enhanced metabolic efficiency favorably affects the mechanism underlying FS.

Cognitive-behavior therapy improves the status of FS patients,[65][66] possibly by reducing metabolic demand via decreased gamma motor activity and decreased skeletal muscle tone. FS patients have increased frequency of urination,[67] as do some hypothyroid patients,[68] possibly due to α-adrenoceptor inhibition of vasopressin secretion by the neurohypophysis[69] or vasopressin action on the cortical collecting tubule or duct.[70] And the cold intolerance of FS patients[71] may result from α-adrenoceptor-induced vasoconstriction[72] and decreased Na-K ATPase activity.[73]

The FS literature gives special attention to three other objective findings. Each, FS researchers believe, may lead to the etiology of FS. Our hypothesis accounts for all three.

Serotonin. The low serotonin levels found in FS patients[9][10][11][12][13][14] would be expected from the model we propose, considering that α_2-adrenoceptors inhibit serotonin synthesis and secretion by serotonergic neurons (see above).[43] Synthesis and turnover of serotonin is decreased in hypothyroid neonatal animals and increased in hyperthyroid animals.[74][75][76]

Thyroxine has been shown to increase serotonin levels in rat skin and ilium,[77] and urinary levels of 5-hydroxy indoleacetic acid (the major metabolite of serotonin) were found to increase in thyrotoxicosis and decrease in hypothyroidism.[78] Tóth and Csaba[79] measured the serotonin levels, minus the blood serotonin content, in brain stems of rabbits that had either been thyroidectomized or fed thyroxine. Brain stem serotonin increased in thyroxine-treated rabbits 56.5% and decreased in thyroidectomized animals 21.7%. Blood content of serotonin increased by the same amount in thyroxine-treated rabbits, but decreased markedly more in the thyroidectomized group. The authors proposed that peripheral symptoms of hyperthyroidism and hypothyroidism are in part the effect of thyroid hormone on CNS metabolism of tryptophan and serotonin.

In the rat brain, 5-HT$_{1A}$ (serotonin) receptors are distributed heterogeneously and in high density in the dorsal raphe nucleus and in limbic tissues such as the cortex and hippocampus.[80] In one study, thyroidectomy caused a decrease in the density of 5-HT$_2$ (serotonin) receptors in the striatum, and large doses of T$_4$ or T$_3$ for seven days increased 5-HT$_2$ receptor density in the cortex and hippocampus in the limbic system.[81] Thyroidectomy did not affect receptor binding in the hypothalamus or receptor density in the dorsal or median raphe nucleus. But at 7 and 95 days after thyroidectomy, there was a regulatory increase of 5-HT$_{1A}$ receptors in the cortex and hippocampus of the limbic system. High doses of T$_4$ for 28 days increased receptor binding in the hypothalamus but not the dorsal raphe nucleus. The authors suggest that a neuromodulatory link exists between the hypothalamic-pituitary-thyroid axis and 5-HT$_{1A}$ receptors in the limbic system.[81] This view is supported by the finding that limbic cells have high levels of expression of the thyroid hormone receptor c-erbAβ₁ gene and all three c-erbAα genes.[82][83]

Growth Hormone. FS patients have low serum somatomedin C (insulin-like growth factor-1) levels, indicating that their growth hormone (GH) levels are low.[84] Bennett suggested that low GH levels in FS patients are due to the loss of slow wave sleep and the absence of the stress of exercise.[85] But if disturbed sleep and lack of exercise contribute to low GH levels,[86][87] they may be doing so only by complicating already existing low levels due to the failure of thyroid hormone to regulate transcription.[88][89][90]

Thyroidectomy induced a 61-65% reduction in hypothalamic growth hormone-releasing factor (GHF-R) mRNA levels. Levels were reversed with T$_4$ replacement. Pituitary GH levels varied parallel to GHF-R after thyroidectomy and T$_4$ supplementation.[91] T$_3$ and T$_4$ increase expression of GH receptor mRNA and potentiate the expression of somatomedin C mRNA in the presence of GH.[92] In the absence of thyroid hormone, GH mRNA synthesis and accumulation drop more than 98%.[88][89][93][94]

Hypothyroidism impairs GH secretion directly through inhibiting the somatotroph cells of the pituitary gland.[95][96] This results in decreased hepatic secretion of somatomedin C and impedes the response of cartilage to somatomedin C.[97]

T$_3$ increases GH mRNA.[88] In fact, measurements of GH mRNA after exposure of chromosomes to T$_3$ provide strong support for the view that the rate of transcription of the GH gene is proportional to the concentration of thyroid hormone occupying thyroid hormone receptors on chromosomes.[98]

Substance P. Substance P, a neuropeptide that is excitatory to nociceptive cells, has been found in increased levels in the cerebrospinal fluid of FS patients.[99] The preprotachykinin-A gene encodes preprotachykinin-A (PPT-A), the precursor of substance P and the cognate receptor, substance P receptor.[100][101] Thyroidectomy largely increased preprotachykinin-A mRNA in the anterior pituitary.[102] T$_4$ replacement after thyroidectomy decreased PPT-A mRNA relative to controls.[103] Excess T$_4$, enough to cause hyperthyroidism, significantly reduced substance P levels.[104]

Hypothyroidism in FS patients. Reports of the similarities between FS and hypothyroidism have been common.[60][105][106][107][108][109][110][111][112][113][114][115][116] Many researchers typically attempt to identify and exclude hypothyroid patients from their FS studies[117][118][119][120][121] because FS symptoms and signs are often seen in hypothyroid patients.

Forslind, Fredriksson and Nived[119] evaluated 25 patients with a diagnosis of primary FS and reevaluated them five years later. At the beginning of the study, 1 patient was diagnosed as hypothyroid. During the subsequent five years, 5 more were diagnosed as hypothyroid. This was a 24% incidence of hypothyroidism in this group. Shiroky and coworkers found that 4 (12%) of 34 FS patients had thyroidal hypothyroidism.[122]

Of Lowe's 38 FS patients,[123] 4 (10.5%) had thyroidal hypothyroidism. Twenty (52.6%) had thyroid function test results consistent with central hypothyroidism (hypothyroidism due to pituitary or hypothalamic dysfunction). Of those 20 patients, 11 (28.9%) had blunted TSH responses to injected thyrotropin releasing hormone (TRH), a finding that suggests pituitary hypothyroidism. Ferraccioli and colleagues[124] reported blunted TSH responses in 5 of 24 FS patients (20.8%), and Neeck and Riedel[105] reported blunted TSH responses in 100% of their 13 FS patients.

Two consensus committees[1][8] have implied that FS and hypothyroidism are concomitant conditions that are etiologically unrelated. The reasoning appears to be that if some FS patients do not have hypothyroidism, then a thyroid hormone deficiency cannot be necessary to the etiology of FS. We agree. A thyroid hormone deficiency is not necessary to generate FS. It is, however, sufficient to generate the syndrome. Moreover, it is also sufficient but not necessary for the generation of FS, that thyroid hormone in normal concentrations fails to exert its regulatory effects at the nuclear level in certain tissues.

Thyroid Hormone Resistance Syndromes (THRS). A recent genetic finding raises the distinct possibility that euthyroid FS results from the same mechanism that mediates most effects of thyroid hormone deficiency—inadequate thyroid hormone regulation of transcription. The finding shows that mutated thyroid hormone receptors prevent normal regulation of transcription.[125] This gives rise to various forms of thyroid hormone resistance syndrome (THRS).

Lowe[126] found that some euthyroid FS patients benefited from the use of T_3 after failing to benefit from T_4, which effectively corrects most hypothyroidism. Lowe reported open trials in which euthyroid FS patients[126] and a central hypothyroid patient[127] markedly improved or recovered from FS symptoms with T_3 therapy. Lowe and colleagues[128] also found in a double-blind placebo-controlled response-driven crossover study that the status of euthyroid FS patients significantly improved during T_3 treatment phases and deteriorated during placebo phases.

As a result, Lowe and coworkers[129] observed four noteworthy phenomena: 1) euthyroid FS patients had hypothyroid-like symptoms, 2) effective doses of T_3 were usually supraphysiologic, 3) these doses typically did not induce thyrotoxicosis, and 4) in some patients, dosages high enough to relieve FS features also caused hypermetabolism in some but not other tissues.

The last feature, variable responsiveness of tissues confirmed by Lowe and colleagues,[128] requires that some euthyroid FS patients use a compromise T_3 dosage that provides satisfactory relief without causing

hypermetabolism of some tissues. The same phenomenon is seen in THRS patients, and is also considered to represent variable tissue responsiveness to T_3.[125]

In the above four respects, euthyroid FS patients resemble those with a form of THRS termed partial peripheral thyroid hormone resistance syndrome (PTHRS). Of 77 euthyroid FS patients in an open trial using supraphysiologic but nontoxic dosages of T_3,[126] the pain thresholds of patients' tender points (the most objective measure of FS status) improved post-treatment (p: 0.01). Of the 58 patients (75%) whose symptom improvement justified continuing T_3, post-treatment tender point scores improved even more significantly (p < 0.0005). Of these patients, 23 (39.66%) had no recurrences of symptoms. Intermittent symptoms were mild in 21 (36.20%), moderate in 11 (18.97%), and severe in 3 (5.17%). Based on this and other open trials,[127][129] Lowe hypothesized that euthyroid FS is a clinical phenotype of PTHRS that selectively involves primarily neuromuscular tissues.[129][130]

PTHRS is characterized by reduced clinical and biochemical manifestations of thyroid hormone action relative to circulating hormone levels.[125] Patients have normal circulating thyroid hormone levels.[131] And because their pituitary thyrotrophs are not resistant (thus the adjective "peripheral"), TSH levels are also normal.[132] Various other tissues, however, are resistant and the normal circulating levels of thyroid hormone are inadequate to maintain normal metabolism in the resistant tissues. In euthyroid FS, we infer that various CNS structures and neuromuscular tissues are resistant to thyroid hormone action.[130]

The genetic basis of the general form of THRS has been established as mutations in the c-erbAβ₁ gene in chromosome 3.[125] The c-erbAβ₁ gene codes for the β₁ isoform of the thyroid hormone receptor. Mutations to date have been located in the nucleotide sequence that codes the T_3-binding domain of the thyroid hormone receptor. Inheritance in most cases is autosomal dominant, occurs in both genders equally, and affects most races.[125]

One PTHRS family, however, is an exception. Patients from this family have a complete deletion of the coding sequences of the thyroid hormone receptor β gene.[133] But they showed clear-cut overstimulation (increased urinary creatine and hydroxyproline, appearance of tremor and cardiac gallop) with higher-end supraphysiologic doses of thyroid hormone, indicating that some functions may be idiosyncratically allocated to the c-erbAα₁ gene,[125] making c-erbAα₁ mutations possibly clinically significant.

Mutant thyroid hormone receptors that are unable to bind T_3 are transcriptionally inactive,[134] showing that transcriptional regulation is a ligand-dependent process. Other mutant receptors can bind T_3 but with greatly reduced affinity. The ability of these mutant receptors to transcriptionally activate or repress target genes in response to T_3 binding is impaired.[134] In PTHRS patients, the thyroid hormone receptors of some tissues but not others are mutated.[125] The c-erbAβ_1 gene of only one well-documented case of PTHRS has been sequenced. No mutations were present.[135] The c-erbAα_1 gene was not sequenced. It is likely, however, that the molecular basis of all forms of THRS is the same, since most steps in the synthesis of thyroid hormone, its molecular integrity, transport, and cellular action (exempting receptor binding) have been eliminated as sources of THRS.[136]

HYPOTHESIS

The basis of euthyroid FS as a hypothyroid-like condition may be PTHRS due to one or more mutations in the c-erbAβ_1 gene, or less likely, the c-erbAα_1 gene. The mutations would be germ line lesions. Selective tissue involvement that gives rise to the clinical phenotypes identified as FS may result from differences in ligand affinity of mutant receptors[134] and/or from differential tissue expression of thyroid hormone receptor subtypes.[137] The resulting mutant β_1 (or α_1) thyroid hormone receptors would bind with low affinity to normal concentrations of T_3.[134] This would result in transcription typical of thyroid hormone deficiency in the involved tissues.

According to this model, euthyroid FS results from failure of normal concentrations of thyroid hormone to normally regulate transcription in select tissues due to mutant thyroid hormone receptors. In affected tissues, the net transcriptional effect of mutant thyroid hormone receptors unliganded due to their low affinity for T_3 would be tantamount to the effect of hypothyroidism:[134] thyroid hormone-activated genes are repressed, and thyroid hormone-repressed genes are activated,[40][41][125][138] resulting in an increase in α-adrenoceptors and a decrease in β-adrenoceptors in some tissues. Increases in phosphodiesterase (that inactivates cAMP[139]) and inhibitory G proteins[140][141][142] (that inhibit cyclic adenylate formation) would also be expected since such increases also result from thyroid hormone deficiency.

Selective Tissue Involvement. The lack of a pathognomonic clinical picture of THRS is consistent with the variable clinical picture of euthyroid FS.

Phenotypes among THRS patients result largely from selective tissue involvement. The tissues involved vary, as attested by the heterogeneity of signs and symptoms.

In the most thoroughly studied form of THRS, the general form, symptoms of inadequate thyroid hormone regulation include:[125] growth and mental retardation, myopathy and myalgia, refractory congestive heart failure, delayed skeletal maturation, hyperbilirubinemia, hypofibrinogenemia, and adrenal insufficiency. Other symptoms, such as recurrent syncopy, headaches, chronic back pain, learning disabilities, somnolence, weight gain, facial puffiness, and fatigue resemble prominent features of FS. The similarity of symptoms in some THRS and FS patients may reflect similar tissue selectivity.

Variations in the Severity of the Clinical Features of FS. It is not clear whether differences in severity of the clinical features of THRS between patients is due to ligand affinity or some other feature of mutant receptor function.[125] However, recent findings may explain the variable severity of clinical features among both THRS and euthyroid FS patients.

Mutant receptors that bind T_3 with low affinity inhibit wild type (non-mutated) thyroid hormone receptors, thus impeding their transcriptional activity.[134][143][144] This dominant negative activity may result from one or a combination of mechanisms:[134] 1) formation of nonfunctional heterodimers between mutant and wild type receptor proteins, 2) competition between mutant and wild type receptors for binding to a common DNA target sequence (the thyroid hormone response element), or 3) sequestering by mutant receptors of a shared accessory factor necessary for wild type receptor modulation of gene transcription.

Differences in the clinical outcome of thyroid hormone receptor mutations may also be related to the ratio of mutant to wild type receptors in select tissues. In one study, minimal dominant negative inhibition of wild types was found at low ratios of mutant to wild type receptors (1:1 or 2:1). But a fourfold excess of mutant receptors caused a 50% inhibition of wild types.[134]

Requirement for supraphysiologic doses of T_3. That most euthyroid FS patients improve or recover only with supraphysiologic doses of thyroid hormone,[126][128] as do THRS patients,[145][146][147][148][149][150][151] supports the likelihood that the underlying condition is PTHRS due to mutant thyroid hormone receptors.

Patients. The usual replacement dose for hypothyroid patients is 25-to-75 μg of T_3.[152] Refetoff, Weiss, and Usala note that a beneficial, anabolic effect in THRS patients may occur only with doses as high as 1,000 µg of T_4 or 500 µg of T_3,[125] although most THRS patients require supraphysiologic doses far below these amounts. Kaplan, Swartz, and Larsen[145] documented the change from hypometabolism to eumetabolism in one PTHRS patient with 500 µg of T_3. Lowe and coworkers[128] found that under blinded conditions, the dosages necessary to relieve signs and symptoms in euthyroid FS patients without evidence of hypermetabolism ranged from 93.75-to-225.00 µg.

In Vitro Findings. An explanation for the supraphysiologic T_3 doses required by FS patients is implied by in vitro findings, where mutant thyroid hormone receptors inhibit counterpart wild type thyroid hormone receptors. The mutant receptor G340R, for example, has no T_3 binding capacity. It is transcriptionally inactive when exposed to low or high levels of T_3, and in either case continues to inhibit wild type receptors.[134] Another mutant receptor, P448H, has a low affinity for T_3, is transcriptionally inactive, and inhibits wild type thyroid hormone receptors when exposed to low levels of T_3. But when exposed to concentrations of T_3 high enough to saturate the receptor, it becomes transcriptionally active, properly stimulating or repressing genes that contain positive or negative thyroid hormone response elements. And at saturation levels of T_3 exposure, the P448H receptor ceases its dominant negative inhibition of wild type receptors so that they become transcriptionally active.[134] Thus, high levels of T_3 appear to override partial resistance of mutant receptors to T_3 and relieve the inhibition of corresponding wild-type receptors. This finding in THRS[143][144] may explain why most euthyroid FS patients recover only with supraphysiologic doses of T_3.

TESTABLE PROPOSITIONS

We propose that molecular biological methods can provide confirmatory or contradictory evidence of a genetic basis of euthyroid FS. The major objective should be to identify mutations in the c-erbAβ₁ gene. Euthyroid patients are now available who have recovered from FS with supraphysiologic dosages of T_3.[128] We recommend sequencing of the c-erbAβ₁ gene from fibroblasts, erythrocytes, or leukocytes from these patients.

If no c-erbAβ₁ mutations are found (none were found in one case of PTHRS), we recommend sequencing of the c-erbAα₁ gene. Although no mutations have been identified in the c-erbAα₁ gene, it is ex-

pressed in virtually all tissues,[153][154] is functional, and is capable of partially substituting for the functions of the c-erbAβ₁ gene. This was shown by clear-cut overstimulation (increased urinary creatine and hydroxyproline, appearance of tremor and cardiac gallop) when members of the PTHRS family with deletion of the entire coding region of both c-erbAβ alleles (see above) took higher-end supraphysiologic doses of thyroid hormone.[155] Even in patients with intact c-erbAβ alleles, some functions may be idiosyncratically allocated to the c-erbAα₁ gene,[125] possibly making c-erbAα₁ mutations clinically significant in FS.

Further support for the view of euthyroid FS as a genetically-based thyroid hormone-related disorder may come from a number of indirect sources. When increased numbers of α_2-adrenoceptors on platelets of euthyroid FS patients are found (as in one study[42]), analyses of α- and β-adrenoceptor balance in various accessible symptomatic tissues should follow. If the balance is typical of hypothyroid status, supraphysiologic doses of thyroid hormone may induce a reversal toward normal adrenoceptor balance.

Serotonin levels should be measured in previously-determined serotonin-deficient euthyroid FS patients who are taking supraphysiologic doses of thyroid hormone. If high levels of thyroid hormone shift transcription so that the density of α_2-adrenoceptors is sufficiently reduced in serotonergic neural membranes, increased synthesis and secretion of serotonin may be obvious in post-treatment testing. Similar testing should be performed with growth hormone and substance P.

While thyroid hormone can exert a profound influence on adrenoceptor balance and cellular responsiveness to catecholamines, adrenoceptors are not the only sites where thyroid hormone impacts cellular metabolism.[156] In thyroid hormone deficiency, the inhibitory effects of increased α-adrenoceptors are compounded by increases in phosphodiesterase (that inactivates cAMP[139]) and G_i proteins[140][141][142] (that inhibit cyclic adenylate formation). Combined, these increases are largely responsible for the hypometabolic effects of hypothyroidism. Deficient thyroid hormone transcription regulation in adipose cells, for example, enhances membrane cAMP phosphodiesterase activity.[139] From adipose cell membranes of FS patients resistant to therapeutic fat depletion regimes (suggesting selective PTHRS of adipose cells), potentially increased low K_m cAMP phosphodiesterase can be studied by chromatography as can cyclic nucleotide phosphodiesterase activity by assay. Also, inadequate thyroid hormone regulation enhances expression of the α subunit of inhibitory G-proteins and G_β-subunits common to all G-proteins and their mRNA levels in adipose cells.[140][141][142] These indices in biopsied fat cell membranes can be measured by techniques such as immunoblotting and solution hybridization probes.

If mutations in the c-erbAβ_1 or c-erbAα_1 gene underlie euthyroid FS, the basis of patients' hypothyroid-like symptoms and objective findings will be established as inadequate thyroid hormone regulation of transcription. Research can then proceed to explore FS as a metabolic manifestation of a molecular aberration.

ACKNOWLEDGMENTS

We wish to extend our gratitude to Dr. Steve Usala for discussions during the evolution of this hypothesis and to Dr. J Eisinger for his comments on the manuscript.

REFERENCES

1. Consensus Document on Fibromyalgia: The Copenhagen Declaration. Myopain '92, Copenhagen, August 17-20, 1992, pp.15-16.
2. Felson, D.T. and Goldenberg, D.L.: The natural history of fibromyalgia. *Arthritis Rheum.*, 29:1522-1526, 1986.
3. Hazleman, B.: Soft tissue rheumatism. *Brit. J. Rheumatol.*, 31:135, 1992.
4. Bengtsson, A., Bäckman, E., Lindblom, V., and Skogh, T.: Long term follow-up of fibromyalgia patients: clinical symptoms, muscular function, laboratory tests—an eight year comparison study. *J. Musculoskel. Pain*, 2(2):67-80, 1994.
5. Cathey, M.A., Wolfe, F., Kleinheksel, S.M., and Hawley, D.J.: Socioeconomic impact of fibrositis: a study of 81 patients with primary fibrositis. *Amer. J. Med.*, 81:78-84, 1986.
6. Henriksson, C.: Living with fibromyalgia. *Scand. J. Rheum.*, 24:179, 1995.
7. Wolfe, F.: Aspects of the epidemiology of fibromyalgia. *J. Musculoskel. Pain*, 2(3):65-77, 1994.
8. Wolfe, F., Smythe, H.A., Yunus, M.B., et al.: The American College of Rheumatology 1990 criteria for the classification of fibromyalgia: report of the multicenter criteria committee. *Arthritis Rheum.*, 33:160-172, 1990.
9. Moldofsky, H. and Warsh, J.J.: Plasma tryptophan and musculoskeletal pain in non-articular rheumatism ("fibrositis syndrome"). *Pain*, 5:65-71, 1978.
10. Russell, I.J.: Neurohormonal aspects of fibromyalgia syndrome. *Rheum. Dis. Clinics North Am.*, 15:149-168, 1989.
11. Russell, I.J., Michalek, J.E., Vipraio, G.A., Fletcher, E.M., and Wall, K.: Serum amino acids in fibrositis/fibromyalgia syndrome. *J. Rheumatol.*, 19(16 suppl.):158-163, 1989.
12. Russell, I.J., Michalek, J.E., Vipraio, J.A., Fletcher, E.M., Javors, M.A., and Bowden, C.A.: Platelet 3H-imipramine uptake receptor density and serum serotonin levels in patients with fibromyalgia/fibrositis syndromes. *J. Rheumatol.*, 19:104-109, 1992.
13. Houvenagel, E., Forzy, G., Cortet, B., and Vincent, G.: 5-Hydroxyindoleacetic acid in cerebrospinal fluid in fibromyalgia. *Arthritis Rheum.*, 33:S55, 1990.
14. Russell, I.J., Vaeroy, H., Javors, M., and Nyberg, F.: Cerebrospinal fluid biogenic amine metabolites in fibromyalgia/fibrositis syndrome and rheumatoid arthritis. *Arthritis Rheum.*, 35:550-556, 1992.
15. Goldenberg, D.L.: Fibromyalgia: treatment programs. *J. Musculoskel. Pain*, 1:71-81, 1993.
16. Carette, S.: What have clinical trials taught us about the treatment of fibromyalgia? *J. Musculoskel. Pain*, 3:133-140, 1995.
17. Wolfe, F., Cathey, M.A., and Hawley, D.J.: A double blind placebo controlled trial of fluoxetine in fibromyalgia. *Scand. J. Rheumatol.*, 23:255-259, 1994.
18. Carette, S., Bell, M., Reynolds, J., et al.: A controlled trial of amitriptyline, cyclobenzaprine, and placebo in fibromyalgia patients. *Arthritis Rheum.*, 37(1):32-40, 1994.
19. Kunos, G., Vermes-Kunos, I., and Nickerson, M.: Effects of thyroid state on adrenoceptor properties. *Nature*, 250:779-781, 1974.
20. Kunos, G. and Ishac, E.J.N.: Mechanism of inverse regulation of α_1- and β-adrenergic receptors. *Biochem. Pharmacol.*, 36:1185-1191, 1987.
21. Ishac, E.J.N., Lazar-Wesley, E., and Kunos, G.: Rapid inverse changes in α_{1B}- and β_2-adrenergic receptors and gene transcripts in acutely isolated rat liver cells. *J. Cell Physiol.*, 152:79-86, 1992.
22. Kunos, G.: Thyroid hormone-dependent interconversion of myocardial α- and β-adrenoceptors in the rat. *Brit. J. Pharmacol.*, 59:177-189, 1977.
23. Kupfer, L.E., Bilezikian, J.P., and Robinson, R.B.: Regulation of alpha- and beta-adrenergic receptors by triiodothyronine in cultured rat myocardial cells. *Naunyn Schmiedeberg's Arch. Pharmacol.*, 334:275-281, 1986.
24. Kunos, G.: Modulation of adrenergic reactivity and adrenoceptors by thyroid hormone. In *Adrenoceptors and Catecholamine Action*. Edited by G. Kunos, New York, John Wiley & Sons, 1981, part A, pp.297-333.
25. Williams, L.T., Lefkowitz, R.J., Watanabe, A.M., Hathaway, D.R., and Besch, H.R., Jr.: Thyroid hormone regulation of β-adrenergic receptor number. *J. Biol. Chem.*, 252:2787-2789, 1977.
26. Sharma, V.K. and Banerjee, S.P.: α-Adrenergic receptor in rat heart. *J. Biol. Chem.*, 253:5277-5279, 1978.
27. Ishac, E.J.N., Pennefather, J.N., and Handberg, G.M.: Effect of changes in thyroid state on atrial α- and β-adrenoceptors, adenylate cyclase activity, and catecholamine levels in the rat. *J. Cardiovasc. Pharmacol.*, 5:396-405, 1983.
28. Preiksaitis, H.G. and Kunos, G.: Adrenoceptor-mediated activation of liver glycogen phosphorylase: effects of thyroid state. *Life Sci.*, 24:35-42, 1979.
29. Malbon, C.C.: Liver cell adenylate cyclase and beta-adrenergic receptors: increased beta-adrenergic receptor

number and responsiveness in the hypothyroid rat. *J. Biol. Chem.*, 255:8692-8699, 1980.

30. Preiksaitis, H.G., Kan, W.H., and Kunos, G.: Decreased α_1-adrenoceptor responsiveness and density in the hypothyroid rat. *J. Biol. Chem.*, 257:4320-4326, 1982.

31. Kunos, G., Mucci, L., and O'Regan, S.: The influence of hormonal and neuronal factors on rat heart adrenoceptors. *Brit. J. Pharmacol.*, 71:371-386, 1980.

32. Baker, S.P.: Effects of thyroid status on beta-adrenoreceptors and muscarinic receptors in the rat lung. *J. Autonom. Pharmacol.*, 1:269-277, 1981.

33. Bahouth, S.W.: Thyroid hormone transcriptionally regulates the β_1-adrenergic receptor gene in cultured ventricular myocytes. *J. Biol. Chem.*, 266(24):15863-15869, 1991.

34. Sharma, V.K and Banerjee, S.P.: β-adrenergic receptors in rat skeletal muscle: effects of thyroidectomy. *Biochimica et Biophysica Acta*, 539:538-542, 1978.

35. Mason, G.A., Bondy, S.C., Nemeroff, C.B., Walker, C.H., and Prange, A.J., Jr.: The effects of thyroid state on beta-adrenergic and serotonergic receptors in rat brain. *Psychoneuroendocrinology*, 12(4):261-270, 1987.

36. Williams, L.T. and Lefkowitz, R.J.: Thyroid hormone regulation of alpha-adrenergic receptors: studies in rat myocardium. *J. Cardiovasc. Pharmacol.*, 1:181-189, 1979.

37. Lazar-Wesley, E., Hadcock, J.R., Malbon, C.C., Kunos, G., and Ishac, J.N.: Tissue-specific regulation of α_{2B}, β_1, and β_2-adrenergic receptor mRNAs by thyroid state in the rat. *Endocrinology*, 29(2):1116-1118, 1991.

38. Brent, G.A., Larsen, P.R., Harney, J.W., Koening, R.J., and Moore, D.D.: Functional characterization of the rat growth hormone promoter elements required for induction by thyroid hormone with and without a co-transfectant β type thyroid hormone receptor. *J. Biol. Chem.*, 264:178-182, 1989.

39. Carr, F.E., Burnside, J., and Chin, W.W.: Thyroid hormones regulate rat thyrotropin β gene promoter activity expressed in GH3 cells. *Mol. Endocrinol.*, 3:709-716, 1989.

40. Brent, G.A., Dunn, M.K., Harney, J.W., Gulick, T., Larsen, P.R., and Moore, D.D.: Thyroid hormone aporeceptor represses T_3-inducible promoters and blocks activity of the retinoic acid receptor. *New Biol.*, 1:329-336, 1989.

41. Damm, K., Thompson, C.C., and Evans, R.M.: Protein encoded by v-*erbA* functions as a thyroid-hormone receptor antagonist. *Nature*, 339:593-597, 1989.

42. Bennett, R.M., Clark, S.M., and Campbell, S.M.: Symptoms of Raynaud's syndrome in patients with fibromyalgia: a study utilizing the Nielsen test, digital photoplethysmography and measurements of platelet α_2-adrenergic receptors. *Arthritis Rheum.*, 34:264-269, 1991.

43. Frankhyzen, A. and Muller, A.: In vitro studies on the inhibition of serotonin release through α-adrenoreceptor activity in various regions of the rat CNS. Abstract of 5th Catecholamine Symposium, 1983, p.137.

44. Benkirane, S., Arbilla, S., and Langer, S.Z.: Newly synthesized noradrenaline mediates the α_2-adrenoceptor inhibition of [3H]5-hydroxytryptamine release induced

by beta-phenylethylamine in rat hippocampal slices. *European J. Pharm.*, 131(2-3):189-198, 1986.

45. Yang, J., Bao, J., and Su, D.F.: Effects of serotonin and norepinephrine on neuronal discharges of the nucleus tractus solitarii in medullary slices. *Acta Pharm. Sinica*, 13(1):42-44, 1992.

46. Trendelenburg, A.U., Trendelenburg, M., Starke, K., and Limberger, N.: Release-inhibiting α_2-adrenoceptor at serotonergic axons in rat and rabbit brain cortex: evidence for pharmacological identity with α_2-autoreceptors. *Naunyn-Schmiedebergs Arch Pharm.*, 349(1):25-33, 1994.

47. Pinchera, A., Martino, E., and Faglia, G.: Central hypothyroidism. In *Werner and Ingbar's The Thyroid: A Fundamental and Clinical Text*, 6th edition. Edited by L.E. Braverman and R.D. Utiger, Philadelphia, J.B. Lippincott Co., 1991, pp.968-984.

48. Bennett, R.M.: Muscle physiology and cold reactivity in the fibromyalgia syndrome. *Rheum. Dis. Clinics North Am.*, 15:135-147, 1989.

49. Henriksson, K.G., Bengtsson, A., Larsson, J., et al.: Muscle biopsy findings of possible diagnostic importance in primary fibromyalgia (fibrositis, myofascial syndrome). *Lancet*, ii:1395, 1982.

50. Kalyan-Raman, U.P., Kalyan-Raman, K., Yunus, M.B., et al.: Muscle pathology in primary fibromyalgia syndrome: a light microscopic, histologic and ultrastructure study. *J. Rheumatol.*, 11:808-814, 1984.

51. Bengtsson, A., Henriksson, K.G., and Larsson, J.: Muscle biopsy in primary fibromyalgia: light-microscopical and histochemical findings. *Scand. J. Rheumatol.*, 15:1-6, 1986.

52. Bengtsson, A., Henriksson, K.G., and Larsson, J.: Reduced high-energy phosphate levels in the painful muscles of patients with primary fibromyalgia. *Arthritis Rheum.*, 29:817-821, 1986.

53. McCain, G.A., Bell, D.A., Mai, F.M., and Halliday, P.D.: A controlled study of the effects of a supervised cardiovascular fitness training program on the manifestations of primary fibromyalgia. *Arthritis Rheum.*, 31:1135-1141, 1988.

54. Eisinger, J., Mechtouf, K., Pauwel, M., et al.: Anomalies biologiques au cours des fibromyalgies: I. lactacidemie et pyruvicemie. *Lyon Méditerranée Med.*, 28:851-854, 1992.

55. Eisinger, J., Plantamura, A., and Ayavou, T.: Glycolysis abnormalities in fibromyalgia. *J. Am. Coll. Nutr.*, 13:144-148, 1994.

56. Is fibromyalgia caused by a glycolysis impairment? *Nutr. Reviews*, 52(7):248-250, 1994.

57. Eisinger, J.: Personal communication with J.C. Lowe. April 25, 1996.

58. Jacobsen, S., Jensen, K.E., Thomsen, C., et al.: 31P magnetic resonance spectroscopy of skeletal muscle in patients with fibromyalgia. *J. Rheum.*, 19:1600-1603, 1992.

59. Ramsay, I.D.: *Thyroid Disease and Muscle Dysfunction.* Chicago, Year Book Medical Publishers, Inc., 1974.

60. Awad, E.A.: Histopathological changes in fibrositis. In *Advances in Pain Research and Therapy*, vol. 17. Edited by J.R. Fricton and E.A. Awad, New York, Raven Press,

Ltd., 1990, pp.249-258.

61. Kunos, G., Vermes-Kunos, I., and Nickerson, M.: Effects of thyroid state on adrenoceptor properties. *Nature*, 250:779-781, 1974.

62. Williams, L.T. and Lefkowitz, R.J.: Molecular pharmacology of alpha adrenergic receptors: utilization of [3H]dihydroergocryptine binding in the study of pharmacological receptor alterations. *Molecular Pharm.*, 13:304-313, 1977.

63. Moldofsky, H. and Scarisbrick, P.: Induction of neurasthenic musculoskeletal pain syndrome by selective sleep stage deprivation. *Psychosom. Med.*, 38:35-44, 1976.

64. Klug, G.A., McAauley, E., and Clark, S.: Factors influencing the development and maintenance of aerobic fitness: lessons applicable to the fibrositis syndrome. *J. Rheumatol.*, 16:30-39, 1989.

65. Nielson, W.R., Walker, C., and McCain, G.A.: Cognitive behavioral treatment of fibromyalgia syndrome: preliminary findings. *J. Rheumatol.*, 19:98-103, 1992.

66. Walco, G.A. and Ilowite, N.T.: Cognitive-behavioral intervention for juvenile primary fibromyalgia syndrome. *J. Rheumatol.*, 19:1617-1619, 1992.

67. Wolfe, F.: Diagnosis of fibromyalgia. *J. Musculoskel. Med.*, 7:54, 1990.

68. Watanakunakorn, C., Hodges, R.E., and Evans, T.C.: Myxedema: a study of 400 cases. *Arch. Intern. Med.*, 116:183-190, 1965.

69. Roman, R.J., Cowley, A.W., Jr., and Lecherie, C.: Water diuretic and natriuretic effect of clonidine in the rat. *J. Pharmacol. Exp. Ther.*, 221:385-393, 1979.

70. Gellai, M. and Ruffolo, R.R., Jr.: Renal effects of selective α_1- and α_2-adrenoceptor agonists in conscious, normotensive rats. *J. Pharmacol. Exp. Ther.*, 240:723-728, 1987.

71. Bennett, R.M.: Muscle physiology and cold reactivity in the fibromyalgia syndrome. *Rheum. Dis. Clinics North Am.*, 15:135-147, 1989.

72. Nichols, A.J.: α-Adrenoceptor signal transduction mechanisms. In *α-Adrenoceptors: Molecular Biology, Biochemistry, and Pharmacology*. Edited by R.R. Ruffolo, Jr., Basal, Karger, 1991.

73. Gambert, S.R.: Environmental effects and physiologic variables. In *Werner's The Thyroid: A Fundamental and Clinical Text*, 6th edition. Edited by L.E. Braverman and R.D. Utiger, Philadelphia, J.B. Lippincott Co., 1991, pp.347-357.

74. Singhal, R.L., Hrdina, P.D., and Rastogi, R.B.: Brain biogenic amines and altered thyroid function. *Life Sci.*, 17:1617-1626, 1975.

75. Rastogi, R.B. and Singhal, R.L.: Influence of neonatal and adult hyperthyroidism on behavior and biosynthetic capacity for norepinephrine, dopamine and 5-hydrotryptamine in rat brain. *J. Pharmacol. Exp. Ther.*, 198:609-618, 1976.

76. Atterwill, C.K.: Effect of acute and chronic triiodothyronine (T₃) administration to rats on central 5-HT and dopamine-mediated behavioural response and related brain biochemistry. *Neuropharmacol.*, 20:131-144, 1981.

77. Spencer, P.S.J. and West, G.B.: Further observations on the relationship between the thyroid gland and the anaphylactoid reaction in rats. *Int. Archs. Allergy Appl.*

78. Haverback, B.J., Sjoerdsma, A., and Terry, L.L.: Urinary excretion of the serotonin metabolite 5-hydroxyindoleacetic acid, in various clinical conditions. *New Engl. J. Med.*, 255(6):270-272, 1956.

79. Tóth, S. and Csaba, B.: The effect of thyroid hormone on 5-hydroxytryptamine (5-HT) level of brain stem and blood in rabbits. *Experientia*, 22:755-756, 1966.

80. Gothert, M.: 5-Hydroxytryptamine receptors: an example for the complexity of chemical transmission of information in the brain. *Arzneimittelforschung*, 2:238-249, 1992.

81. Mason, G.A., Bondy, S.C., Nemeroff, C.B., Walker, C.H., and Prange, A.J., Jr.: The effects of thyroid state on beta-adrenergic and serotonergic receptors in rat brain. *Psychoneuroendocrinology*, 12:261-270, 1987.

82. Bradley, D.J., Young, W.S., III, and Weinberger, C.: Differential expression of α and β thyroid hormone receptor genes in rat brain and pituitary. *Proc. Natl. Acad. Sci. (USA)*, 86:7250-7254, 1989.

83. Cook, C.B. and Koenig, R.J.: Expression of erbAα and β mRNAs in regions of adult rat brain. *Mol. Cell Endocrinol.*, 70:13-20, 1990.

84. Bennett, R.M., Clark, S.R., Campbell, S.M., and Burckhardt, C.S.: Low levels of somatomedin C in patients with the fibromyalgia syndrome. *Arthritis Rheum.*, 35(10):1113-1116, 1992.

85. Bennett, R.M.: Beyond fibromyalgia: ideas on etiology and treatment. *J. Rheumatol.*, 16(suppl 19):185-191, 1989.

86. Hartley, L.H.: Growth hormone and catecholamine response to exercise in relation to physical training. *Med. Sci. Sports*, 7:34-36, 1975.

87. Karagiorgos, A., Garcia, J.F., and Brooks, G.A.: Growth hormone response to continuous and intermittent exercise. *J. Appl. Physiol.*, 11:302-307, 1979.

88. Seo, H., Vassart, G., Brocas, H., and Refetoff, S.: Triiodothyronine stimulates specifically growth hormone mRNA in rat pituitary tumor cells. *Proc. Natl. Acad. Sci. (USA)*, 74:2054, 1977.

89. Seo, H., Refetoff, S., Martino, E., Vassart, G., and Brocas, H.: The differential stimulatory effect of thyroid hormone on growth hormone synthesis and estrogen on prolactin synthesis due to accumulation of specific messenger ribonucleic acid. *Endocrinology*, 104:1083, 1979.

90. Nogami, H., Yokose, T., and Tachibana, T.: Regulation of growth hormone expression in fetal rat pituitary gland by thyroid or glucocorticoid hormone. *Amer. J. Physiol. Endocrin. Metabol.*, 31(2):E262-E267, 1995.

91. Miki, N., Ono, M., Murata, Y., et al.: Thyroid hormone regulation of gene expression of the pituitary growth hormone-releasing factor receptor. *Biochem. Biophys. Res. Comm.*, 217(3):1087-1093, 1995.

92. Brameld, J.M., Weller, P.A., Saunders, J.C., Buttery, P.J., and Gilmour, R.S.: Hormonal control of insulin-like growth factor-1 and growth hormone receptor mRNA expression by porcine hepatocytes in culture. *J. Endocrinol.*, 146(2):239-245, 1995.

93. Martial, J.A., Baxter, J.D., and Goodman, H.M.: Regulation of growth hormone messenger RNA by thyroid and

glucocorticoid hormones. *Proc. Natl. Acad. Sci.*, 74:181-186, 1977.

94. Shapiro, L.E., Samuels, H.H., and Yaffe, B.M.: Thyroid and glucocorticoid hormones synergistically control growth hormone mRNA in cultured GH-1 cells. *Proc. Natl. Acad. Sci.*, 75:45, 1978.

95. Valcavi, R., Dieguez, C., Preece, M., Taylor, A., Portioli, I., and Scanlon, M.F.: Effect of thyroxine replacement therapy on plasma insulin-like growth hormone releasing factor in hypothyroid patients. *Clin. Endocrinol.*, 27:85, 1987.

96. Williams, T., Maxon, H., Thorner, M.O., and Frohman, L.A.: Blunted growth hormone (GH) response to GH-releasing hormone in hypothyroidism resolves in the euthyroid state. *J. Clin. Endocrinol. Metab.*, 61:454, 1985.

97. Snyder, P.J.: The pituitary in hypothyroidism. In *Werner and Ingbar's The Thyroid: A Fundamental and Clinical Text*, 6th edition. Edited by L.E. Braverman and R.D. Utiger, Philadelphia, J.B. Lippincott Co., 1991, pp.1040-1044.

98. Yaffe, B. and Samuels, H.H.: Hormonal regulation of the growth hormone gene: relationship of the rate of transcription to the level of nuclear thyroid hormone-receptor complexes. *J. Biol. Chem.*, 259:6284, 1984.

99. Vaerøy, H., Helle, R., Øystein, F., Kåss, E., and Terenius, L.: Elevated CSF levels of substance P and high incidence of Raynaud phenomenon in patients with fibromyalgia: new features for diagnosis. *Pain*, 32:21-26, 1988.

100. Mendelson, S.C. and Quinn, J.P.: Characterization of potential regulatory elements within the rat preprotachykinin-A promoter. *Neuroscience Letters*, 184(2):125-128, 1995.

101. Too, H.P., Marriott, D.R., and Wilkin, G.P.: Preprotachykinin-A and substance P receptor (NK1) gene expression in rat astrocytes in vitro. *Neuroscience Letters*, 182(2):185-187, 1994.

102. Jonassen, J.A., Mullikin-Kirkpatrick, D., McAdam, A., and Leeman, S.E.: Thyroid hormone status regulates preprotachykinin-A gene expression in male rat anterior pituitary. *Endocrinology*, 121:1555-1561, 1993.

103. Lam, K.S., Lechan, R.M., Minamitani, N., Segerson, T.P., and Reichlin, S.: Vasoactive intestinal peptide in the anterior pituitary is increased in hypothyroidism. *Endocrinology*, 124:1077-1084, 1989.

104. Jones, P.M., Ghatei, M.A., Wallis, S.C., and Bloom, S.R.: Differential response to neuropeptide Y, substance P, and vasoactive intestinal polypeptide in the rat anterior pituitary gland to alterations in thyroid hormone status. *J. Endocrinol.*, 143:393-397, 1994.

105. Neeck, G. and Riedel, W.: Thyroid function in patients with fibromyalgia syndrome. *J. Rheumatol.*, 19:1120-1122, 1992.

106. Beetham, W.P., Jr.: Diagnosis and management of fibrositis syndrome and psychogenic rheumatism. *Med. Clin. North Am.*, 63:433-439, 1979.

107. Golding, D.N.: Hypothyroidism presenting with musculoskeletal symptoms. *Ann. Rheumatic Dis.*, 29:10-14, 1970.

108. Bland, J.H. and Frymoyer, J.W.: Rheumatic syndromes

of myxedema. *New Eng. J. Med.*, 282:1171-1174, 1970.

109. Wilke, S.W., Sheeler, L.R., and Makarowski, W.S.: Hypothyroidism with presenting symptoms of fibrositis. *J. Rheumatol.*, 8:627-630, 1981.

110. Hochberg, M.C., Koppes, G.M., Edwards, C.Q., Barnes, H.V., and Arnett, F.C., Jr.: Hypothyroidism presenting as a polymyositis-like syndrome: report of two cases. *Arthritis Rheum.*, 19:1363-1366, 1976.

111. Delamere, J.P., Scott, D.L., and Felix-Davies, D.D.: Thyroid dysfunction and rheumatic diseases. *J. Royal Soc. Med.*, 75:102, 1982.

112. Fessel, W.J.: Myopathy of hypothyroidism. *Ann. Rheumatic Dis.*, 27:590-596, 1968.

113. Wilson, J. and Walton, J.N.: Some muscular manifestations of hypothyroidism. *J. Neurol. Neurosurg. Psychiat.*, 22:320-324, 1959.

114. Awad, E.A.: Pathological changes in fibromyalgia. First International Symposium on Myofascial Pain and Fibromyalgia, Minneapolis, May 9, 1989.

115. Sonkin, L.S.: Endocrine disorders and muscle dysfunction. In *Clinical Management of Head, Neck, and TMJ Pain and Dysfunction*. Edited by B. Gelb, Philadelphia, W.B. Saunders Co., 1985, pp.137-170.

116. Lowe, J.C.: A case of debilitating headache complicated by hypothyroidism: its relief through myofascial therapy. *Dig. Chiro. Econ.*, Nov/Dec:73-75, 1988.

117. Kravitz, H.M., Katz, R.S., Helmke, N., Jeffriess, H., Bukovsky, J., and Fawcett, J.: Alprazolam and ibuprofen in the treatment of fibromyalgia: report of a double-blind placebo-controlled study. *J. Musculoskel. Pain*, 2(1):3-27, 1994.

118. Jacobsen, S., Danneskiold-Samsøe, B., and Andersen, R.B.: Oral S-adenosylmethionine in primary fibromyalgia: double-blind clinical evaluation. *Scand. J. Rheum.*, 20:294-302, 1991.

119. Forslind, K., Fredriksson, E., and Nived, O.: Does primary fibromyalgia exist? *Brit. J. Rheumatol.*, 29:368-370, 1990.

120. Becker, K.I., Ferguson, R.H., and McConahey, W.M.: The connective-tissue diseases and symptoms associated with Hashimoto's thyroiditis. *New Eng. J. Med.*, 268(6):177-280, 1963.

121. Nørregaard, J., Harreby, M., Amris, K., Bangsbo, J., Bartels, E.M., and Danneskiold-Samsøe, B.: Single cell morphology and high-energy phosphate levels in quadriceps muscles from patients with fibromyalgia. *J. Musculoskel. Pain*, 2(2):45-51, 1994.

122. Shiroky, J.B., Cohen, M., Ballachey, M-L., and Neville, C.: Thyroid dysfunction in rheumatoid arthritis: a controlled prospective survey. *Ann. Rheumat. Dis.*, 52:454-456, 1993.

123. Lowe, J.C.: Thyroid status of 38 fibromyalgia patients: implications for the etiology of fibromyalgia. *Clin. Bull. Myofascial Ther.*, 2(1):47-64, 1996.

124. Ferraccioli, G., Cavalieri, F., Salaffi, F., et al.: Neuroendocrinologic findings in primary fibromyalgia (soft tissue chronic pain syndrome) and in other chronic rheumatic conditions (rheumatoid arthritis, low back pain). *J. Rheumat.*, 17:869-873, 1990.

125. Refetoff, S., Weiss, R.E., and Usala, S.J.: The syndromes of resistance to thyroid hormone. *Endoc. Rev.*, 14:348-

399, 1993.

126. Lowe, J.C.: Results of an open trial of T₃ therapy with 77 euthyroid female fibromyalgia patients. *Clin. Bull. Myofascial Ther.*, 2(1):35-37, 1996.

127. Lowe, J.C.: T₃-induced recovery from fibromyalgia by a hypothyroid patient resistant to T₄ and desiccated thyroid. *J. Myofascial Ther.*, 1(4):26-31, 1995.

128. Lowe, J.C., Garrison, R.L., Reichman, A.J., Yellin, J., Thompson, M., and Kaufman, D.: Effectiveness and safety of T₃ therapy for euthyroid fibromyalgia: a double-blind placebo-controlled response-driven crossover study. *Clin. Bull. Myofascial Ther.*, 2(2/3):31-57, 1996.

129. Lowe, J.C., Eichelberger, J., Manso, G., and Peterson, K.: Improvement in euthyroid fibromyalgia patients treated with T₃ (tri-iodothyronine). *J. Myofascial Ther.*, 1(2):16-29, 1994.

130. Lowe, J.C.: *The Metabolic Treatment of Fibromyalgia.* Tulsa, McDowell Publishing Co., 1999.

131. Weiss, R.E., Marcocci, C., Bruno-Bossio, G., and Refetoff, S.: Multiple genetic factors in the heterogeneity of thyroid hormone resistance. *J. Clin. Endocrinol. Metab.*, 76:257-259, 1993.

132. Refetoff, S.: Thyroid hormone resistance syndromes. In *Werner's The Thyroid: A Fundamental and Clinical Text*, 5th edition. Edited by S.H. Ingbar and L.E. Braverman, Philadelphia, J.B. Lippincott Co., 1986, pp.1292-1306.

133. Takeda, K., Sakurai, A., DeGroot, L.J., and Refetoff, S.: Recessive inheritance of thyroid hormone resistance caused by complete deletion of the protein-coding region of the thyroid hormone receptor-β gene. *J. Clin. Endocrinol. Metab.*, 74:49-55, 1992.

134. Krishna, V., Chatterjee, K., Nagaya, T., Madison, L.D., Datta, S., Rentoumis, A., and Jameson, J.L.: Thyroid hormone resistance syndrome: inhibition of normal receptor function by mutant thyroid hormone receptors. *J. Clin. Invest.*, 87:1977-1984, 1991.

135. Usala, S.J.: Personal communication with J.C. Lowe. Oct. 4, 1994.

136. Refetoff, S.: Thyroid hormone resistance syndromes. In *Werner's The Thyroid: A Fundamental and Clinical Text*, 6th edition. Edited by L.E. Braverman and R.D. Utiger, Philadelphia, J.B. Lippincott Co., 1991, pp.1280-1294.

137. Usala, S.J.: Personal communication with J.C. Lowe. Feb. 14, 1996.

138. Chatterjee, V.K.K., Nagaya, T., Madison, L.D., Datta, S., Rantoumis, A., and Jameson, J.L.: Thyroid hormone resistance syndrome: inhibition of normal receptor function by mutant thyroid hormone receptors. *J. Clin. Invest.*, 87:1977-1984, 1991.

139. Goswami, A. and Rosenberg, I.N.: Effects of thyroid status on membrane-bound low K_m cyclic nucleotide phosphodiesterase activity in rat adipocytes. *J. Biol. Chem.*, 260:82-85, 1985.

140. Milligan, G., Spiegel, A.M., Unson, C.G., and Saggerson, E.D.: Chemically induced hypothyroidism produces elevated amounts of the α subunit of the inhibitory guanine nucleotide binding protein (G₁) and the β subunit common to all G-proteins. *Biochem. J.*, 247:223-227, 1987.

141. Rapiejko, P.J., Watkins, D.C., Ros, M., and Malbon, C.C.: Thyroid hormones regulate G-protein β-subunit mRNA expression in vivo. *J. Biol. Chem.*, 264:16183-16189, 1989.

142. Ros, M., Northup, J.K., and Malbon, C.C.: Steady-state levels of G-proteins and β-adrenergic receptors in rat fat cells. *J. Biol. Chem.*, 263:4362-4368, 1988.

143. Usala, S.J., Tennyson, G.E., Bale, A.E., et al.: A base mutation of the c-erbAβ thyroid hormone receptor in a kindred with generalized thyroid hormone resistance: molecular heterogeneity in two other kindreds. *J. Clin. Invest.*, 85:93-100, 1990.

144. Sakurai, A., Takeda, K., Ain, K., et al.: Generalized resistance to thyroid hormone associated with a mutation in the ligand-binding domain of the human thyroid hormone receptor β. *Proc. Natl. Acad. Sci. (USA)*, 86:8977-8981, 1989.

145. Kaplan, M.M., Swartz, S.L., and Larsen, P.R.: Partial peripheral resistance to thyroid hormone. *Am. J. Med.*, 70:1115-1121, 1981.

146. Gershengorn, M.C. and Weintraub, B.D.: Thyrotropin-induced hyperthyroidism caused by selective pituitary resistance to thyroid hormone: a new syndrome of "inappropriate secretion of TSH." *J. Clin. Invest.*, 56:633-642, 1975.

147. Bantle, J.P., Seeling, S., Mariash, C.N., Ulstrom, R.A., and Oppenheimer, J.H.: Resistance to thyroid hormones: a disorder frequently confused with Graves disease. *Arch. Intern. Med.*, 142:1867-1871, 1982.

148. Refetoff, S.: Personal communication with J.C. Lowe. April 27, 1992.

149. Linde, R., Alexander, N., Island, D.P., and Rabin, D.: Familial insensitivity of the pituitary and periphery to thyroid hormone: a case report in two and a review of the literature. *Metabolism*, 31(5):510-513, 1982.

150. Novogroder, M., Utiger, R., and Boyar, R.: Juvenile hyperthyroidism with elevated thyrotropin (TSH) and normal 24 hour FSH, LH, GH, and prolactin secretory patterns. *J. Clin. Endocrinol. Metab.*, 45:1053-1059, 1977.

151. Elewaut, A., Mussche, M., and Vermeulen, A.: Familial partial target organ resistance to thyroid hormones. *J. Clin. Endocrinol. Metab.*, 43:575-581, 1976.

152. De Visscher, M.: The therapy of hypothyroid states. In *Recent Progress in Diagnosis and Treatment of Hypothyroid Conditions.* Edited by P.A. Bastenie, M. Bonnyns, L. Vanhaelst, Amsterdam, Excerpta Medica, 1980, pp.105-114.

153. Hodin, R.A., Lazar, M.A., and Chin, W.W.: Differential and tissue-specific regulation of the multiple rat c-erbA messenger RNA species by thyroid hormone. *J. Clin. Invest.*, 85:101-105, 1990.

154. Sakurai, A., Nakai, A., and DeGroot, L.J.: Expression of three forms of thyroid hormone receptor in human tissues. *Mol. Endocrinol.*, 3:392-399, 1989.

155. Refetoff, S., DeGroot, L.J., Benard, B., and DeWind, L.T.: Studies of a sibship with apparent hereditary resistance to the intracellular action of thyroid hormone. *Metabolism*, 21:723-756, 1972.

156. Bilezikian, J.P. and Loeb, J.N.: The influence of hyperthyroidism and hypothyroidism on α- and β-adrenergic receptor systems and adrenergic responsiveness. *Endoc. Rev.*, 4:378-388, 1983.

Effectiveness and Safety of T₃ (Triiodothyronine) Therapy for Euthyroid Fibromyalgia: A Double-Blind Placebo-Controlled Response-Driven Crossover Study

John C. Lowe, M.A., D.C.
Richard L. Garrison, M.D.
Alan J. Reichman, M.D.
Jackie Yellin, B.A.
Mervianna Thompson, R.N., M.S.N., A.P.N.
Daniel Kaufman, M.D.

This article originally appeared in the *Clinical Bulletin of Myofascial Therapy*, 2(2/3):31-57, 1997.
It is reprinted with permission of Haworth Medical Press.

ABSTRACT. *Background.* Clinical features of fibromyalgia syndrome (FMS) resemble those of hypothyroidism although some patients have normal thyroid function tests results. The hypothyroid-like FMS features of these patients may result from partial cellular resistance to thyroid hormone. We treated euthyroid FMS patients with T₃ to see if they would respond as do patients with peripheral thyroid hormone resistance syndrome: significant therapeutic effects with supraphysiologic dosages, without target tissue responses typical of thyrotoxicosis.

Methods. Seven patients were alternately treated with T₃ and placebo over an 8-month period. Phase crossover was response-driven, based on changes in measures of mean tender point sensitivity by algometry, mean symptom intensity by visual analog scales, and mean pain distribution by the percentage method and the ACR criteria. Testing for adverse responses to supraphysiologic dosages of T₃ was performed for heart, bone, muscle, and liver.

Results. Significant therapeutic effects were shown in T₃ phases compared to placebo phases on all measures of FMS status. Effective T₃ dosages were supraphysiologic, and ranged from 93.75-to-150 mcg. Available patients had maintained improvement at 2-month follow-up. Tests showed no clinically significant cardiac, osseous, muscle, or hepatic adverse effects.

Conclusions. In this study, supraphysiologic dosages of T₃ were safe and significantly effective in the treatment of euthyroid FMS. Though these dosages produced thyroid function test results indicative of hyperthyroidism, our patients had no clinically significant adverse target tissue effects. Results suggest that euthyroid FMS is a clinical phenotype of partial peripheral resistance to thyroid hormone. We recommend that further studies be done to answer the questions: Are euthyroid FMS patients partially resistant to thyroid hormone? And if so, what are the molecular mechanisms of the resistance? Further testing is also necessary to establish the long-term safety of T₃ therapy.

KEY WORDS. Fibromyalgia, hypothyroidism, euthyroid, thyroid hormone resistance, T₃

INTRODUCTION

Fibromyalgia syndrome (FMS) is the most common condition of chronic widespread musculoskeletal pain with a poor prognosis, and is accompanied by chronic stiffness and fatigue.[1][2] The incidence in the U.S. is 2%, with 90% female.[3] Symptoms and objective findings of FMS are so similar to those of hypothyroidism that numerous authors have noted the resemblances.[4][5][6][7][8][9][10][11][12][13][14] However, not all FMS patients are hypothyroid. Lowe found that of 38 consecutive FMS patients, 10.5% had primary hypothyroidism.[15] This is close to the 12% found by Shiroky,[16] and the 10% found by Eisinger[17] and Gerwin.[18] Thyroid function test results consistent with central hypothyroidism in FMS have been reported by three research groups.[15][19][20] Lowe reported this test result in 52.6% of 38 consecutive, unselected FMS patients.[15]

Lowe also found that 36.8% of his FMS patients were euthyroid.[15] The euthyroid status of some FMS patients led two committees to the implicit conclusion that hypothyroidism is only a concurrent condition in some FMS patients with no etiologic relation to FMS.[1][2] Lowe and colleagues have proposed, however, that the hypothyroid-like features of euthyroid FMS patients may result from the same fundamental mechanism as in hypothyroidism: inadequate thyroid hormone regulation of gene transcription.[21] In hypothyroid FMS, inadequate regulation of transcription may result from a frank thyroid hormone deficiency. In euthyroid FMS, inadequate regulation may result from low affinity mutant thyroid hormone receptors diminishing the transcriptional regulatory effects of normal circulating levels of thyroid hormone.[21] All symptoms and objective findings in FMS may be explained by increases in three molecular by-products of inadequate regulation of gene transcription by thyroid hormone: phosphodiesterase, inhibitory G proteins, and α-adrenoceptors.[21] If tissue hyposensitivity to thyroid hormone were confirmed, euthyroid FMS would properly be classified as a syndrome of partial resistance to thyroid hormone.

The results of two open systematic trials using T_3 therapy for euthyroid FMS support this view.[22][23] Patients in these studies resembled patients with documented thyroid hormone resistance syndrome in four ways: 1) they had hypothyroid-like symptoms despite normal thyroid function test results, 2) effective doses of T_3 were supraphysiologic, 3) in most cases, these dosages did not induce thyrotoxicosis, and 4) in some patients, supraphysiologic dosages high enough to relieve features of FMS also induced indications of mild hypermetabolism of some tissues but not others, indicating a differential responsiveness of target tissues to T_3 and requiring a compromise dosage that sustained benefits but avoided tissue catabolism. Our purpose in this study was to determine: 1) whether the status of euthyroid FMS patients significantly improved with T_3 compared to placebo, 2) if so, whether physiologic or supraphysiologic dosages were necessary for improvement, and 3) if supraphysiologic dosages of T_3 were required, whether peripheral target tissues were adversely affected.

METHODS

Patients

The institutional review board of the Fibromyalgia Research Foundation approved the protocol, and written informed consent was obtained from all patients before the study. Each patient acknowledged her understanding of the effects of overstimulation by thyroid hormone explained in the document. The twelve female patients who began the study ranged in age from 33-to-60. They had responded to a newspaper advertisement soliciting study participants. Repondents who met the entry criteria were sequentially enrolled in the study. Each patient met the 1990 American College of Rheumatology (ACR) criteria for FMS[1]: widespread pain for at least three months and 11 of 18 possible tender points. To more objectively quantify tender point sensitivity, we measured 16 of the 18 tender points with an algometer (a calibrated force gauge) and entered a patient in the study only if the mean pressure/tenderness threshold of her tender points was below 3 kg/cm² (normal is arbitrarily considered to be 4 kg/cm²).[1] All patients were classified as euthyroid on the basis of normal thyroid function test results (third generation basal TSH assay, T_4, T_3 uptake, and FTI). None had previously been treated with thyroid hormone. Patients had no other health conditions that resembled or overlapped with the features of FMS. According to the protocol described by Lowe and colleagues,[4][22][23] patients were permitted to continue medications they were taking to control their FMS symptoms until our measures indicated improvement in FMS status. Then, they were to stop all medications other than T_3. Patients agreed to engage in exercise to tolerance and to take nutritional supplements (especially B vitamins) daily through all phases of the study. Clinical experience has suggested that nutrition supplements augment the therapeutic effects of T_3 in euthyroid FMS patients.[23] Of the twelve patients who began the study, five were lost through protocol violations and subsequent dismissal from the study (see Results section). Seven patients completed the study.

Study Design

This study was a double-blind placebo-controlled response-driven crossover investigation. Identical sets of color-coded capsules were prepared. One set contained various amounts of T_3, the other, lactose as a placebo. All patients and all investigators were unaware of capsule content during all phases. The crossover design was used to show reproducibility of results from phase-to-phase. The response-driven feature enabled marked improvement in FMS status to trigger crossover to an alternate phase. It also served the humanitarian purpose of terminating with a crossover, a phase during which FMS status severely worsened.

Instruments

We used five measures to assess change in FMS status: algometer measurements of tender points, pain distribution drawings, symptom intensity surveys using visual analog scales (VASs), the Fibromyalgia Impact Questionnaire (FIQ), and Zung's Self-Rating Depression Scale (Zung's).

Bennett wrote in 1994,[24] "Criteria for poorly defined diseases are not set in stone and it is already apparent that the 1990 ACR criteria [for diagnosing and assessing FMS] will need to be revised." Littlejohn agreed.[25] In line with the effort to improve FMS assessment, we modified three of the five standard assessment methods. The modifications enabled greater precision at quantifying changes in patient status.

Modification 1: Algometry to Assess Tender Point Sensitivity. Tender point assessment according to the ACR entails applying 4 kg of pressure with a finger to 18 predictable tender point sites. The patient meets the tender point criterion if he or she reports tenderness upon pressure at 11 or more of the 18 tender points.[1] Recently, however, Fisher demonstrated that experienced clinicians were not able to subjectively gauge 4 kg of pressure when not observing a meter. He concluded that reliable FMS diagnosis requires quantification of pressure by algometry.[26] The algometer reliably measures the sensitivity of FMS tender points,[27][28] and its measurements correlate well with pain distribution reported by patients on body drawings.[29] In this study, we quantified tender point sensitivity with algometry at every assessment—the higher the pressure/tenderness threshold, the lower the sensitivity.

Modification 2: Pain Distribution. The ACR diagnostic criteria for FMS include widespread pain, defined as 1) above and below the waist, 2) on the right and left sides of the body, and 3) over an axial area such as the anterior chest or spine. This definition permits a pain distribution score of one-to-four units (0-1-2-3). We assessed changes according to this method, but we also used an alternate method adapted from the "rule of nines" for adult burn victims which describes the percentage of body surface burned.[30][31] The modified rule of nines method for assessing pain distribution has not been previously reported in FMS research. We tested for correlation between changes in widespread pain measured by the ACR method and this percentage method.

Modification 3: Extended Symptom Intensity Scales. We extended the number of 100 mm visual analog scales (VASs) from the usual 1-to-4 to include the 13 most common associated FMS symptoms.[1][32][33] Assessment of symptom intensities, especially pain, using VASs is customarily employed in FMS studies.[34][35][36][37] Scott and Huskisson report

that VASs are the best available procedure for measuring pain.[38] The 13 symptoms we included were pain, fatigue, stiffness, headache, sleep disturbance, bowel disturbance, depression, cognitive dysfunction (poor memory and concentration), anxiety, coldness, paresthesias (numbness and tingling), Sicca symptoms, and difficulty exercising.

We used two other standard methods of FMS assessment: the Fibromyalgia Impact Questionnaire and Zung's Self-Rating Depression Scale.[39] The FIQ is a brief, self-administered instrument with demonstrated validity and reliability, and it is widely used for assessing the impact FMS has on a patient's daily life.[40] It measures physical function, work status, depression, anxiety, sleep, pain, stiffness, fatigue, and well-being. Zung's is an easily self-administered, well-validated measure with acceptable sensitivity and specificity.[41] It correlates significantly with other measures of depression, including the Beck Depression Inventory.[42]

Procedure

Patients were randomly assigned by number and off-site to either an initial placebo or initial T₃ phase. Matching was not necessary because each patient served in alternate phases as her own control. Baseline testing for all patients included algometry, pain distribution, VASs, FIQ, Zung's, and ECG.

Patients were evaluated at one-to-two week intervals with a brief examination (pulse rate, blood pressure, and Achilles reflex), an interview, and an FMS assessment. Three sets of FMS measurements were taken repeatedly throughout all study phases: 1) a tender point examination by one of the investigators (quantified by algometer measurements as the mean of 16 tender points), 2) a pain drawing of the patient's pain distribution since the previous examination (quantified as a percentage of 36 body divisions containing pain), and 3) completion of visual analog scales (VASs) for symptom intensities of the 13 most common symptoms (see above) associated with fibromyalgia (quantified as a mean score from all 13).

After each reevaluation, the mean tender point score, the pain distribution expressed as a percentage, and the mean symptom intensity were applied as data points (for that evaluation date) to graphs for each measure. Successive data points in each graph showed the trend of each measure during each phase. At each evaluation, the examining clinician used the graphs (with data from the current evaluation and previous ones in the same phase) and his global assessment (see below) of the patient to judge when it was appropriate to alter the patient's T₃ dosage or to cross her to the next phase.

At each evaluation, the examining clinician made a global assessment of the patient's status. This assessment considered several factors: 1) results of the physical exam, particularly the resting pulse rate and Achilles reflex, 2) the patient's answers to questions about her status since the last evaluation, and 3) the clinician's impression of the patient's status based on her appearance and attitude. The clinician's judgment as to whether the patient's dosage should be altered was based on consideration of his global assessment of her status, and the trend of her data points in the line graphs for FMS measures in the current phase of the study. Thus, decisions regarding dosage adjustments were clinical judgments. The judgments were based partly on the outcome of the objective FMS measures, partly on signs observable by the clinician, and partly on the patient's subjective report. Depending on the outcome of the evaluation, a patient's daily dosage was kept the same or altered.

If a patient's fibromyalgia status deteriorated according to the examining clinician's judgment, the patient's dosage was increased by 6.25, 12.5, or 25 mcg. If a patient's fibromyalgia status stayed the same or slightly improved, but her ECGs showed no evidence of overstimulation and there was no other clinical evidence of thyrotoxicosis, then her dosage was increased. In any phase, if there were signs of overstimulation, a patient's dosage was backed down by 6.25 mcg decrements until all signs of overstimulation were gone. Serial ECGs were performed on all patients throughout the study to assure awareness at any point of cardiac thyrotoxicosis. (No instance was ever found in this study.)

If a patient reached a dosage of 175 mcg without further improvement through at least two evaluations, the patient was crossed to the next phase and given alternate number-coded capsules. When in the judgment of the examining clinician, a patient's improvement had plateaued, she too was crossed to the next phase.

At the end of each phase, the mean tender point sensitivity, mean symptom intensity, and pain distribution expressed as a percentage were taken along with three other measures: pain distribution according to the ACR method,[1] the Fibromyalgia Impact Questionnaire (FIQ),[40] and Zung's Self-Rating Depression Scale (Zung's).[41] The FIQ is a brief, self-administered instrument with demonstrated validity and reliability, and it is widely used for assessing the impact FMS has on a patient's daily life.[40] It lists ten common daily

activities that patients rate according to their ability to perform, and ten VASs for FMS symptoms that patients mark to indicate severity. The range of possible scores is 0-to-80. Zung's is an easily self-administered, well-validated measure with acceptable sensitivity and specificity.[41] It contains twenty questions about activities or symptoms that indicate depression, and patients rate each according to its presence and severity. The range of raw scores is 20-to-80. The raw score is converted to one of four clinical categories, ranging from "none" to "severe" depression. The FIQ and Zung's forms from this study were number-coded and independently scored off-site.

Treatment

Daily during all phases, patients took combinations of capsules of four different colors. Each color represented a different dose, either 6.25, 12.5, 25.0, or 75 mcg. The lactose capsules patients took during placebo phases were identical in appearance to the T₃ capsules taken in treatment phases. Patients and investigators were instructed to assume that all number-coded bottles in every phase contained T₃.

All patients were educated before the study began about the effects and indications of overstimulation from thyroid hormone. At every assessment, any symptoms or signs of overstimulation were evaluated by investigators. Propranolol (20 mg tablets) was issued to every patient at the beginning of the study because of its usefulness in reversing tachyarrhythmias to normal sinus rhythm.[43] It was to be taken only if a patient felt some threat from overstimulation by the capsules, and upon consultation with one of the investigators. All patients and all investigators were unaware of any patient's actual capsule content during all phases, as the bottles were prepared and coded off-site using patient numbers rather than names.

At the time of any crossover, a patient received a new set of four number-coded bottles prepared off-site (with no knowledge of the outcome of exams or of any patient's individual status or code number). The patient turned in the bottles with the remaining capsules for the phase just completed and picked up bottles for the phase she was about to enter. In any new phase, a patient began by taking 75 mcg (presumed in every phase to be T₃), despite the dosage she had been taking when her previous phase ended.

Safety Testing

After the study was concluded, all patients continued to use supraphysiologic doses of T₃ daily, and at the end of two months, safety testing was performed.

Tests of possible adverse effects of supraphysiologic doses of T$_3$ included serial ECGs throughout all study phases (prior to most dosage increases) and at 2-month follow-up. Urinary N-telopeptides, creatinine, calcium, and phosphorus; serum creatinine, calcium, phosphorus, and alkaline phosphatase; and bone densitometry of the lumbar spine, Ward's triangle, femoral neck, and trochanter with either CT scans or dual photon absorptiometry were evaluated at 2-month follow-up.

Statistics

Statistical analysis was performed using the Statistical Package for the Social Sciences (SPSS, Chicago). Paired-samples *t*-tests were used to test for significant differences between scores in placebo and T$_3$ phases. The Pearson correlation coefficient was used to test for correlations between ACR and percentage methods for assessing pain and between Zung's and VAS scores for depression.

Table 1. Measures of Fibromyalgia Status

Measure	Worst Possible	Best Possible	Placebo Mean	T$_3$ Mean	Outcome	Significance Level
Mean Tender Point Sensitivity[1]	< 1 kg/cm^2	> 4 kg/cm^2	1.98 kg/cm^2	3.07 kg/cm^2	Improved	P < 0.0005
Pain Distribution[2] (ACR Method)	3	0	2.75	1.83	Improved	P = 0.05
Pain Distribution[2] (% Method)	100%	0%	43.49%	21.04%	Improved	P = 0.015
Mean Symptom Intensity[3]	10	0	5.42	2.30	Improved	P < 0.0005
Fibromyalgia Impact Questionnaire	80	0	50.21	21.15	Improved	P = 0.003
Zung's Self-Rated Depression Scale[4]	80	20	54.83	46.50	Improved	P = 0.022

1. Pressure/pain thresholds assessed with algometry.
2. There was a positive correlation between the two methods during placebo phases (*r*=0.601; P=0.039) and during T$_3$ phases (*r*=0.699; P=0.011).
3. Mean of 13 common fibromyalgia symptoms (0-to-10 point visual analog scale).
4. Zung's scores in placebo phases were positively correlated with scores on the VAS for depression, but did not reach significance (*r*=0.54, P=0.073). Zung's scores in T$_3$ phases were also positively correlated with scores on the VAS for depression and were significant (*r*=0.80, P=0.002).

RESULTS

Twelve patients began the 8-month study. Seven completed it. Of those seven, five patients completed two placebo and two T$_3$ phases, and two patients completed one placebo and one T$_3$ phase. The high significance levels on most FMS measures despite the small number of patients indicates T$_3$'s strong therapeutic impact on euthyroid FMS status.[76,pp.257-258] Effective dosages of T$_3$ for the seven patients were

93.75, 112.50, 112.50, 125.00, 131.25, 137.50, and 150.00 mcg. The confidence factor was figured at 95% and 99%, with no difference in results. Group measurement results appear in Table 1.

Five patients were lost through protocol violations and subsequent dismissal from the study. Two of the five patients informed investigators late in the study that they had not been taking the required nutritional supplements throughout the study period. Since this study was a test of a full treatment regimen, the necessity for all subjects to be taking supplements required the dismissal of those who did not. One patient had to drop out because of the probable heart rate accelerating effect of the combination of her cyclobenzaprine and amitriptyline with the first set of study capsules. The high resting heart rate she had since she began taking tricyclic drugs accelerated more after she began taking study capsules (presumably containing T_3). She declined to stop the tricyclics because of previous experience with rebound sleep disturbance upon discontinuing them, and thus was dismissed from the study. The last two patients were simply unable to continue to come for the frequent reevaluations required.

Table 2. Changes in Fibromyalgia Symptoms (VASs)

Symptoms	Outcome	Significance Levels
Pain	Improved	P = 0.002
Fatigue	Improved	P = 0.001
Stiffness	Improved	P = 0.002
Headache	Improved	P = 0.006
Sleep Disturbance	Improved	P = 0.001
Bowel Disturbance	Improved	P = 0.006
Depression	Improved	P = 0.004
Cognitive Dysfunction	Improved	P = 0.001
Anxiety	Improved	P = 0.004
Coldness	Improved	P = 0.011
Paresthesia	Improved	P = 0.006
Sicca Symptoms	Improved	P = 0.043
Difficulty Exercising	Improved	P < 0.0005

Algometer Measurements of Tender Points

Tender point sensitivity assessed by algometry was significantly greater in placebo phases than in T_3 phases. The difference was highly significant ($P<0.0005$). The mean algometer score for placebo phases was 1.98 kg/cm² (the lower the score, the higher the sensitivity). The mean for T_3 phases was 3.07 kg/cm².

Pain Distribution

Patients' pain distribution was markedly higher during placebo phases and lower in T_3 phases. Using the ACR method for assessing pain distribution, the mean distribution for placebo phases was 2.75 and for T_3 phases was 1.83. Using the percentage method, the mean for placebo phases was 43.49%, and for T_3 phases was 21.04%.

The difference between phases using the ACR method was significant ($P=0.05$). The difference using the percentage method, however, was more significant ($P=0.015$). This difference in significance levels indicates that the percentage method is a more sensitive measure of pain distribution. There was a high level of positive correlation between the two methods during placebo phases ($r=0.601$; $P=0.039$) and during T_3 phases ($r=0.699$; $P=0.011$).

Symptom Intensities

Mean symptom intensity was significantly lower during T_3 phases and higher during placebo phases. The difference was significant ($P<0.0005$). These symptoms are listed in Table 2 with the levels of significant difference between placebo and T_3 phases. The mean placebo score was 5.42. The mean T_3 score was 2.30.

Fibromyalgia Impact Questionnaire

The range of possible scores on the FIQ is 0-to-80. Scores were higher (worse) in placebo phases and lower (better) in T_3 phases. The mean placebo score was 50.21 and the mean T_3 score was 21.15. The difference is significant ($P= 0.003$).

Zung's Depression Inventory

Results on the Zung's were significantly different in placebo and T_3 phases ($P= 0.022$). This result reflected decreased depression during T_3 phases reported by patients on the VAS. The mean placebo score was 54.83, and the mean T_3 score was 46.50. Zung's scores in placebo phases were positively correlated with placebo scores on the VAS for depression, but did not reach significance ($r=0.54$, $P=0.073$). Zung's scores in

T_3 phases were also positively correlated with T_3 scores on the VAS for depression and reached significance (r=0.80, P=0.002).

Measures of Peripheral Tissue Status (Table 3)
Weight

Patients' weights remained stable (mean placebo weight: 133.32 lbs; mean T_3 weight: 131.95 lbs) with no significant difference between phases (P=0.233).

Cardiac Effects

ECGs and Heart Rate. Mean heart rate significantly increased from 67.88 bpm in placebo phases to 83.96 bpm in T_3 phases (P=0.003). The range of pulse rates in placebo phases was 42-to-92 bpm, and in T_3 phases was 72-to-96 bpm. No patient developed tachycardia. PR intervals shortened in T_3 phases, but the difference was not significant (P= 0.121). QRS intervals lengthened in T_3 phases, but the difference was not significant (P= 0.166). QT intervals significantly shortened during T_3 phases (P= 0.010). The mean QT interval in placebo phases was 0.40, and in T_3 phases was 0.36. All QT intervals were within the normal limits of 0.30-0.46. All ST segments were within normal limits in all phases.

Table 3. Measures of Peripheral Tissue Status

Measure	Placebo Mean	T₃ Mean	Outcome	Significance Level
Weight	133.32 lbs	131.95 lbs	No change	P = 0.233
Heart rate	67.88 bpm	83.96 bpm	Increased (but stayed within normal range)	P = 0.003
PR interval	0.15	0.14	No change	P = 0.121
QRS interval	0.043	0.05	No change	P = 0.166
QT interval	0.40	0.36	Shortened (but stayed within normal range)	P = 0.01
ST segment	N/A	N/A	No change	N/A
Systolic pressure	117.25	115.92	No change	P = 0.684
Diastolic pressure	77.50	74.25	No change	P = 0.416

During a placebo phase eight days after crossover from the previous T_3 phase, one patient had a non-specific ST-T wave change with a prolonged QT interval. The values, however, were within normal limits. Her pulse rate at this time had decreased from 83 during the previous phase to 62.

Blood Pressure. There was no significant difference in systolic pressures between T_3 and placebo phases (P= 0.684). The range of systolic pressures in placebo phases was 108-to-138, and the mean was 117.25. The range of systolic pressures in T_3 phases was 100-to-130, and the mean was 115.92. There was also no significant difference in diastolic pressure between phases (P = 0.416). The range of diastolic pressures in the placebo phases was 64-to-98, and the mean was 77.50. The range in T_3 phases was 60-to-90, and the mean was 74.25.

Follow-Up Testing (Table 4)
Thyroid Function Tests

Baseline TSH, T_4, T_3 uptake, and FTI were within the normal range for all patients. At 2-month follow-up, these values as well as the free T_4 and free T_3 were in the range typically associated with thyrotoxicity due to excessive exogenous T$_3$ intake. Low values included a mean TSH concentration of 0.05±0.04 µU per milliliter, a mean total T$_4$ of 3.05±0.66 µg per deciliter, a mean FTI of 0.78±0.15, and a mean free T$_4$ of 0.46±0.08 ng per deciliter. The mean T$_3$ uptake of 25.25% was within the normal range. The mean free T$_3$ of 8.05±3.77 pg per milliliter was high.

Muscle Effect

At 2-month follow-up, mean urinary creatinine was slightly low (980.50±50.56 mg per 24 hours), indicating mild reduction in muscle mass. Serum creatinine was normal (0.8±0.115 mg per deciliter).

Osseous Effects

At follow-up, mean urinary calcium (255.70±71.46 mg per 24-hours) and phosphorus (913.00±289.60 mg per 24-hours) were normal. Mean urinary N-telopeptides was high (165±33.72 nMole of bone collagen equivalents per µMole of creatinine), indicating increased bone turnover. Mean serum phosphorus (4.03±0.78 mg per deciliter) and alkaline phosphatase (55.75±16.92 IU per liter) were normal. Compared to reference standards, bone densitometry showed normal bone density. Density of the trochanter was 99±6.08% of age matched controls, the femoral neck was 98.67±5.13%, Ward's triangle was 101.33±10.50%, and the lumbar spine was 101.13±7.43%.

Liver Function Tests

Significant elevations in serum alanine aminotransferase (ALT) and γ-glutamyl transpeptidase (GGPT) have been reported in subclinical hyperthyroidism.[44] At follow-up, our patients had normal values for mean ALT (25.50±13.40 U per liter) and GGPT (13.25±9.25 U per liter). Other liver function test results were also within normal limits, including mean aspartate aminotransferase (26.75±10.24 U per liter), total bilirubin (0.73±0.22 mg per deciliter), alkaline phosphatase (55.75±16.92 IU per liter), A/G ratio (1.43±0.15), globulin (2.93±0.33 g per deciliter), albumin (4.13±0.35 g per deciliter), total protein (7.05±0.58 g per deciliter), and LDH (157.25±30.70 U per liter).

DISCUSSION

During T$_3$ phases compared to placebo phases, patients showed significant improvement according to five measures of FMS status. These measures were tender point sensitivity (quantified by algometry), pain distribution (quantified by both the ACR method and a modified "rule of nines" percentage method), symptom intensity (quantified by 13 VASs), the Fibromyalgia Impact Questionnaire, and Zung's Self-Rating Depression Scale. Improvement had been maintained in the four patients available for a 2-month follow-up evaluation. Patients' improved status in T$_3$ phases was associated with their use of T$_3$ dosages that were clearly supraphysiologic. These dosages, however, caused no clinically significant adverse peripheral target tissue effects. Results imply that in our euthyroid patients, FMS features were the clinical manifestation of partial peripheral resistance to thyroid hormone (with consequent inadequate thyroid hormone regulation of gene transcription), and that supraphysiologic dosages of T$_3$ exerted therapeutic effects by overriding that resistance. These results support the hypothesis that euthyroid FMS is a clinical phenotype of partial peripheral resistance to thyroid hormone.[21]

Ross has written that adverse effects of subclinical hyperthyroidism (low TSH with normal thyroid hormone levels) include cardiac abnormalities and reduced bone density in premenopausal women.[45] To avoid adverse effects, he recommends that patients' TSH levels should be within the normal range. In our euthyroid FMS patients, however, low serum TSH levels were not associated with thyrotoxicity. At follow-up, our patients had TSH levels lower than normal, but cardiac monitoring and follow-up biochemical and densitometry testing showed no clinically significant adverse effects. Thyroid hormone surplus in non-thyroid hormone resistant individuals is associated with excessive protein catabolism, tissue wasting, and weight loss.[44,46] Our patients' weights did not differ between T$_3$ and placebo phases, indicating absence of catabolism despite use of supraphysiologic dosages of T$_3$.

The cardiovascular system is sensitive not only to overt hyperthyroidism,[47] but also to small increases in thyroid hormone levels within the normal range that suppress TSH levels.[45] Even subclinical hyperthyroidism may aggravate angina pectoris or congestive heart failure.[45] In conditions of thyroid hormone overstimulation such as T$_3$-thyrotoxicosis, cardiac abnormalities may include atrial fibrillation, premature ventricular beats, paroxysmal supraventricular tachycardia, atrial flutter, and congestive heart failure.[43] In thyrotoxicosis, there are no specific identifiable electrocardiographic changes.[47] Nonspecific changes may include elevated ST segments, shortened QT intervals,[48] prolongation of PR intervals, Wolf-Parkinson-White syndrome, and complete right bundle-branch

Table 4. Follow-Up Testing

Measure	Outcome	Mean & Standard Deviation
TSH	Suppressed	0.05±0.04 µU/mL
Total T_4	Low	3.05±0.66 µg/dL
FTI	Low	0.78±0.15
Free T_4	Low	0.46±0.08 ng/dL
T_3 uptake	Normal	25.25±3.1%
Free T_3	High	8.05±3.77 pg/mL
Urinary calcium	Normal	255.70±71.46 mg/24-hours
Urinary phosphorus	Normal	913.00±289.60 mg/24-hours
Urinary N-telopeptides	Elevated	165±33.72 nMole bone collagen equivalents/µMole creatinine
Urinary creatinine	Slightly low	980.50±50.56 mg/24-hours
Serum creatinine	Normal	0.8±0.115 mg per deciliter
Serum alkaline phosphatase	Normal	55.75±16.92 IU/L
Serum phosphorus	Normal	4.03±0.78 mg/dL
Densitometry of trochanter	Normal	99.00±6.08% of age matched controls
Densitometry of femoral neck	Normal	98.67±5.13% of age matched controls
Densitometry of Ward's triangle	Normal	101.33±10.50% of age matched controls
Densitometry of lumbar spine	Normal	101.13±7.43% of age matched controls
Alanine aminotransferase	Normal	25.50±13.40 U/L
γ-Glutamyl transpeptidase	Normal	13.25±9.25 U/L
Aspartate aminotransferase	Normal	26.75±10.24 U/L
Total bilirubin	Normal	0.73±0.22 mg/dL
Alkaline phosphatase	Normal	55.75±16.92 IU/L
A/G ratio	Normal	1.43±0.15
Globulin	Normal	2.93±0.33 g/dL
Albumin	Normal	4.13±0.35 g/dL
Total protein	Normal	7.05±0.58 g/dL
LDH	Normal	157.25±30.70 U/L

block.[49] Half of thyrotoxic patients have sinus tachycardia. One tenth of hyperthyroid patients have persistent atrial fibrillation.[50][51] None of the seven patients who completed the study had any detectable adverse cardiac effects from exogenous dosages of T_3. All ECGs were normal throughout the 8-month study and at 2-month follow-up. This finding suggests partial resistance of cardiac regulatory mechanisms to thyroid hormone.

Reports that slightly TSH-suppressive doses of thyroid hormone significantly reduce bone density[52][53][54][55][56][57][58] are contradicted by other studies.[59][60][61][62][63][64] Nonetheless, possible reduction of bone density remained a concern with the supraphysiologic T_3 dosages our patients used (ranging from 93.75-to-150.00 mcg). The higher end dosages would be expected to induce bone resorption in individuals whose tissues are normally responsive to thyroid hormone. Histomorphometric studies indicate that replacement dosages of thyroid hormone result in osteoclastosis of trabecular and cortical bone within the first month of treatment, with decreased bone mass.[53][58] But with our available patients at 2-month follow-up, bone densitometry of the lumbar vertebrae, femoral neck, Ward's triangle, and trochanter with CT scan in one patient and dual photon absorptiometry in three others showed normal bone density. The increase in urinary N-telopeptides, therefore, was not associated with low bone density in our patients (see next paragraph). This finding suggests partial osseous resistance to thyroid hormone.

At 2-month follow-up, testing showed abnormal values for some biochemical markers. The slightly low urinary creatinine suggests reduced muscle mass, and the increased cross-linked N-telopeptides shows increased bone turnover. However, the patients' unchanged weight and normal bone density support the view that such abnormal biochemical markers may be clinically insignificant.[65] Other researchers have also found normal bone density despite abnormal biochemical markers.[66] De Rosa reported that while TSH-suppressive dosages of thyroid hormone can activate bone turnover, they constitute neither an actual risk factor for bone loss nor for osteoporotic fractures.[63] The cumulative evidence supports this conclusion, at least for premenopausal women.[67] Tremollieres and colleagues reported that positive biochemical markers for bone turnover and reduced bone density found during the first year of exogenous thyroid hormone use were followed by a complete recovery of normal values during the second year.[68] They proposed that "transitory" bone loss might result

from temporary "hypersensitivity" of hypothyroid bone to thyroid hormone. The same may be true of peripheral tissues previously hypometabolic due to partial resistance to thyroid hormone. Long-term follow-up, however, is warranted for patients taking TSH-suppressive dosages of T_3.

Target organ resistance to thyroid hormone is diverse, giving rise to different clinical phenotypes. Predominant clinical features vary among different patients with thyroid hormone resistance[69][70] (as do features among FMS patients). Based on the results of this study, and similar results by Sonkin[71] and by Lowe and colleagues,[22][23] euthyroid FMS appears to be another clinical phenotype of partial thyroid hormone resistance. Our patients are properly classified as having partial *peripheral* resistance to thyroid hormone, as distinct from the general or pituitary forms,[69][72] because their suppressed TSH levels showed that their pituitary glands were not resistant. Our patients resembled in several respects the only other well-documented case of peripheral thyroid hormone resistance.[70] With supraphysiologic doses of T_3, patients had essentially unchanged weight, blood pressure, serum calcium, cholesterol, and alkaline phosphatase, but T_4 was low and T_3 and pulse rate increased (within normal range, and no patient had tachycardia). In addition, their clinical status improved significantly only with supraphysiologic dosages of T_3.

The usual dosages of T_3 required to maintain euthyroidism in athyreotic patients have been given variously as 25-to-75 mcg[73] and 50-to-75 mcg per day.[70] Patients in this study had significant therapeutic responses only to dosages ranging from 93.75-to-150 mcg. These dosages were sufficient to cause low TSH, FTI, and total and free T_4, and high levels of free T_3, even in the patient taking the smallest amount of T_3. This pattern of laboratory values in patients taking exogenous T_3 has been interpreted as T_3-toxicosis.[74] Our patients, however, did not have clinical symptoms or signs indicative of thyrotoxicosis. Moreover, the results of electrocardiography, bone densitometry, and most laboratory tests were not those expected from thyrotoxic patients, but were within normal range.

Mutations in the c-erbAβ₁ gene with resultant mutant β₁ thyroid hormone receptors are the molecular bases of most cases of partial thyroid hormone resistance.[69] Mutant thyroid hormone receptors regulate transcription only when exposed to high concentrations of T_3. At low concentrations of T_3, for example, the P448H mutant thyroid hormone receptor has dominant negative activity and represses transcription. At high T_3 concentrations, the receptor becomes transcriptionally active.[75] Our patients' requirement for high T₃ dosages may also have been due to mutated thyroid hormone receptors.[21] We recommend that sequencing of the c-erbAβ₁ gene be performed to determine whether mutations are present in chromosome 3 in euthyroid FMS patients.

Clinical Decisions in this Study

Decisions to change T₃ dosages and to cross patients from one phase to another in this study were response-driven; that is, a patient's response in each phase was the basis of the clinical decisions made during that phase. A patient's "response" consisted of changes in objective FMS measures, the patient's subjective estimate of her status, results of a physical examination, and nonquantified changes in the patient observed by the clinician. The repeatability of this study in the future will critically depend upon researchers making proper use of all these factors.

Our methodology is likely to be criticized because patient management was based in part on a clinician's judgment of patient response (though, both clinician and patient remained blinded). In the best of circumstances in clinical trials, assessment of patient status is reduced to easily measurable criteria. Long-term clinical use of the protocol tested in this study, however, has shown that this is not entirely possible at this time. As most fibromyalgia patients undergo treatment with thyroid hormone, some changes that are difficult to quantify may be obvious to varying degrees to the experienced clinician who is familiar with the individual patient. The changes typically signify improving patient status, and their failure to occur may indicate the need to titrate the T₃ dosage. When considered with the outcome of the objective measures, these phenomena may contribute substantially to proper clinical decisions. We will mention a few of these changes that occurred in the patients in this study.

One was a change from a slow relaxation phase of the Achilles reflex to a speed roughly equal to the contraction phase. Although the speed of the reflex can be objectively measured, we did not do so. Nevertheless, as Sonkin wrote, the change is obvious to the clinician experienced at testing the reflex.[15] Other, more difficult to define responses were: a change from a torpid and pensive facial expression to a zestful expression, and a distinct change in the eyes from a dull, listless appearance to an energetic, alert appearance. Another response that many clinicians are likely to imprudently ignore or reject is a pronouncement by the patient that she is well. These changes occur and persist in many, although not all, FMS patients who

benefit from thyroid hormone therapy. When a patient responds in such ways, it is judicious for the clinician to note the responses and calculate them into judgment of the patient's FMS status. To ignore or otherwise exclude such phenomena from patient assessment is to forfeit one of the richest sources of data upon which to base sound clinical judgment. The blinded clinical decisions in this study were based partly on such patient responses.

We also used line graphs to observe trends in data points that represented mean scores from FMS measures. These provided objective data to calculate into therapeutic decisions. Although clinical judgment of a patient's status influenced clinical decisions, decisions were primarily data-driven by the scores on the objective measures.

CONCLUSION

Whether or not mutant thyroid hormone receptors underlie the clinical features of our euthyroid FMS patients' remains to be determined. But supraphysiologic dosages of T₃ significantly improved their FMS status. Though these dosages produced thyroid function test results indicative of hyperthyroidism, our patients had no clinically significant adverse target tissue effects. We conclude that for these patients during this study, T₃ was effective and safe as a treatment for euthyroid FMS. (Further testing is necessary to establish the long-term safety of T₃ therapy.) Results suggest that euthyroid FMS is a clinical phenotype of partial peripheral resistance to thyroid hormone. We recommend that further studies be done to answer the questions: Are euthyroid FMS patients partially resistant to thyroid hormone? And if so, what are the molecular mechanisms of the resistance?

ACKNOWLEDGMENTS

We are indebted to thyroidologist Stephen J. Usala, M.D., Ph.D., for reading and commenting on the contents of this manuscript, James Bray, Ph.D. and Irene Easling, Ph.D. of Baylor University College of Medicine and to the Department of Family Medicine at Baylor for assistance with methodology and statistical analyses, and to Samuel Pegram, M.D. for providing bone densitometry. We thank EquiMed Corporation for its contribution of ECGs, and Scott W. Carlson, President of EquiMed, for independent scoring. We are especially grateful to our study patients for enduring placebo phases.

REFERENCES

1. Wolfe, F., Smythe, H.A., Yunus, M.B., et al.: The American College of Rheumatology 1990 criteria for the classification of fibromyalgia: report of the multicenter criteria committee. *Arthritis Rheumatol.*, 33:160-172, 1990.

2. Consensus Document on Fibromyalgia: The Copenhagen Declaration. Copenhagen, Myopain '92, 17-20 August, 1992. *J. Musculoskel. Pain*, 1(3/4):295-312, 1993.

3. Wolfe, F.: Aspects of the epidemiology of fibromyalgia. *J. Musculoskel. Pain*, 2(3):65-77, 1994.

4. Lowe, J.C.: T₃-induced recovery from fibromyalgia by a hypothyroid patient resistant to T₄ and desiccated thyroid. *J. Myofascial. Ther.*, 1(4):26-31, 1995.

5. Beetham, W.P., Jr.: Diagnosis and management of fibrositis syndrome and psychogenic rheumatism. *Med. Clin. North Am.*, 63:433-439, 1979.

6. Golding, D.N.: Hypothyroidism presenting with musculoskeletal symptoms. *Ann. Rheumatic. Dis.*, 29:10-41, 1970.

7. Bland, J.H. and Frymoyer, J.W.: Rheumatic syndromes of myxedema. *N. Eng. J. Med.*, 282:1171-1174, 1970.

8. Wilke, S.W., Sheeler, L.R., and Makarowski, W.S.: Hypothyroidism with presenting symptoms of fibrositis. *J. Rheumatol.*, 8:627-630, 1981.

9. Hochberg, M.C., Koppes, G.M., Edwards, C.Q., Barnes, H.V., and Arnett, F.C., Jr.: Hypothyroidism presenting as a polymyositis-like syndrome: report of two cases. *Arthritis Rheum.*, 19:1363-1366, 1976.

10. Delamere, J.P., Scott, D.L., and Felix-Davies, D.D.: Thyroid dysfunction and rheumatic diseases. *J. Royal Soc. Med.*, 75:102, 1982.

11. Fessel, W.J.: Myopathy of hypothyroidism. *Ann. Rheumatic Dis.*, 27:590-596, 1968.

12. Wilson, J. and Walton, J.N.: Some muscular manifestations of hypothyroidism. *J. Neurol. Neurosurg. Psychiat.*, 22:320-324, 1959.

13. Awad, E.A.: Histopathological changes in fibrositis. In *Advances in Pain Research and Therapy*, vol. 17. Edited by J.R. Fricton and E.A. Awad, New York, Raven Press, 1990, pp.249-258.

14. Sonkin, L.S.: Endocrine disorders and muscle dysfunction. In *Clinical Management of Head, Neck, and TMJ Pain and Dysfunction*. Edited by B. Gelb, Philadelphia, W.B. Saunders Co., 1985, pp.137-170.

15. Lowe, J.C.: Thyroid status of 38 fibromyalgia patients: implications for the etiology of fibromyalgia. *Clin. Bull. Myofascial Ther.*, 2(1):36-41, 1997.

16. Shiroky, J.B., Cohen, M., Ballachey, M-L., and Neville, C.: Thyroid dysfunction in rheumatoid arthritis: a controlled prospective survey. *Ann .Rheumat. Dis.*, 52:454-456, 1993.

17. Eisinger, J., Arroyo, P.H., Calendini, C., Rinaldi, J.P., Combes, R., and Fontaine, G.: Anomalies biologiques au cours des fibromyalgies: III. Explorations endocriniennes. *Lyon Méditerranée Méd.*, 28:858-860, 1992.

18. Gerwin, R.: A study of 96 subjects examined both for fibromyalgia and myofascial pain. *J. Musculoskel. Pain*, 3:(Suppl.)1:121, 1995.

19. Ferraccioli, G., Cavalieri, F., Salaffi, F., et al.: Neuroendocrinologic findings in primary fibromyalgia (soft tissue chronic pain syndrome) and in other chronic rheumatic conditions (rheumatoid arthritis, low back pain). *J. Rheumatol.*, 17:869-873, 1990.

20. Neeck, G. and Riedel, W.: Thyroid function in patients with fibromyalgia syndrome. *J. Rheumatol.*, 19:1120-1122, 1992.

21. Lowe, J.C., Cullum, M., Graf, L., Jr, and Yellin, J.: Mutations in the c-erbAβ₁ gene: do they underlie euthyroid fibromyalgia? *Med. Hypotheses*, 48(2)Feb.:125-135, 1997.

22. Lowe, J.C., Eichelberger, J., Manso, G., and Peterson, K.: Improvement in euthyroid fibromyalgia patients treated with T₃ (tri-iodothyronine). *J. Myofascial Ther.*, 1(2):16-27, 1994.

23. Lowe, J.C.: Results of an open trial of T₃ therapy with 77 euthyroid female fibromyalgia patients. *Clin. Bull. Myofascial Ther.*, 2(1):35-37, 1997.

24. Bennett, R.M.: Literature reviews. *J. Musculoskel. Pain*, 2(2):101-112, 1994.

25. Littlejohn, G.O.: A database for fibromyalgia. *Rheum. Dis. Clinics North Am.*, 21(2):527-557, 1995.

26. Fischer, A.A., DeCosta, C., and Levy, H.: Diagnosis of fibromyalgia by manual pressure is unreliable: quantification of tender point sensitivity by algometer is necessary in clinical practice. *J. Musculoskel. Pain*, 3(1):139, 1995.

27. Putick, M., Schulzer, M., Klinkhoff, A., Koehler, B., Rangno, K., and Chalmers, A.: Reliability and reproducibility of fibromyalgic tenderness, measurement by electronic and mechanical dolorimeters. *J. Musculoskel. Pain*, 3(4):3-14, 1995.

28. Rasmussen, J.O., Smidth, M., and Hansen, T.M.: Examination of tender points in soft tissue: palpation versus pressure-algometer. *Ugeskr Laeger*, 152(21):1522-1526, 1990.

29. Lautenschlager, J., Seglias, J., Bruckle, W., and Muller, W.: Comparisons of spontaneous pain and tenderness in patients with primary fibromyalgia. *Clin. Rheumatol.*, 10(2):168-173, 1991.

30. Wilkins, E.W., Dineen, J.J., Moncure, A.C., Gross, P.L., and Fitzgerald, C.P.: *MGH Textbook of Emergency Medicine*, 2nd edition. Baltimore, Williams & Wilkins, 1983, pp.624-627.

31. O'Boyle, C.M., Davis, D.K., Russo, B.A., Kraf, T.J., and Brick, P.D.: *Emergency Care: The First 24 Hours*. Norwalk, Appleton-Century-Crofts, 1985, pp.332-333.

32. Joos, E., Meeusen, R., and De Meirleir, K.: Measurement of physical capacity in fibromyalgia. *J. Musculoskel. Pain*, 3(Suppl 1):87, 1995.

33. Nielson, W.R., Grace, G.M., Hopkins, M., and Berg, M.: Concentration and memory deficits in patients with fibromyalgia syndrome. *J. Musculoskel. Pain*, 3(Suppl 1):123, 1995.

34. Clark, S., Tindall, E., and Bennett, R.M.: A double-blind crossover trial of prednisone versus placebo in the treatment of fibrositis. *J. Rheumatol.*, 12:980-983, 1985.

35. Goldenberg, D.L., Felson, D.T., and Dinerman, H.: A randomized, controlled trial of amitriptyline and naproxen in the treatment of patients with fibromyalgia. *Arthritis Rheumat.*, 29(1):1371-1377, 1986.

36. Jacobsen, S., Danneskiold-Samsøe, B., and Andersen, R.B.: Oral S-adenosylmethionine in primary fibromyalgia: double-blind clinical evaluation. *Scand. J. Rheumatol.*, 20:294-302, 1991.

37. Goldenberg, D.L., Marskīy, M., Mossey, C., Ruthazer, R., and Schmid, C.: The independent and combined efficacy of fluoxetine and amitriptyline in the treatment of fibromyalgia. *Arthritis Rheumat.*, Suppl 38:S229, 1995.

38. Scott, J. and Huskisson, E.C.: Graphic representation of pain. *Pain*, 2:175-184, 1976.

39. Zung, W.W.K.: A self-rating depression scale. *Arch. Gen. Psychiatry*, 12:65-70, 1965.

40. Burckhardt, C.S., Clark, S.R., and Bennett, R.M.: The fibromyalgia impact questionnaire: development and validation. *J. Rheumatol.*, 18(5):728-733, 1991.

41. Naughton, M.J. and Wiklund, I.: A critical review of dimension-specific measures of health-related quality of life in cross-cultural research. *Quality Life Res.*, 2(6):397-432, 1993.

42. Rehm, L.P.: Assessment of depression. In *Behavioral Assessment: A Practical Handbook*. Edited by M. Hersen and A.S. Bellack, Oxford, Permagon Press, 1976, pp.246-295.

43. Vlase, H., Lungu, G., and Vlase, L.: Cardiac disturbances in thyrotoxicosis: diagnosis, incidence, clinical features, and management. *Endocrinologie*, 29(3-4):155-160, 1991.

44. Gow, S.M., Caldwell, G., Toft A.D., et al.: Relationship between pituitary and other target organ responsiveness in hypothyroid patients receiving thyroxine replacement. *J. Clin. Endocrinol. Metab.*, 64:364, 1987.

45. Ross, D.S.: Subclinical hyperthyroidism. In Werner and Ingbar's *The Thyroid: A Fundamental and Clinical Text*, 6th edition. Edited by L.E .Braverman and R.D. Utiger, Philadelphia, J.B. Lippincott, 1991, pp.1249-1255.

46. Tepperman, J. and Tepperman, H.M.: *Metabolic and Endocrine Physiology*, 5th edition. Chicago, Year Book Medical Publishers, 1987.

47. Dillman, W.H.: The cardiovascular system in thyrotoxicosis. In Werner and Ingbar's *The Thyroid: A Fundamental and Clinical Text.*, 6th edition. Edited by L.E .Braverman and R.D. Utiger, Philadelphia, J.B. Lippincott, 1991, pp.759-770.

48. Hof, F.M., San, J.F.Y., and Lowrey, R.D.: The electrocardiogram in thyrotoxicosis. *Am. J. Cardiol.*, 8:893, 1960.

49. Muggia, A.L., Stjernholm, M., and Houle, T.: Complete heart block with thyrotoxic myocarditis. *N. Engl. J. Med.*, 283:1099, 1970.

50. Agner, T., Almdal, T., Thorsteinsson, B., and Agner, E.: A reevaluation of atrial fibrillation in thyrotoxicosis. *Dan. Med. Bull.*, 31:157, 1984.

51. Ciaccheri, M., Cecchi, F., Arcangeli C., et al.: Occult thyrotoxicosis in patients with chronic and paroxysmal isolated atrial fibrillation. *Clin. Cardiol.*, 7:413, 1984.

52. Paul, T.L., Kerrigan, J., Kelly, A.M., Braverman, L.E., and Baran, D.T.: Long term L-thyroxine therapy is associated with decreased hip bone density in premenopausal women. *J.A.M.A.*, 259: 3137-3141, 1988.

53. Coindre, J-M, David, J-P, and Riviere, L.: Bone loss in hypothyroidism with hormone replacement. *Arch. Intern. Med.*, 146:48, 1986.

54. Ross, D.S., Neer, R.M., Ridgeway, E.C., and Daniels, G.H.: Subclinical hyperthyroidism and reduced bone density as a possible result of prolonged suppression of the pituitary-thyroid axis with L-thyroxine. *Am. J. Med.*, 82:1167-1170, 1987.

55. Taelman, P., Kau, F.M., San, J.M., Jansenns, X., Vandecauter, H., and Vermeulen, A.: Reduced forearm bone mineral content and biochemical evidence of increased bone turnover in women with euthyroid goitre treated with thyroid hormone. *Clin. Endocrinol.* (Oxf), 33:107-117, 1990.

56. Ribot, C., Tremollieres, F., Pouilles, J.M., and Louvet, J.P.: Bone mineral density and thyroid hormone therapy. *Clin. Endocrinol.* (Oxf), 33:143-153, 1990.

57. Krolner, B., Vesterdal-Jorgensen, J., and Pors-Nielsen, S.: Spinal bone mineral content in myxoedema and thyrotoxicosis: effects of thyroid hormone(s) and antithyroid treatment. *Clin. Endocrinol.*, 18:439-446, 1983.

58. Fallon, M.D., Perry, H.M., and Bergfeld, M.: Exogenous hyperthyroidism with osteoporosis. *Arch. Intern. Med.*, 143:442-444, 1983.

59. Salmon, D., Rendell, M., and Williams, J.: Chemical hyperthyroidism. *Arch. Intern. Med.*, 142:571, 1982.

60. Fish, L.H., Schwartz, H.L., and Cavanaugh, J.: Replacement dose, metabolism, and bioavailability of levothyroxine in the treatment of hypothyroidism. *N. Engl. J. Med.*, 316:764, 1987.

61. Pearce, C.J. and Himsworth, R.L.: Total and free thyroid hormone concentrations in patients receiving maintenance replacement treatment with thyroxine. *Br. Med. J.*, 288: 693, 1984.

62. Bayer, M.F., Kriss, J.P., and McDougall, I.R.: Clinical experience with sensitive thyrotropin measurements: diagnostic and therapeutic implications. *J. Nucl. Med.*, 26:1248, 1985.

63. De Rosa, G., Testa, A., Maussier, M.L., Calla, C., Astazi, P., and Albanese, C.: A slightly suppressive dose of L-thyroxine does not affect bone turnover and bone mineral density in pre- and post-menopausal women with nontoxic goiter. *Hormone Metab. Res.*, 27(11):503-507, 1995.

64. Chabert-Orsini, V., Conte-Devolx, B., Thiers-Bautrant, D., et al.: Bone density after iatrogenic subclinical long-term thyrotoxicosis: measurement by dual photon absorptiometry. *Presse Med.*, 19:1709- 1711, 1990.

65. Hamburger, J.I.: Strategies for cost-effective thyroid function testing with modern methods. In *Diagnostic Methods in Clinical Thyroidology*. Edited by J.I. Hamburger, New York, Springer-Verlag, 1989, pp.63-109.

66. Faber, J., Overgaard, K., Jarlov, A.E., and Christiansen, C.: Bone metabolism in premenopausal women with nontoxic goiter and reduced serum thyrotropin levels. *Thyroidology*, 6(1):27-32,1994.

67. Bartalena, L., and Pinchera, A.: Effects of thyroxine excess on peripheral organs. *Acta Medica Austriaca*, 21(2): 60-65, 1994.

68. Tremollieres, F., Pouilles, J.M., Louvet, J.P., and Ribot, C.: Transitory bone loss during substitution treatment for hypothyroidism: results of a two-year prospective study. *Revue du Rhumatisme et des Maladies Osteo Articulaires*, 58(12):869-875, 1991.

69. Refetoff, S., Weiss, R.E., and Usala, S.J.: The syndromes of resistance to thyroid hormone. *Endocrine Rev.*, 14:348-399, 1993.

70. Kaplan, M.M., Swartz, S.L., and Larsen, P.R.: Partial peripheral resistance to thyroid hormone. *Am. J. Med.*, 70:1115-1121, 1981.

71. Sonkin, L.S.: Myofascial pain due to metabolic disorders: diagnosis and treatment. In *Myofascial Pain and Fibromyalgia.* Edited by E.S. Rachlin, St. Louis, Mosby, 1994, pp.45-60.

72. Refetoff, S.: Thyroid hormone resistance syndromes. In Werner and Ingbar's *The Thyroid: A Fundamental and Clinical Text,* 6th edition. Edited by L.E. Braverman and R.D. Utiger, Philadelphia, J.B. Lippincott, 1991, pp.1280-1294.

73. De Visscher, M.: The therapy of hypothyroid states. In *Recent Progress in Diagnosis and Treatment of Hypothyroid Conditions: Proceedings of the XVth International Congress of Therapeutics,* Amsterdam, Excerpta Medica, 1980, pp.105-114.

74. Ladenson, P.W.: Diagnosis of thyrotoxicosis. In Werner and Ingbar's *The Thyroid: A Fundamental and Clinical Text,* 6th edition. Edited by L.E. Braverman and R.D. Utiger, Philadelphia, J.B. Lippincott, 1991, pp.880-886.

75. Krishna, V., Chatterjee, K., Nagaya T, et al.: Thyroid hormone resistance syndrome: inhibition of normal receptor function by mutant thyroid hormone receptors. *J. Clin. Invest.,* 87:1977-1984, 1991.

76. Norušis, M.J.: *The SPSS Guide to Data Analysis for SPSS/PC+™,* 2nd edition. Chicago, SPSS Inc., 1991.

The Process of Change During T₃ Treatment for Euthyroid Fibromyalgia: A Double-Blind Placebo-Controlled Crossover Study

John C. Lowe, M.A., D.C.

Alan J. Reichman, M.D.

Jackie Yellin, B.A.

This article originally appeared in the *Clinical Bulletin of Myofascial Therapy*, 2(2/3):91-124, 1997. It is reprinted with permission of Haworth Medical Press.

ABSTRACT. *Methods.* Comparative effects of placebos and T₃ were tested on four euthyroid fibromyalgia patients over a period of nine months. Each patient completed alternately two T₃ phases and two placebo phases, the sequence depending on the medication with which each was randomly assigned to begin. The ABAB single subject crossover design enabled each patient to serve as her own control. Phase crossover was response-driven, based on changes in measures of mean tender point sensitivity by algometry, pain distribution by the percentage method, and mean symptom intensity by visual analog scales. Changes were evaluated by visual inspection of graphs and single subject statistical analyses. Traditional group comparison statistics were performed for changes on the Fibromyalgia Impact Questionnaire, the Zung's Depression Scale, and pain distribution according to the ACR criteria.

Results. Quantitative analysis of trends of repeated measures across phases showed significant improvement in fibromyalgia status in T₃ phases compared to baseline and placebo phases. Testing throughout the 9-month study and at 4-month follow-up showed no clinically significant adverse target tissue effects. No patient met the diagnostic criteria for fibromyalgia by the end of the study.

Conclusion. Repeated administration and withdrawal of T₃ corresponded to significant improvement and deterioration in fibromyalgia measures during this study. It is highly probable, then, that improvement in fibromyalgia status of our four patients was functionally related to their use of supraphysiologic dosages of T₃ (effective range: 118.75-to-162.50 mcg). These dosages were shown to be safe at 4-month follow-up. Further testing is necessary to establish long-term safety.

KEY WORDS. Fibromyalgia, hypothyroidism, euthyroid, thyroid hormone resistance, T₃

INTRODUCTION

Fibromyalgia syndrome (FMS) is the most common condition of chronic widespread musculoskeletal pain, stiffness, and fatigue.[1][2] There is a 2% incidence in the U.S., and 90% of patients are female.[3] FMS patients have largely failed to benefit long term from any treatment in common use (such as tricyclic antidepressants).[4]

The clinical features of FMS and hypothyroidism are remarkably similar,[5][6][7][8][9][10][11][12][13][14][15] and there is a high incidence of hypothyroidism in FMS patients. Compared to the 1% incidence of primary hypothyroidism in the population at-large,[16] the incidence among FMS patients has been reported as 10%,[17][18] 10.5%,[19] and 12%.[20] Compared to the 0.00021% incidence of central (hypothalamic or pituitary) hypothyroidism in the population at large,[16] the incidence indicated by thyroid function testing in one group of 38 FMS patients was 52.6%.[19] Preliminary results from a multicenter study of fibromyalgia patients show a 14.3% incidence of primary hypothyroidism and a 40.0% incidence of central hypothyroidism.[62] Test results consistent with central hypothyroidism in FMS patients have also been reported by other researchers.[21][22]

The incidence of euthyroid status among fibromyalgia patients has been reported as 36.8%[19] and 45.7%.[62] Previously, the euthyroid status of some FMS patients led to the implicit conclusion that while hypothyroidism is a concurrent condition in some patients, it is not etiologically related to FMS.[1][2]

Lowe and his coauthors proposed, however, that the hypothyroid-like features of euthyroid FMS may result from failure of normal concentrations of thyroid hormone to properly regulate gene transcription.[23] Inadequate transcription regulation in hypothyroid FMS would result from a frank thyroid hormone deficiency. In euthyroid FMS, inadequate regulation may result from mutant thyroid hormone receptors having low affinity for thyroid hormone. Each clinical feature of FMS may be explained by increases in three "inhibitory" molecular by-products of inadequate regulation of gene transcription by thyroid hormone: α-adrenoceptors, phosphodiesterase, and G$_i$ proteins. Euthyroid FMS, according to this putative mechanism, is a syndrome of cellular resistance to thyroid hormone.[23]

This hypothesis is supported by the results of two systematic, open trials and one double-blind placebo-controlled study using T$_3$ therapy for euthyroid FMS.[24][25][26] In the blinded study, traditional group comparison statistics showed that according to five measures, FMS status significantly improved in T$_3$ phases and significantly worsened in placebo phases. Therapeutic effects occurred only with supraphysiologic T$_3$ dosages, and without adverse effects on heart, liver, muscle, or bone at four month follow-up.[26]

The first purpose of the current study was to determine whether four euthyroid FMS patients would respond to T$_3$ as did those in the previous blinded study, and as have patients with proven thyroid hormone resistance. The response would be improved clinical status with supraphysiologic dosages of T$_3$ without adverse target tissue effects.[27] The second purpose was two-fold: 1) to use single subject quantitative analyses of data to determine whether patients' FMS status improved in T$_3$ phases and worsened in placebo phases, and 2) if measures differed between T$_3$ and placebo phases, to show (by line graphs) the *process* of change in three FMS measures across the phases.

METHODS

Subjects

The institutional review board of the Fibromyalgia Research Foundation approved the protocol and required that it be used in this study with a maximum of four patients, due to funding restrictions. Ten patients responded to a newspaper advertisement soliciting individuals with FMS symptoms to participate in the study. Interviewing ceased after the fourth individual who met the participation criteria was

sequentially enrolled. All patients signed a written informed consent document before the study began; each patient acknowledged her understanding of the effects of overstimulation by thyroid hormone explained in the document. The four patients ranged in age from 30-to-41. Each met the 1990 American College of Rheumatology (ACR) criteria for the diagnosis of FMS[1]: widespread pain for at least three months, and 11 of 18 possible tender points. The pressure/pain threshold of 16 of the 18 tender points was measured with an algometer (calibrated force gauge). A patient was enrolled only if the mean of her tender points was below 2.5 kg/cm^2, 1.5 kg/cm^2 below the ACR's arbitrary normal of 4 kg/cm^2. All patients had normal thyroid function test results, and none had previously been treated with thyroid hormone. No patient had another health condition with clinical features resembling or overlapping those of FMS. Each patient agreed to stop any medication she was taking to control her FMS symptoms at least two weeks (for a washout time) prior to the start of the study. Each also agreed to engage in exercise to tolerance and to take nutritional supplements (especially B vitamins) daily through all phases of the study. Patients were randomly assigned by number and off-site to either an initial placebo or initial T$_3$ phase.

Treatment

During all phases, patients took combinations of capsules of four different colors. Each color represented a different dose, either 6.25, 12.5, 25.0, or 75 mcg. The lactose capsules patients took during placebo phases were identical in appearance to the T$_3$ capsules taken in treatment phases. Patients and investigators were instructed to assume that all number-coded bottles in every phase contained T$_3$. Propranolol tablets (20 mg) were issued to all patients, but were to be taken only if they felt some threat from overstimulation by the capsules, and upon consultation with one of the investigators. All patients and all investigators were unaware of any patient's actual capsule content during all phases, as the bottles were prepared and coded off-site using patient numbers rather than names.

At the time of any crossover, a patient received a new set of four number-coded bottles prepared off-site (with no knowledge of the outcome of exams or of any patient's individual status or code number). The patient turned in the bottles with the remaining capsules for the phase just completed and picked up bottles for the phase she was about to enter. In any new phase, a patient began by taking 75 mcg (presumed in every phase to be T_3), despite the dosage she had been taking when her previous phase ended.

Assessment

Assessment measures from our previous double-blind study were appropriate for testing the treatment protocol, so we used them in this study. Patients were evaluated at one-to-two week intervals with a brief examination (pulse rate, blood pressure, and Achilles reflex), an interview, and an FMS assessment. Three sets of FMS measurements were taken repeatedly throughout all study phases: 1) a tender point examination by one of the investigators (quantified by algometer measurements of 16 tender points), 2) a pain drawing of the patient's pain distribution since the previous examination (quantified as a percentage of 36 body divisions containing pain[26]), and 3) completion of visual analog scales (VASs) for symptom intensities of the 13 most common symptoms associated with fibromyalgia (quantified as a mean score from all 13). These symptoms were pain, fatigue, stiffness, headache, sleep disturbance, bowel disturbance, depression, cognitive dysfunction (poor memory and concentration), anxiety, coldness, paresthesias (numbness and tingling), Sicca symptoms, and difficulty exercising.

After each reevaluation, the mean tender point score, the pain distribution expressed as a percentage, and the mean symptom intensity were applied as data points (for that evaluation date) to graphs for each measure. Successive data points in each graph showed the trend of each measure during each phase. At each evaluation, the examining clinician used the graphs (with data from the current evaluation and previous ones in the same phase) and his global assessment (see below) of the patient to judge when it was appropriate to alter the patient's T_3 dosage or to cross her to the next phase.

At each evaluation, the examining clinician made a global assessment of the patient's status. This assessment considered several factors: 1) results of the physical exam, particularly the resting pulse rate and Achilles reflex, 2) the patient's answers to questions about her status since the last evaluation, and 3) the clinician's impression of the patient's status based on her appearance and attitude. The clinician's judgment as to whether the patient's dosage should be altered was based on consideration of his global assessment of her status, and the trend of her data points in the line graphs for FMS measures in the current phase of the study. Thus, decisions regarding dosage adjustments were clinical judgments. The judgments were based

partly on the outcome of the objective FMS measures, partly on signs observable by the clinician, and partly on the patient's subjective report. Depending on the outcome of the evaluation, a patient's daily dosage was kept the same or altered.

If a patient's fibromyalgia status deteriorated according to the examining clinician's judgment, the patient's dosage was increased by 6.25, 12.5, or 25 mcg. If a patient's fibromyalgia status stayed the same or slightly improved, but her ECGs showed no evidence of overstimulation and there was no other clinical evidence of thyrotoxicosis, then her dosage was increased. In any phase, if there were signs of overstimulation, a patient's dosage was backed down by 6.25 mcg decrements until all signs and symptoms of overstimulation were gone. Serial ECGs were performed on all patients throughout the study to assure awareness at any point of cardiac thyrotoxicosis. (No instance was ever found in this study.)

If a patient reached a dosage of 175 mcg without further improvement through at least two evaluations, the patient was crossed to the next phase and given alternate number-coded capsules. When in the judgment of the examining clinician, a patient's improvement had plateaued, she too was crossed to the next phase.

At the end of each phase, the mean tender point sensitivity, mean symptom intensity, and pain distribution expressed as a percentage were taken along with three other measures: pain distribution according to the ACR method (pain above and below the waist, on the right and left sides of the body, and axial pain),[1] the Fibromyalgia Impact Questionnaire (FIQ),[27] and Zung's Self-Rating Depression Scale (Zung's).[28] The FIQ is a brief, self-administered instrument with demonstrated validity and reliability, and it is widely used for assessing the impact FMS has on a patient's daily life.[27] It lists ten common daily activities that patients rate according to their ability to perform, and ten VASs for FMS symptoms that patients mark to indicate severity. The range of possible scores is 0-to-80. Zung's is an easily self-administered, well-validated measure with acceptable sensitivity and specificity.[28] It contains twenty questions about activities or symptoms that indicate depression, and patients rate each according to its presence and severity. The range of raw scores is 20-to-80. The raw score is converted to one of four clinical categories, ranging from "none" to "severe" depression. The FIQ and Zung's forms from this study were number-coded and independently scored off-site.

Safety Testing

After the study was concluded, all patients continued to use supraphysiologic doses of T_3 daily. At the end of four months, safety testing was performed. Tests of possible adverse effects of supraphysiologic doses of T_3 included serial ECGs throughout all study phases (prior to each dosage increase) and at 4-month follow-up. Urinary N-telo-peptides, creatinine, calcium, and phosphorus; serum creatinine, calcium, phosphorus, and alkaline phosphatase; and bone densitometry of the lumbar spine, Ward's triangle, femoral neck, and trochanter with dual photon absorptiometry were evaluated at 4-month follow-up.

Study Design

This was a double-blind placebo-controlled response-driven crossover investigation. The study consisted of a single subject design. Single subject designs involve the study of single individuals by repeated measurements, and by the systematic administration and withdrawal of a treatment and/or placebo.[29][30] Data from this design, also termed "time-series," "small-N," and "single system," are depicted as data points on graphs. The data are visually inspected and analyzed with quantitative methods. Matching of patients is not necessary because each patient serves as her own control in alternate phases. As well as end point outcome, the process of change in and across phases is studied in single subject designs.[29]

Eight pretreatment baseline measures provided a basis for comparison of data from subsequent T_3 and placebo phases. The ABAB design used in this study is considered powerful because causal inferences can be drawn from its results: repeatedly administering and withdrawing a treatment permits assessment of a possible functional relationship between the therapeutic intervention and the measures of clinical status.[29]

Data Analysis

Visual Inspection. Graphic analysis and visual inspection are used extensively in applied behavioral research.[29] They provide visual summaries of data, permit valid analysis of data from a small number of patients, allow the systematic inclusion of all patient measurements over time, provide information about possible functional relationships, and show the process of change as well as the outcome. In line graphs, data are converted into changes in level, variability, trend, and slope of curves.[29] Moreover, the insensitivity of

visual inspection to slight changes in measures is considered a strength, in that use of an insensitive form of analysis reveals only changes of clinically important magnitude.[31] To avoid perceptual distortion and misrepresentation of graphed data, we scaled y-axes and x-axes in this study to the recommended 2:3 ratio.[31][32]

A disadvantage of this method is that there are no formal decision rules regarding visual inspection. This encourages subjectivity and inconsistency in interpreting graphed data.[32] This shortcoming has led to the development of methods of statistical analysis to supplement visual inspection.[29] Statistical analysis can detect treatment effects so slight that they are easily overlooked with visual inspection of graphs, avoiding the equivalent of a Type II experimental error.[29]

Quantitative Analysis Based on the Trendline Method. Trend, the direction in which a series of data points progresses, is indicated by a celeration line. The celeration line shows whether a series of data points is stationary, accelerating, or decelerating. It is formed by dividing baseline data points into two groups, determining the median of each, and projecting a line that intersects both median points to the right through the intervention phases of the graph.[29] Our null hypothesis was that during T_3 phases, the proportion of data points above or below the celeration line would not significantly vary from the proportion in baseline phases. However, if T_3 or placebo caused a change in FMS measures, the proportion of data points above or below the celeration line would reflect the change in measures in that phase. The change in the proportion of data points was the basis for statistical comparison across phases.[29]

Data points in all phases were tested for autocorrelation by the autocorrelation coefficient.[33] Data points in the first two intervention phases (a placebo and a T_3 phase) were tested for difference from the 8 baseline data points with two methods.

The first method is reference to a probability table.[34] Reference to the probability table was made to determine the number of data points above or below the celeration line in intervention phases necessary for statistical significance ($P<0.05$), determined by use of the one-tailed test.[34]

The second method is the two standard deviation band method (2SD).[29] This method is based on computation of the standard deviation for baseline data. Because statistical significance is computed directly from the standard deviation of the value of baseline data points, the values *per se* rather than the number of data points is the central factor. The greater the variability in baseline values, the greater the band width outside which data points must fall in intervention phases for statistical significance to be reached. These two methods are viewed as judgment aids that provide a measure of quantitative confidence to results obtained through visual inspection of graphs.[29]

Statistical Analysis. Statistical analyses of group data from the FIQ, Zung's, and pain distribution according to the ACR criteria were performed with the Statistical Package for the Social Sciences (SPSS). Mean scores from these three measures, taken at the end of each T_3 and placebo phase (before crossover to an alternate phase), were analyzed with paired-samples *t*-tests.

RESULTS

Visual Inspection of Graphs

Figures 1 through 3 contain four graphs each, one for each patient. The y-axis shows the magnitude of each measurement, and the x-axis shows the evaluation number. Intervals between evaluations varied (depending on patient availability or symptoms) through the 9-month span of the study. But in no case were evaluations spaced more than two weeks apart. Each graph contains five labels indicating whether a division represents a baseline, placebo, or T_3 phase. Each data point represents the patient's score for that graph's measure at each evaluation, and the series of points in each graph shows the change in that measure across phases. The data points in the graphs of Figure 1 represent the mean pressure/pain threshold (algometer score) of 16 tender points at each evaluation. The data points in the graphs of Figure 2 show the percentage of 36 body divisions that contained pain at each evaluation. The data points in Figure 3 represent mean symptom intensity at each evaluation.

Visual inspection of each patient's graphs shows improved FMS status in T_3 phases and deteriorated status in placebo phases. In T_3 phases, each of the three repeated measures progressed in a positive direction, indicating improvement in FMS status. In placebo phases, repeated measures progressed in a direction indicating deteriorating patient status. The lines connecting the series of data points in each graph show the *process* of change in the three FMS measures.

Extreme variation in measures for some patients suggests rebound phenomena. This was apparent in some placebo phases following T_3 phases. All patients reported severe subjective worsening of their FMS status during these placebo phases. This is best depicted in the pain distribution graph for patient 4 (Figure 2). In her two placebo phases, worsening of pain distribution over baseline was statistically significant according to the 2SD band method. The data points in these phases show that immediately after withdrawal of T_3, an FMS measure may worsen relative to its baseline values. A similar rebound may have occurred in the pain distribution of patient 2 (Figure 2). The data points in her last T_3 phase indicate that administration of T_3 following withdrawal may produce improvement that exceeds the previous level attained with T_3. This is also seen in the tender point threshold of patient 3 in the second T_3 phase (Figure 1), and the mean symptom intensity of patient 2 in the second T_3 phase (Figure 3).

The lengths of time for the four patients after withdrawal of T_3 before measures worsened, and before subjective status became insufferable, were 7, 9, 10, and 30 days. Patients were crossed to the next phase if they requested it because of their subjective discomfort.

The null hypothesis being tested was that during T_3 phases, the proportion of data points above or below the celeration line would not significantly vary from the proportion in baseline phases. This null hypothesis is rejected based on the results of the graphed data.

Single Subject Analyses

Statistical analysis proved useful because the baseline trends in four graphs were accelerating and in five were decelerating. Statistical analysis helped determine that changes in data point trends in intervention phases were greater than what would have been predicted by continuation of the baseline trend.[35] Analyses also showed that the increased variability of data points indicated by visual inspection in the first placebo phases compared to baseline in eight graphs was not statistically significant.[32] (The eight are: the graphs of patients 1, 2, and 3 in Figure 1, patients 1, 2, and 3 in Figure 2, and patients 1 and 2 in Figure 3.) Testing for autocorrelation showed that no phase had a significant level of serial dependency, meaning that predictability of changes in data points was not significant.[29][33] Therefore, no data transformations were necessary before use of the two-standard deviation band method and reference to the probability table.

Statistical analyses involved: (1) the trend line method with reference to a probability table, and (2) the 2SD band method. Analysis of data contained in the graphs indicates statistically significant improvement in mean tender point sensitivity, pain distribution, and mean symptom intensity in T_3 phases, and worsening of these measures during placebo phases. This pattern of significant measures makes highly probable a functional relationship between the patients' use of supraphysiologic dosages of T_3 and improved FMS status.

There were two limitations, however, to the two methods of analysis used. First, a minimum of six data points per phase defines a stable trend, which is necessary to determine significance at the 0.05 level with the probability table.[32] If possible, a degree of stability should be established before the patient moves from one phase to the next.[29] In placebo phases following T_3 phases, however, 3 of 4 patients reported rapid and severe worsening of their FMS status, and this required a rapid cross back to a T_3 phase. This brief sojourn in placebo phases following T_3 phases did not allow accumulation of enough data points to establish a stable trend of changing FMS measures. However, Kazdin has pointed out that a trend of measures in one phase opposite to the direction expected by the trend in the previous phase still permits inferences to be drawn about the effects of treatment.[36]

Second, the brief time patients spent in placebo phases following T_3 phases did not allow data points for some measures to regress back within the 2SD band. Thus, although the trend during the placebo phase was back toward the 2SD band, data points remained outside the band. Because two successive data points outside the 2SD limit are considered significant, the data points during these phases would be misleading without use of visual inspection. A return of data points back to baseline, however, is not a requirement of the single subject design.[37] Even a leveling off of measures in placebo phases contrasted with favorable trends in active treatment phases is considered indicative of a therapeutic effect.[29] According to Hayes, if visual inspection indicates that measures improve faster during treatment phases than during withdrawal phases, this is evidence for a therapeutic effect.[37]

Tender Point Pressure/Pain Thresholds (Figure 1). Patients 1, 2, and 3 had been randomly assigned to a placebo phase following their baseline phases. According to the probability table, the proportion of data points above or below the celeration line in each patient's first placebo phase did not significantly differ from the proportion in baseline phases. In the first T_3 phase for patients 1, 2, and 3, the proportion of data points above the celeration line significantly differed

(P<0.05) from those in the baseline phase, showing an increase (improvement) in pressure/pain threshold. Patient 4 had been randomly assigned to a T_3 phase after her baseline phase. The proportion of her data points above the celeration line during the T_3 phase varied significantly (P<0.05) from that in the baseline phase, showing a significant increase in pressure/pain threshold. None of the subsequent phases for any of the patients contained a sufficient number of data points to make further proper use of the probability table.

For significance using the two standard deviation band method, two successive data points in a phase must fall outside the width of two standard deviations (−2SD to +2SD). According to this criterion, the data points in the first placebo phase of patients 1, 2, and 3 did not differ from those in the baseline phase. The points in the following T_3 phase did significantly differ (P<0.05), showing a significant increase in threshold. In the following placebo phase, data points of patients 2 and 3 did not fall outside the 2SD band, indicating a decrease in threshold. The two data points in this phase for patient 1 were above the +2SD limit, but visual inspection indicates a decline back toward the 2SD band. The second T_3 phase for patients 1, 2, and 3 were above the +2SD limit, indicating a significant increase in threshold. For patient 4, data points in both the first and second T_3 phases were outside +2SD, indicating a significant increase in threshold. Data points in both placebo phases did not show a significant difference from those in her baseline phase.

Pain Distribution (Figure 2). According to the probability table, data points did not significantly vary from baseline points in the first placebo phase for patients 1, 2, and 3. In the following T_3 phase, the proportion of data points below the celeration line was enough to reach statistical significance, indicating reduced distribution of pain. The number of data points below the celeration line in the first T_3 phase for patient 4 was sufficient to indicate statistically significant reduction in pain distribution. Other phases for the four patients did not contain enough data points for proper use of the probability table.

According to the 2SD band method, data points in the first placebo phase for patient 2 did not differ from those in baseline. However, for patients 1 and 3, data points fell below the −2SD limit, indicating reduced pain distribution. But during this phase, data points returned to the 2SD band. In the subsequent T_3 phase, data points for patients 1, 2, and 3 fell and remained below the −2SD limit. In the following placebo phase, data points for patients 2 and 3 reentered the 2SD

Patient 1

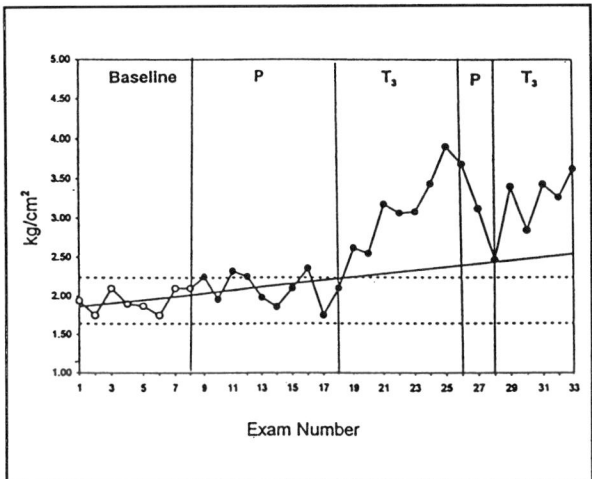

Patient 2

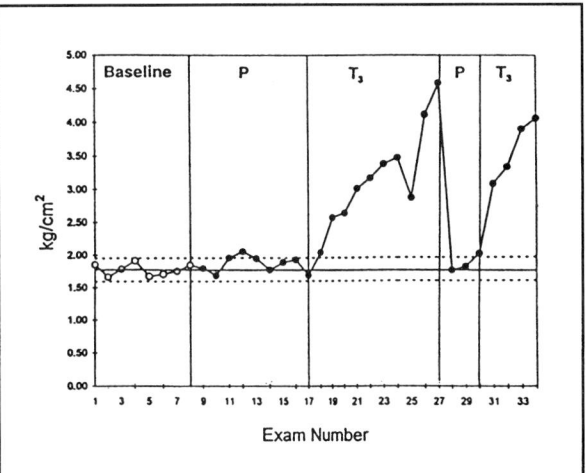

Patient 3

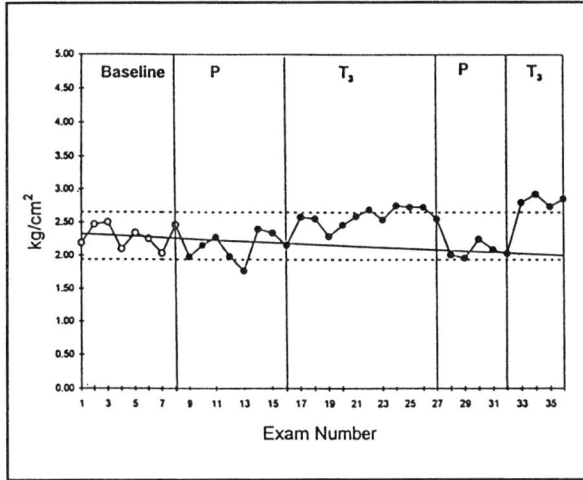

Patient 4

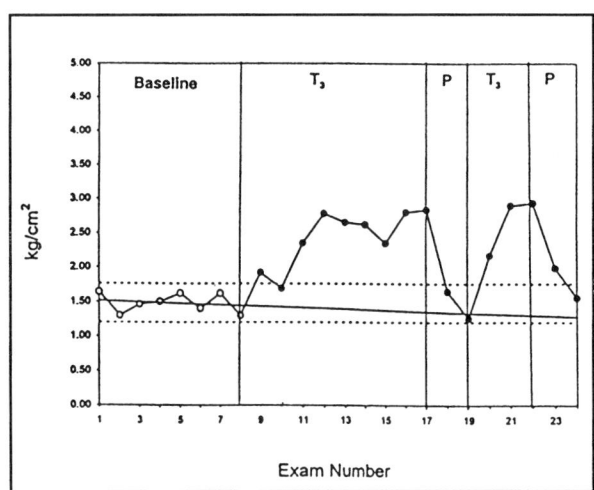

Figure 1. *Circles show the mean pressure/pain threshold of tender points in kg/cm² (higher kg/cm² is better, lower kg/cm² is worse) at each exam during baseline, T₃, and placebo (P) phases.* The straight solid line (the celeration line) in each graph represents the trend of data points through intervention phases predicted from the values of data points in the baseline phase. The two dotted lines represent the two standard deviation (2SD) band calculated from the values of data points in the baseline phase. Statistical significance during intervention phases was determined by the proportion of data points above or below the trend line or outside the 2SD band.

band. Data points for patient 1 in this placebo phase were just below the -2SD limit. For patient 4, data points in both T_3 phases were below the lower limit of the -2SD band, indicating reduced pain distribution, and in placebo phases were above the +2SD band, indicating increased pain distribution. Data points in the second T_3 phase for all patients dropped well below the -2SD band, indicating significantly reduced pain distribution.

Mean Symptom Intensity (Figure 3). In the first placebo phase for patients 1, 2, and 3, too few data points fell below the celeration line to reach significance. In the following T_3 phases, however, sufficient data points were located below the celeration line to indicate a decrease in mean symptom intensity that was significant at the 0.05 level. For patient 4, enough data points fell below the celeration line in her first T_3 phase to indicate a significant reduction in mean symptom intensity compared to baseline. No other phases contained enough data points to make further use of the probability table.

Not enough data points in the first placebo phase of patients 1, 2, and 3 fell outside the -2SD limit to indicate a significant reduction in mean symptom intensity. In the following T_3 phase, however, a sufficient number of data points fell below the -2SD band to show a significant reduction in mean symptom intensity. Data points in the second T_3 phase of each of these patients also fell below the -2SD limit, showing a significant reduction once again in mean symptom intensity. The data points in the second placebo phase for each of these three patients was also below the -2SD limit. While this indicates significance, the reverse direction of data points in the placebo phases from the previous and following T_3 phases for all three patients is strong evidence favoring an increase in mean symptom intensity during the placebo phases. For patient 4, enough data points in the first and second T_3 phases fell below the -2SD band to show a significant reduction in this measure. Data points in her two placebo phases were within the 2SD band, indicating no significant difference from baseline data points.

Group Comparison

Each patient completed two placebo and two T_3 phases. The highly significant difference in the mean values for the FIQ, Zung's, and pain distribution according to the ACR criteria, despite the small number of patients,[68,pp.257-258] indicates T_3's strong therapeutic impact on euthyroid FMS status. Effective dosages of T_3 for the four patients were 118.75, 131.25, 137.50,

and 162.50 mcg. All patients continued their use of T_3 after the last phase, through the time of follow-up, and after follow-up.

Fibromyalgia Impact Questionnaire and Zung's Self-Rating Depression Scale. Table 1 shows the group comparison results (all four patients) for the FIQ and Zung's measures. Mean values for T_3 phases indicate highly significant improvement on both measures when compared to mean values for placebo phases.

ACR Criteria for Pain Distribution. Pain distribution was markedly higher during placebo phases and lower in T_3 phases according to the ACR method for assessing pain distribution (possible scores are 0-1-2-3). Mean scores appear in Table 1.

Safety Assessment. WEIGHT. Patients' weights significantly decreased during T_3 phases (P=0.033). Mean placebo weight was 136.00 lbs, and mean T_3 weight was 133.19 lbs.

CARDIAC EFFECTS. Mean heart rate significantly increased from 68.56 bpm in placebo phases to 83.94 bpm in T_3 phases (P=0.022). No patient developed tachycardia. PR intervals shortened in T_3 phases, but the difference did not reach significance (P= 0.291). QRS intervals lengthened in T_3 phases, but the difference was not significant (P= 0.351). QT intervals significantly shortened within the normal range during T_3 phases (P= 0.027). The mean placebo QT interval was 0.39 sec; the mean T_3 interval was 0.35 sec. All ST segments were within normal limits in all phases. There was no significant difference in systolic blood pressures between T_3 and placebo phases (P= 0.763), and no difference in diastolic blood pressures (P=0.709).

THYROID FUNCTION TESTS. Baseline third-generation TSH, T_4, T_3 uptake, and FTI were within the normal range for all patients. At 4-month follow-up, these values as well as the free T_4 and free T_3 were indicative of T_3-toxicosis (though these patients clearly did not have clinical features of thyrotoxicosis). Low values included a mean TSH concentration of 0.13±0.13 μU per milliliter, a mean total T_4 of 3.60±0.52 μg per deciliter, a mean FTI of 0.93±0.13, and a mean free T_4 of 0.56±0.07 ng per deciliter. The mean T_3 uptake of 27.00±2.94% was within the normal range. The mean free T_3 of 8.50±3.44 pg per milliliter was high.

MUSCLE EFFECT. At 4-month follow-up, both mean serum (0.90 ±0.082 mg per deciliter) and urinary creatinine (1010.00±54.14 ng per 24 hours) were normal, indicating normal muscle mass.

OSSEOUS EFFECTS. At follow-up, mean urinary calcium (234.75±75.55 mg per 24-hours) and phos-

Patient 1

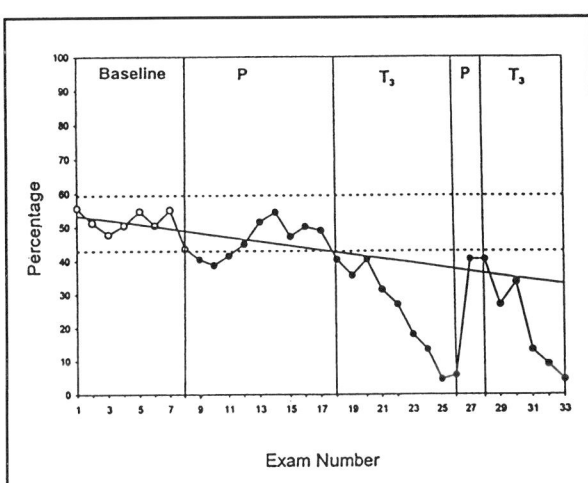

Patient 2

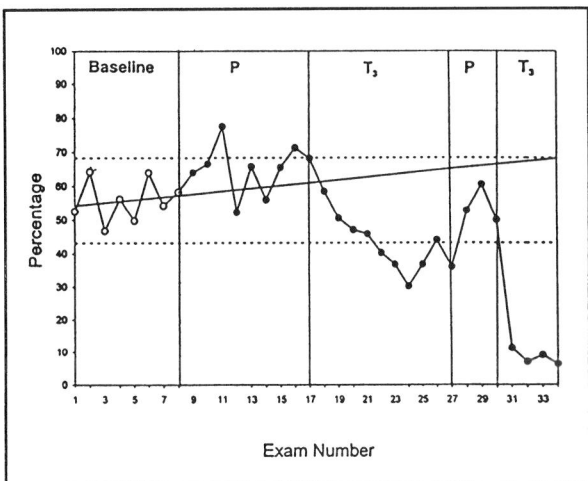

Patient 3

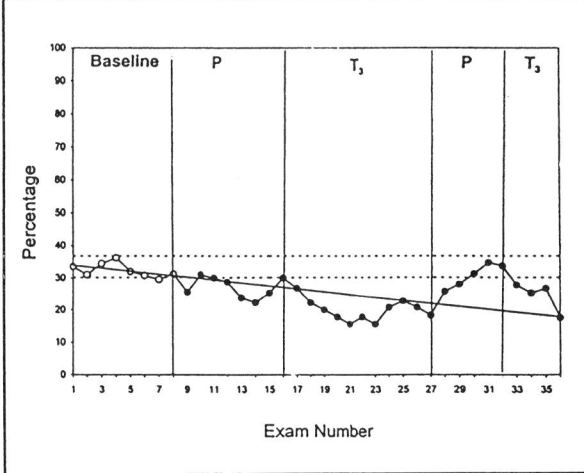

Patient 4

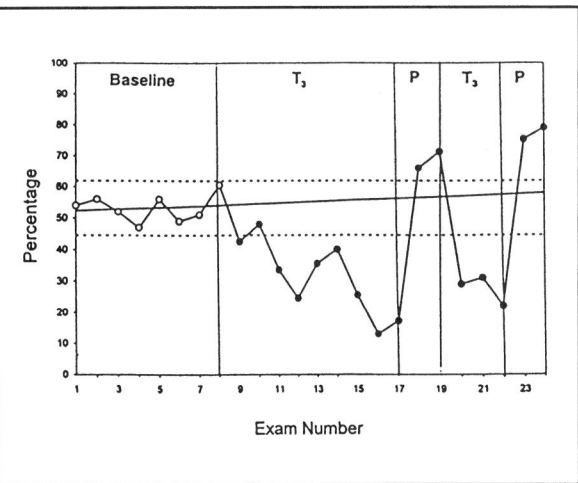

Figure 2. *Circles show the percentage of 36 body divisions containing pain (range: 0%-to-100%) at each exam during baseline, T₃, and placebo (P) phases.* The straight solid line (the celeration line) in each graph represents the trend of data points through intervention phases predicted from the values of data points in the baseline phase. The two dotted lines represent the two standard deviation (2SD) band calculated from the values of data points in the baseline phase. Statistical significance during intervention phases was determined by the proportion of data points above or below the trend line or outside the 2SD band.

phorus (845.25±247.87 mg per 24-hours) were normal. Mean urinary N-telopeptides (121±52.34 nMole of bone collagen equivalents per μMole of creatinine) was high, indicating increased bone turnover. Mean serum phosphorus (3.73±0.61 mg per deciliter) and alkaline phosphatase (57.25±21.00 IU per liter) were normal. Compared to reference standards, bone densitometry showed normal bone density. Density of the trochanter was 100.53±3.90% of age matched controls, the femoral neck was 101.35±6.68%, Ward's triangle was 101.25±9.43%, and the lumbar spine was 101.95±6.74%.

LIVER FUNCTION TESTS. At follow-up, our patients had normal values for mean ALT (27.50±14.82 U per liter) and GGPT (17.50±15.09 U per liter). Other liver function test results were also within normal limits.

DISCUSSION

We conclude that FMS status in our four euthyroid patients, compared to their baseline status, significantly improved with supraphysiologic dosages of T$_3$ and significantly deteriorated with T$_3$'s withdrawal during placebo phases. Both visual inspection and quantitative analyses of the data justify a causal inference regarding T$_3$ therapy and improved FMS status in these patients. Traditional group statistics showed significant improvement in mean scores for the FIQ, Zung's, and pain distribution according to the ACR method. These statistics confirm the outcome of Lowe's previous study showing effectiveness of T$_3$ therapy for euthyroid FMS.[26] By the end of the study, none of the four patients met the diagnostic criteria for FMS.

The ABAB single subject design provided strong evidence of therapeutic responses by each patient. This design is considered "very powerful" because causal inferences, based on results, can be drawn.[29,p.91] The inferences that can be drawn from the results of our study are that it is highly improbable that chance improvement and deterioration in FMS measures coincidentally matched repeated application and withdrawal of T$_3$.[29,p.46] According to the logical principle of Mills' method of concomitant variation,[67,p.393] application and withdrawal of T$_3$ can be inferred to have "caused" the improvement and deterioration in our patients.

After a stable baseline, FMS measures changed in T$_3$ and placebo phases in different directions. Favorable changes in FMS status occurred with administration and readministration of T$_3$. Unfavorable

changes occurred with withdrawal and rewithdrawal of T$_3$ during placebo phases. This pattern, shown through both visual and quantitative analyses, makes it highly probable that improvement in FMS status was functionally related to patients' use of T$_3$, and deterioration of FMS status was functionally related to withdrawal of T$_3$.[29] The probability that this conclusion is correct is expressed in Barlow and Hersen's "principle of unlikely successive coincidences."[38] With each successive pattern of change corresponding to administration and withdrawal of T$_3$, it becomes increasingly unlikely that any change in status can be attributed to coincidence or extraneous variables.[29] The similar response pattern in all four patients increases the likelihood that the pattern was real and not an artifact of the patient or setting. Individual graphs for different measures show that all patients responded in a similar fashion, although the magnitude of improvement varied between patients.

Our data show that withdrawal or readministration of T$_3$ therapy may be followed by a rebound in some measures. With withdrawal, measures may worsen compared to the patient's baseline values. And with readministration, measures may improve beyond the level previously attained with T$_3$.

Adverse Target Tissue Effects

Ross has written that to avoid adverse effects of thyroid hormone overstimulation, such as cardiac abnormalities and reduced bone density in premenopausal women,[39] patients' TSH levels should be kept within the normal range. However, our results and those of Lowe and colleagues[26] indicate that this may not be true of euthyroid FMS patients. Our patients continued to use T$_3$ after the last phase of the study. At 4-month follow-up, they had TSH levels lower than normal, but cardiac monitoring and follow-up biochemical and densitometry testing showed no clinically significant adverse effects.

Heart. Overt hyperthyroidism may profoundly affect the heart,[40] resulting in tachyarrhythmias[41] and dysrhythmias.[42] Thyroid hormone overstimulation, as in T$_3$-thyrotoxicosis, may lead to atrial fibrillation, premature ventricular beats, paroxysmal supraventricular tachycardia, atrial flutter, and congestive heart failure.[43] In thyrotoxicosis, there are no specific identifiable electrocardiographic changes.[40] Nonspecific changes, however, may include elevated ST segments, shortened QT intervals,[44] prolonged PR intervals, Wolf-Parkinson-White syndrome, and complete right bundle-branch block.[45] Half of thyrotoxic patients have sinus tachycardia. One tenth of hyper-

Patient 1

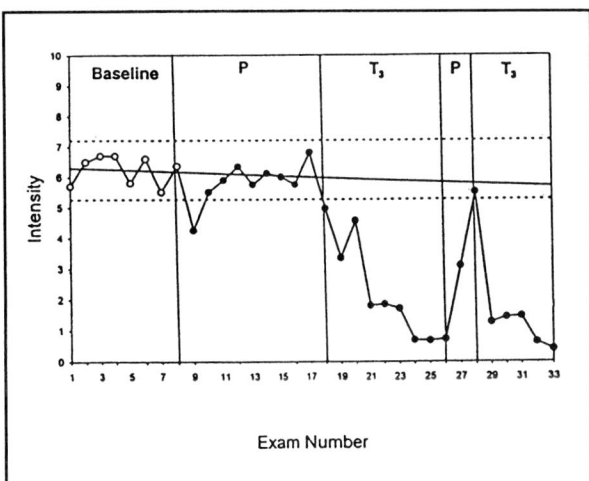

Patient 2

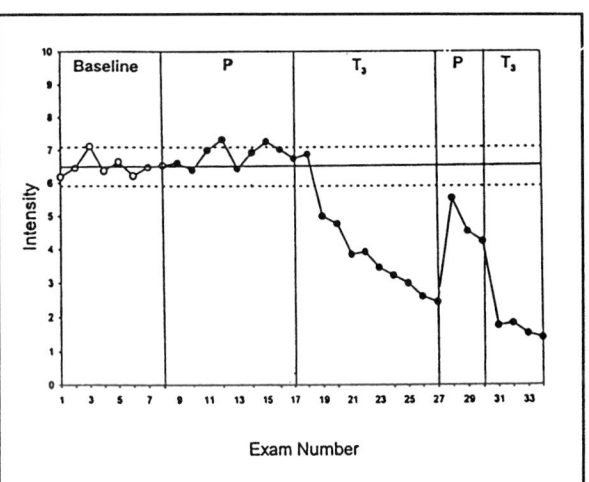

Patient 3

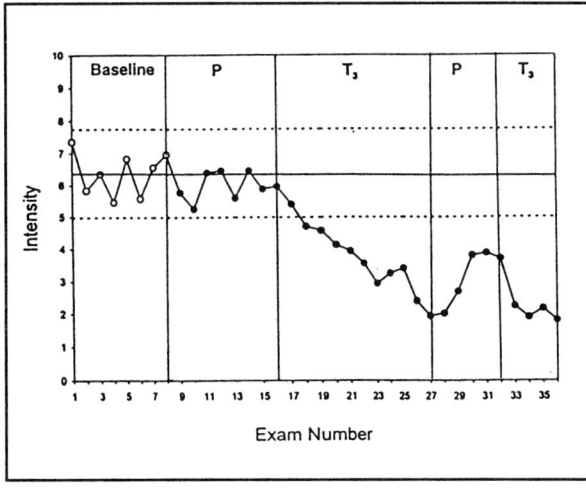

Patient 4

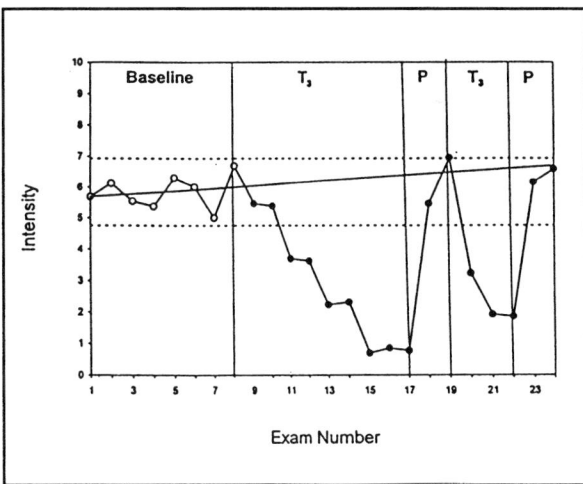

Figure 3. *Circles show the mean intensity of FMS symptoms, 0 (best)-to-10 (worst) VAS scale, at each exam during baseline, T₃, and placebo (P) phases.* The straight solid line (the celeration line) in each graph represents the trend of data points through intervention phases predicted from the values of data points in the baseline phase. The two dotted lines represent the two standard deviation (2SD) band calculated from the values of data points in the baseline phase. Statistical significance during intervention phases was determined by the proportion of data points above or below the trend line or outside the 2SD band.

thyroid patients have persistent atrial fibrillation.[46][47] Even small increases in thyroid hormone levels within the normal range that suppress TSH levels may adversely affect the heart.[39] Subclinical hyperthyroidism, for example, may aggravate angina pectoris or congestive heart failure.[39] None of our four patients had any detectable adverse cardiac effects from supraphysiologic dosages of T_3. All ECGs were normal throughout the 9-month study and at 4-month follow-up. This finding suggests partial resistance of cardiac regulatory mechanisms to thyroid hormone.

Muscle. Thyroid hormone surplus in non-thyroid hormone resistant individuals is associated with excessive protein catabolism, tissue wasting, and weight loss.[48][49] Our patients' weights did significantly differ between T_3 and placebo phases (P=0.033). Their serum and urinary creatinine were normal, indicating absence of catabolic effect on muscle despite use of supraphysiologic dosages of T_3. The mean weight loss of 2.81 lbs may represent fat loss. This is likely because the patients, according to their protocol agreement, began exercising to tolerance during the first phase of the study.

Bone. Studies indicate that slightly TSH-suppressive dosages of exogenous thyroid hormone do not correlate with loss of bone mineral density.[50][51][52][53][54][55] However, possible adverse osseous effects are of concern when patients are taking highly TSH-suppressive dosages. Dual photon absorptiometry of our four patients showed normal bone density even though they had been taking TSH-suppressive doses of T_3 for several months. This indicates that their bones may be among the tissues resistant to thyroid hormone, and demonstrates that, at 4 month follow-up, their supraphysiologic doses of T_3 had not adversely affected their bones.

At 4-month follow-up, testing showed slightly abnormal values for only one biochemical marker. Increased cross-linked N-telopeptides indicate increased bone turnover. However, our patients' normal bone densities support the view that such abnormal biochemical markers may be clinically insignificant.[63] Other researchers have also found normal bone density despite abnormal biochemical markers.[64] De Rosa reported that while TSH-suppressive dosages of thyroid hormone can activate bone turnover, they constitute neither an actual risk factor for bone loss nor for osteoporotic fractures.[54] The cumulative evidence supports this conclusion, at least for premenopausal women.[65] (All patients in our study were premenopausal.) Tremollieres and colleagues reported that biochemical markers and reduced bone density found

during the first year of exogenous thyroid hormone use were followed by a complete recovery of normal values during the second year.[66] They proposed that "transitory" bone loss might result from temporary "hypersensitivity" of hypothyroid bone to thyroid hormone. The same may be true of peripheral tissues previously hypometabolic due to partial resistance to thyroid hormone.

The N-telopeptide results in our patients can be used as baseline measures for one-year and two-year follow-up. Long-term follow-up is warranted for all patients taking TSH-suppressive dosages of T_3.

Liver. Despite our patients' use of supraphysiologic dosages of T_3, they did not show the significant elevations in serum alanine aminotransferase (ALT) and γ-glutamyl transpeptidase (GGPT) that have been reported in subclinical hyperthyroidism.[48]

Implications for the Pathophysiology of FMS

Our four patients significantly improved according to five FMS measures, without adverse target tissue effects, only with supraphysiologic doses of T_3. Be-cause of this, these patients resemble patients with thyroid hormone resistance syndromes due to muta-tions in the c-erbAβ₁ gene in chromosome 3.[56]

There are a variety of clinical phenotypes of thyroid hormone resistance syndrome with distinguishing clinical features resulting from differential target tissue resistance to thyroid hormone.[56][57] The results of this study and similar results by Sonkin[15] and by Lowe and colleagues[24][25][26] raise the possibility that euthyroid FMS is another clinical phenotype of thyroid hormone resistance. The patients in this study would be classified as having *peripheral* resistance to thyroid hormone rather than pituitary or general resistance.[56][58] This distinction is based on suppression of TSH levels in our patients by supraphysiologic dosages of T_3, showing that their pituitary glands are normally responsive to the hormone. However, recent convention defines hormone resistance as conditions caused by defects at the site of hormone action or at the receptor level.[56,p.349] Because of this convention, determination of thyroid hormone resistance in our four patients would depend on the results of evaluation by molecular biological techniques.

Dosages of T_3 necessary for eumetabolism in athyreotic patients have been given variously as 25-to-75 mcg[59] and 50-to-75 mcg per day.[57] Significant therapeutic improvement occurred in our patients only with dosages ranging from 118.75-to-162.50 mcg. In all patients, these dosages induced low TSH, FTI, and total and free T_4, and high levels of free T_3. This pattern of laboratory values in patients taking exo-genous T_3 has been defined as T_3-toxicosis.[60] Our patients, however, exhibited no clinical features of thyrotoxicosis. In addition, the results of their electro-cardiography, bone densitometry, and most laboratory tests were within normal range.

General resistance to thyroid hormone is due to mutations in the c-*erb*Aβ_1 gene in chromosome 3.[56] Mutant thyroid hormone receptors properly regulate transcription only when they are exposed to high levels of T_3. To illustrate, the mutant receptor P448H,

has a low affinity for T_3, is transcriptionally inactive, and inhibits normal thyroid hormone receptors when exposed to low levels of T_3. But when exposed to high levels of T_3, the P448H receptor becomes transcriptionally active, and ceases its dominant negative inhibition of normal receptors so that they also become transcriptionally active.[61] It is possible, then, that mutant thyroid hormone receptors are responsible for our patients' therapeutic response only to high T_3 dosages.[23] This can only be determined, however, with sequencing of the c-*erb*Aβ_1 gene from these patients.

Table 1. Fibromyalgia Measurement Group Results

All Patients	Worst Possible	Best Possible	Mean Placebo	Mean T_3	Significance
Fibromyalgia Impact Ques.	80	0	54.97	13.71	$P < 0.0005$
Zung's Depression Scale	80	20	43.75	31.75	$P < 0.0000$
Pain Distribution (ACR)	3	0	3.00	1.75	$P = 0.0190$

Clinical Decisions in this Study

Decisions to change T_3 dosages and to cross patients from one phase to another in this study were response-driven; that is, a patient's response in each phase was the basis of the clinical decisions made during that phase. A patient's "response" consisted of changes in objective FMS measures, the patient's subjective estimate of her status, results of a physical examination, and nonquantified changes in the patient observed by the clinician. The repeatability of this study in the future will critically depend upon researchers making proper use of all these factors.

Our methodology is likely to be criticized because patient management was based in part on a clinician's judgment of patient response (though, both clinician and patient remained blinded). In the best of circumstances in clinical trials, assessment of patient status is reduced to easily measurable criteria. Long-term clinical use of the protocol tested in this study, however, has shown that this is not entirely possible at this time. As most fibromyalgia patients undergo treatment with thyroid hormone, some changes that are difficult to quantify may be obvious to varying degrees to the experienced clinician who is familiar with the indivi-

dual patient. The changes typically signify improving patient status, and their failure to occur may indicate the need to titrate the T_3 dosage. When considered with the outcome of the objective measures, these phenomena may contribute substantially to proper clinical decisions. We will mention a few of these changes that occurred in each of the four patients in this study.

One was a change from a slow relaxation phase of the Achilles reflex to a speed roughly equal to the contraction phase. Although the speed of the reflex can be objectively measured, we did not do so. Nevertheless, as Sonkin wrote, the change is obvious to the clinician experienced at testing the reflex.[15] Other, more difficult to define responses were: a change from a torpid and pensive facial expression to a zestful expression, and a distinct change in the eyes from a dull, listless appearance to an energetic, alert appearance. Another response that some clinicians are likely to imprudently ignore or reject is a pronouncement by the patient that she is well. These changes occur and persist in many, although not all, FMS patients who benefit from thyroid hormone therapy. When a patient responds in such ways, it is judicious for the clinician to note the responses and calculate them into judgment of the patient's FMS status. To ignore or otherwise exclude such phenomena from patient assessment is to forfeit one of the richest sources of data upon which to base sound clinical judgment. The blinded clinical decisions in this study were based partly on such patient responses.

We also used line graphs to observe trends in data points that represented mean scores from FMS measures. These provided objective data to calculate into therapeutic decisions. Although clinical judgment of a patient's status influenced clinical decisions, decisions were primarily data-driven by the scores on the objective measures.

Implications for Clinical Practice

During the treatment of euthyroid patients with T_3, objective FMS measures of some patients show favorable trends in FMS status before the patients are subjectively aware of improvement, and before any of the responses mentioned above are obvious to the clinician. With other patients, subjective changes precede those of objective measures. The pattern for any particular patient becomes apparent only as therapy progresses. In any case, there is little temporal discrepancy between the two types of data, and therapeutic decisions are best made by considering both.

The empirical feedback from graphed single subject data provides a high level of control in patient management, and aids judgment regarding T_3 dosage adjustments. By referring to established patterns of therapeutic response such as those shown in the graphs from this study, the clinician can formulate proper expectations regarding clinical outcome. The graphs can help him or her determine whether a particular patient is responding with a pattern that represents therapeutic change.

CONCLUSION

The visual and quantitative outcomes of this ABAB single subject study lead to a highly probable inference: that repeated improvements in the FMS status of our four patients was a function of their repeated use of T_3, and that repeated deterioration in their FMS status was a function of their repeated alternate use of a placebo. We therefore conclude that in these four euthyroid patients, the use of supraphysiologic doses of T_3 significantly improved FMS status. By the end of the study, all four patients no longer met the diagnostic criteria for FMS. No medications other than T_3 were necessary. Safety testing at

4-month follow-up showed no clinically significant indications of thyrotoxicosis, though all patients had continued their use of T_3. The absence of adverse target tissue effects, and normal pituitary responsiveness shown by TSH suppression, suggests that in these patients, FMS is a clinical phenotype of partial peripheral resistance to thyroid hormone.

The process of change when T_3 was administered and withdrawn repeatedly is depicted on line graphs. These graphs may serve as guides to proper patient responses to the administration and withdrawal of T_3 therapy. The use of similar graphs can serve as an aid to clinicians in deciding proper T_3 dosage adjustments, and can maintain patient progress along a data-driven path.

ACKNOWLEDGMENTS

The authors would like to thank David G. Simons, M.D. for his suggestion on methods for quantitative analysis of single subject data, and Richard L. Garrison, MD for his recommendation of the response-driven crossover design. We would also like to thank our two consultant peer-reviewers for providing independent blinded reviews of this paper. We give special thanks to our study patients for enduring placebo phases.

REFERENCES

1. Wolfe, F., Smythe, H.A., Yunus, M.B., et al.: The American College of Rheumatology 1990 criteria for the classification of fibromyalgia: report of the multicenter criteria committee. *Arthritis Rheumatol.*, 33:160-172, 1990.
2. Consensus Document on Fibromyalgia: The Copenhagen Declaration. Copenhagen, Myopain '92, 17-20 August, 1992. *J. Musculoskel. Pain*, 1(3/4):295-312, 1993.
3. Wolfe, F.: Aspects of the epidemiology of fibromyalgia. *J. Musculoskel. Pain*, 2(3):65-77, 1994.
4. Carette, S.: What have clinical trials taught us about the treatment of fibromyalgia? *J. Musculoskel. Pain*, 3:133-140, 1995.
5. Lowe, J.C.: T_3-induced recovery from fibromyalgia by a hypothyroid patient resistant to T_4 and desiccated thyroid. *J. Myofascial. Ther.*, 1(4):26-31, 1995.
6. Beetham, W.P., Jr.: Diagnosis and management of fibrositis syndrome and psychogenic rheumatism. *Med. Clin. North Am.*, 63:433-439, 1979.
7. Golding, D.N.: Hypothyroidism presenting with musculoskeletal symptoms. *Ann. Rheumatic. Dis.* 29:10-41, 1970.
8. Bland, J.H. and Frymoyer, J.W.: Rheumatic syndromes of myxedema. *N. Eng. J. Med.*, 282:1171-1174, 1970.
9. Wilke, S.W., Sheeler, L.R., and Makarowski, W.S.: Hypothyroidism with presenting symptoms of fibrositis. *J. Rheumatol.*, 8:627-630, 1981.

10. Hochberg, M.C., Koppes, G.M., Edwards, C.Q., Barnes, H.V., and Arnett, F.C., Jr.: Hypothyroidism presenting as a polymyositis-like syndrome: report of two cases. *Arthritis Rheum.*, 19:1363-1366, 1976.

11. Delamere, J.P., Scott, D.L., and Felix-Davies, D.D.: Thyroid dysfunction and rheumatic diseases. *J. Royal Soc. Med.*, 75:102, 1982.

12. Fessel, W. J.: Myopathy of hypothyroidism. *Ann. Rheuma-tic Dis.*, 27:590-596, 1968.

13. Wilson, J. and Walton, J.N.: Some muscular manifestations of hypothyroidism. *J. Neurol. Neurosurg. Psychiat.*, 22:320-324, 1959.

14. Awad, E.A.: Histopathological changes in fibrositis. In *Advances in Pain Research and Therapy*, vol. 17. Edited by J.R. Fricton and E.A. Awad, New York, Raven Press, 1990, pp.249-258.

15. Sonkin, L.S.: Endocrine disorders and muscle dysfunction. In *Clinical management of Head, Neck, and TMJ Pain and Dysfunction*. Edited by B. Gelb, Philadelphia, W.B. Saunders Co., 1985, pp.137-170.

16. Hershman, J.M.: Hypothalamic and pituitary hypothyroidism. In *Progress in the Diagnosis and Treatment of Hypothyroid Conditions*. Edited by P.A. Bastenie, M. Bonnyns, and L. VanHaelst, Amsterdam, Excerpta Medica, 1980, pp.41-50.

17. Eisinger, J., Arroyo, P.H., Calendini, C., Rinaldi, .JP., Combes, R., and Fontaine, G.: Anomalies biologiques au cours des fibromylalgies: III. Explorations endocriniennes. *Lyon Méditerranée Méd.*, 28: 858-860, 1992.

18. Gerwin, R.: A study of 96 subjects examined both for fibromyalgia and myofascial pain. *J. Musculoskel. Pain*, 3:(Suppl.)1:121, 1995.

19. Lowe, J.C.: Thyroid status of 38 fibromyalgia patients: implications for the etiology of fibromyalgia. *Clin. Bull. Myofascial.Ther.*, 2(1):36-41, 1997.

20. Shiroky, J.B., Cohen, M., Ballachey, M-L., and Neville, C.: Thyroid dysfunction in rheumatoid arthritis: a controlled prospective survey. *Ann .Rheumat. Dis.*, 52:454-456, 1993.

21. Ferraccioli, G., Cavalieri, F., Salaffi, F., et al.: Neuroendo-crinologic findings in primary fibromyalgia (soft tissue chronic pain syndrome) and in other chronic rheumatic conditions (rheumatoid arthritis, low back pain). *J. Rheumatol.*, 17:869-873, 1990.

22. Neeck, G. and Riedel, W.: Thyroid function in patients with fibromyalgia syndrome. *J. Rheumatol.*, 19:1120-1122, 1992.

23. Lowe, J.C., Cullum, M., Graf, L., Jr, and Yellin, J.: Mutations in the c-erbAβ₁ gene: do they underlie euthyroid fibromyalgia? *Med. Hypotheses*, 48(2)Feb.:125-135, 1997.

24. Lowe, J.C., Eichelberger, J., Manso, G., and Peterson, K.: Improvement in euthyroid fibromyalgia patients treated with T₃ (tri-iodothyronine). *J. Myofascial Ther.*, 1(2):16-27, 1994.

25. Lowe, J.C.: Results of an open trial of T₃ therapy with 77 euthyroid female fibromyalgia patients. *Clin. Bull. Myofascial Ther.*, 2(1):35-37, 1997.

26. Lowe, J.C., Garrison, R.L., Reichman, A.J., Yellin, J., Thompson, M., and Kaufman, D.: Effectiveness and safety of T₃ therapy for euthyroid fibromyalgia. *Clin. Bull. Myofascial Ther.*, 2(2/3):31-57, 1997.

27. Burckhardt, C.S., Clark, S.R., and Bennett, R.M.: The fibromyalgia impact questionnaire: development and validation. *J. Rheumatol.*, 18(5):728-733, 1991.

28. Naughton, M.J. and Wiklund, I.: A critical review of dimension-specific measures of health-related quality of life in cross-cultural research. *Quality Life Res.*, 2(6):397-432, 1993.

29. Ottenbacher, K.J.: *Evaluating Clinical Change: Strategies for Occupational and Physical Therapists.* Baltimore, Williams & Wilkins, 1986.

30. Bloom, M. and Fischer, J.: *Evaluating Practice: Guidelines for the Accountable Professional.* Englewood Cliffs, Prentice-Hall, 1982.

31. Parsonson, B.S. and Baer, D.M.: The analysis and presentation of graphic data. In *Single Subject Research: Strategies for Evaluating Change.* Edited by E.R. Kratochwill, New York, Academic Press, 1978.

32. Kazdin, A.E.: *Single-Case Research Designs: Methods for Clinical and Applied Settings.* New York, Oxford Univer-sity Press, 1982.

33. Jones, R.R., Weinrott, M.R., and Vaught, R.S.: Effects of serial dependency on the agreement between visual and statistical inferences. *J. Appl. Behav. Anal.*, 11:277-283, 1978.

34. Bloom , M.: *The Paradox of Helping: Introduction to the Philosophy of Scientific Practice.* New York: Macmillan, 1982.

35. De Prospero, A. and Cohen, S.: Inconsistent visual analysis of intrasubject data. *J. Appl. Behav. Anal.*, 12;573-579, 1979.

36. Kazdin, A.E.: Methodological and interpretive problems of single case experimental designs. *J. Consult. Clin. Psychol.*, 46:629-642, 1978.

37. Hayes, S.C.: Single case experimental design and empirical clinical practice. *J. Consult. Clin. Psychol.*, 49: 193-211, 1981.

38. Barlow, D.H. and Hersen, M.: Single-case experimental designs. *Arch. Gen. Psychiatry*, 29:319-325, 1973.

39. Ross, D.S.: Subclinical hyperthyroidism. In Werner and Ingbar's *The Thyroid: A Fundamental and Clinical Text*, 6th edition. Edited by L.E .Braverman and R.D. Utiger. Philadelphia, J.B. Lippincott, 1991, pp.1249-1255.

40. Dillman, W.H.: The cardiovascular system in thyrotoxicosis. In Werner and Ingbar's *The Thyroid: A Fundamental and Clinical Text.*, 6th edition. Edited by L.E .Braverman and R.D. Utiger, Philadelphia, J.B. Lippincott, 1991, pp.759-770.

41. Unger, J., Mavroudakis, N., Lipski, A., and van Coevorden, A.: Treatment of supraventricular tachyarrhythmias associated with hyperthyroidism by radioiodine, amiodarone, and propylthiouracil. *Thyroidology*, 3(2):85-88, 1991.

42. Symons, C. and Colquhoun, M.C.: Asymptomatic thyroiditis and atrial dysrhythmias. *Recent Progress in Diagnosis and Treatment of Hypothyroid Conditions.* Edited by P.A. Bastenie and M. Bonnyns, L. Vanhaelst, Amsterdam, Excerpta Medica, 1980, pp.137-143.

43. Vlase, H., Lungu, G., and Vlase, L.: Cardiac disturbances in thyrotoxicosis: diagnosis, incidence, clinical features,

and management. *Endocrinologie*, 29(3-4):155-160, 1991.

44. Hof, F.M., San, J.F.Y., and Lowrey, R.D.: The electrocardiogram in thyrotoxicosis. *Am. J. Cardiol.*, 8:893, 1960.

45. Muggia, A.L., Stjernholm, M., and Houle, T.: Complete heart block with thyrotoxic myocarditis. *N. Engl. J. Med.*, 283:1099, 1970.

46. Agner, T., Almdal, T., Thorsteinsson, B., and Agner, E.: A reevaluation of atrial fibrillation in thyrotoxicosis. *Dan. Med. Bull.*, 31:157, 1984.

47. Ciaccheri, M., Cecchi, F., Arcangeli C., et al.: Occult thyrotoxicosis in patients with chronic and paroxysmal isolated atrial fibrillation. *Clin. Cardiol.*, 7:413, 1984.

48. Gow, S.M., Caldwell, G., Toft, A.D., et al.: Relationship between pituitary and other target organ responsiveness in hypothyroid patients receiving thyroxine replacement. *J. Clin. Endocrinol. Metab.*, 64: 364, 1987.

49. Tepperman, J. and Tepperman, H.M.: *Metabolic and Endocrine Physiology*, 5th ed. Chicago, Year Book Medical Publishers, 1987.

50. Salmon, D., Rendell, M., and Williams, J.: Chemical Hyperthyroidism. *Arch. Intern. Med.*, 142: 571, 1982.

51. Fish, L.H., Schwartz, H.L., and Cavanaugh, J.: Replacement dose, metabolism, and bioavailability of levothyroxine in the treatment of hypothyroidism. *N. Engl. J. Med.*, 316:764, 1987.

52. Pearce, C.J. and Himsworth, R.L.: Total and free thyroid hormone concentrations in patients receiving maintenance replacement treatment with thyroxine. *Br. Med. J.*, 288: 693, 1984.

53. Bayer, M.F., Kriss, J.P., and McDougall, I.R.: Clinical experience with sensitive thyrotropin measurements: diagnostic and therapeutic implications. *J. Nucl. Med.*, 26:1248, 1985.

54. De Rosa, G., Testa, A., Maussier, M.L., Calla, C., Astazi, P., and Albanese, C.: A slightly suppressive dose of L-thyroxine does not affect bone turnover and bone mineral density in pre- and post-menopausal women with nontoxic goitre. *Hormone Metab. Res.*, 27(11):503-507, 1995.

55. Chabert-Orsini, V., Conte-Devolx, B., Thiers-Bautrant, D., et al.: Bone density after iatrogenic subclinical long-term thyrotoxicosis: measurement by dual photon absorptiom-etry. *Presse Med.*, 19: 1709-1711, 1990.

56. Refetoff, S., Weiss, R.E., and Usala, S.J.: The syndromes of resistance to thyroid hormone. *Endocrine Rev.*, 14:348-399, 1993.

57. Kaplan, M.M., Swartz, S.L., and Larsen, P.R.: Partial peri-pheral resistance to thyroid hormone. *Am. J. Med.*, 70: 1115-1121, 1981.

58. Refetoff, S.: Thyroid hormone resistance syndromes. In Werner and Ingbar's *The Thyroid: A Fundamental and Clinical Text*, 6th edition. Edited by L.E. Braverman and R.D. Utiger, Philadelphia, J.B. Lippincott, 1991, pp.1280-1294.

59. De Visscher, M.: The therapy of hypothyroid states. In *Recent Progress in Diagnosis and Treatment of Hypothyroid Conditions: Proceedings of the XVth International Congress of Therapeutics*, Amsterdam, Excerpta Medica, 1980, pp.105-114.

60. Ladenson, P.W.: Diagnosis of thyrotoxicosis. In Werner and Ingbar's *The Thyroid: A Fundamental and Clinical Text*, 6th edition. Edited by L.E. Braverman and R.D. Utiger, Philadelphia, J.B. Lippincott, 1991, pp.880-886.

61. Krishna, V., Chatterjee, K., Nagaya T, et al.: Thyroid hormone resistance syndrome: inhibition of normal receptor function by mutant thyroid hormone receptors. *J. Clin. Invest.*, 87:1977-1984, 1991.

62. Lowe, J.C., Reichman, A.J., Honeyman, G.S., and Yellin, J.: The thyroid status of fibromyalgia patients. *Clin. Bull. Myofascial Ther.*, 3(2):35, 1998.

63. Hamburger, J.I.: Strategies for cost-effective thyroid function testing with modern methods. In *Diagnostic Methods in Clinical Thyroidology*. Edited by J.I. Hamburger, New York, Springer-Verlag, 1989, pp.63-109.

64. Faber, J., Overgaard, K., Jarlov, A.E., and Christiansen, C.: Bone metabolism in premenopausal women with nontoxic goiter and reduced serum thyrotropin levels. *Thyroidology*, 6(1):27-32,1994.

65. Bartalena, L., and Pinchera, A.: Effects of thyroxine excess on peripheral organs. *Acta Medica Austriaca*, 21(2): 60-65, 1994.

66. Tremollieres, F., Pouilles, J.M., Louvet, J.P., and Ribot, C.: Transitory bone loss during substitution treatment for hypothyroidism: results of a two year prospective study. *Revue du Rhumatisme et des Maladies Osteo-Articulaires*, 58(12):869-875, 1991.

67. Copi, I.M.: *Introduction to Logic*, 4th edition. New York, Macmillan Pub. Co., Inc., 1972.

68. Norušis, M.J.: *The SPSS Guide to Data Analysis for SPSS/PC+*™, 2nd ed. Chicago, SPSS Inc., 1991.

Metabolic Therapy for Hypothyroid and Euthyroid Fibromyalgia: Two Case Reports

Gina S. Honeyman, DC

This article originally appeared in the *Clinical Bulletin of Myofascial Therapy*, 2(4):19-49, 1997.
It is reprinted with permission of Haworth Medical Press.

ABSTRACT. Fibromyalgia syndrome (FMS) is characterized by widespread pain and abnormal tenderness. The pain must be above and below the waist, on the right and left sides of the body, and in some axial region, all for longer than 3 months. I report the successful metabolic treatment of a hypothyroid FMS patient and a euthyroid FMS patient. Before beginning treatment, both patients met the American College of Rheumatology (ACR) criteria for FMS. By the 8th week of treatment, the euthyroid patient no longer met the ACR criteria; by the 14th week of treatment, the hypothyroid patient no longer met the criteria. The treatment protocol is multidisciplinary. Recovery of these two patients, managed at an independent clinical site, supports the effectiveness of the treatment itself for both hypothyroid and euthyroid FMS. The outcomes of the two cases are consistent with those reported in three systematic open trials and three double-blind trials. The metabolic therapy protocol developed by researchers at the Fibromyalgia Research Foundation appears to be a highly effective treatment for both euthyroid and hypothyroid FMS.

KEYWORDS. Fibromyalgia, hypothyroid, euthyroid, metabolic therapy, T_3, T_4, iron deficiency

INTRODUCTION

The American College of Rheumatology (ACR) established diagnostic criteria for fibromyalgia syndrome (FMS) in 1990.[1] The condition is characterized by widespread pain with abnormal tenderness in at least 11 of 18 specific body sites. The finding of low serotonin levels in FMS patients,[2][3][4][5][6][7] gave rise to the use of tricyclic antidepressant drugs for the condition. These drugs have provided only slight, brief improvement with a minority of patients. Long-term, these drugs have proven no more effective than placebos.[8][9][10][11][12] A recent report that a combination of fluoxetine (Prozac) and amitriptyline was effective in the treatment of FMS involved only short-term use of the drugs,[13] providing no evidence that this combination is any more effective than other antidepressants.

Lowe and colleagues argue that the low serotonin levels and all other symptoms and objective findings in FMS may result from inadequate thyroid hormone regulation of gene transcription.[14] Their hypothesis is supported by the outcome of three systematic open trials,[15][16][17] three double-blind trials,[18][19][20] and a case-control (long-term follow-up) study.[21] The metabolic treatment protocol tested in these studies involves the use of T_3 for euthyroid FMS patients, and T_4 for most hypothyroid FMS patients. The hormones, however, are used by patients only within the context of a broader-spectrum regimen designed to improved the patient's metabolism. Treatment is multidisciplinary, and may involve the use of myofascial therapy and chiropractic adjustments.

I report here the use and outcome of this metabolic protocol by a euthyroid FMS patient and a hypothyroid FMS patient. The euthyroid patient responded in a rapid and smooth fashion, but the hypothyroid patient's course of recovery was more complicated. These cases illustrate the use of the metabolic protocol and the variations in the course of patients' recovery. The complete relief of all features of FMS in these two patients is in line with the treatment outcome reported by Lowe and colleagues, and typifies the outcome with FMS patients in my practice. Such results support the hypothesis that FMS in most patients is caused by inadequate thyroid hormone regulation of transcription, regardless of the patient's laboratory thyroid function test results.

The descriptions below illustrate 1) the diagnostic and therapeutic aspects of the metabolic treatment protocol, and 2) the use of systematic monitoring of FMS status.

ASSESSMENT

The two patients I report here met the ACR criteria for FMS.[1] These criteria require that the patients have widespread pain with abnormal tenderness in at least 11 of 18 specific body sites. The patients must have pain above and below the waist, on the right and left sides of the body, and in some axial region for at least 3 months. For more precise quantification of the patients' FMS status, I also used the modified methods reported by Lowe and coworkers.[15][16][17] Specifically, I used algometry to quantitatively measure the pressure/pain threshold of potential tender points on the body (as outlined by the ACR).[1] Algometry provides greater accuracy and reliability than manual palpation of tender points.[29] I measured the patients' pain distribution as a percentage of 36 body divisions containing pain. This is a modification of the "rule of nines" method for assessing the percentage of the body affected in burn patients.[24][25] This method has been used in several recent FMS studies.[18][19][20][23] I measured the intensity of FMS symptoms as the mean score of 13 visual analog scales (VASs). I also used the FMS Impact Questionnaire[26] (which assesses the impact of FMS on a patient's life), and Zung's Self-Rating Depression Scale.[27][28]

Graphed Data. Scores from the five FMS measures were posted as data points to graphs (Figures 1-10). In the graph depicting tender point measurements, each data point represents the mean of the pressure/pain thresholds of the 16 points tested with algometry at each evaluation. In the graph for symptom intensity, each data point represents the mean intensity of 13 common FMS symptoms: pain, fatigue, stiffness, headache, sleep disturbance, bowel disturbance, depression, cognitive dysfunction (poor memory and concentration), anxiety, coldness, paresthesias (numbness and tingling), Sicca symptoms, and difficulty exercising. The patients indicated the intensity of each symptom by marking a 100 mm VAS, with 0 representing absence of the symptom and 10 representing extreme intensity. In the pain distribution graph, each data point represents the percentage of 36 body divisions containing pain. In the FIQ and Zung's graphs, each point represents the total score on each evaluation date.

Other Tests. I tested the Achilles reflex to assess the effect of thyroid hormone on each patient's neuromuscular system. The relaxation phase of the reflex is usually slow in hypothyroid patients[30] and in patients with euthyroid hypometabolism.[31] As Sonkin noted, the reflex is extremely useful for assessing the

metabolic effects of thyroid hormone therapy.[32] I also performed electrocardiograms (ECGs) on both patients before they began thyroid hormone therapy. And according to proper protocol, each FMS patient is tested for thyroid status before therapy. If a patient's suspected hypothyroid profile is within normal range, a TRH stimulation test is performed to test the function of the hypothalamic-pituitary-thyroid axis. Each patient is diagnosed as having either hypothyroid or euthyroid FMS.[22][34] I ordered a suspected hypothyroid profile for each patient, and a TRH stimulation test for patient #1, whose profile results were normal.

Proper Protocol. It is important to emphasize that the systematic monitoring I report here is *essential* to the effective use of the metabolic treatment protocol. The five FMS assessment measures, and the tests of peripheral indices of metabolic status (such as changes in resting pulse rate and in speed of the Achilles reflex), are indispensable tools for making strategic therapeutic decisions during the use of this protocol.[34] Because of the metabolic effects, patients undergoing this treatment are required to exercise regularly and to take nutritional supplementation. If a patient is not taking nutritional supplements at the first evaluation, I provide an instruction sheet explaining the necessary vitamins and minerals with the appropriate doses. I encourage patients to start with light exercise and gradually increase exertion as their metabolism improves after beginning exogenous thyroid hormone.

PATIENT #1: A CASE OF EUTHYROID FIBROMYALGIA

Patient History. Patient #1 was evaluated for FMS on February 12, 1997. She is a 43-year old homemaker, and she has not worked outside the home in 4 years because of the severity of her FMS. She complained of muscle and joint pain, stiffness, extreme fatigue, and daily headaches for 5 years. Sleep disturbance was severe: her sleep was usually non-restorative and she was often awakened by pain. She had a history of disturbed bowel function, with alternating constipation and diarrhea. Depression was diagnosed by her psychiatrist several months before she consulted me. Prozac had decreased her depression but had not affected her other symptoms. She had excessive cold sensitivity in most areas of her body, but her extremities were the most severely affected. She had constant numbness and tingling of her extremities and scalp. Her mucous membranes and skin were extremely dry. Poor memory and concentration had been severe. She had suffered from these symptoms for 5 years.

Her primary care physician diagnosed chronic fatigue syndrome in 1992. A rheumatologist diagnosed her with FMS in 1996 and prescribed tricyclic antidepressants, which she refused to take because of a disinclination to take medication. Her psychiatrist agreed with the diagnosis of FMS. He believed her depression was situational, but because he was concerned by the potential for suicide, he prescribed Prozac. Although the Prozac reduced her depression, she was tearful while I took her history, and she expressed a sense of desperation regarding her health and lifestyle.

Except for the decrease in depression with the use of Prozac, a range of conventional medications had failed to provide relief from her FMS symptoms. Her medications at the time of my initial exam included 20 mg Prozac daily; 2 mg Estrace administered on a monthly basis; 10 mg Ambien each night; and 500 mg Parafon forte, digestive aids, and Gaviscon as needed (prn). She has received chiropractic care from another chiropractic physician every 2 months for several years. She reported that this care temporarily increased her sense of well-being.

Patient Evaluation. The patient met the ACR criteria for FMS. In addition, she had a low mean tender point pressure/pain threshold, a high mean intensity of the 13 FMS symptoms, pain in 100% of 36 body divisions, a high FIQ score, and a slightly high Zung's score indicating mild depression. Table 1 shows the values of her five FMS measures at the initial evaluation, along with the range of possible scores.

I ordered a hypothyroid battery. Because the values were within normal range, I ordered a TRH stimulation test to rule out possible central hypothyroidism. This result was also normal.[22][34] Table 2 shows the ranges of normal and all of this patient's thyroid function test results.

Based on her FMS evaluation and thyroid function test results, I diagnosed patient #1 as euthyroid fibromyalgic. For treatment purposes, I considered the patient hypometabolic although euthyroid, in line with the theoretical position[14] and experimental findings[15][16][17][18][19][20][21] of Lowe and colleagues. A baseline ECG revealed normal sinus rhythm. The patient's height was 5 ft 2½ in; her weight was 186 lbs. Her blood pressure was 122/78 in the right arm (while sitting), and her resting pulse rate was 72 bpm. The relaxation phase of her Achilles reflex was visibly slow compared to the contraction phase.

When patients undergo metabolic therapy for FMS, weekly monitoring is necessary for those patients taking the more metabolically active form of

thyroid hormone, triiodothyronine or T_3. The purpose of this monitoring is to assess tissue response to both the thyroid hormone and the other aspects of the treatment protocol. I perform an algometry exam and check the patient's reflexes; the patient fills out the pencil and paper forms. I graph all the patient's scores in order to visually track changes in the patient's clinical status, and also for help in making decisions regarding dosage adjustments.

Table 1. Results for patient #1 at her initial exam on the five FMS measures (used for diagnosis and in monitoring for change during treatment).

Test	Range of Normal	Normal Cut-Off	Result
Mean Symptom Intensity	0-to-10		7.78
Pain Distribution	0-to-100%		100%
Fibromyalgia Impact Questionnaire	0-to-80		55.24
Mean Algometer Score		4 kg/cm² or above*	1.18 kg/cm²
Zung's Self-Rating Depression Scale		< 50	51

*In the past, the normal mean threshold was arbitrarily considered 4 kg/cm². Experimental results[18][19] and my clinical experience show that recovered patients, according to subjective assessment and other objective measures, often have mean thresholds below this value.

Treatment. Because euthyroid FMS patients typically do not benefit from thyroxine (T_4), patient #1 was treated with Cytomel (T_3). Her initial dose, started on 3/9/97, was 75 μg—the amount most euthyroid FMS patients of her size begin with.[34] She took the T_3 once per day on an empty stomach. She continued to take Prozac, Estrace, Ambien, and digestive aids. After two days, she experienced overstimulation in the form of irritability and fine tremors of her hands. Her resting pulse rate ranged between 88 and 92 bpm. Her dosage was reduced to 62.5 μg. On 3/13/97, four days after beginning the T_3, she again reported possible overstimulation with the same signs and symptoms as before. Her heart rate was still accelerated. She took a

20 mg propranolol tablet as a test. This reduced her heart rate to 80, and her tremors and irritability stopped. So, her dose was decreased to 50 µg. She had no symptoms of overstimulation at this dosage, which she has continued. On 3/21/97, she reported that she had discontinued the use of Prozac. She stated that she stopped the medication because she did not want to take it in the first place, and her depression had improved enough that she decided she did not need it. On this date, her Zung's score had not changed from its initial value, indicating mild depression. However, at her next evaluation on 4/2/97, her Zung's score decreased below the cut-off point for normal, indicating no depression. At subsequent evaluations, her Zung's scores decreased further into the range indicating no depression.

Table 2. Thyroid function test results for patient #1.

Thyroid Function Test	Range of Normal	Result
T_4	5.3-11.5 µg/dL	9.1 µg/dL
Free T_4 index	5.6-10.8	7.7
T_3 uptake	33.5-44.7%	33.9%
Basal TSH	0.4-5.5 µU/mL	2.7 µU/mL
TRH stimulation:		
—Baseline TSH	0.4-5.5 µU/mL	5.23 µU/mL
—30 min post-injection TSH, minus baseline	8.5-20.0 µU/mL[22]	19.43 µU/mL

Patient #1 used nutritional supplements as I had directed. These included antioxidants, B complex vitamins, minerals, and trace elements. On 4/2/97, she noted that her energy level had markedly increased while doing household activities. As her energy level rose further, she included walking regularly and strenuous housecleaning as exercise. Her exercise tolerance progressively increased during her metabolic treatment.

She has received chiropractic care from another physician every two months for several years. She continued this care at the same frequency during her metabolic treatment for FMS. I recommended myofascial therapy, and her other chiropractic physician has agreed to provide this. She no longer takes pain medication, including over-the-counter preparations. She has continued to take Ambien nightly to help her sleep, but states that she will discontinue its use as she can.

After each evaluation, scores for the five FMS measures were posted to the relevant graphs as data points. These are illustrated in Figures 1-5.

Results. Patient #1 responded very favorably to metabolic therapy. She no longer meets the criteria for the diagnosis of FMS, and she considers herself well. Table 3 shows the date of each evaluation and the score for each measure on each date.

TENDER POINTS. Figure 1 shows changes in the mean pressure/pain threshold of the patient's tender points, measured with algometry. The mean threshold increased from 1.18 kg/cm^2 on her initial visit before she began treatment, to 3.23 kg/cm^2 at her eighth evaluation (a 274% increase). We do not consider her FMS body sites abnormally tender now. In the past, the normal mean threshold was arbitrarily considered 4 kg/cm^2. Experimental results[18][19] and my clinical experience show that many patients who consider themselves recovered according to their subjective assessment, and according to other objective measures, still have mean tenderness values somewhat below 4 kg/cm^2. (See Figure 1)

MEAN SYMPTOM INTENSITY. This patient's mean intensity of the 13 most common FMS symptoms decreased from 7.78 to 1.57 out of a possible score of 10 (a 79.84% decrease). Figure 2 is her graph for symptom intensity.

PAIN DISTRIBUTION. On her initial visit to my office, this patient had pain in 100% of her body (all 36 divisions on the pain drawing). On her fifth visit about two months later, her pain distribution had decreased to 9%. She no longer met the ACR requirement for widespread pain. At her last three evaluations, she had no pain. Figure 3 shows her percentage of 36 body divisions containing pain at each evaluation.

FIQ. Patient #1's initial FIQ score was 55.24; her final score was 7.20 (a 86.96% decrease). The decreased score corresponds to her increase in functional abilities. Figure 4 shows her graphed scores on the FIQ.

ZUNG'S. At her initial evaluation, her Zung's score indicated mild depression. She reported that the Prozac she had taken for several months had diminished what had apparently been severe depression. No objective test results, however, were available to quantify her previous levels of depression. After 4 weeks of metabolic therapy, her Zung's score decreased into the normal range, indicating no depression. The score decreased further through the remainder of the her treatment (see Figure 5).

Outcome. Particularly important to this patient is that fatigue is no longer a problem for her. Her husband now complains he cannot keep up with her activity level. A high energy level was normal for her prior to the onset of FMS. She still has occasional gastric disturbance, but she is using a nutritional approach for this problem. She states that this approach has decreased the frequency of her GI symptoms. Rarely, she has a mild headache. Memory and concentration have noticeably improved. At her initial evaluation, she marked 7 (where 10 is the worst) on the visual analog scale for memory and concentration;

at her last visit, she marked 3. Her tolerance for exercise has also improved. This is shown by the change in her activity level. Before metabolic treatment, she was able to engage only in minimal activity. She and her husband have just returned from the first vacation she has consented to in several years. During this vacation, she engaged in snorkeling, swimming, hiking, and shell-collecting without any adverse consequences. She reported that in the past, barometric pressure changes associated with flying increased her pain. On this vacation, however, she had no pain during the flight from Tulsa to Hawaii.

Table 3. Score for patient #1 on each FMS measure at each evaluation.

Date	Mean kg/cm²	Mean Symptom Intensity	% of Body in Pain	FIQ	Zung's
2/12/97	1.18	7.78	100.00	55.24	51
3/14/97	1.13	7.66	86.25	53.94	51
3/21/97	1.34	7.00	57.00	32.47	51
4/02/97	2.00	4.41	31.50	16.39	41
4/09/97	2.48	2.46	9.00	7.77	35
4/17/97	2.81	2.92	0.00	5.63	29
5/05/97	2.99	1.21	0.00	2.83	29
5/22/97	3.23	1.57	0.00	7.20	29

It is noteworthy that this patient recovered from her FMS symptoms on 50 μg of T₃. Euthyroid FMS patients usually recover only with dosages considered supraphysiologic (75 μg to 160 μg of T₃[18][19]). According to Lowe,[33] rare euthyroid FMS patients recover only after reaching a daily dosage of 300 μg. On the other hand, a small percentage who had failed to benefit even from supraphysiologic doses of T₄ or desiccated thyroid have then improved or recovered with dosages as low as 25 μg of T₃.[33]

It is also worth noting that for four days during week 5 of her treatment, patient #1 mistakenly took 25 μg tablets rather than 50 μg tablets each day. Prior to this, she had experienced subjective improvement in

her FMS symptoms. By the time she realized she had taken only 25 μg tablets for four days, her subjective status had worsened. It improved again promptly after resuming the 50 μg dose.

At end of the systematic monitoring of this patient, her weight had decreased from 186 lbs to 162 lbs, her resting pulse rate was 76 bpm, and the relaxation phase of her Achilles reflex was equal in speed to that of the contraction phase.

I have released her from regular care as recovered, but will evaluate her status at monthly intervals. She will continue chiropractic care on a prn basis with her other physician.

PATIENT #2: A CASE OF HYPOTHYROID FIBROMYALGIA

Patient History. Patient #2, a 51-year old registered nurse, was evaluated for FMS on 12/6/96. She reported that her diffuse pain began 15 years ago. The etiology was unknown. She has had extreme fatigue for 7 years, also of unknown etiology. She reported a history of iron deficiency anemia, and she believed this was a contributing factor in her fatigue. She had occasional headaches, severe sleep disturbance, and mild stiffness in the mornings. Moderate depression was also a problem. She is perimenopausal and has had frequent heavy bleeding for several months. This patient also had a history of mitral valve prolapse which caused occasional dysrhythmia, primarily sinus tachycardia. She stated that maintaining a full-time administrative position with a home health care agency depleted her energy to the point that she no longer exercised.

Patient #2 had Lyme disease in 1991. This is a tick-transmitted, spirochetal, inflammatory infectious disorder.[39, p.1251] Infected patients usually have symptoms that may continue for weeks and that overlap

Table 4. Results for patient #2 at her initial exam on the five FMS measures (used for diagnosis and in monitoring for change during treatment).

Test	Range of Normal	Normal Cut-off	Result
Mean Symptom Intensity	0-to-10		6.20
Pain Distribution	0-to-100%		58.75%
Fibromyalgia Impact Questionnaire	0-to-80		50.45
Mean Algometer Score		4 kg/cm² or above*	1.36 kg/cm²
Zung's Self-Rating Depression Scale		< 50	51

*In the past, the normal mean threshold was arbitrarily considered 4 kg/cm². Experimental results[18][19] and my clinical experience show that recovered patients, according to subjective assessment and other objective measures, often have mean thresholds below this value.

Table 5. Thyroid function test results for patient #2.

Thyroid Function Test	Range of Normal	Result
T₄	5.3-11.5 µg/dL	11.3 µg/dL
Free T₄ index	5.6-10.8	11.3
T₃ uptake	33.5-44.7 %	40.0%
Basal TSH	0.4-5.5 µU/mL	0.06 µU/mL
TRH stimulation: —Baseline TSH	0.4-5.5 µU/mL	0.06 µU/mL
—30 min post-injection TSH, minus baseline	8.5-20.0 µU/mL[22]	0.01 µU/mL

with FMS. These include malaise and fatigue, headache, stiff neck, and myalgias. But Lyme disease can be distinguished from FMS by other features, such as an initial tick bite, characteristic skin lesions, nausea, vomiting, sore throat, lymphadenopathy, and arthralgias. Lyme disease is usually distinguished from rheumatoid arthritis by the absence of morning stiffness. This may also help distinguish Lyme disease from FMS, in that 77% of FMS patients report morning stiffness.[40] Lyme disease was not responsible for initiating this patient's FMS because her FMS preceded the Lyme disease. However, Lyme disease may have exacerbated her FMS for a time.

At her first evaluation, her medications included 75 mg Effexor tid, 2.5 mg Estrol bid, 1 tablet Norgesic qid, 10 mg Ambien nightly, and 0.15 mg Synthroid (T₄). Prior to switching to the T₄ on November 16, 1996, she had used 2 grains of Armour desiccated thyroid for approximately 1½ years. The Armour thyroid had no positive effect on her fibromyalgia symptoms. She was on a good regimen of nutritional supplements that included vitamins C, B-complex, E, D, calcium, iron, chromium, and other trace minerals. She also used 50 mg DHEA at the suggestion of her family practice physician. She has had chiropractic adjustments in the past with brief favorable results.

Patient Evaluation. This patient met the ACR criteria for FMS. She had a low mean pressure/pain threshold of her tender points, a high mean intensity of the 13 FMS symptoms, pain in over half the 36 body divisions, a high FIQ score, and a slightly high Zung's score indicating mild depression (see Table 4). Her height was 5 ft 7 in, her weight was 184 lbs, and her blood pressure was 140/78. The relaxation phase of her Achilles reflex was slow.

In anticipation of my evaluation, this patient's family practice physician ordered a suspected hypothyroid battery, and performed a TRH stimulation test two days prior to the patient's initial visit with me. The previous thyroid function test results that had established her primary hypothyroidism were not available. As a result of the diagnosis, she had taken desiccated thyroid (2 grains) or T_4 (0.15 mg) for a total of 1½ years. Although the TRH stimulation test can confirm primary hypothyroidism, it is not necessary when the condition is evident from the results of the hypothyroid laboratory profile.[34] The family practice physician, however, had already performed the TRH stimulation test result before the patient consulted me. According to the current paradigm in endocrinology, based on her basal TSH level and her 30-minute post-TRH injection TSH level, this patient's T_4 dosage would have been considered excessive. This conclusion, however, would have been erroneous (see below, THE USE OF TSH-SUPPRESSIVE DOSES OF T_4).

Table 6. Score for patient #2 on each FMS measure at each evaluation.

Date	Mean kg/cm^2	Mean Symptom Intensity	% of Body in Pain	FIQ	Zung's
12/06/96	1.36	6.20	58.75	50.45	51
12/26/96	1.68	4.23	13.25	*	*
1/08/97	1.52	4.77	28.50	42.81	51
1/17/97	1.75	5.85	39.25	20.39	51
1/31/97	2.18	2.61	14.50	23.02	41
2/19/97	2.88	1.72	13.50	7.99	35
3/06/97	2.61	1.70	4.50	10.86	29
3/20/97	2.52	3.00	4.50	27.98	29
4/08/97	2.62	3.61	17.75	44.67	43
4/16/97	3.93	4.45	5.50	49.40	46
4/30/97	3.65	2.45	2.00	24.15	38
5/14/97	4.01	2.07	0.00	12.79	30
5/28/97	3.77	1.84	4.50	16.70	35

* Note: The patient did not complete this form on this date.

Treatment. Patient #2 was taking 0.15 mg of T_4 at the time of my initial evaluation. Despite this dosage, she had signs and symptoms of hypometabolism: the phenotype referred to as FMS. Because of this, I recommended to the prescribing clinician that her T_4 dosage be increased to 0.20 mg. After 3 weeks (at her second evaluation), her mean symptom intensity decreased slightly, her pain distribution decreased substantially, and her mean tender point pressure/pain threshold increased slightly. The patient reported that she had less fatigue and that her pain, which was reduced in intensity, seemed less generalized. The pain localized to her neck and low back. The relaxation phase of her Achilles reflex remained slow.

Because 3 weeks is usually sufficient time for measurable changes in FMS status due to a dosage increase in hypothyroid fibromyalgia patients previously using T_4,[34] her dosage was increased to 0.30 mg. She tolerated this dosage well, and over the next 14 weeks, her subjective status improved. Her FMS

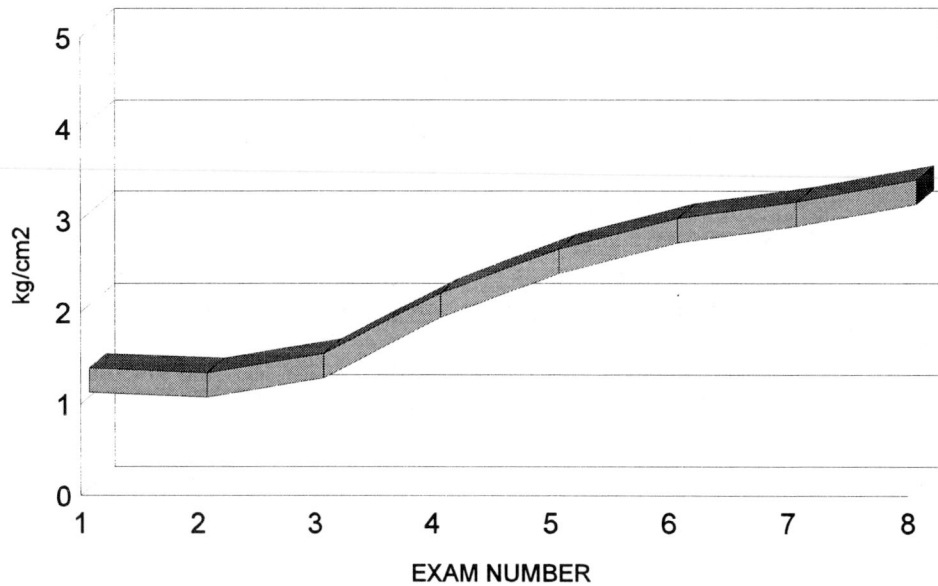

Figure 1. At each evaluation of patient #1, the mean of the pressure/pain thresholds of the 16 tender points was calculated and posted to the graph for that exam. The ribbon represents the trend of changing mean thresholds. The thin line at 4 kg/cm^2 represents the arbitrary cut-off point for normal. Scores below 4 kg/cm^2 were believed to be abnormal, and those above, normal.

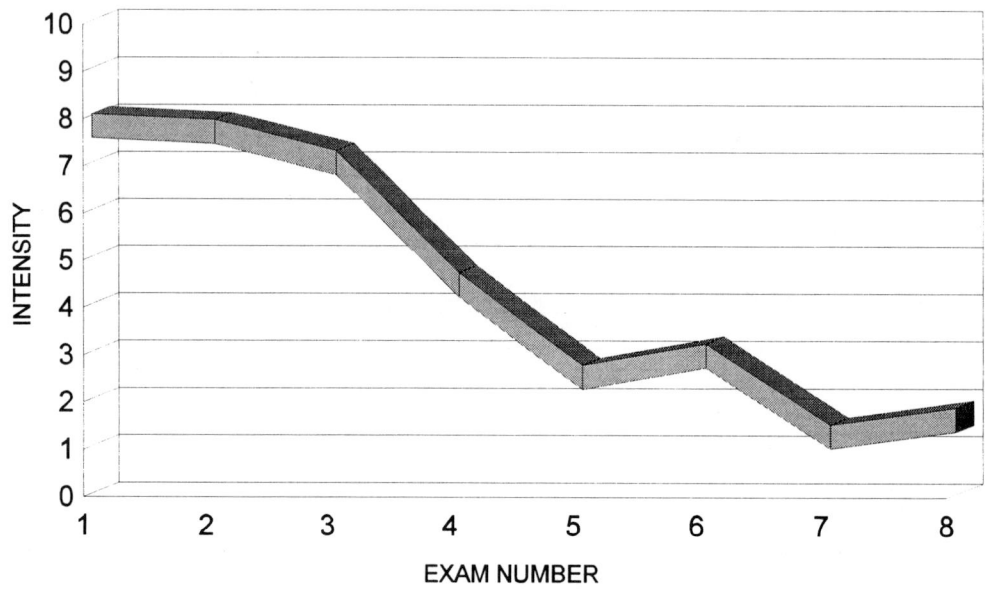

Figure 2. At each evaluation of patient #1, the mean intensity of 13 FMS symptoms (assessed by visual analog scales) was calculated and posted to the graph for that exam. The ribbon represents the trend of changing mean intensities.

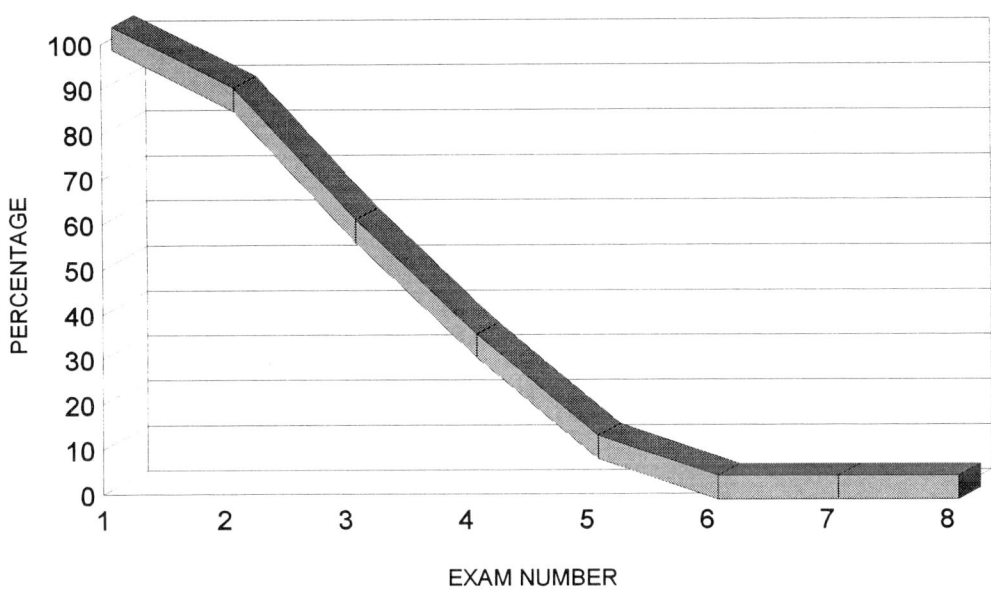

Figure 3. At each evaluation of patient #1, the percentage of 36 body divisions that contained pain (determined by the patient's pain drawing) was posted to the graph. The trend of changing percentages is shown by the ribbon.

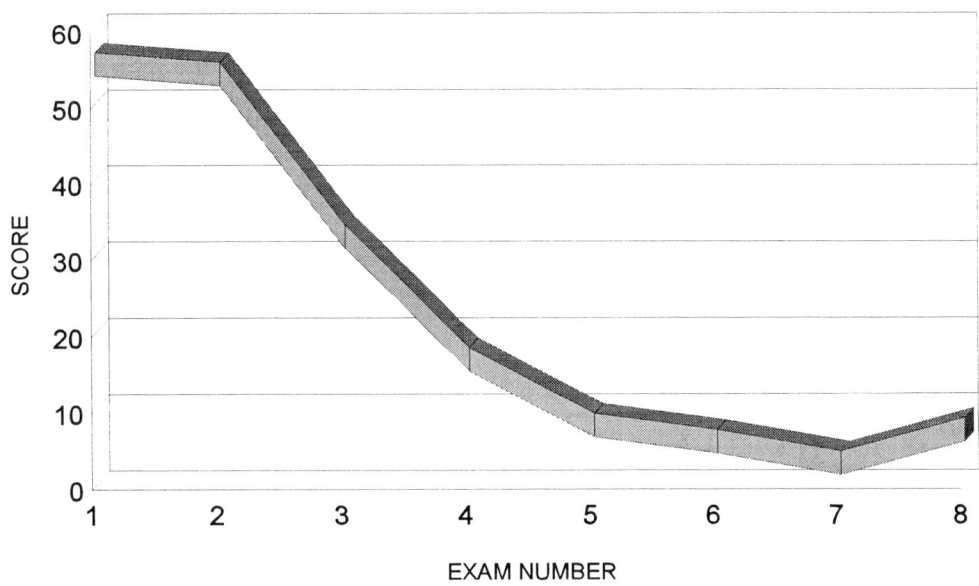

Figure 4. At each evaluation of patient #1, the total score for the Fibromyalgia Impact Questionnaire was posted to the graph. The ribbon shows the trend of changing scores.

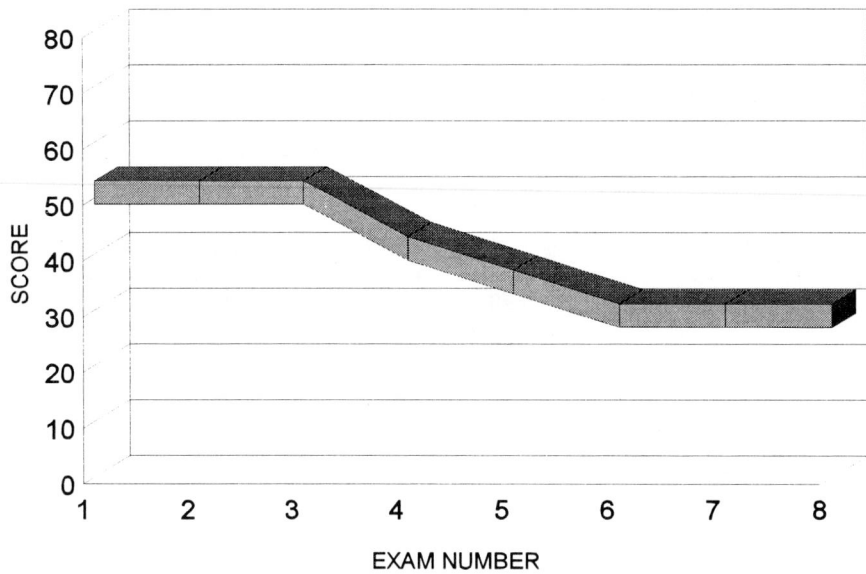

Figure 5. At each evaluation of patient #1, the raw score from the Zung's Self-Rating Depression Scale was posted to the graph. The ribbon shows the change in trend of the scores. The thin line at raw score 50 is the cut-off point for normal. Any score below 50 indicates that the patient had no depression.

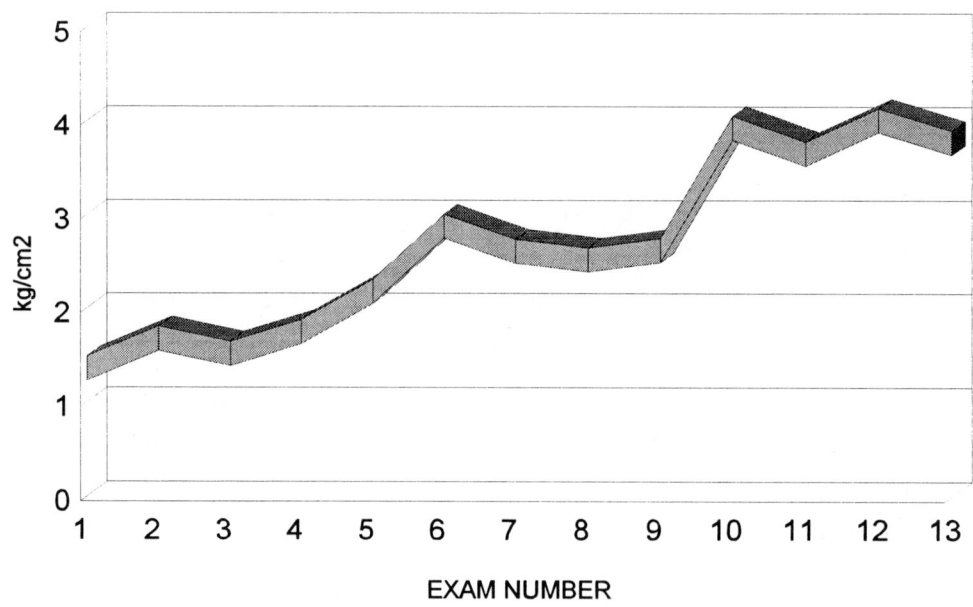

Figure 6. At each evaluation of patient #2, the mean of the pressure/pain thresholds of the 16 tender points was calculated and posted to the graph for that exam. The ribbon represents the trend of changing mean thresholds. The thin line at 4 kg/cm^2 represents the arbitrary cut-off point for normal. Scores below 4 kg/cm^2 were believed to be abnormal, and those above, normal.

measures changed substantially in directions indicating improvement. On April 8, 1997 (exam number 9), however, she reported having mild symptoms of overstimulation. She experienced a pulse rate of 100-to-110 bpm 3-to-4 times per day, and tremors of her calf muscles. I recommended to the prescribing clinician that this patient's dosage be reduced to 0.275 mg. However, the patient did not comply with the prescribing physician's instruction, and during my reevaluation of her on April 16, 1997 (exam number 10) she still had tachycardia. She admitted using Tenormin (prescribed by the physician) several times in the week prior to April 16. She then complied with the physician's instruction, and on her evaluation of April 30, 1997 (exam number 11) she reported that she had had tachycardia only twice per week. This was the previous frequency associated with mitral valve prolapse. After this, her status improved steadily.

THE USE OF TSH-SUPPRESSIVE DOSES OF T_4. When patient #2 consulted me, she was taking 0.15 mg of T_4. Her basal serum TSH level of 0.06 µU/mL was suppressed (normal range: 0.4-5.5 µU/mL). TSH suppression was confirmed by the result of the TRH stimulation test. At 30 minutes post-TRH injection, her TSH level increased to 0.07 µU/mL, only 0.01 µU/mL above the baseline value of 0.06 µU/mL. A normal increase in TSH level 30 minutes post-injection ranges from 8.5-20 µU/mL.[22] The current paradigm in endocrinology stipulates that a patient's T_4 dosage should be adjusted so that the TSH level remains within the limits of what is considered the normal range. This concept, introduced in 1973,[41][42] was based on the speculation that altered laboratory and other test results in patients taking TSH-suppressive doses of T_4 indicated thyrotoxicosis and constituted a health risk. Recent studies, however, show that this speculation was not correct—except possibly for post-menopausal women not taking estrogen supplements (see Lowe [34] for an extensive review of the relevant literature). In addition, it has been established that thyroid function test results are of no value in determining the adequacy of dosage in patients taking T_4.[35] Because the tests are of no value for this purpose, ordering them with the intent of monitoring for adequacy of T_4 dosage is an unnecessary expense.[35] It is probable that if the dosage of patient #2 had been reduced to raise her TSH level, her FMS status would have worsened. Had her T_4 dosage not been raised despite the low TSH levels, she would not have recovered from FMS.

TRANSIENT WORSENING OF FMS STATUS. It appears that a dosage of 0.3 mg of T_4 was excessive for this patient. She indicated that she did not want to comply

initially with the instruction by the prescribing physician to reduce dosage because she was apprehensive that she would resume her previous high level of fatigue. She did decrease the dosage to 0.275 mg for four days after instructed to do so, but seeing no change in her symptoms attributed to overstimulation, she increased her dosage again. I explained to her that changes in status from alterations of T_4 dosage may take weeks instead of days. The period of overstimulation was accompanied by worsening scores on the mean symptom intensity, FIQ, and Zung's (Figures 7, 9, and 10). It is interesting that the exacerbation was not reflected in the mean tender point algometer scores (Figure 6). There was a minor increase in pain distribution (Figure 8). The increase, however, did not qualify as widespread pain according to the ACR criteria.[1] After decreasing her dosage to 0.275 mg, this patient continued to improve throughout the evaluation period.

During the patient's exacerbation, I considered the possible role of iron deficiency anemia. The patient reported having a history of iron deficiency anemia, a mechanism that could account for her fatigue and weakness without an increase in her pain distribution. Her CBC of April 10th was negative for anemia or infection. Her chemistry revealed a total iron of 47 µg/dL (normal range: 50-150 µg/dL), and her family practice physician prescribed an iron supplement.

The patient also had been taking supplemental estrogen to treat an apparent imbalance due to perimenopause. Her biweekly heavy bleeding had subsided by April 8, possibly due to her increased dosage of T_4.[36][37][38] It is possible, of course, that the estrogen therapy or a combination of T_4 and estrogen was responsible.

As part of the treatment protocol, the patient continued her nutritional regimen and began daily stretching and a weight-training program using light weights (2-3 lbs). I treated her with myofascial therapy and chiropractic adjustments on a weekly basis for the first month of her treatment. Subsequently, I treated to coincide with the monitoring of her FMS status.

Results. This patient's improvement was not as smooth a course as that of patient #1. Her progress was more gradual because T_4 has a longer latency of action than T_3. Changes in patient status occur more slowly after T_4 dosage adjustments than do changes with T_3 dosage adjustments. But by the 14th week of treatment, patient #2 no longer met the ACR criterion for pain distribution. At the 20th week her mean tender point algometer score reached 3.93 kg/cm^2 (close to the arbitrary normal of 4 kg/cm^2). At this time, she

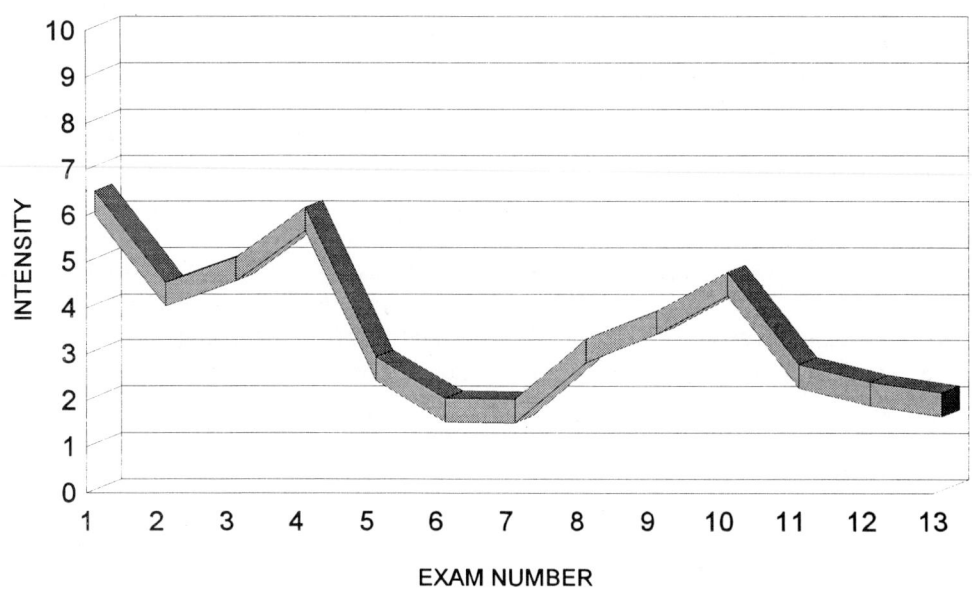

Figure 7. At each evaluation of patient #2, the mean intensity of 13 FMS symptoms (assessed by visual analog scales) was calculated and posted to the graph for that exam. The ribbon represents the trend of changing mean intensities.

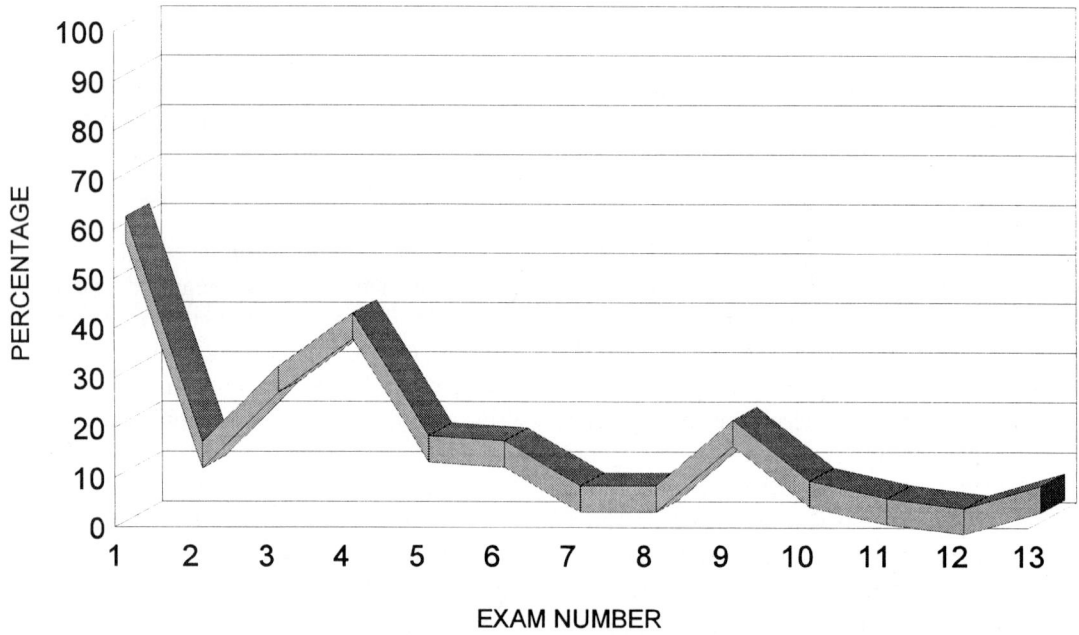

Figure 8. At each evaluation of patient #2, the percentage of 36 body divisions that contained pain (determined by the patient's pain drawing) was posted to the graph. The trend of changing percentages is shown by the ribbon.

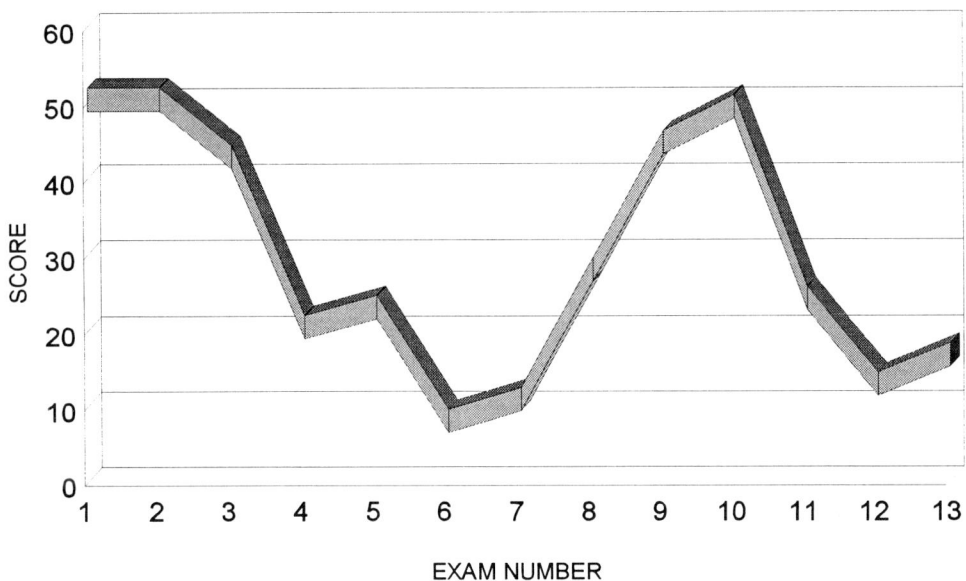

Figure 9. At each evaluation of patient #2, the total score for the Fibromyalgia Impact Questionnaire was posted to the graph. The ribbon shows the trend of changing scores.

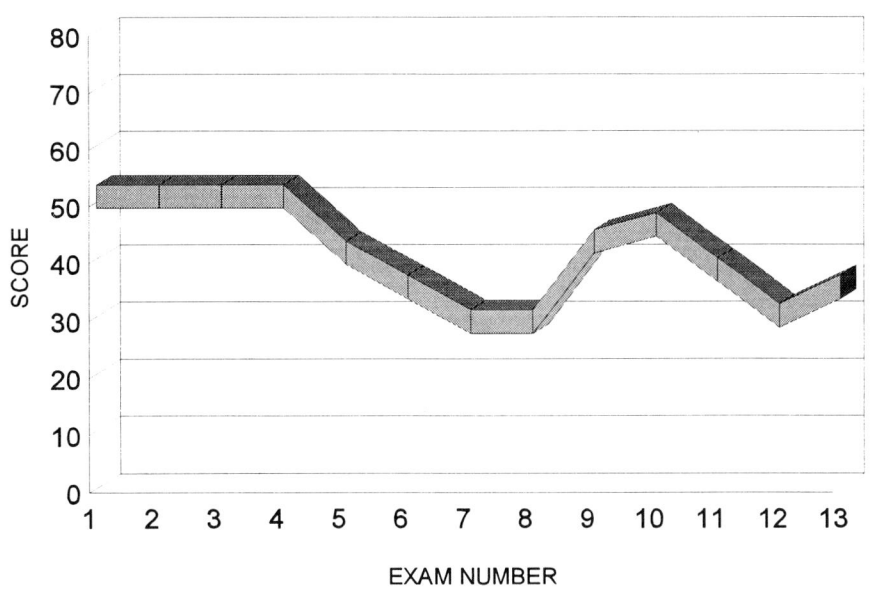

Figure 10. At each evaluation of patient #2, the raw score from the Zung's Self-Rating Depression Scale was posted to the graph. The ribbon shows the change in trend of the scores. The thin line at raw score 50 is the cut-off point for normal. Any score below 50 indicates that the patient had no depression.

no longer met the ACR tender point criterion for FMS.

Because she had a history of tachycardia associated with mitral valve prolapse, it was not clear whether the tachycardia she initially experienced during the period of exacerbation was associated with the valve prolapse or with the T_4. But the frequent tachycardia, weakness, and occasional tremors of her lower extremity muscles (when standing on her toes) were all relieved by the reduced dosage of 0.275 mg. All FMS measures improved during the course of treatment.

TENDER POINTS. Figure 6 shows changes in the mean pressure/pain threshold of this patient's tender points, measured with algometry. Her threshold increased from 1.36 kg/cm^2 on her initial visit before she began treatment, to 3.77 kg/cm^2 on her thirteenth evaluation (a 277% increase). She does not consider her FMS body sites abnormally tender now. Although previously, the normal threshold was arbitrarily considered 4 kg/cm^2, experimental results[18][19] and my clinical experience show that recovered patients often have mean thresholds below this value, and do not consider their body sites tender. See Figure 1.

MEAN SYMPTOM INTENSITY. The mean intensity of the 13 most common FMS symptoms decreased from 6.20 to 1.84 (a 70.33% decrease). See Figure 7.

PAIN DISTRIBUTION. On her initial visit to my office, patient #2 had pain in 58.75% of her body (all 36 divisions on the pain drawing). On her seventh visit, three months later, the distribution had decreased to 4.50% (a 92.34% reduction). See Figure 8.

FIQ. Her initial FIQ score was 50.45 and her final was 16.70 (a 66.89% decrease). The decreased score corresponds to her increase in functional abilities. See Figure 9.

ZUNG'S. At patient #2's initial evaluation, a Zung's score of 51 indicated mild depression. She reported that the Prozac she had taken for several months had diminished her depression. No objective test results were available to quantify her previous levels of depression. After 11 weeks of metabolic therapy, her Zung's score decreased below 50 and into the normal range at 35, indicating no depression. Her score decreased further through the remainder of her treatment monitoring (see Figure 10).

Outcome. At the end of the systematic monitoring of patient #2, her resting pulse rate was 78 bpm and her Achilles reflex was of equal brisk speed in both the contraction and relaxation phases. Her weight decreased by 10 lbs during the treatment, due at least in part to her improved diet. I will monitor her FMS status once per month for three months, and provide chiropractic care on a prn basis.

DISCUSSION

It is impossible to conclusively rule out a placebo response in open trials. For a number of reasons, however, it is unlikely that placebo responses account for the recovery of the two patients reported here. In response to placebos, FMS patients have been reported to improve not at all[7,p.1375] or only slightly.[8][9] But no FMS patients have been reported to respond to placebos in the manner the two patients reported here did to the metabolic protocol: complete recovery from FMS symptoms with normalization of all objective measures.

In one systematic open trial,[15] FMS patients were monitored at 1-to-2 week intervals for one year, during which they maintained their improvement with T_3 therapy. One year is sufficient time to rule out placebo responses. Lowe, Reichman, and Yellin conducted a case-control study of euthyroid FMS patients treated with T_3, hypothyroid FMS patients treated with T_4, and matched untreated FMS patients.[21] At 1-to-5 year follow-up, FMS measures of treated patients indicated significant improvement over their baseline measures. For untreated patients, FMS measures at follow-up were not significantly different from baseline measures, indicating no improvement. Also at follow-up, treated patients were significantly improved compared to untreated patients. The study demonstrates that the benefits of metabolic therapy for both hypothyroid and euthyroid FMS patients were sustained from a period of 1-to-5 years. This makes it highly improbable that the improvement of treated patients was due to placebo responses. The two patients reported here resemble in all relevant respects patients in the Lowe case-control study. Because of this, it is unlikely that improvement in my patients was due to placebo responses.

CONCLUSION

The two patients reported here, treated at an independent clinical site, were relieved of all FMS symptoms and signs with the use of the metabolic treatment protocol reported by Lowe and colleagues.[15][16][17][18][19][20] The therapeutic outcome in these two patients supports the reported effectiveness of the protocol for both hypothyroid and euthyroid FMS patients. The metabolic treatment protocol is a highly effective and economical treatment for FMS.

REFERENCES

1. Wolfe, F., Smythe, H.A., Yunus, M.B., et al.: The American College of Rheumatology 1990 criteria for the classification of fibromyalgia: report of the multicenter criteria committee. *Arthritis Rheum.*, 33:160-172, 1990.
2. Moldofsky, H. and Warsh, J.J.: Plasma tryptophan and musculoskeletal pain in non-articular rheumatism ("fibrositis syndrome"). *Pain*, 5:65-71, 1978.
3. Russell, I.J.: Neurohormonal aspects of fibromyalgia syndrome. *Rheumat. Dis. Clin. North Am.*, 15:149-168, 1989.
4. Russell, I.J., Michalek, J.E., Vipraio, G.A., Fletcher, E.M., and Wall, K.: Serum amino acids in fibrositis/fibromyalgia syndrome. *J. Rheumatol.*, (16 suppl.), 19:158-163, 1989.
5. Russell, I.J., Michalek, J.E., Vipraio, J.A., Fletcher, E.M., Javors, M.A., and Bowden, C.A.: Platelet 3H-imipramine uptake receptor density and serum serotonin levels in patients with fibromyalgia/fibrositis syndromes. *J. Rheumatol*, 19:104-109, 1992.
6. Houvenagel, E., Forzy, G., Cortet, B., and Vincent, G.: 5-Hydroxyindoleacetic acid in cerebrospinal fluid in fibromyalgia. *Arthritis Rheum.*, 33:S55, 1990.
7. Russell, I.J., Vaeroy, H., Javors, M., and Nyberg, F.: Cerebrospinal fluid biogenic amine metabolites in fibromyalgia/fibrositis syndrome and rheumatoid arthritis. *Arthritis Rheum.*, 35:550-556, 1992.
8. Goldenberg, D.L.: Fibromyalgia: treatment programs. *J. Musculoskel. Pain*, 1:71-81, 1993.
9. Carette, S.: What have clinical trials taught us about the treatment of fibromyalgia? *J. Musculoskel. Pain*, 3:133-140, 1995.
10. Wolfe, F., Cathey, M.A., and Hawley, D.J.: A double blind placebo controlled trial of fluoxetine in fibromyalgia. *Scand. J. Rheumatol.*, 23:255-259, 1994.
11. Carette, S., Bell, M., Reynolds, J., et al.: A controlled trial of amitriptyline, cyclobenzaprine, and placebo in fibromyalgia patients. *Arthritis Rheum.*, 37(1):32-40, 1994.
12. Goldenberg, D.L., Felson, D.T., and Dinerman, H.: A randomized, controlled trial of amitriptyline and naproxen in the treatment of patients with fibromyalgia. *Arthritis Rheum.*, 29(1):1371-1377, 1986.
13. Goldenberg, D.L., Marskīy, M., Mossey, C., Ruthazer, R., and Schmid, C.: The independent and combined efficacy of fluoxetine and amitriptyline in the treatment of fibromyalgia. *Arthritis Rheum.*, Suppl 38:S229, 1995.
14. Lowe, J.C., Cullum, M., Graf, L., Jr, and Yellin, J.: Mutations in the c-*erb*Aβ₁ gene: do they underlie euthyroid fibromyalgia? *Med. Hypotheses*, 48(2):125-135, 1997.
15. Lowe, J.C., Eichelberger, J., Manso, G., and Peterson, K.: Improvement in euthyroid fibromyalgia patients treated with T₃ (tri-iodothyronine). *J. Myofascial Ther.*, 1(2):16-27, 1994.
16. Lowe, J.C.: T₃-induced recovery from fibromyalgia by a hypothyroid patient resistant to T₄ and desiccated thyroid. *J. Myofascial. Ther.*, 1(4):26-31, 1995.
17. Lowe, J.C.: Results of an open trial of T₃ therapy with 77 euthyroid female fibromyalgia patients. *Clin. Bull. Myofascial Ther.*, 2(1):35-37, 1997.
18. Lowe, J.C., Garrison, R.L., Reichman, A.J., Yellin, J., Thompson, M., and Kaufman, D.: Effectiveness and safety of T₃ therapy for euthyroid fibromyalgia: a double-blind placebo-controlled crossover study. *Clin. Bull. Myofascial Ther.*, 2(2/3):31-58, 1997.
19. Lowe, J.C., Reichman, A.J., and Yellin, J.: The process of change during T₃ treatment for euthyroid fibromyalgia: a double-blind placebo-controlled crossover study. *Clin. Bull. Myofascial Ther.* 2(2/3):91-124, 1997.
20. Lowe, J.C., Garrison, R.L., Reichman, A.J., and Yellin, J.: Triiodothyronine (T₃) treatment of euthyroid fibromyalgia: a small-N replication of a double-blind placebo-controlled crossover study. *Clin. Bull. Myofascial Ther.* 2(4):1997.
21. Lowe, J.C., Reichman, A.J., and Yellin, Y.: A 1-to-5 year follow-up of fibromyalgia patients treated with metabolic therapy: a comparison of treated and untreated matched patients. In press, 1997.
22. Lowe, J.C.: Thyroid status of 38 fibromyalgia patients: implications for the etiology of fibromyalgia. *Clin. Bull. Myofascial.Ther.*, 2(1):47-64, 1997.
23. Wigers, S.H., Skrondal, A., Finset, A., and Götestam, K.G.: Measuring change in fibromyalgic pain: the relevance of pain distribution. *J. Musculoskel. Pain*, 5(2):29-41, 1997.
24. Wilkins, E.W., Dineen, J.J., Moncure, A.C., Gross, P.L., and Fitzgerald, C.P.: *MGH Textbook of Emergency Medicine*, 2nd edition. Baltimore, Williams & Wilkins, 1983, pp.624-627.
25. O'Boyle, C.M., Davis, D.K., Russo, B.A., Kraf, T.J., and Brick, P.D.: *Emergency Care: The First 24 Hours.* Norwalk, Appleton-Century-Crofts, 1985, pp.332-333.
26. Burckhardt, C.S., Clark, S.R., and Bennett, R.M.: The fibromyalgia impact questionnaire: development and validation. *J. Rheumatol.*, 18(5):728-733, 1991.
27. Zung, W.W.K.: A self-rating depression scale. *Arch. Gen. Psychiatry*, 12:65-70, 1965.
28. Naughton, M.J. and Wiklund, I.: A critical review of dimension-specific measures of health-related quality of life in cross-cultural research. *Quality Life Res.*, 2(6):397-432, 1993.
29. Fischer, A.A., DeCosta, C., and Levy, H.: Diagnosis of fibromyalgia by manual pressure is unreliable: quantification of tender point sensitivity by algometry is necessary in clinical practice. *J. Musculoskel. Pain*, 3(1):139, 1995.
30. Klein, I.: Metabolic, physiologic, and clinical indexes of thyroid function. In *The Thyroid: A Fundamental and Clinical Text*, 6th edition. Edited by L.E. Braverman and R.D. Utiger Philadelphia, J.B. Lippincott Co., 1991, pp. 486-492.
31. Goldberg, M.: Diagnosis of euthyroid hypometabolism. *Am. J. Obst. & Gynec.*, 81(5): 1057-1058, May, 1961.
32. Sonkin, L.S.: Endocrine disorders and muscle dysfunction. In *Clinical Management of Head, Neck and TMJ Pain and Dysfunction.* Edited by B. Gelb, Philadelphia, W.B. Saunders Co., 1985, pp.137-170.
33. Lowe, J.C.: Personal communication, March 11, 1997.
34. Lowe, J.C.: *The Metabolic Treatment of Fibromyalgia.* Tulsa, McDowell Publishing Co., 1999.
35. Fraser, W.D., Biggart, E.M., O'Reilly, D. St. J., Gray, H.W., McKillop, J.H., and Thomson, J.A.: Are biochemical tests of thyroid function of any value in monitoring patients receiving thyroxine replacement? *Br. Med. J.*, 293: 808-810, 1986.
36. Wilansky, D.L. and Greisman, B.: Early hypothyroidism in

patients with menorrhagia. *Am. J. Obstet. Gynecol.*, 70: 789, 1987.

37. Higham, J.M. and Shaw, R.W.: The effect of thyroxine replacement on menstrual blood loss in a hypothyroid patient. *Br. J. Obstet. Gynaecol.*, 99:695, 1992.

38. Rotmensch, S. and Scommegna, A.: Spontaneous ovarian hyperstimulation syndrome assocated with hypothyroidism. *Am. J. Obstet. Gynecol.*, 160:1220, 1989.

39. Berkow, R. and Fletcher, A.J.: *The Merck Manual of Diagnosis and Therapy*, 15th edition. Rahway, Merck, Sharp & Dohme Research Laboratories, 1987.

40. Wolfe, F.: Diagnosis of fibromyalgia. *J. Musculoskel. Med.*, 7:54, 1990.

41. Evered, D., Young, E.T., Ormston, MG., Menzies, R., Smith, P.A., and Hall, R.: Treatment of hypothyroidism: a reappraisal of thyroxine therapy. *Br. Med. J.*, iii:131-134, 1973.

42. Stock, J.M., Surks, M.I., and Oppenheimer, J.H.: Replacement dosage of L-thyroxine in hypothyroidism. *N. Engl. J. Med.*, 290:529-533, 1974.

Triiodothyronine (T$_3$) Treatment of Euthyroid Fibromyalgia: A Small-N Replication of a Double-Blind Placebo-Controlled Crossover Study

John C. Lowe, MA, DC
Richard L. Garrison, MD
Alan Reichman, MD
Jackie Yellin, BA

This article originally appeared in the *Clinical Bulletin of Myofascial Therapy*, 2(4):71-88, 1997. It is reprinted with permission of Haworth Medical Press.

ABSTRACT. *Background.* In a previous study, T$_3$ was found to be highly effective compared to placebos in the treatment of euthyroid fibromyalgia. In this replication study, the comparative effects of placebos and T$_3$ were tested with 4 euthyroid fibromyalgia patients. A randomized double-blind placebo-controlled crossover design was used.

Methods. Patients completed alternately 2 T$_3$ phases and 2 placebo phases. The sequence for each patient depended on the medication with which she was randomly assigned to begin. Crossover from one phase to another was response-driven, based on changes in 3 measures of fibromyalgia status: mean tender point sensitivity by algometry, mean symptom intensity by visual analog scales, and pain distribution by the percentage method. Measurements taken repeatedly during each phase were used to determine when a patient's scores warranted a crossover. Patients also completed the Fibromyalgia Impact Questionnaire and Zung's Self-Rating Depression Scale at the end of each phase.

Results. Paired-samples *t*-tests showed a highly significant difference between scores in placebo and T$_3$ phases. Serial ECGs throughout the 8-month study, and urine and serum calcium, phosphorus, creatinine, serum alkaline phosphatase, and bone densitometry at 6-month follow-up revealed no adverse effects from T$_3$.

Conclusion. The highly significant difference between fibromyalgia measures in placebo and T$_3$ phases, despite the small N, indicates a powerful therapeutic effect of supraphysiologic dosages of T$_3$. Despite low TSH and free and total T$_4$ levels, and high free T$_3$ levels, there was no evidence of thyrotoxicosis. Long-term safety of T$_3$ use by euthyroid fibromyalgia patients has not yet been established.

KEYWORDS. Fibromyalgia, hypothyroidism, euthyroid, thyroid hormone resistance, triiodothyronine, T$_3$

INTRODUCTION

Fibromyalgia syndrome (FMS) is the most common condition of chronic widespread musculoskeletal pain, stiffness, and fatigue.[1][2] Commonly used medications such as tricyclic antidepressants are ineffective for FMS patients.[4] The clinical features of FMS closely resemble those of hypothyroidism,[5][6][7][8][9][10][11][12][13][14][15] and there is a high incidence of both primary and central hypothyroidism in FMS.[16][17][18][19][20][21][22]

In a study of 38 consecutive FMS patients, 36.8% were euthyroid.[19] Lowe and colleagues proposed, however, that the hypothyroid-like features of euthyroid FMS may result from failure of normal concentrations of thyroid hormone to properly regulate gene transcription.[23] Whereas inadequate transcription regulation in hypothyroid FMS would result from a frank thyroid hormone deficiency, in euthyroid FMS inadequate regulation may result from "cellular resistance" to thyroid hormone. All clinical features of FMS may be explained by increases in 3 "inhibitory" molecular by-products of inadequate regulation of gene transcription by thyroid hormone: phosphodiesterase, G$_i$ proteins, and α-adrenoceptors.[3] These by-products can occur in both hypothyroidism and cellular resistance to thyroid hormone.

This hypothesis is supported by the results of 2 open systematic trials and 2 double-blind placebo-controlled studies using T$_3$ therapy for euthyroid

FMS.[24][25][26][59] In the blinded studies, according to 5 FMS measures, FMS status significantly improved in T$_3$ phases and significantly worsened in placebo phases. Therapeutic effects occurred only with supraphysiologic T$_3$ dosages, but without adverse effects on heart, liver, muscle, or bone. The current study is a replication of the first blinded study with a group-comparison design.[26] Our purpose was to determine whether 4 other euthyroid FMS patients would respond to T$_3$ as did those in the previous blinded study, and as do patients with proven thyroid hormone resistance: improved clinical status with supraphysiologic dosages of T$_3$, without adverse target tissue effects.[27]

METHODS

Subjects. The institutional review board of the Fibromyalgia Research Foundation approved the protocol. Written informed consent was obtained from patients before the study. Each patient acknowledged her understanding of the effects of overstimulation by thyroid hormone explained in the consent document.

Eleven patients applied to participate in the study after reading a newspaper advertisement soliciting individuals with FMS symptoms. The study was restricted to participation by 4 subjects due to limitations on funding. Six consecutive applicants of the 11 who applied were interviewed and evaluated for fibromyalgia; interviewing ceased after 4 who met the participation criteria were sequentially enrolled.

The age range of participants was 35-to-44 years. All subjects met the 1990 American College of Rheumatology (ACR) criteria for FMS:[1] widespread pain for at least 3 months and 11 of 18 possible tender points. An algometer (calibrated force gauge) was used to measure the pressure/pain threshold of tender points, and a patient was enrolled only if the mean of her tender points was below 2.5 kg/cm^2 (1.5 kg/cm^2 below the arbitrary normal of 4 kg/cm^2). All patients had normal thyroid function test results, had never used exogenous thyroid hormone, and had no other health condition with clinical features resembling or overlapping those of FMS. Two weeks before the study began, patients stopped any medication they were taking to control FMS symptoms. Each patient agreed to engage in exercise to tolerance, and to take nutritional supplements (especially B vitamins) daily through all phases of the study. This was required of the patients because clinical experience indicates that the therapeutic effects of T$_3$ in euthyroid fibromyalgia patients are partly contingent on the patients simul-

taneously using nutritional supplements. Ceasing the supplements after recovering from fibromyalgia symptoms can result in the reinstitution of fibromyalgia symptoms.[25]

Study Design and Data Analysis. This study used a double-blind placebo-controlled response-driven crossover design. Group comparison analysis was performed to determine whether end point measures for T$_3$ and placebo phases significantly differed from one another. Statistical analysis was performed using the Statistical Package for the Social Sciences (SPSS, Chicago). Paired-samples *t*-tests were used to test for significant differences between scores in placebo and T$_3$ phases.

Treatment. During all phases, patients took combinations of capsules of 4 different colors. Each color represented a dose of 6.25, 12.5, 25, or 75 μg. The lactose capsules patients took during placebo phases were identical in appearance to the T$_3$ capsules. Patients and investigators were instructed to assume that all coded bottles in every phase contained T$_3$. Propranolol tablets (20 mg) were issued to all patients because of its usefulness in reversing tachyarrhythmias to normal sinus rhythm.[43] The tablets were to be taken only if a patient felt some threat from overstimulation by the study capsules and upon consultation with one of the investigators. All patients and all investigators were unaware of actual capsule content during all phases, as the capsule bottles were prepared off-site using code numbers instead of names.

At the time of any crossover, a patient received a new set of 4 number-coded bottles prepared by an investigator who had no knowledge of the outcome of exams or of any particular patient's FMS status or code number. The patient turned in the bottles with the remaining capsules for the phase just completed and picked up bottles for the phase she was entering. In any new phase, a patient began by taking 75 μg (presumed in every phase to be T$_3$), despite the dosage she had been taking when her previous phase ended. Seventy-five μg is the usual starting replacement dosage for euthyroid FMS patients.[24][26]

T$_3$ was used because previous studies indicated that most euthyroid FMS patients do not benefit from T$_4$, even at supraphysiologic dosages, but improve on FMS measures with the use of T$_3$.[24][25][26][59] In the early studies,[24][25] it was suspected that the patients did not monodeiodinate T$_4$ to T$_3$. But extensive laboratory testing with euthyroid patients did not produce evidence consistent with failed deiodination: none of the tested patients had elevated reverse T$_3$ levels or low total T$_3$ levels. Also, none had an elevated 24-hour urinary cortisol level, eliminating the possibility of cortisol-induced (and therefore, possibly stress-induced) inhibition of deiodination.[29] In these respects, euthyroid FMS patients resemble patients with peripheral thyroid hormone resistance.[54]

Instruments and Assessment. We used 5 measures to assess changes in FMS status: algometer measurements of tender points, pain distribution drawings, symptom intensity surveys using visual analog scales (VASs), the Fibromyalgia Impact Questionnaire (FIQ), and Zung's Self-Rating Depression Scale (Zung's). Bennett[63] and Littlejohn[64] recently expressed the need to revise and improve the methods for diagnosing and assessing FMS. We modified 3 of the 5 standard assessment methods. The modifications enabled greater precision at quantifying changes in patient status.

MODIFICATION 1: ALGOMETRY TO ASSESS TENDER POINT SENSITIVITY. Tender point assessment according to the ACR entails applying 4 kg of pressure with a finger to 18 predictable tender point sites. A patient meets the tender point criterion if he or she reports tenderness upon pressure at 11 or more of the 18 tender point sites.[1] Recently, however, Fisher demonstrated that experienced clinicians were not able to subjectively gauge 4 kg of pressure when not observing a meter. He concluded that reliable FMS diagnosis requires quantification of pressure by algometry.[65] The algometer reliably measures the sensitivity of FMS tender points,[66][28] and its measurements correlate well with pain distribution reported by patients on body drawings.[67] We quantified tender point sensitivity with algometry at every assessment—the higher the pressure/tenderness threshold, the lower the sensitivity.

MODIFICATION 2: PAIN DISTRIBUTION. The ACR diagnostic criteria for FMS include widespread pain, defined as pain 1) above and below the waist, 2) on the right and left sides of the body, and 3) over an axial area such as the anterior chest or spine. This definition permits a pain distribution score of 1-to-4 units (0-1-2-3). We assessed changes according to this method, but we also used an alternate method we adapted from the "rules of nine" for adult burn victims that describes the percentage of body surface burned.[68][69] The research team of the Fibromyalgia Research Foundation reported the use of this method in 2 previous studies, and almost simultaneously, a version of the method was devised, employed, and reported by another research group in Norway.[62] The modified rules of nine method for assessing pain distribution has not been reported in FMS research prior to 1997.

MODIFICATION 3: EXTENDED SYMPTOM INTENSITY SCALES. As in the previous study[26] (of which this study is a replication), we extended the number of 100 mm visual analog scales (VASs) from the usual 1-to-4 to include the 13 most common associated FMS symptoms.[1][70][71] The symptoms we included were pain, fatigue, stiffness, headache, sleep disturbance, bowel disturbance, depression, cognitive dysfunction (poor memory and concentration), anxiety, coldness, paresthesias (numbness and tingling), Sicca symptoms, and difficulty exercising. Assessment of symptom intensities, especially pain, using VASs is customarily employed in FMS studies.[72][73][74][75] Scott and Huskisson report that VASs are the best available procedure for measuring pain.[76]

We used 2 other standard methods of FMS assessment: the Fibromyalgia Impact Questionnaire[30] and Zung's Self-Rating Depression Scale.[77] The FIQ is a brief, self-administered instrument with demonstrated validity and reliability. It is widely used for assessing the impact FMS has on a patient's daily life. It measures physical function, work status, depression, anxiety, sleep, pain, stiffness, fatigue, and well-being. Zung's is an easily self-administered, well-validated measure with acceptable sensitivity and specificity.[31] It correlates significantly with other measures of depression, including the Beck Depression Inventory.[78]

Procedure. Patients were randomly assigned by number (and off-site) to either an initial placebo or initial T_3 phase. Matching was not necessary because each patient served in alternate phases as her own control. Baseline testing for all patients included algometry, pain distribution, VASs, FIQ, Zung's, and ECG.

Patients were evaluated at 1-to-2 week intervals with a brief examination (pulse rate, blood pressure, and Achilles reflex), an interview, and an FMS assessment. Three sets of FMS measurements were taken repeatedly throughout all study phases: 1) a tender point examination by one of the investigators (quantified by algometer measurements as the mean of 16 tender points), 2) a pain drawing of the patient's pain distribution since the previous examination (quantified as a percentage of 36 body divisions containing pain), and 3) completion of visual analog scales (VASs) for symptom intensities of the 13 most common symptoms (see above) associated with fibromyalgia (quantified as the mean of the 13 VAS scores).

After each reevaluation, the mean tender point score, the pain distribution expressed as a percentage, and the mean symptom intensity were applied as data points (for that evaluation date) to graphs for each measure. Successive data points in each graph showed the trend of each measure during each phase. At each evaluation, the examining clinician used the graphs (with data from the current evaluation and previous ones in the same phase) and his global assessment (see below) of the patient to judge when it was appropriate to alter the patient's T_3 dosage or to cross her to the next phase. Graphing of data points and the use of the graphs in therapeutic decisions are described in detail in a previous publication.[59]

At each evaluation, the examining clinician made a global assessment of the patient's status. This assessment considered several factors: 1) results of the physical exam, particularly the resting pulse rate and Achilles reflex, 2) the patient's answers to questions about her status since the last evaluation, and 3) the clinician's impression of the patient's status based on her appearance and attitude. The clinician's judgment as to whether the patient's dosage should be altered was based on consideration of his global assessment of her status, and the trend of her data points in the line graphs for FMS measures in the current phase of the study. Thus, decisions regarding dosage adjustments were clinical judgments. The judgments were based partly on the outcome of the objective FMS measures, partly on signs observable by the clinician, and partly on the patient's subjective report. Depending on the outcome of the evaluation, a patient's daily dosage was kept the same or altered.

If a patient's fibromyalgia status deteriorated according to the examining clinician's judgment, the patient's dosage was increased by 6.25, 12.5, or 25 µg. If a patient's fibromyalgia status stayed the same or slightly improved, but her ECGs showed no evidence of overstimulation and there was no other clinical evidence of thyrotoxicosis, then her dosage was increased. In any phase, if there were signs of overstimulation, a patient's dosage was reduced by 6.25 µg decrements until all signs of overstimulation were gone. Serial ECGs were performed on all patients throughout the study to assure detection of cardiac thyrotoxicosis. (No instance was ever found in this study.)

If a patient reached a dosage of 175 µg without further improvement through at least 2 evaluations, the patient was crossed to the next phase and given alternate number-coded capsules. When in the judgment of the examining clinician, a patient's improvement had plateaued, she too was crossed to the next phase.

At the end of each phase, the mean tender point sensitivity, mean symptom intensity, and pain distribution expressed as a percentage were determined along with 3 other measures: pain distribution according to the ACR method,[1] the Fibromyalgia Impact Questionnaire (FIQ),[30] and Zung's Self-Rating Depression Scale (Zung's).[31] The FIQ and Zung's forms from this study were number-coded and independently scored off-site.

Safety Testing. After the 8-month study was concluded, all patients continued to use supraphysiologic doses of T_3 daily, and at the end of 6 more months, safety testing was performed. Tests of possible adverse effects from supraphysiologic doses of T_3 included serial ECGs throughout all study phases (prior to most dosage increases) and at 6-month follow-up. Urinary N-telopeptides, creatinine, calcium, and phosphorus; serum creatinine, calcium, phosphorus, and alkaline phosphatase; and bone densitometry of the lumbar spine, Ward's triangle, femoral neck, and trochanter with either CT scans or dual photon absorptiometry were evaluated at 6-month follow-up.

RESULTS

Each patient completed 2 placebo and 2 T_3 phases. The high significance levels on most FMS measures despite the small number of patients indicates that T_3 had a strong therapeutic impact on the FMS status of these euthyroid patients. Effective dosages of T_3 for the 4 patients were 106.25, 118.75, 125.00, and 137.50 µg.

Fibromyalgia Assessment. Table 1 shows the group comparison results (all 4 patients) for the fibromyalgia assessment measures. Sixteen tender points were measured with algometry, pain distribution was measured by the ACR method and the percentage method, and 13 FMS symptoms were measured with VASs. Mean values for T_3 phases indicate highly significant improvement on all measures when compared to mean values for placebo phases.

Safety Assessment. WEIGHT. Patients' weights significantly decreased during T_3 phases (P=0.022). Mean placebo weight was 124.69 lbs, and mean T_3 weight was 123.10 lbs.

CARDIAC EFFECTS. Mean heart rate significantly increased from 68.50 bpm in placebo phases to 83.00 bpm in T_3 phases (P=0.001). No patient developed tachycardia. PR intervals shortened within the normal range in T_3 phases, but the difference did not reach significance (P= 0.570). QRS intervals lengthened within the normal range in T_3 phases, but the difference was not significant (P= 0.275). QT intervals shortened within the normal range during T_3 phases, but did not reach significance (P= 0.190). All ST segments were within normal limits in all phases. There was no significant difference in systolic blood pressures between T₃ and placebo phases (P= 0.291), and no difference in diastolic blood pressures (P=0.410).

THYROID FUNCTION TESTS. Baseline third-generation TSH, T₄, T₃ uptake, and FTI were within the normal range for all patients. At 6-month follow-up,

these values as well as the free T_4 and free T_3 were consistent with values generally considered "thyrotoxic" due to excessive exogenous T_3 intake. Low values included a mean TSH concentration of 0.19±0.20 μU/mL, a mean total T_4 of 3.05±0.67 μg/dL, a mean FTI of 0.84±0.11, and a mean free T_4 of 0.48±0.09 ng/dL. The mean T_3 uptake of 30.00±3.92% was within the normal range. The mean free T_3 of 9.28±3.79 pg/mL was high.

Table 1. Fibromyalgia Measurement Group Results

All Patients	Worst Possible	Best Possible	Mean Placebo	Mean T_3	Significance
tender points	< 1 kg/cm²	> 4 kg/cm²	1.81 kg/cm²	3.29 kg/cm²	P < 0.0005
pain distribution: ACR method	3	0	3.00	2.00	P = 0.001
pain distribution: % method	100%	0%	69.75%	10.53%	P < 0.0005
symptom intensities (VASs)	10	0	7.03	1.69	P < 0.0005
Fibromyalgia Impact Questionn.	80	0	54.00	16.38	P = 0.001
Zung's Depression Inventory	80	20	55.50	40.75	P = 0.001

MUSCLE EFFECT. At 6-month follow-up, both mean serum (0.92 ±0.20 ng/24-hr) and urinary creatinine (1044.50±109.28 ng/24-hr) were normal, indicating normal muscle mass.

OSSEOUS EFFECTS. At follow-up, mean urinary calcium (253.25±71.84 mg/24-hr) and phosphorus (575.12±378.48 mg per 24-hours) were normal. Mean urinary N-telopeptides (98.09±65.37 nMole of bone collagen equivalents/μMole of creatinine) was high, indicating increased bone turnover. Mean serum phosphorus (3.67±0.47 mg/dL), calcium (8.16±2.82 mg/dL), and alkaline phosphatase (53.10±18.91 IU/L) were normal. Compared to reference standards, bone densitometry showed bone density slightly above that for age-matched women for 3 structures, and slightly below for one. Density of the trochanter was 100.70±0.89% of age-matched controls, the femoral neck was 100.75±3.01%, Ward's triangle was 101.76±3.56%, and the lumbar spine was 99.91±3.41%.

LIVER FUNCTION TESTS. At follow-up, our patients had normal values for mean ALT (26.25±11.70

U/L) and GGPT (28.00±8.83 U/L). Other liver function test results were also within normal limits.

DISCUSSION

FMS status in our 4 euthyroid patients was significantly improved in T_3 phases (using supraphysiologic dosages of T_3) compared to placebo phases. This result is consistent with that recently reported by Lowe and colleagues.[26] The significant difference between measures in T_3 and placebo phases, despite the small number of patients participating, indicates that the use of T_3 had a potent therapeutic effect on the patients' fibromyalgia status.

Because of the response-driven design, we cannot rule out regression toward the mean in alternate phases. It is not likely, however, that regression accounts for the substantial changes in FMS status in alternate phases. Any regression would be minimal, considering the natural history of FMS: epidemiological studies show that patient status changes little over prolonged periods, and natural short-term fluctuations in the intensity of FMS[32][33][34][35][36] are not of the magnitude of the measured changes between phases in this study. In addition, the FMS status of the 4 patients deteriorated and improved in concert with repeated crossovers from T_3 to placebo to T_3 phases. That these were chance occurrences is highly improbable[60] in light of Barlow and Hersen's "principle of unlikely successive coincidences."[61]

Adverse Target Tissue Effects. Ross has written that adverse effects of exogenous thyroid hormone can be avoided only if patients' TSH levels are kept within the middle of the normal range.[37] The results of this study and that of Lowe and colleagues[26] indicate that this is not true of euthyroid FMS patients. At 6-month follow-up, our euthyroid FMS patients had low TSH levels, but cardiac monitoring and follow-up biochemical and densitometry testing showed no clinically significant adverse effects. None of the adverse cardiac effects,[38][39][40][41][42][43][44][45] tissue catabolism or weight loss,[46][47] or elevations in serum alanine aminotransferase (ALT) and γ-glutamyl transpeptidase (GGPT)[46] reported in hyperthyroidism and thyrotoxicosis occurred in our 4 patients. All ECGs were normal throughout the 8-month study and at 6-month follow-up. This finding suggests partial resistance of cardiac regulatory mechanisms to thyroid hormone.

Our patients' weights did significantly differ between T_3 and placebo phases, but their mean serum and urinary creatinine was normal, indicating absence of catabolic effect on muscle despite use of supraphysiologic dosages of T_3. The mean weight loss of 2.81 lbs may represent fat loss. This is likely because the patients, according to their protocol agreement, began exercising to tolerance during the first phase of the study.

Slightly TSH-suppressive dosages of exogenous thyroid hormone in premenopausal women do not correlate with loss of bone mineral density.[48][49][50][51][52][53] However, the use of TSH-suppressive dosages of T_3 may raise concern. Dual photon absorptiometry of our 4 patients showed normal bone density even though they had been taking TSH-suppressive doses of T_3 for several months. Their bone cells may be partially resistant to thyroid hormone. The elevated N-telopeptides indicated increased bone turnover, but are not correlated with osteoporosis or increased fracture rate in patients taking thyroid hormone. Long-range adverse effects, however, can only be ruled out by long-term follow-up safety testing.

Implications for the Pathophysiology of FMS. Our

4 patients significantly improved according to 5 FMS measures, without short-term adverse target tissue effects and only with supraphysiologic doses of T_3. The patients' elevated free T_3 levels at follow-up indicated that the lack of tissue thyrotoxicosis was not due to increased hepatic clearance of thyroid hormone. Rather, the lack of tissue thyrotoxicosis was indicative of a blunted target tissue response to T_3. In this way, our patients resemble patients with thyroid hormone resistance syndromes due to mutations in the c-erbAβ gene in chromosome 3.[27]

There are a variety of clinical phenotypes of thyroid hormone resistance syndrome with distinguishing clinical features resulting from differential target tissue resistance to thyroid hormone.[27][54] The results of this study, and similar results by Sonkin[15] and by Lowe and colleagues,[24][25][26][59] indicate that euthyroid FMS is another clinical phenotype of thyroid hormone resistance. The patients in this study are properly classified as having *peripheral* resistance to thyroid hormone[27][54][55] because their suppressed TSH levels indicate that each patient's pituitary gland was normally responsive to T_3.

Dosages of T_3 reported to maintain normal metabolism in patients without functional thyroid glands have been given variously as 25-to-75 μg[56] and 50-to-75 μg per day.[54] Patients in our study had significant therapeutic responses only to dosages ranging from 106.25-to-137.50 μg. These dosages caused low TSH, FTI, and total and free T_4, and high levels of free T_3 in all patients. This pattern of laboratory values in patients taking exogenous T_3 has been described as T_3-toxicosis.[57] Our patients, however, did not have clinical features of thyrotoxicosis. Moreover, the results of electrocardiography, bone densitometry, and most laboratory tests were within normal range.

Mutations in the c-erbAβ$_1$ gene of chromosome 3 are responsible for general thyroid hormone resistance in most patients studied.[27] Only when exposed to high concentrations of T_3 do mutant T_3-receptors properly regulate transcription. At low concentrations of T_3, for example, the P448H mutant T_3-receptor inhibits normal T_3-receptors and inhibits the normal transcriptional activity of the target gene to which the mutant receptor is bound. At high T_3 concentrations, the mutant receptor becomes transcriptionally active.[58] Our patients' requirement for high T_3 dosages may also have been due to mutated T_3-receptors.[23] Because our research group has accumulated a substantial body of euthyroid fibromyalgia patients who have recovered with the protocol tested in this study, the Fibromyalgia Research Foundation is in the planning stages of an extensive project to sequence both the c-*erb*Aβ and c-*erb*Aα genes from these patients for possible mutations.

CONCLUSION

The FMS status of these 4 euthyroid patients significantly improved with the use of supraphysiologic doses of T_3. No other medications were necessary. The absence of thyrotoxic target tissue effects at 6-month follow-up raises the possibility that in these patients, FMS is a clinical phenotype of partial peripheral resistance to thyroid hormone. More follow-up testing is necessary to determine whether patients' long-term use of supraphysiologic dosages of T_3 is safe.

REFERENCES

1. Wolfe, F., Smythe, H.A., Yunus, M.B., et al.: The American College of Rheumatology 1990 criteria for the classification of fibromyalgia: report of the multicenter criteria committee. *Arthritis Rheumatol.*, 33:160-172, 1990.
2. Consensus Document on Fibromyalgia: The Copenhagen Declaration. Copenhagen, Myopain '92, 17-20 August, 1992. *J. Musculoskel. Pain*, 1(3/4):295-312, 1993.
3. Lowe, J.C.: *The Metabolic Treatment of Fibromyalgia*. Houston, McDowell Publishing Company, 1999.
4. Carette, S.: What have clinical trials taught us about the treatment of fibromyalgia? *J. Musculo-skel. Pain*, 3:133-140, 1995.
5. Lowe, J.C.: T_3-induced recovery from fibromyalgia by a hypothyroid patient resistant to T_4 and desiccated thyroid. *J. Myofascial. Ther.*, 1(4):26-31, 1995.
6. Beetham, W.P., Jr.: Diagnosis and management of fibrositis syndrome and psychogenic rheumatism. *Med. Clin. North Am.*, 63:433-439, 1979.
7. Golding, D.N.: Hypothyroidism presenting with musculoskeletal symptoms. *Ann. Rheumatic. Dis.* 29:10-41, 1970.
8. Bland, J.H. and Frymoyer, J.W.: Rheumatic syndromes of myxedema. *N. Eng. J. Med.*, 282:1171-1174, 1970.
9. Wilke, S.W., Sheeler, L.R., and Makarowski, W.S.: Hypothyroidism with presenting symptoms of fibrositis. *J. Rheumatol.*, 8:627-630, 1981.
10. Hochberg, M.C., Koppes, G.M., Edwards, C.Q., Barnes, H.V., and Arnett, F.C., Jr.: Hypothyroidism presenting as a polymyositis-like syndrome: report of two cases. *Arthritis Rheum.*, 19:1363-1366, 1976.
11. Delamere, J.P., Scott, D.L., and Felix-Davies, D.D.: Thyroid dysfunction and rheumatic diseases. *J. Royal Soc. Med.*, 75:102, 1982.
12. Fessel, W. J.: Myopathy of hypothyroidism. *Ann. Rheumatic Dis.*, 27:590-596, 1968.
13. Wilson, J. and Walton, J.N.: Some muscular manifestations of hypothyroidism. *J. Neurol. Neurosurg. Psychiat.*, 22:320-324, 1959.
14. Awad, E.A.: Histopathological changes in fibrositis. In *Advances in Pain Research and Therapy*, vol. 17. Edited by J.R. Fricton and E.A. Awad, New York, Raven Press, 1990, pp.249-258.
15. Sonkin, L.S.: Endocrine disorders and muscle dysfunction. In *Clinical management of Head, Neck, and TMJ Pain and Dysfunction*. Edited by B. Gelb, Philadelphia, W.B. Saunders Co., 1985, pp.137-170.
16. Hershman, J.M.: Hypothalamic and pituitary hypothyroidism. In *Progress in the Diagnosis and Treatment of Hypothyroid Conditions*. Edited by P.A. Bastenie, M. Bonnyns, and L. VanHaelst, Amsterdam, Excerpta Medica, 1980, pp.41-50.
17. Eisinger, J., Arroyo, P.H., Calendini, C., Rinaldi, .JP., Combes, R., and Fontaine, G.: Anomalies biologiques au cours des fibromyalgies: III. Explorations endocriniennes. *Lyon Méditerranée Méd.*, 28: 858-860, 1992.
18. Gerwin, R.: A study of 96 subjects examined both for fibromyalgia and myofascial pain. *J. Musculoskel. Pain*, 3:(Suppl.)1:121, 1995.
19. Lowe, J.C.: Thyroid status of 38 fibromyalgia patients: implications for the etiology of fibromyalgia. *Clin. Bull. Myofascial.Ther.*, 2(1):36-41, 1997.
20. Shiroky, J.B., Cohen, M., Ballachey, M-L., and Neville, C.: Thyroid dysfunction in rheumatoid arthritis: a controlled prospective survey. *Ann .Rheumat. Dis.*, 52:454-456, 1993.
21. Ferraccioli, G., Cavalieri, F., Salaffi, F., et al.: Neuroendocrinologic findings in primary fibromyalgia (soft tissue chronic pain syndrome) and in other chronic rheumatic conditions (rheumatoid arthritis, low back pain). *J. Rheumatol.*, 17:869-873, 1990.
22. Neeck, G. and Riedel, W.: Thyroid function in patients with fibromyalgia syndrome. *J. Rheumatol.*, 19:1120-1122, 1992.
23. Lowe, J.C., Cullum, M., Graf, L., Jr, and Yellin, J.: Mutations in the c-*erb*Aβ₁ gene: do they underlie euthyroid fibromyalgia? *Med. Hypotheses*, 48(2)Feb.:125-135, 1997.
24. Lowe, J.C., Eichelberger, J., Manso, G., and Peterson, K.: Improvement in euthyroid fibromyalgia patients treated with T_3 (tri-iodothyronine). *J. Myofascial Ther.*, 1(2):16-27, 1994.
25. Lowe, J.C.: Results of an open trial of T_3 therapy with 77 euthyroid female fibromyalgia patients. *Clin. Bull. Myofascial Ther.*, 2(1):35-37, 1997.
26. Lowe, J.C., Garrison, R.L., Reichman, A.J., Yellin, J., Thompson, M., and Kaufman, D.: Effectiveness and safety of T_3 therapy for euthyroid fibromyalgia. *Clin. Bull. Myofascial Ther.*, 2(2/3):31-58, 1997.
27. Refetoff, S., Weiss, R.E., and Usala, S.J.: The syndromes of resistance to thyroid hormone. *Endocrine Rev.*, 14:348-399, 1993.
28. Rasmussen, J.O., Smidth, M., and Hansen, T.M.: Examination of tender points in soft tissue: palpation versus pressure-algometer. *Ugeskr Laeger*, 152(21):1522-1526, 1990.
29. Nicoloff, J.T., Fisher, D.A., and Appleman, M.D.: The role of glucocorticoids in the regulation of thyroid function in man. *J. Clin. Invest.*, 49:1922, 1970.
30. Burckhardt, C.S., Clark, S.R., and Bennett, R.M.: The fibromyalgia impact questionnaire: development and validation. *J. Rheumatol.*, 18(5):728-733, 1991.

31. Naughton, M.J. and Wiklund, I.: A critical review of dimension-specific measures of health-related quality of life in cross-cultural research. *Quality Life Res.*, 2(6):397-432, 1993.

32. Felson, D.T. and Goldenberg, D.L.: The natural history of fibromyalgia. *Arthritis Rheum.*, 29:1522-1526, 1986.

33. Hazleman, B.: Soft tissue rheumatism. *Brit. J. Rheumat.*, 31:135, 1992.

34. Cathey, M.A., Wolfe, F., Kleinheksel, S.M., and Hawley, D.J.: Socioeconomic impact of fibrositis: a study of 81 patients with primary fibrositis. *Amer. J. Med.*, 81:78-84, 1986.

35. Bengtsson, A., Bäckman, E,. Lindblom, V., and Skogh, T.: Long term follow-up of fibromyalgia patients: clinical symptoms, muscular function, laboratory tests—an eight year comparison study. *J. Musculoskel. Pain*, 2(2):67-80, 1994.

36. Henriksson, C.: Living with fibromyalgia. *Scand. J. Rheum.*, 24:179, 1995.

37. Ross, D.S.: Subclinical hyperthyroidism. In Werner and Ingbar's *The Thyroid: A Fundamental and Clinical Text.*, 6th edition. Edited by L.E .Braverman and R.D. Utiger, Philadelphia, J.B. Lippincott, 1991, pp.1249-1255.

38. Dillman, W.H.: The cardiovascular system in thyrotoxicosis. In Werner and Ingbar's *The Thyroid: A Fundamental and Clinical Text.*, 6th edition. Edited by L.E. Braverman and R.D. Utiger, Philadelphia, J.B. Lippincott, 1991, pp.759-770.

39. Unger, J., Mavroudakis, N., Lipski, A., and van Coevorden, A.: Treatment of supraventricular tachyarrhythmias associated with hyperthyroidism by radioiodine, amiodarone, and propylthiouracil. *Thyroidology*, 3(2):85-88, 1991.

40. Symons, C. and Colquhoun, M.C.: Asymptomatic thyroiditis and atrial dysrhythmias. *Recent Progress in Diagnosis and Treatment of Hypothyroid Conditions.* Edited by P.A. Bastenie and M. Bonnyns, L. Vanhaelst, Amsterdam, Excerpta Medica, 1980, pp.137-143.

41. Vlase, H., Lungu, G., and Vlase, L.: Cardiac disturbances in thyrotoxicosis: diagnosis, incidence, clinical features, and management. *Endocrinologie*, 29(3-4):155-160, 1991.

42. Hof, F.M., San, J.F.Y., and Lowrey, R.D.: The electrocardiogram in thyrotoxicosis. *Am. J. Cardiol.*, 8:893, 1960.

43. Muggia, A.L., Stjernholm, M., and Houle, T.: Complete heart block with thyrotoxic myocarditis. *N. Engl. J. Med.*, 283:1099, 1970.

44. Agner, T., Almdal, T., Thorsteinsson, B., and Agner, E.: A reevaluation of atrial fibrillation in thyrotoxicosis. *Dan. Med. Bull.*, 31:157, 1984.

45. Ciaccheri, M., Cecchi, F., Arcangeli C., et al.: Occult thyrotoxicosis in patients with chronic and paroxysmal isolated atrial fibrillation. *Clin. Cardiol.*, 7:413, 1984.

46. Gow, S.M., Caldwell, G., Toft, A.D., et al.: Relationship between pituitary and other target organ responsiveness in hypothyroid patients receiving thyroxine replacement. *J. Clin. Endocrinol. Metab.*, 64: 364, 1987.

47. Tepperman, J. and Tepperman, H.M.: *Metabolic and Endocrine Physiology*, 5th ed. Chicago, Year Book Medical Publishers, 1987.

48. Salmon, D., Rendell, M., and Williams, J.: Chemical hyperthyroidism. *Arch. Intern. Med.*, 142: 571, 1982.

49. Fish, L.H., Schwartz, H.L., and Cavanaugh, J.: Replacement dose, metabolism, and bioavailability of levothyroxine in the treatment of hypothyroidism. *N. Engl. J. Med.*, 316:764, 1987.

50. Pearce, C.J. and Himsworth, R.L.: Total and free thyroid hormone concentrations in patients receiving maintenance replacement treatment with thyroxine. *Br. Med. J.*, 288: 693, 1984.

51. Bayer, M.F., Kriss, J.P., and McDougall, I.R.: Clinical experience with sensitive thyrotropin measurements: diagnostic and therapeutic implications. *J. Nucl. Med.*, 26: 1248, 1985.

52. De Rosa, G., Testa, A., Maussier, M.L., Calla, C., Astazi, P., and Albanese, C.: A slightly suppressive dose of L-thyroxine does not affect bone turnover and bone mineral density in pre- and post-menopausal women with nontoxic goitre. *Hormone Metab. Res.*, 27(11):503-507, 1995.

53. Chabert-Orsini, V., Conte-Devolx, B., Thiers-Bautrant, D., et al.: Bone density after iatrogenic subclinical long-term thyrotoxicosis: measurement by dual photon absorptiometry. *Presse Med.*, 19: 1709-1711, 1990.

54. Kaplan, M.M., Swartz, S.L., and Larsen, P.R.: Partial peripheral resistance to thyroid hormone. *Am. J. Med.*, 70:1115-1121, 1981.

55. Refetoff, S.: Thyroid hormone resistance syndromes. In Werner and Ingbar's *The Thyroid: A Fundamental and Clinical Text,* 6th edition. Edited by L.E. Braverman and R.D. Utiger, Philadelphia, J.B. Lippincott, 1991, pp.1280-1294.

56. De Visscher, M.: The therapy of hypothyroid states. In *Recent Progress in Diagnosis and Treatment of Hypothyroid Conditions: Proceedings of the XVth International Congress of Therapeutics*, Amsterdam, Excerpta Medica, 1980, pp.105-114.

57. Ladenson, P.W.: Diagnosis of thyrotoxicosis. In Werner and Ingbar's *The Thyroid: A Fundamental and Clinical Text,* 6th edition. Edited by L.E. Braverman and R.D. Utiger, Philadelphia, J.B. Lippincott, 1991, pp.880-886.

58. Krishna, V., Chatterjee, K., Nagaya T, et al.: Thyroid hormone resistance syndrome: inhibition of normal receptor function by mutant thyroid hormone receptors. *J. Clin. Invest.*, 87:1977-1984, 1991.

59. Lowe, J.C., Reichman, A.J., and Yellin, J.: The process of change during T_3 treatment for euthyroid fibromyalgia: a double-blind placebo-controlled crossover study. *Clin. Bull. Myofascial Ther.*, 2(2/3):91-124, 1997.

60. Ottenbacher, K.J.: *Evaluating Clinical Change: Strategies for Occupational and Physical Therapists.* Baltimore, Williams & Wilkins, 1986.

61. Barlow, D.H. and Hersen, M.: Single-case experimental designs. *Arch. Gen. Psychiatry*, 29:319-325, 1973.

62. Wigers, S.H., Skrondal, A., Finset, A., and Götestam, K.G.: Measuring change in fibromyalgic pain: the relevance of pain distribution. *J. Musculoskel. Pain*, 5(2):29-41, 1997.

63. Bennett, R.M.: Literature reviews. *J. Musculoskel. Pain*, 2(2):101-112, 1994.

64. Littlejohn, G.O.: A database for fibromyalgia. *Rheum. Dis. Clinics North Am.*, 21(2):527-557, 1995.

65. Fischer, A.A., DeCosta, C., and Levy, H.: Diagnosis of

fibromyalgia by manual pressure is unreliable: quantification of tender point sensitivity by algometer is necessary in clinical practice. *J. Musculoskel. Pain*, 3(1):139, 1995.

66. Putick, M., Schulzer, M., Klinkhoff, A., Koehler, B., Rangno, K., and Chalmers, A.: Reliability and reproducibility of fibromyalgic tenderness, measurement by electronic and mechanical dolorimeters. *J. Musculoskel. Pain*, 3(4):3-14, 1995.

67. Lautenschlager, J., Seglias, J., Bruckle, W., and Muller, W.: Comparisons of spontaneous pain and tenderness in patients with primary fibromyalgia. *Clin. Rheumatol.*, 10(2):168-173, 1991.

68. Wilkins, E.W., Dineen, J.J., Moncure, A.C., Gross, P.L., and Fitzgerald, C.P.: *MGH Textbook of Emergency Medicine*. 2nd edition. Baltimore, Williams & Wilkins, 1983, pp.624-627.

69. O'Boyle, C.M., Davis, D.K., Russo, B.A., Kraf, T.J., and Brick, P.D.: *Emergency Care: The First 24 Hours*. Norwalk, Appleton-Century-Crofts, 1985, pp.332-333.

70. Joos, E., Meeusen, R., and De Meirleir, K.: Measurement of physical capacity in fibromyalgia. *J. Musculoskel. Pain*, 3:Suppl 1:87, 1995.

71. Nielson, W.R., Grace, G.M., Hopkins, M., and Berg, M.: Concentration and memory deficits in patients with fibromyalgia syndrome. *J. Musculoskel. Pain*, 3:Suppl 1:123, 1995.

72. Clark, S., Tindall, E., and Bennett, R.M.: A double-blind crossover trial of prednisone versus placebo in the treatment of fibrositis. *J. Rheumatol.*, 12:980-983, 1985.

73. Goldenberg, D.L., Felson, D.T., and Dinerman, H.: A randomized, controlled trial of amitriptyline and naproxen in the treatment of patients with fibromyalgia. *Arthritis Rheumat.*, 29(1):1371-1377, 1986.

74. Jacobsen, S., Danneskiold-Samsøe, B., and Andersen, R.B.: Oral S-adenosylmethionine in primary fibromyalgia: double-blind clinical evaluation. *Scand. J. Rheumatol.*, 20:294-302, 1991.

75. Goldenberg, D.L., Marskīy, M., Mossey, C., Ruthazer, R., and Schmid, C.: The independent and combined efficacy of fluoxetine and amitriptyline in the treatment of fibromyalgia. *Arthritis Rheumat.*, Suppl 38: S229, 1995.

76. Scott, J. and Huskisson, E.C.: Graphic representation of pain. *Pain*, 2:175-184, 1976.

77. Zung, W.W.K.: A self-rating depression scale. *Arch. Gen. Psychiatry*, 12:65-70, 1965.

78. Rehm, L.P.: Assessment of depression. In *Behavioral Assessment: A Practical Handbook*. Edited by M. Hersen and A.S. Bellack, Oxford, Permagon Press, 1976, pp.246-295.

Thyroid Status of Fibromyalgia Patients

John C. Lowe, MA, DC
Alan J. Reichman, MD
Gina S. Honeyman, DC
Jackie Yellin, BA

This article originally appeared in the *Clinical Bulletin of Myofascial Therapy*, 3(1):69-70, 1998.
It is reprinted with permission of Haworth Medical Press.

ABSTRACT. In a previous retrospective study,* thyroid function tests were used to classify 38 fibromyalgia patients according to thyroid status. Results were consistent with euthyroidism (normal thyroid status) in 14 patients (36.8%), primary (thyroidal) hypothyroidism in 4 patients (10.5%), and central (hypothalamic or pituitary) hypothyroidism in 20 patients (52.6%). In this prospective study, an additional 54 patients were tested. Results were consistent with euthyroidism in 26 patients (48.1%), primary hypothyroidism in 8 patients (14.8%), and central hypothyroidism in 20 patients (37.0%). All patients from both studies were combined into a group of 92 to obtain the total percentage in each classification. Results were consistent with euthyroidism in 40 patients (43.5%), primary hypothyroidism in 12 patients (13.0%), and central hypothyroidism in 40 patients (43.5%).

There was no statistical difference in either study for the mean intensity of fibromyalgia symptoms (measured by visual analog scales) or the mean tender point score (measured with algometry) between any of the categories of patients. In the study of 54 patients, there was also no statistical difference for pain distribution (measured by the percentage of 36 body divisions containing pain), functional ability (measured by the Fibromyalgia Impact Questionnaire), or depression (measured by Zung's Self-Rating Depression Scale) between the three categories of patients.

In both studies, the percentages of patients with primary and central hypothyroidism were extremely high compared to those in the general population (see table below). Of the 92 patients, 52 (56.5%) had laboratory test results consistent with hypothyroidism. Contrary to anecdotal reports, hypothyroidism is extraordinarily common among fibromyalgia patients.

* Lowe, J.C.: Thyroid status of 38 fibromyalgia patients: implications for the etiology of fibromyalgia. *Clin. Bull. Myofascial. Ther.*, 2 (1):47-64, 1997.

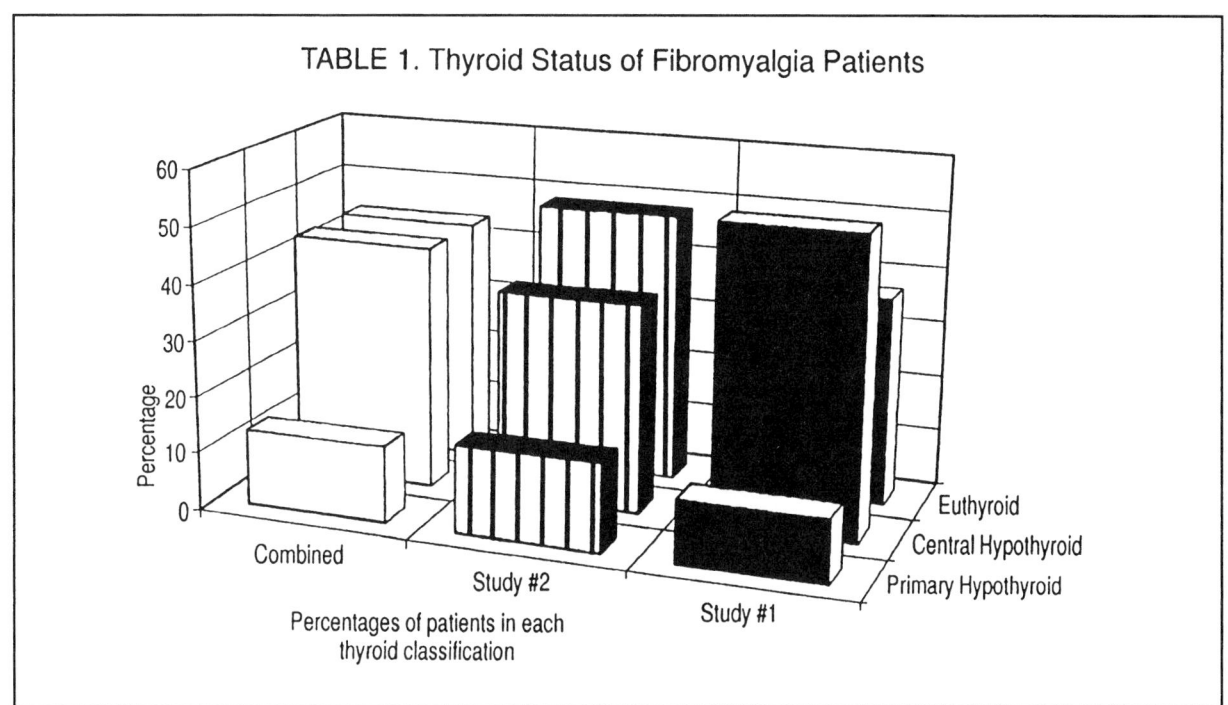

TABLE 1. Thyroid Status of Fibromyalgia Patients

A Case-Control Study
of Metabolic Therapy for Fibromyalgia:
Long-Term Follow-Up Comparison
of Treated and Untreated Patients

John C. Lowe, MA, DC
Alan J. Reichman, MD
Jackie Yellin, BA

This abstract originally appeared in the *Clinical Bulletin of Myofascial Therapy*, 3(1):23-24, 1998.
It is reprinted with permission of Haworth Medical Press.

ABSTRACT. The long-term effectiveness of metabolic therapy for fibromyalgia syndrome (FMS) involving the use of exogenous thyroid hormone was evaluated. Twenty treated FMS patients were compared with 20 matched evaluated but non-treated FMS patients. Treated patients successfully underwent metabolic therapy and were released as significantly improved or recovered between 1991 and 1995. Untreated patients were evaluated during this same time frame, but were not able to undergo treatment because of insufficient or absent insurance coverage. Patients were contacted by mail; they each filled out and returned a questionnaire with forms used to evaluate FMS status. Treated patients were matched with untreated patients based on time since initial evaluation, sex, and thyroid status. In each group, 10 (50%) patients had been classified as euthyroid, 6 (30%) as primary hypothyroid, and 4 (20%) as central hypothyroid. Of treated patients, all but 1 euthyroid patient used T_3, and all but 1 hypothyroid patient used T_4.

Both groups were compared at baseline and follow-up using *chi* square analysis for discontinuous variables. These included age, employment, thyroid status, duration of illness, and use of medications and other forms of treatment. Groups were also compared using analysis of variance for continuous variables at baseline and follow-up. These included pain distribution by the percentage and the ACR methods, mean symptom intensity, and scores on the Fibromyalgia Impact Questionnaire (FIQ) and Zung's Self-Rating Depression Scale (Zung's). Because some patients were not available for physical examination at follow-up, mean algometer scores of tender points for the two groups were compared only for the initial evaluation. There were no significant differences at baseline between treated and untreated groups.

At follow-up, Wilcoxon Matched Pairs Signed Rank Test showed that treated patients had decreased their use of antidepressants and NSAIDS; untreated patients had increased their use of antidepressants and anxiolytics. Comparison of baseline measures with follow-up measures for each group by *t*-tests showed that treated patients improved on all FMS measures, while untreated patients improved on none. Multivariate analysis of variance showed significant differences between the two groups on FMS measures ($F < 0.0005$). Univariate analysis of variance revealed that at follow-up, compared to the untreated group, the treated group significantly improved specifically in pain distribution via the ACR method ($F = 0.0002$) and in pain distribution via the percentage method, mean symptom intensity, FIQ, and Zung's ($F < 0.00005$).

We conclude that at 1-to-5 year follow-up, the FMS status of euthyroid and hypothyroid patients who underwent metabolic therapy, including the use of exogenous thyroid hormone, significantly improved compared to matched untreated FMS patients. (See Table 1.) The continuation of improved FMS status for 1-to-5 years effectively rules out a placebo effect as the mechanism of improvement.

Table 1. Comparisons of FMS measures: treated and untreated groups.

COMPARISON	SIGNIFICANT	NOT SIGNIFICANT
treated versus untreated groups, at baseline		X
treated versus untreated groups, at follow-up	X	
treated group, baseline versus follow-up	X	
untreated group, baseline versus follow-up		X

Facilitating the Decrease in Fibromyalgic Pain During Metabolic Rehabilitation: An Essential Role for Soft Tissue Therapies

J.C. Lowe, G. Honeyman-Lowe

This article originally appeared in the *Journal of Bodywork and Movement Therapies*, 2(4):208-217, 1998. It is reprinted with permission of Harcourt Brace & Co. Ltd.

Abstract Recent evidence indicates that fibromyalgia (FMS) is a manifestation of impaired metabolism. In most cases, the cause is inadequate thyroid hormone regulation of cell function. The measurable features of FMS can be improved or relieved in most patients through therapy that is best termed "metabolic rehabilitation." For some patients undergoing metabolic rehabilitation, however, FMS pain scores normalize only after soft tissue treatment controls or eliminates noxious neural input from the musculoskeletal system to the central nervous system (CNS). Our studies and clinical experiences convince us that effective soft tissue therapy can expedite the typical patient's improvement or recovery. Neglecting to use such therapy can hinder recovery, even when the patient undergoes expertly conducted metabolic rehabilitation. This paper describes the probable mechanisms by which musculoskeletal lesions can sustain FMS pain, and gives guidelines for treating the FMS patient's soft tissues to facilitate the reduction of pain during metabolic rehabilitation.

Introduction

Recent studies of patients with fibromyalgia syndrome (FMS) provide strong evidence for three conclusions. First, FMS is a condition of metabolic insufficiency in select tissues. Second, in most cases, the insufficiency is a result of hypothyroidism or cellular resistance to thyroid hormone. Third, treatments that cause or encourage a sustained increase in metabolism are effective in improving or relieving FMS symptoms. In view of this, does the bodyworker doing soft tissue treatment have a role to play in the care of FMS patients? Definitely. For most patients, soft tissue treatment provides palliative relief during the process of metabolic rehabilitation. More importantly, the use of soft tissue treatment is necessary in many cases if patients are to fully recover from the most distinguishing symptom of FMS: chronic widespread pain. We describe the modifications in technique that are advisable for treating most FMS patients.

Fibromyalgia

Fibromyalgia syndrome (FMS) is the most common condition of chronic widespread musculoskeletal pain, stiffness, and fatigue. The incidence in the U.S.A. is roughly 2%; 90% of patients are female (Wolfe 1994). Diagnostic criteria, established by the American College of Rheumatology (ACR), include widespread pain and abnormal tenderness at predictable anatomical sites (Wolfe et al 1990) (Box 1). Some evidence indicates, however, that although the diagnosis is currently being made more often, most clinicians are still not familiar with the formal diagnostic criteria (Buskila et al 1997). They make the diagnosis when a female patient reports chronic pain and fatigue, and no objective signs are obvious (Marin & Connick 1997). In this paper, when we refer to FMS patients, we mean those who meet the ACR criteria.

Results of conventional drug treatments for FMS are so poor that a majority of patients seek care from alternative practitioners (Bennett 1997). Clinical trials show that conventional FMS treatments, such as tricyclic antidepressants, are no more effective than placebos (Carette 1995). The widespread use of antidepressants is based on the hypothesis that FMS is a manifestation of serotonin deficiency (Russell et al 1992a). Researchers conjectured that antidepressants, by increasing the amount of serotonin at synapses, would improve or alleviate FMS symptoms. The failure of antidepressant treatments to do so makes it unlikely that FMS results from a primary serotonin deficiency. The symptoms and signs of FMS must instead stem from another mechanism—one that causes the serotonin deficiency as well as all the other features of the condition. The available evidence indicates that the most likely mechanism is inadequate thyroid hormone regulation of cell function. This is caused by a deficiency of thyroid hormone, partial cellular resistance to thyroid hormone, or both.

Box 1

The **definition of fibromyalgia syndrome (FMS)**, according to the 1990 American College of Rheumatology (ACR) criteria (Wolfe et al 1990), is:

(1)   widespread pain* for at least 3 months, and
(2)   11 of 18 possible tender points (9 on each side of the body).

*Widespread pain is defined as pain above and below the waist, on the left and right sides of the body, and axial pain (either on the anterior or posterior aspect of the torso).

Associated symptoms include:

● fatigue ● stiffness ● headaches ● disturbed sleep ● depression ● disturbed bowel function ● cognitive disturbance ● anxiety ● paresthesias ● coldness ● dry mucous membranes ● exercise intolerance ● dysmenorrhea

The associated symptoms are not essential to the diagnosis (Wolfe et al 1990), but the probability that a patient has FMS is increased if the patient has one or more of them (Lowe, 1999).

FMS as a manifestation of hypothyroidism or cellular resistance to thyroid hormone

The clinical features of FMS and hypothyroidism are virtually the same (Wilson & Walton 1959, Fessel 1968, Bland & Frymoyer 1970, Golding 1970, Hochberg et al 1976, Wilke et al 1981, Delamere et al 1982, Sonkin 1985, Awad 1990, Lowe 1995). The 13 most common FMS symptoms are also common symptoms of hypothyroidism. (We have listed these with bullets in Box 1.) Moreover, every objectively verified abnor-

mality in FMS can be explained by inadequate thyroid hormone regulation of cell function (Lowe 1999a, Lowe 1999b). These include the low serotonin (Russell et al 1992a) and high substance P (Vaerøy et al 1988) levels that may mediate the chronic widespread pain and pressure sensitivity of FMS patients. Inadequate thyroid hormone regulation can plausibly explain both low serotonin secretion (Frankhyzen & Muller 1983) and high substance P levels (Yellin 1997). We discuss these abnormalities in detail below.

Hypothyroidism in FMS

There is an extraordinarily high incidence of hypothyroidism in FMS patients. The incidence of primary hypothyroidism (thyroid hormone deficiency due to impaired thyroid gland function) in the general U.S.A. population is about 1% (Hershman 1980). The incidence of primary hypothyroidism among FMS patients has been reported as 10% (Eisinger et al 1992, Gerwin 1995), 10.5% (Lowe 1997a), 12% (Shiroky et al 1993), and 13.0% (Lowe et al 1998b). The incidence of central hypothyroidism (thyroid hormone deficiency due to hypothalamic or pituitary dysfunction) in the population at-large is about 0.00021% (Hershman 1980). We found an incidence among FMS patients of 52.6% (Lowe 1997a) and 43.5% (Lowe et al 1998b). Ferraccioli et al (1990) and Neeck & Riedel (1992) reported similarly high incidences of central hypothyroidism among FMS patients. Thus, the incidence of primary hypothyroidism among FMS patients may be some 10 times higher than in the population at-large; the incidence of central hypothyroidism, some 250,000 times higher.

Euthyroid hypometabolism in FMS (partial cellular resistance to thyroid hormone) (Box 2)

We found that 36.8% (Lowe 1997a) and 43.5% (Lowe et al 1998b) of FMS patients were euthyroid (had normal laboratory thyroid function test results). What could cause hypothyroid-like symptoms in these patients? Any factor that impedes the same metabolic pathways as those impeded by thyroid hormone deficiency. Examples of such factors are folic acid deficiency and beta-adrenergic blocking drugs. But our studies and clinical experiences indicate that euthyroid FMS is most often a result of cellular resistance to thyroid hormone. Symptoms and objective abnormalities resulting from cellular resistance are virtually the same as those resulting from thyroid hormone deficiency.

Box 2 The hypometabolism hypothesis of fibromyalgia

Scientific studies and years of related clinical experiences have led to several conclusions about the pathogenesis of FMS and its treatment:

● In most cases, FMS is caused by, or related to, inadequate thyroid hormone regulation of cell function. The inadequate regulation results from one of two phenomena: (1) thyroid hormone deficiency, or (2) partial cellular resistance to the hormone.

● Other metabolism-impairing factors may also induce and sustain symptoms that lead to a diagnosis of FMS if those factors impede the metabolism of the tissues from which FMS symptoms and signs arise. Such factors include B complex vitamin deficiencies, the use of beta-receptor blocking drugs, and deconditioning. Whereas one such factor may not be enough to induce FMS symptoms, combinations of them may be sufficient. (Lowe 1999a, Lowe 1999b).

● The metabolism-impeding factors responsible for FMS must be controlled or eliminated before a patient can significantly improve. When FMS results from inadequate thyroid hormone regulation, thyroid hormone is indispensable if the patient is to improve or recover.

● For most patients, nutritional supplements are also essential. They synergistically interact with thyroid hormone to cause a sustained increase in metabolism (Lowe 1997b). As thyroid hormone accelerates metabolism, the body's requirement for nutrients—especially B complex vitamins—increases. Not taking vitamin supplements may result in vitamin deficiency or cardiomyopathy (Travell & Simons 1983). Taking supplements can avert such adverse effects and facilitate a thyroid hormone-induced increase in metabolism.

● For most patients, exercise to tolerance is necessary. Exercise enables patients to capitalize on the increased metabolic capacity provided by thyroid hormone and nutritional supplements (Lowe 1997b). Resistance exercises contribute to the increase in metabolism by increasing lean tissue mass, which has a higher metabolic rate than fat tissue (Pratley et al 1994). Aerobic exercise contributes by increasing the metabolic rate of the lean tissues (Shinkai et al 1994).

Only one cause of thyroid hormone resistance, mutations in the c-erbAβ gene on chromosome 3, has been proven (Refetoff et al 1993) to date. It is possible that such mutations underlie the hypothyroid-like symptoms and objective findings in euthyroid FMS patients (Lowe et al 1997d). At this time, we conclude that a patient has cellular resistance to thyroid hormone when several conditions are met; when the patient:

1. is euthyroid before beginning to use thyroid hormone;
2. recovers from hypothyroid-like FMS symptoms and signs with "supraphysiologic" (higher than normal) dosages of T_3, the metabolically active thyroid hormone;
3. after beginning treatment, has an "abnormally"

high blood T_3 level; and
4. has no tissue overstimulation (thyrotoxicosis) due to the high T_3 levels, according to the results of EKGs, and laboratory and bone density tests.

We find this pattern in virtually all our euthyroid patients who benefit from metabolic rehabilitation. And according to these criteria, we have documented the presence of thyroid hormone resistance in FMS patients in several double-blind, placebo-controlled, crossover studies (Lowe et al 1997a, Lowe et al 1997b, Lowe et al 1997c). It appears, then, that the hypothyroid-like FMS symptoms and signs of many—and perhaps most—euthyroid FMS patients are a result of cellular resistance to thyroid hormone (Lowe 1999a, Lowe 1999b).

That FMS in most patients is a result of inadequate thyroid hormone regulation is further supported by an important study completed last year (Lowe et al 1998a). *Its results are the first to demonstrate long-term effectiveness of an FMS treatment.* The study was a 1-to-5-year follow-up comparing patients treated with metabolic therapy to untreated patients. Twenty FMS patients who underwent metabolic treatment were matched with 20 FMS patients who did not. Patients were matched by sex, thyroid status, and the time since their initial evaluations. All patients were initially evaluated 1-to-5 years before the follow-up study began. In each group, 10 (50%) patients had been classified as euthyroid, 6 (30%) as primary hypothyroid, and 4 (20%) as central hypothyroid. Before 20 of the patients began treatment, there was no statistical difference on any measure between them and the 20 patients who were to have no treatment. At follow-up, analyses showed that treated patients had decreased their use of antidepressants and NSAIDS; untreated patients had increased their intake of antidepressants and anxiolytics. Comparison of baseline measures with follow-up measures for each group showed that treated patients improved on all FMS measures; untreated patients improved on none. The conclusion is that at 1-to-5 year follow-up, the FMS status of euthyroid and

hypothyroid patients who underwent metabolic therapy significantly improved compared to matched, untreated FMS patients. The continuation of improved FMS status in treated patients for 1-to-5 years effectively rules out two possible mechanisms of improvement: a placebo effect, and a tendency to improve over time (regression toward the mean).

Possible causes of inadequate thyroid hormone regulation

To what do we attribute the inadequate thyroid hormone regulation in FMS? Hypothyroidism in adults results most frequently from autoimmune thyroiditis, but it often occurs following radiation exposure, surgical removal of part of the thyroid gland, or pituitary failure (Oertel & LiVolsi 1991). For some FMS patients, contamination with dioxins or polychlorinated biphenyls (PCBs) may be the source of interference with normal thyroid hormone regulation. These environmental contaminants are nearly ubiquitous in our environment and are abundantly present in human breast milk, fat, and blood (McKinney & Pedersen 1987). The contaminants cause the liver to eliminate thyroid hormone at an abnormally rapid rate (Van den Berg et al 1988). They also displace thyroid hormone

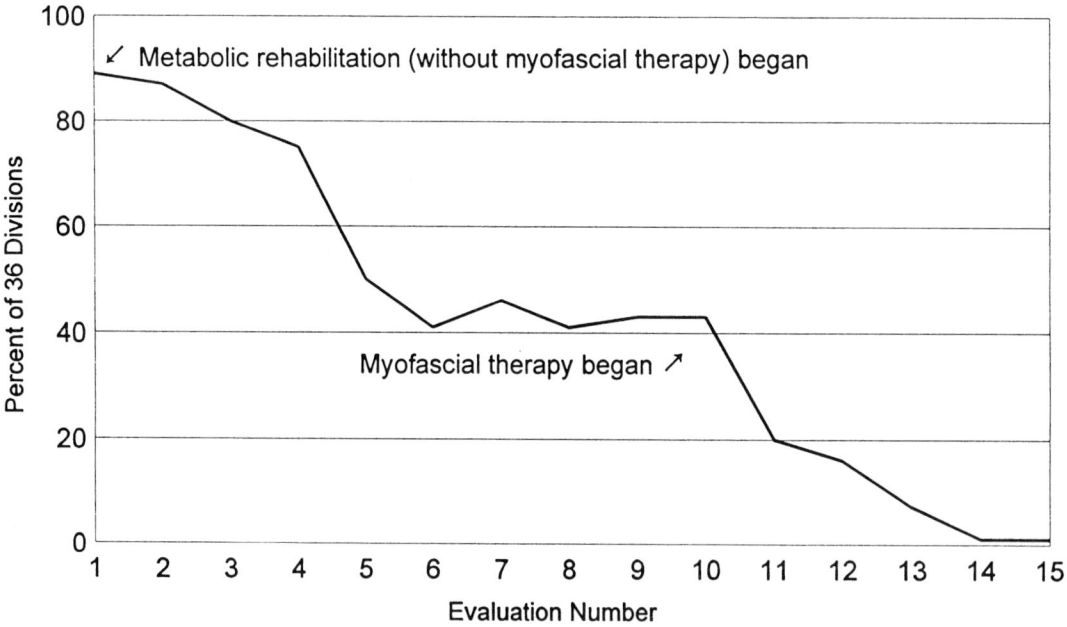

Figure 1. The line in the graph shows the decreases in an FMS patient's pain distribution during treatment. The pain distribution is the percentage of 36 body divisions containing pain, indicated by her on her pain drawing. Her pain distribution decreased during the first 6 weekly evaluations. The distribution did not decrease further until soft tissue treatment was begun, at the time of the 10th evaluation, to desensitize several myofascial trigger points.

from the protein (transthyretin) that transports it into the brain, possibly reducing the concentration of the hormone in the brain (Lans et al 1993). PCBs and dioxins also appear to interfere with the binding of thyroid hormone to its receptors on genes. This interference alters transcription patterns and produces hypothyroid-like effects (McKinney & Pedersen 1987).

Measures of FMS status

To understand the importance of soft tissue treatment for improving the pain status of FMS patients, it is helpful to understand how we measure the graded changes in patients' pain status. In line with the views of Bennett (1994) and Littlejohn (1995), we found it necessary to modify the 1990 ACR criteria. Modification was essential if we were to sensitively detect and precisely quantify changes in pain status and improve statistical analysis of the changes during studies of metabolic therapy (Lowe et al 1997a, Lowe et al 1997b, Lowe et al 1997c). According to our modifications, during a patient's treatment we repeatedly assess pain status with three objective measures. We score the measures and post the scores to line graphs. The graphs depict the trend of changes in pain status as treatment progresses. The line graph in Figure 1 shows the decrease in an FMS patient's pain distribution during treatment. The patient's pain distribution decreased during the first 6 weekly evaluations. The distribution did not decrease further toward normal, however, until soft tissue treatment was begun (at the time of the 10th evaluation) to desensitize several myofascial trigger points.

The most sensitive gauge of pain status is the pain distribution expressed as the percentage of the patient's body in pain. Our research team (Lowe et al 1997a, Lowe et al 1997b, Lowe et al 1997c) and another team in Norway (Wigers et al 1997) simultaneously confirmed the high sensitivity of this method. At each evaluation, the patient shades a body drawing to show where pain has been present since the last evaluation. We quantify the distribution of pain by calculating the percentage of 36 body divisions containing shading for that evaluation.

On a second evaluation form, the patient estimates the intensity of pain since the last visit by placing a mark along a 100mm visual analog scale (VAS). The VAS is divided into 10 units: 0 indicates no pain; 10 indicates severe pain. As a third pain assessment, we use an algometer (calibrated pressure gauge) to measure the amount of pressure (expressed as kg/cm²) that

induces discomfort at each of the 18 fibromyalgia tender point sites.

The objective during metabolic rehabilitation is to help the patient repeatedly adjust metabolism-altering practices until the three measures of pain progress to normal. For the rare patient who has no musculoskeletal source of pain, scores progress to normal as the patient's metabolic rate sufficiently increases. But if a patient has a musculoskeletal source of pain such as a chronically active trigger point, the pain scores are not likely to completely normalize solely with an adequate increase in metabolism. Scores on other measures of FMS status (Box 3) may continue to normalize, producing an apparent disparity with the pain scores. In most cases, however, when the musculoskeletal source of pain is effectively treated, FMS pain scores will also progress toward normal.

It is essential to our protocol that the clinician repeatedly quantify the patient's FMS status. The reassessments must be at 1-to-4 week intervals, and the scores at each reassessment must be posted to line graphs (as in Figure 1). The trend in scores over time makes it clear whether the patient's status is static, worsening, or improving. The positive or negative effects of previous treatment decisions become obvious.

Box 3 Fibromyalgia assessment methods

(1) **Pain Distribution** is quantified by the percentage of the patient's body in pain according to a pain drawing the patient completes at each visit.

(2) **Symptom Intensity** (0-to-10 Visual Analog Scale). One VAS for each of the 12 associated symptoms is marked by the patient. A 13th VAS is for the patient's estimate of pain intensity. The average of the 13 scores is posted to a graph.

(3) **Tender Point Sensitivity** (the pressure/pain threshold) at each of the 18 tender points is measured with an algometer (calibrated force gauge). The average for the points is calculated.

(4) Functional capacity is assessed through the **Fibromyalgia Impact Questionnaire**.

(5) Depression is quantified with the **Zung's Self-Rating Depression Scale**, which grades the presence and degree of depression.

This approach avoids guesswork and enables the clinician to intelligently guide the patient toward improved status or recovery.

Soft tissue treatment

In the early 1980s, I (JCL) worked hard to provide my FMS patients with the type of care that worked well for my non-FMS patients. I soon observed, however, that few FMS symptoms were alleviated with nutritional therapy, soft tissue treatment, spinal manipulation, or physiotherapy. At best, my FMS patients derived minimal benefit, and some, no benefit at all. I accepted on principle that any disease may be worsened by factors such as poor nutrition and chronic musculoskeletal sources of pain. In line with this, I continued to work with FMS patients to free them from as many factors as possible that might have worsened their condition. I influenced them to improve their diet, take nutritional supplements, exercise to tolerance, and undergo physical treatment for soft tissue and articular lesions—as these practices alone can favorably affect FMS patients. This may be why a high percentage of FMS patients patronize alternative practitioners, especially chiropractors and massage therapists (Pioro-Boisset et al 1996). But while alternative care is of value to FMS patients, such care does not appear to improve overall FMS status. For example, Fitzcharles and Esdaile (1997) recently reported that alternative treatments for 6 months did not improve patients' pain or functional impairment.

This report is consistent with our clinical experiences and experimental findings. Except in rare instances, FMS status does not improve solely with alternative treatments. Instead, a patient's metabolism must undergo a sustained acceleration partly by the use of the proper dosage of thyroid hormone. We say "partly" because thyroid hormone alone is not sufficient to enable the typical patient to improve or recover. Patients must also take an active part in normalizing their metabolic rates—at minimum, they must take nutritional supplements and engage in exercise to tolerance. But in addition, most FMS patients should also undergo treatment to control or eliminate musculoskeletal sources of pain, particularly soft tissue abnormalities such as trigger points. Otherwise, their FMS pain scores may remain in the abnormal range.

Pain in FMS

Pain in FMS is a product of two main factors: impaired central nervous system (CNS) pain modulation and the volume of noxious musculoskeletal input to the CNS. The fact that pain scores normalize only with soft tissue treatment in the majority of FMS patients raises a question of the responsible mechanism. The exact mechanism is not known, but general principles of pain physiology provide an approximate understanding. The perception of pain involves an interaction between two factors:

1. the CNS pain-modulating system, and
2. the volume of noxious signals entering the CNS via type C and A delta (nociceptive) nerve fibers.

Spinal cord pain-inhibiting system

The pain modulating system involves a group of neurons and the chemicals they secrete (Figure 2). One system of neurons descends from the brain stem to secrete norepinephrine in the dorsal horns, and another descends to secrete serotonin. When these substances are secreted, they set off a sequence of chemical events that cause dorsal horn neurons to secrete opiates (Dubner & Bennett 1983, Hammond 1985, Hammond 1986). The opiates exert analgesic influences in two ways. First, they inhibit the endings of afferent neurons transmitting signals into the dorsal horns. In addition to blocking signal transmission, the opiates also block the release of substance P from the afferent terminals at the dorsal horns. (Release of substance P would sustain the noxious sensory input.) Second, the opiates inhibit spinothalamic nerves within the spinal cord that would otherwise transmit the noxious afferent signals to the brain.

Impaired pain-inhibiting system in FMS and noxious musculoskeletal input to the CNS

Normally, this pain-inhibiting system prevents afferent signals below a certain volume from inducing pain perception. Consider for illustration a person who has both a normal CNS pain-modulation system and an actively referring trigger point. In this person, signals transmitted by type C and A delta nerve fibers from the trigger point are properly modulated at the dorsal horns of the spinal cord. To induce pain perception, the signals must enter the cord in sufficient quantities to overcome the blocking effects of the system. Low-level transmission registers as mild, intermittent pain. High-level transmission will exceed the ability of the CNS pain-modulation to inhibit incoming afferent signals, resulting in the perception of severe, persistent pain.

In FMS patients, however, the CNS pain-inhibiting system appears to be impaired. Studies indicate that the FMS patient secretes too little serotonin and norepinephrine (Russell et al 1992b). This may reduce the amount of opiates released in the dorsal horns, so low-level afferent signals easily enter the CNS. In addition, FMS patients secrete too much substance P (Vaerøy et al 1988). This probably sustains the noxious afferent flow to spinothalamic neurons, and in turn, to the brain. Relatively low-level afferent signals may then easily enter the CNS and register as severe, persistent pain. Because of this, FMS patients experience pain from even minor sources of musculoskeletal afferent input. Muscle hypertonicity, myofascial trigger points, spinal joint fixations—all may cause great pain. Even the minimal mechanical pressure of lying against a treatment table may be a source of intense discomfort.

Improvement in FMS patients' pain through metabolic rehabilitation

The use of a high enough daily dosage of thyroid hormone appears to be fundamental to normalizing the pain-inhibiting system in FMS patients. Too little thyroid hormone regulation of serotonergic neurons inhibits secretion of serotonin (Frankhyzen & Muller 1983), and inadequate thyroid hormone regulation of a particular gene results in a striking increase in substance P levels (Yellin 1997). Just as too little thyroid hormone regulation can cause low serotonin and high substance P, adequate regulation by the hormone can bring the levels back to normal. Thus, inadequate thyroid hormone regulation (due either to hypothyroidism or cellular resistance to thyroid hormone) may alone account for the impairment of the CNS pain-inhibiting system in FMS. And metabolic rehabilitation, including the use of thyroid hormone, increases serotonin levels and decreases substance P levels. This is indicated by the improved pain modulation with relief of chronic widespread pain in FMS patients who have undergone metabolic rehabilitation (Lowe et al 1994, Lowe 1995, Lowe et al 1997a, Lowe et al 1997b, Lowe et al 1997c, Lowe et al 1998a).

Physical treatment necessary for most patients

For most FMS patients as they undergo metabolic rehabilitation, pain scores improve to some degree

even without soft tissue treatment. Tender point sensitivity decreases, and the estimated pain intensity and pain distribution decrease. But for many patients, these pain measures will indicate maximum pain relief only after the patients undergo effective soft tissue treatment. In most cases, the soft tissue treatment must loosen hypertonic muscle and restricted fascia, and especially must desensitize myofascial trigger points. Less often, soft tissue treatment, manipulation, or physiotherapy are needed to resolve chronic musculoskeletal conditions that are sources of noxious neural input to the CNS. Among the most common of such conditions are chronic shoulder and spinal joint dysfunction.

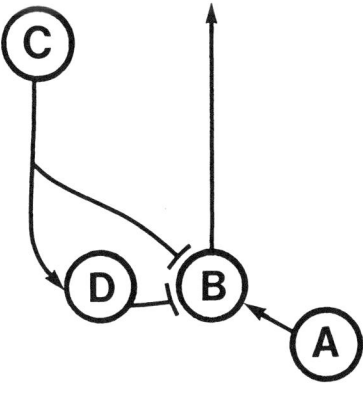

Figure 2. Primary sensory nerves (A) transmit noxious or nociceptive sensory signals (those that can give rise to the perception of pain) into the dorsal horns of the spinal cord. In the dorsal horns, the sensory nerves release chemicals such as glutamate and substance P. These chemicals induce spinothalamic nerves (B) to conduct the signals to the brain where they influence pain perception. Descending nerve fibers may release serotonin and norepinephrine in the dorsal horns. These neurotransmitter chemicals directly inhibit spinothalamic nerves (B). They also stimulate interneurons (D) to release opiate chemicals that in turn inhibit spinothalamic nerves. Serotonin and norepinephrine thus have an inhibiting effect on the transmission of noxious nerve signals to the brain.

When soft tissue treatment is effective, the FMS patient's pain scores usually proceed further toward normal. Figure 3 shows the progressive decreases in pain distribution in a euthyroid FMS patient who completely recovered from the condition (Honeyman 1997). I (GH-L) guided the patient through metabolic rehabilitation, and from the beginning of her care, I treated her with myofascial therapy and spinal adjustments. Compare the smooth descent of her pain distribution with the descent in Figure 1. In Figure 1, the improvement stalled until soft tissue treatment was begun at the time of the 10th evaluation.

Possible neuromuscular mechanism of continuing pain despite effective metabolic rehabilitation

One local muscle mechanism that may sustain FMS pain is the contractures of actin and myosin filaments. Contractures in hypothyroidism are well-documented (Ramsay 1974). Travell and Simons (1983) noted that hypothyroidism can sustain the energy deficiency contractures that underlie trigger points. The trigger points tend to remain treatment-resistant until the hypothyroidism is corrected; even then, some of the trigger points continue to refer pain until locally treated with physical methods. Our clinical experiences indicate that the same is true of trigger points housed in contractures maintained by muscle cell resistance to thyroid hormone.

During inadequate thyroid hormone regulation of skeletal muscle cells, actin and myosin filaments become contractured because of two biochemical abnormalities: decreased production of adenosine 5'-triphosphate (ATP) (Davis 1991), and reduced activity of the enzyme calcium-adenosine triphosphatase (ATPase) (Warnick et al 1991). Rigor mortis is perhaps the most dramatic display of energy deficiency contractures resulting from decreased ATP and reduced calcium-ATPase activity. The stiffening of the corpse, sometimes accompanied by limb or torso movements, is caused by the severe muscle contractures that occur following death, when ATP production and calcium-ATPase activity completely cease.

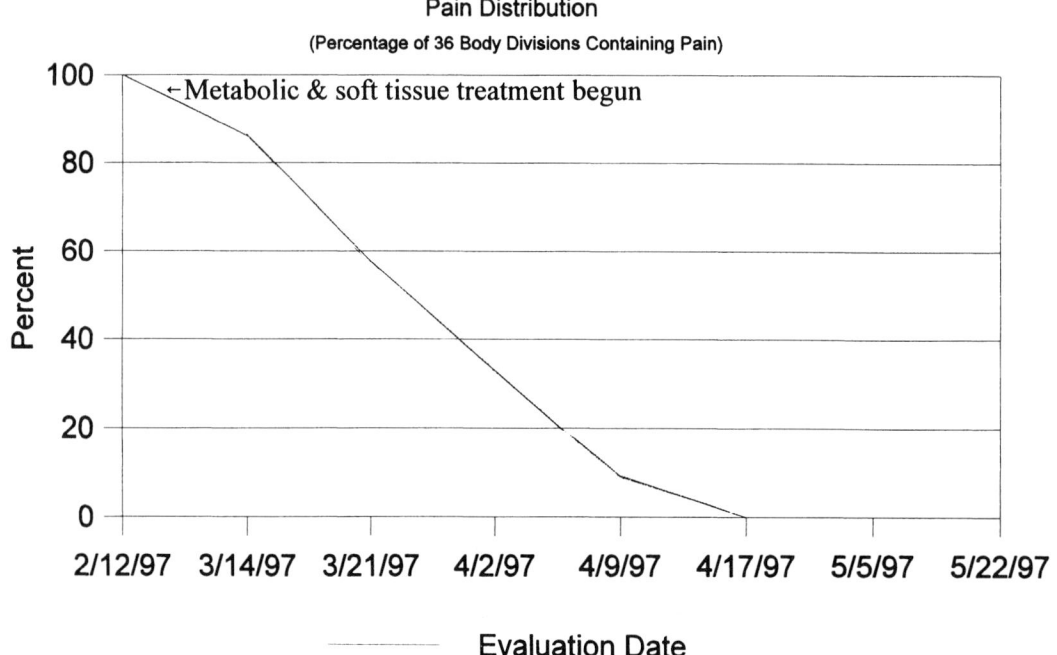

Pain Distribution
(Percentage of 36 Body Divisions Containing Pain)

Figure 3

An adequate supply of ATP molecules and sufficient calcium-ATPase activity are essential to muscle fiber relaxation. When a nerve impulse spreads over and into muscle cells, calcium ions are released from the sarcoplasmic reticulum. The ions attach to the troponin complex on actin filaments. This causes a conformational change in the actin filaments that exposes active sites where the heads of myosin filaments can attach. When the myosin heads attach to the sites, the actin and myosin filaments rachet. This shortens the muscle fiber. As long as the active sites stay exposed—due to the presence of the calcium ions—the myosin heads continue attaching, further shortening the fiber. This occurs when inadequate thyroid hormone regulation reduces the activity of calcium-ATPase, the enzyme responsible for transferring calcium ions from the sarcoplasmic fluid back into the sarcoplasmic reticulum (Guyton 1991).

Once myosin heads attach to actin filaments and shorten the muscle fiber, they detach and move back to attach at other sites only if energy is available. Normally, the energy is derived from the cleaving of a phosphate radical from an ATP molecule. If too few ATP molecules are present, as during a thyroid hormone deficiency, the myosin heads remain attached to active sites on the actin filaments. The muscle fiber then stays locked into a shortened state.

The chronic shortening of muscle fibers due to low ATP and reduced calcium-ATPase activity is termed a contracture. Contractures are biochemically based and independent of the motor nerve supply. Research by Awad (1990) indicates that contractures occur in the muscles of FMS patients. He biopsied lesioned muscle from FMS patients and found papillary projections of the sarcolemmal membranes. He wrote that the projections resulted from the coiling of myosin filaments due to the severe shortening of the muscle fibers. His view was that these findings are the same as those in hypothyroid muscle (E.A. Awad, personal communication, April 6, 1992).

When the use of thyroid hormone increases ATP production and calcium-ATPase activity, most skeletal muscle fibers relax. Some contractures, however, can become locally self-sustaining and may persist even after the thyroid hormone inadequacy is corrected. Studies have shown that localized ischemia causes significant changes in human muscle energy metabolism, and that metabolic recovery is sluggish in conditions with reduced muscle blood flow (Hands et al 1986). So, even when the patient takes enough thyroid hormone to increase ATP production and calcium-ATPase activity in most muscle, regions of muscle so severely contractured that arterial flow into them is impeded or completely blocked would maintain their energy-deficiency contractures. If these regions contain trigger points, noxious signals would likely be transmitted from them and keep nerve cells in the CNS facilitated. The effect of these reflex actions is to intensify the neurovascular activities at the involved region of muscle, further increasing the afferent barrage of the CNS. The flow of noxious signals from contractured muscle, then, may sustain the perception of pain despite improved function (caused by the thyroid hormone) of the CNS pain-modulating system. For FMS patients left with self-sustaining contractures, direct physical treatment for the contractures is necessary.

Soft tissue treatment

Whether arterial flow is reduced or completely blocked, soft tissue treatment techniques are likely to correct the neuro-circulatory abnormality. In doing so, they are also likely to reduce or eliminate the noxious signal transmission from the muscle region. We would expect the reduced noxious input to the CNS to reduce or eliminate CNS facilitation. The resulting reduction in noxious signals from the musculoskeletal system (combined with the increased pain-inhibiting ability of the CNS due to the use of thyroid hormone) relieves the patient's pain. This will be reflected in improved FMS pain scores.

Box 4   Pointers on bodywork techniques for treating clients with fibromyalgia

---

● Be flexible in positioning for maximum client comfort.

● Your FMS client's CNS is impaired in its ability to modulate down incoming sensory signals from mechanoreceptor afferents. Therefore, temper technique and pressure so that your client's threshold for pain is not exceeded.

● Do not use pressure sufficient to induce a catecholamine release. (Instead of cross-frictioning, for example, you may want to use stretching and ultrasound.)

● Aim to relieve your client's pain. Understand, however, that until your client's metabolic status is improved, manual therapies may be capable of providing only slight, and perhaps brief, pain relief.

It is important, in light of the proposed mechanism, that soft tissue treatment be strategically used so as not to exacerbate the patient's pain (Box 4). The most important consideration is that the FMS patient's myofascial mechanoreceptors are hyper-responsive and, if the patient is not undergoing metabolic rehabilitation with thyroid hormone, the CNS pain-modulating system may be impaired. The therapist should apply soft tissue techniques gently. The goal is to increase circulation through the involved muscle regions, but at the same time avoid further increasing noxious signal output from the mechanoreceptors. As the FMS patient progresses through metabolic rehabilitation, more forceful technique may be applied without adverse effects.

Until then, however, the practitioner should keep one qualification in mind: the fibromyalgia patient is likely to benefit from any soft tissue technique the practitioner customarily uses with patients who do not have fibromyalgia. But with most clients, the practitioner must use less mechanical force than with non-FMS clients. How much the force should be reduced depends upon how excessively sensitive to pressure the individual client is. A useful method is to instruct the client to verbally indicate how much discomfort the pressure is causing, on a scale of 0-to-10. With the typical FMS client, post-treatment discomfort can be avoided by keeping the discomfort level during treatment between 1 and 5.

REFERENCES

Awad EA 1990 Histopathological changes in fibrositis. In: Fricton JR, Awad EA (eds). Advances in Pain Research and Therapy, Vol. 17. Raven Press, New York: 126-132.

Bennett RM 1994 Literature reviews. Journal of Musculoskeletal Pain 2(2):101-112.

Bennett RM 1997 Fibromyalgia review. Journal of Musculoskeletal Pain 5(1):91-104.

Bland JH, Frymoyer JW 1970 Rheumatic syndromes of myxedema. New England Journal of Medicine 282:1171-1174.

Buskila D, Neumann L, Sibirski D, Shvartzman P 1997 Awareness of diagnostic and clinical features of fibromyalgia among family physicians. Family Practice 14(3):238-241.

Carette S 1995 What have clinical trials taught us about the treatment of fibromyalgia? Journal of Musculoskeletal Pain 3: 133-140.

Davis PJ 1991 Cellular actions of thyroid hormones. In: Braverman LE, Utiger RD (eds). Werner's The Thyroid 6th Edn. JB Lippincott, New York: 190-203.

Delamere JP, Scott DL, and Felix-Davies DD 1982 Thyroid dysfunction and rheumatic diseases. Journal of the Royal Society of Medicine 75:102.

Dubner R, Bennett GJ 1983 Spinal and trigeminal mechanisms of nociception. Annual Review of Neuroscience 6:381.

Eisinger J, Arroyo PH, Calendini C, Rinaldi JP, Combes R, Fontaine G 1992 Anomalies biologiques au cours des fibromylalgies: III. Explorations endocriniennes. Lyon Méditerranée

Médicine 28: 858-860.

Ferraccioli G, Cavalieri F, Salaffi F, et al 1990 Neuroendocrinologic findings in primary fibromyalgia (soft tissue chronic pain syndrome) and in other chronic rheumatic conditions (rheumatoid arthritis, low back pain). Journal of Rheumatology 17:869-873.

Fessel WJ 1968 Myopathy of hypothyroidism. Annals of Rheumatic Disease 27:590-596.

Fitzcharles MA, Esdaile JM 1997 Nonphysician practitioner treatments and fibromyalgia syndrome. Journal of Rheumatology 24(5):937-940.

Frankhyzen A, Muller A 1983 In vitro studies on the inhibition of serotonin release through α-adrenoreceptor activity in various regions of the rat CNS. Abstract of 5th Catecholamine Symposium: 137.

Gerwin R 1995 A study of 96 subjects examined both for fibromyalgia and myofascial pain. Journal of Musculoskeletal Pain 3(Suppl.)1:121.

Golding DN 1970 Hypothyroidism presenting with musculoskeletal symptoms. Annals of Rheumatic Disease 29:10-41.

Guyton AC 1991 A Textbook of Medical Physiology, 8th Edn. WB Saunders, Philadelphia.

Hammond DL 1985 Pharmacology of central pain-modulating networks (biogenic amines and nonopioid analgesics). In: Fields HL, Dubner R, Cervero F (eds). Advances in Pain Research and Therapy, Vol. 9. Raven Press, New York: 499-511.

Hammond DL 1986 Control systems for nociceptive afferent processing: the descending inhibitory pathways. In: Yaksh TL (ed). Spinal Afferent Processing. Plenum Press, New York: 363-390.

Hands LJ, Bore PJ, Galloway G, Morris PJ, Radda GK 1986 Muscle metabolism in patients with peripheral vascular disease investigated by 31P nuclear magnetic resonance spectroscopy. Clinical Science 71:283-290.

Hershman JM 1980 Hypothalamic and pituitary hypothyroidism. In: Bastenie PA, Bonnyns M, VanHaelst L (eds). Progress in the Diagnosis and Treatment of Hypothyroid Conditions. Excerpta Medica Amsterdam.

Hochberg MC, Koppes GM, Edwards CQ, Barnes HV, Arnett, FC Jr 1976 Hypothyroidism presenting as a polymyositis-like syndrome: report of two cases. Arthritis & Rheumatism 19: 1363-1366.

Honeyman GS 1997 Metabolic therapy for hypothyroid and euthyroid fibromyalgia: two case reports. Clinical Bulletin of Myofascial Therapy 2(4):19-49.

Lans MC, Klasson-Wehler E, Willemsen M, Meussen E, Safe S, and Bouwer A 1993 Structure-dependent, competitive interaction of hydroxy-polychlorobiphenyls, -dibenzo-*p*-dioxins and -dibenzofurans with human transthyretin. Chemico-Biological Interactions 88(1):7-21.

Littlejohn, GO 1995 A database for fibromyalgia. Rheumatic Disease Clinics of North America 21(2):527-557.

Lowe JC 1995 T_3-induced recovery from fibromyalgia by a hypothyroid patient resistant to T_4 and desiccated thyroid. Journal of Myofascial Therapy 1(4):26-31.

Lowe, JC 1997a Thyroid status of 38 fibromyalgia patients: implications for the etiology of fibromyalgia. Clinical Bulletin of Myofascial Therapy 2(1):36-41.

Lowe, JC 1997b Home page, website: http://www.DrLowe.com

Lowe JC 1999a Speeding Up to Normal: Metabolic Solutions to Fibromyalgia. McDowell Publishing Company, Tulsa, OK.

Lowe JC 1999b The Metabolic Treatment of Fibromyalgia. McDowell Publishing Company, Tulsa, OK.

Lowe JC, Eichelberger J, Manso G, Peterson, K 1994 Improvement in euthyroid fibromyalgia patients treated with T_3 (tri-iodothyronine). Journal of Myofascial Therapy 1(2):16-29.

Lowe JC, Garrison RL, Reichman AJ, Yellin J, Thompson M, Kaufman D 1997a Effectiveness and safety of T_3 (triiodothyronine) therapy for euthyroid fibromyalgia: a double-blind placebo-controlled response-driven crossover study. Clinical Bulletin of Myofascial Therapy 2(2/3):31-58.

Lowe JC, Reichman AJ, Yellin J 1997b The process of change during T_3 treatment for euthyroid fibromyalgia: a double-blind placebo-controlled crossover study. Clinical Bulletin of Myofascial Therapy 2(2/3):91-124.

Lowe JC, Garrison RL, Reichman AJ, Yellin J 1997c Triiodothyronine (T_3) treatment of euthyroid fibromyalgia: a small-n replication of a double-blind placebo-controlled crossover study. Clinical Bulletin of Myofascial Therapy 2(4):71-88.

Lowe JC, Cullum ME, Graf LH Jr, and Yellin J 1997d Mutations in the c-*erb*Aβ_1 gene: do they underlie euthyroid fibromyalgia? Medical Hypotheses 48(2):125-135.

Lowe JC, Reichman AJ, Yellin J 1998a A case-control study of metabolic therapy for fibromyalgia: long-term follow-up comparison of treated and untreated patients (abstract). Clinical Bulletin of Myofascial Therapy 3(1):23-24.

Lowe JC, Reichman AJ, Honeyman GS, Yellin J 1998b Thyroid status of fibromyalgia patients (abstract). Clinical Bulletin of Myofascial Therapy 3(1):69-70.

Marin R, Connick E 1997 Tension myalgia versus myoadenylate deaminase deficiency: a case report. Archives of Physical Medicine and Rehabilitation 78(1):95-97.

McKinney JD, Pedersen LG 1987 Do residue levels of poly-

chlorinated biphenyls (PCBs) in human blood produce mild hypothyroidism? Journal of Theoretical Biology 129:231-241.

Neeck G, Riedel W 1992 Thyroid function in patients with fibromyalgia syndrome. Journal of Rheumatology 19:1120-1122.

Oertel JE, LiVolsi VA 1991 Pathology of thyroid diseases. In: Braverman LE, Utiger RD (eds). Werner and Ingbar's The Thyroid: A Fundamental and Clinical Text, 6th Edn. JB Lippincott Co, New York: 601-644.

Pioro-Boisset M, Esdaile JM, Fitzcharles MS 1996 Alternative medicine use in fibromyalgia syndrome. Arthritis Care and Research 9:13-17.

Pratley R, Nicklas B, Rubin M, et al 1994 Strength training increases resting metabolic rate and norepinephrine levels in healthy 50-to-65-year-old men. Journal of Applied Physiology 76 (1):133-137.

Ramsay, I 1974 Thyroid Disease and Muscle Dysfunction. Year Book Medical Publishers, Chicago.

Refetoff S, Weiss RE, Usala SJ 1993 The syndromes of resistance to thyroid hormone. Endocrine Reviews 14:348-399.

Russell IJ, Michalek JE, Vipraio JA, Fletcher EM, Javors MA, Bowden CA 1992a Platelet 3H-imipramine uptake receptor density and serum serotonin levels in patients with fibromyalgia/fibrositis syndromes. Journal of Rheumatology 19:104-109.

Russell IJ, Vaeroy M, Jabors M, Nyberg F 1992b Cerebrospinal fluid biogenic metabolites in fibromyalgia/fibrositis syndrome in rheumatoid arthritis. Arthritis & Rheumatism 35:550-556.

Shinkai S, Watanabe S, Kurokawa Y, Torii J, Asai H, Shephard R.J 1994 Effects of 12 weeks of aerobic exercise plus dietary restriction on body composition, resting energy expenditure, and aerobic fitness in mildly obese middle-aged women. European Journal of Applied Physiology and Occupational Physiology 68(3):258-265.

Shiroky JB, Cohen M, Ballachey M-L, Neville C 1993 Thyroid dysfunction in rheumatoid arthritis: a controlled prospective survey. Annals of Rheumatic Diseases 52:454-456.

Sonkin LS 1985 Endocrine disorders and muscle dysfunction. In: Gelb B (ed). Clinical Management of Head, Neck, and TMJ Pain and Dysfunction. WB Saunders Co, Philadelphia.

Travell JG, Simons DG 1983 Myofascial Pain and Dysfunction: the Trigger Point Manual, Vol. 1. Williams and Wilkins, Baltimore.

Vaerøy H, Helle R, Øystein F, Kåss E, Terenius L 1988 Elevated CSF levels of substance P and high incidence of Raynaud phenomenon in patients with fibromyalgia: new features for diagnosis. Pain 32:21-26.

Van den Berg KJ, Zurcher C, Brouwer A 1988 Effects of

3,4,3',4'-tetrachlorobiphenyl on thyroid function and histology in marmoset monkeys. Toxicology and Applied Pharmacology 41:77-86.

Warnick PR, Davis PJ, Davis FB, Cody V, Galindo J Jr, Blas SD 1991 Rabbit skeletal muscle endoplasmic reticulum Ca^{2+}-ATPase activity: stimulation in vitro by thyroid hormone analogues and bypyridines. Biochemical Pharmacology 45:1091.

Wigers SH, Skrondal A, Finset A, and Götestam KG 1997 Measuring change in fibromyalgic pain: the relevance of pain distribution. Journal of Musculoskeletal Pain 5(2):29-41.

Wilke SW, Sheeler LR, Makarowski WS 1981 Hypothyroidism with presenting symptoms of fibrositis. Journal of Rheumatology 8:627-630.

Wilson J, Walton JN 1959 Some muscular manifestations of hypothyroidism. Journal of Neurology, Neurosurgery, and Psychiatry 22:320-324.

Wolfe F, Smythe HA, Yunus MB, et al 1990 The American College of Rheumatology 1990 criteria for the classification of fibromyalgia: report of the multicenter criteria committee. Arthritis & Rheumatism 33:160-172.

Wolfe F 1994 Aspects of the epidemiology of fibromyalgia. Journal of Musculoskeletal Pain 2(3):65-77.

Yellin J 1997 Why is substance P high in fibromyalgia? Clinical Bulletin of Myofascial Therapy 2(2/3):23-30.

Appendix C

DEBATE WITH MICHAEL WEINTRAUB, M.D.

In October of 1992, the *American Journal of Pain Management* (*AJPM*) published a paper by neurologist Michael Weintraub in which he reported the results of a "study" of chronic pain patients he had recently conducted. His paper was titled *Litigation-Chronic Pain Syndrome—A Distinct Entity: Analysis of 210 Cases*. I immediately prepared a rebuttal paper, working closely with Jackie Yellin to refine it so that the Editor of *AJPM* would not request a rewrite. We sent the paper to the journal within two weeks of the publication of Weintraub's paper. Other members of the American Academy of Pain Management (AAPM) wrote letters to the Editor protesting Weintraub's conclusions and the *AJPM* publishing his paper when it was so fraught with irrationality and erroneous conclusions. The Editor sent the paper to peer reviewers. After the Editor received their comments on the paper, he asked me to rewrite it, incorporating the reviewers' suggested changes. Some of the recommendations were acceptable, but many were not—they were directed toward softening to the point of ineffectiveness my arguments against Weintraub's faulty study protocol, reasoning, and conclusions. Had I rewritten the paper as recommended, the paper would no longer have been a rebuttal. When we sent the revised paper to the Editor of *AJPM*, he again sent it to peer reviewers, and we went through another round of the same process. Again, I received recommendations that would have nullified the effectiveness of my arguments, had I incorporated them into the paper. After Jackie and I struggled to rewrite the paper again, making concessions to the reviewers and the Editor but insisting that we maintain the effectiveness of my arguments, the paper was finally published—9 months after Weintraub's paper appeared in *AJPM*. In the meantime, protests from members of AAPM continued. Out of frustration at having my rebuttal inexplicably held up from publication for this extraordinary length of time, I wrote the following paper that was published in the *Chiropractic Journal*. The paper that finally appeared in *AJPM* also follows. Soon after the series of papers and letters were published in *AJPM*, the AAPM held a conference at which Michael Weintraub and a rheumatologist debated in front of the members of the Academy who were in attendance the issues raised in Weintraub's paper. One of these members was Dr. Janet Travell. The live debate at the conference ended the discussion.

Litigating Pain Patients:
Just Greedy Neurotics?

John C. Lowe, MA, DC

This article originally appeared in *The Chiropractic Journal,* May 1993, pp.27 & 43.
It is reprinted with permission of the publisher, Terry A. Rondberg, D.C.

In October of last year (1992), the *American Journal of Pain Management* (*AJPM*) published a paper by neurologist, Michael Weintraub[1] in which he reported the results of a "study" he had recently conducted. Weintraub's erroneous conclusions—an outrageous example of specious science—were repeated in the *New York Times* and other newspapers. His conclusions may show up in testimony against your litigating chronic pain patients. Patients with fibromyalgia and myofascial pain syndromes are most likely to be victimized.

The *AJPM* is the official publication of the American Academy of Pain Management (AAPM). Some members of AAPM, myself among them, were outraged to read Weintraub's paper in *AJPM*.[2][3] The Academy is predicated on the humanitarian style of Dr. Janet Travell. Her life's work represents the relief of pain and suffering. Yet, in October, 1992, the powers-that-be at the Academy awarded Weintraub for his contributions to the pain management literature. News of this shocked me.

GIVING LAWYERS AMMO

What's wrong with Weintraub's conclusions? Under the guise of science, he expressed his prejudicial and pejorative opinions of litigating chronic pain patients. His opinions are whips that insurance claims adjusters and lawyers may use to beat these patients out of fair compensation.

The most notorious of Weintraub's predecessors was a psychiatrist and company doctor named Henry Miller.[4][5] Miller's opinions, like Weintraub's, were published as a "study." Lawyers used them to deprive litigating patients of just benefit or settlements. Now these suffering humans have Weintraub's "study" to add to their woes. Some may cave in when lawyers club them on their litigating heads with Weintraub's counterfeit science.

For two years during his "study," Weintraub examined litigating pain patients. In his report, he claimed that 63% had "psychogenic" (mentally-caused) pain. They suffered from "unconscious, neurotic behavior," he says, tainted by profit-motivated faking.

QUESTIONABLE SCIENCE

What evidence did Weintraub give for his conclusions? He used physical tests, the interpretations of which are subject to his dripping bias. Merskey explained this about Weintraub's clinical tests back in 1988.[6] But Weintraub still uses them.

He also used MRIs, CT scans, and EMGs to rule out a limited number of organic lesions. But he neglected the most common source of pain—myofascial lesions such as trigger points.[7][8] Worse yet, although his prose is slippery and often eludes comprehension, he seemed to question the very existence of myofascial trigger points!

Some of his patients wore collars and corsets and doctor-shopped. Then they asked him to tell their lawyers they weren't doing well. He considered this evidence of psychogenic pain. Absurd? You bet. Nevertheless, the *AJPM* published his undocumented statements, outlandish suppositions, illogical conclusions, and pseudo-scientific gobbledygook!

The fact that the journal published his "study" legitimizes his erroneous conclusions, especially for the purposes of insurance claims adjusters and defense lawyers working for insurance companies. And far *worse*, the AAPM gave him that award, further validating his unscientific anti-patient babble.

If I were to cast my vote, the publication of Weintraub's paper would go down in medical history as one of the greatest acts of poor judgment by a peer reviewed journal. The fact is, according to his report in the *AJPM*, Weintraub did two things in his "study": (1) he made clinical observations of his patients, and (2) expressed his opinions about them. The *AJPM*'s peer reviewers should have required Weintraub to state *only* that. Instead, they let him misrepresent his opinions as legitimate scientific results.

In short, in his "study," Weintraub failed to use the stringent protocol of modern clinical science; used mainly subjective tests; ruled out only a few lesions through objective tests; ignored the most common source of pain; and expressed scorn for litigating chronic pain patients. In addition, by offering his paper for publication, he lent his "authority" to the disreputable purposes of many insurance companies.

A student in freshman logic could easily see the faulty thinking screaming from Weintraub's paper. Why did this travesty of science reach print? I don't know. But I do know one thing from past experience. Defense lawyers representing insurance companies will not turn a deaf ear to Weintraub's transgressions against reason. They'll make good use of this "study" from a reputable scientific journal. With it, they'll try to discredit chronic pain patients by making them out to be greedy, bellyaching neurotics in need of psychotherapy rather than benefits or a settlement.

Why do I respond in a trade journal instead of the *AJPM*? Within two weeks of reading Weintraub's paper when it came out in *AJPM*, I wrote a lengthy, point-by-point, well-documented rebuttal of his false conclusions. In spite of my alacrity and the *AJPM*'s multi-disciplinary input, my paper somehow hasn't made it into two subsequent issues of the *AJPM*. I've been assured it will appear. However, too much time has passed since Weintraub's paper appeared.

The *AJPM* has published one rebuttal letter to the Editor, by well-known rheumatologist Thomas Romano.[9] Yet, in the same issue, the Editor let Weintraub respond to Romano with the same convoluted misapplications of logic as he used in his paper, along with one hilarious misquote of the scientific literature.

For a copy of my as-yet-unpublished manuscript, please phone my office. By the way, I thank *The Chiropractic Journal* for giving me a forum for rebutting Weintraub's bad and potentially harmful "science." If peer-reviewed journals don't give us a fair shot at dialogue, our trade journals do.

REFERENCES

1. Weintraub, M.I.: Litigation-chronic pain syndrome—a distinct entity: analysis of 210 cases. *A.J.P.M.*, 2(4):198-204, 1992.
2. Romano, T.J.: Personal communication, Jan.1993.
3. Stiller, J.: Personal communication, Feb.1993.
4. Miller, H.: Accident neurosis: Lecture I. *Brit. Med. J.*, 1:919-25, 1961.
5. Miller, H.: Accident neurosis: Lecture II. *Brit. Med. J.*, 1:992-998, 1961.
6. Merskey, H.: Regional pain is rarely hysterical. *Arch. Neurol.*, 45:915-18, 1988.
7. Lowe, J.C.: The neglected mechanism. *Dyn. Chiro.*, Aug.29, 1990, p.35.
8. Lowe, J.C.: The most common source of pain. *North Carolina Chiro. J.*, Aug. 1992, pp.26-27.
9. Romano, T.J.: Letter to the Editor. *A.J.P.M.*, 3(1):4, 1993.

Litigating-Chronic Pain Syndrome: Weintraub's Unproven Entity

John C. Lowe, MA,DC

This article originally appeared in the *American Journal of Pain Management*, 3(3):131-136, 1993.
It is reprinted with permission of the publisher, *A.J.P.M.*

SOME OF THE AUTHOR'S ORIGINAL WORDING WAS REMOVED OR REPLACED BY THE EDITORS OF *A.J.P.M.*
COMPLETE SENTENCES OF THE ORIGINAL WORDING ARE INCLUDED BELOW IN BRACKETS
IMMEDIATELY AFTER THE WORDING THAT WAS PRINTED IN THE JOURNAL.
WHERE JUST A FEW WORDS WERE DELETED, THEY ARE ALSO INCLUDED IN BRACKETS.

Abstract: This article is written in response to Dr. Michael I. Weintraub's article "Litigation-Chronic Pain Syndrome—A Distinct Entity: Analysis of 210 Cases" (AJPM 1992;2:198-204). Weintraub's conclusions are significant because of their potential for misuse. His conclusions, as has been the pattern established by the legal community, may be used to the disadvantage of litigating patients with physically-based chronic pain. [His conclusions, like similar ones in the past, may be used by attorneys to the disadvantage of litigating patients with physically-based chronic pain.] Weintraub has based his conclusions on a 2-year observation of litigating chronic pain patients. There are, however, conceptual and methodological problems with his study. The magnitude of these problems is sufficient to invalidate his conclusions. Weintraub's conclusions should not be generalized to litigating chronic pain patients at-large.

Descriptors. chronic pain, hysterical conversion reaction, litigation, tort law, trigger points.

Received: 10-19-92; Accepted: 5-21-93

INTRODUCTION

An unknown percentage of accident victims, in pursuit of potential profit, claim they have chronic pain when they do not. These people are costly to society, and society would be best served to identify them and give them their non-monetary due. To identify these individuals, the health care community must use methods that differentiate objectively three classes of patients: (1) those with physically-based chronic pain, (2) those with psychogenic chronic pain, and (3) those who do not have pain but claim they do. Weintraub did not do this in his study.[1] Instead, the approach he reports in his paper muddies the diagnostic waters, clouding the distinctions between these three classes of patients.

Weintraub reported that (1) he identified physical lesions as the cause of pain in 37% of his patients, (2) 63% had psychogenic pain (a form of hysteria), (3) hysteria-based pain is mixed with some degree of malingering (i.e., faking pain for financial profit) and is fueled by desires for financial or interpersonal gain, and (4) the prevalence of litigating patients with hysterical pain is "clearly quite high," warranting tort and insurance reform. Thus, Weintraub reaches a disparaging conclusion about the pain of most litigating chronic pain patients. It results, he writes, from subconscious, neurotic behavior driven to some degree by an ulterior profit motive.

A REBUTTAL

It is important to point out the fallacies in Weintraub's conclusions. Based on these conclusions, he proclaims an "entity" that opposing attorneys may use to discredit pain patients' claims, regardless of whether their claims are legitimate. The defense attorney often tries to convince jurors that the chronic pain patient is goldbricking—even when the patient has verified physical injuries. The attorney then predicts that the only effective analgesic will be a financial settlement. Mendelson wrote,[2]

Appearing as an expert witness in cases involving a psychiatric illness developing after a compensable injury, I have been almost invariably asked by counsel representing the side opposing the claimant the question (or one of its variants): "Doctor, is it not true that the plaintiff will improve, become free of symptoms and return to work within a few weeks of the settlement of this claim?" My answer in the negative, based on clinical experience, was usually met with a reference to Miller's "study."

The "Miller Study"[3] is actually two articles summarizing Henry Miller's memories, reflections, and opinions of patients he examined in his capacity as a company doctor. The term "study," often used by defense attorneys, erroneously implies that Miller conducted a systematic investigation of his patients.

Defense attorneys also often imply or assert that litigating chronic pain patients will return to work symptom-free upon receiving a financial settlement. Kelly conducted a study to determine the truth of the assertion. He concluded, "For this statement, which has often been accepted without question in the courts, and on which many final settlements have been based, we have been able to find no authority beyond the oft-repeated remark 'it is common knowledge'. . . ."[4,p.275] It is merely assumed that the patient's pain terminates with a settlement.

In his paper, Weintraub provides fuel to continue this assumption. To wit, he writes (italics mine) there is no long-term documentation, but "*anecdotal and personal observations* reveal 'miraculous' cures after litigation has ceased."[1,p.202] "It *appears* that, in all too many cases, the advantages of illness far outweigh the advantages of health."[1,p.202] "The prevalence of psychogenic pain and litigation is *unknown but is clearly quite high.*"[1,p.202] ". . . there is an *impression* of conscious malingering in many of these patients when they make comments such as, 'Tell my lawyer that I am not doing well'."[1,p.202] "Many now *believe* that litigation undermines the long-term therapeutic benefits of various modalities . . . ."[1,p.202] And ". . . it is *apparent* . . . that (hysteria) is a common problem faced by other clinicians, as well as society."[1]

What scientific evidence does Weintraub offer to support his presumptions? None except, like Henry Miller, his clinical impressions. His study—which boils down to his clinical observations—logically permits no conclusions that any of his litigating chronic pain patients had psychogenic pain. His reasoning is presumptive, pejorative, and *a priori*. As such, it is a threat to the cause of justice for many patients with long-standing pain.

Weintraub took several faulty steps to arrive at his conclusions. They are outlined as follows.

Scientific Validity

On methodological grounds, there are at least two reasons that Weintraub's conclusions do not follow logically from the evidence he presents.

No Control Group

Subjects included in his study had to meet two criteria: (1) symptoms of chronic pain for at least six months and (2) involvement in active, pending litigation. He points out that he used no control subjects, and he states, "notwithstanding this minor criticism, the conclusions of this study seem to coincide with the rising skepticism of many clinicians regarding the validity of complaints in litigation."[1] His concurrence with others' opinions does not compensate for his lack of controls. This fault invalidates his conclusion that hysteria and a desire for gain lie behind most of his study subjects' litigation. [This fault invalidates his conclusion that hysteria and a desire for gain lie behind most chronic pain patients' litigation.]

A control group may have revealed three phenomena reported by other investigators. First, compensation and non-compensation pain patients have a similar incidence of psychological disturbance.[4][5][6][7][8] Second, organic and non-organic symptoms occur in similar proportions in compensation and non-compensation patients.[9] Third, symptoms continue in many patients after claims are settled or without claims being a factor.[10][11][12][13]

Weintraub studied 210 litigating chronic pain patients. If he now studies 210 non-litigating chronic pain patients using the same protocol, he might find no significant statistical difference between the two groups.

A pertinent question is, do some types of psychological disturbance cause patients to litigate, while other disturbances do not? To answer this question, at least two requirements must be met. First, psychological problems peculiar to litigating pain patients must be isolated. This can be done only by comparing them with non-litigating pain patients. Second, the comparisons must be based on legitimate psychological assessments. Weintraub's study meets neither of these criteria. Nevertheless, he concludes there is a link between psychogenic pain and litigation.[1] This conclusion is not warranted based on his study. [This conclusion is not warranted based on his limited observations.]

No Independent Verification
of Examination Findings

Weintraub's exam findings were not independently verified by a second examiner. Examination of study subjects by one evaluator—the same one who will reach and publish conclusions about those subjects—does not assure impartial judgment. The evaluator's conclusions may inadvertently coincide with his preconceived notions. This is a classic fault with unblinded studies. Korr commented on the popular view that researchers are indifferent to the issues they study. "Nothing could be further from the truth. It's precisely their prejudices that researchers investigate; otherwise there would be no passion in science."[14] It is controls that enable the scientist to reach truthful conclusions, untainted by his personal prejudices. The historical example of The Miller Study is cause enough to question Weintraub's expert opinion, and to insist upon—at least in matters of litigation—the more stringent criteria of modern clinical science.

[In short, the methodological shortcomings of Weintraub's study disallow generalizing his conclusions to chronic pain patients at-large. The following sections argue that his conclusions do not apply even to the subjects in his study.]

Methods of Assessing
Physical Sources of Pain

Weintraub lists several methods he used to assess his patients for physical sources of pain. He first lists expert opinion regarding disability and significance of complaints. In addition, he used several objective methods, such as magnetic resonance imaging (MRI), that detect a limited range of physical lesions.[1]

He concedes that the methods he used may not detect organic dysfunction, but emphasizes, "focal examination findings should suggest organic pathology."[1] Yet he did not report examining his patients for what may be the most common focal lesion mediating musculoskeletal pain—myofascial trigger points. In fact, he questions the very existence of myofascial syndromes. Some features of TrPs, however, are objectively verifiable.[15][16]

Some studies suggest that much chronic pain is myofascial in origin. Myofascial TrPs were the culprits in 31% of patients with pain complaints (10% of all patients) in an internal medicine group study.[17] Fifty-five percent of some 300 chronic head and neck pain patients at a dental clinic were diagnosed as suffering from myofascial pain syndromes.[18] And most significantly, in a comprehensive pain center study,

85% of 283 patients were assigned a primary diagnosis of myofascial pain syndrome.[19]

Traditionally, some clinicians have not been able to determine the mechanism of pain in a sizable percentage of neck and low back pain patients.[20][21] One report claims that 28% of chronic low back pain patients have no organic findings when examined.[22] This is so common in clinical practice that a special diagnostic label was created for these patients—chronic intractable benign pain (CIBP).[23]

In the pain center study cited above,[19] clinicians examined CIBP patients. The clinicians found trigger points in the low back muscles of almost 97% of patients with low back pain. They found TrPs in the cervical paraspinal muscles of 100% of patients with neck pain. Many of these patients had decreased ranges of motion, non-dermatomal sensory abnormalities and hypertonic muscles—all common features of myofascial pain syndromes. This study raises the possibility that chronic pain patients whose pain may be blamed on psychogenic mechanisms may be suffering from myofascial lesions.

No patient's chronic pain should be considered psychogenic when myofascial sources have not been ruled out by objective measure. There is high interrater reliability between palpators who are trained and experienced at diagnosing myofascial trigger points.[24] Moreover, features of these lesions can be reliably demonstrated with both algometry[5][6][14][25][26][27][28][29] and thermography.[30][31][32] Weintraub did not rule out this common physical cause of chronic pain in his patients. This is significant because, as he points out, a diagnosis of hysteria is not legitimate unless physical causes have been excluded.[1]

Did Weintraub's Patients
Have Psychogenic Pain?

Weintraub did not demonstrate that his patients had psychogenic pain. The error in his conclusion derives from his proposition that the patients' responses to sensory and motor tests were incompatible with anatomic and physiologic principles. Myofascial TrPs and other organic conditions could account for the patients' test responses.

The criteria for diagnosis of psychogenic pain, now termed somatoform pain disorder in the DSM-III-R,[33] are (1) pain for six months or more and either (2a) failure of a proper evaluation to reveal organic pathology or a pathophysiological mechanism or (2b) when organic pathology is present, pain perception or impairment is out of proportion to that expected from the pathology. Weintraub met the first of these criteria by requiring pain of at least six months for admission to his study. He did not demonstrate that his patients met either of criterion (2a) or (2b).

Weintraub's protocol for determining whether his patients had psychogenic pain involved:

- Observing their sensory responses to pinprick, touch, vibration, and position sense. He noted as indicative of hysteria (1) hyposensitivity in non-anatomic areas, (2) glove-stocking changes, (3) midline splinting, and (4) reduced vibratory sense when bone conduction was normal.
- Observing their motor performance in injured and uninjured extremities. He considered as evidence of hysteria (1) reserve strength, (2) give-away weakness, and (3) absence of signs of atrophy or trophic changes in injured tissues.
- Examining for organic lesions via MRIs, CATs, EMGs, and myelograms.

Weintraub considered that the patient displayed only hysterical conversion symptoms (Group I) if (1) results of sensory and motor tests indicated hysteria and (2) the imaging procedures were negative for organic lesions. He considered the patient to have mixed hysterical and organic findings (Group II) if (1) results of the sensory and motor tests suggested hysteria and (2) imaging procedures were positive (e.g., fracture, herniated disk, spinal stenosis, denervation).

Therefore, Weintraub's diagnosis of hysteria hinges on the patient's responses to physical exam procedures being inconsistent with the responses predictable from presumed anatomic and physiologic principles. He has written elsewhere that this approach is rational and provides positive evidence of hysteria.[34] His approach is dubious, however, on several counts. [His approach, however, is highly dubious on several counts.]

Merskey has addressed each of Weintraub's physical exam procedures for diagnosis of hysteria.[35] Specifically, Merskey pointed out: (1) hyposensitivity may be secondary to organic disease, (2) glove and stocking paresthesias and other non-anatomical sensory symptoms are often caused by organic disease, (3) give-away weakness is not reliable and may just as well indicate pain inhibition as hysteria, and (4) evidence indicates that we cannot accept regional pain or its associated motor changes as indicative of hysteria. Gould and colleagues evaluated the validity of seven purported indications of hysteria, including the tests Weintraub used. They concluded that if these indications are considered specifically indicative of hysteria, misdiagnoses of the condition can easily occur.[36]

Thus, the validity of the sensory and motor tests Weintraub used to diagnose hysterical pain is in question. [Thus, it is doubtful whether there is any validity to the sensory and motor tests Weintraub used to diagnose hysterical pain.]

In addition, despite the high degree of reliability of the imaging and electrophysiologic procedures Weintraub used, they do not rule out all lesions that can mediate abnormal responses to sensory and motor tests. A myofascial trigger point is one such lesion. Pain originating from TrPs may not conform to dermatomal,[19][37] myotomal,[38] or sclerotomal[39] patterns of innervation.[40] Trigger points may also be associated with sensory loss in the absence of hysteria[41][42] and also weakness without atrophy of the affected muscles.[43] Merskey points out that basing a psychiatric diagnosis on the putative absence of physical disease is imprudent.[35] As Hachinski states, "Absence of proof is no proof of absence."[44]

Because of these considerations, Weintraub does not meet either of the second criteria for the diagnosis of somatoform pain disorder. It is questionable whether his patients had psychogenic pain. [He did not demonstrate that his patients had psychogenic pain.]

Is Financial Gain the Primary Motive of Litigating Chronic Pain Patients?

"Financial incentives," Weintraub writes, "have long been thought to have significant and negative effects on symptoms as well as therapeutic response."[1] Probably referring only to patients whose pain he attributes to hysteria, he also states, ". . . symptoms arise because the patient wishes to obtain some gain (financial or interpersonal)."[1]

This corresponds to the view expressed in The Miller Study.[3] Some defense attorneys have use this "study" as a whip to beat injured patients out of settlements. The attorney role-casts the patient as a sly, devious neurotic or feigner. The attorney accuses the patient of faking pain and conniving to grasp as much as he can from the litigative cookie jar.[45]

Such abuse by attorneys stimulated a series of studies spanning the past 30 years. Virtually every one of these studies shows that many patients' pain does not end when they have been compensated.[2][4][7][8][46][47][48][49][50][51][52][53][54] Gotten studied 100 pain patients and reported that after their claims were settled, most of them (88%), were "largely recovered."[48] Macnab felt that Gotten's statement misrepresented the actual outcome of his study. Macnab clarified that five years after the 100 claims were settled, 34% of the patients still had minor discomfort.[52] A noteworthy 12% had serious disability, and 3% were still losing time from work. Romano found that 71% of 14 post-traumatic fibromyalgia syndrome (PTFS) patients returned for treatment repeatedly after their claims were settled.[53] Romano's PTFS patients required more treatment when exposed to conditions known to exacerbate pain in other fibromyalgia patients. Other investigators report similar findings.[54][55] From these studies, it is reasonable to conclude that removing the putative profit motive does not relieve the chronic pain of a significant percentage of patients.

Sources of Chronic Pain
Other than Financial Profit
[. . . Other than Greed]

There are numerous reasons, other than financial motives, that cause a patient to continue to have pain. Recognizing these may help preserve the chronic pain patient's dignity. The list includes at least five categories.

Iatrogenesis
Macnab, writing of whiplash patients, makes an important point. The clinician often does not recognize a patient's pain as legitimate [and treat him properly]. By failing to do so, the clinician may iatrogenically provoke psychological problems. Whether the patient receives adequate treatment or not may depend on the clinician's preconceived notions about the type of injury involved. Macnab argues that, by failing to treat whiplash adequately, the physician [himself] may be responsible for producing some of the so-called litigation neurosis.[52] Macnab's viewpoint is reinforced by the recent report of a National Academy of Sciences Committee.[56] The Committee notes that chronic pain patients are psychologically impacted when their condition goes undiagnosed and untreated. Resulting depression may exacerbate their pain. This also applies to chronic pain patients whose clinicians, like Weintraub, fail to rule out myofascial lesions as the source of pain and attribute the pain to [unverifiable] mental abnormalities.[57]

Systemic Conditions
Numerous systemic conditions (e.g., borderline estrogen or thyroid deficiency) can escalate minor trauma into states of major pain and disability.[58][59][60][61][62]

Direction of Impact and Occult Injuries
Whether a minor impacting force causes severe or long-lasting pain depends partly on its direction. Extension trauma occurring when the cervical spine is slightly rotated may cause damage and pain that seems inordinate.[52] A driver's torso is more likely to be injured when the driver is hit broadside while sitting face-forward in his car. When hit in this manner —from the driver's most vulnerable side—the injury may be worse than expected from the force of impact.[27] In such cases, injury may not be obvious with a clinical exam, and the clinician may attribute the patient's pain to hysteria. Damage to lumbar facet joints in automobile accidents may not be visible on plain x-rays.[27] Trauma-induced intracranial hemorrhages, severed neurons, and diffuse microscopic lesions may not be detectable from clinical exams, but are detectable at autopsy. Such lesions show that nervous system damage may occur yet not be obvious during a clinician exam.[29]

As Weintraub concedes, modern imaging techniques may also not detect organic lesions.[1] One reason for this is the small dimensions of some lesions. Ommaya and Yarnell subjected monkeys to experimental whiplash. The monkeys survived without neurological deficit, yet they had brain surface hemorrhages. The investigators point out that the larger human brain is much easier to damage. They advise the clinician to "bear in mind that a small amount of subarachnoid hemorrhage can produce very marked headaches and stiff neck, two common complaints after whiplash injury which are usually attributed to injury of musculoskeletal structures."[63]

Adversarial System of Evaluation
Reed writes that the adversarial system of court procedure is harmful to the psychological well-being of disabled workers. Repeated interviews and examinations by lawyers and doctors with biases confuse and oppress many patients and reinforce and extend their symptoms.[64] Tait, Chibnall and Richardson studied 201 chronic pain patients and concluded, "Among workers' compensation patients, the decision to retain an attorney clearly was associated with reports of less distress, suggesting that the decision to hire an attorney was an effective coping response to the stresses that they faced."[65]

Littlejohn has stated that patients may enter litigation to try to prove the reality of their pain through the legal process.[26] In this author's experiences with litigating chronic pain patients, litigation has often been stimulated by insurance adjusters and independent medical examiners (IMEs). He has commonly heard accident victims say insurance adjusters expressed contempt toward them and accused them of deceit. What is worse, the IME who takes referrals from insurance companies may do an "exam" that even the patient knows is bogus. Yet the IME concludes there is no physical basis for the patient's complaints. The typical patient finds this unnerving and offensive. Realizing the adjuster and IME are prejudiced against his claims, the patient hires an attorney as a buffer between himself, the adjuster, and the IME.

Psychological stresses associated with our adversarial system may be the predominant factor in some patients' decisions to litigate. This mechanism is different, however, from attributing patients' decisions to subconscious, neurotic processes or to fraudulent simulation for financial gain.

Psychosocial Factors

Chronic pain may disrupt the equilibrium of the patient's family dynamics and cause discord between the relatives. This may lead the patient into depression and despair, all of which may militate against his recovery.[25] Littlejohn points out that individuals other than family members may sway pain patients in directions that contribute to their suffering.[26] [. . . in directions that continue their suffering. "This group of patients," he writes, "feeds an industry which preys on the suffering of such individuals."[26]] A patient may find himself painfully sliding down a social gutter to the courthouse, greased by the personal agendas and attitudes of those about him. These people include family, plaintiff and defense lawyers, insurance adjusters, IMEs, and clinicians. Such influences, however, are more a matter of practical environmental pressures than psychodynamic processes.

CONCLUSION

Weintraub writes, "pain and suffering will continue to dominate the large percentage of awards, unless there is meaningful tort and insurance reform."[1] Why should there be such reform? According to Weintraub, because awards are too often given to profit-seeking patients with hysteria-based and malingering-tainted pain. Weintraub does not provide objective evidence for his claim that 63% of his litigating patients had psychogenic pain. Specifically, he (1) used no controls in his study, (2) did not provide independent verification of his exam findings, (3) did not examine his patients for possibly the most common musculoskeletal source of pain, and (4) used a dubious protocol for

diagnosing psychogenic pain. [. . . (4) used highly dubious criteria for diagnosing an undocumented construct as the cause of his patients' chronic pain. Consequently, both his methods and conclusions are as subjective as the pain perceptions of chronic pain patients.]

Because of these conceptual and methodological faults, Weintraub's study does not justify the conclusion that any of his patients had psychogenic rather than organic pain. Furthermore, his observations do not provide evidence that psychogenic pain is common in litigation. There may be real reasons for recommending tort and insurance reform, but Weintraub's erroneous conclusions are not among them.

REFERENCES

1. Weintraub, M.I.: Litigation-chronic pain syndrome—a distinct entity: analysis of 210 cases. *Am. J. Pain Manag.*, 2:198-204, 1992.
2. Mendelson, G.: Not "cured by a verdict." *Med. J. Austral.*, 2:132-134, 1982.
3. Miller, H.: Accident neurosis: Lecture I. *Brit. Med. J.*, 74:275-277, 1981.
4. Kelly, R. and Smith, B.N.: Post-traumatic syndrome: another myth discredited. *J. Royal Soc. Med.*, 74:275-277, 1981.
5. Pelz, M. and Merskey, H.: A description of the psychological effects of chronic painful lesions. *Pain*, 14:293-301, 1982.
6. Merskey, H. and Woodforde, J.M.: Psychiatric sequelae of minor head injury. *Brain*, 95:521-528, 1972.
7. Hohl, M.: Soft-tissue injuries of the neck in automobile accidents: factors influencing prognosis. *J. Bone Joint Surg.* (Am)56-A:1675-1682, 1974.
8. Mendelson, G.: Compensation, pain complaints, and psychological disturbance. *Pain*, 20:169-177, 1984.
9. Leavitt, F., Garron, D.C., McNeill, T.W., and Whisler, W.W.: Organic status, psychological disturbance, and pain report characteristics in low-back pain patients on compensation. *Spine*, 7:398-402, 1982.
10. Kelly, R.E.: Chronic post-traumatic pain. *Pahlavi Medical Journal*, 3:530-547, 1972.
11. Taylor, A.R.: Post-concussional sequela. *Brit. Med. J.*, 3:67-71, 1967.
12. Durand-Wever, A.M.: Die commotio cerebri und ihre bewertung. *Munch. Med. Wschr.*, 76:1879, 1929.
13. Mayer, E.: Die commotio cerebri und ihre bewertung. *Munch. Med. Wschr.*, 76:2135, 1929.
14. Korr, I.M.: Lecture on the autonomic nervous system. Canadian Memorial Chiropractic College, Toronto, Canada, Aug. 1983.
15. Lowe, J.C.: *Documentary Evidence: The Chiropractic Care of Myofascial Patients.* Houston, McDowell Publishing Co., 1991, pp.33-36.
16. Lowe, J.C.: You can't measure pain, can you, doctor? *Chiro. J.*, 7:37, 1993.
17. Skootsky, S.: Incidence of myofascial pain in an internal

medical group practice. Presented to the American Pain Society, Washington, D.C., November 6-7, 1986.

18. Fricton, J.R., Kroening, R., Haley, D., and Siegert, R.: Myofascial pain syndrome of the head and neck: A review of clinical characteristics of 164 patients. *Oral Surg.*, 60: 615-623, 1985.

19. Rosomoff, H.L., Fishbain, D.A., Goldberg, M., Santana, R., and Rosomoff, R.S.: Physical findings in patients with chronic intractable benign pain of the neck and/or back. *Pain*, 37:279-282, 1989.

20. Biering-Sorensen, F.: Physical measurements as risk indicators for low-back trouble over a one year period. *Spine*, 9:106, 1984.

21. Roland, M. and Morris, R.: A study of the natural history of back pain. *Spine*, 8:141-150, 1983.

22. Naliboff, B.D., Cohen, M.J., Swanson, G.A., Bonebakker, A.D., and McArthur, D.: Comprehensive assessment of chronic low back pain patients and controls: Physical abilities, level and activity, psychological adjustment and pain perception. *Pain*, 23:121-134, 1985.

23. Crue, B.L. and Pinsky, J.J.: An approach to chronic pain of non-malignant origin. *Postgrad. Med. J.*, 60:858-864, 1984.

24. Schiffman, E., Fricton, J., Haley, D., and Tylka, D.: A pressure algometer for myofascial pain syndrome: reliability and validity testing. In *Proceedings of the Vth World Congress on Pain*. Edited by R. Dubner, G.F. Gebhart, and M.R. Bond, Elsevier Science Publishers, 1988, pp.408-413.

25. Rickarby, G.: Compensation-neurosis and the psycho-social requirements of the family. *Br. J. Med. Psychol.*, 52:333-338, 1979.

26. Littlejohn, G.: Medicolegal aspects of fibrositis syndrome. *J. Rheumatol.*, 16(suppl.19):169-173, 1989.

27. Pattimore, D., Thomas, P., and Dave, S.H.: Torso injury patterns and mechanisms in car crashes: an additional diagnostic tool. *Injury*, 23:123-126, 1992.

28. Twomey, L.T., Taylor, J.R., and Taylor, M.M.: Unsuspected damage to lumbar zygapophyseal (facet) joints after motor-vehicle accidents. *Med. J. Australia*, 151:210-217, 1989.

29. Oppenheimer, D.R.: Microscopic lesions in the brain following head injury. *J. Neurol. Neurosurg. Psychiat.*, 31: 299-306, 1968.

30. Fischer, A.A. and Chang, C.H.: Temperature and pressure threshold measurements in trigger points. *Thermology*, 1: 212-215, 1986.

31. Diakow, P.R.P.: Differentiation of active and latent trigger points by thermography. Minneapolis: First International Symposium on Myofascial Pain and Fibromyalgia, May, 9, 1989, p.41.

32. Weinterstein, S.A. and Weinstein, G.: The results of trigger point injection (a thermographic photo-essay). Minneapolis: First International Symposium on Myofascial Pain and Fibromyalgia, May, 9, 1989, p.95.

33. American Psychiatric Association: *Diagnostic and Statistical Manual of Mental Disorders*, 3rd edition. Washington, D.C., American Psychiatric Association, 1987.

34. Weintraub, M.: Hysteria: A clinical guide to diagnosis. *Clin. Symposia*, 29:1-31, 1977.

35. Merskey, H.: Regional pain is rarely hysterical. *Arch.*

Neurol., 45:915-918, 1988.

36. Gould, R., Miller, B.L., and Goldberg, M.A.: The validity of hysterical signs and symptoms. *J. Nerv. Ment. Dis.*, 174:23-28, 1986.

37. Bonica, J.J.: Myofascial syndromes with trigger mechanism. In *The Management of Pain*. Edited by J.J. Bonica, Philadelphia, Lea and Febiger, 1953, pp.1150-1151.

38. Kendall, H.O., Kendall, F.P., Wadsworth, G.E., Gould, R., Miller, B.L., and Goldberg, M.A,: The validity of hysterical signs and symptoms. *J. Nerv. Ment. Dis.*, 174:23-28, 1986.

39. Inman, V.T., Saunders, J.B., and deCamp, M.: Referred pain from skeletal structures. *J. Nerv. Ment. Dis.*, 99:660-667, 1944.

40. Travell, J.G.: Referred somatic pain does not follow a simple "segmental" pattern. *Red. Proc.*, 5:106, 1946.

41. Jaeger, B. and Skootsky, S.A.: Letter to the editor. *Pain*, 29:263-264, 1987.

42. Fishbain, D.A. and Rosomoff, H.: Letter to the editor. *Pain*, 29:265, 1987.

43. Travell, J.G. and Simons, D.G.: *Myofascial Pain and Dysfunction: The Trigger Point Manual*, Vol. 1. Baltimore, Williams and Wilkins, 1983.

44. Hachinski, V.: The nature of regional pain. *Arch. Neurology*, 45:918, 1988.

45. Kennedy, F.: The mind of the injured worker: its effects on disability periods. *Compens. Med.*, 1:19-24, 1946.

46. Balla, J.I. and Moraitis, S.: Knights in armour: a follow-up study of injuries after legal settlement. *Med. J. Austral.*, 2:355-361, 1970.

47. Thompson, G.N.: Post-traumatic psychoneurosis: a statistical survey. *Am. J. Psychiatry*, 121:1043-1048, 1965.

48. Gotten, N.: Survey of 100 cases of whiplash injury after settlement of litigation. *J.A.M.A.*, 162:865-867, 1956.

49. Melzack, R., Katz, J., and Jeans, M.E.: The role of compensation in chronic pain: analysis using a new method of scoring the McGill Pain Questionnaire. *Pain*, 23:101-112, 1985.

50. Schutt, C.H. and Dohan, F.C.: Neck injury to women in auto accidents: a metropolitan plague. *J.A.M.A.*, 206(12): 2689-2692, 1968.

51. Macnab, I.: Acceleration injuries of the cervical spine. *J. Bone Joint Surg.*, 46A:1797-1799, 1964.

52. Macnab, I.: The whiplash syndrome. *Clin. Neurosurg.*, 20: 232-241, 1972.

53. Romano, T.J.: Clinical experiences with post-traumatic fibromyalgia syndrome. *W. Vir. Med. J.*, 86:198-202, 1990.

54. Braaf, M.M. and Rosner, S.S.: Symptomatology and treatment of injuries of the neck. *N.Y. J. Med.*, 55:237-242, 1955.

55. Thiemeyer, J.S., Duncan, G.A., and Hollins, G.G.: Whiplash injuries of the cervical spine. *Vir. Med. Monthly*, 85: 171-174, 1958.

56. Institute of Medicine: *Pain and Disability: Clinical, Behavioral, and Public Policy Perspectives*. Washington, D.C., National Academy Press, 1987.

57. Simons, D.G. and Simons, L.S.: Chronic myofascial pain syndrome. In *Handbook of Chronic Pain Management*. Edited by C.D. Tollison, Baltimore, Williams and Wilkins, 1989, pp.509-529.

58. Sonkin, L.S.: Endocrine disorders and muscle dysfunction.

In *Clinical Management of Head, Neck and TMJ Pain and Dysfunction.* Edited by H. Gelb, Philadelphia, W.B. Saunders, 1985, pp.137-170.

59. Lowe, J.C.: *The Purpose and Practice of Myofascial Therapy.* (Audio-cassette program) Houston, McDowell Publishing Co, 1989, sides 6 and 7.
60. Lowe, J.C.: Oral contraceptives and myofascial pain. *Chiropractic Economics*, 100-101, Nov/Dec, 1991.
61. Lowe, J.C.: Myofascial pain and "the pill". *J. Nat. Ass. Trig. Pnt. Myother.*, 5.1:5-6, 1992.
62. Lowe, J.C.: Treatment-resistant myofascial pain syndromes. In *Functional Soft Tissue Examination and Treat-ment by Manual Methods, The Extremities.* Edited by W. Hammer, Gaithersburg, Aspen Publishing Co., 1991, pp.222-234.

63. Ommaya, A.K., Fass, F., and Yarnell, P.: Whiplash injury and brain damage: an experimental study. *J.A.M.A.*, 204: 285-289, 1968.
64. Reed, J.L.: Compensation neurosis and Munchausen syndrome. *Br. J. Hosp. Med.*, 19:314-321, 1978.
65. Tait, R.C., Chibnall, J.T., and Richardson, W.D.: Litigation and employment status: effects on patients with chronic pain. *Pain*, 43:37-46, 1990.

Appendix D

CONVERSIONS:
T₄, T₃, AND DESICCATED THYROID

Conversions: T_4, T_3, and Desiccated Thyroid

Mathematical conversions are of minimal use in switching a patient from one form of thyroid hormone to another. This is especially true when switching the patient from either T_4 or T_3 to desiccated thyroid or a product containing both T_4 and T_3, or from desiccated thyroid or a combination of T_4 and T_3 to either T_4 or T_3 alone. A useful strategy in switching the patient in such cases is to use mathematical conversion but to correct the dosage based on the use of clinical indicat-ors. The patient's effective dosage must be determined on an individual basis, with the patient and physician closely cooperating. To find that dosage, the patient's fibromyalgia status should be objectively measured repeatedly (see Chapter 4.1), and so should certain physical measures such as the Achilles reflex and pulse rate (see Chapter 4.3). It is critically important to remember that the patient's TSH level is of no value in determining the proper dosage.

Table 1. Equivalent amounts of T_4, T_3, and desiccated thyroid.

T_4	$T_3 \div 4$*	ARMOUR THYROID	ARMOUR[†] CONTENT OF T_4	AND	T_3
0.025 mg (25 µ)	6.25 µ	¼ gr (15 mg)	9.5 µ		2.25 µ
0.05 mg (50 µ)	12.5 µ	½ gr (30 mg)	19 µ		4.5 µ
0.075 mg (75 µ)	18.75 µ	¾ gr (45 mg)	28.5 µ		6.75 µ
0.1 mg (100 µ)	25 µ	1 gr (60 mg)	38 µ		9 µ
0.125 mg (125 µ)[γ]	31.25 µ	1¼ gr (75 mg)	47.5 µ		11.25 µ
0.15 mg (150 µ)[‡]	37.5 µ	1½ gr (90 mg)	57 µ		13.5 µ
0.175 mg (175 µ)[‡]	43.75 µ	1¾ gr (105 mg)	66.5 µ		15.75 µ
0.2 mg (200 µ)	50 µ	2 gr (120 mg)	76 µ		18 µ
0.225 mg (225 µ)	56.25 µ	2¼ gr (135 mg)	85.5 µ		20.25 µ
0.25 mg (250 µ)	62.5 µ	2½ gr (150 mg)	95 µ		22.5 µ
0.275 mg (275 µ)	68.75 µ	2¾ gr (165 mg)	104.5 µ		24.75 µ
0.3 mg (300 µ)	75 µ	3 gr (180 mg)	114 µ		27 µ
0.35 mg (350 µ)	87.5 µ	3½ gr (210 mg)	133 µ		31.5 µ
0.4 mg (400 µ)	100 µ	4 gr (240 mg)	152 µ		36 µ
0.45 mg (450 µ)	112.5 µ	4½ gr (270 mg)	171 µ		40.5 µ
0.5 mg (500 µ)	125 µ	5 gr (300 mg)	190 µ		45 µ
0.55 mg (550 µ)	137.5 µ	5½ gr (330 mg)	209 µ		49.5 µ
0.6 mg (600 µ)	150 µ	6 gr (360 mg)	228 µ		54 µ

*T_3 is considered to be four times more potent on a µg by µg basis. Thus, when switching a patient from T_4 to T_3, the dosage should theoretically be divided by four. When switching the patient from T_3 to T_4, the dosage should be multiplied by four.
[†]Armour Thyroid and other forms of desiccated thyroid, in compliance with the USP, contain 38 µ T_4 and 9 µ of T_3.
[γ]A dosage of 127 mg of exogenous T_4 was found to suppress the TSH response to injected TRH (Hennessey, J.V., Evaul, J.E., Tseng, Y.-Y., et al.: L-thyroxine dosage: a reevaluation of therapy with contemporary preparations. *Ann. Internal. Med.*, 105:11-15, 1986).
[‡]TSH suppression has been reported to occur in patients taking a mean of 0.145 mg of T_4 (Korsic, M., Cvijetic, S., Dekanic-Ozegovic, D., Bolanca, S., and Kozic, B.: Bone mineral density in patients on long-term therapy with levothyroxine. *Lijec Vjesn*, 120(5):103-105, 1998), and in patients taking a mean of 0.171 mg of T_4 (Fowler, P.B., McIvor, J., Sykes, L., and Macrae, K.D.: The effect of long-term thyroxine on bone mineral density and serum cholesterol. *J. R. Coll. Physicians Lond.*, 30(6):527-532, 1996).

Most hypothyroid fibromyalgia patients benefit only from dosages of thyroid hormone equivalent to 200-to-400 µg of T_4 (0.2-to-0.4 mg). Few patients benefit from the equivalent of the 100-to-200 µg of T_4 that most clinicians restrict them to. Some writers have stated that one grain (65 mg) of desiccated thyroid provides the equivalent of 80 micrograms of T_4. How-ever, desiccated thyroid contains both T_4 and T_3. One grain of Armour Thyroid contains 38 µg of T_4 and 9 µg of T_3. T_3 is often reported to be four times more potent than T_4, µg for µg. Thus, in terms of potency, the 9 µg of T_3 is roughly equivalent to 36 µg of T_4 (9 x 4 = 36). So it can be argued that the total potency of the thyroid hormone in one grain of Armour Thyroid is equivalent to about 74 μg of T_4 (38 μg from T_4 + 36 μg from T_3 = the potency equivalent of 74 μg of T_4).

From this consideration, one might assume that to benefit from Armour Thyroid, a patient must take enough to equal the potency of 200-to-400 μg of T_4. If this were true, it would be necessary to take between 2½ and 5 tablets of Armour per day. (2½ tablets would have a potency roughly equivalent to 200 μg of T_4; 5 tablets would have a potency roughly equivalent to 400 μg of T_4.) But this assumption might be incorrect. Most hypothyroid fibromyalgia patients improve on lower dosages of Armour than this. The likely explanation is that the potency of the T_3 in the Amour is actually equivalent to more than four times the potency of T_4. Some recent publications suggest that T_3 may be 10 times more potent than T_4, μg for μg. The response to desiccated thyroid, therefore, is difficult to predict simply through mathematical conversions.

Glossary with Acronyms and Symbols

Acetylcholinesterase inhibitor: Acetylcholinesterase is an enzyme that breaks down acetylcholine (the neurotransmitter secreted by parasympathetic nerves) by hydrolysis. By breaking down the transmitter, acetylcholinesterase prevents excessive parasympathetic innervation of tissues. Substances called acetylcholinesterase inhibitors prevent the enzyme from breaking down acetylcholine, with the result that tissues are excessively innervated by acetylcholine. Essentially, the inhibitors cause parasympathetic dominance, producing symptoms such as lethergy, fatigue, and inability of the heart rate and cardiac output to increase appropriately during exercise and other stresses. Excess acetylcholine also causes excessive stimulation at motor end plates and the autonomic ganglia.

ACR: American College of Rheumatology.

Adrenergic neuron: A nerve that synthesizes and secretes a catecholamine such as epinephrine.

Adrenergic receptor: The adrenergic receptor is a protein in cell membranes that catecholamines bind with to initiate changes in cell metabolism. Also termed "adrenceptor." There are α- and β-isoforms of the adrenergic receptor.

α-Adrenergic receptor: An isoform of adrenergic receptor that, in general, influences cellular metabolism in such a way as to have inhibitory effects on physiological and psychological processes. Also termed "α-adrenoceptor."

β-Adrenergic receptor: An isoform of adrenergic receptor that, in general, influences cellular metabolism in such a way as to have excitatory effects on physiological and psychological processes. Also termed "β-adrenoceptor."

Adrenergic receptor antagonist: Adrenergic receptor antagonists are commonly called "blockers": either "α-blockers" or "β-blockers," depending on the type of adrenergic receptors for which the chemicals are antagonists. An antagonist preferentially binds to a receptor, preventing the binding of the receptor's natural ligand. Binding prevents activation of the chemical processes normally stimulated by the receptor and its natural ligand. Because of its successful competition for binding, an antagonist is said to "competitively bind" to the receptor. Thus, the antagonist is useful because it has a higher affinity for the receptor than do the natural ligands of the receptor. (See Adrenoceptor agonist.) The following is a partial list of such antagonists:

> **α-adrenoceptor antagonist:** phenoxybenzamine
> **α_1-adrenoceptor antagonists:** prazosin, doxazosin, indoramin, phentolamine
> **α_2-adrenoceptor antagonists:** yohimbine, idazoxan, piperoxane, atipamezole, rauwolscine, phentolamine

> **β-adrenoceptor antagonist:** atenolol
> **β_1-adrenoceptor antagonists:** metoprolol, propranolol
> **β_2-adrenoceptor antagonist:** propranolol

Adrenoceptor: Abbreviated version of the term "adrenergic receptor." Adrenoceptors are the proteins in cell membranes to which the catecholamine hormones epinephrine and norepinephrine bind. Binding of adrenergic receptors to catecholamines initiates changes in cell metabolism. Binding of catecholamines to α- and β-isoforms of the adrenoceptor initiates different cellular responses.

Adrenoceptor agonist: Also termed adrenergic receptor activator or stimulant. An adrenergic receptor agonist preferentially binds to a receptor, blocking binding of the natural ligand for the receptor. Binding of the agonist and the receptor stimulates the processes controlled by the receptor and its natural ligand. The following is a partial list of such agonists: (See Adrenergic receptor antagonist.)

> **β-adrenoceptor agonist:** isoproterenol (synonym for isoprenaline)
> **β_1-adrenoceptor agonist:** prenalterol
> **β_2-adrenoceptor agonist:** salbutamol
> **α_1-adrenoceptor agonists:** methoxamine, phenylephrine
> **α_2-adrenoceptor agonists:** clonidine, rilmenidine, epinephrine, norepinephrine, medetomidine, tizanidine, dexmedetomidine

Afferent: Toward a center, or in a centripetal direction. Denotes that arteries, veins, and lymphatics conduct fluids toward a center and that nerves conduct impulses toward a center. [< L. afferens, to bring to] See Sensory nerve. See Efferent.

Aldosterone: A steroid hormone synthesized and secreted by the zona glomerulosa of the adrenal cortex. It is the chief mineralocorticoid. Its main function is to facilitate the exchange of potassium for sodium in the distal kidney tubules. It induces sodium reabsorption (from the tubules into the blood) and potassium and hydrogen loss in the urine. See Mineralocorticoid.

Allele: One of a pair of genes in the same position on a pair of chromosomes. The pair of genes controls hereditary traits.

Allodynia: Literally means pain that differs from normal pain (the prefix "allo" is from the Greek *allos* meaning other; the suffix "dynia" is from the Greek *odynè* meaning pain). In common parlance, pain induced by a stimulus that ordinarily does not evoke pain. See Hyperalgesia.

Allosteric change: There are at least two distinct types of binding locations on enzymes and receptors: allosteric and active sites. Each of the sites binds other molecules. Binding of a hormone to an allosteric site on a receptor alters the three-dimensional shape of the receptor's active site. The active site binds a ligand specific to the receptor. (The active site of an enzyme binds substrates, substances acted upon and changed by the enzyme.) As examples, the T_3-receptor binds T_3 and adrenergic receptors bind the two catecholamines norepinephrine and epinephrine; T_3 and the catecholamines are the ligands of their respective receptors. The change in the structural conformation of the active site has one of two effects: it prevents the receptor from binding to its ligand or enables it to do so. Which effect the conformation has depends on the molecule that binds to the allosteric site. Binding of a molecule to an allosteric site either decreases or increases the affinity of the receptor's active site for its ligand.

Amiodarone: An effective medication for angina and cardiac arrhythmias. Induces either thyrotoxicosis or hypothyroidism in most patients who use it. Hypothyroidism may develop within a year of amiodarone use, and in some cases, the hypothyroidism is severe.

Anabolism: Chemical processes that convert small molecules to larger ones.

Ankylosing spondylitis: An arthritic condition of the spine that resembles rheumatoid arthritis. The condition may progress to bony ankylosis of the spine with prominent lipping of vertebral margins. Ankylosing spondylitis is more common among males. Synonyms: Marie-Strümpell disease and rheumatoid spondylitis.

Anomaly: A deviation from the general rule or what is expected. The term is derived from the Greek word for "irregularity." In science, anomaly refers to a finding that is inconsistent with the main concept of the accepted paradigm. Science progresses by research within a paradigm producing anomalous findings that cannot be explained by the concepts of the paradigm. Accumulating anomalies eventually lead to the formation of new concepts to account for the anomalies. That new concept that is more generally accepted by researchers in the field of study becomes the guide to research within the new paradigm.

Anovulation: Failure to ovulate during the menstrual cycle.

Anxiolytic: Decreasing anxiety.

Apoenzyme: The protein component of an enzyme, as distinct from the nonprotein component, the coenzyme.

Armour®: Tablets containing thyroid hormone synthesized naturally by the pig thyroid glands. Each grain contains 38 µg of T_4 and 9 µg of T_3. Inactive ingredients include calcium stearate, dextrose, and mineral oil. Forest Pharmaceuticals, Inc.

Arteriole: The small, distal end of a large artery. The arteriole is constructed mostly of one or two layers of smooth muscle cells. Collectively, the muscle layers are called the tunica media. The arteriole is continuous with the capillary network that leads the collecting veins. Arterioles are the main site of resistance to blood flow. Constriction of the arteriole increases resistance to blood flow, and dilation increases blood flow. Activation of α-adrenergic receptors on arterioles induces constriction. Activation of β-adrenergic receptors on the arterioles counteracts the vasoconstriction induced by α-adrenergic receptors, causing arteriolar dilation.

Arthropathy: Any disease of joints.

Assay: A procedure or test that detects and quantifies the amount of a substance in a system, such as the amount of T_3 in blood plasma.

Ataxia: Impaired ability to coordinate the muscles during voluntary movements. Incoordination.

Atresia: The normal process by which a primordial ovarian follicle with its ovum dies, degenerates, and ends in closure by the formation of fibrous tissue. The follicle is said to be atretic.

Autoradiograph: A picture that shows the presence of radioactive material. The film is positioned directly on the object containing the radioactive material.

Autoreceptor: A receptor on a presynaptic neuron that, upon binding to its specific neurotransmitter, alters release of a chemical transmitter the neuron secretes.

bid: b.i.d.; twice daily. L. *bis in die*.

Blood brain barrier: Many substances are barred from entry into the brain by the tight junctions of the endothelial cells of brain capillaries. This constitutes the blood brain barrier. The barrier contains transport systems for a number of substances that become cerebral substrates. Systems that transport these substances across this barrier are located in the plasma membranes of epithelial cells of brain capillaries. They transport substances across the barrier.

Blood flow: Blood flow is the quantity of blood that passes any point in the circulation during a given time. Flow through the vessel is determined completely by (1) the difference in pressure between the two ends of the vessel, which forces the blood through the vessel, and (2) resistance to the movement of the blood through the vessel.

Blood pressure: Usually termed the arterial pressure. Arterial pressure is equal to cardiac output times total vascular resistance. (See Cardiac output.)

***Borrelia burgdorferi*:** The spirochete responsible for Lyme disease.

bpm: Beats per minute.

Bradycardia: Slow heart rate. Some sources define bradycardia as a heart rate of 60 or fewer beats per minute. Other sources define it as 50 or fewer beats per minute.

Brain stem: The earliest evolved part of the brain, located between the spinal cord and the cerebral cortex. Brain stem centers regulate autonomic functions such as breathing and the urination reflex.

Brand names, thyroid hormone:

Table 1. Thyroid hormone products by brand name and hormone content.*

CONTENTS	BRAND NAME
Synthetic T_4	Levothroid®, Levoxine®, Levoxyl®, Synthroid®
Synthetic T_3	Cytomel® (oral use), Triostat™ (injectable)
Synthetic T_4 & T_3	Thyrolar®
Naturally-derived T_4 & T_3	Armour Thyroid®, Westhroid®, Naturethroid, S-P-T

*See individual brand names for more detailed descriptions of products.

C: Centigrade (degrees). A temperature scale. The boiling point of water on the scale is 100°. The freezing point of water on the scale is 0°. Synonymous with the Celsius scale.

Ca^{++}: Calcium ion.

Ca^{2+}: Calcium ion.

Calorie: Small calorie. The amount of heat that raises the temperature of 1 mL of water 1° Celsius. See Kilocalorie.

Calorigenesis: Metabolic stimulation of heat. The term "calorie" derives from the Greek term *calor* for heat, and the term "genesis" derives from the Greek term for production. See Thermogenesis.

Candida albicans: A species of fungus that is a constituent of the flora of the human gastrointestinal tract. Under some conditions that cause an imbalance in the intestinal flora, such as prolonged antibiotic use, *Candida albicans* may overgrow to the degree that it becomes pathogenic. Clinical features vary from widespread skin and mucous membrane infections to conditions that may prove fatal, such as septicemia, meningitis, or endocarditis.

Cardiac output: Equal to the heart rate times the blood volume of each stroke of the left ventricle (stroke volume).

Cardiorespiratory: Refers to functions that involve interaction of the heart and lungs. Often used to refer to heart and

lungs interaction in providing oxygen and other nutrient delivery to tissues during exercise. Synonymous with cardiopulmonary.

Catabolism: Chemical processes that convert large molecules to smaller ones.

Catecholamine: A compound consisting of a pyrocatechol moiety (the root of the catecholamine hormones) with an alkylamine side chain. The catecholamines of interest in this book are dopamine, epinephrine, and norepinephrine.

Catecholaminergic: Associated with the catecholamine neurotransmitters: dopamine, epinephrine, norepinephrine.

CBC: Complete blood count.

cDNA: See Cloned DNA.

Central hypothyroidism: Decreased thyroid gland synthesis and secretion of thyroid hormones because of decreased thyroid gland stimulation by thyroid stimulating hormone (TSH; thyrotropin). Decreased TSH stimulation of an intrinsically normal thyroid gland may result from deficient synthesis or secretion of TSH by the anterior pituitary gland. In this case, the terms "pituitary hypothyroidism" or "secondary hypothyroidism" are appropriate. Deficient TSH secretion may also result secondarily from insufficient stimulation of the anterior pituitary gland due to a deficiency of the hypothalamic hormone called thyrotropin-releasing hormone (TRH). In this case, the terms "hypothalamic hypothyroidism" or "tertiary hypothyroidism" are proper.

Central nervous system: The brain and spinal cord. Abbreviated as CNS.

Centrifugal: Movement away from a center. Used to denote nerve signals being conducted away from the central nervous system.. Synonyms: Motor nerve signals and efferent nerve signals.

Centripetal: Movement toward a center. Used to denote nerve signals being conducted toward the central nervous system.. Synonyms: Sensory nerve signals and afferent nerve signals.

Cerebellum: A large posterior brain structure. It is located beneath the posterior part of the cerebrum and above the medulla and pons of the brain stem.

Cerebral ventricles: Four cavities in the cerebral hemispheres that contain cerebrospinal fluid. Each cavity contains a choroid plexus that secretes and absorbs cerebrospinal fluid. (See Choroid plexus.)

Cerebrum: The largest part of the brain. It consists of the two cerebral hemispheres (collectively termed the cerebral cortex) that are divided by the deep longitudinal fissure and the basal ganglia. Generally considered to include all parts of the brain except the cerebellum, the medulla, and the pons. From the Latin term for brain.

CFS: Chronic fatigue syndrome.

CFIDS: Chronic fatigue immune dysfunction syndrome.

Cholinergic: Associated with the neurotransmitter acetylcholine. Cholinergic nerves secrete acetylcholine.

Choroid plexus: A blood vessel network in each of the four cerebral ventricles. Most of the cerebrospinal fluid is formed in the choroid plexuses, especially in the lateral ventricles. The plexuses regulate the pressure in the ventricles by absorbing or secreting cerebrospinal fluid. (See Cerebral ventricles.)

CK: See Creatine kinase.

Clinical assessment: Evaluation of a patient's status based on his or her history, symptoms, and signs. The clinician may supplement the evaluation with the results of technical procedures such as laboratory tests, electrophysiological measures, and imaging methods. (See Clinical medicine.)

Clinical medicine: The practice of medicine in which the clinician makes use of a wide range of methods to make diagnostic and treatment decisions. The clinician uses the patient's history and symptoms, and the results of physical exam procedures and technical test methods. The clinician and patient usually have a collaborative relationship. (See Clinical assessment.)

Clinical phenotype: A characteristic manifestation of an underlying disease process, or the combined manifestation of several different underlying disease processes. The underlying disease process may be distinguished from others on the basis of a sufficiently distinctive clinical phenotype. An underlying disease may give rise to different clinical phenotypes in different patients. Thus, the phenotype for one patient with inadequate thyroid hormone regulation of cell function will be elevated circulating lipids we diagnose as idiopathic hyperlipidemia, while the phenotype for another may be the widespread pain, tenderness, and sleep disturbance that we diagnose as fibromyalgia.

Cloned DNA: A DNA copy of an RNA, made by reverse transcription. Usually abbreviated cDNA.

cm: Centimeter.

CNS: Abbreviation for central nervous system. See Central nervous system.

CO_2: Carbon dioxide.

Consecutive: Term used in clinical research in regard to

study subjects. For example, each new patient who qualifies for participation in a study is enrolled consecutively or in sequence.

Corticosterone: The steroid hormone most abundantly secreted by the adrenal cortices in rats.

Cortisol: The steroid hormone that is most abundantly secreted by the adrenal cortices in humans. Cortisol is a product of cortisone and is also called hydrocortisone. Increased cortisol secretion is a part of the physiological process of stress.

Creatine kinase: An enzyme important in muscle contraction that catalyzes the transfer of a phosphate from phosphocreatine to ADP. Transfer of the phosphate to ADP forms ATP.

Cyclic-AMP: A cyclic nucleotide inside cells that is part of the metabolic machinery of cells. When some hormones bind to their receptors on cell membranes, reactions within the cell membrane cause the formation of cyclic-AMP inside the cell. Cyclic-AMP then stimulates other intracellular activities.

Cynomel®: Name for Cytomel® sold in Mexico as an over-the-counter product.

Cytomel®: Brand name for synthetic T_3. Jones Medical Industries, Inc.

Cytoplasm: The total substance of the cell contained within the outer or plasma membrane but excluding the nucleus. Cytoplasm is made up of the colloidal protoplasm that contains organelles of the cells such as the mitochondria.

Cytosol: The cytoplasm of the cell excluding the mitochondria and the various membranes such as the endoplasmic reticulum.

Dehydrogenase: An enzyme that catalyzes oxidation of a substance, causing it to release its hydrogen.

Deiodination: Removal of an iodine atom from a molecule. In the case of thyroid hormones, deiodination is the removal of an iodine atom from an iodothyronine molecule. 5'-Deiodination is the removal of an iodine atom from the phenolic ring of the molecule, producing T_3. 5-Deiodination is removal of the tyrosyl ring, producing reverse-T_3. This latter reaction liberates iodide from the molecule and enables it to be recycled.

Dermopathy: Any disease of the skin. Also dermatopathy.

Dimer: A protein consisting of a complex of two polypeptides. If the two peptides are the same, the protein is called a homodimer. If they are different, the protein is called a heterodimer.

Dimerization: Combining of two proteins to form a single molecule. The thyroid hormone receptor dimerizes by binding various auxiliary proteins, such as retinoid X receptors.

Diuresis: Production of unusually large volumes of urine. Results from deficient vasopressin secretion by the posterior pituitary. May also result from the influence of increased numbers of α-adrenergic receptors on the posterior pituitary, brain stem centers, and the bladder during inadequate thyroid hormone regulation of the adrenergic genes.

Dopaminergic: Associated with the neurotransmitter dopamine. Dopaminergic neurons secrete dopamine.

Down-regulation: A decrease in the availability of receptors specific for a particular ligand. Down-regulation may involve a decrease in the affinity of the receptors for the binding substances or an actual decrease in the number of the receptors. Down-regulation occurs upon repetitive exposure to a pharmacological or physiological substance that binds to the receptors. Cells with down-regulated receptors are less responsive to the ligand that naturally binds to the receptors.

Dysphoria: An unpleasant mood state. May include overall discomfort, dissatisfaction, restlessness, depression, or anxiety.

ECG: Electrocardiography.

Efferent: Away from a center, such as an organ. Denotes the outward flow of arteries, veins, and lymphatics from a center, or transmission of nerve impulses away from a center. [< L. *efferens*, to bring out] See Afferent.

Ehlers-Danlos syndrome: Several similar inherited diseases in which connective tissues are excessively elastic and fragile. The connective tissues of the skin, joints, and blood vessels are particularly affected. The excessive elasticity and friability of the connective tissues result from a subnormal amount or quality of collagen.

Elastin: The main connective tissue protein of flexible structures, such as large blood vessels. Elastin is a yellow elastic fibrous mucoprotein.

Empirical: In reference to treatment, based on practical experience rather than objective scientific study.

Endogenous: Produced within the body. The opposite of exogenous.

Endometrium: Mucous membrane of the inner layer of the uterus. It is made up of columnar epithelium and a layer containing tubular uterine glands. The endometrium becomes thicker and more vascularized under the influence of estrogen during the first or follicular phase of the menstrual cycle.

Enzyme: A protein that catalyzes chemical reactions at rates hundreds-to-thousands of times faster than would occur in its absence. The reactions catalyzed by enzymes regulate cell metabolism, the assembly of larger molecules from smaller ones (anabolism), and the breakdown of large molecules to smaller ones (catabolism).

Euthyroid hypometabolism: Refers to hypometabolism despite normal thyroid function laboratory test results. The underlying mechanism of euthyroid hypometabolism may be related to thyroid hormone, as in cellular resistance to normal levels of thyroid hormone. However, the mechanism(s) may be unrelated to thyroid hormone. See Euthyroid hypometabolism, thyroid hormone-related. Also see Euthyroid hypometabolism, non-thyroid hormone-related.

Euthyroid hypometabolism, non-thyroid hormone-related: Hypometabolism due to some underlying mechanism that is independent of the patient's thyroid status. Common mechanisms of non-thyroid hormone-related euthyroid hypometabolism are adrenal insufficiency, various B complex vitamin deficiencies, physical deconditioning, and chronic use of high-dosage β-adrenergic blocking drugs.

Euthyroid hypometabolism, thyroid hormone-related: Hypometabolism despite normal thyroid function test results, but involving failure of normal concentrations of thyroid hormone to properly regulate cell function.

Exogenous: Produced outside the body. The opposite of endogenous.

Exophthalmos: Protrusion of one or both eyeballs. Protrusion is bilateral when caused by thyroid disease.

F: Fahrenheit (degrees). A temperature scale. The boiling point of water on the scale is 212°. The freezing point of water on the scale is 32°.

Facilitation: See Segmental facilitation.

Fibromyalgia: A clinical phenotype of inadequate thyroid hormone regulation of cell function, due either to hypothyroidism or partial cellular resistance to thyroid hormone.

Follicle stimulating hormone: One of the two gonadotropin hormones secreted by the gonadotroph cells of the anterior pituitary gland. Abbreviated as FSH. FSH stimulates the maturation of the ovarian follicle during the follicular phase of the menstrual cycle. See LH.

FMS: Fibromyalgia.

Free thyroxine index: The free T_4 index.

FSH: Follicle stimulating hormone. See Follicle stimulating hormone.

Galactorrhea: A white milk-like discharge from the nipples.

Genome: The complete complement of genes of a set of chromosomes.

Genomic: Concerning the genome. In this book, genomic effects refer to those mediated by the regulation of gene transcription. For example, the increase in the cell membrane density of β-adrenergic receptors is a genomic effect of T_3.

Glomerular filtration: The selective excretion of water and dissolved substances in the glomeruli of the kidneys. The water and other substances from the blood pass from the capillaries into the kidney tubules. As dictated by exposure to various hormones and their receptors, some of the water and other substances are reabsorbed into the blood. The tubules transport the rest to the ureters, and the ureters transport them to the bladder from which they are excreted as urine. See Glomerulus.

Glomerulus: A network or plexus of interjoining capillaries at the starting point of the tubules of the kidneys. The plexus is surrounded by a capsule called Bowman's capsule. The structure in the kidney is specifically termed the malpighian glomerulus. Derived from a Latin term for ball of yarn. Plural: glomeruli. See Glomerular filtration.

Glucose intolerance: Impaired metabolism, excretion, or disposal of glucose. Clinicians use the glucose tolerance test to determine whether a patient processes glucose normally. An abnormal elevation of blood glucose during the test indicates that the patient does not properly process glucose; that is, she is glucose intolerant. Adverse health effects are associated with glucose intolerance.

Glycoprotein: A compound composed of polysaccharide (usually the amino sugar hexosamine) and protein. A water-binding constituent of connective tissues. Glycoproteins contain up to 95% polysaccharide. Fibroblasts increase their synthesis and secretion of glycoproteins when exposed to too little T_3 (as in hypothyroidism) and when T_3-receptors in fibroblasts are mutated and have a low affinity for T_3 (as in thyroid hormone resistance). In either case, localized excess water binding develops, producing myxedema. See Glycosaminoglycan.

Glycosaminoglycan: General term for glycoprotein complexes. New term for mucopolysaccharide.

gm: gram.

GnRH: Gonadotropin-releasing hormone. The hormone synthesized and secreted by hypothalamic neurons that stimulates secretion of the gonadotropins (follicle stimulating hormone and luteinizing hormone) by anterior pituitary cells.

Goiter: Chronically enlarged thyroid gland that is not caused by a neoplasm. Occurs endemically in some geographic regions and sporadically in others. French term from the Latin word *guttur* for throat.

Goitrogen: A substance such as cabbage, rapeseed, and soy that induces goiter.

Gonad: An organ that produces sex germ cells. The female gonad, the ovary, produces ova. The male gonad, the testicle or testis, produces sperm.

gr: grain.

Granulosa cells: The wall of cells of the ovarian follicle that secrete estrogen in response to FSH.

Growth hormone-releasing factor: The hypothalamic hormone that stimulates growth hormone secretion by the pituitary somatotroph cells.

hCG: Human chorionic gonadotropin. A glycoprotein produced by trophoblastic cells of the placenta and present in the urine of pregnant women. During the first trimester of pregnancy, hCG stimulates secretion of estrogen and progesterone by the ovaries. Secretion of these two hormones is necessary for the integrity of the embryo and its supporting membrane. During the second and third trimesters of pregnancy, the placenta provides estrogen and progesterone, and hCG plays no further role in their provision.

Head-up tilt test: A test in which patients are changed from a recumbent to a vertical posture. The test is used to assess adaptation of a patient's cardiovascular system to the change in position.

Hepatocyte: A parenchymal (see Parenchyma) liver cell.

Heterodimer: See Dimer.

Heterozygote: A hybrid organism containing genes, in the same position on a pair of chromosomes, for unlike characteristics.

Heterozygous: Dissimilar pairs of genes, in the same position on a pair of chromosomes, for any hereditary characteristic.

Hg: Hydrargyrum; the symbol for mercury.

Homodimer: See Dimer.

Homozygote: An organism with identical pairs of genes with respect to any given pair of hereditary characteristics.

Homozygous: An identical pair of genes, in the same position on a pair of chromosomes, for any pair of hereditary characteristics.

Hormone: A substance produced by one tissue, transported through the circulating blood, and affecting the biochemical and/or physiological activity of another tissue. Most hormones are either peptides or steroids.

HPA axis: Abbreviation for hypothalamic-pituitary-adrenal, as in reference to the HPA axis.

Hyperalgesia: Extreme sensitivity to painful stimuli. In auditory hyperalgesia, the individual has a painful reaction to noises that are not ordinarily noxious. Synonyms: Hyperalgia and allodynia. See Allodynia.

Hyperthyroidism: Elevated thyroid hormone blood levels due to increased thyroid gland production of the hormones. Hyperthyroidism is *not* synonymous with thyrotoxicosis. (See Thyrotoxicosis.) Many published studies I describe in this book contain statements to the effect that researchers rendered animals "hyperthyroid" for experimental purposes. I have used their wording, although it is not clear from many of the published reports whether the researchers meant that they raised the animals' thyroid hormone blood levels above normal or produced tissue thyrotoxicity. In using the researchers' wording, I have complied with convention in the literature. However, the reader should bear in mind the distinction between the terms hyperthyroidism and thyrotoxicosis.

Hypothalamic hypothyroidism: See Central hypothyroidism.

Hypothyroidism: Subnormal circulating thyroid hormone levels due to decreased synthesis and secretion of thyroid hormones by the thyroid gland.

Hypovolemia: A subnormal amount of blood in the body.

Iatrogenic: Doctor caused.

Index: Strictly, the ratio of a given measurement to a fixed standard. Used in this book to refer to indirect measures of metabolic status compared to what is considered normal. Indices can be considered objective, quantified signs.

Interstitial cystitis: Inflammation of the small spaces between the connective tissues of the bladder (called the "interstitium").

Intrathecal: Within a sheath, as the membranous sheaths of the spinal cord. In studies, intrathecal injections refer to injection of substances into either the subarachnoid or subdural spaces of the spinal cord.

Isoform: The term isoform, like subtype, is a term of classification. I use the term isoform in reference to variations of a receptor type. "Iso" is a combining form meaning "equal." In this book, I use the terms α- and β-adrenergic receptors to mean different forms of proteins that bind catecholamines. Used in this way, I make no implication that one form of the receptor is a subtype of the other. On the other hand, "sub," as in receptor subtype, is a combining form meaning "under" in one sense, "in small quantity" in another, and "less than" in another. It is often used as a synonym for "hypo." I use the term "receptor subtype" in this book to refer to variations of a particular receptor isoform. For example, α_1- and α_2- subtypes of the α-adrenergic receptor isoform.

IU: International Unit.

Joule: A unit of energy intended to replace the calorie. Equal to 0.239 calorie. One calorie (small calorie) equals 4.186 joules.

kb: Kilobase.

Kilocalorie: Kilogram calorie. Kilocalories are the equivalent of the popular "Calories." The quantity of heat required to raise the temperature of 1 liter of water 1° C. One thousand times the value of the small calorie. Equal to 4.186 kJ. There are 0.239 kcal/kJ. See Kilojoule. (Different dictionaries and textbooks give different relations of kcal to kJ. The values here are arbitrarily selected.)

Kilojoule: Equal to 1000 joules, or .239 kcal.

Levothroid®: Brand of synthetic T_4 (levothyroxine sodium tablets). Forest Pharmaceuticals, Inc.

Levoxine®: Brand of synthetic T_4 (levothyroxine sodium tablets). Inactive ingredients include lactose, cellulose, starch, magnesium stearate, and different combinations of color additives that vary in tablets of different strength. Provided in tablets of twelve different dosages. Jones Medical Industries, Inc.

Levoxyl®: Brand of synthetic T_4 (levothyroxine sodium tablets). Inactive ingredients include lactose, cellulose, starch, and magnesium stearate. Except for tablets of one dosage, tablets of different strengths contain single or different combinations of color additives. Provided in tablets of eleven different dosages. Daniels Pharmaceuticals, Inc.

Leydig cells: Cells of the testicles that produce testosterone.

LH: Luteinizing hormone. See Luteinizing hormone.

Ligand: Any molecule that specifically binds to a cell receptor, and by doing so alters some function of the cell. From the Latin term for "that which binds." Ligands may be hormones, neurotransmitters, antigens, synthetic drugs, or peptides. See Receptor.

Lipid: A group of organic compounds that are greasy to the touch. They are insoluble in water and soluble in alcohol, ether, and other fat solvents. The term lipid does not refer to a specific chemical compound but instead to the solubility characteristic of being extracted from cells by fat solvents. Fat solvent extractable lipids include fatty acids, glyceride, phospholipids, alcohols, waxes, and the fat soluble vitamins A, D. and E. In this book, in most instances, lipid breakdown (lipolysis) refers to the hydrolysis of fats such as triglycerides and cholesterol.

Locus ceruleus: A brain stem structure near the cerebral aqueduct. The structure contains neurons that synthesize norepinephrine. The axons of the noradrenergic neurons contain and secrete norepinephrine. The axons are widely distributed to structures in the brain, including the cerebral cortex, cerebellum, and hypothalamus.

Luteinization: Formation of the corpus luteum. Conversion of the mature graafian follicle in the ovary into a corpus luteum after ovulation.

Luteinizing hormone: One of the two gonadotropin hormones secreted by the gonadotroph cells of the anterior pituitary gland. Abbreviated as LH. LH stimulates the final maturation of the ovarian follicle, rupturing of the follicle to release the ovum, and conversion of the follicle into the corpus luteum. See FSH.

Mean: An average or arithmetic mean.

Menorrhagia: Excessive menstrual bleeding.

Mesentery: A double layer of peritoneal connective tissue that attaches to the abdominal wall. Its folds enclose abdominal organs and serve as a matrix embedding the blood vessels and nerves that supply the organs.

Metabolism: 1. The total of all chemical changes that occur in tissue involving two classes of changes. First is anabolism: chemical changes that convert small molecules into larger ones. Second is catabolism: changes that convert large molecules into smaller ones. 2. Complete chemical processing of a compound in the body.

mg: Milligram (one-thousandth of a gram: 1/1,000 g).

mg/dL: Milligrams per decaliter (milligrams per ten liters).

Microbe: Term used for both microscopic and ultramicroscopic organisms, such as bacteria, spirochetes, rickettsiae, mycoplasmas, and viruses.

Millijoule: A unit of energy equal to one thousandth of a joule. (See Joule.)

Mineralocorticoid: A steroids hormone secreted by the adrenal cortex that regulates the metabolism and blood and urine levels of sodium and potassium. See Aldosterone.

ml: Milliliter (one-thousandth of a liter).

mm Hg: Millimeters of mercury. The value used in the measurement of blood pressure. The values of the systolic pressure and diastolic pressure are given as the number of mm of mercury the pressure would move in a vertical column.

Monomer: A molecule that forms a polymer by binding to similar molecules.

Motor drive: The capability and inclination of an organism to engage in physical activity through muscular contractions.

Motor nerve: A nerve that generates and conducts impulses that induce muscles to contract. A motor nerve is an efferent nerve in that it transmits impulses outwardly from a center. See Efferent.

Motor response: The overt, and thus measurable, reaction of an organism to a stimulus.

mU/L: milliunits per liter.

Mucopolysaccharide: See Glycosaminoglycan.

Muscarinic receptor: A type of receptor that binds to acetylcholine after its release from postganglionic parasympathetic nerve endings. Upon binding acetylcholine, muscarinic receptors mediate parasympathetic effects in tissues such as smooth muscle. For example, when muscarinic receptors in the smooth muscle lining of the bladder bind to acetylcholine, the muscle lining contracts, expelling urine from the bladder.

Myoglobin: A protein that transports oxygen in skeletal muscle. Also termed "muscle hemoglobin." Myoglobin contains only one heme compared to the four of hemoglobin, and its molecular weight is only about 25% of that of hemoglobin. Confers the dark red color of type 1 or red muscle fibers (see Type 1 fibers).

Myometrium: Muscular wall of the uterus.

Myxedema: Non-pitting edema, usually localized to different skin tissue sites, associated with hypothyroidism. Myxedema was the first recognized sign assumed to represent thyroid hormone deficiency. During the early part of the twentieth century, clinicians used myxedema to diagnose hypothyroidism. The mechanism of the edema is the accumulation of water-binding compounds in the ground substance of the involved connective tissue. The compounds are variously termed mucopolysaccharides, glycoproteins, and glycosaminoglycans. The main constituent is hyaluronic acid. The latter compound is elevated in some hypothyroid and fibromyalgia patients.

Neuron: Any of a variety of nerve cells that conduct electrochemical impulses. Most neurons consist of a nucleated cell body with one axon and one or more dendrites. The axon conducts impulses away from the cell body, and the cell body and dendrite(s) respond to impulses generated by receptors or by other neurons. Neurons constitute most of the brain, spinal cord, and peripheral nerves.

Neuropathy: Any disease of nerves; particularly a disease involving the cranial or spinal nerves. Different mechanisms may cause neuropathy. In entrapment neuropathy, a region of a nerve is subjected to pressure. The sustained external pressure from an adjacent anatomical structure induces inflammation of the nerve (neuritis). This occurs in carpal tunnel syndrome when the tendons around the wrist become swollen (as in hypothyroidism). Neuropathy may be caused by biochemical factors. For example, mononeuropathies and polyneuropathies may develop in nerves of hypothyroid and euthyroid hypometabolic patients because of impaired nerve metabolism.

Neurotransmitter: A substance, such as norepinephrine, that transmits nerve signals across a neuronal synapse.

nm: Nanometer. One-billionth of a meter.

Nociceptive: Capable of appreciating pain or transmitting nerve signals that give rise to the perception of pain. The nervous system component of the nociceptive system of the body detects injurious or potentially injurious stimulation and notifies the central nervous system of the location and intensity of stimulation. Nociceptors are nerve receptors that respond to noxious (potentially injurious or actually injurious to tissues) stimuli.

Noradrenergic neuron: A nerve that synthesizes and secretes norepinephrine.

Nucleus: 1. The organelle in the cell that contains the genomic material. 2. A cluster of cell bodies. May refer to a group of nerve cells as in the sympathetic ganglia, or may refer to a mass of gray matter in the brain.

Nucleus of the solitary tract: See Solitary tract nucleus.

Oligomenorrhea: Scanty or infrequent menstrual bleeding.

Ophthalmopathy: Any disease of the eye.

Orthomolecular: Refers to substances that are natural to the body and necessary for health. Vitamins and thyroid hormone are orthomolecular substances.

Orthostatic hypotension: A sudden drop in blood pressure upon assuming an erect posture. Synonymous with postural hypotension.

Orthostatic intolerance: Abnormal blood pressure and circulation and associated adverse effects from an abruptly assumed erect posture.

Osteocalcin: A vitamin K-dependent noncollagenous protein. It is synthesized by bone cells and circulates in blood. Circulating levels are altered in certain metabolic bone diseases. Osteocalcin appears to reflect bone formation rather than bone resorption. The level tends to vary directly with the degree of osteoblastic activity. Its level usually correlates with the alkaline phosphatase level.

Palpation: Examination through touch. The clinician touches the body part being examined with his fingers, thumbs, or hands.

Paradigm: A conceptual model accepted by researchers in a field of study. Researchers who conduct studies within the paradigm test hypotheses derived from the concepts of the paradigm.

Paravertebral: Beside a vertebra or the vertebral column. For example, the paravertebral sympathetic ganglia are positioned immediately adjacent to the anterolateral aspect of the spinal column.

Parenchyma: The parenchyma is the aggregate of cells of a gland or organ that are specific to its function. Parenchymal cells constitute the unique feature that distinguishes a gland or organ from others. They are distinguished from the cells and tissues, such as fat and connective tissues, that provide anatomical support for the parenchymal cells. These latter tissues are termed the stroma of the gland or organ. See Stroma.

PET: Positron emission tomography. Imaging method for assessing the metabolism of tissues.

***P*-chlorophenylalanine:** Para-clorophenylalanine is a selective inhibitor of tryptophan hydroxylase, the rate limiting enzyme for the synthesis of serotonin. *P*-chlorophenylalanine competes with tryptophan for attachment to the enzyme and binds irreversibly to it. This permanently inactivates the enzyme and interferes with serotonin synthesis. Administering *p*-chlorophenylalanine, through inhibition of the enzyme, inhibits synthesis of serotonin.

Peri-: A prefix indicating around or about some specified time. Perinatal, for example, is around the time of birth. Perimenstrual is around the time of menstruation.

Peripheral tissues: Used in two different senses. 1. Tissues outside the central nervous system; distinguished from central tissues. 2. Tissues other than that of the pituitary gland. When used in this sense, the brain and spinal cord are considered peripheral tissues.

Periphery: Refers to peripheral tissues as distinct from tissues contained within the central nervous system. See Peripheral tissues.

pg: Picogram (on trillionth of a gram).

Pineal gland: A small, flattened gland with a shape that resembles a pine cone. Its anterior end attaches to the posterior commissure below the corpus callosum. It is made up of follicles that contain epithelioid cells and lime concretions termed "brain sand." Although the gland is attached to the brain, it is exclusively innervated by nerve fibers from the peripheral autonomic nervous system. The gland synthesizes and secretes melatonin. Also termed the "epiphysis cerebri."

Pituitary hypothyroidism: See Central hypothyroidism.

Plummer's disease: Hyperthyroidism caused by a toxic nodular goiter.

Polymenorrhea: Abnormally high frequency of menstruation.

Polymer: A substance formed by a combination of molecules (monomers) of the same substance. The number of monomers making up a polymer may number from two-to-millions.

Portal system: A system of blood vessels that transmits substances from one structure to another. The blood passes through one capillary bed and is then conducted through another capillary bed. The portal system of the liver conducts blood from the intestines to the liver sinusoid. In the hypothalamic-pituitary portal system, hormones released by hypothalamic cells enter a capillary plexus in the anterior aspect of the median eminence (on the inferior portion of the hypothalamus). The hormones then descend in the portal vessels to the anterior pituitary gland where they are secreted into the general circulation.

Post hoc ergo propter hoc: Literal interpretation is "After, therefore because of." The inference that one event is the cause of another merely because the first occurs earlier than the second. This logical fallacy is often committed by patients and clinicians when they conclude that a drug was effective because some symptom ceased after the drug was taken.

Postsynaptic: See Presynaptic.

Postural hypotension: A sudden drop in blood pressure upon assuming an erect posture. Synonymous with orthostatic hypotension.

Presynaptic: An adjective that describes the neuron terminal that releases a neurotransmitter substance into a synapse (synaptic cleft). The neurotransmitter "transmits" a nerve signal from the presynaptic neuron to another neuron. The neuron whose cell body or dendrites receive the signal is termed the postsynaptic neuron. The presynaptic neuron is at the proximal end of the synaptic cleft, and the postsynaptic neuron is at the distal end.

Primary hypothyroidism: Decreased synthesis and secretion of thyroid hormones due to a disorder of the thyroid gland, resulting in subnormal circulating levels of thyroid hormones. Synonymous with "thyroidal hypothyroidism."

Propylthiouracil: An antithyroid compound used to inhibit the synthesis of thyroid hormones. Used in the treatment of hyperthyroidism and to induce hypothyroidism in experimental animals. By suppressing the synthesis of thyroid hormones, propylthiouracil, like methimazole (Tapazole®), typically results in increased TSH secretion. A sustained increase in TSH level may result in hypertrophy of the thyroid gland, a condition termed goiter. Because goiter may result from chronic use of propylthiouracil, the compound is classified as a goitrogen. When increased TSH secretion is sustained by administration of propylthiouracil, anterior pituitary and thyroid gland neoplasms may develop. See Tapazole®.

Proteoglycan: See Glycoprotein.

Range of normal: The range of values for a laboratory test considered to represent absence of the disease the test is intended to detect.

Receptor: A cellular molecule that binds ligands. Receptors are made up of one or more proteins, and they occupy either the outer cell membrane, the cytoplasm, or sites on DNA molecules. See Ligand.

Reference range: See Range of normal.

Replacement dosage, thyroid hormone: Dosages of thyroid hormone, usually T_4, that keep the basal TSH and thyroid hormone levels within the normal reference ranges. Considered by conventional clinicians to be an amount sufficient to meet the needs of tissues for metabolic stimulation. Recent evidence indicates that replacement dosages of T_4 (1) do not provide normal amounts of T_3 within the cells of many tissues, (2) do not maintain normal tissue metabolism, and (3) are a common cause of symptoms diagnosed as "new diseases" such as fibromyalgia and chronic fatigue syndrome.

Reverse-T_3 (rT_3): The product of the enzymatic removal of an iodine atom from the tyrosyl ring of T_4. Production of rT_3 is considered an inactivating step in the metabolism of thyroid hormone because rT_3 has no apparent calorigenic or thyromimetic activity.

Segmental facilitation: A reduced threshold for activation of neurons in a specific segmental level of the spinal cord. Facilitation of a segment develops in response to chronic sensory input to the spinal cord from a peripheral tissue site, such as a trigger point.

Sella turcica: The saddle-like prominence in the middle of the cranial fossa on the upper surface of the sphenoid bone. The sella turcica houses the pituitary gland. Enlargement of the sella turcica suggests enlargement of the pituitary gland.

Sensory nerve: A nerve that conducts impulses toward or into the central nervous system. Sensory nerves are afferent nerves in that they transmit impulses inwardly from the peripheral structures toward a body center. See Afferent.

Serotonergic: Associated with the neurotransmitter serotonin. Serotonergic neurons secrete serotonin.

Sicca syndrome: Generally used to refer to dry mucous membranes. See Sjögren's syndrome.

Sign: A manifestation of a disease or dysfunction that can be observed or measured by another person such as a clinician. Signs are objective evidence of disease or dysfunction. Signs are distinguished from symptoms, which are subjective impressions of the patient. In this book, the term index (*pl.* indices) is used to refer to a sign that is measured and quantified against a fixed quantified standard (see Index).

Sjögren's syndrome: Presumably a connective tissue disease. Inflammation of the conjunctiva and of the cornea with dryness of muscous membranes and decreased tears (keratoconjunctivitis sicca). The patient may also have dryness of mucous membranes of the mouth (xerostomia). Lacrimal, parotid, and salivary glands may be enlarged bilaterally due to lymphocytic infiltration of the glandular tissues. The patient may also have dilation of small or terminal blood vessels (telangiectasia) and Raynaud's phenomenon. Menopausal women, especially those with rheumatoid arthritis, are most prone to develop the condition. Also termed sicca syndrome. Some researchers describe the dryness of the mucous membranes in fibromyalgia patients as a sicca-like symptom.

Sodium-potassium pump (Na⁺/K⁺ pump): There are four components of the pump. The first component is carrier protein within the cell membrane. The second component is three receptor sites for binding sodium on the part of the protein that protrudes into the inside of the cell. The third component is two receptor sites for binding potassium on the portion of the protein that protrudes outside the cell. The fourth component is the Na-K-ATPase activity of the portion of the protein inside the cell, near the sodium binding sites. When three sodium ions bind to the inside portion of the protein, and two potassium ions bind to the outside, the ATPase becomes activated. The ATPase activity splits away one molecule of phosphate, reducing the molecule to ADP. The split frees the energy of a high-energy phosphate bond. The energy causes a conformational change in the carrier protein. This change transports the sodium ions out and the potassium ions into the cell, leaving the interior with a more negative charge. The difference in charge between the inside and outside of the membrane is the electrical potential that enables discharge.

Solitary tract nucleus: The major brain stem center that coordinates autonomic function. The nucleus of the solitary tract receives sensory input from most major organs of the body. By means of the input, the nucleus modulates autonomic function. Subnuclei of the nucleus receive sensory fibers from the heart, lungs, and gastrointestinal tract. These fibers then connect to autonomic motor neurons that control effector tissues. The nucleus also coordinates homeostatic adjustments by transmitting signals to both higher and lower brain regions. From these signals, integrated signals necessary for complex autonomic control are then relayed back to the nucleus. Visceral sensory signals from a variety of tissues terminate in the nucleus. These are then transmitted to many brain stem and forebrain nuclei. These nuclei transmit signals back to the nucleus of the solitary tract and other brain stem nuclei. Signals from these nuclei are then transmitted to autonomic output nuclei (such as the dorsal vagal nucleus and the sympathetic preganglionic nuclei) for the gastrointestinal system.

Somatomedin: A hormone synthesized and secreted by liver, kidney, and other peripheral cells in response to growth hormone. Somatomedins mediate the effects of growth hormone on tissues and increase protein and glycoprotein production. Somatomedin stimulates the sulfation of mucopolysaccharides. Synonym for insulin-like growth factor.

Somatomedin C: Synonym for insulin-like growth factor-I. See Somatomedin.

SPECT: Single photon emission computed tomography. Imaging method for assessing blood flow.

S-P-T®: Capsules containing oil-suspended thyroid hormone from pigs. In processing, fresh pig thyroid glands are processed to remove connective tissue and fat. The remaining substance is suspended in soybean oil and encapsulated in gelatin. The ratio of T_4 to T_3 in the capsules is approximately 2.5 to 1. Provided in 1-to-5 grain capsules. This product may be more effective for hypothyroid patients with partial cellular resistance to thyroid hormone than other thyroid products containing a T_4 to T_3 ratio of 4:1. Fleming and Company.

Stroke volume: Synonymous with stroke output. The volume of blood pumped out of a heart ventricle in a single beat.

Stroma: The colorless sponge-like supporting framework of cells. Also, the supporting framework of the tissues of an organ or gland that supports the parenchyma (see Parenchyma). Stroma typically consists of fat and connective tissue.

Subtype: See Isoform.

Superior cervical sympathetic ganglion: The uppermost and largest of the ganglia of the sympathetic trunk. The ganglion lies near the base of the skull between the internal carotid artery and the internal jugular vein. It provides sympathetic fibers to certain structures in the skull such as the hypothalamus.

Supplement, thyroid hormone. A thyroid hormone supplement implies less than a replacement dosage of exogenous thyroid hormone, taken as an addition to endogenous thyroid hormone.

Supraspinal: Above the spine; the brain stem or brain.

Symbols:

α: Greek symbol for alpha.

β: Greek symbol for beta.

γ: Greek symbol for gamma.

kcal: See Kilocalorie.

kj: See Kilojoule. Equal to 1000 joules, or .239 kcal.

μ: Greek symbol for micro.

μg: microgram (one-millionth of a gram: or 1/1,000,000 gram).

μU/mL: Microunit per milliliter.

<:   Less than.

>:   More than.

≥:   Greater than or equal to.

≤:   Less than or equal to.

±:   Plus or minus; denoting the probable error associated with a calculated figure.

Ψ: Lycopene is Ψ,Ψ-carotene, the red pigment of the tomato. It is considered the parent compound from which all natural carotenoid pigments are derived. Its chemical structure is similar to carotene.

^{131}I: A radioactive iodine isotope. Used as a tracer in thyroid hormone studies and as a treatment in hypothyroidism and thyroid cancer.

Sympathetic ganglia: The chain of autonomic nervous system cell bodies situated at the anterior-lateral aspect of the spine. Cell bodies in the intermediolateral column of the thoracic and upper lumbar spinal cord send preganglionic motor fibers to the ganglia. Some of the fibers synapse with cells in the ganglia; others pass to internal structures and synapse there with ganglia.

Sympatholytic: Inhibition of sympathetic nervous system activity or its effects mediated by adrenergic receptors. See also Adrenergic receptor antagonist.

Sympathomimetic: Imitating of action of the sympathetic system. For example, caffeine binds to adenosine receptors and inhibits the action of the enzyme phosphodiesterase. Both actions mimic the effects of sympathetic nervous system stimulation. From the Greek word for imitating.

Symptom: A perception by a patient of a variation from normal structure or function that indicates dysfunction or disease.

Synapse: The region of contact between the axon of one neuron and the dendrite or cell body of another neuron. Synapse also refers to the region of contact between an axon and a target tissue such as muscle or a sensory receptor cell.

Neurotransmitter substances (such as norepinephrine, dopamine, and acetylcholine) transmit nerve signals across synapses, typically in only one direction. The substance is released by a presynaptic nerve terminal into the synaptic cleft. (See Presynaptic.)

Synaptosome: A membrane-bound sac that contains synaptic vesicles that may hold neurotransmitters. Synaptosomes separate from the axon terminal under conditions such as homogenization of brain tissue.

Synthroid®: Brand of synthetic T_4 (levothyroxine sodium tablets). Inactive ingredients include acacia, confectioner's sugar, lactose, starch, magnesium stearate, providone, talc, and single or different combinations of color additives that vary in tablets of different strength. Provided in tablets of eleven different dosages. Knoll Pharmaceutical Company.

T_3: Triiodothyronine.

T_4: Tetraiodothyronine (thyroxine or levothyroxine).

Tachycardia: Rapid heart rate. Tachycardia is defined as a heart rate of 100 beats per minute or more.

Tapazole®: Brand of methimazole, a compound that inhibits synthesis of thyroid hormones. As orally consumed tablets, used to treat hyperthyroidism. Less consistent than but 10 times more potent than the anti-thyroid compound propylthiouracil. Jones Medical Industries, Inc.

Technocratic medicine: The practice of medicine based, usually implicitly, on a philosophy of medical technocracy. Medical technocracy is advocacy of reforming medical practice so that it is conducted according to the reported findings of technologists. In this form of practice, diagnostic and treatment decisions are based solely on the outcome of objective tests. Typically, the practitioner of technocratic medicine disavows the methods of clinical medicine. He tends to devalue the patient's symptoms and signs and communication with the patient. Commonly, the practitioner has an extremist faith in the outcome of objective measures peculiar to his specialty. Patients and medical generalists typically do not have the background education to comprehend some of the measures and the rationale for their use. The technocratic practitioner's specialized knowledge tends to give rise to a sense of superiority that alienates both patients and practitioners of clinical medicine.

Thermogenesis: Heat generation. The term "thermo" is derived from the Greek term for heat, and the term "genesis" derives from the Greek term for production. See Calorigenesis.

Thyroid hormone products, brand names: Products are available that contain only synthetic T_4, only synthetic T_3, synthetic T_4 and T_3, and T_4 and T_3 derived from animal thyroid glands. See Brand names, thyroid hormone: Table 1.

Thyroid response element: A distinct DNA sequence that interacts with the T_3-receptor to control gene expression. The interaction increases or decreases the rate of mRNA synthesis. Also termed the T_3 response element. With either term, often referred to as a TRE.

Thyroid state: A term used with apparently different meanings in the thyroidology research literature. Some authors use the term to refer to the functional status of the thyroid gland: hyperfunction (hyperthyroidism), normal function (euthyroidism), or hypofunction (hypothyroidism). Other authors use the term to refer to the amount of thyroid hormone cells or a tissue are exposed to in an experimental medium.

Thyroidectomy: Surgical removal of the thyroid gland. Often used as an adjective, as in "thyroidectomized rats."

Thyrolar®: Product that contains synthetic T_4 and T_3. The ratio of T_4 to T_3 is 4:1. Available in five potencies. Tablets contain several inactive ingredients including dyes. Forest Pharmaceuticals, Inc.

Thyrotoxicosis: The syndrome resulting from tissue overstimulation by thyroid hormone. May be used to refer to single tissue overstimulation, such as cardiac thyrotoxicosis. Thyrotoxicosis is *not* synonymous with hyperthyroidism. See Hyperthyroidism.

Thyrotrophs: Anterior pituitary gland cells that synthesize and secrete TSH. Activity of the thyrotrophs is under the control of both TRH and thyroid hormones.

Thyrotropin-releasing hormone: Hormone secreted by the hypothalamus that stimulates pituitary thyrotroph cells to synthesize and secrete TSH. Abbreviated as TRH.

tid: t.i.d.; three times per day. L. *ter in die.*

Tone, vascular: In this text, I refer to vascular tone as the degree of contraction of blood vessels, particularly the arterioles. Vascular tone is regulated by a number of different influences. Norepinephrine released from sympathetic nerves binds to α-adrenergic receptors and induces vasoconstriction. Serotonin released from serotonergic neurons binds with 5-HT receptors and induces vasoconstriction. In such cases, vascular tone is increased. In contrast, inhibiting of sympathetic nerve activity results in vasodilation, which is a decrease in vascular tone. During vasoconstriction, or increased vascular tone, resistance to blood flow increases, resulting in decreased flow. During vasodilation, or decreased vascular tone, resistance to blood flow decreases, with an increase in flow. (See Tonic.)

Tonic: From the French word *tonos*, meaning tone. 1. Used in one sense as a state of persistent action. For example, tonic vasoconstriction refers to continuous constriction of blood arteries. 2. Used in another sense, tonic refers to a remedy that is energizing or invigorating. In the 1950s, for example, some pharmaceutical companies advertised T_3 as a tonic.

TRH: Abbreviation for thyrotropin-releasing hormone.

Triostat™: Injectable synthetic T_3. Used to treat myxedema coma or precoma. More recently used to treat various cardiac conditions, especially during surgery. Because of rapid onset of action of T_3, low dosages (10-to-20 μg) may be appropriate for patients with suspected cardiovascular disease. As with other thyroid hormone products, treatment for adrenal insufficiency should precede or occur simultaneously with the initiation of treatment with Triostat™. Jones Medical Industries, Inc.

Trophoblast: The surface cells of the blastocyst, the single, spherical layer of cells that encloses the hollow, central cavity containing the developing embryo. Trophoblast cells fuse with, erode, and penetrate the endometrium, and thereafter serve as a conduit for delivery of nutrients from the uterine lining to the embryo. Trophoblast cells do not enter the embryo itself, but contribute to formation of the placenta.

Type 1 fibers: The "slow-twitch" or "red" muscle fibers of skeletal muscle. Type 1 fibers predominate in muscles that are required to sustain contraction such as the postural muscles of the trunk. Skeletal muscle consisting largely of red muscle fibers is often referred to as "red muscle." Red muscle contains a high percentage of small dark fibers. The dark color is conferred mainly by the high concentration of myoglobin compared to that of white muscle (see Myoglobin). Compared to white muscle, red muscle also contains abundant mitochondria. See Type 2 fibers.

Type 2 fibers: The "fast-twitch," "white," or "glycolytic" muscle fibers of skeletal muscle. Type 2 fibers predominate in muscles that are required to contract rapidly such as the limb muscles. Skeletal muscle consisting largely of white fibers (as opposed to red fibers) is often referred to as "white muscle." White muscle, compared to red muscle, contains few mitochondria and little myoglobin. The low concentration of myoglobin (see Myoglobin), which confers a reddish color to muscle, largely accounts for the pale color of white muscle. See Type 1 fibers.

Up-regulation: An increase in the number of receptors on a cell membrane when not exposed to a pharmacological or physiological substance that binds the receptors, or an increase in the affinity of the receptors for the substance.

USP: Abbreviation for the United States Pharmacopeia. A publication first published in 1820 that describes agents used for treatment, the standards for their potency and purity, and their formulations. The National Food and Drugs Act of 1907 rendered the USP the legal standard in the United States.

Vascular tone: See Tone, vascular.

Vasoconstriction: Decrease in the caliber of blood vessels due to hypermyotonia of the smooth muscle lining of the vessels.

Vasodilation: Increased caliber of blood vessels due to relaxation of the smooth muscle lining of the vessels.

Vasospasm: Acute spasm of the smooth muscle lining of blood vessels with vasoconstriction.

Viscera: Plural for viscus. (See Viscus.)

Visceral: Related or referring to a viscus or viscera.

Viscus: A hollow organ in the respiratory system, digestive system, or urogenital system that has a multilayered wall. The heart, spleen, stomach, intestines, and urinary bladder are examples.

VO$_2$ max: Abbreviation for the rate of oxygen usage during maximum aerobic metabolism.

Index

Note: Words followed by t refer to tables, and words followed by f refer to figures. "FMS," used in this Index, refers to fibromyalgia.

E

N